Critical Thinking Challenges

Home and Community Care Displays

Toxicity Alerts

Clinical Pharmacology and Nursing Management

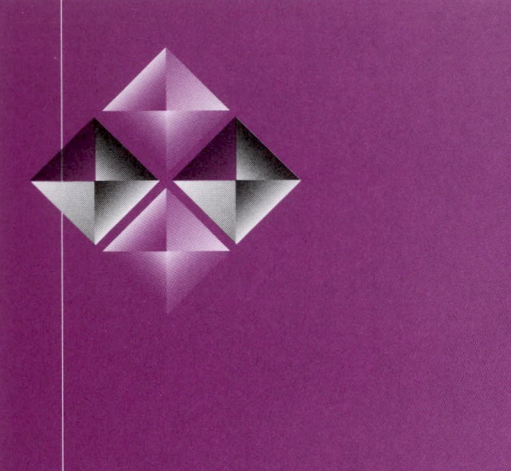

Laurel Eisenhauer, RN, PhD, FANN

Professor of Nursing
Boston College School of Nursing
Chestnut Hill, Massachusetts

Lynn Wemett Nichols, RN, MSN

Doctoral Student
School of Nursing
University of Rochester
Rochester, New York

Associate Professor, Ret.
Department of Nursing
State University of New York College at Plattsburgh
Plattsburgh, New York

Roberta Todd Spencer, RN, MS

Associate Professor, Ret.
Department of Nursing
State University of New York College at Plattsburgh
Plattsburgh, New York

Frances West Bergan, RN, MSN

Director, Hospital Administration
University Hospital
SUNY Health Sciences Center
Syracuse, New York

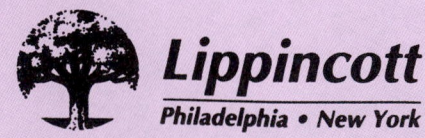

Lippincott
Philadelphia • New York

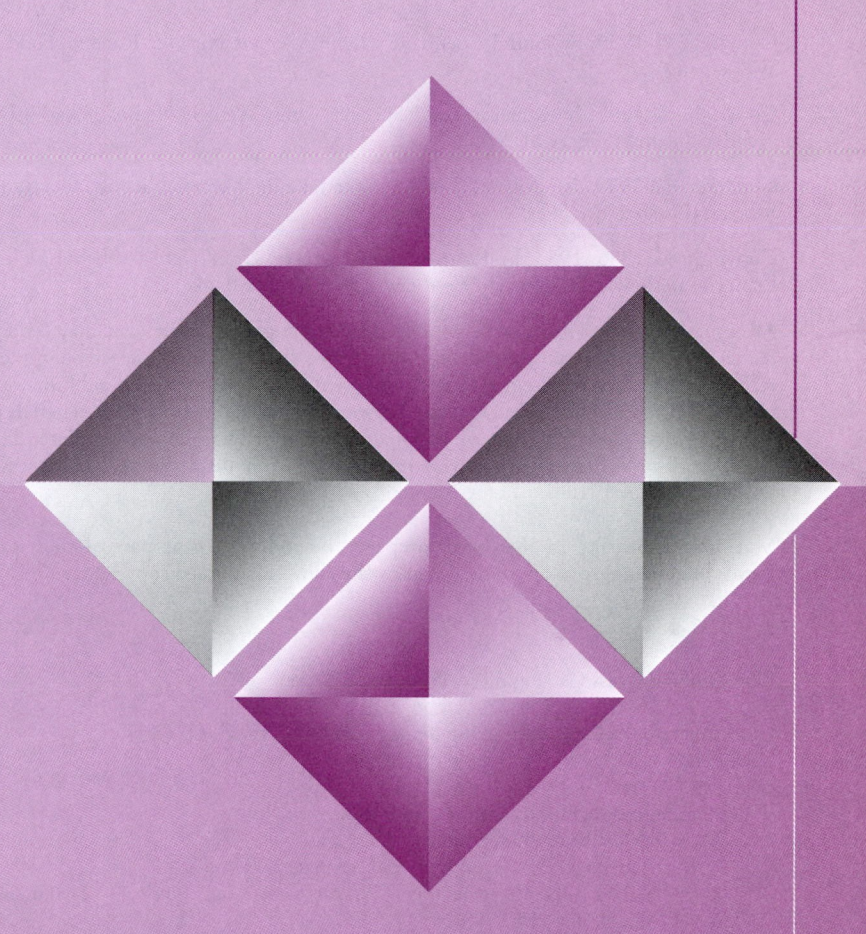

FIFTH EDITION

Clinical Pharmacology and Nursing Management

Acquisitions Editor: Margaret Zuccarini
Developmental Editor: Deedie McMahon
Associate Managing Editor: Barbara Ryalls
Senior Production Manager: Helen Ewan
Production Coordinator: Patricia McCloskey
Design Coordinator: Nicholas Rook
Indexer: Katherine Pitcoff

5th Edition

9 8 7 6 5 4 3 2 1

Library of Congress Cataloging-in-Publication Data

Clinical pharamcology and nursing management. — 5th ed. / [Laurel
    Eisenhauer . . . et al.]
        p.   cm.
    Includes bibliographical references and index.
    ISBN 0-397-55329-3 (alk. paper)
    1. Pharmacology.   2. Nursing.   I. Eisenhauer, Laurel A.
        DNLM: 1. Pharmacology, Clinical—nurses' instruction.   2. Nursing
Care.   QV 38 C6415 1988]
RM300.C526   1998
615'.1'024613—dc21
DNLM/DLC
for Library of Congress   97-8454
                                                                CIP

Care has been taken to confirm the accuracy of the information presented and to describe generally accepted practices. However, the authors, editors, and publisher are not responsible for errors or omissions or for any consequences from application of the information in this book and make no warranty, express or implied, with respect to the contents of the publication.

The authors, editors and publisher have exerted every effort to ensure that drug selection and dosage set forth in this text are in accordance with current recommendations and practice at the time of publication. However, in view of ongoing research, changes in government regulations, and the constant flow of information relating to drug therapy and drug reactions, the reader is urged to check the package insert for each drug for any change in indications and dosage and for added warnings and precautions. This is particularly important when the recommended agent is a new or infrequently employed drug.

Some drugs and medical devices presented in this publication have Food and Drug Administration (FDA) clearance for limited use in restricted research settings. It is the responsibility of the health care provider to ascertain the FDA status of each drug or device planned for use in their clinical practice.

The meaning of the word *dedication* may include setting apart and devoting to a special purpose or addressing to another as a token of respect or affection. In accord with these definitions, we would like to once more dedicate this volume to nursing clients, through its use by students and faculty of schools of nursing and practicing nurses, and to our families and friends with thanks for their understanding and support.

Contributors

Contributors to the Fifth Edition

Deborah Adams Cassidy, RN, PhD
Assistant Professor
Boston College School of Nursing
Chestnut Hill, MA
Chapter 11

David G. Curry, RN-C, MSN
Clinical Nurse Practitioner, PrimeCare Consulting
Plattsburg, NY
Chapter 39

Nancy Fairchild, RN, MS, CAES
Associate Professor
Boston College School of Nursing
Chestnut Hill, MA
Chapters 17, 19, 34

Barbara Wolfe, RN, CS, PhD
Clinical Nurse Specialist
Department of Psychiatry Nursing Service
Beth Israel-Deaconess Medical Center
Boston, MA
Assistant Professor
Department of Psychiatry
Harvard Medical School
Boston, MA
Chapter 20 (supported in part by
USPHS grant KO7 MH00965
from the National Institute of Mental Health)

Laurel Eisenhauer: Chapters 12, 13, 18, 28 29, 37, 41,
42, 43*
Lynn Wemett Nichols: Chapters 5, 6, 21, 22 23, 24, 25,
26, 27, 30, 35, 36, 38, 40, 43,* 44, 45, 46, 47
Roberta Todd Spencer: Chapters 1, 2, 3, 4, 7, 14, 15,
16, 30, 31, 32, 33, 48, 49, 50
Frances West Bergan: Chapters 8, 9, 10

*An asterisk indicates chapters authored by more than
one contributor.

Contributors to previous editions:
Frances Brown Anderson, RN, PhD
Mary X. Britten, RN, EdD
Martha Fortune, RN, MS
Helen Sabo Henderson, RN, MEd
Martha Hryzak Lind, RN, MS
Gladys B. Lipkin, RN, MS
Charlotte Shimmons Torres, RN, EdD

Reviewers

Frances A. Brown, RN, MSN, MSEd, CS
Professor and Chair Department of Nursing
Community College of Southern Nevada
Las Vegas, NV

Jan Boundy, RN, PhD
Associate Professor
St. Francis Medical Center College of Nursing
Peoria, IL

Carolyn Chodak, RN, MSN
Adjunct Faculty
Boston College School of Nursing
Chestnut Hill, MA

Joyce H. Cirrito, RN, MS
Instructor
St. Joseph's Hospital Health Center School of Nursing
Syracuse, NY

Kathryn H. Kavanaugh, RN, PhD
Associate Professor
School of Nursing, University of Maryland at Baltimore
Baltimore, MD

Patricia A. Stockert, RN, MS
Assistant Professor,
St. Francis Medical Center College of Nursing
Peoria, IL

Janice K. Wittman, RN, PhD
Program Director, Evenings
St. Petersburg Junior College
St. Petersburg, FL

Preface

Knowing about pharmacology is but one important aspect of the nurse's knowledge base. Knowing how to wisely incorporate that knowledge into clinical judgment is equally important.

As more and more drugs enter the marketplace, the challenge to the nurse—and especially to the nursing student—is to incorporate essential pharmacologic concepts, critical thinking activities, and clinical judgment skills so that drug therapy is as safe and appropriate as possible for clients and for nurses. As in previous editions of *Clinical Pharmacology and Nursing Management*, this text provides the most useful information for nursing students beginning to study pharmacology. In this thoroughly updated edition, the authors' objective is to support the acquisition of sound clinical knowledge of pharmacology by presenting frequently used, essential information that is based on the concepts needed to make appropriate and wise clinical judgments.

Now in its 5th edition, *Clinical Pharmacology and Nursing Management* typifies sound clinical judgment. The text skillfully incorporates pharmacology content and nursing concerns into a nursing process format. Two of the most highly praised characteristics of *Clinical Pharmacology and Nursing Management* have been the nature and quality of the nursing application of pharmacology theory and the high-quality content *written by nurses for nurses*. Not only have these characteristics been maintained in this new edition, they also have been strengthened—retaining the best of the old and incorporating the most reliable new drug information and latest research and understanding of drug actions, interactions and effects.

Drug therapy, whether prescribed by a healthcare professional or self-prescribed by the client, has unique effects on each person's health and well-being. Understanding these effects is an essential component of the nursing role. The 5th edition of *Clinical Pharmacology and Nursing Management* encourages nursing students to integrate their growing knowledge of pharmacology with their knowledge of each client to support safe clinical practice and to promote optimal therapeutic effects for the client.

What's New

This edition has been extensively updated and revised to incorporate the most current information on new drugs, such as biologic response modifiers and immune system modulators, and trends in health care. There is increased content and emphasis on:

- Home and community care
- Critical thinking in nursing strategies
- Client education
- Alternative therapies
- Current drug therapy regimens
- Nonprescription, over-the-counter medications
- Integration of theory and practice.

Easy-to-Follow, Logical Organization

Text Organization

The text has 50 chapters organized into 14 units.

❑ Unit I, Introduction to Pharmacology, includes three chapters that present a brief history of pharmacology in relation to nursing. Highlights include:

- Legal controls over drug production and use
- Harmful effects of chemical exposure
- Nursing process as it pertains to drug therapy.

❑ Unit II, Therapy with Drugs, includes three chapters that present scientific concepts underlying the medicinal use of drugs: pharmacodynamics and pharmacokinetics, adverse reactions, and drug–drug and drug–food interactions.

❑ Unit III, Administration of Medications, includes three chapters that discuss the theoretical basis of nursing principles and applies them to strategies for administering drugs, promoting therapeutic alliance and adherence, and recognizing the multicultural aspects of drug therapy. The unit offers new perspectives on nursing care and ethnomedicine.

❑ Unit IV, Developmental Considerations in Drug Therapy, includes three chapters that cover variations in client responses and special considerations related to drug therapy in special populations: children, older adults, and pregnant and lactating women.

❑ Unit V, Pharmacology in Community-Based Nursing, focuses on appropriate and inappropriate use of drugs in home and community-based settings. Topics include substance abuse, toxicology, and alternative medicine. Also included are clear, detailed discussions of self-medication, self-care at home, and implications for the nursing care of clients using alternative or complementary medicine.

❑ Units VI through XIV contain drug-focused chapters that are organized by body systems. These units make up the core of the book. Chapters in these units are organized according to therapeutic or pharmacologic drug classification. Each chapter contains a review of key physiologic and pathophysiologic concepts needed for understanding drug actions and effects and a thorough presentation of the nursing management for drugs within each class. Of particular note, because more and more pathogens tend to resist antibiotic and other antiinfective agents, the unit on infection-fighting drugs has been expanded to provide more in-depth coverage of antimicrobial, antiviral, and antiparasitic medications.

Chapter Organization

Each of the 35 drug chapters are organized systematically to present easily accessed information. They follow a systematic and reliable format:

- Outline—presents an overview of the chapter contents.
- Physiology and pathophysiology—reviews essential concepts necessary to understand the actions of the chapter's drug class.
- Key pharmacologic content—provides in-depth explanations of major drug classifications and the prototype drugs within the classifications and then progresses consistently under headings ranging from pharmacodynamics, pharmacokinetics, and therapeutic uses through dosage and administration, adverse effects, drug interactions, and precautions and contraindications. Drug interactions detail currently known interactions of drugs with other drugs, foods, and laboratory tests.
- Nursing management—clearly presents the connection between drug theory and therapy and each step of the nursing process: assessment, nursing diagnosis, planning, intervention, client education, and outcome evaluation.

Nursing Process: The Basis for Sound Clinical Judgments

The nursing process—the systematic delivery of individualized care that distinguishes professional nursing—is introduced early in the text and is used to focus chapter content on the management of clients receiving specific drug therapy.

The responsibilities of the nurse are defined broadly, encompassing those that are inherent in evolving roles: in primary care, in community settings, and in client advocacy.

Nursing Process Features

Within the nursing management sections, the text presents numerous features that enhance student learning and promote sound clinical judgment:

- Detailed clinical examples assist in expanding the text presentation and making it real.
- Client education highlights the importance of the nurse's responsibility to empower clients to self-administer drugs and to recognize, report, and manage side effects that are closely associated with drug therapy. Teaching clients about drug therapy is a major nursing role and a major focus of this text.
- Checklist of nursing actions emphasizes the key aspects of nursing responsibilities in administering drug therapy.

New Chapters

Two new chapters are included in this edition:

- Chapter 39, Drugs that Affect the Eyes and Ears, provides systematic coverage of agents used to treat ophthalmic conditions including glaucoma, ophthalmic infections and inflammations and allergic responses.
- Chapter 40, Drugs that Affect the Integumentary System, presents the full range of agents that are used topically, including antibiotics, antipsoriatics, antifungals and topical corticosteroids.

Special Features

Prominent icons identify special pedagogical features:

Critical Thinking Challenges advance the student's application of knowledge. Because critical thinking is an integral part of clinical thinking and the nursing process, *Clinical Pharmacology and Nursing Management*, 5th edition, employs a variety of features to stimulate developing thinking skills. These skills will help the student understand the impact of drug therapy on the client and and develop and implement appropriate nursing interventions. The text supports the development of such cognitive skills as explanation, analysis, interpretation, inference, evaluation, and self-regulation in a variety of case, issues, and research analyses. More than 50 of these challenges, based on actual acute care and home care situations, ask the student to develop solutions to daily thought-provoking problems, pose new questions and debates about current issues and concerns, or require the student to refer to supplementary resources or research studies. The challenges are posed as:

- *Case analyses* invite students to think inventively about typical clients in real-life situations and to apply knowledge and creative problem-solving throughout the nursing process.
- *Issues analyses* encourage students to explore the pros and cons of issues in drug therapy, to analyze advertising claims, and to consider the ethics or legal consequences of various drug therapy regimens.
- *Research analyses* require students to analyze and critique published drug research findings or ongoing studies.

Home and Community Care guidelines and displays respond to the expanded emphasis placed on the nurse's role in health care in the home and community setting. Independent nursing interventions that supplement each client's therapeutic regimen are underscored.

FOCUS ON Focus On tables highlight similarities and differences of drugs within major drug classifications and encourage the student to think first about drugs in terms of likenesses within a pharmacological classification and then to consider how specific drugs differ from the commonalities. This approach helps to simplify and organize what initially appears to be a vast and overwhelming puzzle of information.

Examples of Nursing Process highlight plans of care for clients receiving selected drugs. These encourage students to apply pharmacological concepts and information to client care.

More Special Features

❑ Toxicity Alerts boldly present hazards of those drugs with a narrow therapeutic range or highly variable effects.

❑ Drug tables present at-a-glance information about specific drugs. Among various features are drug names (generic and brand), including Canadian brand names, dosages and routes of administration, pregnancy risk categories, and other essential information and nursing implications.

❑ Illustrations, diagrams, figures and photos visually represent key concepts in pharmacology and nursing care.

❑ The Glossary, which defines more than 350 common drug-related terms, is a convenient and time-saving reference for student use.

❑ References and bibliography sources for additional information are provided at the end of each chapter.

❑ Extensive index of drugs by generic and brand names, related disease or disorders, and other topics is provided to facilitate quick access to drug information.

❑ FREE Content Review Disk. Each textbook includes a computer disk containing a review system by which students can self-test their knowledge of each chapter's content. NCLEX-style review questions provide rationale for all correct and incorrect answers.

Teaching–Learning Package

Teaching and learning enhancement materials for the 5th edition of *Clinical Pharmacology and Nursing Management* are readily available for students and for faculty.

For Students:

❑ FREE Content Review Disk in each textbook provides a review system by which students can self-test their knowledge of each chapter's content. NCLEX-style review questions provide rationale for all correct and incorrect answers.

❑ Student Workbook (separate bookstore purchase) is organized according to the chapters in the book and offers the student a variety of exercises to promote learning and application of pharmacology. The exercises begin with short answer, true-false, or multiple choice questions and advance to more challenging crossword puzzles, matching questions, essay questions, and additional suggested learning experiences. Answers are provided in the back of the book to facilitate self-learning.

For Faculty:

❑ The Instructor's Manual provides class objectives and content outline as well as teaching-learning strategies for classroom use (eg, small group discussions or projects).

❑ Overhead Transparency Masters are included in the Instructor's Manual, providing enlarged texts, diagrams, and illustrations to support classroom teaching.

❑ Computerized Test Bank provides more than 750 completely new NCLEX-style test items for use in evaluating student learning. These are in addition to those provided in the student workbook and on the student review disk.

❑ Printed Test Bank provides a convenient hard copy of the more than 750 NCLEX-style test items found on the computerized test bank.

Complementary Materials Available as a Separate Purchase

❑ Medication Basics Set (Lippincott's Clinical Skills Series: VHS Video Tapes) provide full motion video showing students how to perform the essential skills. Set includes: Understanding Medication Guidelines, Administering Oral and Inhalation Medications, Administering Injectable Medications, Administering Topical Medications.

❑ Medication Administration (Lippincott's Interactive Skills Series: Interactive Video Disc) provides self-paced, one-on-one learning for mastering this clinical skill.

We believe that this book provides the nursing student with both the pharmacology content and the basis for clinical judgment skills necessary to deliver safe and effective drug therapy to clients. Along with this content are the pedagogical features and other teaching and learning resources that supply the student with sound approaches to learning and thinking about drug therapy. These strategies are designed to serve nursing students in their initial learning as well as during their ongoing professional development.

The Authors
Laurel A. Eisenhauer
Lynn Wemett Nichols
Roberta Todd Spencer
Frances West Bergan

About the Factual Content of this Textbook

The authors, contributors, and editors of this book have expended considerable time and effort to ensure that the facts and opinions offered in the text and tables of this book are in accordance with official standards and with the consensus of foremost authorities at the time of publication.

However, drug therapy is a very dynamic branch of medicine, marked by the continual marketing of new drugs and the discontinuation and withdrawal (often without notice) of older drug products. In addition, the Food and Drug Administration (FDA) constantly orders changes in the labeling of even well-established drug products, on the basis of ongoing studies of their safety and efficacy. For this reason, no claims are made that statements made here concerning the current status of these drugs will continue to reflect the views of the drug industry or the FDA or that the data presented in tabular form are, or will remain, complete and correct in every detail.

The most important aspect of this problem lies in the area of dosage recommendations. Every effort has been made to check that statements made in the tables are, within the limits of space, precisely correct. However, dosage schedules are frequently ordered changed in accordance with accumulating clinical experience.

For this reason, we urge that *before administering any drug, you check the manufacturer's latest dosage recommendations* as presented in the package insert that accompanies each unit of every drug product.

Acknowledgments

The preparation of a textbook requires the involvement of many people who support and complement the work of the authors. This book is no exception. It would be impossible to name everyone who contributed to its publication. However, we would like to acknowledge with gratitude the contributions of the Boston College School of Nursing and the following individuals to this fifth edition:

Contributors: Deborah Adams Cassidy, David N. Curry, Nancy Fairchild, Barbara Wolfe

Editors: Margaret Zuccarini, Deedie McMahon, Barbara Ryalls

Contents

Introduction to Pharmacology

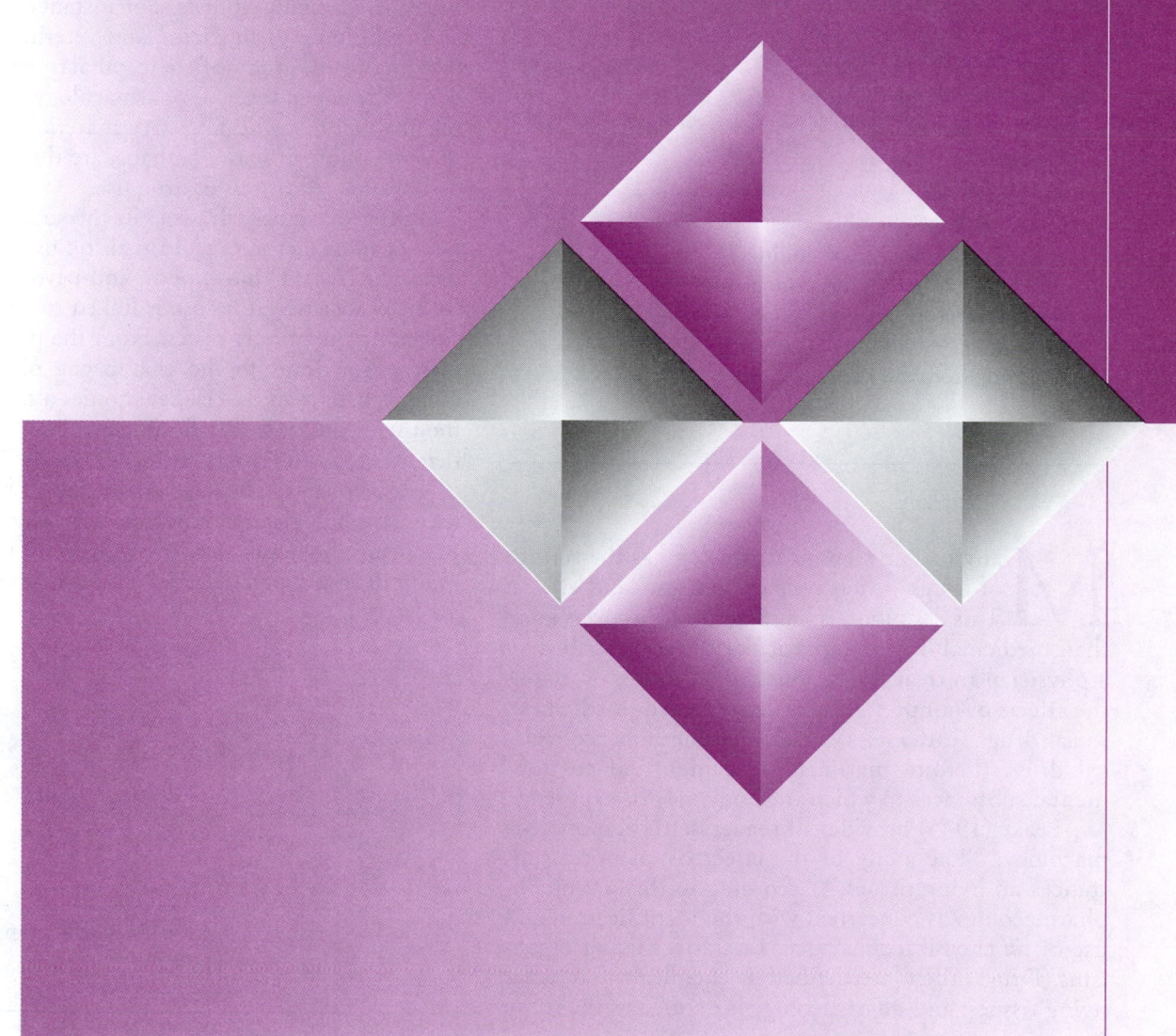

1

Orientation to Pharmacology

Many people view pharmacology as the science of drugs—their preparation, use, and effects. This definition is limiting. It rarely covers more than medicinal drugs, in particular those prescribed by a physician to treat illness. Such a definition overlooks the effects of nonprescription drugs (patent medicines), social drugs (caffeine, alcohol, nicotine, tobacco), illegal drugs (heroin, marijuana, cocaine), and environmental substances to which the body may be exposed.

Leake (1975) provides a broader definition of pharmacology: "The study of the effect of chemical substances on living tissues." According to this definition, pharmacology is concerned with the identification and use of *all* chemical substances that affect living organisms. Drugs, then, are defined as chemicals that affect living tissues, and pharmacology is defined as the study of the physiologic effects and social implications of medicinal drugs, poisons, pharmacologically active foods, and pollutants (Box 1-1).

Scope of Pharmacology

Of the traditional sciences, chemistry is most closely related to pharmacology. Chemical analysis is essential to identifying active drug substances. Moreover, inorganic, organic, and molecular chemistry and biochemistry are all involved in studying drug properties. The chemist determines the relationship of molecular structure to biologic activity, modifies chemicals to change their drug properties, and synthesizes new molecules to be used as drugs.

Other disciplines, particularly biology, botany, geology, microbiology, genetics, nutrition, and animal and human physiology, contribute to identifying active drug substances as well. Because modern drugs are derived from many sources (eg, minerals, plants, microbial cultures, and animal and human tissues), their extraction and manufacture depend on knowledge of many scientific disciplines. For instance, the principles and techniques of medicine and veterinary science are essential to the study of chemical actions in living animals. The dependence of pharmacology on the material sciences (ie, those dealing with material phenomena) is obvious. More obscure, perhaps, are the social and psychologic ramifications of drug use.

Drugs have played a role in the socioreligious practices of most cultures. The ritualistic use of sacramental wine, the "sacred" mushroom, and peyote are examples. In many societies, drug use is linked to and largely controlled by the priestly castes. From the peace pipe of the Native Americans to the champagne of modern weddings, religious and social ceremonies also have involved the use of drugs. Cultural influence is a powerful factor that affects attitudes and practices associated with drugs.

Because drugs have so many medicinal and social uses, psychologic dynamics, social customs, religious practices, and legal controls influence individual and group drug-use practices. In modern times, many psy-

Box 1-1
What is Pharmacology?

Pharmacology is the study of the effects of chemical substances on living tissue, including:

- The study of medicinal drugs
- The study of chemicals with toxic properties
- The study of the use of chemicals for psychotropic or social purposes

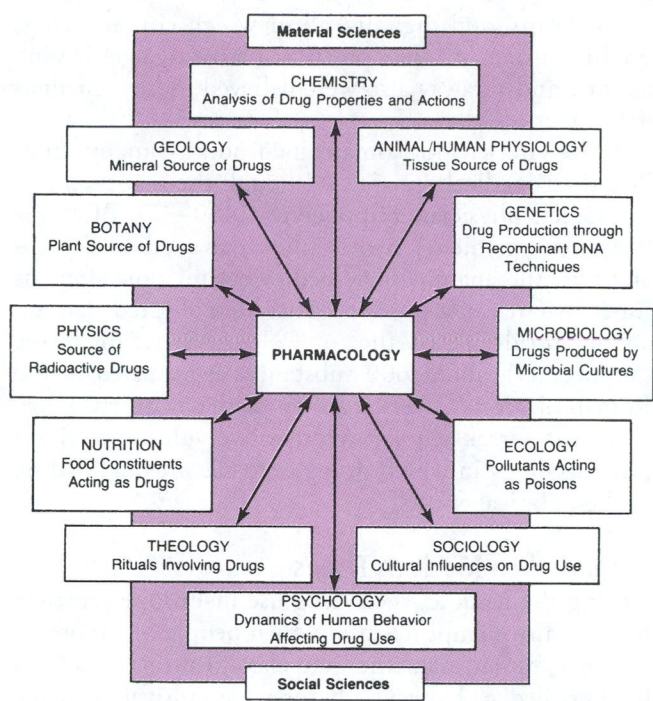

Figure 1-1. The scope of pharmacology.

In its broadest sense, pharmacology is an interdisciplinary study that crosses the boundaries of the physical, biologic, and social sciences to incorporate knowledge of body functions, the nature of matter, pollution, food and nutrition, and human behavior. A comprehensive study of the subject requires a multidisciplinary background (Fig. 1-1).

History of Pharmacology

Pharmacology is one of the oldest sciences (Fig. 1-2). The first person who tasted a strange plant in the hope that it was nutritious was conducting an experiment in both nutrition and pharmacology. If the plant did no harm, nourishment might be extracted from it. If it was poisonous, illness or death could result. Natural healing substances were typically discovered by chance. The history of harmful and helpful effects was transmitted orally from generation to generation.

Prehistoric Era

Every known culture has used certain active substances for their effects on living beings. Tribal traditions of prehistoric and ancient cultures include many drugs used for various effects. These practices were often quite sophisticated and relied on chemicals that modern healers have only recently begun producing for use in current medical therapy.

Salt, for example, is a chemical long recognized as essential to health. Like animals that are herbivorous,

chotropic (mind-altering) chemicals have been developed that can change human behavior, dispel inhibitions, and alter mental functions. These effects pose difficult moral and ethical problems. Pharmacology, therefore, involves not only the biologic sciences but the social sciences as well.

Figure 1-2. Time line of development of pharmacology

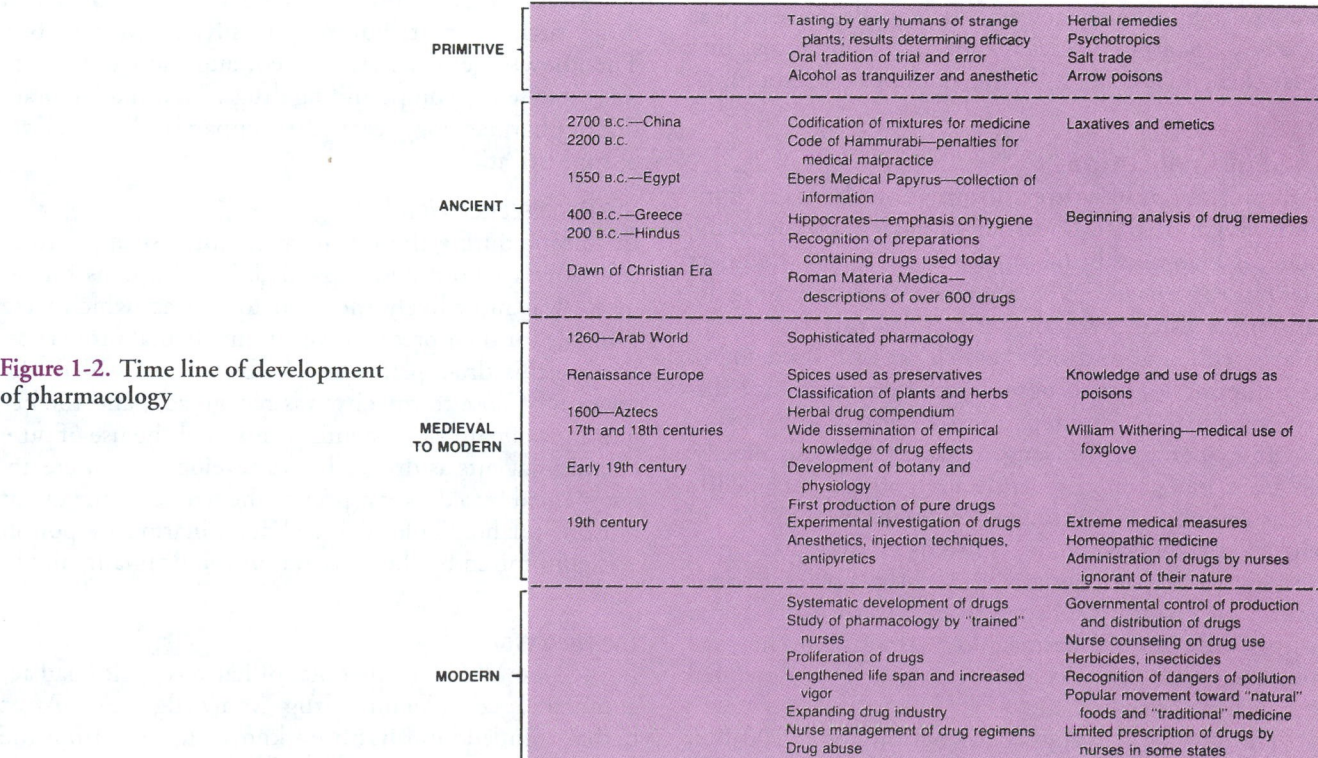

PRIMITIVE		Tasting by early humans of strange plants; results determining efficacy Oral tradition of trial and error Alcohol as tranquilizer and anesthetic	Herbal remedies Psychotropics Salt trade Arrow poisons
ANCIENT	2700 B.C.—China 2200 B.C. 1550 B.C.—Egypt 400 B.C.—Greece 200 B.C.—Hindus Dawn of Christian Era	Codification of mixtures for medicine Code of Hammurabi—penalties for medical malpractice Ebers Medical Papyrus—collection of information Hippocrates—emphasis on hygiene Recognition of preparations containing drugs used today Roman Materia Medica—descriptions of over 600 drugs	Laxatives and emetics Beginning analysis of drug remedies
MEDIEVAL TO MODERN	1260—Arab World Renaissance Europe 1600—Aztecs 17th and 18th centuries Early 19th century 19th century	Sophisticated pharmacology Spices used as preservatives Classification of plants and herbs Herbal drug compendium Wide dissemination of empirical knowledge of drug effects Development of botany and physiology First production of pure drugs Experimental investigation of drugs Anesthetics, injection techniques, antipyretics	 Knowledge and use of drugs as poisons William Withering—medical use of foxglove Extreme medical measures Homeopathic medicine Administration of drugs by nurses ignorant of their nature
MODERN		Systematic development of drugs Study of pharmacology by "trained" nurses Proliferation of drugs Lengthened life span and increased vigor Expanding drug industry Nurse management of drug regimens Drug abuse	Governmental control of production and distribution of drugs Nurse counseling on drug use Herbicides, insecticides Recognition of dangers of pollution Popular movement toward "natural" foods and "traditional" medicine Limited prescription of drugs by nurses in some states

human vegetarians must have salt to maintain essential electrolytes in the body. Some of the earliest known trade routes were developed to meet the need for this substance by populations located far from the sea or from natural deposits of the mineral.

Alcohol also was known and used by most cultures. A byproduct of carbohydrate fermentation, alcohol had particular value as a tranquilizer and anesthetic. Most cultures developed alcoholic beverages from local foods, such as grapes (wine), potatoes (vodka), rice (sake), and other sweet or starchy materials. However, the need for mood-altering drugs was not completely met by alcohol alone. Historically, the psychotropics that various cultures have used include marijuana, opium, coca, tobacco, peyote, coffee, tea, agaric, chocolate, kava, and betel. Few, if any, people in the world lack drugs that ease the difficulties of life or allow a temporary escape from the problems of daily existence.

Another class of drugs was useful in hunting animals. Smeared on arrowheads and other hunting implements, these substances were toxic and were used to stun or kill animals. Such poisons were sometimes used in warfare against enemy tribes. South American natives used curare (from a plant) in this way.

Still other drugs were used specifically for their medicinal effects. Most early civilizations understood the use of laxatives and emetics (preparations that induce vomiting). Plants such as rauwolfia (from a root) were used in cardiovascular and psychiatric illnesses. Folk remedies included practices such as poulticing with moldy bread (a crude topical antibiotic). Most remedies were mixtures of substances in which one or several active ingredients were accompanied by others that were totally ineffective except as placebos (pharmacologically inactive substances that cause changes in the body by the power of suggestion).

Ancient Civilizations

Early collections of written information about drugs include a Chinese codification (about 2700 BC), the Code of Hammurabi (about 2000 BC), and the Ebers Medical Papyrus of Egypt (about 1550 BC). Among the substances listed were rhubarb and senna (laxatives), hyssop, ephedra, and beer, which are still used today. Remedies no longer recognized as effective include rhinoceros horn (a reputed aphrodisiac), pomegranate, and animal excreta. Ginseng, a favorite Chinese remedy, has been investigated recently for possible therapeutic use as an antidepressant. The Egyptians were interested particularly in preservative substances that could prevent decay of the body after death; however, their records also identify substances used to treat the living. In this early era of pharmacology, the use of chemical substances was shrouded in mystery, a closely guarded secret of the priestly caste.

Hindu pharmacology, dating from about 200 BC, recognized such preparations as colchicum, gentian,

castor beans, and digitalis, all of which contain drugs used in current medical practice. Flavoring agents such as anise and caraway also were believed to have medicinal properties.

The Greeks and Romans incorporated many drugs into their medical practice. Although the treatments of the Greek physician Hippocrates (460–377 BC) emphasized hygienic regimens rather than medicinal preparations, the analysis of remedies began soon after his time. In Greece, a pupil of Aristotle collected data on about 500 drugs. By the time Nero reigned in Rome (54–68 AD), about 600 substances were listed in the Roman *Materia Medica*. In the same century, Dioscorides, a Greek scholar, wrote a five-volume work on pharmacology in which drugs were classified according to their clinical effects.

Medieval to Modern Times

During the Middle Ages, drug use in Europe returned to a primitive empiricism in which people relied on experience, rather than emerging classifications, as a basis for knowledge. However, herbs were cultivated in the gardens of monasteries for their medicinal properties, and the harmful effects of certain substances (eg, mushrooms, smutty rye) were recognized. Isolated centers of learning preserved some of the older knowledge, and indigenous drug lore was exploited. A few new remedies evolved, including the ashes of sponges for goiter and alcohol as an antiseptic.

The Eastern World

In the Arab world, pharmacology continued to advance. A compendium appearing in 1260 AD listed drugs such as ergot, borax, quicksilver, and cinnabar. The knowledge was systematized, and meticulous care was exercised in compounding drugs. The Arabian practice of pharmacology reached a comparatively high level of sophistication.

The Renaissance World

In Europe during the Renaissance, interest in pharmacology was reborn and expanded. The impetus for renewal was most likely the need for spices, which were valuable for their preservative and medicinal properties. During this time, plants and herbs were classified, the relation of dose to toxicity was recognized, and the beginnings of empirical chemistry fostered the use of pure chemical agents as drugs. These developments were accompanied by a darker aspect of the science—the use of poisons for homicide. Political assassination by poison was epitomized by the activities of the Borgia family in Italy.

The New World

In the New World, the peoples of Latin America had accumulated considerable drug knowledge. An Aztec herbal compendium has been known to exist from the mid-16th century. These New World natives used coca, chili, balsam, castor oil, jalap, sarsaparilla, and tobacco. Cihuapatli (an oxytocic agent that induces uterine contractions) was known as "women's medicine." In religious rites, hallucinogens such as mushrooms, peyote, and morning glory were also used. Latin American natives used quinine and curare, the former to treat fevers, the latter as an arrow poison.

Modern Times

During the 17th and 18th centuries, empirical knowledge of drug effects grew steadily. As world travel and trade developed, this knowledge was disseminated. The stimulating properties of tea, coffee, and cacao were recognized. Quinine from the New World, ginseng from China, and casein, cinchona, and ipecac from India were added to the compendia of the European nations.

In the late 18th century, the medicinal uses of foxglove (the source of digitalis, a heart stimulant) were described by an English physician, William Withering. The Royal Society of London fostered scientific investigation in many areas significant to the emerging science of pharmacology. Drugs were highly regarded and widely used by physicians and laypeople alike.

In the 19th century, scientists began to analyze, classify, and systematize drug data by a process we now call the scientific method. Simultaneously, the development of chemistry, botany, and physiology enabled pharmacologists to extract the active chemicals from plants and animals and to study their actions in the body. For the first time, the active ingredients in opium, colchicum, and other remedies were available in pure form. New techniques for administering drugs (eg, by injection) and for evaluating their effects provided extensive data on drug effects. As quantitative chemistry and systematic biology were established, modern pharmacology emerged. The emphasis of 19th-century pharmacology was on the organ and tissue effects of chemicals. Among the discoveries of this period were anesthetics, injection techniques, and antipyretic analgesics (medicines to treat fever and pain), such as aspirin.

Medical therapy in the 19th century was characterized by extreme measures designed to force the body to resume normal functions. Patients were subjected to violent purges, sweating, emetics, and bloodletting. For many, the treatment was more harmful than the disease it was intended to cure. Homeopathic medicine arose in reaction to these practices. Characterized by the use of crude drugs in markedly reduced (diluted) dosages, homeopathy was concerned with helping the body to heal itself. Although the weak medicinal preparations administered by homeopathic practitioners had doubtful pharmacologic effects, they acted as placebos and caused little harm. The sympathetic support of the physician undoubtedly aided the natural recuperative powers of the body. Homeopathy provided an alternative to the heroic medicine of the era and is still practiced in some areas.

The World of Today

Pharmacology has evolved into a complex science associated with a burgeoning drug industry. Purified chemicals are prepared from all conceivable natural materials: minerals, plants, animal tissues, and microbial cultures. Increasingly, drugs are developed, modified, and tailor-made through chemical synthesis. Our compendium of drugs is vast and includes both therapeutic medications and mind-altering compounds. Virtually every body function can be enhanced, suppressed, or manipulated by chemicals. A multitude of antiinfective agents controls bacterial infections that in the past killed many people. Drugs have enabled modern medicine to lengthen human life expectancy and increase vigor during the additional years.

Adverse Effects of Chemical Development

The ready availability of chemicals with powerful effects on the mind and body has cured many illnesses, but it has also contributed to such problems as drug abuse, pollution, and health-related expenses. Psychotropic drugs appear initially to relieve the stresses of modern living. However, they may pose other problems, such as chemical dependence or acute overdose, that are difficult to treat.

Modern technology has also fostered multitudes of chemical substances for use in industry and agriculture. These agents include herbicides, insecticides, fuels, solvents, and a bewildering variety of toxins. Exposure to many of these pollutants is associated with an increased incidence of cancer, allergy, and poisoning.

Return to Nature

One response to chemical- and drug-related problems is a resurgent interest in nature, including natural foods and "traditional" medicine. Various persons and groups are interested in investigating and preserving folk medicine. Many of these people practice and teach herbal medical techniques and publish their findings (Aikman, 1977).

Impact of Managed Care

As medicine and pharmacology have advanced, so have the costs of health care. In response, regulatory groups, including governmental and corporate agencies (Medicare, Medicaid, and private insurance companies) have undertaken the charge to "manage" care and control costs. To the healthcare personnel administering drugs and the clients purchasing drugs, managed care means learning new ways to provide and obtain medications and related services responsibly and in accord with specific economic guidelines. For example, many public and private insuring bodies refuse to reimburse the expense of a drug ordered by its trade name but will reimburse for the same drug ordered by its lower-costing generic name. These agencies rarely, if ever, reimburse the cost of drugs used for cosmetic effects (such as Retin-A for pigmented spots or wrinkles) or of drugs available without a prescription (over-the-counter [OTC] drugs such as aspirin and acetaminophen), even when ordered by a physician. Nor do they reimburse the cost of vitamins or any drug regimen considered experimental. If the use of the drug for the specific diagnosis has not been approved by the federal Food and Drug Administration (FDA), payment is likely to be refused. More and more drugs are being categorized as OTC by the FDA, at which point coverage for their costs is withdrawn by prescription insurance plans. The third-party payers decide which drug costs will be paid, and their judgment is difficult to appeal except through court action. In the case of life-threatening illness, legal action may come too late to benefit clients who cannot afford to pay for treatment out of their own pockets (see Critical Thinking Challenge: Issue Analysis).

Another significant aspect of the managed-care movement is the trend to provide treatment at home rather than in hospitals or nursing homes. In the home setting, drugs are usually administered by the recipient or a family member. For seriously ill clients, drug therapy may require learning how to administer injections or set up intravenous infusions. Substances commonly administered intravenously include total parenteral nutrition preparations and relatively toxic chemotherapeutic agents.

Future Concerns

Many problems challenge the medical and pharmaceutical communities. Viral and fungal infections do not respond well to currently available medicines. Many aspects of the immune system still mystify scientists in their quest to prevent or control allergy, autoimmune diseases, and transplant rejection. Gene therapy, now in its early stages, may one day offer a cure for genetic diseases such as cystic fibrosis. However, the use of drugs to treat illness and relieve suffering must be balanced with controls to prevent toxicity and user dependence and to enhance quality of life without poisoning people, animals, or the environment. Humans are likely to continue to produce more chemicals in their quest for progress. The importance of pharmacology as a guide to wise use of chemical substances will increase proportionately. It will remain a critical area of study for future generations.

CRITICAL THINKING CHALLENGE
Issue Analysis

Debate the following:

Resolved: The present system of managed care as it applies to drug therapy is acceptable as a cost-containment measure.

Pros

Controlling the money spent on drugs is an important cost-containment measure. Without some control on expenses, health care can bankrupt governmental and private insurance programs.

The generic drugs approved by medical insurers for cost reimbursement are less expensive than brand-name drugs and are just as effective because they contain the same active ingredients.

In the absence of constraints, many physicians take little care to minimize prescription drug costs, especially when third-party payers (insurers) reimburse those costs.

Government agencies and medical insurance companies can make decisions about costs more objectively than can the physician, who has a close one-on-one relationship with the client.

The cost of over-the-counter preparations, deemed safe enough for clients to manage for themselves, should not be reimbursed by third-party payers.

When physicians prescribe a drug for a purpose not yet approved by the federal Food and Drug Administration, the cost of this experimental use should not be underwritten by insurance companies or government agencies.

Cons

Managed care is a form of rationing, which is unacceptable to North Americans. A rationing program would be impossible to administer fairly. Some people who need more medication than allotted will die or suffer needlessly if they are denied medication.

In the past, certain generic drugs have not had the same effect as brand-name drugs, due to differences in absorption, pH, or the chemical makeup of the drug molecule (eg, acetate or hydrochloride salts).

Cost should not constrain physicians from specifying the particular drug preparations they think are best for the client, whether or not the drug is the least costly one available.

There is a clear conflict of interest between the duty of third-party payers to ensure good medical care for the consumer while containing the cost of that care. For private insurers, the conflict of interest is compounded by the responsibility to produce a profit for the stockholders.

Many over-the-counter drugs are critical to the treatment of serious diseases; if they are prescribed by the physician, their cost should be reimbursable.

The freedom of physicians to use medications to treat conditions that are likely to benefit from the medications is crucial to advancing medical science. Only by such clinical trials can all the benefits of a new drug be explored and its proper uses established.

1. Which of these arguments do you judge to be valid?
2. Discuss why you think they are valid.
3. What changes would you make in the current system to achieve the benefits of cost control without the risks suggested by the cons cited above?

■ SUMMARY

Pharmacology is the study of the effects of chemical substances on living tissues. It is one of the oldest sciences known to humanity. Originating as a trial-and-error method of survival, modern pharmacology has become more sophisticated and proven but is still imperfect. Today, pharmacology is an interdisciplinary study that involves all sciences in an amalgam of physical (ie, material) and social knowledge.

Every culture has studied plants and has developed a system of medicine founded on the use of plants. Many of these ancient herbs and chemicals are still used; many others have been revived in modern medicine.

The role of nurses in pharmacology involves promoting the responsible use of chemicals to enhance health and minimize detrimental effects. This requires knowledge and understanding not only of the physical and social sciences but also of ethical and legal issues pertaining to nursing care.

In carrying out drug therapy, nurses must be skilled in the procedures required to handle, control, and administer drugs safely. They must be able to work cooperatively in developing care plans and drug regimens that are acceptable to the client, physician, and society at large. The supervision and administration of medicinal therapy is an art as well as a science.

Developing a Personal Knowledge Base

Because knowledge is growing so rapidly and its communication is possible so quickly and in so many forms, each nurse must develop a personal knowledge base to keep abreast of trends in pharmacology and nursing practice. To do this, the student nurse must master knowledge pertaining to the activities of chemicals in the body. An understanding of pharmacokinetics (the general mechanisms influencing drug absorption, transport, metabolism, and excretion) and pharmacodynamics (the drug's effects on the body) is essential for administering and managing drug therapy with good judgment (see Chap. 4).

Drug-Related Nursing Responsibilities

The nurse is responsible for knowing about anything that affects nursing care in relation to drug use. Nursing concerns may include timing of doses, special techniques for administration, precautions to take before administering a drug, assessment of toxicity and side effects, the potential for tolerance or addiction, legal constraints on the use of the drug, and so forth. Only in recent years have nursing implications appeared in drug reference sources to a significant extent. Because this is an area of nursing knowledge that needs further development, many practitioners keep a record of verbally communicated information from experienced nurses as well as data from published sources.

The nursing student must master the techniques of drug administration to ensure accurate, safe, and effective delivery of the prescribed medication to the proper body tissues. Once the basic skills and knowledge are acquired, the nurse is ready to begin practice with clients.

The number of drugs in current use is far too vast for anyone to memorize. However, the nurse must know or be able to locate reliable information pertaining to any and all drugs a particular client is using. Student nurses soon learn the facts about drugs in common use. They should also appreciate the benefits of thoroughly learning about the drugs most frequently prescribed in their field of practice. In the pressures of clinical practice, time to look up required drug data may be limited.

Required Drug Knowledge

Data pertaining to specific drugs should include the drug's name and family (or class); physiologic actions; therapeutic uses; adverse effects; potential interactions; data about administration, metabolism, and elimination; and nursing implications. The nurse must know:

- The name of the drug, which may be its generic, trade, or chemical name or a generally recognized abbreviation (see Table 2-2 in Chap. 2)
- The drug's family or families, which may indicate its chemical derivation (eg, heavy metal, xanthines, steroids), mechanism of action (eg, central nervous system depressant, anticholinergic), or route of administration (eg, oral, topical, parenteral). The nurse must know the general properties and characteristics of each classification.
- The drug's mechanisms of action, which are its effects on body cells or tissues. They include desirable (therapeutic) actions and those causing undesirable effects. It is insufficient to know that a drug is a laxative; additional necessary data denote how the drug acts (eg, by lubrication, stimulation, saline catharsis, alteration of surface tension, or formation of bulk in the stool). In the case of analgesics, pain relief may be accounted for by antagonism of prostaglandins, central nervous system depression, inhibition of inflammation, and so forth. To make sound judgments, the nurse must understand how a medication affects function at the cellular or molecular level if possible.
- Side effects, which are desirable or undesirable physiologic effects exerted by the drug other than the intended therapeutic effect. Because some drugs have a multitude of side effects, the nurse must know about serious side effects (no matter how rare) and common side effects (no matter how benign). When rare side effects cause concern, referring to a comprehensive drug reference book usually clarifies the relation of the side effect to the

drug regimen. Virtually all drugs have side effects, the number and range of which may indicate the relative toxicity of a given medication (see Chap. 5).

- Adverse reactions, which are undesirable effects apparent in the recipient (eg, toxic, teratogenic, carcinogenic, paradoxic, allergic). If an antidote or emergency treatment is recommended, it should be included.
- Drug interactions, which are effects caused by the simultaneous presence of a drug and another chemical that are not seen with the drug alone. There are several types: drug–drug, drug–food, drug–pollutant, and drug–laboratory test agent.
- Precautions and contraindications. *Contraindications* are conditions or symptoms that alert the healthcare practitioner to potential dangers of the drug. For example, glaucoma is a contraindication for anticholinergics (which dilate the pupils and may precipitate an acute episode of glaucoma). Some prescribers may, with good reason, prescribe drugs despite contraindications. In these situations, the nurse should clarify the drug order with the physician to be sure the prescriber is aware of the contraindications. In such a case, the prescriber may order drugs or treatment to reduce the risk. *Precautions* are measures taken to prevent or reduce adverse effects.
- Dosage range and route, which must be specified for each method of drug administration. Many factors require a dosage to be adjusted, including body mass (weight), nutritional status, pathologic condition, and the client's ability to metabolize and excrete the drug. If a drug order prescribes an unusual dosage, the nurse must verify and clarify the order with the prescriber. Errors in dosage are not uncommon, especially in the case of verbal orders. It is the nurse's responsibility to alert the prescriber to the possibility of error.
- Drug elimination, which involves the physiologic mechanisms by which a drug is deactivated and eliminated from the body. The efficiency of these processes affects the efficacy and potential for toxicity of a given medication. Many drugs are deactivated by microsomal enzymes in the liver and excreted by the kidneys. Clients whose liver or kidneys function abnormally are at increased risk for complications related to drug therapy.

Reliable Sources of Information

Because no single source provides all the drug information needed by the nurse in a given clinical situation, the student must become familiar with a variety of publications, using each for the particular information it best provides. Types of publications include pharmacopeiae, textbooks, reference books, journals, subscription services, computer data bases, and literature from pharmaceutical firms.

Pharmacopeiae

Pharmacopeiae are collections of drug data considered standard by the group developing them (eg, medical or pharmaceutical societies, governmental task forces) or by some other authority. In most modern countries, one or more pharmacopeiae are adopted by governmental action to indicate that country's "official" drugs. In the United States, an official drug is one that is included in the official compendium *The United States Pharmacopeia & National Formulary* (*USP&NF*). In the United Kingdom, official drugs are listed in *The British Pharmacopoeia* (*BP*). Canada uses *The Canadian Formulary* as well as the *USP&NF* and the *BP*.

Pharmacopeiae are written by committees of experts (pharmacologists, physicians, and pharmacists) designated by the sponsoring government or private agency. They usually include information vital to the preparation, compounding, and dispensing of drugs. Revised periodically (usually every 5 years), new editions exclude drugs that have fallen into disuse or disrepute and add new drugs considered acceptable. The information in an official pharmacopeia is more useful to pharmacists than to other healthcare personnel because there is little medical and no nursing information incorporated in them. A pharmacopeia is usually available in college libraries and hospital pharmacies.

Textbooks

Drug textbooks are written for students of nursing, medicine, or pharmacy. Traditional nursing textbooks provide a general background in pharmacology, specific instruction on the preparation and administration of drugs, and drug data on medications in common use. They function, therefore, not only as textbooks on nursing functions but also as reference sources for drug information. Nursing textbooks are usually available in college and hospital libraries; a nurse may purchase one as a student and may keep an up-to-date text in a personal library.

Medical textbooks are written for medical students and physicians and emphasize therapeutic considerations in the prescribing of drugs. Most include detailed discussions and comprehensive data concerning drug action, pharmacokinetics, drugs in common use, and the treatment of poisoning. These texts tend to be excellent sources of background information concerning the physiologic dynamics of drug therapy and adverse reactions to medication, but they do not apply this information to nursing practice. Examples of standard medical textbooks are *Goodman & Gilman's The Pharmacological Basis of Therapeutics* and *Goth's Medical Pharmacology*.

Books written for pharmacy students (eg, *Remington's Pharmaceutical Sciences*) emphasize information needed for accurate compounding and dispensing of drugs, as well as the clinical applications of drug treatments. Chemical data concerning drugs are extensive, and information about compatibility and interactions is detailed. Pharmacy textbooks are not generally available except in the libraries of colleges of pharmacy.

Journals

Journals are valuable sources of information when a specific topic is to be researched in detail. Pertinent articles may be located through the appropriate indices, the *Index Medicus* and *Cumulative Index to Nursing and Allied Health Literature.*

A survey of the literature should begin with the most recent publications and continue backward until the relevant material appears to be exhausted. This time period varies with the topic, but 5 years is the average.

Many nurses regularly read the periodicals most pertinent to their areas of practice. Various nursing journals and periodicals feature departments that regularly publish drug information, and articles dealing with special drug problems appear from time to time. Although journal articles may be written several months in advance of publication, they still tend to be more current than books and pharmacopeiae.

Journals limited to drug information (eg, *The Medical Letter on Drugs and Therapeutics*) are also available for general use. They may be published monthly or biweekly.

Subscription Services

Subscription services provide current drug information for healthcare agencies. They provide a basic text (sometimes in looseleaf format) and regularly publish revisions to be incorporated in the reference volumes. The drug data are detailed and comprehensive. However, the material is organized according to therapeutic use, and pages may not be numbered consecutively, presenting difficulties in locating needed information efficiently. Because these publications tend to be expensive, they are not generally available. However, many hospital pharmacies maintain one copy, and some college libraries also subscribe. Three major subscription services are *Drug Information*, published by the American Hospital Formulary Service by the authority of the American Society of Health-System Pharmacists; *Compendium of Pharmaceuticals*, published by the Canadian Pharmaceutical Association; and *Drug Facts and Comparisons*, published by Drug Facts and Comparisons.

Electronic Data Bases and Internet

When available, computer programs on drugs can furnish comprehensive, up-to-date information. These data should be evaluated in accordance with the questions listed in Box 1-2. Selected Internet sites and guidelines for evaluating health information on the Internet are located inside the back cover.

Package Inserts and the Physicians' Desk Reference

Pharmaceutical firms publish a great deal of information about their medicinal products. The content is controlled in part by national legislation, which forbids claims of therapeutic efficacy not supported by research data and requires inclusion of certain information concerning

Box 1-2
How to Evaluate Drug References and Resources

When selecting and evaluating a drug reference, ask the following questions:

- What is the source of the data? How accurate is it? Does the author represent any particular point of view or have a vested interest in the effect the information may have on the reader?
- For whom is the information written? Material published for physicians or pharmacists may assume knowledge that the nurse lacks or may emphasize aspects of limited use to the nurse while omitting data of particular value in nursing practice.
- Are pertinent data readily available and generally understandable? Appropriate organization and indexing help the nurse locate information. Clear, concise writing is essential. Print should be large enough for easy reading.
- How pertinent is the material to nursing? The best sources include comprehensive information relative to nursing practice and exclude irrelevant material.
- Is the information current? Textbook material may be 2 or more years old when published. Journal articles tend to involve several months of preparation. The frequency of revision and updating of pharmacopeiae and subscription services affects the usefulness of their data.
- Is availability of the reference limited by its cost? Price influences which references a person, institution, or library purchases. For example, some facilities may buy an inexpensive volume rather than a superior but more costly subscription service.
- Is the format of the publication appropriate and convenient? Pocket-sized volumes are useful for clinical reference; looseleaf formats with discrete entries facilitate updating of material.

drug toxicity, side effects, and adverse reactions. Within these constraints, however, drug firms can and do slant the descriptive material to promote the use of their products. The information must be interpreted with this bias in mind.

Data concerning individual drugs usually are included as a package insert when the medicine is marketed. These brochures are written for prescribing physicians and assume that the reader has a wide knowledge of pharmacology. For this reason, references and allusions may seem cryptic to the nonphysician reader.

The most widely used drug information reference in the United States, the *Physicians' Desk Reference* (*PDR*), is a compilation of selected package inserts, arranged by drug manufacturers and trade names. Drug firms are charged for the listings by the publisher, who then markets the book to physicians and other health professionals. The volume is revised yearly, with supplements published during the year. It can be used to identify the generic drugs contained in new trade-name preparations. The section containing color photographs of various drugs and dosage forms allows identification of unlabeled drugs by their appearance. It is commonly the only easily available source listing a new proprietary drug. Once the generic constituent of a drug is identified, however, the reader is likely to find data in other references that are more objective and comprehensive than the *PDR*.

The Pharmacist

Inevitably, situations arise in which information cannot be obtained from available publications. The nurse may then consult the pharmacist who dispensed the drug; he or she may provide a brochure or other information. As an expert in drug therapy, the pharmacist is a valuable member of the healthcare team and should be involved in client care in ways other than as a consultant of last resort; see the discussion in Chapter 7 on the pharmacist's role. However, the nurse should not burden the pharmacist by requesting information available from other sources.

Drug Firms

When drug information cannot be obtained from any other source, the manufacturer may be contacted directly by telephone. Most firms maintain a toll-free number, and some accept collect calls. There may be different listings for general product, medical, and pharmaceutical information; for reporting side effects; and for after-hours emergencies. Current telephone numbers may be obtained from the telephone company's information service or from listings in the *PDR* or the *Compendium of Pharmaceuticals*.

Supplementary Information

Ideally, students become familiar with as wide a range of references as possible, adopt sources that are most useful and convenient, and guard against undue reliance on any one reference. Periodically consulting supplementary sources helps prevent a systematic bias that may influence a nursing judgment. In this as well as other areas of nursing expertise, the student must develop sound scholarship habits.

▪▪ SUMMARY

Before administering a drug, the nurse must know certain facts about the substance: its names, drug family or families, desired effects and mechanism of action, side effects, adverse reactions, toxic effects, interactions, precautions and contraindications, dosage range and administration routes,

elimination, and nursing implications. Nursing students must understand the general mechanisms of drug action and must practice the techniques of drug administration before applying pharmacology to clinical practice. Because no single source can provide all this information, the nurse should become familiar with many sources of information: pharmacopeiae, textbooks, journals, subscription services, electronic data bases, pharmaceutical firms, and the pharmacist. The student should acquire sound habits of scholarship from which to develop and maintain an adequate, up-to-date knowledge base.

Approaches to Drug Therapy

Modern drug therapy evolved from three major areas:

- Tribal traditions (the magical approach)
- Experience, observation, and analysis of cultural traditions in the use of environmental elements (the empirical approach)
- Development of chemical and biologic research and methodology (the scientific rational approach).

Magical Approach

The use of medicines and the development of basic health customs in different cultures emerged from the practices of spiritual persons, witches, medicine men, and other tribal healers who responded to people's fear of illness and disease. Without clear knowledge of what caused infections or metabolic diseases, healers implemented treatments that today are considered magical and ritualistic. It is difficult to separate the influence of magic from the development of empirical science. The belief in magic inhibited progress toward a scientific rational approach to medicine, but at the same time it facilitated the experimental use of natural elements.

Empirical Approach

Empiricism as an approach to pharmacology attempted to relate drug use to experience. Empirics believe that certain substances are useful in specific circumstances, but they cannot account rationally for their therapeutic effectiveness. Empirical knowledge arises from trial and error. As scientific explanations for drug actions develop, the empirical approach yields to a more rational one. This is not an all-or-none phenomenon: some actions of a given drug may have a theoretical explanation at a given time.

Rational Approach

For centuries, healers attempted to mold empirical protopharmacology into a systematic compendium of information on known remedies throughout the world.

This led to the development of a logical approach to drugs and treatment by the end of the 18th century. The rational approach depended on the development of methods for evaluating crude drugs and chemical compounds. Logical decisions about the use of drugs could be made once science could provide answers to questions regarding the chemical and biologic effects of various compounds.

The rational approach to pharmacologic research and drug therapy now relies on chemical analysis and biologic assay performed by chemists, pharmacologists, clinicians, and other experts. Theories regarding the action of drugs are tested to determine the relation between the molecular structure of chemicals and their biologic effects. This theoretical base allows pharmacologists, in many cases, to alter chemical structure to achieve predicted effects on biologic activity.

■ SUMMARY

Lack of knowledge about cause and effect gave rise to a magical approach to healing based on fear or wishful thinking concerning the use of natural products and persons involved with healing. The empirical approach arose from this as it became clear that certain substances were useful in particular circumstances, although the healer did not know why the substance was helpful. Some systematic methods evolved under empiricism. The rational approach appeared at the end of the 18th century as scientists developed a methodologic evaluation of crude drugs and chemical compounds. Systematic experimentation developed slowly, eventually leading to the problem-solving methodology of modern pharmacology (Box 1-3).

Box 1-3
Development of Modern Drug Therapy

- Magical approach—development and oral transmission of tribal traditions (eg, the practices of spiritual persons, witches, medicine men, and other tribal leaders)
- Empirical protopharmacologic approach—experience, observation, and analysis of cultural traditions in the use of environmental elements (eg, the use of plants and minerals as remedies)
- Scientific rational approach—development of chemical and biologic methodologies (eg, antibiotics specific for certain microorganisms)

Nursing Implications

Healthcare practices today continue to reflect magical, empirical, and rational orientations in client and healthcare provider behaviors. Until recently, clients generally pursued health care only after they became ill or incapacitated. They sought care to cure the malady or to relieve its symptoms. Clients become frustrated when they do not receive medication. Most hope that the medication will be the cure (magical approach). Physicians may accede to the request for medication, even when they have no rational basis for prescribing a drug. The magical powers of medicine are further exemplified through the use of placebos. A visit to a healthcare professional is often considered wasted or unacceptable unless a prescription is written.

Physicians often prescribe medications and use devices in the delivery of health care on an empirical basis only. For example, the intrauterine device has long been used without a clear understanding of how it actually prevents pregnancy, although there are several theories regarding its mechanism of action. Diethylstilbestrol, aspirin, and antihistamines are examples of drugs whose mechanisms of action are still questionable or not fully understood. Empirical evidence also serves as a basis for the continued use of home remedies in the face of information that contradicts their therapeutic value.

Scientific investigations using rational approaches underlie the development of many modern drugs. The pharmaceutical chemist determines the molecular properties associated with therapeutic action and side effects and may construct a drug with the most desirable combinations of these properties.

The administration of drugs was one of the first medical functions delegated by physicians to nurses. Initially, medication was tightly controlled by the physician, and the nurse remained ignorant about the drugs that were administered. Over time, however, increasing responsibility was given to the nurse, who was then expected to exercise judgment in managing drug therapy. Today's nurse must have a knowledge of drug actions and the ability to detect therapeutic and adverse reactions in the client.

Assuming Greater Responsibilities

In accordance with protocols developed jointly with physicians, today's nurses have greater latitude in modifying drug regimens. They are expected to counsel clients on managing drug regimens for optimal effect on health. In some clinical situations, specially skilled nurses can prescribe medications. Thus, the once-dependent nursing function related to prescribed drug therapy has a new and independent dimension not only in administering drugs but also in teaching and health promotion.

In caring for acutely ill clients, the nurse usually administers required medications. This function is demanding because of the proliferation of new drugs and the complexities of multiple-drug therapy. The safety and efficacy of drug therapy at this level depends on an accurate assessment of the client's response to the treatment agents. The nurse must detect early signs and symptoms of toxicity, adverse reactions, and drug interactions as well as therapeutic response; he or she must work closely with the prescriber to revise the drug regimen for optimal effect.

Teaching and Health Promotion

Nurses have always taught people about using drugs, particularly nonprescription drugs. However, as chemical substances proliferate in modern society, this teaching has expanded to include poison control, the nonmedicinal use of drugs, and drug abuse and addiction. Education about drugs is an important part of health promotion and a key to preventing drug-related disease. The nurse may contribute to illness-prevention efforts by compiling pertinent data on the effects of environmental chemicals and medicinal agents on humans.

Convalescing clients require education and assistance to resume control of their lives and to maximize their health potential. In many cases, clients must take medications over the long term to control chronic disease, and they must learn to manage the drug regimen and other aspects of self-care. In addition, the client or family members responsible for administering drugs or using complex equipment need considerable nursing support and guidance to learn the required procedures and precautions and to adjust emotionally to the responsibilities involved in such treatment.

When teaching clients with chronic illness, the nurse's teaching and care plans must take into account the fact that medications used to prolong the life span and ease suffering may precipitate other problems that may call for value judgments about the quality of life. As in other aspects of health care, the nurse should respect the client's right to self-determination. The passive recipient role of the past has been replaced by the active involvement of the client (and family or other responsible caregivers) in determining the therapy to be chosen and the regimen by which it will be carried out.

Case Finding and Referral

Early detection of drug-related problems in otherwise healthy persons involves case finding and referral. The nurse seeks early evidence of drug-related problems such as dependence, toxicity, or adverse reactions from the use of drugs (medicinal or nonmedicinal) and detrimental effects of exposure to chemicals. Then the nurse works with clients to improve self-care practices and, when necessary, refers the person to a proper treatment source.

Continuing Education

Almost all areas of nursing require a knowledge of pharmacology. Beginning students must learn the rudiments of the science and acquire the skills needed in clinical practice. Providing safe, effective nursing care involves not only the accurate administration of medications but also the exercise of sound judgment. Nursing judgments must be based on a broad background of knowledge, including pharmacology.

Nurses must know how to supplement this knowledge quickly and efficiently with additional data when required by the clinical situation, because time is limited in most clinical settings. Nursing students as well as those in clinical practice should allocate time for the regular study of drug data, focusing on the drugs encountered in their own clinical setting. All available references should be used, and new publications should be explored as they appear. The mass of material is expanding so rapidly that computers increasingly are being used to retrieve pertinent information quickly. In the meantime, only continuing study enables a nurse to maintain safe drug therapy practice.

Learning From the Client

The nurse can never be sure that he or she has all the facts (even the known facts) about all the drugs used in work with clients. The nurse should not be discouraged, however, because the client is a key source of knowledge in any situation. The client should be observed and assessed to determine the therapeutic and adverse reactions to the drugs involved. For example, if the client is on antihypertensive drugs, the blood pressure should be checked regularly. A drop in blood pressure toward normal indicates a therapeutic response. Hypotension (or a rapid drop) and symptoms suggestive of hypovolemic shock warn of toxicity. Even without using a sphygmomanometer, blood pressure may be estimated by palpating the pulse; the amplitude of the pulse reflects the systolic pressure.

Many specific observations are recommended for certain drugs (eg, pulse rate for digitalis preparations, respiratory rate for narcotics). In addition to these individual assessments, a global assessment should be made. These data may be acquired quickly. Posture and activity, skin color, facial expression, and vocal expression should be observed. A general impression formed by listening to and observing the client provides many clues to changes that may be related to drugs. Any unusual or unexpected changes in emotional affect, physiologic function, mental ability, or comfort levels should be investigated with that possibility in mind. The nurse who checks to see if the client's signs and symptoms might be drug-related may detect many adverse reactions to medications that otherwise would remain undisclosed.

References

Aikman L. (1977). Nature's healing arts: From folk medicine to modern drugs. In *Folk medicine: An enduring art*. Washington, DC: National Geographic Society.

Leake CD. (1975). *An historical account of pharmacology to the 20th century*. Springfield, IL: Charles C. Thomas.

Bibliography

American Medical Association. *Drug evaluations.* (Subscription service.) Chicago: American Medical Association.

Clark WG et al. (1992). *Goth's medical pharmacology*, 13th ed. St. Louis: CV Mosby.

Coulter CR. (1986). *Portraits of homeopathic medicines: Psychophysical analyses of selected constitutional types.* Washington, DC: Center of Empirical Medicine.

Gennaro AR, ed. (1990). *Remington's pharmaceutical sciences*, 18th ed. Easton, PA: Mack Publishers.

Hardman JG, Limbird LE, et al, eds. (1996). *Goodman & Gilman's The pharmacological basis of therapeutics*, 9th ed. New York: McGraw-Hill.

Krantz JC. (1967). *Profiles of medical science and inspired moments.* Baltimore: John D. Lucas.

*Krogh CM, ed. *Compendium of pharmaceuticals and specialties.* Ottawa: Canadian Pharmaceutical Association. (Published yearly.)

Krogh CM, Carruthers-Czyzewski, eds. (1992). *Self-medication*, 4th ed. Ottawa: Canadian Pharmaceutical Association.

Li CP. (1974). *Chinese herbal medicine.* (Pub. No. NIH75-732). Washington, DC: U.S. Department of Health, Education and Welfare.

Long JW, Rybacki JJ. (1994). *The essential guide to prescription drugs.* New York: Harper & Row.

Lyons A, Petrucelli RJ. (1978). *Medicine: An illustrated history.* New York: Harry N. Abrams.

*McEvoy GK, ed. (1996). *Drug information '96.* Bethesda: American Hospital Formulary Service, American Society of Health-System Pharmacists. (Published yearly with quarterly updates.)

The medical letter on drugs and therapeutics. (A biweekly newsletter.) New Rochelle, NY: Medical Letter, Inc.

Medicines Commission for Her Majesty's Stationery Office. (1980). Cambridge: University Printing House. (With yearly addenda.)

*Navarra T. (1990). Drug therapy: The history of a love affair. *American Journal of Nursing 90*, 91.

Olin BR, ed. *Drug facts and comparisons.* Chicago: Drug Facts and Comparisons. (Published yearly with monthly updates.)

Physicians' desk reference. (1997). Oradell, NJ: Medical Economics Books.

Prescribers' Journal. (A bimonthly publication.) London: National Health Service.

Riddle JM. (1985). *Dioscorides on pharmacy and medicine.* Austin: University of Texas Press.

Thorndike L. (1929). *A history of magic and experimental science during the first thirteen centuries of our era*, vol. 1. New York: Columbia University Press.

Thorndike L. (1963). *Science and thought in the fifteenth century.* New York: Hafner Press.

The United States pharmacopeia & national formulary. (1995). Rockville, MD: The U.S. Pharmacopeia.

USAN and the USP dictionary of drug names. (1993). Rockville, MD: U.S. Pharmacopeial Convention.

*Recommended for further reading.

For more information and sample tests and activities, refer to Chapter 1 in the Student Workbook for Clinical Pharmacology and Nursing Management, 5th edition, available through your bookstore.

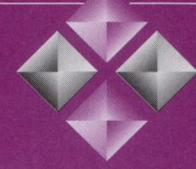

2

Drug Preparations, Controls, and Standards

Substances used for a pharmacologic effect must usually undergo some kind of preparation before medicinal use. Rarely, if ever, are the raw materials containing pharmacologically active chemicals found in a chemically pure form. To eliminate extraneous substances, the active chemical is usually extracted from the raw source, purified, and incorporated in a formulation designed to deliver the drug to the appropriate tissues. Because the process of drug purification is so complex and subject to variables, regulations to ensure purity and safety have been instituted worldwide. This chapter discusses drug preparations and the controls and standards that govern their use and production.

Characteristics of Medicinal Preparations

Among the features that characterize drugs are their sources, components, dosage forms, and names.

Drug Sources

Drugs are developed from a wealth of natural resources, including plants, animal tissues, and organic and inorganic minerals. They are also synthesized chemically.

Plants

Plants were one of the earliest sources of therapeutic agents. Seeds, bark, roots, stems, fruit, and sap were all used for medicinal purposes. Because most of these preparations contained inert ingredients or multiple active ingredients, they were called *crude drugs*. As refined techniques were developed for extracting the active ingredients from plants, *pure drugs* emerged.

Animals

Animal tissues are also sources of crude drugs (eg, liver extract). In modern practice, most tissues are refined to a considerable degree. Animals are the source of drugs such as hormones (eg, insulin from the pancreatic cells of pigs and cows) and vitamins (eg, vitamins A and D from fish oil). Slaughter is not always necessary; for example, vaccines may be produced from cultures grown in eggs, and antitoxins from horse serum.

Minerals

Commonly used mineral products include metallic and nonmetallic compounds, acids, bases, and salts. Coal tar is a source of many drugs such as sulfonamides and salicylates (eg, aspirin).

Synthetic Chemicals

Substances that do not occur naturally may be developed in a pure form in laboratories. Sophisticated equipment and highly skilled personnel are required. Except for simple substances such as inorganic salts, complete synthesis of a drug is relatively rare. More commonly, a substance derived from natural sources is manipulated chemically to produce an improved drug with increased specificity or reduced toxicity. Promising opportunities for drug synthesis are offered by genetic engineering involving recombinant DNA techniques. Although manufactured, these preparations incorporate biologic components such as genes, viruses, or protein fragments.

Drug Components

A medicinal preparation is made of one or more active ingredients and various additives chosen to alter certain properties of the final formulation (Table 2-1).

Active Ingredients

The active ingredients of a drug preparation are responsible for drug action and the desired drug effects. Pharmacologic agents vary considerably in their chemical structure and are systematically classified according to their physical and chemical composition. Major classes include salts, alkaloids, glycosides, polypeptides, and steroids. When a preparation contains only one active ingredient, it is known by the name of that substance. Combinations of more than one ingredient are rarely used for prescription drugs but are commonly used in over-the-counter preparations. As a matter of convenience, multidrug combinations are often known by their trade names.

Salts are compounds consisting of a positive ion other than hydrogen and a negative ion other than hydroxyl. Solid salts tend to form crystals. In solution, a certain proportion of their molecules separate, releasing ions that are electrically charged and (usually) chemically active. Pharmacologic activity is usually confined to either the cation (positively charged ion) or the anion

Table 2-1. Components of Drugs

Component	Form	Examples	Points of Note
Active ingredients: Responsible for producing the action of the drug; categorized according to physical and chemical properties	Salts	Morphine sulfate, potassium chloride	Ionize when placed in solution
	Alkaloids	nicotine, atropine	Contain nitrogen
			Form salts when they react with acids because of basic properties
			Constitute a major source of drugs
			Have names ending in "-ine"
	Glycosides	digitalis	Yield glucose- or carbohydrate-containing molecule
	Polypeptides	insulin	Include high-molecular-weight proteins
			Are destroyed by hydrolysis during digestion
			Include enzymes and hormones
Additives: Impart desired characteristics to drug formulations; must be compatible with the active ingredients and with one another	Vehicles	water, oils, cocoa butter, petroleum jelly	Give form and substance to preparations
			May change the physical and chemical properties of the preparation
	Fillers	dextrose, lactose, starch	Remain relatively inert
			May alter dissolution of the active principle
			May cause adverse reactions in recipients
	Diluents	vehicles and fillers	Reduce the concentration of the active ingredient
	Binders	dextrose, lactose	Improve cohesiveness of the drug ingredients
	Disintegrators	starch	Facilitate disaggregation and dissolution of solid preparations
	Lubricants	cocoa butter, petroleum jelly	Reduce friction
	Flavorings	cherry, raspberry, licorice syrups	Improve palatability
	Dyes	tartrazine (FDA yellow No. 5)	Make products attractive
	Preservatives	antibacterials, chemical stabilizers	Prevent microbial growth or chemical breakdown

(negatively charged ion). Compounds that contain drug ions with like charges tend to be chemically compatible, whereas drug ions of unlike charges tend to form inactive precipitates when combined.

Among major drug sources are the salts formed when alkaloids react with acids. Alkaloids are organic compounds that contain nitrogen and have a basic pH. They exist in the seeds, roots, leaves, or bark of certain plants (eg, the opium poppy, tobacco, cinchona bark). Examples of drugs derived from alkaloids are atropine (a powerful anticholinergic), opiates such as codeine and morphine, and strychnine, a dangerous poison. Most drugs whose names end in *-ine* are alkaloid derivatives.

Glycosides are substances derived from plants. When hydrolyzed (decomposed chemically), glycosides yield a sugar and one or more other products. Sugars derived from glycosides are usually glucose (from glucosides) or galactose (from galactosides). A major glycoside drug is digitalis, a cardiotonic derived from the foxglove plant.

Polypeptides are high-molecular-weight protein compounds. Although polypeptide molecules do not ionize, they usually are amphoteric (ie, they exhibit electric charges at two or more sites on the molecule). Polypeptides used for a systemic effect must be administered parenterally because they are easily hydrolyzed by proteases in the digestive tract. Many enzymes (eg, pancrelipase) and hormones (eg, insulin) are polypeptides.

Steroids are compounds characteristically structured in one pentagonal and three hexagonal carbon rings:

Naturally occurring compounds having a steroid nucleus include cholesterol and the adrenocortical hormones. Steroids used as drugs include estrogen, testosterone, cortisone, and the digitalis glycosides. These medications are usually unaffected by digestion and may be administered orally.

Additives

Among the substances commonly added to drug formulations are vehicles, fillers, diluents, binders, disintegrators, lubricants, flavorings, dyes, and preservatives. Each imparts a desired property to the medicinal preparation. Additives must be nontoxic and compatible with the active drug as well as with each other.

Vehicles are substances added to a formulation to carry or transport the active ingredient by giving it form and substance. Common vehicles include solvents (eg, water, oils, syrups) and solids (eg, cocoa butter, petrolatum). Vehicles may have a significant effect on the drug's physical and chemical properties.

Fillers are powders (eg, dextrose, lactose, starch) added to dry drugs to provide the bulk needed for producing a solid preparation and a uniform dose. Most fillers are relatively inert. Hydrophobic fillers (fillers that do not dissolve readily in water) are sometimes used to delay dissolution of the medication, achieving a timed-release effect. Some people may be intolerant of certain fillers; for instance, persons with a deficiency of the enzyme lactase experience digestive upset when given a product containing lactose.

Diluents are substances that increase the bulk of the formulation, thereby reducing the concentration of the active ingredient. Both vehicles and fillers act as diluents.

Binders are substances added to solid formulations to improve the cohesiveness of dry ingredients so that they may be shaped into durable dosage forms. Dextrose and lactose act as binders.

Disintegrators (eg, starch) facilitate disaggregation and dissolution when solid medications are placed in water.

Lubricants (eg, talc, stearates, hydrogenated vegetable oils) prevent solid tablets and caplets from adhering to compression machinery during production.

Flavorings are added to formulations (usually liquids or chewable tablets) to improve palatability. Common flavoring agents are cherry, raspberry, chocolate, and licorice syrup.

Dyes are added to drug formulations to make products more attractive and to facilitate identification of drugs involved in overdose or poisoning. Colors used in drugs, foods, and cosmetics are scrutinized by the United States Food and Drug Administration (FDA). Some dyes (eg, certain reds) have been banned as carcinogenic. Tartrazine (FDA Yellow No. 5) is known to cause allergic reactions in sensitive persons (mainly asthmatics who are prone to nasal polyps and who are allergic to aspirin).

Preservatives are added to drug formulations to prevent bacterial contamination and chemical decomposition.

Types of Preparations

Pharmaceutical preparations are available in various forms designed to facilitate drug administration. The therapeutic effects of the drug's active ingredients are usually determined by the type of preparation and its dosage. Factors that influence formulation include the route of administration, the rapidity of the response desired, suitability and acceptability for the client, and the specific properties of the drug itself (eg, solubility, stability, bioavailability). Drugs can be in solid, liquid, or gas form.

Solids

Tablets are small disklike masses of medicinal powder that have been compressed sufficiently to maintain their shape. The term *pill* is sometimes used to refer to spherical or pellet-shaped tablets. Most tablets and pills are administered orally. The buccal form of tablet is designed to lodge in the mouth between the cheek and gum until dissolved and absorbed. The sublingual form is designed to be placed beneath the tongue until dissolved and absorbed. The enteric-coated form contains an outside layer that does not dissolve until the tablet reaches the small intestine. The coated form has an outside layer, usually of sugar or chocolate. The effervescent form contains a mixture of sodium bicarbonate and an acidulant, such as citric acid, that generates carbon dioxide when added to water. The prolonged-action or timed- or sustained-release form is designed to be released and absorbed gradually or in stages.

Caplets are tablets shaped like capsules. Hard compressed caplets or tablets do not dissolve readily. Because solubility affects bioavailability, the manufacturer tests the degree to which tablets disintegrate and dissolve. As tablets (particularly pills) age, they tend to dry out (become "case-hardened") and become less soluble.

Capsules are gelatin cases used to enclose solid drugs. Capsules melt and release their solid drug very quickly after ingestion. If the capsule contains powder, the drug tends to dissolve and be absorbed rapidly. If the capsule contains beads, some of the beads may have an enteric coating, causing this form of the drug to remain undissolved until it reaches the small intestine. Common terms for this prolonged effect include *sustained release* and *timed action*. Capsules are more easily tampered with after manufacturing than are caplets or tablets.

Troches (lozenges) are disc-shaped or cylindrical medications consisting chiefly of medicinal powder, sugar, and mucilage. They are designed to be placed in a body cavity for absorption by the mucous membrane. Lozenges are oral preparations; troches may be oral or vaginal.

Pellets are small pills or balls of medication. They are made of materials that are absorbed slowly from muscle or subcutaneous tissue after surgical implantation.

Needles are long, thin cylinders. Like pellets, they are surgically implanted for sustained-release effect.

Patches, which resemble small adherent dressings, contain medication in a central area surrounded by an adhesive rim. The drug may be imbedded in the adhesive ring or in the central area. When applied to the skin, the medication is released gradually and absorbed transdermally.

Powders are measured doses of solid medication in pulverized form. They are usually dissolved in water before ingestion.

Granules are dry medications that resemble powders, but their particles are larger than those in powders. Granules may be prepared as single-dose packets or packaged in bulk.

Dusts are very fine powders. They may be applied topically to the skin or mucous membranes or administered by inhalation as a mist (eg, cromolyn administered by inhalation to control asthma).

Semisolids

Suppositories are cylindrical or cone-shaped medications whose vehicles (eg, cocoa butter) melt at body temperature. They are molded to conform to the contours of body cavities (eg, the rectum, vagina, or urethra).

Pastes are thick, gelatinous substances usually intended for topical application to the skin. Vehicles and fillers used in pastes include oils, waxes, and starch.

Ointments are fatty, soft substances applied to the skin or eyes. Ointments may be insoluble in water (based in petrolatum, lard, or lanolin) or soluble in water. Other terms synonymous with ointment are *salve*, *unction*, and *unguent*.

Creams are topical preparations that are less viscous than ointments but more viscous than lotions. Creams tend to hold their shape when undisturbed but can be easily spread.

Foams are mixtures of finely dispersed gas bubbles in a liquid (eg, contraceptive vaginal foams).

Liquids

Solutions are mixtures of two or more substances dissolved in another substance. In solutions, the molecules of each solute disperse homogenously but do not change chemically. Although solutions may be gaseous, liquid, or solid, medicinal solutions are mainly liquids. Solutions may be administered orally, rectally, topically, by injection, or as a mist by inhalation. They can also be instilled in the eye, nose, and ear and used as sprays or irrigations.

Lotions are liquids with a creamy consistency that are applied topically to the skin (eg, calamine lotion).

Liniments are liquids containing an alcoholic, oily, or soapy vehicle. They are rubbed on the skin and usually act as counterirritants.

Elixirs are clear liquids containing water, alcohol, sweeteners, and flavors (eg, elixir of phenobarbital). They are usually administered orally.

Tinctures are alcoholic extracts of vegetable or animal substances (eg, tincture of belladonna, tincture of benzoin). Tinctures may be administered topically or orally. The usual dose of an oral tincture is 1 dram (1 teaspoon). Potent drugs are dispensed as 10% concentrations, less potent drugs as 20%. Tinctures often contain tannic acid.

Extracts are concentrated solutions prepared by dissolving the active principle of a substance in alcohol or water and evaporating part or all of the solvent. The drug is then dissolved or diluted with an alcoholic solvent. An extract is usually several times stronger than the crude drug. Fluid extracts are alcoholic solutions of 100% concentration—in other words, each milliliter of solution contains 1 gram of pure drug.

Aromatic waters are saturated aqueous solutions of volatile substances (eg, spearmint "oil," peppermint "oil").

Syrups are solutions of sugar and water, usually flavored, to which a drug is added. Syrups are used for palatability, especially in pediatric medications (eg, syrup of ipecac).

Suspensions are mixtures of a solid and liquid in which the solid particles do not dissolve.

Gels and magmas are viscous suspensions of mineral precipitates in water (eg, aluminum hydroxide gel, milk of magnesia). These mixtures tend to separate on standing and must be shaken well before use.

Oils are viscous, greasy liquids that are insoluble in water. There are two types: volatile and fixed. Volatile oils evaporate easily, leaving no greasy residue; fixed oils do not evaporate readily. Oils may act as drug agents (eg, castor oil) or may be used as vehicles to dissolve other drugs (eg, pitressin tannate in oil).

Emulsions are mixtures of two liquids (usually oil and water) that are not mutually soluble. When thoroughly shaken, the oil divides into globules that disperse throughout the mixture. Emulsions tend to separate on standing but can be stabilized by adding an agent that reduces surface tension. Medications dispensed in the form of emulsions may contain oils having little palatability. The emulsion alters the greasy consistency of the substance and tends to disguise its flavor.

Gases are administered by inhalation. Many are used as general anesthetics.

Drug Nomenclature

A single drug may be designated by a number of names: chemical, generic, official, and proprietary (or trade). It may also be identified by an abbreviation or as a member of several drug families, also known as drug classes (Box 2-1).

Chemical Name

A drug's chemical name indicates its atomic and molecular structure. It may be given as a chemical formula or accompanied by a diagram of its structure. These names are of particular interest to the chemist and research pharmacist. They are not capitalized. Chemical names are usually so long and complicated that they are unsuitable for general use. For example, aspirin's chemical name is acetylsalicylic acid ($C_6H_4COOHOCOCH_3$), and its chemical structure is:

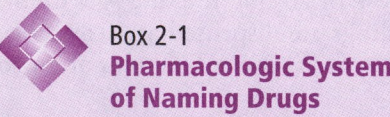

Generic Name

Strictly speaking, the term *generic* should signify a chemical derivation. However, in common usage, it is used to denote the nonproprietary name of a compound used medicinally. For clarity and convenience, generic names should be concise and distinctive. These names are usually proposed by the company that first develops the drug. Like chemical names, generic names are not capitalized. The generic name for acetylsalicylic acid is aspirin. In the United States, a generic name or U.S. Adopted Name is selected by the U.S. Adopted Name Council, a body sponsored by the American Medical Association, the U.S. Pharmacopeial Convention, Inc., and the American Pharmaceutical Association in consultation with a representative of the FDA.

Official Name

Official names are those adopted by bodies authorized to do so by a governing body. In the United States, these names are chosen by a Committee of Revision of the U.S. Pharmacopeial Convention, comprising pharmacists, physicians, and pharmacologists who donate their services. An official name may be identical to the drug's generic name and is not capitalized. Official names are found in the *U.S. Pharmacopeia and National Formulary* (*USP&NF*).

Trade Name

Trademarks, trade names, brand names, and proprietary names are interchangeable terms used to identify the drugs manufactured by various drug companies. Thus, a specific generic drug may have many different trade names. The symbol ™ or ® after the trade name indicates that the trade name is registered. The use of the name is restricted to the manufacturer who owns it. Although all trade name preparations of a particular generic or official drug must contain the indicated drug chemical, formulations may vary in the type and number of additives used.

Trade names may be chosen to denote the drug's chemical structure, to identify the company responsible for manufacturing the drug, or to represent some property of the drug. Names can be easily confused if several different drugs have similar names because of a similarity in chemical makeup or medicinal properties, or if

---

Box 2-1
Pharmacologic System of Naming Drugs

Chemical name

Generic name

Official name

Trade name (trademark, brand name, proprietary name)

Abbreviations

Table 2-2. Some Names of Common Drugs

Generic Name	Chemical Name	Trade Name(s)	Commonly Used Abbreviation
aspirin	acetylsalicylic acid	Ecotrin, Bufferin	ASA
milk of magnesia	magnesium hydroxide	Phillips' Milk of Magnesia	MOM
tetracycline	hydrochloride of 4-(dimethylamino)-1,4,4a,5,5a,6,11,12a-octahydro-3,6,10,12,12a-pentahydroxy-6-methyl-1,11-dioxa-2-napthacenecarboxamide	Achromycin, Tetracyn, Panmycin	
prednisone	11β,17,21-trihydroxypregna-1,4-diene-3-20-dione	Deltasone, Meticorten	
repository corticotropin injection	adrenocorticotropic hormone	Cortigel, Cortrophin gel	ACTH
chlorothiazide	6-chloro-2H-1,2,4-benzothiadiazine-7-sulfonamide 1,1-dioxide	Diuril	CTZ
chlorthalidone	2-chloro-5-(2,3-dihydro-1-hydroxy-3-oxo-1H-isoindol-1-yl) benzenesulfonamide	Hygroton	
hydrochlorothiazide	6-chloro-3,4-dihydro-2H-1,2,4-Benzothiadiazine-7-sulfonamide 1,1-dioxide	Esidrix, Hydro-Diuril, Oretic	HCTZ
ethacrynic acid	[2,3,-dichloro-4(2-methylene-1-oxobutyl)-phenoxy]acetic acid	Edecrin	

different drugs are given similar names indicative of the company of origin.

A single drug product may have many different trade names; for example, aspirin may be known by the trade names Arthritis Pain Formula, Ascriptin, Bayer Aspirin, Bufferin, Easprin, and Zorprin. Trade names are capitalized.

Abbreviations

Drugs in frequent use may be ordered by abbreviated names adopted for expediency. These vary from locality to locality and are rarely standardized or authorized by any official procedure. Abbreviations are often acronyms containing the initial letters of a multiword name (eg, MOM for milk of magnesia) or prominent letters from the generic name (eg, HCTZ for hydrochlorothiazide). An abbreviation often used to designate aspirin is ASA. Abbreviations should not be used unless they have been formally adopted and standardized in the written policies of a healthcare agency. Table 2-2 lists nonproprietary (generic, chemical) and trade (proprietary, brand, trademark) names and abbreviations.

Drug names are significant because they describe the drug as succinctly as possible. For example, hydroxyzine may be called Vistaril or Atarax or described as an antihistamine, antiemetic, antipruritic, or tranquilizer or sedative. Similarly, atropine, a belladonna alkaloid, may be classified as an anticholinergic, antispasmodic, anhydrotic or mydriatic.

Drug Family Name

Drugs with similar characteristics are often grouped together in families or classes (Box 2-2). The family or class name may denote chemical structure (eg, barbiturate), mode of action (eg, antacid), physiologic action (eg, diuretic), or therapeutic effect (eg, anticonvulsant, analgesic). One drug may be listed under more than one classification. For example, aspirin may be classified as an analgesic, antipyretic, and antiinflammatory drug that acts as a prostaglandin inhibitor.

▪ SUMMARY

Drugs may be derived from plants, animals, or minerals. They may also be produced synthetically in the laboratory. Many drugs of natural origin are

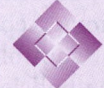

Box 2-2
Drug Families (Classes)

Chemical structure (eg, barbiturates, phenols, aminoglycosides)

Mode of action (eg, antacid, central nervous system stimulant)

Physiologic action (eg, diuretic, anticholinergic)

Therapeutic effect (eg, anticonvulsant, analgesic)

altered chemically to produce semisynthetic drugs with more desirable medicinal properties.

For pharmacologic use, drugs are identified according to chemical name, generic name, official name, and trade name. Chemical names denote the atomic and molecular structure. Generic names are concise names adopted for permanent use. Official names are those authorized by governmental units for use in official compendia; they may be the same as the generic names. Trade names indicate preparations manufactured by a specific pharmaceutical firm. Abbreviations usually are unauthorized and may vary from place to place.

Drug families or classes are groups of drugs with similar chemistry, action, or effect. A single drug may belong to several drug families or classes.

Drug Controls

Just as every society has discovered and used pharmacologically active substances (see Chap. 1), so does each society control their use. The earliest limitations on drug use stemmed from religious practices and social mores. For example, in primitive societies, the use of substances affecting the central nervous system was usually restricted to religious rituals. The effects of the substances were treated as mystical or spiritual experiences. Poisons used for killing animals were carefully applied to the hunting tools in ceremonial fashion. Drug use thereby became sacred; casual use was forbidden. Certain practices were outlawed by taboos, which if broken could bring severe punishment.

Today, legislation formally restricts drug use in most societies, and religious and social controls continue to exert an influence. For example, some religions prohibit alcohol use, and social customs typically restrict acceptable use of alcohol to late afternoon and evening rather than morning. Social mores can be more effective than laws in influencing behavior; for example, U.S. laws prohibiting the manufacture of alcohol in the 1920s failed to eliminate drinking, and in the 1960s, marijuana use was widespread even though it was illegal.

Many modern societies have elaborate and strict legislative controls governing drug use. Laws in most countries restrict the production, distribution, prescription, and administration of drugs. Many medicinal substances are not available legally to the general population except through licensed health professionals. Formal controls on the use of active substances range from the policies of individual institutions to governmental legislation. Drug laws exist at the international, national, state or provincial, and local levels. Healthcare institutions impose further controls. Generally, restrictions become more severe as the unit becomes smaller, with each organization abiding by the restrictions of the larger units of which it is a part while adding to the constraints and specifying in greater detail the procedures for enforcement.

International Controls

International drug controls are based on treaties among national governments established through diplomatic conferences. Whereas these agreements focus mainly on controlling substance abuse, promoting consumer safety by establishing standards for drug purity, nomenclature, labeling, and statistics reflects a growing concern. Under present conventions (the Single Convention on Narcotic Drugs), several bodies within the United Nations are involved in drug control. The Commission on Narcotic Drugs is authorized to make recommendations for implementing or amending the provisions of the convention. An expert body, the International Narcotics Control Board, supervises the workings of the treaties regarding both the licit and illicit drug trade. In addition, three secretariats within the United Nations provide controls for substance abuse: the United Nations Division of Narcotic Drugs, the International Narcotics Control Board Secretariat, and the World Health Organization Drug Dependence and Alcoholism Secretariat.

One important international agreement, the Declaration of Helsinki, offers recommendations for conducting experiments using human subjects (Box 2-3). They were adopted by the 18th World Medical Assembly in Helsinki in 1964 and revised by the 29th World Medical Assembly in Tokyo in 1975. These recommendations apply to studies of drug effects involving human subjects in which the essential object is purely scientific and without therapeutic value to the subject. The Declaration of Helsinki protects the rights of human subjects by requiring informed consent, discontinuation of the research if harm to the subject may occur, and conformity of the research to "generally accepted scientific principles."

Without administrative or judicial structures for enforcement at the international level, controls must depend on voluntary cooperation among nations.

National Controls

Legislative guidelines for drug controls exist largely at the national level. The severity and complexity of these laws vary from country to country and are not necessarily correlated. Countries with the most severe penalties for infractions may make fewer distinctions and exceptions in their laws. Penalties for drug infractions in many countries are much more severe than in the United States. For example, possession of marijuana, considered a misdemeanor in many states, is punishable by long prison sentences in some European and Eastern countries.

Early U.S. Legislation

In the United States, federal legislation began with the 1906 passage of the Food, Drug, and Cosmetic Act. Although largely concerned with food purity, this law also designated official standards for drugs (the USP&NF), empowering the federal government with enforcement.

Box 2-3
Basic Principles of the Helsinki Declaration

1. Clinical research must conform to moral and scientific principles and should be based on generally established facts (eg, from laboratory and animal experiments).
2. The design and performance of research procedures should be approved by an independent committee.
3. Only qualified persons supervised by a qualified medical clinician should conduct research.
4. The importance of the objective should be proportional to the inherent risk to the subject.
5. Risks in comparison to foreseeable benefits should be carefully assessed before research activities.
6. The right of the subject to safeguard his or her integrity should always be respected; privacy must be protected. Special caution is required when the personality of the subject is likely to be altered by experimental drugs or procedures.
7. Research should cease if hazards appear to outweigh benefits.
8. Accuracy of results must be preserved during publication.
9. Researchers must obtain an informed consent from prospective subjects.
10. If subjects are in a dependent relationship to the investigator, informed consent must be obtained by a physician who is not engaged in the investigation and who is completely independent of this relationship.
11. If the subject is legally incompetent, informed consent should be obtained from the legal guardian.
12. Research protocols should contain a statement of the ethical considerations involved and indicate that the principles of this Declaration are complied with.

The law required that the strength and purity of drugs conform to the claims made for them by manufacturers and that labels indicate the kinds and amounts of narcotic ingredients in preparations. The Shirley amendment of 1912 prohibited fraudulent therapeutic claims for drug preparations, laying the legal foundation for quality control. However, this aspect of the law was not enforced for decades.

In 1914, the first federal controls on habit-forming drugs were established. The Harrison Narcotic Act classified certain drugs believed to be habit-forming as *narcotics* and regulated their importation, manufacture, sale, and use. Included in this category were marijuana, opium, cocaine, and all their compounds and derivatives, as well as certain synthetic analgesics. Although this legislation has been superseded by the Controlled Substances Act of 1970, it remains historically significant because it was the first narcotic control act passed by any nation.

Later Legislation: Food, Drug, and Cosmetic Act of 1938

In the 1930s, more than 100 people died as a result of ingesting a solution of the antibacterial drug sulfanilamide that had been prepared with a toxic solvent, diethylene glycol. The poisonous properties of the vehicle had not been investigated before use. This incident poignantly illustrated the need for more stringent regulation of drug production. As a result, the Federal Food, Drug, and Cosmetic Act of 1938 was passed (Box 2-4). This law required the government to approve new drugs as safe before they could enter interstate commerce. The law also specified requirements for labeling and conferred official status on drugs listed in the *Homeopathic Pharmacopeia of the United States.*

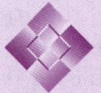

Box 2-4
Provisions of the Federal Food, Drug, and Cosmetic Act of 1938

1. Standards acceptable for drug preparations include those outlined in *The United States Pharmacopeia, The National Formulary,* or the *Homeopathic Pharmacopoeia of the United States.*
2. Before new drugs may be marketed outside the state of origin, the preparation must be approved by the FDA as safe for use as recommended by the manufacturer.
3. Labels on drugs must conform to the following specifications:

   Contents of the preparation must be accurately stated.

   The official or (for nonofficial drugs) usual name of the drug(s) must be specified.

   Certain substances (alcohol, bromides, atropine, digitalis, and others) must be indicated, and quantity and proportion specified. All habit-forming drugs must be noted, with a statement warning of their habit-forming potential.

   The name and address of the manufacturer, packer, or distributor must be included.

   Adequate directions for use and warnings against unsafe use must be included. Recommendations must be for dosage levels and frequency that are not dangerous to health.

   New drugs not yet approved for interstate commerce must bear the statement: "Caution: New Drug—Limited by Federal Law to Investigational Use."

   Statements on the label must not be false or misleading in any way.

In 1945, this act was amended by a law that provided for certification of certain drugs through testing by the FDA of each batch produced. This measure opened the door for government involvement in the direct supervision and inspection of pharmaceutical production.

Prescription and Nonprescription Drugs. The Durham-Humphrey Amendment of 1952 distinguished between prescription (legend) and nonprescription (over-the-counter) drugs and specified the procedures governing the distribution of prescription drugs. As a result of the power given to it by this law, the FDA classified most of the efficacious therapeutic drugs (which, because of their potency, tend to be somewhat toxic) as legend drugs (Box 2-5).

Safety and Efficacy. In the 1950s, two instances alerted the public to the potential for harm of drug substances. The Salk vaccine, the first poliomyelitis immunization, was rushed into production in 1954 in an attempt to forestall the usual summer epidemic of this paralyzing and life-threatening disease. Certain batches of the drug caused permanent paralysis among recipients. In Europe, the use of the drug thalidomide was responsible for the birth of many children afflicted with phocomelia (congenital absence or severe deformity of the limbs). During this same period, widespread abuse of both legal and illegal drugs was extensively publicized by the media, and exposés of the huge profits earned by drug companies provided impetus for new drug legislation.

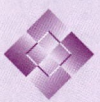

Box 2-5
Provisions of the Durham-Humphrey Amendment of 1952

1. The dispensing of certain (legend) drugs by the pharmacist is limited to prescription by licensed health professionals. Prescriptions may be written or, for certain drugs, verbal (oral or telephone). Substances classified as legend drugs include:

   Hypnotic, narcotic, or habit-forming drugs and their derivatives
   Drugs considered unsafe for unsupervised use because of their toxicity or the method by which they are administered
   New drugs considered unsafe for use by laypersons or those limited to investigational use

2. Refilling of prescriptions without authorization of the prescriber is prohibited.
3. Drugs limited to prescription use must be labeled "Caution: Federal Law prohibits dispensing without prescription."

Box 2-6
Provisions of the Kefauver-Harris Amendment of 1962

1. The Food and Drug Administration (FDA) was empowered to supervise drug production to ensure good manufacturing practices. Included are requirements for:

   Annual registration of persons and firms involved in the drug industry
   Inspection of every registered establishment at least every 2 years
   Withdrawal of approval of drugs when substantial doubts arises as to their safety or effectiveness

2. Statements in advertisements of prescription drugs must be truthful as to effectiveness, side effects, and contraindications.
3. Manufacturers must report adverse reactions attributed to new drugs and antibiotics promptly to the government.
4. The effectiveness of new drugs must be established by substantial evidence before marketing.
5. Safety and effectiveness of all antibiotics for human use must be certified by the government.
6. Official names for drugs are to be established by the FDA.
7. Greater controls are to be exercised over investigational drugs, including adequate preclinical studies before testing on humans.

The Kefauver-Harris Amendment of 1962 attempted to ensure greater drug safety and effectiveness and to improve the dissemination of necessary information about drugs (Box 2-6). It delegates broad powers to the FDA to regulate the manufacture, distribution, and sale of drugs.

Effectiveness of Therapeutic Claims. The National Research Council of the National Academy of Sciences evaluates data supporting therapeutic claims for the FDA, rating effectiveness according to the following scale:

- *Ineffective*: There is no substantial evidence of effectiveness.
- *Ineffective as a fixed combination*: The product is not effective in fixed-dosage combinations for reasons of safety or because one or more components lack substantial evidence of effectiveness.
- *Possibly effective*: Effectiveness may be shown eventually, but at present little evidence of efficacy is available.
- *Probably effective*: Some evidence of effectiveness is available, but it is insufficient to establish drug effectiveness.

- *Effective*: There is substantial evidence of effectiveness.
- *Effective but*: Although effective, there is a qualification or restriction imposed on the drug until completion of further studies, or the drug is effective for some recommended uses but not for all and hence a change in labeling is required.

Data acceptable as evidence of efficacy must be derived from well-controlled scientific and clinical investigations by qualified experts. Observations or testimonials based on inadequate controls are unacceptable. Once evaluated, a drug must include its official rating on its label.

The federal government also collects data on reactions to drug therapy. Reports from healthcare professionals are accepted by the division of Epidemiology and Drug Experience (HFD-210), FDA, 5600 Fishers Lane, Rockville, MD 20857 (see Appendix for MedWatch Report Form).

Reports from healthcare providers have led to changes in the labeling of drugs by revealing adverse reactions not previously reported by manufacturers. One example of how this practice helps consumers is illustrated by the oral antimicrobial drug temafloxacin (Omniflox) first marketed in 1992. During the first 3 months of its use, temafloxacin was associated with 50 serious adverse reactions, including three deaths. At that time, the drug was being used in six countries besides the United States. Before its approval, it had been tried in 4000 clients. Even so, the reports of healthcare providers resulted in the drug's being withdrawn from the market less than 4 months after its approval.

The FDA evaluates drugs in relation to their safety and effectiveness for specific clinical uses. Formal approval granted for using a substance to treat a given condition is indicated on medication labels and package inserts. Physicians may use the drug to treat other conditions; this is one avenue of research for expanding knowledge of medical therapy. However, governmental agencies and medical insurance plans may refuse to pay for such "experimental" treatment, even when the drug is the only hope for effective treatment.

Drug Abuse and Drug Dependence. In the 1960s, increasing public concern about the problems of drug abuse and dependence led to the passage of the Comprehensive Drug Abuse Prevention and Control Act of 1970 (also known as the Controlled Substances Act). This legislation outlined strict controls on the manufacture and distribution of habit-forming drugs and established government programs to promote the prevention and treatment of drug dependence (Box 2-7).

Although specific procedures for controlling harmful drugs may be spelled out in more detail by state legislation, the Controlled Substances Act provides a basis in federal law for at least minimal administration of these regulations. Under this law, possession of a controlled substance without a written prescription is unlawful. Exceptions for possession are made to licensed personnel only when necessary for medical practice. Nurses and other professionals handling controlled substances such as narcotics must keep accurate, detailed records that account for each dose of these drugs.

It is a crime to transfer any drug listed in schedules II, III, or IV to persons other than the client for whom the drug was ordered or prescribed. In many states, narcotics must not be administered except under the direction of a professional licensed to prescribe them. Unused narcotics must be returned to the source from which they were obtained (eg, the pharmacy) or to an office of the state agency responsible for narcotic regulation. Violation of the Controlled Substances Act is punishable by a fine, imprisonment, or (for health professionals) revocation of the license to practice. Enforcement of the Controlled Substances Act is delegated to the Drug Enforcement Administration in the Department of Justice.

Canadian Legislation

Canadian drug laws include the Canadian Food and Drugs Act (originally passed in 1953 and amended yearly) and the Canadian Narcotic Control Act of 1961 (amended periodically). The Canadian Food and Drugs Act provides for the regulation of the manufacture and sale of drug substances (Box 2-8). The Canadian Narcotic Control Act of 1961 restricts the sale, possession, and use of opiates, coca, and marijuana. Amendments to the act extended the controls to methadone. The law restricts possession of these drugs to authorized persons: licensed dealers, healthcare professionals, persons licensed to work with these materials for scientific purposes, members of the Royal Canadian Mounted Police (when necessary in connection with their employment), and persons for whom a narcotic drug is prescribed. Persons in possession of these drugs must ensure their security, promptly report any loss or theft, and maintain complete records of the disposition of the drugs. Narcotic drugs may be dispensed only by prescription and must be labeled with the symbol *N*. Administration of the Canadian Narcotic Control Act is delegated by the Department of National Health and Welfare to the Royal Canadian Mounted Police.

Legal possession of narcotics by a nurse is limited to times when a drug is administered to a client according to a physician's order, when the nurse is acting as the custodian of narcotics in a healthcare agency, or when a narcotic has been prescribed for medical treatment of the nurse.

State Controls

In the United States, state laws regulating drugs must be compatible with federal laws. They may not refute federal restrictions, but they may impose additional ones. Some state regulations specify in great detail the proce-

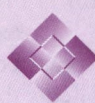

Box 2-7
Provisions of the Controlled Substances Act of 1970

- Definitions of drug dependence were established as follows:

  Drug-dependent person: "A person who is using a controlled substance (as defined in the Controlled Substances Act) and who is in a state of psychic or physical dependence, or both, arising from the use of that substance on a continuous basis. Drug dependence is characterized by behavioral and other responses, which include a strong compulsion to take the substance on a continuous basis in order to experience its psychic effects or to avoid the discomfort caused by its absence."

  Drug addict: "Any individual who habitually uses any narcotic drug so as to endanger the public morals, health, safety, or welfare, or who is so far addicted to the use of narcotic drugs as to have lost the power of self-control with reference to his addiction."

- Funds were provided for:

  The development and dissemination of educational material on drug use and abuse
  The development and evaluation of programs for drug abuse education
  The development of treatment programs for drug-dependent persons

- The Secretary of Health, Education and Welfare (now Health and Human Services) was directed to work with professional groups to develop guidelines for treating narcotic addicts.
- A Commission of Marihuana* and Drug Abuse was established to study marijuana use and abuse.
- The authority and responsibility for drug controls by federal agencies were redistributed in the following manner:

  The responsibility for enforcing drug controls was transferred from the Treasury Department to the Department of Justice, under the Attorney General. The Department of Health, Education and Welfare was assigned responsibility for scientific evaluation of drugs and for final decisions on which drugs should be controlled.

- All persons involved in experimentation with or the manufacture and sale of controlled drugs were required to register with the Bureau of Narcotics and Dangerous Drugs. Controls were imposed to guard against diversion of controlled substances to unauthorized channels.
- **Controlled drugs were classified according to the following schedules:**

  Schedule I: drugs that currently do not have accepted medical use, have a high potential for abuse, and lack accepted safety measures for use (eg, LSD, peyote, heroin)
  Schedule II: drugs that have medical use and a high potential for abuse; those that tend to cause severe dependence (eg, morphine, secobarbital, amphetamines, methadone)
  Schedule III: drugs used in medical practice with less potential for abuse than schedule II drugs; those that tend to cause moderate or low physical dependence or high psychological dependence (eg, nalorphine, drug combinations containing small amounts of narcotics such as codeine)
  Schedule IV: drugs that have medical use and lower potential for abuse than schedule III drugs; those that tend to cause limited physical or psychological dependence (eg, meprobamate, chlordiazepoxide, diazepam)
  Schedule V: drugs that have medical use and lower potential for abuse than schedule IV drugs; those that tend to cause less physical or psychological dependence (eg, mixtures of limited quantities of narcotics such as cough syrups containing codeine)

- Prescriptions of controlled drugs were regulated as follows:

  Each prescription must include the recipient's full name and address, the date, and the name, address, registration number, and signature of the practitioner issuing it.
  Prescriptions dispensed to nonhospitalized clients must be labeled with date of filling, pharmacy name and address, serial number of prescription, prescribing practitioner's name, directions for use, and cautionary statements.
  Prescriptions for schedule II drugs can be filled only once; refills are prohibited; for hospitalized patients, not more than 7 days' supply may be dispensed at one time. Possession of schedule II drugs by institutionalized patients before administration is prohibited.
  Prescriptions for schedule III and IV drugs are limited to five refills. These prescriptions expire 6 months after the date of issue. For hospitalized patients not more than a 33-day supply or 100 dosage units (whichever is less) is to be dispensed at one time, and possession by the institutionalized patient before administration is prohibited.
  Prescriptions for schedule V drugs can be refilled as authorized on the prescription.
  Records of the recipient and dispensing of controlled drugs must be kept (and made available to authorized persons) by pharmacists for at least 2 years.

*The alternative spelling of marijuana was used in the legislation.

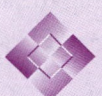

Box 2-8
Major Provisions of the Canadian Food and Drugs Act

- The sale of contaminated, adulterated, or unsafe drugs is prohibited.
- The sale of drugs whose labels are false, misleading, or deceptive is prohibited.
- Drugs must comply with professed standards under which they are sold, or the standards prescribed by recognized pharmacopeiae and formularies. Recognized compendia include *Pharmacopoeia Internationalis, The British Pharmacopoeia, The United States Pharmacopeia, Pharmacopée Française, The Canadian Formulary, the British Pharmaceutical Codex,* and the *Compendium of Pharmaceuticals and Specialties.*
- The process and conditions of manufacture of such drugs as parenteral and radioactive preparations must be approved before the medicines may be sold.
- Safety approval of batches is required for such drugs as arsphenamines and sensitivity disks and tablets.
- The sale of certain drugs (eg, thalidomide) can be forbidden absolutely.
- Certain drugs such as antibiotics, hormones, and tranquilizers can be sold only on prescription; refills must be specified by the prescriber and are limited to 6 months. The symbol PR must be placed on containers of these drugs to designate that a prescription is required.
- Certain drugs (amphetamines, barbiturates, methaqualone, pentazocine, and phenmetrazine) are termed *controlled;* prescriptions cannot be refilled unless the refills are ordered on the original prescription, with specific directions for time intervals between refills.
- The prescription of certain drugs is limited to use in specific conditions unless special permission is obtained. Such "designated" drugs include amphetamines and metrazines. Their uses are limited to the treatment of narcolepsy, hyperkinesis in children, minimal brain dysfunction, epilepsy, parkinsonism, and anesthesia-induced shock.
- The sale of hallucinogens is prohibited, but research on them is allowed by qualified investigators authorized by the Minister of Health and Welfare.
- Sample drugs may be distributed only to duly licensed persons (physicians, dentists, or pharmacists).
- Prescription and controlled drugs cannot be advertised to the general public.
- The information required to be on drug labels is delineated.
- Specific regulations to control the safety and efficacy of certain drugs or drug doses are described.

dures required for complying with drug-control legislation.

Some states have laws regulating the sale of drugs not controlled by federal legislation. For example, laws controlling the sale and use of alcoholic beverages vary from state to state, as do the legal penalties for the possession, use, or sale of illegal drugs such as marijuana. Many states impose restrictions, similar to the national restrictions on opiates, on additional drugs, notably the barbiturates.

In practical terms, this means that the lists of drugs that must be monitored in healthcare institutions vary from state to state. As evidence accumulates about the habit-forming potential of newer drugs, more drugs are likely to be added to these lists.

In many states, drug-control agencies spell out compliance procedures in detail. These regulations specify such things as the number of locks required on narcotic storage areas in hospital units, the number of people allowed access to such storage areas, the information required on controlled-substance records, and even the type of signature required on drug-count sheets. To enforce state regulations, agents inspect establishments that handle controlled substances. These inspections may be more frequent than federal inspections and are usually at times other than those conducted by federal officials.

Local Regulations

County and town (borough) drug regulations usually involve restrictions on the sale or use of alcohol or tobacco. Some areas ("dry" towns or counties) prohibit the sale of alcoholic beverages. In a few areas, the sale of cigarettes and other tobacco products is forbidden.

Institutional Controls

Healthcare institutions' policies on the handling and control of drug substances may vary greatly, although they must conform to federal, state, and local regulations. Institutional policies generally are more restrictive than governmental controls. They are designed to prevent health problems stemming from drug use and to minimize technical violations of existing drug controls. For example, many healthcare institutions adopt policies requiring periodic renewal of orders for drugs not controlled by state or federal law. Commonly, orders for antibiotics or corticosteroids are discontinued automatically after a certain number of days of treatment (usually 10 to 14 days). Such policies help to prevent the problems of drug-resistant infections or toxic syndromes that tend to develop with prolonged medication regimens. Prescribers may continue medication by renewing the order, but it is less likely that drug treatment will be inadvertently prolonged. As another example, in states with laws requiring a renewal of narcotic orders for hospitalized patients every 72 hours, hospital policy may require renewal every other day. This prevents lapsing of the order, which could occur with a 3-day renewal policy if a prescriber orders the drug early in the first day but renews it at a later hour on the third day.

Individual Control

At a personal and family level, a client's practices influence drug use greatly. These practices are established in accord with personal beliefs about and attitudes toward drug use. By giving or withholding consent to treatment and by complying or not complying with the drug regimen, the client exerts the final control on drug use.

Therefore, healthcare personnel must assess the client's drug attitudes and practices and then tailor the regimen of care accordingly. If a need to change old habits is identified, clear explanations must be given, along with explicit descriptions and directions for the drug regimen. If a competent client then refuses to adhere to the treatment plan or refuses drug therapy and treatment altogether, the nurse and other healthcare personnel must respect that decision.

■ SUMMARY

All societies develop controls over drug use. The earliest controls from religious practices and social mores continue to influence the use of drugs today. Formal controls range from simple institutional policies to governmental legislation (local, state or provincial, national, and international). Generally, restrictions become more severe as the unit of administration becomes smaller. The client has final control over drug use, as it is he or she who gives or withholds consent to drug treatment and determines compliance.

Drug Standards

Standards are the yardsticks by which drug preparations are judged. In primitive societies, the potency and safety of drug preparations depended on the preparer's skill and the purity of the product's source. Techniques for preparing and handling potions were transmitted orally through an apprentice system. Today, technology offers sophisticated techniques for determining the chemical composition and biologic effects of drugs and for defining standards of purity and effectiveness (efficacy).

Standards for drug quality are generally established and enforced by the government. Many standards are outlined in official pharmacopeiae; others are established by bureaucratic regulation. Standards are particularly valuable because medications can vary considerably in their purity, strength, bioavailability, efficacy, and safety. To be effective, standards for these or other properties must provide a method for measuring the attribute to be evaluated, as well as stating an acceptable level or range for these measurements.

Purity

A truly pure drug contains only one specific chemical agent and no contaminating ingredients. Few substances sold on the open market approach this level of purity.

Impurities from the raw materials used for manufacturing drugs often remain in medicinal materials. Even if a pure substance is developed during production, other ingredients may need to be added to facilitate formulation of a dosage form or to manipulate drug absorption. Such additives include solvents, fillers, disintegrators, buffers, waxes, dyes, inks, and plastics. In addition, dusts and other contaminants may find their way into a batch of drugs. Standards for purity, therefore, rarely require that the substance be 100% drug chemical. Instead, they tend to specify the type and concentration of extraneous substances allowed to be in the drug product. Generally, pure drugs are more easily controlled in terms of dosage, and they generate fewer side effects.

Potency

The strength (potency) of a drug is measured by assay techniques. Chemical analysis is used when possible to determine the ingredients in a preparation and their relative amounts. Chemical analysis cannot be applied to preparations when the active ingredients are unknown or when techniques for measuring the ingredients are unavailable. In such cases, the relative strengths of various preparations are determined by testing in laboratory animals. Standards are established by specifying a definite, measurable effect on a suitable laboratory animal as the unit of measurement (bioassay). When reliable chemical tests become available for drugs measured by bioassay, they are usually adopted and the substance is labeled in terms of absolute measure of the active ingredient. Common drugs that are still marketed in preparations whose strengths are measured in biologic units include insulin and heparin. Penicillin, which was originally assayed biologically, is now usually measured in milligram doses.

Bioavailability

Bioavailability is the degree to which a drug can be absorbed and transported by the body to its site of action. Bioavailability may be influenced by the particle size, crystalline structure, solubility, and polarity of the drug compound. Bioavailability is commonly determined by measuring the blood or tissue concentration of the drug at a specified time after administration of a dose.

Efficacy

Efficacy, the effectiveness of a drug in treatment, is difficult to measure in absolute terms. Animal studies provide some objective data for certain drugs. Clinical trials compare the clinical progress of people given the drug against that of others given placebos or against reference standards. Such trials must be carefully controlled to generate reliable data. Because clinical status cannot always be measured in objective terms and the desirability of various clinical responses involves value judgments, interpretation of such data is often subjective.

Safety Versus Toxicity

Safety (or its opposite, toxicity) is measured by the incidence and severity of reported adverse reactions after drug use. As with efficacy, controlled tests are required to generate data pertinent to this quality. Some harmful effects (eg, carcinogenicity) may not appear until considerable time has elapsed. For this reason, a complete assessment of safety or toxicity is not always possible before a new medicine is marketed. Safety standards evolve: they are continuously clarified as deficiencies of past standards become apparent and new measurement techniques develop.

Testing Standards

Standards for drug quality depend on testing procedures. These tests are ideally quick, easy to perform, economical, and valid for the uses of the drug tested (Table 2-3). Chemical assays, when available, are usually economical in cost and time. Bioassays are more costly and time-consuming. Clinical trials tend to be expensive and lengthy. Tests for efficacy and safety performed on animals or other laboratory models may not be valid for humans. For example, a test for mutagenicity performed on bacterial cultures (the Ames test) is believed to reflect carcinogenicity in humans, but the degree to which it actually does so has not been proven.

■■ SUMMARY

Drug preparations are evaluated in light of standards for purity, potency, bioavailability, efficacy, and safety or toxicity. Procedures for testing drugs may involve chemical assay, bioassay, or trials on laboratory models, animals, and human subjects. Chemical assays are the most objective of the three tests.

Nursing Management

The nursing functions related to drug therapy are both independent and dependent. Because the nurse is usually the health professional with the most frequent and prolonged client contact, he or she is the one who can best help clients manage their drug regimens. The entire healthcare team collaborates to develop a suitable regimen of prescription drugs and to help clients select nonprescription remedies appropriately. In institutional practice, nurses are usually responsible for preparing and administering doses of prescribed drugs. In all settings, nurses must abide by the constraints of legal and institutional regulations relating to drugs.

Independent Nursing Functions

The drug industry produces a vast array of medicinal preparations and advertises their benefits extensively, and clients sometimes need equally extensive drug information to manage their own medications safely. Although available drug data are too massive for anyone to master completely, the nurse can memorize appropriate data and become skilled at obtaining additional data as needed from reliable resources (see Chap. 1).

Client Education

An important nursing responsibility involves educating clients about the drug regimen. The nurse begins by considering clients' perceptions and acceptance of medication, their level of knowledge compared with that required for safely managing the drug regimen, and any physical or mental limitations affecting safe administration. The nurse also counsels clients about drug use and treats minor side effects of therapeutic drugs that are amenable to nursing interventions. As appropriate, the nurse refers clients needing treatment for problems such as drug abuse to appropriate facilities and personnel.

Table 2-3. Comparing Features of Tests for Drug Quality

Test	Advantage	Disadvantage
Ideal test	*Quick, easy to perform, economical, valid*	*None*
Chemical assays	Usually objective, reasonable in time and cost	Tests not available for all drugs
Bioassays	Allow assessment of potency of substances of unknown composition	Tests are costly and time-consuming.
Tests on animals or lab models	Pose no risk to human subjects	Results may not be valid in humans.
Clinical trials	Yield data relative to effects on human subjects	Tests are expensive and lengthy and involve risk to human subjects.

Client Monitoring

Another nursing responsibility is monitoring clients for responses to drugs (medicinal and nonmedicinal), both favorable and unfavorable. This requires familiarity with the drugs involved and continuous assessment of responses, both before and after drug therapy. Key features of ongoing assessment include monitoring for therapeutic effect, side effects, toxicity, and any other change in status apparently associated with drug use. Responses requiring involvement of the prescriber for adjustment of the drug regimen call for collaborative functions.

Safety and Accuracy

When preparing and administering drugs directly to clients, the nurse must take all necessary precautions to ensure accuracy and safety, providing the right drug in the right amount to the right client, by the right route, at the right time (see Chap. 7).

One factor that influences efficacy and safety is a drug's formula. This is why when problems arise in the use of a particular drug formula or preparation, another preparation of the same drug may sometimes be substituted appropriately. However, certain substitutions may be hazardous. For example, care must be taken when a preparation designed for one route of administration is ordered to be administered by a different route. Many intravenous solutions are too irritating to be infused subcutaneously or intramuscularly. Moreover, solutions intended for subcutaneous or intramuscular injection can seldom be given intravenously because they are too concentrated, or because they contain ingredients (such as lipids) that would be harmful, even lethal, if administered intravenously. Occasionally, injectable solutions are administered by inhalation, but solutions prepared for inhalation administration are inappropriate for injection. Some injectable drugs may be effective when administered orally, but others may be degraded by digestion.

Many institutions strongly recommend that all medicinal preparations be limited to one active ingredient. Rare exceptions are made for the few agents that must be administered with other chemicals to have the desired effect or that are unsafe to give without another protective agent. Bioavailability may vary from one trade name preparation to another of the same generic drug; low bioavailability may lead to treatment failure.

Accuracy and safety involve verifying the drug order before administering the drug. If the name on the prescription and the one on the drug label are not the same, the nurse must verify that the two names refer to identical drugs before the medication can be given. Medication errors may arise from inaccurately transcribed drug orders or from inconsistencies in the drug nomenclature used by the physician and pharmacist. Because accuracy in prescribing, transcribing, and administering drugs is all-important, many healthcare institutions require the use of one system of nomenclature (eg, generic drug names). If abbreviations are commonly used, written policies should clearly identify the acceptable abbreviations and their meanings. Nurses should actively participate in developing institutional policies and procedures governing the use of drug names.

Professional and Lawful Practice

Nurses must remain familiar with regulations affecting drug use in the area where they practice. When moving from one jurisdiction to another, the nurse should review current laws in the new area. If information is unavailable in public or healthcare institution libraries, it may be obtained from the institution pharmacy or directly from the state drug-control agency. The nurse should also review pertinent practice guidelines established by the state board of nursing.

Practicing nurses can stay informed about changes in state drug regulations by consulting officials from the state regulatory agency. Additional updates may be offered by in-service programs for healthcare staff. Nurses also must know and follow the policies of the institution or agency where they work; these policies may vary greatly from institution to institution.

Nurses must abide by the drug-control laws within their practice areas. When advising clients on medication usage, they must avoid recommending illegal substances or providing drugs without the proper authorization (order or prescription). In practice, nurses must ensure the security of controlled substances at all times to prevent diversion to unauthorized persons. For example, in healthcare institutions, medications are commonly locked up during storage, and some drugs must be kept under double locks. When handling medications, the nurse should keep unlocked drugs under direct observation and control and maintain careful records of the disposition of each dose of certain drugs, such as opiates.

Similar precautions apply for nurses practicing in community settings. Although nurses are involved in the handling and administration of controlled substances when functioning as healthcare professionals, this privilege does not extend to their nonprofessional lives. When unnecessary for professional practice, the possession of such drugs or drug paraphernalia without a personal prescription is as much a crime for a nurse as for any other citizen. In addition to the usual penalties for such a drug offense, the nurse's license to practice may be suspended or revoked.

Collaborative Nursing Functions

In collaborative situations, physicians and nurses work together to design a drug regimen to meet the client's needs. Both monitor the client's response to drugs, although nurses usually have more monitoring opportunities because of their frequent and prolonged contact with clients. Nurses, like pharmacists, must consult the prescriber whenever a prescription does not conform with the recommended dosage ranges or when there are contraindications for drug use. This is an additional safeguard for clients. Nurses must be able to recognize the potential for harm from an inappropriate drug order and suggest acceptable alternatives to the prescriber.

❖ NURSING PROCESS

According to Carpenito's model of bifocal clinical practice (1995), clinical problems related to medication regimens may be classified as either nursing diagnoses or collaborative problems. The nurse is usually the primary prescriber in situations involving educating clients about drug use. The physician is the primary prescriber in problems arising from medications requiring a prescribed modification of the drug regimen.

If the drug regimen is a high priority of therapy (as in many cancer therapies), adverse reactions and considerable toxicity may be tolerated to continue treatment. In such a situation, nurses treat problems arising from drug effects as nursing diagnoses. If adverse effects threaten survival or pose intolerable, permanent effects on the client's health, the situation then becomes a collaborative problem requiring consultation with the physician.

ASSESSMENT

A complete drug history is a key portion of the health history. The nurse must identify accurately all chemical substances used by the client, as well as any chemical pollutants to which he or she is exposed. The labels of medication containers usually list the active drug or drugs in the preparation (by generic or trade name); if they do not, or if the label is illegible, the nurse should contact the pharmacist directly to determine the therapeutic agent or agents. The list of drugs thus compiled should be analyzed to ensure there are no duplicate preparations, as may happen if identical preparations are labeled with different names (eg, ibuprofen and Motrin are the same drug).

The nurse should investigate any allergic or other adverse reactions that may be related to exposure to chemicals (foods, drugs, pollutants) and should take a family history of reactions to drugs or chemicals as well, because the types of reactions and the substances causing reactions tend to be similar in relatives.

The client's response to drug regimens should be carefully appraised. If the client has used more than one trade name preparation of a generic drug, the time intervals between their use should be documented. Data on client response to drug therapy should be analyzed

to determine whether the response to different trade name drugs is quantitatively or qualitatively different. When a trade (brand) name drug is formulated, its chemical composition and additives may differ from those of another trade name formula for the same generic drug (eg, ibuprofen by the name of Motrin and ibuprofen by the name of Nuprin). By the same token, bioavailability and therapeutic response or adverse reactions may also vary.

NURSING DIAGNOSIS

The most common nursing diagnosis for clients on drug therapy is:

- Knowledge Deficit, related to medication use

Other nursing diagnoses depend on the drug involved. A few common examples are:

- Body Image Disturbance (common with hormone therapy)
- Diarrhea (sometimes a side effect of antibiotic therapy)
- Fatigue (an adverse reaction to various drugs)
- Altered Sexuality Patterns (when drugs impair potency or sexual response)
- Sleep Pattern Disturbance (when drugs cause insomnia or increased somnolence)

Nursing diagnoses involving a drug reaction should indicate the nature of the response and the specific formulation that triggers it.

PLANNING

Common goals of nursing care may include:

- Client education to improve management of the medication regimen (to decrease exposure to harmful chemicals, to reduce the risk of chemical dependence)
- Prevention (prompt detection and treatment) of adverse drug reactions
- Alleviation of adverse signs and symptoms of drug reactions
- Adjustment of the drug regimen for optimal response and safe use

INTERVENTION

Various nursing interventions are specific to drug therapy and related to drug controls and standards. They involve monitoring and assessment, teaching, and promoting client safety and comfort.

Monitoring each client for his or her response to drug therapy and for contraindications to continued drug use is an integral part of drug safety. Each time he or she prepares a drug dose, the nurse should ensure that the client's condition warrants administration of that dose. To do this, the nurse reassesses the client's condition in relation to drug effects (eg, therapeutic response to previous doses, the presence or absence of side effects, any clinical developments that may increase the risk of undesirable effects from continued dosage). It is vital to monitor for adverse or toxic effects (especially when the drug has a narrow margin of safety) because the earlier adverse reactions are detected, the easier it is to treat them.

Medications likely to produce an adverse reaction should not be administered without consulting the prescriber, who may change the drug order or take precautions to reduce the severity of adverse reactions. The nurse should also consult the prescriber when a client develops a health problem suggesting an adverse drug reaction. Moreover, the nurse should withhold additional drug doses until the prescriber decides what to do.

Nursing measures to reduce signs and symptoms of unavoidable drug reactions and nursing measures to relieve adverse drug reactions must be related to the nursing diagnosis.

When nurses are involved in clinical drug trials in humans, meticulous ongoing assessments are required to protect the human subjects from serious harm related to the unproven drug and to collect valid data for evaluating the experimental substance. Usually in clinical trials, some subjects receive the active drug and others receive a placebo or reference standard. Before entering a clinical trial, subjects must be aware that they may be given an inactive substance instead of the experimental drug. Neither the subjects nor the staff conducting the trials know which subjects receive which substance; hence, such trials are known as *double-blind*. The information identifying the experimental and control subjects must be maintained securely and secretly until data collection is complete, or else the validity of the results may be compromised.

Client Education. Nurses provide drug teaching appropriate to their clients' needs. Teaching may be related to chemical exposure, the use of social drugs, the use of pharmacologically active foods, or medication regimens. The nurse may need to consult the physician or pharmacist to clarify a drug regimen so that the client can be taught clearly what drugs have been prescribed and how to use them. A client who has experienced adverse reactions to a given drug or drug source should be urged to inform medical personnel of such problems and to wear medical identification naming the problem. The nurse should help the client to the limit of his or her expertise and should serve as a resource person when additional information is required.

OUTCOME EVALUATION

Evaluating the success of client education requires assessing the client's knowledge or behavior changes indicating that he or she applied such measures. The client's ability to carry out the drug regimen accurately and his or her response to drug therapy should improve after the teaching plan is completed.

Other data for measuring outcomes include the incidence or absence of errors in self-medication and a reduction in undesirable responses to the drug regimen. Criteria for evaluation should identify the anticipated outcomes selected before intervention.

❖ CHECKLIST OF NURSING ACTIONS

❑ Participate in developing institutional policies and procedures that promote accuracy in medication.

❑ Promote the development of written policies that define common abbreviations used for drug names.

❑ When taking a drug history, identify all medications accurately by both generic and trade names.

❑ Assess and document the client's response to drugs.

❑ Identify any drug intolerances and allergies the client may have.

❑ Analyze the client's drug history to detect possible duplication of drug preparations and multiple prescriptions for similar drugs.

❑ Consult prescribers and pharmacists as necessary to clarify the drug regimen and to develop a regimen tailored to meet the client's needs.

❑ Teach clients appropriate information about their drug regimen.

❑ Serve as a resource person to obtain further information about drugs for the client.

❑ When administering each dose of medication, ensure accuracy in preparation and delivery; assessing whether that dose is appropriate for the client's current status.

❑ Consult the prescriber for verification of or change in orders before administering a new drug that poses a high risk for an adverse reaction.

❑ Teach clients who are allergic to drugs to inform medical personnel of this fact and to wear medical identification that names the allergies.

Reference

Carpenito LJ. (1995). *Nursing diagnosis: Application to clinical practice*, p. 28. Philadelphia: JB Lippincott Co.

Bibliography

Food and Drugs Act and Regulation, 1972, with Amendments to Food and Drugs Act and Regulation to January 1982. (1982). Department of National Health and Welfare. Ottawa: Queen's Printer and Controller of Stationery.

Gennaro AR, ed. (1990). *Remington's pharmaceutical sciences*, 18th ed. Easton, PA: Mack Publishers.

Mosby's medical, nursing and allied health dictionary, 4th ed. (1993). St. Louis: CV Mosby.

Narcotic Control Act and the Narcotic Control Regulations. (1982). Department of National Health and Welfare. Ottawa: Queen's Printer and Controller of Stationery.

Ninety-first Congress. (1972). Public Law 91-513. Washington, DC: US Government Printing Office.

Thomas L. (1993). *Taber's cyclopedic medical dictionary*, 17th ed. Philadelphia: FA Davis.

For more information and sample tests and activities, refer to Chapter 2 in the Student Workbook for Clinical Pharmacology and Nursing Management, 5th edition, available through your bookstore.

3

Nursing Process: Management of Clients With Drug-Related Problems

Assessment
  Data base
  Analysis
Nursing diagnosis
Planning
Intervention
Outcome evaluation
Critical pathways

The primary concern of nurses is the health care of clients and families. Because chemicals are so prevalent in health care, nurses must clearly understand their impact—both medicinal and nonmedicinal—on health. Medicinal substances include prescription and over-the-counter (OTC) drugs and home and herbal remedies. Nonmedicinal substances that can affect health include social and illegal drugs, pollutants, and poisons. The nurse uses the nursing process to promote the client's optimal response to chemicals, to decrease the risk of adverse reactions, and to help clients achieve optimal health through the proper use of drugs.

This chapter deals primarily with the nursing process, the method by which the nurse treats human responses to changes in health status. Specifically, this chapter deals with the independent functions of the nurse in treating clients receiving prescription drugs. Dependent nursing functions related to drug therapy are numerous, and responsibilities relating to them may be critical, particularly in institutional settings; these aspects of care are addressed in Chapter 7.

The nursing process provides the framework for logical scientific problem-solving in nursing care. This process involves assessment, diagnosis, planning (including outcome identification), intervention or implemen-

tation, and outcome evaluation (Box 3-1). The nursing process is applicable to the care of clients receiving prescription medications, to those using nonprescription drugs, and to those exposed to nonmedicinal chemicals.

Assessment

Initial assessment of the client involves taking a drug history and evaluating the client's physical and psychologic responses to previous chemical exposure. The scope of the history varies with the setting and situation.

Data Base

The drug history and the results of the physical examination and related findings form the data base from which the nursing process proceeds.

History

A complete drug history includes:

- Chemicals to which the client is currently exposed
- Past chemical use and exposure
- Responses to drug use and chemical exposure
- The client's practices for handling and storing drugs and other chemicals
- Precautions for minimizing the risk of poisoning (or toxicity) or other adverse reactions
- Problems perceived by the client as being drug or chemically related
- The client's attitude toward the use of drugs and other chemicals.

The particular aspects to be included depend on the circumstances. For example, when treating a client for drug overdose, the most important information to obtain is what substance or substances he or she took; most other data are irrelevant until the emergency situation is resolved. Data about the conditions of drug storage may not be pertinent in an institutional setting but would be in the home. Information related to self-dosage may not be pertinent in settings where medications are administered by professionals. Occupational exposure would be important when assessing noninstitutionalized adults.

The nurse should consider such questions as: What drugs have been used in the past? For what purposes? How frequently? In what dosages? With what success? What problems occurred? Which drugs were prescribed by a physician or dentist? Which were self-prescribed? To what toxic, or potentially toxic, chemicals has the client been exposed? What nonmedicinal drugs has the client used in the past or is using currently? How often? In what quantities? What happens when habitual use of a substance is interrupted? Use of alcohol, tobacco, caffeine, and illegal substances should be assessed specifically.

Clients may be reluctant to give information about social or illegal use of drugs. If questions relating to specific drugs are delayed until the end of the interview, the client may have developed enough trust in the nurse

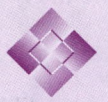

Box 3-1
The Nursing Process in Drug Therapy

I. Assessment
  A. Drug history (specific aspects vary with the situation)
    1. Previous drug use
       a. Prescription drugs ordered to treat illness
       b. Self-prescribed drug substances
       c. Nonmedicinal drugs and chemicals
       d. Drugs taken within the recent past
    2. Responses to drug use
       a. Therapeutic response
       b. Adverse reactions
       c. Idiosyncratic reactions
       d. Allergic reactions
       e. Tolerance and dependence
    3. Family history of unusual drug reactions
       a. Idiosyncratic
       b. Allergic
    4. Attitudes toward drugs and their use
  B. Analysis
    1. Identification of contraindications for drug use, or factors indicating the need for unusual caution
    2. Evaluation of the risk of undesirable drug interactions
    3. Assessment of physical and physiologic responses to previous drug exposure
    4. Comparison of drug data and client data to identify potential problems in the planned drug regimen
    5. Evaluation of factors affecting administration of drugs of self-medication by the client
    6. Comparison of the client's knowledge needed for optimal participation in the drug regimen
    7. Evaluation of the client's attitude toward drug use

  C. Outcome identification
    1. Formulation of criteria for successful outcome
    2. Establishment of measurable parameters, including a defined time frame
II. Nursing diagnosis
  A. Identification of actual problems arising from drug regimen
  B. Identification of potential problems arising from drug regimen
III. Planning
  A. Objectives of nursing care
    1. Prevention of drug-related problems
    2. Amelioration of symptoms
    3. Correction of abnormal states
    4. Improvement of function
  B. Goals
    1. Minimization of side effects
    2. Prevention of drug dependence
    3. Prompt detection and treatment of adverse reactions to drugs
    4. Withdrawal from a dependency-producing chemical
    5. Reduction in (or promotion of) drug use
IV. Intervention
  A. Psychological care measures
  B. Physical care measures
  C. Consultations with physician or pharmacist regarding changes in drug regimen
  D. Client teaching
V. Outcome evaluation
  A. Collection of evaluative data
  B. Comparison of evaluative data with predetermined, measurable criteria for success

to provide candid answers. The sequential listing of drugs should proceed from medicinal substances and generally accepted drug practices to more sensitive topics, leaving illegal and generally unacceptable drug practices to the last. Throughout the interview, the nurse should maintain a uniform, matter-of-fact, nonjudgmental demeanor. Some clients respond more freely if they are asked to complete a written questionnaire.

How does the client feel about the use of drugs? The client's expressed attitude should be compared with the nurse's objective assessment of the client's emotional response during the taking of the drug history. The client may not freely admit heavy use of or dependence on drugs due to the social stigma attached to such behavior.

The nursing history should also record allergies and diseases that have affected the client. The drugs used and the symptoms for which they were taken offer clues to previous and present illnesses. Much of this informa-

tion also appears in the general nursing history and may be duplicated by the physician. Comparing the nursing and medical histories may disclose discrepancies, indicating that one or both histories may be incomplete or inaccurate. Clients may relate information to one health professional that they would hesitate to reveal to another about sensitive topics such as the use of illegal drugs, alterations of drug dosage schedules, and the use of proprietary drugs, obsolete prescriptions, home remedies, "borrowed" prescription drugs, or drugs ordered by other prescribers.

Physical Examination

When examining the client, the nurse should be alert to findings related to previous exposure to drugs or reactions to current medications. When anticipating a new drug regimen or a change in drug orders, the nurse must collect specific data pertaining to the substances involved.

When these data include contraindications for using specific drugs, they must always be reported to the physician or other healthcare provider responsible for prescribing drugs. Although the primary responsibility for determining the appropriateness of the prescription rests with the prescriber, the nurse who detects a contraindication and fails to inform the prescriber will share the responsibility for harmful results.

Analysis

The nurse analyzes data from the history and physical examination to determine actual and potential problems related to drug use. Then the nurse examines the conditions or circumstances that contraindicate the drugs in use or under consideration and identifies factors requiring dosage alterations or precautionary measures. Although the primary responsibility for these safeguards rests with the prescriber, the nurse is also responsible for evaluating the risks involved in administering specific drugs. Additional nursing considerations include whether the client needs assistance in carrying out the prescribed drug regimen, how the client's attitude may affect medication use, and what teaching needs, if any, relate to the drug regimen.

Precautions and Contraindications

Persons with impaired organ systems involved in metabolizing and excreting drugs may require reduced dosages or preferential selection of drugs that are eliminated by the system or systems in best condition. The nurse should compare the assessment data with the pharmacokinetics of the medications (the processes by which chemicals enter the body, circulate through the tissues, are stored and metabolized by the body, and are subsequently eliminated through excretory pathways). Such a comparison helps the nurse determine the likelihood of difficulty in drug excretion. In problems with drug excretion, medications may remain in the body longer than usual and pose a risk of toxicity. These drugs should be identified.

Specific precautions are also listed in such drug data as package inserts and drug reference books. The nurse can compare the client's data base with medication data to determine which precautions are needed to safeguard the client. For example, glucocorticoids are not administered for long periods to clients with a history of exposure to tuberculosis unless antimycobacterial drugs are administered to prevent active infection. Precautions may reduce the risk of drug therapy to an acceptable level, even when contraindications exist.

Certain conditions increase the risk of adverse reactions to specific drugs. These contraindications are listed in drug references. Predisposition to serious adverse reactions common to the drug, specific disease conditions, organ impairment, and pregnancy and lactation are frequently cited as contraindications. Pertinent drug data and assessment data should be compared to determine whether the drugs in question are likely to be safe for the client to use.

Adverse Reactions

Information regarding usual response to drugs should be studied to determine whether the client has experienced adverse reactions such as allergies, toxicities, or failure of therapeutic effect. A client history that discloses no adverse effects despite a family history of allergies and other problems may be considered suggestive of potential problems. Responses to drugs are affected by body metabolism, biochemistry, integrity of organ function, and allergic tendencies. These variables are significantly influenced by genetic factors. A family history of adverse reactions to certain chemicals should alert healthcare personnel to an increased risk for adverse reactions if these or related compounds are prescribed.

Drug Interactions

Certain drug combinations pose obvious risks for adverse interactions. If the list of substances to be considered is long, a pharmacist may need to analyze the list for potentially harmful interactions. Drugs that the client has used in the recent past, as well as current medications, must be included because drug residues may interact with newly prescribed medications.

Tolerance and Dependence

The nurse evaluates data on the client's response to drugs for evidence of tolerance or dependence. Either one can affect the client's response to related substances and can influence the choice of drugs appropriate for treatment. Clients with an existing dependence will experience alterations in function if drugs are withdrawn. For those who have recovered from dependence, repeated use of the substances involved may cause renewed dependence.

Compliance Ability

Factors influencing the client's ability to adhere to a prescribed drug regimen include emotional acceptance of the need for drug therapy, financial resources to pay for the prescriptions, physical and mental abilities necessary for properly administering medications, knowledge of what constitutes appropriate self-care, and functional capacity to make the adjustments required for managing the regimen. The success of a drug program may hinge on obscure data such as difficulty in swallowing or inability to manipulate bottle caps or medication syringes.

Need for Teaching

Once drug therapy is prescribed, the nurse compares the client's knowledge about the drugs involved with the knowledge required for adhering to the desired regimen. Discrepancies between the two indicate a need for teaching. All clients must understand the plan of care, but those who will manage their drug regimens independently need more detailed teaching than do more

Text continues on page 40.

Model Nursing Care Plan Illustrating Use of the Nursing Process

Assessment

Selected Data from the Nursing History and Examination

The client, Thomas, is a 17-year-old high school student with retinitis following thermal injury to both eyes resulting from an atempt to view a solar eclipse through sunglasses. The physician has prescribed prednisone, 40 mg every other day. The drug treatment is expected to last 6 months to 1 year. Thomas' growth and development is essentially normal. He is 5 feet 6 inches tall and weighs 150 pounds. (His father and older brother are both over 6 feet tall.) Thomas denies taking drugs except for a daily multivitamin tablet (maintenance strength) and an occasional dose of aspirin (325 mg) for minor aches and pains, mainly headaches. He has had no allergic or other adverse reactions to drugs; family history is also negative for drug reactions. One aunt has diabetes mellitus. Thomas states that he "eats everything" and likes food from fast-food restaurants (hamburgers and milkshakes).

Thomas likes sailboating and spends much time studying and playing the saxophone. He does not engage in competitive sports but participates regularly in extracurricular activities (club and social events) at school. He also is active in the "big brother" program of the local boys' club. His "little brother" has been ill recently and is being treated for tuberculosis.

Thomas states that the physician discussed prednisone treatment with him and his parents, and he understands that the drug may limit further growth in height. He remarks, "That is a small price to pay to safeguard my sight." He also states that he knows nothing about prednisone except that it will help to limit his loss of vision.

Selected Data on Prednisone from Drug References

Prednisone is a glucocorticoid antiinflammatory drug used to control harmful inflammation and minimize scarring. Usual adult dosage is 5–60 mg daily; alternate-day regimens usually provide for 2 days' dosage to be taken as a single dose every other day. The drug is dispensed as oral tablets. It is metabolized by the liver and excreted through the kidneys.

Side effects and toxic effects of prednisone include:

Fluid and electrolyte imbalance (retention of sodium and water and depletion of body potassium)
Hypertension related to hypervolemia
Hyperglycemia (diabetes mellitus in susceptible persons)
Peptic ulcers in susceptible persons
Changes in fat distribution (sometimes causing "moon face" or "buffalo hump")
Negative nitrogen balance (protein loss, striae, skeletal muscle atrophy, and osteoporosis)
Immunosuppression
Inhibition of cell division (stunting of growth, delayed healing)
Increased coagulability of blood (with increased risk of thromboemboli)
Central nervous system stimulation
Inhibition of the pituitary secretion of corticotropin, causing adrenal atrophy

Among the precautions and contraindications are:

Glucocorticoids are contraindicated for growing children unless the benefits of therapy outweigh the risk of retarded growth.
Persons with a history of exposure to tuberculosis should be given concomitant antimycobacterial therapy.
Recipients with diabetes mellitus should be monitored carefully for glucose imbalance.
Those at high risk for this disease should be monitored for signs and symptoms of diabetes mellitus.
Prophylactic antiulcer therapy should be considered for persons susceptible to peptic ulcer.

Side effects and toxic effects of aspirin include:

Aspirin's antiplatelet effect increases the risk of bleeding.
Aspirin is irritating and can cause tissue breakdown.
The use of aspirin by children and young adults increases the risk of Reye's syndrome associated with infectious disease.

Analysis

Because Thomas has not yet completed his adolescent growth spurt, the administration of prednisone may prevent him from attaining the maximum height he otherwise would. Thomas has discusssed this with the physician and his parents and has accepted it as necessary for the protection of his sight. However, this may be only the first of several factors disturbing to his self-image. As drug therapy progresses, changes characteristic to glucocorticoid excess (so-called cushingoid appearance) are likely to develop. In addition to his altered physical appearance, Thomas may find his emotional affect changing in inappropriate ways in response to the stimulating effects of the drug.

(continued)

Model Nursing Care Plan Illustrating Use of the Nursing Process (Continued)

Assessment (Continued)

Prednisone treatment will reduce Thomas' natural protection against infection. He also has had a recent exposure to tuberculosis and could be harboring an initial infection.

The ulcerogenic property of prednisone will act synergistically with that of aspirin to increase Thomas' risk of peptic ulcer.

Thomas' use of aspirin increases his risk of Reye's syndrome and bleeding.

Because of a family history of diabetes mellitus, Thomas is at increased risk for the development of this disease while on prednisone treatment. Other adverse reactions likely to develop as a result of the drug regimen include hypertension, hypokalemia, which predisposes to constipation, and weakening of the bones.

Because his muscles will tend to atrophy and weaken, Thomas may have problems with muscle coordination. If an accident occurs, his weakened bones would be more vulnerable than normal to fractures. Fat embolus, a complication of long-bone fractures, could be especially serious in Thomas because of the increased coagulability of his blood. Wound healing will be delayed. Therefore, Thomas is at increased risk for accidental injury and for complications of such injuries.

Prednisone is stimulating to the central nervous system and may cause difficulty in sleeping, especially on the day the medication is taken.

Thomas will be receiving glucocorticoid therapy in large doses for a prolonged period of time. Because prednisone inhibits pituitary production of ACTH, atrophy of the adrenal glands will probably occur. This produces a physiologic dependence on the drug and reduces the body's compensatory response to stress.

Thomas' healthcare practices appear to have been adequate but will need to be changed to help prevent complications from the drug therapy. He knows little about the drug he will receive.

Nursing Diagnosis*	Outcome Planning Objective of Nursing Care	Outcome Evaluation Criteria for Evaluation	Interventions	Evaluative Data
1. Risk for Situational Low Self-esteem, related to physical and mental changes secondary to prednisone therapy	Promotion of positive self-image *Goals:* a. Continued participation by Thomas in social activities b. Maintenance of a positive self-concept throughout drug therapy	In discussions with the nurse, after 3 months of drug therapy, Thomas will report no net decrease in the number of social contacts with his peers. Thomas will continue to maintain a neat, well-groomed appearance. Thomas will continue to exhibit good posture and maintain eye contact when conversing with the nurse. When Thomas speaks about himself, positive comments will outnumber negative ones.	Establish good rapport with Thomas, conveying warm acceptance of him as a person. Compliment him appropriately on his appearance and accomplishments. Refer him for advice concerning personal grooming and attire if changes in appearance cause a decrease in physical attractiveness (eg, hair styling to minimize the round appearance of the face, clothes that will make body contours appear more normal). Encourage Thomas to continue to socialize with classmates and friends.	During visit with the nurse 3 months after initiation of drug therapy, Thomas described his social life as being "as active as ever." Thomas' appearance during this visit showed some cushingoid changes, but he was well-groomed and well-dressed. Thomas sat erectly and maintained eye contact with the nurse. During the interview, Thomas made one negative comment about himself and two positive ones.

*Collaborative problems that should be differentiated from the nursing diagnoses include: Potential complications: cardiovascular (hypertension, thrombi, thromboemboli), hyperglycemia, hypernatremia, hypokalemia, immunodeficiency, GI bleeding, pathologic fractures, active tuberculosis infection.

(continued)

Model Nursing Care Plan Illustrating Use of the Nursing Process (Continued)

Nursing Diagnosis*	Outcome Planning Objective of Nursing Care	Outcome Evaluation Criteria for Evaluation	Interventions	Evaluative Data
2. Risk for Infection, related to altered immune response secondary to prednisone therapy	Freedom from serious infection *Goals:* a. Identification by Thomas of risk factors that are associated with potential for infection b. Practice by Thomas of precautions to prevent infection c. Absence of overt signs of infection	Thomas will seek early medical attention and treatment for infectious illness. Minor wounds will heal without developing purulent drainage. Signs and symptoms of tuberculosis will not develop.	Caution Thomas to avoid exposure to people with known infections while on prednisone therapy. Advise Thomas to treat minor wounds carefully to prevent the development of infection. Teach Thomas hand-washing and avoidance of contact with "little brother's" sputum, towels, or other contaminated objects.	Thomas had no infectious illnesses during the first 3 months of drug therapy. Thomas reported that he had sustained two minor injuries: a knife cut to his hand and contusions and abrasions from a fall from his bicycle; each had healed with no signs of infection. Thomas has no cough or weight loss (absence of fever is not a reliable sign, because prednisone inhibits febrile reactions).
3. Risk for Fluid Volume Excess, related to sodium and water retention secondary to prednisone therapy	Maintenance of normal fluid and electrolyte balance *Goals:* a. Maintenance of normal sodium and water balance b. Identification by Thomas of causative factors and methods of preventing edema	Edema will not develop to a significant degree. Thomas' diet reflects his understanding of the role of sodium in the development of fluid retention.	Teach Thomas how to reduce sodium intake; suggest herbs and spices as seasoning substitutes.	Thomas shows no discernable swelling of soft tissues at his weekly visits. Diet as recorded by Thomas is low in salt.
4. Risk for Constipation, related to hypokalemia secondary to prednisone therapy	Prevention of constipation; prompt treatment of constipation should it develop *Goals:* a. Absence of discomfort from fecal elimination b. Prompt resolution of constipation, should it develop	By the third week of therapy, Thomas will state that he has no discomfort with fecal elimination. If constipation occurs, it will be promptly relieved by the use of a laxative.	Teach Thomas measures to prevent constipation, including use of nonirritating foods that are rich in potassium Advise Thomas to use a mild laxative such as milk of magnesia to relieve constipation, if it develops.	Three weeks after the initiation of therapy, Thomas stated, "I have no problem with constipation." During the third visit with the nurse, Thomas stated he had used milk of magnesia once at bedtime, and that evacuation the next morning relieved his discomfort.

*Collaborative problems that should be differentiated from the nursing diagnoses include: Potential complications: cardiovascular (hypertension, thrombi, thromboemboli), hyperglycemia, hypernatremia, hypokalemia, immunodeficiency, GI bleeding, pathologic fractures, active tuberculosis infection.

(continued)

Model Nursing Care Plan Illustrating Use of the Nursing Process (Continued)

Nursing Diagnosis*	Outcome Planning Objective of Nursing Care	Outcome Evaluation Criteria for Evaluation	Interventions	Evaluative Data
5. Risk for Injury, related to musculoskeletal changes secondary to prednisone therapy	Prevention of serious injury, especially skeletal fractures *Goals:* a. Promotion of muscle and bone strength through establishment of a regular exercise regimen b. Increase in Thomas' safety awareness and improvement in his safety practices	By the fourth week of therapy, Thomas will describe his exercise regimen; this should involve daily activity that requires weight-bearing. Thomas will describe appropriate safety practices as taught by the nurse. Thomas will report appropriate changes in his safety practices.	Advise Thomas to engage in regular exercise (such as walking) that involves weight-bearing to stimulate bone regeneration. Caution Thomas to avoid hazardous activities and to seek help when engaging in activities requiring muscular strength to maintain safety (eg, he probably should not sail his boat alone, but should take a companion along who can help maneuver the equipment).	Two weeks after the initiation of drug therapy, Thomas reported to the nurse that he had begun swimming regularly at the local YMCA pool. The nurse pointed out that swimming does not involve weight-bearing. Two weeks later, Thomas reported walking daily one-half mile each way to and from school. On the fourth weekly visit following initiation of drug therapy, Thomas could describe accurately the recommendations of the nurse. On this visit, Thomas stated that he takes a companion with him (his father or his best friend) when he goes sailing. He also stated that he uses special kitchen devices to immobilize food he wishes to cut to minimize the risk of injury.
6. Risk for Sleep Pattern Disturbance, related to central nervous system stimulation secondary to prednisone therapy	Maintenance of adequate rest and sleep *Goal:* a. Maintenance of average daily sleep equal to Thomas' usual duration of sleep	Total sleep over a 2-day span will equal twice the usual daily sleep duration prior to initiation of prednisone therapy.	Teach Thomas techniques to promote rest and sleep.	On the fourth weekly visit with the nurse, Thomas reported that his sleep on the night following medication with prednisone usually lasts 5 hours. On alternate days, sleep usually lasts 9 hours. Thomas normally sleeps 7½ hours per day. This criterion has not been met.

*Collaborative problems that should be differentiated from the nursing diagnoses include: Potential complications: cardiovascular (hypertension, thrombi, thromboemboli), hyperglycemia, hypernatremia, hypokalemia, immunodeficiency, GI bleeding, pathologic fractures, active tuberculosis infection.

(continued)

Nursing Diagnosis*	Outcome Planning Objective of Nursing Care	Outcome Evaluation Criteria for Evaluation	Interventions	Evaluative Data
7. Risk for Pain: Epigastric Discomfort, related to hyperacidity secondary to use of prednisone and aspirin	Prevention or prompt treatment of epigastric discomfort (heartburn) *Goals:* a. Absence of heartburn b. Prompt treatment of heartburn should it occur	By the third weekly visit with the nurse, Thomas will report that he uses acetaminophen instead of aspirin. By the third weekly visit with the nurse, Thomas will identify foods that act as gastric irritants that he has eliminated from the diet. Thomas' complaints of epigastric discomfort will decline from the second weekly visit to the 3-month visit.	Teach Thomas the following adjustments in self-care: a. Substitution of acetaminophen (a nonulcerogenic analgesic) for aspirin for the treatment of minor aches and pains b. Elimination of gastric irritants from the diet c. Use of an antacid containing calcium salt for occasional heartburn d. The need to report persistent heartburn	During the third weekly visit, Thomas stated that he purchased a supply of acetaminophen but has not needed to use it. During the third weekly visit, Thomas reported that he had to eliminate highly spiced pizza and spaghetti sauce from his diet. On the second weekly visit, Thomas reported four episodes of epigastric discomfort (heartburn). During the 3-month visit, he reported only one episode the previous week. He stated that he uses Tums (a calcium salt antacid) to relieve heartburn.
8. Knowledge Deficit related to: a. Adverse reactions likely to develop with prednisone therapy b. Hygiene measures to decrease the risk of adverse reactions c. Health supervision and monitoring d. Management of the dosage regimen e. Age-related contraindication for aspirin use	Reduction in or elimination of knowledge deficit concerning: a. Adverse reactions likely to develop with prednisone therapy b. Hygienic measures to decrease the risk of adverse reactions c. Health supervision and monitoring d. Management of the dosage regimen e. Use of aspirin and acetaminophen	By the third weekly visit with the nurse, Thomas will be able to describe accurately (with appropriate rationale) the recommendations regarding diet, signs and symptoms that should be reported to the physician, and measures to control and manage stress. By the first weekly visit with the nurse, Thomas will be wearing an appropriate medical identification device.	Teach Thomas the following adjustments in self-care: a. Diet limited in sodium, moderate in calories, and rich in protein, potassium, and calcium b. Stress-management techniques to prevent sudden increases in stress for which the body might be unable to compensate c. The importance of wearing medical identification stating that he is receiving prednisone Teach Thomas about glucocorticoid excess: a. Changes in appearance and mild central nervous system stimulation are acceptable. b. Changes to report are persistent and marked hyperglycemia, pronounced weakness, and bone pain Warn Thomas not to stop medication or reduce dosage without consulting physician. Explain need to discontinue dosage gradually to avoid harmful effects. c. Advise Thomas to use acetaminophen instead of aspirin to avoid the risk of Reye's syndrome.	During the third weekly visit, Thomas successfully described the recommendations for self-care. On the first weekly visit, Thomas was carrying a wallet card indicating that he was receiving prednisone. He had ordered a Medic-Alert bracelet, but it had not arrived.

*Collaborative problems that should be differentiated from the nursing diagnoses include: Potential complications: cardiovascular (hypertension, thrombi, thromboemboli), hyperglycemia, hypernatremia, hypokalemia, immunodeficiency, GI bleeding, pathologic fractures, active tuberculosis infection.

dependent clients in institutional settings. When developing a teaching plan, the nurse considers the client's attitude toward current drug therapy and the client's experience with drug therapy in the past. A reluctance to take drugs or an undue reliance on drug use may interfere with optimal drug therapy.

The nurse compares a client's expressed attitude with the nurse's objective assessment of the client's emotional responses during the drug history interview. Proper assessment of clients' attitudes toward drugs can help nurses identify learning needs and select an optimal approach to teaching clients about their drug regimens.

Nursing Diagnosis

A nursing diagnosis is the statement of an actual or potential health problem. The identified problem focuses on the human response of a person or group for which the nurse is responsible and accountable for identifying and treating independently.

In nursing pharmacology, nursing diagnoses identify undesirable changes that are secondary to drug therapy and that can be treated by nursing measures. Some examples of appropriate diagnoses are "Activity intolerance related to fatigue secondary to antihypertensive medication" and "Anxiety, related to knowledge deficit concerning anticoagulant therapy." In both of these diagnoses, the diagnostic statement identifies a problem and a cause that are amenable to nursing intervention.

When developing the appropriate nursing diagnoses, the assessment data may indicate an actual or potential health problem (complication) that focuses on the pathophysiologic response of the body and for which interventions must be carried out in collaboration with the physician. Some examples of collaborative problems include cardiac arrhythmias secondary to potassium deficiency and hypertension related to amphetamine therapy. Because these complications require intervention in collaboration with a physician, they are identified in this text as collaborative problems and are listed separately from the nursing diagnoses.

The list of official nursing diagnoses of the North American Nursing Diagnosis Association (NANDA) is available from NANDA, 1211 Locust St., Philadelphia, PA 19107.

Planning

For the most part, the general objectives of nursing care in drug therapy are to enhance drug action, prevent drug-related problems, ameliorate symptoms of adverse reactions, correct abnormal states, and improve function. Specific goals may be to minimize side effects, prevent drug dependence, detect and treat adverse reactions promptly, promote withdrawal from a dependency-producing chemical, reduce or promote drug use (depend-ing on the client's attitudes and needs), and teach clients to manage their drug regimens independently.

Planning must include outcome identification, the formulation of criteria for successful nursing care. The criteria must be measurable and have a defined time frame. An example of outcome identification is "Within 1 week the client will exhibit a steady gait while ambulating and will report an absence of dizziness or vertigo."

Intervention

Nursing interventions include psychologic and physical care to reduce the need for drugs, to enhance the effectiveness of the drug regimen, and to prevent or ameliorate adverse reactions to medications. Nurses may also influence the drug regimen by suggesting to physicians or requesting from them orders for drugs that they believe are appropriate. Teaching clients about medications is another primary concern. Education may be designed to help clients derive the greatest benefit from the drug regimen while in an acute care setting, or it may prepare them or their families to manage their drug regimens at home.

The Iowa Nursing Intervention Classification (NIC) Project has developed labels and descriptions of nursing interventions (McCloskey and Bulechek, 1992). Of these, many are directly related to drug therapy (Box 3-2). Because the terminology is planned to be comprehensive, reflecting practice at all levels of nursing, some of the listed interventions are not within the scope of practice of many nurses. This is a continuing and evolving project, and there may be many valid nursing interventions that are not yet listed.

Outcome Evaluation

The success of nursing interventions should be measured by comparing client data after the administration of care to predetermined criteria (outcome identification) established as goals in the planning stage. Skill in the development of appropriate criteria is acquired with experience. If the criteria are stated in measurable terms, progress can be assessed even when the criteria are not fully met. Some examples of evaluative data and criteria for success are given in Table 3-1.

Critical Pathways

Critical pathways are standardized interdisciplinary plans for the care of patients with common medical conditions. They have been developed to guide the planning, implementation, and evaluation of medical care. All health professionals involved in patient care follow the same plan of care and record data pertinent to evaluation. The pathways include criteria for evaluation. Reasons that the criteria were not met must be

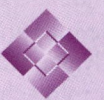

Box 3-2
Iowa Nursing Intervention Classification (NIC) Project: Interventions Related to Drug Therapy

Analgesic administration

Anesthesia administration

Chemotherapy management

Epidural analgesia administration

Family planning: Contraception

Immunization/vaccination administration

Intravenous therapy

Medication administration

    Enteral
    Interpleural
    Oral
    Parenteral
    Topical

Medication management

Pain management

Patient-controlled analgesia (PCA) assistance

Prescribing

Substance abuse prevention

Substance abuse treatment

    Alcohol withdrawal
    Overdose

Teaching: Prescribed medication

Prevention and treatment of medication side effects

    Allergy management
    Bleeding precautions
    Bowel management
    Constipation or impaction management
    Diarrhea management
    Electrolyte management
    Fluid management
    Infection protection
    Neurologic monitoring
    Respiratory monitoring
    Urinary elimination management

Source: McCloskey JC, Bulechek GM (eds). (1992). *Nursing interventions classification.* St. Louis: CV Mosby.

Table 3-1. Examples of Outcome Identification (Criteria) and Data for Outcome Evaluation

Criteria	Evaluation
For Client Receiving Iron	
Stools will be soft and client will state that defecation is free of discomfort.	Soft, formed stool is passed after breakfast. Client states that there was no problem with bowel elimination today.
For Client on Anticoagulant Therapy	
Client will consistently wear a medical identification device warning of anticoagulant use.	Client reports that Medic-Alert tag bearing the words "on anticoagulant therapy" is worn constantly; appropriate Medic-Alert bracelet is observed on client's wrist.
For Client on Diuretic Therapy	
Client will take medication regularly as shown by a tablet count within two of the appropriate number when prescription is half used.	Tablet count on the 15th day of use of a new prescription was 16 (amount dispensed—30; prescribed dosage—1 tablet daily).

cited. Currently, critical pathways are distinctive to individual institutions, but they may evolve into standardized plans of care adopted throughout the health-care industry.

Advantages of critical pathways include:

- The care provided by health professionals from various disciplines is more consistent when all use the same plan of care.
- Outcome criteria are measurable and include defined time frames.

- The pathways define the specifics of care required to meet the client's needs within the expected length of stay (in institutions) in accordance with diagnosis-related groups (DRGs).
- Listing reasons for failure to meet criteria can identify problems in care delivery.
- Wide adoption of standard critical pathways could promote more uniform delivery of health care.

The disadvantage of critical pathways is that the care outlined in the pathway is designed to meet the needs of the average client, rather than the unique needs of each client; nonetheless, health professionals may accept the care plan as appropriate and complete for meeting the needs of all clients. A standardized nursing care plan is integrated into critical pathways. However, unless supplemented by additional plans for individualizing nursing care, it is unlikely that the client's needs will be fully met. These additional plans must be consistent with the critical pathway. Inconsistencies must be resolved by consultation among the health professionals involved in care.

■ SUMMARY

The nursing process is applicable to all nursing care situations. The nurse should diagnose (or rule out) problems arising from exposure to toxins, drug treatment regimens, and inappropriate use or abuse of drugs. Goals are to eliminate the inappropriate use of drugs, to detect and treat adverse reactions to therapeutic drugs promptly, and to teach clients to manage their self-care appropriately as it relates to drugs. Evaluation requires ongoing monitoring of clients for drug effects.

Bibliography

*Carpenito LJ. (1995). *Nursing diagnosis: Application to clinical practice*, 6th ed. Philadelphia: JB Lippincott.

McCloskey JC, Bulechek GM (eds). (1992). *Nursing interventions classification*. St. Louis: CV Mosby.

*Recommended for further reading.

For more information and sample tests and activities, refer to Chapter 3 in the Student Workbook for Clinical Pharmacology and Nursing Management, 5th edition, available through your bookstore.

Therapy
With Drugs

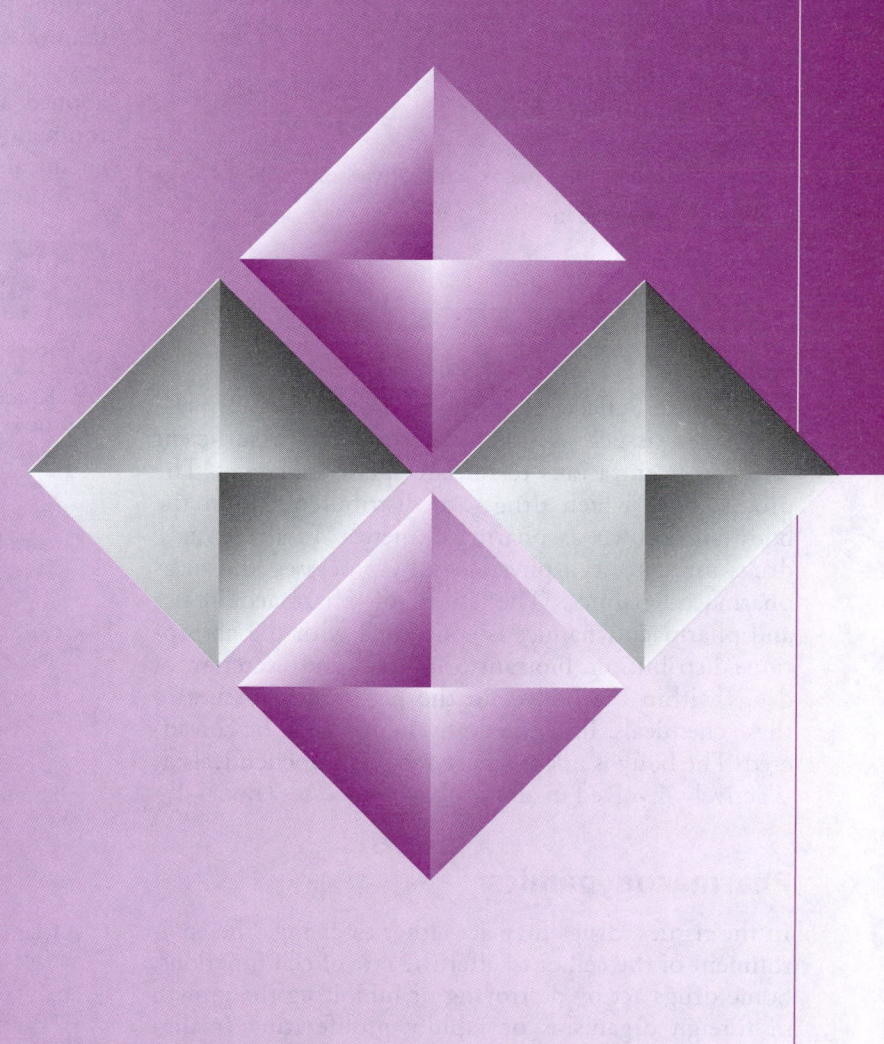

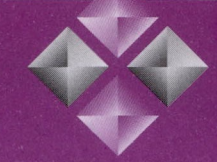
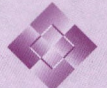

4

Pharmacodynamics and Pharmacokinetics

Pharmacodynamics
   Alteration of cellular environments
   Provision of substrate material
   Alteration of cell functions
   Agonist–antagonist interaction
   Alteration of genetic material

Pharmacokinetics
   Drug absorption
   Drug distribution
   Drug biotransformation
   Drug excretion
   Interaction of pharmacokinetic processes

Nursing management

To exert effects on the body, drugs must reach target tissues in suitable forms and in sufficient concentrations to initiate specific changes. The processes by which drugs are distributed within the body are known as pharmacokinetics. In the tissues, drugs influence cell physiology by processes known as pharmacodynamics. The study of pharmacokinetics and pharmacodynamics is concerned with the absorption, distribution, biotransformation, and excretion of drugs within the body and the response of tissues to these chemicals. Individual physiology must be considered. The body is not a passive recipient of chemicals; it is actively involved in all the above processes (Box 4-1).

Pharmacodynamics

In the tissues, drugs may act either to change the environment of the cell or to alter the rate of cell functions. Some drugs act by destroying or inhibiting the growth of foreign organisms or rapidly proliferating (malignant) cells. Other drugs may protect cells from the influence of physical or chemical agents, promote cell function by providing substances needed for metabo-

---

> **Box 4-1**
> **Definitions**
>
> *Pharmacodynamics*—the processes by which drugs influence cell physiology
>
> *Pharmacokinetics*—the processes by which drugs are distributed within the body

lism, or speed or slow cell processes. To date, no approved drugs can alter cell process. Successful "gene therapy" may accomplish this, however, by adding to or changing the genetic material within cells so that cells lacking normal genes may perform normal functions.

Alteration of Cellular Environments

Drugs change the environment of body cells by physical or chemical processes. Physical actions may involve all the processes of physics, from lubrication to ionizing radiation (Table 4-1). Individual drugs may exert more than one effect. For example, many lubricants also impose a lipid barrier between the tissues to which they are applied and irritating substances. The chemical environment of cells is changed when drugs react with other chemicals, producing changes in the constituents of

Table 4-1. Processes by Which Drugs Alter the Physics of Cell Environments

Process	Examples
Imposition of barriers	Applying petroleum jelly to skin of diaper area of babies to prevent contact with urine
	Applying tincture of benzoin to protect skin from friction of sheets or clothing
Lubrication	Applying sunscreen lotions to prevent sunburn
	Covering skin folds with cornstarch to reduce friction
Osmosis	Initiating saline cathartics
	Administering mannitol intravenously to stimulate osmotic diuresis
	Using saturated magnesium sulfate soaks to reduce tissue edema
Adsorption	Giving Kaopectate to absorb toxins that cause diarrhea
	Administering activated charcoal orally to reduce the absorption of harmful chemicals in cases of poisoning
Alteration of surface tension	Using surfactant stool softeners
	Using quaternary compounds as antiseptic cleaners
Ionizing radiation	Using radioactive tracers in diagnostic tests
	Administering radioactive iodine to ablate thyroid tissue in hyperthyroidism

body fluids (Table 4-2). Drugs that affect body chemistry also may act by more than one mechanism. For example, electrolytes such as chlorides not only change serum levels of individual ions but also influence the pH of body fluids. A drug may act physically and chemically, as do intravenous (IV) fluids that influence the serum osmotic pressure and the chemical makeup of the blood.

Provision of Substrate Material

Many chemicals that act as substrate for metabolism are classified as nutrients and are not considered true drugs. However, because they affect living tissue, they fall into the general classification of drugs. Recent findings by nutritional researchers indicate that food constituents, such as amino acids, are pharmacologically active. Increasingly, specific nutrients are formulated as drugs and used for pharmacologic effect.

Alteration of Cell Functions

Drugs that alter cell function interact with one or more structures of the cell. Such interactions may be general, altering cell membranes or cellular processes, or they may be specific, affecting specialized regions of the cell. General mechanisms of drug–cell interaction include interference with or facilitation of cell membrane functions and alteration of metabolic processes (Table 4-3). The specialized cellular structures with which some drugs interact are called *receptors.*

Receptor Theory of Drug Action

According to the receptor theory of drug action, specific macromolecules in cells interact with certain chemicals because of the nature of their respective three-dimensional structures. If three or more sites on the molecular surfaces match in such a way as to promote chemical bonding, the drug attaches to the cellular structure. These drugs are visualized as "fitting" the receptor as a key fits a lock. Receptors are usually cellular proteins or nucleic acids but can also be enzymes, carbohydrate residues, and lipids.

Table 4-3. General Processes of Drug–Cell Interaction

Process	Examples
Facilitation of membrane transport	Moving glucose across cell membranes by insulin in treating diabetes mellitus
Inhibition of membrane function	Reducing nerve and muscle irritability by ionized calcium salts in treating tetany
	Depressing nerve cell membrane permeability with general anesthetics to produce unconsciousness
Support of energy metabolism	Enhancing energy metabolism by administering oxygen
	Restoring energy metabolism by administering glucose to treat hypoglycemia
Inhibition of energy metabolism	Inactivating mitochondrial cytochrome oxidases with cyanide (in instances of poisoning)
Precipitation of cellular protein	Damaging microorganisms with alcohol used as an antiseptic

A drug that directly alters the functional properties of the receptor with which it interacts is termed an *agonist.* To function as an agonist, a chemical must have affinity for the target tissue (a propensity to locate at the receptor site) and efficacy (the ability to initiate biologic activity). According to the receptor theory of drug action, the agonist forms bonds with the receptor on at least three sites, locking the two molecules together.

The electromagnetic forces produced by these bonds tend to distort the molecular configuration of the receptor molecule, changing its biochemical properties. It is believed that some receptor molecules extend from the outside of the cell membrane to the inside. Occupation of the exterior site by an agonist distorts the portion of the molecule on the interior surface of the cell membrane, thereby altering its ability to interact with intracellular compounds, including enzymes active in metabolic processes (Fig. 4-1).

Experts think receptors evolved to interact with endogenous biologic compounds. Some of these compounds have been identified and studied. For example, certain brain enkephalins and endorphins interact with opiate receptors on nerve cells, causing the same pain reduction and emotional euphoria characteristic of opiate administration. These chemicals are released from the brain as a result of various stimuli, such as vigorous exercise (eg, running) and the expectation that pain will be relieved because some therapeutic action has occurred (placebo effect).

Receptors themselves are subject to external influences. Continued stimulation may result in a decrease in receptor response. This process is termed *desensitization*; the end state is termed *refractoriness.* Desensitization involves a reduction of receptors on cell membranes or a change in existing receptors. If a chronic level of re-

Table 4-2. Processes by Which Drugs Alter the Chemical Environment of Cells

Process	Examples
Alteration of pH	Neutralizing stomach acid with antacids
	Inhibiting bacterial or fungal growth in the vagina by vinegar douches
Detoxification of toxins and poisons	Inactivating diphtheria toxin by antitoxin
	Precipitating opiates by potassium permanganate gastric lavages in instances of opiate poisoning
Alteration of body fluid chemistry	Restoring fluid and electrolyte balance by intravenous therapy
	Interfering with coagulability of blood by administering heparin

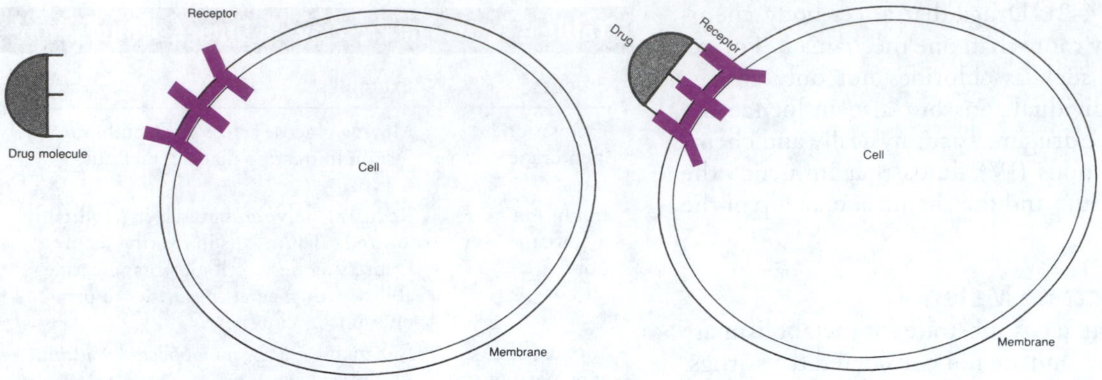

Figure 4-1. The interaction of a drug with a target cell at the cell receptor site. The distortion of the receptor molecule alters its function within the cell

ceptor stimulation is reduced, a state of supersensitivity or hyperreactivity may develop. This effect reflects a restoration of receptors to a responsive state or the synthesis of additional receptors.

A drug is usually classified according to its most prominent effect, its most usual therapeutic effect, or the actions thought to be the basis of these effects. This practice tends to obscure the fact that every drug produces a spectrum of effects. When a drug is administered for a single purpose, the extraneous results are termed *side effects*. Side effects may be desirable and helpful, neutral, or undesirable and potentially dangerous. The relation between the dosages required to produce a therapeutic response and those that produce adverse reactions is termed *therapeutic index, margin of safety,* or *specificity*. No drug produces only a single effect, and few are selective enough to be described as specific.

Therapeutic indices are derived from findings in animal research and clinical trials in humans during the development of new drugs by pharmaceutical firms. A single drug may have several therapeutic indices, one for each therapeutic effect under investigation. Although these indices do not always apply to humans, they do indicate the relative safety of a drug. A therapeutic index of 1 indicates that a drug is as likely to harm as to help the recipient.

Agonist–Antagonist Interaction

Antagonist drugs reduce the physiologic effect of other drugs and are often used as antidotes for drug toxicity. An antagonist's site of action may be the same as that of the agonist (eg, a cell receptor site), or it may be at a distinctly different anatomic site. For example, anticholinesterase insecticides and nerve gas inhibit the enzyme that breaks down acetylcholine at synapses and neuromuscular junctions. As a result, acetylcholine persists and continues to stimulate the nerves and muscles on whose receptors it acts; seizures are one of its effects. Atropine relieves these seizures and other manifestations of anticholinesterase toxicity, but not by exerting any effect on either the anticholinesterase or the excess acetylcholine. Instead, atropine blocks the nerve and cell receptors stimulated by acetylcholine.

The action of atropine is an example of competitive inhibition. The agonist and antagonist bind with the receptor equally well and compete to occupy the receptor site. When the agonist binds more tightly to the receptor than the antagonist, the action of the antagonist is relatively weak. When the antagonist binds more tightly than the agonist to the receptor, the action of the antagonist is relatively strong. Some antagonists are degraded or excreted more rapidly than the agonists they oppose. Therefore, their actions are short-lived and they must be administered repeatedly to prevent the recurrence of toxic signs and symptoms.

Alteration of Genetic Material

Researchers are beginning to correct genetic defects by introducing into the cells normal genes produced by recombinant gene processes. Reports from initial clinical trials are promising.

■ SUMMARY

Drugs either change the cellular environment or alter the rate of cellular function; in the future, gene therapy may be able to alter cell functions. Changes in environment are brought about by physical action or chemical reactions; a drug may have one action or both. Drugs interact with one or more cellular structures to alter cell functions. Such interactions may be general or specific. The specialized structures with which some drugs interact are called receptors. Receptors are most often cellular proteins or nucleic acids. A drug that directly alters the functional properties of the receptor with which it interacts is termed an agonist. A compound inhibiting the action of an agonist is called an antagonist. Continual stimulation of a receptor may result in desensitization, a decrease in receptor response. If the stimulating drug is then removed, a state of supersensitivity or hyperreactivity may develop. A drug is usually classified according to its most prominent effect, but every drug produces a spectrum of effects.

Pharmacokinetics

The effect of drugs is markedly influenced by their form and concentration in the tissues. The study of absorption, distribution, biotransformation, and excretion of drugs in the body is termed *pharmacokinetics*.

Drug Absorption

Drugs applied for their local effect usually act superficially on the surface. Most drugs, however, must penetrate the body to be effective. If a systemic effect is desired, the drug enters the blood and is distributed widely throughout body tissues. Absorption of chemicals conforms to the scientific laws affecting the kinetics of matter. Absorption strongly influences drug efficacy and toxicity.

Mechanisms of Absorption

Chemicals migrate through tissues by water or lipid transport and by active transport mechanisms. Water-soluble drugs are carried by body fluids wherever the passageways (blood vessels, lymphatic vessels, interstitial spaces, or pores in membranes) are large enough for solute particles to penetrate. Where membranes whose pores are impermeable to the solute separate compartments, the drug molecule may cross by diffusion, active transport, or pinocytosis (Fig. 4-2).

Diffusion requires dissolution in the lipid portion of the membrane and is available only to nonpolar, or nonionized, particles. Although diffusion requires no energy, it depends on concentration gradients from one side of the membrane to the other. Passive mechanisms of transport operate in both directions across membranes. Transfer speed depends on and directly relates to the degree of dissolution, the drug concentration, and the area of membrane–drug exposure. It is inversely related to ionization (and hence polarization) of the drug chemical. Both drug dissolution and ionization are affected by pH values in body solutions.

Active transport mechanisms can transfer molecules against concentration gradients. In this process, the drug molecule combines temporarily with a chemical in the membrane that facilitates passage across the membrane, then releases the drug on the other side. The rate of active transport is limited by the capacity of the carrier mechanism. Below the level at which the carrier mechanism is saturated, the rate of transport is proportional to the drug concentration. Active transport requires the expenditure of energy to accomplish its work. Both passive and active transport mechanisms play a role in the excretion as well as the absorption of drugs (Table 4-4).

Pinocytosis involves the transport of a particle across a membrane while it is enclosed in a fragment of the membrane. The particle is enveloped by a pouchlike fold of the membrane that subsequently breaks away from the surface, crosses the membrane, and melds with the opposite surface, freeing the particle.

Routes of Absorption

Drugs are absorbed by several routes: skin, mucous membranes, oral ingestion, inhalation, and injection.

Skin

The skin is less permeable to chemicals than most other ports of entry. Because the epidermis acts as a lipid barrier, only lipid-soluble substances are absorbed through the intact skin. Abraded skin permits penetration by many substances because the dermis is freely permeable to many solutes. Hair follicles and other dermal structures alter the absorption rate, and the skin can also metabolize (biodegrade) drugs. The skin does not present a uniform barrier to drug absorption.

Most drugs applied to the skin are topical remedies used for a local effect. Historically, when systemic absorption was desired, the medicinal chemical was suspended in an oily vehicle and rubbed into the skin, a process known as *unction*. Metallic salts were administered by unction for treating diseases, including syphilis. The transdermal route has been consistently used for over-the-counter (OTC) remedies containing methylsalicylate (oil of wintergreen). The salicylate is systemically absorbed and may provide effective analgesia for arthritic pain.

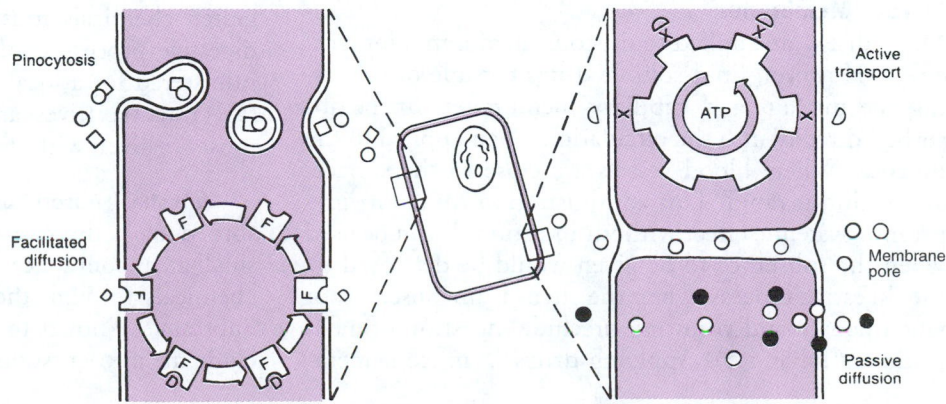

Figure 4-2. Schematic view of physiologic membranes and mechanisms of drug transport.

Table 4-4. Comparing Passive and Active Drug Absorption, Distribution, and Excretion

Elements of Transport	Passive Transport	Active Transport
Rate of transport	Proportional to concentration gradient between the involved cell compartments	Proportional to concentration of drug available until carrier mechanism becomes so saturated that it cannot accommodate an increase in transport
Capacity of transport system	Limited only by the area of the membrane	Limited by the number of carrier units, which are molecules acting as carriers
Molecular movement	Movement from areas of high concentration to areas of low concentration of drug molecules; molecules move across membranes in both directions	Drug molecules can move against the concentration gradient; direction of transport is usually "one way."
Energy requirements	Energy not required, other than the kinetic energy of brownian movement	Consumes energy in work performed by carrier
Diffusability	Many kinds of drug molecules can diffuse. Usually the molecule's size determines its ability to diffuse. Drugs that can exist in charged and noncharged forms approach state of equilibrium primarily by transfer of the noncharged particles across the membrane.	Only specific or similarly chemically structured molecules are transported; similar chemicals compete for transport.

In the past, the skin was rarely a route for administering prescription drugs. However, topical vasodilators, estrogens, and antiemetics have been marketed, indicating renewed interest in the transdermal route for systemic medication.

Systemic toxicity can occur when substances are absorbed through the skin. Salicylate poisoning has been reported with overuse of the OTC arthritis preparations described above. Oily solutions of insecticides have caused poisoning by skin contact alone. The drug hexachlorophene, used widely at one time for cleaning skin and treating acne, was absorbed from the skin in sufficient quantity to cause neurotoxicity. Because of this risk, it can no longer be obtained without a prescription.

Mucous Membranes

Many drugs are applied to mucous membranes for local effect. However, lipid-soluble drugs capable of traversing the mucous and capillary membranes can be absorbed directly into the circulation when applied to the mucosa. Where blood vessels are close to the surface, absorption is rapid. This administration route provides prompt systemic effect without injection. It can be used when the substance to be given would be destroyed by the digestive process, when the client is unconscious, or when nausea and vomiting preclude ingestion of medications (Table 4-5). Applying drugs to mucous membranes may produce toxic symptoms if absorption is very rapid. Mucous membranes commonly used include the sublingual, buccal, nasal, conjunctival, vaginal, and rectal mucosa.

Many topical drugs applied to mucous membranes are irritating and may injure the mucosa if used repeatedly. After drug absorption, the site should be rinsed with water to remove drug residue. If drugs are administered regularly by this route, sites should be rotated if possible.

Oral Ingestion

Because it is comfortable, convenient, and economical, the oral route is used for administering many medications. Drugs to be swallowed may be prepared as solutions, suspensions, powders, tablets, or capsules. Ingested chemicals must be resistant to degradation by digestive processes. Although a few drugs may be administered for a local effect within the gastrointestinal (GI) tract (laxatives, antacids, adsorbent antidiarrheals), most are given with the expectation of systemic effect.

Intestinal Absorption. A few drugs are rapidly absorbed by a discrete segment of the intestine. These small areas contain carrier substances that move specific chemicals through the membrane by active transport. Substances known to be absorbed by this process include the nutrients sodium, potassium, vitamins, amino

Table 4-5. Drugs Commonly Applied to Mucous Membranes

Site of Membrane	Examples
Sublingual	Nitroglycerin for rapid relief of anginal symptoms Isoproterenol to dilate the bronchi in asthma
Buccal	Pitocin to stimulate uterine contractions during labor and delivery
Nasal	Pitressin for controlling diabetes insipidus Decongestant nose drops for local effect, although drug can be absorbed, causing systemic side effects
Conjunctival	Miotic, mydriatic, or antiinflammatory drops for local effect, although drug can be absorbed from conjunctiva, the tear duct lining, or nasal mucosa, causing systemic side effects
Vaginal	Estrogen to alleviate atrophic vaginitis (can be absorbed by vaginal mucosa of the recipient or the genital tissues of male sex partner, causing systemic effects in either)
Rectal	Bisacodyl suppositories to relieve constipation by local stimulation of reflex peristalsis; aspirin suppositories to reduce fever by systemic action

acids, and simple sugars; uracil; thymine; bile salts; and the drugs 5-fluorouracil and 5-bromouracil.

Intestinal absorption of most drugs depends on passive diffusion. Therefore, the rate of absorption is affected by dissolution and ionization of the drug. Solubility depends on the drug particle's size and chemical form. Solid dosage forms such as tablets or capsules must first disintegrate to expose large surface areas of the chemical to the gastric or intestinal juices. As the drug deaggregates, it begins to dissolve in the fluid medium. Drug forms that ionize readily (usually salts) go into solution more rapidly than nonelectrolytes. To facilitate dissolution, disintegrators and chemical buffers may be added to the formulation. Disintegrators are relatively inert substances (eg, starch) that dissolve readily, causing the solid drug to fragment rapidly when moistened. Buffers promote immediate dissolution during the initial stages of disintegration without significantly changing the pH of gastric or intestinal fluids (Figs. 4-3 and 4-4).

Because they are largely nonionized in the acid medium of gastric secretions, acidic drugs are absorbed rapidly by the gastric mucosa. Basic drugs normally remain ionized in this compartment and are not absorbed until they reach the intestines, where the pH is higher. In the stomach, foods or antacids that raise the pH tend to retard absorption of acid drugs and may initiate absorption of basic drugs in this organ.

Although absorption of some drugs may be delayed by foods, overall drug uptake is usually maximal regardless of the timing of the drug dose in relation to meals. This occurs because of the large surface area for absorption provided by the gut and the long time required for intestinal transit. Immediate absorption is not always desirable: blood concentrations may rise rapidly enough to reach toxic levels. Prolonging the absorption time also produces a steadier serum drug level.

The rate of drug absorption is influenced by the speed of transit through the GI tract. Rapid stomach-emptying accelerates the absorption of basic drugs because they more rapidly reach the small intestine, where they are then absorbed. Acidic drugs may not be completely absorbed in the stomach if they are propelled prematurely from that organ. Usually, drugs ingested with food are absorbed more slowly and gradually than are drugs taken on an empty stomach.

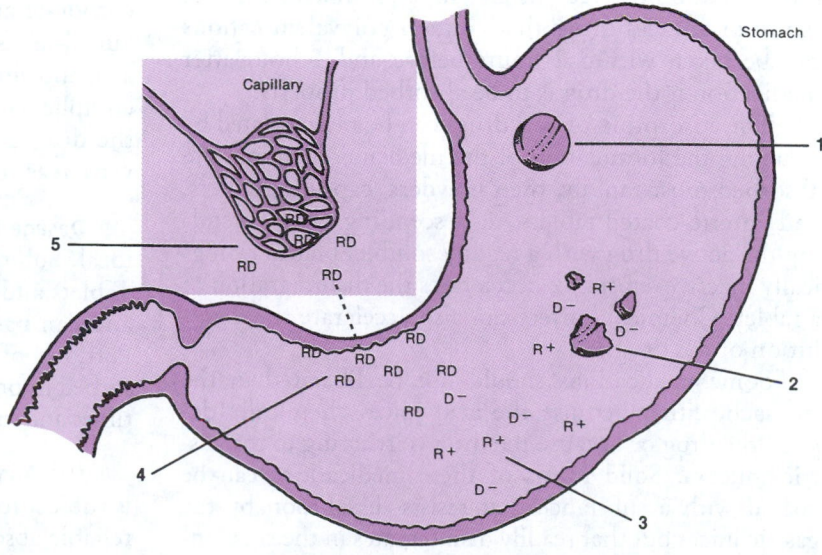

Figure 4-3. Steps in the absorption of solid tablets, acid salts: (1) Solid tablet enters stomach. (2) Tablet begins to disintegrate. Base buffer in tablet promotes dissolution. (3) Charged ions diffuse into the large pool of stomach juices whose pH has not been raised by small amount of buffer in tablet. (4) In acid medium, ions reunite forming nonpolarized compound. (5) Nonpolarized particles diffuse readily through lipid membranes. (D, drug radical; R, nondrug radical)

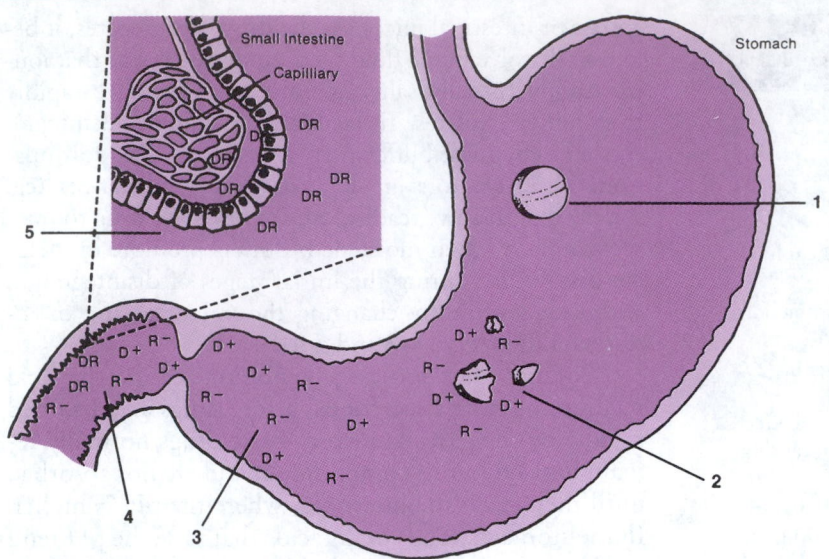

Figure 4-4. Steps in the absorption of solid tablets, basic salts: (1) Solid tablet enters stomach. (2) Tablet begins to disintegrate. Acid medium of stomach favors rapid dissolution of basic salts. (3) Ions remain dissociated in low pH of stomach. (4) Pancreatic juice enters duodenum, raising pH. Drug ions reunite, forming nonpolarized compound. (5) Nonpolarized particles diffuse readily through lipid membranes. (D, drug radical; R, nondrug radical)

Abnormal Digestion and Drug Absorption. Abnormal digestion can markedly affect the absorption of drugs from the digestive tract. Achlorhydria (the absence of hydrochloric acid in the stomach) retards gastric absorption of acid drugs and dissolution of basic drugs. Deficiencies of pancreatic and intestinal secretions may completely prevent the dissolution of enteric-coated tablets, causing them to be excreted unabsorbed in the feces. (Enteric coatings are designed to disintegrate only in the small intestine.) Vomiting and diarrhea tend to propel drugs from the tract before absorption can be completed (Table 4-6).

Manipulation of Drug Absorption. Mixing drugs with food can impair absorption if the drug forms a nonabsorbable complex with elements in the food. For example, tetracycline combines chemically with polyvalent cations (calcium, magnesium, iron, aluminum) to form complexes that cannot be broken down by digestion but are excreted unabsorbed in the feces. Such drugs must be administered on an empty stomach. Neither food nor antacid drugs that contain polyvalent cations can be taken within 2 hours before and 1 hour after medication if the drug is to be absorbed properly.

The absorption of oral drugs can be manipulated by changing the formulation of the medicine. Solutions are absorbed most rapidly, then powders, capsules, tablets, and enteric-coated tablets, in descending order. Blending the active drug with a readily soluble, pharmacologically inactive substance accelerates the disintegration of a tablet. Chemical buffers can also accelerate the dissolution of the drug.

Some medications should not be liberated in the stomach, either because the acid juices chemically destroy the drug or because the drug is irritating to the gastric mucosa. Solid forms of these medications can be coated with a substance that resists dissolution by the gastric juices but that readily disintegrates in the small intestines. Some coatings are soluble only in a basic medium; others are broken down by digestive enzymes specific to the small intestine. Such an enteric coating provides a barrier between the drug and the stomach, preventing damage to either by the other. Enteric-coated preparations should not be crushed, because this will destroy the coating and liberate the drug inappropriately in the stomach. Medications coated with an acid-resistant substance should not be administered with drugs or foods that raise the pH of stomach contents, because this could cause dissolution of the coating in the stomach.

Sustained-release formulations prolong the action period of single-dosage forms. These preparations contain two or more forms of a drug with different absorption times. To prolong absorption, the drug may be encapsulated, enteric-coated, or combined with waxes or fats, ion-exchange resins, colloids, or porous plastics. Sometimes a tablet is prepared in a manner that retards disintegration. To achieve a minimally effective serum level promptly, many sustained-release preparations incorporate an initial dose that is rapidly absorbed. Sustained-released formulations reduce the frequency of dosage, allowing uninterrupted sleep and improving client compliance. A disadvantage is that client exposure to the drug cannot be terminated promptly when an adverse reaction such as allergy develops.

Dosage Formulations. No one formulation of drug is ideal. Solutions and powders are typically unpalatable. Tablets and capsules may fail to disintegrate or dissolve and can pass unabsorbed from the body in the stools. Portions of sustained-release preparations may be absorbed improperly, producing toxic serum levels at certain times and inadequate blood concentrations at others.

Oral Administration. Although GI absorption of drugs is subject to many factors, oral dosage regimens provide reliable absorption for most drugs and remain the most

Table 4-6. Factors Influencing Absorption of Oral Drugs

Factors	Possible Effects on Drug Absorption
Client-Related Factors	
State of Digestive Function	
Peristalsis	Vomiting and diarrhea remove drug from body before complete absorption.
Secretions	Changes in pH of gastric acid or pancreatic secretions alter absorption of drugs requiring specific pH or enzyme for absorption.
Food in the GI tract	Food reacts with some drugs, forming nonabsorbable complexes. Food in the stomach delays stomach emptying and absorption of most drugs.
Antacids in the stomach	Antacids react with certain drugs, forming nonabsorbable complexes. Antacids increase pH of gastric juice, altering absorption of acidic and basic salts and dissolving the protective coating of some enteric-coated preparations.
Method of Taking Drug	
Fluid intake	Inadequate fluid taken with oral medications can cause medication to lodge in the esophagus, delaying transit to the area of absorption.
Crushing, chewing tablets	Crushing and chewing reduce particle size and tend to accelerate absorption. They may also disrupt enteric coating, releasing drugs inappropriately in the stomach (gastric irritation or destruction of the drug may occur).
Medication-Related Factors	
Dosage Formulation	
Physical state of drug	Amorphic drugs dissolve more rapidly than crystals and are absorbed more rapidly. Solutions are absorbed more rapidly than solid drugs, powders more rapidly than tablets.
Inactive ingredients in formulation	Disintegrators and buffers accelerate absorption.
Enteric coating	Enteric coating delays dissolution of drug until it reaches intestine, retarding absorption.

convenient, comfortable, and economical method of administering systemic drugs (Box 4-2).

Inhalation

The lungs provide a large surface for the absorption of gaseous chemicals. The total blood volume traverses the lungs, and rich capillary networks close to the alveolar surface provide a ready reservoir for drug absorption. Inhaled compounds diffuse rapidly from the alveolar space to the bloodstream. Because absorption of inhalant drugs is not compromised by circulatory shock, this route is sometimes used in emergencies.

To be tolerated by the lungs, substances administered by inhalation must not interfere with respiration (the exchange of oxygen and carbon dioxide). Therefore, drugs for inhalation must be in gas or fine-mist forms. Most mists (aerosols) are generated from aqueous solutions, but sometimes a solid drug in fine-powder form may be used (Table 4-7). Devices used to propel medications into the alveolar tree include pressure tanks for dispensing gases, ultrasonic or nebulizer mist generators, and hand-operated inhalers.

Drugs requiring the use of ventilators are usually administered by respiratory therapists, the acknowledged experts in managing these machines. Because the inhalant anesthetics have a narrow safety margin, they are commonly administered by physicians and qualified nurse-anesthetists. Nurses are commonly responsible

only for administering oxygen, drugs delivered by hand-operated inhalers and nebulizers, and aromatic spirits of ammonia, a first-aid remedy for fainting.

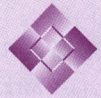

Box 4-2
Drug Absorption by Oral Ingestion

- Oral ingestion is the most convenient, comfortable, and economical method of administering systemic drugs.
- Ingested chemicals must be resistant to degradation by the digestive process and liver metabolism.
- The rate of drug absorption is influenced by the speed of transit through the tract.
- Abnormal digestion can markedly affect absorption of drugs.
- Some foods impair absorption of certain drugs.
- Absorption of drugs can be manipulated through changes in the formulation of the medicine.
- Drugs that are not to be liberated in the stomach are enteric-coated.
- Sustained-release formulations prolong the period of action.
- The absorption of drugs is influenced by their acidity or alkalinity and the pH of the gastrointestinal contents.

Table 4-7. Substances Commonly Absorbed by Inhalation

Drug	Physical Form(s)	Effect(s)
Therapeutic Agents		
Oxygen	Gas	Enhancement of oxygen transport to the tissues in hypoxia
Anesthetics: ether, nitrous oxide, halothane	Gases and volatile liquids	Loss of consciousness and insensitivity to pain during surgery
Cromolyn	Aqueous solutions and dry powder	Prevention of asthma by inhibition of release of autocoids such as histamine
Mucolytics: acetylcysteine (Mucomyst), deoxyribonuclease	Aqueous solutions	Thinning of respiratory secretions
Bronchodilators: salmeterol	Aqueous solutions	Bronchodilation, central nervous system stimulation
Aromatic spirits of ammonia	Volatile drug in aqueous solution	Respiratory stimulation, elevation of blood pressure
Pollutants and Substances of Abuse		
Carbon tetrachloride, paint thinner, industrial solvents, glue	Volatile liquids and volatile substances in solution	Intoxication, emotional disturbance, hallucinations (with chronic exposure, liver damage)
Anesthetics: ether, nitrous oxide, halothane (Fluothane) inhaled by OR staff	Gases and volatile liquids	Excitation, emotional disturbance, unconsciousness (in the case of chronic exposure to Fluothane: increased risk of birth defects and spontaneous abortion)
Poisons		
Carbon monoxide	Gas	Hypoxia and asphyxiation

Injection

Systemic drugs can be injected into various tissues of the body when other administration routes are inappropriate or contraindicated. This administration method generally provides more rapid absorption than either topical application or ingestion. Drugs may be injected into virtually every tissue, including bone (Table 4-8).

When local rather than systemic effects are desired, drugs are injected directly into or near the target tissue. Medicines may also be delivered to divisions of the body by means of extracorporeal perfusion or intra-arterial infusion. In all of these methods except extracorporeal perfusion, the drugs eventually escape from the target tissues and are absorbed by the general circulation. Their concentration in the general tissues, however, is lower than otherwise possible because they diffuse from the target tissue to the blood rather than the reverse.

Systemic drugs are commonly injected into subcutaneous tissues, muscles, or veins. Absorption and distribution are most rapid from veins, then from muscles, and, slowest of all, from subcutaneous tissue. The risk of tissue damage by the drug is greatest with subcutaneous injection. Muscle tissue tolerates many irritating substances that cannot be administered by hypodermic injection (injection beneath the skin). Some substances that are too irritating for intramuscular use can be administered intravenously, although they tend to induce phlebitis.

Because of the speed of distribution, the IV route has the greatest potential for serious toxicity and infection. Doses cannot be retrieved nor absorption delayed because absorption and distribution are virtually immediate. The absorption of drugs administered subcutaneously and intramuscularly can be slowed by constricting or occluding blood vessels in the area, thus reducing local circulation. Among the techniques available are applications of cold (ice packs), local injection of epinephrine, or the intermittent application of a tourniquet (if the injection site is in an extremity).

Absorption from Subcutaneous Sites. Drugs deposited in subcutaneous tissue are normally in aqueous solution. Depot preparations (drugs combined with substances such as oils that delay absorption) and irritating drugs usually are not administered by this route because they tend to cause tissue damage, by forming sterile abscesses or by sloughing. Volumes up to 1 mL can be administered in a single injection to most adults with minimal discomfort. To reach the bloodstream, they must cross the extracellular compartment to a capillary and diffuse across the blood vessel membrane. Movement through the tissues is impeded by hyaluronic acid, an adhesive that cements the cells together. For this reason and because the blood supply to subcutaneous tissue is relatively poor, absorption is relatively slow. If the peripheral circulation is impaired (as in shock), the drug may remain in the tissue site for prolonged periods.

When large amounts of fluid must be absorbed by the subcutaneous route, hyaluronidase (an enzyme that breaks down hyaluronic acid) can be administered into the injection site. This medication is usually prescribed when fluids are ordered by hypodermoclysis (the slow infusion of aqueous solutions into the tissues beneath the skin). As the amount of hyaluronic acid in the tissue

Table 4-8. Routes for Drug Delivery by Injection

Route	Site of Drug Delivery
For Systemic Effect	
Subcutaneous	Subcutaneous tissue or pocket
Intramuscular	Muscle tissue
Intravenous	Venous blood
Central venous catheter	Superior vena cava or right atrium of the heart (used when solutions must be rapidly diluted to prevent damage to the blood)
Intraosseous	Bone marrow
For Local Effect	
Intradermal	Skin
Intra-articular	Joint space
Intrathecal	Cerebrospinal fluid
Intraperitoneal	Peritoneal cavity
Intrapleural	Pleural cavity
Intra-arterial	Arterial blood (used when drug effect at high or toxic levels is desired in a localized area)
Extracorporeal perfusion	Isolated circulation of a segment of the body, commonly an extremity (drug and blood circulate through a perfusion circuit; drug may be removed and fresh blood infused when procedure is completed)
Epidural	Spinal nerves or a segment of the spinal cord

decreases, passageways become available between the cells, allowing rapid dispersal of the fluid through tissue planes. When small amounts of medicine are administered subcutaneously, massage of the tissue site after injection accelerates absorption.

Absorption from Muscle Sites. Drugs administered intramuscularly include solutions, suspensions, and complexes of drugs and various inactive substances that alter the rate of absorption. Ingredients of intramuscular medications include oils and other irritating chemicals, which are not well tolerated by subcutaneous tissue and which may be dangerous if injected directly into veins. Volumes that may be injected safely and comfortably vary with the mass of tissue available at the injection site. Volumes up to 2 mL are easily tolerated; volumes up to 5 mL are sometimes injected into large muscles of adult clients.

As with subcutaneous injection, drugs administered intramuscularly must reach a capillary and diffuse through the blood vessel wall. Muscle tissue, however, is more richly supplied with blood vessels, and the journey is relatively short. Movement through the tissues is accelerated by massaging the injection site and exercising the muscles containing the drug. Hence, the more active the muscle used for injection, the more rapid is absorption.

When gradual absorption of an intramuscular medication is desired, substances are added to the drug that form nonabsorbable or poorly absorbed complexes. Such preparations provide a depot of drug in the tissues that dissipates gradually as biochemical processes in the tissues break down the complex. Depot medications decrease the number of injections required to supply the drug over a prolonged time and sustain a steadier blood level of drug.

Intravenous Injection. Intravenous injection delivers chemicals directly into the vascular system, thus minimizing the onset of action time. In general, only aqueous solutions may be administered by IV injection. One exception is the IV administration of a fat emulsion during parenteral feeding. As mentioned previously, drugs administered intravenously are potentially toxic. Blood levels rise rapidly, and the drug cannot be retrieved once it has been administered. Intravenous lines are a reliable route for drug delivery when the client is very ill and when peripheral circulation is compromised.

One way to reduce the risk for toxicity is to control the speed with which the drug is delivered into the veins. This may be accomplished by slow infusion over time. When a bolus of drug is to be administered by the IV push technique, the nurse must inject it slowly, usually over a period of minutes. Irritating drugs are best tolerated when injected by the IV route. They require gradual administration to minimize vein irritation, which can cause inflammation and subsequent loss of the IV site.

Drug Distribution

When a systemic effect is desired, the drug enters the blood through absorption and is then distributed throughout body tissues. Drugs pass more readily between the intravascular and interstitial compartments than between other compartments of the body. The vascular membrane offers little resistance to dissolved particles unless they are large (colloid) or are bound to serum proteins. The leakiness of the blood vessel wall may be related to the intracellular cement in that tissue or to water-filled microapertures (pores). The speed of distribution can be measured in terms of *distribution half-life*, the time required for blood levels of the drug to drop by half because of migration into tissues, including tissue depots.

Assuming that the drug moves freely from the blood vessel to the extracellular fluid, the concentration of drug at any specific site would depend on the density of blood vessels in the tissue, the degree of local vasodilation or vasoconstriction, and the rate of general circulation of the blood.

Tissues with a minimal blood supply, such as bone or the middle ear, are relatively poorly perfused, and delivery of adequate drug concentrations is difficult. Factors influencing the tissue distribution of drugs include exercise and warming or chilling, which change local circulation dynamics. Other factors include changes in cardiac pumping, blood pressure, and blood volume, which impair or enhance general circulation.

Because drugs cross lipid membranes by diffusion, chemicals move in both directions. Drugs administered by injection, therefore, may appear in the intestinal secretions, sputum, saliva, semen, breast milk, and vaginal secretions, having diffused outward from the blood vessel to those compartments. Volatile substances such as alcohol are excreted by the lungs by this mechanism.

Movement of drugs to and from the vascular compartment is not entirely free, however. Certain tissues pose barriers to drug passage, whereas other tissues tend to trap drugs in various ways.

Blood-Brain Barrier

Transcapillary exchange within the central nervous system is highly selective. Water-soluble nutrients and metabolites pass through readily, but larger water-soluble molecules penetrate little or not at all. The blood-brain barrier is believed to result from the compact organization of a one-cell-thick lining of the inner walls of the cerebral capillaries. The spaces between these cells are filled by proteins that virtually occlude the openings (pores) that would otherwise allow large molecules to enter. Fat-soluble compounds can cross this barrier by dissolving in the lipid portion of endothelial cell membranes (Box 4-3).

The blood-brain barrier is an important protective mechanism because it safeguards the brain from ready disturbance by chemical changes in body fluids. It poses problems, however, when drugs must be delivered to central nervous system tissue. In some cases, such as dopamine, a pro-drug (levodopa) can be developed that can cross the blood-brain barrier. (A pro-drug is a pharmacologically inactive chemical that is converted by the body to an active drug substance.) Once inside the brain, metabolic processes transform the pro-drug into the desired agent. Other approaches that remain experi-

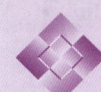

Box 4-3
The Blood-Brain Barrier

- The blood-brain barrier is an important protective mechanism for the brain.
- The blood-brain barrier is a compact layer of cells that line the cerebral capillaries.
- The blood-brain barrier excludes certain chemicals from the brain. It can also prevent therapeutic drugs from reaching the central nervous tissues.
- Very small molecules and fat-soluble substances cross the blood-brain barrier more readily than do large molecules and water-soluble compounds.

mental include joining a drug to a fat-soluble chemical, thereby producing a fat-soluble drug complex; linking a drug to an antibody, which is then absorbed by the capillary cell and transported to the brain; and using chemicals that open the pores in the cerebral capillary wall. Sometimes drugs must be injected intrathecally to bypass the blood-brain barrier.

For some time, a similar barrier was hypothesized for the placenta. However, later studies of the effects of maternal drugs on the fetus indicated that the placenta acts as a simple lipoidal membrane and is not highly selective.

Tissue Trapping

Certain tissues bind or collect drugs temporarily or permanently, converting them to inactive forms. Until these storage depots are saturated, the level of free drug available for pharmaceutical effect may remain low. Some drugs bind with specific tissues in the body. Metallic ions tend to be deposited in bone and hydrocarbons in fatty tissue. Iodine is stored in the thyroid, and B-complex vitamins are stored in the liver.

Plasma proteins bind many substances. Acidic drugs and endogenous bilirubin bind with albumin; basic drugs bind to α_1-acid glycoproteins.

Below the saturation level, stored (bound) drug and free drug maintain a dynamic equilibrium between their levels. If this is disturbed, the drug moves freely from one form to the other to establish a new balance. In the interval between dosages and after administration is discontinued, the chemical moves from the storage depot into the serum as free drug, thus prolonging the physiologic effects.

Drugs, endogenous chemicals, and drug metabolites often compete for binding sites and can displace each other from them. This process is the cause of many drug interactions requiring dosage adjustment when two drugs sharing the same binding sites are administered together (Box 4-4).

Box 4-4
Tissue Trapping

- Certain tissues bind or collect drugs, rendering them inactive (bound drug).
- When drugs leave the tissue-binding site, they again become physiologically active (free drug).
- Drugs, endogenous chemicals, and drug metabolites often compete for binding sites and can displace each other from them. This process is the cause of many drug interactions.

Movement of Drugs Across Membranes

Not all drugs cross the membranes dividing body compartments with equal facility. A few drugs cannot cross the vascular wall. Others (eg, bromides) cannot cross cell membranes. Many drugs cannot penetrate the blood-brain barrier. The cells that secrete milk, tears, saliva, sweat, bile, joint fluid, and gastric, pancreatic, and intestinal juices are permeable to some substances but not to others. Although it is not highly selective, the placenta excludes some substances. Exudates and capsules around abscesses or tumors are barriers of particular significance for antibiotic and antineoplastic chemotherapy. Although blood is the most efficient vehicle for transporting drugs to tissue sites, many operating mechanisms produce differential distribution. Many substances disseminate unevenly throughout the body, and the concentration of a drug may vary markedly from one organ to another. Moreover, the tissue to be treated by the medicine is not necessarily the area that attains the highest concentration of the drug.

Gene Transfer Methods

Currently, two vectors are under study for use in transferring genes into targeted body cells: liposomes (biodegradable lipid droplets) and viruses. When deoxyribonucleic acid (DNA), the genetic material of all organisms, is introduced into liposomes and administered to the subject, the liposome fuses with the cell membrane, allowing the DNA to enter the cell. Genes administered in this way appear not to be incorporated in the nucleus but function as cytoplasmic genes. DNA introduced into viruses is delivered directly into the cell. Adenoviruses do not transfer their genetic material into the cells' chromosomes, but retroviruses do. For this reason, therapy using adenoviruses does not permanently correct the genetic defect but is used as continuing treatment (eg, for cystic fibrosis). Therapy with retroviruses has a potential for permanent cure but requires dividing cells for successful insertion (Wheeler, 1995).

Gene therapy may be administered by several techniques. Cells may be removed from the body, cultured, treated with DNA, and returned by intravenous infusion, or vectors carrying DNA may be infused intravenously or (in the case of cystic fibrosis) administered by inhalation (Wheeler, 1995).

Drug Biotransformation

Like other chemicals within the tissues, drugs are subject to multiple biochemical processes by which they are changed to different compounds. Most of these metabolic processes are mediated by enzymes. Metabolites, the products of these reactions, have properties that differ from those of the original drugs. Their biologic activity may be increased, decreased, or eliminated (Table 4-9). Lipid-soluble compounds may become water-soluble substances. As such, their molecules usually polarize (acquire electric charges on their surfaces), and they tend to ionize (split into charged particles). The general trend of these metabolic processes is to render foreign chemicals less biologically active, less prone to tissue binding, and easier to excrete. Overall, biotransformation serves to break down, detoxify, and remove biologically active chemicals from the body.

However, some active metabolites play an important role in chemically induced liver injury. An example is the metabolite *N*-acetyl-*p*-benzoquinone imine, which is thought to be responsible for acetaminophen-induced hepatotoxicity. This metabolite, enhanced by cytochrome P-450, binds to liver protein to produce toxicity.

Various chemical processes are involved in biotransformation: oxidation, reduction, hydrolysis, and synthesis. Multiple enzymes may be involved in each type of reaction. For example, oxidative enzymes include oxidases, peroxidases, dehydrogenases, and transaminases. Examples of synthetic processes are alkylation, acetylation, methylation, and conjugation with glucuronic or mercapturic acid. Each class of reaction has its favored substrate (eg, water-soluble compounds are usually oxidized), and each produces characteristic changes (as conjugation increases water solubility).

Transformational metabolic pathways may be serial or parallel. In serial transformation, a given molecule undergoes several changes, one after the other:

$$A \rightarrow B \rightarrow C \rightarrow D$$

Parallel transformation indicates that a given substance may undergo several kinds of changes, yielding different products:

$$A \rightarrow B$$
$$A \rightarrow C$$
$$A \rightarrow D$$

By either pathway, a single compound gives rise to several different metabolites. Generally, several metabolites are produced as the body breaks down a given drug. Although knowledge of biotransformation has in-

Table 4-9. Biotransformation and Changes in Pharmacologic Action

Drug	Type of Transformation	Metabolite
L-dopa (inactive pro-drug)	Activation (by brain tissue)	dopamine (active neurotransmitter)
fluoroacetic acid	Toxication (by citric acid cycle)	fluorocitric acid (toxic rodenticide)
codeine (narcotic analgesic)	Toxication (by the liver)	morphine (more potent narcotic analgesic)
heroin (narcotic analgesic)	Alteration with unchanged activity (by liver)	morphine (narcotic analgesic)
epinephrine (sympathetic hormone)	Partial deactivation (by liver)	metanephrine (less potent sympathomimetic)
cyanide (a poison disruptive of internal respiration)	Detoxification by inactivation (by liver)	thiocyanate (pharmacologically inactive compound)

creased rapidly, metabolic processes are extremely complex, and much remains to be explored.

Biotransformation by the Liver

Virtually every tissue in the body is capable of biotransformation. Biochemical processes of this type have been described in the lungs, blood, skin, and brain, but the liver is the most important organ performing this function. This biochemical powerhouse is the major site for oxidation and reduction reactions. Hydrolysis and conjugation also occur at significant rates. Lipid-soluble compounds, a class that includes many important drugs, are transformed by enzymes in the endoplasmic reticulum of liver cells. This arrangement is fortuitous because it protects the body from many toxic substances ingested with food. Much of the material absorbed by the intestinal tract enters the portal circulation, which traverses the liver before mixing with the general circulation. This first pass through the liver allows for degradation of harmful chemicals before they are widely distributed in the tissues. However, it also reduces the proportion of oral therapeutic drug doses reaching the bloodstream.

Factors in Biotransformation

Factors influencing the biotransformation of drugs include genetic differences, physiologic status, and environmental elements.

Genetic Differences

Genetic differences include species, sex, and familial traits. Enzyme systems involved in biotransformation in one species may be completely absent in others; this is why certain animals thrive on foods that are lethal to other species. These differences limit the ability to apply the results of pharmaceutical research involving animals to humans.

Males of certain rat species have a greater capacity to degrade certain chemicals than do females of the same species, and the reverse is true in other species. These differences may reflect differences in the genes located on the X and Y chromosomes. Because each en-

zyme relates to a specific gene on a chromosome, metabolic patterns are more likely to be similar within families than between unrelated persons. Genetic differences render some persons very sensitive to small doses of certain drugs and may explain why others fail to respond to large doses of certain drugs.

An important principle of genetic influence on biotransformation is that each person, by virtue of his or her unique genetic makeup, metabolizes chemicals in a unique way.

Physiologic Status

Features of physiologic status that affect biotransformation include age, hormone status (including that related to pregnancy), nutrition, and disease. Very young children lack the full capacity to metabolize chemicals. Their immature metabolisms cannot handle either the range or total quantity of chemicals that adult systems can. Older adults also have a limited capacity to handle drugs. Although impaired excretory capacity is one reason for this decrease, reduced biotransformation also plays a role. To what degree this loss is attributable to natural aging or to disease and decreased nutrition remains unknown.

Hormones are degraded by the same metabolic processes as drugs. To some degree, these compounds compete with each other in biotransformation. Either may also stimulate or inhibit certain metabolic pathways, altering the system's capacity. Influences of hormones on drug metabolism may underlie the observed fluctuations of drug efficacy and toxicity with diurnal rhythms.

As with all body processes, drug metabolism depends on adequate nutrition for proper cell function and generation of biochemicals. The enzymes involved in biotransformation are protein substances and cannot be produced optimally in malnourished persons. Some foods also may influence enzyme activity because many nutrients are metabolized by biotransformation systems.

Any disease that impairs organ function can interfere with drug metabolism. Liver pathology has the greatest potential for limiting biotransformation. In many cases, persons with impaired liver function cannot process normal doses of drugs, and certain drugs can be toxic in any amount.

Environmental Factors

Certain environmental factors may decrease or increase biotransformation. Stress affects metabolism by altering hormone levels and neural activity in the body. Toxic influences such as ionizing irradiation or poisons that impair tissue function can reduce biotransformation. Cigarette smoking enhances the hepatic metabolism of many drugs. Such alteration in the rate of liver enzyme activity is an important mechanism by which environmental agents affect drug metabolism.

Chemicals may either stimulate or inhibit liver enzymes. A few exhibit a diphasic effect, initially decreasing and then later increasing enzyme activity. Enzyme inducers stimulate proliferation of the endoplasmic reticulum. An increase in microsomal protein content indicates hyperplasia of the structures involved in biotransformation. Many chemicals that affect the enzyme system are drugs. With repeated doses, a drug may stimulate the enzyme pathways for its own metabolism, resulting in an apparent decline in potency of succeeding doses. Enzyme induction or inhibition underlies many drug–drug interactions in which one drug appears to increase or decrease the effect of a second.

Drug Excretion

Drugs are excreted from the body both as intact molecules and metabolites. Elimination occurs by respiration, urination, fecal elimination, and exocrine secretion. Efficient drug excretion depends on the proper functioning of the physiologic systems involved with general excretion: the cardiovascular system (required to transport wastes to the excretory organs), lungs, kidneys, liver, intestines, and sweat, salivary, and mammary glands.

The rate of removal of drug from the body is termed *clearance*; *half-life* ($t_{1/2}$) is another term frequently used to estimate how fast a drug leaves the body. As noted above, half-life is the length of time necessary for the concentration of drug in a specific area of the body to decrease by half. Clearance and half-life vary greatly from one drug to another. For example, in humans, penicillin has a serum half-life of less than 1 hour, whereas that of digitoxin is about 1 week. The excretion rate varies with the concentration and increases gradually as serum levels rise. A steady state is reached when the rate of excretion reaches the rate at which drug enters the system. If the rate of loss fails to match the rate of absorption, serum drug levels will continue to rise gradually, a phenomenon called *cumulation*.

Due to their long half-lives, certain drugs (eg, digitoxin) tend to cumulate in most recipients, posing an increased risk of an adverse reaction such as toxicity. A second factor influencing adverse reactions is the margin of safety. The narrower the margin of safety, the greater the likelihood of toxicity. Drugs such as digitoxin that have a long half-life and a narrow margin of safety are most likely to produce toxic reactions and are typically described as cumulative drugs. Serum levels of cumulative drugs should be allowed to rise gradually to avoid producing toxicity. Loading doses (high initial doses used to saturate tissue depots) are unwise except if a prompt therapeutic response is required.

When a drug is discontinued, the rate of excretion declines exponentially in proportion to the declining serum levels (Fig. 4-5). The serum half-life of some drugs is about 6 hours or less. Thus, a period of 2 to 3 days is generally sufficient to eliminate significant levels of these drugs from the serum. Drugs with longer half-lives may require a few weeks for dissipation. A few drugs with large storage depots remain in the body for much longer periods.

Excretion Processes

The most important and common route for drug excretion is the urine. However, the lungs, intestinal tract, and exocrine glands can excrete some substances as well.

Lungs

The lungs are the favored route for excretion of gaseous and volatile compounds. Agents administered by inhalation, such as general anesthetics, are largely eliminated by this route. In addition, ingested substances such as ethanol (ethyl alcohol, also called grain alcohol) may diffuse from the blood into the lungs and be subsequently exhaled. Excreted alcohol accounts for the breath odor characteristic of persons drinking alcoholic beverages. Respiratory excretion may damage the lungs, as in kerosene poisoning. Excretion of this hydrocarbon through the lungs may cause a life-threatening lipoidal pneumonia.

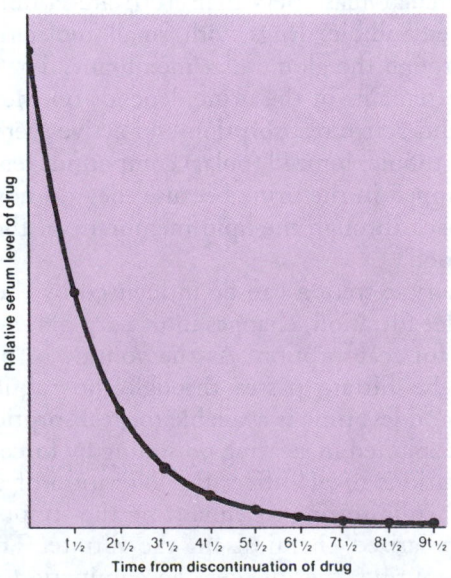

Figure 4-5. General pattern of drug elimination.

Support and stimulation of respiration promote the excretion of volatile drugs. This is the principle underlying the effectiveness of postoperative "stir-up" regimens used in postanesthesia care units. Stimulation alone does not change the level of brain function, which is controlled by drug levels in the central nervous system. However, repeated deep breathing accelerates the excretion of these volatile gases, hastening the return to full consciousness.

By their presence in air exhaled from postoperative clients, anesthetic gases pollute the ambient air in recovery suites. Unless these areas are well ventilated, hospital personnel can experience vertigo or syncope from inhaling these gases. The staff should avoid face-to-face contact with clients, which increases exposure.

Exocrine Glands

Exocrine glands excrete lipid-soluble drugs that cross cell membranes readily. The excretion of chemicals in the saliva often causes characteristic tastes in the mouth. If the saliva is swallowed, the drug will not be lost from the body but may reenter it by intestinal absorption. Sweat containing drugs sometimes alters body odor, and evaporation of perspiration may leave a film (frost) of solid drug that can irritate the skin. This occurs rarely and mainly in toxic states when drug levels are very high. Elimination of drugs through the mammary glands of a nursing mother is a matter of special concern because the chemicals may be absorbed by the nursing infant.

Normally, exocrine glands do not eliminate large quantities of drugs from the body. They can become important pathways for excretion if a primary excretory organ (eg, the kidneys) is not functioning properly.

Kidneys

The kidneys are the most important organs for excreting drugs. Most water-soluble compounds of low relative molecular mass (less than 100) are eliminated in the urine. Soluble drugs with small molecules filter freely through the glomerular membrane. The proportion that remains in the urine depends on the level of passive and active reabsorption and active secretion by the renal tubule. Ionized (polar) compounds tend to become trapped in the urine because they do not readily diffuse back through the lipid membrane of the tubule to the blood.

Urinary excretion can be influenced by the rate of glomerular filtration, changes in urinary pH, and competition for reabsorption. As the volume of urine increases, the filtrate passes through the tubule more quickly, and less time is available for reabsorption. This effect is exploited in treating poisoning by forced diuresis. Alterations in pH affect the ionization of drugs in the urine, minimizing or enhancing the "trapping" effect of polarized chemicals in the filtrate. The more acidic the urine, the quicker the elimination of basic drugs. Acid drugs are more readily excreted in basic urine. If a drug (eg, penicillin) is actively secreted by the renal tubule, the administration of a compound (eg, probenecid) that competes for the active transport mechanism will reduce excretion.

Renal failure greatly prolongs the serum half-life of most drugs. Dosages of therapeutic agents must be reduced and intervals between drug dosages lengthened in clients with poor kidney function. In clients treated by dialysis, the drugs removed by dialysis should be administered after the treatment.

Liver and Intestines

Drugs or drug metabolites with a relative molecular mass exceeding 100 (eg, glucuronides) are excreted largely by the biliary system. Not all the drug secreted by the liver is eliminated at once; a portion is reabsorbed in the intestinal tract. This enterohepatic cycle allows only a portion of bile constituents to escape in the feces, thereby promoting gradual elimination. Excretion of such drugs may be hastened by administering laxatives or cathartics to stimulate peristalsis and reduce bowel transit time.

Interaction of Pharmacokinetic Processes

Once a drug enters the body, the processes of absorption, distribution, transformation, and excretion are carried out simultaneously. Therefore, the quantity and distribution of drug in various compartments are changing constantly. The relations between these processes and their effect on drug levels are illustrated in Figure 4-6.

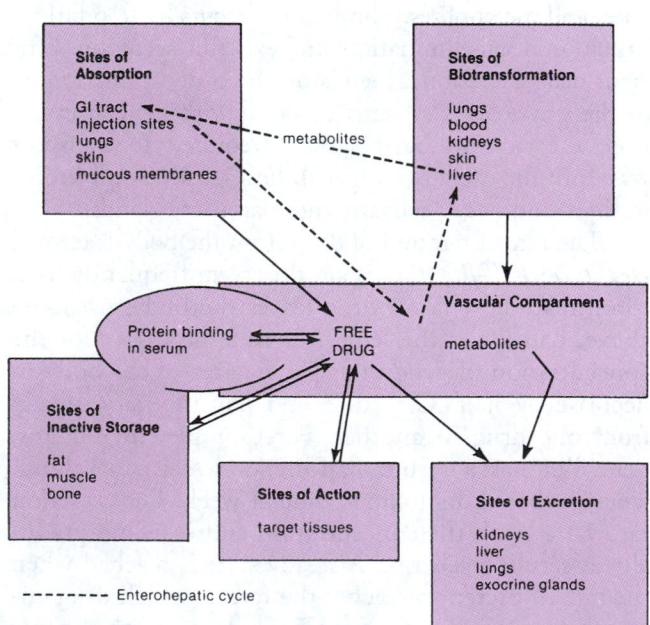

Figure 4-6. Drugs administered for systemic effect move from sites of absorption into the vascular compartment. They are then transported throughout the tissues. There, they may initiate drug action, enter storage depots, undergo biotransformation or leave the body. Because pharmacokinetic processes are ongoing and simultaneous, the volume and distribution of drug in various body compartments change continuously.

Movement of drugs into and out of storage areas affects the plasma half-life and can produce biphasic and triphasic half-life times. The initial $t_{1/2}$ is shorter than the $t_{1/2}$ after saturation of storage depots. The plasma $t_{1/2}$ is increased by movement of drug out of storage depots after intake is discontinued. When storage depots are exhausted, the plasma $t_{1/2}$ drops.

Drug administration schedules are designed to maintain a steady state of drug within the therapeutic range. Single doses of medication produce blood and tissue drug levels similar to those shown in Figure 4-7. Repeated doses are required to raise drug concentration as free drug is lost from the system (Fig. 4-8). The frequency of dosing also affects drug concentrations (Fig. 4-9). When constant blood levels are required, a continuous IV infusion is generally preferred (Fig. 4-10).

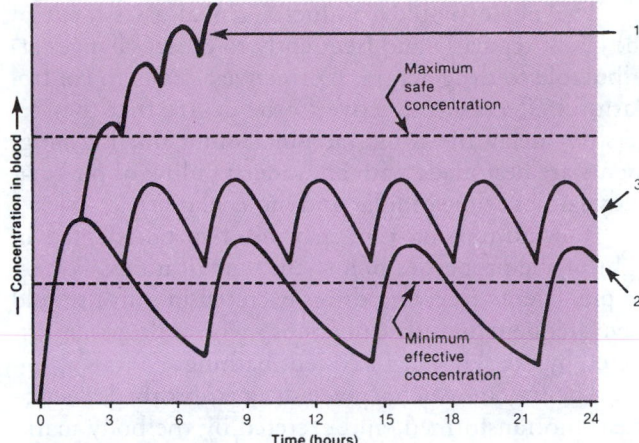

Figure 4-9. Effect of dosage intervals on drug concentration. The objective of the multiple-dosage regimen is to maintain the patient's blood level with maximum and minimum concentrations as shown in the figure. The dosage interval is too short in *curve 1*, too long in *curve 2*, and ideal in *curve 3*. The initial dose used for this simulation is 33% more than the maintenance dose. (Notari BE: Biopharmaceutics and Pharmacokinetics. 4th ed, p 248. New York, Marcel Dekker, 1987.)

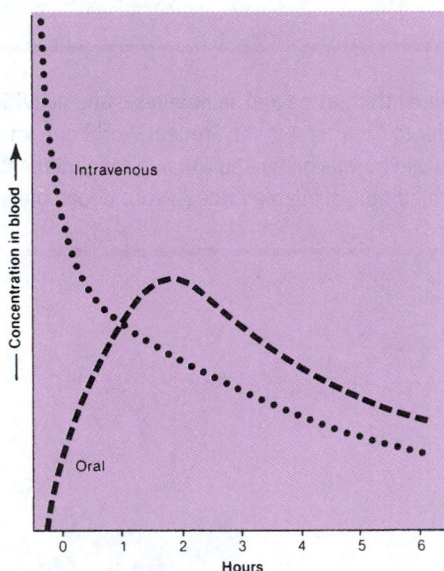

Figure 4-7. Drug levels after single-dose administration. The figure shows the time course for a drug in blood after oral and intravenous doses (dashed line, oral drug; dotted line, IV drug).

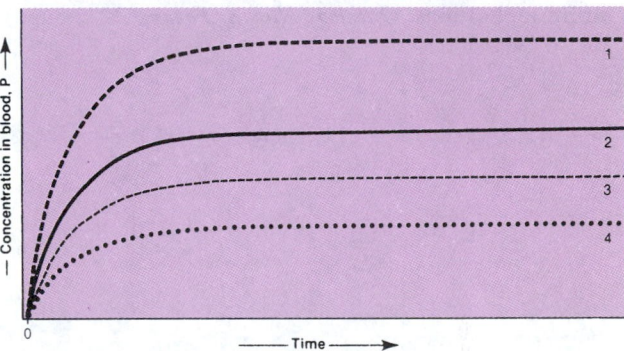

Figure 4-10. Blood concentrations following intravenous infusion. Steady-state blood levels achieved by constant-rate intravenous infusion of drug. The steady-state levels are proportional to the infusion as follows: 10 (*curve 1*), 6.6 (*curve 2*), 5 (*curve 3*), and 3.3 (*curve 4*). (Notari BE: Biopharmaceutics and Pharmacokinetics. 3rd ed, p 100. New York, Marcel Dekker, 1980.)

▪ SUMMARY

Blood levels of drugs are affected by absorption rates, storage in inactive tissue depots, biotransformation, and excretion. Each process is influenced by genetic, physiologic, and environmental factors. The tissue concentration of drugs, therefore, can vary greatly from person to person and from time to time within the same person.

Nursing Management

A knowledge of drug action helps guide monitoring and corrective actions for adverse drug reactions. A drug's mechanism of action affects its therapeutic uses, side effects, and toxic manifestations.

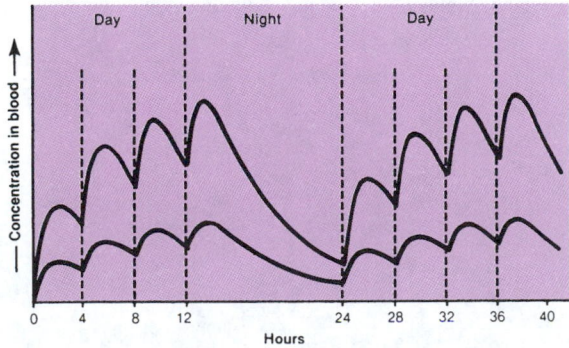

Figure 4-8. Blood levels of drugs with intermittent dosage. A typical regimen or oral dosage four times a day on a schedule of 10-2-6-10 or 9-1-5-9. Two different doses are illustrated over the first and second day of the regimen. (Notari BE: Biopharmaceutics and Pharmacokinetics. 4th ed, p 254. New York, Marcel Dekker, 1987.)

The nurse should conduct a global assessment of the client regularly and frequently to detect changes attributable to drug action. Corrective actions to control harmful effects are effective to the degree that they reverse or delay the drug's action. Sound nursing judgments are best made with an understanding of pharmacodynamics at the cellular and molecular level.

Routine nursing care may need to be adapted in light of the properties of a client's medications. For example, clients receiving drugs excreted in saliva should have frequent mouth care; those whose drugs are excreted by the skin need frequent bathing.

The way in which a given drug is absorbed, distributed, biotransformed, and excreted by the body markedly changes its potency, efficacy, and toxicity. Nurses must understand the pharmacokinetic processes influencing drug concentration and must also monitor clients carefully for responses to drugs that may indicate individual differences in the way their bodies transport, metabolize, and eliminate those drugs.

Reference

Wheeler VS. (1995). Gene therapy: Current strategies and future applications. *Oncology Nursing Forum, 22* (2 Supp): 20–26 (March).

Bibliography

Notari BE. (1987) Biopharmaceutics and pharmacokinetics, 4th ed. New York: Marcel Dekker.

Pickler RH, Munro CL. (1995). Gene therapy for inherited disorders. *Journal of Pediatric Nursing, 10* (1):40–47 (Feb).

Welling PG, Balant LP (eds). (1994). *Pharmacokinetics of drugs.* New York: Springer-Verlag.

For more information and sample tests and activities, refer to Chapter 4 in the Student Workbook for Clinical Pharmacology and Nursing Management, 5th edition, available through your bookstore.

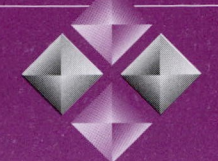

5

Adverse Drug Reactions

ADRs develop over different times—some occur immediately and others take weeks or months. They can affect any body tissue or organ. They are easier to identify and confirm if the client is taking only one drug.

Risk Factors

Clients who receive newer drugs are at greater risk for ADRs, because the newer the drug, the greater the risk of unknown effects. However, ADRs can occur at any time during treatment, even with drugs that have been well tolerated for extended periods (Box 5-1). Additional risk factors for ADRs include:

- The client is undergoing treatment by two or more physicians at the same time.
- The client has intercurrent illness (temporary or permanent, medical or dental).
- The client's ability to metabolize or excrete the drug has changed.
- The client takes several prescription drugs.
- The client uses over-the-counter (OTC) preparations.
- The client takes a drug intermittently, which may contribute to drug allergy.
- The client or a close relative has a history of allergies.
- The client's history discloses previous ADRs.
- The client's long-term use of a drug may promote cumulation leading to toxicity.
- Age (very old or very young), body size (very thin or obese), and impaired hepatic and renal function are other risk factors.

Most drug-related side effects are minor. About 30%, however, are serious, causing severe injury—even death. As many as 140,000 deaths each year can be blamed on adverse drug reactions (ADRs), as can about 1.5 million hospitalizations. Of persons hospitalized for other reasons, about 30% experience an ADR (O'Donnell, 1992).

Overview

Simply stated, ADRs are undesired responses to a drug. These undesired responses vary considerably in form and intensity. They range from iatrogenic reactions to adverse side effects, toxic reactions, and allergic (or immunologic) reactions. Other kinds of ADRs include carcinogenicity, chain reactions, cumulative reactions, idiosyncratic reactions, teratogenicity, and tolerance and dependence.

Box 5-1
Drugs Most Likely to Cause ADRs

Drugs in the following categories are among those most often associated with adverse drug reactions (ADRs).

- *Anticoagulants:* heparin, warfarin
- *Antimicrobials:* cephalosporins, penicillins, sulfonamides
- *Bronchodilators:* sympathomimetic drugs, theophylline
- *Cardiovascular agents:* antihypertensives and diuretics, digoxin, quinidine
- *Central nervous system agents:* analgesics, anticonvulsants, neuroleptics, sedative–hypnotics
- *Diagnostic agents:* radiopaque contrast media
- *Hormones:* corticosteroids, estrogens, insulin

Predictability

Several kinds of ADRs are predictable, including overdose, side effects (eg, postural hypotension from vasodilators, dry mouth from antihistamines), and drug interactions (eg, those between drugs, between drugs and foods, and between drugs and diseases). These kinds of ADRs are usually dose-dependent.

Unpredictable kinds of ADRs are unusual and unexpected. They include those with a known or presumed immunologic basis and those known as idiosyncratic (determined genetically). Such ADRs are usually dose-independent.

Iatrogenic Effects

Every physiologically active drug can cause an undesirable reaction that may induce illness in the recipient. Such an effect is called *iatrogenic* (arising from the treatment).

For an iatrogenic effect to be identified, the drug causing the effect usually must be in therapeutic use for 10 to 20 years. Even then, some problems may remain unrecognized as drug-related. For example, aspirin was widely used for decades before its detrimental effects were acknowledged. Many new drugs are marketed each year, and clients have never been exposed to some of the chemicals used in these new drugs. This can contribute to some unusual reactions; for example, about 15% of clients taking angiotensin-converting enzyme (ACE) inhibitors develop a cough.

An iatrogenic effect has potentially serious consequences, ranging from further or new illness (Table 5-1), delayed recovery, or even death, to increased expense for the client and the healthcare system at large.

Side Effects

Just as iatrogenic effects are induced by drug treatment, so side effects are an offshoot of treatment. Side effects are the actions or effects that are not specifically intended in treatment. Although they are usually considered adverse effects, they may be desired effects as well.

In any case, no drug exerts a single effect on the body; rather, a spectrum of effects occurs. For example, a drug administered in one instance for a particular purpose may be used in another for a different effect. Which action is considered therapeutic and which is considered a side effect depends on the situation.

Desired Effects

Many drugs are prescribed to exploit their desirable side effects. For example, diazepam (Valium) is both a tranquilizer (or antianxiety agent) and a skeletal muscle relaxant. When administered to reduce anxiety, the relaxant properties of diazepam are considered side effects. When used to treat spasms and low-back pain, diazepam's antianxiety property is considered a side effect. In the case of back pain, the tranquilizing side effect is desirable because it helps clients cope with immobility and discomfort.

Table 5-1. Drugs That May Induce Health Problems

Health Problem	Drugs
Bone marrow suppression	antineoplastics, carbamazepine, immunosuppressants, phenytoin
Cardiovascular reactions	antihypertensives, doxorubicin, daunorubicin
Cutaneous reactions	ACE inhibitors, cefaclor, heparin, propylthiouracil, warfarin
Electrolyte imbalance	antibiotics, corticosteroids, diuretics, heparin, laxatives, lithium, vitamin and mineral supplements (eg, potassium)
Endocrine effects	corticosteroids
Gastrointestinal irritation	nonsteroidal antiinflammatory drugs (NSAIDs)
Hepatotoxicity	acetaminophen, erythromycin, valproate, isoniazid
Nephrotoxicity	NSAIDs, analgesic combinations, aminoglycosides
Neurotoxicity	
Tardive dyskinesia	butyrophenones: haloperidol; phenothiazines: chlorpromazine
Acute dystonic reactions	prochlorperazine
Sedation	antihistamines: diphenhydramine, promethazine
Ototoxicity	aspirin, cinchona alkaloids, loop diuretics, cisplatin, aminoglycosides
Respiratory effects	opioid analgesics
Superinfection	broad-spectrum antimicrobials, combinations of antimicrobials, second- or third-generation antimicrobials
Hyperuricemia	thiazide diuretics: triamterene/hydrochlorothiazide, chlorothiazide, hydrochlorothiazide
Hyperglycemia	thiazide diuretics, corticosteroids

Adverse Effects

Side effects may be adverse effects, mild or severe. The ones that are less troublesome to clients may remain undiagnosed, or they may be diagnosed but be manageable and tolerable in the interest of a therapeutic outcome from continued use of the drug. Side effects may lessen in degree over time as the client uses the drug. However, some adverse effects may persist and be serious enough to warrant stopping or postponing drug treatment. In this text, "adverse reaction" is an umbrella term that includes desirable and adverse side effects on a continuum from tolerable to dangerous. Table 5-2 identifies common signs and symptoms of ADRs.

Alopecia

Clients with cancer who receive an antineoplastic drug commonly experience alopecia (hair loss). Other drugs such as antibiotics, anticoagulants, anticonvulsants, and hormones also can cause alopecia. These agents damage the DNA of the stem cells, which atrophies (shrinks or wastes) the hair follicle. The result is weak, brittle hair that breaks at the skin surface or is expelled spontaneously from the hair follicle. The dose and duration of exposure to the drug determine the degree and duration of hair loss. Alopecia may range from thinning and partial baldness to loss of all body hair. Hair loss usually occurs 2 or 3 weeks after drug therapy begins. The loss may be gradual or sudden.

Nurses must reassure clients that their hair will regrow when drug therapy stops, although the new hair may be a different color or texture. Scalp hair usually grows about a half inch each month.

Bone Marrow Suppression

Anemia (abnormal decrease in red blood cell, hemoglobin, or hematocrit values), thrombocytopenia (reduced platelets), and neutropenia (decrease in neutrophils) are the three most clinically significant manifestations of bone marrow suppression (myelosuppression).

With anemia, the client may experience fatigue and hypoxia. When thrombocytopenia occurs and the platelet count is under 50,000/mm^3, the client is at risk for

Table 5-2. Signs and Symptoms of Common Adverse Drug Reactions

Reaction	Signs and Symptoms
Allergy	
Anaphylaxis	Itching of palms, chin, throat; a sensation of swelling in the throat; apprehension, lacrimation, wheezing, dyspnea, hypotension, and cardiovascular collapse
Arthralgia	Joint pain, difficulty in ambulation, impaired manual dexterity
Skin eruption	Erythema, itching, rash
Bone marrow suppression	
Anemia	Weakness, dyspnea, headaches, syncope, unusual tiredness or weakness
Neutropenia	Fever, chills, sore throat, dry nonproductive cough, malaise, redness or pain in a body area
Thrombocytopenia	Petechiae, ecchymoses, unusual bleeding following minor trauma or from mucous membranes, hemorrhage
CNS	
Confusion	Forgetfulness, disorientation, inappropriate verbal responses, anxiety
Excitation	Restlessness, talkativeness, irritability, insomnia, anxiety
Sedation	Sleepiness, lethargy, coma
GI irritation or bleeding	Dysphagia, anorexia, stomatitis (dryness or cracking of lips, swelling and redness of mouth tissues, soreness to burning pain of mouth tissues, mouth odor), nausea, vomiting, abdominal pain, bloody or black tarry stools, diarrhea
Hepatotoxicity	Anorexia, malaise, fatigue, nausea, jaundice, fever, hepatic tenderness, enlargement of the liver, elevated liver enzymes, dark urine, light-colored stools
Nephrotoxicity	Decrease in urination (oliguria to anuria); edema; unusual weight gain; hematuria, albuminuria, or crystalluria; progressive azotemia
Ototoxicity	Abnormal ringing or other noises in the ear (tinnitus), increased sensitivity to noise, difficulty in understanding speech, audiograms showing loss of perception, particularly of high tones

bleeding. When the count drops below 20,000/mm³, the client is at severe risk and may require platelet transfusions.

The longer neutropenia persists and the more pronounced it becomes, the more susceptible the client is to infection from endogenous and exogenous microbes. A serious risk of infection occurs when the neutrophil count drops below 500/mm³. Most chemotherapeutic agents create a high risk for generalized bone marrow suppression and neutropenia. See Chapter 46 for more information .

Cardiovascular Effects

A side effect affecting the cardiovascular system is sometimes called *cardiotoxicity*. This negative effect on heart function appears as alterations in the heart's conduction system or damage to cardiac tissue.

Respiratory Effects

Respiratory depression is an adverse effect of many drugs. Its severity depends on the degree of depression. The effect results from drug action on the brain stem's respiratory mechanism. Opioid analgesic agents are the most common cause of respiratory depression in all age groups. They slow the respiratory rate, which leads to hypoventilation and a rise in the alveolar carbon dioxide level. The increase in carbon dioxide may be tolerated well, or it can have devastating effects, especially if the client has increased intracranial pressure or chronic obstructive pulmonary disease (Shannon, Wilson, Stang, 1995).

Cutaneous Effects

Cutaneous reactions are adverse effects that appear as eruptions and lesions of the skin and mucous membranes. They occur in up to 3% of hospital clients. Esti-

Table 5-3. Cutaneous Reactions Associated with Drugs

Reaction	Signs and Symptoms	Drugs Commonly Responsible	Time From Start of Drug Therapy to Reaction Onset
Stevens-Johnson syndrome	Related to erythema multiforme; erosive stomatitis with involvement of other mucous membranes (nasal, genitalia, eyes); disseminated dusky macules, with darker center or center blister	penicillins, sulfa drugs, cotrimoxazole, carbamazepine, hydantoins, allopurinol, others	1–3 wk
Toxic epidermal necrolysis	Greater than 30% loss of epidermis due to necrosis, skin appears scalded; initially resembles Stevens-Johnson syndrome but evolves to necrolysis in a few days; similarities between histopathologic findings and drugs responsible suggest conditions are part of single process; mortality rate (principally from sepsis) about 30%. Nursing care in ICU or burn unit focuses on pain control, fluid replacement, nutritional support, aseptic handling, antibacterial treatment, and skin care.	penicillins, sulfa drugs, cotrimoxazole, carbamazepine, hydantoins, allopurinol, others	1–3 wk
Hypersensitivity syndrome	Skin rash with fever, hepatitis (51% of cases), arthralgias, lymphadenopathy or hematologic abnormalities	phenytoin, carbamazepine, phenobarbital, sulfa drugs, allopurinol	2–6 wk
Drug-induced vasculitis	Involves small vessels; palpable purpuric papules usually on the lower extremities (but any site possible); process may involve kidneys, GI tract, or nervous system and be life-threatening	allopurinol, penicillin, sulfa drugs, thiazide diuretics, pyrazolones, hydantoins, propylthiouracil (associated with vasculitis of face and earlobes)	1–3 wk
Serum sickness or similar reactions	Type III hypersensitivity reaction; erythema on sides of fingers, toes, and hands; fever, arthralgia, and arthritis not uncommon	IV proteins, beta-lactam antibiotics	8–14 d
Anticoagulant-induced skin necrosis	Rare; occlusive thrombi in vessels of skin and subcutaneous tissue of areas with large quantities of adipose tissue such as breasts, buttocks; with warfarin, people with hereditary deficiency of anticoagulant protein C are at greatest risk	warfarin	3–5 d
		heparin	5–10 d
Angioedema	Hypersensitivity reaction marked by swelling of the feet, hands, face, neck, lips, larynx, viscera, or genitalia; may be life-threatening	penicillin, cephalosporins, contrast media, anesthetics	a few minutes to a few hours
		NSAIDs	1–7 d
		ACE inhibitors	<4 wk

mates suggest that one of every 1000 clients has a serious cutaneous drug reaction (Roujeau, Stern, 1994). Because of the relatively low frequency of severe reactions, these effects are unlikely to be detected in premarketing clinical drug trials.

Not all cutaneous reactions develop rapidly; some occur after prolonged exposure. Serious drug-induced cutaneous reactions include Stevens-Johnson syndrome, toxic epidermal necrolysis, hypersensitivity syndrome, small-vessel vasculitis, serum sickness or similar symptoms, anticoagulant-induced necrosis, and angioedema (Table 5-3).

A reasonably rapid cutaneous reaction is photosensitivity, which occurs when the client's skin is exposed to sunlight for a time. A photoallergic reaction appears as a papular eruption on sun-exposed skin. It probably occurs because the drug forms an antigen (in a process involving the absorption of sunlight) and subsequently combines with a skin protein. A phototoxic reaction is characterized by a severe sunburn caused by a photosensitizing drug.

Gastrointestinal Irritation

Among the most common adverse effects are gastrointestinal (GI) problems, such as anorexia, nausea, vomiting, diarrhea, and constipation. These occur with many oral drugs and result from local irritation of the GI tract. Some drugs also cause more serious effects, such as gastric ulceration or bleeding (signaled by black tarry stools).

Hepatotoxicity

Hepatotoxic reactions are relatively rare but potentially life-threatening. Because the liver is responsible for metabolizing most drugs, the liver is susceptible to drug-induced injury. In addition, liver damage impairs the biotransformation of many drugs. Consequently, these drugs may accumulate in the body and cause adverse effects. Examples of drug-induced liver damage include active metabolite formation (acetaminophen), intrahepatic cholestasis (carbamazepine, haloperidol, imipramine, and many others), virallike hepatitis (dantrolene, isoniazid, mercaptopurine, and more), and depletion of intracellular substance (valproic acid). Intrahepatic cholestasis is marked by fever, liver enlargement, hyperbilirubinemia, dark urine and eosinophilia.

Nephrotoxicity

Some drugs can cause kidney damage; various histologic changes and functional defects can occur. The incidence of acute renal failure due to nephrotoxicants approaches about 15%. Potentially nephrotoxic agents include some antimicrobials (aminoglycosides, amphotericin B), some ACE inhibitors, nonsteroidal antiinflammatory drugs, lithium, cyclosporine, and certain antineoplastics (cisplatin, cyclophosphamide). In addition, underlying renal dysfunction can cause ADRs when drugs are eliminated primarily through the renal system. Cumulation of the drug could occur. In some cases, reduction of drug dosage may help avoid nephrotoxic effects.

Neurotoxicity

The autonomic, peripheral, and central nervous systems can be harmed by drugs. Effects on the autonomic nervous system include constipation, abdominal pain, paralytic ileus, and bowel obstruction. Peripheral nervous system toxicity may be apparent in decreased deep tendon reflexes, paresthesias of the hands and feet, ataxia, slapping gait, and foot drop. Additional symptoms include cranial nerve deficits, such as ptosis, diplopia, and vocal cord paralysis.

The most common effects on the central nervous system (CNS) are excessive depression with sedation or, conversely, excessive stimulation and agitation. Some drugs trigger ADRs in one or more nervous systems; for instance, vincristine, an anticancer agent, affects all three nervous systems.

Ototoxicity

Many drugs are potentially ototoxic—capable of damaging the inner ear or one or both branches of the auditory nerve (Box 5-2). Damage can occur in any of the three areas of the inner ear: the cochlea, which collects sounds, and the vestibule and semicircular canals, which help maintain balance (Haybach, 1993). Signs and symptoms of cochlear toxicity are tinnitus and sensorineural hearing loss (also called nerve deafness). The hearing loss may not be recognized initially, but it usually progresses from higher to lower frequencies. If the client is receiving cisplatin, which destroys cochlear hair

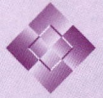

Box 5-2
Ototoxicity: Risk Factors and Toxic Drugs

Whether cochlear or vestibular toxicity resulting from drug use is irreversible or reversible, it is uncomfortable for the client and may pose safety problems as well. Risk factors for ototoxicity include:

- Age (very young and very old)
- History of hearing loss
- Renal or hepatic insufficiency or disease
- Dehydration
- Bacteremia or osteomyelitis
- Previous exposure to loud noises
- Previous cranial irradiation
- Previous use of potentially ototoxic drugs, use of ototoxic and nephrotoxic drugs, or use of two or more potentially ototoxic drugs

cells and directly attacks the cochlear nerve, deafness can occur after a single dose. Common ototoxic drugs include salicylates (aspirin), loop diuretics, cinchona alkaloids (quinidine, quinine), and aminoglycosides. With aspirin, for example, tinnitus usually begins when the serum level exceeds 18 mg/L.

Signs and symptoms of vestibular toxicity include feelings of lightheadedness and weakness, vertigo, horizontal nystagmus, nausea and vomiting, and a spinning or rocking sensation while sitting still.

Toxic Reactions

Although all the reactions identified as adverse reactions could be termed toxic in the general sense of the word (ie, exerting deleterious effects), toxic states are defined more narrowly here: they refer to the effects that characteristically result from high doses of a drug. These effects may be associated with excessive dosage or hyperresponsiveness to the drug.

The likelihood of toxicity is inversely related to the safety margin of a substance. For instance, toxicity rarely occurs with substances such as water-soluble vitamins, which must be administered in huge doses to precipitate harmful effects. However, when drugs with a narrow safety margin, such as digitalis or insulin, are used, the therapy must be closely monitored and carefully managed to avoid toxicity. Some drugs have no safety margin and are dangerous even in therapeutic doses. No desirable drug is completely devoid of toxic potential, because to be effective a substance must either change physiologic function or exert an external influence on body function. If this change reaches sufficient magnitude, harm can result.

Allergic and Immunologic Reactions

Interactions between drugs and the immune system occur as inadvertent consequences of the protective function of the immune system (Rieder, 1993). ADRs mediated by the immune system may account for 10% to 50% of all ADRs and for a disproportionate number of serious or even fatal reactions. The mechanisms of immune involvement have been described in detail for a few drugs but are not fully understood for others (Table 5-4). Other ADRs appear to have an immune component that does not correspond to the four types of drug hypersensitivity (eg, lupuslike reaction to procainamide, halothane hepatitis).

Allergic reactions do not occur during the first exposure to a drug. Initially, a person may be exposed unknowingly to a drug allergen, particularly antibiotics, as these drugs are often used to treat livestock that provide milk and meat. Allergic reactions to drugs are more common in people who have allergies or whose close relatives have allergies.

Although some ADRs mediated by the immune system occur with equal frequency among adults and children, others appear to be more common among children. One factor may be the differences in drug

Table 5-4. Types of Hypersensitivity in Drug Therapy

Type	Mechanism	Signs and Symptoms	Possible Causes
I	Interaction between an antigen and antigen-specific IgE on mast cell receptors, characterized by the release of mediators such as histamine, leukotrienes, and platelet-activating factors	Rhinitis and sneezing, rashes, urticaria, anaphylaxis	Beta-lactam antibiotics (penicillins)
II	Antigen-specific antibodies, usually IgG but sometimes also IgM, directed against antigens present on the cell surface	Symptoms characteristic of hemolytic anemias. (Drug is on surface of red blood cell; antibodies to drug are produced and coat the red blood cell; red blood cell lysis follows.)	Penicillins (high-dose therapy), quinine
III	Mediated by immune complexes formed when antigens interact with antibodies	Serum sickness (lymphadenopathy, arthralgia, fever, rash)	Penicillins and cephalosporins (which are chemically similar to penicillin), barbiturates, isoniazid, phenytoin, NSAIDs, captopril, hydralazine, sulfonamides
IV	Mediated by T cells, takes about 12 hours to develop	Rash	Topical drugs such as neomycin or parabens (rare with systemic drugs)

forms for children (suspensions or syrups rather than tablets or capsules).

Allergic reactions involving the cardiovascular and respiratory systems are life-threatening. The reaction called anaphylaxis or anaphylactic shock is systemic and is characterized by dyspnea, bronchospasm, laryngeal edema, cough, cyanosis, angioedema, pulse variations, hypotension, unconsciousness, acute cardiovascular collapse, and sometimes urticaria and convulsions. The reaction results from the contraction of smooth muscles and increased vascular permeability. A drug that triggers anaphylactic shock should never again be administered to the client.

Carcinogenicity

A few drugs are known to cause cancer. Carcinogenicity apparently results from drug-induced alterations in cellular DNA. A drug's carcinogenic potential is defined by a complex process of animal studies extrapolated to humans.

The difficulty in determining a drug's carcinogenic potential is compounded by the complex nature of many cancers and the latency period between exposure to a carcinogen and the development of cancer. The carcinogenic potential of a medication may be unknown until it has been used clinically for a long time. Cyclophosphamide is an antineoplastic agent known to induce transitional cell carcinoma of the bladder. However, this cancer may not be detected for years after treatment with cyclophosphamide. Other carcinogenic drugs include azathioprine, diethylstilbestrol, and melphalan.

Chain Reactions

Medications are often added to a drug regimen to control the side effects of therapy, and this can initiate a chain reaction. For example, some side effects of corticosteroid therapy may be hypertension, ulcers, diabetes,

and reactivation of arrested tuberculosis. In such a case, additional medications, such as diuretics, antacids or histamine (H_2) antagonists, insulin, or an antitubercular agent, may be prescribed to treat the side effects. If the client receives the antitubercular agent isoniazid, vitamin B_6 may be needed to prevent a deficiency that can be induced by isoniazid. If the client receives an antacid, such as aluminum hydroxide (Amphojel), a stool softener may be required to offset its constipating effects. Thus, the initiation of corticosteroid therapy can result in a chain of events necessitating the prescription of many more drugs (Fig. 5-1). Any proliferation of drug use causes a geometric increase in the risk for undesirable effects and interactions.

Cumulative Reactions

Drugs may accumulate in the body whenever the amount of drug absorbed exceeds the amount the body can metabolize or excrete or both. Because the efficiency of metabolism and excretion is determined by various factors, a drug can accumulate unexpectedly, producing a cumulative reaction. The client may experience no discernible symptoms until drug concentrations reach toxic levels. Cumulative reactions are most likely when the therapeutic margin of safety is narrow or the client has used the medication (eg, digoxin) for a long time.

Idiosyncratic Reactions

An unexpected, abnormal response to a drug may occur because of a difference in the client's genetic composition. This idiosyncratic, or pharmacogenetic, reaction may take the form of extreme sensitivity to low doses or extreme insensitivity to high doses of the drug. It may also be a paradoxical response (an effect opposite to that desired), such as agitation rather than tranquility after taking a sedative. Identification and treatment of these reactions frequently depend on the alertness of healthcare personnel.

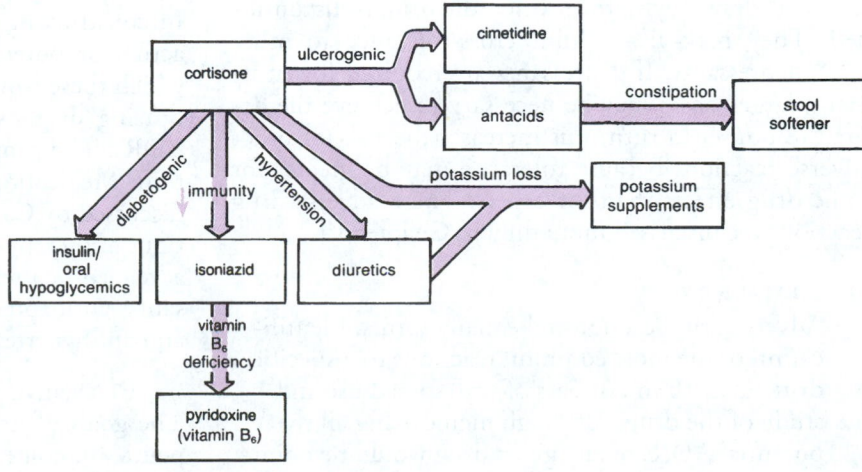

Figure 5-1. Multiple drug prescriptions may be required to treat a chain of side effects initiated by one medication.

An example of such a reaction is the hemolytic anemia that affects 10% of African American males when they receive primaquine. These men have an inherited enzyme deficiency of erythrocytic glucose-6-phosphate dehydrogenase. In these clients, the antimalarial drug primaquine diminishes the metabolic processes of erythrocytes. Vital functions can no longer be carried out, and alterations in the blood cell membranes result in lysis of the cells. This deficiency also affects some Greeks and Iranians.

Teratogenicity

Teratogenicity is the ability of a substance to cause abnormal fetal development. Drug groups such as analgesics, diuretics, antihistamines, antibiotics, and antiemetics include identified teratogens. The determination of a drug's teratogenic potential is conducted with animal studies and extrapolated to human beings. Drug-induced teratogenesis is most likely during the first trimester of pregnancy, but structural and functional teratogenesis can be induced by drugs later in pregnancy.

To guide decisions on drug therapy during pregnancy, the Food and Drug Administration (FDA) established a system for classifying drugs according to their probable risks to the fetus. This system is outlined in Appendix A. Drug use in pregnancy is further discussed in Chapter 10.

Tolerance and Dependence

Tolerance is a condition of decreased responsiveness to a drug after repeated exposure to it or one closely allied to it in pharmacologic activity. Habitual use of drugs can produce dependence. In the case of drug dependence, the client develops signs and symptoms of illness when the drug is withdrawn. Withdrawal is uncomfortable and can be dangerous.

Many drugs induce both tolerance and dependence. For example, clients who have taken heavy doses of opioid analgesics over prolonged periods may experience withdrawal symptoms when the drug is discontinued. They may also exhibit cross-tolerance to other CNS depressants. If depressants are required for treatment, larger doses may be necessary to achieve the desired response. In turn, this increases the risk for other adverse reactions because tolerance may be greater for some drug effects than for others. These adverse drug reactions are discussed more fully in Chapter 14.

■ S U M M A R Y

Adverse drug reactions take many forms. Identification of the most common reactions to a specific drug takes 10 to 20 years of widespread use and study of the drug. Although memorizing all the potential ADRs of any given drug would be point-less, nurses must understand that any drug regimen carries potential problems. With this in mind, nurses should regularly update their knowledge data base by referring to pharmacology texts and standard references for current information on specific drugs.

❖ NURSING MANAGEMENT: ADVERSE DRUG REACTIONS

As the healthcare practitioner with the most prolonged contact with the client, the nurse has a key responsibility for protecting the client from ADRs (Box 5-3).

NURSING PROCESS

ASSESSMENT
A detailed medication history is an essential part of the nursing assessment. This helps the nurse identify clients at high risk for ADRs. Many clients, either by choice or medical necessity, are treated by two or more physicians at the same time. This situation may promote ADRs, especially when one physician is unaware of the medication regimen prescribed by the others.

Data Collection. In taking the client's history, the nurse should assess risk factors for ADRs and elicit information about the existence and management of other temporary or permanent health (medical or dental) problems. The nurse should also determine which prescription and OTC drugs the client uses. Allergic and other adverse reactions to previously used medications should be identified and the client's chart and other records flagged or notated, according to hospital policy regarding drug allergies. The usual dose required when drugs are used (as compared with the usual therapeutic range) may indicate the client's responsiveness to drugs in general.

Analysis. The nurse compares information on the client with data about the drugs prescribed to determine the risk of problems stemming from the drug regimen.

NURSING DIAGNOSIS
In constructing nursing diagnoses, the nurse identifies actual or potential ADRs and the drug or drugs to which these would be related. Carpenito has outlined a nursing diagnosis approach to help nurses deal with ADRs. The proposed diagnosis is Potential Complication: Medication Therapy, Adverse Effects. Prototypes discussed by Carpenito include the potential complications of therapy with anticoagulants, antianxiety agents, adrenocorticosteroids, antineoplastic agents, anticonvulsants, antidepressants, antiarrhythmics, antipsychotics, and antihypertensives (Carpenito, 1995).

PLANNING
The goals of drug therapy are to maximize the therapeutic outcome, minimize the risk for ADRs, and de-

tect and treat promptly any undesired effects that may develop. Measurable criteria for outcome evaluation should be developed during the planning stage.

INTERVENTION

The nurse anticipates ADRs when therapy begins and when dosage increases. When drug therapy starts, the nurse must ensure that an antidote (if any) is at hand. Emergency drugs and equipment must be readily available as well. In addition, the healthcare staff must be proficient in treating emergencies such as respiratory or cardiac arrest and anaphylaxis.

Client Education. Nursing management strategies include teaching the client about prescribed medications. The client must know why he or she is taking the drug, how and when to take it, how it works, and what its expected therapeutic and possible adverse effects

---

Box 5-3
Nursing Interventions for Common Drug-Induced Adverse Effects

Iatrogenic disease syndromes arising from drug therapy require collaborative interventions by the healthcare team. Conditions such as ulcers or Cushing's syndrome do not significantly differ from comparable states that occur naturally, but the client will need skilled nursing care to help control symptoms. The following interventions may aid clients experiencing drug-related problems.

Cardiovascular Reactions

Many drugs used for managing hypertension cause postural (or orthostatic) hypotension by impairing the normal vasoconstriction response to changes in position as a person rises. In postural hypotension, rapid movement causes vertigo or a feeling of faintness.

- Show the client how to rise gradually, sitting for a time before standing, to provide time for adaptation.
- To prevent falls, have someone assist the client as needed while ambulating.
- Urge the client to drink ample fluids to maintain hydration, unless otherwise contraindicated, because hypovolemia accentuates the problem.

Cutaneous Reactions

Itching is a major symptom of allergic hypersensitivity. When hypersensitivity is suspected, the prescriber may decide to substitute another drug for the offending medication. Occasionally, there is no therapeutic alternative and therapy must be continued. Antihistamines may be prescribed to reduce symptoms. Several nursing actions can help.

- First, report the signs of allergic reaction to the prescriber.
- Teach the client to press on the affected areas rather than scratching them. Pressure inhibits the transmission of sensation, whereas scratching contributes to inflammation and increases itching.
- Apply cold compresses locally to reduce discomfort. Cold decreases sensation and can even produce numbness.
- Suggest activities to distract the client, because distraction can reduce the perception of itching.

- Finally, avoid general overheating (warm clothing and bed covers), which may stimulate itching.

Gastrointestinal Reactions

As much as possible, clients should be spared unpleasant sights, sounds, and odors that may contribute to an inability to eat.

- Serve food in attractive surroundings and in small quantities.
- Offer between-meal snacks to increase intake.
- As prescribed, administer antiemetics prophylactically before meals rather than later, after nausea and vomiting have developed.
- To help the client tolerate food, suggest that family or friends bring meals from home if the client finds institutional food unappealing. If this is not possible, find out which foods the client tolerated in the past when eating was difficult, and arrange for these foods to be served.

Common side effects of medication include constipation or diarrhea. Both conditions are uncomfortable and potentially dangerous.

- To ameliorate constipation, encourage a greater intake of dietary fiber, full hydration, increased ambulation, and prompt defecation when the urge is felt. A stool softener may be recommended as well.
- To ameliorate diarrhea, advise the client to avoid foods with laxative effect (eg, rhubarb, prunes, pears, raisins). Medications such as loperamide (Imodium, Kaopectate) may be used. Be sure hydration remains adequate to replace fluids lost in the stools.

Neurotoxicity

Drugs may produce euphoria, depression, loss of inhibitions, drowsiness, increased or decreased libido, confusion, and excitement. Adverse reactions can mimic neuroses, psychoses, or senility. Often such symptoms are treated by adding antipsychotics to the drug regimen. A more rational approach would be to identify the cause(s) of the client's mental and emotional changes. If medication is the cause, the drug regimen should be altered.

may be. The client must learn the signs and symptoms that signal a potentially dangerous ADR. The nurse must discuss possible drug interactions that may produce an ADR and advise the client to consult the physician or another responsible healthcare professional before taking any OTC medications.

The nurse encourages the client to report unusual responses so that they may be evaluated in relation to the medications prescribed. In many instances, a client neglects to report a rash or other adverse reaction until the signs and symptoms are fully developed and require emergency treatment. Had the first sign been reported, the ADR may have been controlled without undue suffering or costly hospitalization.

Ensuring Safety. The nurse is often in a position to suggest that duplicate or excessive drugs be eliminated from the therapeutic regimen—the fewer the drugs, the lower the chance of an ADR. The nurse may suggest that the prescriber order blood tests to evaluate therapeutic or toxic effects. Such tests may include liver and kidney function tests to detect possible organ toxicity, in which altered laboratory values, including blood urea nitrogen, serum creatinine, and liver enzyme levels, are key signs.

Promoting Comfort. In caring for the client who reports unpleasant drug side effects such as dry mouth, nausea, diarrhea, dizziness, and other discomforts, the nurse can offer encouragement and suggestions.

Reporting Adverse Effects. Once an ADR is confirmed, nursing interventions include reporting it appropriately. To meet the standards set by the Joint Commission on Accreditation of Healthcare Organizations (JCAHO), a healthcare organization such as a hospital must have an ADR reporting program in place. The hospital's pharmacy and therapeutics committee must review "all significant untoward drug reactions" to ensure quality client care (O'Donnell, 1992). According to JCAHO, a significant reaction is one in which the drug suspected of causing the reaction must be discontinued, the client requires treatment with another drug (eg, an antihistamine, a steroid, or epinephrine), or the client's hospital stay is prolonged.

The FDA launched a similar safety program—MedWatch—in 1993. According to the FDA, an adverse event is any undesirable experience associated with the use of a medical product in a client. "Products," in FDA parlance, include drugs; biologic and therapeutic sera, toxins, antitoxins, blood, and blood components or derivatives; medical devices such as heart valves, latex gloves, and kidney dialysis machines; and medical foods such as dietary supplements and infant formulas. The event should be reported when the client outcome is death, a life-threatening condition,

hospitalization (initial or prolonged), disability, or congenital anomaly. If use of the product requires intervention to prevent permanent impairment or damage, that too should be reported. Examples of reportable events are pacemaker failure, infusion pump failure, anaphylaxis, pseudomembranous colitis, bone marrow suppression that appears drug-related, cerebrovascular accident due to drug-induced hypercoagulability, and hepatotoxicity due to acetaminophen overdose (Box 5-4).

OUTCOME EVALUATION

Hospitalized clients should be monitored closely for drug effects. In addition to observing the degree of therapeutic response, the nurse must also watch for side effects characteristic of specific drugs and record these observations promptly and in detail. Unusual complaints by the client must be heeded even if the complaint does not agree with the nurse's knowledge of a drug's specific effects—the complaint may signal an idiosyncratic reaction or an as-yet-unrecognized effect of the drug. The nurse pays special attention to the client receiving multiple drugs, particularly as drugs are added or discontinued.

To assess and evaluate drug effects, nurses must be informed about the drugs they are administering. They must understand the indications and goals of therapy for each drug prescribed, as well as the possible adverse effects. A major challenge in controlling ADRs is recognizing them when they occur. Professional responsibility for updating personal knowledge about drugs cannot be overemphasized. Physicians, nurses, and pharmacists should be involved together in conferences and workshops on pharmacology. Drug administration should be a shared responsibility, and drug information resources must be readily available for healthcare providers.

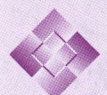

Box 5-4
Reporting ADRs to the FDA

FDA Desk Guides for Adverse Event and Product Problems Reporting are available from:

Food and Drug Administration
MedWatch
5600 Fishers Lane
Rockville, MD 20852-9787

The FDA protects the identity of voluntary reporters because of its belief that confidentiality is a key to encouraging health professionals to report serious adverse drug experiences.

Reports from such healthcare professionals as nurses who witnessed the adverse event are reliable and usually the first warning that a problem exists. (MedWatch form is located in Appendix B.)

❖ CHECKLIST OF NURSING ACTIONS

Before Initiating a Medication Regimen

☐ Take a complete drug history, which should include all drugs currently and recently used, as well as a personal and family history of unusual or adverse reactions to medications.

☐ Compare the client data with data about the drugs ordered by the physician.

☐ Identify potential problems related to the drug regimen.

☐ Use nursing measures to reduce the need to medicate, to reduce the risk of adverse reaction, to detect adverse reactions promptly, and to ameliorate symptoms that may develop.

☐ Teach the client about the drug regimen, including the most likely adverse reactions. Stress the need to contact the healthcare practitioner if unexpected symptoms occur while following a drug regimen.

☐ When necessary, consult the physician for a change in the medication order or for orders for medical treatment of adverse reactions.

Throughout Drug Therapy

☐ Maintain an ongoing evaluation of the client's responses to medication.

☐ Take appropriate action if a delayed adverse reaction to medication develops.

References

Carpenito LJ (1995). *Nursing diagnosis: Application to clinical practice,* 6th ed. Philadelphia: JB Lippincott.

Haybach PJ. (1993). Tuning in to ototoxicity. *Nursing '93, 23* (6):34–41.

O'Donnell J. (1992). Understanding adverse drug reactions. *Nursing '92, 22*(8):34–40.

Rieder MJ. (1993). Immunopharmacology and adverse drug reactions. *Journal of Clinical Pharmacology, 33*(3):316–323.

Roujeau JC, Stern RS. (1994). Severe adverse cutaneous reactions to drugs. *New England Journal of Medicine, 331*(19): 1271–1285.

Shannon MT, Wilson BA, Stang CL. (1995). *Govoni and Hayes' drugs and nursing implications,* 8th ed. Norwalk, CT: Appleton & Lange.

Bibliography

Amdur MO, Doull J, Klaassen CD, eds. (1991). *Casarett and Doull's toxicology: The basic science of poisons,* 4th ed. New York: Pergamon Press.

Ganzini L, Millar SB, Walsh JR. (1993). Drug-induced mania in the elderly. *Drugs and Aging, 3*(5):428.

Hardman J, Limbird LE, et al. (eds). (1996). *Goodman and Gilman's the pharmacological basis of therapeutics,* 9th ed. New York: McGraw-Hill.

Kessler DA. (1993). Using MedWatch: A better way to report adverse events. *Nursing '93, 23*(11):49–50.

Kessler DA. (1993). Introducing MedWatch: A new approach to reporting medication and device adverse effects and product problems. *Journal of the American Medical Association, 269*(21):2765.

Konig St. A, et al. (1994). Severe hepatotoxicity during valproate therapy: An update and report of eight new fatalities. *Epilepsia, 35*(5):1005–1015.

Leonard MS. (1993). Genetically determined adverse drug reactions involving metabolism. *Drug Safety, 9*(1):60.

Liebelt EL, Shannon MW. (1993). Small doses, big problems: A selected review of highly toxic common medications. *Pediatric Emergency Care, 9*(5):292.

Malseed RT, Goldstein FJ, Balkon N. (1995). *Pharmacology: Drug therapy and nursing considerations,* 4th ed. Philadelphia: JB Lippincott.

Meyer UA. (1992). Drugs in special patient groups: Clinical importance of genetics in drug effects. In KL Melmon, HF Morrelli, BB Hoffman, Nierenberg W (eds). *Clinical pharmacology: Basic principles in therapeutics,* 3d ed. New York: McGraw-Hill.

Montella KR, Powrie R. (1994). Critical illness in pregnancy: 4. Pharmacological considerations. *Emergency Medicine, 26*(1):99.

Olin BR, ed. (1995). *Drug facts and comparisons.* St. Louis: Facts and Comparisons.

Rieder MJ. (1994). Mechanisms of unpredictable adverse drug reactions. *Drug Safety, 11*(3):196–212.

For more information and sample tests and activities, refer to Chapter 5 in the Student Workbook for Clinical Pharmacology and Nursing Management, 5th edition, available through your bookstore.

6

Drug Interactions

When an interactant chemical modifies the anticipated therapeutic results of a drug, a drug interaction has occurred. The interactant may be another drug or a combination of drugs, natural or artificial dietary components, environmental pollutants, endogenous body chemicals, or chemicals used for diagnostic tests.

Kinds of Drug Interactions

Among the kinds of drug interactions are pharmacodynamic, pharmacogenetic, and pharmacokinetic interactions.

Pharmacodynamic Interactions

Pharmacodynamic interactions, which have been studied less than pharmacokinetic ones, are difficult to classify. They may occur at similar or different receptor sites. They may be inhibitory as well, taking the form of pharmacologic antagonism (as occurs between carbidopa and amoxapine). They also may promote toxicity. A less direct example of a pharmacodynamic interaction occurs between nonsteroidal antiinflammatory drugs (NSAIDs) and diuretics. Because sodium retention is a pharmacologic effect of NSAIDs, hypertensive clients receiving thiazide diuretic and NSAID therapy may exhibit some loss of blood-pressure control with concurrent NSAID therapy.

Pharmacogenetic Interactions

One of the problems in pharmacotherapy is interindividual variability in response to drugs. In the 1950s, experts first suggested that exaggerated (unusual) responses to drugs may result from genetically determined enzyme deficiencies. Several of these deficiencies that lead to abnormal drug reactions have been described. Genetic abnormalities can increase the effects of drug therapy at normal dosage levels and, therefore, may increase the hazard of specific drug–drug interactions. Persons with an abnormal genetic makeup may experience relatively more and more serious drug–drug interactions. For example, if a client with an enzyme deficiency concurrently receives two drugs that are normally metabolized by the same enzyme, a high concentration of one or both drugs may occur.

If a drug is eliminated by two routes (eg, by renal excretion and hepatic metabolism), then the genetically determined defects in drug metabolism may have only a minor impact, as the intact renal function can compensate for them. If, however, a client has renal failure and a genetically determined lack of metabolic enzyme as well, both routes of excretion are impaired and serious consequences may arise. Some of the drugs associated with pharmacogenetic drug interactions are succinylcholine, mercaptopurine, tricyclic antidepressants, and phenothiazines.

Pharmacokinetic Interactions

Pharmacokinetic interactions are the most prevalent. They occur during drug absorption, distribution, biotransformation, or excretion. Whether pharmacodynamic, pharmacogenetic, or pharmacokinetic, a drug interaction may occur between drugs or between drugs and foods. Throughout this chapter, the word *food* refers to both food and beverages. A drug interaction may alter laboratory test results as well.

Clinically Desirable Interactions

In discussing drug interactions, the emphasis is usually on problems created by drug combinations. However, drug interactions are also induced either to enhance a beneficial drug effect or to mitigate a detrimental one.

A beneficial, synergistic interaction—one in which the effect of one drug is enhanced by another drug—occurs between the antimicrobial combination of trimethoprim and sulfamethoxazole (Bactrim, Septra, and others). This combination works against bacterial infections by blocking two steps in the bacterial synthesis of folic acid. Trimethoprim inhibits the bacterial enzyme called dihydrofolate reductase. Sulfamethoxazole blocks the synthesis of dihydrofolate by inhibiting bacterial utilization of para-aminobenzoic acid to form dihydropteroic acid.

Similarly, the interaction between carbidopa and levodopa (Sinemet) has proved helpful in managing Parkinson's disease. Levodopa used alone to treat Parkinson's disease is rapidly decarboxylated to dopamine by peripheral dopa decarboxylase. To ensure that an adequate amount of levodopa reaches the brain rather than the peripheral tissues, large doses must be administered, and consequently adverse effects may occur. Carbidopa, a peripheral dopa decarboxylase inhibitor, interacts with levodopa to diminish the decarboxylation of levodopa in peripheral tissues. This produces higher plasma concentrations of levodopa and prolongs the drug's half-life, allowing more levodopa to cross the blood-brain barrier to the site of action in the brain. Because of this interaction, the dose of levodopa can be reduced, minimizing or eliminating adverse effects.

Subsequent chapters about specific drug families include additional examples of clinically desirable interactions. One purpose of this chapter is to convey the concept that drug interactions have positive as well as negative effects, and that there are many of them, not just an isolated few. For example, the combination of aluminum hydroxide and magnesium hydroxide (as in Maalox, Gelusil, and Mylanta) is a common and useful drug interaction. Aluminum hydroxide is constipating, and magnesium hydroxide has a laxative effect. The purpose of combining the two agents is to have one cancel out the undesirable effect of the other. Magnesium hydroxide is fast-acting and aluminum hydroxide is slow-acting, so the combination also increases total buffering time.

Drug–Drug Interactions

Drug–drug interactions may be beneficial or detrimental. They may vary from person to person, and they may be clinically significant or insignificant. Chances that a drug interaction will occur increase with the number of drugs a client takes, the number of prescribers a client consults, and the variety of medications prescribed. The best preparation for managing an actual or potential drug interaction is to understand their basic mechanisms. Drug–drug interactions are usually pharmacokinetic: one drug affects the absorption, distribution, biotransformation, or excretion of another.

Interactions and Absorption

Interactions during absorption result in an increase or decrease in the relative rate of absorption, the total amount of drug absorbed, or both. A drug may be absorbed too slowly to reach an effective serum level or the onset of action may be significantly delayed when prompt action is needed to relieve acute symptoms (eg, pain).

Direct Interactions Involving Decreased Absorption

An example of a direct interaction between drugs and one that decreases the amount of drug absorbed occurs after the simultaneous administration of the salts of divalent or trivalent metals (calcium, magnesium, iron, and aluminum) and tetracycline antibiotics. The tetracycline forms relatively insoluble chelates with the metallic ions; antacids, laxatives, and certain foods contain these salts.

Tetracycline is probably absorbed through passive diffusion, and the formation of the metallic complex interferes with the tetracycline molecule's passage through the intestinal wall. The formation of the metallic complex depends on pH. At low pH, little complex forms; at high pH, the complex increases. (This interaction occurs as a drug–food interaction when tetracycline is coadministered with whole milk, buttermilk, and cottage cheese, which contain calcium.) Two of the tetracyclines—doxycycline (Vibramycin) and minocycline (Minocin)—are affected to a lesser extent if taken with foods containing calcium. However, if taken concurrently with aluminum-containing antacids (eg, Amphojel, Basaljel), they still lose some effectiveness because of decreased absorption (Hussar, 1993).

Another example of decreased absorption occurs in the interaction between the antiinfective fluoroquinolones, such as ciprofloxacin (Cipro) and enoxacin (Penetrex), and metallic cation-containing drugs such as antacids. The reduced absorption may result from adsorption of the quinolone molecule to insoluble particles of the antacid or from altered solubility of the quinolone. Another mechanism of the interaction may involve the formation of chelates. Interaction with antacids also reduces absorption of isoniazid, phenytoin, digoxin, chloroquine, cimetidine, quinidine, and NSAIDs.

Cholestyramine (Questran) is an antilipemic that is not absorbed from the gastrointestinal (GI) tract. Cholestyramine exchanges chloride ions for bile acids, which it binds into insoluble complexes that are subsequently excreted in the feces. It can also bind with drugs. Through the exchange mechanism, cholestyramine can interfere with the intestinal absorption of thyroxine, anticoagulants, and various digitalis preparations if these drugs are given concurrently.

Another factor that affects absorption is the drug form, which may affect the release of active ingredients. For example, chewable tablets must be chewed adequately to release the active ingredient, because the tablet may not contain the disintegrators needed to maximize dissolution. Swallowing the tablet whole may interfere with absorption.

A drug's dissolution rate (the time required for a drug to disintegrate and dissolve) changes when a drug is adsorbed onto the surface of a solid. For example, kaolin-pectin suspension (eg, Kaopectate, an adsorbent antidiarrheal) interacts with digoxin and tetracyclines to inhibit the amount and rate of their absorption.

Drug interactions that affect GI motility may affect absorption by changing the residence time of the drug at the site of dissolution. Metoclopramide (Reglan) stimulates gastric emptying, which increases the absorption rates of acetaminophen, levodopa, and lithium. Codeine, morphine sulfate, atropine, and chloroquine delay gastric emptying, which depresses the rate of absorption of other drugs.

Avoiding Drug Interactions That Alter Absorption
Most authorities agree that most drug interactions during the absorptive phase can be avoided or significantly reduced by not giving the drugs simultaneously. The doses of the interactant drugs should be separated by 2 to 4 hours (Hussar, 1993).

Interactions and Distribution
Many drugs bind to plasma proteins, primarily albumin, for transport to the site of metabolism, and some drugs may bind to tissue sites as well. Drugs must be in equilibrium with their binding sites. If free drug is removed (eg, by glomerular filtration), then bound drug will dissociate from its binding sites. It is generally accepted that the bound fraction has no pharmacologic activity; the therapeutically important concentration is that of the free, unbound drug.

Displacement Mechanisms
The bound drug concentration depends on the amount of binding materials in the plasma and tissues and the affinity of the drug for these materials and sites. In the past, experts recognized that some drugs could displace other drugs from their binding sites. This phenomenon was considered a major reason for drug–drug interactions. Some experts think that the importance of protein-binding displacement interactions has been exaggerated.

Certain drugs do compete with other drugs for drug-binding sites on albumin and can displace albumin-bound drugs. However, the body's clearance rate for drugs is proportional to the fraction of drug unbound in the plasma. After displacement, the drug's rate of clearance increases. In most cases, the compensatory increase in clearance reduces the transient increase in free drug concentration to proportions that are clinically insignificant.

Secondary Mechanisms
Because free drug concentration usually remains essentially unchanged after protein-binding displacement, no major drug interactions should result from displacement alone. Therefore, interactions thought to result from displacement may be due to a second mechanism.

An example of an interaction caused by displacement and a second mechanism is that which occurs between methotrexate and aspirin. While aspirin displaces methotrexate, a second mechanism operates simultaneously. The second mechanism involves excretion. Methotrexate and aspirin (or its metabolites) are excreted primarily by the kidney. Aspirin competes with and inhibits the renal secretion of methotrexate, resulting in an increase in the serum methotrexate level. Because of the narrow margin between the therapeutic and toxic effects of methotrexate, this interaction can produce toxic levels of methotrexate.

Phenylbutazone and warfarin bind extensively to plasma protein albumin. Phenylbutazone has the greater affinity for the binding sites. Normally, 98% of warfarin is bound. If phenylbutazone is given concurrently with warfarin, the bound portion of warfarin drops to 96%, thereby doubling (from 2% to 4%) the pharmacologically active concentration of warfarin, and hemorrhagic crises have occurred. The interaction occurs soon (within hours or days) after administering the drug combination. The problem reverses when one drug is withdrawn. This interaction was formerly thought to result from displacement, but experts now think it results from phenylbutazone's inhibition of the metabolism of warfarin.

Sodium valproate or valproic acid raises the free phenytoin concentration between 50% and 100% when the two drugs are given concurrently. Phenytoin toxicity may occur. The rise in free phenytoin concentration is due partly to displacement of phenytoin from tissue-binding sites. However, inhibition of phenytoin metabolism is probably the more important mechanism.

Interactions involving tissue-binding displacement have more potential for adverse effects than do interactions involving plasma protein-binding displacement. However, to date, laboratory methods have not been available to study this mechanism thoroughly.

Interactions and Biotransformation
Many drugs must be metabolized, usually by the liver, before they are excreted from the body, usually through the kidneys. The hepatic mono-oxygenase enzyme system is involved in the biotransformation of many lipid-soluble drugs. These drugs circulate through the liver and the enzymes gradually convert them to water-soluble metabolites. The metabolites may or may not remain pharmacologically active. Interactions related to biotransformation either inhibit drug metabolism or accelerate it (Table 6-1).

Inhibitory Mechanisms and Interactions
One drug may inhibit the metabolism of another drug or of a hormone, neurotransmitter, or other endogenous compound. This means it can block or slow the metabolic breakdown of these substances, thereby increasing their plasma concentration, possibly to the point of toxicity. Drugs that reduce the metabolism of

Table 6-1. Examples of Drug Interactions Related to Biotransformation

Inhibition of Metabolism		Acceleration of Metabolism	
Inhibitor	Drug Metabolism Inhibited	Inducer	Drug Metabolism Accelerated
MAOIs	amphetamines, ephedrine, phenylephrine, tyramine	polycyclic hydrocarbons (in tobacco smoke)	theophylline, imipramine, antipyrine, pentazocine, chlorpromazine, diazepam, chlordiazepoxide, propoxyphene
erythromycin	digoxin, warfarin, theophylline, carbamazepine	phenytoin	hydrocortisone, dexamethasone, prednisolone, methylprednisolone
cimetidine	diazepam, chlordiazepoxide, carbamazepine, theophylline, labetalol, warfarin, phenytoin, propranolol	rifampin	methadone

other drugs are called *inhibitors.* Conversely, drugs that increase the metabolism of other drugs are called *inducers* or *accelerators* (Box 6-1 and Box 6-2).

Inhibition usually arises from competition between one drug and an interacting drug for the active site on an enzyme. Drug-metabolizing enzymes have multiple forms, and drugs may be metabolized by more than one form. Inhibition of metabolism occurs only if both drugs bind to the active site of the same form of the enzyme. In some cases, inhibited drug metabolism may be desired. An example is the interaction of a cholinesterase inhibitor and acetylcholine, which increases the effectiveness of acetylcholine at neuromuscular junctions.

An interaction that inhibits metabolism may also produce undesired effects. For example, monoamine oxidase inhibitors (MAOIs) include isocarboxazid, pargyline, phenelzine, and tranylcypromine. These MAOIs inhibit the enzyme monoamine oxidase (MAO), which normally metabolizes catecholamines, such as norepinephrine. If MAO is inhibited, the body will store more norepinephrine than usual at receptor sites in adrenergic neurons. A client taking an MAOI should avoid another drug, such as a sympathomimetic (ephedrine, phenylephrine, and phenylpropanolamine), that may release this norepinephrine, causing severe headache, hypertensive crisis, cardiac arrhythmias, or intracranial bleeding. Some interacting sympathomimetics are contained in nonprescription medications such as diet, cough and cold, sinus, and hay fever preparations. Examples include Robitussin-PE (contains phenylephrine), Vicks Formula 44D Decongestant Cough Mixture (contains pseudoephedrine), and Alka-Seltzer Plus Cold Medicine (contains phenylpropanolamine).

More commonly prescribed enzyme inhibitors include erythromycin, cimetidine, and allopurinol. Allopurinol inhibits the oxidation of purine to uric acid by inhibiting the enzyme xanthine oxidase. This enzyme is

Box 6-1
Selected Enzyme Inhibitors

Drug Classes

fluoroquinolone antimicrobials

oral contraceptives

psoralen dermatologics

tricyclic antidepressants

Drugs

allopurinol

amiodarone

cimetidine

erythromycin

ethanol

isoniazid

propoxyphene

propranolol

sodium valproate

Box 6-2
Selected Enzyme Inducers

The following enzyme inducers are associated with accelerated metabolism and, therefore, decreased drug effect:

- carbamazepine, phenytoin, primidone (anticonvulsants)
- cigarette smoke
- ethanol
- griseofulvin
- rifampin

important in metabolizing mercaptopurine and azathioprine (Imuran). If xanthine oxidase is inhibited by
allopurinol therapy, the effects of mercaptopurine or
azathioprine may increase to a dangerous level.

Cimetidine, a histamine H_2 antagonist, is a potent
inhibitor of hepatic enzyme activity. Delayed clearance
and increased effects of most benzodiazepines (eg, diazepam), chlordiazepoxide, carbamazepine, theophylline,
chlormethiazole, labetalol, warfarin, phenytoin, and propranolol result from interaction with cimetidine. Serious
unwanted effects may occur. For example, the sedative effect of the benzodiazepine may be increased. However,
cimetidine is unlikely to affect the activity of lorazepam,
oxazepam, and temazepam because it does not alter glucuronide conjugation, which is how these drugs are metabolized. Perhaps one of those three drugs could be substituted for diazepam. Another alternative would be to
substitute famotidine, nizatidine, or ranitidine for cimetidine, because these histamine H_2 antagonists are unlikely to inhibit hepatic enzyme systems.

Accelerant Mechanisms and Interactions

The amount of hepatic drug-metabolizing enzymes
may be increased by interactions that stimulate their
synthesis. Several hundred compounds (known as inducers or accelerators) have been identified as being
able to induce the synthesis of these enzymes. The inducer may cause a drug administered concurrently to be
metabolized and excreted faster than normal, thereby
reducing its effects.

Smoking appears to speed the metabolism of several
drugs by stimulating hepatic drug-metabolizing enzymes. Studies suggest the polycyclic hydrocarbons in
the cigarette smoke increase enzyme activity, which
lowers blood levels and reduces the therapeutic effects
of the drug involved. The enzyme-inducing effect appears to be long-lasting, persisting for up to 3 months
after the person stops smoking. Moreover, there may be
a relation between the number of cigarettes smoked per
day and the significance of the smoking–drug interaction. Smokers of more than one pack of cigarettes a day
tend to experience drug interactions more often than
those who smoke less. Reports show lowered blood levels of diazepam, theophylline, imipramine, and pentazocine in smokers. When a smoker on theophylline is
admitted to the smoke-free environment of the hospital, the serum theophylline level will rise, possibly to a
toxic level.

Enzyme inducers such as the barbiturates, phenytoin, and rifampin may increase the metabolism rate and
reduce the effects of cyclosporine, possibly resulting in
therapeutic failure. In opiate-dependent clients treated
with methadone, introduction of rifampin for tuberculosis treatment has resulted in withdrawal symptoms.
Rifampin decreases plasma concentrations of methadone and increases the urinary excretion of its major
metabolite.

Combined Mechanisms and Interactions

Some drugs are involved in interactions due to both inhibition and acceleration.

Drugs that inhibit warfarin metabolism include disulfiram, metronidazole, allopurinol, tricyclic antidepressants, clofibrate, phenylbutazone, chloramphenicol, propoxyphene, and some sulfonamide preparations, such
as cotrimoxazole (trimethoprim and sulfamethoxazole).
Inhibition of warfarin metabolism increases circulating
anticoagulant levels, and hemorrhage may occur.

Because they induce enzyme synthesis, barbiturates,
rifampin, dichloralphenazone, and carbamazepine interact with warfarin, accelerating its metabolism and
necessitating higher doses of warfarin for suitable anticoagulation. A hemorrhagic crisis can occur if the maintenance dose of warfarin is not lowered when the interacting agent is withdrawn.

Other drugs commonly involved in both inhibition
and acceleration reactions include theophylline, sulfonylureas, cyclosporine, ethanol, and sulfinpyrazone.

Interactions and Excretion

Most drugs and drug metabolites are excreted through
active and passive mechanisms by the renal system. The
hepatobiliary route is also an important excretion route,
particularly for ampicillin, digitoxin, and glutethimide.
Drugs are excreted to a lesser and more variable extent
by the lungs, through the skin, and in saliva, breast
milk, and sweat.

Excretion by the kidney occurs at a rate proportional
to the amount of drug in the body. Excretion occurs by
passive glomerular filtration of the fraction of the drug
not bound to plasma proteins, or by active tubular secretion, using one carrier mechanism for weak acids and another for weak bases. The main location of drug secretion in the kidney is the proximal convoluted tubule.

Any change in the pH of the urine influences excretion, and any change in the urinary flow rate affects
both reabsorption and the pH, thereby influencing
drug excretion via the kidney. Although hundreds of
possible drug interactions may occur during excretion,
only a few are clinically significant. The drug interactions that seem to be the most important during excretion involve certain diuretics, probenecid, and quinidine. Drugs that alter urinary pH include the alkalizers
sodium bicarbonate and acetazolamide and the acidifier
ammonium chloride.

Most drugs are weak organic acids or bases. Usually
the ionized portion of the drug molecule is water-soluble and can thus be excreted by the kidney. Urine having a pH that supports the drug primarily in the ionized
form reduces the possibility for passive reabsorption.
Urine having a pH that supports the drug in the nonionized form enhances the possibility for passive reabsorption. Weak acids are excreted more rapidly in alkaline urine; weak bases are excreted more rapidly in acid
urine. In an alkaline urine, weak bases are more nonion-

ized and less water-soluble, whereas acidic drugs are more ionized and thus more prone to excretion.

Alkalinization of urine increases the rate of excretion of acidic drugs (eg, acetazolamide, phenobarbital, salicylates, sulfonamides). Likewise, acidification of urine increases the urinary excretion of basic drugs (eg, amphetamines, quinidine, tricyclic antidepressants).

Weak Acid Interactions

Interference in the urinary excretion of drugs is important if the fraction of the drug excreted unchanged is large. Furosemide is a weak acid, and 90% of the absorbed fraction is eliminated by the kidney in unchanged form. Both indomethacin and aspirin weaken the diuresis obtained with furosemide if they are used with it. Studies indicate the furosemide–aspirin interaction involves competition for the same carrier mechanism in the tubular cell.

Weak Base Interactions

When quinidine is coadministered with digoxin, an interaction occurs involving approximate doubling of the serum digoxin concentration (Abernethy and Andrawis, 1993). Two different mechanisms may be at work. Quinidine apparently displaces digoxin from peripheral tissue-binding sites in striated muscle without affecting binding to cardiac receptors. In addition, it competes with digoxin for carrier-mediated excretion in the proximal tubule. By these mechanisms, digoxin levels may rise to twice the normal level. The client may experience cardiac arrhythmias and other symptoms of digitalis toxicity.

■ SUMMARY

Drug–drug interactions may be either detrimental or beneficial and may affect the absorption, distribution, biotransformation, or excretion of drugs. Drug interactions may be of major clinical significance or of no clinical significance at all.

❖ NURSING MANAGEMENT: DRUG–DRUG INTERACTIONS

As the healthcare practitioner with close and prolonged client contact, the nurse assumes responsibility for protecting the client from drug–drug interactions (Table 6-2). Memorizing all the potential interactions of any given drug would be too time-consuming to be practical. It is enough to understand that potential problems may occur with any drug regimen. Then the nurse can regularly consult pharmacology texts and references for information on drug–drug interactions.

NURSING PROCESS

ASSESSMENT

A detailed medication history is an essential part of the nursing history. This assessment process helps the nurse identify clients at risk for drug–drug interactions. Many

Table 6-2. Understanding Selected Drug–Drug Interactions

Drug	Other Drug	Mechanism	Possible Outcome	Nursing Interventions
tetracyclines	antacids containing aluminum, calcium, or magnesium	Decreased absorption of tetracycline	Decreased anti-infective effect	Give antacid 3 hours after tetracycline preparation.
digoxin	quinidine	Displacement of digoxin from peripheral tissue-binding sites and reduced digoxin excretion	Digoxin toxicity	Monitor serum levels of digoxin. Observe for signs and symptoms of digoxin toxicity.
cimetidine	diazepam, phenytoin, propranolol, theophylline, others	Cimetidine inhibits hepatic enzyme activity so that metabolism of affected drugs is inhibited.	Increased effect of interactant drug	Monitor serum levels of interactant drug. Observe for signs and symptoms of toxicity of interactant drug.
cholestyramine	thyroxine, anticoagulants, digitalis preparations	Decreased absorption of thyroxine and other affected drugs	Decreased effectiveness of bound drug	Give all medications 1 hour before cholestyramine or 4 hours after cholestyramine. Assess cardiac glycoside level if both drugs are used.
penicillins	probenecid	Decreased excretion of penicillin	Higher and more sustained serum antibiotic level	No action necessary. This principle is applied deliberately to treat gonorrhea and other serious infections.

people (either by personal choice or medical necessity) are treated by two or more physicians at the same time. Such a situation may lead to drug interactions if one physician is unaware of the other's prescriptions.

In compiling the history, the nurse must identify temporary or permanent medical or dental problems and their treatment. Additional responsibilities include compiling a list of every drug the client has taken in the previous 2 weeks, including any over-the-counter (OTC) preparations—specifically, vitamins and minerals, analgesics, antihistamines, antacids, antidiarrheals, cough preparations, laxatives, and sedatives. Some nurses ask the client or responsible others to bring in all medications for review.

Adverse reactions and interactions to medications in the past should be explored (see the "Critical Thinking Challenge: Case Analysis").

In some settings, the nurse may find that using a computerized drug-interaction screening program may help prevent adverse reactions and drug interactions. These programs have identified the drugs most responsible for interactions: antacids, warfarin, digoxin, aspirin, steroids, propranolol, phenytoin, aminophylline, prochlorperazine, quinidine, and penicillin.

After compiling these assessment data, the nurse can analyze the history and the client's current drug regimen to determine the risk for drug-related problems.

NURSING DIAGNOSES

Nursing diagnoses should identify actual or potential interactions among drugs the client is receiving.

PLANNING

The goals and expected outcomes include reducing the risk of adverse drug–drug interactions and promptly detecting and treating any reactions that develop. Measurable criteria for evaluation should be developed during the planning stage.

INTERVENTION

Observations must be recorded and shared with prescribers, pharmacists, and other appropriate members of the healthcare team. Anticipating, preventing, recognizing, and managing drug interactions is the responsibility of the whole team. Each member of the team brings a unique perspective to the subject.

Client Education. Clients and their families should learn why drugs are needed, how they work, what effects to expect, and what possible adverse interactions may occur. Nurses must teach clients how to take the drug correctly to avoid potential interactions. Clients must be encouraged to report any unusual response so that it may be evaluated in relation to the medications being taken. Written and verbal instructions must be supplied. The instructions should identify all signs and symptoms to be reported immediately.

CRITICAL THINKING CHALLENGE
Case Analysis

Mr. Arthur, an overweight 63-year-old manager of a busy retail computer store, has been admitted to your unit. He has severe viral gastroenteritis with diarrhea, and an IV infusion has been started. During the history part of the nursing assessment, you learn that he lives in an adjacent rural community with his wife and two teenage sons. He commutes 40 miles round-trip daily to work, and he eats lunch in the fast-food restaurants near his workplace. He smokes one pack of cigarettes daily and has a history of multiple chronic health problems, for which he takes the following medications:

- digoxin (Lanoxicaps) 0.125 mg qd (he had a myocardial infarction 2 years ago, has coronary artery disease, and has reported symptoms of mild congestive heart failure)
- furosemide (Lasix) 20 mg bid (to treat symptoms of mild congestive heart failure)
- ibuprofen (Motrin) 600 mg tid (to treat osteoarthritis)
- antacid (Maalox) 15 mL 1 hour after meals and at bedtime (to treat symptoms of a hiatal hernia)
- ferrous sulfate 300 mg tid (for mild anemia)
- kaolin-pectin (Kaopectate) 15 mL qid prn (for current diarrhea)

Meals on the hospital unit are served at 8 AM, noon, and 5 PM.

1. What additional data do you need to construct an applicable care plan for Mr. Arthur? What lifestyle factors must you take into consideration? Of what importance are they to Mr. Arthur and his family? What questions might you raise about Mr. Arthur's medication regimen?
2. Suggest possible nursing diagnoses for Mr. Arthur.
3. Discuss some interventions to perform to help Mr. Arthur prevent drug–food and drug–drug interactions in the future.
4. How would you schedule administration of Mr. Arthur's medications, based on your knowledge of drug interaction mechanisms?
5. Construct a teaching plan and a time frame for its completion.

OUTCOME EVALUATION

The nurse should measure the client's progress toward meeting the established evaluation criteria. Data required for evaluation include evidence of the presence or absence of a drug–drug interaction.

Drug–Food Interactions

Usually, the drug–food interactions that concern healthcare staff are associated with the medications, fluids, and foodstuffs ingested every day by most people (Box 6-3). However, other kinds of drug–food interactions, such

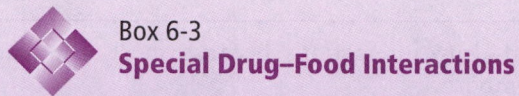

Box 6-3
Special Drug–Food Interactions

Although drug–food interactions occur and vary among people, some interactions may be avoided. Nurses and clients alike should be acquainted with some special interactions.

Tyramine and MAOIs

Found in many foods, tyramine is usually harmless because it is rapidly oxidized by the enzyme monoamine oxidase (MAO). This enzyme normally metabolizes catecholamines such as norepinephrine. When tyramine is not oxidized, it is freely absorbed.

In clients taking a monoamine oxidase inhibitor (MAOI), tyramine circulates through the blood to the adrenergic nerve endings where there is an accumulation of norepinephrine resulting from the effect of the MAOI. Tyramine causes the release of this surplus norepinephrine. The result may be cardiovascular problems, such as an acute hypertensive crisis signaled by severe occipital headache, palpitations, stiff neck, nausea, vomiting, and in some cases fatal cerebral hemorrhage.

Common MAOIs include phenelzine (Nardil) and tranylcypromine (Parnate). Intake of tyramine-rich foods increases the possibility that the tyramine will cause the release of the surplus norepinephrine. Common tyramine-containing foods are red wines (such as Chianti), fava beans, broad bean pods, and any food that is aged, fermented, overripe, spoiled, or simply old. Cheeses such as Camembert, cheddar, Stilton, and Roquefort are usually dangerous to consume with an MAOI, whereas moderate amounts of very fresh cheese, sour cream, yogurt, cream cheese, cottage cheese, ricotta cheese, pickled herring, sausage, and chopped liver may be safe. Likewise, alcoholic beverages other than red wine are probably safe in moderate amounts.

MSG, Caffeine, and MAOIs

The effects of MAOIs can also be enhanced by concurrent intake of caffeine and monosodium glutamate (MSG), a flavor enhancer (Kuhn, 1993). In many restaurants, particularly Chinese restaurants, food is prepared with MSG, so clients taking an MAOI should be cautioned not only to avoid caffeine but also to read prepared-food labels and order restaurant meals carefully.

Grapefruit Juice and Calcium Channel Blockers

A chance finding that grapefruit juice interacts with felodipine, a calcium channel blocker, was also found to be valid for nifedipine (Bailey et al, 1994). Researchers think that this food–drug interaction is probably not limited to this class of drugs and that it has potential clinical importance because citrus juices are often consumed with breakfast, when drugs are also taken.

Researchers think that grapefruit juice increases the rate and the extent of systemic availability of felodipine by inhibiting first-pass metabolism in the small intestinal wall and liver. Because an interaction has not been identified between felodipine and orange juice, the researchers think that the interaction is caused by a substance specific to grapefruit juice. Symptoms of the interaction include significantly reduced blood pressure and acute vasodilation-related effects, such as headache, facial flushing, and lightheadedness. Enhancement of felodipine bioavailability by grapefruit juice has the potential to increase both efficacy and toxicity.

Cruciferous Vegetables and Acetaminophen

Cruciferous vegetables, including cabbage, broccoli, brussels sprouts, and cauliflower, contain several indole derivatives. Studies indicate that cabbage and brussels sprouts increase the glucuronidation and metabolic clearance of acetaminophen in healthy subjects.

Charcoal-broiled Meat and Theophylline

The polycyclic aromatic hydrocarbons produced when meats are charcoal broiled are similar to those found in cigarette smoke. These hydrocarbons are products of incomplete combustion produced when meat drippings fall onto the hot coals. The drippings are volatilized and redeposited on the meat and act as inducers for the metabolism of certain drugs, such as theophylline, thereby decreasing the drug half-life and effectiveness.

Licorice and Antihypertensives

Licorice (which contains glycyrrhizic acid) reduces the effectiveness of antihypertensive drugs. Licorice is related to, and acts like, aldosterone, which enhances sodium retention and potassium excretion in the distal tubule of the kidney, thereby elevating blood pressure (Kuhn, 1993).

Alcohol and Disulfiram

Disulfiram (Antabuse) and alcohol interact, causing the acetaldehyde syndrome when beverages or foods containing alcohol are consumed by persons taking disulfiram. About 15 minutes after alcohol consumption, the person experiences flushing and headache, followed by nausea and vomiting and in some people chest or abdominal pain. The threat of this identified interaction is the intent of prescribing disulfiram for alcoholics who take the drug to prevent continued drinking. The acetaldehyde syndrome results from increased aldehyde concentration in the body. Acetaldehyde is produced by the oxidation of ethanol by the alcohol dehydrogenase of the liver. Disulfiram inhibits aldehyde dehydrogenase irreversibly. Other drugs that can cause the acetaldehyde syndrome when alcohol is consumed are metronidazole, chlorpropamide, griseofulvin, tolazoline, and procarbazine.

as those between drugs and enteral feeding solutions, concern healthcare providers also. Like drug–drug interactions, many drug–food interactions are pharmacokinetic in nature.

Food and Pharmacokinetic Interactions

A drug's effect may be altered by foods during their absorption, biotransformation, and excretion. Absorption is probably the most common mechanism associated with food–drug interactions because most drugs are taken by mouth.

Interactions and Absorption

Foods have active ingredients with physiologic effects on the body (Table 6-3). Food may increase, decrease, delay, or have no effect at all on drug absorption. In general, any drug that has a narrow therapeutic index and well-defined therapeutic serum levels or that may need to be titrated according to a client's condition is

Table 6-3. Pharmacologic Properties of Common Foods

Food	Active Component	Action/Effect
Potatoes	solanin, oxalate, arsenic, tannin, nitrate	When consumed in moderation, none; in large quantities, poisonous
Rutabagas, turnips, cabbage, kale, rape, Chinese cabbage, brussels sprouts, broccoli, kohlrabi, peaches, raisins, lettuce, celery, radishes, green peppers	goitrogens	Inhibition of thyroid function
Spinach, beet tops, Swiss chard, lamb's quarters, poke, purslane, rhubarb	oxalic acid	Decrease in intestinal absorption of calcium; laxative
Tea	tannin	Astringent and antidiarrheal; animal and human carcinogenicity
Berries	various astringents	Astringent and antidiarrheal
Bran	fiber	Laxative
Pears, prunes	sugars and intestinal irritants	Laxative (sugars pull water into the intestine osmotically; irritants stimulate peristalsis)
Sour milk, yogurt	lactobacilli	Maintenance of the natural flora of the digestive tract
Wheat, sesame seed, soybeans	phytates	Binding of zinc, calcium, and other minerals, decreasing their absorption in the intestines
Raw egg whites	avidin	Binding of biotin, decreasing its absorption
Orange peel	citral	Antagonism of vitamin A
Blackberries, black currants, red beets, brussels sprouts, red cabbage, raw fish, seafood	thiaminase	Destruction of thiamine
Legumes	lathyrogens	Changes in collagen maturation and subsequent skeletal and skin abnormalities, (in animals) dissecting aneurysms
"Diet" salad dressings	mineral oil	Interference with intestinal absorption of fat-soluble vitamins
Pickles, ham, bacon, saltine crackers, potato chips	sodium	Water retention, rise in blood pressure
Soups, bananas, orange juice, apricots	potassium	Increased relaxation of cardiac muscle during diastole; reduction of force of cardiac muscle contraction during systole
Beans	trioses (nondigestible sugars)	Increased fermentation and gas production in the intestine
Cranberries, plums, prunes, meats, cereals	acid salts (in metabolic residue)	Decreased pH of urine
Milk, most fruits and vegetables	alkaline salts (in metabolic residues)	Increased pH of urine
Milk	tryptophan	Increases brain levels of serotonin; decreases pain and promotes sleep
Beverages	water	(In large quantities) water diuresis
Citrus fruits	water, vitamin C	Reduced symptoms of the common cold
Garlic	oils	Inhibition of coagulation, reduction of blood levels of low-density lipoproteins, increased levels of high-density lipoproteins

likely to have clinical consequences when absorption is altered. An example of an interaction involving food is the increased absorption of the lipid-soluble drug griseofulvin with a meal containing fat. Enhanced bile acid activity induced by dietary fat is believed to be the mechanism.

Any delay in drug absorption caused by food does not necessarily mean that less of the drug is absorbed, but that more time elapses until a drug reaches its peak blood level after a single dose. When a high serum drug level is needed quickly, as in antibiotic therapy, a delay in the absorption rate may be significant. If drugs are sometimes taken on a full stomach and sometimes on an empty stomach, drug absorption may be erratic.

Dissolution Factors

Dissolution of dosage form and gastric emptying time are two major factors affecting the absorption of drugs (see the earlier discussion of absorption in the section on drug–drug interactions). Most oral drugs must disintegrate and dissolve before they can be absorbed through the intestinal mucosa. The rate at which a drug dissolves into solution from tablets or capsules is an important step in drug absorption. The dissolution rate is affected by the vehicle that delivers the drug to the stomach and by the stomach pH. When foods alter the pH, the rate and degree of breakdown may also change. Food and fluids may promote the disintegration of some tablets and improve the dissolution of some drugs (Box 6-4). For example, the acidity of gastric fluid favors the nonionized form of carbamazepine and phenytoin, thereby enhancing their absorption. Food in the stomach often raises the intragastric pH from 2 (the usual pH of stomach acid) to 5.

Gastric Motility Factors

Food in the stomach delays gastric emptying, which can have a significant effect on drug absorption. The rate at which a drug leaves the stomach depends on whether it is adsorbed to dietary fiber or suspended or dissolved in the fluid contents of the stomach. Slowed gastric emptying times may promote absorption of some drugs because it permits more drug to be dissolved in the stomach before passing on to the small intestine to be absorbed. On the other hand, longer retention in stomach acid may destroy some drugs. Gastric emptying may be retarded by the ingestion of heavy meals, meals containing fat, hot foods, solutions with a high viscosity, and to a lesser extent meals containing mainly carbohydrates. Drugs usually leave an empty stomach quickly (Table 6-4).

Mineral Factors

Minerals are important components of food. Among the various drug–food interactions associated with absorption are drug–mineral interactions (Box 6-5). These

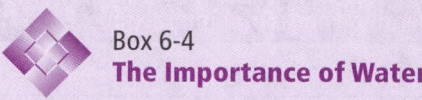

Box 6-4
The Importance of Water

Impaired drug dissolution and absorption may result from insufficient ingestion of a solvent such as water at the time of drug administration. Adequate fluid intake (about 8 oz for adults) is needed to promote disintegration and absorption of a drug's active ingredients.

Nurses must recognize that some clients, particularly older adults on diuretics or those with bladder function problems, try to take medications with as little fluid as possible. This practice can delay drug absorption.

In general, it is a good idea to advise clients to take drugs with water rather than soft drinks, acidic fruit or vegetable juices, or caffeinated beverages, which may alter absorption or contribute to a drug–food interaction.

interactions involve malabsorption of the mineral or drug or both, mineral depletion and retention, and several drug–mineral interactions. Six major minerals and 15 minor or trace elements are considered essential for normal biologic processes. Because of their relative abundance in foods, sodium, potassium, magnesium, calcium, phosphorus (as phosphate), iron, and zinc are frequently involved in drug interactions. Deficiencies in calcium and magnesium, for example, impair the rate of drug metabolism.

Many drug–mineral interactions are inconsequential; however, they are more significant when they occur in elderly clients, clients with poor nutrition, or clients on chronic medication therapy.

Interactions and Biotransformation

Proteins and fats are food components typically involved in drug–food interactions involving metabolism. Hepatic metabolism can be classified on the basis of biotransformation reactions into phase 1 or phase 2, whose net result is to decrease the pharmacologic activity and increase the excretability of drugs.

Phase 1 reactions are those most influenced by dietary manipulation. High-protein, low-carbohydrate diets can accelerate the metabolism of drugs by the liver. For example, theophylline and propranolol have shorter half-lives in clients who have a high-protein diet. In clients whose diet is low in protein, the metabolism of allopurinol seems reduced.

Fat-free diets or diets deficient in essential fatty acids also impair drug metabolism. On the other hand, high-fat meals can substantially increase the plasma level of free fatty acids. These molecules bind to plasma albumin at the same binding sites as numerous drugs. As

Table 6-4. Preventing Food–Drug Interactions: Drugs to Administer with Food or on an Empty Stomach

Drug Class	Drugs	Nursing Management
Drugs to Administer on Empty Stomach (to Promote Absorption)		
Antacids	aluminum hydroxide, calcium carbonate, magnesium hydroxide	Give 1 to 3 hr after meals and at bedtime.
Angiotensin-converting enzyme (ACE) inhibitors	captopril	Give 1 hr before meals.
Antimicrobials	amoxicillin, ampicillin, erythromycin, penicillin G	Give with 8 oz water.
	cephalexin, didanosine nafcillin,	
	metronidazole	Avoid use of alcohol during therapy.
	tetracycline	Avoid giving with fluids, foods, or drugs containing calcium.
Cardiotonics	digoxin	Avoid taking with high-fiber meal.
Laxatives	bisacodyl, mineral oil	Give with 8 oz water 1 hr after meal.
NSAIDs	acetaminophen, aspirin, ibuprofen	
Xanthines	theophylline	Avoid concurrent use of caffeine-containing foods and fluids.
Drugs to Administer with Food (to Enhance Absorption)		
Anticoagulants	warfarin	Limit vitamin K-rich foods.
Anticonvulsants	carbamazepine, phenytoin	Food minimizes GI side effects.
Antihypertensives	hydralazine, propranolol, reserpine	Food minimizes GI side effects.
Antilipemics	lovastatin	Administer with evening meal.
	cholestyramine	Administer with meal, but other drugs are to be given 1 hr before or 4–6 hr after this drug.
	nicotinic acid	Give with meal or just after meal.
Antimicrobials	griseofulvin	Meals with high fat content enhance absorption.
	isoniazid, ketoconazole, metronidazole	Food decreases GI side effects.
	nitrofurantoin	Food increases absorption.
Antineoplastic agents	busulfan, cyclophosphamide, hydroxyurea, melphalan, mercaptopurine, methotrexate, procarbazine, thioguanine	Give on full stomach, but withhold food if nausea and vomiting occur. Force fluids.
Diuretics	hydrochlorothiazide, spironolactone	Food increases absorption.
Histamine H$_2$ antagonists	cimetidine, famotidine, nizatidine, ranitidine	Do not give concurrently with antacids. The drugs impair iron absorption.
Minerals	iron, potassium	Food minimizes GI side effects.
NSAIDs	aspirin, ibuprofen, indomethacin	Food minimizes GI side effects but delays absorption.
Oral hypoglycemics	chlorpropamide, tolbutamide	Food minimizes GI side effects.
Psychoactive drugs	diazepam	
	lithium	Food minimizes GI and other side effects, such as laxative effect.
	phenothiazines	Food minimizes GI side effects.
Sedative–hypnotics	chloral hydrate	Food minimizes nausea and vomiting. Also administer with 8 oz fluid.
Steroidal hormones	cortisone, dexamethasone, methylprednisolone, prednisone	Food promotes more consistent blood drug levels.

a result, competitive binding and displacement occur when both drug and nutrient are present. The outcome is that high-fat meals displace some drugs from albumin enough to increase their pharmacologic and toxicologic properties.

Interactions and Excretion

The kidneys are the primary route for excretion of drugs and their metabolites. Excretion of acidic and basic salts varies depending on urinary pH. Because they are more soluble and more highly ionized in an acid medium, ba-

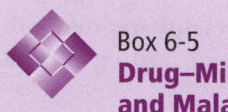

Box 6-5
Drug–Mineral Interactions and Malabsorption

Some drug–mineral interactions result in the malabsorption of minerals. The interaction may prevent the absorption of one or more minerals, or it may interfere with the absorption, disposition, or metabolism of an initial nutrient needed to absorb the mineral.

Mechanisms That Prevent Mineral Absorption

In drug-induced mineral malabsorption, the drug directly prevents the absorption of one or more minerals. Two modes of action are responsible for this phenomenon: 1) direct binding with the nutrient through chemical complexing, as in chelation, and 2) direct adverse action or damaging effect by the drug on the mucosal wall of the small intestine.

Aspirin and other acidic drugs can induce mucosal damage that alters the GI tract's ability to absorb minerals, particularly iron and calcium. Other drugs involved in primary malabsorption interactions are aluminum hydroxide, bisacodyl, cholestyramine, colchicine, lithium carbonate, methotrexate, methyldopa, mineral oil, neomycin, penicillamine, phenolphthalein, phenytoin, and tetracyclines.

Mechanisms That Interfere With Nutrient Absorption

Drugs can interfere with the absorption, disposition, or metabolism of a nutrient needed for absorbing a mineral. The adverse effect of a drug on vitamin D, which may result in calcium malabsorption, is an example of interference. Other drugs involved in interference with mineral absorption include prednisone, glutethimide, phenobarbital, phenytoin, and primidone.

sic drugs are excreted more readily in acid urine. The reverse is true of acidic drugs. For this reason, excretion of basic drugs is enhanced by the consumption of acid ash foods, whereas excretion of acidic drugs is enhanced by the consumption of alkaline ash foods.

Interactions Associated With Enteral Feeding

Several factors make concomitant enteral feeding and drug administration advantageous, especially for very sick and very old or frail clients (Box 6-6). A primary factor is the significantly decreased cost, because oral drug forms are usually less expensive than intravenous forms.

Medications may be administered via enteral feeding systems in two ways: by bolus or by placing the medication in the feeding container. The bolus method allows medications to be given on a schedule similar to that for oral drugs. This method favors such drugs as antihypertensives, because delivering such a drug in a continuous enteral feeding may not provide adequate blood-pressure control.

Altered Concentration

The bolus method presents problems due to the extremely high osmolalities of medications and the osmolality of the enteral formula. In general, enteral formulas that exceed 500 to 600 mOsm/kg should be diluted to avoid inducing osmotic diarrhea resulting from a hypertonic solution. When a hypertonic solution is given, the pyloric sphincter may constrict to maintain the physiologic osmolality of the stomach contents. In some

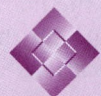

Box 6-6
Guidelines for Administering Medications and Enteral Feedings

Potential drug–food interactions may be prevented in some clients by following these guidelines:

- Administer a liquid form of medication, if possible. Avoid syrups; these cause clumping.
- Give crushed tablets only when no alternatives are available. Crush them completely; incomplete crushing can block holes of feeding tube with tablet particles.
- Do not crush enteric-coated or sustained-release preparations. Crushing the sustained-release form results in a high initial peak serum concentration and a later subtherapeutic concentration.
- Administer each drug separately. Do not mix medications; this helps avoid drug interactions. Flush the feeding tube with at least 5 mL of water between medications.
- Flush the feeding tube with at least 30 mL of warm water before and after giving medication. This clears the tube for giving the medication and helps deliver the drug to the intestine.
- Dilute drugs that are hypertonic or irritating to the GI mucosa with at least 30 mL of water to avoid GI irritation and diarrhea. Discontinue the feeding temporarily if more water is necessary for dilution.
- When it seems necessary to add medication to the enteral feeding bag, check first to see if it is recommended to give the medication this way; medications may be physically or chemically unstable in enteral feeding preparations or may interact with the preparation.
- When adding medication to the enteral feeding bag, add slowly and stir the mixture vigorously. Then observe for any precipitation, creaming, clumping, or flocculation. This helps detect any unanticipated interaction.

clients, the combination of a bolus of hypertonic medication and the residual volume of enteral feeding can be sufficient to cause gastric distention, nausea, and vomiting. To prevent this problem, the nurse may need to dilute the medication to lower the osmolality.

However, dilution may not provide an adequate solution to the problem. For example, flushing a dose of potassium chloride elixir with 10 to 20 mL of fluid through a feeding tube would still present the GI tract with a hypertonic bolus (Miyagawa, 1993). On the other hand, dilution with larger volumes, such as 8 oz of water or juice, may disrupt the feeding schedule when the diluted drug must be administered over 2 to 3 hours. An alternative is to place the medication dose in an enteral feeding bag. This alleviates problems associated with hypertonicity, but another problem may arise: maintaining the physical and chemical stability of the medication in the feeding container. Despite the many formulas and medications on the market, data on the chemical and physical stability of most medications in each enteral formula are unavailable.

Formulation

Drugs available as elixirs, solutions, and suspensions are easiest to administer by feeding tube. The most problematic liquid preparations are the syrups, specifically syrups that are either strongly acidic or buffered to a pH of 4 or below. Adding one of these syrups to an enteral formula results in immediate clumping and increases viscosity, particle size, and tackiness. Drugs in capsules at times may be administered by opening the capsule and reconstituting the contents with 10 to 15 mL of diluent.

Inaccurate drug delivery may stem from a physical incompatibility between the liquid drug form and the feeding tube. Undiluted carbamazepine suspension, for example, may adhere to the walls of a polyvinyl-chloride feeding tube, thereby decreasing drug delivery to the client. Diluting the carbamazepine, or diluting the drug and irrigating the tube, should alleviate the problem.

Altered Absorption

The absorption of phenytoin and warfarin is affected when they are used with enteral formulas. When the feeding tube empties directly into the small intestine and when phenytoin is followed by continuous feedings, GI residence time may not be adequate for total phenytoin dissolution, and the overall phenytoin bioavailability is correspondingly compromised. In addition, there may be a binding interaction between phenytoin and one or more components of the enteral formula. In such a case, the plasma phenytoin level must be carefully monitored because of phenytoin's narrow therapeutic index.

In clients receiving warfarin via enteral feedings, an interaction involving vitamin K in the formula may counter the anticoagulant effect of warfarin. To avoid this problem, drug administration and feeding times should be staggered. Continuous feedings should be discontinued 2 hours before and after drug administration. Theophylline and ciprofloxacin are two other drugs know to interact with enteral feeding formulas (Sacks and Brown, 1994).

■ SUMMARY

Foods and their components may influence the action of drugs by altering pharmacokinetic or pharmacodynamic processes. They may increase, decrease, or delay absorption. Drug–food interactions can involve alteration of complex enzymatic metabolic processes. Drug excretion may also be affected by the effects of foods on urinary pH.

❖ NURSING MANAGEMENT: DRUG–FOOD INTERACTIONS

The Joint Commission on Accreditation of Healthcare Organizations requires that drug–nutrient interaction counseling be provided to clients when appropriate. Implementation of this counseling usually involves nursing staff. As the healthcare practitioner with the closest and most prolonged contact with the client, the nurse plays a major role in protecting the client from drug–food interactions.

NURSING PROCESS

ASSESSMENT

A detailed dietary and food history must accompany a detailed medication history. Components of this part of the nursing history must include any history of adverse reactions to foods or food components. The nurse can compare these baseline data with data identifying potential interactions of the specific drugs with various foods.

NURSING DIAGNOSES

Nursing diagnoses identify actual or potential interactions between foods and drugs.

PLANNING

Identified outcomes or goals include reducing the risk of adverse food–drug interactions and promptly detecting and treating any reactions that develop. Measurable criteria for evaluation should be developed during the planning stage.

INTERVENTION

The nurse should schedule drug administration apart from mealtime, as appropriate.

Client Education. In teaching the client about the medication regimen, the nurse should explain the rationale for avoiding specific foods that pose a risk of adverse interaction with the client's medication. Additional teaching points include controlling the amount and timing of meals and snacks to prevent or minimize the risk of interaction.

OUTCOME EVALUATION

The nurse should measure the client's progress toward meeting the identified outcomes. Data required for evaluation include evidence of the presence or absence of drug–food interactions.

Drug–Laboratory Test Interactions

The goal of the clinical laboratory is to produce accurate and precise diagnostic results. Endogenous or exogenous compounds in body fluids may alter the results of laboratory tests. Major internal (endogenous) factors that affect laboratory test outcomes are lipemia, bilirubinemia, and proteinemia.

Exogenous Interferents

Major external (exogenous) interferents are medications. Exogenous interferents may produce a positive or negative bias in the test result. A positive interference increases the value of the result to greater than the true concentration of the analyte; a negative interference acts in the opposite direction.

Drugs are thought to be as important as age or excess weight in terms of their potential impact on laboratory test values. An early study found the percentage of laboratory tests affected by interference was 7% when the client took one drug and rose to 100% when the client took five drugs (Knoll and Elin, 1994). Such results are important because they may affect the care given the client and may increase healthcare costs.

Any medication given to any client by any route can alter a laboratory test result. Because medications are biologically active, they have a high probability of reacting with analytes or reagents. Cephalothin and cefoxitin, for example, cause positive interference with the Jaffe method for creatinine measurement. Ascorbic acid causes negative interference with glucose oxidase methods for determining glucose levels.

More than 150 drugs may alter the number and function of platelets. Therefore, blood tests in a client taking these drugs may inaccurately detect thrombocytosis, thrombocytopenia, and impaired platelet function. Thrombocytosis, or increased platelet counts, may result from corticosteroid use. Drugs that may cause thrombocytopenia are the cephalosporins, rifampin with ethambutol, aminosalicylate sodium (PAS), isoniazid, trimethoprim–sulfamethoxazole, gold salts, certain NSAIDs, valproic acid, carbamazepine, phenytoin, digitoxin, cimetidine, thiazide diuretics, quinine, quinidine, and colchicine.

The drug best known to impair platelet function is acetylsalicylic acid (aspirin); it prolongs bleeding time by inhibiting the release of endogenous adenosine diphosphate (ADP), adenosine triphosphate (ATP), and other substances, thereby hindering platelet aggregation. This effect lasts throughout the whole life of circulating platelets (4–7 days).

Metabolites

Metabolites of drugs may alter test findings as well. Some drugs are converted to metabolites that can be more reactive than the parent drug. Two different outcomes can occur with regard to interference: the metabolite has a different pharmaceutical function but reacts in the analytical system similar to the parent drug, or the parent drug does not react in the analytical system but the metabolite does.

Test results in clients taking phenytoin provide an example. Phenytoin and its major metabolite create false-positive results in tests measuring barbiturates. In another example, furosemide by itself does not interfere with the Jaffe test for creatinine determination, but in high doses a metabolite may form that causes negative interference.

Additives and Test Materials

Other examples of exogenous interferents are additives and test materials. Additives may be added to the blood collection tube to prevent coagulation, to inhibit glycolysis, and to seal the stopper. All the common additives for anticoagulation (heparin, EDTA, citrate, and oxalate) interfere with findings for many test specimens. In addition, control, calibration, and proficiency survey materials used with instruments in the laboratory may contain added substances that interfere with analysis. For instance, when salicylate is added to proficiency survey material, a falsely elevated theophylline value results.

❖ NURSING MANAGEMENT: DRUG–LABORATORY TEST INTERACTIONS

In compiling assessment data and reviewing test results, the nurse must remain alert to the possibility of drug–laboratory test interactions. Identifying and resolving interference with laboratory test findings calls for collaboration with the physician and laboratory personnel.

NURSING PROCESS

ASSESSMENT

A detailed medication history is part of the nursing history. The process of identifying interference by drugs with laboratory tests usually starts when the laboratory's monitoring system indicates a problem or the client's nurse or physician calls the laboratory because of an unusual laboratory result.

Interference due to an endogenous compound is usually detected by laboratory personnel and is identified as part of the report. A drug taken by the client is usually the exogenous compound interfering with the result. Laboratory personnel are key analysts when faced with a suspected drug–laboratory test interaction.

NURSING DIAGNOSES

Nursing diagnoses identify actual or potential interactions between drugs the client is taking and laboratory tests he or she is undergoing.

PLANNING

The nursing goals are to reduce any actual or potential detriment to the care of the client related to drug–laboratory test interactions and to prevent the added costs related to such interference.

INTERVENTION

Reviewing the medication history and current drug regimen is essential if a drug–laboratory test interaction is suspected. A follow-up discussion with the client's physician is equally important if the process has not been initiated by the physician. A confirmed drug–laboratory test interaction must be documented in the medical record. The information should be shared with the client and family for future reference.

OUTCOME EVALUATION

The nurse should examine the client's condition and record for evidence of problems related to drug–laboratory test interactions.

References

Abernethy DR, Andrawis NS. (1993). Critical drug interactions: A guide to important examples. *Drug Ther, 10*: 15–16.

Bailey DG, Arnold JMO, Spence JD. (1994). Grapefruit juice and drugs. *Clin Pharmacokinet 26*(2):91–98.

Hussar DA. (1993). Reviewing drug interactions. *Nursing '93, 9*:50–57.

Knoll MH, Elin RJ. (1994). Interference with clinical laboratory analyses. *Clinical Chemistry, 40*(11):1996–2005.

Kuhn M. (1993). Drug interactions and their nursing implications. *J NY State Nurses Assoc, 24*(2):10–16.

Miyagawa CI. (1993). Drug–nutrient interactions in critically ill patients. *Crit Care Nurse, 13*(5):69–72.

Sacks GS, Brown RO. (1994). Drug–nutrient interactions in patients receiving nutritional support. *Drug Ther, 3*:35–42.

Bibliography

Clark-Schmidt AL, Garnett WR, Lowe DR, et al. (1990). Loss of carbamazepine suspension through nasogastric feeding tubes. *Am J Hosp Pharm, 47*:2034–2037.

D'Arcy PF, McElnay JC, Welling PG (eds). (1996). *Mechanism of drug interactions.* New York: Springer-Verlag.

Davis JR, Sherer K. (1994). *Applied nutrition and diet therapy for nurses,* 2d ed. Philadelphia: WB Saunders.

Deppermann KM, Lode H. (1993). Fluoroquinolones: Interaction profile during enteral absorption. *Drugs, 45*(Suppl 3):5–72.

Fleischer D, Sheth N, Kou JH. (1990). Phenytoin interaction with enteral feedings administered through nasogastric tubes. *J Parent Enteral Nutr, 14*:513–516.

Lewis RJ, Sr. (1989). *Food additives handbook.* New York: Van Nostrand Reinhold.

Martin JE, Lutomski DM. (1989). Warfarin resistance and enteral feedings. *J Parent Enteral Nutr, 13*:206–208.

Mehta M (ed). (1995). *PDR guide to drug interactions, side effects, indications,* 49th ed. Montvale, NJ: Medical Economics Data Production Co.

Metcalfe DD, Sampson HA, Simon RA (eds). (1991). *Food allergy: Adverse reactions to foods and food additives.* Boston: Blackwell Scientific Publications.

Miyata M, Schuster B, Schellenberg R. (1992). Sulfite-containing Canadian pharmaceutical products available in 1991. *Can Med Assoc J, 147*(9):1333–1337.

Murray JJ, Healy SR. (1991). Drug–mineral interactions: A new responsibility for the hospital dietitian. *Perspectives in Practice, 91*(1):66–73.

Olin BR (ed). (1995). *Drug facts and comparisons.* St. Louis: Facts and Comparisons.

Siest G, Galteau MM. (1988). *Drug effects on laboratory test results, analytical interferences and pharmacological effects.* Littleton, MA: PSG Publishing Co., Inc.

Smith HT, Jokubaitis LA, Troendle AJ, Hwang DS, Robinson WT. (1993). Pharmacokinetics of fluvastatin and specific drug interactions. *Am J Hypertension, 6*(11, Part 2): 375S–382S.

Spatzenegger M, Jaeger W. (1995). Clinical importance of hepatic cytochrome P450 in drug metabolism. *Drug Metab Rev, 27*(3):397–427.

Teresi ME, Morgan DE. (1994). Attitudes of healthcare professionals toward patient counseling on drug–nutrient interactions. *Ann Pharmacother, 28*:576–579.

Tollefson GD. (1993). Adverse drug reactions/interactions in maintenance therapy. *J Clin Psychiatry, 54*(8, suppl):48–58.

Wells PS, Holbrook AM, Crowther NR, Hirsh J. (1994). Interactions of warfarin with drugs and food. *Ann Intern Med, 121*(9):676–683.

Williams L, Davis JA, Lowenthal D. (1993). The influence of food on the absorption and metabolism of drugs. *Med Clin North Am, 77*(4):815–829.

Young DS. (1990). *Effects of drugs on clinical laboratory tests,* 3rd ed. Washington, DC: AACC Press.

For more information and sample tests and activities, refer to Chapter 6 in the Student Workbook for Clinical Pharmacology and Nursing Management, 5th edition, available through your bookstore.

Administration of Medications

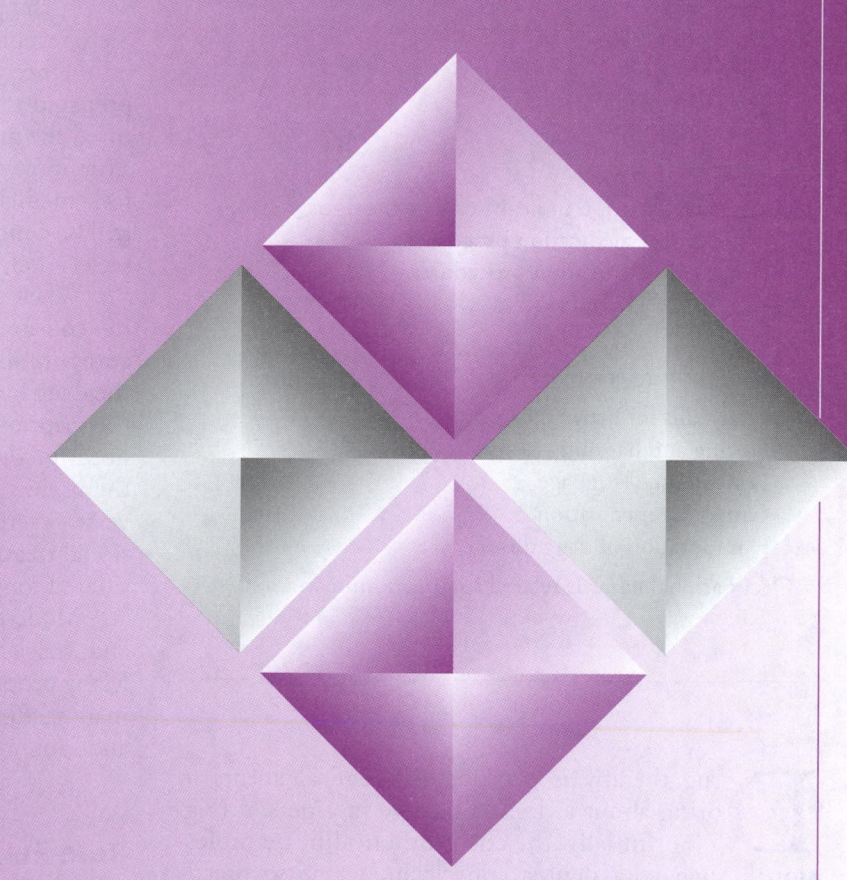

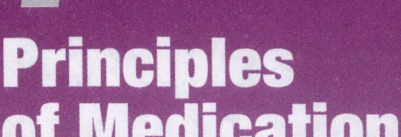

7

Principles
of Medication

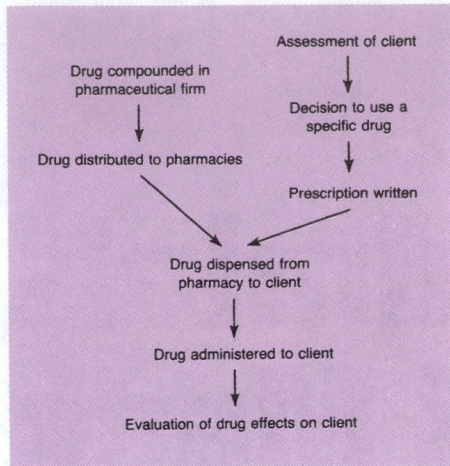

Figure 7-1. Series of events in drug therapy.

Drug therapy is the use of chemical agents to bring about a desired change in a person (Fig. 7-1). Initially, the client or a healthcare professional, such as a dentist, physician, or nurse practitioner, decides that the use of drugs is appropriate. A recommendation for a specific substance with directions for its use is called a *prescription*. Next, the required chemical is compounded or prepared. Most modern drugs are compounded in factories by large-scale production techniques. Distribution of a supply of drug is termed *dispensing*. From such supplies, individual doses are measured and delivered to the tissues of the client to be treated. Finally, the effects of the drug are determined.

In the past, one person customarily assumed complete responsibility for drug treatment. Healers decided on the needed treatment, gathered medicinal substances, prepared the dose, administered it to the client, monitored the drug's effects, and cared for the client until the situation was resolved. Today, for situations in which folk medicines are being used, the entire process may still be controlled by nonprofessionals—the person who seeks relief, relatives or acquaintances, and herbalists.

When over-the-counter (OTC) preparations are used, the consumer controls all steps in the process except for compounding and dispensing, which are performed by the drug industry and the pharmacist, respectively. If no prescription is required, consumers can determine their need for the drugs, purchase them, administer them to themselves, and monitor the results. Only if some adverse reaction occurs must the consumer seek professional treatment. Many potent drugs, however, are considered too dangerous for unsupervised lay use.

Modern medical care is characterized by complexity and specialization, and drug therapy is no exception. Many people are involved in the processes required for the manufacture, distribution, prescription, administration, and monitoring of drugs used to treat human diseases.

Role Functions Related to Drug Therapy

Within the formal healthcare system, stringent control is exercised over those who perform the steps in the drug therapy process. Among the healthcare professionals who can be involved in this process are pharmacists, physicians, dentists, physician's assistants, nurses, and technicians such as respiratory therapists.

Pharmacist

No matter what the setting, the preparation and distribution of drugs require the knowledge and expertise of trained professionals. The pharmacist is the professional licensed to compound and dispense drugs. Pharmacists' education involves a detailed study of drugs, their chemical, physical, therapeutic, and toxic properties, and the precautions required for their safe use. Pharmacists work in many settings, from the laboratories of drug firms to the pharmacies of healthcare agencies and the retail drugstore. The nurse works with these professionals primarily in the last two settings.

Pharmacists employed by large drug firms help develop manufacturing processes to convert raw medicinal materials into suitable dose units. They work with clients primarily in experimental situations that involve human testing of new substances for treatment. Pharmacists who work in healthcare agencies or drugstores are less frequently involved in the compounding of drugs because most drugs arrive from the manufacturer ready for consumption. Pharmacists may have to add solvent to substances that deteriorate after dissolution or mix solutions for intravenous (IV) infusion, but these processing procedures are usually a minor part of the preparation. Proper storage of drugs under safe and secure conditions is an important part of their responsibility. The pharmacist spends much of his or her time dispensing drugs, or packaging individual prescriptions with appropriate labels and directions for use.

The pharmacist's current role may include increased emphasis on the initial selection and monitoring of drug therapy. In institutional settings, this role may include dosage computations (including loading doses) and adjustments based on serum drug concentrations and pharmacokinetic principles. These professionals are eminently qualified to recognize actual and potential problems related to drug interactions, toxicities, and adverse reactions. Increasingly, pharmacists are required to provide client education. They are available for professional consultation with nurses and physicians. These broad clinical roles are also apparent in retail drugstores, where pharmacists commonly maintain drug profiles (or histories) for each client who purchases prescription drugs. These profiles help the pharmacist advise clients about measures to enhance therapeutic drug effects and reduce the risk of adverse reactions. When data on the profiles alert the pharmacist to potentially harmful drug interactions, he or she consults the prescriber, who may change the prescription.

Physician, Dentist, and Veterinarian

Diagnosis of diseases and prescription of drugs are limited by law in some states to physicians, dentists, or (for animals) veterinarians. Within the appropriate parameters of the field, each professional is responsible for determining the state of the subject's health, identifying disease processes, and deciding what treatment is required. When drug therapy is appropriate, the professional writes a prescription, known as an order, for the desired preparation. In compliance with the order, the pharmacist dispenses the drug to the client or the person responsible for the client's care. The professional who prescribes the drug also is responsible for modifying the treatment regimen as necessary and diagnosing and treating significant drug reactions, including toxicity. Physicians, dentists, and veterinarians retain the legal right to compound, dispense, and administer drugs when appropriate.

Paraprofessionals

The extension of medication privileges to paraprofessionals is recent. The right of technical personnel to prescribe or administer drugs may be specified by law. The drugs to be used and the situations appropriate for implementation by the paraprofessional are usually precisely defined.

Pharmacy Technician

Technically trained personnel are often assigned to large pharmacies to assist in the nonprofessional activities needed for the administration of this busy department. In some hospitals, technicians also administer certain medications, such as scheduled antibiotics. The pharmacist bears the responsibility for tasks he or she delegates to these staff members.

Physician's Assistant

The legal status of the physician's assistant varies from state to state, but in many states this healthcare practitioner is permitted to prescribe drug therapy in certain situations following established protocols. The safety of the practice depends on the supervision exercised over the assistant by the physician, a factor that varies by circumstances and from state to state. Because the right to prescribe, in some states, is limited by law to the physician or dentist, the propriety of delegating this responsibility has been challenged by nurses who have refused to follow the orders of a physician's assistant, arguing that in those states, nursing practice and licensing regulations designate only physicians and dentists as professionals whose prescriptions they may carry out. Because nurses are held legally responsible for any drug order they carry out, every nurse should challenge any drug order or any part of a drug order that is questionable. Nurses must know who is legally permitted to prescribe drug therapy according to the law regulating prescriptive authority in the state where they practice.

Practical or Vocational Nurse

Until recently, the administration of drugs by registered practical and vocational nurses was limited to chronic care facilities or private duty care (in which the nurse was directly supervised by the physician). Now, in acute care facilities, these nurses are being assigned to administer medicines, provided the individual nurse demonstrates the knowledge and skill needed for accurate and safe completion of the procedure. A similar demonstration of proficiency is also required of registered nurses (RNs). The administration by practical or vocational nurses of oral, topical, subcutaneous, and intramuscular medications is common in many agencies. Increasingly, they are also responsible for IV procedures, including drawing blood and establishing IV access.

Respiratory Therapist

Except for anesthetics, many substances given by inhalation are administered by the respiratory therapist. This practitioner is a recognized expert in the use of the special machines that deliver such drugs to the lungs. Drugs delivered by inhalation include gases (air, oxygen), humidifiers (saline solution), mucolytics (acetylcysteine), and decongestants (terbutaline, metaproterenol). These substances are readily absorbed from the alveolar membrane and may produce systemic side effects.

Unit Clerk and Unit Manager

Certain clerical aspects of drug therapy are often delegated to nonprofessional members of the unit staff. Transcribing orders, preparing medication administration records, the Kardex, or treatment sheets, ordering drugs from the pharmacy, and collecting information about clients' drug allergies are activities most often assigned to these assistants.

Professional Nurses

The traditional role of the professional RN in drug therapy in institutional settings is to administer medications prescribed by the physician. In its broadest sense, the term *administration* includes all activities related to safe drug use. Assessing the risk to a client of a new drug order, delivering the drug dose to the proper body tissues, assessing the client's response to drug therapy, treating adverse reactions to drugs, consulting with the physician about adjusting the prescribed regimen, and educating the client about the proper use of drug substances are all the RN's responsibilities. Thus, the nurse is directly concerned with every aspect of drug treatment. Even in the areas of prescribing and dispensing, the nurse verifies the accuracy of the actions taken by other professionals.

Trends in Role Assignments

Prescribing

Traditionally, the right to diagnose disease and prescribe treatment has been reserved for physicians and dentists. More recently, some physicians have delegated the choice of drug regimen to a physician's assistant or nurse practitioner. However, such prescriptions or orders may need to be countersigned by the physician.

The current trend toward granting limited prescribing privileges to nonphysicians has been influenced by: 1) better educational preparation of these healthcare professionals (pharmacists, physician's assistants, and nurses), 2) increased pressures for containing healthcare costs, and 3) decontrol of many prescription drugs by reclassification as OTC medications. Unfortunately, many insurance companies that reimburse their clients for prescription drugs no longer do so when the drugs are given OTC status. It has been argued that consumers who understand the drug regimens recommended by their physicians can manage their own care over the long term with the guidance and assistance of other healthcare professionals.

A number of states have granted limited prescription privileges to certain nurses who have advanced credentials, such as certified nurse practitioners. These privileges may be limited to specific drugs and approved protocols. In some cases, prescribing nurses must be supervised by physician overseers. The trend is toward gradual extension of these privileges.

Physician's assistants may also be given broader choices of drug treatment. Technically, assistants are directed and supervised by the physicians who employ them. In actual practice, the assistants assess clients and prescribe treatment (in accordance with standard protocols) with minimal physician involvement. In healthcare institutions, they renew medication orders and may order other drugs.

In the community setting, pharmacists have long recommended appropriate OTC preparations for treating minor or self-limiting conditions. With the recent decontrol of several drugs to OTC status, the number and effectiveness of agents available for such treatment have increased.

Compounding

Most drugs used as therapeutic agents are compounded by pharmaceutical firms. These firms supply convenient standardized dose forms of relatively pure drugs. However, the right to compound is retained by physicians, dentists, and pharmacists. Although unusual, a medication prepared by one of these professionals is perfectly legal to use.

Dispensing

Only physicians, dentists, and pharmacists have the legal right to dispense drugs for treating human disease. Nurses are not trained to dispense and cannot legally undertake this function.

Administering

At one time, physicians jealously guarded their prerogative to administer drug dosages. When nurses were first delegated this task, they were not informed what substances were being used, because medicines were identified by number rather than by name. Gradually, nurses gained more responsibility and authority in drug therapy. Today, hospital nurses are expected to administer oral and topical drugs, as well as parenteral drugs, including those injected directly into the vascular system. In many institutions, the management of IV therapy is recognized as a nursing specialty that requires advanced training. Oncology nurses sometimes administer intra-arterial or intrathecal medication. The administration of anesthesia by nurses is restricted legally to specially qualified persons. In other settings, such as physicians' offices, specialty functions include intralesional injection and the administration of hazardous drugs, such as allergenic extracts.

Only recently has anyone other than a professional nurse been allowed to administer medicines in acute healthcare institutions. Because the administration of drugs by vocational or practical nurses and respiratory therapists has proved efficient and relatively safe, it is likely that technical personnel will increasingly be used for this purpose. With proper training, physiotherapists could administer muscle relaxants or analgesics before treatment, and laboratory technicians could administer many diagnostic agents.

In the community, clients (or their caregivers) usually are responsible for administering medications. Increasingly, care is provided at home rather than in the hospital. Clients discharged from acute care settings to home care often have complex medication regimens. They may receive parenteral drugs by injection or infusion delivered through an implantable central venous catheter or an epidural line. Their lay caregivers must learn the techniques necessary for safe, effective drug administration.

In healthcare institutions, self-medication is less common, although clients are allowed to administer some of their own drugs. Topical preparations, such as ointments or lotions, commonly are left at the bedside for the client's use. Drugs such as cough syrups, antacids, and nitroglycerin also may be left at the bedside, provided the physician writes an order to this effect. Proposals that clients be given total responsibility for self-medication in these settings have not been well received, probably because physicians and nurses fear losing control over drug use. Before discharge from acute care settings, however, some clients may practice supervised self-medication to learn how to manage long-term medication regimens. Clients also may manage administration of opioid medication for acute pain by means of equipment that allows dosage up to the maximum prescribed by the physician. This procedure is termed *patient-controlled analgesia*. In such situations, accurate documentation must be maintained by the nursing staff. Drug, dosage, and route of administration are recorded. The times of specific doses are not monitored or recorded. Client response to medication (both therapeutic and adverse) must also be documented. The form of the medication record varies from agency to agency.

■ SUMMARY

Many healthcare professionals share the responsibility for drug therapy. The nurse's ongoing responsibilities continue to expand. In addition to administering drugs, some specially qualified nurses, such as nurse practitioners, have limited prescription privileges.

❖ NURSING MANAGEMENT

The trend toward delegating professional functions to personnel with less than professional preparation is not without risk. The safety of such practices depends on proper training and adequate supervision.

Nurses must be familiar with current state laws about prescriptions and should consult their state nurses' association for recommendations about the legal status of prescriptions issued by such nonphysicians as physician's assistants and nurse practitioners. Unless the status of these prescribers is legally clarified by state law, it is probably unwise to accept and carry out an order by such a practitioner without verification by the attending physician. When verification is omitted, the nurse may have no legal protection should a malpractice suit result from administering a drug. Regardless of legal status, the nurse should not hesitate to consult the physician about questionable orders.

When vocational or practical nurses, unlicensed assistive personnel (UAPs) and ward managers or clerks are assigned tasks related to drug therapy, the responsibility for their actions remains with the professional nurse. Nurses must allocate sufficient time and skill to train and supervise the personnel who operate under their jurisdiction. Nurses must also resist attempts to assign to personnel functions beyond the scope of their competence. Inappropriate responsibilities are sometimes delegated to ward clerks or pharmacy clerks. Nurses should protest such practices and work to strengthen institutional controls on role functions. The proper procedure is to document incidents that cause concern and present recommendations for administrative action through the existing chain of command to nursing service administration. Recommendations should be supported by evidence documenting the problem and a rationale for the change.

An example of inappropriate use of professional nurses is the request that supervising nurses dispense a supply of drugs from the institution's pharmacy "when necessary." This practice is most likely to occur in smaller healthcare institutions when not enough pharmacists are available to staff this department on a 24-hour basis. Because nurses do not receive the specialized training required for dispensing, and they are not licensed to do so, they should not accept such assignments. The issue may be resolved by calling in the pharmacist when needed or by securing drugs from a commercial pharmacy. Single doses may be given legally by the nurse from supplies in the pharmacy, as from any stock bottle.

NURSING PROCESS

ASSESSMENT

Before administering any medication, the nurse determines client risk factors that contraindicate use of the prescribed drug. Then the drug order should be evaluated to verify that it completely and appropriately relates to the client's condition and to reference data related to proper drug use.

NURSING DIAGNOSIS

Nursing diagnoses may relate to client problems that complicate implementing the drug regimen. For example, the client may have difficulty swallowing oral drugs, or tissue perfusion may be inadequate for the absorption of subcutaneous or intramuscular injections. In addition, the client may need education about the drug regimen.

PLANNING

The goal of care is to resolve problems related to drug therapy.

INTERVENTION

When problems with the drug order or with contraindications to drug administration arise, the nurse must consult the physician. If the consultation settles the nurse's concern about the order, the drug may be given, following the procedures adopted by the healthcare agency.

When drugs are ordered in a healthcare institution, certain clerical procedures are carried out to obtain the drug and to ensure its delivery to the client. The nurse usually is responsible for accurately transcribing drug orders and obtaining supplies from the pharmacy. The legal responsibility for these functions is the nurse's, although the actual tasks may be delegated to a unit secretary or another staff member. If these tasks are delegated, the nurse must provide proper supervision.

Drug Administration. In most healthcare institutions, the nurse (professional, practical, or vocational) is responsible for administering drug doses to clients or residents. Opinion is divided on whether only professional nurses should administer doses. Licensed practical or vocational nurses are taught the procedures of drug administration and perform them well in selected situations. Some healthcare agencies are considering delegating the dosing procedure to technicians with even less preparation in health sciences. Once the client's condition is properly assessed and the decision is made to give a particular drug, preparing the dose is primarily a matter of accuracy. The major concern is that the right drug be given to the right person, at the right time, by the right route, in the right amount. This process is facilitated by modern unit-dose drug delivery systems.

Some argue that dosing is a technical procedure that can be carried out by people with limited preparation. However, delivery of doses is not the simple activity it appears to be. For example, problems in administering the dose often arise. Clients with impaired gag reflexes may aspirate oral drugs if special precautions are not taken; injection sites must be chosen to facilitate appropriate absorption. Psychologic factors that influence the client's response to drugs are altered by the manner in which the medications are given: the attitude and skill of the person who administers the dose can enhance or diminish the client's response. For these reasons, the person who gives medication to a client should have the appropriate training and experience. The fact that a client's condition may change in the interim between professional assessment and technical administration of medications is another reason for having professional nurses retain the function of administering drug doses, especially in acute care situations. In such a case, the professional nurse could reconsider the decision to give a drug, whereas a technician may not detect the significant change.

In addition to executing the physician's drug orders, nurses influence the drug regimen in other ways. They may suggest to physicians or request from them orders for drugs that they think are appropriate. Nursing care includes psychologic and physical care measures to reduce the need for drugs and to enhance the effectiveness of the drug regimen.

Client Education. To grant legal consent to treatment, clients must be informed about the drug regimen. Indeed, safe treatment requires the client's intelligent cooperation. Teaching clients about treatment is a primary concern of the nurse. This education may be aimed at helping clients derive the greatest benefit from the drug regimen while in the acute care setting, or it may prepare them to manage their own drug regimens after discharge.

Nurses provide appropriate information to the client about drugs and plans for treatment. They help clients integrate their drug regimens into their daily routines. These nursing functions apply to OTC preparations and nonmedicinal drugs as well as to prescription medications. Proper instruction about drugs may reduce the client's need for drugs or enhance the effect of those taken. In addition, clients must be reassured about minor side effects and learn techniques for minimizing them. Clients should learn the precautions that accompany accurate drug preparation and administration. They also must learn the signs and symptoms of adverse reactions (including toxicity) so they can judge when to contact the physician and whether to stop taking drug doses pending changes in the regimen.

Effective client education requires that the nurse be knowledgeable about drugs and drug therapy and be skilled in teaching techniques. In addition to offering the client accurate pharmacologic information, nurses must be able to judge the client's readiness to learn and to choose appropriate teaching approaches and materials.

Documentation. All data pertaining to medication procedures and client response to drugs must be recorded on the client's chart. The information should be precise and accurate. All doses should be entered with complete details, including the drug name, dose, route of administration, and exact time of administration. The common practice of charting a dose as if it had been given precisely at the time scheduled, when drugs are actually administered as much as 20 to 30 minutes before or after the hour, is potentially dangerous. It may be crucial in some instances to determine whether a drug ordered for 10 AM was actually given at 9:30 AM or 10:30 AM. Moreover, the reliability of the medical record as a legal document is placed in question when careless documentation becomes evident in court.

An accurate chart is an invaluable tool in assessing clients for drug-related problems. It provides the data needed to establish relations between medication and the emergence of signs and symptoms of adverse reactions. It can establish whether the desired therapeutic response is occurring. Accumulated data in charts are also a valuable resource for research by healthcare professionals.

OUTCOME EVALUATION

A critical responsibility of the professional nurse is monitoring: assessing, reporting, and recording the client's response to drug therapy. The quantity of drugs prescribed for the client is only an educated approximation based on the physician's estimate of the client's needs. In accordance with the client's size, age, health status, and drug history, the physician selects an agent and a drug dosage likely to accomplish the desired therapeutic result. Whether the anticipated effect will in fact occur remains unknown until the client's response is evaluated. The following factors may influence the result.

- The dose actually administered may not correspond exactly to the ordered dose written by the physician. In manufacturing doses, drug firms are allowed to deviate from the designated dose level, often as much as 10%. When fractional doses must be prepared, a further deviation up to 10% may be acceptable. This deviation is dictated by the limitations of measuring devices and the inexactitude of mathematical computations used in converting from one measurement system to another. In extreme instances, when both deviations are maximal, the actual dose given may be as much as 20% above or below the dose the physician ordered.
- The client may absorb the drug more slowly or more rapidly than anticipated. Occasionally, the dose may not be absorbed at all.

- The drug may be transported or stored in the body in unexpected ways, causing more or less of the drug than anticipated to be available to metabolic processes.
- Due to individual differences in metabolism and enzyme systems, the recipient may degrade the drug more or less rapidly than expected.
- Excretion of the drug may vary due to abnormal function of the organs involved in degrading and eliminating the drug.
- An altered state of health may change the recipient's sensitivity to the effects of the drug.
- Allergy may alter the drug's effect or cause harmful reactions.

The initial administration of a drug involves giving an approximate dose to a client whose physiologic response to the substance is at best estimated and at worst completely unknown. Physicians are aware of these uncertainties in therapy and rely on the client or nurse to report significant data about the client's response. Using this information, they can make necessary adjustments and refinements in the drug regimen to achieve the desired therapeutic results.

In assessing the client's response to therapy, the nurse verifies the improvement that is expected from drug action and detects adverse reactions. Then the nurse judges which responses require medical interaction and should be reported to the physician and which indicate minor responses amenable to nursing intervention. Assessment of a client's response to drug therapy is carried out systematically and conscientiously. In the acute care setting, the nurse is responsible for recording these evaluations and promptly reporting data useful to other caregivers. Because they are the professionals who have the most frequent contact with clients, nurses are responsible for observing and reporting clients' responses to drugs. The nurse determines when the physician should be consulted and may temporarily suspend the drug regimen or initiate emergency action when required. Sound professional judgment is required for this critical aspect of drug therapy.

As the responsibility for administering drugs is disbursed among various healthcare personnel, the risk of inadequate evaluation of a client's response increases. Nurses must be aware of all drugs taken by the client, must assess the client regularly and comprehensively for therapeutic response and adverse reactions, and must intervene when necessary to ensure optimal drug therapy.

Evaluation of drug-related care must consider not only client outcomes but also the proper implementation of nursing interventions. In other words, the nurse must ask if the nursing plan was implemented as projected and if the interventions produced the desired effect. To determine the accuracy and consistency with which the nursing plan was carried out, the nurse should consider such questions as: Was a proper drug history taken? Were the effects of the drug treatment assessed regularly and systematically? Was the physician consulted when appropriate? Were the prescribed drugs delivered to the client accurately? Were nursing measures designed to augment the drug treatment or reduce side effects carried out as ordered? Was the teaching program implemented as planned?

To determine the results in terms of the client's outcome, appropriate questions might be: Did the client's symptoms subside? Were side effects detected and controlled? Were drug reactions treated appropriately? Did the client demonstrate an adequate understanding of the prescribed regimen? Did the client emotionally accept the treatment plan? Did the client comply with the prescribed regimen at home? Did the client consult the physician appropriately? Data accumulated during this evaluation are incorporated in the assessment phase of the nursing process as care is continued.

Delivery of Drug Doses

Once a decision for medication is made, the skill with which the medication is prepared and administered becomes paramount. No matter who prepares the dose or where it is administered, the accuracy of five factors must be ensured: the right drug, the right dose, the right client, the right route, and the right time (Box 7-1).

The Right Drug

To ensure that the right drug is administered, the nurse checks the drug label, the Kardex, and the medication administration record. Nurses should prepare the medications they give. They should not deliver to clients drugs prepared by someone else, because the person who administers the medication is held responsible. If a client questions the medication, the nurse should recheck the order, label, and medication card. A mentally alert client will notice a change in medication or may mention problems that have arisen from the medication. Nurses should never ignore these statements and questions.

All doses are best prepared from the original container. It is impossible to read the package label as rec-

ommended if the medicine has been removed from the original container. Medication should never be poured in the dark, and clients should not be allowed to take medication in the dark. Good illumination is necessary for positive identification. Always read drug labels three times (Fig. 7-2). Caution clients about using unlabeled pillboxes, such as the decorative porcelain, purse-sized cases. Also discourage the practice of mixing supplies of several tablets or capsules in a single container from which doses are selected on the basis of appearance alone.

The Right Dose

To obtain the right dose, measure the medicine carefully (Fig. 7-3). Measurement is fairly easy with dry capsules or tablets. If the client requires half a tablet, split scored tablets into two pieces with a knife, or fold the tablet in clean paper and break it with the fingers. Give the two halves of a tablet in successive doses, so that any deviation from the prescribed dose due to uneven breakage levels out as quickly as possible. It is unwise to break all the tablets available and mix the halves. Although this method may appear efficient and convenient, undue fluctuation in the doses is likely. For example, all the larger halves may be taken first, causing overmedication during the first half of the course of treatment and undermedication during the second half. Do not attempt to split unscored tablets or divide the dose of a single capsule (see the Critical Thinking Challenge: Case Analysis).

Measure liquid medications into a container with a scale that has a mark corresponding to the ordered dose. Inexpensive plastic medicine cups or spoons may be purchased for accurate measurement of liquids. If these are unavailable, kitchen measuring spoons are preferable to tablespoons, which may vary considerably in volume. Some liquid medicines are marketed with a measuring utensil, such as a scaled dropper. Figure 7-4

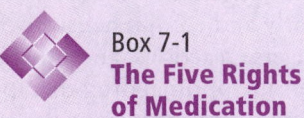

Box 7-1
The Five Rights of Medication

1. The RIGHT drug
2. The RIGHT dose
3. The RIGHT client
4. The RIGHT route
5. The RIGHT time

CRITICAL THINKING CHALLENGE
Case Analysis

The following is based on an actual experience that occurred when the medication prescribed below had just been approved for general use. How would you resolve this situation to derive the greatest benefit for the client with the least risk?

A client was beginning hemodialysis treatment for renal failure. The physician ordered cimetidine, 150 mg, PO, q6h. The pharmacy delivered cimetidine tablets containing 300 mg each. The tablets were not scored. They appeared to have a lustrous coating. The pharmacy had no other preparation of the drug and said this was the only form of the drug marketed at the time.

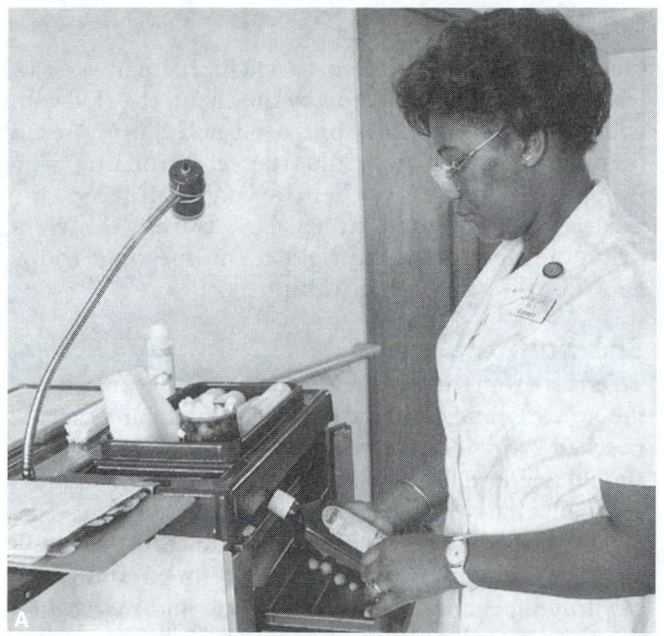

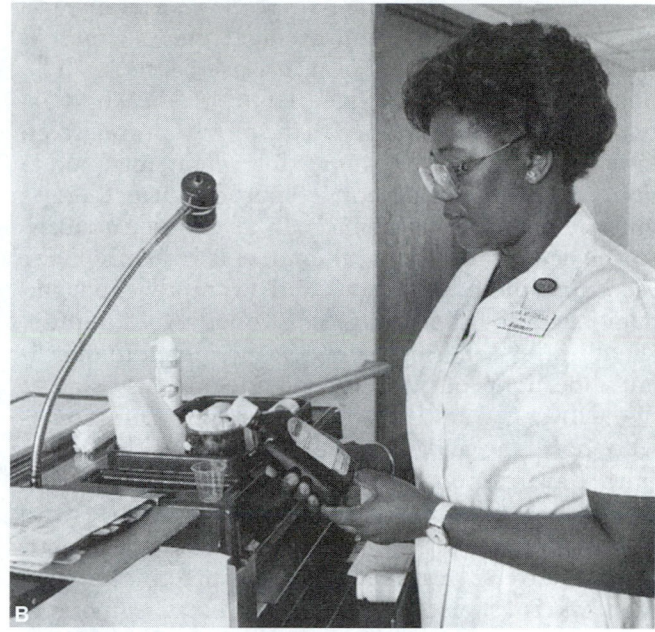

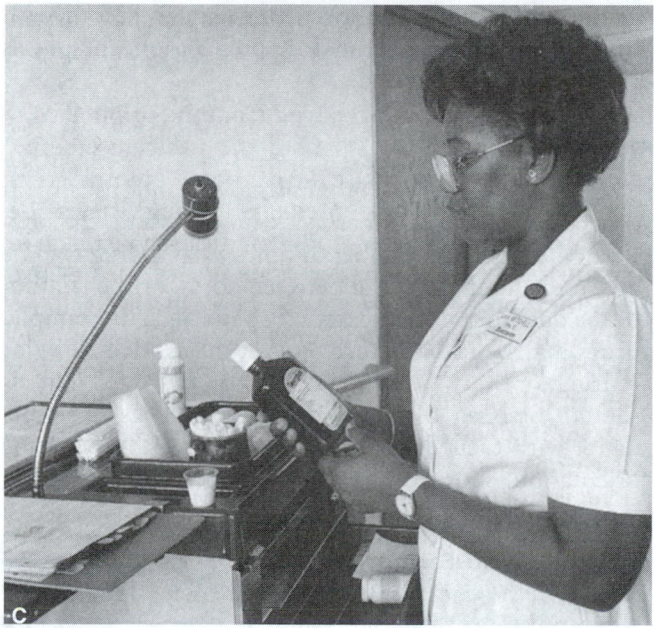

Figure 7-2. Medication labels should be checked (**A**) when removed from the shelf; (**B**) before pouring or measuring; (**C**) when returned to the shelf. Copyright © B. Proud

illustrates several measuring devices for liquids; Figure 7-5 illustrates the correct method for measuring liquids in a cup.

The Right Client

Making sure the right client receives the right drug is rarely a problem outside of institutions. Relatives and lay attendants are likely to know the recipient very well. However, medicines recommended or prescribed for one person are sometimes offered or given to another. This practice can be dangerous. Even if both people are suffering from the same medical condition, a drug suitable for one person may be totally unsuitable for the other.

Drugs should be given only to the person for whom they are prescribed or recommended. Figure 7-6 illustrates how nurses in an agency identify clients by checking their identification bracelets.

Within single households or family groups, it is sometimes necessary to medicate several members for an identical condition. For example, contagious illness is likely to be shared in such close groups. Related members may be subject to familial ailments and respond similarly to drugs. Even in these situations, the physician should be consulted before using one person's prescription for another. The drug best suited for one person may be ineffective or even dangerous when

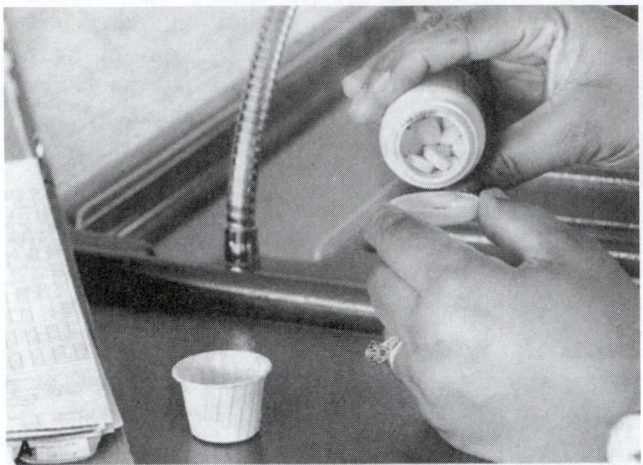

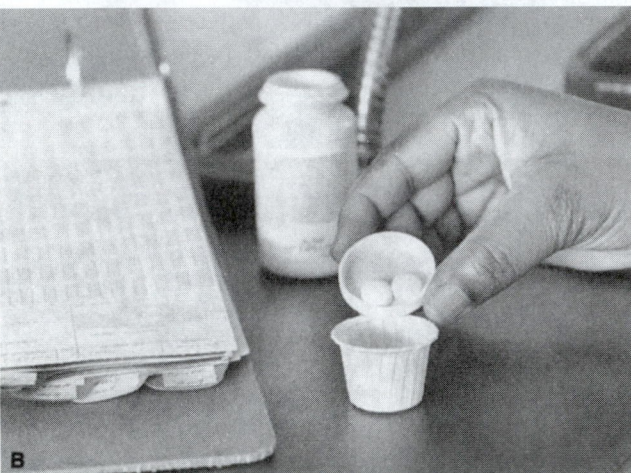

Figure 7-3. The proper technique for pouring solid drugs, such as capsules and tablets. To minimize handling of drugs, the required number of units in the dose are first **(A)** poured into the container's cap and then **(B)** poured from the cap to the medication cup. Copyright © B. Proud

given to another. If a physician does wish to treat more than one person with a drug, it is preferable to write individual prescriptions for each. In the rare situation that involves dosing of more than one person from a single drug supply, written records should be kept to ensure accurate medication.

The Right Route

The right route must be used for drug delivery. Outside of healthcare institutions, most medicines are taken orally or by topical application. The client must clearly understand how the drug is to be taken. Sublingual or chewable tablets should not be swallowed whole. If swallowing is difficult, oral drugs should be crushed or taken in liquid form. However, sustained-release oral products must not be crushed.

Clients who must use parenteral drugs require careful training in injection techniques. Procedures for the application of topical drugs should also be demonstrated to clients and practiced by them. Nurses in institutions must be aware of the usual routes for adminis-

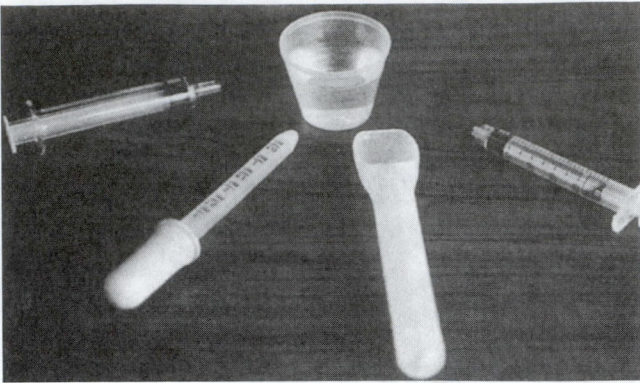

Figure 7-4. Devices used to measure liquid medication accurately: (*left to right*) oral syringe, dropper, medicine cup, spoonlike device, injection syringe without needle.

tering medications. Giving medication by the wrong route can cause death, and the person who administers the drug is held responsible. The nurse should check the physician's orders and the Kardex to verify the medication route. If the route specified is not in accord with that recommended for the drug preparation, the physician should be consulted.

The Right Time

The right time for drug administration is not usually indicated by the physician as clock time. Instead, the physician indicates the number of times a day a drug is to be given, the hourly interval between doses, or the relation of the dose to the client's activity patterns. For example, drugs may be taken before or after meals, on arising or retiring, or every 4 hours, 6 hours, or 12 hours. Clients should establish the times for taking drugs in accordance with their daily routine. Clients with poor time orientation, short-term memory defects, or distracting

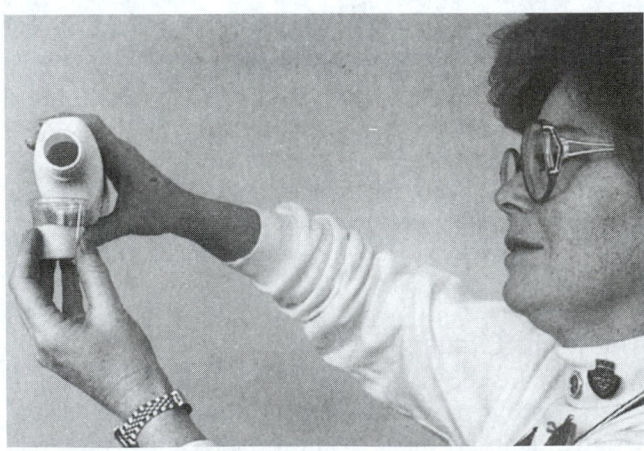

Figure 7-5. To pour a liquid medication, the nurse places a thumbnail at the marking on the medication cup to indicate the dose ordered for the client. The glass and medication bottle are held at eye level so that the meniscus is clearly visible, and the bottle label faces the nurse's palm so that the solution does not drip on the label. Copyright © B. Proud

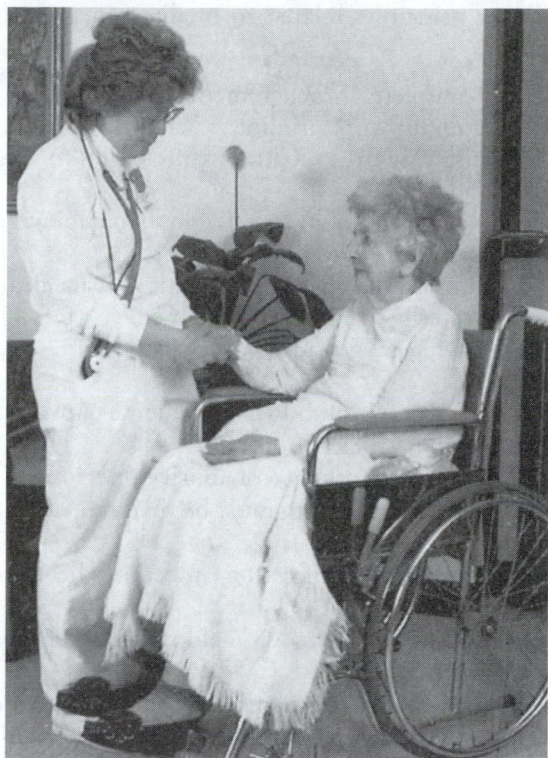

Figure 7-6. The client's name on his or her identification bracelet is checked with the name on the medication card in the nurse's hand. This check is essential to avoid errors.

activity schedules need some system for guiding them in self-medication. Many clients find it helpful to dispense the doses required for the day at one time, labeling each dose with the date or day of the week and the hour it is to be taken. Nursing personnel in hospitals and other institutions set up routines for intervals and times for medication. The effects of drugs may vary greatly at different times in different clients (eg, over the diurnal biologic cycles [Byers and Noll, 1995]). Each medication nurse must be familiar with classes of medications and the appropriate times for administering them.

Drug Administration in Healthcare Institutions

The current trend toward self-medication by clients is best illustrated in health-related facilities, where clients have been controlling their drug regimens for some time. Skilled nursing facilities and acute care agencies have been slower to adopt this practice, even in situations in which clients are alert, responsible, and energetic enough to take their own drugs.

In some acute care institutions, however, self-medication may be started before discharge as part of client education in the management of the medical regimen at home. For the most part, however, medicines are controlled and administered by the nursing staff. The system that is used depends on the organizational pattern of the nursing service.

When total client care is given by one person, such as with a private duty nurse, this person should administer the client's medications for the entire work shift. In primary nursing, one nurse controls all care but shares caregiving activities with other staff members. Either the primary nurse or an associate nurse may administer drugs in this system. When team nursing is the pattern of care, a variety of assignment patterns may be used. Qualified team members may be assigned to give medications to clients whose care is their responsibility. Clients assigned to aides or (in some institutions) practical or vocational nurses must be assigned to qualified personnel for medication. Often one team member is assigned to medicate all clients cared for by the team. In units with functional assignments, one nurse administers drugs to all clients in the unit; usually this is the only duty assigned to this nurse.

From the standpoint of continuity and comprehensive client care, medications should be administered by the nurse most familiar with the client. However, such a method of assignment involves many people in handling drugs. In a typical nursing unit, medication activities are limited to a small room centrally located in the unit and to the medication cart, which moves from client unit to client unit. Use of these areas by many people results in congestion and confusion. Accuracy, efficiency, and drug security are difficult to maintain. Indeed, in some states, regulations prohibit the use of the narcotic key by anyone other than the staff member responsible for controlled drug security and require that drugs be recounted each time a different person takes the key. To avoid these problems, many institutions use some form of functional assignment for medications.

Under the functional method, one nurse per unit or team is assigned to give drugs to all clients cared for by that unit or team. In some cases, one nurse is assigned to administer routine drugs (those given repeatedly at regular intervals) and another staff member gives all other medications (such as one-time-only doses or drugs given as needed to control symptoms). Such a system divides the workload (which may be too great for one person) and reduces the number of interruptions of routine medications. It also usually shortens the intervals between requests by clients for symptom-relieving drugs and their delivery.

Policies about who is allowed to give drugs vary from institution to institution. It is increasingly recognized that basic nursing education cannot provide the beginning practitioner with a high degree of skill in all procedures of all specialties in practice. Acute care facilities may restrict medication assignments to RNs who have demonstrated proficiency in these skills. Staff members must pass a proficiency test or complete a special course of study before they are allowed to administer drugs. Certain procedures, usually IV medication, may be restricted to specially skilled staff members. Other hospitals assign licensed practical or vocational nurses to give medications, provided they have completed a training program. In skilled nursing facilities, medications usually are administered by practical or vocational nurses.

No matter what method of assignment is used or what the criteria are for personnel, standard procedures are adopted for administering medications. Two systems can be used, one relying on medication cards and another using medication carts. Drugs for either system may be dispensed from stock bottles or packaged in unit doses. The trend is moving toward unit-dose packaging, individual client supplies, and the use of medication carts.

Institutional Medication Procedures

Elaborate procedures have been developed for delivering drug doses in institutions. Ritualistic precautions ensure accuracy and avoid errors. Despite these precautions, medication errors continue to be a serious problem for many reasons. Probably the most significant is the tendency for practitioners to depart from routine precautions to one or the other extreme, either ignoring the details of prescribed routines (cutting corners) or relying slavishly on ritual without exercising judgment. Carefully observing routine precautions provides many safeguards to avoid error, but the principles that underlie the steps in the routine must be clearly understood. Then, adherence to these principles guides the practitioner when he or she must deviate from the set routine.

Details of medication administration procedures may vary from institution to institution, but the fundamental principles remain the same. For example, to ensure that the correct drug is given, drugs should be identified with a correctly written label at all steps in the procedure. This principle underlies the following rules followed by most institutions:

- Drug containers are labeled only in the pharmacy by the pharmacist. A container with a soiled or illegible label should be returned to the pharmacy for relabeling.
- Several different drugs may be poured out into one cup for one client, provided that none is a controlled drug and that the names of all the drugs are indicated in some way. If the client does not take all the drugs mixed in this way, all must be discarded and the required drugs repoured, because individual drugs cannot be identified by appearance alone for removal from the group.
- Narcotics must always be specifically identified by a written label. Because narcotics must be carefully accounted for, they are usually returned to the hospital pharmacy if they have been poured and subsequently not used.

Other principles related to medication procedures include:

- Neat, completely stocked medication areas and organization of work promote safety and efficiency in administering drugs. Clutter contributes to confusion and error.
- Original orders are more reliable than copies, which are subject to copying errors.
- To minimize the chance of infection, drug cleanliness or sterility must be maintained.
- Careful, repeated reading of labels promotes accuracy.
- Unnecessary use of multiple medicine cups is costly and inefficient.
- To minimize the chance of abusive or erroneous drug use, drug security must be maintained at all times.
- Careful client identification procedures help prevent errors.
- Drug doses should be withheld if likely to harm the client.
- Written notes are more reliable than mental ones.
- Accurate charting is essential to guide treatment and nursing care and to ensure reliable documentation for legal purposes.
- Accurate evaluation of the client's responses is needed to guide treatment management.

The nurse should study the medication procedure before attempting to administer drug doses. Rather than memorizing steps or specifics of the procedures, which may vary from situation to situation, the nurse must develop the capacity to evaluate the principles underlying a given procedure. Then revisions may be suggested or adaptations safely made to improve practice in a given situation.

Home Care Medication Procedures

In the home setting, nursing care focuses on teaching clients or their families (or both) to manage the drug regimen. Nurses also may be responsible for procedures such as inserting IV needles or catheters or preloading syringes for self-medication (eg, for clients with impaired visual or manual dexterity). In addition to teaching clients to monitor drug effects, the nurse must always make independent assessments of their response to medication.

Medication Errors

The National Coordinating Council for Medication Error Reporting and Prevention has established a working definition of the term *medication error*: "any preventable event that may cause or lead to inappropriate medication use or patient harm, while the medication is in the control of the healthcare professional, patient, or consumer." Such events may be related to professional practice or healthcare products, procedures, and systems, including prescribing, order communication, product labeling, packaging, and nomenclature, compounding, dispensing, distribution, administration, education, monitoring, and use.

This definition is comprehensive and may be useful for minimizing events that adversely affect clients receiving medications. However, it covers many situations beyond the nurse's control. Therefore, the following discussion focuses only on situations in which the nurse is responsible for measuring and delivering drug doses.

Causes

Despite the elaborate rituals used for administering drugs, medication errors continue to be a serious problem in many institutions. Statistics on errors vary and are affected in part by the criteria used to determine what is an error. Allowable margins are often arbitrarily determined in relation to the five "rights" of correct administration.

There is no question that an error has occurred when a drug is administered to the wrong client or when the wrong medication is given. However, the use of an inappropriate route is not always so clearly delineated. It may be difficult to determine whether a drug ordered for subcutaneous delivery actually enters muscle tissue if the needle selected was disproportionately long for a client's thin layer of subcutaneous tissue. Inadvertent IV injection may be difficult to substantiate if it was caused by shifting of the position of the needle tip in the tissues during the drug's injection. Most institutions have clear policies that require a written physician's order for injecting a drug previously given by mouth. Guidelines may be less definite about changing a parenteral to an oral drug form when a client regains the ability to ingest medication. In such situations, erroneous administration routes tend to be underreported.

Errors in timing, on the other hand, are often overreported. Definitions of such errors tend to be narrow, often specifying that medications given more than 20 or 30 minutes before or after the designated hour are in error. The validity of this timetable is questionable, because the actual hours are assigned arbitrarily by the nursing staff and the intent of the physician's order may be carried out properly with much greater tolerance for deviation.

For most drugs, a deviation of as much as 10% is allowed between the dose ordered and the dose received by the client. Some of the discrepancy arises from the conversion of doses from one system of measurement to another. True discrepancies arise when the physician's order specifies doses that cannot be measured precisely by the tools available to the nurse in charge of medication. Certain drugs, such as antineoplastics, insulin, heparin, and certain cardiac drugs, are considered so potentially dangerous that doses are expected to be more exact, and the 10% deviation is not allowed.

Although medication error statistics must be interpreted in relation to recording procedures and criteria, potentially harmful errors occur too frequently in healthcare institutions. Mistakes in drug administration may arise at any step in the process from the physician's order to the delivery of the dose to the client. The following discussion points out errors and suggests ways to avoid them (Box 7-2).

Recording and Transcribing Orders

Whenever possible, orders should be written by the physician. Telephone orders and verbal orders under certain circumstances (eg, if the physician is scrubbed for a surgical procedure) may be written by a nurse, provided they are countersigned by the physician as soon as possible. Exceptions in some states are orders for schedule II controlled substances, which cannot be transmitted legally by telephone. The nurse who takes a spoken order should always read it back to the physician for verification. If pronunciation is unclear, the drug name should be spelled to ensure accuracy. Drug orders should always include the name of the client, the name of the drug, the dose, the route of administration, and the frequency or timing of doses. The nurse should ask the physician to verify the route desired if no route has been specified. Although physicians tend to omit the route when oral drugs are ordered, it is not safe to assume that the oral route was intended. Policies that govern the role of student nurses in taking verbal orders vary from agency to agency. In general, a licensed nurse (instructor or staff member) listens to the orders with the student and cosigns the order written by the student. As with all verbal orders, the physician must countersign the order written by the nurse as soon as possible.

The handwriting of many physicians is illegible. If doubt about any element of a drug order exists, oral verification must be sought from the physician involved. Written orders also occasionally contain errors in dose, drug form, or other elements. If any part of the order appears inappropriate, the physician should be contacted and given the opportunity to correct any mistakes that may have been made.

Labeling of Drugs

Sometimes, pharmacy labels on drug containers do not use the same terms as the physician's order. For example, the physician may have ordered the drug by its trade name, but the pharmacy dispensed it by its generic name. Most pharmacists label preparations with metric doses, whereas some physicians still use apothecary doses. Discrepancies in terms must be reconciled. After verifying the drug name or dose, the nurse may add the terms used on the pharmacy label to the entry on the medication record and Kardex. Such additions are usually enclosed in parentheses.

Box 7-2
Sources of Medication Errors and Precautions

Inaccurate Recording and Transcribing of Order

1. Orders should be written by the prescriber.
2. Some telephone and verbal orders may be written by a nurse provided they are countersigned by the prescriber as soon as possible.
3. The nurse who takes a verbal order should read it back to the prescriber.
4. Drug names should be spelled out if they are unclear.
5. Drug orders should include name of client, name of drug, dose, route of administration, and frequency or timing of doses.
6. If any part of the order seems inappropriate or illegible the prescriber should be contacted and given the opportunity to make corrections.

Unclear or Erroneous Labeling of Drugs

1. Discrepancies in terms (eg, generic and trade name) and measurement systems must be clarified. Nurses may add equivalent terms in parentheses on medication card or Kardex.
2. Liquid medicine bottles should be held with label facing the palm of the hand to prevent soilage of label.
3. If labels are damaged, bottles must be returned to the pharmacy for relabeling.

Misidentification of Client

1. If the client has no identification band, the nurse asks the client to give his or her name; the client's name is not used. The nurse avoids saying "Is your name Pat?" Rather, the nurse says "Can you please give me your name?"
2. A method that encourages cooperation rather than causes sarcasm or confusion should be used.
3. Clients who cannot respond with their names should wear a visible name label at all times, as should clients who cannot hear.
4. Recent photographs of the client are useful in some institutions.

Incomplete Delivery of Drugs

1. Injection sites must be selected with absorption in mind.
2. Drugs are best given by IV or inhalation route to clients in shock.
3. Topical drugs must contact the affected tissue.
4. Topical applications must be protected from friction that will remove them.
5. With oral administration, the nurse must verify that the client swallows the drug with a sufficient amount of fluid.
6. With clients who have problems swallowing, the nurse should inspect the client's mouth after administration to be sure the medicine was swallowed.
7. Solid medications (excluding sustained-release preparations) can be crushed for ease in swallowing, or liquid preparations can be given.
8. If the client is truly incompetent, medications may have to be forced. This action jeopardizes the nurse–patient relationship.

Verification Errors

1. The nurse must make a conscious effort to concentrate on thorough verification of orders.
2. Written materials must be compared; reliance on memory is risky.
3. Dose must be labeled for identification between pouring and administration.

Use of Inaccurate Knowledge or Inadequate Knowledge Base

1. Reliance on memory should be eliminated whenever possible.
2. Facts should be verified in reference sources.

Time and Performance Pressures

1. Workload should be appropriate for the skill and efficiency of the medication nurse.
2. Creative approaches and sound nursing judgment are needed to maintain accuracy and efficiency.

Labels on liquid drugs may become soiled if the solution drips on the label during pouring. To keep the label clean, the nurse should hold the bottle with its label facing the palm of the hand while measuring the drug. If labels are damaged or soiled, the bottle should be returned to the pharmacy for relabeling.

Identifying the Client
Occasionally, a client who requires medication is not wearing an identification band. The band may have been removed temporarily to facilitate IV infusion or some other procedure, or it may have been removed permanently due to the client's allergic hypersensitivity to its materials. In these situations, it is best to ask the client his or her name. Do not ask, "Is your name Pat Doe?" Clients who do not understand what has been said may answer affirmatively merely to acknowledge the communication. Misunderstandings of this type are especially likely during night and early morning hours, when clients are sleepy and are not using their hearing aids or eyeglasses. If a client is unfamiliar to the nurse, he or she may be asked, "What is your name?" This question may evoke a facetious answer or provoke unwillingness to respond if the client believes that the

nurse should know him or her. In such cases, the question, "Would you mind telling me your name?" is usually more effective. It invites the client to cooperate in the identification ritual without implying that the nurse has forgotten the previous contacts.

Clients who cannot respond with their names due to disorientation, expressive aphasia, or an altered level of consciousness should wear a visible name label at all times. When the standard device is unsuitable, ingenuity may be required to devise a satisfactory substitute. Only as a last resort, and only as a temporary measure, should the nurse rely on personal identification by staff members.

In long-term care facilities, resident rather than client status should be promoted. Some institutions of this kind do not use identification tags. Although the relative stability of resident and staff population reduces the risk of mistakes in identification, the danger of errors is not eliminated. Recent photographs of clients are useful for identification. The development of reliable and satisfactory identification procedures within this context is a challenge for creative nursing personnel.

Incomplete Delivery of Drugs

Drugs must reach the site of action to be effective. For many reasons, some or all of the dose given may fail to complete this journey. Problems may be due to factors beyond the nurse's control, such as malabsorption in the intestine, poor circulation in the injection site, or abnormally rapid metabolism and excretion. However, other problems stem from lack of skill in delivery techniques.

An injection of parenteral drugs must deliver the medication to tissues that have adequate perfusion if the substance is to be absorbed rapidly into the systemic circulation. Selecting poor injection sites, such as edematous, hypoxic, or scar tissue, results in inadequate or delayed absorption. When clients are in shock, drugs are best administered IV or by inhalation. IV lines established for the purpose of medication are often vital to proper treatment of the seriously ill or injured client. Intramuscular or subcutaneous injections should not be given to such clients until adequate circulation has been restored.

Topical drugs must contact the affected tissue to exert a therapeutic effect. The presence of tissue debris or excessive exudate in a wound may prevent any response to local medication. Crusts or scales impose a similar barrier to topical applications. Once applied properly, topical applications must be protected from friction or other physical forces that remove them prematurely from the site. Judicious use of materials or devices such as dressings, stockinettes, plastic sheeting, or cradles can offer such protection.

When giving drugs orally, the nurse should ensure that the medicine is swallowed along with enough fluid to propel the dose into the stomach. Clients affected by dysphagia or impaired levels of consciousness may not swallow the dose quickly or easily. For such clients, the nurse should inspect the mouth carefully after giving drugs orally to ensure the tablet or capsule has actually been swallowed. Solid medicines that remain in the mouth often appear hours later in the bedding or on the floor. This problem may be solved by crushing the solid medication or by substituting a liquid preparation. Again, oral sustained-release preparations must not be crushed.

Occasionally, clients refuse to swallow drugs or spit out drugs. Others hide solid medications in the mouth and remove them after the nurse leaves. Some suicidal clients may accumulate a lethal cache of drugs by saving doses retrieved in this way. With some clients, such behavior stems from belligerence or hostility toward the staff; this, in turn, is the outward expression of natural and normal psychologic responses to illness, such as anxiety or despair. Clients with ambivalent feelings may accept liquid medications given by mouth. Open recognition of the client's right to refuse treatment, including medication, may resolve the conflict. Continued rejection of vital treatment raises difficult issues for the healthcare team; ethically and legally, the competent client may not be coerced.

Medication may be forcibly administered to clients who have been legally certified as mentally incompetent (due to delirium, mental impairment, or minor status) or who are a "clear and present danger to themselves or others." Because forcing medication is likely to destroy the therapeutic nurse–client relationship, the nurse should strive to convey an attitude of caring while helping the client to accept help. A show of strength (eg, bringing two or more staff members to the bedside) may discourage active resistance to medication administration. If possible, open conflict and physical struggle should be avoided.

Many thorny legal and ethical questions arise when treatment is imposed on an unwilling client. In most situations, the issues are not black or white. For example, few would question the need to administer glucose or glucagon by force to a belligerent client whose resistance stems from a temporary hypoglycemic state. Differences of opinion are far more likely when clients whose mental competence is uncertain resist treatment. In some cases, a legal determination of competence may have been made; in most instances, it has not. Such decisions afford a measure of legal protection to the nurse (clients may charge staff members who assist in forced treatment with assault and battery), but rarely if ever do they resolve all moral issues. The nurse is confronted with many difficult ethical questions while caring for a resistant client.

Verifying Procedures

Medication procedures customarily include a number of steps designed to detect errors so that they can be corrected before the drug is administered. These steps include comparing the orders on the Kardex with the original orders written by the physician, comparing the client's name on written records with the identification band, and repeatedly reading the drug labels. These routines tend to become rituals and often are carried out automatically with little attention to or perception of their significance.

Preparing ("pouring") drugs is monotonous. If the nurse allows habit to control behavior, the motions of checking may be carried out without integrating the sensory stimuli that enter the brain. It is possible to scan a drug label without comprehending what the eyes have seen. The likelihood of mechanical behavior increases if the nurse's attention wanders. Interruptions and distractions must be eliminated as much as possible. The nurse must make a conscious effort to concentrate on the task at hand if routine checks are to be effective.

When data are compared for accuracy, relying on memory is risky. Printed materials must be placed side by side for comparison. In practical terms, therefore, the medication card or Kardex must be viewed simultaneously with the physician's order sheet. The medication card should be placed next to the client's identification band to verify identification. If there is any interval between pouring and administering the drug, the dose must be labeled for complete and certain identification. Careful observance of such practices helps ensure accuracy.

Using a Faulty Knowledge Base

Relying solely on memory for facts needed to administer drugs safely should be avoided whenever possible. Pharmacologic information needed by the medication nurse has expanded so rapidly in recent years that it is unrealistic to expect anyone to remember all the facts needed every time.

Knowledge frequently used is retained in reliable detail and may safely be used without verification. Information used irregularly tends to be forgotten, and the details that are recalled are unreliable. Although a well-stocked memory is a valuable resource, any fact about which the nurse is unsure must be verified in reference sources, which should be provided for this purpose. Useful references include encyclopedic volumes that contain drug data, charts that provide accurate metric–apothecary equivalents, compatibility tables that warn against incompatible drug mixtures, and any other visual materials considered appropriate to a given situation. It is much safer (and may be quicker) to look up such information than to attempt to recall it.

Yielding to Time Constraints

The sheer number of doses to be given in a limited time may preclude the careful attention to detail needed to eliminate errors. Time is needed for gathering basic drug data, reading labels, and checking identification. Only practiced and efficient nurses can maintain the pace required in many situations. Less skilled personnel either cut corners (eliminate some of the steps) or fall hopelessly behind schedule (an error in itself).

Clearly, the problem of medication errors is complex and its resolution difficult. Creative approaches and sound nursing judgment are needed to establish reliable procedures and precautions for accurate and effective drug therapy in a given situation. No perfect procedure and no one right way can be recommended.

Reporting an Error

When a given medication violates one of the five "rights" (the wrong drug, the wrong dose, the wrong client, the wrong route, or the wrong time), an error in medication procedure has occurred and the nurse must report it immediately. In this way, the nurse and the client are protected. The medication error may be harmless, or it may pose a serious threat to the client. Fast reporting of medication errors means that emergency measures can be taken and undesirable complications prevented.

▪ SUMMARY

The administration of drugs involves complex procedures and many different healthcare professionals. Safety requires thorough training of personnel in the techniques and procedures appropriate for their role function and accuracy in regard to the five "rights" of medication. The nurse is responsible for monitoring clients' responses to drugs and for supervising paraprofessionals in their drug-related tasks. The nurse collaborates with the physician to adapt the drug regimen to meet clients' individual needs.

Special Skills for Drug Administration

Effective drug therapy depends on delivering accurate doses of active chemicals to the body tissues at the appropriate site of action for the drug involved. To complete this process successfully, the nurse must master certain technical skills, including proper storage and handling of drugs, command of the language used in drug therapy, accurate computation of drug doses, and techniques used in delivering drugs by specific routes to specific sites.

Storing and Handling Drugs

Drug substances require careful storage and handling to maintain their safety and potency. All medicines should be kept in a special place and secured from access by unauthorized people.

Preservation

To preserve most drugs, storage areas should be kept cool and dry. Chemical deterioration is hastened by heat, moisture, and in some cases light. Water can dissolve solid drugs, and heat can melt the waxy bases of suppositories and ointments. Sterile substances must be protected from bacterial contamination. Drugs in damaged containers should be discarded. Stocks should be reviewed periodically, and any drugs whose recommended shelf life has expired or that have changed in appearance, indicating possible deterioration, should be discarded. Unusable drugs should be destroyed by incineration, although controlled drugs must be returned to the dispensing pharmacy for disposal. Besides providing the proper conditions for preserving chemicals, storage areas should be kept clean and orderly.

Containers

Drugs keep best in their original containers. Their labels are more accurate, because copying may result in transcription errors. Original containers are effective in protecting their contents; for example, light-sensitive compounds are packaged in amber bottles or containers that filter out much of the harmful radiation. Transfer of sterile substances from container to container should be minimized because of the increased probability of contamination. When drugs are handled, the container should be protected from soiling so that the label may remain legible. Safe drug use requires that medicines have clear, accurate labels at all times.

Childproof Caps

Many drugs are dispensed in containers with childproof caps that require complex dexterity to be opened. This increases the time required for children to gain access to the drug and reduces the chance of accidental ingestion. Although these special containers have lowered the incidence of drug poisoning in children, they are very difficult to open for clients with impaired manual dexterity or grip. Regular, easily opened containers can be requested when the drug is dispensed, but special precautions must be taken to prevent access by children.

Tamperproof Packaging

Several incidents of lethal cyanide poisoning from OTC analgesics occurred in the United States in the 1980s when poison was added to the product after it reached store shelves. To prevent these problems, manufacturers package most drugs in tamper-resistant, sealed containers. Tamper-resistant containers typically have an aluminum foil inner seal and either a plastic outer ring around the cap or shrink-wrap around the entire package. Some preparations are packaged as unit doses in individually sealed packets. The U.S. Pharmacopeial Convention has published a pamphlet ("Tips Against Tampering") designed to help consumers detect tampering (Box 7-3).

Whenever a medicine, its container, or its package appears unusual, the drug should be returned to the pharmacy that dispensed it. If tampering is evident, the pharmacist can report it to the Drug Product Problem Reporting Program, which is coordinated by the federal Food and Drug Administration in cooperation with the

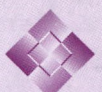

Box 7-3
Clues to Tampering

- Discrepancy between lot numbers on container and numbers on outer wrapping or box
- Breaks, cracks, or holes in outer wrapping, cover, or seal
- Disturbance in outer covering
- Distorted or stretched shrink band around top of bottle
- Slits in or retaping of shrink band
- Looseness of bottle cap
- Glue or paper fragments on rim of an unsealed bottle
- Discolored or disarrayed cotton plug
- Overfilled or underfilled container
- Unusual appearance of medication
- Unusual odor or taste of medication
- Broken seals on tops of tubes or bottles

U.S. Pharmacopeia and the American Society of Health-System Pharmacists.

Medication containers may be damaged accidentally, as well. In such cases, the integrity of containers should be verified before preparing the dose to be given. This is crucial in the case of injectable drugs, when sterility is required.

Storage in the Home

In the home, drugs should be kept under lock and key wherever feasible. The standard bathroom medicine chest is an inappropriate storage area for two reasons: it rarely has a lock, and the bathroom air is usually too humid. A locked container in the bedroom or linen closet would be better. Suppositories and multiple-dose injectable drugs should be refrigerated; they should be enclosed in plastic or other airtight containers to protect them from humidity and food residues. Locking refrigerated drugs is rarely practical, but the drugs should be placed away from children. Drugs should not be stored near the cooling elements of the refrigerator because freezing may damage them.

Storage in Institutions

In healthcare institutions, most nursing units have a medication room where drugs are prepared for use. At the very least, a locked cabinet is needed for storing medicines. Narcotic and other legally restricted drugs are kept in a special locked compartment. Many states specify that such drugs be kept under double lock.

Stock drugs are those supplied in bulk containers, and clients' doses are measured from this single supply. Stock preparations for internal use should be segregated from preparations for external use. Although a few drugs still may be provided in stock bottles, most are dispensed in smaller quantities for the specific client.

Table 7-1. Abbreviations and Symbols for Orders, Prescriptions, and Labels

Abbreviation	Meaning	Derivation (Latin or Greek)	Abbreviation	Meaning	Derivation (Latin or Greek)
aa	of each	*ana*	O S	left eye	*oculus sinister*
a c	before meals	*ante cibum*	OTC	over the counter	
ad	to, up to	*ad*	O U	each eye	*oculus uterque*
ad lib	as freely as desired	*ad libitum*	oz	ounce	*uncia*
Aq	water	*aqua*	PB	piggyback	
Aq dest	distilled water	*aqua destillata*	p c	after meals	*post cibum*
b i d	two times a day	*bis in die*	per	through or by	*per*
b i n	two times a night	*bis in nocte*	Pil	pill	*pilula*
c or c̄	with	*cum*	P O	by mouth	*per os*
caps	capsule	*capsula*	P R N	when required	*pro re nata*
comp	compound	*compositus*	*q d	every day	*quaque die*
D₅W	5% dextrose in water		q h	every hour	*quaque hora*
dil	dilute	*dilue*	q 2 h	every two hours	
elix	elixir	*elixir*	q 3 h	every three hours	
ext	extract	*extractum*	q 4 h	every four hours (and so on for any hourly interval)	
fld or Fl	fluid	*fluidus*			
Ft	make	*fiat*			
g, gm	gram	*gramma*	q i d	four times a day	*quater in die*
gr	grain	*granum*	q s	sufficient quantity	*quantum satis*
gtt	drop	*gutta*	R	right	
H	hypodermic		Rₓ	take thou	*recipe*
h	hour	*hora*	s or s̄	without	*sine*
h s	at bedtime	*hora somni*	S or Sig	write (on the label)	*signa*
I M	intramuscularly		S C	subcutaneously	
I V	intravenously		S L	beneath the tongue	*sub linguam*
L	left		Sol	solution	
M	mix	*misce*	S O S	if necessary (once only)	*si opus sit*
μ or min	minim	*minimum*	sp	spirit	*spiritus*
μg or mcg	microgram		ss or s̄s̄	one half	*semis*
mEq	milliequivalent		stat	immediately	*statim*
mg	milligram		Syr	syrup	*syrupus*
mist or mixt	mixture	*mixtura*	t i d	three times a day	*ter in die*
mL	milliliter		t i n	three times a night	*ter in nocte*
Noct	at night	*nocte*	TO	telephone order	
non repeat	do not repeat	*non repetatur*	tr or tinct	tincture	*tinctura*
NS	normal saline (0.9% sodium chloride)		*U	unit	
			ung	ointment	*unguentum*
½NS	0.45% sodium chloride		×	times	
O	pint	*octarius*	vin	wine	*vinum*
O D	right eye	*oculus dexter*	VO	verbal order	
*o d	every day	*omni die*	>	more than	
*o h	every hour	*omni hora*	<	less than	
ol	oil	*oleum*	=	equal to	
o m	every morning	*omni mane*	↑, ↗	increase, increasing	
*o n	every night	*omni nocte*	↓, ↙	decrease, decreasing	
os	mouth	*os*			

*Abbreviations that are *not* recommended because they are easily misread or misinterpreted. Daily, nightly, hourly, and unit should be written out.

This system requires that each client's drugs be kept in a separate area. Typically, drug carts or cabinets provide a drawer for each client's supply. If drugs are charged to the client when dispensed, unused supplies must be returned to the pharmacy for crediting. Borrowing doses from one client's supply for use by another should be avoided because it increases the risk of error and, if different brand name drugs have been ordered, bioavailability may differ. When necessary, repayment (in drugs or credit) should be made.

Refrigerators are standard equipment in most medication rooms. Drugs that require refrigeration include suppositories with low melting temperatures, insulin, sera, vaccines, and certain antibiotics. To prevent contamination of drugs, avoid storing food in these areas.

Medication rooms and narcotic cabinets should be locked whenever they are not in use. Ideally, the key to the controlled drugs remains in the possession of one nurse, the one who signed for the drugs at the beginning of the work shift. Propping open the door to the medicine room and lending narcotic keys to coworkers may allow unauthorized access to harmful substances and may break down the secure control of drug supplies.

Insulin

Insulin storage presents a special problem. Because this drug is dispensed in multiple-dose, sterile vials, bacterial contamination is possible due to multiple punctures and prolonged time of use. Refrigeration would minimize the risk of bacterial growth; however, insulin should be administered at room temperature to reduce the risk of tissue damage at the injection site. A preservative is added to the insulin formulation to retard microbial growth, so vials in current use should be kept at room temperature. Before use, vials should be inspected carefully for changes in color or clarity that might indicate bacterial contamination. If the solution has an abnormal appearance, the vial should be discarded. If insulin happens to be refrigerated, the cold vial should be removed and allowed to warm to room temperature at least 1 hour before administering the dose.

Learning the Language

For convenience and efficiency, physicians use a system of abbreviations when writing drug orders and prescriptions. The same abbreviations are used by healthcare personnel who dispense and administer drugs. Nurses must know the terminology used in their practice setting to administer drugs accurately and efficiently.

Certain abbreviations are so common that they are generally recognized and accepted (Tables 7-1 and 7-2). These should be memorized. Sometimes abbreviations that are not generally accepted are used habitually in a particular institution. These must be specified by written policy as required by the Joint Commission on Accreditation of Healthcare Organizations so there is no question of their meaning. Each institution should is-

Table 7-2. Commonly Used Abbreviations for Drug Names

Abbreviation	Drug
ASA	aspirin (acetylsalicylic acid)
CO_2	carbon dioxide
CTZ	chlorothiazide
$FeSO_4$	iron sulfate
HCTZ	hydrochlorothiazide
KCl	potassium chloride
$MgSO_4$	magnesium sulfate
MO	mineral oil
MOM	milk of magnesia
m s	morphine sulfate
O_2	oxygen
SSE	soap suds enema
SSKI	saturated solution of potassium iodide
TWE	tap water enema

sue a list defining all abbreviations acceptable for use. Certain abbreviations that are easily misread or misinterpreted should not be used (Table 7-3). Abbreviations not included on official lists should be questioned consistently for clarification until they are incorporated into the written policy. Assuming the meaning of an order leaves a nurse open to error and legally vulnerable.

Orders for Medication

Proper orders for medication convey clear directions that specify the client to be medicated, the chemical to be used, the dose to be given, the route of administration, and the timing of drug doses. The procedure used depends on the setting and the situation. Orders may be written for medications to be administered once only, repeatedly at designated time intervals, or when needed. One-time doses may be ordered to be given immediately (stat), at a designated hour in the future, when in-

Table 7-3. Examples of Abbreviations Commonly Misread or Misinterpreted

Abbreviation	Drug	Misinterpretation
ARA-A	vidarabine	cytarabine (ARA-C)
CPZ	Compazine	chlorpromazine
DIG	digoxin	digitoxin
HCl	hydrochloric acid	potassium chloride (KCl)
HCTZ	hydrochloro-thiazide	hydrocortisone (HCT)
MTX	methotrexate	mustargen (mechlorethamine HCl)
MVI	Multiple vitamins *without* fat-soluble vitamins	Multivitamins *with* fat-soluble vitamins

dicated by the physician at some time in the future (on call), or only if needed (SOS). Drugs to be administered repeatedly may be ordered at specified hourly intervals (eg, q3h, q4h, q6h) or in relation to activity patterns (ac, pc, hs), or the number of doses per day may be indicated (bid, tid, qid).

Standing orders are the usual orders that physicians wish to have carried out on clients in designated situations, unless specifically countermanded. For example, a physician might wish all clients receiving parenteral fluids by hypodermoclysis to have hyaluronidase added to the infusion. Standing orders are limited to the clients of the physician writing the order and should always be available in written form to the nurse carrying out the orders. Protocols are standing orders that outline the steps to be taken in a given situation and the criteria for identifying the situation (eg, regular insulin coverage q6h in accord with urine glucose tests: trace or 1+, no insulin; 2+, 5 units; 3+, 10 units; 4+, 15 units).

Institutional Settings

In institutional settings, physicians' orders may be recorded on a special sheet on the client's chart or in a special drug order book. These orders are then relayed to the pharmacist and the nursing staff for their action. The nurse (or unit secretary) who transcribes orders must read and copy the information accurately. The order must not be changed in any way. If there is reason to think that an error has been made, the physician should be consulted.

If, after consulting the physician, the nurse decides that the order as transmitted is likely to harm the client, he or she must decline to carry it out, in which case the physician must be notified. In this situation, a conflict between physician and nurse can develop; a suggestion by the nurse that the physician prepare and administer the dose personally may resolve it. (A nurse who questions the safety of an order may wish to consult a pharmacology reference, experienced colleagues, or both before refusing to carry out a medication order, particularly if he or she is a new practitioner or is working in an unfamiliar clinical situation.)

When the transcription is completed, this fact should be noted on the order sheet. The written record of orders provides legal protection for everyone involved in the use of medicines—the nurse, physician, pharmacist, and client.

Verbal orders may be necessary in emergencies, when the physician is in sterile garb, or when an oral or telephone order is needed. These orders are written by the nurse on the usual record, with a notation that it was an oral or telephone order. The nurse should sign the entry after entering the physician's name. Such orders must be countersigned by the physician as soon as possible.

Verbal orders place the nurse in legal jeopardy if the physician fails to verify the order. The nurse rather than the physician may be held liable for harm caused to the client as a result of the drug order. If the physician repudiates the order, the nurse might even be charged with practicing medicine without a license. Verbal orders should be avoided whenever possible. When unavoidable, the physician should countersign them promptly.

Prescriptions

Drug orders for clients outside healthcare institutions are written as prescriptions. Drugs deemed by the Food and Drug Administration or Health Protection Branch to require a physician's supervision for their effective and safe use ("legend" drugs) can be obtained only by prescription. Prescriptions are written directions for the dispensing of drugs by a pharmacist. They are composed of the following parts:

- Superscription: the client's name, age, and address, the date, and the symbol ℞ (*recipe*, which means in Latin "take thou")
- Inscription: the name of the drug, the dosage form, and the amount of the dose
- Subscription: directions to the pharmacist about preparing the drug and the number of doses to dispense
- Signature: headed by the abbreviation *S* or *Sig* (*signa*, which means in Latin "write on the label"). Following this are directions for the client and the name of the drug to be placed on the label.

In addition, prescriptions may designate whether a generic drug equivalent may be dispensed and the number of refills allowed. The physician's name, address, and telephone number are usually printed on the prescription blank. The physician must sign the prescription. If a drug listed in the Controlled Substances Act is included in the prescription, the physician's DEA registration number must also be added.

Figure 7-7 is an example of a completed prescription.

Computation of Drug Doses

To compute drug doses and measure medication accurately, the nurse must understand several systems of measurement. Systems commonly used today developed at different periods. The earliest measures were defined in commonly available units—the human hand, finger, foot, arm span, pace, handful, a grain of wheat. Although they provided a rough approximation of quantity, such methods obviously varied with the size of the person or the grain sample used as a standard. Specifying the person (often the reigning king) whose anatomic measures were to be adapted helped refine the system. Eventually, standard measures became generally accepted, although confusing variations tended to persist (eg, a ton varies depending on whether it is mea-

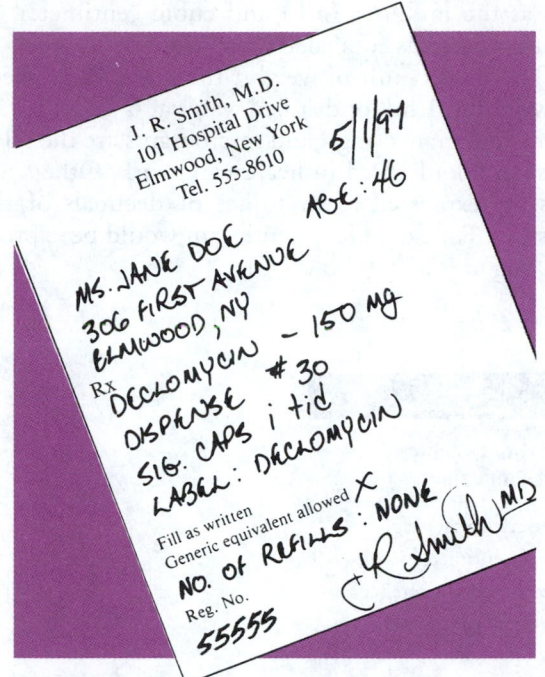

Figure 7-7. Sample of a completed prescription.

sured by troy or avoirdupois weight). Measurement systems that evolved from these historical models tend to be cumbersome. Any schoolchild struggling to convert inches to feet and feet to miles can testify to the complexity of the computations.

Not until the late 18th century was a deliberate attempt made to devise a system of weights and measures that would provide not only a single, unalterable standard but also a mathematical scale to make computation easier. The international standard (System Internationale or metric) system was the result. Although it was adopted early by the scientific community, its acceptance by commerce and industry has been more gradual. Today, most nations of the world either have adopted or are in the process of converting to the metric system as the official standard of measurement. The United States is a conspicuous exception: to date, Congress has recommended but not required the adoption of the metric system.

The metric system is used most often for drug therapy in institutional settings, although the apothecary system is used on occasion. When a medicine is to be self-administered, the household system is sometimes used. In Canada, only the metric system is used.

Metric System

The basic unit of length in the metric system is the meter, which represents one ten-millionth of a quarter of the earth's circumference measured across the pole. The standard of measurement for this length is a platinum bar deposited in the French Archives, which serves as a model for meter measures intended for actual use. Duplicates of the measure used as working standards are retained by the governments of participating nations. Conditions such as temperature, which affect the volume of these models, are held constant when measures are taken. The meter is about 1 yard long (39.37 inches).

The designated unit for capacity or volume is the liter (L) and that for weight is the gram (g). These units bear a specific relation to the meter.

To facilitate computation, basic measures in the system may be either subdivided or multiplied by 10, 100, 1,000, or other multiples of 10. Greek or Latin prefixes designate the degree of subdivision or multiplication. *Deci* means ten; thus, a decimeter is one tenth of a meter, a deciliter is one tenth of a liter, and a decigram is one tenth of a gram. *Kilo* means 1,000; thus, a kilometer equals 1,000 meters, a kiloliter 1,000 L, and a kilogram 1,000 g. The prefixes used and their relation to the unit in question are listed in Table 7-4.

Table 7-4. Subdivisions of the Metric System

Prefix	Meaning	Example(s)	Nonmetric Equivalent
Kilo	1,000	1 kilogram = 1,000 grams (g)	2.2 pounds (lb) or 35.2 ounces
Hecto	100	1 hectogram = 100 grams (g)	3.5 ounces (oz)
Deca	10	1 decaliter = 10 liters (L)	2.6 gallons (gal)
	1	1 gram	about 1/30 oz
		1 liter	about 1 quart (qt)
		1 meter	about 39 inches (in)
Deci	0.1	1 deciliter = 0.1 liter (L)	about 3⅓ ounces (oz)
Centi	0.01	1 centimeter = 0.01 meter (m)	about ½ inch (in)
Milli	0.001	1 milligram = 0.001 gram (g)	grains (gr) 1/60
Micro	$0.000001 \ (10^{-6})$	1 microgram = 0.000001 gram (g)	grains (gr) 1/60,000
		1 micrometer = 0.000001 meter (m)	about 1/30,000 inch (in)
Nano	$0.000000001 \ (10^{-9})$	1 nanogram = 0.000000001 gram (g)	grains (gr) 1/60,000,000
Pico	$0.000000000001 \ (10^{-12})$	1 picogram = 0.000000000001 gram (g)	grains (gr) 1/60,000,000,000

The metric unit of capacity, the liter, is defined as the contents of a cube whose sides measure 1 dm (10 centimeters). Originally intended to be exactly the same as the cubic decimeter, the liter actually varies slightly from this quantity because of the intricacies of measurement. This variation is so small that it is important only in precise measurements. In practice, however, the liter is considered equal to the cubic decimeter. Corresponding units of capacity and cubic linear measurement, such as the milliliter (mL) and cubic centimeter (cc), are also treated as equivalent (Table 7-5).

The metric unit of weight, the gram, is defined as the weight of 1 mL of distilled water at 4°C. Kilograms, grams, milligrams (mg), and micrograms are the related units commonly used in healthcare work. Other quantities are expressed as multiples or decimals of these measures. For example, a centigram would be expressed as 10 mg or 0.01 g (Table 7-6).

Table 7-5. Metric Capacity Measurements

Abbreviation	Unit of Measurement*	Relation to Liter	Approximate cubic Metric Equivalent
mL	milliliter	1/1,000 liter (L)	1 cubic centimeter (cc)
cL	centiliter	1/100 liter (L)	10 cubic centimeters (cc)
dL	deciliter	1/10 liter (L)	100 cubic centimeters (cc)
L	liter	1 liter (L)	1,000 cubic centimeters (cc)

*Units containing multiple liters (decaliter, and so on) are not in common usage.

Table 7-6. Metric Weight Measures

Abbreviation	Unit of Measurement*	Relation to Gram	Nonmetric Approximation
pg	picogram	0.000000000001 gram (g)	grain (gr) 1/60,000,000,000
ng	nanogram	0.000000001 gram (g)	grain (gr) 1/60,000,000
mcg	microgram	0.000001 gram (g)	grain (gr) 1/60,000
mg	milligram	0.001 gram (g)	grain (gr) 1/60
cg	centigram	0.01 gram (g)	grain (gr) 1/6
dg	decigram	0.1 gram (g)	grains (gr) iss
g or gm	gram	1 gram (g)	grains (gr) xv
dkg	decagram	10 grams (g)	⅓ ounce (oz)
hg	hectogram	100 grams (g)	3½ ounces (oz)
kg	kilogram	1,000 grams (g)	2.2 pounds (lb)

Table 7-7. Household Measures of Fluid Volume

Abbreviation	Quantity	Recommended Tool for Measurement
t or tsp	1 teaspoon (4–5 mL)	The teaspoon from a standard set of measuring spoons used for cooking
T or Tb	1 tablespoon (3 teaspoons, 12–16 mL)	If available, a tablespoon from a standard set of measuring spoons used for cooking or three standard teaspoons
oz	1 fluid ounce (2 tablespoons, 30–32 mL)	Measure as above for one tablespoon, or use a standard medication cup (plastic cups are available and relatively inexpensive)
c	1 cup; 1 glass (8 fluid ounces, 240 mL)	A translucent measuring cup
gtt	1 drop (0.06–0.07 mL for watery liquids)	The dropper dispensed with the specific medication to be taken.* (Most liquid medications measured in this unit are packaged with droppers.)

*The size of a drop varies with the density and viscosity of the liquid and the size and configuration of the dropper tip.

Table 7-8. Apothecary Measurements

Symbol/Abbreviation	Quantity	Recommended Tool for Measurement
Units of Weight		
gr	grain	Apothecary balance scales (rarely needed because medicines measured in grains are almost universally prepared in small dose forms, such as tablets, capsules, or liquid preparations measured by volume)
ʒ	dram (60 grains or gr lx)	Apothecary balance scales
ʒ̄	ounce (480 grains or gr xxd)	Apothecary balance scales
Fluid (Volume) Measure		
♏	minim	Minim glass
f ʒ	fluidram (60 minims or min lx)	Minim glass, fluid ounce measure, or standard calibrated medicine glass
f ʒ̄	fluid ounce (8 fluidrams or F ʒ viii, 480 minims or µxxd)	Fluid ounce measure or standard calibrated medicine glass
pt	pint (16 fluid ounces or ʒ xvi)	Standard calibrated graduate or pitcher
qt	quart (2 pints or pt)	Standard calibrated graduate or pitcher
gal	gallon (4 quarts or qt)	Standard calibrated graduate or pitcher

The metric system has many advantages. All standard units bear a simple relation to the fundamental unit and to each other. The use of decimal multiples simplifies mathematical computation and conversion from one unit to another.

Household Measures

To laypeople, household measurements are the most familiar system of measuring. This system uses quantities handled in familiar household containers such as teaspoons, cups, pints, and quarts. However, not all common utensils found in the home are equal in measure. Teaspoons and cups vary in size. Scales on pint and quart containers may be inaccurate. Canning jars usually are not calibrated at all. Moreover, it makes a difference how a dry substance is measured. The amounts in a level, rounded, and heaping spoonful vary greatly. Experienced cooks recognize the value of standard measuring tools and the need to level off measurements. A client who measures potent drugs for self-treatment should exercise just as much care.

In the United States, a standard cup contains 8 oz of volume. Measuring spoons are available in sets that include one eighth of a teaspoon, one fourth of a teaspoon, one half of a teaspoon, and 1 teaspoon. Directions on liquid prescriptions used in the home commonly designate household measurements such as a teaspoon or a cup. Clients should be directed to use standard measuring utensils to determine the correct amounts. Typical household measurements and recommended utensils for measuring them are listed in Table 7-7.

Apothecary System

The apothecary system of measurement was introduced into the United States from England during the colonial era. It was the prevailing system for medications until recent times. Although the current trend is toward adopting the metric system, apothecary doses are still sometimes used, particularly by older physicians.

The basic unit of weight in the apothecary system, the grain, originally meant the weight of one grain of wheat. Other units of weight derived from the grain are the dram, the ounce, and the pound. The unit of fluid measurement, the minim, is approximately the quantity of water that would weigh a grain. Fluid measures derived from the minim include the fluidram, fluid ounce, pint, quart, and gallon. Distinctive symbols are used for the apothecary units of measurement (Table 7-8).

When symbols are used, the quantity is expressed as a small Roman numeral placed after the symbol. For example, one grain is written as gr i; 10 minims as ♏x. Arabic numerals are used to express most fractions, although one half is often abbreviated ss (*semis*, Latin for one half).

Conversion From One Measurement System to Another

As long as the use of household and apothecary measurements persists, nurses must be proficient in converting values from one system to another. As noted above, equivalents are not exact, only approximations. A study of the metric—apothecary table reveals many discrepancies (Tables 7-9 and 7-10). For example, if 1 fluid oz is equivalent to 30 cc, 1 quart (32 oz) is more

Table 7-9. Approximate Equivalents for Household Measures

Household Measure	Equivalent
1 drop	1 minim (min)
1 teaspoon	1 dram (dr) or 4–5 mL
1 dessert spoon	2 drams (dr) or 9 mL
1 tablespoon	1/2 ounce (oz) or 15 mL
1 teacupful	6 ounces (oz) or 180 mL
1 cup or glassful	8 ounces (oz) or 240 mL

Table 7-10. Approximate Equivalents for Metric and Apothecary Measures

Metric Measure	Apothecary Equivalent	Metric Measure	Apothecary Equivalent
Weight		**Weight**	
0.1 mg	grain (gr) 1/600	2 g	grains (gr) xxx
0.12 mg	grain (gr) 1/500	3 g	grains (gr) vl
0.15 mg	grain (gr) 1/400	4 g	grains (gr) lx
0.2 mg	grain (gr) 1/300	5 g	grains (gr) lxxv
0.25 mg	grain (gr) 1/250	6 g	grains (gr) xc
0.3 mg	grain (gr) 1/200	7.5 g	drams (ʒ) ii
0.4 mg	grain (gr) 1/150	10 g	drams (ʒ) iiss
0.5 mg	grain (gr) 1/120	15 g	drams (ʒ) iv
0.6 mg	grain (gr) 1/100	30 g	ounce (oz or ʒ) i
0.8 mg	grain (gr) 1/80		
1 mg	grain (gr) 1/60	**Capacity**	
1.2 mg	grain (gr) 1/50	0.03 mL	min (♏) ss
1.5 mg	grain (gr) 1/40	0.05 mL	min (♏) ¾
2 mg	grain (gr) 1/30	0.06 mL	min (♏) i
3 mg	grain (gr) 1/20	0.1 mL	min (♏) iss
4 mg	grain (gr) 1/15	0.2 mL	min (♏) iii
5 mg	grain (gr) 1/12	0.25 mL	min (♏) iv
6 mg	grain (gr) 1/10	0.3 mL	min (♏) v
8 mg	grain (gr) 1/8	0.5 mL	min (♏) viii
10 mg	grain (gr) 1/6	0.6 mL	min (♏) x
12 mg (0.012 g)	grain (gr) 1/5	0.75 mL	min (♏) xii
15 mg (0.015 g)	grain (gr) 1/4	1 mL	minims (♏) xv or xvi
20 mg (0.02 g)	grain (gr) 1/3	2 mL	minims (♏) xxx
25 mg (0.025 g)	grain (gr) 3/8	3 mL	minims (♏) vl
30 mg (0.03 g)	grain (gr) ss	4 mL	fluidram (fʒ) i
40 mg (0.04 g)	grain (gr) 2/3	5 mL	fluidrams (fʒ) 1¼
50 mg (0.05 g)	grain (gr) 3/4	8 mL	fluidrams (fʒ) ii
60 mg (0.06 g)	grain (gr) i	10 mL	fluidrams (fʒ) iiss
75 mg (0.075 g)	grain (gr) 1¼	15 mL	fluidrams (fʒ) iv
			fluid ounce (fʒ) ss
100 mg (0.1 g)	grain (gr) iss	30 mL	fluid ounce (ʒ) i
125 mg (0.125 g)	grains (gr) ii	50 mL	fluid ounce (fʒ) 1¾
150 mg (0.15 g)	grains (gr) iiss	90 mL	fluid ounces (fʒ) iii
200 mg (0.2 g)	grains (gr) iii	100 mL	fluid ounces (fʒ) iiiss
250 mg (0.25 g)	grains (gr) iv	120 mL	fluid ounces (fʒ) iv
300 mg (0.3 g)	grains (gr) v	200 mL	fluid ounces (fʒ) vii
400 mg (0.4 g)	grains (gr) vi	250 mL	fluid ounces (fʒ) viii
500 mg (0.5 g)	grains (gr) viiss	500 mL	1 pint (pt)
600 mg (0.6 g)	grains (gr) x	750 mL	1½ pints (pt)
750 mg (0.75 g)	grains (gr) xii	1,000 mL	1 quart (qt)
1 g	grains (gr) xv		
1.5 g	grains (gr) xxii		

nearly 960 cc than the 1 L (1,000 cc) given as its equivalent. Using the equivalent gr iss to 100 mg, a grain would be equivalent to 66.7 mg, a considerable variance from the 60 mg listed in many charts. In actual practice, equivalents of 60, 64, 65, or 66⅔ mg are all used for converting grains to milligrams (or the reverse procedure) (Table 7-11). The practitioner can choose the equivalent that allows easy computation without generating fractions or involved decimals. Although the freedom to choose an equivalent is convenient, the nurse must bear in mind the error that is always introduced by this process and should minimize the number of conversions.

The most reliable way to convert a quantity from one system of measurement to another is to look up its equivalent on an accurate conversion table. The accuracy of any table should be verified before it is used, as printing errors sometimes occur. Because most tables

Table 7-11. Deviant Equivalents Commonly Used for Conversion Computations*

Metric	Apothecary
Weight	
60, 64, 65, or 66 ⅔ mg	grains (gr) i
300, 325 mg	grains (gr) v
600 or 650 mg	grains (gr) x
Liquid	
1 mL	drops (gtt) xv or xvi†; minims (℩) xv or xvi
4 or 5 mL	dram (ʒ) i
240 or 250 mL	ounces (oz or ℥) viii
480 or 500 mL	1 pint

*When official conversion factors have been adopted by a health care institution or system, they should be used by the nurse.
†The standard drop should not be confused with the size of a drop in an IV administration set. Although some sets use a drop equivalent to ⅕ mL, others use drops of other sizes (eg, ¹⁄₆₀, or ¹⁄₂₀ mL). The drop factor is included in the package label information and must be used to compute IV flow rates.

are incomplete or abbreviated, the specific quantity in question may not be listed, and multiplication or division using the appropriate equivalent is necessary. Special texts and workbooks are available to provide instruction and practice in the computation of doses.

Although frequently used equivalents will be memorized, it is best to check a table of equivalents to be certain, especially if conversion skills are infrequently used. Confusion of equivalents is common and can have disastrous consequences for the client. An accurate table of equivalents should be readily available in all areas where medications are prepared. Pocket-sized plastic cards with abbreviated tables of equivalents for personal use are available at no cost from several U.S. pharmaceutical manufacturers.

In preparing medications, it is common practice to equate drops and minims, drams and teaspoons, and grams and milliliters, but these are not equal measures. A minim is a specific quantity, whereas the size of drops varies in accordance with several factors: the viscosity of the liquid; the size, composition, and configuration of the dropper used; and the angle at which the dropper is held. The standard teaspoon is not equal to a dram (6 teaspoons is considered equivalent to 1 oz, whereas 8 drams equals 1 oz). Only in the case of water is a milliliter equivalent to a gram. The more the density of a substance differs from that of water, the greater the deviation in measurement if milliliters are equated with grams. Although significant clinical problems do not appear to arise often as a consequence of such practices, in part this is due to the dose safety margin characteristic of most drugs. Also, most of the solids involved are crystalline substances that are fairly close to water in density. However, the nurse must recognize the error inherent in such practices and should use the indicated measure whenever possible.

Having various containers is useful for accurate measurement of drugs. Unfortunately, the equipment available in healthcare institutions may not promote strict accuracy in measurement. Apothecary scales and minim glasses, once standard equipment in medication areas, are rarely provided in modern institutions. Graduated containers also are unlikely to be readily available.

The nurse often must function as well as possible with the tools at hand. The standard medicine glass is scaled to measure household, apothecary, and metric units of an ounce or parts of an ounce. Smaller quantities may be measured with the minim or milliliter scale on injection syringes. Graduated specimen jars (eg, sterile urine specimen containers) provide a metric scale for 100 to 200 mL. Stainless-steel graduated containers measuring liter quantities may be available from the central supply department. If possible, use a scale that measures the particular units being used, thereby avoiding conversions. For example, measure drams on the dram scale on a medicine glass; do not convert to milliliters. If a measuring device is provided with the drug, use it. For example, liquids prescribed in small volumes are often packaged with a special dropper scaled for precise measurement. If makeshift measurements or involved conversions are frequently necessary, the nurse should initiate appropriate changes to eliminate them; new equipment, new prescription policies, or a change in medication dosage form may be needed.

Verifying Computed Dosage

Most medications are dispensed in forms that provide the correct dosage in one or two units—that is, only one or two tablets or capsules are normally required for a single medication. Liquid preparations are also often labeled in quantities appropriate for single doses. For this reason, whenever a dosage computation yields an unusual answer (Box 7-4), the answer is suspect and the computations should be checked carefully for errors. The first time such a drug is given, it is wise to ask another nurse to verify the accuracy of the dosage. In children, medication often requires the computation of fractional doses. These dosages should also be verified. Nurses who administer drugs

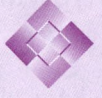

Box 7-4
Unusual Drug Doses That Require Verification

- Fractional parts of a tablet other than 1/2
- Three or more tablets or capsules
- More than 2 mL of injectable solution
- More than 1 unit dose of liquid oral medication
- More than 1 ounce of liquid oral medication

must be able to compute accurately and measure without error, because mistakes may be harmful, even fatal.

Occupational Hazards Related to Drug Administration

Exposure to drugs, including the preparation and administration of drug dosages, increases the risk of certain health problems in the healthcare practitioner. These conditions include chemical dependence, adverse reactions to contact with toxic substances, antibiotic-resistant infections, blood-borne infection, and allergic sensitivity to drug agents.

Chemical Dependence

Physicians and nurses are at increased risk for developing dependence on psychoactive drugs. Factors contributing to the high incidence of dependence include knowledge about the effects of central nervous system drugs, easy access to psychoactive substances, and conditioning through clinical experience to regard these drugs as appropriate agents for the treatment of pain or depression. A reluctance to confront dependent colleagues contributes to delay in treatment.

Adverse Reaction to Toxic Substances

Some drugs are toxic in therapeutic concentrations, so that contact during preparation of doses must be avoided. For example, alkylating antineoplastics are caustic to the skin, and oncology nurses who administer these drugs frequently must take special precautions (eg, wearing rubber gloves) to prevent contact. Chronic exposure to fluothane, an inhalant anesthetic, increases the risk of abortion in female members of the operating room staff. Atropine can cause vision problems, so if the nurse's hands become contaminated while preparing injections of this drug, small amounts of the solution may be transferred inadvertently to the eye; the pupil dilates and vision blurs. Nurses should avoid inhaling drug powders. Serious lung malfunction and asphyxiation have occurred from inhaling the bulk laxative methylcellulose (Table 7-12).

Antibiotic-Resistant Infections

Infectious organisms present in healthcare institutions may become resistant to antibiotics if these treatment agents are allowed to pollute the environment. Nurses whose clothing or skin contacts antibiotics tend to develop a flora of resistant organisms. As a result, those

---

Table 7-12. Selected Agents That May Affect Healthcare Staff

Substance/Drug	Effect on Personnel (Protective Measures)
Antineoplastic drugs	
Alkylating agents/antimetabolites	Irritation at contact sites
	Allergy
	Dizziness, headache, coughing, nausea, hair loss
	Mutagenic changes, increased risk of miscarriage (pregnant women and nursing mothers should avoid all contact; doses should be prepared under vertical laminar flow hoods)
Anesthetics	
halothane	Psychomotor impairment, vertigo, fainting
	Increased risk of miscarriage (operating rooms and recovery rooms should be ventilated by efficient scavenger units)
Sterilizing agent	
ethylene oxide	Anemia, nausea, vomiting, diarrhea, headache, irritation at contact sites
	Possibly carcinogenic, mutagenic, and teratogenic (personnel responsible for gas sterilization require special training in ventilating units and handling articles exposed to ethylene oxide)
Anticholinergics	
atropine	(On eye contact) blurred vision, widely dilated pupil
Antibiotics	
broad-spectrum agents	Normal microbial flora becomes antibiotic-resistant.
Human blood	Exposure to blood-borne infection such as AIDS and hepatitis B virus (Precautions include careful disposal of contaminated equipment, universal blood/body fluid precautions, avoidance of "sticks" by used needles.)

nurses and their families are at increased risk for infections caused by antibiotic-resistant microorganisms.

Blood-Borne Infections

Equipment used to administer medications parenterally is universally contaminated with the client's body fluids. Healthcare personnel accidentally injured by used equipment, such as needles, become inoculated with any systemic infectious agents harbored by the client. Infections known to be transmitted in this way include hepatitis and AIDS. These diseases are serious and can be fatal. To minimize the risk of transmission of blood-borne disease to healthcare personnel, used equipment is deposited directly into special containers. Equipment should be handled as little as possible, healthcare staff should wear protective gloves, used needles should not be recapped, and healthcare staff should observe precautions in accordance with agency policies.

Allergy

Contact with even minute quantities of chemicals while handling drugs may induce an allergy to these substances. Drugs known to be allergenic, such as penicillin, are frequent offenders, but a nurse with a tendency toward allergy could develop antibodies to any chemical agent.

Nursing Considerations

To decrease the risk of occupational illness from drug administration, nurses should adhere to policies and practices designed to control contact with medications and contaminated injection equipment. For example, the nurse should take care not to scatter or inhale powders and granules. When preparing medications, spillage into the environment and personal contact should be avoided. If drugs are spilled, they should be cleaned up immediately and discarded into trash that will be incinerated.

Used injection equipment should be handled carefully to prevent needle sticks. Used needles should not be recapped but should be deposited into special receptacles that are subsequently incinerated. Discarded drugs (except controlled substances, which are returned to the pharmacy for disposal) should be incinerated.

References

Byers JF, Noll ML. (1995). Chronotherapy in acutely ill patients with respiratory disorders: Part I. Respiratory chronobiology and chronopathology. *AACN Clinical Issues, 6*(2): 316–321.

Tips against tampering. (1991). Rockville, MD: The United States Pharmacopeial Convention.

Bibliography

Boyer MJ. (1994). *A pocket guide to dosage calculation and drug preparation*, 3d ed. Philadelphia: JB Lippincott.

*Cohen MR. Medication errors. (A regular feature published monthly, *Nursing '94*.)

Henke G. (1995). *Med-math: Dosage calculation, preparation, and administration*, 2d ed. Philadelphia: JB Lippincott.

Jacobson E. (1990). Hospital hazards: Part two: How to protect yourself. *Am J Nurs 90, 20*(4):48–53 (April).

Thrombolytic therapy is more effective when MI is less likely. (1995). *Geriatrics, 50*(4):13–14.

*Recommended for further reading.

For more information and sample tests and activities, refer to Chapter 7 in the Student Workbook for Clinical Pharmacology and Nursing Management, 5th edition, available through your bookstore.

8

Strategies to Promote Therapeutic Alliance

A client's response to drug therapy is influenced by both physiologic and psychologic factors. Understanding pharmacodynamics and pharmacokinetics helps to explain the physiologic responses, which are unique to each person. As discussed in Chapter 4, the client's age, sex, hormones, nutritional status, disease, and interaction with other chemical substances are factors that affect his or her physiologic response to medications. Of equal concern to the healthcare worker is the need to recognize psychologic factors that may influence the therapeutic outcome of medication use.

Although the physiologic responses can be explained, more subtle interpersonal issues must be explored to promote client adherence or to explain nonadherence to a medication regimen. Management of the clinical interventions and resulting outcomes is particularly challenging when these subtle psychologic variables interfere with the care plan. This chapter explores the significance of establishing a therapeutic alliance between the client and the healthcare provider and its influence on promoting successful therapeutic outcomes.

Developing a Therapeutic Alliance

A therapeutic alliance may best be described as a reciprocal relationship between the healthcare provider and the client. It focuses attention on the interactive nature of the relation-ship, rather than the failure of the client to carry out the provider's directives (usually referred to as noncompliance).

Much information about noncompliance in the literature focuses on clients with chronic mental or physical illnesses, including schizophrenia, tuberculosis, and age-related diseases. Regardless of the cause of the illness, the client's willingness and ability to follow through with the medication regimen are significant. Estimated rates of noncompliance in the United States average up to 40% in the general population (DiMatteo, 1995) and up to 75% after 2 years among chronically ill schizophrenics (Weiden et al., 1994). The clinical and economic impact of noncompliance is significant.

Factors Affecting a Therapeutic Alliance

A nursing diagnosis such as "Ineffective management of therapeutic regimen: Noncompliance" should be considered when lack of evidence of the desired clinical outcome, or an inconsistent outcome, is noted. To understand these outcomes, the nurse should recognize which factors affect compliance. A more contemporary psychosocial view of noncompliance points to the significance of individual values and environmental barriers as the key elements of concern. Understanding these elements is fundamental to developing a therapeutic alliance.

When a client values the medication regimen, there is an overall commitment that motivates him or her to overcome barriers. Such a client is more likely to overcome barriers associated with cost, convenience, social stigma, and adverse medication effects when he or she:

- Is well educated about the benefits of the medication
- Understands the disease process
- Associates adherence to the therapeutic regimen with overall well-being or recovery
- Becomes an active participant in the decision to begin treatment.

When clients view their relationship with the provider as strong, caring, and interactive, the treatment outcomes are generally positive. In this therapeutic alliance, clients tend to invest in their plan of care, understand what to expect during the course of illness and treatment, and remain hopeful about the outcome (Olfson et al., 1993).

Behavioral Responses to Drugs

The values a client brings to the therapeutic alliance are influenced by his or her fundamental attitudes, motivation, and the overall meaning attached to taking the medications. These factors combine to determine the beliefs about and overall commitment to the drug regimen.

Attitudes

Attitudes are initially influenced by genetic factors. In interaction with social and environmental variables, these factors influence perceptions about and interactions with the environment. Attitudes and behavior patterns evolve from the biologic and learned social experiences that dominate the person's family, culture, religion, education, socioeconomic status, and health beliefs.

Motivation

Motivation can be described as drive, incentive, and need. Drive stems from psychologic and biologic needs and is geared toward activating behavior. An incentive directs the behavior toward achieving a specific goal (satisfaction of need). Incentives are learned or recognized over time through interactions with others and with the environment.

Specific behaviors that satisfy need or result in pleasure are repeated and, thus, reinforced. These behaviors may evolve through trial and error or through direct imitation of others. Therefore, motivation is associated with need, incentive, and drive in the client's response to drugs and drug-taking.

Meaning Attached to Drugs

The meaning or significance the drug or therapeutic regimen has for the client affects his or her response to drug treatment. Therefore, the nurse must be aware of and correctly identify the client's emotional state in addition to his or her health status. Feelings of dependency, anger, resentment, hostility, security, well-being, and anxiety can contribute to the client's response to a particular medication or to medications in general.

Dependency

All of us experience feelings of dependency in the course of living. However, some persons always experience dependency in response to experiences. Such a person is said to have a dependent personality. Unable to use skills to meet his or her needs independently, this person may use other people, alcohol, or drugs to help replace a sense of inadequacy with temporary feelings of power and security. However, doing so may create an ever-expanding circle of dependence on such aids or crutches as larger or stronger amounts of a drug (Fig. 8-1). By virtue of their positions as authority figures and decision-makers, healthcare professionals may sometimes foster these feelings of dependency in their clients.

Resentment, Anger, and Hostility

A client with a dependent personality may also resent and feel hostile toward significant others, including members of the healthcare team. These angry feelings arise with the change in health status and the alterations in daily living. Underlying the angry response may be feelings of powerlessness in controlling his or her body or life. This is especially true when the client's needs are being met through dependence on a drug, alcohol, or the sick role. The conflict that arises over attaining physical health and meeting dependency needs may

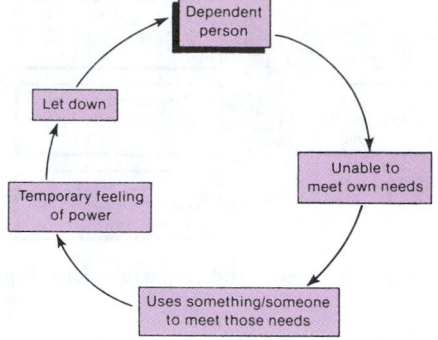

Figure 8-1. The dependent person's use of a crutch may create a repetitious cycle.

result in adverse reactions to medication and an increase in physical symptoms (Fig. 8-2). Just as the appropriate mental state and belief in the therapeutic benefits of a drug enhance a drug's effectiveness, so can anger and hostility reduce or negate its effectiveness.

If the client uses the sick role to gain attention or control of others, the drug therapy may well be sabotaged by the client or family. For such a client, the degree of satisfaction experienced from maintaining this role far outweighs the possible benefits of the drug. The client is not inclined to jeopardize his or her position by getting well and losing the secondary gains or benefits of being sick. Likewise, the family may focus on the client to escape acknowledging or working on difficulties in family roles and relationships. If the client were to get well, family members would need to find another focus or be confronted with their own unsatisfactory and usually dysfunctional relationships. This constitutes too great a threat to maintaining family unity and, as such, is avoided by preventing the client from getting well.

In such a case, the client may adhere to the drug regimen but develop other symptoms or become increasingly ill, may take enough of the drug to feel somewhat better without having to give up the sick role, or may refuse to take the drug at all (Fig. 8-3). Family members may "forget" to administer or purchase the drug. They may tell the client that he or she is well enough to do without the drug, or they may criticize the healthcare providers and the healthcare system as well.

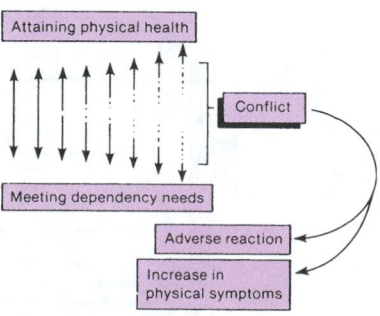

Figure 8-2. The hostile and resentful client's conflicts influence drug effectiveness.

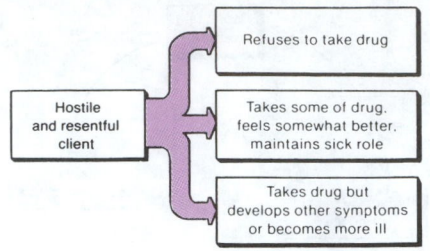

Figure 8-3. The hostile and resentful client response.

Anger has a strong motivating effect on behavior. The resulting behavioral activities can be passively or actively hostile. The nurse should be alert for the strong anger response that results when a client feels less control over his or her body and life.

Security and Well-Being

Some persons gain a feeling of security or well-being from a daily intake of particular medications, whether prescribed or sold over the counter (OTC). These persons view medications as basically helpful. However, some of these same people do not think of OTC preparations as drugs. Vitamin C (to prevent colds), aspirin (for various symptoms), or daily laxatives are commonly overused drug products.

Other prescribed medications may provide the client with a feeling of security, even though they cause adverse reactions. One of the most common of these drugs is digitoxin. The client may suffer from digitoxin toxicity but would not consider contacting the physician or stopping the drug until extremely ill. Belief in the health professionals and the efficacy of the drug regimen is so ingrained that the client does not link harmful reactions to such helpful drugs. In fact, some clients undermine the therapeutic effectiveness of a drug by taking it more often than indicated, by taking it for longer than necessary, or by taking several drugs concurrently without knowledge of drug interaction (Fig. 8-4).

Anxiety and Image

On the other hand, some persons need to maintain a self-image of strength. They resent being sick and fear dependency on drugs and other people. Resentment and fear can lead these clients to strike out in anger. Often,

such attitudes center on role change or loss of role function. These clients may deny their illness and deny the need for drug therapy. With the current emphasis on natural foods, some persons are apprehensive about taking anything into their bodies that may be potentially harmful or may upset the body's balance. The strong value society places on having an attractive body causes even more fear of the deleterious side effects of some medications.

Some of the fears held about drugs pertain to tolerance, addiction, routes of administration, increased or decreased sexual desires, sexual impotence, and side effects. These fears are seldom voiced but become firmly established and remain hidden in the client's mind, causing anxiety. Here there is potential for the client to undermine the effectiveness of drug therapy by taking a smaller dosage than prescribed, by taking the drug less often than needed, by discontinuing the drug before the course of therapy is completed, or by refusing to take the drug at all (Fig. 8-5).

Power of Suggestion

The power of faith, along with a biologic readiness, has led to some spectacular results. Faith can be in a religion or it can be in a person, a particular drug, or the healthcare system in general. A case in point involves the drug laetrile, which has engendered much controversy over its alleged effects. Its effectiveness in treating cancer remains unvalidated and, in fact, has been repudiated by most researchers. Some clients and their families, however, have great faith in it and vouch for its curative power.

Drugs also tend to be more effective when the client has been assured consistently of the benefits of the drug and has a positive attitude toward health personnel and the healthcare system.

Positive Responses

Enhanced drug effectiveness is manifested by a positive response beyond what is usually expected. When penicillin was first marketed, it was hailed as a wonder drug with unlimited therapeutic benefit. People still view antibiotics in this light, although with more caution because of adverse side effects. The power of suggestion strongly affects the therapeutic value of a drug.

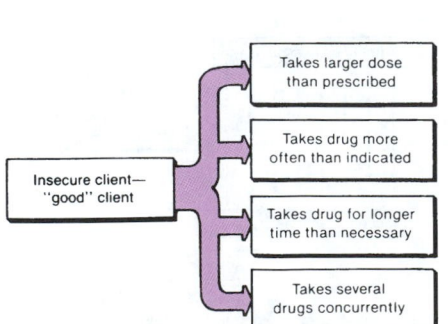

Figure 8-4. The insecure client response.

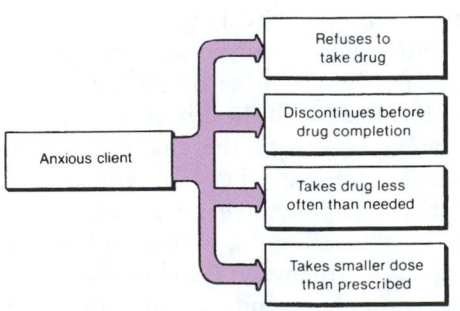

Figure 8-5. The anxious client response.

Placebos are pharmacologically inert substances administered for positive responses in the absence of direct chemical activity. They are given in the form of distilled water, normal saline solution, or sugar. The client believes, however, that a drug has been administered and experiences relief. The mechanisms by which this psychologic response triggers physiologic effects are not well understood. In the case of placebos for pain, researchers think that production of endorphins in the brain is stimulated through this treatment. Placebos have been highly effective in alleviating pain and anxiety, sleeplessness, and allergic reactions. They also can enhance the action of other drugs. Nevertheless, consideration must be given to the ethical aspects of administering something different from what the client expects to be receiving.

Adverse Responses

The power of suggestion can also cause adverse reactions. Occasionally a client complains of nausea, itching, or headaches shortly after taking one drug that resembles another drug that produced such symptoms in the past. The client may have symptoms similar to those of a friend or relative who takes the same drug. The expectation that a drug will produce a specific reaction can, in fact, produce such a reaction. Some healthcare providers erroneously use this as a reason not to educate clients about the adverse reactions and side effects of drugs. Nurses are cautioned to investigate thoroughly any claim of hypersensitivity or other adverse reactions. Whether psychologic or physiologic in origin, the results can be disastrous.

Type of Illness

The type of illness affects the client's psychologic response to treatment. If the illness is chronic, with a prognosis for minimal or no recovery, the response will be different than if the illness is acute and short-term with prospects for a quick recovery. In other words, it is easier for a person to respond positively when the course of the illness is short and drug therapy is brief.

Often in chronic illness, and especially with a terminal disease, Elisabeth Kübler-Ross's stages in dying are seen: denial, anger, bargaining, depression, and acceptance (Kübler-Ross, 1973). The mechanism of denial is common. Although components of denial occur throughout the illness, it is usually strongest during the first stage. Denial of illness may lead to denial of treatment. Sometimes the client, in a state of defiance or anger directed inward, refuses further drug therapy. A behavioral response of this kind may actually stem from fear of dependency or pain, a need to regain some control over one's life, or a fear of dying. In the other stages, the client may refuse drug therapy because of a feeling of hopelessness and helplessness during depression or from anger and the need to strike out at others in the environment. Refusing to go along with the prescribed therapeutic regimen is an attempt to maintain control and to decrease the psychologic pain.

Strategies to Promote Adherence

The client's perceptions and attitudes must be assessed early in the development of the therapeutic alliance. Rating the client's potential for compliance is one strategy. A scale such as the Rating of Medication Influence (ROMI) has been developed for use with the schizophrenic client, but its basic compliance domains may help the clinician assess the potential compliance of any client with any condition. The scale identifies disease features, client–clinician interactions, physiologic and psychologic factors, client characteristics, and therapeutic regimen features (Weiden et al., 1994). Such a scale can be useful in comprehending the client's behavioral responses to medication use as well. However, specific training is required for the administration and interpretation of the scale.

Some concepts to keep in mind for promoting therapeutic adherence are:

- Healthcare providers and the client must clearly understand each other's goals and expectations.
- A treatment regimen that is not "user-friendly" will probably not be followed.
- The healthcare provider must communicate empathy and understanding about the client's emotional as well as physical needs.
- Verbal and nonverbal cues convey sensitivity to the client's concerns and promote trust.

The importance of effective client–clinician communication cannot be overemphasized. Modern pharmacotherapy has the potential to enhance quality outcomes, but failure to comply with prescribed regimens undermines this opportunity.

DiMatteo (1995) summarizes ways to enhance compliance (Box 8-1), recognizing today's changing healthcare delivery systems. Given that the length of hospital stays is continuing to decrease, clients must develop consistent, trusting relationships with primary providers and community-based team members, including nurses and pharmacists, to promote the therapeutic alliance between the client and the healthcare team.

The Nurse's Behavioral Response

The client's response to medication is also affected by the behavioral response of the nurse who administers the drug (Fig. 8-6). The nurse's attitude toward the client and the drug can create a positive or a negative atmosphere. Experts estimate that the nurse's attitude can increase the effectiveness of a drug by as much as 40%. For example, a caring nurse who can instill trust can in-

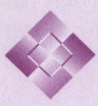

Box 8-1
Enhancing Adherence: Steps to Improve Communication

1. Inform the client, in general terms, about the diagnosis and discuss its possible causes.
2. Listen to the client's fears and frustrations. Encourage questions and descriptions of his or her expectations for treatment outcomes, including the effect of treatment on lifestyle.
3. Answer the client's questions. Address unrealistic expectations.
4. Suggest a treatment approach that may fit the client's expressed preferences. Explain the rationale for the choice, including expected benefits and costs, risks, and expected outcomes. Contrast the chosen treatment with other possible courses of action, including no treatment.
5. Obtain client feedback concerning belief in benefits and efficacy of treatment along with understanding and acceptance of risk. Devise methods to address concerns.
6. Discuss precisely how the client will implement treatment (eg, when and how to take the medication). Correct misunderstandings.
7. Work with the client to elicit a commitment to following the treatment regimen. If the client appears hesitant to make a clear commitment, return to step 2. Client commitment is necessary before a focus on practical issues can be successful. Simplifying and reminding will not help a client follow a regimen he or she does not believe in.
8. After the client makes the commitment, work with him or her to build supports (eg, support groups, reminders) and reduce barriers (eg, frequent medication dosing, prohibitively expensive medication, side effects) to the regimen. Revisit the issue of when and how the regimen will be implemented, and attempt to anticipate problems and suggest solutions.

Adapted with permission from DiMatteo MR. (1995). Patient adherence to pharmacotherapy. *Formulary, 30:*596–605.

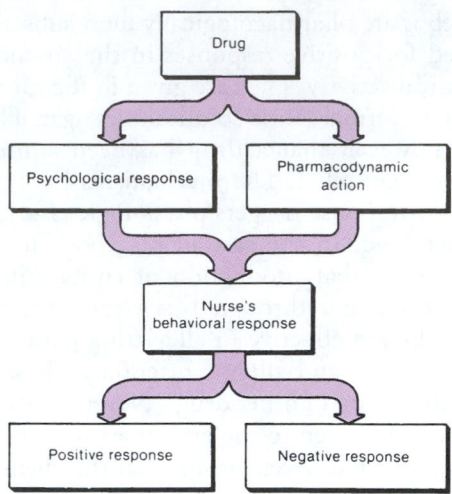

Figure 8-6. The nurse's behavioral response further influences drug effectiveness.

toward the drug and the emotional response of the client. Part of this encompasses perception of role, function, and satisfaction of personal need. A particular style of interaction with clients is assumed according to the nurse's needs. Periodic self-evaluation enables the nurse to monitor his or her own actions by asking: Do I voice rejection of the drug's beneficial properties? Do I feel angry about the client's refusal to take a medication? Do I project defiance or defensiveness at being questioned about a drug? Do I show pity or rejection of the client?

CRITICAL THINKING CHALLENGE
Issue Analysis

Consider the opportunities to develop a therapeutic alliance in the following scenarios.

- A client was recently diagnosed as having cancer. Chemotherapy will begin within the week.
- A client has moderate hypertension and must take an antihypertensive drug for life.
- A client on a course of antibiotic therapy for an acute ear infection receives the original dosage intramuscularly.
- A client receives a mild analgesic for monthly menstrual discomfort.

1. For each situation, identify your responses to the drug therapy.
2. What attitudes affect your responses? Identify the differences among these attitudes and describe the impact they may have in promoting compliance.
3. How do the length of time, degree of threat to life, type of medication, or route of administration influence your behavior?

crease compliance in schizophrenic clients. This trust is important in overcoming a client's lack of confidence in drug therapy.

Nursing actions can increase drug effectiveness. The degree of effectiveness achieved depends on the nurse's knowledge of the disease process, knowledge of the drug administered, and skill in using this knowledge in interacting with the client and family.

The nurse's attitudes, emotions, and drives are developed and reinforced through his or her social experiences. In approaching clients to administer a drug, the nurse should be aware of personal values and attitudes

CRITICAL THINKING CHALLENGE
Case Analysis

You are a new staff nurse being oriented to the mental health unit in your hospital. On rounds, you observe a client with bipolar disorder interacting with the primary nurse who is administering medication. In reading the chart, you note that the patient's lithium levels are not in the therapeutic range. You observe the following:

Nurse: Here, Bill, it's time for your medicine. It's your lithium.

Client: I don't want to take it now. I feel fine. Besides, I never take it at this time of day.

Nurse: Don't give me a hard time, Bill. Just take it like the doctor ordered.

Bill puts out his hand and takes the medication. The nurse hands him a glass of water and walks to the next client's room.

1. What assessment factors and medication administration practices are significant in this situation?
2. Consider the interaction style of the nurse and analyze what emotional responses he or she may be communicating to the client.
3. Describe the nurse's role as a potentiator of drug effectiveness.

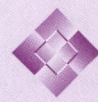

Box 8-2
Nurses as Potentiators of Effective Adherence With Drug Therapy

To promote maximal effectiveness of drug therapy, the nurse can:

- Understand the relation between physical and psychological responses
- Recognize the influence of attitudes and values on the response to drug therapy
- Develop an awareness of personal attitudes to drugs and client response
- Use knowledge of motivation in planning and implementing care
- Identify the meaning of drugs to the client and the impact the ensuing feelings have on drug effectiveness
- Actively involve the client in the development of the care plan
- Understand the power of suggestion in enhancing, decreasing, or negating drug effectiveness
- Begin client education with the initial contact and continue teaching through discharge
- Be knowledgeable about the drugs administered and observant of the client's physiologic and psychological responses to drug therapy
- Differentiate responses to types of illnesses; for example, examine whether one's response differs depending on the client's diagnosis.

Nurses, as potentiators of drug effectiveness, must recognize their own feelings and attitudes and must be alert in identifying the client's ability to cope. The observant nurse, recognizing emotional factors, uses knowledge and skill in reinforcing positive responses to drug therapy and in helping the client develop acceptable alternative responses. Drug therapy is enhanced when the client has faith in the efficacy of the drug and faith in the power of healthcare personnel to help (Box 8-2).

■ SUMMARY

Pharmacotherapy can have little impact on the client if the prescribed medications are not taken in accordance with the care plan. Clients have physiologic and psychologic responses to prescribed drug therapy.

The ability of healthcare providers to promote compliance is enhanced if they can recognize the client's point of view and values and the potential impact of perceived barriers to therapeutic adherence. The degree of compliance is a function of the client's perception that a trusting, caring, mutual therapeutic alliance has been established and will be maintained throughout treatment.

As a member of the healthcare team, the nurse has a significant role as a facilitator of therapeutic relationships. In addition, such nursing responsibilities as assessment, client education, and therapeutic interventions set the stage for the therapeutic alliance to develop. As coordinators of care, nurses facilitate continuation of the alliance beyond the hospital setting and into the community. The behavior and attitudes of nurses and other healthcare providers toward drug therapy also influence client compliance.

References

*DiMatteo MR. (1995). Patient adherence to pharmacotherapy: The importance of effective communication. *Formulary, 30*:596–605.

Kübler-Ross E. (1973). Letter to a nurse about dying. *Nursing '73, 3*:11.

*Olfson M, Glick I, Mechanic D. (1993). Inpatient treatment of schizophrenia in general hospitals. *Hospital and Community Psychiatry, 44*:40–44.

*Weiden P, Rapkin B, Mott T, Zygmunt A, Goldman D, Horvitz-Lennon M, Frances A. (1994). Rating of medication influences (ROMI) scale in schizophrenia. *Schizophrenia Bulletin, 20*(2):297–310.

*Recommended for further reading.

Bibliography

Frank E, Kupfer DJ, Siegel LR. (1995). Alliance not compliance: A philosophy of outpatient care. *Journal of Clinical Psychiatry, 56*(Suppl 1):11–16.

Gabbard GO. (1994). Psychodynamic psychiatry in clinical practice (DSM-IV edition). Washington, DC: American Psychiatric Press, 105–151.

Morris LS, Schulz RM. (1993). Medication compliance: The patient's perspective. *Clinical Therapeutics, 15*:593–606.

Stanitus M, Ryan J. (1982). Noncompliance, an unacceptable diagnosis? *AJN, 82*:941–942.

For more information and sample tests and activities, refer to Chapter 8 in the Student Workbook for Clinical Pharmacology and Nursing Management, 5th edition, available through your bookstore.

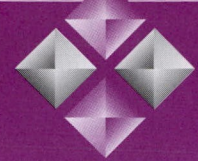

9
Cultural Aspects of Drug Therapy

Ethnomedicine
    Cultural diversity and pharmacotherapy
    Racial diversity and pharmacotherapy
African Americans
    Health and illness beliefs
    Remedies
Hispanic Americans
    Health and illness beliefs
    Remedies
Asian Americans
    Health and illness beliefs
    Remedies
Native Americans
    Health and illness beliefs
    Remedies
European Americans
    Health and illness beliefs
    Remedies
Ethnopharmacology
    Preparation and use of herbs
Nursing management

In recent decades, sociopolitical influences on Western culture have generated a renewed interest in naturalism, ecology, and the study of cultural heritage. The desire to exert more responsibility for and control over one's body and lifestyle has led to a resurgence in self-care practices. These self-treatments are often influenced by folk remedies and the use of medicinal plants for maintaining health and treating common illnesses.

The variety of ethnic backgrounds in the United States has contributed to a wealth of ethnocultural folk practices that have been passed down through generations. Each of the four major ethnic population subgroups in American society (African American, Hispanic American, Asian American, and Native American) has a

---

Box 9-1
Variety of Treatment Regimens

- Use of traditional herbal remedies exclusively
- Combined use of ritual and prayer with vegetable drugs
- Use of Western medical practices exclusively
- Combined use of Western medical practices and folk practices
- Adherence to various dietary and environmental guidelines

---

wide range of practices that influence beliefs and interventions related to health and illness.

Choices between traditional options and Western medical interventions vary within and across ethnic groups, and these choices are not subject to consistent application. At any given time, in any given group and its subgroups, treatment may involve the use of traditional herbal remedies exclusively, a combination of ritual and prayer with the use of vegetable drugs, customary dietary and environmental practices, or the application of Western medical practices alone or as an adjunct to folk practices. From traditions rooted in folklore for using medicinal plants, to recent scientific studies of the effects that certain botanical drugs have in regulating or diminishing the body's response to diseases, a merging of folk beliefs and science is reviving interest in the efficacy of botanical drugs. The science of ethnopharmacology attempts to bridge the gap between traditional uses of medicinal plants and their appropriate role in today's healthcare practice (Box 9-1).

Ethnomedicine

Factors that influence choices of cures are bound to cultural beliefs about the causes of illness. Ethnomedicine sees the ill client as a composite of psychosocial, cultural, physiologic, and spiritual forces that interact with the environment. This view contrasts with Western medical practices, which diagnose disease by categorizing the pathophysiologic deviations in body systems exhibited as symptoms of illness. The holistic approach of ethnomedicine may be considered an appealing departure from the Western rationale. Exploration of folk beliefs and practices in the African, Hispanic, Asian, and Native American populations reveals similarities among these groups' responses to illness. Those with traditional views within a group may respond to illness with the spiritual and ritualistic practices that are basic to the religious expressions of the population (Box 9-2). The response of others may reflect the discontinuity between existing sociocultural norms and the manner in which

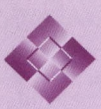

Box 9-2
Determinants of Health and Illness Practices of All Ethnic Groups

- Cross-cultural influences and within-group variations
- Socioeconomic status
- Language facility
- Strength and significance of kinship ties
- Degree to which one accepts beliefs, values, and practices of the dominant culture

illness and therapeutic practices have been expressed from generation to generation.

The following discussion is intended to represent a composite of the beliefs and folk practices in the cultures of different ethnic populations. It is not meant to stereotype various groups; rather, it attempts to develop a historical perspective and promote culturally sensitive health care by describing how culturally diverse persons deal with health and illness. Indeed, as people migrated from the Far East, Middle East, Europe, and Africa over centuries, customs and practices blended, accounting for the similarities that cross cultural boundaries.

Cultural Diversity and Pharmacotherapy

Cross-cultural similarities and differences reveal the epidemiologic differences in morbidity for a particular problem. This fact may indicate the culturally specific significance placed on certain diseases. Thus, the same problem may be handled in culturally unique ways. Responses differ from time to time: what is perceived as a problem in one instance may not be so at another time. These different responses may stem from a specific cultural value orientation. What is common and unavoidable may be considered insignificant; what is unacceptable symptomatic behavior, regardless of the cause, may be denied. Therefore, societal differences in the style of health and illness practices influence both the degree to which a person is aware of body symptoms and the decision to act on these symptoms.

Racial Diversity and Pharmacotherapy

In addition to the cultural influences on drug therapy, biologic variations among racial groups (eg, varying rates and mechanisms of metabolism) affect medication use. Alcohol, psychotropic drugs, antihypertensives, and neuroleptic medications affect racial groups differently. Therefore, consideration should be given to the roles that pharmacokinetics and the environment may play in response to using chemical substances. For example, some studies suggest that Asians and Native Americans do not metabolize alcohol as efficiently as European Americans or African Americans. Consequently, there is

a greater incidence of side effects (eg, flushing of the face, heart palpitations) when these persons use alcohol (Keltner and Folks, 1992). Similarly, psychotropic and neuroleptic drug reactions differ among races. Asians require lower doses to achieve therapeutic serum blood levels and metabolize the drugs more slowly than do European Americans or African Americans. This is especially true for the Chinese, although Indian and Pakistani groups are also affected.

African Americans
Health and Illness Beliefs

The African American population in the United States is estimated to exceed 32 million, according to the U.S. Bureau of Census (1994). Many among this ethnic group in North America carry the traditional health beliefs of their African heritage. Health beliefs are congruent with the holistic principles of ethnomedicine (ie, health denotes harmony with nature of the body, mind, and spirit). Illness is seen as a state of disharmony that results from natural causes or divine punishment. The desire to restore harmony and thereby the sense of self is the focus of folk practices. The person, the family, and the community are essential components of this model.

Survival depends on restoring and maintaining balance and harmony. The practices common to the art of healing and restoring balance stem from a fundamental belief that such power is a divine gift. Traditional healing practices may include treatments with herbs, consultation with voodoo practitioners, and rituals known empirically to restore health. Folk practices of Native Americans and European Americans have also been integrated into current ethnomedical practices. Specific healing forms include using home remedies, obtaining medical advice from a physician, and seeking spiritual healing.

Remedies

There are no universal rules for selecting the most appropriate provider or the most efficacious form of intervention. In fact, simultaneous use of various practitioners is not uncommon. For example, a family member, friend, or neighbor may possess the gift of healing. Usually, the self-treatment practices recommended through this lay referral system must be exhausted before initiating further consultation. If the client knows and trusts these practitioners, more timely consultation with a physician is likely.

Home remedies and medicines that are natural (made from plants) are important aspects of the treatment process. The first line of traditional intervention is generally prayer, alone or in conjunction with rituals, and the practice of laying on of hands. Magic rituals frequently include wearing charms or amulets to protect against evil spirits and disease. Folk practices that have

Table 9-1. Selected Home Remedies Used Among African Americans

Common Malady	Home Remedy
Cold, congestion	Hot toddy, a hot drink prepared with tea, lemon, honey, peppermint, and alcohol Vicks VapoRub, used as a rub but sometimes ingested Hot camphorated oil rubbed on chest and covered with warm flannel or similar cloth Hot lemon, water, and honey beverage blended with garlic, onion, and parsley
Fevers	Onions applied raw to the feet and wrapped in a warm blanket Herbs, brewed into teas
Worms	Turpentine and sugar mixed together and taken orally
Wound infection and inflammation	Potato poultice made of raw sliced or grated potatoes placed in a bag and applied to affected area; as the potatoes rot, the affected area improves, probably as a result of the mold produced as the potato spoils Cornmeal and cooked peach leaf poultice applied to inflamed area; fermentation process creates bactericidal enzymes
Open wounds	Ground bluestone, a mineral thought to prevent inflammation, is crushed and applied to wound Salt pork placed in a cloth and applied to wound Poultice of stale bread soaked in sour milk and wrapped in cloth applied to wound
Boils	Raw egg shell membrane removed from inside egg shell and placed on boil to draw it to a head

withstood the test of generations provide reasonable interventions and comfort measures. For example, the use of hot baths and warm compresses for rheumatism and the use of herbal teas for respiratory illnesses have been validated by their positive results. Kitchen condiments are often used to prepare home remedies. Substances such as lemon, vinegar, honey, saltpeter, alum, salt, baking soda, and Epsom salt are familiar ingredients in folk remedies. Goldenrod, peppermint, sassafras, parsley, yarrow, and rabbit tobacco are a few of the herbs used as medicinal ingredients. Table 9-1 lists some home remedies used in the African American community.

Many African Americans are well versed in the use of home remedies, and reliance on them reflects a belief in their curative properties. It is likely that recognizing, valuing, and accommodating the choices of clients who seek care from the modern healthcare system and who also practice folk medicine will facilitate a return to harmony in the client's mind, body, and soul.

Hispanic Americans

The U.S. Bureau of Census estimates that about 22 million Hispanic Americans live in the United States (1994). Eighty percent of the Hispanic population has its origins in Mexico, Puerto Rico (a U.S. territory), and Cuba. The remaining 20% has its origins in other Spanish-speaking regions, such as Central and South America. This discussion focuses on the beliefs and practices of Mexican American and Puerto Rican cultural groups, as they represent the largest segments of this group.

Health and Illness Beliefs

As with other ethnic groups, the health and illness practices of Hispanic Americans are socially and culturally determined. The acceptance or rejection of traditional folk beliefs depends on individual influences, the person's socioeconomic status, his or her language facility, the strength and significance of kinship ties, and the degree to which the person subscribes to the beliefs and values of the dominant population. Hispanic cultural influences encompass European, Spanish, South American, and Indian folk beliefs (including Mayan, Aztec, and other Native American beliefs). The use of folk healers, medicinal herbs, and magic, accompanied by religious ritual and ceremonies, represents the rich and varied customs of Hispanic Americans.

Fatalism is a dominant characteristic of the belief system. A healthful state of being exists when the psychosocial, biologic, and spiritual natures are holistically balanced in relation to the environment. Traditional Hispanics believe that God is responsible for allowing health or illness to occur. Wellness may be viewed as good luck, a reward for good behavior, or a blessing from God. Praying, using herbs and spices, wearing religious objects such as medals, and maintaining a balance in diet and physical activity are considered appropriate ways to prevent evil or poor health.

The view that health is a state of equilibrium, with illness resulting from physical causes or conditions, reflects the naturalistic concept of disease etiology subscribed to by many Puerto Rican Americans. Maintaining a balance between hot and cold is characteristic of the naturalistic belief system. On the other hand, some

Puerto Rican Americans, for example, credit metaphysical forces, such as supernatural spirits, with causing psychosomatic or incurable illnesses. This belief stems from a personalistic concept of disease etiology.

For traditional Hispanic Americans, including those with origins in Puerto Rico, maintaining a balance between hot and cold forces is basic to promoting wellness. Illness is often categorized as either hot or cold, and the required treatment is determined by the use or removal of hot or cold elements to counterbalance the disease type. To restore the body's balance, cold treatments are required for hot diseases and vice versa. The classification of diseases also reflects imbalances between wet and dry elements. The characterization of body fluids reflects these attitudes (Spector, 1991):

Blood: hot/wet

Yellow bile: hot/dry

Black bile: cold/dry

Phlegm: cold/wet

An application of this belief is the use of chili, considered a hot substance, to treat pneumonia, a cold disease. Other beliefs related to maintaining balance include wetting the head to avoid a sore throat from wet feet, abstaining from pork (a cold food) after childbirth (a hot experience), and using penicillin (a hot drug) to treat pneumonia (a cold disease).

Illness (*enfermedad*) generally is classified as physical when it has to do with the body and natural when it has to do with emotional or natural forces. Symptoms of physical illness may include fever (*calentura*), pain (*dolor*), nausea or vomiting (*basca*), cough (*tos*), or rash (*erupcion*). Physical illness is thought of as benign or mild, temporary or grave. Hispanic Americans may categorize emotional illnesses as mental or moral (Table 9-2).

In addition to physical or emotional illnesses that result from body imbalances, external supernatural or magic causes, envy, or intense emotional states, a fifth cause exists. This category reflects the belief that dislocation of body parts can cause illness. For example, a depressed anterior fontanelle in an infant is thought to result from touching the area (usually by medical personnel). The healthcare provider examining an infant should be alert to this interpretation. Recognizing the interrelationships between folk beliefs and traditional health and illness practices is essential to understanding the cultural implications of drug use in remediating disease.

The range of diseases recognized by a person and the choice of interventions depend on the degree of acculturation in Euroamerican society. Folk beliefs and traditional ethnopharmacologic practices may be person-specific: what may be common practice for treating an illness in one family may be contraindicated, or simply unheard of, in another.

Remedies

Assessing an illness to determine its identity and severity is a systematic, almost scientific, practice carried out by many Hispanic women. They methodically consider signs and symptoms and balance them against what is believed to be health. A strong dichotomy between biophysical and supernatural illnesses does not seem to exist in Hispanic ethnomedical practices. Folk illnesses tend to represent the core group of ailments, but it is not uncommon to mix remedies that may be magical and biophysical to cure a single illness. Hispanic ethnopharmacology is notably more complementary to, rather than competitive with, Western medical practices.

After the illness is identified, appropriate treatment follows. Three options commonly are available: home remedies (*remedio caseros*), which use medicinal vegetables and herbs; over-the-counter patent medicines, such as Alka-Seltzer, Pepto-Bismol, or aspirin; and physician-prescribed medications. Herbs may be collected, dried, and stored by each household, or they may be purchased in local herb stores (*botanicas*). Most remedies take the form of teas, infusions, or poultices to cure mild illnesses. Digestive problems may be relieved by drinking a mild mint tea. Colic may be treated with anise, rosemary, or camomile tea. A cough may be treated with oregano tea.

Ailments commonly identified with folk medicines are stomach ache, menstrual disturbances, pneumonia, sores, and whooping cough. Ethnopharmacologic treatments used by some Hispanics to cure these conditions are applied in various forms, either as a single agent or as a combination of ingredients in a designated preparation.

Remedies for stomach aches are usually prepared as teas that include wormwood, rue, sweet basil, cinnamon, purple sage, horehound, and coriander, as well as the ingredients already mentioned. Garlic is sometimes eaten raw for this problem, and a poultice made of bloodworm, egg, corn tortilla, or other foods may be applied topically for relief.

Table 9-2. Kinds of Emotional Illness Among Hispanic Cultures

Causes of Illness	Examples
Mental illnesses	
Heredity	Epilepsy, mental retardation
Hex	Witchcraft, evil eye
Derangement from worry	Pressure, anxiety
Derangement from fright	Nervous breakdown, hysteria
Derangement from head injury	Craziness, amnesia
Moral illnesses	
Vice	Addiction to drugs, marijuana user
Weak character	Alcoholism, kleptomania
Emotions	Jealousy, rage

Menstrual disturbances may be treated with a tea brewed from borage, bush pepper, rosemary, camomile, rose petals (rue), or cinnamon and aspirin. Sores are treated with remedies prepared in baths featuring olive oil, sunflower, and copperleaf. Sores may also be cured by using herbs prepared in poultices that use sweet basil, onion, swallow wort, gum plant, or sunflower oil and butter. Black burro's milk or teas brewed from purple sage are used in treating whooping cough. Pneumonia may be treated with teas made from mallow or mint.

With options from both ethnomedicine and conventional medicine, the choice of remedies seems to be influenced by several factors, including personal experience, the severity of the illness, and the degree to which symptoms are accommodated in known folk-treatment modalities.

Treatments for hot or cold illnesses, for example, require substances that counterbalance the hot or cold quality of the disease (Box 9-3). Common cold conditions, such as respiratory infections or menstruation, require hot remedies, such as chocolate or alcohol, and spicy or hot foods, such as onions or garlic. Hot conditions, including ulcers, constipation, or diarrhea, respond to treatment with cold or cool substances, such as fruits.

Nurses and other healthcare practitioners should be sensitive to these cultural practices. Table 9-3 describes conditions and behaviors characteristic of clients who have a naturalistic approach to illness. A client who seeks a solution to health problems may use both traditional and conventional healthcare systems.

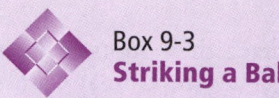

Box 9-3
Striking a Balance

In seeking natural harmony and balance, some Hispanic American groups treat what are known as cold conditions and diseases with hot remedies. Hot conditions are treated with cold remedies.

Cold (Frio) Conditions, Hot Remedies

Among diseases and conditions classified as cold are arthritis, colds, *firaldad del estomago* (cold stomach), menstruation, joint pain, and chills and shakiness (*pasmo*). These conditions are treated with hot medicinal, herbal, and food remedies. Among hot medicines and herbs are alcoholic beverages, anise, aspirin, cinnamon, iron tablets, penicillin, rue, vitamins, and tobacco. Among hot food products are castor oil, cod liver oil, chili peppers, chocolate, coffee, cornmeal, evaporated milk, garlic, kidney beans, onions, and peas.

Hot (Caliente) Conditions, Cold Remedies

Among diseases and conditions classified as hot are constipation, diarrhea, rashes, tenesmus (*pujo*), and ulcers. These conditions are treated with cold or cool foods, medicines, or herbs. Cold foods include avocados, bananas, coconut, lima beans, sugar cane, and white beans; cool foods include bottled milk, chicken, fruits, honey, raisins, salt cod, and watercress. Cool medicines and herbs are bicarbonate of soda, mannitol (*mana de manito*), magnesium carbonate (*magnesia boba*), milk of magnesia, linden flowers, mastic bark, nightshade (*yerba mara*), orange flower water, sage, and barley water.

Table 9-3. Characteristic Health Behaviors of Adherents to Hot–Cold Practices

Client's Condition or Situation	Health Behaviors
Common cold, arthritis, joint pains	Client will not take cold-classified foods or medications but will accept those classified as hot.
Diarrhea, rash, ulcers	Client will not take hot-classified medications and uses cool substances as therapy.
Condition requiring a diuretic as part of a treatment regimen and supplementation of potassium intake with bananas, oranges, raisins, or dried fruit	Client will not eat these cold-classified foods with a cold or other cold-classified condition (for female patients this includes the menses).
Condition requiring penicillin or any other hot medication, particularly on an ongoing basis	Client will stop taking hot medicine when suffering any hot-classified symptoms (eg, diarrhea, constipation, rash).
Infant requires formula, which contains hot-classified evaporated milk	Mother will put baby on cold-classified whole milk or will, after feeding formula, "refresh" the baby's stomach with various cool substances, some of which are diuretic.
Pregnancy	Women avoids hot medicine and hot foods and takes cool foods and medicine frequently.
Postpartum and menstruation	Woman avoids cool foods and medicines, particularly those that are acidic.

Asian Americans

Americans of Asian descent have their roots in Japan, the Philippines, Korea, Laos, Hawaii, China, Cambodia, Vietnam, and Thailand. The total Asian American population is estimated to be about 8 million.

Folk medicine practices and traditional beliefs about health and illness are similar because of the ancient philosophies and practices shared by most Asian cultures. These practices include meditation, special nutritional programs, herbology, and martial arts. A major difference between Eastern and Western cultures is the practice of health promotion and illness prevention. Groups with Asian origins tend to practice prevention; groups with Western European origins tend to emphasize illness intervention and treatment. These different values are reflected in varying degrees in the United States. Many Chinese people who emigrated in the 1920s still practice traditional healing and prevention and continue to influence family health practices. First, second, and subsequent generations of Asian Americans blend Western medicine with aspects of traditional folk beliefs.

Health and Illness Beliefs

For Asian Americans, harmony with nature is essential for physical and spiritual well-being. Universal balance depends on harmony between the elemental forces: fire, water, wood, earth, and metal. These forces are continually interacting, creating the natural balance of elements in the world.

Regulating these universal elements are two forces that maintain physical and spiritual harmony in the body, the *yin* and the *yang*. The characteristics of yin and yang are described in Table 9-4. These forces provide the energy for cosmic control. Imbalance between yin and yang is thought to be the cause of physical disease or natural disaster.

According to tradition, some Chinese physicians receive payment for their efforts to promote health and maintain the body's state of balance. Illness is viewed as a failure by the physician, who is not likely to collect a fee for treatment. Therapeutic options available to the traditional Chinese physician include prescribing herbs, meditation, exercise, nutritional changes, or acupuncture. Potential body imbalances may be diagnosed through inspection of the client's appearance, a history-taking or assessment of the problem through interviewing, palpation of deep and superficial pulses to determine the severity of the condition, or the use of hearing and smell to determine the client's general condition. The treatments recommended may require consultation with an herbalist, a spiritual healer, an acupuncturist, or a Western physician.

The importance of health maintenance in the Chinese healthcare system is based on the belief that the body is a gift from one's ancestors and, as such, should be revered and maintained in good repair throughout the life cycle.

Remedies

Maintaining or restoring yin and yang uses the principles of energy flow and balance of the body's vital organs for health. If the practices discussed previously are insufficient to prevent illness, herbology is used to bolster the body's natural healing forces. Vegetable medicines enjoy a long and significant history in the traditions of Chinese folk remedies. Knowledge about the utility of specific agents for healing has been handed down through generations; this knowledge has been systematically studied, observed, experimented with, theorized about, and recorded. The earliest recordings of medicinal herb use are believed to be more than 2000 years old. Since 1949, scientific analysis of Chinese medicinal herbs has isolated several valuable chemically active compounds (Table 9-5). The herb's classification is based on its active pharmacologic ingredients. The most common types of ingredients are (Lewin et al., 1994):

- Volatile oils, called ethereal or essential oils, are odorous ingredients that evaporate.
- Resins are chemical ingredients that include esters, alcohols, and tannols.
- Alkaloids are alkaline, organic ingredients.
- Glycosides are compounds containing both carbohydrate and noncarbohydrate components.
- Fixed oils are long-chain fatty acids and alcohols.

Cultivation of herbs is supported by the Chinese government, and techniques for growing and harvesting are explicit. The potency and utility of herbs are influenced by the part of the plant collected, the life cycle of

Text continues on p. 129.

Table 9-4. Characteristics of Yin and Yang

Yin	Yang
Female	Male
Negative energy	Positive energy
Emptiness	Fullness
Darkness	Light
Cold	Warm
Inside of the body	Surface of the body
Front of the body	Back of the body
Body organs: heart, liver, lungs, kidney, spleen	Body organs: stomach, small and large intestines, gallbladder, bladder
Winter and spring diseases	Summer and fall diseases
Control of body pulses	Control of body pulses
Stores essential life strength	Protects body from outside attacks
Certain foods (eg, watercress, winter melon)	Certain foods (eg, ginger root, chicken)

Table 9-5. Pharmacology of Traditional Chinese Herbs

Chinese Name	Botanical Name	Plant Family and Plant Part Used	Active Ingredients	Properties/Actions
Huai-niu-hsi or *Sun-niu-hsi*	*Achyranthes bidentata*	Amarantaceae	Calcium oxalate crystal, saponin, oleonolic acid, glucuronic acid, k-salt ash	Decreases blood pressure, peristalsis of the duodenum; causes strong uterine contractions in high doses; in alkaloid form, causes blood hemolysis and denatures protein
Fw-tze or *Wu-tow*	*Aconitum carmichaeli*	Ranunculaceae	Alkaloids of aconine and aconitine	Painkiller
Pin-liang-hua or *Fu-she-tsao*	*Adonis amurensis*	Ranunculaceae: whole plant	Cymarin	Slightly toxic, bitter taste; direct action on cardiac muscle, causing contractions, dilation of coronary blood vessels to increase blood flow; useful as diuretic and tranquilizer
Che-hsi	*Alsima plantago-aqua-tica*	Alismataceae: tuber stem with partial root	Volatile oil, plant sterols, alkaloids, resins, proteins, fatty acids, sugars	Nontoxic, slightly bitter taste; antibacterial agent; lowers blood pressure, blood glucose, and serum cholesterol
Tang-Kuei	*Angelica sinensis*	Umbellifera: main and branch roots	Angelicone, angelic acid, vitamin E, sucrose	Dried roots are sweet, aromatic; prepared in water extract—causes uterine contractions; prepared in ethyl alcohol—causes uterine muscles to relax; reverses vitamin E deficiency symptoms; produces calming effect on cerebral nerves
Tung-Kua or *Tung-Kua-jen*	*Benincasa hispida*	Cucurbitaceae: seed meal, whole plant	Urease, hispidamin, purine, trigonelline	Nontoxic; diuretic; treatment of coughs in infants
Chia-hu	*Bupleurum chinese*	Umbelliferae: dried root	Fatty oils, lignoceric acid, volatile oils	Nontoxic, slightly bitter taste; reduces fever; in extract preparation, used to treat malaria
Hung-hua	*Carthamus tinctorius*	Compositae: flower	Carthamiolin (after chemical treatment)	Nontoxic, slightly bitter taste; used as wound treatment that decreases pain and helps healing
Chi-kow or *Chi-shih*	*Citrus aurantium* (bitter-orange)	Rutaceae: fruit, leaves	Aurantiamanic acid, hesperidin, organic acids, linonene, vitamin C	Aids digestion, decreases gas pain by antispasmodic action; sedative
Shau-chu-yu	*Cornus officinalis*	Cornaceae: dried fruit	Cornin, garlic acid, malic acid, vitamin A, saponin, tannin	Chewy, acidic, slightly bitter taste; diuretic action; decreases blood pressure
Yan-hu-so	*Corydalis bulbosa*	Papaveraceae: tuber	Corydaline, protopine, corybulbine, captisine	Odorless, bitter taste, slightly toxic; improves circulation; reduces pain; tranquilizing effects
Pa-tou	*Croton tiglium*	Euphorbiaceae: dried seeds	Crotin, alkaloids, fatty acids, protein ash	Very toxic; strong cathartic that irritates skin and mucous membrane
Yu-chin	*Curcuma aromatica*	Zingiberaceae: tuber stem, root ends	Camphene, camphor, curcumene	Slightly aromatic; used to treat epileptic convulsions and circulatory disorders
Shan-yao	*Dioscorea batatas*	Dioscoreaceae: tuber roots, tubers above ground	Starch with amylase, saponin, allatonin, mucin	In dried powdered form, used as soothing paste for external application
Kan-sui	*Euphorbia sieboldiana*	Euphorbiaceae: tuber root	Palmitic acid, citric acid, oxalic acid, tannin, resin, glucose, sucrose, starch	Toxic, bitter taste, strong odor; used to treat edema, constipation

(continued)

Table 9-5. (Continued)

Chinese Name	Botanical Name	Plant Family and Plant Part Used	Active Ingredients	Properties/Actions
Kan-tsao	*Glycyrrhiza uralensis*	Leguminosae: root, lower stem	Glycyramarin, liquiritin, mannitol, glucose, starch, sucrose	Mild odor, sweet taste; an additive for herbal remedies; acts like adrenocortical hormones; used to treat duodenal and stomach ulcers
Shih-chi-ching or *Tung-ching*	*Iiex chinensis*	Aquifoliaceae: seed, leaves, bark	Tannin, volatile oil	Low toxicity; antiseptic agent used locally to treat burns
Mao-tung-ching	*Iiex pubescens*	Aquifoliaceae: roots, leaves	Theobromine, ilicin	Nontoxic, slightly bitter taste; acts on coronary artery by reducing blood pressure, increasing flow to cardiac muscle
Chuan-chiung	*Ligusticum wallichii*	Umbelliferae: underground tuber stem	Alkaloid, lactone derivative, ferulic acid	Bitter taste, aromatic; used to treat local pain and swelling; extract preparation used to control central nervous system activities
Hou-pu	*Magnolia officinalis*	Magnoliaceae	Alkaloids, saponin, volatile oil	Slightly bitter taste, aromatic; for treatment of respiratory tract
Chuan-lien-pi	*Melia toosendan*	Meliaceae: stems, bark, roots	Margosine, neutral resins, tannin	Very bitter taste; used to treat parasites
Pe-hua-she-shih-tsao	*Oldenlandia diffusa*	Rubiaceae: whole plant	Hydrocarbons, ureolic acid, stigmasterol, β-sitosterol, *p*-hydroxycinnamic acid	Used as diuretic, anti-infective; to treat heat stroke
Pe-shou	*Paeonia lactiflora*	Ranunculaeae: dried root	Volatile oil, benzoic acid, paeoniflorin, paeonol, paeonine, tannin, fatty oil, resin, starch	Odorless, slightly bitter taste; used as general tonic
Jen-seng	*Panax ginseng*	Araliaceae: dried root	Triterpenic saponosides, essential oils, a triester, panaxatriol	Regulates blood pressure; stimulates central nervous system; counteracts fevers; useful as general tonic to produce long life, strength, and happiness
Huang-pai or *Huang-pi-show*	*Phellodendron chinese*	Rutaceae: inside layer of dried tree bark	Berberine, palmatine, phellodendrine, magnoflorine, obakunone, dictamnolide	Bitter taste, slight odor; decreases fever in the treatment of dysentery; used to treat jaundice
Pan-hsia	*Pinellia ternata*	Araceae: tuber stem	β-sitosterolglucoside, choline, volatile oil, sterols, saponin, starch, fatty acid	Essentially tasteless, odorless; used for respiratory congestion; for relief of gas pain and vomiting during pregnancy
Fu-lin	*Poria cocos*	Polyporaceae: fungal growth on the roots of old pine trees	Pachymic acid, polysaccharide, ergosterol, choline, phospholipids, proteins, resins, fats, enzymes	Diuretic used to treat edema; soothes coughs; used as a tranquilizer
Tao-jen	*Prunus persica*	Rosaceae: dried seeds	Fatty oil, amygdalin	Nontoxic, slightly bitter taste; mild cathartic; used to treat general digestive tract problems
Di-huang	*Rehmannia glutinosa*	Scrophutariaceae: tuber root	Mannitol, glucose, rehumannin	Odorless, sweet taste; decreases fever; diuretic action; decreases blood sugar
Ta-huang	*Rheum tanguticum*	Polygonaceae: dried root stem	Glucosides, tannin, quinone derivatives, resins, dextrin, starch, sugar	Aromatic, bitter taste; used to treat occasional constipation
Dan-seng	*Salvia miltiorrhiza*	Labiatae: dried root	Tanshinone I, II, cryptotanshinone	Slight odor, mildly bitter taste; used to treat insomnia; circulatory problems; enlargement of the liver or spleen; hypertension

(continued)

Table 9-5. (Continued)

Chinese Name	Botanical Name	Plant Family and Plant Part Used	Active Ingredients	Properties/Actions
Di-yu	Sanguisorba officinalis	Rosaceae: tuber root	Tannin, sanguisorbin	Slight odor, slightly bitter taste; used to stop bleeding; externally used to treat burns, insect or snake bites
Mu-hsiang	Saussurea lappa	Compositae: dried root	Volatile oil, resin, sugars, camphorene, saussurine, philladrene	Strong taste, aromatic; general health tonic
Huang-chen	Scutellaria baicalensis	Labiatal	Baicalin, wogonin	Odorless, bitter taste; reduces fever; diuretic action; prevents miscarriages; decreases blood pressure; increases blood sugar
Pu-kung-yin or Kung-yin	Taraxacum mongolicum	Compositae: whole plant, roots	Taraxacin, choline, taraxacerin, pectinum	Used to treat external wounds
Lang-yu	Ulmus parvifolia	Urticaceae	Starch, tannin, ergosterol, sterols	Nontoxic, bitter taste; external dressing for wounds
Chiang or Kan-Chiang	Zingiber officinale	Zingiberaceae: underground stem	Volatile oils, resin, zingirol, starch	Hot taste

the plant at the time of harvest, the time of day and the season of harvest, and the processing the plant must undergo. The cleaning process is important to ensure efficacy, increase or decrease potency, reduce toxicity, and enhance storage.

Commonly, a client presents a prescription to the herbalist, who measures the required ingredients and directs the client to prepare the herb by boiling it for a prescribed amount of time in a nonmetal container. It is then drunk as an extract or tea.

Body imbalances may also be treated through *moxibustion*, the application of heat to traditional acupuncture points using the burning herb moxa (*Artemisia vulgaris*). The herb's potency is determined by its age; it is thought to be most effective if older than 9 years. Acupuncture is viewed as a cold treatment, moxibustion a hot treatment.

Native Americans

The Native American population in the United States includes about 300 tribes, in addition to the Eskimo and Aleutian peoples. Together, they number nearly 2 million. Tribes of significant size include the Navajo (Dine), Cherokee, Sioux (Lakota), Chippewa, Pueblo, Lumbee, Hopi, Choctaw, Apache, Iroquois, Zuni, and Creek. Because each Native American community has unique cultural beliefs and language, any overview of traditional practices runs the risk of misrepresenting or stereotyping the entire population. The following information is intended to identify a cross-section of traditional beliefs and folk practices. They may be characteristic of some tribes, but not of others.

As aborigines, Native Americans survived in harsh regions of the country by understanding the environ-ment. With the introduction of diseases, environmental changes, and health practices, the Spanish and European colonists influenced the Native Americans' existence, which originally included gathering wild plants and hunting animals for food and a strong system of spiritual healing. Later, Native Americans developed an agricultural livelihood. As the Europeans began to colonize North America, Native Americans increasingly migrated west; California, Oklahoma, Arizona, and New Mexico have the largest numbers of Native Americans today.

Health and Illness Beliefs

The theme of total harmony with nature is fundamental to traditional Native American beliefs about health. The human body is both one with and interdependent with the universe. Health for each person depends on maintaining a state of equilibrium among the physical body, the mind, and the environment. Health practices reflect this holistic approach to health and illness.

Illness may be believed to be purposeful in response to social problems (ie, disruptions in the social system). It is accepted as a fact of life that happens in relation to a past or future event. The external event, rather than the illness itself, must be handled to effect improvement. Health or illness is thought to result from variations in the balance between positive and negative body energies and is thought to be controlled by spiritual means. Interventions depend on a fundamental belief in the principle of cause and effect.

A state of unhappiness, sickness, or imbalance may result from several factors, such as tampering with the spirits, a disruption in the elements of nature, neglecting or misusing ceremonial rituals, or witchcraft (Spector,

1991). The method of healing is determined traditionally by the medicine man, who diagnoses the ailment and recommends the appropriate intervention. In the diagnostic phase, the spiritual cause of an illness is identified by using medication, herbs, and divination. Treatment may be accomplished with chants determined through divination. Recommendations are then made to correct the illness. Treatment may include heat, herbs, sweat baths, massage, exercise, diet changes, or other interventions performed in a curing ceremony.

For some Southwestern tribes, diagnosis through stargazing is a learned ritual. Beams of light are believed to determine both the reason for the problem and the prognosis for recovery. The healer asks the star spirit to identify the cause of an illness.

In the hand-trembling ritual, the practitioner's hands move while he or she chants. While thinking of a variety of diseases, the practitioner moves the hands in a set pattern. An involuntary change in hand motions indicates that the practitioner has thought of the correct disease.

A third type of divination is listening. The ceremony resembles stargazing, except that the diagnosis is heard rather than seen. Certain sounds represent specific ailments.

Diagnosis of an illness involves a consultation among the entire family and the medicine man that focuses on the client's condition and the treatment necessary for recovery. Whether an ailment is caused by a breach of tribal taboos or by sorcery, the psychological influence of ceremonies and rituals for curing is significant to the family. These traditions provide personal attention, often for several days, which inspires faith in the predictions made by the medicine man.

Prevention of illness is also valued. Methods used to maintain health include wearing charms, purification through sweat baths, protection from extremes of temperature, dancing, and using herbal decoctions.

Remedies

Traditional folk practices reflected the belief that a person is one with nature and that every person is first part of a community. The practice of total body purification, achieved through immersion in water or through other rituals, was believed essential to restoring or maintaining harmony. As hunters, gatherers, and farmers, Native Americans developed knowledge about the local vegetation. This information became an integral part of their health beliefs, and herbs were used in purification and healing rituals. Minor illnesses with obvious causes were treated by empirically validated folk remedies. When the ailment was thought to be of supernatural origin, the tribe-specific remedies would be sought from the

Table 9-6. Herbal Remedies Used by Some Traditional Native American Tribes

Ailment	Herbal Remedy	Plant Part Used	Active Ingredients	Preparations
Skin wounds, cuts, sores	Balsam fir	Gum, underbark	Tannins and oleoresins have astringent and antiseptic properties.	Underbark used as dressing; gum or saliva mixed with bark after chewing applied to affected area
	Spruce	Bark		
	Pine	Bark		
	Juniper	Bark		
Bleeding wounds	Tobacco plant	Leaves	Tannins provide mild antiseptic, astringent action.	Cuts covered with leaves
	Spikenard			
	Pokeweed			
Infected cuts and burns	Birch	Bark	Methyl salicylate; alkaloids have antibacterial action	Poultice applied to area
	Bloodroot	Bark		Underbark applied to wound
	Balsam fir	Underbark	Tannins and volatile oils have astringent, antiseptic, and odor-masking properties.	
	Cedar	Underbark		
Headache	Skunk cabbage	Plant	Tannins, aloe–emodin, chrysophanole, rheine	Snuff prepared from dried plant parts
	Rhubarb	Root		
	Buttercup	Leaves		
Cough	Wild cherry	Bark	Volatile oils have analgesic, diaphoretic, and stimulant properties.	Expectorant made from tea
Constipation	Butternut	Bark	Contains irritant substances	Teas
	Dock	Root		
Nausea	Bittersweet	Root	Solanine, solanaceous alkaloids	Teas
Stomach ache	Milkweed	Root	Cyanogenetic glycosides, volatile oils, parasorbinic acid, malic acid, sugars	Teas, syrups, extracts
	Mountain ash	Fruit		
	Birch	Inside bark		
Decreased lactation	Dandelion, *Euphorbia* species	Milky latex in leaves, roots	Flavonoids, amino acids, alkanes, triterpenoids, alkaloids	Toxic; sometimes ingested after giving birth; also applied topically to nipples

medicine man. The contributions of Native Americans to the development of pharmacology are seen in the *United States Pharmacopeia & National Formulary* and other drug directories, which cite more than 200 botanical medicines used by different tribes.

Experts in the medicinal use of native plants or animals were usually herbalists. Herbalists were different from medicine men, although both were believed to have healing powers. Superstition was a factor in determining who was gifted with healing powers. A common practice in herbal medicine was the "doctrine of signatures," a belief that "like cures like." Under this doctrine, the selection of a particular plant was based on its odor, shape, or color. For example, the dandelion stem contains a milk, which was used to stimulate increased lactation. Red plants were used for blood-related problems, and yellow plants were considered appropriate for treating jaundice. Numerous medicinal herbs are still commonly used by traditional Native Americans (Table 9-6).

The process of herb collection is prescribed and is based on cultural beliefs and values. An herb's efficacy depends on collecting rituals that take into account the season of the year, time of day, direction of the sunlight, and phase of the plant's life cycle. Autumn is generally thought to be the best time to harvest herbs for drying. The remedial power of a plant is believed to be the result of solar energy, with the early morning rays the strongest. Therefore, a plant part with the benefit of an eastern exposure is preferable. Respect for nature requires the use of only what is essential.

The traditional ways of coping with health and illness remain the first course of action for Native Americans, who have a rich heritage based on respect for self, others, and nature. The isolation and deprivation caused by the conflict of these values with Western values in medical care are taking their toll. The knowledge of traditional medicine is slowly being lost as access to, and the availability of, culturally supportive programs are limited.

European Americans
Health and Illness Beliefs

For European Americans, home treatments are often the front-line interventions used before seeking help from a modern healthcare practitioner. Traditional remedies practiced by European Americans for health promotion, health maintenance, or treatment of an ailment are based on the magical or empirically validated experience of ancestors. These cures are frequently practiced in combination with religious rituals or spiritual ceremonies. For example, an American of Catholic, French Canadian descent may wear camphor around the neck for protection from evil spirits, recite prayers for good health, or place a gold wedding ring on an infected eye and make the sign of the cross three times as a treatment for the problem (Spector, 1991).

Remedies

Remedies often represent rational approaches to uncomplicated problems. Household products, herbal teas, and patent medicines are familiar preparations used in home treatments (eg, salt-water gargle for a sore throat, Vicks VapoRub applied to the nostrils for congestion, or cough syrup made from honey and whiskey). Applying cold, wet tea bags to a sunburned eyelid and using baking soda and water for indigestion are also common home remedies (Spector, 1991).

Ethnopharmacology

"Ethnopharmacology is a multidisciplinary area of research concerned with the observation, description, and investigation of indigenous drugs and their biological activities" (River and Bruhn, 1979). The outcome of this scientific research can be a better understanding of the use of herbs in treating diseases. Studies may uncover information about the chemical structure of the biologically active components of plants, and such data could aid in the synthesis of effective vegetable drugs. For example, empirical evidence based on traditional folk remedies may suggest that an extract of a substance is therapeutic, whereas use of the isolated active ingredient could be toxic.

Scientific investigation can also help standardize doses and specify preparations that produce predictable outcomes. It is thought that some of the side effects of chemically active synthetic products could be more easily controlled or decreased by using medicinal plants. Drugs derived from plants clearly hold a place in both traditional folk medicine and modern health care. Today, the continuing availability and viability of plant-derived drugs are threatened. Given that as much as 80% of the world's population relies on medicinal plants as their primary source of health care, any decline in species availability will affect these practices.

It is estimated that 60,000 species will become extinct by the year 2050 if current trends continue. Pollution, deforestation, and the destruction of tropical rainforests are clearly affecting the ecosystem. Depletion of medicinal plants is inevitable. In developing countries, where most people rely on medicinal plants for their drug needs, industrial encroachment threatens the productivity, variety, and character of the plant species available. Loss of folk knowledge about plant and herbal remedies goes hand in hand with these changes because the native people in the tropical rainforests are also disappearing. Conservation strategies to prevent the disappearance of forests and plant species and a concurrent development of botanical gardens are underway in response to these trends.

Several medicinal plants and herbal remedies have been discussed in relation to the ethnocultural value system in which they are used. Recognition of the active ingredients contained in the plants offers information

CRITICAL THINKING CHALLENGE
Issue Analysis

Is the use of folk remedies and medicinal plants a greater problem for the healthcare system or the consumer?

The issue of compliance is often a challenge for health-care providers, particularly when the client's health be-haviors are grounded in custom and folk medicine. Al-though traditional healthcare systems and professional education programs acknowledge the need to respond to culturally diverse populations, there is still incompatibility between the provider's beliefs and the sick role clients are expected to assume. The client, on the other hand, may have conflicts about continuing to use traditional treat-ments that have succeeded in the past, taking a new di-rection in seeking health care from the established sys-tem of the dominant culture, or combining both types of practices.

1. Consider how the development of a therapeutic al-liance might promote the desired outcomes for both client and care provider, in contrast to focusing solely on compliance issues.
2. Explore the consequences of such conflicts and their impact on the care provider, the delivery system, and the client.
3. Analyze the barriers to successful outcomes that this issue may create.
4. Describe interventions you might devise to promote greater sensitivity to cultural values. How could you incorporate these values into the care plan?

about their potential use in health care. As noted earlier, plants may contain vitamins essential for good health, nitrogenous organic compounds (alkaloids) that act on the vascular and central nervous systems, antibiotics that attack microorganisms, and essential oils, heterosides (glu-cides or sugars), acids, or minerals that interact chemi-cally to affect certain body organs. The chemical prop-erties, drug action, and folk use of several medicinal plants are described in Table 9-7.

Several other medicinal plants are also significant. The purple foxglove (*Digitalis purpurea*) has been rec-ognized for its effectiveness as a diuretic in treating cer-tain forms of heart failure. Its active ingredients include the glycosides digitalin, gitoxin, and digitoxin, which act on the cardiac muscle. The potency and potential for toxicity of this herb are well recognized. Other plants used in treating heart ailments are hawthorn (*Crataegus oxyacantha*), which contains flavonoids and leucoantho-cyanidins; American hellebore (*Veratrum viride*), which contains a glycoside and alkaloids and has hypotensive actions; and rauwolfia (*Rauwolfia serpentina*). The main ingredient of rauwolfia is reserpine, which has hypoten-sive and sedative actions.

Several medicinal plants have been examined as pos-sible cancer cures, including American mandrake root (*Atropa mandragora*), meadow saffron or autumn crocus (*Colchicum autumnale*), and periwinkle (*Catharanthus roseus*). Periwinkle contains the alkaloids vinblastine and vincristine, which are used to treat cancers charac-terized by the proliferation of white blood cells. Pacli-taxel (Taxol), from a variety of the yew tree, is in use as an anticancer agent, particularly for ovarian cancer.

Mandrake contains a highly irritating resin that has been used by Native Americans as a purgative, an emetic, and a treatment for condyloma acuminatum (venereal warts). The latter is an officially recognized use of this plant today. Meadow saffron contains the active ingredient colchicine, which prevents the division of cells. It is highly toxic and has been used to treat certain forms of leukemia, as well as to alleviate the pain of acute gout and arthritis.

Many medicinal plants are recognized for their soothing qualities. The opium poppy (*Papaver somnif-erum*) is one of the oldest and best known of the pain-relieving herbs. This plant is chemically complex, with more than 25 alkaloids, fatty oils, lecithin, and albumin. The pain-relieving and sedative qualities of the opium poppy are found in its morphine and narcotine alkaloids. Henbane (*Hyoscyamus niger*), common lettuce (*Lactuca virosa*), and cocaine, an alkaloid from the leaves of the *Erythroxylon coca* plant, are also used to reduce pain or to promote sedation. Henbane is a toxic plant with the ac-tive ingredients of several alkaloids, including scopola-mine, hyoscyamine, and atropine. Its pharmacologic pro-perties produce analgesia and sedation.

Cocaine is one of the oldest known anesthetics. It was the first effective local anesthetic. Today, it is more commonly used as a topical anesthetic in certain clinical procedures or for minor surgery of the eye, nose, ear, throat, rectum, or vagina. Folk use of cocaine in general tonics was common because the alkaloids acted as cen-tral nervous system stimulants.

Common lettuce (not the salad variety) is a toxic plant that contains several chemically active elements found in the bitter white latex exuded when the plant is cut. The latex in dried form is brown and contains the bitter compounds lactupicrine and lactucine, which have hypnotic and sedative actions and have been used in lozenges for the relief of coughs.

Table 9-8 gives more information on herbal prepa-rations and their toxic effects.

Preparation and Use of Herbs

Ethnopharmacology is the study of the proper collec-tion, use, and storage of medicinal plants. The rules for plant collection are tailored to the plant part that con-tains the drugs. For example, to avoid insect infestation, flowers are best collected immediately on opening and should be dried in an airy, dry, dark environment. Leaves are gathered for drying before and during the flowering season; larger leaves are hung and smaller ones are laid out in a dry, airy place. Seeds require little special treatment; *Text continues on p. 135.*

Table 9-7. Common Medicinal Plants

Herb (Part Used)	Botanical Name	Properties	Active Components	Folk Uses
Alfalfa, lucerne (leaves, seeds)	*Medicago sativa*	Antihemorrhagic, anti-anemic, nutritive, stimulant	Leaves contain vitamins A, C, D, E, K, calcium, potassium, iron, phosphorus	Healing ointment, arthritis, strength-giving
Aloe (leaves)	*Aloe vera*	Laxative	Arthracenosides	Externally for healing wounds and treatment of burns; internally for chronic constipation
Anise (seed)	*Pimpinella anisum*	Diuretic, gastric stimulant, relieves flatulence and cramps, galactogenic	Essential oils of anethole and estragol, fatty oil, choline	Dry cough, flatulence
Bayberry (bark)	*Myrica carolinensis*	Emetic, general stimulant, astringent	Tannin	Gargle, mouth rinse for bleeding gums, douche
Blessed thistle	*Cnicus benedictus*	Appetite stimulant, diaphoretic, emetic, expectorant, diuretic (in high doses—causes burns of esophagus and mouth and may cause diarrhea)	Tannin, mucilage, essential oil, sesquiterpenoid lactone	Digestive problems, reduces fevers, breaks up congestion
Bugleweed (flowers)	*Ajuga reptans*	Astringent, tranquilizer, sedative	Tannin	Treatment of sore throat, coughs, appetite stimulant, relieves pulmonary bleeding
Catnip, wild catmint (leaves)	*Nepeta cataria*	Antidiarrhetic, diaphoretic, antispasmodic	Essential oil with thymol, caroacrol, nepetol, nepetalactone	Chronic bronchitis, diarrhea
Camomile (whole plant)	*Anthemis nobilis*	Antispasmodic, gastric stimulant	Chamazulene, coumarin, flavonic heterosides	Internally for migraines, gastric cramps, anxiety; externally for treatment of wounds, ulcers, conjunctivitis
Cayenne pepper (fruit, seeds)	*Capsicum frutescens*	Stimulant, irritant, toxic in large doses	Aromaticamide, capsaicine, capsanthine	Stimulant, burn treatment, wound treatment, relief of toothaches
Chestnut, horse (fruit, bark)	*Aesculus hippocastanum*	Narcotic, astringent, outer skin of fruit is toxic	Saponins, tannins, glycoside, flavones	Fluid extract of fruit used for sun protection, bark used for fevers
Chicory, wild succory (root, leaves)	*Chichorium intybus*	Tonic, diuretic, gastric stimulant, cholagogic (including flow of bile), laxative	Inulin, intybin	Digestive tract problems, gout, stimulates bile secretion
Comfrey	*Symphytum officinale*	Emollient, sedation, wound healing	Allantoin, alkaloid, consolidine, choline, tannin, sugar, mucilage, starch, asparagine	Poultice for treatment of wounds, ulcers, cuts; gargle for tonsillitis
Dandelion (root)	*Taraxacum officinale*	Diuretic, gastric stimulant, tonic, cholagogic	Lactupicrine, tannin, inulin	Frequently found in patent medicines; treatment of liver and kidney disorders
Elder (bark, flowers)	*Sambucus nigra*	Mucilage, diaphoretic, antispasmodic	Terpenes, glucoside, mucilage, tannin	Used for fevers, chills; gargles for tonsillitis, pharyngitis
Ergot (fungus, not an herb)	*Claviceps purpurea*	Sedative, uterine stimulant	Ergotoxine, ergotamine	Menstrual problems, hemorrhage, migraine
Eucalyptus (leaves)	*Eucalyptus globulus*	Antibiotic, respiratory disinfectant, antimuculatic	Tannin, flavonoid pigment, bitter resin, essential oils	Decreases respiratory secretions, cough suppression, topical treatment for wounds

(continued)

Table 9-7. (Continued)

Herb (Part Used)	Botanical Name	Properties	Active Components	Folk Uses
Fennel (seeds)	*Foeniculum vulgare*	Stimulant, gastric stimulant, diuretic, antispasmodic, carminative, expectorant	Essential oils with anethole, fenchone, fatty oil	Enhances lactation; for treatment of colic, flatulence, gout
Garlic (juices)	*Allium sativum*	Mucosal irritant, vermifuge, antispasmodic, intestinal antiseptic, diuretic, expectorant, antihypertensive	Essential oil of allicine, allyl sulfide, enzymes, vitamins A, B_1, B_2, nicotylamide	Cold treatment, antiseptic, diuretic
Ginseng	*Panax ginseng*	Febrifuge, decreases cholesterol level, CNS stimulant	Essential oils, panaxatriol, saponosides	Tonic, weak aphrodisiac, blood-pressure regulation
Goldenrod (leaves)	*Solidago virgaurea*	Stimulant, diuretic, expectorant, antidiarrhetic, wound healing properties, aromatic	Saponin, flavonoids, essential oil, tannin, bitter compound	Treatment of kidney disorders, rheumatism, general discomfort, sore throat, eczema
Grapevine (leaves, roots)	*Vitis vinifera*	Laxative, diuretic	Potassium bitartrate, calcium bitartrate	Heart tonic
Hollyhock	*Althea rosea*	Diuretic	Mucilage, pectin, sugar	Chest problems
Horehound	*Marrubium vulgare*	Expectorant	Marrubine, tannin, essential oil	Respiratory problems, gastrointestinal disorders
Hound's-tongue (roots, aerial parts)	*Cynoglossum officinale*	Antidiarrhetic, toxic to some animals	Tannin, alkaloids	Diarrhea treatment
Ivy (leaves)	*Hedera helix*	Antispasmodic, berries are toxic, irritant	Saponin, hederagenine, acid	Treatment of rhinitis, cataracts
Juniper (berries)	*Juniperus communis*	Gastric tonic, diruetic	Essential oil containing alphapinene, cadinene, camphene, terpineol, organic acids, sugar	Stomach tonic, enhances appetite and digestion, diuretic, disinfectant of urinary tract
Licorice (root)	*Glycyrrhiza glabra*	Demulcent, expectorant, antispasmodic, diuretic	Saponoside, glycyrrhizin, flavonoids, steroid hormones	Soothes cough, prevents thirst, treatment of stomach ulcers
Lily of the valley (flowers)	*Convallaria majalis*	Powerful cardiotonic, antispasmodic, purgative, diuretic	Cardenolides, saponoside	Headaches, treatment of heart conditions, but may be toxic
Mandrake (roots)	*Atropa mandragora*	Diuretic, sedative, mydriatic	Alkaloids, scopolamine and hyoscyamine	Fertility aid
Marigold (leaves, flowers)	*Calendula officinalis*	Choleretic, antiphlogistic, vulnerary properties, diaphoretic	Resin, essential oil, saponin	Relief of muscle tension, enhances wound healing
Mistletoe (leaves)	*Viscum album*	Peripheral vasodilator, diuretic, hypotensive, narcotic, antispasmodic, toxic in large doses, cardiotonic	Saponoside, amyrines, viscotoxin	Treatment of hysteria, epilepsy, relieves menstrual cramps, sleeping agent
Mullein (flowers)	*Verbascum thapsus*	Expectorant, soothing gargle	Saponins, lanceolate	Smoked as decongestant, sedative as tea
Mustard (whole plant)	*Sisymbrium officinale*	Sedative, gastric stimulant, diuretic, cooling	Sulphur compounds, cardenolides	Purgative, expectorant, treatment of hoarseness
Nightshade (leaves, roots)	*Atropa belladonna*	Highly toxic, spasmolytic, sedative, diuretic, mydriatic	Hyoscyamine, scopolamine	Stimulates circulation, treatment of eye diseases, decreases smooth muscle activity
Parsley (seeds, leaves)	*Petroselinum crispum*	Diuretic, gastric stimulant, carminative, expectorant	Essential oil with apiol and myristicin, flavones, apiine, pinene, vitamin C	Jaundice, coughs, asthma, amenorrhea, dysmenorrhea, conjunctivitis

(continued)

Table 9-7. (Continued)

Herb (Part Used)	Botanical Name	Properties	Active Components	Folk Uses
Peppermint (leaves)	*Mentha piperita*	Antispasmodic, carminative, tonic, stimulant, aromatic	Essential oil with menthol menthone, jasmone, alcohol, aldehydes, tannins	Nervousness, insomnia, cramps, dizziness, coughs
Rosemary (leaves)	*Rosemarinus officinalis*	Stimulant, antispasmodic, stimulates bile secretion (toxic in large quantities), astringent	Essential oil with eucalyptol, borneol, ester, pinene	External: in ointment to soothe rheumatism, sprains, wounds, bruises, eczema; internal: gastric stimulant, relieves flatulence, stimulates bile release from gallbladder, relieves colic
Saffron (flowers)	*Crocus sativus*	Appetite stimulant, regulates menstruation, sedative, diaphoretic	Glycoside (picrocrocine)	Amenorrhea, hysteria, used as an abortive agent, dysmenorrhea
Sarsaparilla (roots)	*Smilax regelii*	Enhances metabolism, enhances absorption, diuretic	Saponosides, essential oil, resin	Skin disorders, rheumatism
Slippery elm (bark)	*Ulmus fulva*	Tonic, astringent	Tannin, mucilage	Soothes stomach; diuretic, diaphoretic, antidiarrhea agent
Soapwort (rhizome, leaves, roots)	*Saponaria officionalis*	Purgative, expectorant, diuretic, detergent	Saponin (saporubine), saponarin, vitamin C	Relief of cough, congestion; to loosen secretions
Sweet violet (flowers)	*Viola odorata*	Expectorant, soothes coughs, antihypertensive	Saponins, alkaloid, aromatic compounds	Expectorants for treating respiratory disorders, purgative, emetic
Thyme (garden)	*Thymus vulgaris*	Antiseptic, deodorant, vermifuge, carminative	Essential oil, tannin, antibiotic and bitter compounds	External: liniment for wounds, in compresses, and as gargle; internal: antidiarrhetic, soothes bronchitis, laryngitis, relief of gastritis, cramps
White willow (bark, leaves)	*Salix alba*	Tonic, febrifuge, antirheumatismal	Glycosides of salicine and salicortine, tannin	To reduce fevers
Woodruff (dried seeds)	*Asperula odorata*	Deodorant, anticoagulant	Coumarin, dicumarol, aromatic compounds	Flavoring wine, to scent linen, blood purifier
Yarrow, milfoil (whole plant)	*Achillea millefolium*	Tonic, antiseptic, astringent, carminative, gastric stimulant, relieves cramps	Essential oils of eucalyptol, proazulene, achilleine	Used for anorexia, dyspepsia

(Leek C. [1975]. *Herbs: Medicine and mysticism.* Chicago: Henry Regnery; Schauenberg P, Paris F. [1977]. *Guide to medicinal plants.* New Canaan, CT: Keats Publishing.)

they do well when air-dried. The whole plant is cleaned of dead foliage or soil and dried by hanging in well-spread bundles. The bark and roots of a plant are best when young plants are used. The process involves washing, cutting into small pieces, and then drying. After cleaning, fruit is dried in a low-temperature oven for a prescribed period of time.

Dried plants may be used for medicinal purposes in various ways. The most common practice is to make a tisane. The recipe is specific and contains several elements:

- The basic remedy (which may have two or more ingredients)
- The adjuvant (to balance or enhance the effect of the basic remedy)
- The complement (added to enhance texture or appearance)
- The correctos (usually aromatic compounds to enhance flavor).

The active ingredients of the plants may be preserved in several ways until they are needed for a tisane: in dried powdered form, as a fluid, or as a solid (pill or suppository form). The methods used to prepare the tisane depend on the physical nature of the ingredients. For example, if the vegetable drug contains mucilage, a maceration is made; this is an aqueous extraction of the product that has been soaking in cold water for 2 to 12 hours. If the flowers, seeds, or leaves of the plant contain the medicinal

Text continues on page 140.

Table 9-8. A Systems-Oriented Approach to Herbal Toxicities

Central Nervous System

Herb Name	Botanical Name	Pharmacologic Principle	Herbalist's Use	Clinical Effects	Toxicity	Miscellaneous
African yohimbe bark	*Corynanthe yohimbe*	Yohimbine	Stimulant, aphrodisiac	Hallucinogen	Increased blood pressure, fatigue, abdominal distress, weakness, paralysis	Smoke or tea
Broom, Scotch broom	*Cytisus scoparius*	Cytisine, scarparin, sarothamonine hydroxytyramine, sparteine, genisteine	Relaxant	Sedative–hypnotic	Vomiting	Smoke, diuretic, cathartic, emetic
California poppy	*Eschscholtzia californica*	Alkaloids, tryamine and glycosides, coptisine, sanguinarine	Euphoriant	Euphoriant		Marijuana substitute, poppy family (opioids)
Cinnamon	*Cinnamon camphora*	Tannin, mannitol, essential oil	Stimulant, carminative, astringent	Stimulant	Local irritant to skin or eye; nausea, vomiting, renal genitourinary irritation	Bark is smoked
Damiana	*Turnera diffusa aphrodisiaca*	Volatile oil, resin, tannin, damianin	Stimulant, purgative, aphrodisiac	Stimulant, purgative, aphrodisiac	Genitourinary irritation	Liquid, pill, smoke; may exacerbate preexisting urinary infection
Hops	*Humulus lupulus*	Lupulinic acid, lupulon, humulene oil	Sedative, antiseptic	Sedative	?Hemolysis	Not wild hops (*Byronia* species is toxic); fruit of plant used as tonic for dyspnea, diuresis
Hydrangea	*Hydrangea peniculata*	Hydragin (glycoside), saponin, cyanogenic glycoside	Stimulant, carminative	Stimulant	Dizziness, chest pain, nausea, vomiting	Decrease bladder calculi, treatment of cystitis, marijuana substitute; smoke
Kava-kava	*Piper methysticum*	Arylethylene pyrone, flavokawain, methysticin, dihydromethysticin, kawain	Sedative	Sedative, hallucinogen	Yellow pigmented skin lesions; sedation	Drowsiness, pigmented lesions, diuretic, genitourinary antiseptic
Kola nut, gotu cola	*Cola nitida*	Caffeine, theobromine, kola catechin (tannin)	Stimulant, diuretic, astringent	Stimulant, decreases fatigue	Insomnia, anxiety, tachycardia, increased symptoms of peptic ulcer disease	Smoke, tea, capsules
Lobelia	*Lobelia inflata*	Lobeline, atropine, scopolamine, pyrridines	Stimulant, depressant	Euphoriant, anticholinergic	Nausea, vomiting, headache, convulsion, coma; hepatotoxin	Marijuana substitute
Mate	*Ilex paraguayensis*	Caffeine; ?pyrrolizidine alkaloids	Stimulant, diuretic	Hallucinogen, laxative, diuretic, diaphoretic	Caffeinism, veno-occlusive disease	Smoke, tea, capsules

Common name	Scientific name	Active constituents	Traditional use	Action	Toxic effects	Route/comments
Mormon tea	*Ephedra nevadensis*	Ephedrine	Stimulant, rheumatism, syphilis, fever	Stimulant, sympathomimetic	Hypertension, tachycardia	Tea
Morning glory	*Ipomea purpurea*	Resin, lysergic acid amide	Hallucinogen, purgative	Hallucinogen	Nausea, diarrhea, confusion, coma	Marijuana-like effect
Nutmeg, mace	*Myristica fragrans*	Myristicin (volatile oil), nutmeg oil, elemicin, eugenol	Hallucinogen, GI disorders, rheumatism, emmenagogue, abortifacient, aphrodisiac	Vomiting	Nausea, vomiting, hypothermia, chest pain, dizziness, headache	Myristicin converted to MMDA; elemicin converted to TMA
Passion flower	*Passiflora caerulea*	Cyanogenic glycosides, harmine alkaloids	Hallucinogen	Hallucinogen, stimulant	Convulsions, decreased blood pressure, temperature, respiratory rate	No report of cyanide poisoning; smoke, tea, capsules
Periwinkle	*Catharanthus roseus*	Indole alkaloids, vinca alkaloids	Euphoriant	Hallucinogen, dry mouth	Drowsiness, nausea, ataxia, hepatotoxicity, seizures, decreased bowel sounds, alopecia	Smoke, tea
Prickly poppy	*Argemone mexicana*	Isoquinolone alkaloids, protopine, berberine	Euphoriant	Euphoriant	Visual difficulties, nausea, vomiting, diarrhea	Smoke seeds
Snake root	*Rauwolfia serpentine*	Reserpine, other alkaloids	Tranquilizer, decreases blood pressure	Decreased blood pressure	Bradycardia, coma, diarrhea, dizziness, hypotension, miosis, nasal congestion	
Thorn apple (sacred datura, jimson weed)	*Datura stramonium*	Atropine, hyoscyamine, scopolamine	Hallucinogen, asthma, dyspepsia	Anticholinergic syndrome	Anticholinergic syndrome, contact dermatitis	Smoke, tea, seeds
Tobacco	*Nicotiana* species	Nicotine	Stimulant	Stimulant	Nicotine syndrome	Cigarettes
Valerian (garden heliotrope)	*Valeriana edulis* *V. officianelias*	Valerine alkaloids and glycosides	Tranquilizer	Tranquilizer	Vomiting, drowsiness	Cigarettes
Wild lettuce	*Lactuca sativa*	Lactucarine nitrates; ?hyoscyamine	Depressant; ?opium substitute; cough medicine, relaxant	Sedative		In cattle, *L. sacriola* causes emphysema after eating immature plants
Wormwood	*Artemisia absinthium*	Absinthol, volatile oil	Relaxant	Sedative, analgesic	Seizures, coma	Smoke, tea; use dried leaves and flowering tops

(continued)

Table 9-8. (Continued)

Herb Name	Botanical Name	Pharmacologic Principle	Herbalist's Use	Clinical Effects	Toxicity	Miscellaneous
Cardiovascular System						
Buchu	Barosoma betulina	Diosphenol (volatile oil)	Diuretic, also genitourinary uses	Diuretic	Nausea, vomiting	
Foxglove	Digitalis purpurea Digitalis lanata	Digitoxin, digoxin, gitoxin	Heart stimulant	Cardioactive	Vomiting, bradycardia, dysrhythmia	Decreases in blood pressure and heart rate
Hellebore	Veratrum viride Veratrum album	Steroidal glycolalkaloids, aconitine veratrum, veratrine, veratrosine	Decreased blood pressure, toxemia of pregnancy	Cardioactive	Vomiting, bradycardia, hypotension	
Oleander	Herium oleander	Oleendroside, other cardioactive glycosides; ?nerioside	Heart stimulant	Cardioactive	Vomiting, diarrhea	Dried root and rhizomes used in tea or made into tincture enemas
Gastrointestinal System						
Black cohosh	Cimicifuga species	Cimicifugin (resin)	Dyspepsia	Dyspepsia, cathartic, emetic	Nausea, vomiting	
Caraway	Carum carvi	Carvone (ketone), terpene (volatine oil), calcium oxalate	Colic	Carminative, flavoring agent	Nausea, vomiting, CNS depression	
Cardamom	Ellettaria cardemonum Amonum cardemonum	Cardemom	Condiment	Carminative, purgative	Nausea, vomiting, diarrhea	
Castor bean	Ricinus communis	Castor oil (fixed oil), lectin (ricin)	Laxative, cathartic	Laxative, cathartic	Nausea, vomiting, bleeding	Phytotoxin, protoplasmic poison
Coconut	Cocos ruficera	Trilaurin	Antihelminthic	Cathartic	Diarrhea	
Dandelion	Taraxacum officinale	Taraxacerin (resin)	Dyspepsia, diuretic	May stimulate gastric secretion	Vomiting	High in vitamin A, C, and niacin; protein, fat, iron
Golden seal	Hydrastis canadensis	Hydrastine, berberine Emetine, cephaline	Dyspepsia, stop postpartum bleeding	Nausea, vomiting	Nausea, vomiting, paresthesia, hypertension, CNS stimulant, respiratory failure	Fatalities; used to mask EMIT urine; toxicology screen for opioids
Ipecac	Cephaelis acuminata Cephaelis ipecacuerha		Emetic	Emetic		

Common Name	Scientific Name	Active Ingredient	Use	Effect	Toxicity
Jalap	*Exogonium purga*	Jalapin glycoside (resin), convolvulin	Cathartic	Watery diarrhea	Volume depletion, excessive catharsis; Wound care
Olive oil	*Olea europoea*	Olein (fixed oil)	Laxative	Emollient	Diarrhea
Peanut oil	*Arachis hypogaea*	Olein	Laxative	Demulcent	Diarrhea; Increases serum cholesterol
Senna	*Cassia acutifolia*, *Cassia angustifolia*	Anthraquinones	Laxative	Watery diarrhea	Abdominal pain
Respiratory System					
Grindelia	*Grindelia camporum*, *Grindelia humilis*, *Grindelia squarrosa*	Balsamic resin	Expectorant, asthma, bronchitis, mild sedative		Renal toxicity, cardiotoxicity
Jimson weed	(See CNS system)		Asthma	Drowsiness, decreases heart rate, mydriasis, increases blood pressure, stimulates expectoration	(See CNS system)
Lobelia	(See CNS system)		Asthma, expectorant	Bronchodilation	
Miscellaneous: Metabolic, Hepatic, and Hematologic					
Heliotrope, Rattlebox, Groundsel, Viper's bugloss	*Crotalaria spectabilis*, *Heliotropium europeaum*, *Senecio species*, *Echium plantagineum*	Pyrrolizidine			Hepatic veno-occlusive disease, hepatic and pancreatic tumors
Gordolobo	*Cephaelis*		Edema, stress		
Ipecac	*Cephaelis ipecacuenha*	Cephaeline, emetine		Emetic	Seizures, GI bleeding
Pennyroyal oil	*Hedeoma pulegioides*	Pulegone	Abortifacient	Menstrual bleeding	Hepatotoxicity
Periwinkle	(See CNS system)		Hypoglycemic	(See CNS system)	

ingredient, an infusion is made by pouring boiling water on the plant parts. This plant steeps in a covered container for 5 to 15 minutes before it is filtered. When the vegetable drug is found in the bark, stems, or roots of a plant, a decoction is prepared by soaking the parts in cold water and then bringing them to a boil gradually. This mixture is cooked for 5 to 20 minutes, depending on the texture of the ingredients used.

Folk practices using medicinal plants are complex processes that require accurate knowledge for safe use (Box 9-4). In the traditional use of herbal remedies, empirical evidence of efficacy was sufficient to sustain the practice of using plants to treat illness. Although herbal medicine is used throughout the world, and is on the rise in the United States, the potentially toxic effects of some species should not be overlooked. The sale and distribution of plants for medicinal use is not currently regulated by the Food and Drug Administration.

Several factors create the potential for poisoning. Huxtable (1990) identified several causes of such poisoning:

- Consumption of plants misidentified as safe
- Unknown toxicity of a plant
- Inability to distinguish which plant parts are in an herbal compound
- Lack of knowledge about substance safety
- Variable chemical composition of a given herbal preparation because of the part of the plant used, time of year harvested, conditions of storage, and problems with adulteration.

With the goal of creating a culturally sensitive healthcare system, the risks and benefits of herbal remedies must be weighed. The client must recognize that just because something is "natural," it is not necessarily safe to consume.

■■ SUMMARY

Our health habits and health-seeking behaviors are a function of our environmental, economic, and cultural background. What we believe and learn is heavily influenced by family practices and historical patterns. Differences and similarities in health practices exist among and within the many major population groups in the United States. The remedies considered therapeutic and the health or illness strategies applied are often steeped in tradition.

Plants and plant derivatives often contain chemically active elements that are or are thought to be therapeutic. Medicinal plants play a significant role in the health practices of many cultural groups.

❖ NURSING MANAGEMENT

Nursing education provides general knowledge about the impact of cultural attitudes on persons who enter the healthcare system. However, each nurse must de-

Box 9-4
Worldwide Ethnopharmacology

In the mid-1900s, increasing awareness of the cultures of developing countries focused attention on the use of traditional medicines. Scientists began exploring the rational use of medicinal plants within the context of the cultural groups using them. The studies aimed to document the pharmaceutical efficacy of certain herbs, the psychosocial value of indigenous cultural healing practices, and the interdependence of mind, body, and the environment for healthful behavior.

In 1978, the World Health Organization (WHO), an arm of the United Nations, set forth criteria for studying and documenting medicinal plants in the developing countries of the world. In doing so, WHO recognized the necessity of using indigenous treatments in providing health care. It became important, therefore, to have accurate information about the actual use of botanical medicines in a given region, accompanied by any available scientific data on their pharmaceutical efficacy.

In the attempt to standardize data gathering and investigations, WHO defined *medicinal plants* ("any plant which in one or more of its organs contains substances that can be used for therapeutic purposes or which are precursors for chemopharmaceutical semisynthesis") and *vegetable drugs* ("part of the medicinal plant used for therapeutic purposes") and established a standard format for investigations. The format covers several categories: general information, ecological investigation, botanical investigation, pharmacognostic investigation, method of use, information on general therapeutic activity, and other data and observations. The agency to contact for further information is the World Health Organization, United Nations, New York, NY 10000; telephone (212) 963-6132.

velop sensitivity to and respect for the beliefs of different ethnic and cultural groups.

Whether cultural beliefs are founded in the realm of magic, spiritualism, empiricism, or rational science, they represent humanity's struggle to come to terms with the limits of the human condition and the complexity of the environment. The nurse should assess each client as an individual and should not ascribe general characteristics based on the client's cultural background. Moreover, each client's cultural background is unique because cultural beliefs and values vary within cultural groups. The understanding of different value systems should not result in cultural stereotyping.

Nursing practice requires careful, objective assessment of the client's health beliefs, traditional practices, and cultural realities to plan interventions that will not

HOME AND COMMUNITY CARE

Guidelines for Using Herbal Remedies

Clients who use herbal remedies must weigh the risks and benefits of such use. Keeping in mind that quality, composition, and preparation are not monitored in these over-the-counter products or harvested substances, the nurse should offer the client the following guidelines:

- Do not take for granted that because a substance is a natural herb or plant product, it is beneficial or harmless.
- Seek medical care when ill.
- When seeking medical care, always inform the provider if herbs are being used.
- Avoid taking herbal remedies if you are pregnant or lactating.
- Be sure that any product package contains a list of all contents.
- Frequent or continual use of large quantities of a given preparation is not advisable.

be antagonistic to the client's values. Nursing interventions should encourage social and psychological support for the client throughout the healthcare system. These interventions should recognize the value of traditional folk practices to the client's well-being. Therapy that accommodates a client's belief in traditional rituals is likely to encourage compliance and to decrease the potential for cultural dissonance or disenfranchisement from the healthcare system.

Of course, clients should always be advised of the potential for chemical interactions between traditional home remedies and prescribed medications. They should be informed of the possible harm that may result if therapies are mixed. Alternative forms of healing must be recognized, however. With this recognition may come the preliminary steps to bridging the gap between the scientific rationalism of medical practices and the client's culture-dependent beliefs about wellness and illness.

References

Huxtable R. (1990). The harmful potential of herbals and other plant products. *Drug Safety, 5*(Suppl 1):126–136.

Keltner NL, Folks DG. (1992). Psychopharmacology update: Culture is a variable in drug therapy. *Perspectives in Psychiatric Nursing, 28*(1):33–35.

Lewin NA, Howland M, Goldfrank LR. (1994). Herbal preparations. In Goldfrank LB, et al. *Goldfrank's toxicologic emergencies*, 5th ed. Norwalk, CT: Appleton & Lange.

River L, Bruhn J. (1979). Editorial. *J Enthnopharmacology 1*(1):1.

Spector R. (1991). *Cultural diversity in health and illness*, 3d ed. New York: Appleton-Century-Crofts.

U.S. Bureau of Census (1994). *Statistical abstracts of the United States*, 114th ed. Washington DC.

Bibliography

Akerele O. (1993). Nature's medicinal bounty: Don't throw it away. *World health forum, 14*:390–395.

Andrews MM, Boyle JS. (1995). *Transcultural concepts in nursing care*, 2d ed. Philadelphia: JB Lippincott.

Anyinam C. (1995). Ecology and ethnomedicine: Exploring the links between current environmental crisis and indigenous medical practice. *Social Science Medicine, 40*(3):321–329.

Bauwens E, ed. (1977). *Ethnic medicine in the southwest*. Tucson: University of Arizona Press.

Centers for Disease Control and Prevention (1995). Self-treatment with herbal and other plant-derived remedies in rural Mississippi, 1993. *MMWR, 11*(44):204–207.

Giger JN, Davidhizar RE. (1995). *Transcultural nursing: Assessment and intervention*, 2d ed. St. Louis: CV Mosby, pp. 128–161.

Helman CG. (1990). *Culture, health and illness*, 2d ed. London: Wright.

McElroy A, Townsend PK. (1985). *Medical anthropology in ecological perspective*. Boulder: Westview Press.

Pachter L. (1994). Culture and clinical care: Folk illness beliefs and behaviors and their implications for health care delivery. *JAMA, 271*(9):690–694.

Secondy MG, ed. (1992). *Trials, tribulations and celebrations: African American perspectives on health, illness, aging and loss*. Yarmouth, ME: Intercultural Press.

Schauenberger P, Paris F. (1977). *Guide to medicinal plants*. New Canaan, CT: Keats Publishing.

Simmonite W, Culpeper N. (1957). *The Simmonite-Culpeper herbal remedies*. London: W. Foulsham.

For more information and sample tests and activities, refer to Chapter 9 in the Student Workbook for Clinical Pharmacology and Nursing Management, 5th edition, available through your bookstore.

IV

Developmental Considerations in Drug Therapy

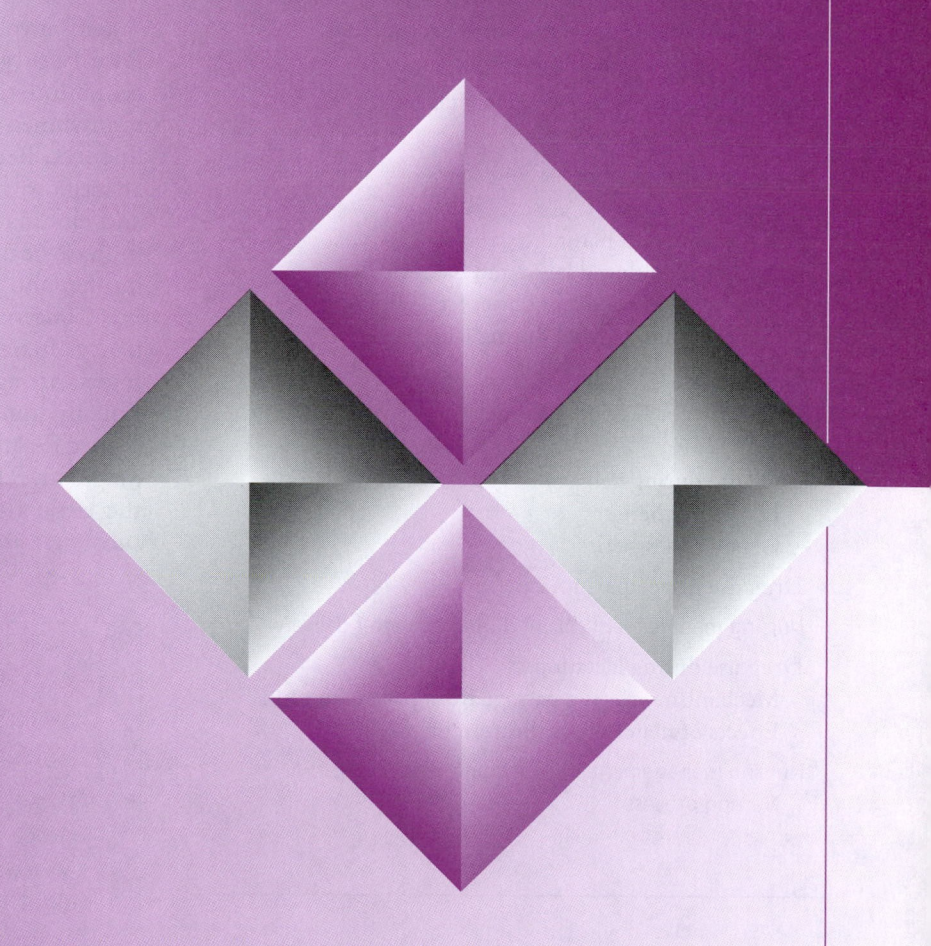

10

Drug Therapy in Maternal Care

From the beginning of pregnancy, the fate of the fetus is tied to that of its mother. Any substance and any drug that the mother ingests, inhales, or receives parenterally may pass through the placenta to the fetus unless it is destroyed or changed on its passage.

Drug Safety in Pregnancy

When a pregnant woman takes a drug, its rate and mechanism of entry are important: a low degree of permeability increases the chance of undesirable agents being inactivated, whereas a high degree of permeability encourages passage. Substances that contain fat-soluble undissociated molecules at physiologic pH ranges are likely to pass through the placenta immediately. The molecular weight of drugs taken by the mother is also important; those weighing less than 600 pass easily, whereas those over 1000 find the placenta almost impermeable.

Substances that cross the placenta usually reach concentrations in the fetus that are 50% to 100% of the concentrations in the mother. A few drugs reach higher levels in the fetus when it excretes the drugs into the amniotic fluid, then later swallows and recirculates them. The waste products from the fetus return to the mother through the two umbilical arteries that pass through the placenta to the mother. This return of wastes (particularly toxic wastes) may be slow because many of the fetal systems involved in detoxification are not fully developed. Positive pregnancy outcomes are directly related to placental functioning because the placenta is the source of nourishment and protection from harmful external influences. Because the physiologic changes of pregnancy affect how drugs are absorbed, distributed, metabolized, and eliminated, maternal education is essential to promote a healthy pregnancy and outcome for both the mother and fetus.

Concerns about the effects of medication during pregnancy often focus on potentially teratogenic effects. (Teratogens are agents that cause congenital fetal anomalies.) Equally important, the drug dosages needed to achieve a specific plasma level may differ when a woman is pregnant. The five major considerations to be used in the evaluation of possible harm to the fetus from any substance are listed in Box 10-1.

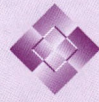

> ### Box 10-1
> ### Considerations in Evaluating a Drug's Potential for Fetal Harm
>
> The amount of the substance that can be expected to reach the embryo or fetus
>
> The gestational age of the embryo or fetus at the time of administration
>
> The duration of the exposure
>
> The genotypes of the mother and embryo or fetus
>
> The expected effects on the embryo or fetus of this substance when combined with other agents in the mother's body

There are three critical periods in pregnancy when environmental agents are more likely to have an adverse effect on fetal development. The first period is fertilization, when fetal development is affected by the quality of the ovum and sperm, the overall condition of the intrauterine environment, and the mother's general health and nutritional status. During the second critical period, from day 18 through 55, exposure to teratogens may result in both structural and functional defects. In the third period, from day 56 through birth, structural defects and fetal growth retardation can occur (Simpson and Creehan, 1996). Table 10-1 identifies teratogenic maternal conditions and infectious agents.

When a drug ordered for the pregnant woman may cause adverse effects in the fetus, the substitution of another medication should be considered. The Food and Drug Administration (FDA) has actually approved only one prescription drug for use during pregnancy: ritodrine (a neurotransmitter that interrupts premature labor). Prescribers, however, can prescribe drugs not specifically approved for use during pregnancy. Drugs that can be safely used during pregnancy fall into a category of "unlabeled use" versus "approved use." However, for the purposes of informed consent, the mother must be given information about the drug's potential effects before using it.

FDA approval does not guarantee a drug's safety for the mother or fetus. It only means that in the FDA's opinion, the benefits to be gained by using the drug outweigh the possible risks. Information gathered by the FDA may cause withdrawal of prior approval. For example, diazepam was reclassified as unacceptable as an antianxiety drug for women in labor because of the adverse effects on the neonate.

FDA Pregnancy Risk Ratings for Drugs

The FDA's "use-in-pregnancy" rating is limited to drugs for which information is available about the fetal risk versus potential maternal benefits. The rating system known as the pregnancy risk category is presented in Appendix A. The FDA pregnancy categories are used throughout this book because pregnant women may require medications for conditions related or unrelated to pregnancy. Knowledge of pregnancy category ratings helps healthcare providers compare the hazard of administering a drug that may place the fetus or neonate at risk with the drug's potential benefit to the mother.

TERIS and Canadian Ratings

An automated teratology resource known as TERIS was developed in Canada, rating the human teratogenicity dangers of 157 drugs frequently prescribed for outpatients in the United States. Of the agents with sufficient data for rating, 92.5% demonstrated minimal teratogenic risk. The information on 83 of the agents was compared to that presented in the FDA pregnancy categories.

The Canadian researchers believe that any information on risks must be modified for all the conditions of exposure, such as dose, route, and timing, to be valid. They disagree with the FDA classifications that combine risk and quality data in a single interpretation for client counseling. Canadians do not offer this type of counseling. They use their own rating system only after

Table 10-1. Potential Teratogenic Maternal Conditions and Infectious Agents

Teratogen	Effects on Fetus
Maternal conditions	
Diabetes mellitus	Affects various systems; caudal dysplasia or caudal regression syndrome; insulin therapy protects fetus
Endocrinopathies	Effects similar to those of administering the hormone; masculinization of female fetus
Phenylketonuria	Fetal death; mental retardation; intrauterine growth restriction
Maternal infections	
Cytomegalovirus	Central nervous system damage; intrauterine growth restriction
Herpes simplex	Central nervous system anomalies; microcephaly; intracranial calcification; eye defects
Rubella virus	Cardiovascular malformation; deafness; mental retardation; cataracts; glaucoma; microphthalmia
Syphilis	Maculopapular rash; hepatosplenomegaly; deformed nails, osteochondritis at joints of extremities; congenital neurosyphilis; abnormal epiphyses; chorioretinitis
Toxoplasmosis	Hydrocephaly; microphthalmia; chorioretinitis
Varicella zoster (chickenpox)	Skin and muscle defects; intrauterine growth restriction; limb and eye defects
Venezuelan equine encephalitis	Hydroanencephaly; microphthalmia; luxation of hip

the client has been exposed to a particular drug, at which time the teratogenic risk to the fetus is considered.

Drug-Related Factors Affecting Pregnancy

Various factors associated with drug use during pregnancy must be considered in any discussion about drug therapy in maternal care: the effects of nutrients, inhaled and ingested environmental and chemical contaminants (eg, alcohol, tobacco smoke, various anesthetic and other gases), and illegal substances.

Maternal Nutrition

One of the first considerations during pregnancy is maternal nutrition. The mother must have a sufficient intake of high-quality foods to encourage proper fetal and placental growth and development. The old fears about maternal obesity that led to severe caloric restrictions have proved detrimental to the fetus. Inadequate nutrition prevents the increase in maternal blood volume needed to vascularize the uterus properly. Without this increase in blood flow, nutrients cannot be carried to the fetus in sufficient quantity to sustain proper growth. The food ingested by the mother must also be as free of contaminants as possible.

Nausea and vomiting are common during the early weeks of pregnancy, affecting 50% to 90% of all pregnant women. If possible, symptoms should be controlled by diet—dry crackers eaten before arising in the morning and several small, easily digested meals during the day. Clients on salt-restricted diets should be instructed to eat unsalted crackers. Antiemetic drugs are generally not used because their safety during pregnancy has not been established. Dietary and nursing measures are safer routes to combat nausea and vomiting.

In response to her body's need to deposit fat for lactation, the mother's appetite increases, as does her absorption of iron and calcium. Inadequate nutrition may not only impede fetal growth, it may also promote teratogenic effects or spontaneous abortion. Maternal consequences of malnourishment may include preterm labor, premature rupture of membranes, or preeclampsia.

If the mother eats properly, she will probably gain 25 lb or more during the pregnancy. Ideally, the neonate should weigh about 8 lb; therefore, the mother should have a daily increase of about 300 to 500 calories, with higher intake necessary if she was underweight before pregnancy. Even overweight women should be instructed to gain at least 15 lb during pregnancy. This gain is important to prevent low infant birth weights, which have a negative effect on the development and survival of neonates.

The source of the additional daily calories consumed by the mother, although important, is not essential to the fetus. If the mother ingests more carbohydrates than proteins, her own muscle tissue breaks down to provide the needed amino acids for the fetus. Whenever possible, the maternal protein intake should increase by 30 g a day (or 60 to 70 g daily) so that her own body is protected and fetal growth ensured.

Because maternal blood volume increases during pregnancy and the fetus must develop its own blood, the need for iron is pronounced. Iron can be supplied by eating red meats, beans, dried fruits, and fortified grain products. If these are unavailable in sufficient quantity, supplementary iron should be taken. The mother requires 30 mg of iron daily to prevent iron deficiency. Absorption of iron can be enhanced by including foods high in vitamin C. Caffeine interferes with iron absorption.

Folic acid, a B vitamin rarely available in sufficient amounts in the diet, must be supplemented to ensure proper cell division of the uterus and of the fetus and to guard against neural tube defects (Wald, 1991). The U.S. Public Health Service recently recommended a daily supplement of 0.4 mg of folic acid for women of childbearing age before conception and throughout pregnancy. In cases of previous neural tube defects, the woman should consult her physician for advice concerning folic acid dosage for a subsequent pregnancy. Foods containing folic acid include dark-green leafy vegetables, whole grains, milk, legumes, and eggs.

Calcium is another mineral required for proper skeletal development in the fetus. To meet the combined needs of the mother and the fetus, 1,200 mg of calcium are needed daily. Women who smoke may require even more, because smoking may cause loss of calcium from the mother's bones. Calcium absorption decreases if phosphorus intake is too high (as when the intake of nuts and grains is excessive). This decrease may cause an electrolyte imbalance and is an important point to make when teaching pregnant women about nutrition. It may be necessary to supplement calcium if the woman's diet does not contain enough dairy products.

Ingested and Inhaled Contaminants

Alcohol ingestion presents major concerns for the fetus, and other substances of particular concern include caffeine, tobacco, various gases, and drugs of abuse.

Alcohol

Alcohol is considered by some to be the most common teratogen affecting humans. About 30% to 45% of pregnant women who drink heavily (six mixed drinks or six cans of beer a day throughout pregnancy, equivalent to 3 oz of absolute alcohol) can be expected to deliver infants with full-blown fetal alcohol syndrome. This condition is characterized by mental and growth retardation, central nervous system (CNS) problems, behavioral and developmental abnormalities, and heart, limb, and facial defects. It has surpassed Down syndrome and spina bifida as the leading cause of mental retardation in the United States.

Fetal alcohol effects, a milder disorder found in children of mothers who do not ingest alcohol as heavily, affect between five and ten times as many children as those who suffer from fetal alcohol syndrome. Because no minimum safe level for maternal alcohol ingestion has been set, the U.S. Surgeon General and the National Council on Alcoholism recommend that a woman abstain from drinking alcoholic beverages from the time she actively seeks to conceive. No matter what stage she has reached in her pregnancy, she should stop drinking, or at least decrease her intake as much as possible, to try to limit the damage to the fetus.

In pregnant women with alcoholism, referrals for professional counseling should be offered. If detoxification is indicated, the woman should be admitted to a treatment facility where the effects of alcohol withdrawal on both the woman and the fetus can be monitored. When medications to control maternal withdrawal symptoms or to treat the alcoholism are prescribed, the possibility of placental transfer and the effects of teratogenicity or carcinogenicity must be considered. For example, researchers think that maternal barbiturate sedation may increase the child's risk of developing cancer when older. Antabuse, helpful in treating alcoholics because it makes them physically ill if they drink, is contraindicated because it affects the pregnancy by inhibiting enzymes. Drugs such as chlordiazepoxide (Librium) and diazepam (Valium), frequently used in alcohol detoxification programs, are also contraindicated due to their possible teratogenic effects.

In the past, alcohol was used as a tocolytic drug. Today it has been replaced by terbutaline or ritodrine, and women are advised not to use alcohol because of its adverse effects on the fetus (see Chap. 18 for more information on alcohol).

Caffeine

Women who consume more than 300 mg of caffeine a day appear to have a higher incidence of first-trimester spontaneous abortion, stillbirth, and premature birth. Clients should be reminded that coffee, tea, cocoa, chocolate, and cola and other carbonated beverages contain caffeine. In addition, prescription and over-the-counter (OTC) drugs should be checked for caffeine content.

Tobacco Smoke

Just as maternal food ingestion affects the fetus, so do inhaled substances. Respiratory functions change in the pregnant woman. Tidal volume increases about 40%, but both vital capacity and respiratory rate remain at about prepregnancy levels. Inspiration increases but expiratory reserve decreases, so that the lung shows greater deflation after expiration. Both residual and total lung volumes decrease.

The alveolar tension of inhaled substances is normally diluted by the residual air volume in the lungs. Because pregnancy results in a decreased reservoir of air to dilute the inhaled air, contaminants are not diluted to the extent that they would have been before pregnancy. This places the mother who breathes impure air at risk for hypoxia. Depending on the ability of the substance to cross the placenta, the inhalant may adversely affect the fetus. The stage of fetal development may determine how the compound affects different cells, causing teratogenesis in immature embryonic cells and carcinogenesis in mature cells.

One of the most common air contaminants is cigarette smoke. Babies whose birth weight is low for gestational age are born twice as frequently to women who smoke as to women who do not smoke. These babies have smaller livers and have a higher rate of hypoglycemia (blood glucose levels < 30 mg/dL), placing the infant at risk for permanent brain damage. The placenta seems vulnerable to maternal smoking. The nicotine in smoke decreases placental perfusion. Pregnant women who smoke have a higher incidence of placental abruption, placenta previa, and bleeding. Long-term studies of children born to mothers who smoke suggest adverse effects on growth, intelligence, and behavior. Retardation is associated with heavy smoking and may result from chronic fetal hypoxia.

Carbon monoxide is one component of cigarette smoke. Normally, pregnant women show a 50% increase in endogenous carbon monoxide production during pregnancy. Smoking not only increases the maternal carbon monoxide level, but it also increases the amount that crosses the placental barrier. The increased carbon monoxide level interferes with the oxygenation of fetal tissue. If carbon monoxide poisoning develops, the child may sustain neurologic problems.

Cigarettes also contain tar and nicotine. Nicotine increases body heat production between 10% and 15%. Whether or not a woman smokes, her basal body temperature increases by 0.3° to 0.6°C after ovulation. This elevated temperature is maintained halfway through the pregnancy, after which it returns to normal. Because excessive heat adversely affects the fetus, the mother may be placing the fetus at additional risk by smoking.

Radioactive Agents; Anesthetic Gases and Other Fumes

Anesthetic gases are usually hazardous to the fetus and the mother, as are radioactive agents and the inhaled fumes of various industrial and environmental chemicals (Box 10-2). Risks include higher-than-normal abortion rates, premature delivery, and fetal and maternal death.

Illegal Substances

Abuse of drugs during pregnancy is often overlooked or not recognized when the client seeks initial prenatal care. Because of stereotypes associated with the use of illicit drugs, healthcare providers may assume that certain clients are not at risk for using these drugs and, therefore, do not include an assessment of illegal substances in the routine health history.

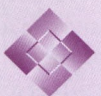

Box 10-2
Workplace Hazards for Healthcare Personnel

Like their pregnant clients, pregnant nurses and other healthcare providers must exercise caution in working with various drugs and chemicals, particularly those prevalent in healthcare facilities. Among substances posing hazards during pregnancy are anesthetic gases, radioactive agents, and heavy metal and chemical vapors.

Anesthetic Gases

According to various studies, pregnant healthcare professionals are at increased risk for problem pregnancies when they work around anesthetic gases. A summary of various studies indicates that spontaneous abortion affects about 38% of pregnant anesthetists and 30% of operating room nurses but only about 10% of general duty nurses. One gas in particular, halothane, a fluorinated hydrocarbon, has been closely linked with spontaneous abortions among female anesthetists.

Anesthetic gases are hazardous for families of healthcare professionals as well. These gases are highly lipophilic and may be excreted in the breath of anesthetists up to 30 hours after their last exposure. Therefore, a pregnant woman in contact with the anesthetist may unknowingly be at risk.

Radiation

Healthcare staff who care for any client receiving radiation therapy should take radiation precautions. These precautions include wearing a monitoring device and a lead-lined apron while involved in direct client care. In indirect care, the nurse or other healthcare worker should stand behind a portable shield. Radiation exposure can be minimized by planning efficient care ahead of time, working quickly, leaving the room as soon as possible, and keeping radioactive specimens in shielded containers. Pregnant nurses should not care for clients with radioactive sources.

Heavy Metals and Chemical Fumes

Industrial chemicals inhaled by pregnant workers can be deadly. Of 95 women who died of beryllium poisoning, 66% were pregnant. Beryllium has also been found in the urine of children whose mothers were exposed to this chemical. Other known inhalant teratogens include benzine, carbon tetrachloride, oxides of nitrogen, paraquat, polychlorinated biphenyls, Malathion, cyanides, and formaldehyde.

Implications for Nurses

Under various right-to-know laws throughout the United States, workers, including nurses, are entitled to know of any hazardous substances that exist in the workplace—now or in the past. In most cases, workers can obtain records on hazardous substances in the workplace through their employer or through local or state departments of health.

Assessment activities that include a discussion about using drugs and substances known to be harmful to the fetus should be an essential component of a thorough prenatal history. A useful approach might be to review substance use across a continuum from familiar substances to illicit substances; in other words, from cigarette smoking and the use of OTC and prescription medications, to alcohol use and, finally, to the use of illegal drugs such as marijuana and cocaine.

In pregnancy, the most frequently used illicit substances are marijuana and cocaine. Marijuana impairs DNA and RNA formation and therefore should be avoided during pregnancy. It also may decrease maternal oxygenation, making less oxygen available to the fetus.

Cocaine, a strong vasoconstrictor, can cause seizures, hypertension, cardiac arrhythmia, respiratory arrest, and cardiac failure in the pregnant woman. Abruptio placentae, resulting from the formation of a blood clot behind the placenta, may also occur and result in fetal death. The pharmacologic actions of cocaine include stimulation of the peripheral nervous system, causing these conditions, along with placental vasoconstriction and uterine contractions. Cocaine abuse in pregnancy can lead to preterm labor, an increased incidence of meconium-stained amniotic fluid, and retarded fetal growth.

Neonates born to cocaine-addicted mothers may show a number of abnormalities at birth, in addition to neurobehavioral problems that may become evident later in life (Kaye and Cashoff, 1993). Such neonates tend to be of lower gestational age at birth than nonexposed neonates. They are smaller and have lower birth weights as well. They tend to be highly irritable and tremulous, cannot sustain eye contact, and often are inconsolable. They may also have genitourinary anomalies and differences in muscle tone. These newborns tend to be highly reactive to stimulation and need interventions to help them regain control and be comforted. Their reactions may affect bonding because of the difficulty the mother usually encounters in calming and comforting them. These behavioral characteristics are often symptomatic of developmental delays that may require periodic assessment to monitor long-term development.

If cocaine use stops in the first trimester, fetal outcomes are improved. Every effort should be made to identify and educate substance-abusing mothers early in pregnancy in a nonjudgmental, compassionate way. Illicit drug use is typically accompanied by other behaviors (eg, alcohol use, poor nutrition, cigarette smoking) that may further complicate the pregnancy and require accurate and timely assessment and interventions.

Therapeutic Drug Use During Pregnancy

Pregnant women are susceptible to the same medical disorders found in the general population. If treatment requires medications, the risk of the drugs on the fetus, as well as the mother, must be considered. Due to increases in maternal blood and plasma volumes during pregnancy, the concentration of maternal serum protein is lower. Therefore, the capacity of the protein to bind drugs in the maternal system decreases, leaving more drugs free to be transferred through the placenta.

Medication may be needed to treat a maternal condition throughout pregnancy and during lactation. The effects on the fetus may be different from those on the neonate. Table 10-2 lists fetal risks from medications given during pregnancy and neonatal risks from drugs given during lactation.

Pharmacokinetics. Many drugs are metabolized in the liver. However, during pregnancy, the hepatic blood flow does not increase, so a minimal degree of centrilobular bile stasis affects the liver. Therefore, drugs may be biotransformed more slowly. On the other hand, the kidneys may excrete drugs more rapidly as a result of the increased renal perfusion and glomerular filtration that occurs during pregnancy.

As discussed earlier, the lower the molecular weight of a substance, the greater the chance it will cross the placenta. Most drugs, with a molecular weight of 250 to 500, can penetrate the trophoblast (the connective and endothelial tissues that divide the circulatory systems of mother and fetus). The changes in the placenta during the third trimester add to the probability of drug transfer through the placenta. Some of the drugs that cross the placenta within minutes after administration include ampicillin, penicillin G, cephalothin, kanamycin, tetracycline, sulfonamides, streptomycin, diazepam, phenytoin, barbiturates, ethanol, meperidine, salicylate, lidocaine, mepivacaine, bupivacaine, and propranolol.

Some substances undergo metabolic changes through oxidation, reduction, dealkylation, or synthesis before crossing the placenta. Certain drugs inhibit or increase the placental enzymes needed for their conversion or for transport mechanisms. Some evidence suggests that most carcinogenic drugs undergo oxidation to cross the placenta.

Once drugs have passed to the fetal side of the placenta, they travel through the umbilical vein to the fetal liver via the portal vein. Some pass through the liver to the ductus venosus, which empties into the inferior vena cava and then into the heart. Traveling through the pathways that are less resistant, the drug-laden blood reaches the brain and heart. From there, more than 50% of the blood goes to the umbilical arteries, then to the placenta, returning to the maternal circulation. The remaining blood diffuses through the fetus. Because the level of protein available to bind drugs is lower in the fetus than in the mother, more of the drug is free to remain in fetal tissues. This process probably increases with gestational age, and some tissues are more receptive than others to certain drugs.

Drug Intervention in Maternal Medical Problems

Medications used to ensure the mother's health must be evaluated for possible toxic effects at various stages of fetal development (Table 10-3). Ongoing monitoring and evaluation of drugs are important. Possible teratogenic effects should be reported to the FDA for correlation with other consumer information.

Chronic maternal medical problems may escalate during pregnancy or may necessitate changes in maternal medications known to affect the fetus. Other maternal conditions may be associated only with pregnancy, requiring medical management to safeguard the mother and fetus. The mother's illness may be well controlled before pregnancy, but her health may deteriorate with the additional burden of pregnancy. Medication taken to control the condition may have to be changed completely or given in a different dosage.

Antihypertensive Therapy

Hypertensive women may become pregnant, or pregnancy-induced hypertension (PIH) may occur in women with previously normal blood pressure. In either situation, prompt diagnosis and treatment are important, because PIH is the third leading cause of maternal death in the United States. PIH can be anticipated in 5% to 7% of pregnancies, a figure that jumps to 25% to 35% for women with chronic hypertension. About one third of women with PIH have a recurrence during a future pregnancy.

Salt restriction and diuretics are no longer considered advisable. The weight reduction or control formerly advised for PIH is now thought to add to fetal problems associated with low birth weights. However, diet is essential. The woman should eat a well-balanced diet with a high daily protein intake (80–100 g) and a normal intake of sodium (6 g). Even if the client has edema, some salt (2–4 g) should be taken daily, with six to eight glasses of fluid per day.

Using medications to regulate PIH is controversial. Clients who took antihypertensive drugs before pregnancy may continue to take them, because the risk of abruptio placentae is greater if PIH is superimposed on hypertension. Sudden discontinuation of diuretics in the

Text continues on page 156.

Table 10-2. Comparative Effects of Selected Drugs on Fetus and Breast-Fed Neonate

Pharmacologic Class	Fetal Risk	Breast-Feeding Data
Antihistamines		
brompheniramine	Congenital defects	Single adverse report, therefore considered contraindicated by one manufacturer
buclizine (also anti-emetic)	Teratogenic in animals; contraindicated in early pregnancy by manufacturer	No data available
chlorpheniramine (also antiemetic)	Possible malformations; more data needed to assess risk	No data available
cimetidine (H_2-receptor antagonist)	Crosses placenta at term but no adverse effects noted	Potential adverse effects on infant (gastric acidity, CNS stimulation), therefore contraindicated
cyclizine (also antiemetic)	Teratogenic in animals but apparently not in humans	No data available
diphenhydramine	No evidence of large numbers of major or minor malformations, but actual risk associated with individual cases needs further assessment	Manufacturer says contraindicated during lactation; American Academy of Pediatrics (AAP) says it is acceptable
hydroxyzine (also tranquilizer)	Manufacturer says contraindicated in early pregnancy; seems safe in labor to relieve anxiety	No data available
meclizine (also antiemetic)	No evidence of large numbers of major or minor malformations, but actual risk associated with individual cases needs further assessment	No data available
pheniramine	Possible association with respiratory, eye, and ear problems	No data available
promethazine (also antiemetic)	No association between use in pregnancy and malformations; when used in labor may impair platelet aggregation in neonate, but less in mother; watch for bleeding in newborn	Accurate assessment unavailable due to rapid metabolism
ranitidine (H_2-receptor antagonist)	Use in labor to prevent gastric acid aspiration does not appear to cause neonatal problems	Contraindicated because it decreases gastric acidity
trimeprazine	No evidence of large numbers of major or minor malformations, but actual risk associated with individual cases needs further assessment	Excreted in breast milk at levels too low to produce effects in baby; considered acceptable while breast-feeding by AAP
tripelennamine	No evidence of association with major or minor malformations	Manufacturer says contraindicated during lactation; AAP says it is acceptable
Anti-infectives		
Aminoglycosides		
gentamicin (antibiotic)	Possibility of eighth cranial nerve toxicity. Possible neuromuscular effect with $MgSO_4$	No data available
kanamycin (antibiotic)	Reports of eighth cranial nerve damage; ototoxicity with hearing losses reported	May affect bowel flora, may interfere with diagnostic culture results, may cause other adverse effects
neomycin (antibiotic)	Potential for eighth cranial nerve toxicity	No data available
streptomycin (antibiotic)	Ototoxicity and eighth cranial nerve toxicity reported	May affect bowel flora, may interfere with diagnostic culture results, may cause other adverse effects
Antifungals		
amphotericin B (antibiotic)	No negative reports	No data available
griseofulvin	Embryotoxic and teratogenic in animals; human data unavailable	No data available
miconazole (antibiotic)	Topical use not associated with congenital malformations; IV effects unknown	No data available
Cephalosporins		
cephalexin } cephalothin }	No defects or toxicity reported	May affect bowel flora, may interfere with diagnostic culture results, may cause other adverse effects

(continued)

Table 10-2. (Continued)

Pharmacologic Class	Fetal Risk	Breast-Feeding Data
Penicillins amoxicillin ampicillin oxacillin penicillin G penicillin V	No relation to major or minor malformations	May affect bowel flora, may interfere with diagnostic culture results, may cause other adverse effects (allergy, sensitization)
Tetracyclines tetracycline (and others in this class)	Adverse effects on teeth and bones; congenital defects; possible association between minor malformations and tetracycline, major and minor malformations between demeclocycline and oxytetracycline	May affect bowel flora, may interfere with diagnostic culture results, may cause other adverse effects; remote possibility of dental staining and inadequate bone growth
Antiviral acyclovir	No controlled study available	No data available
amantadine	Animal studies: embryotoxic, teratogenic in animals in high doses	Potential for vomiting, skin rash, urinary retention; hence, contraindicated
Sulfonamides sulfapyridine	No relation to major or minor malformations; potential for toxicity in newborn; therefore, should not be administered near term	Apparently no risk to healthy, full-term newborn; do not administer if neonate is premature, has hyperbilirubinemia or glucose-6-phosphate dehydrogenase deficiency
Urinary Germicides nalidixic acid	No defects observed	One case of hemolytic anemia in neonate with glucose-6-phosphate dehydrogenase deficiency reported
nitrofurantoin	No reports of congenital defects; however, manufacturer cautions against use near term because it may cause hemolytic anemia if neonate's red blood cells are deficient in reduced glutathione, or if neonate has glucose-6-phosphate dehydrogenase deficiency	Infants with glucose-6-phosphate dehydrogenase deficiency may develop hemolytic anemia
Autonomics **Parasympathomimetics (Cholinergics)** neostigmine	No defects reported	Insufficient data
Parasympatholytics (Anticholinergic) atropine	No relation to major or minor malformations	No adverse effects reported
belladonna	Associated with malformations when administered in first trimester	No adverse effects reported
scopolamine	No relation to malformations; however, when given at term, may cause fetal tachycardia, decreased heart rate, deceleration, and variability	No adverse effects reported
Sympathomimetics (Adrenergic) albuterol (tocolytic)	No relation to congenital anomalies reported, even with continuous IV use for 17 weeks to prevent premature labor; may cause fetal tachycardia, hypoglycemia, and increased serum insulin (can be prevented with glucose); lower risk of respiratory distress syndrome	No data available
ephedrine	Some association of first-trimester use with minor defects, inguinal hernias, clubfoot; may cause fetal tachycardia and beat-to-beat variability	One case of irritability, disturbed sleep, and excessive crying reported (reversed within 12 hours after breast-feeding stopped)
epinephrine	Some association of first-trimester use with major and minor defects	No data available

(continued)

Table 10-2. (Continued)

Pharmacologic Class	Fetal Risk	Breast-Feeding Data
ritodrine (tocolytic)	Manufacturer says contraindicated before 29th week of gestation; fetal heart rate may increase to 200/min; ketoacidosis with fetal death has occurred; lower risk of respiratory distress syndrome	No data available

Sympatholytics (β-Adrenergic Blockers)

acebutolol (cardioselective)	No malformations reported; should be observed for β-blockade if used near delivery (blood pressure and heart rate down); no data about use in first trimester or long-term exposure	Observe for signs or symptoms of β-blockade
atenolol (cardioselective)	Resembles acebutolol but lower birth weight	Resembles acebutolol; considered acceptable for breast-feeding by AAP
metoprolol (cardioselective)	Resembles acebutolol	Resembles atenolol
propranolol (nonselective)	Oxytocic effects after IV or extra-amniotic injections or high oral doses; may be related to intrauterine growth retardation; fetal and neonatal toxicity may occur; observe for β-blockade if used near delivery; no data on long-term exposure	Resembles atenolol

Cholesterol-lowering Agents

lovastatin	Contraindicated in pregnancy because cholesterol is needed for the synthesis of steroids and cell membranes essential for fetal development	Manufacturer says it is contraindicated

Coagulant/Anticoagulant

Anticoagulants

coumarin derivatives	Multiple defects noted, with 30% of the infants born with abnormalities	Only warfarin and dicumarol (bishydroxycoumarin) considered acceptable with breast-feeding
heparin	No links with congenital defects reported; may cause indirect adverse effects on fetus, including lethal problems	Not excreted in breast milk

Thombolytics

streptokinase	No association with congenital defects	No data available

Cardiovascular Drugs

Cardiac Drugs

digitalis, digitoxin, digoxin (cardiac glycosides)	No association with congenital defects	Digoxin only cardiac glycoside reported as excreted in breast milk; considered acceptable for breast-feeding by AAP
quinidine (antiarrhythmic)	No association with congenital defects; has been used to treat fetal tachyarrhythmia	Excreted in breast milk; considered acceptable for breast-feeding by AAP

Antihypertensives

acebutolol, atenolol, metoprolol, propranolol	Discussed previously	

Central Nervous System Drugs

Analgesics and Antipyretics

acetaminophen	Appears safe for short-term use in therapeutic dosage range; no association with large categories of major or minor malformations; may be associated with congenital dislocation of the hip and clubfoot	Excreted in breast milk; considered acceptable for breast-feeding by AAP
aspirin	Increased perinatal mortality, intrauterine growth retardation, antepartum hemorrhage or bleeding complications after birth	Potential risk of adverse effects on platelet function

(continued)

Table 10-2. (Continued)

Pharmacologic Class	Fetal Risk	Breast-Feeding Data
Narcotic Analgesics		
codeine	Not associated with large categories of major or minor malformations; however, first-trimester use is linked to some defects, including respiratory defects; second-trimester use is linked to alimentary tract defects; use in labor is linked to respiratory depression in the newborn	In breast milk in small amounts; considered acceptable for use while breast-feeding by AAP
meperidine	Not associated with large categories of major or minor malformations; use in labor linked to respiratory depression in the newborn	In breast milk, decreasing after 24 hours; considered acceptable for use while breast-feeding by AAP
Narcotic Antagonists		
naloxone	Should not be given before delivery, unless definite evidence of narcotic toxicity is present	No data available
Nonsteroidal Antiinflammatory Drugs		
ibuprofen	No association with congenital defects reported; however, theoretical possibility of constriction in utero of ductus arteriosus	Considered safe while breast-feeding by AAP
indomethacin (analgesic and tocolytic)	May cause premature closure of ductus arteriosus when used in pregnancy; a few defects reported	Too few data available
Anticonvulsants		
bromides (also sedative)	No association with large categories of major or minor malformations; however, may be related to congenital defects (more data needed); newborns exposed in utero should be monitored for serum bromide concentrations	Contraindicated for mothers taking medications that contain bromide (intake of 5.4 g/day leads to rash, weakness, absence of cry)
carbamazepine (tricyclic)	Anomalies that have been observed may be due to the disease process (epilepsy) rather than to the medication; more data needed; this drug has been prescribed as the drug of choice for women who may become pregnant, requiring anticonvulsant therapy for the first time	Considered safe while breast-feeding by AAP
magnesium sulfate (also cathartic, tocolytic)	No association with congenital defects; should not be given with aminoglycoside antibiotics because the combination may cause neonatal respiratory depression; if magnesium sulfate is given near delivery, neonate should be observed for signs of neurologic depression	Considered safe while breast-feeding by AAP
phenobarbital (also sedative)	May result in minor congenital defects, addiction, hemorrhage at birth; should be used at lowest possible effective dose to control epileptic seizures; does not appear to cause defects when used by nonepileptic mothers	Infant should be watched for sedation, and phenobarbital levels should be monitored to prevent toxicity; considered safe while breast-feeding by AAP. One case of methemoglobinemia reported.
phenytoin	Fetal hydantoin syndrome may occur in varying degrees, causing craniofacial or limb malformations; teratogen effects vary; may also be a human transplacental carcinogen, with the possibility of tumor development occurring several years later; hemorrhages may occur within 24 hours after birth and may cause death; regardless of these adverse effects, it may be necessary to administer to the mother to prevent convulsions	Keeping the maternal level within the therapeutic range should not increase the risk to the infant; considered safe while breast-feeding by AAP; one case of methemoglobinemia reported

(continued)

Table 10-2. (Continued)

Pharmacologic Class	Fetal Risk	Breast-Feeding Data
primidone (structural analog of phenobarbital)	Anomalies similar to those in fetal hydantoin syndrome; hemorrhages may occur, as well as tumors; hyperactivity may also be present	The conversion of primidone to phenobarbital may lead to sedative effects in the infant; considered safe while breast-feeding by AAP
valproic acid	Anomalies similar to those in fetal hydantoin syndrome	No association with adverse effects; considered safe while breast-feeding by AAP
Antidepressants		
amitriptyline	Possibility of limb reduction anomalies	Considered safe while breast-feeding by AAP
imipramine	Symptoms of withdrawal in neonate may occur; not a major cause of congenital limb anomalies	Considered safe while breast-feeding by AAP
nortriptyline	Reports of limb reduction anomalies; observe neonate for urinary retention	Effects of chronic exposure unknown
SSRIs		
fluoxetine	Insufficient controlled studies exist; animal studies found an increase in mortality, declining birth weight, and survival rates	Excreted in breast milk; cautious use is advised
paroxetine	As above	As above
sertraline	As above	As above
Tranquilizers		
chlorpromazine (propyl-amino phenothiazine)	Possibility of delayed ocular damage; use during labor should be discouraged due to possibly dangerous drop in maternal blood pressure	Observe breast-fed infant for sedation, lethargy; considered safe while breast-feeding by AAP
lithium	Possible association with congenital defects, particularly of the cardiovascular system; frequent reports of toxicity in the newborn, becoming normal within 1 or 2 weeks	Effects of long-term exposure unknown; considered safe while breast-feeding by AAP, but manufacturer says it should not be used
Sedatives and Hypnotics		
amobarbital (barbiturate)	Possibility of congenital defects	No data available
chlordiazepoxide (benzodiazepine)	High potential for severe congenital anomalies but not linked to large classes of malformations	No data available
diazepam	Greater incidence of oral defects, inguinal hernia; use during labor does not seem harmful	May accumulate in breast-fed neonates, so should not be used while breast-feeding
ethanol	Teratogenic effects leading to fetal alcohol syndrome associated with as little as 1 oz of absolute alcohol daily (two drinks); growth retardation also associated with alcohol withdrawal; alcohol combined with hydantoin may be carcinogenic in utero and require long-term follow-up	Considered safe while breast-feeding by AAP, even though adverse effects have been noted, including drowsiness, diaphoresis, sedation, weakness, decrease in linear growth, abnormal weight gain
Diuretics		
acetazolamide (carbonic anhydrase inhibitor)	No association with congenital defects or large categories of major or minor defects reported	Watch for suppression of lactation; no data available
furosemide	Can be used to assess fetal kidney functions during pregnancy; should not be used during pregnancy except for treatment of maternal cardiovascular disorders	Manufacturer says breast-feeding should be discontinued if drug is used

second to third trimesters may lead to rebound edema, with a 10- to 14-pound weight gain within a week. All medications should be decreased to the lowest possible effective dose; a combination of hydralazine and methyldopa is preferred for maximum efficacy and fewer side effects. Methyldopa alone may lead to maternal sedation, a rare hemolytic anemia, and a positive Coombs' test. Hydralazine may cause maternal tachycardia and headaches. Fetal effects for both drugs are negligible. Nife-

dipine, a calcium channel blocker, appears to be helpful in treating PIH, particularly severe preeclampsia. Few neonatal complications have been noted with its use. Maternal side effects appear to be minor and include hot flushes and headaches controlled with analgesics. In some instances, intravenous (IV) magnesium sulfate is given before the nifedipine, then stopped 24 hours after the blood pressure stabilizes. Nifedipine can then be administered orally as long as needed (Fenakel et al., 1991).

Table 10-3. Maternal Drugs That Exert a Pronounced Effect on Fetal Tissues

Receptive Tissue	Specific Drugs
Heart	digoxin, phenytoin, isotretinoin
Skeleton	tetracycline, warfarin
Red blood cells	sulfonamides
Central nervous system	diazepam, ethanol, narcotics
Platelets	aspirin
Adrenal gland	sex steroids, phenytoin
Müllerian duct, vagina	diethylstilbestrol, gentamicin, kanamycin (aminoglycosides)
Otic nerve	streptomycin
Brain, ears	isotretinoin

The use of beta-adrenergic blocking agents is associated with fetal growth retardation, neonatal respiratory distress, hypoglycemia, and bradycardia. Discontinuation of such a drug a day before delivery prevents it from remaining in the neonate. Of course, the neonate should be observed for signs of distress in the nursery.

A 1991 study found that 60 to 150 mg of aspirin taken daily in the last two trimesters of pregnancy helped prevent PIH in 65% of the participants and reduced the number of births of severely low weight babies by 44%. The aspirin selectively inhibits the synthesis of platelet thromboxane A_2. At the low dose, it did not cause maternal or fetal bleeding. Higher doses of aspirin are inappropriate and are contraindicated during antiplatelet therapy (Imperiale et al., 1991).

Diabetes Therapy

Maternal hyperglycemia acts as a teratogen during the first trimester, resulting in congenital malformations, including neural tube defects, caudal regression syndrome, atrial and ventricular septal defects, and holoprosencephaly. If present in the second or third trimester, it is associated with neonates that are large for gestational age and that have hypoglycemia, hypocalcemia, and respiratory problems.

Ideally, a woman who has diabetes should have complete control of her blood glucose levels before conceiving. Glucose crosses the placenta, but insulin does not. The fetus starts to manufacture insulin at about the 12th week of pregnancy. By the 28th week, it produces sufficient insulin to keep its blood glucose at a normal level. The excess glucose received from the mother results in hypertrophy of the beta cells in the fetal pancreas. The fetus produces the additional insulin needed because of the excessive glucose received from the mother. Fetal glycogen and fat stores then increase, leading to fetal obesity.

The most effective way to evaluate maternal glucose levels is with home blood glucose monitoring. Although it requires maternal compliance, this type of monitoring is usually more acceptable to clients than urine monitoring. Tests should be conducted on fasting and postprandial blood. Ideally, blood glucose levels should be maintained at 60 to 90 mg/dL before meals and less than 120 mg/dL about 2 hours after meals. For women with type I diabetes, insulin requirements may change, with larger amounts and different types needed. More frequent blood glucose testing may also be necessary. Three well-balanced meals are needed each day, plus snacks (particularly at bedtime) to maintain the proper blood glucose level.

The client's emotional needs must be considered, because pregnancy and the stringent requirements for glucose control may increase her level of stress. Exercise, rest, and psychosocial support are important factors to consider (Leff et al., 1991).

To control blood glucose levels, pregnant diabetics have had to rely on multiple injections of insulin, using short- or intermediate-acting insulin, according to the glucose level. A continuous subcutaneous insulin infusion pump is believed to provide greater control of the maternal glucose level. It can be programmed to deliver insulin in small amounts throughout the day, along with larger doses preprandially.

Because insulin requirements may vary considerably during pregnancy, decreasing early in pregnancy and rising thereafter, insulin requirements must be individualized. On average, the insulin requirement may increase two to three times the prepregnancy dosage in the second and third trimester, but it levels off during the last month of pregnancy. Similarly, insulin requirements of women in labor are based on the client's needs. After delivery, the amount needed drops precipitously. By the third postpartum day, only two thirds of the prepregnancy dose is required. Usually, the dose at the end of the first postpartum week is the same as before pregnancy.

The American Diabetes Association (ADA) has prepared a position statement on gestational diabetes mellitus, defined as carbohydrate intolerance of variable severity with onset or first recognition during the present pregnancy. It is estimated that 40% of women diagnosed during pregnancy with gestational diabetes mellitus will go on to develop type I (insulin-dependent) or type II (non–insulin-dependent) diabetes within 10 years (Arias, 1993). The ADA recommends that all pregnant women be screened for gestational diabetes between 24 and 28 weeks with a random 50-g, 1-hour oral glucose challenge test. If the plasma glucose level exceeds 140 mg/dL at 1 hour, no further testing is needed. If the level is less than 140 mg/dL (nonfasting) or 135 mg/dL (fasting), the ADA recommends proceeding with the 3-hour glucose challenge test. The definitive diagnosis is made if two or more of the venous plasma glucose concentrations meet or exceed the following levels: fasting, 105 mg/dL; 1 hour, 190 mg/dL; 2 hours, 165 mg/dL. Fasting levels above 105 mg/dL or postprandial levels above 120 mg/dL result in the greatest risk for intrauterine or neonatal death. Women who maintain normal glucose levels, with optimal obstetric care, place the fetus at lower risk than do those who are uncontrolled.

Any degree of gestational diabetes places the fetus at significant risk for macrosomia, hypoglycemia, hypocalcemia, and hyperbilirubinemia. Monitoring of maternal capillary blood or venous plasma for increased fasting or postprandial glucose levels is imperative. (Monitoring of maternal urinary glucose is no longer considered adequate.) Insulin may be ordered if diet does not control the glucose level, using only highly purified human insulin (a recombinant DNA product) with self-monitoring of blood glucose levels.

The ADA also encourages breast-feeding by women with gestational diabetes. It advises that these women be further evaluated at the first postpartum visit by having a 2-hour oral glucose tolerance test and that they should be monitored carefully to ensure early detection of diabetes in the future.

Cardiovascular Drugs

To protect the fetus, the client with well-controlled cardiovascular disease may require changes in medication during pregnancy. Propranolol, an effective beta blocker, may have been used to control hypertension and tachyarrhythmia, but it can induce premature labor or result in neonatal problems (Rayburn and Marsden, 1993). Procainamide and disopyramide, used in treating arrhythmia, should be avoided in pregnancy because of their potential to initiate uterine contractions. Warfarin (Coumadin), an anticoagulant, is also contraindicated in pregnancy because it may result in CNS abnormalities in the neonate or lead to stillbirth. Heparin does not have the same effect on the fetus and is the only anticoagulant recommended for use in pregnancy. Diuretics, such as thiazides or furosemide, may result in maternal hypovolemia, which reduces placental perfusion and causes low-birth weight infants. Diuretics may also cause symptomatic hyponatremia in the newborn. Therefore, diuretics are used only in pregnant women who have congestive heart failure or pulmonary edema.

Some cardiovascular medications can be used safely during pregnancy. They include quinidine (antiarrhythmic; 200–400 mg PO qid) and digoxin (a cardiac glycoside useful in congestive heart failure; 0.125–0.75 mg PO daily). Some sodium restriction may be necessary for women with fluid retention. If a thiazide diuretic has been used before pregnancy, it must be tapered off carefully to prevent rebound edema. Thiazide diuretics may lead to thrombocytopenia and electrolyte disturbances in mother and fetus and therefore should not be administered. If the pregnant client requires digitalization, an initial dose of 0.25 mg of digoxin may be administered IV and repeated at 4- to 6-hour intervals until 0.75 to 1.0 mg has been given. Oral delivery may be the preferred route, with 1.0 to 1.5 mg administered in divided doses. The maintenance dose is 0.125 to 0.375 mg daily. Digoxin levels should be checked monthly. Side effects may include nausea and vomiting, headaches, and neurologic problems. Arrhythmia may occur and can be controlled with a beta-adrenergic blocker, chiefly propranolol (Rayburn and Marsden, 1993), if the maternal benefits outweigh the risks to the fetus.

Rh Factor Therapy

Isoimmunization for women with Rh-negative blood is administered by injection within 72 hours of delivery. For a discussion of diagnosis and treatment of Rh-negative women during pregnancy, see Chapter 35.

Asthma Therapy

Asthma is probably the most common medical problem during pregnancy. Maternal hypoxia or acidosis may necessitate the use of oxygen therapy during an acute gestational asthma attack to prevent impaired fetal oxygenation.

It appears that asthmatic women who are identified early in pregnancy and treated appropriately are probably at no greater risk of important perinatal complications than those without asthma. If possible, antigen immunotherapy should be avoided if systemic reactions are anticipated, because these reactions are associated with abortions. If needed, allergen immunotherapy should be continued carefully during pregnancy for women who are already receiving it and who are unlikely to have systemic reactions. Women on maintenance therapy may have to receive a lower dose to decrease the chance of a systemic reaction. For women on an increasing antigen schedule, it may be necessary to stabilize the dose or increase the dose conservatively. Women who were not previously on immunotherapy should not start such treatment during pregnancy and should not be skin-tested, because systemic reactions may occur in response to the tests. Drugs used during pregnancy must be evaluated for the possibility of teratogenic or other effects on the fetus, as well as for effectiveness in the treatment of maternal asthma.

Anticonvulsant Therapy

Anticonvulsant therapy is necessary for pregnant women who would experience seizures without its use. Major seizures may precipitate hypoxia, leading to fetal damage or death. Anticonvulsant drugs have teratogenic effects, with an increase in the number of microcephalic children born to women on these drugs. Women taking anticonvulsants should be educated about the increased risk (two to three times) of fetal anomalies and mental retardation.

Because the anticonvulsant drug level may drop during pregnancy, seizure control may be lost. Drug levels should be checked monthly. Women on short-acting drugs must maintain a certain drug level to prevent seizures during delivery, as seizures may result in anoxia in the neonate (Rayburn and Marsden, 1993). One anticonvulsant, valproic acid, is associated with neural tube defects. Other anomalies noted in the children include misshapen craniofacial features and hypoplasia of the distal phalanges. Mental retardation and nonfebrile seizures are more common in these offspring. During labor, these women may receive IV phenytoin as prescribed to prevent intrapartum or postpartum seizures. The neonate should be observed for generalized depression or drug withdrawal. Some experts recommend prophylactic oral folic acid (1 mg daily) throughout pregnancy to offset any folic acid antagonism caused by anticonvulsant drugs, and oral vitamin K (5–10 mg daily) in the last month of pregnancy to prevent neonatal coagulopathy. The blood level of anticonvulsants may increase slowly after delivery and should be monitored weekly to detect early toxicity (Rayburn and Marsden, 1993).

Treatment for Sexually Transmitted Diseases

Routine screening tests for sexually transmitted diseases, such as syphilis and gonorrhea, alert healthcare providers to these diseases so that proper treatment can be instituted to protect mother and fetus. Other sexually transmitted diseases also require treatment during pregnancy to prevent complications for mother and fetus.

Perhaps the greatest health fears are generated by AIDS. In 1990, 2,628 cases of the disease had been reported in children (with over 700 new cases in 1990) and a mortality rate of 61%. By 1995, the number of pediatric AIDS cases increased to 6,948 (National AIDS Hotline CDC Case Reporting, 1995). About 80% of the children under age 13 who are diagnosed with AIDS were infected perinatally. The rate of maternal fetal transmission is estimated to range from 13% to 43%. (Regan et al., 1993). These numbers will increase as the number of women with AIDS expands from its present 11% of all AIDS clients, increasing the likelihood of transmission of the disease to the fetus.

To prevent maternal–fetal transmission of HIV and thereby prevent the spread of AIDS, a regimen of zidovudine (azidothymidine/AZT) is given beginning between the 14th and 34th weeks of gestation. The therapy continues throughout labor and is administered orally to the newborn after birth. The maternal dose is 100 mg orally five times a day until labor. Then IV AZT 2 mg/kg is administered over 1 hour, followed by a continuous infusion of 1 mg/kg/hr until the umbilical cord is clamped. The newborn then receives 2 mg/kg orally every 6 hours starting within 12 hours after birth through age 6 weeks (Drug Facts and Comparisons, 1996).

Healthcare personnel should follow the procedures discussed in Chapter 31 when caring for clients with AIDS throughout pregnancy and delivery. The neonate should be aspirated with a bulb syringe or gentle mechanical suction, never with a mouthpiece-type suction, to prevent aspiration or ingestion of the newborn's secretions. Placing mother and infant in a private rooming-in unit facilitates carrying out blood and secretion precautions for both.

Antimicrobial Therapy

If toxoplasmosis is acquired during pregnancy (usually through contact with the feces of an infected cat or from eating inadequately cooked meat), the organism causes congenital defects, particularly cataracts, in the newborn. Normally, active toxoplasmosis is treated with a combination of pyrimethamine and sulfadiazine or with sulfa drugs. Pyrimethamine is not used in pregnant women because it is a teratogen. Therefore, sulfa alone is used for treatment during the first trimester.

Drug Intervention in Fetal Medical Problems

Because certain medications given to the mother cross the placenta and reach a specific fetal organ, and other drugs introduced directly into the amniotic fluid are then swallowed by the fetus, researchers are finding ways to treat fetal medical problems that are amenable to drug therapy. Nurses should be aware of findings in these areas so they can help clients understand various treatment suggestions (Table 10-4).

The fetus, rather than the mother, may demonstrate cardiac problems. Intrauterine treatment of fetal tachycardia (>200 beats per minute) can be accomplished by medicating the mother, in some cases, with procainamide, propranolol, digoxin with propranolol, or digoxin with verapamil. Achieving and maintaining adequate fetal blood levels is imperative to prevent fetal or neonatal congestive heart failure. The daily dosage for the mother must be regulated to keep her serum level at the point at which the fetal tachycardia is controlled.

Both mother and fetus must be observed for toxicity or other side effects of the drugs. Digoxin is the drug used most frequently. It has been used successfully alone

Table 10-4. Drugs Administered During Pregnancy for Therapeutic Effect on the Fetus

Fetal Condition	Cause	Therapeutic Drug
Heart failure	Severe anemia	digoxin
Hypothyroidism	Maternal use of propylthiouracil	sodium levothyroxine
Exposure to syphilis	Maternal syphilis	penicillin
Biotin dependency	Genetic disorder	biotin
Candidate for neonatal development of respiratory distress syndrome	Anticipation of neonatal prematurity	glucocorticoids
Rh incompatibility, jaundice, hydrops	Rho(D)-negative mother with a Rho(D)-positive fetus	Rho(D) immune globulin

or in combination with other drugs. Propranolol may have adverse effects in the fetus or neonate (eg, intrauterine growth retardation, postnatal bradycardia, hypoglycemia, respiratory depression after delivery) and should be used only if the expected benefits outweigh possible fetal or neonatal risk. If used, it should be withdrawn before the onset of labor. Verapamil, a calcium channel blocker, requires care in attaining and maintaining adequate maternal levels. Procainamide may cause maternal hypotension, which can lead to uteroplacental insufficiency. This drug may also cause problems in the neonate because it is eliminated slowly, with resultant higher levels in the neonate than in the mother.

Implications: Benefits and Risks

Because the teratogenic effects of most medications are unknown, to be safe, only drugs that are necessary should be used, and even then only with the permission of a knowledgeable practitioner. Ongoing research may prove that some abortions, miscarriages, and birth defects are unwittingly caused by maternal use of certain drugs. Some of these effects are due to one drug, others to the synergistic action of combinations of drugs. Either effect may be influenced by the genotypes of mother or fetus, which increase or decrease vulnerability.

Animal research on the safety or teratogenicity of drugs cannot be applied with certainty to humans because of the differences between species in drug reactions. For example, the initial laboratory studies of thalidomide on rats did not indicate the possibility of deformities in humans, although later studies on monkeys and rabbits did disclose this problem. Using more recent research techniques, scientists have tried to find the appropriate animal species to be used in the testing process. Again, fetal safety cannot be completely ensured for humans using results from animal studies. Some drugs taken by the mother, although not necessarily teratogenic or carcinogenic, may cause other adverse effects on the embryo, fetus, or neonate. The potential harm that a specific drug poses to the fetus must be weighed against its benefits to the mother.

■ SUMMARY

Exposure to some substances during the first 3 weeks after conception can be so destructive to the embryo that spontaneous abortion occurs. Major malformations are most likely to occur between weeks 3 and 10 of gestation, when the organs are being formed. From week 11 through delivery, exposure mostly slows growth or creates physiologic deficits in the fetus or neonate.

❖ NURSING MANAGEMENT: THE PREGNANT CLIENT

Once pregnant, a woman must be aware of the effects that her lifestyle and any medications she uses have on herself and on the fetus. For many people, lifestyle alterations are difficult. For the pregnant woman, adjusting to a change in body image, they may be especially difficult. To help the client make informed choices during pregnancy, the nurse can offer support and information about the effects of various substances on the client and the fetus. Instruction and educational materials about tobacco, caffeine, alcohol, OTC medications, dietary supplements, and, possibly, illicit drugs should be part of the comprehensive nursing care plan. The nurse must recognize the woman's needs while helping her to work through the feelings associated with pregnancy and parenthood.

NURSING PROCESS
ASSESSMENT

A woman who had medical problems before pregnancy may have to modify the drug regimens that kept her functioning well because the medications may be contraindicated for the fetus. Other women may develop medical problems during pregnancy and may have to take medications or follow diets that make them feel uncomfortable. Some women may be reluctant to discuss their feelings or anxieties, fearful of disapproval from others if they are not fully committed to doing everything that is best for the fetus. In accumulating assessment data, the nurse must be nonjudgmental and supportive, in some cases acting as a sounding board for the woman's feelings.

Obstetric care incorporates wellness care, as most pregnant women are in good health. It is a time for health teaching that can provide a basis for family care throughout life. Assessments should therefore include information about the client's lifestyle, nutrition, responses to stress, and health practices.

The history is important, especially the history of prescribed or OTC medications, tobacco, and other drugs, including alcohol. For example, the client's history of alcohol consumption (quantity, frequency, kind, such as wine, beer, or grain alcohol), as well as any history of fetal alcohol syndrome in other family members, may be significant in instances of suspected alcohol abuse. Tact must be used in obtaining additional data so that the client does not feel diminished or defensive. A social history may reveal more about the client's attitudes about pregnancy and her coping mechanisms.

NURSING DIAGNOSIS

Using the data collected during the assessment, the nurse can determine the areas in which the client needs help, including:

- Knowledge Deficit, concerning maternal, fetal, or neonatal harm that may result from the medical status or medication regimen of the client
- Knowledge Deficit, concerning maternal and fetal requirements, including nutritional needs, such as caloric requirements and food choices
- Anxiety, related to the stress of pregnancy and pre-existing or new conditions requiring medication

PLANNING

Because most pregnant clients are well and capable of determining their own care, any desired changes should be presented as options rather than requirements. Incorporating the client as a full partner in care planning tends to promote therapeutic alliance.

If the client must carry out certain medical regimens, including drug therapy (eg, a diabetic client), the nurse should help her plan time and learn skills to accommodate whatever has to be done. The client must feel that she is participating in setting the goals for her own care.

INTERVENTION

Whatever is done must take the mother as well as the fetus into consideration. If medications taken before pregnancy must be changed to protect the fetus, full explanations are necessary.

Client Education. Some pregnant women may be unaware that the drugs they take may affect the fe-

tus. The general public believes that OTC preparations are safe, or that all physicians are aware of fetal reactions to drugs prescribed for maternal conditions unrelated to the pregnancy. As a result, nearly 20% of pregnant women use some systemic medication during the first trimester. Pregnant women should be advised to inform any healthcare professionals of their pregnancy before accepting any medications or taking any OTC drugs.

The client's cooperation in adhering to the medication regimen to prevent or cure fetal or neonatal disorders is necessary. The client should be instructed in all aspects of medication therapy, including the possible risks and benefits to herself and the fetus. For example, the pregnant woman with syphilis must take a course of penicillin not only to treat her own disease, but also to prevent congenital syphilis in the newborn.

OUTCOME EVALUATION

Any intervention must be judged by its value to both mother and fetus. Medications that may cause problems for the neonate at birth may have to be discontinued or modified before labor. At the same time, medications that may help the fetus but potentially harm the mother during labor may also have to be changed. Plans for stress reduction should be evaluated in light of the mother's behavior during labor and the postpartum period. Plans for eliminating or reducing drug use (including alcohol) during pregnancy can be objectively evaluated by determining intake during pregnancy.

Drug Use During Labor

A normal pregnancy lasts about 280 days (40 weeks, 9 calendar months, or 10 lunar months). Normally, labor begins about 280 days after conception. However, the full mechanism of labor remains obscure. Sometimes labor starts prematurely, posing a risk to the fetus. About 85% of infant deaths that are not related to birth defects are due to prematurity.

Premature Labor

Before the 1970s, treatment of premature labor focused on bed rest in the Trendelenburg position, adequate nutrition, avoidance of sexual activity, and sedation. Hospitalization was used when needed. At that time, neither preventive nor adequate treatment measures existed for the most serious neonatal complication, respiratory distress syndrome, then referred to as hyaline membrane disease.

In the mid-1970s, an additional treatment modality was added: 10% alcohol (ethanol), usually as an IV drip, was given as a tocolytic (contraction-inhibiting) agent. Although the alcohol was somewhat effective in terminating contractions, clients complained of uncomfortable side effects (headaches, nausea, hangover). The fetus was also affected, appearing intoxicated and lethargic and showing signs of hypotonicity.

Since that time, various tocolytic agents have been used. There are four classes of tocolytics: beta-sympathomimetics, magnesium sulfate, calcium antagonists, and prostaglandin inhibitors. Home uterine activity monitoring systems are used to detect uterine contractions that lead to preterm labor. The monitor has a sensor that is placed against the mother's abdomen for an hour, twice a day. The information is transmitted via telephone to a perinatal nurse, usually at a perinatal center. This information permits early diagnosis of labor and the use of tocolytic drugs if needed.

Ritodrine Hydrochloride

In 1981, the U.S. government approved a tocolytic drug, ritodrine hydrochloride (Yutopar). It is a potent beta-sympathomimetic agent specifically useful as a uterine relaxant. Approval came after many clinical trials, with thorough records that documented maternal, fetal, and neonatal outcomes. Ritodrine is discussed here in some detail; other drugs used for similar purposes (terbutaline, magnesium sulfate, calcium channel blockers, and prostaglandin inhibitors) are discussed as well.

Pharmacodynamics. Ritodrine relaxes the smooth muscles of the uterus, bronchial tree, and arterioles. Its effectiveness is greatest between 20 and 36 weeks of gestation, when there is no evidence of fetal distress, and the membranes have not ruptured.

Pharmacokinetics. Treatment is initiated with an IV infusion during the acute phase of preterm labor. The dose is titrated and continued until contractions are suppressed for at least 12 hours. About 30 minutes before IV therapy stops, oral therapy begins. The tablets are usually taken several times a day, with reintroduction of IV therapy if labor starts again. Oral therapy is usually terminated by the 38th week of gestation, because delivery by then should produce a neonate capable of maintaining life.

Therapeutic Uses. Ritodrine is used to inhibit labor so that parturition is delayed until the fetus is mature enough to sustain vital functions.

Adverse Reactions. Infusion therapy required by ritodrine induction can cause fluid volume excess and maternal pulmonary edema, especially when combined with glucocorticoid medication (McCombs, 1995). Maternal and fetal heart rate and blood pressure increase with ritodrine therapy. Cardiac and CNS stimulation is common. Hyperglycemia may develop. Although ritodrine presents one approach to the problem of preterm labor, it also carries significant risks.

Drug–Drug Interactions. Ritodrine and atropine may cause increased systemic hypertension. Ritodrine's action is inhibited by beta blockers, and its use with corticosteroids should be avoided because the combination increases the risk for pulmonary edema. Combined with sympathomimetic drugs, such as albuterol or dopamine, ritodrine may increase cardiac side effects.

Drug–Lab Test Interactions. In blood tests, ritodrine can elevate plasma insulin and glucose levels and decrease potassium concentrations.

Precautions and Contraindications. Ritodrine is contraindicated before 20 gestational weeks and in women with pre-existing conditions such as hypovolemia, uncontrolled hypertension, and cardiac arrhythmias. Before administering ritodrine, the utmost consideration should be given as to whether it is truly needed. If fetal lung maturity is adequate, it may be better to allow delivery, because infants in this situation usually have an uncomplicated course after birth. Fetal lung maturity can be evaluated by a sonogram to determine fetal age, by the lecithin-sphingomyelin rate in the amniotic fluid, or both. Contractions should be regular, occurring at least every 10 minutes and lasting at least 30 seconds, the fetal weight should be less than 2,500 g, and cervical effacement should be less than 80%, with dilation less than 4 cm. Ultrasonography may help distinguish women who are in premature labor with changes in the cervix and lower uterine segments from those who are having contractions without changes.

Because ritodrine therapy poses risks primarily to the mother, it must be monitored carefully. Contractions and fetal heart rate and maternal vital signs should be checked frequently (eg, every 15 minutes during titration and then every 30 minutes during maintenance therapy). Maternal fluid balance must be monitored to prevent overhydration, particularly if used in combination with corticosteroids. Fluid intake should be limited to 90 to 100 mL hourly; output should be measured every hour during contractions and then every 4 hours.

Multiple gestations and administration of ritodrine IV for more than 24 hours may increase the risk of pulmonary edema. Maternal serum glucose and potassium levels should be checked twice a day during IV administration. Although the many effects of ritodrine do not appear to result in clinical problems, neonates should be observed for changes in their renal, electrolyte, and fluid levels (McCombs, 1995).

Ritodrine should never be used in women with cardiac arrhythmia, pulmonary hypertension, bronchial asthma (treated with beta agonists, corticosteroids, or both), hyperthyroidism, or pheochromocytoma. Fetal contraindications include chorioamnionitis, fetal death, or conditions incompatible with neonatal survival. See the Critical Thinking Challenge: Issues Analysis.

Terbutaline

Terbutaline (Brethine, Bricanyl) is another beta-mimetic drug with tocolytic effects. It is administered IV

CRITICAL THINKING CHALLENGE
Issues Analysis

Consider the issues confronting the client and clinician when deciding on interventions for preterm labor. The following information points out the advantages and disadvantages of tocolytic drug therapy.

Advantages of Tocolytic Treatment

- Used over as few as 48 hours, allows healthcare provider to medicate fetus, via mother, with corticosteroids to promote fetal pulmonary maturation
- Retards premature labor, which buys time to transfer client to a high-risk obstetric facility with a neonatal intensive care unit
- May stop premature labor altogether, permitting pregnancy to reach term or fetus to become viable

Disadvantages of Tocolytic Therapy

- Does not decrease prenatal mortality or reverse respiratory disorder in neonates
- Cannot be used in women with arrhythmia, pulmonary hypertension, bronchial asthma treated with beta agonists or corticosteroids, hyperthyroidism, or pheochromocytoma
- May be responsible for maternal increase in blood pressure and cardiac and CNS stimulation
- In women taking corticosteroids, may result in pulmonary edema and hyperglycemia
- Cannot be used in conditions incompatible with neonatal survival, chorioamnionitis, or fetal death
- May cause increases in the following:

  —Fetus: heart rate, blood pressure, cardiac and CNS stimulation, hyperglycemia, bilirubin level (with neonatal icterus), plasma renin activity

  —Neonate: weight increase at age 6 days (possibly from fluid retention) and urinary excretion of vasopression for several days after birth

1. Keeping these issues in mind, consider the cost of the treatment choice in terms of potential fetal outcome and treatment of the neonate in a neonatal intensive care unit.
2. What impact might the cost of the treatment choice—to use tocolytic therapy or not—have on the healthcare provider's counseling and teaching and the client's decision?

When the client cannot be maintained on oral therapy, parenteral therapy is started in the hospital for 48 hours, and then the client is treated on an outpatient basis. In conjunction with home uterine activity monitoring, a miniature portable terbutaline infusion pump is used to provide a continual amount of terbutaline through a tube threaded beneath the skin. The subcutaneous site is usually in the upper abdomen and is changed every 3 days. The client receives instruction on operating the pump, caring for the infusion site, and monitoring the fetal heart rate. The infusion rate is adjusted to keep the uterine contractions under four per hour. For most clients, about 80% of the contractions usually occur over a 6-hour period in the evening. With this system, about 3 mg or less of terbutaline is required daily, as opposed to 40 to 60 mg daily orally or 60 mg per day IV. Treatment continues until term or until hospitalization is required again (Freda, 1991).

The perinatal nurse may be responsible for adjusting the dose of terbutaline according to the information received over the telephone from the home uterine activity monitor and registered on a computerized device in the healthcare facility. Agency protocols must be determined and followed for this procedure to meet safety standards.

Terbutaline, unlike ritodrine, does not have FDA approval for use as a tocolytic drug. Although both drugs prolong gestation—a factor in increased birth weights—a landmark 1988 study (King et al.) noted that neither drug reduced perinatal mortality or severe respiratory disorders in neonates. Several cases of maternal deaths have been associated with these tocolytic drugs, usually due to fluid overload. In interaction with certain anesthetic gases, such as halothane or cyclopropane, there is the potential for cardiac arrhythmias.

The positive aspect of tocolytic drug use is the time they provide for transferring the client to a high-risk obstetric facility with a neonatal intensive care unit. In addition, the extra time can be used to administer glucocorticoids to enhance fetal lung maturation.

Magnesium Sulfate

Magnesium sulfate ($MgSO_4$) has traditionally been used in pregnancy to treat preeclampsia. Although the mechanism of action is unknown, $MgSO_4$ is also used in treating preterm labor. Experts think that $MgSO_4$ interferes with calcium uptake by the myometrial cells, which need it to contract. The usual regimen for IV use is a loading dose of 4 g, followed by maintenance doses of 2 to 4 g/hr until the desired results are achieved or signs of toxicity are noted (Gilbert, 1993).

Adverse reactions include side effects related to the loading dose and include nausea, hot flashes, vomiting, blurred vision, and drowsiness. Signs of toxicity include a respiratory rate less than 12, absence of deep tendon reflexes, severe hypotension, and extreme muscle relax-

initially in the hospital, 5 mg in dextrose 5% in water (or other compatible IV solution), 500 mL at 10 µg/min, increased every 10 minutes until contractions stop (limit 80 µg/min). The dose is then reduced to the lowest effective level. Terbutaline may also be given subcutaneously. Once stabilized, the client can be discharged on oral doses of 2.5 mg every 4 hours the first day, then every 6 hours until term (McCombs, 1995).

ation. Women receiving $MgSO_4$ for preterm labor need close monitoring (Box 10-3). If the maternal serum level is maintained below 8 mEq/L, neonatal side effects are rare.

Calcium Channel Blockers

These drugs may interfere with the transport of extracellular calcium into the calcium channels of the cells and thus prevent contractions. Nifedipine (Procardia) and nicardipine (Nicardipine) are used in Europe as tocolytic agents, but their use in the United States is limited.

Prostaglandin Inhibitors

Naturally occurring prostaglandins cause uterine contractions and cervical ripening. Indomethacin as an oral prostaglandin inhibitor to suppress uterine activity in preterm labor is an unlabeled use of the drug. The initial loading dose of 100 mg by rectal suppository is most common. The maintenance oral dose is 25 mg q4h for up to 48 hours.

Prostaglandin inhibitors have the potential for serious side effects. Beyond 34 weeks' gestation, indomethacin use increases the risk of fetal pulmonary hypertension, premature closure of the ductus arteriosus, and oligohydramnios. Indomethacin is contraindicated in clients sensitive to salicylate.

Term Labor and Natural Oxytocin

Although the full triggering mechanism for the beginning of labor remains unknown, it is known that the posterior pituitary secretes oxytocin, a hormone with the power to stimulate uterine contractions. The myometrium of the uterus is most sensitive to this stimulation toward the end of the pregnancy. As the cervix effaces and dilates, additional oxytocin is released. This release stimulates additional contractions of the uterine fundus, resulting in greater cervical effacement and dilation. The oxytocin level seems to peak during the second (expulsive) stage of delivery.

Nonpharmacologic induction of labor has occurred with breast self-stimulation to ripen the cervix. Gentle massage of the nipples with a warm, moist washcloth for 1 hour, three times daily, showed statistically significant changes in the amount of cervical effacement and dilation. Tetanic contractions and other adverse contractions were not present, making this technique one to be considered when induction is necessary. Electrostimulation of the nipples has also been used, as it can be controlled more exactly than the washcloth massage (Tal et al., 1988). For either method of stimulation, the cervix must be inducible and the client must be monitored for signs of decreased fetal heart rate or prolonged uterine contractions, with intervention if either occurs.

Artificially Induced Labor and Oxytocic Drugs

In cases of fetal postmaturity, gestational diabetes, maternal diabetes mellitus, PIH, or any other maternal or fetal condition that warrants induction of labor, the

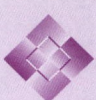

Box 10-3
Monitoring Magnesium Sulfate Use in Preventing Preterm Labor

1. Check vital signs frequently, paying close attention to changes in blood pressure and respiration.
2. Monitor deep tendon reflexes hourly. If significantly depressed, may be a sign of impending respiratory suppression.
3. Monitor hourly intake and output. Output should be at least 30 mL/hr.
4. Check $MgSO_4$ serum levels daily. Levels of 10 mEq/L or more can lead to toxicity.
5. Avoid administering narcotics or sedatives. Simultaneous use could lead to respiratory depression.
6. Keep calcium gluconate (1–2 g) available as an antidote.
7. Restrict fluids to 2,500 mL/daily.

Adapted from Gilbert ES, Harmon JS. (1993). *Manual of high-risk pregnancy and delivery*. St. Louis: Mosby, p. 440.

client is hospitalized and a synthetic oxytocic drug is given.

Pharmacodynamics. Oxytocic drugs are synthetic peptides. They have the same properties as the naturally occurring oxytocin in the posterior lobe of the pituitary gland. They work via a selective action on the smooth muscle of the uterus, stimulating contractions or increasing the forcefulness of existing contractions. Oxytocics must be administered with care to ensure the proper level of contractile activity.

Pharmacokinetics. Oxytocin (Pitocin, Syntocinon) may be administered as a nasal spray, buccal tablet, intramuscular (IM) injection, or IV infusion. The preferred administration route is IV via a controlled infusion device, which allows discontinuation of the drug at any time. When administered IV, a dose of 10 units of the oxytocic drug is given in 1,000 mL of normal saline (0.9% sodium chloride) solution. The initial dose should be limited to 1 to 2 mU/min and may be gradually increased at a rate of no more than 1 to 2 mU/min until a contraction pattern occurs that resembles normal labor. The peak uterine contractile response is reached in 40 minutes. The infusion should be discontinued immediately if uterine hyperactivity or fetal distress occurs. Because the half-life is 3 to 5 minutes, the effects subside quickly after discontinuation. With the IM route of administration, uterine response should start within 3 to 5 minutes and should persist for 2 to 3 hours.

Oxytocic drugs are distributed throughout the extracellular fluid and may reach the fetus as well. They are excreted from the plasma by the kidney and liver.

Therapeutic Uses. Oxytocic drugs can be used in controlled situations to induce or reinforce labor and to control postpartum bleeding or hemorrhage.

Adverse Reactions. Oxytocic drugs have an antidiuretic effect, with the possibility of water intoxication and pulmonary edema when they are administered continuously IV and the client is taking fluids by mouth. Oxytocics can cause hypertonic or tetanic contractions and therefore must be carefully monitored. For the mother, the risk of uterine rupture, hypertension, subarachnoid hemorrhage, postpartum hemorrhage, anaphylaxis, cardiac arrhythmia, afibrinogenemia, and pelvic hematoma exists. Intense uterine contractions decrease the flow of oxygenated blood to the fetus, creating the possibility of fetal damage, particularly to the brain, or death. Arrhythmia, neonatal jaundice, and a low Apgar score at 5 minutes may also occur.

Drug Interactions. Interaction between oxytocics and sympathomimetic drugs increases the potential for postpartum hypertension. When oxytocic drugs are used with vasoconstrictors and regional anesthetics, severe hypertension has occurred.

Precautions and Contraindications. Oxytocics should never be used to induce labor for any reason other than medical necessity. The convenience of the client or healthcare provider is an unacceptable reason for induction.

The cervix must be ripe (inducible) for the drug to be effective. Topical prostaglandin (PGE$_2$) applied to the cervix has been found to help ripen the cervix if applied the night before attempting an induction of labor with oxytocin. These drugs should never be used if significant cephalopelvic disproportion is present, an indication that the fetal position or other problem will preclude vaginal delivery, if hypertonic uterine patterns are evident, or if hypersensitivity to the drug is indicated. Prolonged use is contraindicated in the presence of uterine inertia, severe toxemia, or fetal distress.

Throughout the administration of oxytocic drugs, the flow must be accurately controlled with an infusion pump or similar device. Fetal monitoring is required to determine the frequency, duration, and force of the contractions, as well as the fetal heart rate. The client should be hospitalized during the procedure, with a physician available at all times.

Artificially Induced Labor After Fetal Demise

Certain prostaglandins that occur naturally in the body stimulate uterine contractions. One form, PGE$_2$, is synthesized by the cervix and is being studied as a way to induce labor because it softens and ripens even an unfavorable cervix. The FDA has approved the use of dinoprostone (PGE$_2$) for expelling a fetus that dies before 28 weeks of gestation, using 20-mg suppositories inserted high in the vagina. Oxytocin is usually administered concurrently. This dose can be repeated every 2 to 4 hours until a maximum dose of 280 mg has been administered. If labor does not ensue within 24 hours, a period of 12 to 24 hours should pass before another attempt is made. The drug should not be given for more than 48 hours and should not be administered to women with active pulmonary, hepatic, cardiac, or renal disease or acute pelvic inflammatory disease.

Hypertension Control During Labor

During pregnancy or labor, a marked elevation of blood pressure may occur. Active intervention is necessary to prevent seizures. Magnesium sulfate is the drug of choice and may be given IM or IV to prevent or control convulsions. Severe CNS depression may occur, requiring IV administration of calcium gluconate. Oral, IM, or IV hydralazine (Apresoline) is also used as a vasodilator with antihypertensive action. Teratogenic effects have been noted when it is used in mice and rabbits, although clinical experience with the drug does not indicate any positive evidence of an adverse effect on the human fetus. Phenobarbital is another drug used as an anticonvulsant. Its disadvantage lies in its ability to cross the placental barrier, resulting in the possible depression of neonatal respiration.

Pain Control During Labor

Pain control during labor is a prime example of conflict between maternal and fetal needs. Relief of pain may be the foremost desire of the mother, whereas the risk of prematurity, slow heart rate, or low level of fetal lung maturity may preclude the use of medication to relieve the mother's pain. For this reason, techniques such as biofeedback, hypnosis, acupuncture, therapeutic touch, and psychoprophylaxis are useful. These help control rather than eliminate pain. The client then requires less medication than she might otherwise request.

Pharmacologic approaches to the management of labor pain include using sedatives, tranquilizers, narcotic analgesics, and anesthetics. Narcotic analgesics in common use include butorphanol (Stadol), meperidine (Demerol), and nalbuphine (Nubain).

Analgesia With Meperidine and Other Drugs

Sometimes, parenteral meperidine hydrochloride is given during labor to produce analgesia and sedation. Because it readily crosses the placenta in appreciable amounts, meperidine use is restricted in late labor because it may cause neonatal respiratory depression. It may be combined with other drugs for additional effects.

Table 10-5. Drugs Used Frequently for Pain Relief During Labor

Drug Name	Usual Dosage	Type/Desired Action	Possible Side Effects			Precaution
			Maternal	Fetal		
Narcotic analgesic*						
butorphanol (Stadol)	IM: 1–2 mg IV: 0.5–1 mg	30–40 times more potent than meperidine	Respiratory and circulatory depression, dizziness, potential respiratory depression	Apnea, CNS depression		Not for use with opioid-addicted mothers. Have Naloxone 0.1 mg/kg for neonatal depression.
meperidine (Demerol)	25–100 mg every 3 to 4 hr	Narcotic/analgesic, increased pain tolerance	Nausea, vomiting, some circulatory and respiratory depression	Respiratory depression in the neonate		Avoid within 2 hours of delivery; found in neonate urine for 3 days
nalbuphine (Nubain)	IM: 5–10 mg IV: 1 mg at 6- to 10-min intervals	Decreased pain	Minimal side effects, does not interfere with labor	Potential respiratory depression		Not for use with opioid-addicted mother
fentanyl (Sublimaze)	IM: 50–100 mg Epidural: 100–200 mg Intrathecal: 25 mg	100 times as potent as meperdine, decreases pain	Increased sedation	Potential respiratory depression		
Sedatives						
pentobarbital (Nembutal)	30 mg	Barbiturate/sedative, sleep inducer	Nausea, vomiting, hypotension, vertigo, restlessness, slow labor	Apnea, CNS depression		Avoid late in labor
secobarbital (Seconal)	30 mg	Barbiturate/sedative	Nausea, vomiting, hypotension, vertigo, restlessness, slow labor	Apnea, CNS depression		Avoid late in labor
Tranquilizers						
diazepam (Valium)	2–10 mg	Tranquilizer/anti-anxiety, potentiates narcotics and barbiturates	Hypotension, vertigo, drowsiness	Hypothermia, CNS depression, may remain active in fetus for 10 days		Decrease narcotics or barbiturates to ½ dose
hydroxyzine (Vistaril)	IM or IV: 5–15 mg	Tranquilizer/anti-anxiety, potentiates narcotics and barbiturates	Hypotension, vertigo, drowsiness	CNS depression		Decrease narcotics or barbiturates to ½ dose
promethazine (Phenergan)	IM or IV: 25–50 mg		Same as above	Same as above		Same as above

*Newborn respiratory depression due to narcotization can be reversed within 2 minutes by IV administration of naloxone hydrochloride (Narcan), a narcotic antagonist. Infant must be watched for subsequent episodes of apnea.

Meperidine hydrochloride may be used with tranquilizers such as hydroxyzine hydrochloride (Vistaril), which improves sedation and acts as an antiemetic during labor. (Its use is contraindicated in early pregnancy.) Promethazine hydrochloride (Phenergan) is sometimes combined with meperidine for its sedative and antiemetic effects. All of these combinations must be administered with the greatest caution because they may cause neonatal respiratory depression. To help the mother rest during prolonged labor, sedatives, such as secobarbital (Seconal) or pentobarbital (Nembutal), were used in the past for their calming effects when delivery was not anticipated for 12 to 24 hours. These drugs are not commonly used today. Depending on the situation, pain relief during delivery may be obtained with a local or general anesthetic. Table 10-5 highlights drugs used to control pain during labor.

■ SUMMARY

Drugs are available to manage premature labor as well as to induce labor. In either situation, the dangers for mother, fetus, or neonate must be considered carefully, and both mother and child must be monitored closely.

❖ NURSING MANAGEMENT: CLIENT IN LABOR

Labor and delivery usually occur safely, but they may be complicated by unexpected situations. Labor may begin before the fetus has attained sufficient maturity to sustain life, or it may be delayed beyond the time that the fetus can be nurtured properly in the uterus. Nurses must be prepared to recognize any adverse effects on the mother or child caused by drugs given to delay or induce labor or to relieve pain.

NURSING PROCESS

ASSESSMENT

The client in labor may present herself in a variety of ways. She may or may not be in control and may or may not be properly prepared for the experience of labor and delivery. She may react to pain stoically, or she may want relief through medication. If an oxytocic is administered, she may need to be guided into using relaxation or other techniques for pain control, in addition to any medication ordered.

Assessments during labor include the duration, forcefulness, and frequency of contractions. Their effect on the fetal heart rate must be carefully observed. This observation becomes even more important when oxytocics are used. The nurse also must assess the amount of support the client needs during labor, whether or not she has a lay coach with her. At times, the coach may need even more support than the mother!

NURSING DIAGNOSIS

Nursing diagnoses likely to be made for clients in labor and delivery include:

- Altered Tissue Perfusion in the Fetus, related to medications or labor
- Risk for Injury, related to complications associated with medications or labor
- Knowledge Deficit, related to expected or unexpected effect of medications used in labor

PLANNING

The primary goal of nursing care during labor and delivery is to provide safety for mother and fetus. In addition, comfort should be considered so that the mother can bond more easily with the infant. (Bonding may be difficult if the mother views the newborn as the cause of insufferable pain and distress.)

INTERVENTION

The mother's antepartum fantasy of labor and delivery should be examined. If it varies greatly from the actual occurrence, help should be given to facilitate acceptance of what took place. In addition to the psychological aspects of care, the physical care throughout labor and delivery should be of the highest caliber to prevent iatrogenic problems. Medications must be prepared and administered accurately, with adequate monitoring of the effects on mother and fetus. Neonatal reactions to the medications should be observed and treated as necessary. See the Critical Thinking Challenge: Case Analysis.

OUTCOME EVALUATION

Nursing care can be considered successful if both client and newborn are in good health throughout labor and delivery or if complications have been skillfully resolved and negative effects reversed to the extent possible.

CRITICAL THINKING CHALLENGE
Case Analysis

Mrs. Anderson is being admitted to the birthing area in your hospital. As you begin your initial assessment, she tells you she has no interest in breathing techniques or other nonpharmacologic methods to reduce pain during labor. Her goal is to be "knocked out" and wake up with the baby born and no recall of pain.

1. Consider the educational needs of this mother and identify the factors that affect the use of analgesics during labor and delivery.
2. What actions would you take to create an effective plan for pain management?
3. Given the advantages and disadvantages of each type of analgesic/anesthetic, what choices might you make in this client's situation, and why?

Drug Use During Delivery

Local anesthetics used in regional anesthesia are listed in Table 10-6. Anesthetics and analgesics are discussed further in Chapter 18. Clients who are otherwise reasonably comfortable may elect to have a local anesthetic if an episiotomy is needed.

Local Anesthetics

Lidocaine hydrochloride (Xylocaine) and procaine hydrochloride (Novocain) are among the drugs used for pudendal or local anesthesia by infiltration. These two are the least toxic of all the local anesthetics. Another advantage of lidocaine is that its action is immediate; thus, it is helpful in an emergency episiotomy. Overdose and too-rapid administration must be avoided with both because these factors may cause adverse effects including anaphylactic reactions, seizures, burning, tissue swelling, and necrosis.

These drugs are also used to provide regional anesthesia, particularly for epidural administration. The popularity of epidural anesthesia has increased. The use of dilute anesthetic concentrations, combined with narcotics, is effective for pain management in the later phases of labor. Previously, epidural anesthesia required doses of local anesthetics, which resulted in loss of motor function. However, by using a continuous infusion device, the dilute anesthetic and narcotic combination successfully relieves pain without significantly blocking motor function. For example, 0.125% or 0.0625% of bupivacaine (Marcaine) with sufentanil (Sufenta) provides the desired pain control, reducing the risk of systemic toxicity by decreasing the total amount of anesthetic required (Creehan, 1996).

Epidural anesthesia eliminates the perception of pain during uterine contractions and also maintains waist-to-toe anesthesia during cesarean sections, allowing the client to remain conscious. However, epidural anesthesia does have drawbacks. Some clients develop severe hypotension, which can result in fetal bradycardia. If this occurs, treatment usually consists of positioning the client on her side, administering oxygen by face mask or nasal cannula, and providing IV fluids. Intravenous ephedrine may also be needed to increase the blood pressure. The lack of sensation also interferes with the client's urge to push, leading to the possibility of ineffective pushing and the need for forceps to aid the delivery. Some clinicians avoid administering epidural anesthesia unless the cervix is dilated 4 cm and contractions are consistent and well established. Otherwise, the mother's inability to push may necessitate a forceps or cesarean delivery. Box 10-4 describes potential complications of epidural anesthesia.

General Anesthetics

Nitrous oxide, a general inhalation anesthetic, was used in the past during the last part of the first stage of labor, during delivery of the baby and the placenta, and during the postpartum internal examination immediately after the birth. Today, other anesthetics are in more common use. Ketamine hydrochloride (Ketaject, Ketalar) is given IV and can be used alone or with nitrous oxide. It is sometimes used as an alternative to thiopental as an induction agent. However, it has a high incidence of adverse effects (particularly unpleasant dreams or hallucinations), making it less satisfactory than thiopental for induction of anesthesia for elective cesarean section.

General anesthesia that causes unconsciousness may be needed for a complicated vaginal delivery or cesarean delivery. Thiopental sodium (Pentothal Sodium) and succinylcholine chloride (Anectine), administered IV, provide short-term total anesthesia. Few contraindications for their use exist, and they can be used safely in almost all cesarean deliveries.

The disadvantages of general anesthesia include a higher incidence of newborn depression, postponement

Table 10-6. Local Anesthetics Frequently Used for Regional Anesthesia

Drug Name	Concentration or Usual Dosage	Onset of Action	Duration of Action	Nerve Block	IV	Uses Infiltration	Caudal	Epidural Peridural	Spinal
bupivacaine (Marcaine)	0.5%–0.25%	5–20 min	2–7 hours			✔	✔	✔	
chloroprocaine (Nesacaine)	1%–3% solution	Fast	30–60 min	✔	✔	✔	✔	✔	
lidocaine (Xylocaine)	0.5%–5% solution	Fast	1–2 hr	✔	✔	✔		✔	✔
mepivacaine (Carbocaine)	1%–2% solution	15 min	3 hr	✔	✔	✔		✔	
procaine (Novocain)	0.2%–2% solution	2–5 min	1 hr	✔		✔			✔
tetracaine (Pontocaine)	up to 15 mg	15 min	3 hr						✔

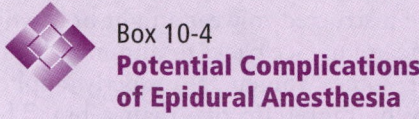

Box 10-4
Potential Complications of Epidural Anesthesia

Although epidural anesthesia is usually safe, the nurse must know and inform the client that some complications may accompany it.

Complications from the Anesthetic

Signs and symptoms of a complication from the local anesthetic itself (eg, lidocaine, procaine) include shivering, hypotension, increased need for cesarean delivery, maternal pyrexia, neonatal hyperthermia, persistent occiput posterior, late decelerations, and seizures.

Complication from the Anesthetic Combined With a Narcotic

In the later stages of labor, the physician may add a narcotic drug to the local anesthetic. In such cases, complications may take the form of respiratory depression, urinary retention, nausea and vomiting, sedation, and pruritus.

Complication from the Procedure

Additional problems may result from the administration of the anesthetic: backache, headache, unilateral anesthesia, migration of the catheter, or accidental puncture of the dura.

Adapted with permission from Creehan, PA. (1996). Pain relief and comfort measures during labor. In Simpson KR, Creehan PA. *AWHONN's perinatal nursing.* Philadelphia: Lippincott-Raven.

of mother–infant contact, and exposure of the mother to the potentially lethal complication of pulmonary aspiration of gastric contents.

Drug Use in Postpartum Care

Once the placenta has been delivered, oxytocin may be administered to increase uterine contraction, thereby preventing or controlling uterine hemorrhage.

Uterine atony can be life-threatening because it leads to severe bleeding after delivery. If the usual use of external uterine massage, IV oxytocin, or IM methylergonovine does not stop the hemorrhage, 15-methyl $PGF_2\alpha$, a synthetic prostaglandin, may prove effective. Uterine contractions should start within 45 minutes after an initial dose of 250 μg IM or by injection into the uterine wall, which can be administered through the abdomen or vagina. The 250-μg dose can be repeated every 90 minutes as needed to a maximum dose of 15 mg. Side effects are usually limited to nausea, vomiting

and diarrhea, variations in blood pressure with a possible diastolic elevation (particularly in preeclamptic women), fever, and flushing. The use of this prostaglandin may obviate the need for a blood transfusion.

Ergonovine, derived from ergot, is particularly useful in the immediate postpartum period. It contracts the uterus, thus lessening the flow of blood from the placental site during the first few days after delivery. Ergonovine maleate (Ergotrate) or methylergonovine maleate (Methergine) is usually administered three or four times daily for 2 to 7 days after delivery. If uterine relaxation recurs later in the puerperium, another course may be given.

Postpartum uterine contractions are usually painless for the primipara; however, they are increasingly painful after each successive pregnancy because the uterine fibers do not have the same ability to contract after subsequent pregnancies. Pain may be controlled with meperidine, hydroxyzine, propoxyphene (Darvon), oxycodone, aspirin, acetaminophen (Tylenol), or various combinations.

Mothers who have Rh-negative blood and who have not received RhoGAM prophylaxis prenatally should receive IM Rho(D) immune globulin (RhIG) within 72 hours after delivery of an Rh-positive infant. If bleeding has been severe, an additional vial of RhIG may be administered to prevent isoimmunization. If the time limit of 72 hours is exceeded, even by as much as 7 days, the American College of Obstetricians and Gynecologists recommends that RhIG still be given. They also suggest that all Rh-negative women be given RhIG after abortions, ectopic pregnancies, second- or third-trimester amniocentesis procedures, and possibly after antepartum hemorrhage, fetal death, sterilization, and transfusions. Some practitioners give all pregnant women with Rh-negative blood RhoGAM at about 28 weeks' gestation for prophylaxis.

While the infant is in the delivery room, its eyes are treated with drops or ointment to prevent gonorrheal infection of the eyes (ophthalmia neonatorum). The drugs of choice are erythromycin 0.5% ophthalmic ointment or tetracycline 1% ophthalmic ointment in a single immediate application. Both are also effective against *Chlamydia trachomatis*, another sexually transmitted disease that may affect the newborn's eyes and cause blindness. Silver nitrate 1% topical solution is effective only for neonatal gonococcal ophthalmia. In addition, most newborns receive an injection of vitamin K (AquaMephyton) to build up their clotting capacity.

■ SUMMARY

Careful consideration must be given to both mother and fetus during the birth. The physical condition of either one may necessitate using a medication with the potential to harm the other. For this reason, any medication must be thoroughly evaluated before use to ensure that the potential benefit outweighs the potential harm to either client.

Nurses should institute comfort measures to decrease maternal anxiety and pain during pregnancy, labor, and delivery. Such intervention may decrease the need for drugs, which have the potential to compromise the health of the mother, fetus, or neonate.

❖ NURSING MANAGEMENT: CLIENT DURING AND AFTER DELIVERY

Clients are increasingly aware that drugs may have negative effects on them or their fetuses and may request additional information before permitting their administration. This active consumerism requires healthcare professionals to be knowledgeable about all medications given to the mother.

Labor and delivery call for a balance between maternal desires and fetal safety. One mother may demand a pain-free amnesiac birth, but her infant's health status may make that impossible. Another mother may want a drug-free experience, with herself fully in control, and that may be impossible because of a maternal or fetal emergency that requires the use of drugs or anesthesia. In either instance, the nurse can help the mother explore her disappointment, perhaps anger, at not having her wishes met. Most importantly, the mother may need a great deal of help to work through her feelings about the birth experience and how it affects her relationship with the infant.

Aside from providing information to the pregnant woman about possible medications to be used during labor and delivery and discussing alternative methods, the nurse's most important responsibility in the labor and delivery room is the careful observation and monitoring of the mother and fetus. The progress of labor must be observed, whether the induction of labor has been natural or artificial. The uterine contractions must be monitored carefully to prevent complications that affect the mother (eg, uterine rupture, cerebral hemorrhage, hypertensive crisis, cardiac arrhythmia, cervical lacerations) or the fetus (eg, cardiac arrhythmia, cerebral damage).

The obstetric nurse must know about the complications of various pain-relief measures, must be able to recognize the signs and symptoms of adverse reactions immediately, and must know what action to take until a physician or anesthesiologist is available.

Comfort measures during labor should include relaxation techniques that lessen the mother's anxiety, fear, and tension. When possible, she should be talked through contractions, decreasing her need for medications to relieve pain. Clients who receive tocolytic drugs should be observed carefully to prevent overhydration, which may lead to pulmonary edema. Those who receive oxytocic drugs should be observed for signs of uterine rupture or fetal distress.

After delivery, the mother who is not planning to breast-feed may be instructed to wear a tight bra, avoid nipple stimulation, and use ice packs to minimize breast engorgement. For some women, a properly applied breast binder may be more effective than a bra. This nonpharmacologic method provides greater safety than any antilactation drug available.

Drug Use During Lactation

It is difficult to obtain accurate information about the excretion of medications in human milk. Published reports include data that are based on limited samples or that have been obtained under poorly controlled conditions. Many medications have been studied only in animals. If more than one report has been made about a given medication, the findings may be contradictory. Thus, care must be taken when any medication is given to the nursing mother.

In general, the administration of medications to the nursing mother is of greater concern when the infant is 1 week old than when the child is 1 year old. One of the body's principal detoxifying mechanisms is the ability to combine potentially harmful materials with glucuronic acid. This mechanism is generally not fully functioning in an infant who is 1 to 2 weeks old. This mechanism is of special importance in the case of chloramphenicol, which is almost exclusively metabolized by glucuronide conjugation. Other studies have shown that the acetylation and oxidation enzyme systems are not fully functioning either at this age. These systems are important in the metabolism of drugs such as sulfisoxazole. Immature enzyme systems and incompletely developed kidney function make the newborn susceptible to accumulations of toxic levels of drugs.

Although the immediate effects of drugs ingested in human milk have been the primary focus of the literature, an additional concern must be the long-term effects of exposure to a medication. For example, if a child nurses until age 2 years and has been exposed for 2 years to a drug excreted in breast milk, are there any consequences that have not yet been recognized? Is it possible that a medication that produces no immediate observable effects could have effects at a later age?

Simply measuring the concentration of the medication in breast milk is meaningless. Although the drug may be present, it may be pharmacologically inactive or destroyed before absorption and, therefore, poses no problems to the infant. Of greater consequence is the amount of drug actually absorbed.

Mechanisms of Drug Passage From Plasma to Milk

Passive diffusion is the most common mechanism by which medications pass through biologic membranes. Substances that diffuse can achieve the same or different concentrations in milk as in plasma. In accord with the principles of passive diffusion, no changes in the milk–plasma (M-P) ratios are noted at different plasma concentrations of the medication or at varying volumes of secreted milk. Back-diffusion can occur when blood levels of a medication are decreasing.

The M-P ratio refers to the concentration of the protein-free fractions in milk and in plasma. Dissimilar M-P ratios reflect differences in the binding of the medications to plasma proteins. A medication with an M-P ratio of 1 has the same concentration in milk as it does in plasma. An M-P ratio of 4 means that the level of the medication in milk is four times higher than the level in plasma.

Substances may compete with medications for binding sites, a process that may result in the displacement of medication or the passage of an increased amount of medication into the breast milk.

The composition of milk goes through three phases, each with a different pH and fat content. Initially, during the first 3 or 4 postpartum days, colostrum is secreted. This substance has a lower carbohydrate and fat content than whole breast milk. After several days, colostrum is replaced by transitional milk, which assumes the characteristics of whole milk by the third week. Thus, the tendency for the same drug to cross the plasma into milk changes as the milk goes through these transitions.

Passive diffusion of larger molecules across membranes depends on their lipid solubility and state of ionization. The lipid solubility of a medication depends in part on the degree to which it is ionized in solution. Medications that are largely nonionized in solution are lipid-soluble and, for this reason, diffuse readily through the membrane. The more lipid-soluble the medication is, the greater and more rapid its absorption across a membrane. Medications with low lipid solubility diffuse rather slowly into milk. Medications such as pentobarbital and secobarbital, which are more lipid-soluble, tend to transfer into milk as its fat content rises. Therefore, an infant is more likely to ingest these medications under certain conditions (ie, when the fat content of the milk is high).

Most medications are weak acids or weak bases. The ionization of these acids and bases depends on the pH of the environment and the dissociation constant of the medication (pKa). The dissociation constant is the pH level at which the concentrations of ionized and nonionized medication are equal. Weak bases become more ionized as the pH decreases. Because the pH of human milk (6.6–7.0) is lower than the pH of plasma (7.4), the ionized component of a weak base increases in milk. The opposite occurs with weak acids. For this reason, lincomycin, erythromycin, antihistamines, alkaloids, and isoniazid, which are all weak bases, can be expected to have concentrations in milk that are equal

to or higher than those in plasma. On the other hand, barbiturates, organic acids, sulfonamides, and diuretics, which are all weak acids, should have concentrations in milk that are equal to or lower than those in plasma (Catz and Giacoia, 1972). The infant, therefore, is likely to ingest more of a medication that is a weak base than a medication that is a weak acid.

Effects of Maternal Medication on the Infant

Several factors should be considered when evaluating the potential effects of a medication to be taken by a mother on her nursing infant. For instance, many drugs pass more easily from plasma into colostrum during the first week after delivery than they do later into milk. Drugs administered IV reach a higher level in the maternal circulation than those given in the same dose IM, and they generally reach a higher level than those taken orally in that dose. Drugs with a molecular weight under 200 pass into the milk more easily than those with higher weights. Furthermore, large molecules that are fat-soluble and nonionized are more likely to enter the milk. The amount of a drug that enters an infant through its mother's milk depends on the volume of milk ingested. The effects of the drug depend on whether it is in an active or inactive form and how it is subsequently detoxified and excreted by the infant. Drugs that are not fully excreted build up in the infant. Toxic levels may be reached, due to accumulation, even though the maternal intake is low.

Therefore, whenever possible, perineal and other discomfort should be relieved by nonmedication measures. Jet hydrotherapy or sitz baths help overcome soreness and promote healing (Aderhold, 1991). Local applications of compresses, ointments, and heat lamps also lessen pain, aid healing, and decrease the need for systemic medications for perineal pain.

During the infant's first week of life, some drugs may compete with bilirubin for protein-binding sites. The resulting unbound bilirubin that remains in the infant's circulation places the infant at risk for kernicterus. This risk is a particular problem for premature infants because their livers are less capable of detoxifying drugs and because they have fewer available binding sites for the drugs or bilirubin.

As infants mature, they are better able to metabolize drugs transported in the milk. Therefore, substances that might have been harmful during the first weeks (eg, the sulfa drugs) may not pose a problem at a later date. One guideline in choosing maternal medications is to evaluate the safety of each medication for the infant and how it is detoxified and excreted at that stage in the infant's life. Another consideration is the length of time that the drug is to be taken; continuing exposure places the infant at higher risk. Long-acting drugs are also more hazardous because they are more likely to accumulate.

No drug can be considered absolutely safe for use during lactation. The maternal need for the drug should be balanced against the drug's possible harm to the infant. The American Academy of Pediatrics and the Swedish National Board of Health have established standards to help practitioners determine the safety of drugs transferred to the infant during breast-feeding. Unless contrary information exists, it can be assumed that any drug absorbed by the mother is excreted to some extent in the milk (Table 10-7).

Analgesics

Among the analgesic (nonnarcotic) drugs, acetaminophen (Tylenol) theoretically should not be given during the immediate postpartum period to lactating women because it is detoxified in the neonate's liver. However, it does not appear to harm the neonate. Although it is excreted in the milk, aspirin rarely affects the neonate unless the mother takes more than the prescribed dose.

Narcotics

Narcotics should be used cautiously, if at all. Oxycodone (Percodan) or propoxyphene (Darvon) can lead to sleepiness in the infant, poor nursing, and a subsequent loss of weight. Codeine or meperidine (Demerol) can build up in the infant, leading to neonatal depression. Morphine or heroin can be addicting to the newborn. Methadone can lead to depression and failure to thrive. Marijuana impairs DNA and RNA formation and may be inhaled by the infant if its mother or other people are smoking during the feeding. The active substance, tetrahydrocannabinol, is secreted in breast milk and, therefore, can be absorbed by the nursing infant, resulting in drowsiness.

Antibiotics

If a mother requires an antibiotic, it is important that she be aware of its possible adverse effects on her infant. It may be appropriate for the mother to discontinue breast-feeding temporarily while taking antibiotics that are highly sensitizing. With the exception of cephalexin (Keflex), cephalothin (Keflin), nystatin (Mycostatin), oxacillin (Prostaphilin), para-aminosalicylic acid (PAS), and penethamate (Leocillin), most antibiotics are excreted in human milk. The following drugs have little, if any, effect on the neonate: colistin (Colimycin), carbenicillin (Pyopen, Geopen), cefazolin (Ancef, Kefzol), demeclocycline (Declomycin), lincomycin (Lincocin), mandelic acid, methenamine, penicillin G, potassium, and sodium fusidate.

Anticoagulants

Heparin is not excreted in human milk, but the infant's partial thromboplastin time should be checked just to be safe. Anisindione (Miradon) is excreted in milk, causing prolonged prothrombin times in the infant; thus, it is contraindicated. Ethyl biscoumacetate (Tromexan) may cause cephalhematoma and hemorrhage around the umbilical stump and is contraindicated. The safest anticoagulants for the infant are the coumarin derivatives bishydroxycoumarin (dicumarol) and warfarin (Panwarfin). The infant's prothrombin times should be checked regularly and the drug discontinued if the infant is scheduled for surgery or has been injured. Vitamin K should be given to the nursing infant while the mother is on a coumarin derivative.

Sedatives

If the mother requires sedation either as a sleeping aid or as an anticonvulsant, the infant receives some of the drug in the milk. Most barbiturates are excreted in milk but do not sedate the infant. Those that are contraindicated include sodium bromide (Bromo-Seltzer and OTC sleeping pills) and phenobarbital (Luminal) in hypnotic doses. However, in usual analeptic doses, phenobarbital appears safe for infants. Pentobarbital (Nembutal) should not be given until it can be detoxified by the infant's liver (normally after 1 week of age), but after that it seems safe in analeptic doses. Barbital (Veronal) and chloral hydrate (Noctec, Somnos) are considered safe for the infant.

Cardiovascular Drugs

When taken by the mother, digoxin and guanethidine (Ismelin) do not affect the infant. Hydralazine (Apresoline) may cause neonatal jaundice, electrolyte disturbances, or thrombocytopenia. Methyldopa (Aldomet) may result in galactorrhea (increased milk production); reserpine (Serpasil) may cause galactorrhea plus diarrhea, nasal stuffiness, and lethargy.

Diuretics

Diuretics given to the mother can cause dehydration and electrolyte imbalances in the infant, or insufficient maternal milk production. The infant's weight should be monitored at intervals, the specific gravity of the urine should be checked, and the number of wet diapers per day should be noted. Furosemide (Lasix) is not excreted in milk. Acetazolamide (Diamox) may cause some dehydration, as do the thiazides (Diuril, Enduron, Esidrix, HydroDiuril). Spironolactone (Aldactone) may cause sodium excretion and potassium retention in infants. The mercurial diuretics (Dicurin, Thiomerin) are not absorbed orally, even though they are present in milk. However, they present a risk of mercury deposits in the infant's tissue.

Autonomic Nervous System Drugs

Atropine sulfate deserves particular consideration because it is found in many prescription as well as OTC drugs. Many mothers are unaware of the presence of this autonomic drug in their systems. Excreted in milk, it may cause atropine toxicity or hyperthermia in the neonate. Other drugs that affect the autonomic nervous

Text continues on page 173.

Table 10-7. Relative Safety of Selected Drugs in Breast Milk

Drug Name	Considered Acceptable*	Use Only With Caution	Unacceptable
Nonnarcotic Analgesic/Sedatives			
acetaminophen (Datril, Paraceta-mol, Tylenol)	✔		
ibuprofen (Advil, Motrin)			✔
phenobarbital (Nembutal)	✔ Watch for symptoms of depression, changes in sleep and feeding patterns		
primidone (Mysoline)			✔
propoxyphene (Darvon)	✔ Watch for poor nursing and sleepiness in infant		
salicylates (aspirin, Empirin, Bufferin, Ecotrin)	✔ Acceptable for single dose; increase maternal vitamin C intake		
sodium bromide (Bromo-Seltzer)			✔
Narcotic Analgesics			
codeine		✔ Build-up can lead to neonatal depression	
heroin			✔
marijuana			✔
meperidine (Demerol)		✔ Build-up can lead to neonatal depression	
methadone			✔
Anticoagulants			
coumarin derivatives (dicoumarol, warfarin)	✔ Check infant's prothrombin time, discontinue before surgery; give vitamin K to infant		
heparin	✔ Check infant's PTT		
phenindione (Hedulin, Dindevan)			✔
Cardiovascular			
digitalis (digoxin, Lanoxin)	✔		
guanethidine (Ismelin)	✔		
hydralazine (Apresoline)		✔ May cause neonatal jaundice, electrolyte imbalance, thrombocytopenia	
methyldopa (Aldomet)	✔ May cause maternal galactorrhea		
propranolol (Inderal)	✔ May cause hypoglycemia or other β-blocking effects		
quinidine	✔ May cause arrhythmia		
reserpine (Serpasil)	✔ May cause maternal galactorrhea; diarrhea; nasal stuffiness, lethargy in infant		
Diuretics†			
acetazolamide (Diamox)	✔ Watch for dehydration		
mercurial diuretics (Dicurin, Thiomerin)			✔
spironolactone (Aldactone)		✔ Watch for sodium excretion and potassium retention	
sulfamoylanthranilic acid (furosemide, Lasix)	✔		
thiazides (Diuril, Enduron, Esidrix, HydroDiuril, Oretic, Thiuretic tablets)	✔ Watch for maternal and infant dehydration		

*There is no "black-or-white" choice on drug acceptability. Before administration of a drug, careful assessment of the mother and infant must be made, considering age, physical conditions, and necessity of medication. Possibility of adverse effects must be discussed clearly with the client before drugs are administered.
†When using any diuretic, monitor infant's weight, number of wet diapers per day, and specific gravity of infant's urine.

(continued)

Table 10-7. (Continued)

Drug Name	Considered Acceptable*	Use Only With Caution	Unacceptable
Central Nervous System			
alcohol		✓ Drowsiness	
atropine sulfate (in prescribed and OTC drugs)		✓ May cause atropine toxicity, hyperthermia in neonate	
caffeine		✓ Excess may lead to irritability	
carisoprodol (Rela, Soma)			✓
cimetidine (Tagamet)			✓
ergotomine (Cafergot)			✓
magnesium sulfate	✓		
neostigmine (Prostigmin)	✓		
Mental Problems			
chlordiazepoxide hydrochloride (Librium)		✓ May accumulate to high levels; may contribute to jaundice	
diazepam (Valium)		✓ May add to neonatal jaundice, hypoventilation, drowsiness, may accumulate to high levels	
haloperidol (Haldol)	Questionable, behavioral problems in animals		
lithium carbonate (Eskalith, Lithane, Lithonate)			✓
phenothiazines:			
chlorpromazine (Thorazine)	✓		
mesoridazine (Serentil)	✓		
thioridazine (Mellaril)	✓ Maternal galactorrhea		
trifluorperazine (Stelazine)	✓		
tricyclic antidepressants:			
amitriptyline (Elavil)	✓		
desipramine hydrochloride (Norpramin, Pertofrane)	✓		
imipramine hydrochloride (Tofranil)	✓		
Antihistamines			
brompheniramine (Dimetane)	✓		
diphenhydramine (Benadryl)	✓ Observe for decrease in milk supply, poor nursing, tachycardia		
tripelennamine (Pyribenzamine)	✓		
Hormones			
carbimazole (Neo-Mercazole)	May cause goiter, depress thyroid		
insulin	✓		
epinephrine (Adrenalin)	✓		
Cathartics			
milk of magnesia, mineral oil, saline cathartics, stool softeners, suppositories, bulk-forming laxatives	✓		
aloin, cascara, rhubarb			✓
phenolphthalein			✓

*There is no "black-or-white" choice on drug acceptability. Before administration of a drug, careful assessment of the mother and infant must be made, considering age, physical conditions, and necessity of medication. Possibility of adverse effects must be discussed clearly with the client before drugs are administered.

system and that can affect the newborn include cariso-prodol (Rela, Soma), which causes drowsiness, hypotonia, and poor nursing, and ergot (Cafergot), used for migraines, which causes ergotism, vomiting, diarrhea, erratic blood pressure, and weak pulse.

Psychotropic Drugs

Clients who require psychotropic or mood-changing drugs should be given those that exert the least possible effect on the infant, in the smallest possible dose, because all these drugs are excreted in milk. The benzodiazepines are among the most frequently prescribed drugs in the United States. Chlordiazepoxide (Librium) usually has little if any effect on the infant, but it may accumulate in the mother in high levels. Diazepam (Valium) may contribute to neonatal jaundice, possibly exerting cumulative effects. It may also lead to hypoventilation, lethargy, drowsiness, and weight loss due to poor feeding.

Other drugs used to treat mental health problems must also be monitored. Haloperidol (Haldol) has caused behavioral problems in animals. Lithium carbonate (Eskalith, Lithane, Lithonate) has been shown to cause cyanosis, poor muscle tone, and changes in the infant's electrocardiogram.

The phenothiazines seem to be safe, creating no apparent symptoms in the infant. They include chlorpromazine (Thorazine), mesoridazine (Serentil), thioridazine (Mellaril), and trifluoperazine (Stelazine). By increasing maternal pituitary prolactin secretion, these drugs can cause maternal galactorrhea when taken in large doses.

The tricyclic antidepressants also appear to be safe for infants, although neonates should be watched for failure to feed or depression. These drugs may also cause maternal galactorrhea through an increase in maternal prolactin secretion. The frequently used medications in this group include amitriptyline (Elavil), desipramine (Norpramin, Pertofrane), and imipramine (Tofranil).

Selective serotonin reuptake inhibitors (SSRIs) is another class of antidepressants whose action is believed to be linked to the inhibition of serotonin uptake. Fluoxetine (Prozac), paroxetine (Paxil), and sertraline (Zoloft) are all found in breast milk. Caution is recommended if SSRIs are used by a lactating mother.

Antihistamines

Antihistamines are also excreted in breast milk, causing a wide variety of reactions. The infant may appear sleepy, feed poorly, or become very active and develop tachycardia. A cumulative effect may occur from long-acting drugs. The frequently used antihistamines are brompheniramine (Dimetane), diphenhydramine (Benadryl), methdilazine (Tacaryl), and tripelennamine (Pyribenzamine).

Cathartics

For the most part, cathartics appear to have no effect on the infant. The exceptions are aloin, cascara, and fresh rhubarb, all of which may cause diarrhea and colic in the infant. The others, which are safe, include milk of magnesia, mineral oil, saline cathartics, stool softeners, suppositories, and bulk-forming laxatives. Phenolphthalein has caused increased bowel activity in some neonates.

Hormones

Hormones are sometimes required for treating maternal conditions. Those that are destroyed in the infant's intestinal tract (corticotropin, epinephrine, and insulin) have no effect on the infant, but other hormones may have negative effects.

Prednisone is considered safe if used in small doses for short periods. Thyroid and thyroxine are considered safe for the infant, but the antithyroid medications may cause hypothyroidism in the infant.

Oral Contraceptives

Further studies are needed on the excretion of oral contraceptives or their metabolites in breast milk. Some effects reported are a diminished milk supply, reduced milk proteins and fats, a marked decrease in all water-soluble vitamins, and possible adverse long-term effects. Development of gynecomastia in male infants and the proliferation of vaginal epithelium in some females have been reported.

Heavy Metals

Because the heavy metals are excreted in milk, the infant and mother must be carefully observed for negative signs, particularly neurotoxicity in infants exposed to lead or mercury. Because lead may or may not cause toxicity at maternal serum levels of 40 µg or more, infants should be observed for symptoms of lead poisoning.

Radioactive Agents and Antineoplastic Drugs

Nursing mothers should avoid certain radioactive agents (gallium-69, iodine-125, iodine-131, and technetium-99). The analysis of data on iodine-125 indicates that a large dose of radioactive iodine is received by the infant—about 0.1 rad. A significant number of thyroid tumors have occurred in people who received radiation therapy for thymic enlargement in early infancy. The risk of cancer resulting from irradiation of the thyroid has been calculated at about 100 per 10,000 rad. Based on this calculation, a dose of 0.1 rad produces a cancer incidence of one out of every 1,000 children irradiated.

The Committee on Drugs of the American Academy of Pediatrics notes that breast-feeding should temporarily cease for varying amounts of time, depending on the radioactive drug being used: technetium-99m for 1 to 3 days, radioactive sodium for 21 to 22 days, iodine-131 for 2 to 14 days, iodine-125 for 12 days, and gallium-69 for 14 days. The committee also notes that antineoplastic drugs, such as amethopterin and cyclophosphamide, are contraindicated in breast-feeding because they may cause immune suppression, have unknown effects on growth, and are possible carcinogens.

Other Substances

Maternal intake of caffeine (eg, coffee, tea, cola, chocolate) may accumulate in the infant, causing the infant to remain wakeful. This effect is particularly evident if the mother also smokes cigarettes, which also produce a stimulant effect. On the other hand, the occasional use of alcohol, which reaches a level in milk equal to that in plasma, may have a calming effect but may be injurious to the infant.

■ SUMMARY

Some maternal conditions require the use of medications that may cause serious effects on the breast-feeding infant; other medications have little or no effect. When considering the administration of medications to the mother, the nurse should question not whether a medicated mother should be allowed to breast-feed but whether a breast-feeding mother needs to be medicated.

❖ NURSING MANAGEMENT: THE LACTATING CLIENT

Nurses should remain informed about the latest research on how drugs given to the lactating woman affect the mother, the neonate, or the older child. Updated information may necessitate discarding or replacing medications previously considered acceptable. Research studies rely on increasingly sophisticated techniques to evaluate medications so that infants can continue to nurse safely even though their mothers require medication.

NURSING PROCESS

ASSESSMENT

Any nurse in contact with a breast-feeding mother should take a thorough medication history, including prescribed medications and OTC drugs. In some cases, the physician is responsible for making the decision; in other cases, the mother and nurse can decide together which is more important, breast-feeding or the medication.

NURSING DIAGNOSIS

Nursing diagnoses likely to arise include:

- Knowledge Deficit, related to the effects on the infant of prescription and OTC drugs conveyed in breast milk, dietary needs during lactation, and the lactation process
- Risk for Injury, related to use of drugs during lactation

PLANNING

Quality care by the nurse can lessen the possibility of undesirable and unnecessary medication of either the mother or the infant. Another goal is to educate the mother about lactation, dietary needs during lactation, and substances conveyed in milk from mother to child.

INTERVENTION

The nurse should encourage the client to verbalize any concerns that she may have about breast-feeding. She should also encourage the client to join her in the planning process, making certain that the client's wishes are incorporated whenever possible.

It is important to plan preventive measures to offset the need for some medications. For example, effective hand-washing and aseptic techniques by staff members are preferable to reliance on antibiotics for mother or child. Mothers should also be taught these techniques. Mothers who experience painful breasts associated with nursing need help in managing that pain or they are unlikely to be relaxed during feedings. The resulting tension is likely to decrease milk production, as well as cause tension and poor sucking by the infant.

If the mother must take medications, the nurse should evaluate the potential for harm to the mother or baby that may be caused by the medication. Some medications may have been taken through the pregnancy without harm to the fetus, but they should not be continued during lactation because of a different effect on the breast-fed baby. Another medication may have to be substituted so that the mother can continue to breast-feed.

When medications are necessary and the mother decides to continue breast-feeding, the nurse should be supportive but should not reassure the mother that no adverse consequences from taking the medication will occur. Once again, recognizing the mother's needs and openly appreciating the new mother as an individual may be major factors in helping her to accept the necessary restrictions while nursing. In addition, accurate information about the effects of maternal medication on the nursing infant helps protect the child from problems that can be avoided.

To provide greater safety for the child, maternal medications should be taken after the infant has been fed so that the least amount of drug is present in the milk at the next feeding. The baby should also be carefully observed for any reactions, such as development of a rash or fussiness, and any changes in responses or feeding or sleeping patterns.

When a medication that may be harmful to the baby cannot be avoided, breast-feeding may have to be discontinued temporarily. By pumping her breasts at regular intervals, a mother continues to stimulate them and should be able to resume breast-feeding after completing the course of medication.

Drugs that are detoxified by the liver should not be given to the lactating mother during the immediate postpartum period because the infant's liver may be too immature to detoxify them. Narcotics should also be avoided because they may build up in the infant and lead to respiratory depression.

Because caffeine taken by the mother may accumulate in her infant, lactating mothers should be discouraged from ingesting coffee, tea, cola, or chocolate. This prevents overstimulation of the infant. Even though alcohol may have a calming effect, its use is not approved because of possible long-term effects on the child, including weakness, decrease in linear growth, abnormal weight gain, and damage to the growing brain.

Client Education. Breast-feeding is an ongoing activity, one in which the mother is responsible for her own food intake and use of drugs (prescribed or self-administered, including alcohol and illicit substances). Compliance will occur only if she agrees with the worth of suggestions that are made and if she is comfortable with the program that is outlined. It is important for the client to understand any changes that are made in her medication regimen from the one prescribed prenatally, including any adverse effects that may occur to herself or the infant, with information as to what to do about them if they materialize.

Client education should include information about foods, medications, and substances that are usually used by the mother, and their safety for mother and child. Dietary concerns are important. Lactation requires an adequate intake of calories and fluids, with a limitation on empty calories (ie, cake, cookies, candy, and other high-calorie snacks that lack nutritional value). The food selection should be varied, with attention to the inclusion of foods high in calcium, protein, and vitamins. Foods that contain contaminants (eg, chemicals, food coloring, artificial sweeteners) should be avoided, because their long-term effects on the child may not be known. The nurse should supply this information if a nutritionist is not available.

Counseling may help the mother overcome her problems, reducing their effects on her milk production and her need for particular medications. Reassurance and relief of tension through good nursing are better for mother and infant than sedation or tranquilizers.

The advantages of breast-feeding and the disadvantages of abrupt weaning should always be foremost in the nurse's mind when teaching and counseling mothers about the use of medications.

OUTCOME EVALUATION

Follow-up care should include evaluation of the mother's perception of how well breast-feeding is proceeding. The breasts and nipples should be healthy, without areas of infection, induration, or fissures. The infant's growth, feeding, sleep and waking patterns, responsiveness, and general comfort level should be within normal limits. The level of maternal–child bonding should also be examined,

including the way the mother holds, comforts, and cares for the baby. The client may need reassurance that she is doing well in her mothering techniques.

References

Aderhold K. (1991). Jet hydrotherapy for labor and postpartum pain relief. *MCN, 16*(2):97–99.

Arias F. (1993). *Practical guide to high-risk pregnancy and delivery,* 2d ed. St. Louis: Mosby.

Catz CS, Giacoia GP. (1972). Drugs and breast milk. *Pediatr Clin North Am, 19*:157.

Creehan PA. (1996). Pain relief and comfort measures during labor. In Simpson KR, Creehan PA. *AWHONN's perinatal nursing.* Philadelphia: Lippincott-Raven, pp. 227–245.

Drug facts and comparisons 1996. St. Louis: Facts and Comparisons, 404b.

Fenakel K, et al. (1991). Nifedipine in the treatment of severe preeclampsia. *Obstet Gynecol, 77*(3):331–337.

Freda M. (1991). Home care for preterm birth prevention. *MCN, 16*(1):9–14.

Gilbert ES, Harmon JS. (1993). Manual of high-risk pregnancy and delivery. St. Louis: Mosby.

Imperiale T, et al. (1991). A meta-analysis of low-dose aspirin for the prevention of pregnancy-induced hypertensive disease. *JAMA, 266*(2):260–264.

Kaye M, Cashoff I. (1993). Substance abuse in pregnancy. In R Knuppel, I Drukker (eds). *High-risk pregnancy: A team approach,* 2d ed. Philadelphia: WB Saunders, pp. 163–179.

King JF, Grant A, Keirse M, Chalmers I. (1988). Beta-mimetics in preterm labor: An overview of the randomized controlled trials. *Br J Obstet Gynaecol, 95*:211–222.

Leff E, et al. (1991). Type I diabetes and pregnancy. *MCN, 16*(2):83–87.

McCombs J. (1995). Update on tocolytic therapy. *Ann Pharmacother, 29*:515–522.

Rayburn WF, Marsden D. (1993). Medications in pregnancy. In R Knuppel, J Drukker (eds). *High-risk pregnancy: A team approach,* 2d ed. Philadelphia: WB Saunders, pp. 149–162.

*Regan AM, et al. (1993). Overview of pediatric HIV infection. In Libman H, Witzburg R. *HIV infection: A clinical manual,* 2d ed. Boston: Little, Brown & Co., pp. 484–485.

*Simpson KR, Creehan PA. (1996). *AWHONN'S perinatal nursing.* Philadelphia: Lippincott-Raven.

Tal Z, et al. (1988). Breast electrostimulation for the induction of labor. *Obstet Gynecol, 72*(4):671–674.

Wald N. (1991). Prevention of neural tube defects: Results of the Medical Research Council's Vitamin Study. *Lancet, 338*:131–137.

Bibliography

Briggs GG, Freeman RK, Yaffe SJ. (1986). *Drugs in pregnancy and lactation,* 2d ed. Baltimore: Williams & Wilkins.

deVeciana M, et al. (1995). Tocolysis in advanced preterm labor: Impact on neonatal outcome. *Am J Perinatol,* July, p. 294.

Fetal alcohol syndrome. (1990). *Mental Health, 7*(5):1–4.

*Recommended for further reading.

Friedman JM, et al. (1990). Potential human teratogenicity of frequently prescribed drugs. *Obstet Gynecol, 75*(4):594–599.

Knuppel RA, Drukker J (eds). (1993). *High-risk pregnancy: A team approach,* 2d ed. Philadelphia: WB Saunders.

Lawrence R. (1989). *Breast feeding: A guide for the medical profession,* 3d ed. St. Louis: CV Mosby.

*Novak JC, Broom BL. (1995). *Ingalls & Salerno's maternal and child health nursing,* 8th ed. St. Louis: CV Mosby.

Nowicki P, et al. (1984). Effective smoking intervention during pregnancy. *Birth, 11*(4):217.

Phillips C. (1996). *Family-centered maternity and newborn care,* 4th ed. St. Louis: CV Mosby.

Physicians' Desk Reference. (1997). Montvale, NJ: Medical Economics Press.

Rayburn WF, Lavin JP Jr. (1986). Drug prescribing for chronic medical disorders during pregnancy: An overview. *Am J Obstet Gynecol, 155*:565–569.

Sherwin L, et al. (1995). *Nursing care of the childbearing family,* 2d ed. East Norwalk, CT: Appleton & Lange.

Zamule E. (1989). Drugs and pregnancy: Often the two don't mix. *FDA Consumer, 23*(5):7—10.

*Recommended for further reading.

For more information and sample tests and activities, refer to Chapter 10 in the Student Workbook for Clinical Pharmacology and Nursing Management, 5th edition, available through your bookstore.

11

Drug Therapy in Pediatric Nursing

The pediatric nurse's ability to prepare and administer children's medications is a skill and an art. It requires not only clinical and pharmacologic expertise but also knowledge of child development and psychology and a healthy dose of creativity and perseverance.

Factors Influencing Drug Responses in Children

Various influences affect how a child responds to drug therapy, including individuality, maturity, metabolism, and developmental factors.

Uniqueness of the Client

Like adults, each child responds uniquely to pharmacologic interventions. However, because infants and children lack the medical and developmental histories of adults, their response is usually unknown. Allergic manifestations and sensitivities occur quickly and without warning. To implement preventive health care, the nurse can educate parents about adverse signs and symptoms, necessary care measures, and access to ongoing and emergency healthcare.

Body System Maturity and Metabolism

Each child has a unique physiologic response to a medication. Research and practice demonstrate that myriad factors affect how a child metabolizes therapeutic agents. Immature organ systems, nutritional status, genetic endowment, and physiologic variations influence drug use and effectiveness for each child.

Neonates, infants, and young children experience differences in such pharmacokinetic parameters as absorption, distribution, protein-binding, metabolism, and excretion related to variables such as age, size, and level of organ maturity.

Absorption

Gastrointestinal absorption of oral medications in infants and young children is generally slower than in adults and can be influenced by several factors. Most oral medications are absorbed in the duodenum. The neutral gastric pH that exists at birth gradually declines to reach adult levels at 2 to 3 years of age. This can enhance the absorption of acid-labile medications such as penicillin. Conversely, delayed absorption with decreased bioavailability of acidic drugs, such as phenobarbital, phenytoin, and acetaminophen, can occur with this age group (Dionne and McManus, 1993; Kraus and Hatzopoulos, 1995; Radde, 1993).

Infants and young children have decreased gastric motility, irregular peristalsis, and a significantly prolonged gastric emptying time, ranging from 6 to 8 hours, until about age 9 months. These factors may increase the absorption of acidic medications; however, they may delay the peak serum concentrations of oral medications. Young children usually have lower levels of intestinal flora; this increases the bioavailability of drugs, such as digoxin, that are usually reduced by bacterial flora (Kraus and Hatzopoulos, 1995).

Distribution

Age-related variations in total body water, fat composition, and the degree of protein-binding for drugs influence the effectiveness of drug distribution in infants and young children. Newborns and infants have relatively higher total body water and percentages of extracellular water than do adults. Neonates and young infants have less skeletal mass and subcutaneous tissue than adults. Infants and young children have decreased plasma protein-binding, possibly resulting from a lower concentration of serum albumin and other binding proteins (ie, lipoproteins, beta-globulins), the presence of fetal albumin, or a decreased plasma pH. In addition, competition for protein-binding sites, because of endogenous substances such as bilirubin, can displace a drug (McLeod and Evans, 1992). Children do not have adult drug-binding capacity before 2 or 3 years of age.

Children with reduced protein-binding affinity may be at risk for an increased concentration of unbound drug. This may decrease the half-life and result in higher free serum concentrations of drugs such as theophylline and phenytoin. This increases the potential for toxicity or adverse reactions and may necessitate larger loading doses of such drugs to maintain therapeutic blood levels (Dionne and McManus, 1993).

Metabolism

In full-term infants, the microsomal enzymes responsible for drug metabolism (specifically, oxidation and glucuronidation of drugs such as phenobarbital and theophylline) are significantly reduced. Thus, immature hepatic function may affect the infant's ability to metabolize drugs efficiently, and it may increase the infant's sensitivity to drugs eliminated predominantly by hepatic metabolism. Significant alterations in the neonate's ability to metabolize drugs with preservative additives is due to the neonate's immature hepatic function.

Because dehydrogenation of alcohol is depressed in neonates, elixirs with a high alcohol content should be avoided in this age group (Dionne and McManus, 1993). Also, solutions containing preservatives to enhance stability and shelf life (eg, benzyl alcohol, propylene glycol) should not be given to premature infants, infants, or young children. Intravenous (IV) fluids, heparin, pancuronium bromide, vitamin K, and hydrocortisone sodium succinate (Solu-Cortef) are commonly used drugs that contain such preservatives. The nurse must exercise caution when administering these solutions.

The cellular action of many pharmacologic agents is not clearly understood, and individual variations in drug metabolism affect drug use in infants and young children. Because of the potential for cumulative toxicity, careful observation by the nurse for adverse reactions, side effects, and alterations in laboratory values can provide vital data for adjusting dosages.

Excretion

The infant's renal system is immature and does not efficiently excrete certain substances. Fewer glomeruli and a diminished blood volume reduce the excretion of pharmacologic agents through the kidneys. Renal blood flow, glomerular filtration rate, tubular secretion, and tubular reabsorption are significantly decreased in infants as well. This reduction, combined with decreased hepatic enzyme activity in infants, can result in a prolonged clearance of renally excreted drugs and extended drug half-lives. Because of such changes, maintenance doses should be adjusted and administered less frequently to this age group. In addition, frequent clinical assessment and therapeutic drug monitoring are key to prevent drug toxicities (Kraus and Hatzopoulos, 1995). Adult levels of renal function are usually reached between ages 9 and 12 months (Levin, 1992).

Physical Growth and Development

Infants have a greater cerebral blood flow than adults. Furthermore, the composition of lower myelin content in the immature brain may increase the permeability of the blood-brain barrier to drugs such as morphine sulfate, chloral hydrate, phenytoin, and phenobarbital, thereby altering drug distribution and possibly rendering infants more sensitive to certain drug effects (Levin, 1992). Thus, drugs used for their central nervous system effects should be administered in reduced dosage (Lehne et al., 1994).

Because the organ systems responsible for regulating drug levels are immature, infants and young children are more at risk for adverse drug reactions and atypically prolonged, intense drug responses. In addition, children's ongoing growth and development can be harmed by elevated serum drug levels. For example, glucocorticoids can suppress growth; tetracycline can stain developing teeth (Byington, 1992).

During rapid physical growth and maturation of organ systems, infants are affected by many substances introduced into their environment. Neonates and breast-fed infants are affected by the mother's intake of potential toxins such as alcohol, drugs, caffeine, or nicotine. Placental transfer or drug consumption through breast milk can alter growth and development. The effect of chemical substances on organ system maturity (eg, teratogenesis, potential neonatal addiction, congenital abnormalities) is an important concern (see Chap. 10). A child's chemical substance intake must be considered before administering any additional pharmacologic substances.

Pharmacologic Toxicity

Many factors influence a child's metabolism of a given substance. Chronic illness, level of hydration, nutritional status, hormonal levels, and heredity may contribute to the cumulative effects of a particular medication. Reactions to specific drugs may vary according to race. For example, isoniazid, a drug used to treat tuberculosis, is more rapidly metabolized by Native Americans, Eskimos, and Asians than by European Americans (Giger and Davidhizar, 1991).

Specific medications can be monitored by measuring the concentration of the drug in blood. Monitoring is useful when caring for children requiring long-term medications for chronic conditions (eg, asthma, seizure disorders) or in acute situations (eg, a drug overdose). The limitations are that 1) therapeutic levels for certain drugs vary widely, 2) concentrations of other medications may be difficult to assess, 3) necessary information may be unavailable, and 4) the multiple venipunctures and invasive procedures for specimen collection may injure the child.

Nursing intervention includes monitoring the child's response to medication and educating parents about the signs and symptoms of drug toxicity, preventive measures, and how to administer medication.

Genetic Endowment

A child's heredity may influence the metabolism and proper use of pharmacologic agents. Underlying conditions, such as sickle-cell disease, disorders of vitamin metabolism, and congenital anomalies, affect a child's health and ability to use certain drugs or treatments. One example of a congenital defect that alters drug dynamics is the hemolytic anemia associated with a deficiency of the enzyme glucose-6-phosphate dehydrogenase. Because this anemia worsens after chemical oxidants are ingested, these agents should be avoided, or the child must be closely monitored during drug therapy. Another example of an inherited problem is thrombocytopenia (decreased or defective production of platelets), which may be triggered by the ingestion of agents such as quinidine, sulfisoxazole, hydrochlorothiazide, or heparin (Waechter et al., 1985).

Chronic Conditions

In many cases, children with chronic illnesses are more susceptible to drug toxicity and interactions. Their altered physical conditions, potential aberrations in nutrition, and alterations in drug metabolism affect the type, dose, and timing of pharmacologic agents. Because chronically ill children commonly need several concurrent medications, the potential for drug interactions increases. The nurse must be aware of and watchful for signs and symptoms of adverse reactions.

Chronic illness also affects a child's psychologic well-being. Resentment about taking medications, being perceived as ill or "different" by peers, and behavioral changes may cause the child to refuse or discontinue necessary medications. The nurse and parents must be aware of these possibilities and must monitor the child's compliance.

Circadian Rhythms

Diurnal patterns are manifested in sleep–wake cycles, vital signs, energy levels, and hormonal activity. Hormonal control affects the use, metabolism, and excretion of pharmacologic products. Sick or hospitalized children often are nutritionally depleted because of their altered health state, and concurrent sleep deprivation is caused by environmental stresses or lack of comfort. Circadian rhythms are affected by illness and environment. Consequently, metabolism of pharmacologic agents may be disturbed by hormone and enzyme levels, leading to adverse reactions or toxicity.

Psychologic Development

The ability of children to comprehend their bodies and their health increases with age, education, and the development of abstract thinking. Young children cannot visualize or perceive illness and thus have difficulty accepting medication that is unpleasant in taste, appearance, or smell or that is administered invasively. The cognitive ability to associate medication with relief of symptoms is an abstract and elusive concept for children (Ormond and Caulfield, 1976). The nurse must be knowledgeable about developmental theory and expert at applying that theory when explaining the therapeutic value of medication to a child. To encourage compliance, it is especially important for chronically ill children to understand and accept medication.

During the initial assessment, the nurse should determine who is the child's primary caregiver. It is not always the biologic parent; instead, it may be a grandparent, sibling, or other responsible person.

To help the child understand and accept medication, family education is essential. Before the nurse administers any drug, the parent or guardian and the child, when old enough to understand, should be informed of the indications, side effects, timing, and contraindications of the medication. The family may or may not be aware of medication administration strategies that have worked in the past. Therefore, offering helpful ideas for medication administration encourages compliance with the treatment plan, which is the goal of family education. Astute relatives often report subtle changes in the child, and these may actually be adverse reactions to medications. Open communication involving the family, the child, and the healthcare provider promotes the discussion of concerns and aids the treatment regimen. Sensitivity, creativity, and a positive approach to the child and family help when giving medications.

Factors in Administering Medications to Children

Some important factors related to administering medications to children are dosage, age and development, and pain level.

Determining the Appropriate Dosage

Although the physician or other prescribers determine the therapeutic dosage of medication, the nurse remains responsible for assessing the accuracy of the dose to ensure it is within a safe range. Most pediatric facilities require that the dosage of highly toxic drugs be double-checked with another professional before the drug is administered. After verifying the dosage, the nurse's goal is to determine a correct and palatable means of having the child accept the medication.

The prescribed administration route affects the dosage calculation. Factors that alter prescribed pediatric dosages include the child's water and fat mass, liver and kidney metabolism, and excretory function (Dionne and McManus, 1993; Kraus and Hatzopoulos, 1995; McLeod and Evans, 1992). Therapeutic dosage ranges are published in various resources. Sometimes physicians use alternate criteria based on body size and organ maturity to calculate therapeutic dosages. Pediatric pharmacists, a growing subspecialty, can help physicians and nurses in scientifically determining therapeutic doses.

Although previous practice recommended the use of formulas such as Fried's and Young's rules, which use

CRITICAL THINKING CHALLENGE
Case Analysis

Calculating a safe dosage range

The pediatrician orders cefotaxime 470 mg IV q8h for your client, a 37-pound, 4-year-old child who has a bacterial respiratory infection. In carrying out this order, you first make sure that the dosage ordered is within the safe and effective IV dosage range for this child, as follows:

Step 1: Convert the child's weight to kilograms (kg) by dividing the child's weight in pounds by 2.2 (1 kg = 2.2 pounds)—37 pounds ÷2.2 = 16.8 kg

Step 2: Consult a reliable pediatric drug reference, such as Harriet Lane Handbook or another formulary, to obtain the recommended safe dosage range for the child's age and weight.

In this case, the Children's Hospital of Boston Formulary recommends that the dosage range for children who are older than 1 month but younger than 12 years and who weigh less than 50 kg can receive cefotaxime 100–200 mg/kg/day in 3 divided doses.

Step 3: Calculate the low and high safe dose range for 24 hours for the 37-pound, 4-year-old child (in this case, using the dosage range from Step 2)—

16.8 kg × 100 mg = 1680 mg/day
16.8 kg × 200 mg = 3360 mg/day
Safe range: 1680–3360 mg/day

Step 4: Calculate the safe amount for each dose administration (3 times/day) and determine whether this falls within the safe, effective range.

1680 ÷ 3 = 560 mg/dose
3360 ÷ 3 = 1120 mg/dose
Safe range of individual dose given every 8 hours: 560–1120 mg/dose)

- Based on your findings, construct Step 5.
- Once you find the individual safe dose, calculate the amount of IV diluent needed and determine the IV flow rate.

Step 5. The ordered dose 470 mg q8h is below safe, effective dosing recommendations. This order should be rewritten by the prescriber.

the child's age to determine the appropriateness of an ordered dose for a specific child, more recent pediatric practice discourages this method because these formulas do not account for changes in body mass (eg, poor nutrition, obesity) and can also be inaccurate (Wink, 1991). For greatest accuracy, a child's dose is calculated on the basis of milligrams per kilogram of body weight (mg/kg) for infants and children who are within normal limits for their age in height and weight. References such as the *Harriet Lane Handbook, Children's Hospital Formulary*, and the pharmacology sections in some pediatric journals provide safe ranges for pediatric dosages (see the Critical Thinking Challenge: Case Analysis).

For children who are extremely tall, short, lean, or obese, or for children receiving chemotherapeutic agents that are potentially toxic, body surface area (BSA), calculated on a milligram-per-square-meter (mg/m²) basis, is the most effective method (Wink, 1991; Levin, 1992; Johns Hopkins University Staff, 1993). Surface area guidelines use body mass as the primary criterion and provide the greatest accuracy for determining a therapeutic and safe dose. After the child's height and weight are measured, an intersecting line is drawn between these two measurements on a scale known as a nomogram. The intersecting point represents the BSA in square meters (Fig. 11-1). To calculate the dose, use the formula:

$$\text{Approximate pediatric dose} = \frac{\text{(child's BSA in m}^2 \text{ [from nomogram] × adult dose)}}{1.73}$$

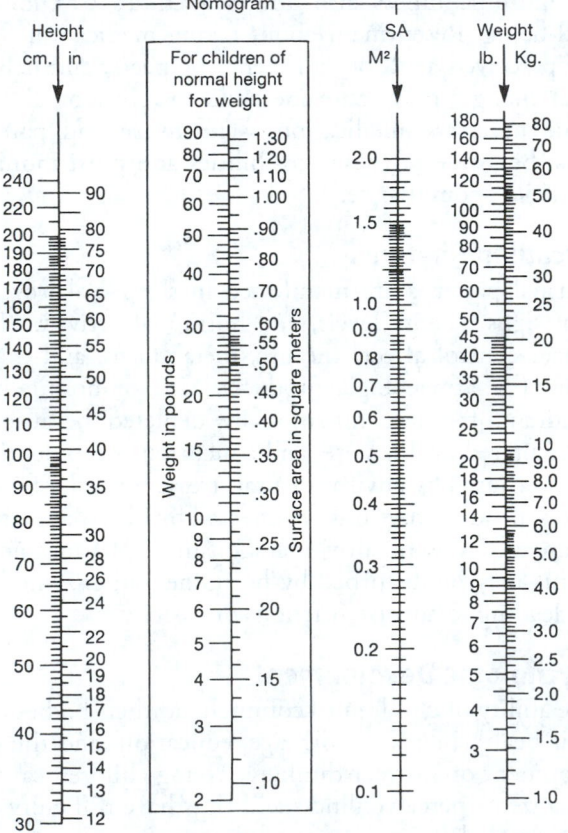

Figure 11-1. The West nomogram for calculating body surface area (BSA). To determine a child's BSA, draw a straight line from the child's height (*left column*) to the child's weight (*right column*). BSA value is at the intersection of the straight line and the column labeled SA, which is calculated in square meters (m²). The formula for estimating a child's dose is:

child's BSA (in m²) × adult dose ÷ 1.73

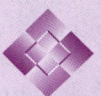

Box 11-1
Detecting Signs of Pain in Children

In many cases, children cannot verbalize pain. Instead, they act it out. The following are nonverbal signs and symptoms to watch for in children suspected of having pain.

- **Infants:** Crying, facial expressions of distress, and muscular rigidity followed by thrashing are some common signs of pain. However, infants have a limited repertoire of responses that serve highly differentiated sensory systems. Therefore, the absence of these signs and symptoms does not indicate a lack of pain.
- **Toddlers:** Like infants, toddlers manifest pain with signs of physical resistance. In fact, because of their mobility, toddlers may show increased physical activity when they feel pain. Because normal toddlers are perceived as restless and very active, pain may be misinterpreted and may go unrecognized.
- **Preschoolers:** These children react to pain with aggressive behaviors, verbal expressions, and need for comfort and support. The nurse should recognize the child's need to be dependent and should provide structure to cope with the painful experience.

- **School-agers:** Increasing verbal ability, the developing interest in body and health, and the desire to learn are important in helping school-age children understand pain. When expressing pain, however, the school-age child may regress and exhibit behaviors characteristic of younger children. Passive methods of dealing with pain such as holding still or bearing the pain may be coupled with aggressive outbursts.

    Children in this age group may describe pain in graphic detail. Despite their ability to communicate, these children may also present nonverbal cues. When an analgesic can be administered as needed (prn), the nurse must be aware that requesting pain medication requires that the child be verbal, assertive, and cognizant of time, which are skills few children can consistently demonstrate when sick and in pain.
- **Adolescents:** In their quest for identity and independence, adolescents react to pain with self-control and, possibly, fear of disclosing pain. Seeking verbal descriptions of pain, using pain assessment tools, and being attuned to nonverbal cues are ways the nurse can help the adolescent collaborate in planning pain-control strategies.

Managing Pain

Administering medications, particularly analgesics, to children is a complex nursing responsibility. Concurrent with assessment, the nurse must explore ways to anticipate and manage pain based on what are usually obvious alterations in anatomic and physiologic integrity in relation to the child's developmental level. With knowledge of the underlying pathophysiology, the routine administration of analgesics to children before procedures and during selected periods after surgery would become acceptable (Eland, 1988). The issue of inadequate blood levels of analgesics due to dosage and timing inaccuracies and the effect this problem has on pain in children remain topics of concern, particularly in nursing research.

Knowing the child's usual behavioral patterns helps the nurse assess pain. Like adults, children manifest pain in different ways based on learned behaviors from previous experiences or from role models and cultural variables. The nurse should interview the family to learn about the child's behavior, responses to pain, and previously successful interventions. Various reliable instruments are available for measuring pain in children. The selection of a particular instrument depends on the nurse's knowledge of the instrument and its interpretation as well as on the child's developmental age and health (Box 11-1).

Clinical practice guidelines on acute pain assessment and management in infants, children, and adolescents undergoing surgical and medical procedures are

available from the U.S. Department of Health and Human Resources. These guidelines recommend routinely administering opiates around the clock or by patient-controlled analgesia (PCA) infusion pumps rather than as needed (PRN) for children 7 years and older (Agency for Health Care Policy and Research, 1992).

■ SUMMARY

Each pediatric client is unique. Administering drug therapy to a child requires knowledge of his or her physiologic, psychologic, and cognitive development. The nurse should strive to develop a therapeutic, trusting relationship with the child and family, based on frequent contact and genuine interest. Adopting creative techniques, understanding usual behavior patterns, calculating safe dosage ranges, administering drugs safely, implementing comfort measures, and educating clients and families are key nursing responsibilities.

❖ NURSING MANAGEMENT

For the child, play is a medium for exploring, contemplating, rehearsing life events, and gradually accepting and integrating a given situation. The value of play cannot be overemphasized when the child needs health care. It allows the child to clarify and develop an understanding of unfamiliar personnel, intrusive procedures, and unpleasant medications.

NURSING PROCESS

ASSESSMENT

The nurse must assess the child's weight, maturity, health status, allergies and previous reactions, and current drug therapy. The calculated drug regimen must be reviewed. Medical problems such as shortness of the intestine, encephalopathy, diarrhea, and liver dysfunction may influence the metabolism and excretion of medications. These data should be assessed by the nurse before medication administration. In addition, assessing the child's level of development and cognitive skills helps the nurse to plan care tailored to the child's developmental level rather than his or her chronologic age. The child's health may affect his or her development. Some children with chronic illness have an advanced knowledge of healthcare procedures, whereas others regress due to the stress of the illness and treatments. Assessing each child for advanced or delayed development allows individualized care planning.

NURSING DIAGNOSIS

The following are examples of nursing diagnoses that may be considered in planning care for pediatric patients and their families:

- Knowledge Deficit, related to drug therapy and procedures or hospitalization
- Risk for Ineffective Management of Therapeutic Regimen, related to insufficient knowledge of drug therapy
- Noncompliance, related to age, complexity of medication regimen, and distastefulness of the drug
- Ineffective Individual Coping, related to invasive procedures associated with drug therapy

PLANNING

One goal of nursing care is to help the child and family understand the reasons for medical and nursing interventions, particularly drug therapy. The impact of an episodic illness on the family may be extensive. Acute hospitalization may cause family dysfunction due to stress, separation, loss of parental income, and sibling and client behavioral problems. Children who are chronically ill are at increased risk for these concerns and others. Peer relationships may be affected because of the child's inability to participate in activities and school. When planning a child's care, the nurse must take into account the child's community (eg, family, school, social and religious activities, cultural background).

INTERVENTION

Developing a trusting relationship with the client and family requires spending time with them. Feeding, bathing, and medicating, as well as monitoring IV infusions, are routines that lend themselves to spending concentrated time with an infant or child (Nugent, 1989).

When administering medication, the nurse may need to use creative techniques such as dissolving or crushing it or mixing it with a more palatable substance. A pharmacist can help the nurse determine whether a change from the original dosage form would alter the drug's pharmacologic properties.

The nurse should ask about the child's concerns, behaviors, coping mechanisms, and rewards for taking medications. Older children, chronically ill children, and adolescents often have routines and preferences for the way their medication is administered.

Administering Medication to Infants. Infants have a natural sucking reflex that is helpful for ingesting liquid oral medications. Liquid elixirs and suspensions are given with a plastic syringe or dropper, placed in the cheek alongside the tongue toward the back of the mouth.

If the child can eat table food, tablets and capsules (with the exception of sustained-action capsules and enteric-coated tablets) can be crushed to a fine powder and mixed with small amounts of applesauce, jam, fruit juice, pudding, or ice cream, provided the drug and food are compatible. Honey and syrup can be used to mix medications for older children but are contraindicated in infants because of the risk of botulism. When in doubt, the nurse can consult the pharmacist to minimize the risk of altering the availability of the drug (Malseed et al., 1995; Wong, 1996).

The medication can be mixed in small volumes of a sweet vehicle to disguise unpleasant flavors, enhance the suspension of drugs that are difficult to dissolve in water, and promote complete ingestion. Distasteful medications should not be mixed with essential foods such as milk and cereal; doing so may lead the child to refuse essential food in the future.

Liquid medications can also be given through an empty nipple placed in the infant's mouth. The infant is then held in a comfortable, upright position to aid swallowing and to control head movements. Medications may be taken more readily if given before feeding times, when the infant is hungry. A small flexible medication cup may be used to retrieve medication that may leak from the child's mouth. Stroking the neck or cheek facilitates sucking and swallowing.

Slow administration of oral medications in small amounts is recommended. Care should be taken not to force medication or inject it rapidly into the mouth, because this can cause choking, aspiration, or oral trauma.

In the event of regurgitation, which is common among infants, a pharmacology reference, the pharmacist, and the child's pediatrician should be consulted to determine whether a specific dose should be repeated. The main criteria for repeating the medication are the medication's potential toxicity and the type of oral medication (tablet, liquid, gel, capsule). A second dose sometimes is administered if the infant regurgitates the first dose immediately or soon after administration. Certain medications, however, should not be repeated, because they are absorbed rapidly through the buccal mucosa (Waechter et al., 1985).

When administering intramuscular (IM) medication to an infant, the nurse should assess factors such as muscle mass, the medication's viscosity and volume, and the frequency of injections. The suggested sites for infants and children under age 3 years are the vastus lateralis and the rectus femoris muscles to prevent sciatic nerve damage. The needle is injected at a 90° angle as the muscle mass is pinched up to prevent hitting nerves, blood vessels, or bones. A minimum of 0.5 mL can be administered to infants in each injection via a 25- to 27-gauge, 0.5- to 1-inch needle (McKenry and Salerno, 1995). For infants over age 3 months, a 1-inch needle is recommended to achieve adequate muscle penetration. After an IM injection, the child needs comforting; often the parent does, too.

For subcutaneous injection of lipid-soluble drugs (eg, diazepam), the dosage must be reduced, because infants have proportionally less subcutaneous fat than older children.

Topical medications should be applied as thinly as possible to the smallest body surface area possible. The skin of neonates and small infants is more permeable because of the thin layer of stratum corneum and the larger ratio of surface area per kilogram of body weight (Byington, 1992; Radde, 1993). A dose adjustment may be required to minimize the potential for toxic systemic drug reactions from topical applications.

As infants grow, their feeding and tactile behaviors change. Between ages 3 and 12 months, infants may require more than one nurse to administer medications because they are more mobile and larger. Plastic syringes and droppers work well with this age group. A small medication cup is helpful, too, because older infants often retain medications in their mouth or spit them out.

Drug palatability can be improved by mixing the medicine with small amounts of soft food. Care must be taken to prevent infants from associating medications with food and possibly rejecting some foods. A bottle or cup of pleasant-tasting liquid after medication administration may comfort the child, dispel the taste, and prevent oral retention of the medication. Cleansing the mouth with water after medication administration is encouraged to remove potentially cariogenic substances from developing teeth. Providing physical and verbal comfort after medication administration is essential for the child's well-being.

Administering Medication to Toddlers. As mobility, agility, and independence increase with age, toddlers pose a special challenge for the nurse administering

medication. Independence is displayed by voluntary lip and tongue control, verbalization, and spitting. When the child spits out a significant amount of drug, the nurse should estimate and readminister that amount, being cautious not to overmedicate the child (Lehne et al., 1994).

The parents should be consulted to determine previously successful medication techniques and the child's preferences or routines. Simple directions immediately before medication administration, disguising medications in palatable foods, praise, and a positive yet firm approach are strategies used with this age group.

Toddlers sometimes display anxiety regarding medications through change in appetite or daily routines. Fear can also be displayed in play sessions. Careful observations by the nurse or a relative can offer the nurse a chance to ease such fears by therapeutic play.

Administering Medications to Preschoolers. Preschoolers often attempt to divert the nurse from administering medication by bargaining and stalling. Simple, concrete directions and explanations are helpful for this age group. Therapeutic play (eg, administering medications to a teddy bear by syringe) enables the child to work through his or her fears about the medication experience. The young and middle-aged child can be held or placed in an upright, sitting position with minimal movement before administering oral medication. To gain the child's compliance when taking distasteful medications, offer water or juice after the drug. Rewards such as stars and stickers for work especially well with this age group (Wong, 1996).

Loss of body integrity produces fear in this age group. Invasive procedures such as surgery or parenteral medications cause the child great anxiety. Reassurance, information, and comfort alleviate the problem of injecting medications.

In preschoolers, fantasy thinking has begun to develop and affects the child's perception of health interventions. Making use of fantasy thinking to describe "magic medicines" and to explain their use in alleviating discomfort is effective. Preschoolers enjoy rituals and routines. The most effective medication administration method should be documented and followed by nurse and parent.

When administering IM injections to children over age 3, either the vastus lateralis or ventrogluteal sites can be used. A 22-gauge, 1-inch needle is preferred. A volume of 1 mL can be injected at each site. Two or more persons are usually required to help restrain the child during the injection. Distracting the child by having him or her wiggle the toes is sometimes effective. Choices about medications are offered if available. Rewards, praise, and physical comfort allay the preschooler's anxiety and encourage cooperative behavior.

Administering Medications to School-Age Children. School-age children demonstrate an active interest in their health or illness and eagerly seek information to maintain a sense of control in times of stress or uncertainty. Of all age groups, school-age children most often engage in play to display concerns and anxieties. They tend to demonstrate a greater degree of cooperation than toddlers or preschoolers when taking medications. The opportunity to help the child express fears is part of the nursing role with this age group.

Although developmentally able to swallow a pill or capsule, a school-age child does not associate medication with symptom relief. Because concrete thinking predominates in this age group, a child may respond as well to a warm cloth to soothe a headache as to an oral analgesic. Control and mastery of situations are sought by school-age children. Offering choices (when available), providing explanations using pictures and diagrams, and giving rewards are helpful measures.

School-age children usually have developed adequate muscle mass to receive IM injections in the gluteus maximus or ventrogluteal muscle. Older school-age children or adolescents may have developed sufficient deltoid muscles for injections. A 22- to 25-gauge, 1- to 1.5-inch needle is preferred. Volumes up to 2 mL can be injected at each site, depending on the child's size. Other considerations include the volume and type of injectate, the frequency of injections, the condition of muscle and skin, and the child's age and diagnosis.

Immediately before giving an injection, the nurse should provide a simple explanation to the child. The child may wish to choose the site or a supportive person to help during the procedure. Adequate restraint during the procedure provides reassurance and safe administration. Praise, comfort measures, and a bandage over the injection site are also helpful.

Illness or hospitalization may cause regression in the child. When regression occurs, the nurse should adapt the strategies for medication administration accordingly.

Administering Medications to Adolescents.
Adolescents are developing identities and roles separate from their parents and family and are more closely linked to their peers. Some adolescents may be concerned about taking any type of medication. Education about prescription or over-the-counter drugs enlarges the adolescent's knowledge base, promotes control, and encourages pertinent questions and evaluations by this budding healthcare consumer. On the other hand, the use of illicit substances often alters a therapeutic regimen, and the nurse must assess the adverse effects of combining prescribed medications and illicit drugs. The concurrent use of alcohol or illegal substances with narcotic analgesics, anticonvulsants, and other medications places the adolescent at additional risk for adverse effects and drug reactions.

Chronically ill adolescents may resist treatment regimens in their quest for identity and control, and their health can suffer during this period. A frank discussion between the client and nurse sometimes elicits feelings of helplessness, vulnerability, concern about addiction, a desire to be like others, and a lack of knowledge. By providing the appropriate information, the nurse can encourage informed decision-making and can enhance the client–nurse relationship, benefiting the client.

After administering medications, the nurse must monitor the response to the medications and continually assess for signs and symptoms of drug toxicity.

Administering IV Medications to Children.
The use of a volume-control device (burette) or retrograde technique is preferred when administering IV medications to infants and children. More recent trends in healthcare centers involve the insertion of a heparin lock device in children for IV drug therapy when additional fluid volume is not required. The heparin lock is flushed according to agency policy (typically with 1–2 mL of 10-unit/mL heparin flush solution after the initial insertion and first drug administration). Patency is then maintained by flushing the device with 1 to 2 mL of preservative-free normal saline solution after completing each medication instillation.

To administer a medication using the burette (most common method), the nurse must refer to dilution manuals to determine the recommended cc/mL dilution and compatibility with the ordered IV fluid for each drug to be given (Box 11-2). Unless otherwise specified, most medications are administered to children over a 30-minute period using an infusion pump. Intravenous drugs should be properly diluted and administered in the smallest possible dose at the slowest possible rate (McKenry and Salerno, 1995). The following formula is used to calculate the IV flow rate for medications infused by tubing that delivers 60 drops (gtt)/cc:

$$\frac{(cc \text{ to be infused} \times \text{drop factor [gtt/cc]})}{\text{time (min) to be infused}}$$

After completing the calculations, the nurse should fill the burette with the recommended amount of IV solution, add the medication through the rubber port at the top of the burette, and gently mix the solution by rolling the burette from side to side between the hands. The recommended IV flow rate is then set and the infusion is initiated. Once the drug is administered, an additional 20 mL of IV fluid is added to the empty burette and infused to clear the tubing of medication.

The retrograde technique is particularly useful for premature infants and infants with compromised cardiopulmonary status or fluid overload because it allows IV administration of a number of selected drugs (ie, an-

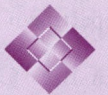

Box 11-2
Determining the Volume of IV Diluent and Infusion Rate

The pediatrician orders cefotaxime 840 mg IV q8h for a 37-pound, 4-year-old child with a bacterial infection and no other health problems. In preparing to administer the medication, the nurse follows certain steps to calculate the volume of diluent and the infusion rate.

Step 1: Refer to unit recommendations for diluting the drug, or consult the pharmacist. For the above child, the recommendation for diluting cefotaxime is 1 mL of dilution solution (diluent) for every 20 to 60 mg of drug per drug dose.

Step 2: Calculate the safe low and high dilution range:

$$840 \text{ mg} \div 20 = 42 \text{ mL}$$
$$840 \text{ mg} \div 60 = 14 \text{ mL}$$

Thus, the drug must be diluted with between 14 and 42 mL of diluent.

Step 3: Consider the child above. Review the child's medical history to evaluate renal status, cardiac status, possible edema, number of medications administered and dilutions required, type and size of IV catheter, and daily maintenance fluid requirements and fluid balance before reaching a decision.

Next, consider how the drug is delivered from the pharmacy. Most pharmacies predilute the drug according to agency protocol. For the child above, assume the drug is delivered in 8.4 mL of solution.

Then consider the safe low and high dilution range. In this case, the drug can be diluted with as little as 14 mL of diluent or as much as 42 mL. Because the child does not have a history of renal or cardiac disease or edema, the nurse could select the lowest amount in the range to prevent overloading. But the nurse may also select an amount of diluent to even out the calculation. In this case, the nurse may reasonably decide on 22 mL.

Step 4: Having selected 22 mL of diluent, the nurse must calculate the IV rate. In many cases, the infusion is through a burette on an infusion pump (drop factor = 60). The equation for delivering medication in a volume of 8.4 mL for a total of about 30 mL (22 + 8.4) over 30 minutes would be:

$$(30 \text{ mL} \times 60 \text{ gtt/min}) \div 30 \text{ min} = 60$$

---

tibiotics) without substantially increasing the child's fluid intake (Zenk, 1986). This method involves setting up IV tubing with two three-way stopcocks placed on each side of the extension tubing with adequate volume, depending on the diluted medication to be administered (typically 1–20 mL). One stopcock is positioned close to the IV insertion site and the second stopcock is placed on the other side of the extension tubing nearest the IV solution bag. The syringe containing the medication is attached to the stopcock closest to the client while an empty displacement syringe of equal size is attached to the other stopcock. With the stopcocks turned off to both the client and the IV solution bag, the appropriately diluted drug is then instilled into the IV line away from the client, displacing the IV solution into the empty syringe. The stopcocks are then repositioned off to the two syringes, new protective covers are attached to both ports, and both syringes are discarded. The drug infusion rate is then set on the pump to infuse the medication over 30 minutes.

The intraosseous route can be used in emergencies to administer drugs to critically ill children who are under age 3 and who have poor IV access. Medications, blood, and IV fluids are infused after inserting a bone marrow needle into the medullary cavity of a long bone.

Use of Play. By encouraging play, the nurse can help the child cope with drug therapy or a difficult procedure. Play enhances the child's sense of control, reflects the child's knowledge of the environment, and allows him or her to become familiar with strange equipment and personnel. Actual equipment can be used, with dolls, puppets, costumes, and dollhouses serving as the healthcare environment and instruments. Children who are usually in the submissive role of "client" may choose to be the healthcare provider in the play scenario. The use of actual or replicated healthcare equipment also stimulates play.

In promoting cooperation and adherence to the medication regimen, the nurse can guide the child's play to recreate an event or elicit feelings about a particular procedure. Guided play involves continuous validation of the nurse's perceptions of the play situation. It is a useful teaching tool, particularly for identifying and correcting the child's misconceptions. The nurse must be knowledgeable about childhood development and must determine each child's tolerance for this type of play. A given play situation may be repeated several times to incorporate it into the child's experience.

Play can also be a random event in which the nurse acts as an observer. Verbal and nonverbal behaviors allow the nurse access to the child's emotions, concerns, and understanding. Watching the child play offers the nurse opportunities for teaching and clarifying events, leading to more formal therapeutic interventions. Knowing the child's developmental level enables the nurse to assess and intervene in a way that can encourage the child's understanding of drug therapy and his or her coping strategies and growth. The nurse may also use books, dolls, drawings, and concrete explanations with a school-age child. Diagrams, models, books, and explanations can help adolescents comprehend the need for medication or interventions.

Client Education. Learning about the options for drug treatment are important issues for children and their families. In the expanding healthcare arena of pharmacology and drug therapy, consumers are increasingly active in determining their treatment plans. They require information as a necessary part of informed decision-making. In this context, the nurse must educate the child and the family by providing information, answering questions, and clarifying treatment options. As the usual advocate and liaison between children, parents, and physicians, the nurse promotes informed consent and disseminates knowledge about pediatric drug therapy for the benefit of the child, the family, and the community.

Because many of the child's reactions to a well-care visit or hospitalization become evident only after the child returns home, the nurse must assess learning readiness and focus family education on developing interventions to help the child cope, if necessary.

Home care instructions should include the drug name, its therapeutic action (explained in simple terms), the correct dose and dosage regimen, administration strategies and route, adverse reactions, and when and how to contact the physician. Information should be reinforced, and the parents should perform a return demonstration of successfully administering the medications to the child at least twice before leaving the healthcare facility.

OUTCOME EVALUATION

A child's response to therapeutic interventions, such as drug therapy and play, may be considered effective if the child's symptoms abate with drug therapy and the child's behavior remains age-appropriate. In addition, parental or caregiver progress may be observed to be positive. In evaluating the nursing care plan, the nurse's communication skills and recognition of the child's developmental level help in devising future plans and interventions. Other outcome measures include determining whether the child feels free to discuss or act out concerns in the healthcare facility or at home. A child may exhibit a behavioral change due to the stress of contact with the healthcare system. Future interactions with the healthcare system may be improved with nursing interventions targeted at the child's behavior after discharge.

References

Agency for Health Care Policy and Research. (1992). *Acute pain management in infants, children, and adolescents: Oper-* *ative and medical procedures* (AHCPR Pub. No. 92-0020). Rockville, MD: Public Health Service, U.S. Department of Health and Human Services.

Byington KC. (1992). The pediatric patient. In Baer CL, Williams BR. *Clinical pharmacology and nursing*, 3d ed. Spring House, PA: Springhouse Corporation, pp. 149–162.

Dionne R, McManus C. (1993). Pediatric critical care pharmacodynamics. *Critical Care Nursing Clinics of North America, 5*(2):367–375.

Eland JM. (1988). Pharmacologic management of acute and chronic pediatric pain. *Issues in Comprehensive Pediatric Nursing, 11*(2-3):93–111.

Giger J, Davidhizar R. (1991). *Transcultural nursing*. St. Louis: CV Mosby.

Johns Hopkins Hospital Staff, KB Johnson (ed). (1993). *Harriet Lane Handbook*, 13th ed. Chicago: Year Book Medical Publishers.

Kraus DM, Hatzopoulos FK. (1995). Neonatal therapy. In Young LY, Koda-Kimble MA (1995). *Applied therapeutics: The clinical use of drugs,* 6th ed. Vancouver: Applied Therapeutics Inc.

Lehne RA, Moore LA, Crosby LJ, Hamilton DB. (1994). Drug therapy in pediatric and geriatric patients. In RA Lehne (ed). *Pharmacology for nursing care*, 2d ed. Philadelphia: WB Saunders.

Levin RH. (1992). Pediatric and neonatal therapy. In ET Herfindal, DR Gourley, LL Hart (eds). *Clinical pharmacy and therapeutics,* 5th ed. Baltimore: Williams & Wilkins.

Malseed RT, Goldstein FJ, Balkon N. (1995). Pediatric pharmacology. In RT Malseed, FJ Goldstein, N Balkon (eds). *Pharmacology: Drug therapy and nursing considerations,* 4th ed. Philadelphia: JB Lippincott, pp. 46–50.

McKenry LM, Salerno E. (1995). *Mosby's pharmacology in nursing,* 19th ed. St. Louis: CV Mosby.

McLeod HL, Evans WE. (1992). Pediatric pharmacokinetics and therapeutic drug monitoring. *Pediatr Rev, 13*(11): 421.

Nahata MC. (1997). Pediatrics. In JT DiPiro, RL Talbert, GC Yee, GR Matzke, BG Wells, LM Posey (eds). *Pharmacotherapy: A pathophysiologic approach,* 3d ed. Stamford, CT: Appleton & Lange, pp. 77–85.

Nugent KE. (1989). Routine care: Promoting development in hospitalized infants. *Am J Maternal Child Nurs, 14*(5): 318–321.

Ormond E, Caulfield C. (1976). A practical guide for giving medications to young children. *Am J Maternal Child Nurs, 1*(3):3320–325.

Pharmacy Committee. (1993). *Formulary of Children's Hospital, Boston, Mass.* Ohio: Lexi-Comp Inc.

Radde IC. (1993). Mechanisms of drug absorption and their development. In Radde IC, MacLeod SM (eds). *Pediatric pharmacology and therapeutics.* St. Louis: CV Mosby.

Waechter EH, Phillips J, Holaday B (eds). (1985). Fluid and drug therapy. In *Nursing care of children.* Philadelphia: JB Lippincott, pp. 197–221.

Wink DM. (1991). Precision and caution: Safety. *MCN, 16*: 317–321.

Wong DL. (1996). *Wong and Whaley's Clinical manual of pediatric nursing,* 4th ed. St. Louis: CV Mosby.

Zenk KE. (1986). Administering IV antibiotics to children. *Nursing '86,* 50–52.

Bibliography

Evans M, Hansen B. (1981). Administering injections to different aged children. *Am J Maternal Child Nurs, 6*(3): 194–199.

Franck LS. (1989). Pain in the nonverbal patient: Advocating for critically ill neonates. *Pediatr Nurs, 15*(1):65–68.

Hick JF, Charboneau JW, Brakke DM, Goergen B. (1989). Optimum needle length for diphtheria-tetanus-pertussis inoculation of infants. *Pediatrics, 84*(1):136–137.

Johnston CC, Strada ME. (1986). *Acute pain response in infants: A multidimensional description. Pain, 24*(3):373–382.

Marino B. (1991). Studying infant and toddler play. *J Pediatr Nurs, 6*(1):16–20.

Pridham D, Adelson F, Hansen M. (1987). Helping children deal with procedures in a clinic setting: A developmental approach. *J Pediatr Nurs, 2*(1):13–21.

Ramirez A. (1989). The neonate's unique response to drugs: Unraveling the causes of drug iatrogenesis. *Neonatal Network, 7*(5):45–49.

Reed MD, Besunder JB. (1989). Developmental pharmacology: Ontogenic basis of drug disposition. *Pediatr Clin North Am, 36*:1053–1074.

Skaer TL. (1991). Dosing considerations in the pediatric patient. *Clin Ther, 13*,(5):526–544.

Stewart CF, Hampton EM. (1987). Effect of maturation on drug disposition in pediatric patients. *Clin Pharm, 6*:548.

Stoklosa MJ, Ansel HC. (1986). *Pharmaceutical calculations.* Philadelphia: Lea & Febiger, pp. 88–94.

Wong DL. (1995). Family-centered care during illness and hospitalization. In DL Wong (ed). *Nursing care of infants and children,* 2d ed. St. Louis: CV Mosby

For more information and sample tests and activities, refer to Chapter 11 in the Student Workbook for Clinical Pharmacology and Nursing Management, 5th edition, available through your bookstore.

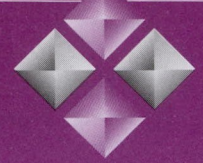

12

Drug Therapy in Gerontologic Nursing

Was 2.3 prescribed medications (Hershman et al., 1995). About 75% of elderly persons in a community take at least one prescription medication, and about two thirds take at least one nonprescription, over-the-counter (OTC) medication (Fillenbaum et al., 1993). In one study, about 14% of urban elderly and 27% of rural elderly adults used four or more OTC drugs daily (Stuck et al., 1994).

An estimated two thirds of physician office visits by elderly clients result in one or more new prescription drugs. An estimated 50% of these prescriptions will not have the desired therapeutic effect, for reasons ranging from improper dosage to failure to fill the prescription (American Medical Association, 1990).

Geriatric clients are more likely to have adverse drug reactions. Adverse drug reactions account for a significant number of hospital admissions of older adults: as many as 28% of admissions are drug-related (11% related to noncompliance and 17% to adverse drug reactions). As many as two thirds of the elderly persons in a community may have at least one drug–drug reaction or drug–alcohol combination associated with a possible adverse reaction (Pollow et al., 1994).

Aging and concurrent diseases interact with social, emotional, and environmental factors to affect the pharmacokinetics of the medications given to elderly clients. It is essential to monitor the client's responses, whether he or she is in the home, the hospital, or a long-term care institution. Factors that interact with each other and with the elderly client to cause a potentially wide range of reactions include:

- Physiologic changes and their potential effects on pharmacokinetics
- Patterns of toxicity that may go unrecognized

CRITICAL THINKING CHALLENGE
Case Analysis

Mrs. Luck is a 78-year-old woman with a long history of gastrointestinal problems (peptic ulcer disease and spastic colon). She takes antacids and cimetidine (Tagamet) when her heartburn flares up. About 12 years ago, amitriptyline (Elavil) was prescribed as an antidepressant, and she took it for 2 years. Her mood and sleeping pattern improved. She takes no other medications on a regular basis. Recently Mrs. Luck's heartburn flared up and she became depressed and had difficulty sleeping. Her physician advised her to begin taking amitriptyline again. This time, however, she became agitated and unable to sleep.

- Develop as many hypotheses as you can that might explain the difference in Mrs. Luck's response to the antidepressant.

W ith the progressive "graying" of society, health-care providers can no longer ignore the many issues related to drug therapy in elderly clients. By the year 2030, about 28% of the U.S. population will be over age 60; more than 8 million people will be over age 85. A continuing proliferation of new drugs, such as potent new antiarrhythmics, nonsteroidal anti-inflammatory agents, biogenetically engineered drugs, and new forms of old drugs, adds to the already overwhelming medical, social, economic, and ethical dimensions of drug therapy in elderly persons.

Elderly persons, currently about 12% of the population, take about 30% of all prescription medications. In a study of urban elderly, the average for each person

- Chronic disease and polypharmacy
- Social and emotional behaviors that may affect the client's perception of or compliance with medication regimens
- Changing resources and the implications for drug therapy

In this chapter we will discuss the implications these factors have on nursing assessment, client advocacy, client teaching, and health management.

Physiologic Changes of Aging

A drug's action is subject to the pharmacokinetics of absorption, distribution, metabolism, and excretion, processes that can be affected by the normal physiologic changes of aging. Table 12-1 summarizes the effects of aging on pharmacokinetics. Although research on the effects of aging has been limited, known aging factors can alter the responses of an elderly adult to drug therapy. Not until the 1990s did the Food and Drug Administration require that clinical trials of drugs include elderly subjects.

Table 12-1. Effects of Aging on Drug Therapy

Physiologic Changes of Aging	Effects on Drug Therapy
Decreased GI motility, decreased gastric acidity	Possible decreased or delayed absorption of acidic drugs; decrease in peak effect
Dry mouth and secretions (xerostomia)	Difficulty swallowing oral drugs
Decreased liver blood flow; decreased liver mass; decrease in microsomal enzymes	Delayed and decreased metabolism of certain drugs; possible increased effect, leading to toxicity of most drugs; no activation of prodrugs
Decreased lipid content in skin	Possible decrease in absorption of transdermal medications
Increase in body fat; decrease in body water	Possible increased toxicity of water-soluble drugs; more prolonged effects of fat-soluble drugs
Decrease in serum proteins	Possible increased effect, leading to toxicity of highly protein-bound drug; increased possibility of interactions of two or more highly protein-bound drugs
Decrease in renal mass, blood flow, and glomerular filtration rate	Possible increased serum levels, leading to toxicity of drugs excreted renally
Changes in sensitivity of certain drug receptors	Increase in drug effects (eg, benzodiazepines, warfarin) or decreased drug effects (eg, beta blockers)

Absorption

Elderly persons tend to have an increased (less acidic) gastric pH and a reduced gastrointestinal (GI) blood flow. In addition, gastric emptying tends to be delayed, and GI motility is reduced. These changes affect how elderly clients absorb drugs, although there is not enough evidence to identify all the implications of these changes. Absorption through the skin may be decreased; this may result in less absorption of topical drugs (eg, transdermal patches).

Distribution

As the body ages, total body water decreases and body fat increases, resulting in a reduction of lean body mass. Weight-related drug doses, whose distribution is affected by body water or fat-free body mass, may, therefore, produce higher blood or tissue concentrations in elderly clients. Fat-soluble drugs also tend to accumulate in the increased body fat, producing prolonged or even toxic effects.

Serum albumin can decrease to such an extent that, in the case of drugs that bind to albumin, less of the drug is bound. Therefore, higher concentrations of unbound drug are available to produce pharmacologic effects, including increased side effects.

Metabolism

The liver is the site where many drugs become inactivated. Changes in liver function, such as decreased hepatic flow, influence the body's ability to metabolize drugs. The microsomal enzymes that regulate the biotransformation of many drugs are decreased. In addition to the obvious pathologic effects of disease on the liver, a wide range of factors (eg, genetic, environmental) can influence liver function. These effects on liver function make it difficult to establish a definitive association between drug metabolism and the physiologic changes of aging.

Excretion

Renal function gradually declines throughout life. Thus, the elderly adult has a decreased glomerular filtration rate, decreased total renal plasma flow, and altered tubular excretory capacity. Therefore, drugs normally eliminated through the kidneys may accumulate in the body tissues.

In elderly adults, the serum creatinine level is less reliable as an indicator of renal function because of the normal reduction of muscle mass. Various formulas taking into account age or age and weight are often used to estimate creatinine clearance (Box 12-1).

Pharmacodynamic Changes

In elderly persons, the sensitivity of drug receptors may be increased or decreased, resulting in more or less of a drug effect.

> ### Box 12-1
> ### Formulas for Estimating Creatinine Clearance
>
> 1. Creatinine clearance (Cockeroft and Gault, 1976):
>
> $$\frac{(140 - age) \times body\ weight\ in\ kg}{72 \times serum\ creatinine\ level} \times 0.85\ for\ women$$
>
> 2. Another formula, which does not use weight, is the Jelliffe formula (Jelliffe, 1973):
>
> $$\frac{98 - (0.8 \times [age - 20])}{serum\ creatinine\ level}$$

Other Physiologic Changes

Elderly persons have a diminished homeostatic response to change. Autonomic nervous system reflexes and the regulation of blood pressure, temperature, vasoconstriction, and vasodilation are less stable than in younger persons. Therefore, the elderly do not rebound as rapidly from changes in sleep patterns, dietary habits, stress levels, and so forth. Because many drugs have excitatory or depressive effects on autoregulatory mechanisms, elderly persons may be predisposed to exaggerated drug responses.

Patterns of Drug Toxicity

Until recently, pharmacokinetic data have been based almost exclusively on healthy young adults. Standard doses are determined by the objective and subjective responses of subjects in clinical trials. However, several age-related factors can alter the predictability of drug responses in elderly persons.

Elderly persons frequently exhibit such signs of drug toxicity as behavioral changes, restlessness, confusion, irritability, anxiety, insomnia, and hallucinations suggestive of mental deterioration. Elderly clients presenting with signs of confusion secondary to drug toxicity may be diagnosed as having acute brain syndrome while the adverse drug reaction goes unrecognized. About 20% of elderly clients treated in emergency departments have symptoms of mental deterioration or pseudodementia. Frequently, the changes are insidious and go unnoticed. Too often, healthcare personnel dismiss such symptoms as part of the aging process without fully assessing the client's medication regimen. Tables 12-2 and 12-3 list drug effects and drugs that may affect cognitive function in the elderly.

Adverse effects from drugs increase rapidly as the number of drugs taken increases. Even physical symptoms such as headache, anorexia, and visual changes are frequently attributed to the natural aging process and are overlooked as possible indicators of drug toxicity. Drug assessment should be performed initially and repeated periodically. An often-overlooked consequence of adverse drug reactions is the economic impact. For example, the cost of one hospitalization for drug toxicity from low-cost generic digoxin (about $10 per month) can easily exceed $10,000 (McCue et al., 1993).

Chronic Disease

Compounding the effects of physiologic aging are the chronic diseases affecting many elderly clients. After age 65, a client is likely to suffer on average one to three

Table 12-2. Adverse Drug Effects as a Cause of Depression

Types of Drugs	Examples of Drug
Histamine-2 blockers	cimetidine, ranitidine
Cardiac medications and antihypertensives	digoxin, procainamide, reserpine, hydralazine, propranolol, methyldopa, guanethidine, clonidine
Antiparkinson agents	levodopa, amantadine
Steroids	corticosteroids, estrogen, progesterone
Analgesics and nonsteroidal antiinflammatory drugs (NSAIDs)	narcotics and ibuprofen, sulindac, indomethacin
Antineoplastic agents	asparaginase, tamoxifen

With permission from Miller CA (1995). *Nursing care of older adults: Theory and practice.* Philadelphia: JB Lippincott.

Table 12-3. Mechanisms of Drug-Induced Mental Changes

Mechanism of Action	Examples of Drugs
Anticholinergic interactions	atropine, scopolamine, antihistamines, antipsychotics, antidepressants, antispasmodics, antiparkinson agents
Decreased cerebral blood flow	antihypertensives, antipsychotics
Depression of respiratory center	central nervous system depressants
Fluid and electrolyte alterations	diuretics, alcohol, laxatives
Altered thermoregulation	alcohol, psychotropics, narcotics
Acidosis	diuretics, alcohol, nicotinic acid
Hypoglycemia	hypoglycemics, alcohol, propranolol
Hormonal disturbances	thyroid extract, corticosteroids

With permission from Miller CA (1995). *Nursing care of older adults: Theory and practice.* Philadelphia: JB Lippincott.

chronic diseases. The most common chronic diseases involve compromised respiratory, cardiovascular, or metabolic functions that alter the body's ability to respond predictably to drug therapy. Chronic disease commonly predisposes the elderly client to excessive drug use for extended periods. The rate of adverse drug reactions is directly proportional to the number of drugs taken. Nursing home residents take an average of four to nine different drugs daily.

Many of the drugs prescribed for common conditions in elderly clients have anticholinergic effects. The combined effects may produce serious cumulative anticholinergic effects and may intensify many of the client's problems (Tables 12-4 and 12-5).

Table 12-4. Mechanism and Consequences of Anticholinergic Effects

Adverse Effect	Receptor Location	Potential Consequences
Central		
Sedation	Unknown (? brain stem)	Accidents, falls, social withdrawal, physical deterioration
Cognitive impairment, disorientation, memory loss	Hippocampus	Reversible dementia, developing into irreversible dementia if not corrected
Ataxia, imbalance	Brain, spinal cord, basal ganglia	Falls, resulting in fracture; fear of falling, resulting in self-imposed activity restriction
Other central symptoms: hallucinations, agitation, tremors, increased susceptibility to tardive dyskinesia	Brain (striatum, hippocampus)	Dementia, psychosis, tardive dyskinesia, stereotypy
Peripheral		
Dry mouth	Salivary glands	Dental caries, denture intolerance, reduced sense of taste, difficult speech, mucosal infection and lesions, dysphagia, dysphasia, anorexia, malnutrition, paresthesias of tongue
Impaired sweating	Sweat glands	Dry skin, fever, heatstroke, increased susceptibility to hyperthermia
Eye effects: dilated, nonreactive pupils; paralysis of accommodation	Iris, ciliary muscle, lacrimal glands	Blurred vision, glare intolerance, precipitate acute angle-closure glaucoma attack, falls, accidents, keratoconjunctivitis sicca, lesions of cornea, contact lens intolerance, blindness
Tachycardia	Sinoatrial node	Increased cardiac workload leading to angina or congestive heart failure
Decreased bowel motility	Smooth muscle of bowel	Constipation, fecal impaction, paralytic ileus
Decreased tone of bladder and increased tone of sphincters	Detrusor muscle and sphincters	Urinary hesitancy: urinary retention leading to renal damage, overflow or stress incontinence
Failure of penile erection	Corpora cavernosa	Impotence, sexual dysfunction
Decreased bronchial secretions	Bronchial glands	Mucous plugs, pneumonia
Drug interactions	Small intestine, stomach	Delayed stomach emptying, slowed absorption of many drugs

Pepper G. (1991). Monitoring the effects of anticholinergic drugs. In Chenitz C, Stone J, Salisbury S (eds). *Clinical gerontological nursing.* Philadelphia: WB Saunders, pp. 377–389.

Table 12-5. Examples of Drugs with Anticholinergic Activity

Drug Class	Selected Examples*
Belladonna alkaloids	atropine, diphenoxylate with atropine (Lomotil), scopolamine, belladonna (Bellergal)
Antipsychotic agents	chlorpromazine (Thorazine), thioridazine (Mellaril), haloperidol (Haldol)
Antiparkinson agents	trihexphenidyl (Artane), benztropine (Cogentin)
Antidepressants	amitriptyline (Elavil), imipramine (Tofranil), amoxapine (Asendin)
Antispasmodics (gastrointestinal)	dicyclomine (Bentyl), propantheline (Pro-Banthine), clidinium (Quarzan), glycopyrrolate (Robinul)
Antispasmodics (genitourinary)	oxybutynin (Ditropan), L-hyoscyamine (Levsin, Cystospaz)
Antihistamines	diphenhydramine (Benadryl), cyclizine (Marezine), chlorpheniramine (Chlor-Trimeton), hydroxyzine (Vistaril)
Ophthalmologic cycloplegics and mydriatics	homatropine, cyclopentolate (Cyclogel)
Antiarrhythmic	disopyramide (Norpace)
Skeletal muscle relaxants	orphenadrine (Norflex), cyclobenzapine (Flexeril)
Analgesics	methotrimeprazine (Levoprome), droperidol (Inapsine, Innovar)

*Some agents include an anticholinergic drug as one component of a multidrug preparation.
Pepper G. (1991). Monitoring the effects of anticholinergic drugs. In Chenitz C, Stone J, Salisbury S (eds). *Clinical gerontological nursing*. Philadelphia: WB Saunders, pp. 377–389.

Polypharmacy

Polypharmacy, the concomitant use of more than one drug, is the result of having multiple diseases and having several different physicians prescribing drugs. It is a sign of poorly coordinated healthcare management. The combination of an aging population, an increase in chronic diseases, and the proliferation of new drugs puts frail, elderly clients at increased risk of polypharmacy. Too often, aches, pains, and other complaints of elderly people are handled by recommending medication. An agitated elderly client may be given a tranquilizer, which compounds his or her arthritic immobility problems, leading to more "complaints" to be treated with more medications. Excessive use of medications in the elderly can create a costly (economically, psychologically, and physiologically) cycle of events from which the client may never fully recover.

Multiple drugs with varying dosages administered at different hours create confusion. Drug reactions that mimic medical complaints are often treated with yet another drug. Polypharmacy increases the risk of drug interactions, increases the potential for administration error, and reduces the level of compliance. Therefore, healthcare providers should thoroughly evaluate all medications being taken by their elderly clients and be knowledgeable about potential interactions.

Social and Emotional Behaviors Affecting Drug Use

Elderly persons may engage in several practices that affect drug therapy. Elderly clients often do not inform physicians or other prescribers about all the medications they are taking, including OTC drugs or home remedies. Nor do they tell prescribers about prescriptions other healthcare providers have given them. In fact, elderly people often report that they do not want to "bother" clinicians with their complaints.

Another significant behavior among aging clients is sharing medications. Many clients relate instances in which they relieved arthritic pain or other ailments by sharing medications with a relative or friend suffering from the same condition. Most elderly clients do not throw away unused prescriptions because they "might need them again." In fact, clients have been known to ask whether they can take prescription medication belonging to a deceased relative who suffered from the same illness. Some elderly clients also hoard medications.

Older adults have an increased risk for harmful drug interactions if they use OTC drugs and home remedies. The most common misuse of self-treatment involves laxatives. Elderly persons commonly become preoccupied with their bowel habits. Frequently, they forget to consider other changes that affect bowel function, such as decreased mobility, decreased appetite, changes in dietary patterns, or the side effects of medication. Using laxatives in combination with other drugs, such as diuretics or cardiovascular drugs, or decreasing fluid intake potentiates the risk of electrolyte imbalance or drug toxicity.

The use and abuse of alcohol can be a problem among the elderly. Alcohol is a drug that can react with many other drugs. Moreover, alcohol abuse can cause alterations in the function of the liver and other organs.

Home remedies are seldom considered to be drugs. For instance, it is not uncommon for elderly clients to use large amounts of sodium bicarbonate to relieve symptoms of gastric distress. However, an increased amount of sodium can be harmful in light of the decreased excretory capacity of the kidneys or the predisposition toward congestive heart failure common in this age group. Use of herbs and other health foods can also alter responses to drug therapy.

Changing Resources of Elderly Clients

The longer a person lives, the greater the possibility of diminishing physical, mental, financial, and social resources and support. All these factors have a direct or indirect impact on drug use and must be taken into account.

Decreased Physical Capacity

To an arthritic adult, physical challenges may be presented by such simple implements as childproof caps on a drug bottle. As a result, a client may skip doses or leave containers open, exposing the medication to air or moisture and increasing the potential for rapid deterioration. Many people are not aware that regular (non-childproof) containers can be requested from the pharmacist. They should be cautioned to store these containers safely away from grandchildren or other youngsters visiting or living with them.

Hearing Impairment

Most elderly persons experience a decrease in hearing acuity as well as in discrimination of words. Frequently, they are embarrassed to ask the physician or nurse to repeat words or instructions. Thus, they misunderstand the dosage regimen. This is compounded by the fact that most prescription bottles do not contain complete instructions for use. Bottles are usually labeled "Take as directed" or "Take three times a day." Without adequate knowledge of the peak action of drugs or the effects of drug–drug or drug–food interactions, clients and their families are left to guess at the proper drug administration.

Vision Impairment

Many elderly persons also have decreased vision (eg, presbyopia, cataracts, macular degeneration). Most prescription and OTC drug containers have fine print that is difficult to read. Special instructions written on separate pieces of paper may also be difficult or impossible to read. Vision problems may make it impossible for the elderly client to match the arrows on a childproof cap.

Dietary Alterations

Diet and fluid intake also become significant problems for many elderly clients. Age-related alterations in taste and smell, loss of natural teeth, and changing nutritional requirements affect food intake. The association between food and fluid intake and drugs (eg, the need for increased potassium with digoxin and for increased fluid intake with diuretics) is well known. A spiraling, downward cycle of depressed appetite from drug effect, decreased thirst sensation, dysphagia, and difficulty in maintaining an adequate diet can lead to increased side effects and decreased benefit of drug therapy.

Memory Changes

Aging is often accompanied by decreased memory, particularly for events in the immediate past. Directions for taking medications are usually given to clients when they are apprehensive about their health. Sometimes when the client finally gets the medication, he or she cannot recall what it is for, when it is to be taken, or when it was last taken.

Financial Circumstances

Diminished finances are frequently overlooked as a deterrent to taking medications. Often the physician prescribes a large number of pills, intended to last several months. This consumes a large portion of the client's monthly budget. Most drugs prescribed for common conditions of the elderly range from $50 to $100 for a month's supply of each drug. Not uncommonly, elderly clients wait 2 or 3 weeks to fill their prescriptions because they need their next pension or government check to pay for the medications. If the medication is changed before all the medication is used, the client may be reluctant to spend money on another prescription.

In many managed care programs, prescription drugs are provided with a small co-payment. Usually, however, only a 30-day supply can be dispensed at a time. Thus, the client taking multiple medications that were prescribed on different dates may be faced with multiple trips to the pharmacy and the need to keep close track of prescription renewals. As more prescription drugs become available OTC, the client will have easier access to many medications; however, they may be more difficult to pay for, because OTC drugs are not covered under most insurance plans.

Before any drugs are prescribed to elderly clients, nonpharmacologic treatments such as behavior modification, diet therapy, exercise, stress management, and biofeedback must be considered. Even though these alternative therapies may not eliminate the need for pharmacotherapy, they may reduce the dose of medication required and probably will have other positive consequences such as additional symptom relief.

■ SUMMARY

Elderly clients have a higher risk of adverse drug reactions than younger clients. Factors contributing to this vulnerability include 1) physiologic changes that influence how the body handles drugs and the way it responds to them, 2) the need for multiple prescriptions, increasing the risk of drug interactions, 3) sensory and perceptual changes that may impair the client's ability to carry out the drug regimen accurately, 4) diminished socioeconomic resources for adjusting to the drug regimen.

The proportion of the population that is age 65 or older has increased rapidly since the 1950s and will continue to do so in the 21st century. For this reason, health concerns of elderly clients will be of increasing importance to nurses and other healthcare professionals.

❖ NURSING MANAGEMENT

Nurses are responsible for assessing the client, administering drugs, and monitoring the client's response to drug therapy. Therefore, nurses can best serve as a client advocate to prescribing clinicians (eg, physicians, nurse practitioners) and other members of the healthcare team.

Nurses can encourage clients to bring all their medications to the prescriber's office for review at the next appointment. Nurses can also ask that prescribers and pharmacists ensure that prescription labels have clear, specific instructions for use and that written information is provided for reference. Likewise, nurses can clearly document facts and observations pertinent to a client's drug therapy for the rest of the healthcare team. In these ways, nurses can represent clients who are reluctant or unable to speak for themselves.

When clients are referred to nurses, they are frequently described as "noncompliant." Noncompliance is considered a client problem. However, some healthcare professionals argue that there is no such thing as a noncompliant client: there are only unrealistic expectations or deficiencies in health teaching by healthcare professionals. It is rare to find a client who will not take his or her heart medication knowing that by doing so, he or she might die. It is not uncommon, however, to find a client who has not taken heart medication because he or she was too weak to get the cap off the bottle of tablets, could not afford to refill the prescription, or was told to take it with breakfast, which he or she never eats.

NURSING PROCESS

ASSESSMENT

The nursing assessment should include a thorough drug history, addressing such questions as, What do you do if you miss a dose? What reminders do you use to take your medication? Do you have any difficulty purchasing or obtaining your medications?

An initial drug history should be taken and placed in the client's record and referred to every time a new drug is prescribed. In addition, the drug assessment should be completely updated on a regular basis. Periodic assessments should include all drugs taken, including OTC drugs and home remedies. Even when an elderly client is in the hospital, family members sometimes bring in nonprescribed drugs (Box 12-2).

NURSING DIAGNOSIS

Most elderly clients may be diagnosed as having a knowledge deficit concerning chronic illness and medication regimens used for treatment. This may be a recurrent nursing diagnosis because medication regimens are usually revised to meet the changing needs of the client and because managing multidrug therapy is complex. Additional nursing diagnoses commonly identified in older clients include:

- Ineffective Management of Therapeutic Regimen, related to short-term memory deficit, insufficient funds for medications, physical mobility limitations, or knowledge deficit
- Altered Thought Processes, related to electrolyte imbalance associated with medication
- Body-image Disturbance, related to dyskinesia associated with side effects of medication
- Altered Sexuality Patterns, related to CNS changes associated with long-term medication for chronic illness
- Self-esteem Disturbance, related to dependence on medication therapy and to chronic illness
- Risk for Injury, related to adverse effects associated with medication therapy, multiple medication therapy, or possible drug interactions

PLANNING

Goals of nursing care focus on alleviating or eliminating adverse drug effects, such as confusion, nausea, and vomiting; enhancing self-image; optimizing role function; resolving fear or anxiety; maintaining tissue perfusion and good nutrition; and educating the client to manage drug regimens safely and effectively.

Box 12-2
Aspects of Nursing Process in Elderly Clients on Drug Therapy

Assessment

- Initial and continuing need for all medications including prescription, OTC, and home remedies
- Physiologic factors that may affect pharmacokinetics and pharmacodynamics: aging, acute and chronic disease
- Variables affecting drug regimen management: vision, hearing, cognition and memory, ability to swallow medications or administer by other routes
- Psychosocial variables: cultural beliefs about illness, its cause and cure; use of home remedies, health insurance, economics, type and level of family or caregiver support
- Environmental variables: access to adequate storage sites for medications and refrigeration if needed
- Effectiveness of drug therapy (eg, effects, adverse effects, degree of compliance) and effect of drug regimen on overall functioning and quality of life

Intervention

- Provide or obtain (from physician or pharmacist) written information in client's language, preferably in large print, about drugs and instructions for use.
- Develop optimal scheduling for drug regimen: fewest doses, fewest number of times drugs must be taken, dosing connected to other daily events.
- Develop with client a method for recording actual administration of the medication.
- Teach client and caregivers about therapeutic regimen. Check adequacy of vision and hearing and provide assistive devices if necessary. Ask clients to repeat back information. Advise clients to take medications as prescribed unless they consult the prescriber. Have clients bring all medications being used to all appointments with prescribing clinician.
- Provide nursing interventions that reduce or prevent the need for the medication.
- Provide nursing interventions to help clients tolerate any necessary side effects and thereby continue with the therapy as prescribed.
- Collaborate with prescriber and all members of the healthcare team to coordinate drug and other therapy to reduce possible adverse effects of drug therapy.

INTERVENTION

The nurse should note the times of drug administration, the route of administration, the client's response, and any changes in the client since the original assessment. The nurse must be particularly alert to behavioral and physical changes that may signal a developing toxicity. Whenever a significant change occurs in the client's condition, or before a new drug is added, all drug therapy should be reviewed.

Nursing interventions should aim to prevent or decrease side effects. Interventions may range from measures to increase dietary bulk to prevent constipation when a patient is receiving a drug with anticholinergic side effects to scheduling a once-a-day medication that has a sedative side effect in the evening if possible. Other nursing interventions must be directed toward enhancing the intended drug effects—for example, by correctly timing drug administration in relation to food or other medications, or by reducing the need for pain medication with comfort measures such as massage or biofeedback.

Client Education. Client teaching must be based on the client's drug history and his or her perception of and compliance with the drug regimen. Teaching must be carried out at a pace that is slow enough for the client to assimilate instructions. For clients with memory impairment, aids can be used to increase compliance. For example, calendars can be marked to show drug administration times, or the nurse can use egg cartons to show clients how to measure specific daily doses. The timing of drug doses should be consolidated as much as possible and tied to routine events such as toileting, eating, or bedtime. Routine activities are not the same for every client: the client's and family's routines must be identified, and teaching must be individualized. Family members must be taught to administer medications correctly and to provide support.

Medication schedules should be simplified as much as possible. Giving a single dose should be considered if possible, because it is less complicated to give or take than two divided doses. If the client is homebound and has a home health aide who works, for example, from 10 AM to noon, it may be easier to schedule as many medications as possible to be taken during this time, when the aide can remind the client.

In the hospital and long-term care settings, the nurse traditionally controls administration of medications. At discharge, however, the client may receive a variety of prescriptions to be filled and self-administered. In this era of short hospitalizations, the nurse must spend time before discharge teaching the elderly client and family members about the drug regimen. In the home, the visiting nurse plays a major role in monitoring the client's responses and correct use of medications, as well as reinforcing the teachings of the nurse, pharmacist, or physician.

Coordination of Services. Improved coordination of services among all members of the healthcare team can reduce many of the risks of drug therapy for elderly clients. The nurse is in a unique position to facilitate this coordination and promote active participation among the healthcare team. This ensures that the total number of drugs prescribed is minimized, that the risk/benefit ratio is carefully weighed before adding any new drug, and that the smallest possible dosage is prescribed. This also ensures that frequent assessments of prescription and OTC drug therapy are made, that home remedies and drug–food interactions are evaluated, that client and family teaching is initiated as early as possible, and that the client and family are encouraged to ask questions and report physical or behavioral changes.

Factors that predispose elderly persons to increased risks point to the need for increased nursing management. Drug therapy for elderly clients must be systematically assessed at periodic intervals. Nurses must act as client advocates, educate the client and family, and coordinate services for clients within a multidisciplinary environment.

OUTCOME EVALUATION

Data required for evaluation are specific to the diagnoses and goals previously established. Data collected during evaluation must be interpreted in relation to the medical regimen and the client's physiologic status (eg, disease conditions and the normal changes of aging).

The effects of altered pharmacokinetics, polypharmacy, and multiple diseases on elderly clients make it difficult to evaluate drug responses. The desired pharmacologic effects may be associated with, or even preceded by, undesirable side effects. Evaluation is further complicated by "ageism"—for example, an 87-year-old person may be considered "confused" on meperidine, whereas a 37-year-old person with the same symptom on the same drug is considered to be having a drug reaction. As persons age, they become more complex and less homogeneous in their physiologic, mental, and emotional responses. Therefore, the nurse must become familiar with the normal status of each elderly client so that subtle departures from the norm may be recognized as possible drug reactions.

References

American Medical Association Council on Scientific Affairs. (1990). American Medical Association White Paper on Elderly Health: Report of the Council on Scientific Affairs. *Arch Intern Med, 150,* 2459–2472.

Cockcroft DW, Gault MH. (1976). Prediction of creatinine clearance from serum creatinine. *Nephron, 16:*31.

Fillenbaum GG, Hanlon JT, Corder EH, Ziqubu-Page T, Hall WE Jr, Brock D. (1993). Prescription and nonprescription drug use among Black and White community-residing elderly. *Am J Publ Health, 83*(11):1577–1582.

Hershman DL, Simonoff PA, Frishman WH, Paston F, Aronson MK. (1995). Drug utilization in the old and how it relates to self-perceived health and all-cause mortality: Results from the Bronx Aging Study. *J Am Geriatr Soc, 43:* 356–360.

Jelliffe RW. (1973). Creatinine clearance: Bedside estimate. *Ann Intern Med, 79:*604.

*McCue JD, Tessier EG, Gaziano P. (1993). *Geriatric handbook for long-term care.* Baltimore: Williams & Wilkins.

*Miller CA. (1995). Medications that may cause cognitive impairment in older adults. *Geriatr Nurs, 16*(1):47.

*Pepper G. (1991). Monitoring the effects of anticholinergic drugs. In Chenitz C, Stone J, Salisbury S (eds). *Clinical gerontological nursing.* Philadelphia: WB Saunders, pp. 377–389.

*Pollow RL, Stoller EP, Forster LE, Duniho TS. (1994). Drug combinations and potential risk of adverse drug reactions among community-dwelling elderly. *Nurs Res, 43*(1):44–49.

Stuck AE, Beers MH, Steiner A, Aronow HU, Rubenstein LZ, Beck JC. (1994). Inappropriate medication use in community-residing older persons. *Arch Intern Med, 154*(19): 2195–2200.

Bibliography

Ali NS. (1992). Promoting safe use of multiple medications by elderly persons. *Geriatric Nursing, 13*(3):157–159.

Alt-White A, Romano E. (1993). An interdisciplinary approach to improving quality of life for nursing home residents. *Nursing Connections, 6*(4):51–59.

American Nurses Association adopts position statement on polypharmacy. *Am J Hosp Pharm, 48*(5):862, May 1991.

Col N, Fanale JE, Kronholm P. (1990). The role of medication noncompliance and adverse drug reactions in hospitalizations of the elderly. *Arch Intern Med, 150*(4):841– 845.

*Conn V, Taylor S, Miller R. (1994). Cognitive impairment and medication adherence. *J Gerontologic Nurs,* July, 41–47.

*Drake AC, Romano E. (1995) Protecting your older patient from the hazards of polypharmacy. *Nursing '95,* June, 35–39.

Esposito L. (1995). The effects of medication education on adherence to medication regimens in an elderly population. *J Adv Nurs, 21:*935–943.

Fielo SB, Warren S. (1993). Medication usage by the elderly. *Geriatr Nurs, 14*(1):47–51.

Fitten LJ, Coleman L, Siembieda DW, Yu M, Ganzell S. (1995). Assessment of capacity to comply with medication regimens in older patients. *J Am Geriatrics Soc, 43:*361– 367.

*Kee CC. (1992). Age-related changes in the renal system: Causes, consequences, and nursing implications. *Geriatric Nurs, 13:*80–83.

*Knox DM, Martof, MT. (1995). Effects of drug therapy on renal function of healthy older adults. *J Gerontologic Nurs,* April, 35–40.

Miller CA. (1995). *Nursing care of older adults: Theory and practice.* Philadelphia: JB Lippincott.

Moore JM, Johnson, JE. (1993). Over-the-counter drug use by the rural elderly. *Geriatric Nurs, 14:*190–191.

Rice PA, Jensen M, Lyons M, Murphy MF. (1994). Medications in well and institutionalized elders. *Geriatr Nurs, 15:*216–218.

*Recommended for further reading.

Schmader K, Hanlon JT, Weinberger M, et al. (1994). Appropriateness of medication prescribing in ambulatory elderly patients. *J Am Geriatrics Soc, 42*:1241–1247.

*Stone J. (1991). Preventing physical iatrogenic problems. In Chenitz C, Stone J, Salisbury S (eds). *Clinical gerontological nursing*. Philadelphia: WB Saunders, pp. 359–375

Wolfe SC, Schirm V. (1992). Medication counseling for the elderly: Effects on knowledge and compliance after hospital discharge. *Geriatric Nurs, 13*:134–138.

*Recommended for further reading.

For more information and sample tests and activities, refer to Chapter 12 in the Student Workbook for Clinical Pharmacology and Nursing Management, 5th edition, available through your bookstore.

V

Pharmacology in Community-Based Nursing

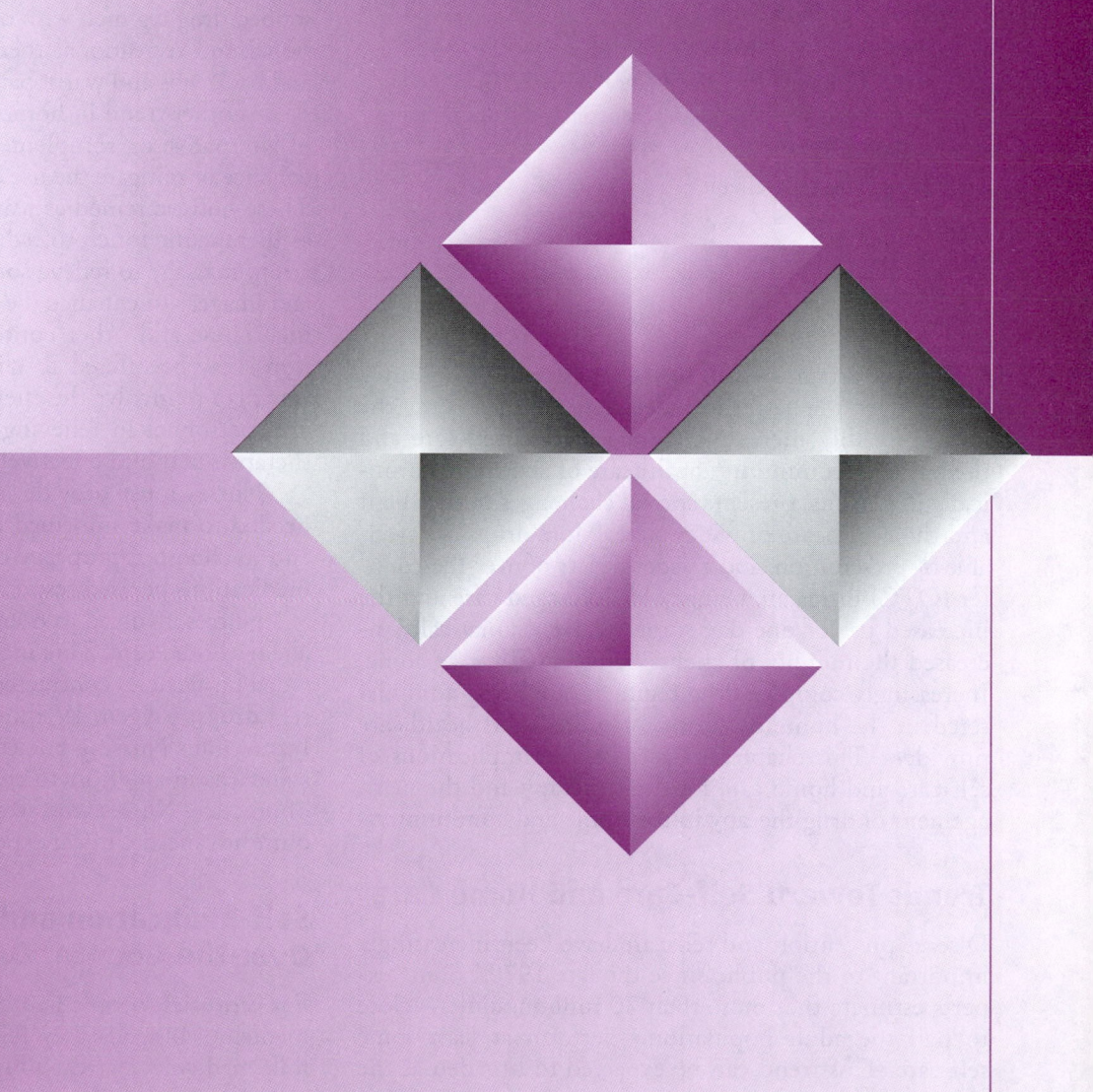

13

Drug Therapy in the Home and Community

The expansion of the pharmaceutical industry over the last three decades, coupled with the steadily increasing trends toward self-care and the home or community healthcare of acute and chronically ill persons, presents special challenges to the client and the healthcare provider alike. More drugs are available by prescription, and a wider variety of over-the-counter (OTC) drugs are being sold. Managed care and the increased use of one-day surgery have dramatically increased the number of clients being cared for at home. Increasingly complex drug regimens are being administered in the home by clients, families, and healthcare providers. This chapter focuses on the implications of self-care and home care for drug therapy and the management of drug therapy in the home and community.

Trends Toward Self-Care and Home Care

Disease prevention and self-care have been increasingly important to the public since the late 1970s. Some experts estimate that more than 70 million adults—close to half the adult population—perform at least some self-care. This trend can be expected to broaden as the public realizes that health insurance increasingly does not cover many healthcare costs, that many diseases cannot be cured, and that care services are limited and expensive.

Since the regulation of for-profit home health agencies in 1985, the change in third-party reimbursement mechanisms, especially managed care, has resulted in the need to adapt hospital-based drug administration policies and procedures to the home. The range of services these agencies can deliver include management of venous access devices; stabilization therapies, such as intravenous (IV) antibiotic delivery and parenteral and enteral feedings; pain management; chemotherapy; and investigational therapies. The treatment of persons with AIDS has led to an expanded population that has learned to provide complex drug treatments safely at home.

The rise in home births and deaths further demonstrates the public's increasing desire to minister to a family member at these two highly charged times. For the terminally ill person in a home hospice care program, the nurse can help generate a safe, client- and family-centered plan of care that incorporates the traditional, prescribed drug regimen with other measures, such as diversional and recreational therapy, music and art therapy, and back rubs and warm baths, where appropriate.

Another trend in home care and self-care is the use of alternative or complementary therapies, which may enhance or mitigate the use of drugs, prescribed or OTC. These holistic remedies feature nursing measures, such as therapeutic touch to reduce pain and promote relaxation, massage to relieve sore muscles, and visualization and imagery to enhance the client's participation in healing. These and other contemporary nursing interventions may be offered to clients as part of the nursing care plan to involve the client, family, and home healthcare personnel in relieving symptoms and using drug therapy safely and effectively.

Nurses must provide clients with the information needed to make informed decisions about their health and to choose appropriate care. Encouraging that OTC medications be used responsibly is essential.

Nurses involved in home health care coordinate the client's home care. This includes technical services provided by agencies contracted to administer such therapy (eg, drugs, oxygen, IV fluids, hyperalimentation). The Intravenous Nursing Society has established home care standards in an effort to control and define their scope of practice. Nurses who work in this expanding area require advanced clinical expertise and experience.

Self-Medication and Over-the-Counter Drugs

For centuries, people had limited access to professional medicine. Instead, they relied on herbal remedies and folk medicine to treat illnesses. During the Industrial

Revolution, when people began to migrate from rural to urban areas, patent medicines became popular. Patent medicines were drug preparations protected by a legal document called a patent. No one other than the person who held the patent could produce or sell the preparation. Patent medicines were readily available, did not require a physician's prescription, and were advertised as cure-alls for even the most serious diseases, including cancer, tuberculosis, and plague.

The self-care movement and the growing availability of nonprescription drugs have led to the increased use of OTC preparations. About six of every 10 medicines in the home are OTC drugs. One survey estimated that four times as many common health problems are treated with nonprescription medicines as are treated by a physician. A national survey showed that almost 54% of 3-year-old children in the United States were given an OTC medication within a 30-day period. Most commonly given were acetaminophen (Tylenol) and cough and cold medicines. Women who were educated, white, and financially stable were more likely to have given their children OTC medications (Kogan et al., 1994).

Economic Issues

As new products are developed and prescription ingredients are deemed safe for OTC use, the number of OTC preparations increases. As people become interested in maintaining health and preventing illness, their use of OTC products also increases. As early as 1989, some sources estimated that by 2000, clients will save $34.1 billion in healthcare costs simply by using OTC drug products. Much of this cost, however, may be borne by the client, because when a drug receives OTC status, most insurance companies do not pay for it. Therefore, some persons whose insurance plans cover prescription drugs may find it less expensive to use prescription drugs than OTC drugs. A study of older adults in Pennsylvania showed that those with prescription coverage were more likely to medicate a problem with prescribed rather than OTC drugs (Stuart and Grana, 1995).

In a study of the availability of OTC vaginal antifungal products, a managed care provider found a 1-year savings of $42,528 in medication costs and as much as $25,729 in costs associated with physician visits. After they were granted OTC status, the number of prescriptions written for these products were reduced by 6.42 per 100 clients (Gurwitz et al., 1995).

Legislative Control

Although OTC drugs can be purchased without a prescription, they are regulated by the federal Food and Drug Administration (FDA). These products contain low doses and often a combination of ingredients. They are used as the purchaser desires and are not supervised by a physician or other healthcare professionals licensed to prescribe drugs. These preparations contain both active and inactive ingredients. Active ingredients are those considered to have therapeutic effects (eg, reduce fever). Inactive ingredients (eg, preservatives, flavorings) do not have therapeutic effect. In general, the fewer the active ingredients, the better.

By the late 1800s, many states had food and drug laws, but the first federal Food and Drug Act was not passed until 1906. The initial focus of federal legislation regarding food and drugs was protective and focused on adulterated products. The law then expanded to include mislabeled products and, finally, safety and effectiveness (Table 13-1). For more information on drug legislation, see Chapter 2.

Table 13-1. Legislation Affecting OTC Drugs

Legislative Act	Date	Provisions Affecting Nonprescription Drugs
Federal Food and Drug Act	1906	Labels must be accurate in describing the strength and purity of drugs and must indicate the kind and amount of narcotic ingredients contained therein.
Shirley Amendment	1912	This law prohibited fraudulent claims, establishing a legal basis for control of drug efficacy.
Federal Food, Drug and Cosmetic Act	1938	New drugs must be approved as safe before they may enter interstate commerce. This act further defined labeling requirements.
Amendment to the Food, Drug and Cosmetic Act	1945	Certain drugs must be certified after batch testing at the manufacturing plant.
Durham-Humphrey Amendment	1952	This law defined prescription and nonprescription drugs and prohibited the sale of prescription drugs without medical authorization.
Kefauver-Harris Amendment	1962	Drugs of doubtful safety or efficacy can be withdrawn from the market. Adverse reactions must be reported to the government. Efficacy of new drugs must be proven before marketing. False or misleading advertising is prohibited.
Over-the-Counter Drug Review	1972	The FDA created 17 advisory panels to study ingredients in over-the-counter drugs to determine their efficacy. Ingredients are classified into Category I (safe and effective), Category II (not recognized as safe and effective), or Category III (insufficient data to classify either as Category I or II).

When the National Research Council of the National Academy of Sciences found that 75% of OTC preparations that it reviewed were not effective for at least one of their intended uses, the FDA established the FDA OTC Drug Review in 1972. Review panels determine whether OTC drugs are safe, effective, and correctly labeled. These panels apply two standards in their reviews: safety and effectiveness. Safety measures include a low potential for harm if the product is misused and minimal occurrence of major side effects or adverse reactions when the product is used in accord with clear directions and precautions. Effectiveness refers to a product's pharmacologic effect. A product is considered effective if it provides the type of relief intended in most of the target population if used as directed. In addition, FDA regulations require that the terminology used on labels be clear and basic enough so that ordinary persons have adequate directions for use and warnings about incorrect and inappropriate use.

The OTC review established various classes of OTC drugs. Included are antacids; antimicrobials I and II; antiperspirants; cold, cough, allergy, bronchodilator, and antiasthmatic preparations; contraceptive and other vaginal drug preparations; dentifrices and dental care preparations; hemorrhoidal preparations; internal analgesics, antipyretics, and antirheumatics; laxatives, antidiarrheals, emetics, and antiemetics; miscellaneous external drug preparations; ophthalmics; oral cavity preparations; sedatives, tranquilizers, and sleeping aids; and vitamins, minerals, and hematinics.

Since the FDA review of OTC products began in 1972, some ingredients (eg, phenacetin) have been removed from the market because they are unsafe. Others (eg, hexachlorophene) have been reclassified as prescription drugs after clinical data revealed serious side effects. Some prescription drugs (eg, some hydrocortisone creams and ibuprofen) have been awarded OTC status.

Characteristics of Over-the-Counter Drugs

Hundreds of OTC products are available, including oral and topical drugs, cosmetics, cleansers, diagnostic agents for in vitro use, and contraceptives. Over-the-counter products are used to prevent or treat many ailments, including indigestion, the common cold, minor injuries, constipation, diarrhea, allergies, skin irritation, obesity, corns, calluses, and muscle aches.

Hundreds of active ingredients can be sold without a prescription, and these are marketed singly or in combination, often for multiple purposes. Because federal regulations limit the dosage of OTC drugs, they tend to

Table 13-2. Interactions and Adverse Effects of OTC Drugs

OTC Drug	Interactions or Adverse Effects*
Acetaminophen	May cause liver damage if taken with alcohol. Increases blood levels of methotrexate and zidovudine (AZT)
Alcohol	Contained in many liquid cough medicines, liquid analgesics, mouthwashes, sleep aids, and vitamins and some homeopathic medications (as a preservative)
	Even small amounts can cause reaction in persons on disulfiram (Antabuse) therapy.
	Increased sedation and CNS depression when used with other CNS depressants
Antacids	May interfere with absorption of antibiotics (eg, tetracyclines)
	May dissolve the enteric coating of oral medications, resulting in gastric irritation
Antihistamines	Most cause drowsiness when taken initially.
	May potentiate sedative effects of other medications, including alcohol
Aspirin, other salicylates	Increase anticoagulant effects of other anticoagulants
	Gastric bleeding may result from irritation of gastric mucosa.
	Avoid in children or adolescents with viral symptoms because of risk of Reye's syndrome.
Bulk laxatives (eg, psyllium)	Swallowing sufficient liquid after administration is necessary to prevent swelling of the bulk in the esophagus.
Cold remedies	Contain multiple ingredients—for instance, cough medicines and cold remedies may contain the same ingredients, leading to overdosing.
	Clients should use a product that treats the symptoms they have, not those they anticipate.
Decongestants	Many products contain drugs with sympathomimetic effects (eg, naphazoline, ephedrine, triprolidine, phenylpropanolamine); may increase blood pressure and counteract effect of antihypertensives
Laxatives	Prolonged use can lead to bowel dependency and fluid and electrolyte disturbances.
Nonsteroidal antiinflammatory drugs	Can cause serious gastric bleeding from GI irritation without symptoms of indigestion, pain, or other warning
Steroids (topical)	Prolonged use, especially on inflamed skin or on mucous membranes, can result in systemic absorption and possible systemic side effects.

*This table presents only some interactions and side effects. See more detailed discussions of these effects in the appropriate chapter.

produce fewer adverse reactions than prescription drugs. They also may have less effect than the same ingredient in a prescription drug because of the lower dose.

General Precautions for Use

Most OTC drugs are used to relieve symptoms rather than cure an underlying disease. Using nonprescription medicines, home remedies, or alternative therapies may delay the diagnosis of a medical problem or may mask serious illness. Moreover, although OTC drugs are available to all age groups, they do not necessarily have the same effect in these groups. For instance, infants have nonuniform biologic maturation, and very old persons have nonuniform biologic deterioration. Age, therefore, influences how a person responds to a product, as well as how the product is absorbed and eliminated.

Therapeutic Uses

Over-the-counter drugs are used to relieve symptoms of minor, self-limiting conditions and to control non-progressive, chronic conditions. Upper respiratory infections; occasional indigestion, constipation, or diarrhea; superficial cuts and abrasions; and minor aches and pains can be treated with OTC preparations with minimal risk. Self-medication for these problems empowers the client and decreases the workload of healthcare personnel and facilities.

Adverse Reactions

Over-the-counter drugs are not guaranteed to be safe even if taken as directed. Persons who use OTC products should be aware of both the therapeutic effects and the adverse effects, including conditions that enhance 1) toxicity, 2) interaction with prescription drugs, and 3) age-related problems. For example, in large doses, acetaminophen can be toxic to a person who consumes more than 3 or 4 oz of alcohol a day. In addition, thousands of products on the market contain the same ingredients, and some products contain combinations of similar ingredients. Consumers should read labels carefully each time they buy a product because the ingredients, directions, warnings, and indications may change.

Drug Interactions

Some ingredients in OTC products may interact with other OTC and prescription drugs. Table 13-2 highlights some interactions and adverse effects. Because hundreds of OTC drugs are marketed every year, identifying all the ingredients becomes crucial. For example, although alcohol has been eliminated from OTC preparations for children, the amount of alcohol in products for adults varies considerably (Table 13-3). Liquid analgesics, cold and cough preparations, decongestants, mouthwashes, sleep aids, and vitamins may contain alcohol. Alcohol may also be contained in homeopathic medicines. Even small amounts of alcohol can cause severe adverse reactions (eg, vomiting, confusion) in

Table 13-3. Alcohol Content of Selected OTC Liquid Drugs

Drug Category	Percentage of Alcohol	Examples of Trade Names
Analgesics	7.0	Tylenol Extra Strength
Cold and cough preparations	25.0	Nyquil
	23.0	Dimetapp DM
	19.0	Medi-flu
Cough preparations	10.0	Vicks 44
	5.0	Benylin DM
	3.5	Robitussin
	2.4	Sudafed cough syrup
Decongestants	10.0	Novahistine DMX, Vicks 44D
	2.3	Dimetapp elixir
Mouthwashes	21.6	Listerine
	67.9	Scope
	14.0	Cepacol
Sleep aids	10.0	Excedrin PM liquid
Vitamins	12.0	Geritol Tonic

persons taking disulfiram (Antabuse) to abstain from alcohol.

Other OTC preparations contain sugars. Diabetics, therefore, must be wary of using OTC preparations and should discuss their use with a healthcare professional.

Interest in Alternative Therapies

A growing trend in healthcare is the use of alternative (nontraditional) therapies to enhance or mitigate the use of drugs, whether prescribed or OTC. Alternative medicine has been described as any medical practice or intervention that lacks sufficient documentation of its safety and effectiveness against specific diseases and conditions. It is not generally taught in U.S. medical schools, and treatment by alternative therapies is rarely covered by health insurance.

Home-Based and Cultural Practices

Alternative therapies include home remedies and cultural health practices (see Chap. 9), as well as modalities such as homeopathy, which may involve the ingestion of substances intended to provide a therapeutic effect. To provide information about possible conflicts among treatment modalities, the nurse must be aware of the client's use of alternative therapies. Many clients do not inform their usual healthcare practitioners about their use of these modalities. One study showed that one third of the clients studied used alternative therapies and that more than 80% used conventional medicines concurrently but did not inform their physicians they were doing so (Eisenberg et al., 1993).

Concerns About Effectiveness. The general public is showing increased interest in natural and alternative therapies, but many professionals have expressed concern about the adequacy of research done on the effectiveness of these therapies. To encourage research in this area, the government established the Office of Alternative Medicine under the National Institutes of Health and provided funding.

The use of unproved therapies can be detrimental. These therapies may be expensive. Health and life may be threatened by possible delays in diagnosing and obtaining treatment for adverse effects of some therapies. On the other hand, many alternative therapies are complementary with conventional medical care; therefore, the term *complementary medicine* has been proposed.

Healthcare Fraud. The FDA defines health fraud as the promotion, advertisement, distribution, or sale of articles intended for human or animal use that are represented as benefiting health or being effective in diagnosing, preventing, treating, curing, or mitigating disease (or other conditions) but that are not proven scientifically to be safe and effective for such purposes (Stehlin, 1996).

Experts have placed the cost of false claims of effectiveness at about $30 billion yearly in the United States (Stehlin, 1996). Increases in the claims for foods as providing health benefits and the increased marketing of OTC drugs and homeopathic preparations are areas of concern. OTC medications are intended for use in self-limiting conditions, not for serious conditions (eg, cancer, diabetes, heart disease) and not for enhancement of the immune system.

Older adults are at high risk of becoming fraud victims because most of them have at least one chronic health problem. Persons with arthritis, cancer, and AIDS are common targets for unproven health remedies as well. Teenagers may fall prey to fraudulent diet pill claims, breast developers, and muscle-building potions. Clients must be informed about how to evaluate such claims. Box 13-1 discusses how to evaluate alternative therapies.

Homeopathy

Homeopathy is a system of medicine founded in the 19th century by the German physician Samuel Hahnemann. It is based on the principle of similars—in other words, the use of substances that cause symptoms and syndromes in high or toxic doses can heal when given in specially prepared and exceedingly small or diluted doses. Widely practiced in India and Europe, homeopathy is used by about 1% of adults in the United States. (Fugh-Berman, 1996). However, the self-care movement has contributed to an increase in marketing of homeopathic remedies and practices.

Conventional practitioners view homeopathy as controversial and unproven. Although some research results support homeopathy, the positive findings are often criticized as the result of poor research designs (Fugh-Berman, 1996).

Homeopathic remedies are considered drugs by the FDA if they are included in the *Homeopathic Pharma-*copoeia of the *United States Formulary.* The legislation authorizing this was the federal Food, Drug, and Cosmetic Act of 1938; this occurred before the legal requirement that drugs be considered effective as well as safe. Homeopathic drugs are available in health-food stores and in some pharmacies. They may be prescribed by those legally authorized to practice medicine (eg, physicians, dentists, veterinarians) and may be used by clients for self-care.

Since homeopathic drugs are very diluted, they seldom interfere with conventional drugs. However, homeopathic liquid drugs may contain alcohol as a preservative. Most conventional medicines are considered detrimental to the effectiveness of homeopathic medicine because they are believed to suppress symptoms without strengthening the person as a whole. Considered particularly detrimental are caffeine, camphor, hormones in birth-control pills, large doses of vitamins, or therapeutically prescribed herbs (Ullman, 1995).

A problem may also occur if the client's symptoms increase. Homeopathic medicine considers the worsening of symptoms after treatment with a homeopathic remedy to be a beneficial "healing crisis." This could result in differing interpretations of the significance of symptoms and could lead to a delay in the medical diagnosis and treatment of serious conditions.

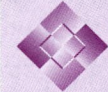

Box 13-1
Deciding to Use Alternative Therapies

The National Institutes of Health (NIH) Office of Alternative Medicine recommends the following before using any alternative therapy:

- Obtain objective information about the therapy. Besides talking with the person promoting the approach, speak with people who have experienced the treatment—preferably both those who were treated recently and those treated in the past. Ask about the advantages and disadvantages, risks, side effects, costs, and results. Find out the time span over which results can be expected.
- Inquire about the training, expertise, and credentials of the person administering the treatment (eg, certification or licensing).
- Consider the costs. Alternative treatments may not be reimbursable by health insurance.
- Discuss all treatments with your primary care provider, who needs this information to have a complete picture of your treatment plan.

Adapted from Stehlin IB. (1996). An FDA guide to choosing medical treatments. Internet, http://www.thebody.com/fda/medical.html

Drug Therapy in the Home

Many more complex drug regimens are being administered in the home today than in the past. The trend toward decreased hospital stays and increased community-based care has increased the responsibility of client, family, caregiver, and nurse to provide accurate, safe medication administration.

Assessment for Home Drug Therapy

Thorough knowledge of a drug includes its method of administration (dose, route, frequency), its intended effects and possible side effects, contraindications, and concurrent effects if the client is taking two or more drugs at the same time. Substance abuse must be monitored carefully to avoid potentially harmful effects. Ideally, the assessment data are gathered over several home visits, although this is not always possible.

Assessing Traditional Drug Use

If possible, the nurse should take a thorough drug history from every client and family visited regularly. When deciding whether an in-depth drug history should be taken, the nurse considers three factors: the client's degree of illness, the amount and types of medication taken, and the client's ability to comply with the drug regimen.

For clients of any age with a chronic illness that requires drug therapy, a thorough drug history is needed. Any client taking one or more prescribed medications should also be interviewed to assess the expected action and effects of the drug.

When an acute or chronic disease that results in changes in bodily functions is newly diagnosed, the nurse must reassess the client for the need to alter the drug regimen. For a client undergoing a stressful experience (eg, a job change, loss of a spouse), the nurse should inquire about any actual or potential changes in drug use.

Assessing Nontraditional Drug Use

Another reason to ask clients about their home drug use is to increase their knowledge of home remedies, OTC drugs, and alternative products. They may not recognize these as drugs, and the assessment process can expand their awareness and appreciation of drugs and increase their sense of responsibility for self-care.

Because the term *drug* is defined in many ways by clients, the scope of drug use in the home setting needs clarification. A drug is any substance that has a beneficial or harmful effect on the body. To obtain an accurate and comprehensive drug history, the following assessment categories are useful. The nurse should assess the use of substances that are:

- Applied (eg, deodorants, cosmetics, depilatories, soaps, detergents, hair rinses and dyes, dentifrices, lotions, ointments, transdermal patches)
- Ingested (eg, tablets, pills, capsules, vitamins, minerals, syrups, house plants, leaded paints, lozenges, herbal teas, bicarbonate of soda, elixirs, alcohol)
- Inhaled (eg, exhaust fumes from buses, tobacco, marijuana, spray cleaners, industrial pollutants, fumes from bleach, ammonia, and other cleaning products)
- Injected (eg, serums, insulin, vitamins, spider bites and bee stings, "hard" drugs, antiallergens, antileukemics, narcotics, hormones, antineoplastics)
- Inserted (eg, suppositories [vaginal and rectal], contraceptives, sublingual preparations, gelatin sponges)
- Instilled (eg, ear, nose, and eye drops, solutions for catheter and wound irrigation).

Items prepared in the home may be subcategories of applied or ingested drugs. Home remedies such as poultices and vegetable or herbal concoctions may be made from family or traditional medicinal recipes. In addition, many constituents used in preparing food products must also be considered drugs (eg, preservatives, additives, monosodium glutamate, vitamins, herbs). Although this information may be difficult to obtain, it can be crucial for both the client and nurse when assessing the total sources of drugs in the home.

Categorizing drugs raises the client's awareness about the products used in daily activities. He or she may not be aware, for example, of the side effects of harsh detergents, hard water, or food additives on bodily functions. Clients taking multiple laxative preparations may be having the drug's intended effects canceled out and thus may be taking them without benefit.

Assessing Drug Misuse

What appears to be abuse may actually be misuse due to misinformation. For instance, clients who seek medical attention from more than one source may be taking multiple prescriptions of similar-acting drugs. Some clients may inadvertently take drugs that potentiate each other, especially when OTC and prescribed drugs are taken together without the prescriber's knowledge. The nurse or client must inform the primary care provider of such situations. The client's pharmacist should also be notified so that the prescriptions can be verified and cross-checked with the prescriber. Some clients may not admit to the use of illicit or recreational drugs because they fear discovery. Other inappropriate uses of drugs include taking a drug intended for someone else or taking a drug prescribed for a different condition.

Assessing Drug Effects

The nurse routinely monitors the intended effect and the side effects of drugs taken at home. First, the nurse must ask general questions about whether the drug is having the desired effect. The nurse may also ask the client what the prescriber and pharmacist, as well as family and friends, have said about the drug. Second, the nurse should ask, in an organized manner, about the specific effects of the drug. Has the client observed any side effects? If so, what actions did the client take, if any? Finally, objective findings that document and measure the effects of the drug should be sought. For a client taking an antihypertensive drug, the nurse should measure the client's blood pressure and compare it with previous data. For a client taking a diuretic, the nurse should look for signs of dehydration (dry skin and mouth) or ankle edema; monitor weight, urine output, and lung sounds; and assess dietary and prescribed potassium supplements.

Side effects are best assessed by systematically posing open-ended but specific questions about any undesirable drug effects. When side effects include altered physical signs, the nurse must assess and record them. Any adverse or undesired drug effects should be noted and explained to the client, and the physician should be promptly notified. Performing this kind of activity in the home can teach clients self-care and enhance awareness of their responsibility for regular and safe self-medication.

Assessing Safety

When reviewing the possible hazards involved in storing drugs, the nurse should remind the client to inspect all OTC drugs at the time of purchase for evidence of tampering (see Chap. 7). In addition, all OTC drugs should be checked for possible contamination (eg, unusual appearance, inconsistent color and odor); if detected, this should be reported to the pharmacist, who may suggest an alternative.

Storage. The nurse should observe how the client stores drugs in the home. Some drugs must be stored away from excessive heat, light, and moisture. Some preparations, such as suppositories, must be refrigerated. The nurse should ensure that all drugs and chemicals are stored out of the reach of children. Drugs must have childproof caps unless the client has a physical handicap (eg, arthritis, paralysis) that prohibits removal of such a cap. The client or prescriber can request the pharmacist to dispense in regular caps. The nurse should stress the importance of labeling each drug correctly and storing it in its own container.

Labeling. When checking prescribed medications, the nurse notes whether they are all from the same physician and the same pharmacy. Additional concerns are the number of pills, tablets, or capsules prescribed versus the number in the bottle (or quantity of liquid). The original quantity dispensed can be verified with the pharmacist by referring to the prescription number on the label. The quantity of pills or liquid remaining should relate to the date when they were prescribed, the dose, and the frequency of intended administration. Any discrepancies should be noted and discussed with the client. If necessary, the prescriber should be informed, with the client's knowledge.

Labels on prescribed medication provide a great deal of information. In some states, expiration dates appear only on OTC products, but most liquid preparations do include them. Some drug labels may include warnings or recommendations such as "Avoid driving," "Take this drug with milk," or "Refrain from using alcohol." The nurse should also note whether the client is taking a generic drug in addition to a similar brand-name drug.

All labels should be legible and waterproof to ensure correct administration by the client. When the nurse or client has been instructed verbally by the prescriber to alter the administration of a drug, the label must be updated to reflect the new regimen. Again, any discrepancies should be pointed out to the client and reported to the prescriber. Any unusual label notations or instructions should be investigated in case the prescriber or pharmacist has made a mistake.

Disposal. A further consideration to the safe use of drugs at home includes the proper disposal of contaminated needles and other objects soiled with bodily wastes. Used needles, syringes, drug vials, IV tubing, and lancets should be placed in a sturdy container—an empty thick plastic detergent bottle or, preferably, a metal coffee can with a tight-fitting lid. When the container is full, the contents should be covered with a solution of 1 part household bleach and 10 parts water. The container is then covered, taped tightly, and placed in two plastic bags. This parcel is then tied securely and thrown into the trash. Naturally, it is important to wash one's hands before and after this procedure. Local communities and states may have their own regulations about the disposal of toxic wastes (eg, cancer drugs) and infectious wastes. Nurses should be aware of and follow agency policies related to safe disposal to protect themselves, their clients, families, the community, and the environment.

Assessing Client Variables

Assessment of client variables is a key tool for promoting safety and compliance as well as a good outcome (Box 13-2).

Health Status. The value of knowing the client's health status cannot be overestimated. Obviously, if the client is pregnant or lactating, any drug use must be carefully considered. For the client taking medications for a chronic health problem such as diabetes, the drug use assessment must include a physical assessment and a history of the disease, the signs and symptoms of hyperglycemia and hypoglycemia, any drug side effects experienced throughout the course of the disease, and the client's use of diet and exercise to offset drug use. The experience of living with chronic illness may also help encourage drug compliance at home.

Clients on a short course of drug therapy for an acute illness after hospitalization or a visit to the physician must be assessed for their ability to take medica-

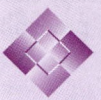

Box 13-2
**Client Variables That Affect
Drug Use in the Home**

Alliance (compliance) with drug regimen

Knowledge of drug

> Administration
> Regimen
> Action effects
> Side effects
> Contraindications

Knowledge of disease process

Mental and emotional status

Motivation

Age

Role in family

Cultural/ethnic background

Socioeconomic status

Attitudes about self-care

Health status

Lifestyle

Attitudes and beliefs about drugs

Previous experience with drugs

Length of time taking drugs

Level of education

Level of intelligence

Language barrier

Sensory and physical impairments

Allergies

One of the first questions to ask when making a drug assessment is whether the client can explain the effect of a drug on the body and on the disease process. This provides the nurse with information about the client's mental state and also gives an idea of the client's vocabulary, knowledge, and intellectual level. When such information is obtained at the beginning of the drug interview, the nurse can develop a framework within which to plan further teaching and interventions.

Age. The older the client, the greater the potential for exposure to various OTC and prescribed drugs and the greater the experience with home remedies and advice from family, friends, and healthcare providers. The younger the client, the greater the chance of accepting drugs (in general) because of the effects of the media, peers, and the proliferation of drugs from the pharmaceutical industry. Older clients may be reluctant to take prescribed medications because they consider drugs harmful, but younger clients may take various drugs for common ailments such as fatigue, stomach ache, and feelings of depression.

The reverse can also be true. Because older clients have witnessed the advent and widespread successful use of drugs, they may accept drug therapy without question on the advice of peers and professionals alike. On the other hand, younger clients may have observed the harmful effects of drugs on their friends or learned about adverse drug effects in school and may, therefore, hesitate to take OTC or prescription drugs. Thus, nurses must avoid stereotyping clients according to a single factor such as age.

Family Role. The client's role in the family often suggests how much responsibility he or she is assuming for self-administering drugs or administering medications to other family members. With an elderly parent, for example, a son or daughter may assume full responsibility for administering medications. On the other hand, the parent of a teenager may be overly cautious about the use of drugs and may not want the teen to assume self-care. The nurse must always encourage appropriate self-care and independent drug administration for the client of whatever age.

Socioeconomic Status. A client's socioeconomic status can have several effects on compliance with the drug regimen. This information, coupled with the client's cultural beliefs about drugs, helps the nurse understand the level of importance that drug-taking behavior has for him or her. Medications may be purchased regularly and self-administered by clients regardless of the financial cost to the family. Some clients, however, believe that a prescribed medication such as an allergy shot is nontherapeutic or a waste of money and may refuse to take it or discontinue it prematurely, even though they can afford it. When the cost of drugs is not reimbursed by health insurance, clients may not fill the prescription or may

tion correctly, particularly if their previous health status was stable and uncomplicated.

The nurse should first establish a rapport and professional relationship with the client. She or he can then obtain an accurate data base, beginning with client variables such as allergies, health status, length of time taking drugs, and knowledge about drug effects.

The nurse may never become fully acquainted with the client as a person with individual beliefs, values, and cultural background, but essential baseline information may be learned while assessing other aspects of the healthcare regimen. For instance, self-care activities such as eating a well-balanced diet, getting regular exercise, and making time for recreation and relaxation may reflect the client's attitude toward self-administering drugs.

Attitudes and Motivation. Over the course of therapy, the astute nurse will ascertain the client's self-concept, especially as it relates to his or her attitude about drugs and level of motivation for following a specific drug regimen.

replace it with a cheaper substitute or home remedy, resulting in possible embarrassment when this substitution is discovered. The nurse then is in the position of having to urge compliance in the face of factors beyond his or her control. The use of less expensive generic drugs has helped to alleviate this situation, but the problem may continue for elderly clients and persons on fixed incomes who have inadequate insurance coverage.

Experience. The nurse must assess the client's previous experience with drugs, especially during hospitalization and as the result of traumatic or chronic illness. A previously successful outcome from drug therapy is likely to enhance compliance with the current drug regimen. The client who understands the expected effect of the drug and believes that it will promote well-being tends to provide accurate drug self-treatment. If previous experience indicates that the client is unwilling to accept the daily responsibility for adhering to drug therapy accurately, the nurse must provide additional home monitoring, teaching, and reassessment. Such clients are often readmitted to the hospital due to exacerbations of their illness that might have been prevented if a reminder or backup system had been provided.

Knowledge and Capability. A language barrier will probably become evident during initial contacts and may be remedied by using family or community translators. The client's level of education and intelligence can be assessed from data gathered during the rapport-building home visits. However, a high level of education does not guarantee the desired level of therapeutic compliance, nor does a low level of education mean the client lacks intelligence. Mitigating factors such as fear of drugs, doubts about their therapeutic effects, insufficient funds, illiteracy, and poor memory can reduce compliance and provide inaccurate assessment findings.

The nurse must be aware of cues indicating that the client understands the drug regimen. One way to obtain this information is to ask open-ended questions about the system used for taking drugs. For less articulate clients, asking them to demonstrate this system can produce a similar outcome.

Other. Questions about sensory and physical impairments are important. If appropriate, ask the client to demonstrate how he or she prepares and administers drugs. In this way, the nurse can detect partial blindness due to glaucoma, cataracts, untreated visual disturbances, or dyslexia. Difficulty in opening a medication container or in pouring a liquid preparation or a glass of water may indicate a psychomotor disturbance (eg, intentional tremors, arthritis, parkinsonian gestures). The nurse should report such signs and symptoms to the physician for further medical workup. In some cases, an alternative system of administering the medication may have to be devised—for example, soliciting the aid of a family member, friend, or neighbor, or using devices that aid in the correct ad-

ministration of drugs. The nurse should periodically check the client in whom an impairment is suspected, preferably at different times of the day and week.

Home Drug Administration and Management

Administering medication is a skilled nursing function. In an acute care setting, it is a frequent, often complex task that requires expertise and specialized techniques. Indeed, administering medicines and monitoring their effects constitute a major part of the nurse's role in the hospitalized client's therapeutic regimen. The acute care nurse is responsible for performing these roles safely and effectively.

When discharged from the hospital, the client and, in some cases, the family assume responsibility for managing the therapeutic regimen. A potential danger lies in the lack of the usual "checks and balances" that exist in the controlled setting of the hospital. Monitoring a client's administration of medication in the home presents a challenge for the home health nurse, who must ensure compliance with the medication regimen and tailor the client's care to the home environment.

Teaching clients and caregivers to administer medications may require teaching aseptic techniques, the administration of suppositories, the preparation and administration of intramuscular or subcutaneous injections, and the management of IV infusions. Clients and caregivers must know what signs, symptoms, or situations indicate the need to contact a healthcare professional immediately. Support from neighbors or other relatives and friends should be in place, as well as a carefully developed written plan for contacting the appropriate healthcare provider if questions arise.

The home healthcare nurse must supervise the home caregiver and related paraprofessionals in reminding the client to self-administer medication. Home care personnel require regular supervision and instruction regarding their role in the plan of care. When the nurse prepours the client's medications on a daily or weekly basis, it may be the function of home health aides to remind the client to take the dose and help him or her to do so. Home health aides can be useful in helping clients who live alone and are forgetful or confused or are too weak or incapacitated to handle drug bottles. The plan of care must indicate that the aide is to remind the client to take medication; this protects the client and the aide and clarifies the aide's role to any family members involved in the home drug regimen.

Compliance/Alliance Issues

The issue of therapeutic compliance—sometimes called therapeutic alliance—is all too familiar to nurses working in the community. Noncompliance is commonly the reason a referral is generated, which with a prescribed drug regimen can have many negative connotations. The term *noncompliance* defines the problem only from the provider's perspective. Failing to adhere to a drug regimen may be viewed as deviant behavior by a healthcare provider, but the client may view it as a cautious approach to self-administering potentially harmful substances. A client may choose not to take a drug as prescribed for various valid reasons (sometimes called *intelligent noncompliance*), or the client may be unaware of the correct dosage regimen. Whatever the reason, the nurse must avoid a one-sided judgmental approach and instead must work with the client to achieve the desired effect of the drug in a manner acceptable to both. See Chapter 8 for a full discussion of noncompliance and strategies to promote therapeutic alliance.

Because the community-based nurse works with the client in the context of family and community, he or she must also view the problem of compliance from a broader perspective. Thus, a thorough drug history must be generated to afford the nurse the greatest amount of information from which to plan interventions and evaluate outcomes of nursing care.

Communication, Referral, and Continuity of Care

Continuity of care within the healthcare system requires faultless communication among healthcare providers. When making a referral to a home healthcare nurse, hospital personnel must provide client data and all relevant medical and nursing background data, medication information, and confirmation that the client understands his or her therapeutic drug regimen. Without this data, the nurse has difficulty assessing the client's home self-care reliably and systematically. One approach to alleviating this interruption in care would be to involve the client more in discharge planning. Providing the client with medication cards that explain how to identify and administer drugs safely is one way to enhance continuity of care, and it can also aid the nurse's home assessment of drug use.

Community Resources

The nurse should know about community resources available to the client, including the location of a reputable pharmacist for reference purposes, drug education classes, and the local poison control center.

A potential resource in some communities is the pharmacy of a teaching or university-based hospital. This department can provide nurses with updated information about current drugs and new or experimental medications. An additional resource is a directory or list of companies that service drug-related equipment and supplies (eg, portable infusion pumps, blood glucose monitors). Nurses may also contact the National Council on Patient Information and Education (666 11th Street, N.W., Suite 810, Washington, DC 20001; 202-347-6711), a coalition of constituent health-related organizations that promotes communication about prescription drugs among clients and healthcare professionals.

Some communities may have a warning system for older clients. In these systems, a bright sticker listing the client's drugs is posted prominently in the house for reference in an emergency such as an overdose or an adverse reaction. In some communities, clients may subscribe to a call-in service. If the client fails to call the service by a particular time each day, the service takes steps to verify that the client is at home. If there is no response, someone will visit immediately. In addition, several electronic alert systems have been developed to link clients instantly to a 24-hour emergency service. Even a bed-bound or partially paralyzed client can enjoy the security such a system can provide. Should the client experience any difficulties or medical problems, he or she activates the device. This signals the emergency service operator, who then calls the client to obtain further information or sends emergency assistance if necessary. Services such as these provide the client with a level of independence while offering some protection against possible harm from unexpected drug effects.

■ SUMMARY

An open nurse–client relationship in the home setting fosters a more thorough drug use assessment. The drug use assessment is best done over several home visits, but when time constraints prevent this, the nurse must take a more formal drug history. A systematic drug history is actually a sharing of information between client and nurse, with the desired outcome being a complete identification and proper administration of all drug forms commonly found in the home.

The home healthcare nurse helps clients manage their drug regimens. The use of prescription and OTC drugs, as well as home remedies, must be monitored. Because clients today are managing serious health problems in the home, the regimens may be complex. The nurse must work closely with the caregivers and must use professional and community resources to ensure safe and effective medication management in the home.

❖ NURSING MANAGEMENT: CLIENTS RECEIVING DRUG THERAPY AT HOME

As role models, nurses should be aware of their own self-medication practices, identify the rationale for such behavior, and change habits that are inappropriate or potentially harmful. Nurses also serve as resources for information about drug preparations. Although many laypeople have access to drug information through the mass media, they still need guidance from healthcare professionals. Laypeople may have little information about the meaning or severity of symptoms. Therefore, they may be unable to make informed choices about which drugs, particularly OTC drugs, and preparations can be used safely and which to avoid or use only with the guidance of a healthcare professional.

CRITICAL THINKING CHALLENGE
Case Analysis

A 32-year-old stockbroker comes to the walk-in clinic of a hospital near her office. She complains of a bad cold and a fever of 99.6°F for the past 3 days. She has a nonproductive cough and reports difficulty sleeping. She says she also has a "really upset stomach" even though she has been taking an antacid. Because of her upset stomach, she has not been eating very much, but she has been drinking lots of fluids, mainly cola beverages. She has been self-medicating with an OTC sustained-action cold remedy. She asks the nurse practitioner for an antibiotic so she can function better at work.

1. What hypotheses do you have about possible causes of the client's upset stomach?
2. If the OTC preparation contained aspirin, what concerns would you have?
3. If the OTC preparation contained acetaminophen, what concerns would you have?
4. What response would you have to the client's request for an antibiotic?
5. What nonpharmacologic measures could you recommend?

Nurses, therefore, must know about the wide variety of OTC products available in their locale. Periodic analysis of these products should include intended therapeutic effect, directions for use, warnings and contraindications, pharmacologic properties of active ingredients, and characteristics of inactive ingredients. The cost and composition of name-brand and generic products also should be considered.

In managing any client's care, the nurse hopes to promote therapeutic compliance as well as client knowledge. To do so, the nurse must determine what the client knows and believes about his or her condition. In managing drug therapy, the nurse determines what the client knows and believes about drug use.

NURSING PROCESS

ASSESSMENT

The client's use of OTC drugs should be included in every drug history. Many clients do not think to mention their use of OTC products to healthcare providers because they do not consider OTC preparations to be medications. A nurse can elicit this information by asking direct questions such as:

- What do you do for a cold?
- What do you do for a headache?
- Do you ever take anything for indigestion?
- Do you take vitamins or minerals?
- What do you use if you have a rash?

In addition to identifying the specific OTC products used by clients, the nurse should list reasons for use and frequency, response to the product, and any adverse reactions experienced. The same information should be obtained for prescription drugs that the client is taking concurrently, particularly because the interaction between OTC and prescription products can be severe.

When analyzing a client's drug history, the nurse should look for the use of drugs that have the same effect, the use of a combination of drugs for the same purpose, and potential adverse reactions to these preparations in addition to their therapeutic effects. The nurse also must assess the client's knowledge of the appropriate use of prescription and OTC products, the therapeutic effects of preparations, the potential side effects, and the expiration date of medication.

The nurse must assess the client's understanding of drug therapy in the therapeutic regimen. In addition to assessing the client's use of OTC drugs, the nurse must also assess compliance with the prescribed drug regimen. For example, if the client is directed to take a medication four times a day, the nurse may investigate how the client remembers to take it—perhaps with breakfast, lunch, dinner, and at bedtime. Or if the medication must be stored out of sight (away from children), the nurse may ask how the client remembers to take it as prescribed.

The nurse also assesses whether the appropriate amount of medication has been taken. Any discrepancy—too much or too little left in the medication container—should cue the nurse to explore the client's compliance. Noncompliance in such cases may result from memory loss, unexpressed fear of drugs, doubts about the effects of the drug, unpleasant side effects, or a decision that the drug's effect was achieved before the supply was exhausted.

With a parent who incorrectly administers medication to a child, the nurse must consider the possibility of child abuse or neglect, document the situation thoroughly and carefully, and report it to the appropriate authority in accordance with the law.

NURSING DIAGNOSIS

Many nursing diagnoses may be appropriate for clients using OTC preparations and for clients receiving drug therapy at home. Many collaborative problems may be noted as well. Examples are:

- Knowledge Deficit, related to unfamiliarity with resources outlining proper use of OTC preparations
- Ineffective Management of Therapeutic Regimen, Noncompliance

Potential complication: GI bleeding related to gastric irritation from use of nonsteroidal antiinflammatory drugs or related to interaction of anticoagulant and aspirin

PLANNING

The aim of nursing care of clients receiving drug therapy at home is to empower them to use OTC and prescribed drugs appropriately and to adhere to the drug regimen for a healthful outcome. Secondary goals of nursing care, therefore, include:

- Teaching clients how to choose appropriate preparations for minor health problems and to eliminate the inappropriate use of such products
- Educating clients about self-medication to reduce the risk of adverse interactions between OTC products and prescription drugs
- Informing clients about healthcare problems for which self-medication is inappropriate
- Teaching clients to identify and manage adverse reactions to OTC preparations.

In planning ways to deal with actual or potential noncompliance, the nurse works with the client to establish a mutual goal of compliance. Then expected outcomes can be identified. Once this contract has been established, strategies can be implemented to achieve the stated objectives. If the client is noncompliant because he or she does not understand the consequences of nonadherence, the nurse states this observation and assessment. If the client agrees with the assessment and sees the relation between noncompliance and emerging health problems, the nurse and client can construct a plan to alter drug-taking behaviors.

INTERVENTION

Nursing interventions for clients receiving drug therapy or clients self-medicating with OTC drugs primarily focus on compliance and client education.

The nurse can promote compliance and trigger memory for forgetful clients in several ways. One way is to initiate a home drug-dispensing system, such as an empty egg carton or ice cube tray for holding pills, tablets, and capsules. A list of all drugs to be taken, including those prescribed on an as-needed basis, can be posted nearby, naming each drug and its action, effects, and dosage schedule. Commercial products are available for this same purpose (eg, a tray divided into seven sections labeled with each day of the week).

The nurse can encourage the forgetful client to link a specific time or favorite snack with the need to take medication. If possible, a family member or friend can be enlisted to provide backup support and to remind the client to take medications on time. The nurse can suggest that the client have his or her pharmacy maintain a drug profile.

Other compliance-promoting activities include organizing or supporting programs to increase public awareness of drugs and home therapy (eg, public service announcements, letters to the newspaper, drug education classes for at-risk groups). Not least among these interventions is the routine practice by hospital, clinic, and community-based nurses of exchanging relevant information about drug therapy issues.

The increasing number of clients of all ages with multiple chronic conditions requiring complex drug therapy has led to a rise in the number of "revolving door" hospital admissions and emergency department visits for apparent lapses in compliance. Although it may be tempting to blame the client in these situations, the reasons for such apparent noncompliance include a host of other factors. Therefore, healthcare providers must be aware of the client's situation and cognizant of interventions that are helpful in either setting. For example, when a newly diagnosed diabetic client reenters the hospital for assessment and treatment of unstable blood glucose levels, the home healthcare nurse, with the client's knowledge, can call the hospital nurse to relate the client's drug-taking regimen at home and to discuss side effects, the client's self-administration practices, and possibly how the client best learns about drugs. When the client is discharged, compliance with the new drug regimen can be encouraged if the hospital nurse provides written, clear instructions for both the client and the home healthcare nurse.

In the client's follow-up care, communication among nurses should continue. This promotes continuity of care, reduces noncompliance, and enhances the client's return to optimal health. This underscores the interdependence of healthcare providers in various settings, emphasizing the need for timely and pertinent communication. The nurse must remain open to trying new interventions, keeping in mind both the goals of the drug therapy and the client. This challenging and often rewarding nurse–client interaction can yield a greater understanding of each other's attitudes about drugs.

Defining the client's unique set of variables, establishing a workable contract, eliminating or reducing barriers to drug taking, and teaching about the effects of drugs should help increase the client's motivation, knowledge, and compliance and thereby yield reliable self-care. Any intermittent support needed should be readily available from the nurse or others. Obviously, if

CRITICAL THINKING CHALLENGE
Issue Analysis

1. After reading this chapter, what do you consider to be the advantages and disadvantages of the increasing use of OTC medications and alternative therapies?
2. Discuss why you think this trend should be encouraged or discouraged.
3. Identify clients or consumers for whom you think self-medication is useful and those for whom you think it is inappropriate. Explain why.

the client does not agree to assume this responsibility, the situations must be reevaluated. In some cases, perfect compliance is never achieved. In others, a compromise may minimize the risks of symptom recurrence and maximize client participation, especially in reporting any side effects that occur.

In any case, the client and nurse must be mutually accountable if a workable solution is to be found and incorporated into the client's drug-taking routine. The nurse must refrain from judgmental attitudes or punitive actions, remembering that, ultimately, taking any drug is the choice of the client or responsible caregivers. Clients' rights must be upheld, and in the broad realm of healthcare, these rights are receiving increasing attention and discussion by clients and professionals alike.

Client Education. It is the nurse's responsibility to educate clients and families about drug therapy, OTC products, and self-medication. It is the client's responsibility, however, to summon the motivation for adhering to therapy and using drug products safely. Nonetheless, the nurse, together with the client's physician and family members, can promote motivation in several ways.

Boosting Motivation. First, the nurse may present—clearly and in a nonthreatening manner—information about the effects of the drugs on the client's condition and the risks of noncompliance. Second, barriers to taking the drugs as indicated can be identified and minimized or eliminated. Barriers may be physical limitations imposed by disease or disabling conditions (eg, a client with arthritis who cannot remove childproof caps and tamperproof seals). Third, the client is included as a partner in the drug regimen. This means that the nurse formulates a plan in which both the nurse and client offer, implement, and evaluate solutions in the context of the same goal. This builds a well-defined concept of how the client can safely and effectively adhere to the drug regimen for the best effect.

Teaching About Safety. The nurse should teach clients how to examine a new package for tampering and to avoid using any product if the tamperproof seal is not intact. A package with a broken seal should be returned to the pharmacy or store where it was purchased and exchanged for one that is intact.

The nurse must explain the importance of checking the product's label and expiration date when purchasing it and also before using it. Using OTC products allows clients to take control of their healthcare. It also decreases healthcare costs and lightens the load on the healthcare system. If the client follows product recommendations, self-medication is usually safe and effective. Product labels are required by law to be accurate and to include warnings about when not to use a preparation and when to seek advice from a healthcare professional. The nurse points out where labels note the intended use of the product, the recommended dosage, potential adverse reactions, warnings, and guidelines for use and storage. The nurse must pro-

vide instructions for handling an adverse reaction, such as stopping use of the drug immediately and taking the actions recommended on the product label. If the adverse reaction is severe (eg, hives, vomiting, bleeding), the nurse advises seeking professional care immediately. The client should also seek professional care if symptoms are not relieved or if they worsen.

Explaining Risks of Self-Medication. Despite the relative safety of self-medication, some risks exist, and the nurse must alert clients to them (Table 13-4). Some clients may self-medicate rather than seek professional care for potentially serious problems. Nurses must emphasize that OTC products should be taken for minor, self-limiting conditions, such as scrapes and abrasions, occasional headaches, the common cold, occasional indigestion, or skin irritations. If problems or symptoms are severe, occur frequently, or are persistent, a healthcare professional should be consulted. The nurse can emphasize that the regular use of OTC preparations may mask symptoms of serious disease and that the client should consult a healthcare provider periodically to avoid this problem.

Over-the-counter drugs (eg, aspirin, antacids) may be used to treat chronic medical conditions (eg, arthritis, coronary heart disease, peptic ulcer); however, this use should be monitored by a healthcare professional.

Nurses also must inform clients that manufacturer-recommended dosages of OTC products may not provide relief or may precipitate unexpected adverse reactions. This can occur because dosages are calculated for persons of average age, height, and weight and because the dosage is usually less than what it would be if it were a prescribed drug. Clients who weigh less than average may experience enhanced, even toxic, drug effects; those who are over the average weight may experience little effect. The very young and the very old, in particular, may need less than the recommended dosage.

Allergic reactions are as likely to occur with OTC preparations as with prescription products. Allergic reactions may be caused by active or inactive ingredients. Some clients may be attracted to OTC products that contain multiple drug preparations, and the nurse must explain that more is not necessarily better: the greater the number of active ingredients, the greater the chances for adverse reactions and the more likely the chance of interactions. In addition, the nurse should warn clients that long-acting or timed-released preparations should be avoided when a new product is used for the first time. If an adverse reaction occurs, it will be prolonged and may be difficult to treat because of continued absorption of the active ingredients.

When discussing OTC products with clients, the nurse should explain not only the uses and properties of specific preparations but also the advantages and disadvantages of self-medication. The nurse should also offer clients guidelines for the appropriate use of OTC products as well (Box 13-3).

Table 13-4. Advantages and Disadvantages of Self-Medicating With OTC Drugs

Advantages	Disadvantages
OTC drugs often relieve symptoms of minor or self-limiting conditions.	Relief of symptoms fosters avoidance or delay in seeking professional care for potentially serious conditions.
Recommended dosages are relatively low, reducing the risk of adverse reactions.	Lack of therapeutic response may lead to use of dosages much greater than recommended.
Self-medication reduces the demand for services from healthcare professionals, freeing them to treat seriously ill persons.	Fixed dosage combinations prevent tailoring of dosage to individual needs.
OTC drugs cost less than prescription drugs.	Use of multiple preparations that may contain the same active ingredients increases the risk of adverse reactions.
	OTC drugs may contain inappropriate or superfluous ingredients.
	OTC drugs may increase toxicity of prescription drugs when used in combination with them.
	Health insurance usually does not cover costs of OTC drugs.

Box 13-3
Self-Medication Guidelines for Clients

Nurses can help clients decide when and how to use OTC drugs by offering these guidelines.

Determining the Need for an OTC Product

1. Are symptoms minor and self-limiting? Do they have an insignificant effect on my functioning? — Yes → Stop. Consider not using any medication to treat symptoms.
2. Do symptoms indicate a possibly serious health problem (eg, fever exceeding 101°F; sudden onset of acute abdominal pain, chest pain, or pain radiating down arm)? — Yes → Consult physician
3. Have my symptoms continued or increased despite my use of OTC or prescription medications? — Yes → Consult physician
4. Am I pregnant or nursing an infant? — Yes → Consult physician
5. Will use of an OTC drug relieve my symptoms, increase my comfort, or increase my ability to perform daily activities? — Yes → Consider using OTC drug

Selecting and Evaluating the Product

Evaluate the product under consideration in relation to:

- Current symptoms and other health problems
- Allergies
- Potential interactions with other drugs currently used
- Concerns about alcohol, sugar, sodium content
- Daily functioning (eg, product may cause drowsiness).
- Active and inactive ingredients
- Indications for use
- Warnings, contraindications and interactions
- Expiration date.

Check the product for:

- Tamper-resistant features
- Name of product

Compare several similar products for:

- Active and inactive ingredients
- Cost (particularly the difference between brand-name and generic products).

Clients also must be aware that some preparations advertised in the media and sold in some pharmacies or other stores may not be approved as drugs by the FDA and therefore may not be effective. In some cases, they may not meet standards of purity. The nurse can teach clients how to evaluate product claims.

OUTCOME EVALUATION

Data required for evaluating the efficacy of OTC preparations include the client's response to the preparation and evidence that the client is using the product appropriately. A client's response to an OTC preparation includes the actual effect of the product, the incidence of adverse reactions, and the subjective report of effectiveness. Evidence that the client is using the OTC product appropriately includes self-reports of how closely the client followed the recommended dosage and instructions and a low incidence of adverse reactions.

Other measures by which to evaluate the outcome of nursing measures include whether the goals shared by the client and nurse were achieved, whether the client adhered to the agreed-on therapeutic regimen, and whether the client's health improved or stabilized (as measured by changes in signs and symptoms).

❖ CHECKLIST OF NURSING ACTIONS

❑ Compile a drug history of the client's use of OTC drugs, home remedies, and alternative therapies. Analyze the history for appropriate practices and adverse reactions.

❑ Assess the client's internal and external exposure to chemicals to determine the risk of adverse reactions. Advise the client how to decrease the risk.

❑ Teach clients to use OTC drugs and other remedies appropriately, safely, and effectively.

❑ Encourage clients to request and maintain an updated drug profile with a pharmacist. The profile should include prescription and nonprescription drugs.

❑ Counsel clients to use OTC preparations only for minor, self-limiting health problems and to discuss their use with a healthcare professional.

❑ Encourage clients who use OTC products regularly, over long periods of time, or in large doses to seek advice from a healthcare provider for supervision of their regimen.

❑ Advise clients to store OTC preparations in a cool, dry, secure place out of reach of persons who could be harmed by them.

❑ Refer clients to a pharmacist if the nurse lacks knowledge or reference materials.

❑ Establish workable contracts, eliminate or reduce barriers to drug taking, and teach about the effects of the drugs to increase motivation, knowledge, compliance, and, ultimately, reliable self-care.

❑ Provide education and reinforce teaching with reference materials.

❑ Provide intermittent support as needed, and assess the client's condition regularly.

❑ Teach the client how to read drug container labels and how to manage side effects.

❑ Refrain from judgmental attitudes or punitive actions, remembering that taking any drug remains the choice of the client or responsible caregivers.

❑ Uphold the client's right to choose to comply or not comply.

The Community as Client

The idea of the community as client is an aggregate approach toward identifying and solving large-scale health problems. The role of the community health nurse (CHN) depends on how a community is defined (eg, a neighborhood composed of census tracts, an ethnic group within a geographic location, or a subpopulation known by their health attitudes, beliefs, or habits). Using epidemiologic methods together with the nursing process, a given community's drug-related problems may be identified and relevant programs planned, implemented, and evaluated. Some ways to assess such problems include:

• Comparing the crime and death rates involving drugs in one community with similar parameters in another community to determine the magnitude of the problem

• Determining the extent to which homeopathy or home remedies are used in a given community versus the use of conventional therapies (OTC and prescribed drugs)

• Examining the effect of toxic industrial effluents (including drug wastes) on the local environment.

Another example of the community as client involves the ethnic or culturally different populations in a given area. When healthcare providers consider the drug-taking practices of these clients, they must be aware of how the clients define a drug, when and how they self-administer drugs, who usually takes drugs, and generally how clients respond to drug therapy. Similarly, the nurse who cares for a client must become familiar with the client's attitudes toward drugs, as well as the common beliefs about health conditions for which drugs are used, especially the major healthcare problems in that community. In some cases, the client may rely on home remedies, homeopathic preparations, and the advice of elders or nonprofessional "specialists" or healers in the community. Knowing who the client is and what resources are available to the community as a whole are important aspects of community-based nursing practice. For further discussion, see Chapter 9.

When drug-related problems occur in a community, the CHN can use specific measures to reduce or eliminate them. These measures include educating the target population, documenting problems to local officials to enhance public awareness and participation, and working with other healthcare professionals to prevent misuse and abuse of drugs in the entire population or in at-risk groups only. Occupational health nurses are often the first to identify drug problems and exposure to harmful chemicals and other environmental pollutants by monitoring employees' healthcare complaints.

Likewise, school nurses may assess a group problem involving drugs by considering variations in students' attendance rates, grades, and absences from school for unexplained reasons. Effective action to solve such community health problems involves a dual approach: the community as a whole and individual members. When drug abuse has been documented in a specific population (eg, early teenagers), parents, teachers, police, and other community leaders may institute a media campaign to publicize the hazards of social drug and alcohol use. In addition to participating in collective action, persons such as the school nurse may also provide one-to-one or small-group education for students who need a personalized approach to drug problems. Community-based nurses should be involved with all members of the community to achieve better health and healthcare for the entire group.

The CHN participates in community programs designed to decrease the incidence of drug abuse and accidental poisoning and to promote the appropriate use of medications in the community.

■ SUMMARY

In response to the increased use of home health care and self-care, nurses are involved with various activities at the local, state, and national level to ensure client access to safe home care. Community health nurses coordinate the client's home care, which may include technical service house calls by contractual agencies to administer drug and other therapies (eg, oxygen, IV fluids, hyperalimentation). The Intravenous Nursing Society has created home care standards in an effort to control and define their scope of practice. Nurses who work in this expanding area require advanced clinical expertise and experience in both high-tech and home care practice. On the national level, nurses are involved in lobbying for clients' access to safe and accountable home health care. The nurse's role as client advocate is crucial in this time of transition from hospital to home-based care, and to managed care.

References

Eisenberg DM, Kessler RC, Foster C, et al. (1993). Unconventional medicine in the United States: Prevalence, costs, and patterns of use. *N Engl J Med, 328*:246–252.

Fugh-Berman A. (1996). *Alternative medicine: What works.* Tucson, AZ: Odonian Press.

Gurwitz H, McLaughlin TJ, Fish LS. (1995). The effect of an Rx-to-OTC switch on medication prescribing patterns and utilization of physician services: The case of vaginal antifungal products. *Health Serv Res, 30*(5):672–685.

Kogan MD, Pappas G, Yu SM, Kotelchuck M. (1994). Over-the-counter medication use among US preschool-age children. *JAMA, 272*(13):1025–1030.

Stehlin IB. (1996). An FDA guide to choosing medical treatments. Internet, http://www.thebody.com/fda/medical.html.

Stuart B, Grana J. (1995) Are prescribed and over-the-counter medicines economic substitutes? A study of the effects of health insurance on medicine choices by the elderly. *Med Care, 33*(5):487–501.

Ullman D. (1995) *The consumer's guide to homeopathy.* New York: Putnam.

Bibliography

Azzarello JD. (1989). Reviewing your patient's medication regimen: A systemic approach. *Home Healthcare Nurse, 7*(6):24–26.

Conn VS, Taylor SG, Messina CJ. (1995). Older adults and their caregivers: The transition to medication assistance. *J Gerontol Nurs, 21*(5):33–38.

Chubon SJ, Schulz RM, Lingle EW Jr, Coster-Schulz MA. (1994). Too many medications, too little money: How do patients cope? *Public Health Nurs, 11*(6):412–415.

Haylock PJ. (1993). Home care for the person with cancer. *Home Healthcare Nurse, 11*(5):16–28.

McPherson ML. (1990). Medicating home health patients: Considerations for the caregiver. *Caring, 9*(1):38–40.

Micozzi MS. *Fundamentals of complementary and alternative medicine.* New York: Churchill-Livingstone.

Ralph IG. (1993). Infectious medical waste management: a home care responsibility. *Home Healthcare Nurse, 11*(3): 25–33.

Starr P. (1982). *The social transformation of American medicine.* New York: Basic Books.

*Recommended for further reading.

For more information and sample tests and activities, refer to Chapter 13 in the Student Workbook for Clinical Pharmacology and Nursing Management, 5th edition, available through your bookstore.

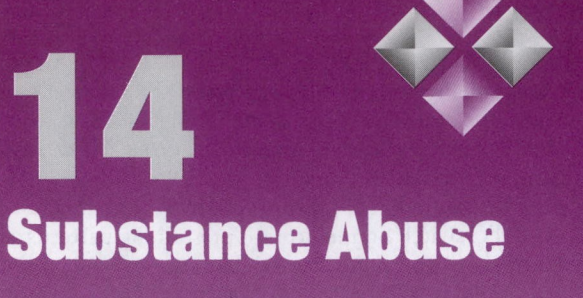

14
Substance Abuse

Throughout history, societies have used pharmacologically active substances for nontherapeutic or recreational purposes. Substance abuse is broadly defined as the use of psychoactive products without medical sanction or contrary to cultural norms. Traditionally, the abuse of substances was motivated by their therapeutic qualities, such as relieving pain or altering mood.

Nature of Dependence and Addiction

To recognize and help substance abusers, one must first understand the use of psychoactive substances in a nontherapeutic way. *Abuse* is the self-directed use of chemical substances for nontherapeutic purposes that does not comply with approved social and cultural norms. Extended abuse tends to interfere with one's biologic, psychologic, and social health. *Addiction* is a behavioral

state characterized by loss of ability to control a drive or craving. Daily life tends to be dominated by the psychoactive agent.

When a person responds to a chemical substance by continuous or sporadic use to experience its pharmacologic effects, the person is said to be dependent on the drug. Two types of dependency exist: psychologic and physical. Psychologic dependence is a compulsion to use a substance to achieve a desired outcome—for example, to avoid anxiety or to feel pleasure. Physical dependence is characterized by an altered physiologic state from continuous use of the psychoactive agent. If use is interrupted, a drug-specific withdrawal or abstinence syndrome results.

When a user must increase the amount of drug taken to achieve the same effects experienced from a previously smaller dose, tolerance to the substance has developed. Tolerance also exists when a specific dose produces a reduced pharmacologic effect (either in intensity or duration) after repeated use. Tolerance does not necessarily mean that the person is physically dependent. According to the *Diagnostic and Statistical Manual of Mental Disorders*, 4th ed (DSM-IV), the diagnosis of substance dependence requires the presence of at least three criteria from the list in Box 14-1.

Cycles of Dependence

With substance abuse, behavior generally reflects a stereotypical pattern of social learning and reinforcement. The rewards of substance use or abuse reinforce and maintain the behavior. Drug use may produce pleasurable effects (a "high"), or it may relieve some unpleasantness, such as high stress or severe pain. In either case, the use of chemical substances is a learned response to certain stimuli. The use persists because it produces a desirable effect. Although drug use seems to help initially, it leads to greater problems and an increased need for more drugs.

The behavior involved in substance abuse becomes a vicious cycle. The person who is vulnerable tries to cope with disequilibrium in social, psychologic, biologic, or environmental influences, but adaptive responses fail to restore balance. The user becomes dependent on drugs to relieve the pain of imbalance. The cycles reflected in drug dependence and addiction may be physiologic, cerebral, social, or psychologic (Fig. 14-1).

The cycle of physiologic dependence and addiction occurs when usual dosages do not have the usual effect and discomfort (physical or psychologic) develops when the substance is withdrawn.

Drugs causing physical dependence cause physiologic imbalance on withdrawal. Abstinence syndromes most often involve signs and symptoms that are the direct opposites of the physiologic effects of the drug of abuse. These effects result from the abnormal physiology that develops in adaptation to the addictive drugs. The effects of withdrawal may be severe enough to be life-threatening.

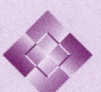

Box 14-1
DSM-IV Diagnostic Criteria for Substance Dependence and Abuse

Substance Dependence

A maladaptive pattern of substance use, leading to clinically significant impairment or distress, as manifested by three (or more) of the following, occurring at any time in the same 12-month period:

1. tolerance, as defined by either of the following:
   a. a need for markedly increased amounts of the substance to achieve intoxication or desired effect
   b. markedly diminished effect with continued use of the same amount of the substance
2. withdrawal, as manifested by either of the following:
   a. the characteristic withdrawal syndrome for the substance
   b. the same (or a closely related) substance is taken to relieve or avoid withdrawal symptoms
3. the substance is often taken in larger amounts or over a longer period than was intended
4. there is a persistent desire or unsuccessful efforts to cut down or control substance use
5. a great deal of time is spent in activities necessary to obtain the substance (eg, visiting multiple doctors or driving long distances), use the substance (eg, chain-smoking), or recover from its effects
6. important social, occupational, or recreational activities are given up or reduced because of substance use
7. the substance use is continued despite knowledge of having a persistent or recurrent physical or psychological problem that is likely to have been caused or exacerbated by the substance (eg, current cocaine use despite recognition of cocaine-induced depression, or continued drinking despite recognition that an ulcer was made worse by alcohol consumption)

Substance Abuse

A. A maladaptive pattern of substance use leading to clinically significant impairment or distress, as manifested by one (or more) of the following, occurring within a 12-month period:
   1. recurrent substance use resulting in a failure to fulfill major role obligations at work, school, or home (eg, repeated absences or poor work performance related to substance use; substance-related absences, suspensions, or expulsions from school; neglect of children or household)
   2. recurrent substance use in situations in which it is physically hazardous (eg, driving an automobile or operating a machine when impaired by substance use)
   3. recurrent substance-related legal problems (eg, arrests for substance-related disorderly conduct)
   4. continued substance use despite having persistent or recurrent social or interpersonal problems caused or exacerbated by the effects of the substance (eg, arguments with spouse about consequences of intoxication, physical fights)
B. The symptoms have never met the criteria for Substance Dependence for this class of substance.

American Psychiatric Association. (1994). *Diagnostic and statistical manual of mental disorders*, 4th ed. Washington, DC: American Psychiatric Association.

The cerebral cycle is the result of central nervous system (CNS) damage from excessive drug use. The damage occurs in the form of reduced mental capacity for regulating and controlling behavior, including a person's ability to make judgments about the drug-taking behavior.

The social consequences of abuse reinforce and maintain drug use. The general social disapproval of drug abuse creates a need to find companions whose moral and social expectations tolerate or reinforce the habit of taking drugs.

Drug abuse often begins with an attempt to relieve psychologic distress. In the psychologic cycle, unpleasant feelings, such as guilt and shame, that result from substance abuse are resolved by taking more drugs. Withdrawal from drugs on which the person is psychologically dependent causes stress that may also produce physical signs and symptoms. These syndromes are general rather than specific to the drug of abuse, and they are usually milder than those caused by physiologic dependence.

Whichever cycle exists—and several may exist simultaneously—the pattern of behavior is predictable and self-perpetuating. Unless intervention is offered, the dependence or addiction worsens.

The likelihood that dependence will develop varies with the person and the situation. Factors contributing to abuse include curiosity, peer pressure, pain, anxiety, fatigue, pleasure-seeking, and boredom. Two recent studies on the use of drugs for the relief of severe, acute pain indicate that dependence is not always inevitable. (The subjects of these studies were veterans of the Vietnam war and victims of physical trauma.) When the source of pain was eliminated, some people no longer needed drugs.

Relation of Potency and Dependence
A positive relation exists between drug potency and addiction. The more potent a dependence-producing agent is and the more pleasure it produces, the more rapidly addiction develops. During the initial period of

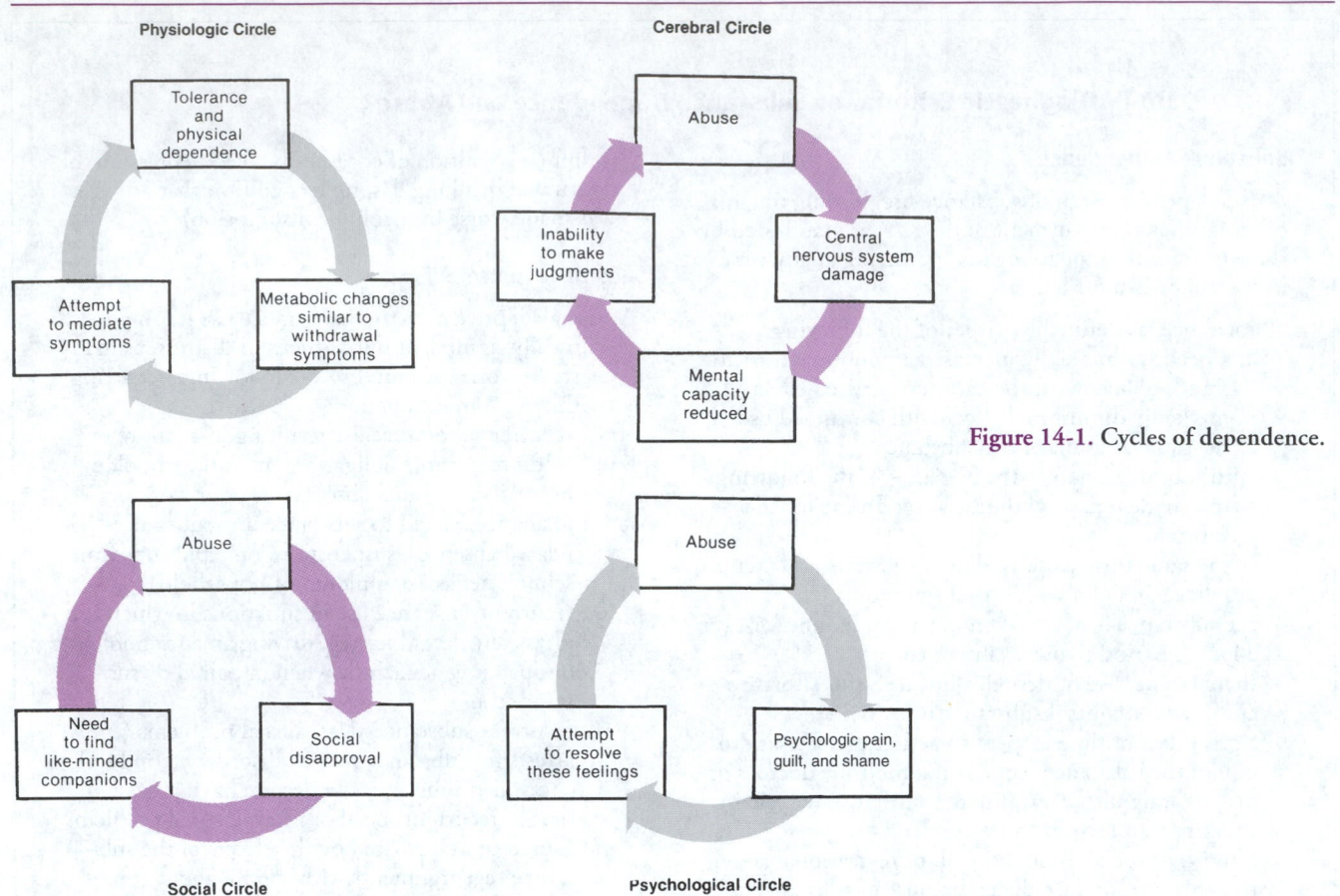

Figure 14-1. Cycles of dependence.

drug abuse, the user can control consumption and the degree of intoxication. Depending on the addictive quality of the substance, the intensity, pattern, and length of time of abuse, and the person's specific psychologic and physical traits, the abuse of a substance can progress to dependence, which then shows the characteristics of a compulsion or craving. Once control is lost through continued abuse, the addiction gains control and dominates the user's life. This fact has implications for treatment because it indicates that removing the "causes" of addiction does not necessarily result in recovery.

Classifications

Dependence and addiction can be classified in various ways. In relation to the manner in which it is acquired, addiction may be therapeutic, epidemic, or endemic.

Therapeutic addiction is a consequence of a medical regimen (iatrogenic), or it is self-established (the client tries to treat his or her own physical or psychologic ailments). This type of addiction commonly occurs among healthcare personnel. Therapeutic addiction is usually not "contagious"—that is, it does not involve others.

Epidemic addiction is the most prevalent addiction in the Western world. It is characterized by direct involvement between an established abuser and a novice.

Epidemic abusers tend to use more than one substance simultaneously.

Endemic addiction occurs when a psychoactive substance is accepted and socially tolerated by the general population. This type of addiction is present within the culture once an addicting substance is generally accepted for pleasure. An example of endemic addiction in the United States is the use of tobacco and alcohol.

Drug abuse may also be classified according to the types of drugs abused. These commonly include CNS depressants (eg, opioids, alcohol) and CNS stimulants (sympathomimetics, hallucinogens, nicotine).

Central Nervous System Depressants

Opioid Analgesics

The primary source of natural narcotics is the poppy *Papaver somniferum*. The milk from unripe seed pods is collected and dried, forming raw opium. Several substances are extracted from opium, two of which fall into the major chemical groups: phenanthrene and benzylisoquinoline. Analgesics and cough suppressants of the phenanthrene group include morphine, codeine, and thebaine; substances in the benzylisoquinoline group do not have the morphinelike effects of the former and are nonnarcotic. Papaverine and noscapine are the major natural alkaloids of the benzylisoquinoline group. Phenanthrenes include opioid analgesics (Table 14-1); their therapeutic use is discussed in Chapter 18.

In addition to natural opioid drugs, several commonly abused semisynthetic and synthetic substances are derived from components of opium or synthesized in the laboratory: heroin, hydromorphone (Dilaudid), oxycodone (Percodan, Percocet), meperidine (Demerol), levorphanol (Levo-Dromoran), and methadone (Dolophine). Although they vary in potency and duration of action, all have effects similar to those of morphine. All but heroin are available for medicinal use.

"Designer drugs" have been developed with heroin-like effects from fentanyl. They include MDMA (Ecstasy), MDE (Eve), MPPP, and MPTP. These substances produce parkinsonian symptoms in some users. MDMA is reported to cause lasting damage to the parts of the brain that produce serotonin.

Illegal (street) drugs are usually marketed as powders diluted with such substances as quinine, starch, sugar, or powdered milk. Potency may vary greatly, a factor in many overdoses when users take their customary dosage of a preparation that is purer than the drugs they habitually use. Sold in small bags, heroin is usually less than 10% pure. Its street names include *scag*, *smack*, *junk*, *horse*, *H*, and *brown sugar*. Morphine is referred to as *cube*, *hocus*, *first-line*, and *morf*.

General Pharmacologic Effects. Opioid analgesics cause short-lived euphoria, drowsiness, lethargy, decreased physical activity, pinpoint pupils, decreased vision, and constipation. The drugs may be taken orally, sniffed, smoked, or injected. Intravenous (IV) injection tends to produce warm flushed skin and a lower abdominal sensation that resembles an orgasm in quality and intensity. This sensation is termed *rush*, *thrill*, or *kick*. The drugs

Table 14-1. Opioid Analgesics

Drug Name	Preparations	Additional Information
Natural Opioids		
morphine	White crystals, injectable forms, hypodermic tablets	One of the most potent pain-relieving drugs available
		Bitter taste, odorless
		Dependence and tolerance develop rapidly.
codeine	Injectable and tablet forms, liquid for antitussive action	Relief of moderate pain
Semisynthetic and Synthetic		
heroin	Bag of powder diluted with quinine, starch, sugar, or powdered milk	White, bitter taste
		Similar in pharmacologic action to morphine
hydromorphone (Dilaudid)	Tablet and injectable forms	Two to eight times more effective than morphine
		Shorter-acting and more sedative effect than morphine
oxycodone (Percodan)	Tablet form; illicitly, tablets are dissolved and injected IV	Relief of pain
		More potent than codeine
		Leads to dependence
meperidine (Demerol)	Tablets, elixir, injectable form	Widely used, effective narcotic analgesic
methadone (Dolophine)	Tablets, liquid, injectable form	Similar in pharmacologic action to heroin and morphine
		Originally an analgesic agent
		Commonly used in drug treatment programs
oxymorphone (Numorphan)	Injectable solution or rectal suppository	As potent as morphine
levorphanol tartrate (Levo-Dromoran)	Oral or parenteral preparation	May produce less nausea and vomiting than morphine
paregoric (Parepectolin)	Liquid tincture	Limited use as antidiarrheal agent
diphenoxylate (in Lomotil)	Tablet and liquid, contains atropine	Definite constipating effect
fentanyl (Sublimaze)	IV injectable	Used only for anesthesia
propoxyphene (Darvon)	Oral preparation	More potent than morphine
		Related to methadone
		Relief of pain

also produce sleep, nausea, vomiting, and respiratory depression. See Chapter 18 for further information about medicinal opioids.

Chronic abusers neglect their health and may become malnourished. Apathy and analgesia lead to untreated injuries and diseases. Sharing injection needles increases the risk of skin abscesses, endocarditis, and blood-borne infections (eg, hepatitis, human immunodeficiency virus [HIV]).

Tolerance and Dependence. Tolerance to opioid analgesics occurs at different degrees of pharmacologic potency. Opioid tolerance is characterized by a generalized decrease in the normal action of the drugs in depressing the CNS. The amount of a drug necessary for a lethal dose is also significantly increased.

The opiate withdrawal syndrome is dramatic to the observer and briefly disabling to the addict. It tends to peak within 72 hours. Provided the user's general physical health is intact, it is probably less serious than that of some other drug groups. However, sudden withdrawal by a person using large doses can be life-threatening. Four phases of the syndrome represent the accelerating intensity of the withdrawal process. Signs and symptoms are both physical and psychological (Box 14-2). Withdrawal is sometimes characterized by tactile hallucinations (the "monkey on your back"). It can cause marked dehydration and weight loss, ketosis, acid–base imbalance, and cardiovascular collapse. The aged and debilitated are at highest risk for death. Withdrawal is immediately reversible by the administration of an opioid. It can be moderated by gradually reducing opioid dosages. Without any treatment, it usually subsides in 7 to 10 days.

Treatment. Detoxification from opioids without drugs ("cold turkey") is not recommended. The Food and Drug Administration (FDA) has developed a legal treatment plan for people addicted to opioids. Medically supervised withdrawal is available in federally designated treatment programs that use methadone. Methadone may also be administered by a physician to a drug-dependent person hospitalized for an illness not related to the addiction. Treatment decreases the severity of withdrawal, but it also prolongs it.

The use of methadone is legal only for detoxification, maintenance, or analgesia. According to FDA regulations, *detoxification* is the use of methadone for medically supervised withdrawal from physical dependence on opioid drugs. Detoxification must be completed within a 21-day period. FDA regulations define *maintenance* as the use of methadone as an oral substitute for morphinelike drugs and heroin for more than 32 days.

Methadone analgesia is designated for clients in advanced stages of illness who suffer intractable pain. These clients must not receive narcotic antagonists or weaker opioid drugs such as pentazocine (Talwin); the administration of such drugs would displace methadone from opioid receptors, causing an increase in perceived pain.

General Central Nervous System Depressants

The psychoactive substances considered to be general CNS depressants are barbiturates, related sedative–hypnotics, benzodiazepines, and alcohol. They promote sleep and reduce anxiety.

Meprobamate (Miltown, Equanil) is commonly used for its antianxiety properties, including muscle relaxation. In addition to its sedative effects, methaqualone (Quaalude, Sopor) has antispasmodic, anticonvulsant, local anesthetic, antitussive, and mild antihistaminic qualities. The benzodiazepines are used to treat alcohol withdrawal syndrome; diazepam (Valium) is the most frequently abused drug in this category. Excluding nicotine, alcohol is the most abused drug available to the public.

General Pharmacologic Effects. The effects of these drugs stem from their depressant action on the CNS. Signs and symptoms of depressant use include sedation, hypnosis, and decreased anxiety. Inhibitions may be reduced before general depression is evident, causing the appearance of stimulation. Toxicity results in stupor and coma. When two or more of these drugs are used together, they interact, heightening the toxic state and possibly causing cardiovascular collapse and respiratory arrest. For example, combining either barbiturates or benzodiazepines with alcohol poses a high risk of death from respiratory failure.

Tolerance and Dependence. Most drugs in this class cause tolerance and dependence (both physical and psychologic). Tolerance may develop rapidly, and the capacity to consume greater dosages reduces the safety

---

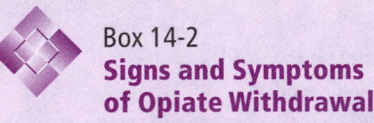

Box 14-2
Signs and Symptoms of Opiate Withdrawal

Phase I: Perspiration, anxiety, restless sleep or insomnia, lacrimation, yawning, rhinorrhea

Phase II: Coryza, severe sneezing, piloerection, abdominal cramps, mydriasis, arthralgia, muscle cramps and twitching, myalgia

Phase III: Nausea, vomiting, anorexia, fever, elevated blood pressure, tachypnea, tachycardia, extreme restlessness

Phase IV: Diarrhea, fetal position, hyperglycemia, dehydration, flushing, hot and cold flashes, insistent drug-demanding behavior

Table 14-2. Barbiturates and Duration of Action

Very-Short-Acting	Short- to Intermediate-Acting	Long-Acting
hexobarbital (Sombulex)	amobarbital (Amytal)	phenobarbital (Luminal)
methohexital sodium (Brevital)	aprobarbital (Alurate)	mephobarbital (Mebaral)
thiamylal sodium (Surital)	butabarbital sodium (Butisol)	metharbital (Gemonil)
thiopental sodium (Pentothal)	pentobarbital sodium (Nembutal)	
	secobarbital (Seconal)	
	talbutal (Lotusate)	

margin between an intoxicating and a fatal dose. Chronic abuse over long periods causes adaptive neuro-physiologic changes (heightened nerve activity) that tend to blunt or negate the effects of the drugs. Abrupt withdrawal results in hyperacuity of all senses and an abstinence syndrome that may be more severe than a narcotic withdrawal syndrome.

Treatment. The life-threatening severity of withdrawal requires gradual, controlled reduction of dosage, using drugs that can stabilize and detoxify the user from the addictive substance. Phenobarbital is the drug of choice to treat abstinence syndromes from all drugs of this class except alcohol.

Barbiturates

Among the drugs classified as barbiturates are pentobarbital (Nembutal), amobarbital (Amytal), and secobarbital (Seconal). They are among the most abused depressants.

General Pharmacologic Effects. Barbiturates exert a calming and sedating effect on the body. They reduce anxiety and motor activity. Depending on dosage, they induce drowsiness, sleep, stupor, or coma. Death may occur from respiratory arrest. Table 14-2 categorizes common barbiturates according to duration of action. Street terms for these drugs include *barbs, blue devils, downers, green dragons, goofballs, yellow jackets, nimbies, pink ladies, rainbows, red devils, reds,* and *stumblers.*

Tolerance and Dependence. Both tolerance and dependence are characteristic of barbiturate abuse. The abstinence syndrome is considered to be one of the most dangerous. Withdrawal is characterized by anxiety, hyperactivity, and seizures (Fig. 14-2).

Treatment. Treatment of overdose focuses on maintenance of vital functions, especially respiration and circulation. Barbiturate abusers should not attempt to detoxify without medical assistance. The drugs must be withdrawn gradually to control the severity of the abstinence syndrome.

Sedative–Hypnotics

Pharmacologic substances in this category (Table 14-3) include chloral hydrate ("knockout drops"), ethchlorvynol (Placidyl), glutethimide (Doriden; street names: *cubes, CD*), meprobamate (Miltown, Equanil), and methaqualone (Quaalude, Sopor; street names: *quads, soapers, sopes*). Most are used medicinally to treat anxiety, insomnia, and muscle spasms. Paraldehyde is a treatment agent for alcohol abstinence syndrome. Chloral hydrate and paraldehyde are seldom used today.

General Pharmacologic Effects. Sedative–hypnotic drugs depress the CNS, including the reticular formation, which maintains wakefulness and alertness. They promote drowsiness and blunted consciousness. They also relieve anxiety. Toxic doses cause stupor, coma, and respiratory depression.

Tolerance and Dependence. Tolerance and both physical and psychologic dependence can develop after repeated use of most of these drugs. Paraldehyde seems to be an exception, but this drug is rarely used on a long-term basis because it is unpleasant to take and causes gastric irritation.

Treatment. Treatment of acute toxicity focuses on maintaining vital functions, particularly respiration. During withdrawal, symptoms such as anxiety, restlessness, and insomnia can be controlled by a gradual reduction in dosage.

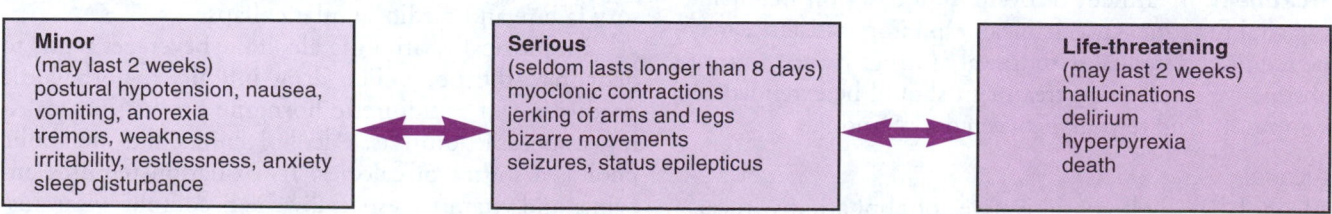

Minor
(may last 2 weeks)
postural hypotension, nausea,
vomiting, anorexia
tremors, weakness
irritability, restlessness, anxiety
sleep disturbance

Serious
(seldom lasts longer than 8 days)
myoclonic contractions
jerking of arms and legs
bizarre movements
seizures, status epilepticus

Life-threatening
(may last 2 weeks)
hallucinations
delirium
hyperpyrexia
death

Figure 14-2. The barbiturate abstinence (or withdrawal) syndrome may be minor or severe, with severe withdrawal leading to possible death.

Table 14-3. Nonbarbiturate Sedative–Hypnotics

Drug Name	Preparations	Additional Information
chloral hydrate	Capsule and liquid	Popular sedative and sleep-inducing drug Combination with alcohol very toxic
ethchlorvynol (Placidyl)	Capsule	Also effective anticonvulsant and muscle relaxant Drug action is rapid and of short duration.
glutethimide (Doriden)	Capsule and tablet	Onset of action is about 30 min and is of long duration (4–8 hr).
meprobamate (Equanil, Miltown)	Tablet	Muscle relaxant; antianxiety agent Anticonvulsant properties
methaqualone (Quaalude, Sopor)	Tablet	Used also as antispasmodic, anticonvulsant, local anesthetic, antitussive, and mild antihistaminic
paraldehyde (Paral)	Colorless liquid	Has been used chiefly in treatment of alcohol abstinence syndromes Unpleasant taste and strong odor make it an unlikely drug to abuse.

Benzodiazepines

Among the benzodiazepines are chlordiazepoxide (Librium), clonazepam (Clonopin), clorazepate dipotassium (Tranxene), diazepam (Valium), flurazepam (Dalmane), and oxazepam (Serax). Newer short-acting benzodiazepines include lorazepam (Ativan), triazolam (Halcion), and alprazolam (Xanax). All benzodiazepines are comparable, but diazepam is the most frequently prescribed by physicians. These drugs are used therapeutically to treat status epilepticus, alcohol withdrawal, and back pain caused by muscle spasm. They are frequently abused for relief of psychologic pain.

General Pharmacologic Effects. The benzodiazepines suppress the CNS, especially the limbic system. They act as anxiolytics, sedatives, and muscle relaxants. Symptoms of intoxication resemble those of alcohol intoxication. Inhibitions are depressed before motor activity. Intellectual function such as foresight and judgment are impaired. As with other CNS depressants, toxic dosages tend to cause stupor, coma, and death from respiratory failure. Cardiovascular collapse can develop.

Tolerance and Dependence. Repeated use of the benzodiazepines causes tolerance and dependence. Diazepam is frequently abused, and dependence may develop from therapeutic use. Withdrawal is characterized by nervousness, tremors, insomnia, and sometimes muscle spasms. Seizures can occur. The signs and symptoms of withdrawal from benzodiazepines tend to be delayed when compared to those from short-acting barbiturates.

Treatment. Treatment of overdose focuses on maintaining vital functions. Mechanical respiratory assistance may be required. Gradual withdrawal of drugs is used to treat abstinence syndromes; treatment should be extended, as symptoms tend to peak between days 5 and 9.

Alcohol

Alcohols are hydroxy derivatives of aliphatic hydrocarbons formed by the fermentation of sugars by yeasts. They are produced naturally from decomposing carbohydrate substances and are well known in history. They have long been used for a variety of purposes, such as foods, medicines, and industrial chemicals. They are useful solvents, fuels, and disinfectants. Ethyl alcohol (ethanol, grain alcohol, ETOH) is the least toxic of the alcohols when taken internally. (For simplicity and consistency in this chapter, the term *alcohol* is used in place of ethyl alcohol, ethanol, or ETOH).

Alcohol is the active pharmacologic component of beer, wine, and other intoxicating beverages. The concentration of alcohol in beverages is sometimes increased by fractional distillation of the ferment, as in the production of whiskey, brandy, and other spirits (Table 14-4). Virtually every human culture has used some form of alcohol in the diet or as a drug. Alcohol is the most prevalent legal drug of abuse of the CNS depressants. Alcoholism is endemic in many countries and is considered one of the most serious public health problems in the United States.

Pharmacodynamics. Alcohol acts primarily as a CNS depressant. It appears to reduce the resting action potential on nerve membranes by decreasing sodium and potassium ion conduction across the cellular membrane. Alcohol first affects the higher functions, particularly learned inhibitions, often producing a temporary increase in activity that has given it an undeserved reputation as a stimulant. In moderate amounts, alcohol functions as a tranquilizer, reducing anxiety and inducing euphoria. As the dosage increases, depression of the CNS is reflected by progressive loss of function: decrease in activity, stupor, coma, and death from respiratory failure and cardiovascular collapse.

Paradoxically, drinking alcoholic beverages tends to dehydrate the body. The drug inhibits hypothalamic production of antidiuretic hormone production, causing noticeable diuresis. Alcohol enters the metabolic pool as a source of calories. Its oxidation requires enzymes and vitamins, especially the B-complex vitamins. Most alcoholic beverages contain few nutrients other than calories, which are generally considered to be

Table 14-4. Composition of Common Alcoholic Beverages

Beverage	Source	Method of Preparation	Alcohol Concentration (Average Range)	Additional Information
Beer	Grain	Treatment with malt to produce sugar, then fermentation with hops (for flavor)	3%–5%	Beer contains carbohydrates and other nutrients. Absorption is relatively slow because of slow gastric emptying.
Wine	Fruits and berries	Fermentation	Up to 14%	Wine contains some vitamins. Dry wines have a higher alcohol content than sweeter wines. Wines made from berries are used as folk remedies for diarrhea.
Sherry wine	Fruits and berries	Fermentation, fortification, addition of brandy, refermentation	18%–20%	
Brandy	Fruits and berries	Fermentation and subsequent distillation	30%–45% (60–90 proof)	Brandy is flavored by volatile substances from the substrates that distill along with the alcohol.
Whiskey (*Spiritus frumenti*)	Grains	Treatment with malt to produce sugar, fermentation, and subsequent distillation	40%–60% (80–120 proof)	Concentration is generally reported as proof, which is equal to twice the percentage of alcohol.
Vodka	Grain or potatoes	Fermentation and subsequent distillation	40%–60%	Vodka was originally produced in Eastern Europe.
Sake (beer)	Rice	Fermentation	14%–16%	Sake was originally produced in Japan.
Sake (liquor)	Rice	Distillation of sake beer	57%–74%	

"empty" calories. Although each gram of alcohol provides 7 kcal of energy, it is not an efficient source of energy. Alcohol increases lipid formation and raises the ratio of high-density lipoproteins to low-density lipoproteins in the blood plasma.

Alcohol is a local irritant and stimulant. Small amounts stimulate intestinal peristalsis and gastric acid secretion. Alcohol is biphasic in many of its reactions. Initially, it lowers the blood pressure by vasodilation (which causes visible flushing). Over time, however, it tends to produce or exacerbate hypertension. Alpha brain waves are slowed and convulsions suppressed immediately, but later, nervous hyperirritability increases the risk of seizures.

Applied topically to the skin or inanimate surfaces, alcohol is an effective disinfectant, provided sufficient time (30 minutes on a clean surface) is allowed for its action. It does not sterilize.

Pharmacokinetics. Alcohol is rapidly absorbed by both the lungs and the gastrointestinal (GI) system. Absorption from the stomach is delayed if ingestion occurs over time ("nursing" a drink) or if there is food in the stomach. Skin absorption is negligible. When infused IV, alcohol is well tolerated. It distributes readily, quickly reaching comparable levels in most tissues of the body. It readily crosses the placenta.

Alcohol is metabolized by the liver, which oxidizes it to acetaldehyde by enzymatic action. Acetaldehyde is rapidly converted to acetyl coenzyme A, which may then enter the citric acid cycle or be used for anabolic reactions that produce cholesterol, fatty acids, and other tissue components. Part of a given dose is metabolized by the microsomal enzymes of the endoplasmic reticulum of the liver. Small percentages (2%–10%) are excreted unchanged by the lungs and kidneys. Alcohol is metabolized at a steady rate that seems not to vary appreciably with changes in the concentration of alcohol in body fluids. A normal adult can metabolize about 10 mL in an hour, roughly the volume in a typical drink (eg, 10 oz of beer, 3–4 oz of wine, 1 oz of whiskey).

Therapeutic Uses. At one time, alcohol was widely used medically as an analgesic, anesthetic, and tranquilizer, but professional use declined with the development of safer and more selective agents. However, alcohol is still used, rarely, to interrupt premature labor, to tranquilize, to sedate or stimulate social interaction in elderly clients, and (in low doses: one drink or less daily) to elevate the level of high-density lipoproteins and decrease the risk of heart disease. Local injections of alcohol are used medically to produce a relatively permanent nerve block to relieve intractable pain or promote peripheral vasodilation (Table 14-5). The drug may be administered IV to boost the caloric value of IV fluids or to suppress chronic severe pain. Alcohol is widely used as a solvent and vehicle for other drugs in the form of elixirs. It is, of course, commonly used by the lay public for its psychoactive effects.

Because all alcohols are organic solvents capable of breaking down toxicodendrol, the molecule responsible

Table 14-5. Medicinal Preparations of Alcohol

Name	Preparation	Administration	Therapeutic Uses
Alcohol for injection	5- and 50-mL vials	Local injection	Long-term nerve block
	5% alcohol with dextrose	IV infusion	Interruption of premature labor
			Control of intractable pain
Elixirs	Aromatic sweetened solutions used as flavored vehicles for medicinal agents	Oral	Depends on medicinal agent involved (eg, elixir of phenobarbital, a CNS depressant used as a sedative)
Tinctures	Alcohol or hydroalcoholic solutions of drugs in 10% or 20% concentration	Oral or topical	Depends on drug involved (eg, tincture of iodine, used as a topical antiseptic)
Fluid extracts	Alcoholic solutions of drugs in 100% concentration	Oral	Depends on drug involved (eg, glycyrrhiza fluid extract, used as a flavoring agent; cascara sagrada extract used as a cathartic)

for the irritant properties of poison ivy, they can be applied topically to treat this condition. Alcohols applied to the intact skin tend to disinfect, dry, toughen, and cool the skin; they are used in preventing pressure ulcers in people with tender moist skin. Mixtures that contain alcohols also act as rubefacients and counterirritants when applied topically.

Adverse Reactions. Like other alcohols, ethanol is a protoplasmic poison that precipitates and dehydrates the protein within cell membranes. It is irritating when applied to denuded skin or mucous membranes. Topical applications of alcohol may also cause undue drying of the skin.

When injected into the tissues, alcohol may cause degeneration of the treated nerves, even when only a temporary nerve block is desired. Concentrated solutions are astringent and can compromise the local blood supply when injected subcutaneously, resulting in tissue necrosis and sloughing. Extravasation of IV solutions is also highly irritating to the tissues.

Systemic cardiovascular effects of alcohol include vasodilation. Conversely, chronic use tends to increase the severity of hypertension. The vasodilating action of alcohol may underlie its aggravation of ear discomfort associated with flying or other reduction of barometric pressure. Nasopharyngeal vasodilation increases congestion in those tissues, blocking the eustachian tube.

The inebriating effects of alcohol are well known. It depresses brain function, abolishing inhibitions and impairing judgment and psychomotor function. In nontolerant people, the clinical effects of alcohol vary proportionately with blood concentration (Table 14-6). People with a tolerance to alcohol may exhibit fewer overt signs and symptoms of intoxication than do naive drinkers with the same blood levels. However, they do

Table 14-6. General Signs of Alcohol Toxicity

Approximate blood alcohol level	Corresponding Urine Levels	Usual Signs and Symptoms
0%–0.10%	0%–0.14%	No overt signs: slight deterioration of performance on tests of specific learned motor and mental skills, decreased feelings of fatigue
0.10%–0.20%	0.14%–0.28%	Alcohol level associated with legal drunkenness; slowing of reaction time, slight incoordination, loss of inhibitions, emotional lability, loss of discrimination
0.20%–0.30%	0.28%–0.40%	Analgesia, staggering gait, slurred speech, confusion, loss of concentration
0.30%–0.40%	0.40%–0.54%	Relative lack of response to stimuli, loss of insight, marked incoordination, stupor
0.40%–0.50%	0.54%–0.66%	Depressed reflexes, coma, anesthesia, subnormal temperature, circulatory collapse
0.50% and above	more than 0.66%	Death by respiratory failure

*The above data apply to nontolerant persons. In tolerant persons, blood levels are characteristically higher before progression of signs and symptoms.

have nervous system impairment, as shown by delayed reaction time, motor incoordination, and abnormal thought processes.

Few overt signs of alcohol toxicity exist until the blood alcohol level reaches 0.10%, the point recognized by most states as legal evidence of intoxication. At this level, motor coordination is impaired. When the blood alcohol level approaches 0.40%, coma occurs; at about 0.50%, respiratory failure tends to develop. Levels above 0.50% are generally believed to be fatal, although these and higher levels are occasionally reported in people with tolerance to the chemical. The IV administration of alcohol can produce intoxication identical to that of oral ingestion.

Except in small doses, alcohol interferes with sexual function and reproduction. Temperate use of alcohol may enhance sexual performance in people unable to function well because of learned inhibitions. However, drinking more than 10 mL hourly tends to erode performance, despite increased sexual desire. Chronic alcoholism alters the balance of sex hormones by increasing estrogen retention and promoting testosterone metabolism. Men become feminized and suffer impotence and relative infertility. Women also experience decreased libido.

Alcohol is teratogenic, and its use by pregnant women seriously endangers the fetus. Because it readily crosses the placenta, the concentration in fetal tissues reflects that in maternal tissues. The drug inhibits embryonic cellular proliferation, causing congenital anomalies and growth retardation. Newborns with full-blown fetal alcohol syndrome exhibit characteristic facial deformities, joint, cardiac, and genital anomalies, and microcephaly. Virtually all such infants suffer permanent mental retardation. After birth, alcohol withdrawal syndrome may be evident in the infant. Alcohol is also carcinogenic: immoderate use increases the risk of developing cancer of the mouth, larynx, esophagus, liver, and lungs.

Adverse Effects in Acute Alcoholism. Pain associated with alcohol ingestion may indicate Hodgkin's disease. The pain occurs at or near the tumor site within minutes of alcohol ingestion. It may be sharp and stabbing or dull and aching. Acute alcoholism is marked by profound CNS depression. Because of the accompanying euphoria, fatigue may be ignored and exhaustion may develop. Convulsions, cardiovascular collapse, and death may occur. Hyperglycemia, acute gastritis, pylorospasm, nausea, vomiting, and dehydration often accompany the acute phase of alcohol abuse. During the subsequent withdrawal (hangover) period, hypoglycemia develops, increasing the headache and malaise caused by residual dehydration and exhaustion. Both alcohol toxicity and withdrawal increase the risk of seizures in epileptics.

Adverse Effects in Chronic Alcoholism. Based on descriptions of the National Institute on Alcohol Abuse and Alcoholism and the National Council on Alcoholism, a person is considered an alcoholic when alcohol use negatively influences or interferes with the activities of daily living in any of the following areas: physical health, emotional health, social health, or employment. Addictive drinking is characterized by an overall loss of control shown behaviorally as preoccupation, compulsiveness, and the tendency to relapse.

Chronic alcoholism shortens the expected lifespan. Leukocyte response to the inflammatory process declines; resistance to infectious disease is reduced. Malnutrition often accompanies this condition, further compromising basic physiologic defenses. The additional calories provided by alcohol may cause obesity. If food intake is reduced to compensate for the calories ingested as alcohol, a general undernutrition can develop. Deficiencies of vitamin B complex are particularly pronounced because the need for these vitamins is increased by alcohol intake. Chronic use of alcohol may also contribute to the loss of bone mass and may promote osteoporosis. Alcoholics may appear many years older than their actual age.

Alcoholism increases the risk of many serious health problems, including gastritis, liver disease, peptic ulcer, pancreatitis, peripheral neuritis, muscle degeneration, hypertension, heart disease, cancer, and dementia (Box 14-3). The liver tends to develop fatty degeneration, with eventual cirrhosis. This process stems from the toxic effect of alcohol and from the nutritional deficiencies that commonly accompany alcoholism. Effects on normal kidneys are less pronounced, but some authorities believe that a high concentration of alcohol in urine damages these organs as well. Alcohol also increases the incidence of seizures in people prone to them. People particularly prone to alcoholism may have a genetic predisposition to dependence because their metabolisms cannot break down alcohol properly.

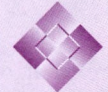

Box 14-3
CNS Syndromes Associated With Chronic Alcoholism

Korsakoff's Syndrome

A personality disorder characterized by amnesia (loss of both long-term and short-term memory), confabulation, psychosis, disorientation, confusion, muttering, delirium, insomnia, illusions, hallucinations, and polyneuritis

Wernicke's Encephalopaphy

An inflammatory, hemorrhagic, degenerative condition of the brain caused by thiamine deficiency and manifested by double vision, involuntary and rapid movements of the eyes, lack of muscular coordination, and decreased mental function

Drug Interactions. Alcohol interacts with many other drugs. Because it stimulates the liver enzyme system, it hastens the metabolism of warfarin anticoagulants and propranolol, decreasing the effectiveness of a given dose. The effects of other CNS depressants are enhanced, particularly in nontolerant persons, causing life-threatening respiratory depression and cardiovascular collapse in naive users. Aspirin and alcohol taken together tend to damage the stomach and can cause active GI hemorrhage. Disulfiram and many medicinal drugs taken concurrently with alcohol can produce a disagreeable reaction characterized by flushing, increased pulse and respirations, nausea and vomiting, headache, dyspnea, and palpitations. Chronic alcoholics are at increased risk of liver damage from acetaminophen.

Precautions and Contraindications. Alcohol should not be applied to extensive or deep wounds because an eschar forms, trapping tissue debris beneath the surface and increasing the risk of secondary infection. Alcohol must be used with extreme caution (if at all) in persons with hypertension, peptic ulcer disease, hepatic disease, extreme obesity, alcoholic myopathy, and pregnancy. People in recovery from alcohol dependency should not receive alcohol. Epilepsy, acute genitourinary infections, and kidney disease are relative contraindications. To avoid wide fluctuations in the blood glucose level, diabetic clients should be cautious in using alcohol.

Alcohol intake in a social setting by normal adults usually does not produce acute intoxication if ingestion is limited to 10 mL or less hourly. When alcohol is administered IV, flow rates must be carefully controlled to prevent inebriation. After an initial loading dose equivalent to 10 mL, the flow rate should be limited to the volume that will deliver 10 mL or less hourly.

Exposure to alcohol fumes should be avoided, because inhalation can deliver a toxic dose to systemic tissues. Death from acute toxicity after exposure to concentrated fumes has been reported.

Tolerance and Dependence. Repeated exposure to alcohol produces tolerance and dependence similar to that of opioid addiction. Alcohol may increase the level of opioid-like alkaloids in the brain. Over time, these produce tolerance or dependence similar to that which develops with prolonged use of opiates. In addition, repeated exposure to alcohol increases the body's capacity to metabolize the substance, thereby requiring higher doses to achieve intoxication. Physical dependence develops when the concentration of alcohol is chronically maintained at high levels.

Tolerance to alcohol produces cross-tolerance to most CNS depressants, including anesthetics. Because large doses of anesthetics are required for surgery, and because of the high incidence of malnutrition and poor resistance to infection, habitual users of alcohol tend to be poor surgical risks.

When alcohol use is suspended, rebound hyperactivity of the CNS precipitates a classic alcohol withdrawal syndrome in predictable stages (Box 14-4). This syndrome, termed "the shakes" by alcoholics, is also known as delirium tremens (DTs).

Treatment. Acute alcohol overdose (most common in naive drinkers) is life-threatening. In addition to support of vital functions, hemodialysis may be necessary to reduce blood alcohol levels rapidly.

Alcohol dependence is treated in two steps: detoxification to eliminate physical dependence and long-term treatment to control psychologic dependence. The primary goal of alcohol detoxification is to prevent or minimize symptoms of the abstinence syndrome. Most treatment programs use some form of drug therapy, usually a benzodiazepine such as chlordiazepoxide or diazepam. Clients who have a history of epilepsy are given phenytoin (Dilantin) to prevent seizures. In addition to drug therapy, diets high in calories, proteins, and fluids are encouraged.

Long-term treatment usually involves group counseling and self-help groups such as Alcoholics Anonymous. Psychologic dependence is much more difficult to manage than physical dependence, and most alcoholics must maintain this treatment for life.

When impulse drinking is a persistent problem, disulfiram (Antabuse) treatment may be used. Disulfiram disrupts the metabolism of alcohol, causing an accumulation of aldehyde in the body. Possibly due to this toxin, the interaction of disulfiram and alcohol causes unpleasant body changes: flushing of the face, throbbing in the head and neck, throbbing headache, hypo-

---

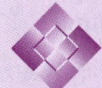

Box 14-4
Stages of Alcohol Withdrawal

Stage 1 develops about 8 hours after beginning abstinence or significantly reducing alcohol use. Symptoms include nausea and vomiting, tremor, a jittery feeling and restlessness, headache, and anxiety.

Stage 2 occurs 8 to 24 hours into withdrawal from alcohol. Symptoms include hyperactivity with more severe tremors, fever, agitation, irritability, and exhaustion. Paradoxically, the client may report insomnia with nightmares, as well as terrifying visual (snakes, bugs) hallucinations. Seizures are most likely to occur in this stage.

Stage 3 begins when the client experiences delirium tremens, a pathologic state of consciousness resulting from interference with brain metabolism and causing confusion and disorientation. Mortality from delirium tremens ranges from 4% to 20%. If the client survives, detoxification lasts 5 to 7 days.

tension, dyspnea and hyperventilation, nausea, vomiting, thirst, chest pain, palpitations, tachycardia, syncope and vertigo, confusion and anxiety, blurred vision, sweating, and weakness. Severe reactions may progress to respiratory depression, cardiovascular collapse, arrhythmias, heart attack, congestive heart failure, coma, seizures, and death. Usually taken daily, disulfiram sensitizes the person to alcohol for 6 to 12 hours. It must never be administered without the client's knowledge. Persons who take disulfiram must avoid contact with any form of alcohol, including vapors (eg, from cosmetic lotions or rubbing alcohol) and cooking ingredients (eg, fermented vinegars, creme de menthe). For more information on disulfiram, see Appendix.

■ SUMMARY

Ethyl alcohol, produced by the fermentation of sugars by yeasts, is the active ingredient in wines and beers. Alcohol is a potent CNS depressant with tranquilizing, hypnotic, and anesthetic properties. Its margin of safety is narrower than that of many newer depressant drugs that have replaced alcohol for most medicinal uses. Alcohol is generally toxic to most tissues and can produce both acute and chronic medical problems. Acute toxicity can cause death from cardiovascular collapse and severe CNS depression. The drug is associated with both tolerance and dependence. Chronic alcoholism predisposes the body to degeneration of the nervous system, liver, pancreas, heart, and other organs. It is an important risk factor for certain forms of cancer, hypertension, and peptic ulcers. Chronic alcoholics tend to develop malnutrition, cirrhosis of the liver, other serious medical problems, and dementia. Alcohol use during pregnancy poses a serious risk of congenital malformations to the fetus as well as mental and growth retardation.

❖ NURSING MANAGEMENT: ALCOHOL ABUSE

Acute Alcohol Toxicity. Acute alcohol toxicity may be life-threatening, especially in a naive drinker with no acquired tolerance to the drug. It is treated with hemodialysis to reduce blood alcohol levels. Vital functions (respiration and circulation) must be supported. In addition, the client may be physically exhausted, chronically malnourished, and overcome by shame and guilt.

As blood alcohol levels decline and the severe CNS depression decreases, the client may exhibit hostility or aggression. Paraldehyde or tranquilizers may be prescribed or restraints used to control the client's behavior. Alcohol blood levels may rise after discontinuation of hemodialysis (due to movement of the drug from tissue depots into the bloodstream), adding to the depressant effects of such medication and increasing the risk of serious depression.

Some clients receiving treatment in acute care facilities for alcohol toxicity may have career, family, and legal problems. For this reason, and because of the guilt and shame associated with alcoholism, clients usually experience considerable stress during treatment. The success of follow-up care may be influenced by the nurse–client relationship developed during the crisis period. The nurse must strive to be nonjudgmental and accepting while meeting the client's many needs for nursing care.

Chronic Alcohol Dependence. Habitual ingestion of alcohol usually results in the development of tolerance and physical dependence. In the absence of psychologic dependence, support through withdrawal corrects the problem. Psychologic dependence is what makes recovery from alcohol dependence difficult.

Chronic alcoholics are likely to have multiple serious health problems. The drinker who maintains a nutritious diet may become obese because his or her total caloric intake is excessive. More often, food intake is reduced and the drinker is chronically malnourished, predisposing him or her to infection (especially pneumonia), cirrhosis of the liver, and central and peripheral nervous system degeneration.

Habitual alcohol users who are treated for acute toxicity are less likely than naive users to exhibit life-threatening depression but are more likely to develop withdrawal symptoms as drug levels decline. During the abstinence period ("drying out"), the client should be observed for tremors, restlessness, agitation, and fright arising from hallucinations. Seizure precautions should be taken. Small frequent doses of mild tranquilizers or treatment with clonidine (Catapres) may be prescribed to control withdrawal symptoms. The client should be weaned gradually from these drugs after the acute phase of withdrawal.

Hidden Alcohol Dependence. Alcohol withdrawal may occur in clients who enter the hospital for treatment of a condition unrelated to alcohol use or abuse. Persons who are alcohol-dependent are usually reluctant to reveal this fact. They may delay hospitalization as long as possible, attempt to take alcohol into the facility, or arrange for it to be brought in by visitors. The nurse should be alert to indications of hidden alcohol dependence: restlessness and agitation that develop after several hours in a controlled setting, or sudden insistence by the client on leaving the facility. Alcoholic beverages in the client's possession on admission may alert the staff to potential problems. (When deprived of alcohol, the dependent person may ingest mouthwash, shaving lotion, or any other substance containing alcohol.) Clients whose behavior changes noticeably after seeing visitors may have received alcoholic beverages during the visit.

Example of Nursing Process and Alcohol Abuse

A 45-year-old female is admitted to the hospital with a primary diagnosis of GI bleeding secondary to alcohol abuse. She presents as a confused, somewhat restless woman who is experiencing periodic hallucinations. No family members accompany her, although she is married. Her physical appearance is that of an undernourished, unkempt woman with dermatitis and petechiae on the face and arms. A strong alcohol odor is evident.

Assessment Data

Alcohol odor

Bleeding attributed to alcohol abuse

Hallucinations

Restlessness

Confusion

Alcohol abuse

Nursing Diagnosis	Intervention	Goals and Outcomes
Altered Perception: Hallucinations, related to CNS overactivity due to alcohol withdrawal	Arrange for someone to remain with the client at all times. Furnish the client with information about her surroundings, explaining that unreal sensory perceptions are the result of drug withdrawal. Offer emotional support and reassurance that the abnormal sensations will not persist indefinitely.	The client will accept the explanation of hallucinations; she will not experience panic.
Ineffective Individual Coping, related to alcohol abuse	When the client's condition is stabilized, explore with her the patterns of and reasons for her alcohol abuse. Advise the client of the risks of continued alcohol use. Advise the client about community resources available for assistance should she decide to decrease her use of alcohol (eg, Alcoholics Anonymous, community treatment programs). Teach the client alternative coping techniques for stressful situations.	The client will accept the need to decrease her reliance on alcohol; she will contact a source of help before discharge from the hospital.

Whenever a chronic alcohol-dependence problem seems likely, the nurse should discuss it openly with the client, stressing that alcohol use in combination with other drugs required for treatment can be dangerous. In addition, withdrawal symptoms should be identified, and the client must be informed that these can seriously complicate recovery. Only if all the facts are known can the healthcare team successfully manage the client's treatment.

When clients are assured that the healthcare team will meet their needs, they are often relieved to acknowledge the problem. In any case, the physician must be alerted to facts that point to dependency as a prob-

lem and must be consulted regarding changes in the treatment regimen.

Alcohol Withdrawal and Follow-up Care.
Acute alcohol withdrawal is treated symptomatically and by administering sedatives, IV fluids, and replacement nutrients (vitamins and minerals). Clonidine may be used to decrease hypertension, heart rate, and nausea and vomiting. Clients in acute withdrawal need constant monitoring and emotional support. To minimize visual hallucinations, the client's environment should be kept lighted.

The nurse who can establish a therapeutic relationship with the alcoholic client is in an excellent position to promote action toward resolution of this health problem. After treatment in a healthcare facility, most clients have gotten through the worst of the withdrawal period. Receptive clients should be referred to available treatment programs. These may range from short-term residential programs to outpatient facilities. Self-help groups modeled after Alcoholics Anonymous are effective in promoting long-term control.

Clients known to have an alcohol-dependence problem need a careful general health assessment, with special attention given to evidence of malnutrition, peptic ulcer disease, cancer, and hypertension. Such clients are at high risk for infections and delayed healing and require excellent physical and psychologic supportive care (see "Example of Nursing Process and Alcohol Abuse").

Alcohol Education Programs. Education of the public about the uses and abuses of alcohol is vital for long-term control of alcohol dependency. Introduction to alcoholic beverages is considered a rite of passage to adulthood in many modern subcultures. Children should be acquainted with the facts about alcohol before they reach the age when they are likely to be introduced to the drug. Although alcohol use by minors is illegal, exposure to alcoholic beverages usually occurs at a relatively early age—often well before puberty. Alcohol education programs, therefore, are more effective when presented in elementary school. Scare tactics should be avoided, and both the beneficial and harmful effects of the drug should be taught. It may be best to include alcohol in a program in which all drugs of abuse are discussed, along with their potential to produce dependency.

Education in parenting skills is of fundamental importance for preventing drug dependence. People who have grown up with a healthy self-image and with self-confidence are least likely to need the chemical crutch of psychotropic drugs.

Nurses and other healthcare personnel must warn women of childbearing age to avoid alcoholic beverages during pregnancy. The risk of fetal alcohol syndrome is directly related to the amount of alcohol used by the mother. Any use of alcohol during pregnancy is considered unsafe.

Abstinence and Temperance. Clients with a family history of alcohol dependence may be at increased risk for dependence because their physiologic reactions to alcohol are more blunted than are those of people not related to alcoholics. They should be alert to the indications of developing dependence. Complete abstinence may be advisable.

Diabetics may include one daily alcoholic beverage in their diet, provided it is computed at the proper exchange value. Because these beverages contain few nutrients and many calories, ample vitamins and minerals should be provided by the rest of the diet.

Management of Hangovers. Clients who seek advice on managing hangovers can be advised to eat food and drink fluids to restore hydration, raise blood glucose levels, and maintain proper nutrition. A mild analgesic such as acetaminophen may be recommended to relieve headache. The significance of hangovers as indications of excessive drinking should be pointed out, and clients should be encouraged to evaluate their use of alcohol critically.

Central Nervous System Stimulants

Central nervous system stimulants include the amphetamines, cocaine, and hallucinogens. Amphetamines and cocaine are sympathomimetic (adrenergic). Street names include *rush, flash, speed, crack, double cross, uppers, pep pills, lightning,* and *truck drivers.*

Amphetamines

Selected amphetamine drugs are listed in Table 14-7. Amphetamine-related stimulants include methylphenidate (Ritalin), benzphetamine (Didrex), chlorphentermine (Pre-Sate), clortermine (Voranil), diethylpropion (Tenuate, Tepanil), fenfluramine (Pondimin), dexfenfluramine (Redux), mazindol (Sanorex), pemoline (Cylert), phendimetrazine (Plegine, Melfiat, Bacarate, Statobex, Tanorex, Trimstat, Trimtabs, Phenzine, Phendiat), phenmetrazine (Preludin), and phentermine (Ionamin, Wilpowr). They are psychostimulant drugs that were

Table 14-7. Principal Amphetamines Available in the U.S.A.

Generic Name	Trade Name	Slang
amphetamine complex (amphetamine and D-amphetamine resin)	Biphetamine	
amphetamine combined	Obetrol, Delcobese	
D-amphetamine plus amobarbital	Dexamyl	
D-amphetamine plus prochlorperazine	Eskatrol	
dextroamphetamine sulfate	Dexedrine, Ferndex	Dexies, oranges, orange hearts
dextroamphetamine hydrochloride	Daro	
dextroamphetamine tannate	Obotan	
methamphetamine hydrochloride (desoxyephedrine hydrochloride)	Desoxyn, Methampex	Meth, crystal whites, speed
racemic amphetamine sulfate	Benzedrine	Bennies, peaches

originally used as nasal decongestants, appetite suppressants, and narcolepsy treatment agents.

In some cases, people become amphetamine abusers after using them sporadically for specific purposes. Dieters use amphetamines to lose weight; students take them to stay awake studying for examinations; truck drivers use them to avoid falling asleep at the wheel. Amphetamines continue to be used therapeutically to treat obesity and in children with hyperkinetic behavior due to minimal brain damage. Amphetamines paradoxically act as calming agents in these children.

General Pharmacologic Effects. Amphetamines and related stimulants raise systolic and diastolic blood pressure and increase heart rate. High dosages can provoke tachyarrhythmia. The drugs can reduce intestinal absorption by slowing peristalsis, causing constipation and delayed gastric emptying. The metabolic rate and oxygen consumption increase, and the CNS is markedly stimulated.

A toxic dose of stimulants leads to anxiety, agitation, fever, and insomnia. Some users react with panic or delirium. Other signs and symptoms include headache, diaphoresis, nausea, vomiting, diarrhea, and abdominal cramps. Excessive cardiovascular stimulation leads to increased heart rate with palpitations, arrhythmia, and hypertensive crises. Death may result under conditions of extreme heat or excessive physical activity. Toxic signs of chronic high-dose stimulant abuse include compulsive and repetitive body movements, bruxism, and facial grimacing. The initial sense of well-being may be replaced with violent, angry, and aggressive behavior. Paranoia and delusions are common, and hallucinations occur. Sleep deprivation from the use of stimulants may cause visual hallucinations.

Tolerance and Dependence. Tolerance to amphetamines develops rapidly, increasing the risk of a toxic reaction. Gross physiologic changes do not occur during withdrawal from stimulants. Symptoms include prolonged lethargy, sleep disturbances, and depression. Withdrawal is not as severe as that from CNS depressants, nor does it produce life-threatening physiologic side effects.

Treatment. Amphetamine toxicity is treated by acidifying the urine to promote excretion. Phenothiazines, haloperidol, or tricyclic antidepressants are used to treat mental problems from chronic abuse.

Cocaine

Cocaine is an alkaloid derived from the leaves of the South American coca plant. It is the strongest natural stimulant available and has become a popular recreational drug. Street names include *big C, coke, crack, flake, gold dust, nose candy, rush, snow,* and *white.*

General Pharmacologic Effects. The paradoxical effects of topical cocaine in blocking nerve transmission make it a medically useful local anesthetic (see Chap. 18).

Systemically, cocaine's initial action on the brain affects the cortex, producing restlessness, excitement, intense euphoria, and heightened mental acuity. It is valued by users for its pleasurable effects and also because it reduces appetite and increases energy. In toxic dosages, cocaine can cause nausea, vomiting, abdominal pain, headache, rapid pulse, uneven respirations, chills and fever, mydriasis, exophthalmos, and formication (a tactile hallucination that ants are moving over the skin). Severe overdose causes delirium, Cheyne-Stokes respiration, seizures, and unconsciousness. Death, when it occurs, is caused by respiratory arrest. The drug is dangerous and frequently leads to acute illness requiring emergency treatment. A few thousand cocaine-related deaths are reported annually.

When abused, cocaine is injected, smoked, or snorted (applied to the nasal membrane). It creates paranoia, anxiety, and agitation. Chronic snorting causes marked local vasoconstriction, inadequate perfusion, and tissue erosion. Because of the anesthetic effect of cocaine, the abuser is unaware of tissue damage. The resultant perforation of the septum is difficult to correct surgically.

Abusers sometimes purify cocaine through heat processing with a solvent such as ether, a process called *freebasing*. Freebasing poses a fire hazard, and abusers have sustained serious burns. A further refinement of freebasing creates a highly purified, inexpensive variety of cocaine known as *crack*. Smoking crack produces euphoria within 8 seconds, followed by depression.

Tolerance and Dependence. Cocaine rapidly promotes dependence and addiction. It is estimated that more than 25 million people have tried cocaine, of whom about 10% have become compulsive users. The cycle of intense highs and crashing depressions reinforces the user's need for increasing the frequency of use. Experts debate whether tolerance to cocaine exists and tend to conclude that it does not.

Treatment. Treatment of cocaine toxicity is similar to that for amphetamine and related drug toxicities. In addition, total body cooling using mechanical methods may be necessary to control high fever. Cocaine is thought to cause no withdrawal symptoms, so the treatment of chronic abusers focuses on reducing psychologic dependence. This does not make treatment easier: generally, psychologic dependence is more difficult to overcome than physical dependence.

Hallucinogens

Hallucinogens alter thoughts and generate perceptions and feelings that are not experienced in any normal state of sleep or alertness. They are also known as *psychedelics* because they can induce a state characterized by distortion of reality. The effects of psychedelics are unpredictable, and responses may vary with each use.

Hallucinogens in common use include mescaline, psilocybin, psilocin, lysergic acid diethylamide (LSD),

2,5-dimethoxy-4-methylamphetamine (DOM, DOA ["dead on arrival"], STP ["serenity, tranquility, peace"]), dimethyltryptamine (DMT), diethyltryptamine (DET), aa3-methoxy-4,5-ethylenedioxyamphetamine (MMDA), phencyclidine (PCP), and cannabinoids. Although some are derived from natural substances, all can be made synthetically.

Mescaline is derived from the peyote cactus (*Lophophora williamsii*) found in Mexico. In natural form, mescaline is produced by slicing the peyote cactus buttons into discs and drying them. The discs are chewed or ground into a powder and ingested. The powder is sometimes made into a tea to make it more palatable. Street names include *beans*, *buttons*, *cactus*, *mesc*, and *mescal*.

Psilocybin and psilocin are natural drugs derived from the mushroom *Psilocybe mexicana*. Slang terms include *magic mushrooms* and *mushrooms*.

The hallucinogen known as STP is a semisynthetic substance that produces hallucinations and also has many of the same effects as amphetamines. It is chemically related to mescaline and amphetamines. One effect of the drug is uncontrolled psychic energy with perceptual distortions.

The hallucinogen DMT is found in plants indigenous to South America and the West Indies. This drug and DET have brief durations of action (about 30 minutes). They are available in a liquid form that is applied to cigarettes, marijuana, or parsley and then smoked.

The hallucinogen MMDA is chemically related to STP, mescaline, and amphetamines. It is available as a powder, tablet, or liquid and may be taken orally, snorted, or injected IV. In street jargon, MMDA is known as "the love drug."

These four substances—STP, DMT, DET, and MMDA—are termed *psychotomimetic* or *psychotogenic* substances because their effects are similar to those of psychosis.

General Pharmacologic Effects. The above group of hallucinogens stimulate the peripheral sympathetic nervous system, resulting in dilated pupils, elevated heart rate, blood pressure, and body temperature, lowering of simple reflex thresholds, muscular weakness, tremor, and nausea. Effects on the brain cause visual illusions, hallucinations, and perceptual changes. Not uncommon is synesthesia, a distortion of perception characterized by 1) displacement of a perception from the site of stimulation to another site, 2) a secondary sensation accompanying an actual perception, or 3) the perception of stimulus of one sense as a sensation of a different sense (eg, a sound produces a sensation of color).

Tolerance and Dependence. Although the repeated use of hallucinogens produces a high degree of tolerance to the behavioral effects of the chemicals, normal sensitivities return after the drug is discontinued. Withdrawal seems to cause no abstinence syndrome, indicating that physical dependence probably does not develop. Users can, however, become psychologically dependent on these drugs.

Treatment. With hallucinogens, treatment is most commonly required when acute toxic reactions precipitate psychotic episodes. Continuous orientation and reassurance are frequently successful in "talking down" a user on a "bad trip." When these methods are unsuccessful, medication with pentobarbital is usually effective.

Lysergic Acid Diethylamide (LSD)

The hallucinogen LSD, a derivative of lysergic acid, is produced by a natural fungus found in rye. The purified drug may be in liquid or tablet form. Amounts as small as 1/700 millionth of a person's body weight can produce psychedelic effects. The drug is 100 times as potent as psilocybin and 4,000 times as potent as mescaline.

Experiences with LSD vary, reflecting the setting and the user's personality. On a "good trip," the most common effects are visual and perceptual changes in light, color, texture, and shape. Time and space also seem altered. The user may experience delusions of grandeur, feelings of omnipotence, or a sense of loss of control. "Bad trips" result in intense anxiety, fear, and traumatic visions.

The LSD experience has three stages:

- CNS overactivity, which may produce discomfort, including anxiety and nausea. This stage may last 2 hours.
- The actual psychedelic experience, lasting 6 to 12 hours
- Waves of normal consciousness, ending with feelings of fatigue and relaxation.

Flashbacks of the psychedelic experience may recur at any time for up to 2 years. Flashbacks are recurrences of the psychedelic effects without renewed exposure to the drug. The phenomenon of flashbacks implies that CNS changes caused by the drug tend to persist. Lysergic acid does not appear to cause physical dependence. Treatment of toxicity is as described for other hallucinogens.

When sold in thin squares of gelatin, LSD is called *windowpane*. When sold on small pieces of paper, it is known as *blotter acid*. Other street terms for LSD include *acid*, *beast*, *blue heaven*, *brown dots*, *California sunshine*, *chocolate chips*, *haze*, *mellow yellows*, *orange mushrooms*, *orange wedges*, *paper acid*, *sugar*, *sunshine*, *white lightning*, and *yellows*.

Cannabinoids

Cannabis is a plant found in the temperate and tropical zones of the world. The pharmacologically active chemical in cannabis is delta-9-tetrahydrocannabinol (THC). All parts of the plant contain cannabinoids, but the flowering tops have the highest concentration. A purified derivative, dronabinol (Marinol) has been approved by the FDA for medicinal use.

Cannabis is sold on the street primarily as marijuana, hashish, or hashish oil. Marijuana, which resembles tobacco, is made by drying and chopping the leaves and tops of the cannabis plant. It is smoked in cigarette form (*joints* or *roaches*) or through pipes, or it may be ingested. Marijuana is known as *Acapulco gold, gold, grass, hay, hemp, J, Jane, Mary Jane, Panama red, pot, reefer, smoke,* and *weed.*

Hashish, the dried resinous secretions from cannabis flowers, is significantly more potent than marijuana: the THC content may be two to 10 times that of marijuana. Hashish is smoked or ingested. It is referred to as *hash, kif, black Russian, quarter moon,* or *soles.* Hashish oil is a concentrated form of cannabis produced by a repeated extraction process that results in a dark viscous oil with a concentration of THC four to 10 times that of hashish. A few drops may be placed on cigarettes and smoked. It can also be mixed with less potent marijuana to enhance its quality. Less common is oral ingestion.

General Pharmacologic Effects. Cannabis in low dosages tends to produce euphoria and a sense of well-being, followed by a dreamy state of total relaxation. Sensory perceptions are altered and enhanced; time and space seem to expand. Visual, auditory, and tactile senses are enhanced. Taste is more acute, and food cravings frequently occur ("the munchies").

In moderate dosages, reactions to THC are intensified, exhibited as rapid emotional changes, impaired memory, alterations in self-image, and dulled or short attention span. Toxic doses may result in panic reaction, hallucinations, loss of personal identity, delusions, and psychosis. Symptoms subside when the drug is eliminated from the body.

Somatic effects of cannabis include bronchodilation, increased heart rate and blood pressure, and markedly injected conjunctivae. Other signs and symptoms include dry mouth, giddiness, loss of coordination, and cold extremities.

Tolerance and Dependence. It is unclear how or if users develop tolerance to cannabis. Some evidence supports the existence of withdrawal symptoms in chronic heavy users. However, no pattern of physical dependence has been well defined. Some users report abstinence symptoms, including loss of sleep, irritability, restlessness, decreased appetite, weight loss, hyperactivity, and diaphoresis.

Treatment. Acute adverse reactions to marijuana are uncommon, but when they occur they are treated as described for other hallucinogens. Chronic users (*pot-heads*) develop a syndrome characterized by intellectual impairment, inability to work, and social dysfunction. To what degree this results from permanent CNS impairment or to lost learning opportunities in youth is unknown; probably both factors are involved. Asiatic countries with long histories of marijuana abuse are now recognizing this as a serious social problem. (Earlier, life expectancy was so short that abusers did not live long enough to develop full-blown chronic toxicity.) Because no effective treatment of this syndrome has been identified to date, these countries are focusing on prevention of marijuana abuse as the only effective remedy.

Phencyclidine (PCP)

Phenycyclidine is a psychogenic drug with both amphetamine- and anesthetic-like properties. Once used as an anesthetic, it fell into disfavor due to frequent negative reactions. It is now used in veterinary medicine. A popular drug of abuse, PCP is easily manufactured. It is a white crystalline solid that can be dissolved in water or alcohol for administration. It may be snorted or smoked (via a treated marijuana cigarette). Street names include *angel dust, peace pill, surfer, killer weed, hog, rocket fuel,* and *elephant tranquilizer.* When sold, it is sometimes misrepresented as THC or mescaline.

Phencyclidine produces both depressant and stimulant effects. Symptoms of intoxication with doses as low as 5 mg include drowsiness, ataxia, nystagmus, flushing, agitation, hyperreflexia, diaphoresis, miotic pupils, catatonic rigidity, and excitability. Moderate doses (5–10 mg) produce stupor, coma, vomiting, fever, repetitive motor activity, and myoclonia. High doses (10 mg or more) result in prolonged coma, which can last from 12 hours to several days. In addition, flushing, fever, diaphoresis, and vomiting may increase. Convulsions, lack of peripheral sensation, and hypertension complete the clinical picture of PCP poisoning.

Opinions vary as to the safest intervention for PCP intoxication. Generally accepted treatment includes gastric lavage, urine acidification, and the use of diazepam for sedation, if required. If a combination anxiety and depression reaction occurs, haloperidol is preferred over diazepam. Although PCP leaves the body in 3 to 4 days, a residual psychotic reaction may persist. Long-term use is thought to dull intellectual functioning, resulting in a "burned-out" personality.

Inhalant Vapors

The inhalation of certain vapors (sniffing) causes intoxication. This practice has been popular among adolescents, possibly because these substances are more readily available to them than are other drugs of abuse. Substances producing intoxicating vapors include gasoline, paint thinner, aerosol sprays, glue (the most frequently used), and solvents such as toluene. The contents of these products vary, and their effects can range from disorientation to coma after prolonged exposure. Effects commonly include lightheadedness, weakness, delirium, nausea, headache, syncope, hypotension, vasoconstriction, and tachycardia.

Volatile nitrites marketed as room deodorizers may also be abused. Referred to as *poppers* because of the sound created by crushing the capsules before inhaling the fumes, these products are sold under such names as *Ban Apple Gas, Toilet Water, Bullet, Rush*, and *Heart-On*. Adverse reactions to chronic abuse of vapors are not well understood, but liver damage has been reported.

Nicotine

Nicotine, the active ingredient in tobacco, is considered the most widespread, costly, and physically addictive substance of abuse in the United States. Despite extensive campaigns to educate the public about the harmful effects of smoking, more than 50 million adults are dependent on nicotine. Nearly half a million deaths annually are attributed to tobacco-related diseases, including lung and heart diseases and cancer. Tobacco is most commonly smoked, but it is also chewed (chewing tobacco) and applied to the mucous membranes (snuff).

General Pharmacologic Effects. Nicotine causes complex changes in the body, with both stimulant and depressant phases of action. The nicotine-stimulated release of epinephrine from the adrenal medulla accelerates the heart rate and elevates the blood pressure. Small amounts of nicotine stimulate the ganglionic cells of the peripheral nervous system; larger doses first stimulate, then block, transmissions.

Nicotine stimulates the CNS and can provoke respiratory excitation and vomiting. Cardiovascular responses to nicotine include vasoconstriction, tachycardia, and an increased cardiac workload. Stimulation of the parasympathetic nervous system increases tone and motor activity in the GI tract, occasionally resulting in diarrhea.

Adverse effects of nicotine on the body include vasoconstriction and stimulation of abnormal (cancer) cell growth. In pregnant women who smoke, constriction of placental blood vessels is believed to underlie the high risk of early labor and low birth weight in newborns. The risk of congenital hearing defects is also higher in babies exposed to nicotine in utero (*Science News*, 1993).

Tolerance and Dependence. Tolerance and dependence develop with chronic nicotine use. On withdrawal, smokers experience such symptoms as irritability, hostility, depression, and difficulty concentrating. These symptoms can last for several days after cessation of smoking but resolve without drug therapy. Cessation of smoking may also be followed by upper respiratory tract soreness caused by the regrowth of cilia that had been destroyed by cigarette smoke. Former smokers report that the craving for tobacco never entirely disappears and is activated by the smell of smoke.

Treatment. Several products are available (either over-the-counter or by prescription) to help reduce the symptoms of withdrawal from nicotine. These products provide controlled dosages of nicotine to wean the user from the drug. A chewing gum containing nicotine has been marketed, but the dosage is difficult to regulate. Most smokers use enough of the gum to provide their usual dosages of nicotine. Topical patches have been more successful. These are marketed in various strengths. The FDA recently approved a nicotine nasal spray.

Caffeine

Caffeine and related xanthines are found in chocolate and in many beverages. Caffeine is the major pharmacologic agent in coffee, tea, and cola beverages. Refined caffeine is added by bottlers to other carbonated beverages, including some derived from natural fruit juices. (The bottlers claim that caffeine enhances flavor, although taste tests do not bear this out.) Caffeine is also marketed in over-the-counter preparations such as No Doz.

Caffeine is not generally recognized as a drug of abuse. However, excessive dosages may be used to maintain alertness (eg, by students cramming for tests and by long-distance truck drivers). Sleep deprivation associated with the use of excessive caffeine may cause visual hallucinations.

Caffeine decreases fatigue, increases alertness, and in low doses enhances the performance of previously mastered psychomotor tasks. In large doses, caffeine impairs psychomotor performance. Irritability, trembling, and insomnia tend to develop. After ingesting a cup of coffee, glycogen is moved from storage and converted into glucose, causing a pronounced rise in blood glucose level and an increase in energy.

Many chronic users become physically or psychologically dependent on caffeine. In some people, an abstinence syndrome develops when use is interrupted. Withdrawal can cause fatigue, sleepiness, and a severe (hypoglycemic) headache. (If coffee is taken only once or twice daily, these headaches tend to occur at the time of day coffee is habitually ingested.) The abstinence syndrome seldom lasts more than 1 or 2 days. No treatment is required, but eating may help resolve the headache.

For more information on caffeine, see the section on xanthine drugs in Chapter 37.

Substance Control

There are no legal controls on caffeine or the substances that generate intoxicating vapors. Controls on alcohol are imposed by local governments (states, towns, or boroughs). Except for legislation regulating the age for drinking alcohol, restrictions vary greatly from place to place. Similarly, legal controls on tobacco are mainly proscriptions on the sale of tobacco products to minors. The federal government has passed several acts to control the use of other drugs of abuse (see Chap. 2).

Substance Abuse and Reproduction

The chronic use of drugs is associated with many reproductive problems. In both sexes, marijuana damages chromosomes, posing a risk of congenital defects in children. Although the body seems able to repair some of the damage when drug abuse is discontinued, it is uncertain to what extent normal gametes are restored.

Children exposed in utero to high levels of drugs causing physiologic dependence are physically dependent at birth. The severity of the withdrawal syndrome is directly related to the drug dosages in the mother before parturition. Neonates exposed to cocaine in utero exhibit signs and symptoms of cocaine toxicity at birth.

Nicotine use during pregnancy increases the risks of premature birth and low birth weight. It is believed that vasoconstriction, an effect of nicotine, damages the placenta and impairs its function. Children of mothers who use alcohol are at risk for fetal alcohol syndrome (see Chap. 10), which is marked by facial deformities and mental retardation.

In addition to the direct effects of drugs on gametes and fetuses, substance abuse is associated with a lifestyle that poses risks of blood-borne and sexually transmitted infections that can affect unborn children.

Drug Abuse and AIDS

No discussion on substance abuse would be complete without mentioning the connection between substance abuse and the international epidemic of human immunodeficiency virus (HIV) infection. The needle-sharing practices of IV drug users are a principal avenue of transmission of this virus and other blood-borne pathogens (eg, those causing hepatitis and bacterial endocarditis). Once users are infected with HIV, whether or not they develop AIDS, they are a source of infection to others with whom they share needles, to sexual partners, and (for women) to their unborn children.

Substance abuse may suppress immune functions, increasing the likelihood that exposure to a given pathogen will produce illness. Thus, a substance abuser who is also HIV-positive is more likely to develop AIDS, and to develop it more quickly, than is a nonuser. The risk of AIDS is thought to be one reason for the increased number of IV drug abusers who are seeking treatment for substance abuse.

■ SUMMARY

Many substances are abused for pleasurable effects. Substance abuse has a major impact on the biologic and psychosocial aspects of the user and society. Acute life-threatening illnesses can result from use by the naive user and by overdose in any user. Chronic abuse increases the risk of many serious diseases. Many drugs of abuse cause physical and psychologic dependence and abstinence syndromes on withdrawal. Chronic abusers of some drugs never cease to crave the substance, even after long periods of abstinence. Intravenous injection by drug abusers is a major risk factor for HIV infection. Recognizing the signs and symptoms of drug abuse and effectively treating it requires an understanding of the cycles of dependence, the pharmacologic effects of drugs, and the treatment modalities available.

❖ NURSING MANAGEMENT: SUBSTANCE ABUSE

Because the nursing needs of a client who willfully or indiscriminately abuses potentially harmful drugs are numerous and complex, nurses must be aware of their values and attitudes toward substance abuse when establishing a therapeutic relationship. In addition, accurate information about current trends in substance abuse, including an understanding of the legal issues that define the scope of the problem, will help facilitate nursing care.

Despite wide-ranging educational campaigns, substance abuse remains a persistent and serious problem. More effective approaches are needed; perhaps promotion of lifestyles that provide natural "highs" is needed. For instance, endogenous opioids are secreted in response to stimuli such as vigorous exercise, exchanges of affection, and successful accomplishments. Of equal importance is the example set by role models. Nurses should encourage parents to be aware of how their behavior influences their children. The drug habits of significant others (parents, peers) are particularly important to adolescents.

Various community resources are available to the drug abuser. Nurses must be familiar with the goals of and acceptance criteria for specific programs so they can refer clients to the most appropriate agencies. Some organizations have outreach workers available to assist clients in acute distress and to establish contact with clients before their discharge from acute care settings.

Many complex and sometimes obscure reasons underlie clients' decisions to change habits that have compromised their health. It may take repeated drug-induced crises or a serious threat to health from excessive alcohol consumption or cigarette smoking before a client is ready to change. Whatever the motivation, a supportive, nonjudgmental nurse-counselor is in a position to provide the impetus for change.

NURSING PROCESS
ASSESSMENT

In acute care institutions, familiarity with the physiologic, psychologic, and social changes that accompany drug abuse enables the nurse to identify abusers or clients who are at high risk for abuse. Accurate nursing histories must include data regarding the client's previous drug exposure, including recent or habitual use of drugs of abuse. Drugs used recently may not have been cleared from the body, posing risks for interactions with prescribed drugs. A client who has abused drugs chronically in the past may be at risk for recurrent dependence if exposed again to these drugs. In addition, hypo- or hypersensitivity to drugs such as anesthetics can be a problem.

Overall assessment of the client's status should include all aspects of the following functional health patterns:

- Health perception/health management (awareness of current health status, factors that influence health behavior, overall history of health practices)
- Physiologic homeostasis (physical examination and general description of the client, including assessment of cardiovascular, neurologic, respiratory, mental, musculoskeletal, integumentary, and GI systems)
- Elimination (daily bowel and bladder practices)
- Nutrition and metabolic condition (appetite, weight, height, normal nutritional intake, status of mucous membranes, dental needs)
- Activity and exercise (usual level of activity, impact of present illness on activities of daily living)
- Sleep/rest (usual sleep patterns, use of sleeping aids)
- Cognitive and perceptual conditions (level of understanding, ability to comprehend, sensory responses and deficits, presence of pain or discomfort)
- Self-perception/self-concept (general appearance, body image, sense of control)
- Roles and relationships (support systems, family constellation, sick role, communication skills, interpersonal relationships)
- Sexuality and reproduction status (reproductive history, incidence of sexual abuse or trauma, history of sexually transmitted diseases)
- Coping and stress tolerance (recent significant life changes, situational and maturational changes, coping strategies—positive/negative)
- Values and beliefs (religious preference, source of strength, life goals, health beliefs).

NURSING DIAGNOSIS

Applicable nursing diagnoses may include:

- Ineffective Individual Coping
- Self-esteem Disturbance
- Body Image Disturbance
- Altered Nutrition: Less than Body Requirements
- Ineffective Breathing Pattern, related to drug-induced respiratory depression
- Sensory/Perceptual Alterations: Visual, Auditory, or Tactile Hallucinations
- Pain, Paresthesia, related to peripheral neuropathy secondary to chronic alcoholism
- Knowledge Deficit, related to substance abuse

PLANNING

The long-term goal is cessation of substance abuse. Physical dependence can usually be resolved within a few days or weeks. Psychologic dependence, however, is persistent and commonly leads to recurrent abuse, often when the client leaves the healthcare setting and returns to the environment and companions associated with substance abuse.

Intermediate nursing care goals are to preserve life during acute overdose, improve coping strategies, improve self-concept, improve nutrition, decrease or eliminate hallucinations, eliminate or alleviate pain, and educate clients about substance abuse.

INTERVENTION

For a listing of interventions for substance abuse, see Box 14-5. These interventions are measurable and can be implemented in the community as well as in institutional settings.

Helping clients cope with drug treatment regimens in acute and long-term rehabilitation programs is a significant role of the nurse. Care involves counseling and supportive interventions for the secondary effects of chronic substance abuse (eg, malnutrition, impaired immunity, skin infections, blood-borne infection).

During acute drug toxicity (including overdose), managing the client's physiologic crisis or physical and behavioral actions can be demanding. When homeostasis or vital functions are disrupted, they must be maintained. A generally calm, soothing, one-to-one interaction in an environment with minimal stimuli is usually effective for stimulant overdose. When more than one drug has been taken, care is complicated by their interaction and by the varying rates at which they are eliminated. The nurse should be able to assess the client's overall condition and implement emergency procedures to reverse toxic reactions and the effects of withdrawal.

With CNS depressants, a primary concern is to support respiration; mechanical respiratory assistance may be required. In CNS stimulant abuse, the client may be at risk for hyperpyrexia. The fever may be high enough to require cooling blankets or other antipyretic treatment.

To prevent accidental injury during psychotic episodes, emotional support, reassurance, and sometimes restraints are needed. Seizures must be prevented or controlled. During such crises, clients require continuous monitoring and individual care.

Follow-up care involves measures to correct nutritional deficits, counseling about substance abuse, and referral to treatment programs or self-help groups, such as Alcoholics Anonymous, for long-term help.

Client Education. In all areas of practice, nurses have the opportunity to provide health information about the long-range and immediate risks to health posed by substance abuse. Information is considered to be most effective when given at an early age, with

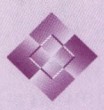

Box 14-5
Nursing Interventions for Substance Abuse

Prevention

- Promotion of good parenting
- Client education
- Family education
- Community education
- Screening for identification and risk
- Advocacy and actions to change policies and legislation

Intervention

- Health, mental status, psychosocial, and addictions assessments
- DSM-IV diagnostic assessments
- Referring clients to treatment based on placement criteria
- Safe detoxification from alcohol and other drugs
- Physical examinations
- School-based interventions

Treatment

- Lecturing on various topics
- Individual counseling
- Group counseling
- Family counseling
- Case management

Aftercare

- Education about and provision of self-help group resources
- Relapse prevention education
- Follow-up
- Community resources for recreation and exercise

Adapted from Allen KM. (1996). *Nursing care of the addicted client.* Philadelphia: Lippincott-Raven Publishers.

emphasis on maintaining a healthy body. Giving literature to clients offers them an opportunity to choose healthy lifestyles and to minimize the risks to health of inappropriate use of chemicals.

OUTCOME EVALUATION

Data required for evaluation relate to the absence or presence of continued substance abuse, resolution of episodes of crisis, coping strategies used by the client, communications about self-concept (including verbal comments and body language), weight as compared to desired weight, complaints of pain, and client ability to repeat information conveyed during teaching sessions.

References

Mom's smoking linked to hearing defect. (1993). *Science News, 144*:23.

Bibliography

*AIDS file: Support urged for needle exchange programs. (1993). *AJN, 93*(12):12.

Antai-Otong D. (1995). Helping the alcoholic patient recover. *AJN, 95*(8):22–30.

*Belcaster A. (1994). Caring for the alcohol abuser. *Nursing '94, 24*:56–59.

*Bower B. (1994). Alcoholism exposes its "insensitive" side. *Science News, 145*:118.

*Bower B. (1993). Smoke gets in your brain: Warning: Cigarettes may be hazardous to your thoughts. *Science News, 143*:46.

*Casey D. (1993). The greatest gift of all. *AJN, 93*(9):46.

*Cigarettes: Are they doubly addictive? (1994). *Science News, 145*:296.

Department of Health and Human Services. (1991). *Drug abuse and drug research III* (DHHS publication No. ADM 91-1704). Washington DC: U.S. Government Printing Office.

*Drugwatch: Alcoholism and cognitive dysfunction. (1995). *AJN, 95*(8):51.

*Ethical dilemmas: Alcohol on the physician's breath. (1995). *AJN, 95*(1):68.

Martinez R. (1990). Alcoholism and society. *Emerg Med Clin North Am, 8*(4):903–912.

*Raloff J. (1994). Threat from passive smoke is upgraded. *Science News, 145*:373.

*Raloff J. (1994). What's in a cigarette? *Science News, 145*:30.

Seachrist L. (1995). Nicotine plays deadly role in infant death. *Science News, 148*:39.

*Seachrist L. (1995). Smoking depletes vitamin C from mom, fetus. *Science News, 147*:310.

*Smoking withdrawal and sleepiness. (1994). *AJN, 94*(8):52.

*Soloway RAG. (1993). Emergency nursing: Street-smart advice on treating drug overdoses. *AJN, 93*(9):65.

*Wilson S. (1994). Can you spot an alcoholic patient? *RN, 57*(1):46–51.

*Recommended for further reading.

For more information and sample tests and activities, refer to Chapter 14 in the Student Workbook for Clinical Pharmacology and Nursing Management, 5th edition, available through your bookstore.

15
Toxicology

Toxicology is the study of the effects of chemicals on biologic systems, with emphasis on the mechanisms of harmful effects of chemicals and the conditions under which harmful effects occur. Although toxicology embraces a variety of specialized fields, environmental, economic, and forensic branches are the major divisions of this science.

Environmental toxicology is concerned with toxic agents that influence the health and safety of people in their environment, in the atmosphere, and in food and drink. Environmental toxicology also studies the effects on humans of exposure to toxic chemicals.

Economic toxicology deals with the effects of toxic chemicals on plants and animals as they affect economic values. Study in this area has led to the development of insecticides, food additives, food preservatives, and pesticides.

Forensic toxicology studies the degree of damage to humans caused by exposure to specific quantities of a toxic substance. This branch of toxicology also deals with legal issues related to chemically induced illness or death.

In all three divisions of this field, scientists study the effect of toxic substances on humans, their environment, and all living creatures. Toxicology has enabled scientists to determine the fine line between a therapeutic dose of a chemical agent and a lethal dose.

Access Routes of Toxic Substances

A chemical's toxicity is determined by the nature of the substance, the dose, the susceptibility of the recipient, biologic factors, genetic factors, and the route of administration. Toxins come in contact with the human organism by various routes, including percutaneous, gastrointestinal (GI), inhalation, and parenteral (Fig. 15-1).

Percutaneous Route

Humans are most commonly exposed to toxins of all kinds through percutaneous, or skin, contact. Toxic matter penetrates the skin more or less rapidly depending on the substance. For example, gases generally pass freely through the skin. Liquids move across the membrane with less ease, and solids that are insoluble in water are least likely to penetrate the epidermal tissue.

Factors such as pH, extent of ionization, molecular size, and water and lipid solubility influence the transfer of chemicals through the skin. Local factors, such as temperature and blood flow to the site, affect the rate of absorption and, therefore, the percutaneous toxicity of potent chemicals.

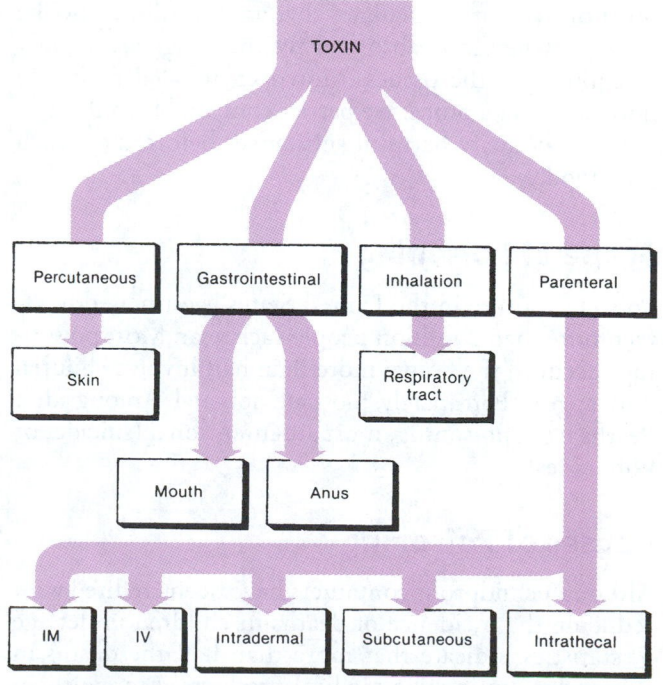

Figure 15-1. Routes by which toxins come in contact with humans.

Gastrointestinal Route

Poisons can enter the body through the GI tract via the mouth or the anus. The level of toxicity depends on the amount of substance absorbed from the mouth or GI tract. Chemicals tend to cause local irritation and tissue damage before exerting a systemic effect. The toxicity of orally ingested chemicals also depends on pre-existing conditions in the GI tract. For example, toxic substances taken when there is food in the stomach tend to be less potent than those taken when the stomach is empty. An additional factor influencing GI toxicity is the nature of pre-existing stomach secretions and the presence of hydrochloric acid. After absorption, the liver detoxifies many substances before they reach the general circulation.

Parenteral Route

Entry by the parenteral route refers to the introduction of substances into the body by means of injections, thereby circumventing body orifices. The most common parenteral routes of administration are intramuscular, intravenous, intradermal, intrathecal, and subcutaneous. Because these methods bypass the body's protective membranes, their potential for toxicity is greater. High tissue concentrations of a chemical can be produced rapidly by parenteral administration, so these are the most hazardous routes for administering medicinal drugs. Natural toxins affecting the body by the parenteral route include insect and snake venoms.

Inhalation Route

Atmospheric toxins enter the body through inhalation. To enter the respiratory tract, poisons must be in the form of gases or particulates that are not filtered by the airways. Chemicals absorbed by the lungs are rapidly distributed to the tissues. Moreover, inhaled toxins do not encounter a protective barrier comparable to the liver that can detoxify harmful substances before they reach the blood.

Scope of Poisoning

Poison exposure in the United States is estimated to affect more than 2 million people each year. Most poisonings occur in the home; more than half involve children under age 6. Fortunately, most are nonfatal. Among adult deaths from poisoning, most are intentional (suicides or homicides).

Causes of Poisoning

Although childproof containers have been credited with reducing the incidence of deaths in children under age 5, statistics indicate that more than half the deaths in this age group involve medical products. Among them are analgesics and antipyretics (eg, aspirin, acetamino-phen), vitamin and mineral supplements (especially therapeutic dosage preparations), and psychotropic drugs (amphetamines, antidepressants, barbiturates, benzodiazepines, cocaine, opioids). The latter are the most common drugs involved in adult nonaccidental ingestions.

Of the numerous nonmedicinal chemicals prevalent in the environment, a small fraction accounts for most episodes of poisoning. The most frequent offenders are household cleaning substances and cosmetics and personal care products. Other common causes of poisoning include heavy metals; toxic plants; paint and stripping agents; insect and snake bites; hydrocarbons (fuels and solvents); bacterially contaminated foods; insecticides and pesticides; art, crafts, and office supplies; gases and vapors; adhesives and glues; deodorizers; and polishes and waxes.

Poison Management

Acute poisoning results from exposure over a short time to toxic amounts of a chemical. It is characterized by signs and symptoms of acute illness and is often life-threatening. Therefore, it is usually a medical emergency that requires accurate knowledge and an immediate response. The basic steps in poison management are to provide first aid, remove and eliminate the poison, administer an antidote, and prevent future poisoning.

Chronic poisoning is the development of illness as a result of prolonged exposure to relatively low levels of a toxin that gradually accumulates in the body. Signs and symptoms are those of chronic illness. Substances causing chronic poisoning include alcohol, tobacco, and heavy metals such as lead and mercury. (Alcohol and tobacco are discussed in Chap. 14).

Poison Control Centers

The science of toxicology and the techniques used in chemical emergencies are constantly evolving, making up-to-date and reliable information essential. The most reliable information about poisoning emergencies is generally available through an established network of regional poison control centers across the United States, Canada, and Mexico. These centers (usually located in medical center emergency care units) maintain telephone hotlines 24 hours a day and serve as resources for emergency medical advice about poison treatment (see Box 15-1 for guidelines on emergency telephone advice). The front pages of most telephone books list local poison information centers with emergency numbers. Lists are also given in *Taber's Cyclopedic Medical Dictionary* (including centers in Canadian provinces and Mexico) and in the *Physicians' Desk Reference*. However, because telephone numbers may change, these reference works do not always contain the most current information.

Poison control centers use various reference sources when responding to inquiries. These include Poisondex

Information System, Drugdex Information System, and Identidex. Poisondex is computerized and provides on microfiche the world's most complete listing of product ingredients. It is updated every 3 months.

Medical Management

First-aid treatment of acute poisoning should be started as soon as possible. Laypersons or emergency medical personnel can, with information and direction from poison control centers, initiate treatment. The client is usually admitted to an emergency care unit for follow-up treatment, where supportive care to maintain vital functions is available. The poison may be removed by such measures as cleansing showers, gastric lavage, catharsis, diuresis, or hemodialysis. Antidotes (if any) are administered. Some toxins (eg, acetaminophen) cause delayed reactions; in such cases, the client is admitted to a hospital unit for further treatment. Finally, causes of the poison episode should be explored and steps taken to prevent recurrences.

■ SUMMARY

Toxins come in contact with the human body through various routes, including percutaneous, GI, parenteral, and inhalation. A poisoning emergency requires accurate knowledge and quick responses. Current information can be obtained from poison control centers maintained in many North American medical centers. First aid is administered as soon as possible, with direction from the poison control center. Vital processes must be maintained. Most poison victims are seen in emergency medical care units; some are admitted to the hospital. Treatment steps include the dilution, removal, and elimination of the poison and the use of an antidote. The key component in the treatment of poisoning is prevention through education.

Lead Poisoning

To illustrate the problems associated with environmental pollutants, lead poisoning is discussed here as a prototype. Exposure to lead in the environment is difficult to avoid. As a heavy metal, lead (Pb) is distributed from automobile emissions, in water supplies, and from industrial pollutants. Lead-based paints were used in households before 1940 and in playgrounds even more recently. Pesticide residues in tobacco and foodstuffs contain lead.

Many older buildings have water systems that use lead pipes; leaching of metal in these systems is enhanced by acid water (a consequence of acid rain). Newspaper print, ceramic glazes, decals used to decorate glass, and urban dust also contain lead. Therefore, although the amount of lead residues in people varies, most people in developed countries are exposed to the metal. Lead in any amount has no positive function in the body.

Lead poisoning is most dangerous in children, due to its harmful effect on the growing brain. This form of poisoning also is most likely to occur in small children, who may ingest substances such as paint, a common source of lead.

Pathophysiology

The amount of lead absorbed into the body depends on the person's general nutritional status and age (younger children absorb lead more than older children) and the size of the lead particles absorbed. The lead level determined through serum analysis represents the balance between the lead present in bones and tissues and that which is excreted. Lead absorbed in the bloodstream may be deposited in the kidney, brain, or bone marrow. Because of its chemical similarity to iron, lead may displace the iron in red blood cells and lead to anemia. Other body systems damaged by lead include the GI tract and the central nervous, reproductive, immune, endocrine, and cardiovascular systems.

Signs and Symptoms

An early sign of lead poisoning (plumbism) is an elevated level of free erythrocyte protoporphyrin (FEP), which represents the final link in hemoglobin synthesis. Normally, the blood level is 50 µg/dL or below. When FEP combines with iron, a red blood cell forms. The relation between iron and lead and hemoglobin synthesis is significant in screening and diagnosing plumbism. If the body is deficient in iron, the FEP level is elevated. A lack of available iron results from poor nutrition, malabsorption, blood loss, or displacement of iron by the chemically similar element lead. Levels of FEP approaching 200 µg/dL generally indicate anemia; levels above 200 µg/dL are caused by lead poisoning.

Symptoms of lead poisoning may range from none to serious ones that reflect the site of tissue absorption of the lead. Mild toxicity causes fatigue, mood swings, loss of appetite, malaise, pallor, restless sleep, irritable behavior, and (in children) developmental delays. Vomiting, abdominal pain, ataxia, weakness, clumsiness, alterations in the level of consciousness, and acute encephalopathy indicate serious lead poisoning.

A positive diagnosis of plumbism exists when:

- Two successive venous Pb levels are 70 µg/dL or more, with or without symptoms
- The FEP level is 250 µg/dL or more and the venous Pb level is 50 µg/dL, with or without symptoms
- The FEP level exceeds 109 µg/dL and there is an elevated venous Pb level (30 µg/dL or more) with symptoms

- The venous Pb level exceeds 49 μg/dL with symptoms and there is evidence of toxicity (eg, abnormal FEP level, positive results from provocative chelation).

Treatment

Chelation therapy is used to mobilize the lead for potential excretion. Three agents used for this purpose are calcium disodium edetate (CaEDTA), D-penicillamine (PCA), and 2,3-dimercaptopropanol or British anti-lewisite (BAL).

Table 15-1 lists the schedule for chelation based on symptoms and lead levels. Chelation injections are painful; therefore, they are usually prepared with procaine to minimize discomfort. An oral medication, succimer (Chemet), may be used for severe lead poisoning in children. The drug is given in a 19-day course in children with blood lead levels exceeding 45 μg/dL.

Lead is removed most easily from the soft tissues of the body, whereas deposits in bone are more resistant to removal. Mobilization of heavy metals from bone is unpredictable. As long as the metal is contained within the

---

Table 15-1. Chelation Choices in Lead Poisoning Based on Symptoms and Lead Level

Clinical Presentation	Treatment	Comments
Symptomatic: encephalopathy present	BAL 450 mg/m²/d CaNa$_2$-EDTA 1,500 mg/m²/d	Start with BAL 75 mg/m² IM every 4 h. After 4 h, start continuous infusion of CaNa$_2$-EDTA 1,500 mg/m²/d. Continue therapy with BAL and CaNa$_2$-EDTA for 5 days. Interrupt therapy for 2 days. Treat for 5 additional days, including BAL if blood Pb remains high. Initiate other cycles depending on blood Pb rebound.
Symptomatic: encephalopathy absent	BAL 300 mg/m²/d CaNa$_2$-EDTA 1,000 mg/m²/d	Start with BAL 50 mg/m² IM every 4 h. After 4 h, start CaNa$_2$-EDTA 1,000 mg/m²/d, preferably by continuous infusion, or in divided doses IV (through a heparin lock). Continue therapy with CaNa$_2$-EDTA for 5 days. Discontinue BAL after 3 days if blood Pb < 50 μg/dL. Interrupt therapy for 2 days. Treat for 5 additional days, including BAL if blood Pb remains > 50 μg/dL. Repeat cycles depending on blood Pb rebound.
Asymptomatic before treatment, measure venous blood lead	BAL 300 mg/m²/d CaNa$_2$-EDTA 1,000 mg/m²/d	Start with BAL 50 mg/m² IM every 4 h. After 4 h, start CaNa$_2$-EDTA continuous infusion, or in divided doses IV (through a heparin lock).
Blood Pb: ≥ 70 μg/dL		Continue treatment with CaNa$_2$-EDTA for 5 days. Discontinue BAL after 3 days if blood Pb < 50 μg/dL. Initiate other cycles depending on blood Pb rebound.
Blood Pb: 56–69 μg/dL	CaNa$_2$-EDTA 1,000 mg/m²/d	Give CaNa$_2$-EDTA for 5 days, preferably by continuous infusion, or in divided doses (through a heparin lock). Alternatively, if lead exposure is controlled, give CaNa$_2$-EDTA as a single daily outpatient dose IM or IV.
Blood Pb: 25–55 μg/dL Perform CaNa$_2$-EDTA provocation test to assess lead excretion ratio (μg Pb/mg EDTA)		Initiate other cycles depending on blood Pb rebound.
If ratio > 0.70	CaNa$_2$-EDTA 1,000 mg/m²/d	Treat for 5 days IV or IM, as above.
If ratio 0.60–0.69	CaNa$_2$-EDTA 1,000 mg/m²/d	Treat for 3 days IV or IM, as above.
Age < 3 years of age		
Age > 3 years of age	No treatment	Repeat blood Pb and FEP, and CaNa$_2$-EDTA provocation test periodically.
If ratio < 0.60	No treatment	Repeat blood Pb and FEP, and CaNa$_2$-EDTA provocation test periodically.

Adapted from Piomelli S, Rosen JF, Chisolm JJ, Graef JW. (1984). Management of childhood lead poisoning. *J Pediatr, 105:*527.

bone tissue, little danger exists, but gradual or intermittent release may occur. For this reason, blood levels of lead must be monitored over time to detect the need for further treatment.

Because chelation may damage the kidneys, clients must be well hydrated and renal function must be monitored throughout treatment. Because this therapy can also deplete the body of calcium, clients must be monitored for signs of hypocalcemia.

The anemia that frequently accompanies plumbism must be treated, but iron-replacement therapy is contraindicated during chelation therapy. Children commonly remain on long-term iron therapy after completing treatment for lead toxicity.

Prevention

Prevention of additional exposure to lead usually requires collaboration by several agencies. Guidelines are delineated locally for the required environmental investigations and interventions. Permanent removal of hazards in the home is of primary importance, especially when children are involved. Clients and family members must learn how to avoid future poisoning episodes.

▪▪ S U M M A R Y

Lead poisoning is a prototype for diffuse environmental pollution and the diagnosis and treatment of chronic poisoning. Lead reaches the environment by many routes and from many sources. Chronic exposure leading to elevated blood levels can cause illness and permanent damage. Like many pollutants, lead is stored in tissue depots and can reenter the blood, posing a continued risk. Clients must be monitored for long periods and may require retreatment. Successful treatment requires education to decrease the risk of repeated toxicity from renewed exposure.

Other Environmental Toxins

In addition to lead, mercury and other metals can contaminate the environment and cause serious poisoning. The organic substance methylmercury is one of the most potent toxins. Its effects in humans are usually permanent, causing irreversible damage to the central nervous system (CNS). Inorganic mercury (Hg) in the form of mercury salts (eg, mercury chloride) is less hazardous because of its low solubility, although it is toxic to the kidneys. Mercury contaminates the environment from natural and industrial sources. Acid rain leaches mercury from the soil into fresh water supplies. From there, it enters the food chain. Although eventually the metal reaches the sea, high concentrations of mercury in ocean waters usually result from industrial pollution.

In addition to heavy metals, a multitude of chemical products—medicines, caustics, solvents, insecticides, herbicides, and plastics—are produced by modern technology. Unless incinerated (a process that destroys some but not all pollutants), these substances are eventually disseminated into the environment and, to some degree, into humans.

Toxins in Healthcare Settings

Chemical hazards to healthcare personnel include disinfectants, laboratory reagents, and medicinal drugs (see Chap. 7 for a discussion of hazardous medicines). In surgical suites, personnel are at risk for chronic toxicity from volatile anesthetics, which increase the incidence of cancer, spontaneous abortion, stillbirth, birth defects, and hepatic and renal disease. Immediately after exposure to these anesthetics, healthcare personnel may experience impaired psychomotor function. To minimize these risks, the National Institute of Occupational Safety and Health has established standards for operating room ventilation exhaust systems.

The use of methylmethacrylate poses other risks for operating room personnel. This gluelike substance is used to bond implants such as hip prostheses. It must be compounded from a liquid and a powder during a surgical procedure just before its use. Employees exposed to the vapors of methylmethacrylate may experience local irritation of the respiratory mucosa and may face an increased risk of cancer.

Ethylene oxide (EtO) is a colorless gas that can be found as a liquid or vapor and has an etherlike odor. In acute care settings, it is used to sterilize items that cannot withstand steam or the intense heat of sterilization. It is highly toxic if inhaled or absorbed systemically or if it comes in contact with skin or mucous membranes. Other hazardous disinfectants include alcohols, halogens (chlorine, iodophor), phenols, quaternary ammonium compounds, and aldehydes (glutaraldehyde, formaldehyde). Exposure to the aldehydes poses the greatest toxic risk.

Prevention of toxic levels of exposure is the key to reducing hazards in the workplace. Systems and procedures designed to reduce environmental levels of offending chemicals must be properly maintained and consistently used.

▪▪ S U M M A R Y

Healthcare personnel and their clients are at risk for toxic exposure to chemicals used for disinfecting and sterilizing the environment and equipment, and for diagnosing and treating disease. Prudence dictates caution, respect, and continued research to minimize risks.

❖ NURSING MANAGEMENT

Nurses active in poison control centers are responsible for responding to calls from the community about first-aid measures, providing information about product contents to identify toxins, and educating the public and other healthcare professionals about poison control and safety. Because many nurses involved in the field of toxicology believe there is a need for specialization, they are designing a curriculum to prepare toxicology clinicians.

During the confusion and emotion of a medical crisis, telephone contact is sometimes disrupted abruptly. For this reason, the healthcare professional answering a call in the poison control center should first obtain the telephone number and address of the caller. If the call is subsequently interrupted, contact can be re-established or emergency medical help dispatched.

In a crisis, the management of poisoned or exposed clients requires poise and skill. Telephone intervention must defuse the crisis and avoid panic. Calm and clear questions and repeated instructions are essential (see Box 15-1).

When initial client contact occurs in the emergency department, healthcare personnel can make first-hand assessments, which are easier than telephone contacts. Conversely, because the client may not have received previous first-aid care, treatment often has been delayed.

Chronic poisoning is likely to present as a collection of sometimes vague symptoms of illness. Seldom is it a medical emergency. However, proper diagnosis and treatment are essential to prevent or minimize permanent damage, which can include severe neurologic impairment.

NURSES' ROLE IN POISON PREVENTION

The public must be informed and aware if the incidence of toxicologic emergencies is to be reduced. Poison control centers provide an assortment of tools that can be used by nurses in various clinical settings. Because many poisonings occur in children under age 5, pediatric nurses in clinics and physicians' offices may be influential in educating parents of young children about ways to decrease accidental poisoning. Many poison control centers offer poison prevention and education materials, such as checklists for poison-proofing a home, illustrated first-aid guidelines, tips for avoiding childhood poisonings, lists of household items that are toxic to children, and other materials useful for public education. Health education materials for poison prevention, such as the comic book *Dennis the Menace Takes a Poke at Poison* and "Officer Ugg" or "Mr. Yuk" stickers are attractive aids to use with the high-risk preschool group.

Community health nurses have an ideal opportunity to demonstrate poison control and safety measures to families in the home. For example, the skull-and-crossbones symbol for poison, which is required on the labels of toxic household products, can be pointed out to children on an exploratory poison-proofing adventure tour through their home. The consciousness-raising efforts of all healthcare professionals with parents and children can reduce the chances of accidental poisoning. Knowledge of community resources available for toxicologic emergencies, client education, accurate first-aid practices, and supportive care are essential for therapeutic intervention during a poison crisis.

NURSING PROCESS: ACUTE POISONING

ASSESSMENT

The nurse who answers calls at a poison control center should assume that callers reporting a case of poisoning or overdose are emotionally distraught. Therefore, she or he must first obtain the caller's name, address, and telephone number so that help can be sent if the call is interrupted. Next, the nurse should ask, "What is the condition of the victim?" If the victim's respiration or circulation is impaired and if the caller is familiar with cardiopulmonary resuscitation, the caller is instructed to start measures to resuscitate the victim and stabilize his or her condition. Then, the nurse must determine whether the situation is life-threatening, stable, or non-threatening. If the nurse determines that the client needs to be observed, arrangements should be made to dispatch an emergency medical team.

Objectivity is lost in a telephone assessment: some experts estimate that 50% of the data taken during a poison crisis may be inaccurate. For this reason, a follow-up telephone call may be needed to ensure compliance with emergency instructions, to determine the client's condition, and to repeat instructions about first-aid measures, if the initial information was not accurately perceived.

Once the victim's condition is stabilized, intervention for the poison can be selected by determining the chemical(s) involved, the route of entry, and the amount of exposure. Usually, the poison control center establishes protocols for giving advice to the caller, depending on the toxic substance involved.

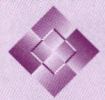

Box 15-1
Telephone Guidelines: First Aid for Poisoning

- Treat the victim, not the poison.
- Obtain caller and victim's name, telephone number, address/location, conditions, age, weight.
- Obtain a poison history: type of poison, route and time of entry, amount of poison.
- Evaluate victim's condition. Is it life-threatening?
- Intervene, basing actions on the victim's assessed condition and the poison's route of entry.
- Direct caller to the nearest treatment facility if the victim's condition warrants emergency care.
- Follow up to evaluate outcome and begin poison prevention education.

When the victim is first seen in the emergency department, assessment is facilitated by face-to-face contact. After administering first aid and obtaining as complete a history as possible, the nurse and other healthcare team members evaluate the client's condition to determine the next steps in treatment. Decisions on treatment approaches include such factors as 1) physiologic parameters (cardiac, respiratory, neurologic, and mental status), 2) poison history (the type, amount, time, and route of poisoning as well as first-aid measures implemented), and 3) the client and family's psychologic support needs. Once the poisoning emergency is resolved, the nurse and others can assess the educational needs to be met to prevent recurrence.

Nursing Diagnosis

Nursing diagnoses relate to the specific agent and its physiologic effects. Examples include:

- Ineffective Breathing Pattern, related to CNS depression secondary to sedative overdose
- Altered Tissue Perfusion: Hypotensive Shock, related to depressant overdose
- Impaired Tissue Integrity, related to chemical burns by corrosive substances
- Risk for Aspiration, related to emesis or gastric lavage
- Anxiety, related to CNS overactivity secondary to stimulant overdose

If toxicity is related to a suicidal episode, additional diagnoses may include:

- Ineffective Individual Coping
- Hopelessness
- Situational Low Self-esteem
- Body-image Disturbance

Many clients and their families exhibit:

- Knowledge Deficit, regarding poisoning and poison prevention

Planning

Appropriate nursing goals include maintaining vital functions, preventing continued absorption of toxic materials, preventing complications related to treatment measures, reducing fear, preventing or minimizing permanent tissue damage, and educating the client about poison prevention. In attempted suicide, the client should be given psychologic counseling to improve coping skills and self-image.

Intervention

First-aid measures should be administered as soon as possible. These are likely to have been delayed if the client is contacted first in the emergency department. In most cases, the victim should be seen in an acute care facility after first aid in the field. If possible, a package containing the toxic substance should accompany the victim.

CRITICAL THINKING CHALLENGE
Case Analysis

Mrs. Scott is a 72-year-old widow who lives alone in a house that is less than 2 miles from the homes of each of her daughters. She has frequent contact with her family, especially with several grandchildren and two preschool-aged great-grandchildren. She manages her life independently with the help of hired assistants for heavy housework and yardwork. Mrs. Scott is on medication for hypertension (hydrochlorothiazide) and chronic congestive heart failure (digitalis). Her physician has also prescribed a potassium supplement and a daily multivitamin and mineral tablet (maintenance dosage). Mrs. Scott stores her medications on an upper shelf of the kitchen cabinet, dispensing each day's doses on arising in the morning. She places the drugs on the dining-room table and takes them after eating breakfast. She sometimes uses acetaminophen for headaches and carries a small bottle of tablets in her purse. She enjoys painting with oils. She keeps a bottle of mineral spirits for cleaning her brushes and palette on a table near her easel. Other chemicals stored in the home include cleaning supplies and bug spray.

1. What additional assessments should be made to determine the risk of toxin-related problems to this client and her family?
2. What should you include in a teaching plan for Mrs. Scott? Explain your choices.

Eliminate the Poison. Steps commonly used in eliminating the poison include washing contaminated skin, emesis, lavage, adsorption by activated charcoal, and catharsis. More active steps may also be required, such as forced diuresis, peritoneal dialysis, hemodialysis, exchange transfusion, or hemoperfusion. These steps would be taken only after thorough evaluation by a physician.

If the poison was inhaled, remove the victim to fresh air. Two toxic gases occurring in the home are chlorine (generated, for example, by the interaction of bleach with other household cleansers) and carbon monoxide (leaking from improperly vented heating systems in poorly ventilated buildings).

If skin contamination occurs, flood the skin with water for 2 or 3 minutes. Placing the victim under a shower is the best method, but other methods can be used in emergencies. Speed in applying water and washing away the chemical is important. Remove the affected apparel when the patient is under the stream of water. After flooding the skin, gently wash the exposed part with soap and water. If the eyes are contaminated, irrigate them copiously with lukewarm water for 15 minutes. The eyelids may need to be held open to wash the eyes thoroughly. Do not use chemicals such as eye drops.

If the poison was ingested and the victim is alert and able to swallow, give milk or water to dilute the swallowed material. Never give liquid to an unconscious person. Removal of the poison is more desirable. Experts are not unanimous in recommending emesis as the treatment of choice. However, vomiting is generally believed to be superior to lavage when there are no contraindications.

Most clinicians consider emesis to be contraindicated if any of the following are present:

- Ingestion of volatile hydrocarbons
- Ingestion of corrosives (strong acids or bases)
- Coma, convulsions, loss of gag reflex
- Frank shock
- Strychnine poisoning.

Unless contraindicated, emesis may be induced on the recommendation of a poison control center. Syrup of ipecac is preferred for this purpose (Box 15-2). To administer an emetic, position the client to avoid aspiration of stomach contents and implement seizure precautions. Syrup of ipecac is contraindicated if strychnine, petroleum distillates, or corrosives such as lye or strong acids have been ingested, if the client is convulsing, or if the client has cirrhosis or thrombocytopenia.

Gastric lavage is used to evacuate stomach contents when emesis is contraindicated but the removal of gastric contents is considered safe and necessary. This procedure, referred to by laypersons as "pumping the stomach," must be performed only by trained personnel. Because not all the toxin is usually removed by lavage, further absorption of poison must be prevented.

Several ingestants can be adsorbed by activated charcoal, a black, powdery substance that is tasteless, odorless, and nontoxic to humans. Contraindications include the presence of caustic acids or alkalis, ileus, and an unprotected airway, posing a high risk for aspiration. The desired dose is mixed with water or a cathartic in a 1:4 or 1:8 charcoal-to-liquid ratio to form a slurry (Box 15-3). It is administered orally or through an orogastric tube. The exact dose is not critical because it is a nontoxic substance. Shortly after the administration of charcoal, it is removed by lavage. Because activated charcoal inactivates syrup of ipecac, it is best administered after emesis.

Cathartics are often used to facilitate the rapid transport of ingestants through the GI tract. This process decreases the absorption of ingestants. The use of oil-based cathartics is discouraged because they can cause aspiration pneumonitis. Unless contraindicated, clinicians commonly use magnesium sulfate (Epsom salts) to promote elimination. The usual adult dose is 10 to 30 g, the usual pediatric dose 250 mg/kg. It may be mixed with a sweet liquid for palatability. A period of 2 to 4 hours is required to produce the desired results. These doses may be given in lesser amounts initially, and once the results are assessed (2–4 hr), the remaining dose

---

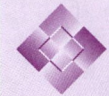

Box 15-3
Activated Charcoal:
Administration Guidelines

Dose for Adult and Child

Initial dose: 1 g/kg body weight or 10:1 ratio of activated charcoal, whichever is greater. Following massive ingestions of drug, 2 g/kg may be indicated; however, doses in excess of 100 g may be difficult to administer.

Repetitive Doses

0.5–1 g/kg body weight every 2–6 hours tailored to the dose and dosage form of drug ingested (occasionally, larger doses and shorter dosing intervals, for example). Repetitive doses of cathartics should not be used routinely.

Procedure

1. Add 4–8 parts of water to chosen quantity of activated charcoal in powdered form. This will form a transiently stable slurry that the patient can drink or receive by an orogastric tube.
2. The activated charcoal can be given in a mixture with the chosen cathartic.
3. If the patient vomits the dose, repeat the dose. Smaller, more frequent, or continuous nasogastric administration may be better tolerated. An antiemetic is sometimes needed.
4. If the client ingested a drug with a small volume of distribution, low plasma protein binding, biliary or gastric secretion, or active metabolites that recirculate, repetitive charcoal doses may be useful.

Box 15-2
Syrup of Ipecac: Dosage Guidelines

Pediatric

Age 6 to 12 months, administer 10 mL orally; age over 1 year, administer 15 mL orally, followed by 1–2 glassfuls of whatever fluid the child will tolerate (ipecac is not effective on an empty stomach). It is important to maintain activity level. Results should occur within 30 min.

Adult

Administer 30 mL. The same procedure as above is applied to the adult victim.

may be given if needed. Magnesium-based cathartics are contraindicated when the client is in renal failure.

Every household should have magnesium sulfate and syrup of ipecac available for the first-aid treatment of poisoning when use is recommended by a poison control center or medically knowledgeable personnel. A gag reflex must be present when using these drugs.

Follow-up contact must be made to evaluate the outcome, especially if the poisoning did not seem serious enough to warrant emergency department treatment. The Rocky Mountain Poison Control Center in Denver recommends 1-hour, 4-hour, and 24-hour follow-up telephone calls.

Administer an Antidote. An antidote is an agent that counteracts the action of a poison. Antidotes may force excretion, promote adsorption, or implement the mechanical removal of the toxic chemical. The choice of antidote depends on the poison and the client's condition. Antidotes act by several mechanisms of action:

- The antidote may form an inert complex with the toxin, which is then excreted.
- The antidote may enhance the detoxification of a poison.
- The antidote may slow conversion of a poison to a more toxic material.
- The antidote may compete with or block essential receptor sites that mediate the toxic effects of the poison.

Specific antidotes are available for less than 2% of all poisonous substances. The antidotes listed on the labels of caustic household chemical products are frequently incorrect. For instance, the use of a weak acid such as lemon juice is often suggested to neutralize the poison or the caustic substance. This procedure is no longer approved because the neutralization process can produce intense heat. The United States Consumer Product Safety Commission, which is responsible for antidotal labeling of poisonous household products, is trying to ensure accuracy on product labels. Poisondex is the most reliable source of information for correct antidotes.

Experts suggest that emergency departments should maintain a cyanide kit containing clear instructions for use and packaged according to the order in which its contents should be used. Several other materials suggested for use in poison emergencies are listed in Box 15-4. This list gives only the basic supplies. Other emergency drugs and specific protocols to be used in the treatment of poisoning are available through poison control centers and the Poisondex system.

Support the Client and Family. Clients and persons close to them need considerable support during treatment for acute poisoning. This is usually a life-or-death situation. Clients and family members are fearful and possibly guilt-ridden. A member of the

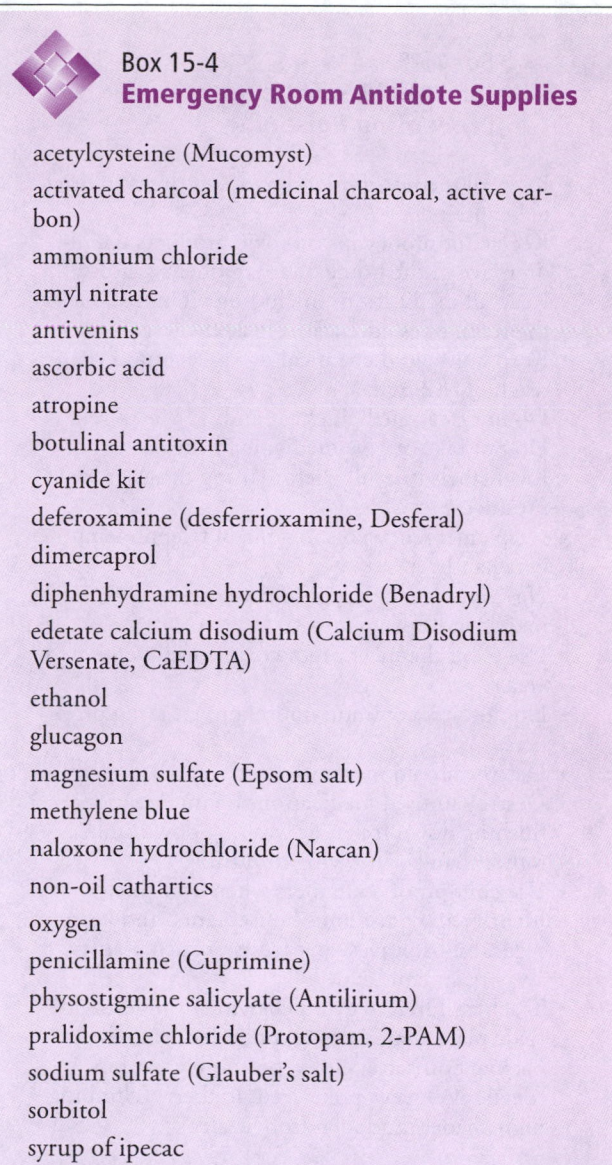

Box 15-4
Emergency Room Antidote Supplies

acetylcysteine (Mucomyst)

activated charcoal (medicinal charcoal, active carbon)

ammonium chloride

amyl nitrate

antivenins

ascorbic acid

atropine

botulinal antitoxin

cyanide kit

deferoxamine (desferrioxamine, Desferal)

dimercaprol

diphenhydramine hydrochloride (Benadryl)

edetate calcium disodium (Calcium Disodium Versenate, CaEDTA)

ethanol

glucagon

magnesium sulfate (Epsom salt)

methylene blue

naloxone hydrochloride (Narcan)

non-oil cathartics

oxygen

penicillamine (Cuprimine)

physostigmine salicylate (Antilirium)

pralidoxime chloride (Protopam, 2-PAM)

sodium sulfate (Glauber's salt)

sorbitol

syrup of ipecac

vasopressors

vitamin K_1

healthcare staff should be responsible for supporting waiting relatives. Treatment should be administered in a caring way and the client accepted warmly and non-judgmentally.

Client Education. When the victim's condition stabilizes, the need for poison prevention education, or for referral for psychologic counseling, should be determined and follow-up care and counseling ensured.

The nurse should explore with the client or family the circumstances and events leading to the toxic exposure. Specific instructions may then be given regarding secure storage of toxins, elimination of pollutants, and avoiding contact with poisons. Parents should be taught the principles for preventing childhood poisonings (Box 15-5).

Box 15-5
Household Safety: Preventing Poisoning

- Keep all medications and toxic products in original containers.
- Keep childproof caps on toxic products if children live in the home or are frequent visitors.
- Keep all medications, including vitamins, out of the reach of children, in a locked chest.
- Keep household chemical products out of the reach of children.
- Do not treat medicines as candy.
- Do not take or give medicine in the dark.
- Read labels carefully before using drugs or toxic products.
- Keep emergency poison control telephone numbers handy.
- Have emergency drugs in the home—syrup of ipecac and Epsom salts.
- Use toxic chemical products in a well-ventilated area.
- Do not mix common household cleaning products.
- Destroy all old medications.
- Destroy unused medications by incineration, flushing down toilet, or washing down sink, rather than by throwing in trash.
- Use childproof containers when available.
- Identify any poisonous houseplants, and keep seeds, bulbs, leaves, and fruits of such plants away from children.
- Teach children to avoid chewing or ingesting toxic plant materials (eg, philodendron, diefenbachia, poinsettia, holly, poison ivy, pothos (devil's ivy), yew, pokeweed, inkberry, climbing nightshade, rhododendron, azalea).

teaching. Ultimately, however, outcome is evaluated by whether or not there is a recurrence of the poisoning episode.

Bibliography

Agent orange: Link to birth defects? (1995). *Science News, 147*:28.

Biomedicine: Cancer and heart risks of dioxins. (1995). *Science News, 148*:399.

*Biomedicine: Endotoxins harm grain workers' lungs. (1994). *Science News, 146*:175.

*Drug watch: TB drug overdose may be rising. (1991). *AJN, 91*(7):52.

*Environment: . . . as lead can [impair fertility] in men. (1994). *Science News, 145*:175.

Environment: Newest estrogen mimics the commonest? (1995). *Science News, 148*:47.

Fackelmann KA. (1993). Panel weighs health impact of herbicides. *Science News, 144*:70–71.

Huston CJ. (1994). Gasoline poisoning. *Nursing '94, 24*(3):33.

*Markiewicz T. (1993). Clinical savvy: Recognizing, treating, and preventing lead poisoning. *AJN, 93*(10):59–64.

*Morelli J. (1993). Pediatric poisonings: The 10 most toxic prescription drugs. *AJN, 93*(7):27–29.

PCBs' legacy can affect next generation. (1995). *Science News, 148*:310.

Raloff J. (1995). AIDS progression fostered by dioxin? *Science News, 147*:214.

*Raloff J. (1993). Ecocancers. *Science News, 144*:10–13.

*Smothered pine trees reveal unseen killer. (1995). *Science News, 148*:134.

*Wojner AW. (1993). Seconds count when a child is poisoned. *AJN, 93*(10):46–52.

*Recommended for further reading.

OUTCOME EVALUATION

Data required for evaluation include serial observations of vital signs, the emotional reactions of the victim and family, and the presence or absence of signs and symptoms of permanent tissue damage after the toxic episode. Client education can be evaluated by the ability of clients to repeat information conveyed during

For more information and sample tests and activities, refer to Chapter 15 in the Student Workbook for Clinical Pharmacology and Nursing Management, 5th edition, available through your bookstore.

VI

Drugs That Affect the Nervous System

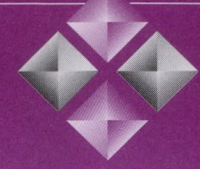

16

Drugs That Affect the Autonomic Nervous System

The automatic nervous system
    Physiology

Adrenergic drugs
    Catecholamines
    Synthetic catecholamines
    Noncatecholamines

Nursing management: clients receiving adrenergic therapy
    Nursing process

Antiadrenergic drugs
    Alpha-adrenergic blockers
    Beta-adrenergic blockers

Nursing management: clients receiving antiadrenergic therapy
    Nursing process

Cholinergic drugs
    Parasympathomimetic agents
    Anticholinesterase agents

Nursing management: clients receiving cholinergic therapy
    Nursing process: cholinergic drugs
    Nursing process: cholinergics and myasthenia gravis
    Nursing process: cholinergics and insecticide poisoning

Anticholinergic drugs
    Atropine
    Scopolamine and semisynthetic antimuscarinics

Nursing management: clients receiving anticholinergic therapy
    Nursing process

Ganglionic stimulants

Ganglionic blockers

The nervous system is a complex information processor and control mechanism. With the endocrine system, it adjusts the body's reactions to internal and external conditions. It controls movement, organ functions, thought processes, and emotions. Chemical substances that influence nerve functions, therefore, have wide-ranging effects on physical functions, emotional states, and mental capacity.

Box 16-1
Categories of the Nervous System

Anatomy

Central nervous system

    Brain
        Cortex
        Brain stem
            Diencephalon (thalamus, hypothalamus)
            Mesencephalon
            Basal ganglia
            Medulla
            Pons
            Midbrain
            Cerebellum
    Spinal cord

Peripheral nervous system

    Voluntary (motor and sensory)
    Autonomic (sympathetic and parasympathetic)

Physiologic Functions

Systems

    Sympathetic, parasympathetic, limbic, spinothalamic

Centers

    Speech, vital functions (eg, breathing, circulation)

Circuits

    Reflex arcs, reverberating circuits

Subunits

    Sensory cortex, motor cortex, inhibitory fibers, excitatory fibers, synapses

Biochemical Neurotransmitters

Excitatory substances

    acetylcholine
    norepinephrine
    dopamine
    serotonin
    L-glutamate
    L-aspartate

Inhibitory substances

    GABA (gamma aminobutyric acid)
    glycine
    histamine
    prostaglandins
    polypeptides

The nervous system is organized into subsystems and organs having various functions and components (Box 16-1). Within these structures, tissues are of two types: gray matter (nerve cell bodies) and white matter (conducting fibers). Their function may be sensory or motor. Nervous system biochemistry is complex and involves many neurotransmitters, only some of which have been identified and studied.

Drugs may affect all or only a part of the system. The more general the action of a drug, the more side effects it causes. Selective drugs tend to generate fewer side effects and have greater clinical utility.

Many nervous system drugs administered systemically affect all body systems to some degree. Locally administered drugs, such as a spinal anesthetic, restrict the drug's action to part of the system. Due to differences in physiologic chemistry, the actions of certain drugs are more pronounced in some tissues than in others. The more selective drugs affect only a small part of the system. For example, cholinergic substances mimic the effects of parasympathetic stimulation; tranquilizers depress the limbic system. In large doses, however, the effects become more widespread, causing increased side effects. Toxic symptoms tend to be similar for the major classes of drugs. Thus, excessive doses of any central nervous system (CNS) depressant tend to cause hypotension, respiratory depression, and coma.

Some drugs that affect the nervous system (eg, opium, alcohol) are among the oldest known drugs. Many traditional substances (eg, reserpine, curare) have been purified and standardized for use in modern medicine. Other drugs are recently discovered or synthesized chemicals. As research into nervous system functions continues, the potential for the development of new drugs that affect this system increases. The advent of new drugs, however, is like a double-edged sword: on one side are promising, more effective treatments for nervous system disorders, and on the other side are greater risks for toxicity and substance abuse.

The Autonomic Nervous System

The autonomic nervous system (ANS) controls vital bodily functions: cardiac action, temperature regulation, fluid and electrolyte balance, metabolism, digestion, and excretion. Through the sympathetic and parasympathetic systems, autonomic nerves influence the homeostasis of the total organism. Somatic and visceral reflexes play a large role in coordinating this control (Fig. 16-1). Autonomic drugs are chemicals that

Figure 16-1. Examples of somatic and visceral reflex pathways. Arrows indicate direction of impulse transmission. Afferent neurons are shown in black; somatic central and efferent neurons are shown in color on the left. Visceral efferent neurons, shown in color on the right are preganglionic (solid lines) and postganglionic (broken lines); synapses occur in either vertebral or prevertebral ganglia.

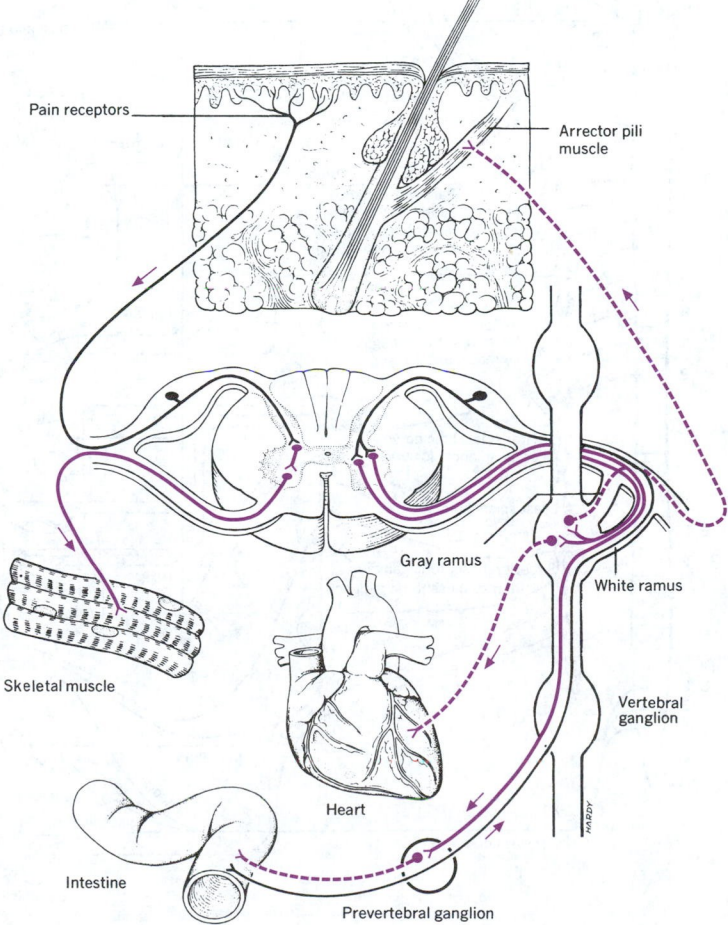

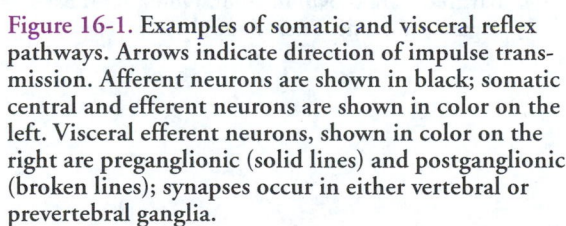

change this balance, either by altering the function of the autonomic system or by augmenting or counteracting its effects. A thorough understanding of autonomic function, therefore, is required for understanding the action and effects of autonomic drugs.

Physiology

The two main divisions of the ANS are the sympathetic (thoracolumbar) and parasympathetic (craniosacral) nervous systems (Fig. 16-2). In each, nerves leave the CNS to synapse with other nerve fibers in ganglia (sympathetic fibers are located close to the spinal cord; parasympathetic fibers are near effector organs). Postganglionic fibers extend to effector organs, where they control organ function. In the synapses of the ganglia and the nerve/organ junction, endogenous chemicals

play a role in transmitting nerve impulses. The synapses are sensitive to the influence of exogenous chemicals (drugs). Therefore, drug effects on the ANS are best understood in relation to their effects on synaptic function.

Chemistry of the Synapse

Synaptic transmission involves the production, storage, and release of chemical neurotransmitters, which stimulate a response in the postsynaptic cell (Fig. 16-3). Chemical substrates needed for the synthesis of neurotransmitters are transported down the axon of the nerve cell. In the nerve terminal, organelles and enzymes control the synthesis, storage, and release of the transmitter. Under normal conditions, the transmitter crosses the short distance that separates the terminal from the postsynaptic

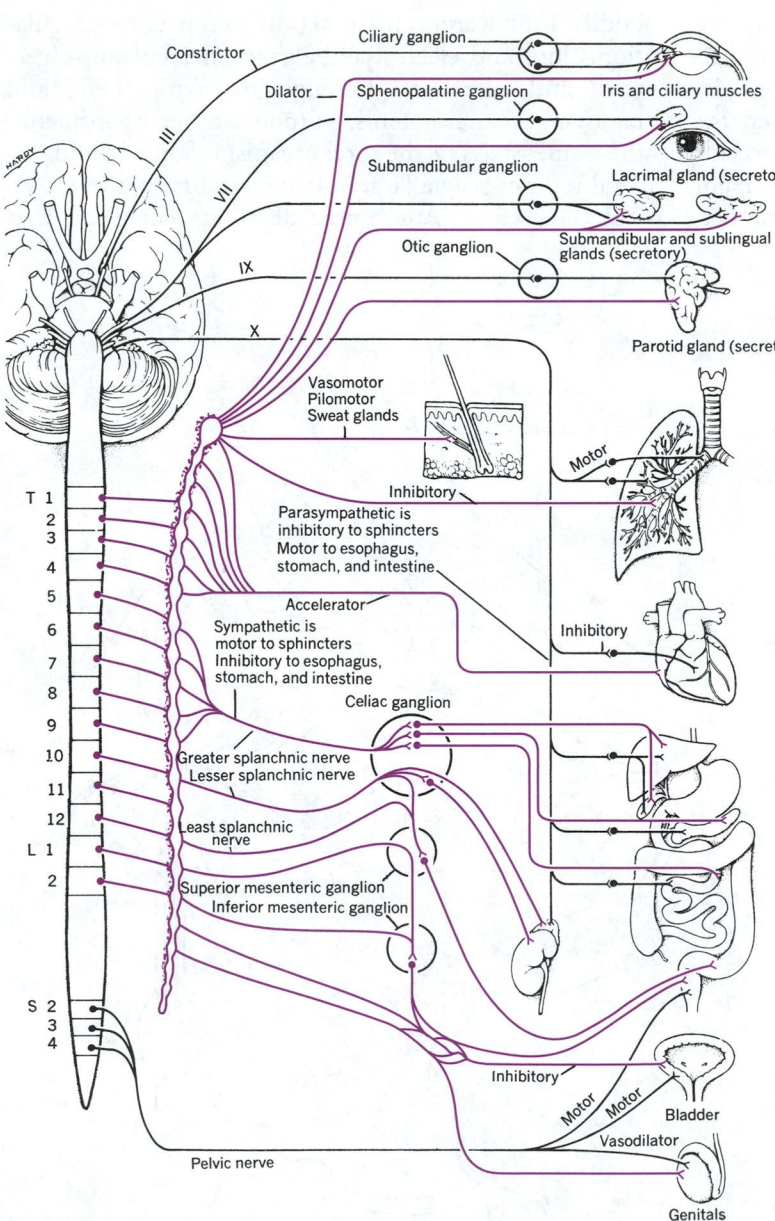

Figure 16-2. Diagram of the autonomic nervous system. Parasympathetic or craniosacral fibers are shown in black. Sympathetic or thoracolumbar fibers are shown in color. Note that most organs have a dual nerve supply.

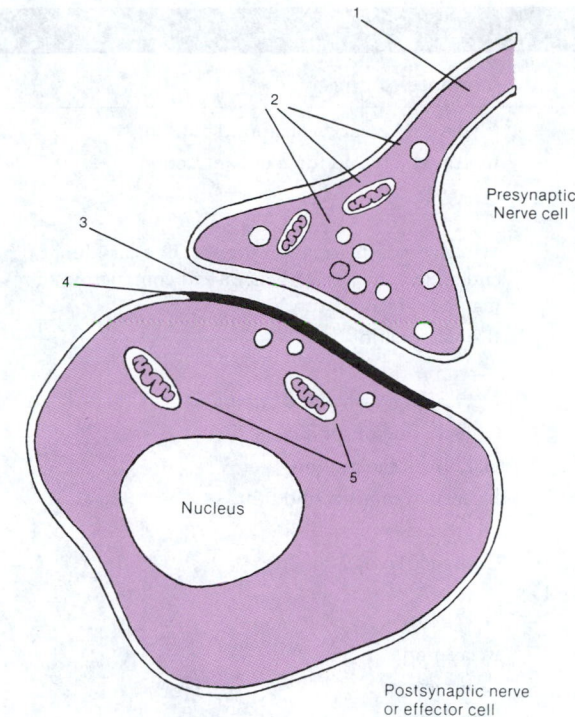

Figure 16-3. Steps in synaptic transmission. 1) Substrate is transported down the presynaptic axon. 2) Organelles and enzymes in the nerve terminal synthesize, store, release and actively re-uptake the transmitter chemical. 3) In the synaptic contact zone, extracellular enzymes catabolize the transmitter chemical. 4) The postsynaptic receptor triggers a postsynaptic cell response to the transmitter chemical. 5) Organelles within the postsynaptic cells respond.

cell, where it interacts with receptors on the cell membrane. When sufficient receptors are activated in this fashion, an action potential is generated in the receptor cell, resulting in a second nerve impulse or effector organ response (eg, muscle contraction, glandular secretion).

Transmitter that has been released from the axon terminal is dissipated by at least two processes. Enzymes in the extracellular space degrade excess transmitter, and the axon terminal actively reuptakes part of the chemical. Theoretically, any step in this process could be modified by drug action. However, most drugs appear to act at the synapse by processes such as augmenting the amount of neurotransmitter, influencing the action of catabolic enzymes in the synaptic cleft, or interacting with receptors on the postsynaptic membrane.

Because of differences in the chemical transmitters and receptors in various parts of the ANS, different drugs modify autonomic response in characteristic fashion. Acetylcholine is the neurotransmitter in ganglionic synapses, postganglionic parasympathetic synapses, and certain postganglionic sympathetic synapses (Fig. 16-4). Norepinephrine activates most postganglionic sympathetic synapses, the main exception being innervation of the sweat glands, which is mediated by acetylcholine. Cholinergic drugs that mimic or augment the effects of

acetylcholine, therefore, increase parasympathetic activity, presynaptic sympathetic activity, and sympathetic stimulation of sweat glands. Sympathomimetics or adrenergic drugs produce the same general physiologic effects as sympathetic nerve stimulation. Certain drugs act only at the neuromuscular junction. The effects of others vary depending on the site of action and, in the case of receptor action, on the specific receptors affected by these chemicals (Table 16-1).

Receptors

Both the sympathetic and parasympathetic systems appear to have two distinct types of receptors (Table 16-2). In the sympathetic system, these receptors are designated by the first two letters of the Greek alphabet, α and β. The alpha receptors mediate responses, such as vasoconstriction; contraction of the uterus, ureters, and nictitating membrane; dilation of the pupil; and inhibition of the gastrointestinal (GI) tract. Beta-receptor activity is characterized by vasodilation, inhibition of uterine contraction, dilation of the bronchi, and stimulation of the heart. Each type is divided further into two subclassifications according to the tissues affected. Drugs that affect one type of receptor but not another have specific actions characteristic of the receptor involved. For example, beta$_1$-sympathetic blocking agents prevent sympathetic stimulation of the heart.

The parasympathetic system also has two distinct types of receptors, nicotinic and muscarinic. These names

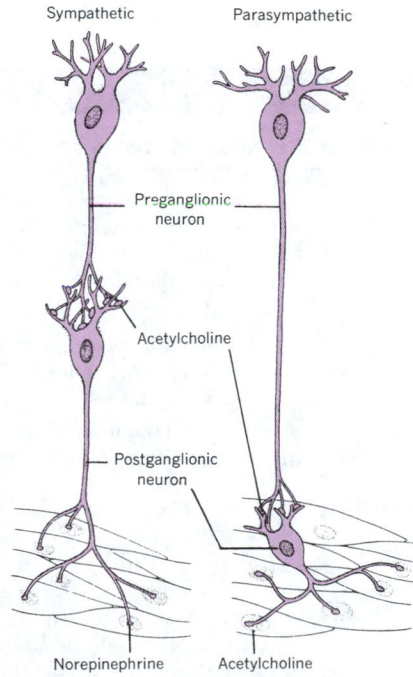

Figure 16-4. The chemical mediators. Acetylcholine is liberated by preganglionic fibers at synapses in all autonomic ganglia and by parasympathetic postganglionic fiber endings. Norepinephrine is liberated at most sympathetic postganglionic fiber endings.

Table 16-1. General Body Responses to Autonomic Activity

Body Part	Cholinergic Activity	Adrenergic Activity
Eye	Mioisis, ciliary contraction	Mydriasis,* ciliary relaxation,† blinking*
Heart	Decreased rate and force of contraction	Increased rate and force of contraction†
	Tendency toward atrioventricular block, progressing to vagal arrest	
Blood vessels	Selective vasodilation (coronary, skin, mucosal, and cerebral arteries)	Selective vasodilation (arteries of the heart, lungs, and skeletal muscles),† generalized constriction of remainder of vasculature*
Lung	Bronchoconstriction	Bronchodilation†
	Increased secretion	
Gastrointestinal tract	Increased motility and secretion	Decreased motility and secretion*
	Relaxation of sphincters	Constriction of sphincters*
	Gallbladder contraction	Gallbladder relaxation
Ureter	Increased motility and tone	Decreased motility and tone*
Urinary bladder	Increased contractility	Decreased contractility†
	Relaxation of sphincter	Constriction of sphincter*
Uterus	Variable, depending on phase of menstrual cycle and hormone state	
Nonpregnant		Relaxation†
Pregnant		Contraction*
Male sex organs	Erection	Ejaculation*
Skin	Generalized perspiration	Pallor and localized perspiration*
Adrenals	Secretion of epinephrine and norepinephrine	
Liver	Glycogen synthesis	Glycogenolysis, gluconeogenesis*†
Fat cells		Lipolysis*†

*Responses mediated by α-adrenergic receptors.
†Responses mediated by β-adrenergic receptors.

Table 16-2. Autonomic Receptors

Receptor Type	Responses Mediated by Receptors
Sympathetic	
α_1	Vasoconstriction, uterine contraction, blinking, ureteral contraction, mydriasis, inhibition of the GI tract
α_2	Presynaptic feedback inhibition
β_1	Increased force and rate of cardiac contractions, increased conduction velocity in the myocardium
β_2	Vasodilation, inhibition of uterine contraction, bronchodilation
Parasympathetic	
Muscarinic	Decreased rate of atrial contraction, selective (and limited) vasodilation, miosis, contraction of the ciliary muscle, increased tone and motility of the GI tract, contraction of the gallbladder and biliary ducts, contraction of the detrusor muscle of the bladder, relaxation of the bladder sphincter
Nicotinic	Transmission in the autonomic ganglia

were given to the two subsystems because their specific actions were first recognized from responses to the chemicals nicotine and muscarine. Nicotinic receptors are found in the ganglia, adrenal medulla, and striated muscle (the neuromuscular junction). Muscarinic receptors are found in the heart, smooth muscle, and glands (see Table 16-2). Many drugs affect one or the other of these receptor systems, but only a few affect both.

Autonomic drugs are best studied in relation to their specific action at the cellular level. Although agents are generally classified as adrenergic (sympathomimetic), cholinergic (parasympathomimetic), antiadrenergic (sympatholytic), or anticholinergic (parasympatholytic), the serious student must further distinguish between muscarinic and nicotinic agents, alpha- and beta-receptor drugs, and the specific site and mode of action of the particular compound.

Adrenergic Drugs

Chemicals that cause an apparent increase in sympathetic nervous activity in the body are called adrenergic, sympathomimetic, or sympathetic drugs. The compounds in this group that contain dihydroxybenzene in their molecular structure belong to the chemical class of catecholamines. Other terms often applied to this group (eg, pressor amines, decongestants) reflect characteristics of their physiologic action (Box 16-2).

Although their individual effects vary somewhat—and these differences are highly significant in clinical practice—most adrenergic compounds share many actions. They generally stimulate the nervous system, constrict peripheral blood vessels, increase the heart rate, dilate the bronchi and pupils, and cause a feeling of psychological tension. They tend to inhibit GI activity and micturition; they also mobilize energy sources in the body by increasing blood glucose and fatty acid levels. The net effect is to prepare the recipient to withstand critically stressful situations by mobilizing the body for necessary action, as described in Cannon's (1939) fright/fight/flight syndrome.

Adrenergic medications tend to cause nervous system overactivity. Signs and symptoms of toxicity include irritability, insomnia, hallucinations, and seizures. The risk of toxic reaction is greatest in children younger than age 6 and in people with diseases characterized by nervous system overactivity, such as hyperthyroidism.

Moreover, tolerance to the effects of adrenergic drugs can develop. Withdrawal may be followed by an exacerbation of the symptoms for which they are used. Such dependence has been documented with decongestant nose drops or sprays: rebound congestion often develops after each dose as soon as the initial decongestant action subsides.

Catecholamines

Two adrenergic drugs used in clinical practice, epinephrine and norepinephrine, are actually natural body hormones. Both drugs must be administered parenterally because they are destroyed by digestion. Their effects are not identical because their action on alpha and beta receptors differs. Synthetic catecholamines are also available for clinical use (Table 16-3).

Epinephrine

Epinephrine is described as a prototype of adrenergic compounds.

Pharmacodynamics. Epinephrine stimulates both alpha- and beta-adrenergic receptors, producing the body responses described in Table 16-1 as characteristic of adrenergic activity. Stimulation of beta cells activates adenylate cyclase, increasing the level of intracellular cyclic adenosine monophosphate. Stimulation of alpha receptors appears to mobilize calcium ions or to increase inositol triphosphate (alpha$_1$ receptors) or to inhibit adenylate cyclase (alpha$_2$ receptors). Desired therapeutic responses depend on the clinical situation and may include vasoconstriction, mydriasis, increased heart rate

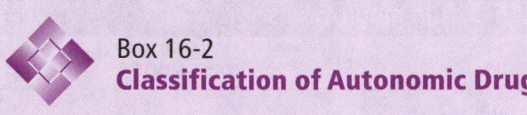

Box 16-2
Classification of Autonomic Drugs

Adrenergic Compounds

Catecholamines
Noncatecholamines

Antiadrenergic Agents

α-adrenergic blocking agents
β-adrenergic blocking agents
Adrenergic neuron-blocking agents

Cholinergic Drugs

Parasympathomimetic agents
Anticholinesterase agents

Anticholinergic Drugs

Ganglionic Drugs

and force of contraction, and bronchodilation. Epinephrine is a potent vasoconstrictor and cardiac stimulant. It also inhibits histamine release in allergic reactions.

Pharmacokinetics. Epinephrine must be administered parenterally or by inhalation because its protein structure is destroyed by digestive enzymes. After inhalation or injection, onset of action occurs within minutes. The drug crosses the placenta and is distributed in breast milk. Epinephrine has a short duration of action because it is rapidly taken up and metabolized in sympathetic nerve endings. The liver and other tissues also metabolize epinephrine, in part by the action of monoamine oxidase (MAO). Metabolites and a small amount of unchanged drug are excreted by the kidneys.

Therapeutic Uses. Intracardiac injection of epinephrine has been a heroic measure used for decades in extreme emergencies. Although more effective resuscitation means are now available, epinephrine is still used occasionally and as an adjunct in treating cardiac arrest.

Epinephrine is the drug of choice for treating anaphylaxis, an acute allergic reaction characterized by cardiovascular collapse and vasogenic shock. Injections of epinephrine reverse most of the pathologic processes of anaphylaxis by constricting the vascular bed, stimulating heart contraction, and correcting the bronchial constriction and secretion associated with this syndrome.

Epinephrine is also a primary agent for relieving acute asthma. It brings about a rapid therapeutic effect by dilating the constricted bronchi and relieving bronchial

Text continues on page 256.

Table 16-3. Adrenergic Drugs

Drug Names	Preparations	Usual Dosage	Clinical Uses
Catecholamines			
β-Adrenergic Receptor Stimulator			
isoproterenol hydrochloride, isoproterenol sulfate (Aerolone, Isuprel, Norisodrine)	Sublingual tablets Solutions for oral inhalation Solutions for injection	*Inhalation:* 100–200 µg, 4–6 times daily *Sublingual:* Adults: 10–20 mg q3–4 h to a maximum of 60 mg/day; children 5–10 mg q3–4 h to a maximum of 30 mg/day PC: C	Alleviating bronchospasm Treating cardiac arrest and arrhythmia (as an adjunct)
β₁-Adrenergic Receptor Stimulator			
dobutamine (Dobutrex)	Vials containing powder for preparing IV infusions	2.5–10 µg/kg body weight/min, adjusted according to heart rate, blood pressure, and urine flow PC: C	Short-term treatment of cardiac decompensation caused by organic disease or cardiac surgery
α- and β-Adrenergic Receptor Stimulator			
epinephrine (Adrenalin, AsthmaHaler, AsthmaNefrin, Bronitin Mist, Bronkaid Mist, EpiPen Auto-Injector, Medihaler-Epi, microNefrin, Nephron, Primatene, S-2, Vaponefrin)	Solutions for injection, inhalation, and topical application Ointment for topical application	Adults: 100–500 µg at intervals of 20 min–4 h (up to 5 mg/day in divided doses); children: 10 µg/kg body weight, to a maximum dose of 500 µg PC: C	Treating acute anaphylaxis (the agent of choice) Treating cardiac arrest (as an adjunct) Local anesthesia (as an adjunct)
α- and β₁-Adrenergic Receptor Stimulator			
norepinephrine bitartrate, levarterenol bitartrate (Levophed)	Solution for IV infusion	Initially: *Adults:* 8–12 µg/min; *children:* 2 µg/min, thereafter: according to blood-pressure response PC: C	Treating hypotensive shock that persists after adequate fluid volume replacement
α- and β₁-Adrenergic and Dopaminergic Receptor Stimulator			
dopamine hydrochloride (Dopastat, Intropin, *Can*: Revimine)	Solution for diluting IV infusion	Initially: 1–5 µg/kg body weight/min, increased by 1–4 µg/kg/min at 10–30-min intervals, until optimal response occurs PC: C	Treating hypotensive shock (including cardiogenic shock) that persists after adequate fluid volume replacement
Noncatecholamines			
β-Adrenergic Receptor Stimulator			
albuterol, albuterol sulfate, salbutamol (Proventil, Ventolin, *Can*: Novo-Salmo, Volmax)	Oral tablets Aerosol spray for inhalation	*Inhalation:* Adults and children age 12 and older: 180 µg/q4–6 h; children under age 12: 100–200 µg qid. *Oral:* Adults and children age 12 and older: 2–4 mg tid or qid (with adjustments in relation to tolerance and response) PC: C	Alleviating bronchospasm Preventing exercise-induced bronchospasm
bitolterol mesylate (Tornalate)	Aerosol solution for inhalation	Adults and children older than age 12: 2 inhalations (370 µg each) q8h; maximum dosage: 1.11 mg (3 inhalations) q6h or 740 µg (2 inhalations) q4h PC: C	Preventing and treating bronchospasm in obstructive pulmonary disease

(continued)

Table 16-3. (Continued)

Drug Names	Preparations	Usual Dosage	Clinical Uses
isoetharine hydrochloride, isoetharine mesylate (Beta-2, Bronkometer, Bronkosol)	Solution for inhalation	Adults: 0.5–1.0 ml of 0.5% solution q4h, diluted 1:3 for nebulizer administration PC: C	Alleviating bronchospasm
metaproterenol sulfate (Alupent, Metaprel)	Tablets and solutions for oral use Solutions for inhalation	Adults and children over age 9 or more than 27.3 kg: 20 mg tid or qid Children ages 6–9 or under 27.3 kg: 10 mg tid or qid Children under age 6: 1.3–2.6 mg/kg body wt/day, divided in 3 or 4 doses *Inhalation:* Adults and children age 12 or older: 2–3 inhalations, q3–4 h (not to exceed 12 inhalations/24 h) PC: C	Alleviating bronchospasm
terbutaline sulfate (Brethine, Bricanyl)	Oral tablets Solutions for subcutaneous injection	*Oral:* Adults: 5 mg tid, administered at 6-hr intervals during waking hours; children ages 12–15: 2.5 mg tid *SC:* Adults: 0.25 mg, repeated once after 15–30 min if necessary; children: 3.5–5 μg/kg body weight PC: B	Alleviating bronchospasm Inhibiting uterine contraction in premature labor

α-Adrenergic Receptor Stimulator

Drug Names	Preparations	Usual Dosage	Clinical Uses
methoxamine hydrochloride (Vasoxyl) phenylephrine bitartrate, phenylephrine hydrochloride (Duo-Medihaler, Neo-Synephrine)	Solution for IM or IV injection Solution for injection Solution for inhalation Solutions for topical application to the nose (with other drugs) Cough syrups (with other drugs)	Adults: *IM:* 5–20 mg; *IV:* 3–5 mg; children: *IM:* 0.25 mg/kg body wt, or 7.5 mg/m² body surface *IV:* 0.08 mg/kg body weight PC: C *IV infusion:* Initial rate of 0.1–0.18 mg/min, thereafter in accordance with blood-pressure levels (usual maintenance dosage: 0.04–0.06 mg/min) *Topical:* 2–3 gtt q4h *Oral:* Adults: 10 mg q4h PC: C	Treating hypotensive shock that persists after adequate fluid volume replacement Treating hypotensive shock that persists after adequate fluid volume replacement Alleviating nasal congestion

α- and β-Adrenergic Receptor Stimulator

Drug Names	Preparations	Usual Dosage	Clinical Uses
ephedrine, ephedrine hydrochloride, ephedrine sulfate (Ectasule Minus, Efedron Nasal, Ephedsol-1%, Nasdro No. 3, Va-Tro-Nol)	Solutions and jelly for nasal application Capsules, syrups, and extended-release capsules for oral use Solutions for injection	*Oral:* Adults: 25–50 mg q3–4 h PRN; children: 2–3 mg/kg body weight/day, divided in 4–6 doses *Parenteral:* Adults: *IV:* 10–25 mg; *IM:* 25–50 mg *Maximum daily dosage:* 150 mg (adults) PC: C	Alleviating bronchospasm Treating hypotensive shock that persists after adequate fluid volume replacement

(continued)

Table 16-3. (Continued)

Drug Names	Preparations	Usual Dosage	Clinical Uses
α- and β₁-Adrenergic Receptor Stimulator			
metaraminol bitartrate (Aramine)	Solution for injection	*SC or IM:* Adults: 2–10 mg; children: 0.1 mg/kg body wt, or 3 mg/m² body surface *IV:* Adults: 0.5–5 mg as a single dose; children: 0.01 mg/kg body weight, or 0.3 mg/m² body surface, as a single dose *IV infusion:* in accordance with blood-pressure levels PC: D	Treating hypotensive shock that persists after adequate fluid volume replacement
β- and (to a Lesser Degree) α-Adrenergic Receptor Stimulator			
mephentermine sulfate (Wyamine)	Solutions for IM or IV injection	*Adults: IM:* 10–80 mg. *IV:* 1–5 mg/min PC: C	Controlling and treating hypotension in selected situations
α- and (to a Lesser Degree) β-Receptor Stimulator			
pseudoephedrine hydrochloride (Cenafed, First Sign, Neofed, Novafed, Sinufed, Sudafed, Sudrin)	Tablets, extended-release capsules, and syrup for oral use	Adults and children age 12 or older: 60 mg q4–6h (maximum daily dosage: 240 mg) Children ages 6–11: 30 mg q4–6h (maximum daily dosage: 120 mg) Children ages 2–5: 15 mg q4–6h (maximum daily dosage: 60 mg) PC: C	Alleviating nasal congestion
Indirect Stimulator α- and β-Adrenergic Receptors			
phenylpropanolamine hydrochloride (Anorexin, Appress, Cenadex, Control, Decongestant-P, Dex-A-Diet, Dexatrim, Dietac, Diet Gard, Nobese, Prolamine, Propagest, Resolution, Rhindecon, Westrim)	Tablets, syrup, capsules, and extended-release tablets and capsules for oral use	*Oral:* (as a decongestant), adults: 20–25 mg q4h (maximum daily dose: 150 mg); children ages 6–12: 10–12.5 mg q4h (maximum daily dose: 75 mg); children ages 2–6: 6.25 mg q4h (maximum daily dose: 37.5 mg) *Oral:* (as an anorectic): 25 mg tid or 37.5 mg bid PC: C	Alleviating nasal congestion Short-term treatment of exogenous obesity

KEY: PC = pregnancy category. (See Appendix A.) *Can:* Canadian trade name.

congestion. It increases vital capacity, respiratory rate, and tidal volume. In addition, its inhibition of histamine release may add to its therapeutic action in asthma.

Historically, epinephrine has been used to treat hypoglycemic episodes in diabetics who receive insulin therapy. The rise in blood glucose level that follows epinephrine administration produces a temporary remission of symptoms. This restores normal physical and mental function and allows the client to achieve a longer-lasting metabolic correction by eating food that replenishes blood glucose. (Spontaneous correction of such insulin reactions has been reported when the victim became angry, a state in which endogenous epinephrine is released into the circulation.) Currently, glucagon is preferred for treating hypoglycemia because it has a more specific action and causes fewer adverse effects.

Epinephrine can be applied topically to control superficial bleeding. It is sometimes used to inhibit uterine contractions in premature labor and to inhibit the formation of intraocular fluid in open-angle glaucoma. Epinephrine has been administered intra-arterially to control severe GI or renal bleeding.

Adverse Reactions. Epinephrine increases sympathetic nervous system activity and frequently causes signs and symptoms of overstimulation (eg, restlessness, headache, tremor, weakness, dizziness, palpitation, pallor, fearfulness, tension, anxiety). Blood glucose levels rise, a response potentially harmful to persons with diabetes mellitus. Blood pressure also rises, an undesirable effect in many clients. The most serious adverse reactions are increased risk of cerebral hemorrhage (one cause of stroke) and cardiac arrhythmia.

Drug Interactions. Physicians and dentists who administer local anesthetics before performing painful procedures exploit an interaction between epinephrine and anesthetic agents. By mixing epinephrine with the anesthetic, the numbing effect of the anesthetic is prolonged without increasing the dose. Epinephrine constricts blood vessels in the area injected, reducing circulation to that site and thereby slowing the rate of absorption and dissipation of the anesthetic. Systemic toxicity from the anesthetic is diminished.

On the other hand, interactions with many therapeutic agents may have dangerous results, especially for clients who are receiving general anesthetics. In these clients, the interaction may be responsible for cardiac arrest. Some authorities believe this adverse interaction may account for many unexplained deaths in anesthetized persons in the past. (See Table 16-4 and also the discussion below of contraindications for MAO inhibitors and tricyclic antidepressants.)

Precautions and Contraindications. Side effects are transient but may be dangerous in clients with hypertension, angina, heart failure, hyperthyroidism, pheochromocytoma, and forms of shock (hemorrhagic, cardiogenic) characterized by compensatory physiologic vasoconstriction. Epinephrine must be used with caution during anesthesia because of the risk of cardiac arrest. When local anesthetics are used to block pain in areas perfused by end arteries (the digits, nose, and penis), only epinephrine-free solutions can be used; local vasoconstriction can compromise circulation and cause hypoxic gangrene.

Adrenergic drugs are contraindicated for clients receiving MAO inhibitors and tricyclic antidepressants because the interaction can cause severe hypertension.

Norepinephrine

Norepinephrine (Levarterenol) differs from epinephrine in that it does not stimulate beta$_2$-sympathetic receptors. It causes vasoconstriction with much less effect on other body systems than epinephrine. Although it does increase stroke volume and coronary blood flow, norepinephrine does not effectively increase cardiac output, probably because of the increase in peripheral resistance in the vascular tree. Its metabolic effects are insignificant when compared to those of epinephrine. Through its hypertensive action, norepinephrine increases mean arterial pressure, glomerular filtration, and urine production. Therapeutically, norepinephrine is used chiefly for treating vasogenic shock characterized by enlargement of the vascular bed disproportionate to the existing blood volume. It is administered by continuous intravenous (IV) drip. This treatment must be strictly controlled because it poses a high risk of severe peripheral vasoconstriction, reduced blood flow to vital organs, increased workload on the heart and myocardial oxygen consumption, and extreme hypertension (which can cause hemorrhage; eg, hemorrhagic cerebrovascular accident or stroke). Extravasation of norepinephrine solutions causes severe local vasoconstriction and reduced perfusion, and tissue necrosis can develop.

Norepinephrine therapy is not a substitute for volume replacement. Blood volume depletion should be corrected before therapy starts. Vital signs must be monitored closely during and immediately after norepinephrine infusion. Care is required to prevent tissue infiltration of norepinephrine IV solutions. Should extravasation

Table 16-4. Interactions of Epinephrine with Other Drugs		
Interacting Drugs	**Physiologic Effect**	**Special Considerations**
Sympathomimetic drugs	Additive effects, causing toxic levels of sympathetic nervous system activity	Allow enough time between doses of sympathomimetic drugs for the effects of each to dissipate.
Digitalis, mercurial diuretics, cyclopropane, halogenated hydrocarbon anesthetics	Sensitization of the myocardium to the effects of epinephrine, increasing the risk of arrhythmia	Do not use epinephrine with chloroform, trichlorethylene, and cyclopropane. Use lidocaine or propranolol prophylactically when epinephrine is to be given with other halogenated hydrocarbon anesthetics to reduce the risk of cardiac arrhythmia.
Thyroid hormone, tricyclic antidepressants	Potentiation of the cardiovascular effects of epinephrine	Reduce the dose of epinephrine and monitor clients closely during therapy.
Monoamine oxidase inhibitors	Potentiation of effects of epinephrine	Do not use concurrently.
Insulin	Decreased efficacy of insulin	Increase dosage of hypoglycemic drugs to meet the needs of diabetic clients when epinephrine is used.
Adrenergic-blocking agents	Reduce some or all of the effects of epinephrine	Use blocking agents to ameliorate epinephrine toxicity.

occur, the injection of phentolamine (5–10 mg diluted in 10–15 mL normal saline solution) directly into the affected tissues helps prevent hypoxic necrosis.

Synthetic Catecholamines

Synthetic catecholamine drugs include isoproterenol, dopamine, and dobutamine (see Table 16-3).

Noncatecholamines

The effects of noncatecholamine adrenergics depend on a combination of direct action on effector cells and the release of norepinephrine from quantities stored in adrenergic nerve terminals. When the former effect predominates, beta-receptor action is apparent. When the latter predominates, alpha activity is apparent. Many noncatecholamines are widely used in clinical conditions that require beta-sympathetic stimulation. Some noncatecholamines are also contained in over-the-counter (OTC) drugs marketed for treating respiratory conditions. The toxic and side effects of these preparations include tachycardia, hypertension, anorexia, nausea, and vomiting, which are characteristic adverse effects of adrenergic drugs. Their unsupervised use by the general public is potentially dangerous.

Ephedrine

Ephedrine, a plant extract, was first used more than 5000 years ago in China. Producing both alpha- and beta-sympathetic effects, the drug acts directly on receptors and indirectly through the release of norepinephrine. The rapid reduction in the effectiveness of repeated doses (tachyphylaxis) is believed to result from depletion of norepinephrine stores. Ephedrine is effective when administered orally and has a long (2–4 hr) duration of action. Its main medicinal uses are in bronchospasm, Adams-Stokes syndrome, narcolepsy, and allergic disorders.

As an ingredient in certain OTC preparations, a botanical source of ephedra is marketed as a dietary supplement for weight loss, energy, and body-building purposes (*FDA Medical Bulletin*, 1994). In most OTC drugs, however, it is used as a mydriatic and nasal decongestant.

Phenylephrine

Phenylephrine exerts powerful alpha-adrenergic stimulation, primarily by direct action on receptors. Central stimulation is minimal. The predominant actions are cardiovascular, causing a rise in blood pressure and reflex bradycardia. Phenylephrine is used therapeutically as a nasal decongestant and mydriatic. Its hypertensive effect is helpful in terminating attacks of paroxysmal atrial tachycardia, and it can be substituted for epinephrine in administering local anesthetics.

Terbutaline Sulfate

One of a group of drugs developed for treating bronchial asthma, terbutaline sulfate shares the selective activity of these drugs on beta$_2$-receptors. This activity relaxes the smooth muscle of the bronchi, the uterus, and the skeletal muscle vasculature. Terbutaline stimulates the heart much less than other sympathetic agents, such as isoproterenol. Terbutaline is effective when given orally. (For information on sympathomimetic drugs used for respiratory conditions, see Chap. 37.)

Amphetamines

Amphetamines exert both alpha and beta actions common to other adrenergic agents. In addition, they are a powerful CNS stimulant. Amphetamines are discussed in Chapter 17, bronchodilators in Chapter 37.

■ SUMMARY

Chemicals that cause responses resembling the signs and symptoms of sympathetic nervous system activity are called adrenergic or sympathomimetic drugs. Generally, they stimulate the nervous system, constrict blood vessels, dilate the bronchi and pupils, and cause psychological tension. They tend to inhibit GI activity and micturition and to mobilize energy sources. In short, they prepare for the fright/fight/flight syndrome. Catecholamine adrenergics may be natural hormones or they may be produced synthetically. Some noncatecholamine adrenergics are used widely in OTC drugs for respiratory conditions. Their unsupervised use by the general public is potentially dangerous.

❖ NURSING MANAGEMENT: CLIENTS RECEIVING ADRENERGIC THERAPY

Adrenergic therapy, such as that provided by epinephrine, requires careful nursing management. Epinephrine therapy often requires repeated dosing because the drug is metabolized quickly and may be degraded before the desired effect occurs. Because repeated doses may produce side effects, the client should be monitored to detect toxicity, should it develop. Undesirable side effects can also occur during prolonged surgical procedures that involve local anesthesia in which epinephrine is used adjunctively.

Injectable epinephrine should be stocked routinely in emergency drug supplies. Nurses who practice in situations where acute anaphylactic reactions are likely and emergency medical care is not immediately available should ensure that a supply of the drug is available. They also must be familiar with its use. Standing orders for treatment in specific situations are also helpful. For example, because anaphylactic reactions to insect bites can be rapidly fatal, camp nurses should be prepared to initiate on-the-spot treatment (see "Example of Nursing Process and Drug Therapy for Allergic Reaction").

Intravenous infusions of adrenergics, such as norepinephrine, dopamine, or dobutamine, should be administered with an infusion pump or controller. The client must be closely monitored and blood pressure must be maintained within the prescribed parameters. Close observation is needed to detect infiltration promptly, should it occur. An adrenergic-blocking agent, such as phentolamine, should be available at the bedside during these treatments as an antidote if the drug solution extravasates into the tissues. The alpha-blocking agent should be injected directly into the infiltrated tissues to prevent and reverse dangerous vasoconstriction.

In cardiovascular disease, serious complications may be precipitated by using adrenergic agents. The potential benefits of the drug must be weighed against the risks of cardiac stimulation, vasoconstriction, and hypertension. The client receiving adrenergics must be monitored for signs of cardiovascular problems, especially when norepinephrine or dopamine is administered IV to maintain circulation. Acute hypertension of lethal proportions may occur. Such a situation requires monitoring vital signs as often as every 2 minutes when the dosage is being altered. Lethal doses vary from 10 to 30 mg. The use of adrenergic drugs to inhibit premature labor also requires close monitoring to detect early signs and symptoms of complications, such as myocardial ischemia, cardiac arrhythmia, hypotension, and pulmonary edema. These adverse reactions are potentially life-threatening. Vital signs should be checked at least every 15 minutes. Parameters to monitor include urinary output and blood glucose levels.

NURSING PROCESS

ASSESSMENT

Before adrenergic drugs are administered, the client's history should be reviewed to rule out contraindications, which include disease states (eg, thyrotoxicosis, hypertension, coronary artery disease, hemorrhagic or cardiogenic shock, occlusive vascular disease, pheochromocytoma) or other drugs being taken (eg, other sympathomimetic agents, tricyclic antidepressants, MAO inhibitors). The physical assessment should include lung and cardiac status, peripheral circulation, and blood chemistries. If hypovolemia, hypoxia, acidosis, hyperglycemia, potassium imbalance, or hypercapnia is present, the physician should be informed so that the condition can be corrected before initiating adrenergic therapy. Throughout therapy, the client must be monitored for signs and symptoms of toxic or adverse effects.

NURSING DIAGNOSIS

Some initial diagnoses that arise from the client's illness include:

- Decreased Tissue Perfusion, related to hypotension
- Impaired Gas Exchange, related to bronchoconstriction

A common collaborative problem is:

Potential Complication: Hemorrhage

Conditions that stem from using adrenergic drugs may include:

- Anxiety, related to severity of illness and to the physiologic effects of adrenergic drugs
- Pain: Discomfort, Perspiration, Sensations of Warmth, related to adrenergic medication
- Altered Nutrition: Less than Body Requirements, related to anorexia or nausea secondary to adrenergic medication
- Self-care Deficit, related to fatigue secondary to adrenergic medication
- Sleep Pattern Disturbance: Insomnia, related to CNS stimulation secondary to adrenergic medication
- Risk for Altered Health Maintenance, related to knowledge deficit concerning the drug regimen and self-care measures for minimizing adverse reactions

PLANNING

Treatment goals may include restored tissue perfusion, increased gas exchange, decreased bleeding or its cessation, reduced anxiety, increased comfort, improved nutrition, improved care by substituting nursing care for self-care, increased rest and sleep, and expanded knowledge about the drug regimen.

INTERVENTION

Dependent nursing care involves administering prescribed drugs by the inhalation or IV route. Verification of the dosage and administration route is crucial, as errors in either may be life-threatening. Interdependent interventions include consulting with the physician about the client's response to treatment and orders that may need to be changed. Independent nursing interventions include monitoring the client for therapeutic and adverse response to the drug regimen (including close monitoring of vital signs), providing physical comfort measures (eg, frequent bathing, cool clothing and lightweight bed covers, positioning for optimal respiration and circulation), promoting appetite and encouraging eating, providing hygienic care that the client cannot complete without undue fatigue, implementing measures that promote rest and sleep (eg, reduction in stimuli, soothing backrubs), and developing and implementing an appropriate teaching plan.

Client Education. If clients receiving adrenergic therapy are too sick to discuss their condition or the drugs used in its treatment, the nurse must provide clear, brief instructions and explanations during treatment. After the crisis resolves, the client's knowledge should be assessed.

Clients who receive therapeutic adrenergics should be warned that they may feel fearful, anxious, tense, and restless, and that they may have difficulty sleeping. Headache, tremor, weakness, dizziness, palpitations, and pallor may occur. Clients may be reassured that feelings of apprehension and tension are direct effects of the chemicals and do not indicate emotional breakdown or mental illness. They should be taught techniques to promote rest and sleep and to relieve muscle tension.

Adrenergic bronchodilators may be prescribed for home treatment, using an air compressor and nebulizer to generate a mist that is inhaled. The client must be taught correct use of the device and the specifics of the drug regimen. The client should be taught how to rinse the mouth to remove drug residues and how to clean the nebulizer (see Chap. 37 for more information on respiratory drugs).

Clients subject to acute anaphylaxis in response to allergens (eg, bee stings, foods such as peanuts) sometimes carry an emergency epinephrine kit. One product, EpiPen, is a preloaded automatic syringe that can be self-administered. The nurse must provide clients and their families (or other responsible parties) instructions for using the emergency kit. After an anaphylactic episode, medical attention should be sought promptly, because the effects of the epinephrine are short-lived.

Nurses also must inform clients to avoid excessive use of OTC drugs that contain adrenergic compounds (marketed as decongestants). Because their effects are temporary and are followed by rebound congestion, they tend to cause dependence. Their short-term use (a few days) is relatively harmless, but medical attention should be sought if they are needed for prolonged periods (more than 2 weeks).

OUTCOME EVALUATION

Data required for evaluating whether goals were achieved include information related to tissue perfusion and oxygenation, amount of bleeding, the client's physical and mental comfort, sleep patterns, and knowledge of the drug regimen and self-care measures for minimizing adverse drug effects. (See Example of Nursing Process.)

❖ CHECKLIST OF NURSING ACTIONS

- ❑ Verify the dosage and route of administration for the prescribed drug.
- ❑ Implement nursing measures to promote sleep and prevent insomnia.
- ❑ Bathe the client frequently.
- ❑ Present food when drug effects are minimal.
- ❑ Provide the client ample opportunities for rest.
- ❑ Monitor the client carefully for signs of cardiovascular problems and sympathetic effects on other body systems.
- ❑ Reassure the client that feelings of apprehension and tension are a result of the drug.
- ❑ Teach the client how to manage long-term medication regimens.
- ❑ Teach the client techniques to promote rest and sleep.
- ❑ Ensure that injectable epinephrine preparations are available for emergency use in the healthcare setting, and become familiar with their use.

Antiadrenergic Drugs

Antiadrenergic drugs (also called adrenergic blockers) reduce sympathetic responses either at the receptor cell site or at the adrenergic nerve level. Sympathetic blocking agents inhibit responses by interacting with the receptor site on the effector cell in a way that prevents interaction of the receptor site with either natural body hormones (epinephrine and norepinephrine) or other sympathomimetic amines. The inhibition is selective; some blockers inhibit only alpha-adrenergic response and others block only beta-adrenergic response. Adrenergic neuron-blocking agents interfere with the normal release of norepinephrine at nerve terminals. They reduce pulse transmission of all peripheral sympathetic fibers, whether alpha or beta receptors are involved, but interfere with neither hormone secretion by the adrenal medulla nor the response to sympathomimetic drugs.

Alpha-Adrenergic Blockers

Alpha-adrenergic blocking agents (Table 16-5) include ergot alkaloids, haloalkylamines (phenoxybenzamine), and imidazole preparations (phentolamine).

Ergot Alkaloids

Ergot is prepared from the dried parts of a fungus (*Claviceps purpurea*) that grows on grains, especially rye. The alkaloids in this natural material are toxic, causing abortion and peripheral vascular insufficiency (due to vasoconstriction) in poisoned mammals. Fungal contamination of grains is most likely to occur during warm moist growing seasons. The toxic potential of moldy grain has been known for centuries, but epidemics of poisoning have occurred as recently as 1953 (in France). In addition to ergot alkaloids, the mold sometimes produces lysergic acid diethylamide (LSD), causing CNS complications (perceptual disorders and hallucinations) in affected persons.

Crude ergot is a complex substance that contains a dozen or more active alkaloids. Pure preparations are preferred for medicinal use. Some drugs in current use are semisynthetic.

Pharmacodynamics. The ergot alkaloids discussed below act by competitive inhibition of alpha-adrenergic receptors. Interaction of the blocking agent with the receptor site does not initiate effector cell stimulation. It also prevents sympathetic hormones and sympathomimetic drugs from doing so. The drugs block such harmful effects of catecholamines as pulmonary edema, reduced plasma volume, pericardial effusion, adrenal cortex necrosis, hyperglycemia, and cardiac arrhythmia. In addition, ergot alkaloids tend to dilate hypertonic blood vessels and constrict hypotonic blood vessels.

Pharmacokinetics. The GI absorption of ergot alkaloids is variable. Dihydroergotamine is not well absorbed and is administered parenterally. The absorption of ergot-

Example of Nursing Process and Drug Therapy for Allergic Reaction

The client, a 12-year-old girl in summer camp, has a history of allergic sensitivity to nuts and chocolate, which cause asthma attacks if she eats them when she has a "cold." She also reacts allergically to bee stings, which have caused skin rash and fever.

The client brought a bee-sting kit with her to camp. The syringe in the kit contains 1 mL of 1:1,000 epinephrine. Her physician instructed her parents to administer 0.3 mL of this solution if she is stung by a bee. The nurse in the physician's office taught her mother how to use the kit. The client says no one has ever told her how to avoid bee stings or use the kit.

Two days before the end of camp, the client is stung on the ankle while hiking with a group. The group counselor administered a dose of epinephrine immediately.

When seen in the infirmary an hour later, the client exhibited no signs or symptoms of allergic reaction, except for redness and swelling at the site of the sting. In mid-afternoon (5 hours after the client was stung) a counselor returned the client to the infirmary because she had "broken out all over with hives." The client had many large wheals on her trunk and extremities; she complained of intense itching. She said she had eaten a peanut butter sandwich, carrot sticks, milk, and an Oreo cookie for lunch.

Assessment Data

History of asthma

History of systemic reaction to bee stings

5-hour-old bee sting treated with 0.3 mL of epinephrine 1:1,000

Urticaria

Complaint of itching

Allergy to chocolate and nuts

Consumption of peanut butter and chocolate cookie

Nursing Diagnosis

Risk for Impaired Gas Exchange and Altered Tissue Perfusion, related to acute allergic reaction to bee stings

Intervention

Advise the client to carry bee-sting kit with her at all times and to inform a member of the camp staff immediately if stung.

Advise the client to avoid using perfume with floral scents and walking in areas where bees are frequently seen.

Advise the client to report any allergic symptoms as soon as possible.

Inform all members of the staff about the camper's allergy to bee stings; demonstrate the kit and instruct the staff in its use.

Ask staff members to inform you as soon as possible if the camper is stung.

Verify that the emergency supplies in the infirmary include syringes, needles, and epinephrine solutions for injection.

Review the standing orders given by the camp physician for treating symptoms of acute allergy.

Goals and Outcomes

The client will not experience dyspnea or hypotension.

Should an allergic reaction occur, it will be detected and treated promptly.

The client will not receive another bee sting.

The client will repeat back to the nurse the information provided in teaching sessions.

The client will avoid floral scents; she will report to the nurse promptly if she experiences signs or symptoms of allergy.

If the client is stung, she will be properly medicated by a staff member.

Staff members will inform the nurse promptly if the camper is stung.

(continued)

Example of Nursing Process and Drug Therapy for Allergic Reaction (continued)

Nursing Diagnosis (continued)	Intervention (continued)	Goals and Outcomes (continued)
Pain, related to altered comfort: Itching from urticaria secondary to allergic reaction to a bee sting	If the standing orders indicate the use of epinephrine for urticaria, **give** the client a second dose; if necessary, consult the physician on call regarding treatment of urticaria. If the physician concurs, give the client an antihistamine, such as chlorpheniramine maleate (Chlortrimeton). **Apply** cold packs to the affected area.	The wheals will fade and disappear. The client will state that the itching is relieved.
Risk for Infection, related to scratching secondary to urticaria and itching	**Apply** phenolated calamine lotion to the wheals; advise client to return for renewal of the calamine lotion after 4 or more hours if itching continues or returns. **Instruct** the client to press on itching areas rather than to scratch them; suggest the use of cold compresses or ice packs for relief, if needed, between applications of calamine lotion. **Arrange** with the kitchen staff for the client to obtain ice if needed.	The client will not scratch the inflamed skin. The client will not develop signs and symptoms of skin infection.
Knowledge Deficit, regarding allergy and self-care measures to prevent allergic reactions	**Advise** the client to avoid all substances to which she is known to be allergic (specifically nuts and chocolate) for a week or more, because reaction to them will exacerbate her reaction to the bee sting. **Prepare** a teaching program for the client's parents that will cover the following: a recommendation that they secure an automatic self-injection kit (EpiPen or EpiPen Junior) for the client's use; emphasize the importance of avoiding all allergens when the client has any signs or symptoms of allergic reaction; discuss techniques for avoiding bees when outdoors and for avoiding food allergens. Educate parents about desensitization treatments, to eliminate or reduce the severity of the client's allergic reactions. On the last day of camp, **meet** with the client's parents and implement the teaching plan. **Arrange** with the staff to substitute allowable treats for the client when treats she must avoid are served. **Monitor** the client for an increase in or recurrence of signs and symptoms of allergic reaction.	The client will relate to the nurse the major points of the content taught. The client will avoid contact with known allergens for the next week. The client will avoid practices that increase the risk of allergic reactions. The client will not experience a severe systemic allergic reaction.

amine tartrate varies, but the drug is administered both orally and rectally. Ergoloid and methysergide are rapidly absorbed orally. Administration with caffeine appears to enhance the GI absorption of ergot alkaloids. Because all these compounds are metabolized by the liver, part of each oral dose is destroyed during the first pass through the liver; in the case of ergoloid, as much as 50% of the dose is involved. Ergot alkaloids are distributed widely in the body, crossing the blood-brain barrier and probably distributing in breast milk in nursing mothers. Plasma half-lives tend to be biphasic, varying from 1.4 to 3.6 hours during the initial phase to almost 24 hours during the late phase. Excretion is by the kidneys.

Therapeutic Uses. Alpha-adrenergic blocking ergot alkaloids are used to improve cerebral circulation. Administered early during migraine and cluster headaches, they often abort the attacks. Some ergot preparations are also used to treat senility caused by cerebrovascular insufficiency.

Adverse Reactions. Common adverse reactions to ergot alkaloids include GI upset (nausea, vomiting, abdominal

Table 16-5. α-Adrenergic Blocking Agents

Drug Names	Preparations	Usual Dosage	Therapeutic Uses
Ergot Alkaloids			
dihydroergotamine mesylate (DHE)	Solution for IM or IV injection	Adults: *IM:* Initially 1 mg, followed by 1 mg/h until relief is obtained (to a maximum dosage of 3 mg); *IV:* Up to 2 mg; maximum weekly parenteral dosage: 16 mg PC: X	Prevention or abortion of vascular headaches, including migraine and cluster headaches
ergoloid mesylate (Deapril-ST, Hydergine, Hydro-Ergoloid, Hydro-Ergot, Hydroloid-G, Niloric, Uni-Gine)	Tablets, capsules, and solution for oral use Sublingual tablets	1–2 mg; maximum daily dosage: 12 mg PC: X	Alleviation of symptoms of senility due to cerebrovascular insufficiency
ergotamine tartrate* (Ergomar, Ergostat, Gynergen, Medihaler Ergotamine, Wigrettes)	Sublingual tablets Solution for oral inhalation In combination with caffeine: oral tablets, extended-release oral tablets, and rectal suppositories	*Oral or sublingual:* Adults: Initially 2 mg, followed by 1–2 mg q30 min to a total of 6 mg (maximum dosage: 6 mg/24 h or 10 mg/wk); children: 1 mg repeated once after 30 min if necessary (safety and efficacy in children have not been established) *Inhalation:* 360 μg (one inhalation) q5min (Maximum dosage: 2.16 mg [6 inhalations]/24 hr or 5.4 mg [15 inhalations]/wk)	Prevention or abortion of vascular headaches, including migraine and cluster headaches (the agent of choice)
methysergide maleate (Sansert)	Oral tablets	Adults: 4–8 mg/day, divided in 3 doses administered with meals. Maximum duration of treatment: 6 mo (3–4 wk intervals must separate treatment periods)	Prevention of severe refractory vascular headaches, including migraine and cluster headaches
Haloalkylamine			
phenoxybenzamine hydrochloride (Dibenzyline)	Oral capsules	Adults: Initially 10 mg qd, thereafter increased by 10 mg daily at intervals of 4 days or more until a response occurs (usual maintenance dose: 20–60 mg/day); children: Initially 0.2 mg/kg body wt, or 5 mg/m², once daily (maximum initial dose: 10 mg; usual maintenance dosage: 0.4–1.2 mg/kg body wt, or 12–36 mg/m², daily) PC: C	Control or prevention of paroxysmal hypertension and sweating in clients with pheochromocytoma Treatment of peripheral vasospastic disorders (as an adjunct)

(continued)

Table 16-5. (Continued)

Drug Names	Preparations	Usual Dosage	Therapeutic Uses
Imidazoline			
phentolamine mesylate (Regitine)	Vials that contain powder for preparing solutions for IM or IV injection	For diagnosis of pheochromocytoma: Adults: 5 mg IV; children: 1 mg IV or 3 mg IM To control hypertension caused by pheochromocytoma: Adults: 5 mg q1–2h; children: 9.1 mg/kg body weight, repeated once if necessary As an antidote for infiltrated norepinephrine: 5–10 mg in 10 mL normal saline, infiltrated into the affected area	Diagnosis of pheochromocytoma Control or prevention of paroxysmal hypertension in clients with pheochromocytoma Prevention of necrosis and sloughing after extravasation of IV norepinephrine

*Also marketed in various combinations with caffeine.
KEY: PC = pregnancy category. (See Appendix A.)

pain) and weakness of the legs. Withdrawal of medication may be followed by rebound headache.

Arterial spasms may cause cold painful extremities with paresthesia (numbness, tingling) and claudication (pain and weakness on walking). Abdominal angina or angina pectoris can occur.

Serious toxic reactions are rare but include gangrene of the extremities and myocardial or enteric infarction. In addition, methysergide can cause fibrosis in retroperitoneal, pleuropulmonary, and cardiac tissues. This condition often regresses and may subside when the drug is discontinued.

Drug Interactions. The interaction between ergot alkaloids and beta blockers may cause circulatory problems such as peripheral ischemia (cold extremities) and, possibly, peripheral gangrene. The interaction between ergot alkaloids and sumatriptan prolongs vasoactive reactions.

Precautions and Contraindications. Ergot alkaloids should be discontinued if signs and symptoms of impaired circulation develop. Contraindications for the use of ergot alkaloids include peripheral vascular disease (severe arteriosclerosis, arteritis, severe hypertension, cardiovascular disease, phlebitis) and allergic hypersensitivity to these substances. They should not be given to persons who have received sumatriptan within the preceding 24 hours. In addition, methysergide is contraindicated for clients with pulmonary disease, collagen disease, fibrotic processes, valvular heart disease, peptic ulcer, impaired hepatic or renal function, or serious infections.

Other Alpha-Adrenergic Blockers

Phenoxybenzamine is the drug of choice for treating pheochromocytoma. It controls or prevents the paroxysmal hypertension and sweating characteristic of this disorder. It is used for clients awaiting surgery to remove the tumor and also for clients for whom surgery is not indicated. Phenoxybenzamine has also been used as an adjunct in treating vasospastic disorders (eg, Raynaud's disease, frostbite damage).

Phentolamine is used to diagnose pheochromocytoma in adults; the test dose temporarily reduces symptoms of norepinephrine overactivity. It is also administered before or during surgery for pheochromocytoma to prevent or control paroxysmal hypertension that may occur because of anesthesia, stress, or tumor manipulation. Phentolamine is an antidote for norepinephrine and should be available at the bedside of any client who is receiving IV norepinephrine (Levophed) to maintain blood pressure.

Beta-Adrenergic Blockers

See the "Focus On Adrenergic Neuron-Blocking Agents: Similarities and Differences." Beta-adrenergic blocking agents are discussed in Chapter 23.

❖ NURSING MANAGEMENT: CLIENTS RECEIVING ANTIADRENERGIC THERAPY

Whenever a physiologic response system is altered, homeostasis may become unbalanced. The sympathetic blocking agents interfere with the normal response to stress mediated by the ANS. This interference can inhibit adaptive compensatory mechanisms and predispose a client to circulatory shock. The nurse should eliminate unnecessary environmental stressors that may affect the client. If unusual stress develops, the client should be carefully monitored for cardiovascular malfunction, particularly hypotension.

A common and annoying side effect of beta-blocker therapy is postural hypotension, which is most evident with rapid changes in posture and exercise. The normal vasoconstrictor response that maintains cerebral circu-

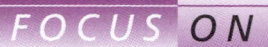

Adrenergic Neuron-Blocking Agents: Similarities and Differences

Similarities

Pharmacodynamics

These agents block chemical mediation at the postganglionic adrenergic nerve endings by depleting neurotransmitter stores and preventing mediator release.

Pharmacokinetics

These agents are stored in adipose tissue, cross the placenta, and are distributed in breast milk. They are metabolized by the liver and excreted primarily in the urine, with some in the feces. The maximum antihypertensive effect is achieved in 1 to 3 weeks.

Therapeutic Uses

These agents are used in the treatment of hypertension.

Adverse Reactions

These include: (CNS) drowsiness, lassitude, fatigue, dizziness, syncope, weakness, depression; (CV) postural hypotension, bradycardia, congestive heart failure; (RESP) nasal congestion; (GI) dry mouth, diarrhea; (SEXUAL) inhibition of ejaculation.

Interactions

Adrenergic blockers enhance hypotensive effects of vasodilators and diuretics.

Contraindications

These agents are contraindicated for people with allergic sensitivity to them.

Precautions

These agents should be gradually discontinued 2 to 3 weeks before surgery and should be used with caution in people with coronary insufficiency, heart failure not due to hypertension, recent myocardial infarction, asthma, cerebrovascular disease, ulcerative colitis, and peptic ulcer.

Nursing Considerations

Monitor pulse and blood pressure frequently for changes; assess client for signs and symptoms of depression; if client is scheduled for surgery, instruct client to notify surgeon and anesthesiologist so drug can be gradually withdrawn over 2 to 3 weeks; instruct client to avoid sudden position changes; institute safety measures to prevent injury; encourage using hard candy, ice chips, or gum to relieve dry mouth; teach client the signs and symptoms of adverse effects and the need to report them; warn client to avoid hazardous activities that require mental alertness; instruct client in drug regimen.

Differences

Guanethidine depletes norepinephrine stores and prevents release of norepinephrine from adrenergic nerve endings.
Reserpine depletes catecholamine and serotonin stores and reduces the uptake of catecholamines by adrenergic neurons.

Guanethidine is incompletely absorbed from the GI tract. It is not known whether guanethidine crosses the placenta, and only negligible amounts are passed into breast milk. Its terminal half-life is 5 days; small amounts are excreted in the feces.
Reserpine is absorbed rapidly from the GI tract. Reserpine elimination half-life occurs in two phases: in the first phase, the half-life averages 4.5 hours; during the second phase, the half-life is 11.3 days.

Reserpine is also used in treating agitated psychoses.

Reserpine may cause extrapyramidal symptoms that resemble Parkinson's disease and increased dreaming.
Guanethidine (prolonged use) may cause hair loss.

Guanethidine increases the risk of hypoglycemia in clients receiving insulin. With cardiac glycosides or procainamide, **guanethidine** increases the risk of cardiac arrhythmias. With MAO inhibitors, **rauwolfia** may produce excitation and hypertension. **Rauwolfia's** antihypertensive effects are enhanced by tricyclic antidepressants; its CNS depressant effects are increased by other CNS depressants. **Rauwolfia** may decrease therapeutic response to levodopa.

Guanethidine is contraindicated in pheochromocytoma.
Reserpine is contraindicated in depression, lactation, and electroconvulsive therapy.

Reserpine should also be used with caution in people with epilepsy, impaired renal function, or a history of gallstones.

Instruct client who is taking **guanethidine** to avoid using over-the-counter cold and allergy medications.

lation is impaired by these drugs, and dizziness and weakness frequently occur. Supervision and assistance in ambulation by nursing personnel is prudent, especially since the clients who receive these drugs are often elderly and the risk of serious injury from falls is high.

NURSING PROCESS

ASSESSMENT

Before the client begins therapy with antiadrenergics, he or she should be screened for risk factors related to adverse reactions to these drugs. For alpha blockers, these include peripheral vascular disease (severe arteriosclerosis, arteritis, severe hypertension, cardiovascular disease, Raynaud's phenomenon, Raynaud's gangrene, phlebitis), pulmonary disease, collagen disease, fibrotic processes, peptic ulcer, or serious infections.

The physical assessment should include a complete evaluation of the client's cardiovascular status, blood analyses, urinary function, and neurologic status. A global assessment of mental and emotional status should be performed and a complete drug history taken.

NURSING DIAGNOSIS

Clients who receive adrenergic blockers usually exhibit knowledge deficits related to their drug regimens. Other diagnoses that arise from alpha-adrenergic blocker therapy include:

- Altered Peripheral Tissue Perfusion, related to vasospasm secondary to drug therapy
- Risk of Impaired Tissue Integrity, related to impaired oxygen transport secondary to drug therapy
- Pain, related to angina resulting from vasospasm or nausea secondary to drug therapy
- Impaired Physical Mobility, related to angina or intermittent claudication secondary to drug therapy
- Activity Intolerance, related to angina secondary to drug therapy

A common collaborative problem that should be differentiated from the nursing diagnoses is:

Potential Complication: Cardiovascular Malfunction, including decreased cardiac output

PLANNING

A major treatment goal is educating the client about the drug regimen and self-care measures to enhance therapeutic response and reduce the risk of adverse drug reactions. Additional goals include alleviating discomfort or pain, promoting tissue perfusion, reducing adverse drug reactions, and promptly detecting and treating drug reactions. For clients who receive alpha blockers, goals include increased mobility and restored tissue integrity.

INTERVENTION

Nursing interventions range from first-aid treatment of acute reactions (eg, severe hypotension) to preparing and implementing a comprehensive teaching plan. An important nursing measure is monitoring the client for early signs and symptoms of adverse drug reactions. Therapeutic response should also be assessed.

Clients who receive alpha blockers should be monitored for impaired peripheral circulation. They should be kept warm to promote peripheral circulation. The extremities, especially, should be kept warm to promote circulation. The use of shawls, gloves, and warm socks is recommended. Severe peripheral vasoconstriction may be treated by IV sodium nitroprusside or intra-arterial tolazoline.

Alterations in comfort, impaired mobility, and activity intolerance are likely to remain chronic problems as long as the underlying cause, altered perfusion, remains uncorrected. The nurse collaborates with the physician to adapt the drug regimen to the client's needs. For example, when symptoms of migraine are first noted, administering an analgesic that contains caffeine and rest in a quiet room may abort the attack and prevent the need for medication with alpha-blocking agents. Changes in drug orders may alleviate toxic or other adverse effects. Comfort measures should be used to minimize adverse reactions such as nausea. The nurse should assist clients with activities of daily living that they no longer can perform because of activity intolerance or impaired mobility.

Client Education. Teaching the client about the drug regimen promotes compliance with drug therapy. To begin, the nurse may explore the client's perceptions of and emotional reactions to the prescribed treatment. If factors such as adverse drug reactions contribute to noncompliance, the physician should be consulted to consider whether a change in the drug regimen could improve the client's response. Of course, when a change is impossible, the client has the right to refuse a medication or specific doses of medicine, and the nurse must accept this noncompliance.

Clients who receive sympathetic blocking agents should avoid stressful situations and should be taught stress management techniques. The nurse can help clients evaluate their coping strategies and identify the need for new approaches or improved coping skills. Clients affected by high stress levels and those with poor stress management skills may be referred to counselors for more specialized help.

When drug therapy begins, clients should be informed that the physiologic side effects, such as fatigue, will soon subside but that postural hypotension tends to persist, although its severity may decline. To prevent loss of balance and accidental injury, clients should be taught to move slowly, especially when getting out of bed or standing from a sitting position. Another teaching point can focus on exercising the legs to help pump blood through the venous system to reduce pooling of blood.

Clients receiving alpha blockers should be taught to protect their feet from trauma and to wear shoes when walking. Special care of the feet includes daily washing and inspection for lesions and applying powder or lotion if needed to maintain skin integrity. Injuries or irritations should be reported to the physician and treated aggressively until they heal.

OUTCOME EVALUATION

Data required for evaluation should measure the client's ability to repeat accurately the information in the teaching plans and to demonstrate self-care measures previously taught. In addition, clients who receive alpha blockers should be asked to report changes in comfort levels (alleviation of migraine headache pain, intermittent claudication, paresthesias in the hands and feet, and chest or abdominal pain). The extremities should be examined regularly for persistent lesions that could become gangrenous.

Clients must be monitored for cardiac arrhythmia, peripheral edema, pulmonary congestion, sudden alterations in blood pressure, and nutritional status. Clients should be questioned about dizziness when suddenly changing positions.

❖ CHECKLIST OF NURSING ACTIONS

- ❑ Eliminate unnecessary environmental stressors that affect the client; help the client control activity, as recommended by the physician.
- ❑ Monitor for cardiovascular malfunction if unusual stress in the client develops.
- ❑ Supervise and assist in ambulation.
- ❑ Teach stress management techniques to clients. Help clients evaluate coping strategies; refer to counselors those who need specialized help in managing stress.
- ❑ Reassure clients that the side effect of fatigue will subside.
- ❑ Teach clients to change position slowly because of postural hypotension.

Cholinergic Drugs

Several classes of drugs act to enhance parasympathetic activity in the body (Table 16-6). Parasympathomimetic agents stimulate cells that have cholinergic receptors. Their effects may be global, but the most useful therapeutic agents are selective in action. Anticholinesterase agents inhibit or inactivate cholinesterase, causing acetylcholine to accumulate at the receptor site and thus prolonging its stimulating effect. Ganglionic stimulators, such as nicotine, are not used therapeutically, but they must be understood because of their effects.

Parasympathomimetic Agents

Chemicals that directly stimulate cholinergic receptors include muscarine, pilocarpine, acetylcholine, and the choline esters methacholine, carbachol, and bethanechol chloride.

Pharmacodynamics. Pilocarpine and muscarine act on muscarinic receptors in peripheral and ganglionic synapses. Acetylcholine stimulates all four classes of cholinergic nerves:

- Cholinergic fibers within the CNS
- Motor nerves that supply skeletal muscle fibers
- Preganglionic autonomic fibers to ganglion cells, which stimulate sympathetic and parasympathetic response
- Postganglionic fibers to parasympathetic effector cells.

Choline esters act with greater selectivity than acetylcholine.

When applied topically to the eye, cholinergic agents constrict the pupil.

Pharmacokinetics. Administered as a drug, acetylcholine penetrates the CNS poorly, and its effects are primarily peripheral. Its action is diffuse, and it is rapidly destroyed in vivo. Choline esters should be administered orally or subcutaneously, never intramuscularly (IM) or IV because rapid absorption is likely to cause toxicity.

Therapeutic Uses. Muscarine is not used medicinally. Ambenonium is the drug of choice for myasthenia gravis. Other cholinergic agents are used topically to induce miosis in glaucoma. Bethanechol is also used as a smooth muscle stimulant to relieve postoperative distention and urine retention.

Adverse Reactions. The side effects of cholinergic agents are typical of increased parasympathetic activity. They include increased perspiration and salivation, blurred vision, bradycardia with decreased cardiac output and hypotension, increased intestinal and ureteral peristalsis, and contraction of the bladder with urinary urgency. Bladder or bowel incontinence may occur. Bronchial secretion and constriction are increased. Use of cholinergic drugs may precipitate acute asthma in susceptible clients. Cholinergic drugs can also cause atrial fibrillation in hyperthyroidism, acute angina in coronary insufficiency, and an exacerbation of peptic ulcer disease.

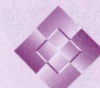

Toxicity Alert: Cholinergic Crisis

Renewed weakness, salivation, perspiration, abdominal cramping, and miosis (pupillary constriction) are signs of toxicity following cholinergic treatment for myasthenia gravis.

Treatment consists of withdrawing cholinergic medication until weakness subsides, providing mechanical respiratory support to maintain respiration, monitoring vital signs, and offering reassurance and emotional support.

Table 16-6. Cholinergic Drugs

Drug Names	Preparations	Usual Dosage	Therapeutic Uses
Parasympathetic Agents			
bethanechol chloride (Duvoid, Mictrol, Myetonachol, Urecholine, Urolax, Vesicholine)	Oral tablets Solution for subcutaneous injection	Adults: *oral:* 40–400 mg daily, divided in 4 doses; *subcutaneous:* 2.5 mg q 15–30 min (for urinary retention) or 7.5–10 mg q4h (for neurogenic bladder) PC: C	Treatment of acute postoperative and postpartum urinary retention Treatment of postoperative distention and postvagotomy gastric retention
Reversible Anticholinesterase Agents			
ambenonium chloride (Mytelase)	Tablets for oral use	*Initially:* Adults: 15–20 mg daily, divided in 3–4 doses; children: 300 µg/kg body weight/day, divided in 3 or 4 doses *Maintenance:* Adults: 45–400 mg daily, divided in 3 or 4 doses; children 1.5 mg/kg body weight/day divided in 3 or 4 doses	Treatment of myasthenia gravis
neostigmine (Prostigmin)	Tablets and powder for oral use Solutions and powder for preparing solutions for injection	*Maintenance in myasthenia gravis:* Adults: 15–375 mg daily, divided in 6–12 doses; children: 0.33 mg/kg body weight or 10 mg/m² 6 times daily PC: C	Diagnosis and treatment of myasthenia gravis (neostigmine is the standard against which newer drugs are compared) Alleviation of postoperative distention and urinary retention Antidote for reversing nondepolarizing neuromuscular blockade after surgery
physostigmine salicylate, eserine salicylate (Antilirium, Isopto Eserine)	Solution for injection Ophthalmic solutions and ointments	Adults: *Parenteral:* 500 µg–2 mg doses repeated as indicated by response PC: C	Treatment of atropine and tricyclic antidepressant toxicity Treatment of glaucoma
pyridostigmine bromide (Mestinon)	Solution, tablets, and extended-release tablets for oral use Solution for injection	*Initially:* Adults: 180 mg daily, divided in 3 doses; children: 7 mg/kg body weight/day, divided in 5 or 6 doses; doses are increased gradually until maximal effective dose is determined *PC: C*	Treatment of myasthenia gravis Reversing effects of neuromuscular blocking agents
tacrine hydrochloride (Cognex)	Oral capsules	*Initially:* 10 mg qid, increasing gradually to a maximum of 40 mg qid	Palliative treatment of mild to moderate primary degenerative dementia of the Alzheimer's type

KEY: PC = pregnancy category. (See Appendix A.) See Chapter 39 for cholinergics in ophthalmic use.

Drug Interactions. Effects are increased in combination with other cholinergic drugs. Cholinergic agents should not be used with ganglionic blocking agents because of the high risk of paralysis and respiratory arrest.

Precautions and Contraindications. Cholinergic medications are potent, and large doses should be avoided. Response to these drugs varies, and some persons experience cholinergic toxicity from therapeutic doses. For this reason, these drugs are administered orally or subcutaneously, not IM or IV.

Cholinergics exacerbate many medical conditions. They should be used with caution in clients with epilepsy, asthma, bradycardia, vagotonia, hyperthyroidism, cardiac arrhythmia, and peptic ulcer. Contraindications for their use include mechanical obstruction of or recent surgery in the GI or genitourinary tract, spastic or inflammatory GI conditions, parkinsonism, and obstructive pulmonary disease (see "Focus On Parasympathomimetic Agents: Similarities and Differences").

The anticholinergic antidote atropine should be readily available when cholinergic drugs are adminis-

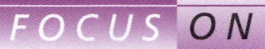

Parasympathomimetic Agents: Similarities and Differences

Similarities

Pharmacodynamics

These agents stimulate cells with cholinergic receptors to simulate the action of acetylcholine at the postganglionic neuroeffector sites.

Pharmacokinetics

The absorption, distribution, metabolism, and excretion of these agents are generally unknown. The onset of action is 10 to 30 minutes, peaking in 2 to 4 hours and lasting 4 to 8 hours.

Therapeutic Uses

These agents are used topically to induce miosis in the treatment of glaucoma. They may someday be used in the treatment of botulism and Alzheimer's disease.

Adverse Reactions

These include: (CNS) dizziness, confusion, hallucinations, muscle weakness; (EENT) miosis, blurred vision, tearing; (CV) bradycardia, decreased cardiac output, hypotension; (RESP) increased bronchial secretions, bronchospasm, bronchoconstriction; (GI/GU) nausea, vomiting, belching, incontinence, urinary urgency; (OTHER) increased perspiration and increased salivation.

Interactions

Sympathomimetic drugs increase the neuromuscular inhibition of aminoglycoside antibiotics, antiarrhythmic drugs, and local and general anesthetics. Atropine antagonizes the muscarinic effects of parasympathomimetic drugs.

Contraindications

These agents are contraindicated in mechanical obstruction or recent surgery of the GI or GU tract, spastic or inflammatory GI conditions, Parkinson's disease, obstructive pulmonary disease, and pregnancy.

Precautions

These agents should be used cautiously in people with epilepsy, asthma, bradycardia, vagotonia, hyperthyroidism, cardiac arrhythmia, and peptic ulcer.

Nursing Considerations

Frequently monitor cardiovascular and respiratory status for changes; institute safety measures to prevent injury; warn client that vision will be temporarily blurred and peripheral vision will be decreased; when giving topically, instruct client to apply finger pressure on the lacrimal sac for 1 to 2 minutes after instillation; instruct client in drug regimen and signs and symptoms of adverse reactions.

Differences

Pilocarpine and **muscarine** act on the muscarinic receptors in the peripheral and ganglionic synapses.
Acetylcholine stimulates cholinergic fibers in the CNS, motor nerves that supply skeletal muscle fibers, preganglionic autonomic fibers that stimulate sympathetic and parasympathetic responses, and postganglionic fibers to parasympathetic effector cells.
Bethanechol chloride directly stimulates cholinergic receptors.

Acetylcholine begins to act within minutes, and its duration of action is 10 to 20 minutes.
Bethanechol chloride is poorly absorbed from the GI tract. Its onset of action is 30 to 90 minutes (PO), 5 to 15 minutes (SC), with a duration of action that lasts 1 hour (PO) and up to 2 hours (SC).

Muscarine is not used medicinally.
Bethanechol chloride is also used as a smooth muscle stimulant to reduce postoperative urinary retention and gastric retention.
Acetylcholine and **carbachol** are used during eye surgery to induce miosis.

Pilocarpine also causes brow pain.
Pilocarpine and **carbachol** also cause myopia; **bethanechol chloride** also causes reflex tachycardia and decreased diastolic blood pressure.

Bethanechol chloride is contraindicated in people with bradycardia, hyperthyroidism, hypotension, epilepsy, cardiac or coronary artery disease, peptic ulcer, and asthma.

Bethanechol chloride should be used cautiously in people with hypertension, vasomotor instability, peritonitis, or other acute GI inflammatory conditions.

Prepare and use solutions of **acetylcholine** immediately because they are unstable; never give **bethanechol** IM or IV because of possible circulatory collapse, severe hypotension, severe abdominal cramps, shock, or cardiac arrest; give parenteral **bethanechol** subcutaneously only; give oral **bethanechol** on an empty stomach to avoid nausea and vomiting associated with food; have bedpan, urinal, or commode within reach of client who is taking **bethanechol;** monitor client's urinary and bowel elimination closely.

tered. Cardiac monitoring, endotracheal intubation, assisted respirations, or cardiopulmonary resuscitation may also be needed.

Anticholinesterase Agents

Pharmacodynamics. Drugs that inhibit or inactivate cholinesterase cause acetylcholine to accumulate at the receptor site, enhancing and prolonging the nerve response to each stimulus. The effects of these agents depend on the speed with which the drug/enzyme complex can be broken down by the body to regenerate active enzyme. Under normal conditions, cholinesterase combines with acetylcholine, forming a complex that is rapidly converted to choline, acetic acid, and regenerated cholinesterase. The reactions between cholinesterase and anticholinesterase compounds are almost identical except that the enzyme/substrate complex is broken down less quickly, keeping the enzyme inoperative for longer times.

Quantitative differences determine toxicity; chemicals that produce "irreversible" binding of cholinesterase are more dangerous. With the more toxic anticholinesterase chemicals, essentially none of the enzyme is regenerated. The accumulated acetylcholine continues to induce neuronal stimulation. Because cholinergic neurons are widespread, body effects are numerous and varied. They are qualitatively similar regardless of the chemical involved.

Anticholinesterases also may exert direct action—either a blocking action or a cholinomimetic effect—at autonomic ganglia. The importance of these direct actions depends on the drug involved, the dose, the application site, and the recipient species.

The pharmacologic properties of anticholinesterases are physiologic release of acetylcholine by nerve impulses and the effector response to this release. These agents can produce muscarine-like cholinomimetic actions at autonomic effector organs, nicotinic effects (characterized by stimulation and subsequent depression of autonomic ganglia and skeletal muscle), as well as stimulation (with subsequent depression) of cholinoreceptor sites in the CNS. Most of these effects accompany toxic or lethal doses. With smaller doses, as in therapeutic administration, actual response depends on the balance between ganglionic and peripheral response and the distribution of drug in various tissues.

Inhibitors of the "reversible" type that are useful drug agents include physostigmine and its derivatives neostigmine, edrophonium chloride, pyridostigmine, and ambenonium chloride. Examples of irreversible cholinesterase inhibitors (the irreversible anticholinesterases) include the insecticides parathion and malathion and the nerve gases tabun, sarin, and soman.

Pharmacokinetics. Little information is available on the systemic distribution or metabolic fate of anticholinesterases used topically for eye conditions. Some

aspects of the systemically administered drugs are also unknown. Physostigmine is readily absorbed from the GI tract, mucous membranes, and subcutaneous injection sites. Ambenonium chloride, neostigmine, and pyridostigmine are administered orally but are poorly absorbed by this route. Edrophonium chloride is administered only by injection. After absorption, these drugs are all widely distributed. Physostigmine readily crosses the blood-brain barrier; edrophonium chloride does so only in large doses. Pyridostigmine, ambenonium chloride (in large doses), and neostigmine cross the placenta.

The duration of action varies. Edrophonium chloride acts only briefly. The duration of action of ambenonium chloride, pyridostigmine, physostigmine, and neostigmine is 4 to 8 hours, 3 to 6 hours, 30 minutes to 5 hours, and 2.5 to 4 hours, respectively. The processes of metabolism and excretion are unknown for edrophonium chloride and ambenonium chloride. The other three drugs are hydrolyzed by cholinesterases. Neostigmine and pyridostigmine are metabolized by the liver and undergo tubular excretion by the kidneys. Only a small amount of physostigmine is eliminated in the urine. What happens to the rest is unknown.

Anticholinesterase insecticides are readily absorbed by the skin, and distressing symptoms may develop from topical exposure (eg, spills on the body).

Therapeutic Uses. Anticholinesterases are used to induce miosis in clients with glaucoma, to stimulate gastric motility and secretion in clients with vagotomy, and to increase the strength of skeletal muscle contraction in clients with myasthenia gravis. In addition, these drugs form the active ingredients of many insecticides and nerve gases.

Adverse Reactions. The toxic and side effects of anticholinesterases are similar to those of cholinergic agents—in other words, the signs and symptoms of parasympathetic activity. Exposure to insecticides, such as DDT and dioxin, can cause pronounced cholinergic effects. Contamination of the skin on an arm or leg may be followed by muscle spasms and paresthesia (prickling pain) that rapidly moves up the extremity. Acute systemic poisoning causes salivation, sweating, tearing, weakness, hypotension, nausea, vomiting, incontinence, ataxia, slurred speech, memory loss, agitation, hallucinations, labile mood, confusion, convulsions, and paralysis.

The effects of chronic poisoning by insecticides are poorly understood. Insecticides are considered carcinogenic and may be mutagenic. Breast-feeding mothers who have been exposed to these pollutants pass them on to their infants in breast milk. Evidence suggests that most, if not all, people have absorbed enough of such chemicals to be detectable in the blood. Because concentrations in storage depots such as fatty tissue are likely to be higher than those in the blood, the threat to public health may be much greater than is generally recognized.

FOCUS ON

Anticholinesterase Agents: Similarities and Differences

Similarities

Pharmacodynamics

These agents block the hydrolysis of acetylcholine by cholinesterase, causing acetylcholine to accumulate at the receptor sites, enhancing and prolonging the nerve response to each stimulus.

Pharmacokinetics

These agents are poorly absorbed from the GI tract. Information about distribution, metabolism, and excretion is generally unknown.

Therapeutic Uses

These agents are used to induce miosis in the treatment of glaucoma, to stimulate gastric motility and secretion in people with vagotomy, and to increase the strength of muscle contraction in people with myasthenia gravis.

Adverse Reactions

These include: (CNS) headache, muscle weakness, confusion, nervousness, dizziness; (EENT) lacrimation, blurred vision, miosis; (CV) hypertension, hypotension, bradycardia, arrhythmia; (RESP) bronchial constriction, tracheobronchial secretion, bronchospasm; (GI) nausea, vomiting, diarrhea, abdominal cramps; (GU) urinary frequency and urgency, enuresis, incontinence; (OTHER) excessive salivation, sweating, pallor.

Interactions

Anticholinesterase drugs tend to prolong the effects of depolarizing muscle relaxants. They antagonize the effects of nondepolarizing muscle relaxants. Atropine antagonizes the muscarinic effects of anticholinesterases.

Differences

Demecarium and **echothiophate** inhibit the enzymatic destruction of acetylcholine.

Neostigmine is metabolized by the liver and excreted in the urine. Its duration of action varies with clients, depending on the degree of physiologic and emotional stress and the severity of the disease. Its elimination half-life varies from 50 to 90 minutes. **Edrophonium** has an onset of action of 30 to 60 seconds when given IV and 2 to 10 minutes when given IM, and a duration of action of 5 to 10 minutes after IV administration and 5 to 30 minutes after IM administration. It may cross the placenta. **Pyridostigmine** has an onset of action of 30 to 45 minutes PO, 2 to 5 minutes IV, and 15 minutes IM; its duration of action is 3 to 6 hours (PO) and 2 to 3 hours (IV). **Pyridostigmine** is excreted in the urine. **Physostigmine** is readily absorbed from the GI tract, mucous membranes, and subcutaneous tissues; onset of action is 3 to 8 minutes (parenterally) with a duration of action of 30 minutes to 5 hours and a terminal elimination half-life of 15 to 40 minutes; it penetrates the blood-brain barrier; it is metabolized by the liver, and small amounts are excreted in the urine.

Demecarium, echothiophate, and **isoflurophate** are used in the diagnosis and initial treatment of convergent strabismus. **Edrophonium** is also used in the diagnosis of myasthenia gravis, evaluation of response to drug regimens for myasthenia gravis, and differentiation of cholinergic and myasthenic crisis. **Edrophonium, neostigmine,** and **pyridostigmine** are used to reverse the effects of neuromuscular blocking agents after surgery. **Neostigmine** is also used to alleviate postoperative distention and urinary retention. **Physostigmine** is also used in the treatment of atropine and tricyclic antidepressant toxicity.

Edrophonium and **ambenonium** can cause respiratory muscle paralysis. **Demecarium** and **echothiophate** can cause dyspnea. **Neostigmine** can cause respiratory depression. **Edrophonium** can also cause muscle fasciculations; **physostigmine** and **pyridostigmine** can cause convulsions. **Pyridostigmine** can also cause thrombophlebitis when given IV.

(continued)

Anticholinesterase Agents: Similarities and Differences (continued)

Similarities (continued)	Differences (continued)
Contraindications These agents are contraindicated in people with mechanical obstruction of the GI or GU tract and people receiving ganglionic blocking agents.	**Neostigmine** should not be given to people with peritonitis. **Physostigmine** is contraindicated in people with asthma, gangrene, diabetes, or cardiovascular disease, or those receiving choline esters or depolarizing neuromuscular blocking agents.
Precautions These agents should be used with caution in people with epilepsy, bronchial asthma, bradycardia, recent coronary occlusion, vagotonia, hyperthyroidism, cardiac arrhythmia, or peptic ulcer. Large doses should be avoided in people with megacolon or decreased GI motility.	**Physostigmine** should be used with caution in people with Parkinson's disease.
Nursing Considerations Administer with food or milk to reduce the GI effects; observe closely for cholinergic reactions, especially when using the parenteral form; have atropine available to reduce or reverse hypersensitivity reactions and to control muscarinic effects of early therapy; instruct client in disease, treatment, drug regimen, compliance, and signs and symptoms of adverse effects; monitor client's muscle strength, function, and mobility status for changes.	Use **edrophonium** to differentiate myasthenic from cholinergic crisis; administer neostigmine to the client with myasthenia gravis before possible periods of fatigue.

Drug Interactions. Anticholinesterases and anticholinergic drugs have additive effects in the body. Atropine is the antidote.

Precautions and Contraindications. Precautions and contraindications for medicinal anticholinesterase compounds are the same as those for cholinergic agents.

When anticholinesterase compounds are used as insecticides, precautions should be taken to avoid contact with the poison. Protective gear is required because both inhalation and skin contact can cause poisoning. The use of many insecticides has been sharply limited by law. Some agents can be used only in special circumstances when other less toxic agents are ineffective, and the use of some agents is limited to specially trained personnel (see "Focus On Anticholinesterase Agents: Similarities and Differences").

SUMMARY

Cholinergic drugs enhance parasympathetic activity in the body. Parasympathomimetic agents stimulate cells with cholinergic receptors, whereas anticholinesterase agents inhibit or inactivate cholinesterase. These drugs are used to treat atony of the intestines or bladder and myasthenia gravis, as well as to maintain miosis in glaucoma. Side effects can be pronounced and may include blurred vision, hypotension or hypertension, bradycardia, bronchoconstriction, nausea, cramping, diarrhea, and excessive salivation or perspiration. Anticholinesterases are the substances used in insecticides and nerve gases.

❖ NURSING MANAGEMENT: CLIENTS RECEIVING CHOLINERGIC AGENTS

Muscarine has no clinical uses, but it is the principal toxin in mushroom poisoning. After ingestion of certain mushroom species, symptoms of parasympathetic overactivity begin within 30 minutes to 2 hours. These include tearing, salivation, nausea, vomiting, headache, blurred vision, colic, diarrhea, dyspnea, bradycardia, hypotension, and shock. Irritability, restlessness, ataxia, anxiety, mania, hallucinations, delirium, and convulsions are indications of CNS stimulation. Some of these effects are desired by persons who use muscarine-containing mushrooms for psychotropic purposes. This kind of mushroom poisoning is treated by administering atropine to reverse the peripheral effects and sedatives to reduce CNS effects.

Client problems with parasympathomimetic drugs depend on the condition for which the drug is given. Response to these medications in a client with myasthenia gravis is quite different from that of the postoperative "normal" client. When neostigmine is used to correct paralytic ileus or urine retention after surgery, the client experiences the full range of side effects. In this situation, the drug is usually administered parenterally. Response occurs within 30 minutes. The problems that result from insecticide poisoning also differ. For this reason, the nursing process for myasthenia gravis and that for insecticide poisoning are discussed separately.

NURSING PROCESS: CHOLINERGIC DRUGS
ASSESSMENT
Before any cholinergic drug is administered, the client must be assessed carefully for contraindications, such as allergic conditions (especially asthma), obstructive pulmonary disease, peptic ulcer disease, inflammatory conditions of the GI tract, mechanical obstructions in the intestinal or urinary tract, recent surgery involving the GI or genitourinary system, cardiac arrhythmia (especially bradycardia), epilepsy, parkinsonism, and hyperthyroidism.

NURSING DIAGNOSIS
Clients for whom occasional doses of cholinergic drugs are ordered are likely to have nursing diagnoses such as:

- Constipation or Obstipation, related to reduced cholinergic response
- Urinary Retention, related to reduced cholinergic response
- Pain, related to altered patterns of elimination

When ophthalmic solutions are prescribed, clients are likely to have:

- Sensory-Perceptual Alteration: Blurred Vision, secondary to instillation of eye drops
- Sensory-Perceptual Alteration: Loss of Vision, secondary to glaucoma

Adverse reactions to cholinergic drugs may cause:

- Pain: Nausea or Abdominal Pain, related to adverse reactions to cholinergic drug therapy
- Risk for Injury, related to blurred vision
- Functional Urinary Incontinence, related to cholinergic drug therapy
- Bowel Incontinence, related to cholinergic drug therapy
- Decreased Tissue Perfusion, related to bradycardia, decreased cardiac output, and hypotension
- Impaired Gas Exchange, related to bronchospasm and increased bronchial secretion or respiratory paralysis

All clients are likely to exhibit:

- Knowledge Deficit, concerning cholinergic drugs

PLANNING
Treatment goals include reducing the risk of adverse drug reactions, restoring normal elimination patterns, eliminating discomfort or pain, conserving vision, prompt detection and treatment of adverse drug reactions should they occur, and client education. Among the goals for treating cholinergic toxicity are improved tissue perfusion and improved gas exchange.

INTERVENTION
Assessment findings before administration of cholinergic medication may reveal one or more contraindications or risk factors for drug use. If so, the nurse must inform the physician, who may decide to change the drug order. If not, the nurse considers the client to be at high risk for an adverse drug reaction.

Atropine should be readily available as an antidote when cholinergic drugs are administered. Epinephrine (Adrenaline) may also be required if the client has a history of allergy. Corrective action should be taken promptly if signs or symptoms of bronchial constriction or excessive secretion (wheezing, dyspnea) develop.

When cholinergic agents are administered systemically, they must be injected subcutaneously, not IM or IV. Rapid absorption of the drug by the latter routes makes a toxic reaction likely. To avoid inducing nausea, systemic doses should be administered before, not after, meals. When solutions are administered topically (usually as eye drops), the nurse can reduce systemic absorption by exerting gentle pressure at the inner canthus of the eye to occlude the tear duct for a few seconds.

When cholinergics are administered systemically, the nurse should supply the client with a bedpan or urinal, because the action of the drug is likely to cause rapid micturition or defecation. A rectal tube facilitates the passage of flatus.

Vital signs should be monitored for indications of respiratory or circulatory impairment. Acute reactions can be life-threatening and cardiopulmonary resuscitation, assisted ventilation, or treatment for shock may be necessary. The nurse should be prepared to inject atropine or epinephrine to counteract the adverse effects of the cholinergic drugs.

Client Education. Before initiating cholinergic medication, the nurse should inform the client about the drug's effects. Clients with glaucoma require long-term therapy with miotic eye drops. Accordingly, the nurse should prepare and implement a teaching plan that focuses on the drug and its therapeutic effects, common side effects, and serious toxic effects. The nurse should also explain measures the client should take if an adverse reaction develops.

OUTCOME EVALUATION

Data required for evaluating the success of nursing care include information about patterns of urinary and bowel elimination, the client's reports of comfort level, visual acuity, adverse reactions, and the time required to detect and treat such reactions. Additional evaluation data include the client's response to treatment and his or her ability to demonstrate procedures taught by the nurse and to repeat information from the teaching sessions.

NURSING PROCESS: CHOLINERGICS AND MYASTHENIA GRAVIS

In clients with myasthenia gravis, an autoimmune disease, acetylcholine apparently fails to interact sufficiently with neuromuscular receptors to produce normal muscle contraction. Although initial muscle response may be normal, it rapidly declines, and the victim cannot maintain voluntary muscle activity for more than brief periods. Administration of an anticholinesterase drug raises the client's response to stimulation and muscle strength toward normal levels, relieving both fatigability and the respiratory depression that is life-threatening in this disease.

When cholinergic therapy is used to control and alleviate the symptoms of myasthenia gravis, nursing care focuses on the problems that stem from the disease. Tolerance to the muscarinic side effects of the drugs develops with long-term use. Until then, anticholinergic drugs such as atropine are used to control these symptoms.

ASSESSMENT

The client's muscle function and strength should be assessed in detail. Muscle tone and strength fluctuate along with drug levels in the blood and should be measured before medication and at the peak of drug action. Orders for cholinergic medication often allow the client to make adjustments according to symptoms. The client's usual schedule should be determined and recorded. The nurse should question the client about drug effects such as urinary urgency, abdominal cramping, dyspnea, wheezing, perspiration, or salivation. Medications or other measures taken by the client to ameliorate adverse reactions should also be identified. Atropine may be prescribed to control these symptoms during the early stage of therapy, before tolerance to the muscarinic effects of cholinergics develops. Asthmatic clients are likely to require maintenance medication with atropine indefinitely to control respiratory symptoms.

NURSING DIAGNOSIS

Diagnoses related to myasthenia gravis include:

- Self-care Deficit
- Self-esteem Disturbance
- Risk for Impaired Gas Exchange
- Risk for Ineffective Airway Clearance
- Sensory-Perceptual Alteration: Diplopia

- Risk for Urinary Retention
- Risk for Constipation

Usually the client has:

- Knowledge Deficit, related to myasthenia gravis and the drugs used to treat the disease

Diagnoses related to cholinergic drugs include:

- Altered Comfort: Excessive Perspiration, Excessive Salivation, Nausea, or Abdominal Cramping
- Risk for Injury, related to blurred vision
- Functional Urinary Incontinence
- Bowel Incontinence

Diagnoses related to cholinergic crisis include:

- Impaired Gas Exchange, related to bronchospasm and increased bronchial secretion or respiratory paralysis
- Impaired Physical Mobility

A collaborative problem that should be differentiated from the nursing diagnoses is:

- Potential Complications: Cardiovascular (eg, decreased cardiac output, bradycardia, heart block)

PLANNING

Treatment goals include improving muscle tone to maintain adequate gas exchange, increasing tissue perfusion, maintaining mobility and self-care, and eliminating diplopia, as well as eliminating urine retention or constipation. Goals related to the drug regimen include reducing the risk of adverse reactions, promptly detecting and treating a drug reaction should one occur, and preventing or correcting side effects such as discomfort, blurred vision, urinary urgency, and incontinence. Other goals include promptly correcting or improving impaired tissue perfusion, impaired gas exchange, and immobility and helplessness engendered by a cholinergic crisis, should one develop. A key goal is informing the client and teaching skills needed to manage myasthenia gravis.

INTERVENTION

When the initial assessment reveals risk factors or contraindications for cholinergic therapy, the nurse must consult the physician to verify that these factors were considered when the drug regimen was determined. It is unlikely that cholinergic therapy will be canceled, because there is no effective alternative for control of myasthenia gravis. However, all healthcare personnel should be informed of the additional risk to the client. Atropine may be ordered to control the muscarinic effects of the cholinergic agents during the first few weeks of therapy. During long-term therapy, most clients develop a tolerance to the muscarinic action of the cholinergics, and the atropine may be slowly withdrawn. Asthmatic clients may require atropine indefinitely to maintain adequate respiration.

Drugs used to treat myasthenia gravis are usually taken orally. Medication is taken in accordance with the signs and symptoms of weakness: for instance, when eyelids cannot be fully opened (lid lag), additional medication is required. Clients with severe disease must receive medication every 2 to 4 hours, during sleeping hours as well as waking hours. Sustained-release preparations are available that allow undisturbed rest for 6 to 8 hours. Medications must be given at the time needed because delay may allow muscle weakness to progress to respiratory arrest.

The client's response to the drug regimen should be monitored closely. Muscle weakness should improve steadily. If an improvement period is followed by renewed weakness, the client should be assessed for signs and symptoms of cholinergic crisis. In this toxic condition, muscle weakness is caused by excessive cholinergic toxicity. Cholinergic crisis must be differentiated from myasthenic weakness because escalating the cholinergic drug dosage increases rather than decreases the symptoms. If the client is not taking atropine, muscarinic effects (eg, salivation, perspiration, abdominal cramping, miosis) should allow the nurse to determine the nature of the client's weakness. Cholinergic drugs, then, are withheld until the crisis resolves. Meanwhile, the client may require mechanical ventilation.

Client Education. When myasthenia gravis is diagnosed, clients require extensive teaching about the disease and its treatment. Instruction related to the drug regimen should focus on the action of the drugs, the expected therapeutic response, common side effects, and the phenomenon of cholinergic crisis. Clients who are beginning long-term therapy experience muscarinic effects until they develop tolerance to these actions. They may be reassured that these side effects usually decrease and subside within a few weeks.

Clients whose illness is complicated by obstructive airway disease (especially asthma) must know that they probably will require atropine indefinitely to control the pulmonary side effects of cholinergic medication. Because both atropine and cholinergic drugs are potent, the dosage must be carefully regulated to maintain the proper physiologic balance. Clients must be taught to repeat cholinergic drugs whenever they experience lid lag. As myasthenia gravis progresses, dosage intervals are likely to shorten. If doses are scheduled for sleeping hours, the client should use a reliable alarm clock to ensure awakening. If an electric clock is used, a manual or battery-operated alarm clock can act as a backup in case of an electrical outage. If a manual clock is used, it must be easily manipulated for setting and winding. If the client is a very sound sleeper, a family member must wake up to verify the client's response to the alarm.

Clients should learn to recognize the early signs and symptoms of urinary and intestinal obstruction and bronchial asthma. They should seek prompt medical attention should any of these symptoms develop.

OUTCOME EVALUATION

Data required for evaluation relate to muscle tone and strength, respiratory rate, skin color, peripheral circulation, mobility, visual acuity, urinary and fecal elimination, and activity and comfort levels.

NURSING PROCESS: CHOLINERGICS AND INSECTICIDE POISONING

Mild poisoning sometimes occurs in persons who lose weight quickly, as the breakdown of fatty tissue releases stored insecticides into the bloodstream. Transdermal absorption of the oily solutions applied to plants or soil may precipitate more serious toxicity. Signs and symptoms of poisoning vary with the blood level of the toxin.

ASSESSMENT

Whenever illness develops during or immediately after using insecticides, poisoning should be suspected. Signs and symptoms may range from initial transitory paresthesia and muscle cramps at the contaminated body site to systemic parasympathetic overactivity (nausea, vomiting, abdominal cramping, wheezing, dyspnea, blurred vision, intestinal cramps, bladder spasm), or to generalized convulsions, cardiorespiratory arrest, and death.

NURSING DIAGNOSIS

Nursing diagnoses may include:

- Knowledge Deficit, related to procedures for safe use of insecticides
- Pain: Abdominal Cramping, Nausea, Vomiting, related to anticholinesterase toxicity
- Impaired Gas Exchange, related to bronchospasm and bronchial hypersecretion secondary to anticholinesterase toxicity
- Risk for Injury, related to blurred vision, secondary to anticholinesterase toxicity

A common collaborative problem that should be differentiated from the nursing diagnoses is:

Potential Complication: Seizures

PLANNING

Goals of treatment include preventing or terminating seizures; improving gas exchange, tissue perfusion, and vision; reducing intestinal cramping and bladder spasm; alleviating discomfort; and teaching the client how to use insecticides safely.

INTERVENTION

When insecticide poisoning is suspected, contaminated clothing should be removed and residues of the solutions washed immediately from the skin at the site of exposure. If seizures or cardiorespiratory collapse occurs, an emergency medical unit should be called to treat the client and provide transportation to an acute care center. Cardiopulmonary resuscitation and continued mechanical ventilatory assistance may be needed. Atropine is the antidote most likely to be ordered. Clients who experience milder systemic disturbances should also seek medical care. Administering oral antimuscarinics (eg, belladonna) can accelerate recovery.

After the acute symptoms resolve, the nurse should develop and implement a teaching program to inform the client of the risks of insecticide exposure and the precautions required for safe use.

OUTCOME EVALUATION

Data required for evaluation relate to the absence or presence of airway obstruction or convulsive muscle movements, respiratory rate, skin color, peripheral circulation, visual acuity, and comfort level. The client should be able to demonstrate procedures taught and to repeat the information given during the teaching sessions (see the "Critical Thinking Challenge: Case Analysis").

CRITICAL THINKING CHALLENGE
Case Analysis

A 20-year-old college student living in an apartment near campus comes to the infirmary with nausea, vomiting, abdominal cramping, and weakness during the last 2 hours. She relates that she and her two apartment mates had decided to spray the apartment with an insecticide to kill flies and silverfish. While filling the sprayer, she spilled solution on her hands, causing prickling sensations up her arms, accompanied by transitory spasms of the small muscles. She cleaned up the insecticide but felt ill and could not complete the spraying. She has not changed her clothes, and there is a faint odor of insecticide on her jeans.

1. Prioritize the actions that must be taken immediately to safeguard the client.
2. Discuss assessment approaches the nurse can take to identify the chemical involved in this toxic reaction.
3. List the medical emergencies that could develop in this client. What can the nurse do to reduce the risk of these conditions?
4. Prepare a plan teaching the client how to prevent future episodes of this kind.

❖ CHECKLIST OF NURSING ACTIONS

Before Cholinergic Therapy

- ❏ Assess client for current or previous obstructive airway disease, peptic ulcer disease, ulcerative colitis, and urinary obstruction.

During Cholinergic Therapy

- ❏ Administer parasympathomimetic drugs before meals.
- ❏ Use a rectal tube to facilitate the passage of flatus.
- ❏ Ensure that facilities for elimination (bedpan, bedside commode, or private bathroom) are readily available.
- ❏ Watch clients for respiratory arrest and cardiovascular collapse; initiate cardiopulmonary resuscitation should they occur.
- ❏ Be prepared to administer atropine or epinephrine if signs or symptoms of bronchial constriction or excessive secretion develop.
- ❏ Monitor urinary output.
- ❏ Administer medications to clients with myasthenia gravis every 2 to 4 hours unless sustained-release preparations are used. Repeat the drug when muscle weakness causes lid lag.
- ❏ Awaken clients with myasthenia gravis during the night to administer scheduled medication.
- ❏ Inform clients about the side effects of cholinergic medication.
- ❏ Help clients with myasthenia gravis to develop dosage regimens to control the signs and symptoms of muscle weakness.
- ❏ Teach clients about the early signs and symptoms of urinary and intestinal obstruction and bronchial asthma. Urge the client to seek medical attention if these signs and symptoms develop.
- ❏ Teach clients exposed to cholinergic drugs or anticholinesterase agents about drug actions, toxic and side effects, and measures to prevent or correct adverse effects.

In Anticholinesterase Poisoning

- ❏ Secure emergency care (atropine, cardiopulmonary resuscitation) for clients with systemic signs and symptoms of anticholinesterase insecticide poisoning.

Anticholinergic Drugs

Drugs that inhibit response to acetylcholine (anticholinergics) relax smooth muscle and reduce stimulation of postganglionic nerves. Their actions are most pronounced in relation to the muscarinic effects of acetylcholine. These drugs have been called antispasmodic, spasmolytic, antiparasympathetic, cholinolytic, and parasympatholytic; these terms reflect their main properties. Because most of these agents have little effect on nicotinic receptor sites, the term "antimuscarinic" is more truly descriptive of their actions (Table 16-7).

Pharmacodynamics. All drugs of the anticholinergic class resemble atropine in their action. They act by competitive antagonism to acetylcholine and other muscarinic agents. Their effects are dose-related, with responses occurring in orderly fashion according to a characteristic progression. Small doses of anticholinergics inhibit salivary, bronchial, and sweat secretions. Larger doses cause mydriasis, inhibit visual accommodation, and increase heart rate. Still larger doses inhibit micturition and intestinal motility. At highest doses, anticholinergics reduce gastric secretion.

Pharmacokinetics. Little information is available about the pharmacokinetics of most anticholinergics. Absorption is variable. Because they are completely ionized, anticholinergics that have a quaternary ammonium group are incompletely absorbed from the GI tract. Scopolamine is well absorbed percutaneously after topical application. Atropine is rapidly absorbed from IM injection sites.

Distribution of most anticholinergics has not been determined. Atropine appears to be rapidly distributed throughout the body. Quaternary ammonium anticholinergics do not readily cross the blood-brain barrier because they are poorly soluble in lipids; atropine and hyoscyamine readily enter the cerebrospinal fluid. Atropine, hyoscyamine, and scopolamine cross the placenta, but whether other anticholinergics do is unknown. It is unlikely that quaternary ammonium anticholinergics enter breast milk, but atropine has been reported to do so.

Information about elimination of anticholinergics is also incomplete. Atropine is apparently metabolized in the liver. Propantheline is hydrolyzed in the upper small intestine. Elimination of anticholinergics is mainly through the kidneys. Substantial amounts of oral doses of anticholinergics (especially quaternary ammonium compounds) may remain unabsorbed and pass from the body in feces. Atropine is apparently not removed by hemodialysis; it is unknown whether the quaternary ammonium compounds can be dialyzed.

Therapeutic Uses. Anticholinergic drugs are used in treating conditions characterized by hypersecretion (asthma, peptic ulcer, parkinsonism), smooth muscle spasm (hypermotility of the bowel, bladder spasms), abnormal parasympathetic activity (toxicity from cholinergic or anticholinesterase drugs and motion sickness), and sinus bradycardia. They are often administered preoperatively to decrease respiratory secretion. Topical preparations are used to dilate the pupils before ophthalmic examinations.

Adverse Reactions. The side effects of anticholinergics vary depending on the purpose for which the drugs are used and the dosage involved. Thus, when atropine is administered in large doses, the client experiences a full range of side effects: dry mouth, visual disturbances, constipation, and an increased tendency for urine retention. A relatively small dose administered as an adjunct to sympathomimetic treatment of asthma may cause only a dry mouth. With drug use over time, sexual dysfunction characterized by impaired tumescence may develop.

Toxic effects include rapid and weak pulse, blurred vision, hyperthermia or hypothermia, ataxia, restlessness, and excitement. The client appears flushed, the iris is virtually obliterated, and the skin feels hot and dry. Hallucinations, delirium, and coma occur in extreme poisoning.

Drug Interactions. The effects of atropine are heightened by many drugs with anticholinergic properties, such as meperidine (Demerol), diphenylate with atropine (Lomotil), flurazepam hydrochloride (Dalmane), diphenhydramine (Benadryl), phenothiazine tranquilizers, and tricyclic antidepressants. Combining two or three of these drugs (eg, atropine, meperidine, and a tranquilizer) in preoperative medication may be a major factor in the development of postoperative delirium.

Precautions and Contraindications. Anticholinergics must be administered with great caution to clients with benign prostatic hypertrophy, because the force of micturition is diminished and acute urinary retention may occur. Extreme caution is also required in clients with GI infections, because the drugs inhibit the protective hypermotility that eliminates organisms and toxins. Other conditions in which the drug may be harmful include glaucoma, hyperthyroidism, hepatic or renal disease, and hypertension. Use of anticholinergics in febrile clients and those exposed to high environmental temperatures increases the risk of hyperthermia. The drugs also may cause drowsiness or blurred vision, a safety hazard in situations that require mental alertness.

Anticholinergics are contraindicated for clients with glaucoma, obstructive uropathy, or myasthenia gravis (except for mitigating the initial side effects of cholinergic medications), and those with allergic hypersensitivity to them.

Atropine

The first anticholinergic substances were natural alkaloids found in the belladonna plant. Atropine is the primary agent of this ancient herb. The drug was first

Text continues on page 280.

Table 16-7. Anticholinergic Drugs

Drug Names	Preparations	Usual Dosage	Therapeutic Uses
Tertiary Amine Compounds			
atropine, atropine sulfate	Oral tablets Solutions for injection	Adults: 400–600 µg q4–6h; children: 10 µg/kg body weight or 300 µg/m² (not to exceed 400 µg) q4–6h	Dilation of the pupil Inhibition of secretion preoperatively Treatment of spastic states, including biliary and ureteral colic and bronchospasm
belladonna, deadly nightshade (*Can:* Belladenal)	Tablet, powder, leaf, and tincture for oral use	Adults: *Extract:* 45–120 mg/day, divided in 3 or 4 doses; *tincture:* 0.6–1 mL tid or qid; *L-alkaloids:* 0.5–1 mg/day, divided in 7 or 8 doses Children: *L-alkaloids:* 0.125–0.5 mg/day, divided in 1–4 doses, *tincture:* 0.1 mL/kg body weight daily, divided in 3 or 4 doses; safety and efficacy of belladonna extract for children have not been established	Treatment of peptic ulcer (as an adjunct) and hypermotility problems of the GI tract Alleviation of ureteral spasm Symptomatic treatment of parkinsonism
dicyclomine hydrochloride (A-Spas, Antispas, Bentyl, Dibent, Dilomine, Or-Tyl, Spasmoject; *Can:* Bentylol)	Oral capsules, tablets, and solutions Solutions for IM injection	Adults: *Oral:* 10–20 mg tid or qid; *IM:* 20 mg q4–6h Children age 1 yr or older: *Oral:* 10 mg tid or qid; children younger than age 1: 5 mg tid or qid PC: C	Treatment of functional disturbances of GI motility, such as irritable bowel syndrome
hyoscyamine, hyoscyamine hydrobromide, hyoscyamine sulfate (Anaspaz, Cystospaz, Levsin, Levsinex; *Can:* Buscopan)	Tablets, capsules, elixir, and solutions for oral use Solution for injection	Adults: *Oral:* 0.375–1 mg/day, divided in 3 or 4 doses Children: 12.5–188 µg q4h (depending on weight) PC: C	Treatment of peptic ulcer (as an adjunct) and hypermotility problems of the GI tract Treatment of infant colic Treatment of hypermotility problems of the urinary tract
Tertiary Amine Compounds			
scopolamine, scopolamine hydrobromide (Triptone; *Can:* Transderm-V)	Tablets and capsules for oral use Solutions for injection Transdermal patches for topical use	Adults: *Oral:* 0.3–0.8 mg tid or qid PRN; *parenteral:* 0.3–0.6 mg up to qid	Inhibition of secretion preoperatively Prevention of motion sickness
Quaternary Ammonium Compounds			
clidinium bromide (Quarzan)	Oral capsules	Adults: 7.5–20 mg/day, divided in 3 or 4 doses Safety and efficacy for children have not been established PC: C	Treatment of peptic ulcer (as an adjunct)
glycopyrrolate (Robinul)	Oral tablets Solution for IM or IV injection	Adults: *Oral: Initial:* 1–2 mg tid; *maintenance:* 1 mg bid (maximum daily dosage: 8 mg); *IM:* 0.1 mg tid or qid PC: C	Treatment of peptic ulcer (as an adjunct)
isopropamide iodide (Darbid)	Oral tablets	Adults: 10–20 mg/day, divided in 2 doses, administered at 12-h intervals Safety and efficacy for children have not been established PC: C	Treatment of peptic ulcer (as an adjunct) and hypermotility problems of the GI tract

(continued)

Table 16-7. (Continued)

Drug Names	Preparations	Usual Dosage	Therapeutic Uses
Quaternary Ammonium Compounds (continued)			
mepenzolate bromide (Cantil)	Oral tablets	Adults: 75–200 mg/day divided in 3 or 4 doses Safety and efficacy for children have not been established PC: C	Treatment of peptic ulcer (as an adjunct) and hypermotility problems of the GI tract
menhantheline bromide (Banthine)	Oral tablets	Adults: 200–400 mg/day, divided in 4 doses, administered at equal intervals Children older than 12 mo: 50–200 mg/day, divided in 3 or 4 doses PC: C	Treatment of peptic ulcer (as an adjunct) Treatment of neurogenic bladder
methscopolamine bromide (Pamine)	Oral tablets	Adults: 10–20 mg/day divided in 4 doses, administered ac and hs Children: 0.2 mg/kg body weight, or 6 mg/m²/day, divided in 4 doses PC: C	Treatment of peptic ulcer (as an adjunct)
oxyphenonium bromide (Antrenyl)	Oral tablets	Adults: 40 mg/day, divided in 4 doses Safety and efficacy for children have not been established PC: C	Treatment of peptic ulcer (as an adjunct)
propantheline bromide (Pro-Banthine)	Oral tablets	Adults: 75 mg/day (15 mg tid ac and 30 mg qd hs) Safety and efficacy for children have not been established PC: C	Treatment of peptic ulcer (as an adjunct) and hypermotility problems of the GI tract
tridihexethyl chloride (Pathilon)	Tablets and extended-release capsules for oral use	Adults: 75–200 mg/day, divided in 4 doses, administered ac and hs Safety and efficacy for children have not been established	Treatment of peptic ulcer (as an adjunct) and hypermotility problems of the GI tract
Antiparkinson Agents			
benztropine mesylate (Cogentin)	Oral tablets Solution for injection	Adults: 1–2 mg/day (maximum daily dosage: 6 mg) PC: C	Treatment of parkinsonism (as an adjunct)
biperiden hydrochloride, biperiden lactate (Akineton)	Oral tablets Solution for IM or IV or injection	Adults: 6–8 mg/day, divided in 3 or 4 doses PC: C	Treatment of parkinsonism (as an adjunct)
procyclidine hydrochloride (Kemadrin, *Can*: Procyclid)	Oral tablets	Adults: 6–60 mg/day, divided in 3 or 4 doses PC: C	Treatment of parkinsonism (as an adjunct)
trihexyphenidyl hydrochloride	Tablets, exilir, and extended-release capsules for oral use	Adults: Initially 1 mg/day, increasing gradually to 6–10 mg/day, divided in 3 or 4 doses (maximum daily dosage: 15 mg) PC: C	Treatment of parkinsonism (as an adjunct)

KEY: PC = pregnancy category. (See Appendix A.)
Can = Canadian trade name.

isolated in the early 19th century; its pharmacology is well understood. Atropine is found in many plants, including deadly nightshade, jimson weed, and thorn apple. Extracts of the deadly nightshade plant that contain atropine were often used to poison enemies during the Middle Ages. Tincture of belladonna owes its clinical activity mainly to its atropine content.

Pharmacodynamics. Atropine stimulates the medulla and higher brain centers. It induces mydriasis, cycloplegia, and photophobia. Respiration is enhanced by bronchodilation and decreased secretion of the respiratory passages. Atropine inhibits vagal activity, thus increasing heart rate and inhibiting gastric secretion and motility. This action is most evident in healthy young adults; little or no effect may occur in infants or elderly persons. Atropine also selectively inhibits CNS centers that stimulate muscle tremor and rigidity.

Pharmacokinetics. Atropine may be administered orally, topically (to mucous membranes), IM, or by inhalation. It is readily absorbed from mucous membranes and the upper small intestine. Transcutaneous absorption is limited. After absorption, atropine is widely distributed in the body. It readily crosses the blood-brain barrier and the placenta. Although evidence is limited, it is believed that the drug is not secreted in breast milk in large quantities. Binding to plasma protein (albumin) equals about 18%. Atropine is metabolized by the liver; metabolites and unchanged drug are excreted in urine. Its plasma half-life is about 2 to 3 hours.

Therapeutic Uses. Atropine is frequently administered preoperatively to inhibit respiratory secretion, to dilate the bronchi, to treat cardiac arrhythmias, such as bradycardia, to reduce the risk of laryngospasm, and as an adjunct in treating asthma.

In the past, an atropine preparation, tincture of belladonna, was prescribed to reduce gastric secretion and motility in clients with symptoms of excessive gastric acid secretion or peptic ulcer disease. In medical practice, its use has been largely supplanted by histamine-receptor inhibitors (eg, cimetidine, ranitidine) and antibiotics. Belladonna's antispasmodic properties have been valued by folk herbalists, who used it to relieve colic and menstrual cramps. Belladonna is useful in treating enuresis in children, urinary frequency in paraplegia, muscle tremor and rigidity in parkinsonism, and hypertonic bladder.

Atropine is a specific antidote for cholinergic toxicity, including poisoning by mushrooms, insecticides, and nerve gas. It is used adjunctively to treat propranolol overdose and to reduce the risk of cardiovascular collapse resulting from vagal nerve stimulation by emetics, such as ipecac.

Adverse Reactions. Atropine is a potent drug (Table 16-8). Excluding dosages for treating cholinergic poisoning, doses for adults are measured in micrograms.

Table 16-8. Effects of Atropine in Relation to Dose

Dose	Effects
0.5 mg	Slight cardiac slowing; some dryness of mouth; inhibition of sweating
1.0 mg	Definite dryness of mouth; thirst; acceleration of heart, sometimes preceded by slowing; mild dilatation of pupil
2.0 mg	Rapid heart rate; palpitation; marked dryness of mouth; dilated pupils; some blurring of near vision
5.0 mg	All the above symptoms marked; difficulty speaking and swallowing; restlessness and fatigue; headache; dry, hot skin; difficulty in micturition; reduced intestinal peristalsis
10.0 mg and more	Above symptoms more marked; pulse rapid and weak; iris practically obliterated; vision very blurred; skin hot, dry, and scarlet; ataxia, restlessness, and excitement; hallucinations and delirium; coma

Hardman JG, Limbird LE, Molinoff PB, et al. (eds) (1996). *Goodman & Gilman's The pharmacological basis of therapeutics*, 9th ed. New York: McGraw Hill.

Adverse effects range from dry mucous membranes to delirium and death. Overdoses can be life-threatening.

Drug Interactions. Phenothiazines and tricyclic antidepressants enhance the anticholinergic effects of atropine. Meperidine adds to atropine's vagolytic action. Diphenhydramine accentuates the inhibition of secretions caused by atropine.

Precautions and Contraindications. Atropine should be used with caution in asthmatics and in elderly men, who are likely to have an enlarged prostate gland. It is contraindicated in acute urinary retention, constipation or obstipation, diarrhea caused by enteric infections, glaucoma, and myasthenia gravis (except for treating asthma or the transitory side effects of cholinergic medication).

Scopolamine and Semisynthetic Antimuscarinics

Like atropine, scopolamine comes from plant sources, including deadly nightshade. Its effects are overshadowed by the more potent atropine when the unrefined plant extract is used. Scopolamine shares many of the properties of atropine and has other distinct ones that are clinically valuable.

Scopolamine depresses the CNS rather than excites it. Its antinauseant properties are useful in combating motion sickness and postoperative nausea. Scopolamine causes drowsiness, euphoria, and amnesia. For these reasons it may be preferable to atropine for preoperative use. It has also been used in obstetric analgesia.

Attempts have been made to develop antimuscarinic drugs with more selectivity of action for use in specific diseases. The drugs developed to date continue to exert most of the effects of the natural anticholinergics, but those with a quaternary ammonium structure are not as well absorbed or widely distributed as atropine. They generally do not cause CNS effects because they pass the blood-brain barrier with difficulty. They are of little value in ophthalmology because penetration of the conjunctiva is poor. Because these drugs are more active ganglionic blockers than atropine, impotence, urinary retention, and postural hypotension are more likely to occur.

The quaternary ammonium compounds in common use include methscopolamine bromide (Pamine) and methantheline bromide (Banthine). They are used primarily to control GI activity in peptic ulcer disease. Use of histamine H_2-receptor antagonists and, most recently, antibiotics for peptic ulcer disease has reduced reliance on the quaternary ammonium compounds.

Synthetic anticholinergics are contraindicated in acute urinary retention and acute glaucoma. Caution is required when they are given to clients with prostatic hypertrophy or chronic glaucoma.

■ SUMMARY

Anticholinergic drugs inhibit response to acetylcholine. They tend to relax smooth muscle and reduce postganglionic stimulation. As a class, anticholinergic drugs are potent and have a high potential for toxicity. They are used to treat asthma, peptic ulcer disease, parkinsonism, motion sickness, and toxicity from cholinergic substances.

❖ NURSING MANAGEMENT: CLIENTS RECEIVING ANTICHOLINERGIC THERAPY

All anticholinergic drugs predispose the client to dry mouth, delayed digestion, constipation, and urinary retention. Frequent mouth care, measures to stimulate the appetite, and precautions to promote regular fecal and urinary elimination are needed.

Atropine is an extremely potent drug, and inappropriate exposure to small amounts can cause adverse reactions. One source of toxicity is mucosal absorption of ophthalmic solutions that have drained into the nose through the tear duct. Systemic poisoning in children has resulted from conjunctival instillation of anticholinergic drugs.

Exposure to atropine is an occupational hazard for nurses. Surgical nurses sometimes experience persistent blurred vision from accidental introduction of minute quantities of atropine into the eye while preparing preoperative injections. To avoid accidental exposure to atropine, nurses must take care to use correct technique when drawing solutions into syringes. The dose should be adjusted exactly before withdrawing the needle from the medicine vial. Accidental ejection of drug from the syringe, either while eliminating air from the syringe or while discarding excess solution, should be avoided. If such a maneuver is necessary, care should be taken to point the needle away from the eyes.

Atropine poisoning can occur in users of OTC preparations that contain scopolamine, such as those used to control motion sickness. The nurse should advise clients not to exceed the recommended dosages of such nonprescription drugs. Ingestion of berries or seeds that contain belladonna alkaloids can also cause adverse reactions. Both adults and children should be warned against ingesting plant materials that have unknown toxic potential.

Symptoms of belladonna poisoning include widespread paralysis of organs innervated by parasympathetic nerves, dry mucous membranes, unresponsive and widely dilated pupils, tachycardia, flushing, fever, and acute mental and neurologic symptoms. Any client with acute onset of bizarre behavior should be assessed for possible drug poisoning. Treatment involves gastric lavage and other measures to limit GI absorption. In extreme cases, physostigmine should be administered. Diazepam may help control seizures and provide sedation.

Atropine as an Antidote. As the specific antidote to nerve gas, atropine is a crucial substance in any military conflict in which gas chemical agents are used. Atropine must be administered at the moment of exposure to nerve gas, before the agent induces convulsions that incapacitate the victim and lead to respiratory arrest.

NURSING PROCESS

ASSESSMENT

Before initiating atropine therapy, the nurse should assess the client for risk factors of adverse reaction to the drug, such as dehydration, a tendency toward hypotension, prostatic hypertrophy or other predisposition to urine retention, glaucoma, cardiac arrhythmia (especially tachycardia), infection of the GI tract, hyperthyroidism, hypertension, and fever.

A complete drug history should be taken, with specific queries about drugs that interact with atropine: meperidine, flurazepam, diphenhydramine, phenothiazine tranquilizers, and tricyclic antidepressants. The nurse should also ask clients if they have taken atropine in the past and, if so, how they responded to it.

NURSING DIAGNOSIS

Diagnoses related to atropine therapy include:

- Altered Comfort: Dry Mouth, Abdominal Distention, and Restlessness
- Altered Tissue Perfusion: Postural Hypotension

- Urinary Retention
- Risk for injury, related to blurred vision
- Sexual Dysfunction, related to impaired tumescence and impotence
- Knowledge Deficit, related to anticholinergic drugs and self-care measures to prevent or ameliorate adverse reactions to them

PLANNING

Treatment goals include improved comfort (relief of dry mouth, abdominal distention, and restlessness), instruction in techniques to minimize the signs and symptoms of postural hypotension, promotion of fecal and urinary elimination, improved vision, correction of sexual dysfunction (or assistance in adopting alternative modes of sexual expression), and instruction about the drug regimen, adverse reactions, and self-care practices to minimize adverse reactions.

INTERVENTION

When anticholinergic drugs are administered for a short time only, the adverse reactions subside on withdrawal of the drugs. Clients should be informed of the cause of such symptoms as dry mouth and blurred vision and should be reassured that they are temporary. Frequent mouth care should be administered and, if allowed, oral fluids may be encouraged. If blurred vision persists, the client should be referred to an ophthalmologist or optometrist.

Nursing measures to promote micturition are appropriate, but if acute retention cannot be relieved, catheterization may be necessary. A rectal tube may relieve abdominal distention.

Postural hypotension, constipation, and sexual dysfunction are more likely to occur with long-term therapy. Nursing measures to minimize dizziness and weakness from postural hypotension include promoting fluid intake and changing the client's position slowly. Adequate hydration and fiber in the diet are important in preventing constipation. The client should also engage in physical activity and develop a habitual pattern of defecation. Moderate use of laxative foods, such as pears and prunes, may be recommended. When sexual dysfunction occurs, the physician should be consulted for a possible change in the drug regimen. If a change in drug is inadvisable, the client should be informed of alternatives to intercourse. Referral to a sex therapist may be desired.

Client Education. When long-term therapy with anticholinergic drugs is prescribed, the nurse should develop and implement a teaching program to inform the client about the drug regimen, adverse effects, and self-care measures that promote therapeutic response and decrease the risk of adverse reactions. Clients should be warned about early symptoms of drug intoxication (see Table 16-8).

Clients should be urged to report any decrease in the strength of the urinary stream (particularly elderly men at risk for prostatic enlargement). Clients also should be taught ways to prevent constipation and to minimize symptoms of postural hypotension.

OUTCOME EVALUATION

Data required for evaluating the outcome of nursing measures include measurement of abdominal girth, amount and patterns of urinary output, patterns of fecal elimination, visual acuity, and statements by the client describing changes in symptoms. Data for evaluating the teaching plan include the client's ability to demonstrate techniques shown and to repeat information conveyed during teaching sessions.

❖ CHECKLIST OF NURSING ACTIONS

- ❑ Warn clients of the toxic potential of berries and seeds that contain anticholinergic alkaloids.
- ❑ Warn clients who use OTC preparations that contain anticholinergics not to exceed the recommended dosages.
- ❑ When sudden, bizarre behavior occurs, assess the client for poisoning, including anticholinergic toxicity.
- ❑ Remember that atropine is extremely potent and toxic.
- ❑ To avoid accidental exposure to atropine, use correct technique when drawing solutions into syringes.
- ❑ When administering eye drops, occlude the tear ducts by external pressure until solutions are completely dispersed over the conjunctival sac.
- ❑ Identify early symptoms of drug intoxication for clients.
- ❑ Tell male clients to report any weakening of the urinary stream to the physician.
- ❑ When sexual dysfunction is a problem, give sexual counseling or refer the client to a counselor for alternatives to intercourse.
- ❑ Advise the client that blurred vision may occur. In long-term anticholinergic therapy, recommend refraction for corrective lenses after the drug dosage is stabilized for maintenance.
- ❑ Monitor clients for toxic and side effects.
- ❑ Alleviate oral dryness by administering frequent mouth care.
- ❑ Encourage oral intake of fluids, when allowed.
- ❑ Report urine retention to the physician promptly.
- ❑ Catheterize as ordered to relieve retention.
- ❑ Teach clients ways to prevent or control adverse drug reactions.

Ganglionic Stimulants

Impulse transmission through autonomic ganglia is more complex than was previously believed. The basic acetylcholine/cholinesterase system is modified by secondary pathways and possibly by an intermediary neuron that uses a catecholamine transmitter. Consequently, drug actions at the ganglion level do not always correspond to the effects predicted by previous theories of cholinergic mechanisms.

Except for nicotine chewing gum and the nicotine patch used to reduce withdrawal symptoms in clients who attempt to stop smoking, no therapeutically useful ganglionic-stimulating drugs exist. However, ganglionic stimulators must be understood because of their toxic effects. Two natural alkaloids, nicotine and lobeline, and several synthetic compounds are useful as experimental tools. For instance, nicotine patches have been reported to relieve the symptoms of ulcerative colitis in some clients.

Because of its nonmedicinal uses and abuses, nicotine is the drug of most interest to healthcare practitioners. It is discussed in Chapter 14.

Ganglionic Blockers

Several drugs block transmission in autonomic ganglia by occupying receptor sites and preventing response to acetylcholine. Two agents are available for medical use: mecamylamine (Inversine), an oral preparation, and trimethaphan camsylate (Arfonad), a parenteral preparation. These drugs reduce vasoconstriction in clients with hypertensive cardiovascular disease or hypertensive crisis. They also produce controlled hypotension for certain surgical procedures in which bleeding in the operative field must be minimized (see the discussion of drugs that affect vascular tone in Chap. 23).

References

Adverse events with ephedra and other botanical dietary supplements. (1994). *FDA Medical Bulletin,* September, p. 3.

Cannon W. (1939). *The wisdom of the body.* New York: WW Norton.

Bibliography

*Carroll P. (1994). Speed: The essential response to anaphylaxis. *RN, 57*:26–35.

*Handerhan B. (1994). Dealing with an anticholinergic overdose. *Nursing '94, 24*:68–69.

*Recommended for further reading.

For more information and sample tests and activities, refer to Chapter 16 in the Student Workbook for Clinical Pharmacology and Nursing Management, 5th edition, available through your bookstore.

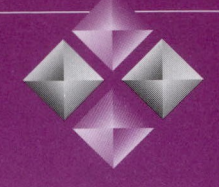

17

Drugs That Stimulate the Central Nervous System

This chapter discusses central nervous system (CNS) stimulants and their implications for nursing management. Among the drugs discussed are amphetamines and similar drugs used to treat attention deficit hyperactivity disorder (ADHD) and narcolepsy; xanthines, most of which are natural stimulants; ana-leptics, which are seldom used but may be encountered in clients with insecticide poisoning; antiparkinson agents such as selegiline, dopaminergics (levodopa), dopamine agonists, and anticholinergics used to treat idiopathic Parkinson's disease and drug-induced parkinsonism; and cholinesterase inhibitors (Alzheimer's drugs) such as tacrine.

Physiology of the Central Nervous System

The CNS includes the organs and tissues enclosed in the cranium and in the spinal column, namely the brain and spinal cord. Its function somewhat resembles that of a computer. Information enters through sensory fibers, is processed by the system, and is then emitted as instructions through motor fibers. The process is continuous, providing for appropriate responses of the organism to changing conditions. The brain also carries out intellectual processes and is responsible for consciousness and subjective awareness.

Many functions of the CNS are spatially distributed (Figs. 17-1 through 17-4). Others, such as memory, seem to be more pervasive. Selectivity of drug action depends on a drug's ability to affect one area or type of tissue more than others. For example, drugs that affect the cerebral cortex tend to influence sensory perceptions, motor activity, and intellectual processes. Drugs with pronounced effects on the limbic system change emotional status.

The distribution of chemicals to the brain is controlled by a mechanism known as the blood-brain barrier. Cells in the cerebral capillaries are tightly joined, almost fused. Because the spaces between these cells lack the slit pores found in other capillary membranes, only tiny molecules pass through these openings. Normally, water, carbon dioxide, oxygen, sodium, chlorine, phosphorus, and lipid-soluble substances penetrate to the brain. The efficiency of the blood-brain barrier is influenced by the condition of its tissues. If the barrier is impaired by an inflammation, such as meningitis, it may allow entry of therapeutic drugs that are normally poorly distributed in the CNS.

Response to CNS drugs depends largely on the client's status. Underlying personality, physiologic function, and emotional status reflect and influence CNS physiology, the milieu in which drugs act. Drug response is also influenced by the client's history and situation. For instance, previous exposure to the drug can produce tolerance or sensitization. Environmental stimuli can alter CNS activity and can promote or inhibit response to pharmacologic agents.

Central nervous system stimulants include amphetamines, xanthines, some of the antiparkinson drugs, and analeptics. Cocaine, khat, betel, and hallucinogens, such as marijuana and LSD, are also CNS stimulants; they are discussed in Chapter 14.

In small doses, these drugs increase mental alertness and capacity for work, improve motor performance, and impart a feeling of well-being. They tend to stimulate the respiratory system, cardiac system, and general metabo-

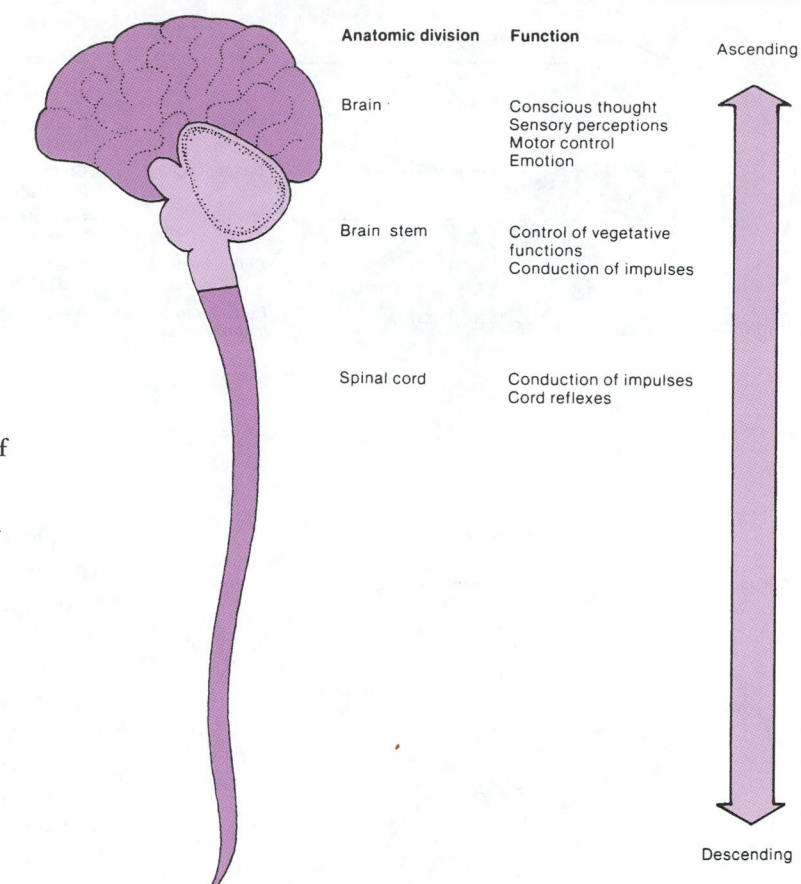

Anatomic division	Function	
		Ascending
Brain	Conscious thought Sensory perceptions Motor control Emotion	
Brain stem	Control of vegetative functions Conduction of impulses	
Spinal cord	Conduction of impulses Cord reflexes	
		Descending

Figure 17-1. Spatial distribution of functions of the central nervous system: divisions of the central nervous system. Functions of the brain are considered "higher" functions, those of the spinal cord "lower" functions. Drugs that exhibit an ascending pattern of activity affect first the function of the spinal cord, then successively higher functions, affecting the brain last of all. Drugs that exhibit a descending pattern of activity affect the cortex of the brain first, then successively lower functions.

Motor area

Central fissure

Sensory area

Inhibition, planning, judgment

Frontal lobe

Parietal lobe

Visual sensory area

Occipital lobe

Temporal lobe

Lateral fissure

Auditory sensory area

Midbrain

Pons

Medulla oblongata

Spinal cord

Transverse fissure

Cerebellum

Figure 17-2. Spatial distribution of cortical function.

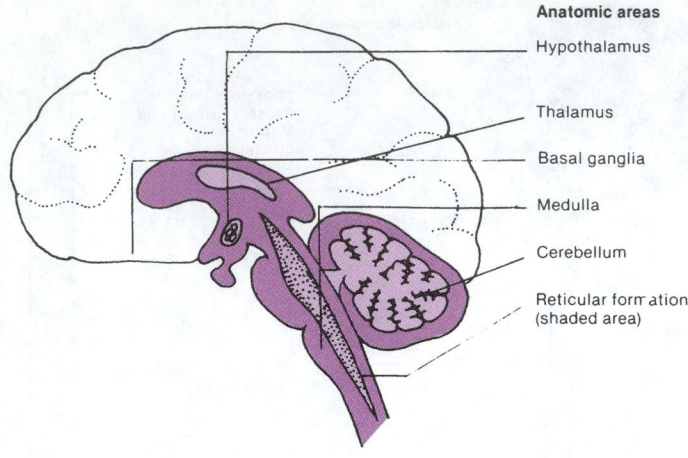

Anatomic areas	Functions
Hypothalamus	Physical expression of emotion; appetite; temperature regulation
Thalamus	Crude sensation of pain; focusing of attention
Basal ganglia	Control of habitual (semiautomatic) motor function
Medulla	Control of vital functions (respiration and blood pressure)
Cerebellum	Muscular coordination and balance
Reticular formation (shaded area)	Wakefulness

Figure 17-3. Spatial distribution of functions of the brain stem. The brain stem controls many vital and automatic or semi-automatic functions.

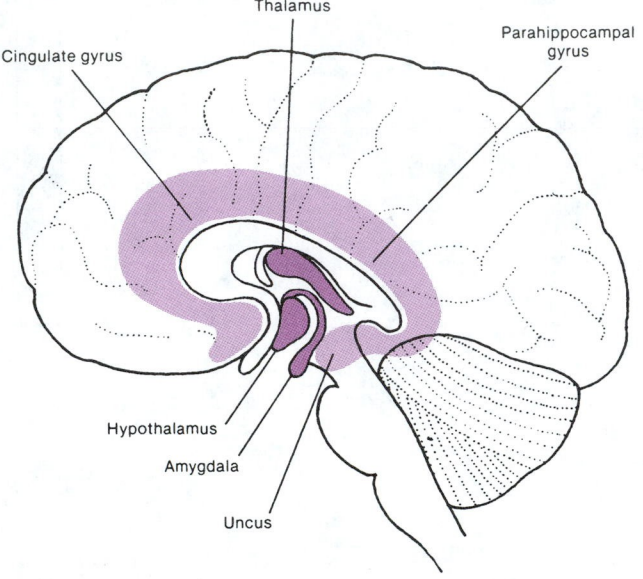

Figure 17-4. Spatial distribution of the limbic system. The limbic system includes the cingulate gyrus, parahippocampal gyrus, uncus, thalamus, hypothalamus, and amygdala. It functions as a storehouse for memories of past emotional experiences (pain, pleasure, sexual activities) and odors and controls emotional responses such as excitement, aggression, and sexual behavior.

lism. In large doses, they cause tremor, restlessness, and insomnia. Motor performance deteriorates. Prolonged use can lead to hypertension and exhaustion. As toxicity increases, hallucinations, seizures, and serious cardiac arrhythmia can develop (Box 17-1). Central nervous system stimulants are used for selected clinical conditions.

Amphetamines

Amphetamine (beta-phenylisopropylamine) is a synthetic derivative of ephedrine. It exerts CNS and peripheral alpha- and beta-adrenergic effects. Several related substances have similar actions (Table 17-1). Because they can produce severe psychological dependence, they are classified as schedule II drugs by the Controlled Substances Act of 1970 (see Chap. 2).

Pharmacodynamics. Amphetamines stimulate the release of neurotransmitters in the brain. The neurotransmitters norepinephrine, dopamine, and serotonin are involved at successively higher doses (Table 17-2). The drugs may also exert a direct agonistic action on central receptors for serotonin. The resulting effects include increased alertness, mood elevation, decreased perception of fatigue, increased ability to concentrate, a reduction in appetite, and an increased capacity for work. Psychologically, initiative and self-confidence increase. Physiologic changes include bronchial relaxation, an increase in systolic and diastolic blood pressure, increased or decreased peristalsis, and increased tone in the urinary bladder sphincters. Rapid-eye-movement (REM) sleep is suppressed. Amphetamines are considered among the most powerful sympathomimetic amines for stimulating the CNS.

Pharmacokinetics. Amphetamines are readily absorbed from the gastrointestinal (GI) tract. They are widely distributed throughout the body, with high concentrations in the brain and cerebrospinal fluid. Varying proportions of the drugs are metabolized, but the sites and mechanisms of metabolism are not well understood. Excretion is by the kidneys and depends on urinary pH. An acidic urine enhances elimination.

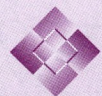

Box 17-1
Action of CNS Stimulants

- Small doses increase mental alertness and capacity for work, improve motor performance, impart a feeling of well-being, and stimulate the respiratory and cardiac systems and general metabolism.
- Large doses cause tremor, restlessness, and insomnia and result in deterioration of motor performance.
- Prolonged use can lead to hypertension and exhaustion.
- Results of toxicity are hallucinations, convulsions, and serious cardiac arrhythmia.

Table 17-1. Amphetamines and Related Substances

Drug Name	Preparations	Usual Dosage	Therapeutic Uses and Additional Information
amphetamine (Benzedrine, "bennies")	Oral tablets and capsules	Adults: 5–30 mg daily, divided in up to 3 doses PC: C	Treatment of narcolepsy, attention deficit hyperactivity disorder (ADHD), and obesity; abused as a stimulant
benzphetamine (Didrex)	Oral tablets	Adults: 25–150 mg/day, divided in 1–3 doses PC: X	Treatment of obesity
dextroamphetamine (Dexedrine, "dexies," Dextrostat)	Oral tablets, capsules, elixir, and extended-release capsules	Adults: 5–60 mg daily, divided in up to 3 doses Children: 2–15 mg daily, divided in 3 doses PC: C	Treatment of narcolepsy, ADHD, and obesity; abused as a stimulant
diethylpropion (Tenuate, Tepanil)	Oral tablets and extended-release tablets	Adults: 25–100 mg/day, divided in 3–4 doses, administered before meals PC: C	Treatment of obesity
fenfluramine (Ponderal, Pondimin)	Oral tablets	Adults: 60–120 mg daily, divided in 3 doses, administered before meals PC: C	Treatment of obesity
mazindol (Mazanor, Sanorex)	Oral tablets	Adults: 2–3 mg/day; a 2-mg dose is administered as a single dose before lunch; a 3-mg dose is divided in 3 doses, administered before meals PC: C	Treatment of obesity
methamphetamine (Desoxyn, Methampex, "speed")	Oral tablets and extended-release tablets	Adults: 5–30 mg daily, divided in up to 3 doses PC: C	Treatment of obesity and ADHD
methylphenidate (Ritalin)	Oral tablets and extended-release tablets	Adults: 20–60 mg daily, divided in 2–3 doses Children age 6 and older: 250 µg/kg body weight/day, divided in 2 doses, administered before breakfast and lunch PC: C	Treatment of ADHD and narcolepsy
pemoline (Cylert)	Oral tablets and chewable tablets	Children: *Initially:* 37.5 mg/day; *maintenance:* 56.25–75 mg/day, administered as a single daily dose on awakening PC: C	Treatment of ADHD in children older than age 6
phendimetrazine (Anorex, Appecon, Bontril, Dyrexan, Melfiat, Plegine, Prelu-2, Weh-Less, Obezine, Phendiet)	Oral tablets, capsules, and extended-release capsules	Adults: 70–105 mg/day, divided in 2–3 doses (extended-release forms administered as a single daily dose on awakening) PC: C	Treatment of obesity
phenmetrazine (Preludin)	Oral tablets and extended-release tablets	Adults: 25–75 mg daily, divided in 2–3 doses PC: C	Treatment of obesity
phentermine (Adipex-P, Fastin, Ionamin, Obephen, Phentrol, Wilpowr, Phentercot, Termin, Zantryl)	Oral tablets, capsules, and extended-release capsules	Adults: 24 mg/day, divided in 3 doses, administered before meals (extended-release forms administered as a single daily dose on awakening) PC: C	Treatment of obesity

KEY: PC = pregnancy category. (See Appendix A.)

Table 17-2. Dose-Related Effects of Amphetamine Drugs

Dose	Effect on Central Nervous System Biochemistry	Physiologic Effects
Low	Release of norepinephrine from nonadrenergic neurons	Increased alertness, decreased appetite, limited locomotor stimulation
Medium	Release of dopamine from dopaminergic neurons in the neostriatum	Increased locomotor activity, stereotypic behavior
High	Release of serotonin from tryptaminergic neurons	Perceptual disturbances, overt psychotic behavior
	Release of dopamine in the mesolimbic system	

Therapeutic Uses. Amphetamines are used for treating narcolepsy, hyperactivity syndrome, and learning disabilities in children affected by ADHD. In narcolepsy, amphetamines prevent sleep episodes and decrease catalepsy. In children with ADHD, treatment with amphetamines or amphetamine-like drugs improves concentration and coordination, lengthens attention span, increases scholastic achievement, and paradoxically has a calming effect.

Using amphetamines as anorectics in treating obesity is controversial. Tolerance develops rapidly to this effect of the drug, and prolonged use is contraindicated. Drug therapy must be accompanied by a prescribed reduction in caloric intake.

Amphetamines are sometimes used in treating enuresis, depressive psychoneuroses, and Parkinson's disease when levodopa cannot be used.

Adverse Reactions. Administration of amphetamines to children can precipitate Tourette syndrome, a neurologic condition characterized by motor tics (eye-blinking, throat-clearing, jaw-jerking, chin-dropping, arm-jerking, hip-turning) and abnormal phonation (snorting and snuffling, humming and panting noises, puppy-like sounds, language outbursts). Uninterrupted amphetamine therapy can retard growth. Muscle stiffness sometimes develops when the drugs are first used, but this subsides with continued treatment. Other undesirable effects of the drugs are largely related to toxic signs and symptoms; their appearance with normal doses of the drug is considered idiosyncratic.

Toxic symptoms occur as dosage increases. Intermediate dosage produces elation, euphoria, talkativeness, increased motor activity, sleeplessness, and restlessness. Libido tends to increase. Systolic and diastolic blood-pressure measurements rise, and reflexes become hyperactive. A metallic taste and dryness in the mouth can occur, as well as a tendency toward anorexia, nausea, vomiting, and abdominal cramps. Sweating and tremor are common. Hyperactivity may cause a rise in body temperature. Incoordination, irritability, headache, palpitations, dizziness, dysphoria, apprehension, anxiety, agitation, and confusion usually occur as toxic levels approach. Confusion, delirium, paranoid hallucinations, and overt psychotic behavior may develop as well. Panic states and suicidal or homicidal tendencies sometimes occur. Cardiac signs and symptoms include arrhythmia and angina. Blood pressure may rise or fall. In extreme toxicity, circulatory collapse, convulsions, and coma precede death. Numerous cerebral hemorrhages are found on autopsy.

Chronic amphetamine toxicity is characterized by psychotic behavior in addition to the signs and symptoms of acute toxicity. The client may have classic symptoms of schizophrenia. Weight loss is common. Dermatitis occurs on occasion. Continuous long-term use by children inhibits growth and may permanently stunt it.

Tolerance to the drug's effects varies. Tolerance can develop rapidly in relation to appetite suppression in clients who take the drug to control obesity, but it is rarely seen in treatment regimens for narcolepsy. The use of chronic high dosages, common in drug abusers, considerably reduces the response to a given dose.

Severe mental depression and fatigue are experienced on withdrawal from prolonged use or use of high doses. To what extent these conditions are due to psychological or physical dependence is uncertain.

Drug–Drug Interactions. The interaction of amphetamines with other adrenergic agents and tricyclic antidepressants results in additive adrenergic effects. Phenothiazines decrease the effect of amphetamines. Amphetamine use with monoamine oxidase inhibitors (MAOIs) can result in hypertensive crisis. Amphetamine use with anticonvulsants, such as phenytoin, may delay the effects of the anticonvulsants. The interaction of amphetamine and antihypertensive agents may antagonize the effects of the antihypertensive drug.

Drug–Food Interactions. Foods that acidify urine can enhance the excretion of amphetamines.

Precautions and Contraindications. Amphetamines should be used with caution in malnutrition, restlessness, and insomnia. They are contraindicated for clients with hypertension, cardiovascular disease, hyperthyroidism, anxiety states, motor tics, or a personal or family history of Tourette syndrome.

Clients who receive amphetamines must have continuing medical supervision. During amphetamine therapy, clients should be monitored for signs and symptoms of overstimulation, such as increased blood pressure, tremor, muscle stiffness, and hyperactive reflexes. They should be assessed for nervousness, sleeplessness, and side effects. After extended use, amphetamine dosages should be reduced gradually to prevent withdrawal symptoms.

Amphetamine therapy for ADHD should be discontinued at the first sign of motor or phonic tics. During long-term treatment of children, medication should be interrupted frequently to allow growth to resume. Growth during these "drug holidays" is usually rapid and sufficient to prevent permanent stunting.

The use of amphetamines to eliminate fatigue and prolong performance is extremely dangerous. Amphetamine-induced hallucinations have been cited as a cause of motor-vehicle accidents. Chronic use is associated with malnutrition and reduced resistance to disease. Homicidal and suicidal behavior can occur. Susceptible persons are thought to be at increased risk for developing schizoid psychoses.

■ SUMMARY

Amphetamines are CNS stimulants used in treating narcolepsy and ADHD. Side effects include hypertension, irritability, and anxiety. Psychotic behavior develops in toxic states. Amphetamines can cause physical and psychological dependence.

❖ NURSING MANAGEMENT: CLIENT RECEIVING AMPHETAMINES

Because amphetamines have been widely abused, they have acquired a reputation of being harmful drugs. Some clients, fearing chemical dependence, are reluctant to take them. Despite continuing controversy, amphetamine therapy has been useful for ADHD, narcolepsy, and obesity.

ADHD. Researchers theorize that ADHD arises from a disruption of norepinephrine metabolism. By stimulating norepinephrine release, amphetamines may alter brain chemistry toward a more normal state. Hyperactivity may be caused by an immaturity of brain tissue that controls selective screening of stimuli and motor inhibition. Stimulation of these brain areas tends to normalize behavior.

Treatment of ADHD is usually established by the family's physician and remains within parental control. Drug therapy may be prescribed after a complete examination and evaluation. Doses are given in the morning and, if a second dose is required, at noon. The second dose may need to be given by the school nurse. In such cases, the nurse works closely with the family, and in accordance with school policies, to coordinate treatment.

Intermittent drug therapy is usually advised to prevent tolerance to medication and to minimize its growth-retarding effect. Drug holidays usually coincide with school vacations. When therapy is initiated (or resumed), the client may develop slight muscle stiffness. With continued treatment, this symptom, which is most noticeable in the neck, tends to subside.

Narcolepsy. Narcolepsy is characterized by the sudden occurrence of hypersomnia and sleep under conditions not usually conducive to sleep. Its onset may be in late adolescence or early adulthood. In some cases diagnosis is difficult because the person may underestimate the frequency and length of sleep episodes or consider them insignificant. The development of cataplexy (sudden collapse due to loss of muscle tone) may prompt the person to seek medical care. Narcolepsy is a safety hazard because sleep episodes are uncontrollable and occur suddenly. Amphetamine therapy can eliminate sleep episodes and lessen the severity of cataplexy. Tolerance to and dependence on the drugs are not problems in this situation. Some clients with narcolepsy respond positively to treatment with tricyclic antidepressants or MAOIs.

Overdose/Toxicity. Amphetamines are frequently abused for psychotropic effect. The effect of the drugs on the user varies widely, depending on the user's physiologic and psychological state at the time a dose is taken. Toxicity is most likely to occur in the neophyte user. Acute overdoses can occur because of the user's increased susceptibility to the drug or because an unusually potent preparation was ingested.

An amphetamine overdose requires emergency measures. As soon as amphetamine overdose is identified, treatment is instituted to promote excretion of the drug and counteract its most serious effects. Ammonium chloride is administered to acidify the urine and promote rapid renal elimination of the drugs. If the blood pressure is high, a rapidly acting alpha-adrenergic blocking agent (phentolamine) is given to reduce blood pressure to the normal range. Fever is managed by cooling procedures. Symptoms related to CNS overstimulation are ameliorated by administering chlorpromazine or a short-acting barbiturate. In addition to treating toxicity, the healthcare team must offer supportive care and counseling to reduce the risk of continued substance abuse and recurrent overdoses.

Educational programs to reduce chemical abuse should be directed to children and adults. For more information, see Chapter 14.

NURSING PROCESS

ASSESSMENT

Factors to assess before amphetamine therapy begins include previous use of and response to stimulant drugs, history and current status of the condition for which amphetamines are prescribed, and history of conditions for which the drugs are contraindicated (hypertension, cardiovascular disease, hyperthyroidism, anxiety states, history of homicidal or suicidal trends, motor tics, and Tourette syndrome). Any family history of Tourette syndrome should be noted as well.

Physical examination should include height and weight measurements and an assessment of GI, cardiovascular, neuromuscular, endocrine, and emotional status. Attention span and speech patterns should be noted.

NURSING DIAGNOSIS

Diagnoses related to the conditions for which drug therapy is prescribed include:

- Altered Growth and Development, related to ADHD and drug therapy
- Ineffective Coping (family, individual, or both), related to shortened attention span and hyperactivity
- Altered Nutrition: More than Body Requirements, related to ingestion of more food than required for activity

Amphetamine therapy increases the risk of:

- Pain, related to muscle stiffness
- Altered Nutrition: Less than Body Requirements, related to anorexia
- Anxiety, related to CNS stimulation
- Sleep Pattern Disturbance: Insomnia, related to hyperactivity and CNS stimulation
- Risk for Injury, related to confusion, dizziness, panic, or suicidal ideation secondary to CNS stimulation

Most clients exhibit:

- Knowledge Deficit concerning the medical use of amphetamines

Some are at risk for:

- Ineffective Management of Therapeutic Regimen: Noncompliance related to lack of knowledge, fear of stimulant drug use, and mistrust of regimen

A common collaborative problem that should be differentiated from the nursing diagnoses is:

Potential Complication: hypertension

PLANNING

Outcomes identified for ADHD treatment include promotion of growth and development, improved family dynamics, and improved individual and family coping. In narcolepsy, a reduction in daytime sleep episodes, improved nighttime sleep, and a reduction in cataplexy are desired. Weight reduction is the goal when the drug is used as an anorexic. Additional goals for all clients who use the drugs include avoiding drug dependence, ameliorating muscle stiffness and pain, maintaining good nutrition, preventing injury, promoting rest and nighttime sleep, and learning about the drug regimen. Prevention or prompt detection and treatment of toxic signs and symptoms such as anxiety, panic, hyperthermia, incoordination, confusion, dizziness, angina, stroke,

and suicidal tendencies is also important. The goal of teaching is to help the client and family manage the drug regimen safely and effectively.

INTERVENTION

When the initial assessment of the client is completed, the nurse should inform the physician of any contraindications for amphetamine use, as well as any evidence of CNS and sympathetic overactivity.

Amphetamines used for extended therapy should be administered with breakfast and, if a second dose is required, with lunch. Amphetamines prescribed for weight control should be taken 30 to 60 minutes before meals. If noontime medication is required for school-age children, the school nurse should work closely with the family to coordinate treatment.

Frequent drug holidays help prevent dependence and stunted growth. The drugs are usually given on school days and at other times when a high performance level is required; drug-free periods may be scheduled for school vacations or other recesses. Drug holidays for adult clients should also be scheduled for periods of relative leisure. Adults do not require as much drug-free time as do children.

Although school performance will probably improve with drug treatment, children with ADHD may need special education to compensate for residual academic deficits. The nurse may refer the child and family for psychological counseling if the family indicates a desire for such services.

If signs and symptoms of withdrawal develop during drug holidays, a weaning schedule may be needed. Caffeine-containing beverages (coffee or cola) can ameliorate withdrawal.

During the first few weeks of treatment, massage and applications of heat (particularly to the neck) help prevent or relieve muscle stiffness. Muscle stiffness and anorexia tend to dissipate with continued treatment.

If the client is not being treated for obesity, appetizing meals of foods favored by the client help maintain food intake.

All clients who receive amphetamines on a long-term basis should be monitored regularly for early signs and symptoms of amphetamine toxicity. If these develop, the physician should be consulted for a reduction in dosage. Frank toxicity requires discontinuation of the drugs and definitive treatment.

Client Education. The nurse must develop and implement a teaching plan to help the client and family manage the drug regimen.

Clients on long-term therapy should be advised to avoid other stimulant substances, including caffeine, except for periods when the amphetamines are temporarily withheld. Doses of the stimulants should be avoided for at least 6 hours before bedtime. Clients who need to lose weight should take the medications 30 to

60 minutes before meals. All clients may be taught measures to promote rest and sleep: a period of quiet activity such as reading before bedtime, retiring at about the same time every night, and adherence to a bedtime ritual. If family members are willing, they may be taught to give the client a soothing backrub at bedtime.

Clients may need to learn how to plan diets to meet their nutritional needs. Caloric requirements may be increased while amphetamines are used. Unless clients are overweight, they should be advised to consume enough food to maintain weight. Clients who need to lose weight should be cautioned to limit use of the drugs to the first 2 to 4 weeks, when their use facilitates adjustment to a reduced food intake. Emphasis should be on the diet rather than the drugs as the cause of weight loss.

Clients should be informed that they may experience muscle stiffness during the first few weeks of treatment and again when treatment resumes after drug holidays. Applications of heat and massage may be recommended, and the techniques for these treatments should be demonstrated. The nurse may recommend monitoring blood pressure, especially if the client is elderly. As appropriate, the nurse can teach the client or family members how to obtain, use, and read a sphygmomanometer or other blood-pressure-measuring devices. Blood pressure should be monitored several times a week.

The nurse can teach clients or family members to recognize the early signs of amphetamine toxicity. Instructions for consulting the prescriber for an adjustment in dosage should include the specific signs and symptoms the prescriber wishes to know about.

Clients who are reluctant to take amphetamines over a long period should be reassured that medical use does not usually lead to psychological dependence. If a mild physical dependence develops, the nurse can explain that gradual weaning from the drug may be effective and produce little or no discomfort.

OUTCOME EVALUATION

Data required for evaluating therapy of children include information related to academic achievement and behavior, physical growth compared to norms for the client's age group, and family interaction and coping. As the child matures, parents and healthcare personnel should evaluate performance during drug-free periods to determine when amphetamine therapy may be discontinued. To evaluate adult clients with narcolepsy, sleep–wake patterns should be assessed, as well as the incidence of cataplexy. Body weight is monitored at regular intervals (usually weekly or biweekly) to evaluate weight-reduction regimens.

The presence or absence of toxic effects and side effects of the drugs (tolerance and dependence, discomfort from muscle stiffness, confusion, inappropriate affect, fever, angina, stroke, and injury) should be ascertained. Food intake should be recorded and compared with appropriate intake for the client. To evaluate client education, the nurse should ask the client and family to repeat information conveyed during teaching and to demonstrate techniques that have been taught.

AMPHETAMINE OVERDOSE

ASSESSMENT

In assessing for possible amphetamine overdose, the nurse evaluates the client's mental and physical status. Amphetamine overdose may be characterized by elation and euphoria or anxiety, agitation and panic, restlessness and hyperactivity, fever, hypertension, hyperpnea, hyperactive reflexes, or GI upset (nausea, vomiting, diarrhea). The client may appear to be suffering from seizure disorder, stroke, or schizophrenia. Physical examination should include a complete neurologic assessment. After resolution of the immediate health crisis, the client's coping skills should be evaluated.

NURSING DIAGNOSIS

Nursing diagnoses related to amphetamine overdose may include:

- Anxiety, related to nervous system overstimulation
- Hyperthermia, related to hyperactivity
- Fatigue, related to hyperactivity
- Sleep Pattern Disturbance: Insomnia and Restlessness, related to nervous system overstimulation
- Risk for Injury, related to seizures or to suicidal ideation
- Impaired Physical Mobility, related to coma and paralysis secondary to stroke
- Impaired Gas Exchange, related to coma and paralysis

Clients who habitually abuse stimulants may have ineffective coping skills.

PLANNING

Goals for treatment include ameliorating anxiety or panic, reducing fever and hypertension, promoting rest, and preventing injury or self-injury. For comatose clients, preventing complications resulting from immobility (eg, hypoxia, pressure ulcers, thrombophlebitis) is important. A long-term client goal is development of more effective coping skills.

INTERVENTION

Hyperactive clients should be removed to a quiet room and protected from unnecessary stimuli. An emotionally supportive environment should be provided. The presence of a supportive relative or friend can be helpful. Seizure and suicide precautions should be instituted. Treatment is largely symptomatic. A cooling blanket may be used to reduce body temperature. Temperature and blood pressure should be monitored closely. Clients with anxiety or panic may benefit from the nurse's reassurance and matter-of-fact attitude.

Clients should be monitored closely for a reversal in symptoms as amphetamine levels decline. A withdrawal period of lethargy, depression, and sleep, characterized by a high amount of REM sleep, is common. This may be severe if depressant drugs have been administered. After resolution of the immediate crisis, drug-dependent clients should be encouraged to enter a drug treatment program that stresses the development of coping skills.

OUTCOME EVALUATION

Data required for evaluating the outcome of nursing measures include assessment of skin color, body temperature, blood pressure, emotional affect, energy level, psychomotor function, incidence of injury, and level of consciousness. To evaluate the client's coping skills after lengthy treatment programs, the incidence of recurrent drug abuse should be determined.

❖ CHECKLIST OF NURSING ACTIONS

- ❏ Assess clients who are to receive amphetamines for contraindications and for risk of adverse drug reactions.
- ❏ Monitor for amphetamine-related changes in appetite, hypertension, hyperactive reflexes, muscle tremors, hyperactivity, and sleep disorders.
- ❏ Emphasize dietary management more than drug therapy as effective treatment of obesity.
- ❏ Advise clients receiving prescribed amphetamines to limit drug dosage to morning and early afternoon hours.
- ❏ Encourage clients on amphetamine treatment to adhere to the prescribed regimen, including specified drug holidays.
- ❏ Teach concerned people about the therapeutic benefits of amphetamine use.
- ❏ Provide a quiet, supportive environment for victims of amphetamine overdose.
- ❏ During emergency treatment of victims of amphetamine overdose, give priority to controlling high fever, hypertension, and seizures.
- ❏ Teach about the problems related to overuse and abuse of amphetamines.
- ❏ Promote parenting skills to increase self-confidence and self-esteem in children as an important factor in preventing amphetamine abuse.

Xanthines

The methylated xanthines—caffeine, theophylline, and theobromine—are natural alkaloids that are structurally related to uric acid. They are found in plant materials and are used in preparing foods and beverages such as chocolate, coffee, tea, and cola. They are descending stimulants that affect the brain before the spinal cord and lower structures.

Pharmacodynamics. The physiologic action of the xanthines is not completely understood, although they increase the turnover of monoamines in the CNS, augment the release of sympathoadrenal catecholamines, inhibit the degradation of cyclic adenosine monophosphate, and decrease the cytosolic concentration of calcium ions. These mechanisms could explain many physiologic effects of the drug family, but cause-and-effect relations remain unknown.

Caffeine increases norepinephrine secretion and enhances neural activity in many brain areas. It is thought that many caffeine and other xanthine effects occur by means of competitive antagonism at adenosine receptors. Adenosine is a neurotransmitter with a pronounced sedative effect. This adaptation to caffeine represents a type of tolerance and could explain the sedation and craving for caffeine that can occur when caffeine is abruptly withdrawn from a habitual user.

General effects of the xanthines in the body include CNS stimulation, constriction of cerebral blood vessels, diuresis, cardiac stimulation, and relaxation of smooth muscles, including those of the bronchi. Xanthines apparently serve as natural insecticides, protecting plants such as coffee, tea, coca, and kola from insect pests.

Pharmacokinetics. The solubility of the xanthines can be increased by formulation of salts such as theophylline ethylenediamine (aminophylline) or other complexes such as caffeine and sodium benzoate. They are absorbed rapidly after oral, rectal, or parenteral administration. Protein binding varies, being highest at 50% with theophylline. The methylated xanthines distribute widely to all tissues, cross the placenta, and pass into breast milk. Relative concentration in the CNS is greater for caffeine than theophylline. Xanthines are deactivated primarily by the microsomal enzymes in the liver. Small amounts are excreted by the kidneys.

Therapeutic Uses. Beverages that contain xanthines are used socially and as part of the diet because of their stimulant properties. They decrease drowsiness and fatigue, increase mental alertness, reduce reaction time, and increase the capacity for physical and intellectual work without appreciably impairing the performance of accustomed tasks.

Caffeine is incorporated in many over-the-counter (OTC) headache remedies. Its vasoconstrictive action reduces blood flow to the brain. When taken at the first symptom of an attack, these preparations sometimes abort migraines, a type of headache associated with cerebral vasodilation and congestion.

Prescription use of the xanthines as CNS stimulants for maintaining vital functions is rare. In the past, xanthines were prescribed because adequate supportive measures to treat respiratory and cerebral depression were unavailable. Caffeine is still occasionally used as an adjunct in treating toxicity related to CNS depressants.

Xanthines are valuable as respiratory stimulants in the treatment of chronic obstructive airway disease in adults (see Chap. 37) and in the treatment of apnea in premature infants. They are particularly useful in obstructive airway disease associated with bronchoconstriction. In infants, plasma levels of theophylline maintained between 2 and 10 µg/mL (11–53 µmol/L) reduce the frequency and length of apneic episodes of undetermined origin.

Caffeine has been suggested as a treatment for hyperactive behavior in children with ADHD when amphetamines are poorly tolerated. Xanthines are also used therapeutically as diuretics and bronchodilators.

Adverse Reactions. Side effects of the xanthines include nervousness, restlessness, insomnia, tremor, and hyperesthesia. Anxiety, nervousness, fear, nausea, restlessness, and panic disorder are increased by caffeine use. Xanthines impair the performance of motor skills that have been imperfectly or incompletely mastered. They are irritating to the gastric mucosa, whether administered orally or systemically. Xanthines increase plasma levels of free fatty acid and glycerol and elevate blood pressure, and they may stimulate cardiac arrhythmia.

The relation between long-term consumption of large amounts of coffee and serum cholesterol appears to be related to something other than caffeine. Evidence linking xanthines to fibrocystic breast disease is controversial. In linking xanthines to heart disease, further research is required.

Excessive intake of caffeine (600 mg or more daily) has been associated with human fetal death and birth defects. Xanthine toxicity can cause focal and generalized seizures. Lethal doses for humans range from 3,000 to 10,000 mg. Theophylline frequently causes toxic symptoms when plasma levels exceed 20 mg/mL. Toxicity from this drug is more difficult to treat than that caused by other xanthines.

Chronic use of caffeine produces both tolerance and dependence in some persons. Withdrawal is characterized by fatigue and sedation; withdrawal from large doses can result in severe headaches and nausea.

Drug Interactions. Xanthines increase the toxicity of other CNS stimulants, including therapeutic drugs such as the amphetamines and theophylline. Xanthines may antagonize the effects of sedative–hypnotics, antidepressants, and antipsychotics. Caffeine increases the renal excretion of lithium, necessitating higher-than-normal dosages of this antipsychotic. If caffeine is suddenly withdrawn without reducing lithium dosages, serum concentrations of lithium may reach toxic levels.

Precautions and Contraindications. Xanthines are contraindicated in hyperthyroidism, pheochromocytoma, peptic ulcer disease, and cardiac conditions in which the risk of serious arrhythmia is increased. They should be avoided when other CNS stimulants (eg, amphetamines) are used. Seizure disorders may be worsened by xanthine use. Xanthines should not be used by stimulant-sensitive persons, in whom they cause restlessness, tremor, and insomnia.

Regular tests for theophylline plasma levels must be performed on clients who receive long-term theophylline therapy. Diazepam should be readily available to treat seizures should a toxic reaction occur.

Xanthine drinks and oral medications should be taken with food to prevent direct irritation of the gastric mucosa.

■ SUMMARY

Xanthines are CNS stimulants in common use as dietary components. They reduce fatigue and improve work performance. Medically, they are used to treat chronic obstructive airway disease and asthma. Xanthines may exacerbate the symptoms of psychotic states, panic disorder, sleep disorders, and fibrocystic breast disease. They also increase the effects of other CNS stimulants and antagonize the effects of CNS depressants. Chronic use can cause a toxic syndrome characterized by restlessness, irritability, and insomnia. Tolerance and dependence can develop in long-term users.

❖ NURSING MANAGEMENT: CLIENT RECEIVING XANTHINES

Xanthine-containing beverages and foods may help control withdrawal symptoms when amphetamines are withheld temporarily from clients on extended therapy. If xanthines are used to prevent exacerbations of symptoms during drug holidays, the physician should be informed so that the evaluation of the client's response to drug withdrawal is accurate. Clients and parents should inform the physician about the client's xanthine-rich diet.

On the other hand, dietary restriction of xanthine-containing beverages and foods is usually ordered by physicians treating clients with thyroid toxicity, pheochromocytoma, heart disease, or peptic ulcer disease. Clients who receive narcotic analgesics should avoid caffeine because it diminishes the effectiveness of these drugs. Decaffeinated products may be used by most of these clients, but even decaffeinated preparations contain some caffeine and should be avoided by clients subject to gastric hypersecretion and cardiac tachyarrhythmia.

Response to caffeine varies among people. Children are generally more sensitive than adults. Most infants cannot metabolize caffeine until they are at least 7 months old, possibly 9 months. Some people have no difficulty sleeping after drinking coffee, tea, or cola; others must avoid even small amounts of caffeine. Chronic use of caffeine may produce tolerance to the stimulant while emphasizing the hyperglycemic and cardiovascular effects of the drug.

The side effects of xanthine-containing beverages and foods stem from substances other than xanthines. Whether decaffeinated or not, coffee increases the rate of glycogenolysis (raising the blood glucose level), stimulates peristalsis, and induces extrasystole in cardiac rhythm. Tea, an astringent, tends to cause constipation. Foods that contain chocolate are usually high in sugar and calories.

NURSING PROCESS

ASSESSMENT

No drug history is complete without a comprehensive evaluation of caffeine intake. In addition to the habitual use of coffee, the use of tea, soft drinks, and chocolate should be explored. Clients who report high levels of caffeine intake and those who receive medicinal xanthines should be assessed for fine muscle tremors and subjective symptoms such as nervousness, headache, irritability, fatigue, and insomnia. Pulse and respirations may be elevated.

NURSING DIAGNOSIS

Diagnoses that derive from social or medicinal use of xanthines include:

- Altered Comfort: Restlessness, related to CNS stimulation
- Disturbance in Self-concept, related to tremulousness, nervousness, and irritability
- Ineffective Individual Coping, related to irritability and fatigue
- Sleep Pattern Disturbance: Insomnia, related to CNS stimulation
- Knowledge Deficit, concerning the health effects of xanthine drugs
- Ineffective Management of Therapeutic Regimen, related to knowledge deficit, mistrust of regimen, or powerlessness

Abrupt withdrawal of xanthines from dependent clients can cause:

- Pain: headache possibly related to hypoglycemia
- Altered Thought Process, related to decreased alertness, depression, and lethargy
- Sensory/Perceptual Alteration: Decreased Sensory Acuity, related to CNS depression

PLANNING

Goals of treatment for clients who receive xanthine medication include increased rest and sleep, reduced fatigue by conservation of energy, and decreased restlessness. For clients affected by excessive dietary use of xanthines, the goal is a reduction of xanthine intake. Improved self-concept, improved coping skills, and increased knowledge about xanthines are appropriate goals for all clients. For clients who experience withdrawal, goals include alleviation of pain (headache) and stimulation to increase wakefulness and sensory acuity.

INTERVENTION

When xanthine medications are used to treat an acute illness such as an exacerbation of respiratory disease, they may be administered intravenously. Because the margin of safety is relatively narrow, the rate of flow must be carefully controlled, preferably by an infusion pump. Regardless of the route of administration, blood levels of the drug should be monitored when repeated doses are required.

Three combination drugs that contain caffeine and ergotamine titrate (Cafergot, caffeine, Cafatine) have been confused with Carafate, a drug used to treat peptic ulcer disease. The nurse must differentiate carefully between drugs such as these with similar trade names. Comparing the generic names (in this case caffeine, ergotamine, and sucralfate) helps clarify these differences. Clients must be monitored closely for early signs of toxicity, such as tremor, agitation, or irregular pulse. The aim of most theophylline regimens is to maintain plasma levels of 10 to 20 µg/mL (55–100 µmol/L); symptoms of toxicity may appear when plasma concentrations approach 20 µg/mL (100 µmol/L). Parenteral preparations of diazepam must be readily available for emergency use if seizures occur.

Clients medicated with xanthines require nursing care to alleviate the side effects of the drugs. Clients who receive xanthine medications require assistance with activities of daily living. They have limited energy, especially if they are affected by pulmonary disease that restricts gas exchange in the lungs. All nursing measures to promote rest and sleep should be used. The nurse should accept client irritability as a manifestation of both hypoxia and adverse drug effects. When long-term use of xanthines is necessary (as in the control of chronic asthma), clients or their families may benefit from psychological counseling to improve self-image and coping skills.

Persons who attempt to reduce xanthine intake need considerable support and assistance during the withdrawal period. The nurse should acknowledge that withdrawal from caffeine can be as distressing as withdrawal from nicotine and other dependence-producing substances. For the first few days, the client may need treatment for headache. Nursing measures for headaches include administering (or recommending) non-opioid analgesics such as acetaminophen (Tylenol), eliminating unnecessary stimuli such as strong light and noise, encouraging rest in a quiet room with subdued light, and applying cold applications to the head. Usual patterns of social behavior (coffee breaks) should be encouraged, with substitution of caffeine-free beverages and foods for regular coffee, tea, and so forth.

Clients should also be encouraged to participate in activities that provide pleasure and enhance their self-image. If energy levels decline or the client feels lethargic, the nurse may recommend increased exposure to light (especially in winter or cloudy climates), stimulating activities such as dancing or other exercise, and alternating hot and cold showers.

Therapeutic communication designed to promote a positive self-concept is appropriate for all clients. Clients who receive xanthine therapy may need counseling to help them adjust to the side effects of treatment. They must learn to cope with limited energy, fatigue, irritability, and restlessness. Clients who are withdrawing from excessive use of caffeine may have used the drug to compensate for inadequate coping skills. They may need help controlling environmental stressors and managing their stress responses.

Client Education. All clients should understand the nature of xanthine drugs, their therapeutic uses, and toxic effects and side effects. Clients who receive xanthine medications should be reassured that the irritability, restlessness, and insomnia are effects of the drugs and subside when drug dosages are reduced. They should be taught relaxation techniques and measures to promote rest and sleep. Clients may seek counseling about using stimulant beverages. In most cases, moderate use in the absence of symptoms probably poses little risk. However, before the nurse reassures the client, an assessment for fine muscle tremors and subjective symptoms should be performed. Many clients do not recognize the association between difficulty in sleeping or "nervousness" and the use of beverages that contain xanthines. The nurse should identify stimulant drinks as possible causes of these problems.

Some clients should be warned not to use beverages and food that contain xanthines. The drugs are relatively contraindicated in peptic ulcer disease, poorly controlled epilepsy, heart disease characterized by irregular heart rhythm, insomnia, severe dysmenorrhea, and "coffee nerve" syndrome. They should be used with caution in gastric hyperacidity.

The nurse must convey to clients that xanthines are not recommended for normal children. They should be used only in moderate amounts by pregnant women and in clients with well-controlled epilepsy or diabetes. Decaffeinated products, beverages prepared from roasted grains, and herbal teas may be recommended for clients not affected by gastric hyperacidity.

Most people recognize the toxic potential of coffee but may not realize that tea, cola and many other soft drinks, and chocolate cause similar problems.

The nurse can teach clients who have difficulty eliminating all such beverages and foods to omit coffee first. If toxic symptoms persist, weak tea may be substituted for stronger brews. Although an infrequent offender, chocolate is not tolerated by some persons. Light use of xanthines early in the day may be better tolerated than larger doses in the evening. Occasionally, sensitivity is so high that no foods that contain stimulants can be used. For such clients, all xanthine-containing beverages and foods, including chocolate desserts and candy, should be avoided.

Clients who receive xanthine medications should be taught the following measures to promote rest and sleep:

Elimination of disturbing stimuli such as strong lights and noise from the environment

Quiet activities for a period before bedtime

Warm nonchocolate milk drinks before retiring

Warm baths or sedative massages.

Consistency in rituals associated with preparing for sleep promotes a better sleep response.

OUTCOME EVALUATION

Data required for evaluating nursing measures related to xanthine use include observations about the length of time clients sleep, statements by clients that they feel rested, an increase in activity of choice by clients, and statements by clients that headache is diminished or gone. Evaluation of programs to decrease intake of dietary xanthines depends on reports from clients that indicate the amounts of xanthine-containing beverages and foods consumed, the incidence or absence of withdrawal symptoms such as headaches, and changes in self-concept. Coping skills may be observed directly if the client appears stressed while talking with the nurse. Teaching is evaluated by asking the client to repeat information conveyed or to demonstrate techniques previously taught.

❖ CHECKLIST OF NURSING ACTIONS

- ❑ When taking a client's drug history, assess his or her use of xanthine-containing beverages and foods. Assess clients who use large amounts of xanthine-containing beverages and foods for signs and symptoms of CNS and sympathetic overstimulation.
- ❑ Counsel clients about the nonmedicinal use of xanthines.
- ❑ When clients wish to decrease their use of xanthines, assist and support them through the withdrawal period; teach clients measures to relieve withdrawal symptoms.

Before Initiating Therapy With Xanthine

- ❑ Screen clients for contraindications to stimulant drugs. Assess clients for signs and symptoms of CNS and sympathetic overstimulation. Consult with the physician to verify the drug order if contraindications or risk factors are found.
- ❑ Administer intravenous solutions of aminophylline slowly, using an infusion pump.
- ❑ Monitor clients for CNS and sympathetic overstimulation.

❑ Monitor clients who are receiving theophylline for excessive blood plasma levels (more than 20 µg/mL).

❑ Use nursing measures to alleviate the side effects of xanthine therapy.

Analeptics

An analeptic is a restorative substance because it stimulates the CNS. This descriptive title has been applied to a group of drugs once widely used to counteract depressed physiologic functions characteristic of sudden severe illness or toxicity. Supportive care to maintain vital functions is currently regarded as much more effective, and the use of analeptics has declined considerably. Common analeptic drugs are listed in Table 17-3.

Strychnine

Strychnine is a vegetable alkaloid derived from the seed of a tree native to India. It acts as a competitive antagonist of glycine at the postsynaptic receptor that inhibits nerve cells on activation. Strychnine is an ascending stimulant that acts first on the lower centers (such as those in the spinal cord). In toxic doses, strychnine causes exaggerated motor reflexes, tetanic convulsions, which are symmetric and coordinated, and respiratory arrest. Face and neck stiffness progresses to spasms that produce characteristic facies called *risus sardonicus*.

Strychnine was formerly used in small doses as a stimulant in nonprescription tonics. Because of its bitter taste, it stimulates intestinal secretion and improves the appetite. Toxic doses are incorporated into pesticides and rodenticides. Strychnine is a major source of accidental poisoning in children. Its only recognized medicinal use is in the treatment of the rare congenital metabolic disorder nonketotic hyperglycemia.

Pentylenetetrazol

Pentylenetetrazol (Metrazol) is a synthetic compound used for its stimulant and convulsant properties. Its mechanism of action is unknown. It may act by reducing neurologic recovery time or by increasing nerve cell permeability to potassium ions. The drug is sometimes used in small doses to increase physical and mental activity in elderly clients. It is also used as a provocative agent in diagnosing epilepsy. Subconvulsant doses activate latent epileptogenic foci, which alter the electroencephalogram tracing in characteristic patterns. In the laboratory, pentylenetetrazol is used as a tool to screen for anticonvulsant drugs.

Ammonia

Ammonia is an irritating chemical that stimulates vital centers in the medulla through peripheral reflexes. The drug may be inhaled or taken orally as a dilute solution. Stimulation of sensory nerves in the pharynx, esophagus, and stomach causes reflex stimulation of respiration and vasoconstriction.

Aromatic spirits of ammonia ("smelling salts") are marketed in ampules. The preparation is used to prevent and treat fainting. The ampule is crushed and held near the nose of the recipient. Whiffs of the vapors are sufficient to produce the desired stimulation. Excessive concentration may cause choking.

Table 17-3. Analeptics

Drug Name	Preparations	Medicinal Uses	Usual Dosage	Additional Information
strychnine	Rat and crow poison	Nonketotic hyperglycemia (a rare condition)	Not used medicinally	Strychnine is a frequent cause of poisoning in children.
picrotoxin ("fish-berries")	None	None	Not used medicinally	Berries of the plant are used to incapacitate fish in East Indies.
pentylenetetrazol (Cardiazol, Leptazol, Metrazol, Pentrazol)	Tablets and elixir for oral use; solution for injection	Stimulant and convulsant	To diagnose epilepsy: 2 mg/kg body weight IV, followed by 1 mg/kg body weight/30 sec until EEG spike activity occurs or a maximum dose of 350 mg is reached. As a stimulant for adults: 100–200 mg tid, orally	This drug is used as a laboratory tool to evaluate anticonvulsant drugs, as a provocative agent to diagnose epilepsy, and (sometimes) to enhance mental and physical activity in the elderly.
ammonia (aromatic spirits of ammonia, "smelling salts")	Mesh-covered ampules to be crushed for administration by inhalation. Oral solution	Prevent or terminate fainting	*By inhalation:* whiffs of the vapors of a 4% solution until a response occurs. *Orally:* (adults) 2–4 mL of a 4% solution well diluted in water	Whiffs are sufficient; excessive concentration may cause choking. In high doses it can be damaging to tissues.

In high doses, ammonia can damage the tissues that it contacts. Exposure to ammonia is an occupational hazard in the refrigeration industry. Environmental pollution can result if a container is accidentally damaged during shipment. Tissues exposed to ammonia should be flushed with copious amounts of water, and emergency medical care should be sought without delay.

■ SUMMARY

Analeptics are chemicals that stimulate central vital centers and thus tend to correct depressed physiology due to illness or toxicity from depressant drugs. They are seldom used in healthcare practice because more effective means of maintaining vital functions are available. Analeptic drugs include strychnine, pentylenetetrazol, and ammonia.

❖ NURSING MANAGEMENT: CLIENT RECEIVING ANALEPTICS

Because analeptics are rarely used in healthcare practice, the nurse seldom encounters them in client care. These drugs are sometimes prescribed to improve function in elderly clients and to help diagnose epilepsy.

Analeptics can stimulate convulsions; the degree of risk is related to the client's seizure threshold. Spirits of ammonia are a stock item in nursing units in healthcare facilities. The drug may be used cautiously to restore consciousness. The cause of the fainting episode should then be determined and appropriate corrective measures taken.

The use of analeptics by laypeople for medical purpose should be discouraged. The drugs are believed to serve no therapeutic purpose when incorporated into nonprescription preparations.

Pesticides that contain strychnine must be carefully controlled to prevent accidental ingestion. Unused portions of such materials should be destroyed promptly, in accord with local waste-disposal regulations.

Treatment of acute strychnine poisoning is similar to that of other CNS stimulants. Gastric lavage reduces intestinal absorption of ingested poison. Solutions for lavage include tincture of iodine (1:250), tannic acid (2%), strong tea, potassium permanganate (1:5,000), or activated charcoal slurry. A quiet environment is essential, as slight stimuli can trigger seizures. Diazepam is administered as an anticonvulsant. The client must be monitored closely for respiratory depression, and mechanical ventilation should be supplied as prescribed.

NURSING PROCESS

ASSESSMENT

Before initiating pentylenetetrazol therapy, the nurse should question the client about previous seizures or a family history of epilepsy. Clients with a positive history are at increased risk for a toxic reaction. Muscle tone and reflexes should be assessed. Increased muscle tone, muscle spasms, and hyperactive reflexes also increase the risk of toxicity.

NURSING DIAGNOSIS

Clients for whom pentylenetetrazol is prescribed are likely to have:

- Self-care Deficits, related to lethargy and fatigue

Those receiving analeptic drugs have:

- Risk for Injury, related to seizures

PLANNING

Goals of treatment are improved self-care, increased energy, and prevention of seizures.

INTERVENTION

Nursing actions include administering the analeptic medication and monitoring the client's response. Seizure precautions should be instituted. Diazepam or another anticonvulsant should be readily available for treating seizures, should they occur. Nursing measures to reduce the risk of seizures include alleviating acute stressors that could stimulate sympathoadrenal response or hyperventilation, encouraging regular meals to prevent hypoglycemia, and eliminating repetitive stimuli from the environment (eg, blinking lights), which can trigger seizures in some clients.

Client Education. Clients should be cautioned against factors that increase the risk of seizures: missed meals, exposure to febrile contagious diseases, excessive sodium intake, alcohol intoxication, and (for diabetics) insulin reactions.

OUTCOME EVALUATION

Data required for evaluating the outcome of therapy include client reports of more energy and less fatigue than before medication, observations that the client participates more fully in activities of daily living, and the absence or decreased incidence of seizures.

❖ CHECKLIST OF NURSING ACTIONS

- ❑ Before initiating analeptic therapy, assess clients for factors that increase the risk of seizures.
- ❑ Monitor clients who receive analeptics for toxic effects and side effects.
- ❑ Be prepared to institute emergency treatment for seizures when pentylenetetrazol is administered.
- ❑ Administer spirits of ammonia sparingly for treating or preventing fainting.
- ❑ Warn clients about strychnine pesticides to prevent accidental poisoning.
- ❑ Advise clients to avoid proprietary remedies that contain analeptics.
- ❑ Advise clients who use nonprescribed analeptics about alternative measures to relieve health problems.

Antiparkinson Agents

Parkinson's disease is a progressive neurologic disorder characterized by a loss of neurons in the substantia nigra that produce dopamine. The balance between dopamine and acetylcholine is responsible for normal motor function, and with dopamine depletion this balance is disrupted. When dopamine is reduced by 80% or more, the characteristic manifestations of Parkinson's disease become apparent. These include resting tremor, which usually stops during voluntary movement, muscular rigidity, bradykinesia (slowness of movement), and postural instability, causing gait disturbances and falls.

Beside physical changes, depressive symptoms and cognitive impairment may also occur. Although the exact cause of Parkinson's disease is unknown, many theories exist, including excessive free radical formation and oxidative damage to the cells of the substantia nigra. Parkinson's disease affects about 1 million adults, primarily the elderly.

Other disorders besides Parkinson's disease may produce parkinsonism. In addition, some common drugs in clinical use may produce parkinsonism. These drugs include antipsychotics (eg, chlorpromazine [Thorazine] and haloperidol) and antiemetics (eg, prochlorperazine and metoclopramide).

Drug therapy is the mainstay treatment of Parkinson's disease. The medications used include MAOIs, dopaminergics, dopamine agonists, anticholinergics, and antihistamines. Levodopa is considered the cornerstone of treatment for Parkinson's disease but not drug-induced parkinsonism. Anticholinergics are more effective in treating parkinsonism caused by drugs (Table 17-4).

Selegiline

Neuroprotective therapy, which slows the progression of the disease, is a relatively recent focus in treating Parkinson's disease. One drug shown to provide neuroprotection in animal studies is selegiline hydrochloride (Eldepryl). Selegiline is currently approved as adjunctive therapy for Parkinson's disease. Investigational studies of clients with newly diagnosed Parkinson's disease showed a slowing in both the rate at which symptoms developed and the need for levodopa therapy. It is unclear whether these results were due to the drug's neuroprotective effect on the substantia nigra neurons or the drug's effect on symptoms; more research is needed.

Pharmacodynamics. Selegiline selectively inhibits monoamine oxidase type B (MAO-B). MAO-B, found predominantly in the brain, oxidizes dopamine and noradrenaline. By inhibiting MAO-B, selegiline may slow the progression of the disease by decreasing the formation of toxic free radicals, allowing dopamine-producing neurons to survive longer.

Pharmacokinetics. Selegiline is well absorbed after oral administration and is widely distributed. Metabolism involves some conversion to amphetamine and methamphetamine. Almost half is excreted as metabolites in the urine.

Therapeutic Uses. Selegiline is currently approved for use as adjunctive treatment in Parkinson's disease. The normal adult dosage is 5 mg twice a day, at breakfast and lunch. Some clients may further divide the dosage (eg, 2.5 mg four times a day).

Table 17-4. Oral Dosages of Primary Drugs Used to Treat Parkinsonism

Dose	Initial Dose	Range of Daily Dose
Neuroprotectives		
selegiline (Eldepryl, Deprenyl)	5 mg bid	2.5–10 mg
Dopaminergics		
carbidopa/levodopa (Sinemet)	25/100 mg bid or tid	200–1200 mg levodopa
carbidopa/levodopa, sustained-release form (Sinemet CR)	50/200 mg bid	200–1200 mg levodopa
amantadine* (Symmetrel)	100 mg bid	100–400 mg
Dopamine Agonists		
bromocriptine mesylate (Parlodel)	1.25 mg bid	3.75–40 mg
pergolide mesylate (Permax)	0.05 mg qd	0.75–5 mg
Anticholinergics		
benzotropine (Cogentin)	1–2 mg qd	2–4 mg
trihexyphenidyl (Artane)	1 mg bid	2–25 mg

*Causes neurons to release dopamine and has a mild anticholinergic effect

Adverse Reactions. The most common adverse effects of selegiline are nausea, abdominal pain, dry mouth, dizziness, confusion, hallucinations, and insomnia.

Drug–Drug Interactions. Selegiline potentiates the action of levodopa, so a reduction in the dosage of levodopa may be required. Severe side effects are possible when selegiline is combined with other drugs, such as fluoxetine and meperidine or other opioids.

Drug–Food Interactions. Severe side effects may also result from an interaction between selegiline and tyramine and other high-pressor amine-containing foods. In addition, hypertensive crisis may result from large amounts of caffeine.

Precautions and Contraindications. Selegiline is contraindicated in peptic ulcer disease and in clients taking fluoxetine, meperidine, or tyramine. It should be cautiously used in dementia, severe psychosis, tardive dyskinesia, or excessive tremor.

Levodopa

Levodopa is a precursor of dopamine in normal body biochemistry. It is used in idiopathic parkinsonism and parkinsonian syndrome to reduce the muscle tremors and rigidity characteristic of these conditions. It is considered the single most effective agent in the treatment of Parkinson's disease.

Dopamine, an intermediate product in the synthesis of norepinephrine from tyramine, is one of the stimulant neurotransmitters involved in brain function. The caudate nucleus and putamen are among the neural structures in the brain that require dopamine for proper function. These structures play a role in integrating stereotyped motor functions, such as backward extension of the head and upper trunk. An adequate level of dopamine in the caudate nucleus and putamen requires normal function of pigmented nerve cells in the substantia nigra. One of the physiologic abnormalities found in Parkinson's disease is a decrease of dopamine in the caudate nucleus and putamen, associated with lesions in the pigmented nuclei of the substantia nigra and locus ceruleus. The disease is considered to involve a relative deficiency of dopamine in brain structures that control unconscious motor activity.

Pharmacodynamics. Levodopa is enzymatically converted to dopamine in the basal ganglia. Administration of the drug elevates the levels of this neurotransmitter in the brain, helping to correct one biochemical manifestation of parkinsonian syndrome. Muscular function and control improve as a result.

Levodopa also stimulates the release of pituitary growth hormone. This effect may potentiate the drug's cerebral effects.

Pharmacokinetics. The administration of dopamine does not result in improvement in parkinsonian syndrome because it cannot cross the blood-brain barrier. On the other hand, levodopa, by means of an active transport system, crosses the blood-brain barrier readily and is converted in the brain to dopamine. However, when levodopa is administered orally, it is so rapidly converted to dopamine in extracerebral tissues that only a small portion of the dose is transported to the CNS. Administered alone, the drug must be given in large amounts for therapeutic effect; with such doses, high levels of extracerebral dopamine cause distressing side effects. To reduce the peripheral use of levodopa and to increase the proportion of each dose available to the CNS, a drug that inhibits decarboxylation of peripheral levodopa may be administered concurrently with levodopa. The main drug used for this purpose is carbidopa, a decarboxylase inhibitor that does not cross the blood-brain barrier. By adding carbidopa, the half-life of levodopa increases slightly, its bioavailability doubles, and the required dose is reduced by 75%. Excretion of levodopa is primarily in the urine in the form of catecholamine metabolites.

Therapeutic Uses. Levodopa is used in managing idiopathic Parkinson's disease. In therapeutic doses, the drug produces symptomatic improvement by reducing tremor and rigidity and improving motor function. It does not alter the course of the disease. With long-term levodopa treatment (4–6 years), only 25% of clients continue to exhibit a positive response to therapy. Motor fluctuations and dyskinesia develop in about 75% of clients who use levodopa over the long term. This "wearing off" phenomenon appears to result from the continued loss of dopamine terminals in the striatum, as well as changes in their response to dopamine. At this stage, other drugs, such as selegiline or dopamine agonists, are used.

Dosage and Administration. Levodopa is available in capsule and tablet forms under various trade names. Doses must be individually titrated, starting with low doses and increasing gradually to optimal levels. The usual initial dosage for adults is 0.5 to 1 g daily, divided into two or more doses. The dose may be increased gradually in increments of 0.75 g or less every 3 to 7 days as tolerated. Total dosage should usually not exceed 8 g daily. Levadopa is also marketed in combination with carbidopa (Sinemet). When used with carbidopa, much smaller amounts are required. The maintenance dosage is 75 to 150 mg of carbidopa with 200 to 1200 mg of levodopa daily, divided into three to four doses.

To minimize gastric irritation, food may be administered shortly after medication. Ingesting food before or with levodopa may retard its effect but may be necessary to decrease GI irritation. Also, large amounts of amino acids in the diet can compete with levodopa for transport across the blood-brain barrier and significantly change its effect. Thus, if levodopa must be taken with food, the client must eat a lower amount of protein.

The therapeutic response to levodopa includes a short-term improvement that occurs after each dose and lasts about 5 hours and a longer-duration improvement that persists for 3 to 5 days after the drug is discontinued. The drug has a narrow margin of safety; slight increases above optimal levels produce toxic symptoms.

Selegiline is sometimes used as an adjunct to levodopa therapy. It prolongs levodopa's duration of action by delaying the breakdown of dopamine. During the early stage of parkinsonism, selegiline alone delays the progression of symptoms and the need for levodopa.

Adverse Reactions. Adverse reactions are frequent. They are usually dose-dependent and reversible. The most serious reactions are choreiform, dystonic, dyskinetic, and other adventitious movements that develop when doses exceed optimal levels. Involuntary movements occur in 50% of clients on long-term therapy.

Nausea and vomiting are common reactions, especially when levodopa is given without a decarboxylase inhibitor. These side effects tend to subside with continued administration of the drug. Other GI effects include constipation, diarrhea, epigastric and abdominal distress, flatulence, dry mouth, dysphagia, hiccups, and changes in taste sensation. Duodenal ulcer and GI bleeding may develop.

Orthostatic hypotension occurs frequently but is usually mild and subsides with continued administration. Other cardiovascular side effects stem from peripheral sympathetic activity and include palpitations, sinus tachycardia, ventricular tachycardia or extrasystole, atrial flutter or fibrillation, and atrioventricular block. Flushing and hypertension may occur.

Central nervous system manifestations are both intellectual and emotional in nature. They may include decreased attention span, memory loss, nervousness, anxiety, agitation, restlessness, confusion, insomnia, nightmares, daytime somnolence, euphoria, malaise and fatigue, depression, dementia, delirium, delusions, hallucinations, and inappropriate or excessive sexual behavior. Respiratory side effects appear as episodic hyperventilation and other alterations in breathing patterns, hoarseness, and excessive nasal discharge. Ocular side effects include blurred vision, diplopia, mydriasis or miosis, widening of the palpebral fissures, and oculogyric crisis. Phlebitis, blood dyscrasias, and convulsions have been reported. The drug may adversely affect glucose balance in diabetic clients.

Drug–Drug Interactions. Levodopa interacts with many other drugs. Hypotension can occur when antihypertensives (eg, methyldopa or guanethidine) are administered at the same time. Reserpine, phenytoin, and papaverine diminish the client's response to levodopa. The risk of cardiac arrhythmia during general anesthesia induced by cyclopropane or halogenated hydro-

carbon agents increases in clients who have received levodopa. When levodopa is administered alone, its therapeutic effects are antagonized by the benzodiazepines chlordiazepoxide (Librium) and diazepam (Valium). Use with MAOIs may result in hypertensive reactions. Use with selegiline or cocaine increases the risk of adverse reactions.

Drug–Food Interactions. Foods and vitamin preparations with pyridoxine (vitamin B_6) reverse the effect of levodopa. However, when a decarboxylase inhibitor (carbidopa) is used, pyridoxine does not reduce levodopa's therapeutic action. In this situation, pyridoxine can be administered to inhibit some of levodopa's undesirable side effects.

Drug–Laboratory Test Interactions. Levodopa may interfere with urine tests for glucose or ketones. Coombs' test results may be false, and results of urine tested by the colorimetric method may falsely indicate an increased uric acid level.

Precautions and Contraindications. Levodopa is contraindicated in clients who are receiving MAOIs, clients with narrow-angle glaucoma, and clients with a known hypersensitivity to the drug. It should not be used in clients with a history of melanoma or in clients with undiagnosed pigmented lesions because it may exacerbate malignant melanoma.

Extreme caution must be used when levodopa is administered to clients with a history of myocardial infarction who have residual atrial, nodal, or ventricular arrhythmia. Caution is required also with clients with bronchial asthma or emphysema who may require sympathomimetic drug therapy. Peptic ulcer disease, severe cardiovascular, renal, hepatic, or endocrine disease, and psychosis are also reasons for caution. During levodopa therapy, hepatic, hematopoietic, cardiovascular, and renal function should be evaluated periodically. Safe use for pregnant women or for children younger than age 12 has not been established. Levodopa should not be administered to breast-feeding mothers because the drug enters breast milk and tends to inhibit lactation.

Drug administration is best initiated in an acute care facility. Intensive coronary care facilities must be available if drug therapy is attempted for clients with cardiac arrhythmia.

■ SUMMARY

Selegiline is thought to offer a neuroprotective effect in treating early Parkinson's disease, thereby delaying the progress of the disease. It is approved as adjunct therapy and is used in combination with levodopa or levodopa and carbidopa to treat Parkinson's disease.

Levodopa, the metabolic precursor of dopamine, is used for the palliative treatment of idiopathic parkinsonism. The drug crosses the blood-brain barrier and is metabolized intracerebrally to dopamine, decreasing the tremor and rigidity characteristic of these conditions.

Levodopa has a narrow margin of safety; drug therapy must be initiated cautiously and monitored carefully. Side effects, some of which are characteristic of sympathetic nervous system activity, affect many body systems.

❖ NURSING MANAGEMENT: CLIENT RECEIVING ANTIPARKINSON AGENTS

During the early stages of levodopa treatment, clients require considerable emotional support. The tremors characteristic of parkinsonism may increase initially before a therapeutic response occurs. Moreover, distressing side effects from drug therapy may develop. Clients may become quite discouraged before a therapeutic response to the drug is evident.

NURSING PROCESS

ASSESSMENT

Before levodopa therapy begins, clients must be evaluated for factors that increase the risk of drug use. A careful history should be taken, with particular attention to the presence of glaucoma, cardiovascular, hepatic, renal, or endocrine disorders, peptic ulcer disease, or chronic obstructive airway disease. The drug history should include information about previous use of levodopa and response to it. Clients should be asked specifically about recent use of MAOIs, antihypertensives, phenytoin, and papaverine.

In adjunctive selegiline therapy, the nurse must assess for peptic ulcer disease, emotional disorders, and tremorous conditions. The nurse must also make certain the client is not taking meperidine or opioid analgesics, because an interaction could be fatal. If the daily dose of selegiline exceeds 10 mg, the client must avoid tyramine-containing foods.

During the physical examination, the nurse should assess for cardiac arrhythmia. If the client is a woman of childbearing age, pregnancy and lactation should be ruled out before drug therapy begins. A complete appraisal of signs and symptoms of parkinsonian syndrome should be made as a baseline for comparison with the client's condition after drug therapy.

NURSING DIAGNOSIS

Diagnoses related to the signs and symptoms of parkinsonism may include:

- Impaired Physical Mobility, related to paralysis and tremor
- Body Image Disturbance, related to involuntary body movement secondary to paralysis and tremor
- Self-esteem Disturbance, related to disability secondary to paralysis and tremor
- Altered Role Performance, related to disability secondary to paralysis and tremor

- Altered Nutrition: Less than Body Requirements, related to difficulties in chewing and swallowing
- Sexual dysfunction, related to paralysis

Nursing diagnoses related to drug treatment are:

- Altered Nutrition: Less than Body Requirements, related to nausea and vomiting, dysphagia, and altered taste sensation
- Constipation
- Diarrhea
- Risk for Injury, related to dizziness secondary to postural hypotension
- Anxiety
- Sleep Pattern Disturbance
- Sexual Dysfunction: Inappropriate or Excessive Sexual Behavior
- Sensory/Perceptual Alteration, related to ophthalmic changes secondary to levodopa therapy

Many clients exhibit:

- Knowledge Deficit, about Parkinson's disease and its treatment with medications

Some clients may demonstrate:

- Ineffective Management of Therapeutic Regimen, related to knowledge deficit, powerlessness, or mistrust of regimen

PLANNING

Goals for treatment include prevention of injury, improved physical mobility, improved body image and self-esteem, resumption of role performance, resumption of usual sexual function, improved nutrition, alleviation of constipation or diarrhea, improved sleep, improved vision, and increased knowledge about drug therapy.

INTERVENTION

Levodopa therapy is initiated with small divided doses that are gradually increased until desired effects occur. If selegiline is added, the levodopa dose is reduced 10% to 30% or more.

Until the dosage is stabilized, clients must be monitored carefully for toxic effects and side effects. Cardiovascular status should be monitored closely, with particular attention to cardiac rhythm. Other significant signs and symptoms include changes in respiratory, renal, liver, and visual function. Transient elevations in levels of alkaline phosphatase, aspartate aminotransferase (AST, formerly SGOT), alanine aminotransferase (ALT, formerly SGPT), lactic dehydrogenase, bilirubin, and blood urea nitrogen may occur. The glucose balance in diabetic clients may be unstable. Any of these changes should be reported promptly to the physician to facilitate correction of the drug dosage.

Clients may need referral to physiotherapy to help them recover normal mobility as nerve function improves. To prevent falls, clients should be supervised and assisted during ambulation.

Clients should be encouraged to maintain an adequate diet, especially those who are already malnourished due to the difficulties in eating that sometimes occur in Parkinson's disease. A soft diet may be required until mastication and swallowing improve. All nursing measures to stimulate the appetite and alleviate nausea should be used. Clients who are also receiving 10 mg or more per day of selegiline must avoid tyramine-containing foods to prevent a hypertensive reaction.

Xanthine-containing foods may aggravate nausea and should be eliminated from the diet. Laxative foods may be offered to clients with constipation. Nursing measures to correct alterations in bowel function should be instituted as needed.

Clients need warm acceptance from healthcare personnel. They should be encouraged to express their feelings about their disabilities. The etiologic role of parkinsonism in these deficits should be pointed out. Healthcare personnel should convey a positive attitude toward the prospect of improvement as a result of treatment. As clients progress, their achievement should be acknowledged and praised.

Inappropriate sexual activity may occur and usually is verbal. Clients may be embarrassed by unintended suggestive comments or allusions. The nurse should inform the client that such behavior is considered a side effect of drug therapy and is not unusual during initial treatment. The client should be encouraged to anticipate a return to usual sexual activity when the drug regimen stabilizes and the signs and symptoms of parkinsonism decrease.

Sleep pattern disturbance and visual changes may subside as the client adjusts to maintenance therapy. Until then, nursing measures to promote rest and sleep are appropriate. The client may need assistance with activities that require visual acuity. Relatives or friends may read to the client. If visual difficulties persist, clients should be referred to an ophthalmologist. A change in glasses may improve acuity.

After the dosage has been established and maintenance levels are prescribed, monitoring should continue for adverse reactions to the drug. Clients who experience epigastric distress should be monitored for GI bleeding because the drug is ulcerogenic. Levodopa has a narrow therapeutic index and can produce toxic effects with minimal increases in serum blood levels.

Client Education. Clients should be cautioned that medications do not cure parkinsonism; the drugs' actions are only palliative. However, a positive attitude should be fostered toward the benefits of therapy (see Home and Community Care: Teaching About Drugs for Parkinson's Disease).

Clients with postural hypotension and GI distress, which may occur initially, should be reassured that they will subside with continued treatment. Clients whose involuntary tremors increase when the drug is first taken should be informed that this effect is temporary. Clients should be told that optimal response to drug therapy may not occur for 6 to 8 weeks.

To minimize dizziness and the risk of falling, clients should wear elastic hose and move slowly and deliberately until this side effect subsides. The nurse should help the client adjust dietary intake to minimize nausea and vomiting and to maintain nutrition.

When emotional, intellectual, or sexual changes occur, the nurse should explain that these are side effects of the drug, which can be reduced or eliminated by adjusting the dosage. Clients should be told that successful therapy requires continued close medical supervision and periodic blood tests.

OUTCOME EVALUATION

Data required for evaluating the effect of drug therapy and nursing measures include the absence or decreased incidence of injury, measurement of activity and mobility, statements by the client indicative of improved self-esteem and body image, and observation of role activities or statements by the client or family about participation in daily activities, including sexual activity.

Nutrition can be evaluated by observing the foods the client eats and by assessing parameters of nutrition such as body weight and integrity of the skin and mucous membranes. Frequency and consistency of stools should be noted. Sleep time can be measured, and clients can be asked if they feel rested. Visual function is tested with wall charts and reading materials. The teaching plan can be evaluated by asking the client about information conveyed during the teaching sessions (see Example of Nursing Process and Treatment with Levodopa).

❖ CHECKLIST OF NURSING ACTIONS

- ❑ Assess clients who are to receive levodopa and selegiline for factors that increase the risk of adverse reactions. Inform the physician if significant factors are present.
- ❑ Monitor clients closely for side effects and toxic effects, especially during the initial 6 to 8 weeks of therapy.
- ❑ Take precautions to prevent falls and accidental injury of clients who experience postural hypotension as a side effect of therapy.
- ❑ Promote dietary intake in clients who experience anorexia, nausea, or vomiting as side effects of therapy.
- ❑ Provide emotional support to clients, especially during the initial stage of therapy before optimal response occurs.
- ❑ Inform clients that side effects are due to the medication and may be ameliorated by continued administration of the drug or a dosage adjustment.
- ❑ Accept the behavioral changes that may occur in response to drug therapy.
- ❑ Advise clients of measures that help minimize side effects (eg, the use of elastic support stockings for

postural hypotension, and dietary modification to promote nutrition).

❑ Advise clients to avoid taking vitamin supplements that contain large doses of pyridoxine.

❑ Teach clients taking selegiline to recognize the signs and symptoms of MAOI-induced hypertensive crisis. Advise them to notify the physician if these signs and symptoms occur. Also urge them to avoid tyramine-containing foods, which produce the same signs and symptoms.

Other Central Nervous System Stimulants for Parkinsonism

Dopamine Agonists

Dopamine agonists are tetracyclic ergot derivatives. Two dopamine agonists available in North America are bromocriptine mesylate (Parlodel) and pergolide mesylate (Permax). A third, lisuride, is available in Europe.

Pharmacodynamics. Dopamine agonists directly stimulate dopamine receptors. Bromocriptine and pergolide have the same effect but differ in the way they stimulate the receptors. Thus, if a client's motor impairments do not improve with one of the agonists, the other one may be tried. These drugs can also bind to other receptors, especially serotonergic receptors.

Pharmacokinetics. Both are well absorbed orally, have a plasma half-life of 3 to 7 hours, and are highly protein bound. Bromocriptine is completely metabolized by the liver; pergolide is highly metabolized by the liver, with the metabolites excreted by the kidneys.

Therapeutic Uses. The most common use of the dopamine agonists is in the treatment of clinical symptoms of Parkinson's disease in combination with carbidopa/levodopa. They are usually used in advanced Parkinson's disease in clients who are experiencing levodopa failure with fluctuations in motor function. The dopamine agonists may also be used as an alternative to levodopa, although they are rarely as effective.

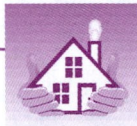

HOME AND COMMUNITY CARE

Teaching About Drugs for Parkinson's Disease

Parkinson's disease is a chronic, progressive disease, and clients must know about their disease and its treatment. They also must participate actively in their care. The nurse can encourage clients to keep a journal.

Because safety is a major concern, an environmental safety assessment should be conducted. Many antiparkinson agents cause orthostatic hypotension, so the client must learn to change position slowly. If medications are to be discontinued, clients need to be aware that they must be discontinued slowly, not abruptly. The following are additional teaching points for specific drugs taken at home.

Dopaminergics

- In advanced Parkinson's disease, clients frequently complain of painful foot cramps. Explain that these can sometimes be decreased by using sustained-release carbidopa/levodopa or a dopamine agonist. Advise clients to consult the physician about this form of medication.
- To decrease gastric irritation, administer food shortly after levodopa. Because large neutral amino acids in the diet can alter levodopa's effects, a low-protein diet is recommended. To ensure adequate protein intake, divide the daily protein among all meals.
- Inform clients that levodopa preparations may darken the urine and sweat.

- Advise the client to avoid vitamin B_6 (pyridoxine) preparations and vitamin-fortified foods containing vitamin B_6 because they can reverse the effects of levodopa.

Anticholinergics

- Inform clients that excessive exercise during warm weather or excessive heat exposure combined with anticholinergic drugs puts them at risk for serious overheating or hyperthermia.
- Forewarn older adults that they may be especially susceptible to anticholinergic side effects: confusion, constipation, dry mouth, and urinary retention (more in men than in women). Some older adults experience paradoxic reactions such as excitement or irritability.

Selegiline

- Tell clients to avoid foods high in tyramine if the daily dose of selegiline is 10 mg or more.
- Inform clients that large amounts of caffeine can cause hypertensive crisis.

Amantadine

- Caution clients that with the long-term use of amantadine, livedo reticularis (reddish-blue, networked mottling of skin) may develop, but it will disappear when medication use stops.

Example of Nursing Process and Treatment with Levodopa

The client, Mr. James, is a 54-year-old man who has been hospitalized for treatment of a stroke with right-sided paralysis and expressive aphasia. In general, recovery has progressed well. He is receiving speech and physical therapy and is ambulating well, and his speech is much improved. He has developed a coarse tremor of the hand that resembles pill-rolling. The neurologist has ordered levodopa 75 mg with carbidopa 150 mg (Sinemet), 1 tablet twice a day. The dosage is to be increased as tolerated until the optimal dosage is determined.

During the first few days of treatment, Mr. James complained that the tremors were worse than before, but with continued therapy these movements subsided and a noticeable improvement occurred.

Mr. James was upset when told he had Parkinson's syndrome. He stated that his grandmother had suffered with this condition for years before her death and that it was a disease he "never wanted to have." He expressed fears that he could not resume employment, his home-maintenance responsibilities, or his hobbies (woodworking and gardening).

Assessment Data

Comment by the client that Parkinson's was a disease he "never wanted to have" because his grandmother "suffered for years with it"

Pronounced tremors

Diagnosis of Parkinson's syndrome (parkinsonism often alters the gait and causes unsteadiness and shuffling gait)

Levodopa therapy (levodopa may cause altered gait, altered taste sensations, altered bowel function, nausea, weakness, dizziness, visual changes, and inappropriate sexual expression.)

Fears that lifestyle will be greatly altered

Unpleasant memories of his grandmother's condition when she had Parkinson's

Muscular tremors

Nursing Diagnosis	Intervention	Goals and Outcome Criteria
Knowledge Deficit, concerning Parkinson's disease and current modes of treatment for it	**Prepare** and implement a teaching plan that explains Parkinson's syndrome and its present treatment. Emphasize that new drugs and other modes of therapy have been developed since his grandmother was alive.	The client will repeat accurately information conveyed during teaching sessions. He will become more cheerful and resume active participation in therapeutic regimens and planning for the future.
Physical Mobility: Resting Tremor of the Hands, related to impaired integrity of tissue in the basal ganglia secondary to Parkinson's syndrome	**Administer** levodopa with carbidopa as ordered. Encourage the client to continue treatment, advising that it takes a little time to establish optimal response to the drugs.	Within 2 weeks, the resting tremor will be decreased or abolished, except when the client is under unusual stress.
Risk for Altered Nutrition: Less than Body Requirements, related to nausea, altered taste sensations, or alteration in bowel elimination secondary to levodopa therapy	**Implement** all possible nursing measures to promote adequate food intake (eg, serve food favored by the client, serve moderate portions of food, offer between-meal snacks, eliminate noxious stimuli at mealtime, make sure food trays are neat and inviting in appearance and that food is at the proper temperature).	The client will not lose weight during the period of dosage adjustment.

(continued)

Example of Nursing Process and Treatment with Levodopa (continued)

Nursing Diagnosis (continued)	Intervention (continued)	Goals and Outcome Criteria (continued)
Body Image Disturbance, related to tremors and memories of his grand-mother	**Explain** to the client that muscle tremors are side effects of the medications he is receiving and that they will subside when dosages are reduced or discontinued. When appropriate, compliment the client (eg, about his appearance, his cooperation with the treatment regimen).	The number of negative comments made by the client relating to self-concept and body image will decrease; the client will begin to say positive things about himself.
Risk for Constipation or Diarrhea, related to nerve stimulation secondary to levodopa	**Monitor** bowel function; if constipation or diarrhea occurs, institute nursing measures to counteract them.	The client will state that he does not experience disabling or discomfiting alterations in bowel function.
Risk for Injury, related to weakness, dizziness, orthostatic hypotension and visual changes secondary to levodopa	**Warn** the client that he may experience visual changes as well as weakness and dizziness when changing position rapidly; teach him to change position slowly, especially when rising from a lying or sitting position. If these symptoms develop, provide assistance for ambulation.	The client will not sustain accidental injury.
Risk for Self-esteem Disturbance, related to inappropriate or excessive sexual expression secondary to levodopa therapy	**Explain** to the client that unusual sexual impulses sometimes occur during the initial stages of levodopa therapy. Assure him that overt sexuality reverts to normal with continued treatment.	The client will accept the temporary changes in sexuality as a side effect of the drug.

Dosage and Administration. Pergolide is much stronger than bromocriptine. Both are given orally. When added to the carbidopa/levodopa regimen, the daily dose of bromocriptine is 2.5 to 30 mg; that of pergolide is 0.75 to 3 mg daily.

Adverse Reactions. The adverse effects are similar to those produced by levodopa: orthostatic hypotension, dizziness, hallucinations or confusion, dyskinesia, somnolence, nausea, constipation, dry mouth, abdominal pain, and rhinitis. Unlike levodopa, both drugs can induce pleuropulmonary and retroperitoneal fibrosis and digital vasospasm.

Drug Interactions. Phenothiazines, metoclopramide, or haloperidol may decrease the effect of pergolide by antagonizing the effects of dopamine. Added hypotensive effects may occur when given with antihypertensives. Bromocriptine causes hypotension when given with antihypertensives and CNS depression when given with antihistamines, alcohol, opioid analgesics, and sedative–hypnotics.

Precautions and Contraindications. Pergolide is contraindicated in lactating women and should be used with caution in clients with arrhythmias or psychiatric disorders. The safety of either drug is not established in pregnancy or in children. Bromocriptine is contraindicated in severe cardiac and peripheral vascular disease and lacta-

tion and should be used cautiously in cardiac disease, mental disturbances, and severe liver impairment.

Anticholinergics and Amantadine

Anticholinergics are the least potent medications used to treat the symptoms of Parkinson's disease. They are prescribed primarily for treating tremors and do little to control bradykinesia. Table 17-4 lists the most common anticholinergics used in treating the symptoms of Parkinson's disease. Amantadine (Symmetrel) is a synthetic tricyclic amine originally developed as an antiviral drug. It is useful for treating rigidity and bradykinesia. Unfortunately, the beneficial effects of amantadine in Parkinson's disease usually decrease within a few months.

Pharmacodynamics. The anticholinergic drugs act to correct the imbalance between dopamine and acetylcholine. The anticholinergic action results from partial blockade of the cholinergic receptors, lowering the excitation of the cholinergic pathways, which arises when the inhibitory control of the dopaminergic pathways is blocked. Depression of the synaptic transmission occurs in the CNS. These agents, which also make more of the dopamine transmitter available to receptors, are anticholinergics, smooth muscle relaxants, and antihistamines. They relieve the spasticity of voluntary muscles by acting on the cerebral motor center. Amantadine has both anticholinergic and dopaminergic properties, but its mechanism of action is unknown.

Pharmacokinetics. These antiparkinson agents are well absorbed from the GI tract, making them suitable for oral administration.

Therapeutic Uses. These antiparkinson agents, which are short-term muscle relaxants, reduce rigidity and tremors. These agents are used to control extrapyramidal effects caused by antipsychotic agents and to treat parkinsonism by relieving spasms, tremors, rigidity, akinesia, and akathisia. Their effectiveness in dyskinesia increases if the symptoms are treated early. Amantadine reduces rigidity and bradykinesia. Although the symptoms of drug-induced parkinsonism are similar to the symptoms of Parkinson's disease, levodopa is ineffective in their treatment.

Dosage and Administration. Drug therapy consists of small doses divided throughout the day. Some clients may tolerate one drug better than another (see Table 17-4). Depending on the drug, the dosage, and the client, relief from extrapyramidal symptoms may occur within a few hours.

Adverse Reactions. All these drugs provoke similar adverse reactions: dry mouth, blurred vision, urinary disturbances, confusion, and dizziness. In addition, probable effects include constipation, fecal impaction, increased ocular tension, tachycardia, dilated pupils, nausea, suppression of perspiration, and nervousness. The antiparkinson agent benztropine, given in small doses, may cause or aggravate glaucoma due to its ability to produce mydriasis. Overdoses of trihexyphenidyl, biperiden, and procyclidine cause cerebral excitement, hallucinations, and delirium. Large doses may produce CNS symptoms of mental confusion, delirium, hallucinations, and ataxia. Amantadine also tends to induce ankle edema and livedo reticularis of the legs.

Drug Interactions. Concurrent administration of antiparkinson agents, tricyclic antidepressants, and antipsychotic agents can lead to additive effects and increased extrapyramidal symptoms. Monoamine oxidase inhibitors potentiate the antiparkinson drugs, intensifying tremors.

Precautions and Contraindications. These drugs should not be given to clients with glaucoma or prostatic hypertrophy.

▪ SUMMARY

Anticholinergics or amantadine are used as antiparkinson agents in treating drug-induced parkinsonism and as monotherapy in early Parkinson's disease to reduce symptoms, especially tremors. Amantadine appears to have both anticholinergic and dopaminergic properties.

❖ NURSING MANAGEMENT: CLIENT RECEIVING ANTICHOLINERGICS OR AMANTADINE

NURSING PROCESS

ASSESSMENT

The nursing history should include past responses to drug therapy and a blood-pressure measurement. Elimination patterns should be noted. Any history of glaucoma, prostate problems, or visual disturbances should be noted.

NURSING DIAGNOSIS

Possible diagnoses are:

- Constipation, Colonic, related to side effects of drug therapy
- Risk for Injury, related to falls due to dizziness and blurred vision secondary to anticholinergic medication
- Knowledge Deficit, concerning the drug regimen

PLANNING

Goals for nursing care include alleviation of constipation and thirst, prevention of injury, and an increase in the client's knowledge about the drug regimen.

INTERVENTION

The client's blood pressure and urinary and bowel habits must be monitored. Because hypotension may occur, monitoring blood pressure is important. It is also important to record fluid intake and output. Urinary hesitancy or retention may occur with drug therapy, and constipation and fecal impaction are common. A high-residue diet, increased fluid intake, and laxatives may be necessary.

Dry mouth can be alleviated with ice chips, hard candies, chewing gum, frequent sips of fluid, and frequent rinsing of the mouth.

If dizziness or blurred vision occurs, the bed side rails may need to be raised, and the client may require supervised ambulation. Visual changes should be reported because the drug can increase intraocular pressure.

Client Education. The client should be cautioned to exercise care when driving a car or operating dangerous machinery while on antiparkinson medication. A teaching plan to prevent further problems with elimination would include dietary changes and increased fluid intake (see Critical Thinking Challenge: Case Analysis).

OUTCOME EVALUATION

Extrapyramidal symptoms caused by drug-induced parkinsonism should decrease or disappear. Tremors should abate in Parkinson's disease. Elimination patterns should return to normal, and dietary changes should be maintained.

CRITICAL THINKING CHALLENGE
Case Analysis

After reading the text and the "Example of nursing process and treatment with levodopa," consider these questions:

1. What advantage do you think the neurologist had in mind by prescribing carbidopa/levodopa (Sinemet) rather than levodopa for Mr. James, the client with Parkinson's syndrome?
2. In constructing a discharge teaching plan that focuses on safety, home care, and self-medication, what would you be sure to emphasize? Why did you select these teaching points?
3. Assume that Mr. James takes carbidopa/levodopa for several years and then experiences an increase in parkinsonian symptoms. His physician prescribes amantadine and bromocriptine and asks you to explain the medication regimen to Mr. James. How will you proceed? What teaching needs do you expect the client will have? Develop some strategies to meet these needs.

❖ CHECKLIST OF NURSING ACTIONS

- ❑ Monitor blood pressure for hypotension.
- ❑ Monitor fluid intake and output.
- ❑ Monitor bowel habits for constipation and fecal impaction. Consider providing a high-residue diet, laxatives, and increased fluids.
- ❑ If dizziness or blurred vision occurs, raise the side rails and supervise ambulation.
- ❑ Alleviate dry mouth with ice chips, hard candies, gum, frequent sips of fluid, and frequent rinsing of the mouth.
- ❑ Caution client about driving a car or operating dangerous machinery until the effects of drug therapy are known.

Alzheimer's Drugs

Tacrine

Tacrine (Cognex) is a cholinesterase inhibitor used in treating Alzheimer's disease, which is characterized by severe atrophy of the cerebral cortex with loss of cortical and subcortical neurons. Tacrine is thought to slow the neuronal degeneration that marks this progressive, irreversible, and incurable disease, which produces cognitive impairment in about 4 million older Americans. With the neuronal loss, there is a marked deficiency in chemical neurotransmitters, especially acetylcholine.

Pharmacodynamics. Tacrine, a potent centrally acting acetylcholine inhibitor, increases the CNS level of acetylcholine by inhibiting its breakdown, thereby improving cognitive function. It appears to be of modest benefit in about one third of clients with mild to moderate Alzheimer's disease.

Pharmacokinetics. Tacrine is one rapidly absorbed following oral administration, with the brain concentration being 10 times higher than the plasma concentration. Tacrine is metabolized by the liver and has a half-life of 2 to 4 hours, with a bioavailability of only 17%. It is excreted in the urine.

Therapeutic Uses. Tacrine is one of the FDA-approved drugs for treating cognitive deficits in clients with mild to moderate Alzheimer's disease.

Dosage and Administration. Tacrine 10-mg orally is administered 4 times a day for 6 weeks. If the client's ALT remains unchanged, the dose is increased to 20 mg 4 times a day. Dosage may be increased every 6 weeks as tolerated, up to a maximum of 160 mg/day (40 mg qid).

Adverse Reactions. Adverse reactions to tacrine may be significant and dose-limiting. They include abdominal cramping, nausea, vomiting, and diarrhea. All have been reported in up to one third of clients. Tacrine may be hepatotoxic: serum transaminases are elevated in up to 20% of clients. This is usually resolved by discontinuing the drug. Other adverse reactions include headache, ataxia, muscle aches, dizziness, bradycardia, and GI bleeding.

Drug–Drug Interactions. Tacrine increases theophylline levels and the risk of theophylline toxicity. It potentiates the effects of succinylcholine and cholinergic drugs. Cigarette smoking decreases the blood level of tacrine; cimetidine increases the blood level of tacrine.

Drug–Food Interactions. Food decreases the absorption of tacrine by 30% to 40%.

Precautions and Contraindications. Caution should be used when administering tacrine to clients with renal or hepatic disease or any history of stroke, subdural hematoma, or CNS tumor. Tacrine is contraindicated in persons hypersensitive to the drug and those with a history of or risk for GI bleeding.

Donepezil Hydrocholoride

Donepezil (Aricept) is a selective anticholinesterase used for improving cognition and function with mild to moderate dementia caused by Alzheimer's disease. It has a better safety profile than tacrine and requires only one daily dose.

Pharmacodynamics. Donepezil is a reversible inhibitor of the enzyme acetylcholinesterase that is responsible for breaking down the neurotransmitter acetylcholine.

This inhibition causes an increase in the level of acetylcholine in the brain, thus improving memory, language, orientation and functioning in ADLs.

Pharmacokinetics. Donepezil is well absorbed orally and not affected by either food or time of administration. The drug is 96% protein bound and the peak plasma levels are reached in 3 to 4 hours. Approximately one half of the drug is excreted unchanged in the urine and the other half is metabolized by the hepatic cytochrome-P450 system.

Therapeutic Uses. Donepezil is FDA approved for improving cognition and functioning in clients with mild to moderate dementia of the Alzheimer's type.

Dosage and Administration. Donepezil 5-mg is given once a day orally. Some clients may benefit from a 10-mg oral daily dose after 4 to 6 weeks of the 5-mg daily dose.

Adverse Reactions. The most common side effects seen with donepezil are nausea, diarrhea, insomnia, vomiting, muscle cramps, fatigue and anorexia. These effects are usually mild and generally subside with continued treatment. There was no evidence of hepatotoxicity so liver monitoring is not required. Donepezil has the potential to cause bradycardia and syncope has been reported.

Drug–Drug Interactions. Thus far few problems have been identified with drug displacement from plasma proteins or increased metabolism related to hepatic enzyme induction.

Precautions and Contraindications. Donepezil has the potential to slow the heart and lead to fainting spells and should be used with caution in clients suffering from cardiac disease.

Other Alzheimer's Drugs

Physostigmine, another cholinesterase inhibitor, showed some promise in treating Alzheimer's disease. Unfortunately, success was limited because physostigmine has a short half-life and tends to produce symptoms of systemic cholinergic excess.

Because the cause of Alzheimer's disease remains unknown, the aim of therapy is to control symptoms. Low doses of neuroleptic drugs, such as haloperidol, are effective in managing agitation and delusions. Antidepressants with low anticholinergic properties (eg, desipramine) and selective serotonin reuptake inhibitors (eg, fluoxetine) may be beneficial for depression. Hypnotics and tranquilizers may also be used. However, benzodiazepines and anticholinergic agents are avoided because they only increase the client's confusion.

Extensive research and clinical trials are ongoing to find a drug that will be effective either in disease prevention or treatment. For example, some researchers are citing evidence that antiinflammatory agents, such as steroids, and nonsteroidal antiinflammatory drugs may protect against Alzheimer's disease. Some epidemiologic studies indicate a lower incidence of this disease in women taking estrogen. First-, second-, and third-generation cholinesterase inhibitors, such as velnacrine and metrifonate, are being evaluated in clients with Alzheimer's disease, as are the neuroprotective agents selegiline and vitamin E. Other drug categories being investigated include potassium channel blockers, calcium channel blockers, and muscarinic cholinergic agonists.

❖ NURSING MANAGEMENT: CLIENT RECEIVING TACRINE OR DONEPEZIL

The goal of drug therapy in clients with Alzheimer's disease is to retard the disease's progression while keeping the client safe and as functional as possible.

NURSING PROCESS

ASSESSMENT

Cognitive functioning before and during therapy should be assessed and documented. Baseline assessment data—vital signs, client orientation, reflexes, liver function test results, and complete blood count—should be compiled.

NURSING DIAGNOSIS

Diagnoses related to signs and symptoms of Alzheimer's disease may include:

- Self-esteem Disturbance, related to disability secondary to disorientation and memory loss
- Altered Role Performance, related to disability secondary to neuronal degeneration

Some nursing diagnoses related to drug treatment include:

- Altered Nutrition: Less than Body Requirements, related to nausea and vomiting, diarrhea, abdominal cramping
- Risk for Injury, related to dizziness or GI bleeding Knowledge Deficit, about Alzheimer's drugs

PLANNING

Goals for nursing care include maintaining adequate nutrition, preventing injury, and aiding compliance with the therapeutic regimen.

INTERVENTION

In addition to education of the client and caregivers about tacrine and its administration, nursing interventions focus on maintaining the client's health and safety. Before and during tacrine therapy, the nurse must ensure that transaminase levels are evaluated and recorded as required. During therapy, tacrine must be administered around the clock on an empty stomach while donepezil is not affected by food. The client should be monitored for therapeutic or adverse effects. Signs of hepatotoxicity need to be assessed with tacrine therapy. If serious adverse effects occur, the physician should be informed so that tacrine therapy can be discontinued gradually.

Client Education. The client and family or other caregivers must be informed about tacrine's potential benefits and side effects and its role as a retardant of, not a cure for, Alzheimer's disease. They must understand the dosage regimen and the need for weekly monitoring, such as blood testing. Other teaching points include assisting the family and client to recognize and report signs and symptoms of serious adverse reactions, including nausea, vomiting, diarrhea, rash, jaundice, or changes in the color of stools. The home-based client must be taught not to stop taking tacrine without consulting the healthcare provider; the drug must be discontinued gradually, not abruptly.

OUTCOME EVALUATION

Reassessment is ongoing. One way to assess the success of nursing management is to compare the client's status before care began with his or her current status, focusing on nutrition, hepatic function, and general daily cognitive functioning.

❖ CHECKLIST OF NURSING ACTIONS

- ❏ Assess for contraindications to medication or factors that increase the client's risk for adverse reactions.
- ❏ Arrange for regular transaminase level determinations before and during therapy.
- ❏ Monitor the client closely for side effects and toxic effects, especially hepatotoxicity.
- ❏ If dizziness occurs, supervise ambulation. Take precautions to prevent falls and accidental injury.
- ❏ Promote dietary intake in clients who experience nausea, vomiting, or diarrhea as side effects of therapy.

Bibliography

*Ahlskog JE. (1994). Treatment of Parkinson's disease. *Postgrad Med, 95*:5(4), 52–69.

Avorn J, et al. (1995). Neuroleptic drug exposure and treatment of parkinsonism in the elderly: A case-control study. *Am J Med, 99*(7), 48–54.

Becker R, et al. (1996). Double-blind, placebo-controlled study of metrifonate, an acetylcholinesterase inhibitor for Alzheimer's disease. *Alzheimer's Dis Assoc Disorders 10*(3), 124–131.

*Calne DB. (1993). Treatment of Parkinson's disease. *New Engl J Med, 329*:14, 1021–1027.

Devoe LD, Murray C, Youssif A, Arnaud M. (1993). Maternal caffeine consumption and fetal behavior in normal third trimester pregnancy. *Am J Obstet Gynecol, 168*(4), 1105–1110.

*Eskenazi B. (1993). Caffeine during pregnancy: Grounds for concern? *JAMA, 270*(24), 2973–2974.

Farlow M. (1994). Management of Alzheimer disease: Today's options and tomorrow's opportunities. *Alzheimer's Dis Assoc Dis 8*(suppl 2), S50–S57.

*Filley C. (1995). Alzheimer's disease: It's irreversible but not untreatable. *Geriatrics 50*(7), 18–23.

Fitzsimmons B, Bunting L. (1993). Parkinson's disease. *Nursing Clin North Am, 28*:4(12), 807–818.

Funk JB, Chessare J, Weaver MT, Exley AR. (1993). Attention deficit hyperactivity disorder, creativity and the effects of methylphenidate. *Pediatrics, 91*(4), 816–819.

Giacobini E (1995). Third International Springfield symposium on advances in Alzheimer's therapy. *Alzheimer's Dis Assoc Dis 9*(3), 160–165.

Greener M. (1993). Perk or poison? *Nursing Times, 89*(49), 36–37.

Hardiman JG, Limbird LE, Molinoff PB, et al. (eds). (1996). *Goodman and Gilman's pharmacological basis of therapeutics*, 9th ed. New York: McGraw-Hill.

Infante-Rivard C, Fernandez A, Gautier R, David M, Rivard G. (1993). Fetal loss associated with caffeine intake before and during pregnancy. *JAMA, 270*(24), 2940–2943.

Levin GM. (1995). Attention-deficit hyperactivity disorder: The pharmacists rule. *Am Pharm, 35*(11), 10–20.

Lynch J, House MA. (1992). Cardiovascular effects of methamphetamine. *J Cardiovasc Nursing, 6*(2), 12–18.

McKim EN, McKim WM. (1993). Caffeine: How much is too much? *Can Nurse, 89*(11), 19–22.

Saint-Cyr JA, et al. (1993). Neuropsychological and psychiatric side effects in the treatment of Parkinson's disease. *Neurology, 43*(suppl 6)(12), 547–550.

Schneider LS, et al. (1996). Effects of estrogen replacement therapy on response to tacrine in patients with Alzheimer's disease. *Neurology 46*(6), 1580–1584.

*Silverstein P. (1996). Moderate Parkinson's disease. *Postgrad Med, 99*(1), 52.

*Silverstone T. (1992). Appetite suppressants: A review. *Drugs, 43*, 820.

*Smitherman CH. (1990). A drug to ease attention-deficit hyperactivity disorder. *MCN, 15*(6), 362–365.

Stacy M, Brownlee HJ. (1996). Treatment options for early Parkinson's disease. *Am Fam Phys, 53*(4), 1281–1287.

*Standaert DG, Stern M. (1993). Update on the management of Parkinson's disease. *Med Clin North Am, 77*(1), 169–183.

*Sweeney P. (1995). Parkinson's disease: Managing symptoms & preserving function. *Geriatrics, 50*(9), 24–31.

*Voo J, Lantz M. (1995). Alzheimer's disease: How to give and monitor tacrine therapy. *Geriatrics, 50*(5), 50–53.

*Recommended for further reading.

For more information and sample tests and activities, refer to Chapter 17 in the Student Workbook for Clinical Pharmacology and Nursing Management, 5th edition, available through your bookstore.

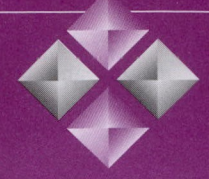

18

Drugs That Depress the Nervous System

Drugs that depress the central nervous system (CNS) are commonly used to control pain. As a drug group, these substances are known as CNS depressants. They tend to slow or reduce general body activities and psychomotor function and produce mild sedation.

Overview of CNS Depressants

The effects of CNS depressants include decreased alertness, apathy, lethargy, sleep, and coma, which occur in succession as CNS depression increases. Vital functions such as heart rate, circulation, respiration, and metabolism are slowed with deep sedation (Box 18-1). Some drugs affect specific functions before general depression becomes apparent. These drugs produce tranquility, analgesia, skeletal muscle relaxation, or amnesia. Such drugs are selective at lower doses, but depression becomes more generalized as doses increase. At toxic levels, all CNS depressants tend to produce coma, cardiovascular collapse, respiratory arrest, and death.

Certain depressant drugs appear to act initially as stimulants, because they first affect the inhibitory functions of the brain. For example, alcohol initially depresses the limbic system and forebrain. This action decreases learned inhibitions, foresight, and judgment. If the recipient has impulses toward "unacceptable" behavior, the elimination of forebrain control may result in acting out that behavior. For this reason, some people become overactive, hostile, garrulous, or otherwise increasingly active after drinking a few alcoholic beverages. As intoxication progresses, activity levels decline, and stupor may appear.

CNS depressants include drugs classified as anesthetics, opioid analgesics, sedatives, hypnotics, anticonvulsants, and tranquilizers. Commonly, combinations of depressant drugs are synergistic. For example, tranquilizers and analgesics in combination provide more relief from pain than either does alone. Analgesics po-

---

 Box 18-1
Action of CNS Depressants

Mild sedation: slowing of psychomotor functions, lessening of inhibitions

Moderate sedation: (in succession) decreased alertness, apathy, lethargy, and sleep

Increasing sedation: slowing of vital functions such as heart rate, circulation, respirations, and metabolism

Toxic levels: coma, cardiovascular collapse, respiratory arrest, and death

tentiate the action of hypnotics when pain is a factor in sleeplessness. CNS depressants are indispensable for anesthesia during surgery, pain relief, and controlling and treating other clinical states.

Despite their positive effects, CNS depressants are major drugs of abuse. Dependencies on opiates, barbiturates, and alcohol are worldwide public health problems. The distribution and use of CNS depressants are strictly controlled in most parts of the world (see Chap. 14 for a discussion of substance abuse).

Because the main uses of CNS depressants are pain relief (analgesia) and loss of sensation (anesthesia), this chapter discusses not only CNS depressant drugs but also the pain and sleep phenomena that these drugs alter.

Understanding Pain

Pain is a subjective sensation involving various physiologic, psychologic, and emotional responses. Pain protects the individual organism by alerting it to harmful environmental influences or to processes in the body and by motivating the individual to eliminate them. The mechanisms of pain involve:

Stimulation of pain receptors

Transmission of impulses to the CNS

Modification of these impulses by certain central structures (eg, the substantia gelatinosa, thalamus, and frontal lobe)

Cortical interpretation of resultant nerve tissue activity as a characteristic pain sensation.

Pain Threshold

The point at which a stimulus of pain receptors is perceived as painful is called the *pain threshold*. Experimental studies indicate that most healthy people have similar pain thresholds; that certain drugs, such as promethazine, lower the pain threshold for some people (McCaffery & Beebe, 1989); and that endogenous analgesics such as endorphins in the brain are likely to influence the pain threshold.

Pain Response

After the pain receptors have been stimulated and the brain interprets the impulses as pain, the individual response depends on many factors: past experiences of pain, learned responses to pain (which can be cultural or familial), the meaning assigned to the pain, and the success or failure of coping mechanisms.

Most people adapt to pain to some degree. An initial response to pain may include gasping, facial grimaces, crying, moaning, muscle tension, perspiration, pallor, and alterations in vital signs. Adaptation to pain involves a reversion back to the prestimulus state, both physiologically and behaviorally. This occurs even if the pain persists. Because fluctuations in pain may cause temporary loss of adaptation, assessment of a client in pain may or may not disclose objective evidence of that pain. Evidence of pain may also be masked by exhaustion or depression.

Pain Syndromes

When pain becomes severe or chronic, pain receptors undergo repeated or prolonged stimulation. This stimulation of the neural pathway alters synaptic function, facilitating the passage of pain impulses and subsequent activation of the nerves by a wider variety of stimuli and by weaker stimuli. Preventing this phenomenon is crucial in caring for the client over the long term because the increased sensitivity forms a basis for the "habit" of pain. Pain habits are thought to contribute significantly to syndromes of chronic, phantom, and intractable pain.

Recent experience in care of terminally ill clients suggests that early, aggressive treatment with large doses of analgesics given at regular intervals can achieve effective pain control. Once the client feels comfortable, the drug dose is reduced gradually to determine the minimal effective amount. In contrast to traditional treatments that rely on increasing drug dosage, this approach promotes more complete pain relief and reduces fear. It also minimizes permanent physical changes in the nervous system that predispose a person to persistent pain or its recurrence, and provides overall control of pain with minimal drugs over the long term.

Pain Management

Strategies for coping with pain vary greatly from person to person. Clients may ignore the pain, use hot or cold packs, drink intoxicating beverages, exert pressure on or massage body areas, engage in diverting activities, meditate, pray, or intellectualize the experience. Coping strategies that were perceived as helpful in the past are used repeatedly and become habitual.

Professional pain management strategies are a joint responsibility of the healthcare team and the client. Nurses can meet the needs of the client in pain by applying nursing techniques and administering prescribed analgesics. Nursing interventions can help prevent or reduce the need for drugs, as well as enhance their intended analgesic effect.

Nurses caring for a client with pain must always bear in mind that pain is a universal experience, but it is also intensely personal and unique to the individual. Not even by recalling one's own pain can an observer relate reliably to another person's pain, because the pain threshold, response to pain, perception of pain, and strategies for coping with pain vary so greatly among persons.

The nurse's role in pain management is to devise, in collaboration with the physician and the client, a regimen of drug administration and nursing care that prevents the client's discomfort from reaching a level that interferes with the recuperative processes of the body, activities of daily living, or mental and emotional well-being. To do this, the nurse must understand the pathologic processes that cause pain as they relate to normal sensation, perception of pain, and response to stress. The nurse also must understand the client to predict the probable pain course and to plan effective interventions for pain control.

Nonpharmacologic Pain Management Measures

Pain can be alleviated by nonpharmacologic measures (eg, relaxation techniques, such as imagery and distraction by music therapy; cognitive/behavioral approaches, such as hypnosis and biofeedback; and physical therapies, such as applications of heat and cold,

exercise, and transcutaneous electrical nerve stimulation).

Pharmacologic Pain Management Measures

Of the drugs used to relieve pain, CNS depressants are commonly used agents. These drugs can eliminate pain by interrupting pain impulses before they reach the CNS; alter awareness and response to pain impulses; or produce unconsciousness.

Pain may be further ameliorated with drugs that reduce the anxiety that intensifies pain or that eliminate memory of past pain (amnesia). Interruption of peripheral pain impulses prevents both the physiologic and psychologic effects of pain. Unconsciousness eliminates pain per se, but it does not prevent the autonomic and hormonal responses to pain stressors: the pain impulse continues to influence subcortical brain processes.

Drugs that relieve pain include local and general anesthetics, opioid analgesics, and nonopioid analgesics, such as the nonsteroidal antiinflammatory drugs (NSAIDs) discussed in Chapter 36. Neuropathic pain may be alleviated by low doses of tricyclic antidepressants. Figure 18-1 illustrates the sites of action of the various types of drugs that relieve pain.

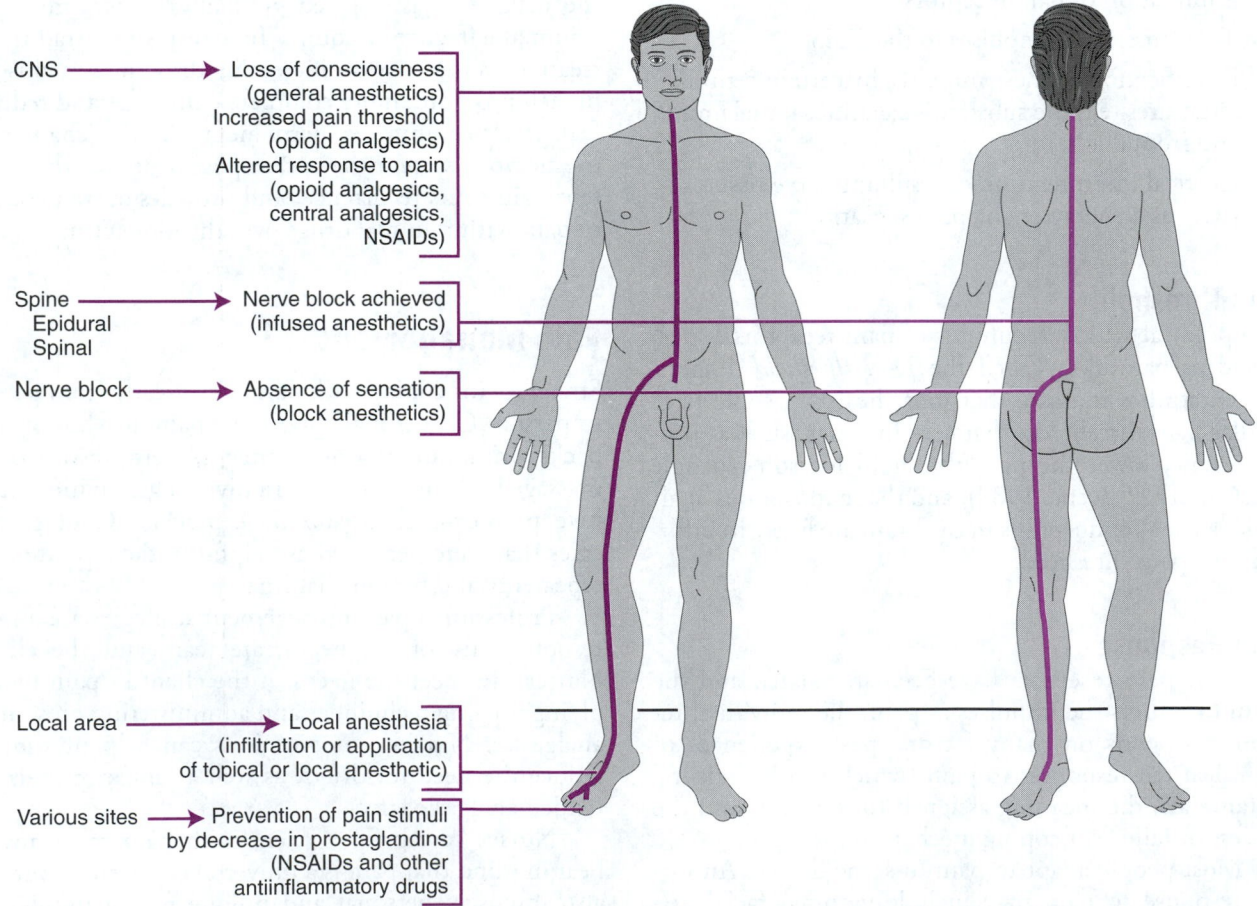

Figure 18-1. Sites and mechanisms of action of drugs used for analgesia.

Analgesic Regimens

The selection of a drug regimen depends on many factors. Drugs that will eliminate the cause of pain are used when available. For example, pain from muscle spasm can be relieved by muscle relaxants; heartburn pain responds to antacids or drugs that suppress gastric acid. However, when the cause of pain cannot be eliminated promptly, analgesic drugs may be used to reduce or relieve the subjective experience of pain. These drug choices range from nonnarcotic analgesics, such as salicylates and acetaminophen, to potent narcotic opioid agents, such as morphine. In choosing a drug, the type of pain to be relieved, its severity, and its expected duration must be considered. The following sections discuss management of acute short-term pain, chronic pain, and pain in clients with terminal illness (Table 18-1).

Analgesia in Acute Short-Term Pain

Acute short-term pain commonly results from accidental or surgical trauma. In some cases, pain immediately after injury may be delayed due to the numbing effects of acute, sudden stress or to the residual effects of anesthetics used during surgery. Afterward, however, pain is commonly regarded as most intense in the beginning, with gradual tapering off as recovery progresses. Pain usually increases when inflammation peaks (usually within 3 days of injury) and during certain activities (ambulation, dressing changes, coughing, and so forth). Pain also fluctuates in a diurnal pattern in relation to hormonal secretion cycles, particularly that of cortisone, which blunts all sensory modalities. Therefore, clients with typical daytime patterns of cortisone production experience more pain in the afternoon, evening, and night, when cortisone levels are lowest.

Opioids, or a combination of opioids and NSAIDs, are the drugs most often ordered for severe, acute pain, such as postsurgical pain that is expected to be brief. Pain changes in quality and degree as convalescence progresses. The opioids relieve initial pain. When the inflammatory reaction peaks and discomfort prevails, opioid analgesics are usually less effective in pain control than drugs such as salicylates. If an NSAID has not been prescribed, the nurse should request an order for one.

In evaluating the client's response to the drug regimen for acute short-term pain, the nurse assesses any unusual pain or pain that deviates from the usual pattern for an injury. Unusual pain may be related to complications (eg, infection, hematoma, intestinal obstruction), a pain habit developed during previous illnesses, or emotional disturbances, such as anxiety or fear, which are powerful potentiators of pain. Administering analgesics without determining the cause of inappropriate pain may mask the symptoms and prevent proper diagnosis. It is the nurse's responsibility to assess pain carefully and completely before administering pain medications.

Failure to control pain from trauma increases the risk of various complications, depending on the client's response to the stress of pain (Table 18-2). Relief of pain is, therefore, essential for the client's physical well-being.

The client may need analgesics intermittently or continuously. This requires conscientious application of all steps of the nursing process. The type and degree of pain perceived by the client, the physical and psychosocial responses of the client, and the orders included in the medical regimen must all be considered before a decision is made regarding drug administration. In acute pain, such as postoperative pain, the AHCPR guidelines recommend administering analgesics on a regular basis initially (eg, for the first 36 hours), then on a PRN basis.

An alternative regimen for controlling acute pain is continuous parenteral infusion of analgesics. This approach facilitates uninterrupted control of pain and titration of dosage to the client's needs.

Table 18-1. Common Drug Regimens For Various Types of Pain

Type of Pain	Etiology	Drug Regimens Frequently Prescribed
Acute short-term pain	Trauma, surgery, or acute medical pathology	Opioid analgesics (optimally a combination of opioid and NSAID) for 3–6 days, often with tapering of doses or progressive prolongation of dosage intervals; opioids may be administered intermittently (PO or by injection), continuously (by parenteral infusion), or by the client (patient-controlled analgesia)
		Substitution of nonopioid analgesics for opioids when acute stage has resolved
Chronic pain	Chronic degenerative disease such as arthritis or neuralgia	Nonopioid analgesics or antiinflammatory drugs (usually PO)
		Dosage intervals may be fixed (by the clock) or flexible (when necessary).
Pain of terminal illness	Life-threatening illness such as cancer or progressive neurologic disease	Nonopioid or opioid analgesics with progressive increases in dosage, shortening of dosage intervals, or movement from less to more potent drugs
		Drugs may be administered intermittently (PO or by injection) or continuously (by parenteral infusion).

Table 18-2. Problems Arising from Unrelieved Trauma Pain

Predominant Response	Clinical Signs and Symptoms	Potential Complication
Sympathoadrenal activity	Increased blood pressure Increased pulse rate	Hemorrhage from injured tissue
Strong reflex vasodilation (likely to occur from deep visceral pain)	Decreased blood pressure	Shock
High cortisone levels	Suppressed immune response	Infection
	Increased renal reabsorption of sodium	Fluid and electrolyte imbalances
	Increased renal excretion of potassium	Hemorrhage
	Increased blood volume	
	Increased blood pressure	

Analgesia in Chronic Pain

The character of chronic pain varies widely: it can range from occasional and mild to constant and severe. Drug regimens for its treatment are equally diverse. In general, the mildest drugs adequate to control discomfort are the ones used initially. They may be given PRN with specified minimal time intervals, or regularly by the clock. When pain persists, using analgesics poses two problems: the risk of drug dependence and the likelihood that a pain habit will develop.

The client who has chronic pain and who takes medications is at risk for developing drug dependence. For this reason, drugs with the least potential for causing dependence are used, and the lowest dose adequate to control pain is prescribed.

The appropriate drug or dose is not always easy to determine. The underuse of analgesics encourages psychologic dependence by allowing the stimulus of pain to arise frequently. Minimizing or eliminating the stimulus of pain requires that ample medication be used to prevent pain or establish early control over it. Then the dosage is reduced gradually until the minimal effective dose is determined. Dependence on drugs can be minimized by carefully titrating the dosage to meet individual needs and by complementing the drug regimen with nursing interventions to minimize the perception of pain. Nursing approaches to pain and medication should not be considered alternatives but rather enhancements that offer the client a way to minimize discomfort. Adequate pain relief is an important factor in reducing iatrogenic drug dependence.

Whenever possible, opioid or narcotic analgesics should be avoided in treating chronic pain of indefinite duration, such as that experienced in conditions that are not life-threatening. The relative potencies of analgesics used for mild to moderate chronic pain are compared in Table 18-3.

The World Health Organization provides a stepped approach to managing cancer pain that aims to relieve pain while minimizing or delaying the development of tolerance and dependence (Fig. 18-2).

Analgesia in Terminal Illness

Terminal illness reorders priorities for care. With cure no longer possible, the client's comfort, function, and quality of life are of primary importance, and drug dependence is rarely a concern. However, the principle of

Table 18-3. Equipotent Doses: Analgesics for Mild to Moderate Pain*

Drug Name	PO Dose (mg)
acetaminophen (Tylenol)	650
aspirin (ASA)	650
codeine	30
meperidine (Demerol)	50
propoxyphene hydrochloride (Darvon)	65
propoxyphene napsylate (Darvon-N)	100
sodium salicylate	1,000

*Expressed in doses approximately equivalent in total effect of aspirin 650 mg. Data from McCaffery M, Beebe A. (1989). *Pain: Clinical manual for nursing practice.* St. Louis: CV Mosby, p. 61.

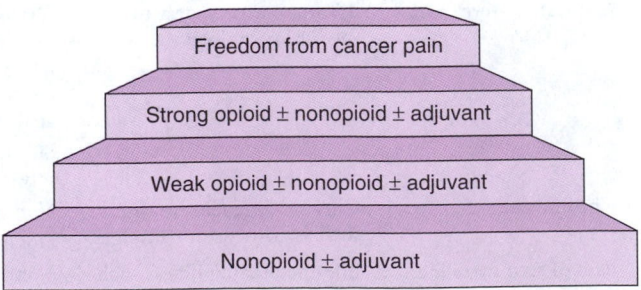

Figure 18-2. WHO 3-step analgesic ladder shows recommended drug regimen for relieving cancer pain (Adapted from the World Health Organization [1986]. *Cancer pain relief.* Geneva: WHO.)

adequately controlling pain with the least amount of drugs is still important if tolerance is to be minimized.

It is appropriate to offer terminally ill clients control over their drug regimens, because only they can determine the quality of life best for them for the time remaining. In general, most clients wish to remain as active and alert as possible with a tolerable level of comfort. To that end, intermittent medication should be given regularly without waiting for pain to develop. If drug administration is controlled by the healthcare staff, it is most effectively provided at regularly timed intervals. Allowing the client to participate in administering drugs helps reduce anxiety and offers a measure of control.

Continuous Parenteral Infusion

An alternative to intermittent medication is continuous parenteral infusion of analgesics. This provides a constant blood concentration of drug and good pain control even for clients for whom regularly scheduled intermittent doses have failed to provide relief. Continuous parenteral analgesia may be administered locally or by intravenous (IV), subcutaneous (SC), intrathecal, or epidural routes. Narcotic analgesics are commonly administered IV or SC; local infusions supply anesthetics or opioids. Drugs can be delivered continuously with external equipment or via an implanted pump whose reservoir is refilled periodically with doses of analgesics.

Continuous parenteral infusion was first used to control the severe pain of malignant tumors refractory to usual analgesic regimens. Now its use extends to acute, severe pain (eg, burns, multiple trauma) and to the initial control of inadequately controlled chronic pain. Continuous therapy provides stable serum drug concentrations and ease in titrating dosage to individual needs. However, it requires familiarity with mechanical devices, such as infusion pumps, to control the flow rate and prevent inadvertent overdoses.

Parenteral doses of analgesics may differ significantly from those administered orally (Table 18-4). Many analgesics are extensively metabolized by the liver, and only part of the oral dose reaches the circulation. Usually, therefore, oral dosage is much higher than parenteral dosage.

Table 18-4. Equivalents for Oral and Parenteral Doses of Opioid Analgesics

Drug	Approximate Equianalgesic Dose		Usual Starting Dose for Moderate to Severe Pain	
	Oral	Parenteral	Oral	Parenteral
Opioid Agonist				
Morphine	30 mg q3–4h (repeat around-the-clock dosing) 60 mg q3–4h (single dose or intermittent dosing)	10 mg q3–4h	30 mg q3–4h	10 mg q3–4h
Morphine, controlled-release (MS Contin, Oramorph)	90–120 mg q12h	N/A	90–120 mg q12h	N/A
Hydromorphone (Dilaudid)	7.5 mg q3–4h	1.5 mg q3–4h	6 mg q3–4h	1.5 mg q3–4h
Levorphanol (Levo-Dromoran)	4 mg q6–8h	2 mg q6–8h	4 mg q6–8h	2 mg q6–8h
Meperidine (Demerol)	300 mg q2–3h	100 mg q3h	N/R	100 mg q3h
Methadone (Dolophine, others)	20 mg q6–8h	10 mg q6–8h	20 mg q6–8h	10 mg q6–8h
Oxymorphone (Numorphan)	N/A	1 mg q3–4h	N/A	1 mg q3–4h
Combination Opioid/NSAID Preparations				
Codeine (with aspirin or acetaminophen)	180–200 mg q3–4h	130 mg q3–4h	60 mg q3–4h	60 mg q2h (IM/SC)
Hydrocodone (in Lorcet, Lortab, Vicodin, others)	30 mg q3–4h	N/A	10 mg q3–4h	N/A
Oxycodone (Roxicodone, also in Percocet, Percodan, Tylox, others)	30 mg q3–4h	N/A	10 mg q3–4h	N/A

Dosages are for adults and children weighing more than 50 kg. Dosages do not apply to clients with renal or hepatic problems. In clients unable to take morphine, hydromorphone, or oxymorphone orally, rectal administration may be used. With opioid analgesics and NSAIDs, aspirin and acetaminophen dosages must be adjusted to client's weight. Codeine doses exceeding 65 mg do not relieve more pain but do increase nausea, constipation, and other side effects. Adapted from Cancer Pain Management Guideline Panel. (1994). *Management of cancer pain.* AHCPR publication 94-0592. Rockville, MD: Agency for Health Care Policy and Research, Public Health Service. U.S. Department of Health and Human Services.

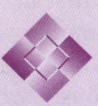

Box 18-2
Kinds of Patient-Controlled Analgesia

Demand dosing: Predetermined fixed dose (bolus) when client pushes the button

Constant-rate infusion plus demand dosing: Continuous background infusion and patient-initiated, demand dosing

Demand infusion: Dosing by infusion instead of bolus

Variable-rate infusion plus demand dosing: Most sophisticated form of patient-initiated dosing in which microprocessor monitors the client's demands and controls infusion rate accordingly

Adapted from Stanton-Hicks M. (1994). Is PCA an effective method of treating postoperative pain? *Curr Rev PACN, 16*(19), 169–176, and Thomas N. (1994). Patient-controlled analgesia. *Elderly Care, 6*(3), 23–26.

Patient-Controlled Analgesia

Certain equipment can be incorporated into the continuous parenteral infusion setup so that the client can self-infuse pain-relieving medication by pressing a button as needed. This drug administration technique is known as patient-controlled analgesia (PCA).

Table 18-5. Comparing Pharmacodynamics and Pharmacokinetics of Fentanyl and Morphine

	Fentanyl	Morphine
Dose (mg)		
IV	0.1	11–20
E	0.1	2–5
Time to peak effect (minutes)		
IV	3	30
E	10–20	30–60
T	14 hours	
Duration (hours)		
IV	1	4
E	2–3	8–24
Lipid solubility (log P)	4.05	0.78
Distribution ½ time $t\frac{1}{2}\alpha$ (minutes)	1.7	1.65
Terminal elimination time $t\frac{1}{2}\beta$ (minutes)	219	100–240

IV = intravenous route; E = epidural route; T = transdermal route; Lipid solubility = the ability of the drug to dissolve in fatty tissues, expressed as log P; Distribution ½ time = the amount of time necessary for a drug to move from blood and plasma to other tissues ($t\frac{1}{2}\alpha$); Terminal elimination time = the time it takes for 50% of the drug to be eliminated from the body ($t\frac{1}{2}\beta$). The lipid solubility, $t\frac{1}{2}\alpha$, and $t\frac{1}{2}\beta$ refer to IV administration. From Willens J. (1994). Giving fentanyl for pain outside the OR. *AJN, 94*(2), 28.

Table 18-6. Recommended IV-PCA Settings for Fentanyl and Morphine

	Fentanyl (μg)	Morphine (mg)
Initial bolus	20–100	5
Background infusion	20–150	1–2
Demand dose	50	1
Lockout interval (minutes)	3–10	6

From Willens J. (1994). Giving fentanyl for pain outside the OR. *AJN, 94*(2), 28.

Studies of PCA indicate that client control of analgesia provides maximal pain control and minimal side effects. In addition, clients usually administer less medication. PCA usually involves IV or epidural routes. Usually a background continuous level of an opioid analgesic is administered through a controlled-demand, push-button drug delivery cassette operated by the client. A timed lockout interval is set to prevent overdosage. Box 18-2 describes various modes of PCA. Morphine and fentanyl are the opiates most commonly used (Tables 18-5 and 18-6).

The nurse must be skilled in preparing and monitoring the PCA equipment to ensure safe functioning and to ensure that delivery catheters remain patent and intact. The client must be monitored, particularly for analgesic effectiveness, respiratory depression, and other side effects.

Impediments to Effective Pain Management

Analgesia is a goal that is sometimes inadequately achieved. Many clients suffer needless discomfort and risk complications because healthcare personnel fail to manage pain effectively. Factors that interfere with effective analgesia include inadequate assessment of pain, inaccurate assumptions about pain, lack of knowledge, biased attitudes, and misapprehensions.

Inadequate Assessment of Pain

Too often analgesics are administered without sufficient information about the client's condition and level of pain. To administer pain control effectively and efficiently, the nurse must interview the client; too often work demands preclude this action. One impediment to collecting adequate assessment data is an excessive workload, which may prompt the medication nurse to administer an analgesic drug automatically without investigating the kind of pain reported. Another potential impediment is a workplace in which unlicensed assistive personnel administer medications. These caregivers may lack sufficient skills to conduct adequate assessments of pain and the effectiveness of analgesic drugs.

Substitution of Inappropriate Drugs for Analgesics

Several drugs, such as sedatives, tranquilizers, and antidepressants, are useful adjuncts to analgesic drugs. Administering a sedative with an analgesic often provides a longer period of comfortable rest or sleep than either provides alone. Tranquilizers and antidepressants are potentiators of analgesics when the two are administered together. Tricyclic antidepressants in low doses have been used to provide effective analgesia in certain types of peripheral neurologic pain.

However, the complete substitution of any of these drug groups for an analgesic can fail to relieve pain and result in undesirable side effects. For example, sedatives should never be substituted for analgesics for pain control. Clients in pain react poorly to sedation alone. They become restless and disoriented, their pain is not reduced despite CNS depression, and the physiologic effects of pain persist.

Invalid Assumptions

The nurse who waits for the client to complain of pain before administering medication makes assumptions that may be invalid. These assumptions include:

The client will know when discomfort becomes pain that should be medicated.

The client knows that pain medication is available.

The client will complain of pain.

The client regards pain relief as desirable and beneficial.

In actuality, many clients are likely to believe that some pain is inevitable and must be endured and that only excruciating pain should be relieved by medication. Other clients may think that the nursing staff will automatically detect pain and take appropriate action. Some clients think that using analgesics (especially opioids) is bad and should be avoided when possible, that enduring pain is virtuous, and that complaining will earn them dislike and disrespect from the staff. Other clients think, for various reasons, that nothing can be done to relieve pain.

Insufficient Knowledge

Because pain is primarily a subjective phenomenon, clients must be educated about available pain relief measures and how to request and use them. They also must understand that adequate pain relief is essential to promoting recovery and avoiding potential complications.

Biased Attitudes

Attitudes toward drugs are usually colored by cultural background, moral training, and social mores. In modern society, these attitudes tend to be polarized—some people are very permissive toward drug use and experimentation, and others are very restrictive.

The proliferation of new and effective therapeutic drugs has contributed to curing and controlling health problems, but it has also contributed to misuse of many drugs (eg, opioid analgesics, sedatives, tranquilizers). Among the public at large and in many healthcare institutions, a bias toward undermedication prevails. The belief that overmedication with analgesics can lead to dependency or oversedation and is therefore hazardous is rarely a clinical reality. Far more real is the failure of analgesia—people suffering needless pain because of reluctance to use analgesics liberally.

Misapprehension of Pain

Healthcare personnel tend to assign a cause to every phenomenon and a blame for every therapeutic failure. A condition that defies diagnosis or fails to respond to treatment is often labeled psychosomatic. This would be accurate if the use of the term denoted its true meaning (involving both mind and body). In practice, however, the term has come to mean "arising from psychologic causes." Many clients with so-called psychosomatic conditions are referred for psychiatric counseling, and physical care may be reduced or discontinued. The client's pain then becomes his or her responsibility.

In such cases, the temptation is to reduce genuine pain medication and administer placebos in the belief that placebos can produce as much or more relief than drugs. Studies of the placebo effect indicate that pain relief associated with this therapy results from the client's production of endogenous endorphins. Placebos are autogenous analgesics that interact with opioid receptors, producing effects similar to those of narcotic analgesics. These effects and the pain relief experienced are abolished when narcotic antagonists are administered. Response to placebos can no longer be regarded as good evidence that the source of pain is mental rather than physical.

The danger in dealing separately with the physical and psychologic aspects of health problems is that one aspect or the other may be neglected. An integrated approach is needed.

❖ NURSING MANAGEMENT: CLIENT WITH PAIN

In caring for clients in pain, nurses must first recognize and clarify their attitudes toward the use of analgesics. Self-knowledge helps eliminate bias and promote objectivity and logic. They also must develop a broad knowledge base to support clinical judgments.

NURSING PROCESS
ASSESSMENT
When pain medication is ordered to be administered intermittently, the nurse should assess the client before each dose. To help the client report the severity of pain accurately, a quantitative scale may be used. Appropri-

ate measurements may be numeric scales (0 to 10 or 0 to 5, with 0 representing no pain and the highest number representing maximal pain) or verbal reports (no pain, small amount of pain, moderate pain, severe pain, excruciating pain). The same scale should be used consistently.

Additional assessment features include factors that alter the client's perception of pain. For example, the client may report increased pain at bedtime when distractions (eg, activity, TV programs, visitors) are decreased or eliminated.

The nurse should also verify that the minimal time between analgesic doses has elapsed, that the source of pain is appropriate to the medication ordered, and that the quality and intensity of the pain are appropriate to the client's condition. Besides this minimal, immediate assessment, the pattern of pain as it is expected to recur throughout the day should be evaluated. Appropriate times for medication and maximal analgesic effect can then be projected for the next 24 hours. This approach helps to maximize pain control and minimize the total amount of drugs required.

The daily cycle of pain should be considered within the context of the probable future course of the client's illness. Anticipating future pain patterns helps the nurse identify unusual developments that may signal complications, adjust the analgesic regimen to maintain adequate pain control, and avoid inappropriate medication.

NURSING DIAGNOSIS

Nursing diagnoses should be tailored to the client's needs and may include:

- Pain, related to nerve stimulation due to malignant tumor growth
- Pain, related to trauma to nerve cells secondary to surgery; contributing factors: refusal of analgesic drugs related to knowledge deficit regarding pain's adverse effects on healing and anxiety related to the outcome of treatment
- Pain, phantom, related to irritation of nerve endings secondary to amputation
- Pain, habit, related to recurrent pain secondary to arthritis; contributing factors: exposure to cold and increased muscle tension
- Pain, related to irritability of nerve cells secondary to withdrawal syndrome during narcotic dependence

PLANNING

Goals of nursing care include preventing, alleviating, or eliminating pain and educating clients concerning the physiologic effects of pain, the use of analgesics, and self-care practices to reduce the perception of pain.

INTERVENTION

Nurses often prepare and administer pain medication. They also implement nursing measures to reduce pain and its perception by the client.

Client Education. A key to effective pain relief measures is client education. Nurses must teach clients

CRITICAL THINKING CHALLENGE
Issues Analysis

It is ethically and professionally permissible to administer morphine to a terminally ill client to relieve pain even though the depression of respiration it produces may accelerate the client's death.

Discuss how you would respond to the following scenario:

A managed care program refuses to pay for oral or continuous IV infusion of morphine because "it costs too much and the client is going to die anyway."

how to administer medication, practice relaxation techniques, evaluate their response to analgesics and pain control techniques, and identify adverse effects to report to the appropriate healthcare practitioner.

OUTCOME EVALUATION

Data required for evaluation include (most importantly) reports from clients describing the level of comfort, discomfort, or pain in terms of the pain scale used for initial assessment. In addition, the nurse should assess physical signs that indicate the presence or absence of pain for the individual client.

❖ CHECKLIST OF NURSING ACTIONS

- ❏ Assess pain by measuring physical changes attributable to pain and by listening to the client's descriptions of pain; use a numeric or verbal scale acceptable to the client to rate pain.
- ❏ Evaluate each client's pain over the diurnal cycle; predict the likely course of pain during the client's illness.
- ❏ If the severity of pain appears inappropriate, given the client's reaction to discomfort and the nature of the underlying illness, evaluate the client carefully for complications.
- ❏ Consult the prescriber when appropriate to request new or different orders for analgesia.
- ❏ Administer analgesics in ample amounts to control pain, reducing dosage to the minimum needed once control is established.
- ❏ Always implement nursing measures to decrease perception of pain.
- ❏ Educate clients about the nature of pain, its adverse effects, and the use of analgesics and self-care measures to reduce its impact.
- ❏ Evaluate the effects of pain control measures by seeking the client's evaluation of comfort levels; monitor physiologic signs that indicate his or her response to pain or its absence.

Analgesics

Analgesics are drugs that relieve or decrease pain without interrupting consciousness. They inhibit the transmission of pain impulses, reduce the cortical response to pain stimuli, or alter nerve activity in areas of the brain (eg, the frontal lobe and limbic systems) that moderate perception of pain. Analgesics include both natural and synthetic compounds. The term "narcotic" is confusing and therefore is not used in this chapter without qualification (Box 18-3).

Nonnarcotic Analgesics

Nonnarcotic analgesics include acetaminophen, NSAIDs such as aspirin and ibuprofen, and other drugs that produce analgesia through more peripheral mechanisms. Chapter 36 provides detailed information about the pharmacology of these agents. They also are discussed in the section on pain management in this chapter.

Opioid Analgesics

Opium is one of the oldest analgesics known. First used in Asia Minor, where the opium poppy (*Papaver somniferum*) is indigenous, substances derived from its juice are termed *opiates*. Because several synthetic substitutes have been developed with opium-like properties, the term *opioid* was coined to designate both opiates and their synthetic substitutes. The active drugs contained in opium are alkaloids of two types: phenanthrene and benzylisoquinoline.

Phenanthrene alkaloids, which include morphine and codeine, exhibit potent analgesic and sedative properties not characteristic of benzylisoquinolines. The ma-

jor alkaloid of the benzylisoquinolines is papaverine, used medicinally as a vasodilator (see Chap. 24).

In addition to the natural phenanthrene derivatives, synthetic phenylpiperidine and diphenylheptane derivatives are available for use as opioid analgesics. Meperidine, fentanyl, alfentanil, and sufentanil are the major phenylpiperidine derivatives; diphenylheptane derivatives used medicinally include methadone and pentazocine (Box 18-4).

Categories of Opioid Analgesics

Opioid analgesics are categorized as agonists, mixed agonist–antagonist, or antagonists according to their activity with the different opioid receptors (Table 18-7). This classification system is useful to know when selecting an analgesic.

Agonists have activity at the mu receptors and possibly the delta receptors. There is no ceiling on their analgesic efficacy. They are used extensively in managing pain and controlling bronchospasm and coughs. *Agonist–antagonist* drugs have mixed activity—agonist activity at certain receptors and antagonist activity at others. There is a ceiling to their analgesic effect. Moreover, they may precipitate a withdrawal syndrome and increased pain if given concurrently with a full opioid agonist. *Antagonists* do not produce agonist activity at any

---

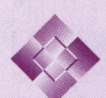

Box 18-4
Active Drugs in Opium and Opioids

Phenanthrene alkaloids (morphine and codeine): exhibit potent analgesic and sedative properties

Synthetic phenylpiperidine derivatives (meperidine, fentanyl): exhibit analgesic and sedative properties

Diphenylheptane derivatives (methadone): mild analgesia; signs and symptoms of methadone withdrawal; they are easier to wean from than other opioids

Benzylisoquinoline alkaloids (papaverine): dilate blood vessels (discussed in Chap. 24)

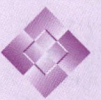

Box 18-3
Clarifying Terminology: Narcotic

Analgesics are commonly described as narcotic or nonnarcotic agents. The use of these terms is unfortunate, because the word *narcotic* has two distinct definitions that tend to be confused.

The original meaning of *narcotic* is a substance that induces sleep or stupor. A secondary meaning stemming from the Harrison Narcotic Act of 1914, however, defines a narcotic as a member of various classes of drugs (opium, coca, and marijuana) believed to be habit-forming. The Act forbade sale or use of these drugs or their derivatives without a medical prescription.

Legally, therefore, a narcotic is a dependency-producing drug, the use of which is strictly controlled by law. Since 1914, prescription controls have been extended to other drugs characterized by dependency, but the term *narcotic* is not usually applied to them.

Table 18-7. Hypothetical Subtypes of Opioid Receptors

Receptor Type	Functions Mediated by the Receptor
μ (mu)	Supraspinal analgesia, miosis, hypothermia, respiratory depression, euphoria, physical depression
κ (kappa)	Spinal analgesia, miosis, hypothermia, sedation, possible respiratory depression
σ (sigma)	Dysphoria, hallucinations, respiratory and vasomotor stimulation
δ (delta)	Alterations of affective behavior, possible respiratory depression

of the receptor sites, but they do block the receptor from interacting with agonist opioids. They are commonly used to block the action of an agonist opioid.

Pharmacodynamics. Opioid agonists interact with receptors in the brain and other tissues at the normal sites of action of endogenous ligands (endorphins and enkephalins), which function to control the pain response and modify the client's mood or psychologic state (Table 18-8). Several subtypes appear to be distinguished by the functions that they mediate and the action of various chemicals that interact with them. Receptors are

Table 18-8. Representative Narcotic/Opioid Agonists

Drug Name	Preparation	Dosage	Additional Information
alfentanil (Alfenta) (*Can*: Rapifen)	Solution for continuous infusion	Adults, *IV:* Initial: 8–50 µg/kg, then increase by 3–15 µg/kg Induction: 130–245 µg/kg, then 0.5–1.5 µg/kg/min	Alfentanil is used for inducing anesthesia or with other drugs during anesthesia.
alphaprodine (Nisentil)	Solutions for IV, SC, or submucosal injection	Adults, *IV:* 0.4–0.6 mg/kg; *SC:* 0.4–1.2 mg/kg; maximum daily dosage: 240 mg PC: C	Alphaprodine should not be administered IM because of erratic absorption. This drug is for moderate to severe acute pain.
codeine (*Can:* Paveral)	Oral tablets Combined with other ingredients: oral tablets and syrups	Adults, *oral, SC, IM:* 15–60 mg q4h as needed Children: 0.5 mg/kg or 15 m² of body surface q4–6h PC: C (D for prolonged use or use of high doses at term)	Codeine is used for mild pain and in cough preparations to suppress cough.
fentanyl (Innovar, Duragesic, Fentanyl, Oralet, Sublimaze)	Solutions for SC or IM injection Transdermal patches Transmucosal lozenges	Adults, *IM:* 0.05–0.1 mg Children 2–12 yr, *IM:* 0.05–0.1 µg/kg *Transdermal:* Titrated according to client; usual initial dose: 25 µg/hr, q72h *Transmucosal:* 5 µg/kg PC:C (D for prolonged use or use of high doses at term)	Fentanyl is used for pain control before or during anesthesia. Transdermal patches are used to manage chronic pain in clients requiring opioid analgesia.
heroin (horse, smack)	Nonmedicinal: powder for oral use: topical application to mucous membranes, or preparation for injection	N/A	Manufacture, sale, and use is illegal in United States.
hydrocodone (Hycodan) (*Can:* Robidane)	Oral tablets	Adults, 5–10 mg q4h as needed	Hydrocodone is used for moderate to severe pain and as an antitussive.
hydromorphone (Dilaudid)	Oral tablets Solutions for SC or IM injection Suppositories	Adults, *oral:* 2–4 mg q4–6h as needed; *SC or IM:* 1–2 mg q4–6h as needed; *Rectally:* 3 mg q6–8h as needed Children over 12 yr: 1 mg q3–4h; 6–12 yr: 0.5 mg q3–4h PC: C (D for prolonged use or use of high doses at term)	Hydromorphone produces minimal hypnotic, euphoric, and GI side effects. Also used in children to control cough.
levomethadyl (ORLAAM)	Oral solution	Adults, Initial: 20–40 mg q48–72 hr and adjusted in 5–10-mg increments until steady state (1–2 weeks) PC: B	Used only in treating narcotic addiction.
levorphanol (Levo-Dromoran)	Oral tablets Solutions for SC or slow IV injection	Adults, *oral* or *SC:* 2 mg q6h as needed PC: C (D for prolonged use or use of high doses at term)	Levorphanol is for moderate to severe pain. Safe use for children or during pregnancy has not been established.
meperidine (Demerol)	Oral tablets and syrup Solutions for SC or IM injection	Adults, *oral, IM,* or *SC:* 50–150 mg q3–4h as needed Children, 1.1–1.8 mg/kg q3–4h as needed (*maximum single pediatric dose:* 100 mg) PC: C (D for prolonged use or use of high doses at term)	Meperidine has limited effects on GI tract.

KEY: PC = pregnancy category (see Appendix A); *Can* = Canadian trade name.

(continued)

Table 18-8. (Continued)

Drug Name	Preparation	Dosage	Additional Information
methadone (Dolophine)	Oral tablets and syrup Solutions for SC or IM injection	Adults, 2.5–10 mg q3–4h as needed; maximum parenteral dose: 10 mg PC: C (D for prolonged use or use of high doses at term)	Preparation used to manage addiction
morphine (MS Contin, RMS, Roxinol; *Can:* Astamorph, Duramorph, Epimorph	Oral tablets, controlled-release tablets Solutions for SC, IM, IV injection, and epidural infusion Rectal suppositories	Adults, *oral:* 10–30 mg q4h as needed; controlled-release tablets: 30 mg q8–12h; *SC or IM:* 5–20 mg q4h as needed; *IV:* 2.5–15 mg over 4–5 min; *rectal:* 10–20 mg q4h as needed; *continuous epidural infusion:* 2–4 mg q24h Children, *SC:* 0.1–0.2 mg/kg q4h as needed; *maximum pediatric dose:* 15 mg PC: C (D for prolonged use or use of high doses at term)	Morphine is the prototype drug for narcotic analgesics and is a standard for comparison of strong analgesic effects of other drugs.
opium (Pantopon, Opium Tincture Deodorized, Paregoric)	Oral solutions Solutions for SC or IM injection	Adults, *oral,* Opium tincture deodorized: 0.6 mL; paregoric (camphorated tincture of opium), 5–10 mL 1–4 times daily, *SC or IM* (Pantopon): 5–20 mg q4–5h as needed Children, *oral* (opium tincture deodorized), analgesia: 0.01–0.02 mL/kg/dose q3–4h; diarrhea: 0.005–0.01 mL/kg q3–4h; paregoric (camphorated tincture of opium): 0.25–0.5 mL/kg 1–4 times daily	Opium currently is used primarily for antiperistaltic effects. *The oral preparations have similar names (tinctures) but have very different dosages.*
oxycodone (Roxicodone) (*Can:* Supeudol)	Oral tablets and solution	Adults, 5 mg q6h as needed PC: C (D for prolonged use or use of high doses at term)	Oxycodone is used for moderate to severe acute pain. It is used also with other mild analgesics (Percocet, Percodan, Tylox).
oxymorphone (Numorphan)	Solution for SC, IM, or IV injection Rectal suppositories	Adults, *IM* (initially): 1–15 mg; *IV* (initially): 0.5 mg (dosage may be increased cautiously until therapeutic response is obtained); *rectal:* 5 mg q4–6h as needed PC: C (D for prolonged use or use of high doses at term)	Oxymorphone causes fewer side effects that does morphine.
propoxyphene HCl (Darvon, Dolene) propoxyphene napsylate (Darvon-N)	Oral capsules, tablets, and suspensions	Adults, *oral:* propoxyphene HCl: 65 mg q4h as needed not to exceed 390 mg/24 h; propoxyphene napsylate: 100 mg q4h as needed not to exceed 600 mg/24 h	Propoxyphene is structurally related to methadone and has half the analgesic potency of codeine.
remifentanil (Ultiva)	Powder for reconstitution for IV infection	Adults, Induction: IV 0.5–1 mcg/kg/min Monitored anesthesia care: Single dose 1 mcg/kg over 30–60 sec given 90 sec before local anesthesia. Continuous: 0.025–0.2 mcg/kg/min PC: C	Used as analgesic component of monitored anesthesia care and for induction and maintenance of general anesthesia.
sufentanil (Sufenta)	Solutions for parenteral administration	Adults (initially), 1–8 μg/kg; additional 25–30 μg/kg PC: C (D for prolonged use or use of high doses at term)	Sufentil is used with nitrous oxide and oxygen for anesthesia.

KEY: PC = pregnancy category (see Appendix A); *Can* = Canadian trade name.

most numerous in the limbic system, thalamus, striatum, hypothalamus, midbrain, and substantia gelatinosa of the spinal cord. They are also present in nerve plexi and exocrine glands of the stomach and intestines.

Opioids may also alter the chemical environment in the brain. For example, morphine decreases the calcium ion concentration in the brain and prevents its uptake in brain cells. Other opioids inhibit the release of acetylcholine and norepinephrine and modify dopamine release. Several central effects result from these and possibly other unknown mechanisms. Activity decreases in the locus ceruleus, the structure responsible for alarm responses, such as panic, fear, and anxiety. The client's perception of pain is inhibited and the reaction to pain or its stimulus is reduced. At the same time, the client's mood improves and some euphoria occurs.

Opioid agonist–antagonists also act as agonists or partial agonists on different opioid receptors, producing some of the same pharmacologic effects as the opioid agonists (Table 18-9). In general, however, the effects are milder, and certain effects (eg, antitussive, gastrointestinal [GI]) may not occur at all. Because they compete with the stronger opioids for placement on the receptor, these drugs can act as antagonists of opioid agonists.

Pharmacokinetics. Opioid analgesics are readily absorbed from the GI and nasal mucosa, the surface of the lungs, and the peripheral tissues after injection. Medicinally, the drugs are administered by oral, rectal, SC, IM, IV, transdermal, and epidural routes. When abused, the compounds may be applied as snuff to the nasal mucosa, smoked, or injected (see Focus On Opioid Agonists: Similarities and Differences on pp. 324–325).

Drugs administered by IV injection take effect immediately. Absorption from SC and IM sites is directly related to lipid solubility. The effectiveness of oral administration varies because many preparations undergo significant first-pass metabolism in the liver immediately after intestinal absorption. Because of the first-pass mechanism, oral morphine and related drugs must be given in higher doses than IV morphine and related drugs. Meperidine, codeine, and methadone are less affected by first-pass metabolism and are relatively more effective when administered orally.

After absorption, agonist opioids are widely distributed in body tissues. Morphine concentrates mostly in parenchymatous tissues (liver, kidney, spleen, lungs) and somewhat less in muscle tissues. About one third binds to plasma proteins. Although relatively little morphine

Table 18-9. Representative Opioid Agonist–Antagonists

Drug Name	Preparations	Usual Adult Analgesic Dosage	Additional Information
buprenorphine (Buprenex)	Solutions for IM and IV administration	0.3–0.6 mg q4–6h PC: C (D for prolonged use or use of high doses at term)	Should respiratory depression develop, give doxapram (Dopram) or naloxone.
butorphanol (Stadol)	Solution for IM or IV injection Nasal spray	*IM:* 1–4 mg q3–4h as needed *IV:* 0.5–2 mg q3–4h as needed PC: B (D for prolonged use or use of high doses at term) Nasal: 1 mg (1 spray) per nostril; repeat in 60–90 min as needed, then 1 mg q3–4h	Butorphanol is used for moderate to severe pain. It is 3.5–7 times more potent than morphine.
dezocine (Dalgan)	Vials, syringes, and multiple-dose vials for IM or IV administration	*IM:* 5–20 mg q3–6h *IV:* 2.5–10 mg q2–4h PC: C	Dezocine's effectiveness is comparable to that of morphine sulfate. Dezocine contains sodium metabisulfate; it is contraindicated for clients with allergic sensitivity to sulfites. Dezocine is too irritating to administer SC.
nalbuphine (Nubain)	Solution for SC, IM, or IV injection	10 mg q3–6h as needed In nontolerant persons, *maximum single dose:* 20 mg; *maximum daily dosage:* 160 mg PC: B (D for prolonged use or use of high doses at term)	Nalbuphine is used for moderate to severe pain. Pharmacologically, nalbuphine is similar to pentazocine and butorphanol.
pentazocine (Talwin)	Solution for SC, IM, or IV injection Oral tablets	30 mg q3–4h as needed 50–100 mg q3–4h as needed PC: C (D for prolonged use or use of high doses at term)	Pentazocine is used for moderate to severe pain. When given orally, a higher dose is required to achieve effects equal to parenteral administration.

KEY: PC = pregnancy category (see Appendix A).

passes the blood-brain barrier in adults, this fraction accounts for its central actions.

Codeine and heroin pass more readily than morphine into the CNS but exert few central effects until converted by the tissues to morphine. Heroin is rapidly metabolized to morphine, but only a small fraction of codeine follows this pathway.

Initially, most methadone binds to plasma proteins. Subsequently, it becomes firmly bound to tissue proteins. This depot is responsible for its accumulation with repeated administration and its prolonged effects in suppressing the withdrawal syndrome in morphine- or heroin-dependent persons. As with morphine, only fractional parts of a methadone dose cross the blood-brain barrier.

All opioid agonists are metabolized by the tissues. Most are deactivated by hepatic microsomal enzymes. Drugs and their metabolites are excreted mainly by renal tubule filtration, but small amounts (10% or less) enter the enterohepatic circulation. Some of the latter is excreted in the feces, but a portion is reabsorbed and prolongs the duration of drug effect.

Opioid agonist–antagonists are administered orally and by injection. After absorption, they are widely distributed in the body—to the brain, into breast milk, and across the placenta. Metabolism is by the liver, and excretion is primarily by the kidneys.

Therapeutic Uses. Opioid analgesics are widely used to relieve pain resulting from acute or terminal illness. Codeine and related compounds are prescribed for moderate pain. Meperidine, morphine, and morphine's relatives are reserved for severe pain. In countries outside the United States, heroin is often preferred for treating intractable pain. Methadone is used mainly in treating withdrawal syndrome in heroin- or morphine-dependent persons and as an oral analgesic for relieving severe pain, particularly that of terminal cancer. Equipotent doses of opioid analgesics are listed in Table 18-10.

In some cases, opioid analgesics have been used to interrupt labor in threatened abortion and to ease induction of anesthesia before surgery (antianxiety agents are gradually replacing their use in surgery). High doses of opioid agonists are sometimes used as primary agents for general anesthesia. Because they produce fewer cardiovascular changes than other general anesthetics, opioids are sometimes used as anesthetic agents in cardiac surgery.

The value of opioid analgesics as antidiarrheals and antitussives is discussed in Chapters 29 and 37. In addition, opioids are used on an empirical basis in such clinical situations as left ventricular failure with pulmonary edema, even though the specific mechanisms involved remain unknown.

The opioid agonist–antagonists can relieve pain that is not responsive to antiinflammatory analgesics and acetaminophen. Their use allows the healthcare provider to postpone administering the opioids, which have a greater abuse potential and carry greater risk for physical dependence.

When used to treat pain, opioids rarely cause psychologic dependence. If the cause of the pain is corrected, most clients respond well to gradual withdrawal schedules and do not abuse the drug after withdrawal is completed.

Administration. Opioids are usually administered by the oral, SC, IM, or IV route. They can also be infused intrathecally or epidurally. The transdermal route is now available for fentanyl. Doses administered IM or SC are not absorbed unless vascular circulation is adequate. Ineffective doses should not be repeated: they remain in tissue deposits and tend to be absorbed simultaneously when circulation is restored, causing a toxic reaction due to overdose. Increasingly, pain medication is administered by PCA equipment, which allows the client to control the drug administration.

Adverse Reactions. Adverse effects of opioid analgesics relate to both the central and peripheral actions of the drugs. They affect many tissues and systems of the body, causing various physiologic responses. Table 18-11 lists common systemic adverse effects. Other adverse effects of opioid analgesics include toxicity, tolerance and withdrawal, idiosyncratic reactions, and allergic reactions.

Toxic effects of opioid agonist–antagonists resemble those of the stronger opioids, although tolerance and dependence seem to develop more slowly. As opioid drug dosages increase, so do the incidence and severity of adverse effects. Higher doses accentuate subjective effects such as euphoria. They also increase the incidence of nausea and vomiting. In addition, respirations become slow and shallow; muscle rigidity and catalepsy

Table 18-10. Doses of Opioid Analgesics With Effects Comparable to Morphine

Drug	Dose Equivalent to Morphine Sulfate 10 mg IM
Agonists	
codeine	130 mg IM
hydromorphone	1.5 mg IM
levorphanol	2 mg IM
meperidine	75 mg IM
methadone	10 mg IM
oxymorphone	1 mg IM
Agonist–Antagonists	
butorphanol	2 mg IM
nalbuphine	10 mg IM
pentazocine	60 mg IM

(Adapted from McEvoy GK, ed. [1991]. *Drug information 91,* p 1153. Bethesda, MD: American Society of Hospital Pharmacists and American Pain Society. [1989], p. 10).

FOCUS ON

Opioid Agonists: Similarities and Differences

Similarities

Pharmacodynamics

These agents act as agonists by interacting with the receptors in the brain and tissue. They act on several sites within the CNS, involving systems of neurotransmitters to produce analgesia by altering the pain perceptions at the spinal cord or higher levels in the CNS. They also alter the person's emotional response to pain.

Pharmacokinetics

These agents are readily absorbed from the GI tract, nasal mucosa, surface of the lungs, and peripheral tissues after injection. They are given orally, rectally, SC, IM, or IV. They are metabolized by the liver enzymes and also by the CNS, kidneys, lungs, and placenta. They are excreted primarily in the urine, with small amounts excreted in feces.

Differences

- **Morphine** decreases the calcium ion concentration in the brain cells.
- **Sufentanil** has a high affinity for opiate receptors.

- **Morphine** must be given in larger doses orally; **meperidine, codeine,** and **methadone** are more effective orally.
- **Morphine** concentrations are greatest in the lungs, liver, kidney, and spleen, with half binding to plasma proteins. Most of **methadone** binds to plasma proteins.
- **Codeine** acts within 15 to 30 minutes (PO or SC). Its effect lasts 4 to 6 hours. Negligible amounts are excreted in feces.
- **Fentanyl** is given parenterally: onset of 7 to 15 minutes, peak of minutes, duration of action 30 to 60 minutes (IV), 1 to 2 hours (IM).
- **Hydromorphone** is given orally, rectally, or parenterally with an onset of 15 to 30 minutes, duration of 4 to 5 hours with no excretion in feces.
- **Levorphanol** is well absorbed orally or SC; peaks in 20 minutes (IV), 60 to 90 minutes (SC), with a duration of 6 to 8 hours and no excretion in feces.
- **Meperidine** peaks in 1 hour (PO), 40 to 60 minutes (SC), 30 to 50 minutes (IM), with a duration of 2 to 4 hours; 60% to 80% is bound to plasma proteins. It crosses the placenta and is found in breast milk. It has a half-life of 2 to 11 minutes and then 3 to 5 hours (elimination half-life is prolonged in people with liver dysfunction) with no excretion in the feces.
- **Methadone** is bound to tissue protein and has a duration of 4 to 6 hours. Morphine peaks in 60 minutes (PO), 20 to 60 minutes (R), 50 to 90 minutes (SC), 30 to 60 minutes (IM), and 20 minutes (IV); small amounts are found in breast milk.
- **Oxycodone** is only given orally; its onset is 10 to 15 minutes, peaks in 30 to 60 minutes, with a duration of 3 to 6 hours with no excretion in the feces.
- **Oxymorphone** can be given rectally, SC, IM, or IV; its onset is 15 to 30 minutes (R), 5 to 10 (IV), 10 to 15 minutes (SC or IM), with a duration of 3 to 6 hours and no excretion in feces.
- **Sufentanil** is given IM or IV with an onset of 1 to 2 minutes (IV); rapidly eliminated from the tissues; with a duration of 40 to 80 minutes (IV), 2 to 4 hours (IM); elimination half-life is 2 to 3 hours. Small amounts have been found to be metabolized in the small intestines.

Therapeutic Uses

These agents are used for temporary analgesia in symptomatic relief of moderate to severe pain, during diagnostic and orthopedic procedures, for preoperative sedation, and as a supplement to anesthesia.

- **Codeine** and **hydrocodone** are used as cough suppressants; **methadone** is used as detoxification and maintenance treatment, as oral substitute for heroin and other morphinelike drugs; **opium** preparations are rarely used for analgesia; tinctures and paregoric are used as antidiarrheals; **morphine** is used to allay anxiety and cardiovascular effects in pulmonary edema and is the drug of choice in relieving the pain of acute myocardial infarction.

(continued)

Opioid Agonists: Similarities and Differences (continued)

Similarities (continued)

Adverse reactions

These include: (CNS) mood elevation, euphoria, lethargy, sedation, dizziness, sleep, coma, weakness, fainting, agitation, nervousness; (CV) postural hypotension, circulatory depression, bradycardia; (RESP) decreased rate and depth, irregular breathing patterns, bronchoconstriction; (EENT) pupil constriction, decreased visual acuity; (GI) nausea, vomiting, constipation, biliary colic; (GU) urinary retention, urgency, fluid retention; (SKIN) flushing, itching, increased perspiration, pruritus at injection site; (MS) increased muscle rigidity; (ENDO) reduced glucocorticoid levels, impotence, decreased libido; (OTHER) tolerance, psychologic dependence, physical dependence (with chronic use), painful plaques with continuous SC infusions.

Drug Interactions

Opioid agonists given with barbiturate anesthetics and other CNS depressants can result in increased respiratory and CNS depression. Cimetidine may contribute to CNS toxicity.

Nursing Considerations

Instruct in disease, drug treatment regimen, adverse reactions, and need for compliance; assess respiratory status and do not administer if rate is less than 12 breaths per minute; monitor skin color; evaluate laboratory results for indication of tissue ischemia; monitor liver and renal function studies; assess pain characteristics, including onset, type, location; assess level of orientation and neurologic status; institute measures to reduce anxiety and stress; help to divert attention from pain; monitor pain relief; instruct in measures to promote bowel elimination, including the use of stool softeners, laxatives as necessary, and high-fiber diet; monitor urinary elimination status, including intake and output; institute safety measures to prevent injury; raise side rails and assist in moving and getting in and out of bed; instruct client to change position slowly; instruct client to avoid driving or activities that require mental alertness until the effects of the drug are known.

Differences (continued)

- **Sufentanil** and **fentanyl** in high doses produce amnesia and loss of consciousness.
- **Sufentanil** can also cause increased airway resistance, apnea, tachycardia, bronchospasm, and chills.

- **Meperidine** should not be given concurrently with or within 14 days of therapy with monoamine oxidase inhibitors. The pharmacologic effects of **meperidine** and **methadone** may be decreased by hydantoins. **Fentanyl** and **droperidol** may cause hypotension and a decrease in pulmonary arterial pressure. **Methadone** plasma levels may be decreased by rifampin. Cardiovascular depression may occur if nitrous oxide is used with high doses of **sufentanil** and **fentanyl**.

- Monitor cough type and frequency when giving **codeine**; do not use **codeine** when cough is helpful in clearing the airway; keep resuscitative equipment available when giving **fentanyl, hydromorphone, levorphanol,** and **sufentanil**; rotate injection sites when giving **hydromorphone** parenterally; give IV **hydromorphone** slowly; warn that **levorphanol** has a bitter taste; administer IV **morphine** slowly and diluted (SC administration is painful); give **methadone** maintenance as an oral liquid—dissolve in 120 mL of orange juice or powdered citrus drink; monitor blood pressure closely when giving **morphine** parenterally; keep in mind that **fentanyl** and **sufentanil** reduce muscle rigidity with neuromuscular blockers.

---

tend to develop. T waves on electrocardiograms appear depressed or inverted. With very high doses of opioids, hypopnea secondary to respiratory impairment occurs. Blood pressure and pulse rate decline, partly from depression of the central vasomotor center and partly from lowered oxygen tension. Bronchoconstriction and convulsions may also develop. Overdose-related death usually results from respiratory failure.

Tolerance and withdrawal problems may arise from chronic opioid use. Tolerance occurs because repeated

Table 18-11. Common Adverse Effects of Opioid Analgesics

Signs or Symptoms	Underlying Mechanism
Respiratory System	
Reduced rate and depth of respirations	Depression of response of the central respiratory center to increased carbon dioxide in the blood
Irregular or periodic breathing	Depression of the medullary and pontine centers that regulate respiratory rhythms
Suppressed cough	Inhibition of cough reflex
Bronchoconstriction and possibly asthma	Release of histamine
Cardiovascular System	
Postural hypotension	Peripheral vasodilation
Skin	
Flushing (with reported sense of warmth and heaviness)	Peripheral vasodilation and histamine release
Increased perspiration	Histamine release
Pruritus (mostly of nose and injection site)	Histamine release
Gastrointestinal System	
Nausea and vomiting	Increased vestibular sensitivity and stimulation of the vomiting center
Delayed passage of stools (constipation)	Increased absorption of water from intestines
	Central sedation
	Decreased secretion of hydrochloric acid, bile, and pancreatic juice
	Increased tone of valves and sphincters
	Changes in peristaltic patterns (decrease in propulsive waves and increase in nonpropulsive waves)
Increased pressure in the biliary system (colic—most likely with morphine, least likely with meperidine)	Spasm at the sphincter of Oddi
Urinary Tract	
Urgency	Increased tone of detrusor muscle
Retention, particularly in postoperative clients and men with prostatic hypertrophy	Increased sphincter tone
	Central sedation that reduces attentiveness to the need to void
Reproductive Tract	
Interrupted or prolonged labor	Decrease in oxytocin-induced hyperreactivity of the uterus
Respiratory depression in the newborn	Depression of the fetal respiratory center by drug that crosses the placenta
Decreased motility of sperm, volume of ejaculate, and testosterone levels in males	Inhibition of luteotropin hormone production by the pituitary
Endocrine System	
Reduced glucocorticoid levels	Inhibition of pituitary production of adrenocorticotropin
Fluid retention	Enhanced antidiuretic hormone release by the pituitary
Musculoskeletal System	
Increased muscle rigidity	Stimulation of the spinal cord
Eye	
Pupillary constriction and decreased visual acuity (characteristic signs of toxicity)	Excitation of autonomic fibers of the oculomotor nerve
Central Nervous System	
Inability to concentrate and think	Depression of the cortex
Lethargy, sedation, or sleep	Depression of the reticular formation
Mood elevation, tranquility, euphoria, and apathy (most obvious after administration of heroin, which quickly converts to morphine)	Depression of the limbic system and brain stem
Decreased temperature	Resetting of the hypothalamic temperature-regulating mechanism
Electroencephalogram changes	Increased voltage and decreased frequency of electrical activity in the brain

opioid/receptor interaction leads to an adaptation of cell physiology that compensates for the presence of the drugs. Adenylate cyclase production increases, bringing cellular levels back to normal and restoring normal cell function. Tolerance is fairly complete to pain relief, sedation, mood elevation, and respiratory effects. Only partial tolerance develops to responses of the GI and male reproductive systems. Eye response does not change with repeated use of drugs, and pupillary constriction provides a reliable index of opioid exposure. If tolerance develops, withdrawal of opioids produces abnormal physiology resulting from overactivity in cells in which the adenylate cyclase level rose abnormally to compensate for the drugs. Signs and symptoms of abnormality are opposite to the usual effects of opioid analgesics and include dysphoria and increased sensation, particularly of pain and touch. Tactile hallucinations ("a monkey on the back") tend to develop. Nasopharyngeal secretions, GI secretions, and propulsive peristalsis increase; rhinorrhea and diarrhea occur. Pupils dilate and photophobia results. When tolerance is highly developed and drugs are withdrawn abruptly ("cold turkey"), these symptoms can be severe.

Idiosyncratic reactions to opioid use vary from person to person and within the same person over time. Nausea, vomiting, dizziness, mental clouding, dysphoria, increased biliary pressure, and diarrhea do not appear invariably or uniformly, but they do tend to emerge in characteristic patterns. Rarely, delirium may occur. Some clients experience an increased sensitivity to pain when the analgesic effect of the drugs subsides. Changes in physiology influence individual drug response. For example, pain may temporarily increase tolerance to the drugs so that sizable doses may be received without side effects. Should the pain subside before the drug effect dissipates, drowsiness and other opioid side effects may occur.

Clients with hypothyroidism, myasthenia gravis, and multiple sclerosis are unusually sensitive to opioids, whereas clients with hyperthyroidism are relatively insensitive. Clients with liver or renal impairment may experience prolonged drug effect because of the body's altered ability to excrete the drugs. Clients with a low blood volume are prone to develop hypotension in response to opioids. Clients with chronic hypercapnia (due to obstructive airway disease, kyphoscoliosis, obesity, or cor pulmonale) are hypersensitive to the depressant effects of opioids on respirations.

Age also plays a role in idiosyncratic responses. Infants are prone to respiratory depression, presumably due to increased permeability of the blood-brain barrier. Clients over age 60 report an enhanced analgesic response to the drugs, perhaps because of their decreased sensitivity to pain.

Allergic reactions to opioids are uncommon and usually signaled by urticaria or a rash. Contact dermatitis has been reported in people occupationally exposed to opioid compounds (nurses, pharmaceutical workers). On rare occasions, IV administration of morphine has produced anaphylaxis.

Drug Interactions. If an opioid agonist–antagonist is given to a client already receiving an opioid agonist, withdrawal symptoms and loss of analgesia occur. When used with other CNS drugs (eg, alcohol, tranquilizers, hypnotics, antihistamines, some antidepressants), opioids tend to enhance the central effects of these drugs and hence their toxicity. Meperidine should not be used in clients taking monamine oxidase inhibitors (MAOIs) or in those who have received these drugs within 14 days. See also Focus On Similarities and Differences in Opioid Analgesics.

Precautions and Contraindications. There are no absolute contraindications to using opioids, provided that equipment, supplies, and trained personnel are available to sustain vital functions and reverse acute adverse reactions. Mechanical ventilation may be required to maintain oxygenation, and opioid antagonists may be needed to reverse the physiologic manifestations of toxicity. Intensive therapy may be required for several hours to resolve life-threatening reactions when opioids are administered to high-risk clients.

In general, administering opioids to clients with head injury or severe obstructive lung disease should be avoided. Clients with brain injury are highly vulnerable to respiratory arrest, and the analgesic and hypnotic properties of the drugs tend to mask signs and symptoms of abnormalities, especially increased intracranial pressure. Great caution must be exercised when opioids are administered to clients with decreased respiratory reserve. When opioids must be used, lower-than-normal doses may be prescribed and the client's respiratory function should be monitored closely because opioids tend to increase hypoxemia. Likewise, hypovolemic clients should be monitored for circulatory shock. Urine output must be assessed carefully in clients prone to urinary retention.

■ SUMMARY

Opioid analgesics and related compounds remain the drugs of choice for alleviating severe pain, especially in terminal illness. When administered orally or by injection, these drugs diminish discomfort and may reduce or abolish the sensation of pain. Tranquility and euphoria enhance the positive response to medication. Undesired side effects include respiratory depression, constipation, and (in some recipients) nausea, vomiting, and dizziness. Toxicity may produce respiratory arrest and convulsions.

Opioids induce both physiologic and psychologic dependency with chronic use (sometimes as little as 2 weeks of regular use). Withdrawal produces a syndrome characterized by dysphoria, increased pain and other sensations, tactile hallucinations, rhinorrhea, and diarrhea. Physical dependence is treated by substituting methadone for other opioids and then gradually withdrawing the methadone. Sustained opioid dependence cure rates are low, possibly due to the persistence of psychologic dependence.

❖ NURSING MANAGEMENT: CLIENT RECEIVING OPIOID ANALGESICS

Nurses caring for clients who receive opioid analgesics must carefully consider issues such as adequate pain control versus drug dependency, management of drug dependence and abuse, protocols for controlled substances, and toxicity.

Pain Control. When opioids are ordered PRN, the nurse is responsible for managing analgesic therapy and ensuring pain relief. Aware of both the need to keep the patient comfortable and the dependence potential of opioids, the nurse may be inclined to administer the least drug possible. However, if the client is not relatively pain-free, this approach can be counterproductive. Recurrent pain that is relieved by medication sets up a stimulus–response–reward sequence that conditions the client to depend psychologically on the drugs. Careful nursing management can prevent pain from developing or increasing and, at the same time, avoid conditions leading to dependence. For instance, providing medication regularly before painful activities (dressing changes, ambulation) reduces client stress and minimizes psychologic dependence. Clients using PCA should be informed of scheduled activities likely to increase discomfort so they can premedicate as needed.

Drug Dependency. Because opioids produce euphoria, they are among the drugs of choice for abuse. Education is an important component of programs aimed at resolving drug-dependence problems. Nurses must help clients understand the nature of opioid substances and the risks inherent in their abuse. Nurses can educate families to recognize signs and symptoms of developing drug dependence so that intervention can be initiated early. Of course, when pain is severe or stems from a progressive terminal illness, some physical dependence is acceptable. Should the illness resolve, this type of dependence is readily resolved by a weaning regimen, provided the client is not psychologically dependent.

Treating chronic opioid dependence during the initial phase requires a controlled environment. Withdrawal symptoms may be minimized first by substituting methadone for the drug in use and then by gradually reducing the dosage. Methadone alleviates the most pronounced withdrawal symptoms and produces less discomfort and physiologic problems. Physiologic function can return to normal and physical dependence can be eliminated within a few weeks or months (2 weeks to 6 months). Psychologic dependence, however, is much more persistent, and relapses are frequent. It is not unusual, for example, for addicts to remain in drug treatment facilities for a year or more. To boost clients' success rates, nurses may help by making referrals to private or community resources, halfway houses, and self-help groups. These offer the client some protection, as well as support from others with similar problems. See Chapter 14 for more information.

Legal Implications. The nursing responsibility of preparing opioids for administration is somewhat complex because narcotic drugs are strictly controlled by law. They are usually stored in cabinets with double locks, the keys to which are retained by only one staff member. An accurate record must be made of the amount of the drug removed from the supply, the name of the client to receive the drug, the time the drug was administered, and the name of the physician and nurse involved.

Toxicity. Toxic levels of opioids may occur in high-risk clients who receive drugs by prescription, but toxicity occurs more often in abusers who overdose. The nurse must be alert for major signs of toxicity, such as respiratory failure. Respiratory support is the first priority of care. An IV line is established for rapid administration of medications and treatment of shock should it develop. Administering opioid antagonists may produce dramatic improvement, but this tends to be short-lived because these drugs are eliminated from the body more rapidly than opioids; repeated doses are usually necessary. The client needs intensive care for at least 24 hours (see Chap. 15 for more information).

NURSING PROCESS
ASSESSMENT

The client receiving opioid analgesics must be assessed carefully to determine the degree of risk in such therapy. The history of previous use or abuse of these drugs and responses to them should be explored. The specific drugs involved and the nature of the reaction should be delineated if the client has experienced adverse reactions. The prescriber must be informed of this history; if a drug to which the client is intolerant has been prescribed, the nurse should consult the prescriber about changing the drug order.

Respiratory function must be carefully assessed. Clients with a history of multiple sclerosis, myasthenia gravis, or other paralytic disorder involving the respiratory muscles, obstructive airway disease, or myxedema are at high risk for acute respiratory depression when opioids are given.

Liver and kidney problems should be investigated, because clients with liver or kidney impairment cannot metabolize opioids at a normal rate. Therefore, drug dosage is usually reduced, or the interval at which drugs are administered is lengthened. Laboratory data should be explored for indications of liver or kidney dysfunction and conditions that impair tissue perfusion (eg, anemia, poor cardiac function).

The client should be examined to assess further risk factors. Obese clients are at high risk for respiratory complications. Respiratory rate and depth and skin color should be noted. Opioids are not usually given to clients with a respiratory rate less than 12/min because further depression of respirations can be dangerous.

A careful pain assessment should be made before *each* dose of medication ordered to relieve pain. Objective signs of distress as well as subjective symptoms should be explored. The location, severity, quality, and intensity of pain should be determined. The purpose for which the drug has been ordered should be specified by the prescriber; the drug should not be given to relieve pain of a different type or in a different location than that for which it was prescribed.

The nurse should determine when the last analgesic medication was administered to the client. All drugs received by the client for the previous 24 hours should be reviewed to determine if substances antagonistic to or synergistic with opioids have been given. If so, the prescriber should be consulted to determine whether a change in dosage is appropriate. For example, if a client receives a combination of droperidol and fentanyl (Innovar) during anesthesia, the dosage of opioid analgesics should generally be cut in half until the Innovar is eliminated from the body.

Immediately before administering opioids, the nurse should count the respirations and note their depth. The degree of pupillary constriction should also be noted. If the effects of previously administered opioids have subsided, the pupils are usually normal. Persistent constriction is an indication of developing tolerance, because the symptoms for which the drug is used are recurring before the drug has been eliminated by the body.

NURSING DIAGNOSIS

Nursing diagnoses related to opioid administration may include:

- Pain, related to trauma
- Impaired Gas Exchange, Risk for: Hypoxia secondary to use of depressant drugs
- Constipation, related to decrease in propulsive peristalsis secondary to use of depressant drugs
- Altered Tissue Perfusion: Cerebral hypoxia related to postural hypotension secondary to use of depressant drugs
- Urinary Retention, related to drug-induced increased sphincter tone and decreased bladder contractility

PLANNING

Nursing management goals include reducing pain, maintaining respirations and gas exchange, preventing or alleviating constipation, maintaining cerebral circulation, reducing urinary retention, and increasing knowledge.

INTERVENTION

Every client in pain should receive intensive nursing care to reduce perception of and reaction to pain and to enhance the analgesic effect of drugs. Measures to reduce anxiety and stress in the client, to promote relaxation, and to divert attention from the pain are crucial.

Drug regimens in progressive conditions usually begin with the least powerful analgesics and progress to more potent preparations. Aspirin, acetaminophen, or NSAIDs may be sufficient in early pain. Propoxyphene or pentazocine may be used next. As pain increases in severity, codeine and eventually meperidine or morphine may be required.

It is the responsibility of the nurse to monitor the client's pain and response to medication so that the drug regimen may be adapted to the client's needs. Response to each dose of the administered analgesic should be carefully evaluated in light of pain control and adverse or toxic effects. If pain relief is inadequate or adverse reactions to the drug are apparent, the prescriber should be consulted about changing the drug order.

If respirations become unduly depressed (less than 12/min), assisted respiration or an opioid antagonist may be needed. Administering an opioid antagonist may temporarily abolish the analgesic effect of previous opioids, and acute severe pain may result. Intensive nursing care to decrease the perception of pain should be instituted. As effects of the opioid antagonist dissipate, analgesic effects resume.

Nursing measures to promote fecal elimination are appropriate but may not be sufficient if the client needs opioids over the long term. In such cases, a stool softener should be used daily. Enemas or stimulant laxatives may also be needed. Care should be exercised to avoid

CRITICAL THINKING CHALLENGE
Case Analysis

Mr. Takano is a 45-year-old computer programmer of Japanese descent. He has been treated conservatively for lower back pain for more than 3 years. When you enter his room, he and his family are sharing jokes and laughing. You observe that he seems relaxed and does not appear to be in pain. He tells you, however, that he is having severe pain and needs a "shot of Demerol."

What are your hypotheses about Mr. Takano's pain?

What further data would you obtain?

constipation or fecal impaction. Nursing measures to promote micturition should be implemented as well to prevent urinary retention. As with constipation, however, these measures may be inadequate, particularly in elderly men who are prone to prostatic hypertrophy. Catheterization may be necessary.

Clients subject to postural hypotension from pain medication should be shown how to change position slowly, especially when arising from a bed or chair. Support hose may be used to minimize pooling of blood in the lower extremities.

Client Education. Many clients know little about opioid analgesics and their use in controlling pain. Although most people are aware of some undesirable aspects of opioid drug use, they may not appreciate the therapeutic value. Moreover, cultural beliefs may affect the client's understanding of pain and its relief.

When opioids are given for relieving pain, the client should be informed of the purpose of the medication. The effect of the drug is usually enhanced by the placebo effect of suggestion. Moreover, clients must know about the drugs they are receiving if their consent to treatment is to be informed and valid.

Occasionally, clients are afraid to use opioid substances. In the absence of a history of opioid dependence or religious or philosophical scruples, this fear is usually unwarranted. Such clients may need instruction about how pain retards healing to provide a rational basis for making a decision for or against taking medication. Clients who wish to avoid drug use should be provided with instructions detailing nonpharmacologic approaches to pain treatment.

Clients on long-term opioid treatment should learn self-assessment techniques to evaluate their need for the drug and to assess their undesirable reactions to the drug. The nurse can show the client how to count and interpret respirations before each dose of medication and how to maintain the dosage schedule. The nurse should also teach the client to recognize signs and symptoms to report, particularly if pain relief is inadequate.

Clients or their families benefit from instruction in techniques to reduce the perception of pain and to enhance analgesic effect. Techniques focusing on relaxation, controlling stressors, and diversion are helpful. Some people benefit from self-hypnosis.

Most clients who receive opioids experience some constipation. They should be cautioned to maintain full hydration, regular exercise, and a diet with adequate fiber. A regular schedule of defecation should be established (daily, if possible). A stool softener such as docusate sodium (Colace) or bulk-forming laxatives such as psyllium hydrophilic mucilloid (Metamucil) may be recommended.

Clients should learn how to store drug supplies safely to prevent inadvertent ingestion, overdose, or theft. Locked containers are recommended.

Under the influence of opioids, psychomotor skills decline and clients tend to be less alert and less proficient than usual. For safety's sake, they should avoid driving, operating machinery, or performing tasks that require coordination and mental alertness while drug effects persist.

OUTCOME EVALUATION

Data required for evaluating nursing measures include client statements reporting comfort or pain relief. Respirations, skin color, and peripheral tissue perfusion should be monitored to evaluate the adequacy of gas exchange. Sufficiency of elimination is judged by consistency and frequency of bowel movements and patterns of micturition. The ability of clients to repeat information conveyed during teaching sessions and their acceptance of appropriate analgesic regimens may be used as measures of teaching effectiveness (see Example of Nursing Process for Adverse Effects of Codeine).

❖ CHECKLIST OF NURSING ACTIONS

- ❑ Assess clients about to receive opioids for history of use or abuse and increased risk of adverse reactions and respiratory impairment.
- ❑ Assess respiratory rate and depth before administering opioid analgesics. Respiratory rate should be 12 or more breaths per minute in adults.
- ❑ Assess the client's response to opioid medication carefully, particularly pain relief, adverse and toxic effects, and signs and symptoms of developing allergy or tolerance.
- ❑ Consult the prescriber about a change of medication if the response is undesirable or complications, such as allergy, develop.
- ❑ Teach clients who manage their own opioid regimens how to monitor their responses to the drugs and to perform self-care to enhance response and reduce side effects.
- ❑ Caution clients who manage their own opioid regimens not to engage in potentially dangerous activities, such as driving a car or operating a power saw, while under the influence of the drugs. Also explain how to store drug supplies securely to prevent inadvertent poisoning.
- ❑ Educate the public about the risks of nonmedicinal use of opioids.
- ❑ Store opioid drugs securely in accord with agency protocol; keep an accurate record of their use and disposition.
- ❑ Monitor clients with opioid toxicity for at least 24 hours, administering opioid antagonists as necessary. Maintain adequate tissue oxygenation during this time.

Example of Nursing Process for Adverse Effects of Codeine

The client is a 50-year-old man discharged from the hospital 4 weeks ago following diagnosis of adenocarcinoma of the lung with metastases to the cervical vertebrae.

The client complains of back pain, stating that the pain pills provided relief until 3 days ago. Now, they "take the edge off the pain" but never make him "really comfortable." His prescription for pain medication specifies codeine 30 mg PO q3h for chest or back pain. He has taken one dose at 6 AM and another at noon. It is now 4 PM. He states he is reluctant to take more of these pills because they "are not working," and he doesn't want to become "addicted."

The client's vital signs (blood pressure, pulse, and respiratory rate) are elevated above his normal range. His pupils are equal and reactive to light.

The client also complains of constipation, which began in the hospital and has not improved much since his discharge.

Assessment Data

Diagnosis of metastatic cancer

Complaints of back pain

Client statement that the pain medication does not promote real comfort

Client takes pain medication infrequently because he doesn't want to become "addicted."

Elevated vital signs

Use of opioid medication

Nursing Diagnosis	Intervention	Goals and Outcome Criteria
Knowledge Deficit, related to severe pain and therapeutic regimens for its relief	**Discuss** with the client the meaning pain has for him, its impact on his quality of life, and the therapeutic use of opioid medications, stressing the adverse effects chronic pain has on health.	The client will accept pain medication.
	Advise the client to take another dose of analgesic immediately.	
Pain: Back pain, related to irritation of pain receptors by metastatic lesions in the vertebrae	**Urge** the client to take the pain medication by the clock until the pain is under control, then to increase gradually the time interval between doses until the optimal dosage schedule is determined.	The client will state that his pain is controlled and that he feels comfortable. The client's vital signs will drop to levels normal for him.
	Recommend that the client contact the physician for a change in medication if the pain is not controlled within 24 hours.	
	Notify the physician about the client's pain and the recommendations given him.	
Constipation, related to increased sphincter tone and decreased propulsive peristalsis secondary to use of opioid medication	**Inform** the client that constipation is a side effect of opioid analgesics and is likely to be a continuing problem.	The client will state that constipation has been alleviated or eliminated.
	Encourage the client to take an over-the-counter stool softener.	
	Advise the client of measures that help to counteract constipation.	
	Recommend using a saline or stimulant laxative of the client's choice.	

Opioid Antagonists

Certain drugs that interact with opioid receptors in the CNS produce little or no agonist effect at these sites. Because they can displace the opioid molecule from the receptor site, they tend to reduce the physiologic effects of these drugs—hence, their designation as *opioid antagonists*. When administered to persons under the influence of opioids, they displace these more active analgesics from the receptor sites, reducing the overall effect. When administered to opioid-dependent persons, they displace residual drug from the receptor site and precipitate withdrawal signs and symptoms.

Pharmacodynamics. Opioid antagonists interact with opioid receptors, producing antagonistic effects (Table 18-12). Without either opioid molecules or opioid tolerance at the site, the physiologic effects exerted by these drugs depend on the degree to which they act as agonists at the sites. Naloxone, naltrexone, and nalmefene appear to exert little or no agonistic action and are considered to be relatively pure antagonists. (See Focus On Opioid Antagonists: Similarities and Differences.)

The physiologic actions of these drugs are substantially different when administered to subjects under the influence of opioid agonists. By displacing the opioid agonist molecule from the receptor site, antagonists either abolish the physiologic effects of opioid agonists or greatly diminish them. The person who suffers from acute opioid toxicity responds to the administration of an opioid antagonist with a decrease in symptoms (eg, respiratory depression). If the client has no underlying physical opioid dependence, physiologic function can return to near normal by the judicious use of opioid antagonists.

Response to these drugs is affected by physical dependence on opioids in the recipient. Whether or not these clients exhibit signs and symptoms of opioid toxicity initially, administration of opioid antagonists tends to elicit the withdrawal syndrome.

Because opioid antagonists reduce analgesia induced by placebos and acupuncture, their therapeutic effectiveness is probably mediated by the production of endogenous chemicals that exert agonistic effects on opioid receptors. These substances, which have been identified as endorphins and enkephalins produced by the CNS, may also be responsible for abolishing the pain perception that occurs in situations involving extreme excitement or stress. They may also be responsible for the reported euphoria experienced by many athletes during vigorous exercise. Chronic exposure to both danger and active exercise appears to have some addictive potential, as indicated by reports of restlessness, degrees of depression, and other mild withdrawal symptoms by athletes during periods of abstinence from exercise.

In brief, the physiologic response to opioid antagonists depends on several factors:

- Presence or absence of opioid agonists at the receptor site
- Presence of endogenous endorphins or enkephalins at the receptor site
- Degree of physical dependence on opioids previously developed by the recipient
- Drug concentration at the receptor site, as determined by dosage.

Pharmacokinetics. Naloxone and nalmefene are administered by injection rather than orally; naltrexone is administered orally. The serum half-lives of these drugs are shorter than are those for opioid agonist drugs. The drugs are excreted by the kidneys.

Therapeutic Uses. Opioid antagonists are used primarily to treat acute opioid toxicity. When given to a person who took an overdose of opioid drugs, they dramatically reduce characteristic respiratory depression and sedation. Vital functions can be stabilized relatively quickly. Because of their short half-lives, opioid antagonists usually must be administered repeatedly when treating overdose.

Opioid antagonists given to the newborn, or preferably to the mother just before birth, prevent or reverse the respiratory depression seen in infants whose mothers received opioid analgesics late in labor. The drugs are best given prophylactically to prevent respiratory depression.

Postoperatively, nalmefene can be used in lower dosage to reverse excessive opioid effects without causing acute pain from a complete reversal. In higher doses, nalmefene produces complete or partial reversal of opioid

Table 18-12. Representative Opioid Antagonists

Drug Name	Usual Dosage	Additional Information
naloxone (Narcan)	Adults, *IV:* 400 μg q2–3 min for up to 3 doses Children, *IV:* 5–10 μg/kg q2–3 min PC: B	Naloxone is a pure antagonist and is considered the drug of choice in most situations that require an opioid antagonist.
naltrexone (ReVia)	Adults, *initially:* 25 mg PO, repeated after 1 h if withdrawal does not occur; *maintenance:* 50–150 mg daily PC: C	Naltrexone is a pure antagonist; it is the first oral narcotic antagonist approved by the FDA to treat narcotic addiction.
nalmefene (Revex)	Opioid overdose, Adults, *IV:* 0.5 mg/70 kg Reversal of postoperative opioid depression: 0.25 μg/kg PC: B	Available in ampules in two different concentrations: 100 μg/mL for postoperative use and 1 mg/mL (10 times as concentrated) for managing overdose.

KEY: PC = pregnancy category (see Appendix A).

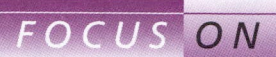

FOCUS ON

Opioid Antagonists: Similarities and Differences

Similarities

Pharmacodynamics

These agents act by displacing the opioid molecule from the receptor site, reducing or abolishing the physiologic effect of opioids. They have no agonist properties. They are thought to act as competitive antagonists at the opiate receptor sites.

Pharmacokinetics

These agents are excreted by the kidneys and metabolized by the liver. It is unknown if they cross into breast milk.

Therapeutic Uses

These agents are used to treat opioid toxicity and overdose. They are also used prophylactically to prevent respiratory depression in infants whose mothers have received opioid analgesics during labor. They can be used to diagnose physical opioid dependence.

Adverse Reactions

These agents exhibit few effects in the absence of opioid use or dependence; however, some nausea and vomiting and tachycardia have been reported.

Contraindications

These agents are contraindicated for clients with a known hypersensitivity to the drug.

Precautions

These agents should be used with caution in clients suspected of opioid dependence.

Nursing Considerations

Assess the client's level of consciousness and neurologic status for signs and symptoms of opioid overdose; assess cardiopulmonary status and have resuscitative equipment readily available; institute CPR as necessary; monitor for signs and symptoms of opioid dependence or withdrawal; check pupil dilation for drug effectiveness; institute measures to combat withdrawal symptoms; inform client of measures to be taken; continue monitoring until physiologic stability persists beyond the duration of activity of the last drug dose; assist in coping with withdrawal signs and symptoms; provide a quiet environment; refer for treatment of drug abuse or dependence as necessary.

Differences

- They have no agonist properties. They are thought to act as competitive and antagonists at the opiate receptor sites.

- **Naloxone** is administered by injection; **naltrexone** is given orally.
- **Naloxone** has an onset of action of 1 to 2 minutes (IV), 2 to 5 minutes (S or IM); its duration of action depends on the dose and route given; it is rapidly distributed into body tissues and fluids and crosses the placenta; its plasma half-life is 60 to 90 minutes for adults and 3 hours for neonates.
- **Naltrexone** is rapidly and completely absorbed from the GI tract; its onset of action is 15 to 30 minutes, peaking in 1 hour with a terminal half-life of 95 hours; it is unknown if it crosses the placenta.
- **Nalmefene** is completely bioavailable after parenteral administration and has a half-life of about 10 hours after an IV dose.

- **Naltrexone** has been used investigationally in the treatment of autistic children.
- **Naloxone** is used to reduce hypertension due to clonidine toxicity.

- **Naltrexone** can cause painful cramps, elevated liver enzymes, hepatotoxicity, nervousness, insomnia, anxiety, lassitude, depression, musculoskeletal pain, rash, and upper respiratory congestion.

- **Naltrexone** is contraindicated for clients with acute hepatitis or liver failure, clients receiving opioid agonists, clients experiencing acute withdrawal, nondetoxified clients or those physically dependent on opioids, and clients who experience opioid withdrawal after the **naloxone** challenge test.
- **Naloxone** should be avoided after the use of opioids in surgery.

- **Naloxone** should be used with caution in clients with preexisting cardiac disease or those receiving potentially cardiotoxic drugs.

Make sure the client is opiate-free before starting **naltrexone**; instruct in using over-the-counter nonopiate drugs for relief of pain, diarrhea, or cough; administer the **naloxone** challenge test before giving **naltrexone**; if there are signs of opiate withdrawal do not give.

Check dosage strength of nalmefene preparations; they come in significantly different strengths.

drug effects; it can also produce acute withdrawal symptoms.

Opioid antagonists are useful in diagnosing physical opioid dependence in a person whose appearance and function appear normal because of residual opioids in the body. Such a person exhibits signs and symptoms of withdrawal after receiving an opioid antagonist. No response is apparent in a nondependent person.

Adverse Reactions. As pure opioid antagonists, naloxone, naltrexone, and nalmefene exhibit few effects in persons who do not use opioids or who are not opioid-dependent. Naloxone and nalmefene sometimes cause nausea and vomiting and can aggravate hypertension, however. Administered for opiate overdose, naloxone may produce an abrupt return to consciousness accompanied by tremor and hyperventilation. Naltrexone can cause adverse GI effects (pain, cramps, nausea, vomiting) and hepatocellular damage in excessive doses. CNS symptoms (nervousness, insomnia, anxiety, lassitude, depression), musculoskeletal pain, rash, and upper respiratory congestion have also been reported. Nalmefene is associated with adverse cardiovascular effects, including pulmonary edema and ventricular arrhythmias, especially during abrupt reversal.

Drug Interactions. The main interaction of the antagonists is with opiate agonists, which is the intended use. However, clients on naltrexone therapy for addiction must be advised to avoid over-the-counter (OTC) products containing opiates (eg, cough or diarrhea medications).

Precautions and Contraindications. Opioid antagonists should be used with caution in persons suspected of opioid dependence if concurrent medical problems make an acute withdrawal syndrome dangerous. Persons receiving naltrexone for narcotic addiction should carry medical identification indicating that they are taking this drug. Naltrexone is contraindicated in clients with acute hepatitis or liver failure.

■ SUMMARY

Opioid antagonists are substances that interact with opioid receptors while exerting little or no agonist effect. By displacing more powerful agonists from these receptors, they reduce the physiologic effects of these drugs. In opioid-dependent persons, opioid antagonists elicit the withdrawal syndrome. Opioid antagonists are used to treat acute opioid toxicity and opioid overdose, as well as to diagnose physical dependence on opioids.

❖ NURSING MANAGEMENT: CLIENT RECEIVING OPIOID ANTAGONISTS

When clients receive opioid antagonists to treat opioid overdose, they must be monitored closely because the duration of effect of the drug involved in the overdose may exceed the length of action of the antagonist; additional doses may be needed. Opioid antagonists do not reverse respiratory depression caused by other drugs that may have been taken concurrently with the opiate.

When opioid antagonists are administered to diagnose opioid dependency, the healthcare staff must be prepared to cope with the acute withdrawal syndrome that may result. The client is likely to experience nausea, rhinorrhea, and diarrhea. In addition, any "high" the user has experienced from recent drug doses is reversed. Because opioid withdrawal causes hypersensitivity to stimuli, a quiet environment should be provided for the test. If the results of the test are positive, healthcare personnel should avoid judgmental or punitive attitudes.

Various opioid antagonists may be stored together in the healthcare facility's stock supplies of emergency drugs. Before administering such an agent, the nurse must take care to identify it accurately and to differentiate among several drugs with similar names.

NURSING PROCESS

ASSESSMENT

Drug overdoses are seen most commonly in emergency departments of acute care facilities. Initial assessment should focus on vital functions and on determining the drug involved. Clients with opioid toxicity are likely to be unconscious and to exhibit decreased blood pressure and pulse and respiratory rates. Clients who are responsive, or the people who accompany them, should be asked to identify the drugs taken and whether or not the client is dependent on opioids.

NURSING DIAGNOSIS

The most common nursing diagnoses are:

- Impaired Gas Exchange, related to respiratory depression secondary to toxicity from CNS depressant
- Altered Tissue Perfusion, related to cardiovascular depression secondary to drug-induced toxicity

If opioid dependence is likely or confirmed, the client will exhibit:

- Pain, related to opioid withdrawal

PLANNING

Immediate goals of nursing care include maintaining vital functions (respiration and circulation) until drug effects are reversed. If the client is opioid-dependent, eliminating dependence is a long-term goal.

INTERVENTION

Cardiopulmonary resuscitation is initiated as necessary. Mechanical respiratory assistance must be instituted immediately for any client with a respiratory rate of 10/min or less. If opioid drugs are the confirmed source of toxicity, an opioid antagonist may be ordered. Repeated injections of the antagonist are usually required because antagonists are metabolized more rapidly than are opioids.

The nurse must monitor the client's condition closely. Pupillary dilation is one indicator of response to the opioid antagonist. The respiratory rate should increase within 1 to 2 minutes after the client receives the opioid antagonist, and a rapid but transitory improvement in general condition should occur. Repeated doses of antagonist may be required before the client's condition stabilizes. During this time, nursing measures should be instituted to ameliorate withdrawal symptoms, if they develop.

Client Education. Clients receiving emergency treatment should be informed of what is to happen, even when they appear unresponsive or comatose. Instructions should be given to help them cooperate with treatment procedures. This is not the appropriate time to discuss the dangers of drug abuse or dependence; the nurse should focus on measures to help the client cope with the immediate situation. After the crisis resolves, clients who experienced pronounced withdrawal may desire a referral for long-term treatment of drug dependence.

OUTCOME EVALUATION

Data required for assessing the outcome of nursing measures include vital signs, particularly respiratory rate and depth, color, peripheral circulation, pupil size, and level of consciousness. The success of referral is judged by evidence of attendance at a drug-treatment facility. Abstinence from drug use in the future determines whether the long-term goal, elimination of drug dependence, is achieved.

❖ CHECKLIST OF NURSING ACTIONS

Treating Opioid Toxicity

- ❑ Give priority to maintaining vital functions, particularly respiration.
- ❑ Inform clients of measures to be taken and ways they can assist in the treatment.
- ❑ Monitor response to opioid antagonist medication closely.
- ❑ Continue monitoring clients until physiologic stability persists beyond the duration of activity of the last dose of opioid antagonist medication.

Diagnosing Drug Dependence

- ❑ Help clients cope with withdrawal signs and symptoms.
- ❑ Provide a quiet environment.
- ❑ Refer clients to treatment facilities for drug abuse or dependency as necessary.

Central Analgesics

Central analgesics are drugs that produce analgesia through effects on the CNS but remain pharmacologically different from opioid analgesics. They are used in managing moderate to moderately severe pain. Examples of these drugs include methotrimeprazine (Levoprome) and tramadol (Ultram).

Methotrimeprazine is a phenothiazine derivative with potent CNS depressant effects. It has analgesic, amnesiac, anticholinergic, antihistaminic, and antiadrenergic effects. It produces analgesia similar to that produced by morphine and meperidine, with marked sedation. Because sedation, orthostatic hypotension, and fainting or dizziness may occur, ambulation, if necessary, must be supervised for at least 6 hours after the initial dose. Otherwise, the client should be kept supine for 6 to 12 hours after injection.

Tramadol is an orally administered central analgesic; its mechanism of action is unknown, but it does bind to the mu opiate receptors. Because it also inhibits the reuptake of norepinephrine and serotonin, it should be used with great caution in clients taking monoamine oxidase inhibitors. Miosis produced by tramadol may interfere with assessing the client for increased intracranial pressure. It may also produce opioid-like dependence and withdrawal symptoms in clients who have taken large amounts of opioid analgesics.

Anesthetic Drugs and Anesthesia

Anesthesia is a state of insensibility or loss of sensation, especially the sensation of pain. Although anesthesia can be achieved by other means (eg, hypnosis, hypothermia, acupuncture), anesthetic drugs are the primary agents used in modern Western medicine. The advent of anesthesia was a great impetus to the practice of surgery. Before the first anesthetics (nitrous oxide and ether) were discovered, surgery was limited to procedures that could be completed quickly. Although pain could be blunted by administering alcohol or opium, the physical and psychic trauma of surgery could be endured only briefly. Speed was a major criterion for successful surgery.

Humanitarian concern was not the only reason for time restrictions. Clients subjected to lengthy procedures did not progress well postoperatively. We now know that acute stress, such as that caused by severe pain, induces hormonal changes that disturb fluid and electrolyte balance, decrease resistance to infection, and delay healing. Most of the surgical procedures performed today would not be possible without the pain control that modern anesthesia affords.

Anesthetic drugs induce two kinds of anesthesia: general and local. General anesthesia abolishes perception of all sensations by quickly rendering the client unconscious, without permanent damage or immediate risk of death. Local anesthesia eliminates pain from a part of the body without affecting consciousness. The anesthetized area feels numb because the sensations of heat, cold, and light pressure are also eliminated. Sensitivity to heavy pressure and motor function may or may not remain.

Whether anesthesia is local or general, the recipient needs protection from injury during this period. The degree of protection needed and the duration of the vulnerable period are directly related to the number of physiologic functions that have been interrupted by the anesthetic drug. Effects may include insensitivity to

pressure, immobility, and depression of vital functions, such as respiration and circulation.

General Anesthetics

Drugs capable of producing general anesthesia include inorganic gases, hydrocarbons, ethers, and barbiturates. The degree to which they induce analgesia and relaxation vary, but all are descending CNS depressants that alter the level of consciousness. A general anesthetic should induce rapid loss of consciousness without causing permanent damage or risk of death (Table 18-13). The ideal drug would be safe for all occupants of the

Table 18-13. Representative General Anesthetics

Drug Name	Preparations	Additional Information
Inhalant Anesthetics		
methoxyflurane (Penthrane)	Liquid in bottles	Nonflammable and nonexplosive in anesthetic concentrations
		Induction slow and associated with excitement
		Recovery period prolonged
		Light planes of anesthesia have little effect on uterine contractions.
		High doses can cause liver and kidney damage.
halothane (Fluothane)	Liquid in unit packages PC: C	Nonflammable and nonexplosive
		Used to maintain anesthesia after induction
		Provides moderate muscle relaxation
		Not recommended for obstetric anesthesia except when uterine relaxation is required
		Can cause hepatotoxicity
		Is suspected of being teratogenic; increased incidence of interrupted pregnancies and birth defects among operating suite staff members reported where halothane is used frequently
nitrous oxide ("laughing gas")	Liquid under pressure in steel cylinders	Produces analgesia and decreased reflexes
		Nonflammable but supports combustion
		Associated with hypoxia; oxygen given during and after anesthesia
Intravenous Anesthetics		
thiopental sodium (Pentothal, "truth serum")	Powder for preparing solutions for IV injection PC: C	May precipitate acute neurologic signs and symptoms in clients with low reserves of vitamin B_{12}
		Used for induction or light general anesthesia
		Rapid induction
		Pleasant emergence with little nausea
propofol (Diprivan)	Ampules containing solution for IV administration PC: D	Rapid onset of action
		Short duration of action
		Relatively little nausea and vomiting during recovery
		Safety during pregnancy or parturition unestablished
		Contraindicated for clients with increased intracranial pressure or decreased cerebral circulation
		Reduced dosages required for elderly, debilitated, or hypovolemic clients
		Reduced dosages required when other CNS depressants are used
Rectal Anesthetics		
paraldehyde	Liquid for rectal administration PC: C	Has sedative and anticonvulsant properties
		Useful for alcoholics, psychotics, and extremely apprehensive candidates for surgery
		Absorption variable

KEY: PC = pregnancy category (see Appendix A).

surgical suite and would be effective and pleasant for the client.

Anesthetics that are chemically unstable are dangerous. They tend to be flammable, explosive, and also corrosive to materials used in the administration equipment.

Compatibility with catecholamines is important for two reasons: anxiety or fear elevates catecholamine levels in most surgical clients, and catecholamine medication may be needed during surgery to stimulate vital functions.

Anesthesia deep enough to produce skeletal muscle relaxation is required for surgical access to deep organs and tissues. Rapid response to changes in dosage is desirable because it allows easy control of the depth of anesthesia.

Of particular concern is an anesthetic's propensity to depress vital functions or to induce cardiac arrhythmia. Some anesthetics, in combination with catecholamine stress hormones, pose a high risk for cardiac arrest. Agents that produce a rapid, pleasant induction are desirable because they prevent pronounced emotional reactions that can disturb hormonal and nervous status.

Inhalant anesthetics should be nonirritating to the mucous membranes so as to limit stimulation of respiratory secretions, which can obstruct breathing. Injectable drugs should not induce phlebitis or damage other tissues. Any tendency to promote capillary bleeding increases blood loss during surgery.

Anesthetic drugs vary somewhat in their properties and physiologic effects. None is ideal. Agents are chosen to provide the characteristics most needed in a given situation: the client's status, the operative procedure, and the expected duration of surgery. Usually a combination of agents is used to achieve the best balance of efficacy and safety. The depth of anesthesia and the degree of muscle relaxation needed for different stages of surgery vary, requiring adjustments in dosage. In addition, analgesics, sedatives, tranquilizers, and other pharmacologic agents are used as adjuncts to promote the effectiveness of anesthetic agents or to counteract their undesired effects.

Pharmacodynamics. The mechanism of action of most general anesthetics is unknown. Some drugs (ethers, aldehydes, halogenated hydrocarbons) are potent in proportion to their lipid solubility. They may alter the nerve cell membrane in such a way as to inhibit impulse transmission. Different classes of drugs probably act in different ways. Some experts think that some anesthetics interfere with biochemical processes such as oxidation, phosphate uptake, and synthesis of acetylcholine and adenosine triphosphate. Why interruptions of such fundamental cell processes fail to harm the tissues permanently remains unknown.

A considerable amount is known about the effects of anesthetic agents, however. Depression of nervous tissue progresses in a generally descending order, affecting cortical and higher brain functions before the lower functions. Vital centers in the medulla are usually spared longest. Progressive nervous system depression during general anesthesia has been categorized into stages (Table 18-14). Progression through these stages is continuous; abrupt changes or physiologic landmarks do not always signal transition from one stage to another. Modern induction techniques move the client so rapidly through stages 1 and 2 that these changes may be imperceptible. Planes 2 and 3 of stage 3 are preferred for most surgical procedures. As plane 3 deepens, the risk increases of entering stage 4, life-threatening toxicity.

Pharmacokinetics. General anesthetics may be administered IV, rectally, or by inhalation. Absorption by the IV or inhalational routes is rapid and dependable; absorption from the rectal mucosa is less reliable. Once in the bloodstream, anesthetics rapidly affect the brain, inducing loss of consciousness. At the same time, the movement of drugs into tissue depots causes a gradual drop in plasma concentration. This redistribution lowers the CNS concentration, necessitating repeated doses to maintain the proper level of anesthesia. Most anesthetics are stored in fatty tissues; thiopental, for example, is also bound by plasma albumin. The longer the surgery, the greater the saturation of such tissue depots. When administration is discontinued and plasma levels of free drug decline, stored drug redistributes into the blood, prolonging anesthesia.

Volatile anesthetics are eliminated mainly by the respiratory tract, with about 15% metabolized by the liver's microsomal enzymes. Thiopental, for example, is largely metabolized by the liver; the remainder is excreted by the kidneys.

Therapeutic Uses. General anesthetics are used principally to control pain and to promote relaxation during surgical procedures. They may also be used to alleviate pain during labor and delivery and to terminate refractory convulsive seizures. Anesthetics are often used with oxygen, muscle relaxants, analgesics, and other anesthetic agents.

Adverse Reactions. General anesthetics are associated with a small but definite risk of death or permanent disability. The margin of safety for most agents is relatively narrow; toxic doses are sometimes only two to four times those required for therapeutic effect. Acute reactions to general anesthetics include cardiac arrest, anaphylaxis, and irreversible progression through the stages of anesthesia to cardiovascular collapse and respiratory arrest.

Anesthetics tend to decrease respiratory and cardiac function. They may elevate or depress blood pressure. By irritating local tissues, agents administered by inhalation stimulate respiratory secretions and predispose the client to laryngospasm. Some drugs increase tissue sensitivity to catecholamines. A few stimulate excitation

Table 18-14. Characteristics of the Stages of General Anesthesia

Physiologic Effects	Stage I	Stage II	Stage III Planes				Stage IV
			1	2	3	4	
Consciousness	Present Altered perceptions Analgesia Euphoria Amnesia	Absent	Absent	Absent	Absent	Absent	Absent
Skeletal muscles	Normal tone	Increased tone	Small muscle relaxation	Large muscle relaxation	Complete relaxation	Complete relaxation	Flaccidity; diaphragmatic paralysis
Eyes							
Lacrimation	Increased with some agents			Decreased	Decreased	Absent	
Pupils	Normal reaction to light	Dilated	Constricted	Partially dilated	Partially dilated	Partially dilated	Fully dilated
Movement	Normal	Increased	Increased	Absent	Absent	Absent	Absent
Reflexes							
Lid	Present	Present	Absent	Absent	Absent	Absent	Absent
Corneal	Present	Present	Present	Absent	Absent	Absent	Absent
Pharyngeal	Present	Present	Absent	Absent	Absent	Absent	Absent
Laryngeal	Present	Present	Present	Absent	Absent	Absent	Absent
Cough	Present	Present	Present	Present	Absent in large bronchi	Absent in small bronchi	Absent
Cutaneous	Present	Present	Present to absent	Absent	Absent	Absent	Absent
Respirations	Normal or somewhat increased and irregular	Rapid, irregular	Deep and regular	Regular, expirations longer than inspirations	Shallow	Depressed	Absent
Cardiovascular function							
Heart rate	Unchanged	Increased	Decreased	Decreased	Decreased	Decreased	Decreased to absent
Blood pressure	Normal	Increased	Normal	Normal	Decreased	Decreased	Decreased to absent
Venous pressure	Normal	Increased	Normal	Normal	Normal	Normal	Increased initially

during induction or delirium during emergence. Muscle pain, nausea, vomiting, and inhibited peristalsis may also occur postoperatively.

Complications resulting from general anesthetics include atelectasis, aspiration pneumonia, urinary retention, paralytic ileus, and liver or kidney damage. Hypersensitivity or anaphylaxis can occur in allergic clients.

Malignant hyperpyrexia or hyperthermia may develop rapidly when halogenated agents are administered to genetically predisposed clients. Malignant hyperthermia results from muscle contraction caused by the abnormal influx of calcium. It affects more clients between ages 3 and 30 than others. It usually occurs in the operating room but can occur 24 to 48 hours later. Symptoms are skeletal muscle rigidity, rising fever (may be a late manifestation), tachycardia, tachypnea, acidosis, and flushing that progresses to cyanosis. Because of improved screening, early detection, and the use of the skeletal muscle relaxant dantrolene, the mortality rate has been reduced from over 70% to about 7%. Nurses working in the operating room and postanesthesia care unit (PACU) must know the protocol for managing malignant hyperthermia and must have rapid access to the malignant hyperthermia cart and cooling equipment (Class, 1991).

Drug Interactions. General anesthetics interact with many other pharmacologic agents in unfavorable ways (Table 18-15). Used with anticholinesterases, atropine, calcium, catecholamines, digitalis, ketamine, potassium, and theophylline, they can trigger malignant hyperthermia.

Table 18-15. Examples of Drug Interactions Involving General Anesthetics

Interacting Drugs	Adverse Reaction
Adrenergics (with halothane and cyclopropane)	Increased risk of cardiac arrhythmia including cardiac arrest
Hormone (oxytocin)	Vasoconstriction and myocardial ischemia
Antihypertensives	Bradycardia, hypotension, and impaired circulation
Opioids, tranquilizers (and other CNS depressants)	Exaggerated CNS depression, hypotension, respiratory depression

Precautions and Contraindications. A discussion of all medical conditions that require special consideration in choosing or administering general anesthetics is beyond the scope of this book. The anesthesiologist or anesthetist is responsible for screening the client for such risk factors and choosing a general anesthetic agent accordingly (Table 18-16).

General anesthetics are not administered to clients with marginal respiratory function, severe anemia, or serious cardiac conditions unless an emergency situation exists. Every effort is made to stabilize the client's condition, to eliminate infectious disease, and to promote a high level of health before surgery is attempted. Among the factors that suggest modifying plans for anesthesia are prior use of drugs that interact with anesthetics, pregnancy, a morbid fear of death, or a personal or family history of malignant hyperthermia. The administration of general anesthetics is reserved for specially trained physicians or nurses. They have primary responsibility for the client's safety and comfort during surgical procedures.

In addition to precautions and contraindications for clients, some precautions apply to healthcare personnel as well. Nurses and other healthcare professionals may absorb anesthetic vapors from the ambient air in operating and recovery rooms, despite the use of closed anesthetic delivery and special ventilation systems. In addition, skin contact with at least one anesthetic (halothane) increases exposure because the anesthetic diffuses through the skin. Occupational exposure is not innocuous. Female operating room personnel have a higher incidence of spontaneous abortion, stillbirths, low-birth weight babies and babies with birth defects (particularly defects in the cardiovascular and musculoskeletal systems), myeloneuropathy, interference with vitamin B_{12} metabolism, cancer, and hepatic and renal diseases. In addition, halothane is linked to elevated serum bromide levels. Chronic exposure to nitrous oxide may alter hormonal cycles and impair fertility. Moreover, subanesthetic levels of anesthetic gas slow individual response times and decrease recent memory. Acute exposure to anesthetics may also cause lethargy, dizziness, fatigue, and nausea.

Table 18-16. Factors That Make General Anesthesia Riskier

Risk Factor	Nature of the Increased Risk
Obesity	Need for increased dosage of anesthetic due to large deposits of fat for drug storage; delayed emergence from anesthesia; decreased vital capacity; difficulty in ambulating postoperatively
Habitual use of alcohol	Cross-tolerance to anesthetic agents that increase dosage requirements for anesthetics and analgesics
Smoking	Impairment of respiration and circulation increases risk of poor vital function during and after anesthesia; inflammation of lung tissues increases risk of respiratory obstruction during anesthesia
Diabetes	Increased likelihood of cardiovascular deterioration and circulatory problems during anesthesia; abnormal blood sugar levels increase risk of CNS malfunction during anesthesia
Respiratory infection	Increased risk of respiratory impairment during anesthesia
Excessive fear	Increased risk of cardiac arrhythmia leading to ventricular fibrillation
Use of glucocorticoids within previous 3 months	Adrenal atrophy that reduces ability of body to withstand stress; tendency toward hypotension
Malignant hyperthermia	Potentially fatal, genetically based reaction to fat-soluble, inhalational general anesthetics, skeletal muscle relaxants, and other drugs

■ SUMMARY

General anesthetics are systemic drugs that prevent or alleviate pain by reducing the level of consciousness. They prevent pain during surgery, reduce the discomfort of labor and delivery, and terminate refractory seizures. They have a narrow margin of safety, tending to produce hypotension, circulatory collapse, and respiratory arrest.

A combination of pharmacologic agents is commonly used to produce a balanced anesthesia characterized by adequate analgesia and muscle relaxation. Because safe administration of anesthetics requires special skills, physicians with specialty training and certified nurse anesthetists are among the few qualified to administer general anesthetics.

❖ **NURSING MANAGEMENT: CLIENT RECEIVING GENERAL ANESTHESIA**

NURSING PROCESS: BEFORE GENERAL ANESTHESIA

ASSESSMENT

The client undergoing general anesthesia must be carefully assessed for factors that increase the risk of this procedure. The nursing history should include data on previous responses to general anesthetics and information on diseases that may lead to complications (eg, poor nutritional status, obstructive airway disease, cardiovascular disease, diabetes, porphyria, myasthenia gravis, liver or renal disease, allergies). Any adverse experiences of family members with anesthesia should be explored to determine the possible risk for malignant hyperthermia. The client should be assessed for any unusual fears about anesthesia or surgery.

The drug history should describe allergies to drugs as well as the use of prescription, nonprescription, social, and illegal drugs. Specifically, the nurse should ask about the use of glucocorticoids within the preceding 3 months and tobacco or alcohol consumption. All drugs used within the preceding 2 weeks should be identified. Of particular importance are hormones (insulin, cortisone, estrogens), antibiotics, sedatives, cardiovascular drugs, sympathomimetics, aspirin, and psychotropics.

Clients should be examined for signs and symptoms of infection of the skin, respiratory tract, and urinary tract. Cardiovascular assessment should rule out abnormalities. Vital signs are recorded to provide a baseline for comparison with postoperative values. The client's emotional state and stress level should also be evaluated. In addition, the nurse should determine the client's knowledge of and experience with surgery and anesthesia.

NURSING DIAGNOSIS

Nursing diagnoses for the client about to receive a general anesthetic include:

- Anxiety, related to impending unconsciousness and surgery
- Risk for Injury, related to dizziness and weakness secondary to depressant medication
- Knowledge Deficit concerning surgery and anesthesia

PLANNING

Treatment goals include reducing anxiety, the risk of injury, and adverse effects as well as educating the client about anesthesia and its effects during and after surgery.

INTERVENTION

Any contraindications or risk factors for adverse reactions to general anesthesia discovered by the nurse during assessment should be reported to the prescriber. In particular, verbal expressions of premonitions about the outcome of surgery must be reported and recorded. Preoperative medications usually include a hypnotic to promote sleep the evening before surgery, as well as a combination of a narcotic analgesic and an anticholinergic or tranquilizer to be given about 1 hour before surgery.

Informed consent for the anesthetic and surgery must be obtained before administering any preoperative medications. Informed consent given after medication with a CNS depressant is not considered legally valid. In addition, drugs used during anesthesia may produce amnesia for events in the perioperative period. Clients may not remember giving informed consent or receiving postoperative instructions if these are done too close to the time of surgery.

Supportive care on the day of surgery must be provided to prevent undue apprehension. The client should not be left alone. Family members or significant others should be encouraged to sit with the client when the nursing staff is not involved in direct care.

Preoperative medication may be ordered to be given about 1 hour before inducing anesthesia. Timing of this medication is crucial because the drug actions should coincide with anesthesia induction. Premature or delayed administration increases the difficulty of induction and the need for higher doses of the initial anesthetic. Delayed administration also increases the risk of CNS depression, because drug action then occurs after anesthesia begins. To enhance the effect of the preoperative medication, the nurse should minimize external stimuli after administering medication and urge the client to relax and rest.

Client Education. Preoperative teaching is a critical part of preparing the client for the experience of anesthesia and surgery. It is also key to eliminating apprehension. Several nursing studies have shown the effectiveness of preoperative teaching in reducing the incidence of postoperative nausea and vomiting. The client undergoing surgery must know what to expect. For example, the client must be informed that he or she will be aware of the environment until induction begins, although premedication will cause drowsiness before transport to the operating room. The client also must know that an IV line will probably be established before surgery.

Older adults often are quite fearful of surgery because they have lived long enough to remember when deaths resulting from general anesthetics and surgical complications were more common. These clients should be reassured that current anesthetic agents are safer and increase the likelihood of a good outcome.

Preoperative teaching is crucial in promoting client cooperation with treatment procedures aimed at preventing complications from a general anesthetic after surgery. With the increasing numbers of clients undergoing same-day surgery and earlier discharges after surgery, teaching must involve the client's family or other caregivers. Ideally, before surgery, clients should learn how to perform deep-breathing, coughing, turning, splinting, and other maneuvers that promote comfort and recovery.

The nurse should inform the client, in terms of the subjective experience, what to expect during surgery. When clients are not admitted until the day of surgery, client teaching may occur by telephone or in special preadmission teaching sessions. Essential teaching should be provided before the day of surgery when conscious sedation or other drugs causing amnesia are to be used. Because of potential retrograde amnesia from some anesthetic agents, any instructions for postoperative care at home should be provided to the client and caregiver in written form.

Clients, their families, and caregivers should learn about the usual postoperative regimens, such as medication for pain relief and pain-reporting methods. A scale for reporting pain (one that is used by all the nursing staff) should be introduced (eg, numbers 1 through 10, with 1 representing slight pain and 10 representing excruciating pain). The client must know that he or she can ask for pain medication early, instead of waiting for pain to become severe. If PCA is to be used postoperatively, its use should be explained to the client.

Clients should be cautioned to remain in bed with side rails up after medication with CNS depressants and to request assistance from the healthcare staff if they need to get out of bed. Lying quietly in bed minimizes the risk of falling and the likelihood of nausea in response to narcotic medications. Head movements tend to augment the stimulation to the CNS centers for nausea and vomiting that may occur after administration of narcotic analgesics.

Clients going home after same-day surgery must have someone accompany them home. The effects of anesthetics, analgesics, and other drugs used during surgery may impair judgment and reflexes to such a degree that clients should refrain from driving or performing other potentially hazardous activities for 24 hours.

OUTCOME EVALUATION

Data required for evaluation include statements by clients that they are more relaxed or less apprehensive about the impending surgery and that they are (or are not) nauseated as a result of receiving an anesthetic. Other data should describe the absence or incidence of accidental injury from falling or cardiac arrest during anesthesia.

NURSING PROCESS:
DURING GENERAL ANESTHESIA

ASSESSMENT

Once in the operating suite, the client should be assessed for signs and symptoms of sympathetic nervous activity that reveal anxiety. In addition, level of consciousness and speech patterns should be monitored to detect the degree of sedation. The chart should be reviewed for previous assessment data and the time of preoperative medication administration. Any signs and symptoms of adverse reactions to the preoperative medication should be noted.

NURSING DIAGNOSIS

Nursing diagnoses may include:

- Anxiety, related to surgery
- Ineffective Breathing Pattern, related to CNS depression secondary to the combined effects of preoperative sedatives and general anesthetics

A common collaborative problem that should be differentiated from the nursing diagnoses is:

Potential Complication: Decreased cardiac output

PLANNING

Goals of treatment include reducing anxiety and reducing the risk of adverse reactions to the anesthetic.

INTERVENTION

Nursing care to minimize the stress response should continue in the operating room. Stimuli should be minimized. Expression of a warm concern for the client and competent execution of procedures provide continued reassurance.

If the preoperative medication was administered at a time other than ordered or if the client seems unusually apprehensive, this fact should be drawn to the attention of the anesthetist or anesthesiologist. When the client is transferred from the stretcher to the operating table, excessive motion, which can exacerbate nausea, should be avoided. Until anesthesia has been induced, clients should be protected from stimulation that could reduce the level of sedation or increase apprehension.

When an IV agent is used to induce anesthesia, the position of the needle in the blood vessel must be carefully checked. Improper placement in the extravascular tissues delays the effect of the drug and can cause tissue necrosis. During induction, the nurse should remember that hearing is the last function to be lost; therefore, staff should avoid talk that may disturb the client.

Once the client is under the influence of a general anesthetic, consciousness is lost and total nursing care appropriate to this state is required. The unconscious person is completely helpless and vulnerable. Vital functions must be maintained, and the client must be protected from injury. In the operating suite, the primary responsibility for monitoring the client and maintaining vital functions belongs to the anesthetist or anesthesiologist, but all members of the healthcare team share in this responsibility.

Safety precautions in the operating room should include eliminating static electricity or other sources of sparks, which can ignite flammable anesthetics and cause an explosion in the client's lungs, as well as injure others. The operating suite is at high risk for fires because of the flammable substances and oxygen used in the area. The area should be well ventilated to minimize the risk of fire and to protect the staff from exposure to anesthetic drugs exhaled by the client.

Client Education. Before the client receives an IV anesthetic, he or she should be forewarned about feeling a slight stinging sensation at the needle site. If a gaseous anesthetic is used, the client should be told about breathing through a mask just before losing consciousness. Children receiving an anesthetic gas may be told to "blow away the smell" to promote deep breathing and rapid induction.

OUTCOME EVALUATION

Notable evaluation data include facial or verbal expressions that show apprehension or discomfort, absence or incidence of adverse reaction to anesthesia, and absence or incidence of fire or explosion during surgery.

NURSING PROCESS:
AFTER GENERAL ANESTHESIA
ASSESSMENT

When the client is transferred to the PACU (or recovery area for ambulatory surgery), charting for the operative period should be complete. The anesthetist, surgeon, or nurse from the operating room should give a comprehensive verbal report to the PACU nurse of the client's current status, drugs administered during surgery, and any unusual events during surgery. The PACU nurse then assesses the client's respiratory and cardiovascular status, level of sedation, responses indicative of pain, and risk factors for postoperative complication, such as hemorrhagic shock, wound dehiscence, pneumonia, or intravascular thrombi (see Example of Nursing Process for Client Who Had a General Anesthetic).

NURSING DIAGNOSIS

Nursing diagnoses may include:

- Ineffective Breathing Pattern, related to potential inability to sustain spontaneous ventilation as a result of general anesthetic agent
- Risk for Injury, related to altered level of consciousness (confusion, delirium) secondary to diminished effect of anesthetic agent
- Pain, related to altered comfort resulting from thirst associated with decreased intake of fluids and preoperative administration of anticholinergic agents, nausea or vomiting related to emergence from anesthesia, and surgical trauma

Common collaborative problems that should be differentiated from the nursing diagnoses include:

Potential Complication: Hemorrhage
Potential Complication: Thrombus formation
Potential Complication: Hypokalemia, hypernatremia

PLANNING

Goals of nursing care include improved gas exchange, reorientation of the client on emergence from anesthesia, prevention of injury, maintenance of IV therapy, reduction in stress, decreased pain, and prevention of hemorrhage and thrombophlebitis (or their prompt detection and treatment, should they develop).

INTERVENTION

The client must be carefully monitored after surgery to ensure that vital functions continue uninterrupted. Oxygen is frequently administered because respirations tend to be depressed, resulting in hypoxemia. This tendency is particularly important to consider if clients have received nitrous oxide, which predisposes them to hypoxia. Clients should be stimulated verbally to breathe deeply to promote elimination of gaseous anesthetics and secretions from the lungs.

Because the events of surgery activate stress hormones, the client retains sodium and fluids, which may lead to hypervolemia, hypertension, and hemorrhage. IV infusions are administered at flow rates that replace fluid losses but do not unduly raise blood pressure.

The nurse should reduce noxious stimuli (especially noise) and other stressors. As much as possible, the emotional tone of the PACU should be that of quiet competence.

Restlessness that persists in the well-oxygenated client is probably from pain, which should be controlled by regular administration of analgesics. Liberal use of drugs prevents severe pain from developing, reassures clients that they are not expected to bear severe pain, reduces their stress, and results in greater analgesic effects with minimal drug use.

Some anesthetics are not potent analgesics, and the client may need pain relief before he or she is fully alert. The drugs used for anesthesia must be reviewed to determine whether the dosage of depressant analgesics should be reduced. If the client is at all hypotensive, vital signs should be monitored closely at least every 5 minutes after administering the analgesic. Hypotension from pain should begin subsiding within 30 minutes of drug administration. If the blood pressure remains low, the anesthesiologist or surgeon should be notified.

Throughout this period, the nurse must monitor the client regularly for signs and symptoms of hemorrhage, shock, and respiratory infection and notify the physician promptly if such signs occur.

Client Education. As the client becomes more alert, the nurse orients him or her to time and place, announces that surgery is over, and repeatedly urges deep breathing and, if allowed, coughing. The client is reminded to begin the postoperative exercises of turning and exercising that were taught before surgery.

OUTCOME EVALUATION

Data required for evaluation include the client's vital signs, color, energy level, rate of wound healing, physical signs of pain, statements by the client indicating the absence or relief of discomfort, the absence or incidence of hemorrhage or thrombophlebitis, and the speed with which these are detected and treated, if they develop.

❖ **CHECKLIST OF NURSING ACTIONS**

- Throughout the perioperative period, protect clients from stress and help them manage stress levels.
- Before surgery, assess clients for factors that increase the risk of adverse reactions to anesthesia.
- Teach preoperative clients what the experience of induction will involve.

Example of Nursing Process for Client Who Had a General Anesthetic

The client, 36, was admitted for elective cholecystectomy. She is 5′5″and weighs 205 pounds. She smokes half a pack of cigarettes daily and drinks socially (one or two drinks) on the weekend. She had the surgical procedure and has been transferred to the postanesthesia care unit. She is responsive to verbal stimuli but sleeps intermittently. Her blood pressure and pulse are within normal limits, but her respirations are 14/min. She lies quietly in bed and offers no complaints of pain.

The client cannot void; the edge of her bladder is palpable three fingers below the umbilicus.

Assessment Data

Client lies quietly in bed, sleeps intermittently

Respiration 14/min

High dose of anesthetic

Inability to void

Bladder palpable three fingers below the umbilicus

Nursing Diagnosis	Intervention	Goals and Outcome Criteria
Risk for Infection: Pneumonia, related to immobility and hypopnea secondary to prolonged effect of anesthesia	**Stimulate** the client to cough and deep breathe at least 2h. Ambulate her as soon as she is alert.	The client will not develop signs and symptoms of pneumonia (fever, cough, cyanosis).
Urinary Retention, related to nervous system depression secondary to prolonged anesthesia	**Use** all nursing measures to promote micturition. If none is effective, consult the physician for an order for catheterization.	The client's bladder will be emptied.
	If necessary, **catheterize** the client to empty the bladder.	

- Teach preoperative clients about measures they can take to promote uncomplicated recovery from anesthesia.
- Alleviate undue apprehension with realistic reassurance about the safety of modern anesthesia. Give personalized, concerned care.
- Promote rest and relaxation before surgery. Administer preoperative medication at the time ordered.
- Protect the anesthetized client from injury and monitor closely for impaired vital functions.
- Stimulate the client who is recovering from anesthesia to breathe deeply to promote excretion of gaseous anesthetic agents.
- Monitor postanesthesia clients for signs and symptoms of complications related to anesthesia.
- Avoid exposure to anesthetic gases exhaled by the anesthetized client.
- Encourage early ambulation and deep breathing postoperatively to minimize complications of anesthesia.

Local Anesthetics

Local anesthesia is the elimination of sensation in a limited region of the body. A local anesthetic interferes with impulse transmission in peripheral or spinal cord nerves. Local anesthesia, which is characterized by absence of pain in a circumscribed part of the body without loss of consciousness, may be produced by several phenomena, including mechanical trauma, low temperature, anoxia, and various chemical agents. Anesthesia may be temporary or relatively permanent. Usually, a return to function is desirable within a short time (eg, soon after a surgical procedure). In certain clinical states (refractory pain), permanent anesthesia may be desired and may be accompanied by some degree of nerve damage.

Typical agents used for local anesthesia include cocaine, phenol, and a variety of ester/amide and amino/amide compounds. An ideal drug for inducing temporary local anesthesia has the following properties:

- A wide margin of safety without local tissue irritation, nerve or muscle damage, or systemic toxicity
- Effectiveness when injected or applied topically
- Appropriate duration of effect, as shown by a rapid onset of action, duration of action appropriate to the clinical use, and rapid elimination from the body when anesthesia is no longer required.

Chemicals with local anesthetic properties generally contain in their molecules both hydrophilic amine and lipophilic (aromatic) structures. These are usually separated by an intermediate alkyl chain. Either an ester or amide linkage may join the aromatic group to the intermediate chain. The nature of this linkage influences both the properties of the drug and the way it is deactivated in the body.

Pharmacodynamics. Most local anesthetics inhibit nerve impulses by impeding sodium influx across the cell membrane during depolarization. The drugs appear to compete with calcium for a receptor site on the internal surface of the cell membrane, which must be unoccupied to allow sodium influx. During normal impulse transmission, calcium leaves its position on the receptor, thus opening the membrane's sodium channel. The anesthetic/receptor interaction results in a blockade of this sodium channel, preventing depolarization.

The interruption of sensory function in a nerve in response to these agents progresses in a definite order. The sensation of pain is usually the first to subside, followed in order by cold, warmth, touch, and response to deep pressure. Motor function is the last to be obliterated.

Pharmacokinetics. To reach their site of action (the neural membrane), local anesthetics must traverse the tissues that surround the nerve and penetrate, in turn, the epineurium, perineurium, and endoneurium, in addition to the connective tissue or myelin sheath that surrounds individual cells. The drugs are injected or applied topically, using various routes (Table 18-17).

Because only a local effect is desired, the spatial distribution of the drugs is critical. Penetration of soft tissues may be hastened by adding hyaluronidase (Wydase) to the drug solution. Systemic absorption may be delayed by various strategies, including the judicious use of tourniquets on extremities, administering vasoconstrictors with the local anesthetic, or positioning the client so that gravity controls drug migration. Eventually, all drugs escape into the systemic circulation and are metabolically deactivated or excreted. Ester/amide drugs are degraded largely by a plasma enzyme, pseudocholinesterase; amino/amide compounds are metabolized by liver enzymes. Excretion of drugs and metabolites is primarily through the kidneys.

Therapeutic Uses. Local anesthesia is used to eliminate pain during surgical procedures, especially when general anesthesia is considered unnecessary or unduly risky. It is commonly used for nose and throat procedures and endoscopy. The anesthetic is applied topically to relieve surface pain or itching. Intractable pain is treated by local anesthetics with relatively permanent effects. Representative agents are listed in Table 18-18.

Administration. Local anesthetics should be administered slowly, and inadvertent IV administration should be avoided. Appropriate techniques should be used to control the systemic rate of absorption, because reactions can be severe and must be treated immediately and aggressively. Resuscitative equipment and agents, such as oxygen and diazepam, must be at hand. Oxygen is required to prevent and ameliorate seizures. Diazepam is the agent of choice for terminating convulsions. An IV line should be established promptly. Fluids are given to prevent or treat shock. Vasopressors may be required in cardiovascular collapse. Endotracheal intubation and respiratory assistance may be required in respiratory collapse.

Adverse Reactions. Adverse effects of local anesthetics usually depend on the agent. For example, phenol irritates tissues; when administered frequently or in large amounts, it may promote tissue damage. No local anesthetic containing preservatives should be used for spinal or epidural anesthesia.

Metals react with local anesthetics, causing release of metal ions that, if injected, can cause severe local irritation. Therefore, any disinfecting agent used on the area designated for local anesthesia should not contain heavy metals.

The effects of ester/amide and amino/amide anesthetics on impulse conduction are not limited to pain fibers or peripheral nerves. Impulse transmission is reduced in the CNS, autonomic ganglia, smooth muscle, neuromuscular junction, and muscle fibers. For this reason, these anesthetic agents can produce a variety of side effects when they are absorbed systemically. In the CNS, inhibitory fibers may be depressed before other structures are affected. This produces signs of paradoxical stimulation (restlessness, tremors, clonic convulsions). If the drug level continues to rise, depression, culminating in respiratory failure, follows. When the systemic concentration of these anesthetic agents rises rapidly, the stimulation phase may be nonexistent or fleeting. Blockade of neuromuscular junctions and ganglionic synapses varies with the preparation. Some compounds reduce the release of acetylcholine by the motor nerve endings and also impair impulse conduction.

Local anesthetics generally decrease the conduction rate, force of contraction, and electrical excitability of the myocardium. (Lidocaine and procainamide, a derivative of procaine, are used as antiarrhythmic drugs to suppress ectopic foci in the myocardium.) Depression of cardiac conduction and response by these agents tends to reduce cardiac output and can induce arrhythmias, including ventricular fibrillation. The drugs also promote arteriolar dilation by reducing sympathetic activity. Several anesthetics (benzocaine, lidocaine, procaine, and prilocaine) have caused methemoglobinemia. The combined effects on the cardiovascular system, especially when the drugs are inadvertently administered IV, can produce cardiovascular collapse or cardiac arrest.

Although the direct effect of these drugs on smooth muscle fibers is depression, paralysis of the sympathetic nervous system may cause a net increase in the tone of the GI mucosa.

The side effects of local anesthetics are commonly manifested as nausea, vomiting, tachycardia, talkativeness, and syncope. Allergic hypersensitivity is most common in relation to the ester/amide compounds. Some

Table 18-17. Routes of Administration for Local Anesthetics

Route	Clinical Uses	Effective Agents	Advantages	Disadvantages
Topical				
Skin	Relieve skin irritations; initial anesthesia before infiltration	cocaine tetracaine dibucaine lidocaine	Limited systemic toxicity	Application and absorption variable
Mucous membranes	Surface anesthesia before instrumentation or infiltration anesthesia			
Infiltration				
Extravascular (intradermal, subcutaneous)	Prevention of pain during dental procedures and minor surgery	procaine lidocaine prilocaine bupivacaine propoxycaine	Rapid onset of action	Prolonged use requires vasoconstrictors
Intravascular (Bier's block)	Prevention of pain during surgery on the arm	procaine chloroprocaine lidocaine mepivacaine prilocaine bupivacaine etidocaine	Reduces dose of anesthetic required; analgesia disappears rapidly with termination of procedure	Produces tissue hypoxia and ischemic pain secondary to the use of occlusive tourniquets to delay absorption of the anesthetic
Peripheral Nerve Blockage (Field Block Anesthesia)				
Minor nerve block (single nerve block)	Relief of pain and relaxation of the extremities, anterior abdominal wall, or neck	procaine lidocaine mepivacaine prilocaine bupivacaine etidocaine tetracaine	Less drug required and greater area of anesthesia than infiltration anesthesia	Motor function is usually eliminated
Major nerve block (multiple nerve or nerve plexus block)	Relief of pain and relaxation of the extremities, anterior abdominal wall, or neck		Minor nerve block: rapid onset of activity Major nerve block: long duration of analgesia	Short duration of effect of minor nerve block Slow onset of action of major nerve block
Spinal Subarachnoid				
Blockade	Surgery on the lower extremities, lower abdomen, and pelvis	tetracaine procaine lidocaine	More rapid onset than epidural administration; area of anesthesia more readily controlled than with epidural administration	Shorter duration of action than with epidural administration
Central Neural Blockade (Epidural/Peridural Anesthesia)				
Cervical	Rarely used medicinally	procaine chloroprocaine lidocaine mepivacaine prilocaine tetracaine bupivacaine etidocaine		
Thoracic	Relief of pain after thoracic or upper abdominal surgery			
Lumbar	Adjunct in surgery of the lower abdomen, pelvis, perineum, lower extremities, and in obstetric procedures		Longer duration of action than with spinal	Slower onset than spinal anesthesia; area of anesthesia less readily controlled than with spinal anesthesia
Caudal	Pelvic and perineal surgery and vaginal deliveries			

local anesthetic preparations contain sulfites or tartrazine (yellow dye no. 5), which can trigger an allergic reaction in susceptible persons. Allergic hypersensitivity reactions may be manifested by dermatitis, bronchoconstriction, or anaphylaxis; the latter can be fatal.

In a few people, local anesthetics fail to produce the desired blockade of pain impulses. This may be related to genetic factors that interfere with the drug's mechanism of action or that promote rapid breakdown of the drug in the body.

Table 18-18. Representative Local Anesthetic Drugs

Drug Name	Preparation	Therapeutic Uses	Usual Dosage	Additional Information
Topical Anesthetics				
Esters				
benzocaine (Anbesol, Americaine, Dermoplast, Lanacaine, Solarcaine)	Oral lozenges, gels, solutions, aerosol sprays, and otic solutions for topical use	Relief of pain that arises from inflamed skin or mucous membrane	Apply q1–2h as needed, for a maximum of 2 days if self-administered	Benzocaine is often added to OTC preparations.
cocaine	Topical solutions Powders and tablets for preparing topical solutions	Surface anesthesia, before superficial surgical procedures or injection of parenteral anesthetics	Depends on area and vascularity of tissue to be anesthetized and individual tolerance; *maximum single dose:* 1 mg/kg	Not recommended for injection or ophthalmic use
Amides				
dibucaine (Nupercaine)	Ointment and cream for topical (including rectal) use	Temporary relief of pain and itching that affects the skin or results from hemorrhoids	Adults: *Maximum dosage:* 1 oz of 1% ointment (containing 300 mg dibucaine)/day Children: 1/4 oz of 1% ointment (containing 75 mg dibucaine)/day	Dibucaine is added to some OTC preparations. Dibucaine is one of the most potent and toxic of local anesthetics.
Miscellaneous				
dyclonine (Dyclone)	Topical solutions	Surface anesthesia before superficial surgical procedures or injection of parenteral anesthetics	Depends on area and vascularity of tissue to be anesthetized and individual tolerance Adults: 200 mg; *maximum dose:* 30 mL of 1% solution (300 mg) PC: C	Adverse reactions from systemic toxicity include CNS and cardiovascular malfunction.
phenol (carbolic acid)	Solution for topical application to the skin	Relief of skin irritation	1% solution applied at intervals of at least 3 h	Phenol is added to some OTC skin preparations. Repeated application may cause painless burns.
Systemic Anesthetics				
phenazopyridine* (Azo-Standard, Baridium, Phenazodine, Prodium, Pyridiate, Pyridium, Urodine)	Oral tablets	Symptomatic relief of discomforts that result from irritation of the lower urinary tract	Adults: 200 mg tid pc Children: 12 mg/kg/day, divided in 3 doses PC: B	Because it is an azo dye, phenazopyridine may interfere with urinalysis based on spectrometry or color reactions. Phenazopyridine colors the urine a bright orange-red.
Parenteral				
Esters				
chloroprocaine (Nesacaine)	Solution for injection	Infiltration anesthesia Block anesthesia	Adults: (with epinephrine) 1 g; (without epinephrine) 800 mg PC: C	Onset of action is more rapid and duration of action longer than procaine.

(continued)

Table 18-18. (Continued)

Drug Name	Preparation	Therapeutic Uses	Usual Dosage	Additional Information
Parenteral				
Esters (continued)				
procaine (Anduracaine, Anuject, Novocain)	Solutions for injection	Infiltration anesthesia Block anesthesia	Adults: *Initially:* up to 1 g PC: C	Procaine acts within 2–5 min; duration of action is about 1 h. Severe allergic reactions may occur. Procaine is painless when injected.
propoxycaine (Ravocaine)	Solution containing a combination of propoxy-caine, procaine, and levo-nordefrin	Dental block	Adults: 9 mL of solution (containing 36 mg propoxycaine and 180 mg procaine) Children: 0.275 mL/kg up to a maximum of 9 mL	Onset of action is the same as that of procaine; duration of action is longer (2–3 h).
tetracaine (Pontocaine)	Powder and solution for injection	Spinal anesthesia	Variable, depending on the site and duration of anesthesia required Adults: 5–15 mg; *maximum dosage:* 20 mg PC: C	Onset of action is delayed up to 15 min in large nerve trunks. Duration of action is about 1.5–3 h.
Amides				
bupivacaine (Marcaine, Sensorcaine)	Solution for injection	Infiltration anesthesia Block anesthesia	Adults: (without epineph-rine) 175 mg q3h; (with epinephrine) 225 mg q3h; *maximum dosage:* 400 mg PC: C	Not recommended for use in children younger than 12 yr
etidocaine (Duranest)	Solution for injection	Block anesthesia	Adults: 225–300 mg q2–3h PC: B	Safe use of etidocaine in children younger than 14 yr has not been estab-lished.
lidocaine (Dolicaine, L-Caine, Lidoject, Nervocaine, Nulicaine, Xylocaine)	Solution for injection	Infiltration anesthesia Block anesthesia	Adults: (without epineph-rine) single doses of up to 4.5 mg/kg; (with epineph-rine) up to 7 mg/kg (or 500 mg) PC: B	Solutions for anesthesia contain no preservatives; they may or may not con-tain epinephrine. Solu-tions for anesthesia must be distinguished from those used to treat cardiac conditions. Lidocaine is the drug of choice for clients allergic to amino/ester anesthetics.
mepivacaine (Carbocaine, Isocaine, Polo-caine)	Solution for injection	Infiltration or block anes-thesia	Adults: *Maximum single dose:* 400 mg; *maximum daily dose:* 1 g Children: 5–6 mg/kg	Mepivacaine has a more rapid onset and longer du-ration of action than lido-caine.
prilocaine (Citanest)	Solution for injection	Infiltration or block anes-thesia	Adults: *Maximum dosage:* 600 mg q2h	Dosage must be reduced for debilitated clients and those with liver impair-ment.

*Although administered orally, this drug exerts its therapeutic effect only in the urinary tract, where it is concentrated on excretion.
KEY: PC = pregnancy category (see Appendix A).

(continued)

Table 18-18. (Continued)

Drug Name	Preparation	Therapeutic Uses	Usual Dosage	Additional Information
Miscellaneous				
alcohol	Solution for injection	Relief of intractable pain	2–4 mL injected around a nerve or ganglion	Anesthesia may last several months.
proparacaine (Alcaine, Ophthetic; *Can:* Ophthaine)	Ophthalmic solutions Topical solution	Prevention of pain during eye surgery Surface anesthetic before injection of parenteral anesthetics for eye or orbital surgery	1–2 drops q 5–10 min for up to 5–7 doses	Rarely, proparacaine can cause a severe allergic keratitis, iritis, or contact dermatitis.
tetracaine (Pontocaine)	Ophthalmic solutions and ointments	Surface anesthesia of the eye, nose, and throat	Apply as necessary; *maximum adult dosage:* 20 mg PC: C	The manufacturer recommends the addition of 0.1% epinephrine solution to tetracaine solutions used to anesthetize the larynx, trachea, or esophagus. Tetracaine is the most potent of amino/ester compounds.

*Although administered orally, this drug exerts its therapeutic effect only in the urinary tract, where it is concentrated on excretion.
KEY: PC = pregnancy category (see Appendix A). *Can* = Canadian trade name.

The topical spray ethyl chloride is highly combustible and can cause serious burns if ignited.

Prilocaine causes methemoglobinemia in up to 15% of recipients. Viscous lidocaine, an oral topical anesthetic, has caused seizures in young children.

Drug Interactions. When administered to clients who are taking beta-adrenergic blockers, local anesthetics may produce a brief hypertensive crisis followed by a drop in heart rate or cardiac arrest. Respiratory difficulties, shock, and convulsions can occur in severe interactions. Local anesthetics may cause additional sedating effects with sedatives used to reduce anxiety during dental procedures.

Ester/amide and amino/amide drugs tend to antagonize physostigmine and add to the effects of curare. Procaine, chloroprocaine, or tetracaine should not be used in clients on sulfonamide therapy because para-aminobenzoic acid is a metabolite and interferes with the action of sulfonamides.

Precautions and Contraindications. Cocaine should not be used to treat clients with a history of dependency on that drug. The ester/amides are contraindicated for clients known to be allergic to one or more of these drugs. Cross-sensitivity is fairly complete. An amino/amide drug should be used or a sensitivity test performed before administering the anesthetic. In a client with a history of unresponsiveness to local anesthetics, a test dose of the drug should be given. Both ester/amide and amino/amide agents may be ineffective. If local anesthesia must be attempted, the client should be observed closely to determine the response to the chosen drug.

Test doses should also be administered to clients who have cardiac, thyroid, or other endocrine diseases to determine tolerance to the drug chosen. The prescriber orders small doses initially, followed by careful comprehensive assessment of client response.

In obstetric procedures, local anesthetics are chosen with consideration of their effects on uterine contraction. Small doses of agents that depress uterine muscle function are acceptable for cesarean surgery but are contraindicated in vaginal delivery.

Topical ethyl chloride should be avoided if heated or electrical apparatus, such as that used in electrocautery, is used.

■ SUMMARY

Agents used for local anesthesia include cocaine, phenol, and various ester/amide and amino/amide compounds. They act by blocking the conduction of impulses along nerve fibers. Anesthetic agents are administered by several techniques designed to limit action to an area or region of the body while preserving consciousness and minimizing systemic absorption. Systemic actions cause side effects that range from nausea and vomiting to convulsions or cardiovascular collapse. Adverse reactions are treated by controlling symptoms and maintaining vital functions during the relatively short time required for metabolic degradation of the compounds.

❖ NURSING MANAGEMENT: CLIENT RECEIVING A LOCAL ANESTHETIC

In preparing solutions for topical application or injection, the usual precautions to ensure accurate medication administration are observed. Additives to the anesthetic drug (vasoconstrictors or hyaluronidase) must be ordered specifically. Solution labels must be read carefully, because concentrations vary and some commercial preparations contain combinations of drugs. Most common are solutions marketed with vasoconstrictors, such as epinephrine, already added to the primary drug. Solutions that contain epinephrine are not used in tissues whose blood supply comes from end arteries—fingers, toes, ears, nose, or penis—because the vasoconstriction can compromise circulation, resulting in gangrene. When helping the physician draw up solutions, the nurse should announce the exact preparation and concentration being used. The label should also be shown to the physician for visual confirmation. Solutions that appear cloudy or that contain solid crystals should not be used.

NURSING PROCESS

ASSESSMENT

The client receiving a local anesthetic should be assessed for factors that increase the risk of the drug. Previous adverse reactions to local anesthetics should be explored, with particular attention paid to lack of response. Possible cardiac or endocrine disease (specifically, thyroid or cortisone imbalance and pheochromocytoma) should be determined, and drugs used currently or in the recent past should be identified. During the history, the nurse can estimate the client's knowledge of local anesthesia.

NURSING DIAGNOSIS

Nursing diagnoses may include:

- Knowledge Deficit concerning effects of local anesthesia
- Risk for Pain, related to inherited refractoriness to local anesthetics

A common collaborative problem that should be differentiated from the nursing diagnoses is:

Potential Complication: Hypovolemic shock

PLANNING

Goals of treatment include teaching the client about local anesthesia and the surgical procedure, reducing the risk of adverse reaction to the anesthetic, maintaining tissue perfusion should an adverse reaction occur, limiting toxic reaction to vasoconstrictors, and preventing pain during the procedure.

INTERVENTION

If the client has a history of adverse reaction or inadequate response to local anesthetics, the physician should be notified promptly.

During surgery with local anesthesia, the nurse monitors the amount of anesthetic used and observes the client for signs of side effects, toxicity, or allergic reaction, such as restlessness, talkativeness, respiratory difficulty, rash, and changes in vital signs. These should be reported to the physician unless they are apparent to the surgical team. The total dose of anesthetic used and the time span elapsed since initiation of anesthesia should also be reported.

The surgical staff must be prepared to administer corrective action should a reaction occur. Oxygen, IV therapy, and assisted respirations may be required. Vasoconstrictors and diazepam should be readily accessible. Endotracheal intubation and cardiopulmonary resuscitation may be necessary.

The nurse must offer the client reassurance and emotional support, keeping in mind that even a sedated client remains aware of the environment. The usual sights, sounds, and smells associated with surgery may be disturbing. If the procedure interferes with the client's ability to talk, a signal should be established whereby he or she can indicate pain or another adverse reaction.

Positioning is crucial to control the spread of the drug when spinal or epidural anesthesia is administered. Rapid changes may be necessary. After surgery, the client should be protected from injury to the anesthetized area until sensation resumes. Clients who have undergone lumbar puncture for regional anesthesia experience paralysis of the lower part of the body until the drug concentration falls. These clients require special nursing care to prevent complications of immobility, especially thrombophlebitis and pressure necrosis. They should be positioned with pillows to maintain body alignment and to distribute pressure to all tissues. Because of leakage through the puncture site, the volume of cerebrospinal fluid may be reduced and spinal headache can occur. The head should be kept flat, but the client need not remain supine. Turning is required at least every 2 hours. The lower back and hips should be massaged frequently. The client should be monitored for headache. Nonopioid analgesics may be given for relief. Prolonged headache usually indicates that spinal fluid is leaking from the puncture site. The physician should be notified if a headache persists for more than a few hours. In some cases, the leakage may be corrected by creating a small hematoma at the puncture site (a small amount of the client's blood is drawn from a vein and injected at the puncture site). Ample fluid intake also hastens recovery from spinal headache by accelerating the regeneration of spinal fluid.

Client Education. The client must be informed that local anesthesia produces numbness but that deep pressure sensation may remain. Warn a client receiving a spinal anesthetic that motor function will be lost temporarily. Because odors from cauterization and sawing or chiseling sounds common in surgery can be disturbing to laypeople, the client should be warned about these. Advise the client to communicate any pain, nausea, restlessness, or difficulty in breathing.

Many clients fear receiving a spinal anesthetic because of rumored subsequent permanent paralysis. These rumors may originate from instances of progressive paralysis in clients who underwent lumbar puncture to diagnose an existing spinal cord disease. An apprehensive client should be informed that the site at which the anesthetic will be injected lies below the level of the spinal cord and is in an area providing ample space for the needle without encroaching on nerve structures. In the rare instance when a nerve is touched by the needle, irritation is limited to one or, at most, a few fibers. Symptoms are therefore confined to one or a few dermatomes. Moreover, nerves usually recover completely from such irritation. The client may need to be reassured that reports of paraplegia after this procedure are not related to the procedure but rather to an existing progressive disease.

After having spinal anesthesia, the client should remain flat in bed for the rest of the day and drink plenty of fluids to promote regeneration of the cerebrospinal fluid. Explain the nursing measures (turning, coughing, and deep breathing) that will be carried out to promote respiration and circulation. Encourage the client to report a headache, if one develops, so that corrective action may be taken.

Caution the client to avoid injuring the anesthetized areas in the interval before numbness subsides and sensation returns. This is particularly important for the client who leaves the healthcare setting before the effects of anesthesia have completely dissipated.

OUTCOME EVALUATION

Data required to evaluate the outcome of nursing measures during local anesthesia include client reports of numbness during surgery, a lack of adverse effects and complications (or quick, effective intervention should they occur), and client communications that indicate he or she understands the purpose and effects of local anesthetics.

❖ CHECKLIST OF NURSING ACTIONS

- ❑ Assess the client undergoing local anesthesia for previous response to local anesthetic agents.
- ❑ Determine whether the client has taken medication recently that may interact with the local anesthetic agent.
- ❑ Assess the client for cardiac or endocrine disease that increases the risk of adverse reaction.
- ❑ Verify the accuracy of medications used for anesthesia.
- ❑ Monitor the amount of local anesthetic used.
- ❑ Inform the client about the effects of the anesthetic and the surgical procedure. Reassure the fearful client that lumbar punctures do not cause permanent paralysis of the lower body.
- ❑ Instruct the client to notify the staff of pain or symptoms of adverse reaction.
- ❑ Monitor the client for lack of response and for signs and symptoms of adverse reaction.

- ❑ Be prepared to control seizures and maintain vital functions if an acute drug reaction occurs.
- ❑ Provide reassurance and emotional support during the procedure.
- ❑ Caution the client to avoid injury to the anesthetized area until numbness subsides.
- ❑ Provide appropriate positioning and fluids for the client who received a spinal anesthetic. This will help prevent headache and other complications.

Alternative Anesthetic Regimens

Monitored anesthesia care refers to the techniques increasingly being used for various inpatient and outpatient procedures. A combination of agents, usually an analgesic, an anxiolytic, and local or regional anesthetics, is used. Various anesthetic regimens are available: conscious sedation, neuroleptanesthesia, dissociative anesthesia, and twilight sleep. Their features are noted in Table 18-19.

Conscious Sedation

Conscious sedation is a type of anesthesia that provides analgesia and amnesia while the client is conscious but sedated. This allows the client to respond to the physician's directions. This type of anesthesia is used for dental surgery and certain types of ambulatory surgery or diagnostic procedures (eg, colonoscopy, implanting pacemakers). The regimen usually consists of an opiate such as fentanyl (Sublimaze), a phenothiazine such as midazolam (Versed), and a local anesthetic. Subanesthetic doses of IV anesthetics such as propofol (Diprivan) may also be used (Smith & White, 1992).

Because of the danger of respiratory depression and respiratory arrest, the client's circulating oxygen level is usually monitored by pulse oximetry. Another person besides the operating surgeon or dentist must be responsible for monitoring the client's vital signs and responses.

Amnesia of the procedure is a desired effect; however, the amnesia may remove memory of some preoperative events, such as instructions and informed consent. All essential postprocedure instructions should be in written form for the client and should also be given to the client's family or caregiver. A client who undergoes conscious sedation and who is discharged directly must not drive home: he or she may appear to be functioning but may not have regained enough judgment and reflexes to be safe.

Neuroleptanesthesia

Neuroleptic compounds are sometimes used with opioid analgesics to produce analgesia during diagnostic procedures or minor surgery. Under the influence of these drugs, clients appear indifferent to the environment. They appear anxiety-free and exhibit reduced motor function. However, they can respond to commands and cooperate with the healthcare staff when

Table 18-19. Alternative Anesthetic Regimens

Characteristics	Neuroleptanesthesia	Dissociative Anesthesia	Conscious Sedation
Effect on recipient	Indifference to surroundings Lack of anxiety Responsiveness to commands retained Residual respiratory depression	Marked analgesia Immobility Sedation Amnesia Mental dissociation from surroundings	Analgesia Amnesia Sedation Ability to respond to commands retained
Agents used	Innovar (a combination of fentanyl and droperidol)	Ketamine (*Can:* Ketalor)	Various combinations of analgesics, amnesics, anxiolytics, local anesthetics, and subanesthetic doses of IV anesthetics
Precautions required (for all three regimens, clients must be protected from injury and watched closely for adverse reactions)	Carefully control rate of administration. Support respirations during and after anesthesia. Reduce dosage of potent analgesics until anesthetic effects are completely dissipated.	Minimize environmental stimuli. Observe and treat for psychic disturbance (nightmares or hallucinations).	Observe for respiratory depression and hypoxemia using pulse oximetry.
Uses	Diagnostic procedures or minor surgery (with opioid analgesics)	Burn dressing changes	Dental and surgical procedures in which client cooperation is needed

necessary. Analgesia may be converted to anesthesia by administering nitrous oxide with oxygen by inhalation.

The agent most commonly used for inducing neuroleptanalgesia is a mixture of droperidol and fentanyl (Innovar). This preparation is diluted in 5% dextrose in water and administered slowly by IV injection. The administration rate must be controlled carefully to prevent adverse reactions, such as excitement and spasms of the larynx and chest wall. If chest wall spasms develop, respirations can be restored by administering succinylcholine.

The induction of neuroleptanalgesia may depress respiration, especially if potent analgesics are used. If this occurs, drug dosage must be reduced and the client's respiratory function monitored carefully.

Dissociative Anesthesia

Certain chemicals produce a state similar to neuroleptanalgesia that is characterized by marked analgesia, immobility, sedation, amnesia, and a strong feeling of disassociation from the environment. The agent most commonly used to induce this type of anesthesia is ketamine (Ketalar). Ketamine acts on the cortex and limbic system rather than on the reticular formation. Administered IM or IV, it induces anesthesia in less than 1 minute. Anesthesia lasts 10 to 15 minutes and may be prolonged by giving additional doses. Analgesia persists for more than 30 minutes, and amnesia is evident for 1 to 2 hours.

A quiet environment is essential for smooth progress of dissociative anesthesia. Muscular movement may occur in response to extraneous stimuli. Ketamine reduces airway resistance and helps maintain an unobstructed airway. It is particularly useful for changing burn dressings on the face and neck. However, night-

mares and hallucinations may occur when the client emerges from anesthesia and may sometimes recur subsequently. Diazepam may be prescribed to reverse the dissociative anesthesia.

Twilight Sleep

Various combinations of potent analgesics and amnesia-inducing agents have been used to alleviate pain during procedures that require some participation by the client. The effect, known as twilight sleep, was popular for managing labor but has fallen out of favor because the medicated client often loses control and cannot cooperate or participate appropriately in the necessary procedures.

Sedative–Hypnotic Drugs

Sedative–hypnotic drugs induce sleep. Natural substances with hypnotic properties, such as alcohol and opium, have been used for centuries to relieve insomnia and to promote rest. Today, however, most sedative–hypnotics are general CNS depressants that have dose-related effects. In small doses, they produce sedation, a state characterized by reduced excitation and activity and increased relaxation and lassitude. Moderate doses promote drowsiness or sleep; large doses induce general anesthesia.

Understanding Sleep

Sleep is a temporary state of altered consciousness characterized by amnesia and reduced perception of and responsiveness to the environment. Unlike unconscious states resulting from disease or the administration of anesthetics, sleep can be interrupted by appropriate stimulation. Sensory and motor activity during sleep are virtually suspended, and body processes slow down. This hiatus provides time for reparative processes to restore tissues and organs to optimal condition.

During sleep, the molecular and cellular biochemical changes that occur in the waking hours are reversed to prepare the body for another cycle of activity. Functionally, the brain appears to use sleeping time for sorting and storing in permanent memory the perceptions of the previous waking period. At the psychologic level, the psyche similarly attends to psychologic perceptions and tensions.

Stages and Patterns of Sleep

Sleep occurs in stages; it is not a steady state. Specific stages of sleep reflect the basic rest/activity cycles (BRACs) that characterize both waking and sleeping hours. BRACs, which last 60 to 120 minutes, are related during wakefulness to fluctuations in efficiency and to spontaneous behaviors such as food-seeking. During sleep, BRACs can be tracked by monitoring brainwave patterns, muscle activity, and vital signs.

Sleep is one of several body functions characterized by rhythmic diurnal or circadian patterns. Physiologic processes characterized similarly include maintenance of body temperature, endocrine hormone secretion, mental alertness, and psychomotor function. Body temperatures, alertness, and activity levels are generally highest during the day and lowest at night. Activity patterns that vary from this norm can, however, induce changes in the chronology of other functions to conform to their rhythms. Adjustment to aberrant schedules usually requires at least 2 weeks.

Stages in the cycles have two main categories: rapid eye movement (REM) sleep and nonrapid eye movement (NREM) sleep. REM sleep, also known as paradoxical or desynchronized sleep, is when most dreaming occurs. NREM sleep, or slow-wave sleep, occurs in four stages.

A complete sleep cycle progresses from stage I through stage IV of NREM sleep, and the sequence then reverses, returning to stage I and a subsequent period of REM sleep (Fig. 18-3). In normal people, the cycle always begins with stage I NREM sleep and progresses through the usual sequence. Interrupting sleep—a return to arousal—causes the cycle to begin again at stage I NREM sleep. People who have been deprived of REM sleep by repeated awakenings before or at the initiation of this phase of the cycle eventually adopt an abnormal sleep pattern characterized by immediate onset of the REM phase on falling asleep. This phenomenon implies that the REM phase is necessary for important functions that cannot be performed adequately during NREM stages.

Sleep patterns vary from person to person and for a given person over time, but divergence is not apparent among normal subjects. NREM sleep tends to predominate during the early hours of sleep, and periods of REM sleep tend to lengthen progressively during later hours.

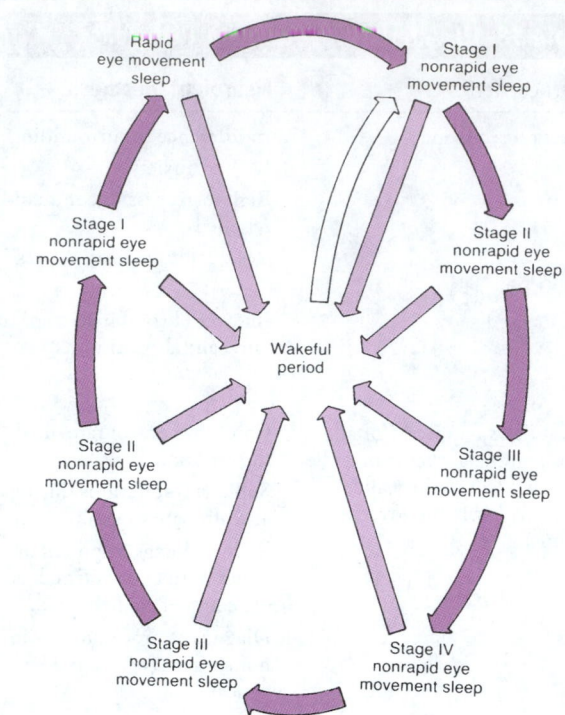

Figure 18-3. Sleep cycles.

Sleep patterns vary with age. Children and young adults experience long periods of stage III and IV NREM sleep, with longer periods of REM sleep as the night progresses. Older adults have little or no stage IV NREM sleep and may have frequent and often lengthy awakenings during the night. Although this pattern is normal in elderly people, it may cause them to seek hypnotics (Kales, 1968).

Sleep disruptions are fairly common. They range in severity from occasional delays in falling asleep to sleep deprivation that leads to psychotic manifestations. Inability to sleep may be caused by an imbalance in brain neurotransmitters, environmental overstimulation, or both. Etiology may be exogenous, endogenous, or a combination of both (Box 18-5). Drugs and foods may also adversely affect the sleep pattern; examples include CNS stimulants, caffeine (in coffee, tea, and soft drinks), theophylline, and alcohol. Usually psychotropic drugs, especially antidepressants, improve sleep pattern disturbances caused by psychiatric disorders. However, some (eg, diazepam) can alter sleep patterns by their effects on REM sleep.

Adequate rest and sleep are essential to health. They are particularly important to tissue regeneration or restoration of physiologic or psychologic equilibrium. For these reasons, promotion of adequate rest and sleep is a matter of concern to healthcare professionals.

The ideal sleep-inducing drug would take effect soon after administration, promote natural sleep without disrupting normal sleep stages, allow sleep to end at the usual time of awakening, and produce no residual (hangover) or undesirable effects. No known chemical con-

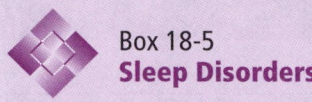

Box 18-5
Sleep Disorders

Dyssomnias Associated with Disruptions of the Diurnal Sleep–Wake Cycle

Phase shift in sleep cycles: a change in cycle induced by rapid travel across time zones ("jet lag") or a change in work schedule ("shift work" syndrome)

Fixed-phase sleep cycle: inconvenient or inappropriate sleep–wake cycle (the "owl" and "lark" syndromes)

Inappropriate length of sleep–wake cycle: a cycle that is shorter or longer than 24 hours. Such a cycle is "out of phase" with normal day–night patterns much of the time

Disorders of Initiating and Maintaining Sleep

Psychophysiologic insomnia: disturbances in sleep due to the presence of unaccustomed cues or other situational stressors

Psychiatric insomnia: sleep disturbances accompanying psychiatric illness that may be due to the psychosis, may contribute to the psychosis, or may be caused independently by the processes underlying the psychosis

Insomnia associated with medical conditions: interruption of sleep by pain, dyspnea, urinary frequency, or other discomfort

Sleep-induced ventilatory impairment: sleep apnea syndromes characterized by brief awakenings stimulated by respiratory embarrassment

Nocturnal myoclonus: brief awakenings after clonic movements of one or both legs

Childhood insomnia: early onset of insomnia usually associated with a positive family history of a similar problem

Insomnia due to drug use: chronic use of CNS stimulants or withdrawal from chronic use of CNS depressants that interfere with sleep by heightening CNS activity

forms to these criteria, but present sedative–hypnotics are as effective as or safer than agents used in the past.

Drugs such as alcohol, bromides, chloral hydrate, paraldehyde, opiates, and barbiturates are sedative–hypnotics. Prescribed drugs to promote sleep are largely limited to sedating tranquilizers (particularly the benzodiazepines), chloral hydrate, paraldehyde, antihistamines, and selected barbiturates. Other drugs have largely replaced barbiturates in treating insomnia. Nonprescription sleeping aids usually contain an antihistamine, most commonly diphenhydramine. Alcohol is a CNS depressant with hypnotic effects, but it is not usually recommended for sleep induction because of its as-

sociation with dangerous interactions, dependency, and adverse effects on sleep patterns.

Pharmacodynamics. The benzodiazepines and barbiturates appear to act by mimicking or enhancing the effects of gamma-aminobutyric acid (GABA) in the brain. The specific effect of the barbiturates is unknown. The benzodiazepines antagonize a protein that inhibits GABA binding to its receptors. Their effects depend on adequate levels of GABA in the tissues. Enhancement of GABA action produces a selective inhibition of postsynaptic impulses in polysynaptic pathways in the CNS. The mesencephalic reticular formation is particularly sensitive.

Hypnotics act as descending CNS depressants. They tend to decrease spontaneous activity and response to afferent sensory input, shorten sleep latency, raise the awakening threshold, and increase total sleep time. Their actions in subjects with neurotic or psychotic disturbances may be greater than and different qualitatively from those in normal people. For example, the benzodiazepines tend to shorten slow-wave NREM sleep in normal people but lengthen the same sleep stages in people subject to neuroses or depression. Because they affect the limbic system, the benzodiazepines exert some sedative effect, whereas barbiturates sedate through general CNS depression.

Pharmacokinetics. Most hypnotics are well absorbed by the GI mucosa. Chloral hydrate, which irritates mucous membranes, is administered in capsules or in olive oil as a retention enema.

Paraldehyde, barbiturates, and benzodiazepines may be administered parenterally. Table 18-20 lists preparations and dosages of various sedative–hypnotics. Paraldehyde is sometimes injected IM. Both IM and IV solutions of the benzodiazepines are available. Barbiturates may be administered IV but are never injected IM because they cause pain and necrosis at the injection site.

After absorption, chloral hydrate, barbiturates, and benzodiazepines are bound to plasma proteins in proportion to their lipid solubility. Binding may range from minimal (as with flurazepam) to 99% (diazepam). These drugs can displace other drugs from protein-binding sites, thereby increasing their physiologic action and accelerating their metabolism and excretion.

Hypnotic drugs are rapidly taken up by the gray matter of the brain. They then redistribute to the white matter and adipose and other body tissues. Eventually, they reach all tissues. Fetal blood levels are comparable to maternal levels, and the drugs are secreted in the breast milk.

Some sedative–hypnotics, notably phenobarbital and the benzodiazepines, circulate in the enterohepatic cycle. Metabolism of hypnotic drugs is carried out mainly by the liver microsomal enzyme system. Many metabolites are physiologically active, and an accumulation of these substances may prolong the action of a

Text continues on page 357.

Table 18-20. Representative Sedative–Hypnotics

Drug Name	Preparation	Usual Dosage	Additional Information
Benzodiazepines			Some benzodiazepines are also used as tranquilizers, sedatives, skeletal muscle relaxants, and anticonvulsants. Benzodiazepine may cause fetal damage when taken during pregnancy.
chlordiazepoxide (Libritabs, Librium, Mitran, Resosans-10) (*Can*: Medilium, Novopoxide)	Oral tablets and capsules Solutions for deep IM or slow IV injection	*Preoperatively:* Adults: 50–100 mg IM 1 h before surgery; children 12–18 yr: 25–50 mg PC: D	Safe use in children younger than 12 yr has not been established.
estazolam (ProSom)	Oral tablets	Adults: 1 mg	Somnolence is a common side effect
flurazepam (Dalmane) (*Can*: Somnol)	Capsules for oral use Oral tablets	Adults: 15–30 mg PC: D	Safe use in children younger than 15 yr has not been established.
lorazepam (Ativan) (*Can*: Novolorazem)	Solutions for IM or IV injection	*Preoperatively:* Adults: *IM:* 0.05 mg/kg at least 2 h before surgery; *IV:* 0.44–0.5 mg/kg 15 min before surgery; *maximum dosage:* 4 mg Insomnia due to anxiety: Adults: 2–4 mg at bedtime PC: D	Lorazepam causes amnesia proportional to dosage. Safe use of oral lorazepam in children younger than 12 yr and of parenteral lorazepam in children younger than 18 yr has not been established.
midazolam (Versed)	Solution for injection	70–80 μg/kg PC: D	Midazolam is used as a preoperative sedative and amnesiac and is also used in conscious sedation. Adverse reactions to midazolam are similar to those of other benzodiazepines.
oxazepam (Serax) (*Can*: Ox-Pam, Zapex)	Capsules for oral use	Adults: 10–30 mg PC: C	Although not approved for use in sleep disorders, oxazepam is preferred by some physicians for the treatment of sleep disorders in elderly people.
quazepam (Doral)	Tablets for oral use	Adults: 15 mg For some clients, dose may be halved after a few nights of therapy PC: X	Long duration of action may prevent withdrawal signs and symptoms when medication is discontinued. Teratogenic; contraindicated during pregnancy. Concurrent use with cimetidine may prolong effects of quazepam. Safety and effectiveness in clients younger than 18 yr are unproven.
temazepam (Restoril)	Oral capsules	Adults: 15–30 mg PC: X	Safe use in children younger than 18 yr has not been established.
triazolam (Halcion) (*Can*: Apo-Triazo, Novo-triolam, Nu-Triazol)	Oral tablets	Adults: 0.125–0.5 mg PC: X	For geriatric clients, the usual adult dosage should be halved. Safe use in children younger than 18 yr has not been established. Triazolam has been used to prevent "jet-lag" upsets in workers on 12-h shift of sleep schedules. May cause anterograde amnesia and rebound insomnia.

KEY: PC = pregnancy category (see Appendix A).

(continued)

Table 18-20. (Continued)

Drug Name	Preparation	Usual Dosage	Additional Information
Barbiturates			Barbiturates as sedatives or hypnotics have been largely replaced by other agents. Barbiturates are also used to prevent cerebral edema after brain injury; to antagonize the unwanted CNS stimulation by other drugs; to reduce jaundice in kernicterus and obstructive liver conditions; and as sedatives, anesthetics, and anticonvulsants.
amobarbital (Amytal) (*Can*: Novanobarb)	Powder for preparing solutions for deep IM or slow IV injection	*IM hypnotic dose for adults:* 65–200 mg *IV hypnotic dose for both adults and children older than 6 yr:* 65–500 mg; *maximum IV dose:* 1 g *IM hypnotic dose for children:* 2–3 mg/kg	Amobarbital should not be used as a hypnotic for longer than 2 weeks. After long-term use, amobarbital should be withdrawn gradually.
aprobarbital (Alurate)	Oral elixir	*Hypnotic dose:* Adults: 40–160 mg PC: D	Aprobarbital should not be used as a hypnotic for longer than 2 weeks. After long-term use, aprobarbital should be withdrawn gradually. Dosage for children has not been established.
butabarbital (Buticaps, Butisol)	Oral tablets, capsules, and elixir	*Hypnotic dose:* Adults: 50–100 mg PC: D	Butabarbital should not be used as a hypnotic for longer than 2 weeks. After long-term use, butabarbital should be withdrawn gradually.
mephobarbital (Mebaral)	Oral tablets	*Oral sedative dose:* Adults: 32–100 mg tid or qid; children: 16–32 mg tid or qid PC: D	Mephobarbital is used primarily for sedation.
phenobarbital (Solfoton, Luminal)	Oral tablets, capsules, and elixir Solution for injection	*Oral sedative doses:* Adults: 30–120 mg/day in 2 or 3 divided doses; children: 8–12 mg *Oral hypnotic dose:* Adults: 100–200 mg *Parenteral sedative dose:* Adults: 30–120 mg/day IM or IV in 2 or 3 doses *Parenteral hypnotic dose:* Adults: 100–320 mg IM or IV PC: D	Phenobarbital should not be used as a hypnotic for longer than 2 weeks.
pentobarbital (Nembutal) (*Can*: Pentogen)	Oral capsules and elixir Solutions for deep IM or slow IV injection Rectal suppositories	*Oral hypnotic dose:* Adults: 100–200 mg *Rectal hypnotic doses:* Adults: 120–200 mg; children 12–14 yr: 60–120 mg; children 5–12 yr: 60 mg; children 1–4 yr: 30–60 mg; children 2 mo to 1 yr: 30 mg *IM hypnotic doses:* Adults: 150–200 mg; children: 2–6 mg/kg or 125 mg/m²; *maximum dose:* 100 mg PC: D	Pentobarbital should not be used as a hypnotic for longer than 2 weeks. After long-term use, pentobarbital should be withdrawn gradually.
Secobarbital (Seconal) (*Can*: Secal)	Powder Oral tablets, capsules, and elixir Solutions for injection	*Oral or IM hypnotic dose:* Adults: 100–200 mg *IM hypnotic dose:* Children 3–5 mg/kg or 125 mg/m²; *maximum dose:* 100 mg PC: D	Secobarbital should not be used as a hypnotic for longer than 2 weeks. After long-term use, secobarbital should be withdrawn gradually.

KEY: PC = pregnancy category (see Appendix A). *Can* = Canadian trade name.

(continued)

Table 18-20. (Continued)

Drug Name	Preparation	Usual Dosage	Additional Information
Miscellaneous Hypnotics			
chloral hydrate (Aquachloral, Noctec, SK-Chloral Hydrate; also called "knock-out drops" or "Mickey Finn" when combined with alcohol)	Crystals Oral capsules and solution Rectal suppositories	*Hypnotic dose:* Adults: 500 mg–1 g, 15–30 min before retiring; children: 50 mg/kg; *maximum dose:* 1 g PC: C	Gastric irritation may be minimized by diluting oral solutions with extra water or taking other oral dosage forms with ample liquids. Chloral hydrate has been found to lose much of its effectiveness for inducing and maintaining sleep after 2 weeks of use.
diphenhydramine (Compoz, Nytol, Sleep-eze, Twi-Lite) (*Can:* Insomnal)	Oral capsules	*Hypnotic dose:* Adults: 50 mg PC: B	May cause gastric irritation. Often used with other ingredients in OTC sleep aids.
ethanol ("alcohol")	Liquid for preparation of drinks (wine, beer, distilled liquors) Solutions for parenteral administration	Adults: 5–15 mL Total abstinence is recommended during pregnancy.	Alcohol has been administered in a social setting in some extended care facilities.
ethchlorvynol (Placidyl)	Oral capsules	*Hypnotic dose:* Adults: 500 mg hs; for awaking in the early morning hours: 100–200 mg PC: C	Ethchlorvynol should not be used as a hypnotic for longer than 1 week. Ethchlorvynol dependence resembles dependence on barbiturates.
glutethimide (Doriden)	Powder Oral capsules and tablets	*Hypnotic dose:* Adults: 250–500 mg hs; *maximum daily dosage:* 1 g PC: C	Tolerance of and dependence on glutethimide resembles that of the barbiturates. Glutethimide should be used as a hypnotic for no longer than 1 week.
methyprylon (Noludar)	Oral capsules and tablets	*Hypnotic dose:* Adults: 200–400 mg, 15 min before retiring; *maximum daily dosage:* 400 mg *Hypnotic dose:* Children older than 12 yr: 50 mg; *maximum dose:* 200 mg PC: B	Safe use of methyprylon during pregnancy and lactation has not been established.
paraldehyde (Paral)	Oral and rectal liquids	*Hypnotic dose:* Adults 4–8 mL orally Children: 0.3 mL/kg orally or rectally PC: C	Paraldehyde is preferred by some physicians for hypnosis in elderly people. Do not administer if a vinegar odor is present or container open more than 24 h. Mix with juice and chill to administer orally. Dilute in 2 volumes of olive oil for rectal use. Paraldehyde reacts to plastics and rubber; measure in glass containers; use only freshly opened containers. IV administration is hazardous; IM administration may cause sterile abscess or tissue sloughing.
zolpidem tartrate (Ambien)	Oral tablets	*Hypnotic dose:* Adults 10 mg PC: B	Cautious use in elderly or debilitated clients or those with hepatic insufficiency.

KEY: PC = pregnancy category (see Appendix A). *Can* = Canadian trade name.

given dose. For this reason, the full drug effect may not be apparent until the medication has been administered for several days. Persistence of active metabolites also contributes to a prolonged residual, or hangover, effect.

Excretion of most sedative–hypnotics is performed by the kidneys. Renal filtration of unchanged drug is inversely proportional to the degree of protein binding and is insignificant for many drugs. Drug metabolites are readily eliminated in the urine, however. Renal excretion of free barbiturates may be increased by alkalinization of the urine (which increases the solubility of the acid salts) and by osmotic diuresis. Small amounts of chloral hydrate and the benzodiazepines are excreted in the feces after their secretion in the bile.

Because many hypnotics persist in the body more than 24 hours, repeated use is accompanied by accumulation and a gradual increase in physiologic effects. Toxicity is likely to develop.

Therapeutic Uses. Sedative–hypnotic drugs are frequently prescribed to promote rest and sleep in ill or insomniac clients. They are also administered preoperatively to prepare clients for anesthesia. They are most useful in ameliorating temporary sleep disturbances that result from short-term illness or unavoidable environmental stimuli.

Adverse Reactions. Sedative–hypnotic drugs alter sleep stages to some degree. The significance of many of the changes is unknown, but reduced REM sleep, a common effect, is generally considered detrimental. Chronic use of hypnotics may produce pronounced REM deprivation. This condition could underlie the personality changes sometimes seen in clients after prolonged use of these drugs. Distortion of sleep phases also can alter daytime perception, with the benzodiazepines sometimes causing "daymares," phenomena analogous to nightmares that occur during sleep. Rebound insomnia, in which clients withdrawing from sedative–hypnotic drugs experience insomnia and nightmares, may be related to decreases in REM sleep; rebound insomnia tends to be less likely with hypnotics that have intermediate or long half-lives.

Side effects of hypnotic drugs include impaired psychomotor and cognitive function and decreased inhibitions. Reaction time increases; weakness, vertigo, and confusion may occur. Behavior resembling that of alcohol intoxication is common with higher dosages.

Some clients, particularly older adults, react paradoxically to hypnotics. They become more wakeful and have increased difficulty in falling asleep. Confusion and delirium have also been reported. Hypnotic drugs may also cause sleep apnea, particularly in obese middle-aged men.

Anterograde amnesia has been reported with some of the benzodiazepines, especially those with short half-lives.

Hypnotics share with other CNS depressants a potential for producing physical dependence. Induction

(stimulation) of liver microsomal enzymes by some sedative–hypnotics accelerates the rate of biotransformation in the bodies of habitual users; to maintain a constant response, an increase in dose is required. Of greater quantitative importance is the homeostatic response to the depression caused by these drugs: an excitatory feedback response compensates by increasing basal CNS activity. This phenomenon is common to all CNS depressants, and cross-tolerance is apparent among these drugs.

Discontinuation of sedative–hypnotic drugs precipitates physical withdrawal syndromes characterized by wakefulness, depression, anxiety, bizarre dreams, agitation, delirium, and psychosis. Seizures, coma, and death may occur, particularly in the case of barbiturate withdrawal. Because their addictive properties make treatment difficult, abuse of hypnotic drugs is a major health problem.

Many tranquilizers have exhibited significant teratogenic effects. Thalidomide belongs to this class. Results from retrospective studies suggest an increased risk of congenital malformations in infants of mothers who received benzodiazepines.

Allergic reactions to hypnotic agents include rashes (from chloral hydrate and barbiturates) and precipitation of acute allergic attacks in clients subject to asthma, urticaria, and angioedema (from barbiturates). Many tranquilizers have some degree of antihistamine action, but paradoxically these agents also can cause allergic reactions in some people.

Among other undesirable effects of hypnotics are nausea and vomiting (most common with chloral hydrate). The barbiturates increase porphyrin and somatotropin production and decrease adrenocorticoid secretion. Both barbiturates and chloral hydrate cause hyperalgesia. Paradoxical excitement occurs in some clients (especially the elderly) who receive barbiturates or benzodiazepines.

Toxicity Alert: Sedative–Hypnotics

Toxicity resulting from sedative–hypnotics is similar to that from other CNS depressants. Somnolence tends to progress to coma. Respiratory depression is especially severe in barbiturate toxicity. Cardiovascular collapse is a relatively late sign.

Drug–Drug Interactions. The effects of sedative–hypnotic drugs and other CNS depressants, including alcohol, are additive and can produce serious toxicity when multiple drugs are used. Antihistamines used with sedative–hypnotics also produce an additive effect. Oral anticoagulant effects may be altered by chloral hydrate, glutethimide, and ethchlorvynol. If chloral hydrate is followed by IV furosemide, sweating, hot flashes, weakness, hypertension, tachycardia, and nausea may occur.

Combinations of barbiturates or tranquilizers with alcohol have been implicated in many deaths from sedative overdose. The effects of barbiturates may be decreased by rifampin and increased by alcohol, monoamine oxidase inhibitors, and valproic acid. Barbiturates stimulate the microsomal enzymes and, therefore, may increase the metabolism and decrease the effects of many drugs (eg, anticoagulants, beta blockers, oral contraceptives, corticosteroids, digitoxin). Barbiturates also decrease serum levels of carbamazepine, clonazepam, doxorubicin, doxycycline, quinidine, theophylline, felodipine, fenprofen, and griseofulvin. The effectiveness of metronidazole, phenmetrazine, and phenylbutazone may be decreased. The renal toxicity of methoxyflurane may be enhanced. When barbiturates are used with hydantoins or narcotic analgesics, the effects of these drugs must be monitored closely because of potential unpredictable variations.

Drug–Food Interactions. Food may interact with zolpidem to delay the onset of sleep.

Drug–Laboratory Test Interactions. Chloral hydrate may interfere with the copper sulfate test for glycosuria and some tests for urinary catecholamines. A single dose of barbiturate may influence BSP and liver function studies.

Precautions and Contraindications. The barbiturates and chloral hydrate are absolutely contraindicated in clients with a history of acute intermittent porphyria. Administration of barbiturates or chloral hydrate is likely to precipitate a life-threatening attack of this disease. Sedative–hypnotic drugs are usually contraindicated for persons with a history of drug abuse, especially when the drugs abused are CNS depressants.

Sedative–hypnotics must be prescribed and administered carefully, taking into account the potential of the client to use them to attempt suicide. Because of the potential for dependence, sedative–hypnotics should be discontinued whenever an increased dose is needed to sustain the therapeutic effect. Because of the dangers of misuse, limited amounts of drugs are prescribed at one time. Precautions should be taken to ensure that clients do not obtain multiple prescriptions from different prescribers.

Clients with chronic obstructive pulmonary disease should take sedative–hypnotics with extreme caution, if at all, and they must be monitored closely when hypnotics are used. Dosages should be minimal, and respiratory function should be assessed frequently.

■ SUMMARY

Sedative–hypnotic drugs are often used to promote rest and sleep when illness or environmental changes temporarily disrupt normal sleep patterns.

Chronic use is undesirable because it disrupts sleep stages to some degree and impairs waking function. Moreover, dependency tends to develop. The benzodiazepine tranquilizers are considered the safest drugs to use in most situations. They are the drugs most commonly prescribed for hypnosis, although chloral hydrate, paraldehyde, selected barbiturates, and other drugs are used occasionally.

Sedative–hypnotic drugs tend to accumulate in the tissues, so toxicity may develop with prolonged use. They often influence the action of other drugs by altering their storage or metabolism in the body. Withdrawal from chronic use of hypnotics produces abstinence syndromes that can be life-threatening, particularly in barbiturate dependence.

❖ NURSING MANAGEMENT: CLIENT RECEIVING SEDATIVE–HYPNOTICS

Promoting rest and sleep is a major nursing concern. Inadequate sleep is associated with many physical and psychologic problems and tends to delay recovery from illness. Inadequate sleep is an appropriate diagnosis for nurses to make because it is a health problem largely amenable to nursing treatment. The use of sedative–hypnotic drugs is an important adjunct to this treatment.

Sleep Patterns. To diagnose inadequate sleep, the nurse must understand normal sleep patterns. Sleep requirements vary but tend to conform to certain normal ranges. Factors such as age and cultural conditioning affect sleep patterns. The need for sleep is highest in the early years of life, decreases gradually throughout childhood, and levels off early in the third decade of life. The number of awakenings after the onset of sleep increases with age. Cultural conditioning and personal preference influence the rest/activity pattern but do not appreciably change the overall need for sleep. People who suffer from disease or trauma need more sleep than usual.

Toxicity. Acute sedative–hypnotic toxicity is a medical emergency. It usually results from accidental or deliberate overdose. The client exhibits signs of severe CNS depression and somnolence or coma. Respiratory depression is the major threat to life. Cardiovascular collapse and convulsions can occur, particularly in severely hypoxic clients. Treatment is supportive. Mechanical respiratory assistance and oxygen administration are required to maintain tissue oxygenation. Adrenergic vasopressors are administered IV to maintain circulation. Cardiotonics may also be required. The stomach is lavaged to remove any residual drug. In severe toxicity, hemodialysis may be instituted to remove the offending drug from the bloodstream. Until toxic drug levels subside, the client requires intensive nursing care appropriate to the comatose condition.

Drug Storage. Schedule II, III, and IV hypnotic drugs such as barbiturates and benzodiazepines must be secured in storage. Double locks and detailed records of the disposition of all doses may be required. All prescribed sedative–hypnotics must be monitored, and careful records should be kept of their use. Automatic expiration of orders for these drugs and special records of the disposition of dispensed supplies are wise precautions to take.

Drug Abuse. Abuse of sedative–hypnotic drugs is a major health problem. Worldwide, more prescriptions are written for CNS depressants than for any other drug class. Illegal use of these compounds is also widespread. Educating clients and the general public to the effects of drugs and the risks of abuse is crucial. The client's general attitude toward the use of chemical agents should be carefully considered when evaluating the risk for habituation.

Counseling and instruction designed to improve self-care and parenting techniques are basic to promoting optimal physical and emotional health. Robust health and competence in coping with minor illnesses and psychologic stress are good insurance against the need for habitual drug use. Self-confidence and a good self-image decrease the need for chemical use as a psychologic crutch. In addition, people need information about the physical and mental effects of drugs and the detrimental effects of dependence to make intelligent decisions about drug use.

NURSING PROCESS

ASSESSMENT

To assess the adequacy of sleep, the nurse compares current data with baseline data from pertinent age and cultural groups and baseline data from the client's health history. A complete sleep history should be taken before drug therapy begins. The client's normal sleep pattern as well as the disturbed sleep pattern should be determined. In addition, the client's perception of feeling rested and alert or fatigued and dull may be most important.

Measures to promote sleep, including use of OTC preparations (eg, Nytol) and the client's response to them, should be explored. The client's usual sleeping environment and bedtime rituals should be determined.

Risk factors that affect the client must be assessed before administering any sedative–hypnotic agent. Of particular significance are habitual or chronic use of sedative–hypnotic drugs and the presence of chronic obstructive airway disease. When chloral hydrate or barbiturates are ordered, the nurse should determine any history of porphyria.

NURSING DIAGNOSIS

The primary nursing diagnosis should be:

- Sleep Pattern Disturbance: Insomnia, related to CNS stimulant effects of therapeutic drugs or fear of impending event, such as surgery

It is useful to delineate the underlying factors for ultimate correction of the sleep disturbance. When hypnotics are used, the following diagnoses may be applicable:

- Ineffective Breathing Pattern, Risk for, related to drug-induced respiratory depression
- Risk for Injury, related to falls secondary to dizziness or sleepiness

PLANNING

Goals of nursing care include promoting sleep, maintaining effective respiration, and preventing accidental injury.

INTERVENTION

If the underlying cause of the sleep disturbance is known and amenable to correction, it should be eliminated. All appropriate nursing measures to promote sleep should be used. General nursing measures can be taken to decrease arousal by reducing cerebral and skeletal muscle activity that interferes with sleep by maintaining arousal. Such measures include eliminating or masking environmental stimuli, promoting muscle relaxation, reducing anxiety, and promoting physical and psychologic comfort.

Before retiring, the client should engage in quiet activities in an environment characterized by reduced sensory stimuli. As much as possible, the client should follow a bedtime ritual (eg, toileting, mouth care, special clothing). Through conditioning, habitual routines become stimuli for relaxation and induction of sleep (Box 18-6).

Any critical judgments required of the client should be made before sedative–hypnotic drugs are administered. The validity of legal documents (eg, informed consent, permission for surgery) is questionable if they were signed under the influence of CNS drugs.

The use of sedative–hypnotics may be effective when factors that interfere with rest cannot be controlled adequately to maintain normal sleep patterns. However, in view of the potential toxicity of such drugs and their effects on the stages of sleep, such use should

Box 18-6
General Nursing Measures to Promote Sleep

- Eliminate or mask environmental stimuli
- Promote muscle relaxation
- Reduce anxiety
- Promote physical and psychologic comfort
- Maintain a regular bedtime ritual for retiring
- Avoid stimulant drugs or food containing caffeine
- Avoid exercise immediately before bedtime

be minimized. Drugs should never be used as a substitute for nursing care that is directed at promoting sleep.

The hypnotic drug may be administered when the client has been made comfortable. If the client tolerates milk and is not at high risk for gastric hyperacidity, warm milk given with oral hypnotics enhances their effects. Tryptophan, an amino acid in milk, is a natural soporific. Cocoa should be avoided; the stimulant xanthines in chocolate tend to excite the nervous system. Malt or vanilla flavoring may be used instead.

Analgesics should usually be administered with the sedative–hypnotic if pain is a problem. Although hypnotic tranquilizers sometimes relieve pain because of their antianxiety effects, other hypnotics have no analgesic properties and may cause hyperalgesia. Pain alters response to sedatives, causing an increased incidence of disorientation and paradoxical excitement. For optimal hypnotic effect, the nurse should manage the administration of analgesia through the day so that a dose is available at bedtime. Sleep induction is enhanced by a soothing backrub given during the latent period required for drug absorption.

Monitoring During Sleep.

Special precautions should be implemented to ensure the safety of the sedated client. Hypnotic drugs impair judgment and psychomotor function. They may produce lightheadedness or dizziness. The nurse can use raised side rails and other measures to remind clients to obtain help if they must leave bed.

The client's sleep should be monitored carefully to evaluate the effectiveness of sleep-promoting measures. Care should be taken to minimize disruption of sleep when observations are made. Shielded flashlights are preferred to overhead lights. The nurse must move quietly and avoid making noise. Gentle touch is used for palpation if the pulse must be monitored. If a required procedure is likely to interrupt sleep, it should be delayed until REM sleep ceases.

During sleep, the client's respirations should be monitored. Although serious respiratory depression is unlikely with therapeutic doses of sedative–hypnotics, it can occur in clients who are unusually sensitive to sedatives, in the obese, and in those with respiratory disease. Respiratory rates in adults should not drop below 12 breaths per minute.

Postmedication Care.

The day after the client receives a sedative–hypnotic drug, the nurse should assess its effectiveness in producing restful sleep or sedation as well as any other residual effects. The client should be questioned about subjective feelings of fatigue or dysphoria and the occurrence of daymares. If significant hangover is evident, the prescriber may need to reduce the dose or change to another drug.

Regular use of hypnotic drugs over long periods should be avoided. If chronic health problems make this impossible, the client must be monitored closely for personality changes that could indicate deprivation of sleep phases such as REM sleep. Such changes, or a decrease in or failure of sedative effect, indicate that the soporific should be discontinued. Hypnotic drugs must be withdrawn gradually from clients who have received them over a period of time. Abrupt withdrawal is likely to precipitate uncomfortable and dangerous abstinence syndromes. During the weaning period, the client should be assessed for wakefulness, restlessness, agitation, or depression. If pronounced symptoms develop, seizure precautions must be taken and the prescriber should be asked to increase the hypnotic dose temporarily or slow the weaning schedule.

Client Education.

Inability to sleep may arise because of erratic activity/rest patterns, daytime naps, high levels of stimulation before retiring, use of stimulating drugs, lack of physical exercise, and excessive stress. The nurse can do much to reduce the need for hypnotic drugs and enhance their effects by teaching clients techniques to promote rest and sleep. Clients may learn to modify their lifestyles in several ways to achieve this goal. The nurse should instruct the client about measures such as:

Techniques of stress management to prevent excessive production of corticosteroids and epinephrine, CNS stimulants

Regular, active exercise during the day; exercise should be completed several hours before bedtime to avoid residual stimulation from the activity.

Avoiding stimulant drugs such as caffeine

Going to bed and arising at regular times, allowing a period of sleep sufficient for the client's needs

Reducing stimuli before bedtime (eg, sedentary activity, absence of bright lights and loud noises)

Comfortable bed and comfortable nightclothes

Adequate ventilation in the sleeping area

Having a warm, protein snack rich in tryptophan (eg, milk) before retiring

Eliminating pain through pain control techniques and, when necessary, the use of a bedtime dose of analgesic

Using routine comfort measures before retiring to avoid interrupting rest

Eliminating disturbing stimuli after retiring by using eye shades and ear plugs

Clients for whom hypnotic drugs are prescribed should be instructed about the risks of use. Supplies of the drugs should not be kept on the bedside table. A place should be chosen that is far enough away from the bedroom so that the client is roused to full alertness before repeating a dose. Clients who take hypnotics can develop amnesia about drug use; it is thought that many cases of sedative–hypnotic overdose arise from repeated doses taken by a client during wakeful periods. Measures should be taken to prevent such automatism. It may be necessary to place drug supplies under the control of a second person.

The client should avoid ambulation after onset of hypnotic drug effect unless assistance is available. Impaired psychomotor function and judgment while under the influence of these drugs increase the risk of accidental injury. Making critical decisions and using power machinery (including cars) should be avoided while drug effects persist.

Some cases of chronic overdose arise because clients receive prescriptions from more than one prescriber, each of whom is unaware of the other's recommendations. Clients should be cautioned to inform each prescriber of all drugs being used. OTC preparations may also increase the effects of hypnotics; use of these drugs should also be disclosed to the nurse and the prescriber. Clients should be warned specifically of the risk of concurrent use of more than one CNS depressant. Of particular importance is the use of opioids, tranquilizers, and alcohol, all of which depress the CNS. Antihistamines also have an additive effect when taken with sedatives. Dangerous combinations of drugs are more likely to be identified if the client purchases all medicines from the same pharmacy. Most pharmacists maintain drug profiles on their clients and monitor the records for inappropriate or potentially dangerous drug combinations.

❖ CHECKLIST OF NURSING ACTIONS

When Sedative–Hypnotics Are Prescribed

- ❑ Use all available nursing measures to promote sleep.
- ❑ Assess the risk of drug use by taking a careful history. Ask specifically about previous use of hypnotics, porphyria, and chronic obstructive pulmonary disease. Note the client's attitude toward the use of sedation.
- ❑ Monitor the client's sleep to evaluate the effectiveness of the drug and to detect hypopnea or other adverse reaction to the drug.
- ❑ Institute safety measures to protect clients from accidental injury while sedated.
- ❑ Evaluate clients during waking hours for residual effects of the drug.
- ❑ Assess clients who use hypnotics over a long term for personality changes or other signs of sleep phase deprivation.
- ❑ Reevaluate the hypnotic regimen if a need for increased dosage becomes apparent.
- ❑ Teach clients who control their own drugs about safe management techniques.
- ❑ To enhance the effects of hypnotics, use nursing measures to promote rest and sleep.

When Overdose and Toxicity Occur

- ❑ Administer care supportive of respiration and circulation.
- ❑ Assist with medical measures to remove the drug from body systems (eg, gastric lavage, hemodialysis).
- ❑ Give supportive nursing care appropriate to the client's condition.

When Drug Abuse and Dependence Are a Risk

- ❑ Teach self-care and parenting skills designed to promote robust physical and emotional health.
- ❑ Inform clients of the properties of sedating drugs and the risks inherent in their use.

References

*Acute Pain Management Clinical Guideline Panel. (1992). *Acute pain management: operative or medical procedures and trauma.* AHCPR Pub. No. 92-0032. Rockville, MD: Agency for Health Care Policy and Research, Public Health Service, U.S. Department of Health and Human Services.

*Class P. (1991). Nursing considerations for the malignant hyperthermia patient. *Curr Rev PACN, 13*(11), 81–88.

Kales A. (1968). Sleep and dreams: recent research in clinical aspects. *Ann Intern Med, 68*, 1078.

*McCaffery M, Beebe A. (1989). *Pain: Clinical manual for nursing practice.* St. Louis: CV Mosby.

Smith I, White PF. (1992). Use of intravenous adjuvants during local and regional anesthesia (monitored anesthesia care). *Curr Rev PACN, 14*(6), 45–52.

Smith I, White PF. (1994). Anesthesia for ambulatory surgery. *Curr Rev Nurs Anesth, 16*(20), 169–180.

Willens JS. (1994). Giving fentanyl for pain outside the OR. *Am J Nurs*, February, 24–28.

Bibliography

Aker J. (1994). A safe approach to monitored anesthesia care. *Curr Rev Nurs Anesth, 17*(12), 113–120.

Berger JJ. (1994) Postoperative pain management. *Curr Rev Nurs Anesth, 17*(11), 101–112.

Brockopp DY, Warden S, Colcough G, Brockoff GW. (1993). Nursing knowledge: acute postoperative pain management in the elderly. *J Gerontol Nurs,* November, 31–37.

*Cancer Pain Management Clinical Guideline Panel. (1994). *Management of cancer pain.* AHCPR Pub. No. 94-0592. Rockville, MD: Agency for Health Care Policy and Research, Public Health Service, U.S. Department of Health and Human Services.

Council on Scientific Affairs, American Medical Association. (1993). The use of pulse oximetry during conscious sedation. *JAMA, 270*(12), 1463–1468.

Ferrell BR. (1993). Pain management. Cancer and the older adult. *Elderly Care, 5*(3), 29–31.

*Recommended for further reading.

Heath ML, Thomas VJ. (1993). *Patient-controlled analgesia.* New York: Oxford University Press.

Idemoto BK. (1995) Propofol: a new treatment in intensive care unit sedation. *AACN Clinical Issues, 6*(1), 135–142.

Lindaman CL. (1995) Talking to physicians about pain control. *Am J Nurs,* Jan, 36–37.

Maxwell L. (1992). Acute pain management: IV patient-controlled analgesia places patient in control. *Canadian Operating Room Nursing Journal,* Sept–Oct, 12–15).

McEvoy GK. (ed). (1991). *Drug information 91,* p. 1153. Bethesda, MD: American Society of Hospital Pharmacists and American Pain Society.

Melzack R. (1990). The tragedy of needless pain. *Sci Am, 262*(2), 27–33.

Miller CA. (1993). Intervention for sleep pattern disturbances. *Geriatr Nurs, 14*(5), 235–236.

National Institutes of Health Consensus Conference. (1990). *Treatment of sleep disorder of older people.* NIH Consensus Statement.

Partridge C. (1994). Pain in the confused patient. *Elderly Care, 6*(5), 19–21.

Ryan P, Vortherms R, Ward S. (1994). Cancer pain: knowledge, attitudes of pharmacologic management. *J Gerontol Nurs,* January, 7–15.

Somerson SJ, Husted CW, Scilia MR. (1995) Insights into conscious sedation. *Am J Nurs,* June, 26–32.

Stanton-Hicks M. (1994). Is PCA an effective method of treating postoperative pain? *Curr Rev PACN, 16*(19), 169–176.

Stoller MK. (1994). Economic effects of insomnia. *Clin Ther, 16*(5),

Thomas N. (1994). Patient-controlled analgesia. *Elderly Care, 6*(3), 23–26.

*Todd KH, Samroo N, Hoffman JR. (1993). Ethnicity as a risk factor for inadequate emergency department analgesia. *JAMA, 269*(12), 1537–1539.

Williams-Russo P, Sharrock NE, Mattis S, Szatrowski TP, Charlson ME. (1995). Cognitive effects after epidural vs general anesthesia in older adults. *JAMA, 274*(1), 44–50.

World Health Organization. (1986). *Cancer pain relief.* Geneva: World Health Association.

*Recommended for further reading.

For more information and sample tests and activities, refer to Chapter 18 in the Student Workbook for Clinical Pharmacology and Nursing Management, 5th edition, available through your bookstore.

19

Drugs That Control Seizures

Anticonvulsant drugs are used to eliminate or reduce seizure activity in persons subject to epilepsy and other seizure disorders. They control seizures by raising the seizure threshold and limiting the spread of neuronal activity from initiating foci.

Pathophysiology of Seizures

Seizures are uncontrollable physiologic responses to abnormal electric discharges in the cerebral cortex. These responses are usually sporadic, synchronous, rhythmic, and self-limiting. Seizure disorders known as epilepsy indicate neuronal hyperexcitability but not the underlying cause for the condition. The seizures are considered symptoms rather than disease entities.

The nervous system normally exhibits a basal level of excitability that increases with nervous system activity. Test results show that whenever the degree of excitability exceeds a critical threshold, called the seizure threshold, electrical impulse transmission becomes pronounced and generalized, stimulating abnormal discharges in nerve cells that would otherwise not be active. In seizure disorders, the seizure threshold is either lower than normal or one or more areas in the brain spontaneously discharge, triggering generalized nerve activity. In some cases, both phenomena occur. If the entire cortex and diencephalon are involved, the person loses consciousness.

The physiologic changes that occur during seizures are unresponsive to the usual inhibitory controls of the nervous system and to voluntary inhibition. Experts think that epilepsy is associated with dysfunction of the brain neurotransmitters, causing an imbalance between the excitatory and inhibitory mechanisms of the central nervous system (CNS). Some endogenous CNS stimulants that have been studied include the amino acids aspartate and glutamate. An important inhibitory substance that has been studied is gamma-aminobutyric acid (GABA), an inhibitory neurotransmitter. When the person experiences a reduction in GABA-mediated inhibition, seizures may occur.

Seizure activity reflects the areas of the nervous system affected by the abnormal electrical discharges. Epileptic seizures are assigned to two broad categories: generalized seizures and partial seizures. Generalized seizures begin simultaneously from both sides of the brain; partial seizures begin in a localized area of the brain. Each category is further differentiated (Table 19-1).

Factors Affecting Seizure Occurrence

Three factors affect the occurrence of seizures:

    Level of the basal seizure threshold
    Presence of foci that initiate abnormal stimuli
    Irritation of nerve cells as a result of biochemical changes in the body.

The basal seizure threshold varies from person to person and is influenced by genetic inheritance and environmental factors. Because nerve function and excitability are affected by the biochemical environment, inherited metabolic patterns that influence brain chemistry play a major part in determining predominant nerve activity patterns and vulnerability to seizures. A low basal threshold predisposes a person to seizure activity and seizure disorders, but it does not by itself determine whether a person will develop epilepsy.

Foci in the nervous system that are hyperirritable tend to initiate abnormal stimuli that can spread to adjacent tissue. These foci may develop because of inflammation, abnormal pressure, or other factors. Often, they represent scars from previous lesions that have contracted or have undergone other changes over time that irritate adjacent tissue.

Changes in body chemistry that increase nerve irritability include hypoxia, hypoglycemia, hypocalcemia, hypomagnesemia, alkalosis, high levels of stimulant hormones (eg, epinephrine), and the use of stimulant drugs. A high fever increases CNS activity and the risk of seizures. Deprivation of oxygen and glucose, two substances essential for normal brain function, also can induce convulsions. Such changes lower the seizure threshold and increase the likelihood of seizure activity.

Theoretically, any one of the above factors may precipitate seizures. Usually, however, more than one factor is

Table 19-1. Classification and Management of Common Seizures

Seizure	Characteristics	Conventional Anticonvulsants	New Anticonvulsants
Partial Seizures			
Simple partial	Diverse manifestations depending on site of cortex Key feature: no loss of consciousness Motor symptoms (jacksonian) Special sensory or somatosensory (jacksonian) symptoms Autonomic symptoms Psychic symptoms	carbamazepine phenytoin phenobarbital primidone valproic acid	gabapentin lamotrigine felbamate topiramate
Complex partial	Impaired consciousness (30 sec–2 min) often accompanied by purposeless movements Cognitive symptoms Affective symptoms Psychosensory symptoms Psychomotor symptoms Mixture of symptoms	carbamazepine phenobarbital phenytoin primidone valproic acid	gabapentin lamotrigine felbamate topiramate
Partial with secondarily generalized tonic-clonic seizures	Simple or complex partial seizure that becomes a tonic-clonic seizure; for example, sustained muscle contractions followed by periods of muscle contraction (tonic), alternating with relaxation (clonic) 1–2 min of loss of consciousness	carbamazepine phenobarbital phenytoin primidone valproic acid	gabapentin lamotrigine
Generalized Seizures			
Absence (petit mal)	Abrupt interruption of consciousness (usually less than 30 sec); may be accompanied by staring, eyelid fluttering, head nodding	clonazepam ethosuximide valproic acid	lamotrigine
Myoclonic	Sudden, violent muscle contractions involving whole body, extremity, part of extremity, or head	valproic acid	
Tonic-clonic (grand mal)	Most common seizure; tonic extremity rigidity followed by massive clonic jerking	carbamazepine topiramate phenobarbital phenytoin primidone valproic acid	topiramate

required. In a given situation, it may be impossible to identify the factors responsible for a seizure. The family health history may or may not identify a pattern of epilepsy. Although seizure patterns indicating an irritable focus imply localized brain damage at some time in the past, the initial insult may not be known. (Among the suspected causes are prenatal or perinatal hypoxia and head trauma.) Internal chemical changes related to emotional reactions or altered metabolism are rarely obvious causes.

As symptoms, seizures suggest some primary neurologic disease (eg, a brain tumor) that must be diagnosed and treated, or they may be the outward manifestation of biochemical imbalance or residual scars from past injury to the nervous system. In either case, abnormal nerve discharges must be controlled. Frequent seizures may cause further brain damage; if prolonged—as in status epilepticus—they are life-threatening.

Treatment With Drugs

Drug treatment of seizure disorders aims to prevent abnormal nerve activity by decreasing the discharge of impulses from initiating foci, thereby inhibiting the spread of impulses. This may be accomplished by inhibiting the movement of sodium, potassium, and calcium ions across the membranes, interfering with amino acid–mediated excitation, decreasing focal activity, or damping the post-tetanic potentiation of synaptic transmission or potentiation of inhibitory pathways in the CNS. These actions stabilize nerve cell membranes and elevate the seizure threshold. Medication can achieve complete seizure control in about 50% of epileptic clients. Another 25% report significant improvement with antiseizure drugs.

The ideal antiseizure drug would prevent seizures and would produce no side effects; unfortunately, no such agent exists. Adverse effects of current drugs range from mild CNS impairment to death from such entities as aplastic anemia or hepatic failure. Sedation is common but may decrease with continued drug therapy. Nystagmus, ataxia, tremor, dizziness, hyperactivity, or behavioral changes may occur, especially in cases of drug toxicity. Long-term phenobarbital therapy, multi-drug therapy, or use of high dosages may impair intellectual function. Gastrointestinal (GI) symptoms may also occur; nausea, vomiting, and diarrhea are most common. If pronounced, they may interfere with retention or absorption of the medications, thereby lowering serum levels and allowing seizures to occur.

To decrease adverse effects and toxicity, seizures are initially treated with a single drug. If this drug does not control the seizures, another drug may be substituted. For clients with several different types of seizures, multiple drugs may be required. When antiseizure medication is initiated, plasma drug levels should be assessed. However, as treatment continues, the plasma level is not always the best indication of the effectiveness of therapy because plasma levels of some drugs do not correlate well with the dose. In such cases, careful clinical assessment of the client affords the most accurate indication of drug effects and toxicity.

Treatment regimens rely heavily on CNS depressant drugs (Table 19-2), although at least one stimulant drug is used to manage absence seizures (petit mal). Among drugs used for controlling epilepsy are the hydantoins, barbiturates, benzodiazepines, succinimides, carbamazepine, and newer agents such as gabapentin and lamotrigine. Oxazolidinediones, magnesium sulfate, and acetazolamide are also used in selected situations (Box 19-1).

Hydantoins

Hydantoin drugs are used primarily to control major motor and psychomotor seizures. They are the most frequently prescribed medications for seizures in the United States. Individual drugs are also effective for other types of epilepsy—for instance, phenytoin for autonomic seizures as well as ethotoin and mephenytoin for focal seizures. Hydantoin drugs are not useful for absence seizures and may actually increase the frequency of these seizures. The hydantoins are not strong CNS depressants and usually do not decrease normal sensory function. Because it is the most frequently prescribed of the hydantoin drugs, phenytoin will be discussed in detail.

Phenytoin

Pharmacodynamics. Phenytoin stabilizes cell membranes and decreases the movement of sodium, calcium, and potassium ions involved in depolarization and propagation of membrane action potentials. Although these effects have not been demonstrated by therapeutic levels of the drug, they may support its therapeutic actions. Phenytoin decreases focal activity in the nervous system, reduces post-tetanic potentiation of synaptic transmission, decreases the spread of the seizure process from an active focus, limits the development of maximal seizure activity, and reduces abnormal hyperexcitability toward a normal level. It causes few sedative or hypnotic effects. In the heart, phenytoin reduces the force of myocardial contraction, depresses pacemaker action, improves atrioventricular conduction (especially when depressed by digitalis), and prolongs the refractory period.

Pharmacokinetics. Phenytoin is absorbed slowly whether administered intramuscularly (IM) or orally. Because the drug precipitates in the tissues, the IM route should be avoided when possible. Phenytoin is sometimes ad-

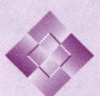

Box 19-1
Drugs Used to Control Seizures

- hydantoins
- barbiturates
- benzodiazepines
- succinimides
- carbamazepine
- valproic acid
- gabapentin
- lamotrigine
- topiramate
- oxazolidinediones*
- magnesium sulfate*
- acetazolamide*

*Used in selected situations.

ministered intravenously (IV). GI absorption is variable. Bioavailability among commercial preparations is also inconsistent. When prompt-release forms are used, plasma drug levels peak in 1.5 to 3 hours, whereas levels of extended-release capsules peak in 4 to 12 hours.

Phenytoin is highly bound to both tissue and plasma proteins; about 90% binds to plasma proteins. The drug distributes widely. Levels in the cerebrospinal fluid (CSF) are equal to levels of unbound drug in the plasma.

Clients vary widely in their ability to metabolize phenytoin. With normal renal function, less than 5% of phenytoin is excreted unchanged by the kidneys. The rest is degraded by the liver's microsomal enzymes, after which it is secreted in bile and becomes part of the enterohepatic cycle. The drug's inactivation by the liver microsomal enzyme system can be altered by other drugs. Eventually, the metabolites are excreted by the kidneys. Metabolism in the liver is a saturable process—thus, small increases in dosage can result in substantial increases in the plasma phenytoin concentration. Plasma half-time ranges from 8 to 60 hours but averages 24 hours.

Therapeutic and toxic effects correlate most closely with unbound serum levels of the drug. Although these levels are not always proportionate to total serum levels, the total serum levels are used most frequently to monitor drug levels. The recommended total phenytoin serum levels for therapeutic effect range from 10 to 20 µg/mL. Drug therapy begins with relatively low doses that are increased gradually until the optimal therapeutic response is obtained.

Therapeutic Uses. Phenytoin is used to control seizures in most forms of epilepsy except absence seizures. Phenytoin is sometimes administered IV as an adjunct in treating status epilepticus. Phenytoin is also used in treating disturbed, nonepileptic, psychotic clients; seizures associated with head trauma and increased

Text continues on page 369.

Table 19-2. Anticonvulsant Drugs

Drug Name	Preparation	Usual Dosage	Additional Information
Hydantoins			
phenytoin (Dilantin, Diphenylan)	Capsules, chewable tablets, and suspension for oral use Extended-release forms Solution for injection	Adults: 300–600 mg/day, divided in 3 doses Children: 4–8 mg/kg, divided in 2 or 3 doses Do not exceed infusion rate of 50 mg/min in adults or 1–3 mg/kg in neonates. PC: C	Therapeutic serum concentrations (10–20 μg/mL) may be achieved more rapidly by giving a loading dose (1 g to adults or 500 mg to children). Initial dosage should be reduced for the elderly, newborns, and others with impaired hepatic function. Phenytoin is frequently used with phenobarbital for the control of major motor seizures. A frequent side effect is gingival hypertrophy. Absorption of IM doses may be erratic due to crystallization of the drug in the injection site.
ethotoin (Peganone)	Oral tablets	Adults: 2–3 g/day, divided in 4 to 6 doses, administered after food Children: 500 mg–1 g/day, divided in 4 to 6 doses, administered after food PC: C	Ethotoin does not have the antiarrhythmic properties of phenytoin. Ethotoin is both less effective and less toxic than phenytoin; it is usually used in conjunction with other anticonvulsant drugs.
mephenytoin (Mesantoin)	Oral tablets	Adults: 200–600 mg/day, divided in 3 equal doses Children: 100–400 mg/day, 3–15 mg/kg/day, or 100–450 mg/m^2/day, divided in 3 equal doses PC: C	Mephenytoin causes greater sedation and risk of serious blood dyscrasias than phenytoin. Mephenytoin is used for the management of grand mal, jacksonian, and psychomotor seizures in persons who are refractory to less toxic anticonvulsants.
fosphenytoin (Cerebyx)	Solutions for IM and IV use	Doses, concentrations and infusion rates are expressed in phenytoin equivalents (PE); in status epilepticus, loading dose of 15–20 mg PE/kg to be administered at 100–150 mg PE/min; in nonemergency situations, loading dose: 10–20 mg PE/kg; initial daily maintenance dosage is 4–6 mg PE/kg/day	Before infusing, dilute in 5% dextrose or 0.9% saline solution to a concentration of 1.5–25 mg PE/mL; should not exceed 150 mg PE/min
Barbiturates and Derivatives			
amobarbital (Amytal)	Powder Oral tablets Powder for preparing solutions for IM injection or IV infusion	(As an anticonvulsant used only to treat acute seizure states) Usual dosage for adults: IV infusion at a *maximum* rate of 100 mg/min (ie, 1 mL of 10% solution over 1 min) For insomnia: 60–200 mg for adults; for children: 2–3 mg/kg For sedation: 60–150 mg daily, divided in 2 or 3 doses for adults; for children: 2 mg/kg/day, divided in 4 doses PC: B	Preparation of solutions: add diluent and rotate; do not shake; use within 30 min. IM doses must be injected deeply to avoid sterile abscesses or tissue sloughing. Do not use for insomnia for more than 2 weeks. After long-term use, wean over at least 5–6 days.

KEY: PC = pregnancy category (see Appendix A).
Can = Canadian trade name.

(continued)

Table 19-2. (Continued)

Drug Name	Preparation	Usual Dosage	Additional Information
Barbiturates and Derivatives (continued)			
phenobarbital (Barbital, Luminal; *Can.* Solfoton)	Tablets, capsules, elixir, solution, powder, and extended-release capsules for oral use Rectal suppositories Solutions and powders for preparing solutions for injection	Adults: 100–300 mg/day, preferably in a single dose at bedtime Children: 3–5 mg/kg daily, in 1 or 2 doses PC: D	Phenobarbital may be used for initial treatment of all forms of epilepsy except petit mal. It is often given concurrently with phenytoin or other anticonvulsants. Phenobarbital may impair intellectual ability.
mephobarbital (Mebaral)	Powder Oral tablets	Adults: 400–600 mg/day, taken as a single dose or in divided doses Children younger than 5 yr: 16–32 mg tid or qid Children older than 5 yr: 32–64 mg tid or qid PC: D	Mephobarbital is metabolized to phenobarbital. Mephobarbital is used in place of phenobarbital in the management of seizures in persons who exhibit undesirable reactions to phenobarbital (excessive drowsiness, hyperexcitability, irritability, or mood disturbance).
metharbital (Gemonil)	Oral tablets	Adults: 100–800 mg/day, divided in 1 to 3 doses Children: 50–100 mg qid or tid; or 5–15 mg/kg/day, in divided doses	Metharbital is used in the management of seizures in persons who have adverse reactions to phenobarbital.
primidone (Myidone, Mysoline)	Chewable tablets and suspension for oral use	Adults and children 8 yr or older: 250 mg tid or qid Children younger than 8 yr: 125–250 mg tid; 10–25 mg/kg/day, in divided doses; or 1.25 g/m²/day, divided in 2 to 4 doses PC: D	Primidone is considered by some physicians to be the drug of choice for the treatment of psychomotor epilepsy. Primidone is partially (15%–25%) metabolized to phenobarbital.
Oxazolidinediones			
paramethadione (Paradione)	Capsules and solution for oral use	Adults: 900–2,400 mg/day, divided in 3 or 4 equal doses Children: 300–900 mg/day and up, depending on the appearance of toxic signs and symptoms PC: D	Paramethadione is used in the management of petit mal (absence seizures) in persons who have not responded to other anticonvulsants (eg, ethosuximide).
trimethadione (Tridione)	Tablets, capsules, and solution for oral use	Adults: 900–2,400 mg/day, divided in 3 or 4 doses Children: 40 mg/kg/day, divided in 3 or 4 doses PC: D	Trimethadione acts selectively to suppress petit mal epilepsy. Trimethadione is used only for refractory absence seizures because of its high toxic potential.
Succinimides			
ethosuximide (Zarontin)	Capsules and solution for oral use	20 mg/kg/day (maximum of 1.5 g for adults or 1 g for children) in divided doses PC: C	Ethosuximide is considered to be the agent of choice for petit mal seizures.
methsuximide (Celontin)	Oral capsules	10 mg/kg/day, in divided doses; or 600 mg/m²/day, in divided doses PC: C	Methsuximide is used in the management of petit mal (absence seizures). Because it does not usually precipitate grand mal (tonic-clonic seizures), it is particularly useful in managing (with other anticonvulsants) combined absence and tonic-clonic seizures.

KEY: PC = pregnancy category (see Appendix A).
Can = Canadian trade name.

(continued)

Table 19-2. (Continued)

Drug Name	Preparation	Usual Dosage	Additional Information
Succinimides (continued)			
phensuximide (Milontin)	Oral capsules	1–3 g/d, divided in 2 or 3 doses PC: D	Phensuximide is the least toxic and least effective of the succinimide-derivative anticonvulsants. Phensuximide is used in the management of petit mal (absence seizures).
Valproate			
valproic acid (Depakene, Depakote; *Can:* Epival)	Capsules, enteric-coated tablets, and solution for oral use	15–60 mg/kg/day, in one or more doses PC: D	Valproate is used to treat absence seizures, both simple and complex. Valproic acid capsules must *not* be chewed (to prevent local irritation to the mouth and throat). GI side effects can be minimized by starting with low doses and increasing gradually. A plasma level of 50–100 µg/mL has been suggested as the therapeutic range.
Benzodiazepines			
clonazepam (Klonopin; *Can:* Rivotril)	Oral tablets	Adults: 1.5–20 mg/day, divided in 2 or 3 doses Children: 0.1–0.2 mg/kg/day, divided in 2 or 3 doses PC: C	Clonazepam is useful in the treatment of petit mal and myoclonic seizures in children. Also used to treat akinetic seizures.
diazepam (Valium)	Solutions for injection	Not used for maintenance In the management of status epilepticus: Adults: 5–10 mg q 10 min up to a maximal dose of 30 mg (this regimen may be repeated q2–4h up to a maximal dose of 100 mg/24 h) PC: D	Diazepam is the drug of choice for initial treatment of status epilepticus (IV route preferred).
Miscellaneous Agents			
carbamazepine (Epitol, Tapazine, Tegretol; *Can:* Apo-Carbamazepine)	Oral tablets and chewable tablets	Adults and children 12 yr or older: 800–1.2 g/day, divided in 3 or 4 doses Children 6–12 yr: 400–800 mg/day, divided in 3 or 4 doses PC: C	Carbamazepine is structurally related to the tricyclic antidepressants. Carbamazepine is extremely toxic to a small percentage of persons and is not used unless other anticonvulsants have been ineffective in controlling seizures.
magnesium sulfate	Solutions for IM or IV injection	Not used for maintenance In the management of seizures due to toxemia of pregnancy: IV: up to 150 mg/min IM: Adults: *Initially:* 8–10 g (as a 50% solution), divided in two doses and administered in the buttocks; thereafter, 4–5 g q4h; dosage is adjusted according to response and must be discontinued as soon as the desired therapeutic effect is obtained PC: B	Magnesium sulfate is useful in the treatment of convulsions of eclampsia or preeclampsia of pregnancy.

KEY: PC = pregnancy category (see Appendix A).
Can = Canadian trade name.

(continued)

Table 19-2. (Continued)

Drug Name	Preparation	Usual Dosage	Additional Information
Miscellaneous Agents (continued)			
acetazolamide (Ak-Zol, Diamox)	Tablets and sustained-release capsules for oral use Powder for preparing solutions for injection	Adults and children: 8–30 mg/kg/day, divided in 1 to 4 doses PC: C	Acetazolamide is used in the management of refractory epilepsy, especially petit mal and grand mal.
gabapentin (Neurontin)	Oral capsules	900–1,800 mg/day in 3 divided doses PC: C	Used as adjunctive therapy in partial seizures with or without secondary generalization; safety and effectiveness in children under 12 not established; false-positive result on Ames N-Multistix SG dipstick for urinary protein has occurred.
lamotrigine (Lamictal)	Oral tablets	Initial dose in adults *not* taking hepatic enzyme-inducing drugs or valproic acid: 50 mg daily for 2 weeks, followed by 100 mg in divided doses for 2 weeks; *maintenance:* 300–500 mg/day in divided doses. In patients taking hepatic enzyme-inducing drugs and valproic acid: initial dose, 25 mg every other day for 2 weeks, followed by 25 mg daily for 2 weeks with a maintenance dose of 100–150 mg daily. PC: C	Indicated for adjunctive therapy of partial seizures in adults over age 16
phenacemide (Phenurone)	Oral tablets	Adults: 2–3 g/day, divided in 3 equal doses Children: 0.75–1.25 g/day, divided in 3 equal doses PC: D	Phenacemide is extremely toxic and is used only when other less toxic anticonvulsants are ineffective in controlling seizures.
topiramate (Topamax)	Oral tablets	Optimal dose in vicinity of 400 mg/day in 2 divided doses	Relatively narrow therapeutic range

KEY: PC = pregnancy category (see Appendix A).
Can = Canadian trade name.

---

intracranial pressure; trigeminal and related neuralgias; and cardiac arrhythmias.

Dosage and Administration. The daily dose phenytoin is divided initially to minimize GI irritation and toxic effects. After the client's condition stabilizes, the use of extended-release phenytoin capsules (one daily) may be considered. IV solutions of phenytoin must be administered slowly to avoid cardiovascular collapse and marked CNS depression. The rate must not exceed 50 mg/min (even slower in elderly clients and those who cannot metabolize the drug at a normal rate). IV phenytoin must be administered with normal saline solution because it is incompatible (forms a precipitate) with dextrose and acidic solutions.

Adverse Reactions. Side effects are generally dose-related, so dosage should be carefully regulated. Adverse reactions to phenytoin are common and can be serious. They vary widely and may involve the GI, cardiovascular, integumentary, lymphatic, hepatic, or hematologic system or the CNS. Nausea, vomiting, constipation,

epigastric pain, difficulty in eating, and weight loss can occur. The drug depresses pacemaker activity in the heart and may cause arrhythmias. Early neurologic changes include nystagmus, ataxia, and visual changes. These may progress to nervousness, dizziness, insomnia, confusion, tremor, and chorea. Moreover, phenytoin can damage the cerebellum, causing permanent ataxia.

Skin reactions range from rashes to serious conditions such as systemic lupus erythematosus or Stevens-Johnson syndrome, a severe form of erythema multiforme. A syndrome resembling mononucleosis may occur. Lymphadenopathy associated with phenytoin may be manifested by lymph node hyperplasia, lymphoma, or Hodgkin's disease. In addition to the liver changes seen in the mononucleosis syndrome, toxic hepatitis or other liver abnormalities may develop. Phenytoin decreases intestinal absorption of folic acid and can cause anemia. Anemia usually responds to folic acid therapy, but bone marrow depression is sometimes fatal.

Phenytoin causes cosmetic changes. A very common side effect (20%–30% incidence), especially in children, is hyperplasia of the gums. This may become so severe that surgical removal is required. Excess hair growth and coarsening of the features may also develop.

Phenytoin is a suspected carcinogen and teratogen. It may cause lymphoma and Hodgkin's disease in recipients. In children exposed in utero, it may cause a fetal hydantoin syndrome, congenital defects such as spina bifida, or malignancies (including neuroblastoma).

When administered IV, phenytoin can cause cardiovascular collapse or CNS depression. The drug irritates blood vessels and may cause phlebitis. Rapid administration tends to cause hypotension and to damage blood vessels. As noted above, phenytoin can damage the cerebellum, causing permanent ataxia.

Drug–Drug Interactions. Phenytoin interacts with numerous other drugs, usually by changing the rate of drug metabolism. It stimulates the metabolic breakdown of the hormones T_3 and T_4, estrogens, and corticosteroids. It can cause signs and symptoms of hypothyroidism in clients with marginal thyroid function, as well as in clients with known hypothyroidism who are taking hormone replacements. Phenytoin also decreases the effectiveness of corticosteroid medications when taken concurrently. The metabolic breakdown of phenytoin decreases (causing blood levels to increase) with concurrent administration of ethanol (alcohol), chloramphenicol, cimetidine, dicumarol, disulfiram, isoniazid, miconazole, or certain sulfonamides. Not only do carbamazepine and theophylline decrease phenytoin levels, but their own levels in the blood are reduced by phenytoin. Cisplatin also lowers serum phenytoin levels.

Interaction between phenytoin and phenobarbital may cause blood levels of either drug to decrease or increase. Mechanisms involved in these changes may include induction of microsomal enzymes in the liver, competition for binding sites on plasma proteins, and changes in intestinal absorption.

Drug–Food Interactions. Phenytoin interacts with folic acid, calcium, and vitamin D, leading to decreased absorption. Phenytoin absorption may be further decreased by enteral nutritional supplements.

Precautions and Contraindications. Phenytoin is contraindicated in clients with allergic hypersensitivity to it and should be discontinued at the first sign of allergic reaction, such as rash or dyspnea. To prevent permanent damage to the cerebellum, the drug should be discontinued at the first sign of ataxia.

When phenytoin is administered IV, vital signs should be monitored. Clients with known cardiac disease, elderly clients, and those with unstable vital signs should be continuously monitored via electrocardiography. Because it is teratogenic, phenytoin should not be used during pregnancy. When its use is necessary, blood phenytoin levels should be monitored closely. Mothers taking phenytoin should not breast-feed (see Focus On Hydantoin Anticonvulsants: Similarities and Differences).

Barbiturates

All barbiturates provide some anticonvulsant activity, but only two—phenobarbital and mephobarbital—are used for suppressing seizure activity. A third agent, metharbital, is now rarely used for seizure control. Because phenobarbital is effective and inexpensive and was thought to be relatively nontoxic, it is discussed here as the prototype barbiturate anticonvulsant.

Phenobarbital

Phenobarbital was the first organic agent found effective in treating seizures. It is still widely used; it has relatively low toxicity and is inexpensive. It has been useful with other anticonvulsants, particularly phenytoin.

Pharmacodynamics. The anticonvulsant activity of phenobarbital is relatively nonselective. It elevates the seizure threshold and limits the spread of seizure activity. These effects appear to stem from the potentiation of inhibitory pathways in the CNS. Phenobarbital stimulates GABA receptors, thereby inhibiting microsomal activity. However, its action on GABA is less than that of other barbiturates with more pronounced sedative properties. (Activation of GABA receptors inhibits neuronal activity.)

Pharmacokinetics. Taken orally, phenobarbital is absorbed slowly but relatively completely (70%–90%). Peak blood levels occur in 8 to 12 hours; peak brain levels occur 2 to 3 hours later. Delayed onset of action is also apparent with IV administration, which requires about 5 minutes for effects to appear. From 40% to 60% of a given dose binds to plasma proteins. Tissue binding, including that in the brain, occurs to a similar degree. Because phenobarbital is relatively nonlipophilic, it penetrates and leaves the brain slowly, resulting in both slow onset and long duration of effect.

Toxicity Alert: Phenytoin

Toxic effects of phenytoin are associated with blood concentrations exceeding the therapeutic range of 10 to 20 μg/mL. Although most clients tolerate blood concentrations under 25 μg/mL, some experience nystagmus, ataxia, and diplopia between 20 and 30 μg/mL; lethargy, drowsiness, and asterixis between 30 and 40 μg/mL; extreme lethargy between 40 and 50 μg/mL, and coma with concentrations exceeding 50 μg/mL. Certain persons with inherited enzyme deficiencies metabolize phenytoin slowly and exhibit toxic effects even with reduced dosages.

FOCUS ON

Hydantoin Anticonvulsants: Similarities and Differences

Similarities

Pharmacodynamics

These agents are thought to stabilize the neuron cell membrane at the cell body, axon, and synapse to limit the spread of seizure activity. They are thought to decrease focal activity, reduce post-tetanic potentiation of synaptic transmission, reduce spread of seizure progress from active focus, limit development of maximal seizure activity, and reduce abnormal hyperexcitability.

Pharmacokinetics

These agents are rapidly absorbed from the GI tract. They are primarily metabolized by the liver and excreted in the urine as metabolites; some are excreted in feces and breast milk, and small quantities are excreted in saliva.

Therapeutic Uses

These agents are used as anticonvulsants in all forms of epilepsy except petit mal seizures.

Adverse Reactions

These include: (CNS) ataxia, slurred speech, dizziness, insomnia, nervousness, nystagmus, behavioral changes, hand trembling; (CV) diminished pacemaker activity; (GI) nausea, vomiting, constipation, epigastric pain, difficulty eating, weight loss, gingival hyperplasia; (HEMA) anemia, bone marrow depression; (OTHER) rash, erythema multiforme, Stevens-Johnson syndrome, exfoliative dermatitis, lymphadenopathy, excessive hair growth.

Drug Interactions

Drug–Drug: Phenylbutazone, disulfiram, isoniazid, chloramphenicol, cimetidine, influenza vaccine, sulfonamides, benzodiazepines, omeprazole, methronidazole, ketoconazole, fluconazole, miconazole, succinamides, and felbamate may cause increase in hydantoin activity and toxicity; alcohol (chronic use), barbiturates, and warfarin may decrease hydantoin's activity; hydantoins may stimulate the metabolism and decrease the effectiveness of digitoxin, oral contraceptives, theophylline and cyclosporin; additive CNS depression with alcohol, antihistamines, antidepressants, narcotic analgesics and sedatives/hypnotics; additive cardiac depression may occur with propranol or lidocaine.

Drug–Food: Hydantoin may decrease absorption of folic acid.

Differences

- **Phenytoin** decreases sodium, potassium, and calcium ion influx into the cell involved in depolarization and propagation of membrane action potentials; it also decreases the force of heart muscle contraction, depresses pacemaker activity, improves atrioventricular conduction, and prolongs refractory period.
- **Fosphenytoin** is the water-soluble prodrug of phenytoin and limits the spread of seizure activity.

- **Phenytoin** is slowly absorbed orally or IM; IM route is not recommended because of erratic absorption; it may be given IV.
- **Phenytoin** excretion is enhanced by an alkaline urine.
- **Phenytoin** has a half-life averaging 22 hours, an onset of 1½–3 hours (4–12 hours with extended-release preparations).
- **Ethotoin** has a half-life of 3–9 hours.
- **Mephenytoin** has a half-life of 7 hours, peaks in 45 minutes to 4 hours with a duration of 24–48 hours.
- After parenteral administration **fosphenytoin** is rapidly converted to phenytoin; has a half-life of 24 hours; peaks in 40 min after IM injection and 15–40 min following IV administration.

- **Phenytoin** is used in treating status epilepticus, disturbed non-epileptic psychosis, trigeminal neuralgia, and cardiac arrhythmias.
- **Topiramate** is efficacious in treating Lennox-Gastaut syndrome.

- **Phenytoin** given IM can cause pain, necrosis, and inflammation at the injection site; IV administration may cause cardiovascular collapse and CNS depression.
- **Fosphenytoin** may cause hypotension, bradycardia (especially with rapid infusion rates), and hepatotoxicity.

- IV **phenytoin** and dopamine may cause severe hypotension and bradycardia; **fosphenytoin** may cause a false increase in serum digoxin levels and may interfere with T3 and T4 levels.

(continued)

Hydantoin: Anticonvulsants: Similarities and Differences (continued)

Similarities (continued)

Contraindications

These agents are contraindicated in persons with hypersensitivity to hydantoins.

Precautions

Use these agents cautiously in persons taking other hydantoins.

Nursing Considerations

Instruct in disease, treatment, drug therapy, adverse effects, and compliance; assess seizure disorder, including characteristics of seizures; never withdraw drug suddenly; warn client to avoid activities requiring mental alertness; monitor complete blood count and platelets initially and at frequent intervals; give drugs with meals to avoid gastric upset; warn that alcohol use may decrease the benefit of drug; evaluate for signs and symptoms of neurologic abnormalities including effects of drug; assist in eliminating or controlling factors that might precipitate seizure activity; begin drug therapy with a low dose, gradually increasing until adequate control is achieved; monitor behavior and neurologic function closely; administer regularly at consistent intervals; assess response to drug therapy; assist in maintaining an acceptable appearance; instruct in measures to diminish the side effects of the drug; and institute safety and privacy measures.

Differences (continued)

- **Ethotoin** is contraindicated in persons with hepatic or hematologic disorders.
- **Phenytoin** IV Is contraindicated in persons with sinus bradycardia, sinoatrial block, second- or third-degree atrioventricular block, or Stokes-Adams syndrome.
- **Fosphenytoin** should not be used in pregnancy or lactation unless seizures are life-threatening.

- Use **phenytoin** cautiously in persons with acute intermittent porphyria, hepatic or renal dysfunction, myocardial insufficiency, or respiratory depression, and in elderly or debilitated clients.
- **Fosphenytoin** should be used with caution in patients with history of cardiovascular disease, hepatic or renal impairment, hematologic disorders, diabetes mellitus, and hypothyroidism.

- When giving **phenacemide,** monitor liver function studies and urinalysis; instruct client to watch for personality changes; increase dosage slowly while other anticonvulsants are being discontinued; and assess for signs and symptoms of jaundice or hepatitis.
- When giving **phenytoin,** mix only with normal saline solution; give within 1 hour of preparation; and administer infusion over 30–60 minutes or as IV bolus at 50 mg/min. Instruct that **phenytoin** may change urine to pink, red, or reddish brown. Administer **phenytoin** into a large vein; avoid using hand veins because of tissue irritation; advise client not to change brands or dosage forms of **phenytoin** once regimen is stabilized.

Phenobarbital crosses the placenta and appears in the breast milk. About 75% of a dose is degraded by the hepatic microsomal enzymes; the rest is eliminated unchanged by the kidneys. Renal excretion is pH-dependent—it is most rapid when urine is mostly alkaline. Plasma half-life in adults is about 90 hours; in children it tends to be shorter and more variable, and in neonates it is longer. To maintain anticonvulsant activity without toxic effects, a serum level of 10 to 25 µg/mL is recommended. Daily maintenance doses may be divided to minimize toxicity.

Therapeutic Uses. Phenobarbital has been a primary agent for treating generalized tonic-clonic and partial seizures. It is ineffective in absence seizures. Phenobarbital is often given concurrently with phenytoin and may be part of a multidrug regimen in treating epilepsy characterized by several forms of seizures. It is used to prevent recurrent seizures in children who have experienced one or more febrile seizures and who are judged to be at high risk for repeated episodes. However, phenobarbital-related sedative effects and behavior disturbances have decreased its use as a primary agent for seizure control in children. Because of its slow onset of action, phenobarbital is seldom used in treating status epilepticus.

Dosage and Administration. The usual oral daily anticonvulsant dose of phenobarbital is 1 to 5 mg/kg (60–250 mg for adults). Several weeks are required to attain a steady plasma level. Loading doses (double dosage for the first 4 treatment days) can shorten the latency period, but these dosages produce marked sedation. Recommended dosages for beginning treatment in children are 3 to 5 mg/kg. Only one daily dose is required because phenobarbital has a long half-life. Dosages are adjusted in accord with the client's response to the regimen until the minimal effective dosage for maintenance is determined.

Plasma levels of phenobarbital may be used as a monitoring measure. Although these do not correspond exactly with therapeutic response, 10 to 25 µg/mL is the recommended therapeutic range. To prevent febrile convulsions, a level of at least 15 µg/mL is required. In most clients, levels of 30 to 60 µg/mL produce signs and symptoms of toxicity.

Adverse Reactions. CNS depression, GI upset, pain, and allergic hypersensitivity are among the adverse effects of anticonvulsant dosages. Other effects include respiratory depression, lethargy, vertigo, headache, nausea, vomiting, diarrhea, myalgia, neuralgia, and arthralgia. Sedation is the most frequent undesired effect, but with prolonged use clients usually become tolerant. Phenobarbital is a suspected teratogen. Doses administered during pregnancy affect the fetus, and barbiturates given to lactating mothers may produce toxicity in the infant.

Allergic hypersensitivity to phenobarbital may produce skin reactions, some of which progress to lifethreatening conditions such as Stevens-Johnson syndrome. Early symptoms of hypersensitivity include headache, fever, stomatitis, conjunctivitis, rhinitis, and urethritis (or balanitis). Phenobarbital also enhances the synthesis of porphyrin. Rarely, blood dyscrasias develop during its use.

Some tolerance develops with continued administration of phenobarbital. The seizure threshold is lowered when the drug is withdrawn; abrupt discontinuation may precipitate status epilepticus (see also Chap. 14). Excitement or confusion can occur when phenobarbital is administered to elderly clients. Children also may exhibit paradoxical excitement and hyperactivity. A disproportionate depression of CNS inhibition by the drug probably accounts for these effects. Subtle personality changes (mood distortions and impaired judgment) also develop in some clients, especially with prolonged therapy.

Drug–Drug Interactions. Phenobarbital stimulates liver microsomal enzymes that inactivate many drugs and change them to metabolites, which are easily eliminated by the body. There is also evidence that the drug stimulates the rate of its own breakdown, which may account in part for the tolerance the client develops to barbiturates. In addition, phenobarbital interferes with absorption or secretion of some chemicals. Drugs whose effects are decreased because of more rapid metabolism by liver enzymes include coumarin, digitalis, corticosteroids, tricyclic antidepressants, doxycycline, and oral contraceptives. Phenobarbital interferes with pituitary secretion of corticotropin.

Drug–Laboratory Test Interactions. A few drugs affect serum levels of phenobarbital. For example, disulfiram and monoamine oxidase inhibitors restrict the metabolism of phenobarbital, prolonging its half-life in the body. Phenobarbital competes with other weak acids for binding to plasma albumin, and displacement of thyroxine from these sites may produce clinically significant increases in free thyroxine levels.

Precautions and Contraindications. Phenobarbital is contraindicated in clients with bronchopneumonia and in clients with known allergic hypersensitivity to the drug. It is not given to persons with a history of porphyria.

Caution should be used in clients with pulmonary insufficiency and children with hyperactivity. The drug should be withdrawn if depression develops. To prevent serious allergic syndromes, the drug should be promptly discontinued if a skin rash develops.

When phenobarbital is prescribed concurrently with known interactant drugs, the dosage of each drug must be carefully regulated to achieve optimal effects. If the dosage of one drug is altered, the dosage of the other may need adjustment.

After prolonged therapy, phenobarbital should be withdrawn gradually (see Focus On Barbiturates: Similarities and Differences).

Oxazolidinediones

The oxazolidinedione class of drugs acts to control absence seizures. They are usually used when other agents do not work. They are ineffective in major motor seizures; rather, they tend to precipitate or exacerbate grand mal epilepsy.

One of the oxazolidinediones, trimethadione, was the first truly selective anticonvulsant discovered. It is discussed below as a prototype of the class.

Trimethadione

Pharmacodynamics. In addition to suppressing petit mal seizures, trimethadione has some sedative activity. It raises the seizure threshold of the thalamocortical system, which appears to be particularly important in the genesis of absence seizures. The drug depresses projection of seizure activity from cortical foci to the thalamus. It does not affect the cortical spread of seizure activity or post-tetanic potentiation in the spinal cord or stellate ganglia.

Pharmacokinetics. Trimethadione is rapidly absorbed from the GI tract, reaching peak plasma concentrations in 0.5 to 2 hours. Although it is uniformly distributed in the tissues, it does not bind to plasma proteins. Trimethadione is readily metabolized by liver enzymes

FOCUS ON

Barbiturates: Similarities and Differences

Similarities

Pharmacodynamics

These agents act as nonselective CNS depressants. They depress the sensory cortex, decrease motor activity, alter cerebral function, and produce sedation and hypnosis. They enhance or mimic the inhibitory synaptic action of GABA. They also decrease the REM phase of sleep.

Pharmacokinetics

These agents are absorbed in varying degrees after oral, parenteral, or rectal administration. They are rapidly distributed to all tissues and fluids. They are primarily metabolized by the liver and excreted in the urine. Their onset occurs in 20–60 minutes for oral administration, slightly faster for IM, and seconds to 5 minutes for IV administration. The average half-life ranges from 24 to 34 hours.

Therapeutic Uses

These agents are used for sedation, hypnosis, insomnia, and preanesthetic sedation.

Adverse Reactions

These include: (CNS) confusion, depression, paradoxical excitement, drowsiness, lethargy, vertigo, headache, CNS depression, hangover effect, impaired judgment and motor skills; (CV) hypotension, bradycardia, circulatory collapse; (RESP) respiratory depression, apnea, laryngospasm, bronchospasm; (GI) gastric upset, nausea, vomiting, diarrhea; (HEMA) megaloblastic anemia, agranulocytosis, thrombocytopenia; (OTHER) exfoliative dermatitis, Stevens-Johnson syndrome, dependence, rash, fever, myalgia, neuralgia.

Drug Interactions

With barbiturates, alcohol and CNS depressants cause additive CNS depression; may increase risk of hepatic toxicity of acetaminophen, MAOIs, valproic acid, or divalproex; may stimulate liver enzymes that metabolize other drugs, which would decrease their effects (including many corticosteroids, oral contraceptives, estrogens, oral anticoagulants, quinidine, theophylline, valproic acid, and some tetracyclines).

Differences

- **Phenobarbital** and **mephobarbital** depress the monosynaptic and polysynaptic transmission in the CNS; they increase the threshold for electrical stimulation of the motor cortex.

- **Mephobarbital** and **phenobarbital** have an average duration of 10–12 hours (PO).
- **Amobarbital, butabarbital,** and **aprobarbital** have an average duration of 6–8 hours.
- **Pentobarbital** and **secobarbital** have an onset of action of 10–15 minutes (PO) and average duration of 3–4 hours (PO).

- **Phenobarbital** and **mephobarbital** are also used as anticonvulsants in treating tonic-clonic or absence seizures.
- **Phenobarbital** and **secobarbital** are used to treat status epilepticus.
- **Primidone** is used for generalized tonic-clonic and complex partial seizures.
- **Mesoridazine** is used as an adjunctive treatment for alcohol depression.

- **Phenobarbital, secobarbital,** and **amobarbital** can cause thrombophlebitis, pain, and tissue damage at the injection site.
- **Primidone** can cause alopecia, impotence, polyuria, edema, and thirst.

- **Amobarbital** may alter the effect of phenytoin.
- **Amobarbital** and **pentobarbital** increase nephrotoxicity of methoxyflurane.
- **Phenobarbital** serum levels and therapeutic and toxic effects are increased with valproic acid.

(continued)

FOCUS *ON*

Barbiturates: Similarities and Differences (continued)

Similarities (continued)

Precautions and Contraindications

These agents are contraindicated in those with known hypersensitivity to barbiturates and in those with bronchopneumonia, status asthmaticus, severe respiratory distress, depression or suicidal ideas, uncontrolled or chronic pain, or porphyria.

These agents should be used cautiously in persons requiring mental alertness to work, and those with renal or hepatic dysfunction.

Nursing Considerations

Assess neurologic status and level of consciousness frequently; check vital signs frequently for changes; assess sleeping patterns before and during therapy to determine drug's effectiveness; institute non-pharmacologic measures to assist with sleep; institute safety measures to prevent falls and injury; anticipate possible rebound excitement; assess bowel and bladder elimination for changes; assist with measures to promote urinary elimination; instruct in measures to promote bowel elimination, including high-fiber diet; monitor blood studies frequently for changes; discontinue slowly to avoid withdrawal symptoms; instruct in disease, drug therapy, treatment, adverse effects, and need for compliance; monitor for signs and symptoms of overdose.

Differences (continued)

- **Mephobarbital** and **primidone** are contraindicated in suspected pregnancy or near-term pregnancy.
- **Parenteral amobarbital, pentobarbital,** and **phenobarbital** should be given cautiously to those with hypotension, severe pulmonary or cardiovascular disease, shock, and uremia.
- **Primidone** and **mephobarbital** should be used cautiously in persons using alcohol, CNS depressants, MAOIs, narcotic analgesics, or anticoagulants.

- Administer IM deep into a large muscle to prevent tissue damage; have resuscitative equipment available when giving IV; do not mix **pentobarbital** with other medications; **secobarbital sodium** injection is not compatible with Ringer's lactate solution; do not mix **secobarbital** with acidic solutions; rotate ampule of **secobarbital,** and do not shake.

---

to an active metabolite, dimethadione, which is responsible for its therapeutic effects. Eventually, dimethadione is excreted by the kidneys. Its half-life ranges from 6 to 13 days.

Dimethadione serum levels are more indicative of therapeutic levels than are trimethadione levels. Therapeutic serum levels of dimethadione range from 700 to 800 µg/mL. Therapy is initiated with low doses that are increased gradually until a therapeutic effect is achieved, a process requiring several weeks.

Therapeutic Uses. Trimethadione controls absence seizures that are refractory to ethosuximide. If the dosage is adequate, up to 80% of clients achieve control of absence seizures. Trimethadione can be used with most other anticonvulsants to treat epilepsy typified by mixed types of seizures.

Adverse Reactions. Trimethadione is a relatively toxic drug. Drowsiness is the most frequent side effect but tends to subside with continued administration. Visual disturbances are fairly common and include hemeralopia (blurred vision in bright or glaring light), di-plopia, and photophobia. Allergic reactions include neutropenia, rashes, hepatitis, nephrotic syndrome, and symptoms resembling myasthenia gravis. Other side effects are alopecia, paresthesias, vaginal bleeding, and changes in blood pressure. Trimethadione may be teratogenic; congenital malformations have occurred in children born to women taking the drug.

Precautions and Contraindications. Trimethadione is used only for absence seizures that fail to respond to other less toxic drugs. It is not recommended for women who are or may become pregnant. The drug is contraindicated in persons known to be allergic to it. Extreme caution is required when trimethadione is prescribed for patients with retinal or optic nerve disease.

Therapy must be closely monitored, especially during the first treatment year. White blood cell counts are monitored regularly and the drug is discontinued if the neutrophil count falls to 2,500/mm^3. If symptoms of nephrosis, hepatitis, or myasthenia gravis occur, the drug is also discontinued. To reduce the risk of precipitating seizures, trimethadione is best withdrawn slowly.

Succinimides

The frequency and severity of toxic reactions to the oxazolidinedione anticonvulsants have limited their usefulness in treating epilepsy. Continued research led to the development of the succinimides: ethosuximide, methsuximide, and phensuximide. Ethosuximide, the primary agent in this group, is used to treat absence seizures. It is more effective than trimethadione and carries a lower risk of serious side effects.

Ethosuximide

Pharmacodynamics. Ethosuximide exhibits frequency-dependent effects on the cortical response to stimuli: response to stimuli occurring at intervals exceeding 200 milliseconds is markedly decreased. Experts suspect that ethosuximide prevents absence seizures by inhibiting T currents in thalamic neurons. Ethosuximide reduces the focal activity that produces spike and wave patterns on electroencephalograms even more effectively than does phenytoin. Its effect in reducing thalamocortical excitation is similar to that of phenytoin.

Pharmacokinetics. Ethosuximide is administered orally, and GI absorption appears to be complete. Peak plasma concentrations occur within 3 hours after administration. The drug does not bind significantly to plasma proteins. It distributes widely and evenly in the tissues, producing concentrations in CSF comparable to those in plasma. Plasma half-life averages 30 hours in children and 40 to 50 hours in adults. A period of 4 to 7 days of treatment is required to achieve steady-state concentrations.

Ethosuximide is largely metabolized by the liver. About 75% is degraded by the microsomal enzymes and subsequently eliminated by the kidneys. Most of the remainder is excreted unchanged by the kidneys. Small amounts appear in bile and feces.

Therapeutic Uses. Many consider ethosuximide the agent of choice in treating absence seizures. Plasma concentration in adults should be 40 to 100 µg/mL. The drug is sometimes used to control myoclonic or psychomotor seizures.

Adverse Reactions. Ethosuximide is associated most often with GI upset. Anorexia (with weight loss), nausea, vomiting, and epigastric distress are among the adverse effects. CNS manifestations include drowsiness, headache, fatigue, dizziness, euphoria, ataxia, irritability, and hiccups. Parkinsonism and photophobia sometimes occur. Myopia, vaginal bleeding, and swollen tongue have also been reported. The most serious complications of therapy are allergic reactions to the drug, blood dyscrasias, and syndromes resembling systemic lupus erythematosus and Stevens-Johnson syndrome. Leukopenia, eosinophilia, agranulocytosis, pancytopenia, and aplastic anemia may occur. Recent reports indicate that ethosuximide, like other anticonvulsants, may be teratogenic.

Drug Interactions. Carbamazepine has been linked to decreased ethosuximide levels; isoniazid, conversely, reportedly increases ethosuximide levels significantly. Levels of both phenobarbital and ethosuximide may be altered with increased seizure frequency.

Precautions and Contraindications. If ethosuximide is used to treat mixed epilepsy, adequate doses of anticonvulsants must also be given to control major motor seizures. The dosage of ethosuximide must be adjusted carefully and slowly. Abrupt withdrawal should be avoided because it may precipitate frequent seizures or petit mal status (prolonged absence seizure).

Blood counts must be monitored regularly to detect changes indicative of bone marrow malfunction. The skin is inspected frequently for lesions and rashes. Ethosuximide must be discontinued if either of these conditions occurs: fatalities have resulted when such side effects have been allowed to progress.

Carbamazepine

Carbamazepine, an iminostilbene, is structurally related to the tricyclic antidepressants and is the second most frequently prescribed antiseizure medication in the United States.

Pharmacodynamics. Like phenytoin, carbamazepine limits seizure propagation by reducing post-tetanic potentiation of synaptic transmission. The drug exhibits sedative, anticholinergic, antidepressant, muscle relaxant, antiarrhythmic, antidiuretic, and neuromuscular transmission-inhibitory actions. It has only slight analgesic properties.

Pharmacokinetics. After oral administration, carbamazepine is slowly and erratically absorbed from the GI tract. About 2 to 4 days may be required to achieve steady-state plasma concentrations. The therapeutic range of plasma concentration is reportedly 6 to 12 µg/mL (8–34 µmol/L). Signs and symptoms of abnormal CNS function are common when concentrations reach or exceed 9 µg/mL.

After absorption, carbamazepine is widely distributed to body tissues and fluids, including the brain, CSF, bile, and saliva. The drug crosses the placenta and accumulates in fetal tissues. It is distributed in breast milk in concentrations 60% of maternal plasma levels. About 75% of carbamazepine is bound to plasma proteins. Less than 3% of carbamazepine is excreted unchanged by the kidneys. The drug is metabolized by microsomal enzymes in the liver to active metabolites and is a liver enzyme inducer. The plasma half-life of the drug is relatively long, reportedly averaging 10 to 20 hours.

Therapeutic Uses. Carbamazepine is a primary drug in managing partial and tonic-clonic seizures. It is sometimes used with phenytoin, phenobarbital, or primidone. Carbamazepine has also been used for treating schizophrenia, bipolar illness that does not respond to lithium, and pain associated with true trigeminal neuralgia.

Adverse Reactions. Carbamazepine shares the toxic potential of the hydantoin-derivative anticonvulsants such as phenytoin. The most common side effects are nausea, vomiting, dizziness, drowsiness, unsteady gait, and blurred vision. In addition, carbamazepine can cause renal, pancreatic, and hepatic impairment, as well as serious hematologic disorders, such as agranulocytosis and aplastic anemia. Genitourinary problems include urinary frequency or retention, oliguria with hypertension, impotence, albuminuria, glycosuria, elevated blood urea nitrogen level, and microscopic deposits in the urine. Acute renal failure has been reported. Inflammation can develop in both the liver and biliary system. Hypersensitivity reactions such as dermatitis, splenomegaly, and lymphadenopathy have occurred. Acute intoxication can lead to stupor or coma, hyperirritability, convulsions, and respiratory depression. A late complication in elderly clients with heart disease is water retention with decreased plasma sodium concentrations and osmolality.

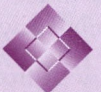

Toxicity Alert: Carbamazepine

Carbamazepine may be extremely toxic to a few recipients. In about 2% of clients, persistent leukopenia may occur, necessitating discontinuing the drug. Clients should be informed of the potential toxicity of the drug. Blood cell studies, liver function test results, and ophthalmic status should be assessed before carbamazepine therapy begins and regularly thereafter. Treatment must be discontinued if bone marrow depression, hepatotoxicity, or eye changes occur.

Drug Interactions. Carbamazepine interacts with several drugs. It increases the metabolism (decreasing blood levels) of phenytoin and valproate. In turn, phenytoin may increase carbamazepine degradation, lowering its blood levels. Propoxyphene, erythromycin, and two calcium blockers, verapamil and diltiazem, inhibit carbamazepine metabolism. Isoniazid increases serum levels of carbamazepine. Carbamazepine accelerates the conversion of primidone to phenobarbital.

Precautions and Contraindications. The initial fear that long-term therapy with this drug would increase the frequency of aplastic anemia has proved to be unfounded: the incidence of aplastic anemia is about one in 200,000. The drug is best withdrawn gradually to prevent abrupt declines in blood levels, which can precipitate seizures.

Clients who perform work requiring mental alertness or physical coordination should be warned about the possible neurologic effects of the drug.

Safe use of carbamazepine in children and during pregnancy and lactation has not been established. Carbamazepine is contraindicated for persons with a history of bone marrow depression or hypersensitivity to the drug or to any of the tricyclic antidepressants. The drug should be administered with extreme caution, if at all, with other drugs that may increase the possibility of adverse reactions.

Valproate (Valproic Acid)

Valproic acid's anticonvulsant properties were discovered when it was used as a vehicle for other compounds tested for anticonvulsant activity.

Pharmacodynamics. The specific mechanism of action of valproic acid is unknown. It appears to affect GABA function at the synapse by inhibiting enzyme degradation of this neurotransmitter or by inhibiting its reuptake by glial cells and nerve endings. This selective increase in synaptic concentration of GABA decreases impulse transmission.

Pharmacokinetics. Valproate is rapidly and almost completely absorbed by the GI tract. Peak plasma concentration occurs 1 to 4 hours after administration of oral doses. Protein binding is as much as 95% and tissue concentrations appear highest in the extracellular fluid. The drug is metabolized by the liver. Little of the unchanged drug is excreted in the urine. Some drug appears in the feces. Plasma half-life is about 15 hours.

Valproic acid treatment begins with low doses that are gradually increased to achieve a therapeutic effect. Therapeutic plasma levels do not correlate well with efficacy, but the therapeutic range is considered to be 30 to 100 μg/mL.

Therapeutic Uses. Valproic acid is particularly effective in treating both simple and complex absence seizures. Although this is the only approved use for the drug in the United States, it has exhibited some therapeutic effect in intractable hiccups and in myoclonic and grand mal seizures. It is less effective in partial seizures.

Adverse Reactions. Valproic acid has a low incidence of side effects. The most common side effects are anorexia, nausea, and vomiting. The drug has caused hepatotoxicity and liver failure. It decreases hepatic conversion of ammonia to urea, causing blood ammonia levels to rise. Valproic acid is irritating to the tissues and can cause stomatitis if dosage forms are chewed. CNS manifestations—sedation, ataxia, and incoordination—occur infrequently. The drug causes thrombocytopenia in some clients. It may also be teratogenic.

Drug Interactions. Valproic acid and phenobarbital used together may result in plasma concentrations of phenobarbital greater than those that occur when phenobarbital is used alone (valproic acid may inhibit the liver enzymes that degrade phenobarbital). When valproic acid and phenytoin are used concurrently, valproic acid may produce either increased or decreased plasma levels of phenytoin. When used with clonazepam, absence seizure status may occur.

Precautions and Contraindications. Hepatic function should be tested before valproic acid therapy begins and every 2 months thereafter as long as the drug is used. The drug should not be used by clients with decreased liver function. If possible, valproic acid should be discontinued if ammonemia or a change in liver function develops. Alternatively, ammonemia may be moderated either by decreasing protein in the diet or by adding arginine or carnitine to it. GI complaints may be minimized by beginning with very low doses and slowly increasing the dose. When valproic acid is used concurrently with phenobarbital or phenytoin, dosage levels must be carefully adjusted for therapeutic effect; if the dosage of one agent is altered, then that of the other may also require adjustment.

Benzodiazepines

A detailed discussion of benzodiazepine drugs appears in Chapter 20. Although many benzodiazepines have antiseizure properties, only two—clonazepam and clorazepate—have been approved in the United States for the long-term management of certain type of seizures. Diazepam and lorazepam are agents of choice for the treatment of status epilepticus.

Clonazepam

Clonazepam is administered orally for prolonged management of absence or myoclonic seizures in children. It acts by facilitating GABA action at the synapses, apparently by increasing the affinity of this neurotransmitter for binding sites. (GABA acts to inhibit nerve impulse transmission.) About half of the clients who take clonazepam develop drowsiness, somnolence, fatigue, and lethargy, but these symptoms usually subside with continued treatment. Muscular incoordination and ataxia are fairly common. Other side effects include hypotonia, dysarthrias, dizziness, anorexia (or hyperphagia), and increased salivation and bronchial secretion. Tolerance can develop after 1 to 6 months of taking the drug. Behavioral problems such as aggression, hyperactivity, irritability, or inability to concentrate may necessitate discontinuation of the drug. See Table 19-3 for more information on adverse effects.

Diazepam

Diazepam is administered parenterally in treating status epilepticus. For adults or older children, a dose of 5 to 10 mg is administered slowly by IV initially. This may be repeated at 10- to 15-minute intervals to a maximal total dose of 30 mg. If necessary, the regimen may be repeated every 2 to 4 hours. No more than 100 mg should be administered in any single 24-hour period. Because diazepam is absorbed by plastic tubing, the therapeutic response to infusions will increase gradually until the tubing is saturated by the drug. Its short duration of action is a disadvantage. Tolerance increases with long-term use of diazepam, and physical dependence may develop.

Other Agents

Several antiseizure drugs are in various stages of clinical trials. These agents act on one of three mechanisms of action: changing the voltage-dependent sodium, calcium, or chloride ion channels, increasing GABA-mediated inhibition, or decreasing glutamate- and aspartate-mediated excitation. Any one of these mechanisms will reduce seizure activity.

Gabapentin

Gabapentin is an antiseizure drug recently approved by the Food and Drug Administration as an adjunct in treating partial seizures, with or without secondary generalization, in epileptic clients over age 12.

Pharmacodynamics. Gabapentin was originally synthesized as a GABA agonist; however, it does not mimic GABA at any known GABA site. It appears to promote the release of GABA by an unknown mechanism. It also alters the transport or metabolism of brain amino acids.

Pharmacokinetics. Gabapentin is absorbed well from the GI tract after an oral dose. Plasma concentrations peak in 3 hours. It is not metabolized and is excreted unchanged primarily in the urine. The half-life ranges from 5 to 9 hours. Gabapentin does not interfere with other antiseizure medications (eg, phenytoin, carbamazepine, phenobarbital, valproate).

Therapeutic Uses. Gabapentin is recommended for partial seizures, with and without secondary generalization, when used concurrently with other antiseizure drugs.

Adverse Reactions. Gabapentin is usually well tolerated. Common adverse effects include somnolence, dizziness, ataxia, fatigue, and nystagmus. These effects are usually transient and range in severity from mild to moderate.

Lamotrigine

Because phenobarbitone and phenytoin have some antifolate properties, scientists investigated the role that folic acid may play in seizure mechanisms. Researchers began developing agents with new and more powerful antifolate properties, and lamotrigine was the result.

Pharmacodynamics. Lamotrigine stops excessive release of excitatory amino acid transmitters (glutamate and aspartate) by interacting with the voltage-dependent sodium channels. The exact mechanism is unknown.

Text continues on page 380.

Table 19-3. Adverse Effects of Commonly Prescribed Anticonvulsants

Drug	Adverse Effects	Toxic Effects
phenytoin (Dilantin, Diphenylan)	*Adults:* Gingival hypertrophy Gastric irritation Hyperglycemia Hirsutism, facial coarsening Increased risk of birth defects when used during pregnancy Inappropriate antidiuretic hormone secretion* Allergy*—fever, rash, exfoliative dermatitis, bone marrow depression, systemic lupus erythematosus *Children:* Unsteady gait, involuntary movements, fatigue, altered emotions Impaired problem-solving and visuomotor skills Short attention span	Nausea and constipation Nystagmus, ataxia, drowsiness, tremor, increased frequency of seizures Hyperactivity, behavioral change, confusion, or dullness Hallucinations After rapid IV administration: cardiovascular collapse, hypotension, and CNS depression Lymphadenopathy
phenobarbital (Barbital, Luminal; *Can*: Sulfoton)	*Adults:* Stevens-Johnson syndrome* Excitation in the elderly and very young* Pain in muscles, nerves, or joints Physical dependence Personality changes Depression and suicidal tendencies* Increased risk of birth defects when used during pregnancy Porphyria in susceptible persons* Inflammation of the mouth, conjunctiva, nose, urethra, and glans penis Allergy*—fever, rash, bone marrow depression, systemic lupus erythematosus *Children:* Lethargy, depressive symptoms Irritability, hyperactivity, sleep disturbance Stubbornness, disobedience Impaired memory Impaired concentration	Sedation GI disturbances Vertigo, headache, depression Nystagmus, ataxia Respiratory depression
trimethadione (Tridione)	*Adults:* Stevens-Johnson syndrome* Hemeralopia, diplopia, photophobia Alopecia, paresthesias, vaginal bleeding Changes in blood pressure Increased risk of birth defects when used during pregnancy Neutropenia, hepatitis, nephrotic syndrome Myasthenia syndrome (muscle weakness) Allergy*—rash *Children:* Drowsiness	Sedation Major motor seizures
valproic acid (Dalpro, Depakene; *Can*: Epival)	*Adults:* Transient hair loss Drowsiness, ataxia, incoordination GI disturbances Inhibition of platelet aggregation Increased risk of birth defects when used during pregnancy Hepatotoxicity and thrombocytopenia *Children:* Drowsiness, lethargy	Coma
ethosuximide (Zarontin)	*Adults:* Headache Epigastric distress Hiccups Myopia Vaginal bleeding Increased risk of birth defects when used during pregnancy Allergy*—urticaria, erythema multiforme, pancytopenia, rash, bone marrow depression, systemic lupus erythematosus *Children:* Drowsiness Minimal deficits in psychosocial function	Anorexia, nausea, vomiting Dizziness, drowsiness, fatigue, euphoria, ataxia, irritability, photophobia Parkinsonism

*Indications for discontinuation of the offending drug.
KEY: *Can* = Canadian trade name.

(continued)

Table 19-3. (Continued)

Drug	Adverse Effects	Toxic Effects
clonazepam (Klonopin, Can: Rivotril)	*Adults:* Stevens-Johnson syndrome* Drowsiness, fatigue, lethargy Muscular incoordination, ataxia Anorexia or hyperphagia Increased risk of birth defects when used during pregnancy Allergy*—rash, bone marrow depression *Children:* Irritability, hyperactivity Antisocial behavior, aggression, disobedience	Thick speech, hypersalivation Excessive bronchial secretions Hypotonia Aggression, hyperactivity, irritability, inability to concentrate
carbamazepine (Epitol, Tegretol, Can: Apo-Carbamazepine)	*Adults:* Bone marrow depression* Aggravation of cardiovascular disease Hepatotoxicity Nephrotoxicity Urinary frequency, retention Impotence Nausea, vomiting, abdominal pain, diarrhea, constipation, glossitis Rash, Stevens-Johnson syndrome*, aggravation of systemic lupus erythematosus, alopecia Chills and fever Arthritis *Children:* Emotional lability Irritability, agitation Insomnia Impaired task performance	Ataxia, dizziness, stupor, opisthotonus, agitation, disorientation, tremor, adiadochokinesis, abnormal reflexes Mydriasis, nystagmus Cyanosis Urinary retention Glycosuria, acetonuria Coma
gabapentin (Neurontin)	*Adults:* Somnolence, dizziness, ataxia, fatigue, nystagmus, hypertension, anxiety, altered reflexes *Children:* Safety and effectiveness not established in children	Sedation Slurred speech
lamotrigine (Lamictal)	*Adults:* Dizziness, headache, ataxia, somnolence, diplopia, blurred vision, rash, photosensitivity, nausea, vomiting *Children:* Not recommended for persons under age 16	Somnolence leading to coma

*Indications for discontinuation of the offending drug.
KEY: *Can* = Canadian trade name.

Pharmacokinetics. Lamotrigine is completely absorbed from the GI tract and is 55% protein bound. It is metabolized in the liver by glucuronidation and excreted primarily in the urine. Plasma concentrations peak in 2 hours and the plasma half-life of a single dose is about 24 hours. When used as adjunctive therapy with phenobarbital, phenytoin, carbamazepine, or another hepatic enzyme inducer, its half-life decreases to about 15 hours. Added to valproic acid, valproic acid concentrations drop by about 25% and the half-life of lamotrigine increases to 48 hours.

Therapeutic Uses. Lamotrigine has been approved as adjunctive therapy for adults with partial seizures, with or without secondary generalized tonic-clonic seizures. Preliminary data indicate that this drug may also be effective as monotherapy for newly diagnosed partial or generalized seizures.

Adverse Reactions. The most common side effects when lamotrigine is added to another antiseizure drug regimen are dizziness, ataxia, blurred or double vision, headache, nausea, vomiting, and rash. These adverse effects are usually transient, subsiding in 2 to 3 weeks. A few cases of Stevens-Johnson syndrome and disseminated intravascular coagulation have been reported.

Felbamate
Felbamate was approved by the Food and Drug Administration in 1993 for treating partial seizures. Since then, several cases of aplastic anemia have been associated with the drug. Felbamate is structurally similar to meprobamate. Its mechanism of action is unknown but it appears to block sustained repetitive neuronal firing, possibly by its effect on sodium channels. The most common side effects are fatigue, nausea, insomnia, headache, anorexia, weight loss, constipation, and diarrhea.

Vigabatrin
Vigabatrim is available in Europe and Australia for treating refractory partial seizures, but it is not available in the United States. Its development resulted from further understanding of the synaptic mechanisms that control seizure thresholds. Vigabatrin blocks the GABA amino-

transferase enzyme, which increases GABA in the brain and CSF. Increasing the GABA level prevents neuronal excitation and thereby decreases seizure activity. The most common side effects are drowsiness, fatigue, dizziness, headache, and weight gain. Less common adverse effects are ataxia, visual disturbances, GI upset, and rash. These effects are usually transient and usually decrease in 2 to 3 weeks. The most serious effects from this drug are psychiatric disorders, including depression and psychosis, which have occurred in a few recipients.

Magnesium Sulfate

The seizures associated with magnesium deficiency and acute eclampsia are best treated with magnesium solutions. The mechanism by which magnesium depresses the CNS is unknown, although magnesium sulfate is known to decrease the amount of acetylcholine liberated by the motor nerve impulse. Magnesium solutions also act osmotically to reduce brain edema, a factor contributing to irritability and lowered seizure threshold.

Magnesium sulfate is the drug of choice for managing convulsive toxemia in pregnancy. It is also used as an anticonvulsant in preventing and controlling severe eclamptic seizures. Adverse effects include flushing, sweating, hypotension, confusion, sedation, cardiac and respiratory depression, and depressed or absent reflexes. Knee-jerk reflexes must be assessed and the drug withheld if they are absent. Cases of hypocalcemia with tetany resulting from magnesium sulfate have been reported. Magnesium sulfate is usually administered by slow IV infusion. Serum magnesium levels are monitored as a guide to dosages. The maximum recommended dosage is 150 mg/min. Excessive use may result in hypermagnesemia (manifested by severe CNS depression).

Acetazolamide

Acetazolamide is sometimes useful as an adjunct to other anticonvulsants in the prophylaxis of certain types of epilepsy, particularly petit mal. It resembles carbon dioxide in its anticonvulsant properties; its inhibition of carbonic anhydrase activity may act by reducing carbon dioxide elimination from glial cells. Elevation of the seizure threshold and selective depression of spinal cord monosynaptic pathways result. Because tolerance to the drug action develops rapidly, acetazolamide has limited therapeutic value.

Topiramate (Topamax)

Topiramate is a drug newly approved by the FDA for the treatment of partial seizures and generalized tonic clonic seizures. It is a weak carbonic anhydrase inhibitor and appears to act by blocking the spread of seizure activity rather than raising seizure threshold. How it does this is not known. The drug is well absorbed after oral administration, with a 75% bioavailability. Peak effect occurs from 2 to 4 hours and it is primarily excreted unchanged in the urine. Adverse effects caused by topiramate have been dose-related and reversible. The most common include: sedation, dizziness/ataxia, paresthesia, visual disturbances, diarrhea, decreased appetite, with weight loss and cognitive dysfunction.

■ SUMMARY

Antiseizure drug therapy aims for a balance between seizure control and adverse effects. Anticonvulsant drugs control seizures by raising the seizure threshold and limiting the spread of neuronal activity from initiating foci. Many anticonvulsants are CNS depressants, and many are relatively toxic. They cause CNS symptoms, GI upset, and various allergic reactions. Most are also teratogenic. Despite the risks of therapy, anticonvulsant drugs allow most epileptic clients to control their seizures and lead relatively normal lives.

❖ NURSING MANAGEMENT: CLIENT RECEIVING ANTICONVULSANTS

Seizures and seizure disorders pose many risks to the affected person. An unexpected seizure can result in serious accidental injury: drowning or near drowning if it occurs while the person is swimming; fractures or head trauma from falling; collision with objects in the environment; or injury by power machinery that the person may have been near at the time of the attack. Status epilepticus is a threat to life and can cause brain injury. In addition, frequent seizures interfere with the normal activities of life (eg, school, work, recreation, socializing).

Many persons lose consciousness during a seizure and report cloudy consciousness for some time afterward, especially after major motor seizures. Moreover, psychomotor seizures can mimic unacceptable behavior, alienating people who are unaware of the true nature of the episode. In addition, failure to control seizure activity may result in legal constraints—specifically, loss of a driver's license. Inability to control the symptoms of the condition also reinforces the stigma attached to the disease, leading to rejection of the afflicted person. The uncontrolled epileptic, therefore, is at a disadvantage in accomplishing critical developmental tasks. Optimal control of seizures is vital for the client's normal development and enjoyment of life.

Fortunately, with current drug therapy, seizures can be virtually eliminated in most clients. The nurse can be instrumental in educating the client about the disorder and drug therapy, helping the client adhere to an effective drug regimen, and helping the client adjust his or her daily activities to enhance safety and social satisfaction. The nurse also works closely with the physician, especially when drug therapy fails to control seizures or when frequent or severe side effects occur. These may indicate inappropriate dosages; the prescriber must be alerted to these so that a revised regimen may be

Example of Nursing Process for Changes in Anticonvulsant Drug Regimen

The client, Donna, is a 19-year-old secretarial school student who is on anticonvulsant drugs for control of psychomotor epilepsy, diagnosed 3 years ago. Her seizures take the form of inappropriate behavior, such as irrelevant answers to questions and apparent failure to pay attention to verbal communication.

During the first week of school after Christmas recess, the client was counseled by her faculty advisor that instructors had reported that her academic performance had deteriorated, that she was not applying herself, and that she was not paying attention to directions. In view of her medical history, the counselor advised the client to consult her physician to rule out seizure disorder as a factor in the change in performance.

In the physician's office, the client appears anxious and defensive. She states, "I'm afraid the school will dismiss me because I am an epileptic." The client was last seen by the physician during the holiday recess, at which time the drug regimen was changed. A low dose of phenobarbital was added to the regimen, and the dosage of phenytoin was increased.

Assessment Data

Anxious appearance

Defensive demeanor

Perception of academic counseling as preliminary to dismissal from school

Behavior suggestive of exacerbation of psychomotor epilepsy

Recent change in medication regimen

Nursing Diagnosis	Intervention	Goals and Outcomes
Fear of dismissal from school related to unusual behavior, possibly secondary to exacerbation of psychomotor seizures	**Remind** the client of her 3-year record of excellent seizure control; reassure her that it is likely that control can be regained; inform her that there are several drugs that can be used if necessary to develop a successful drug regimen for her. **Point** out that the school advisor has recommended medical attention; the client should view this as a positive sign that the school administration regards epilepsy as a medical problem amenable to medical treatment.	Signs and symptoms of anxiety will decrease and the client will appear more relaxed.
Knowledge Deficit, related to knowledge deficit regarding the new drug regimen	**Examine** the client's medication bottles, count the remaining doses and compare the number taken with the number required for compliance with the new drug regimen. Ask the client how and when she is taking the drugs. **Explore** reasons for noncompliance, if appropriate. **Intervene** as necessary to promote improved compliance. **Schedule** a return visit by the client for reevaluation of the new regimen.	The client will take the drugs accurately, in accord with the prescribed regimen. An accurate evaluation of the new drug regimen will be made.

established (see Example of Nursing Process for Changes in Anticonvulsant Drug Regimen).

NURSING PROCESS

ASSESSMENT

Because of the stigma still attached to epilepsy, clients sometimes try to conceal seizure disorders. Gingival hypertrophy, a side effect of phenytoin, may be a clue that the client is re-

ceiving therapy for a seizure disorder. Another clue is depression, a result of prolonged barbiturate therapy. If these signs are apparent, the nurse should ask specifically about seizure disorders when taking an initial health history.

Some affected clients may be unaware of seizure episodes; their only clues may be an unexplained lapse of time. Only when incontinence or mental clouding occurs can many clients detect episodes. A family member may be able to give more accurate information regarding the frequency of seizures. The nurse should determine what clients know about their seizures.

Data required for assessment include a history of the seizure disorder: the type of seizures experienced, including behavior before, during, and after; the pattern of progression of the seizure; precipitating circumstances; the presence and type of aura; whether any seizures (and how many) have occurred recently; the usual anticonvulsant treatment regimen; and the client's acceptance of and adaptation to therapy.

During the physical examination, the nurse should evaluate the client for signs and symptoms of neurologic abnormality, as well as for toxic and side effects of anticonvulsant drugs. Skin integrity, level of consciousness, and signs and symptoms of allergy should be assessed, as should blood test results for abnormalities related to the drug regimen. The reproductive status of a female client (ie, plans to have children in the near future, pregnancy, or lactation) should be determined.

NURSING DIAGNOSIS

Diagnoses may include:

- Risk for Injury, related to drug-induced side effects or seizure activity not controlled by medication
- Body Image Disturbance, related to cosmetic effects of medication and to the seizure disorder
- Risk for Impaired Skin Integrity, related to side effects of anticonvulsant drugs
- Impaired Social Interaction, related to cosmetic side effects of anticonvulsant drugs, the stigma of epilepsy, and negative self-image
- Risk for Altered Growth and Development in breast-fed infants of female clients taking anticonvulsant, CNS depressant medication
- Knowledge Deficit concerning seizure conditions and treatment regimens
- Risk for Injury, related to seizures secondary to inappropriate drug dosages or to noncompliance with the drug regimen

A common collaborative problem that should be differentiated from the nursing diagnoses is:

Potential Complication: Congenital defects

PLANNING

Nursing goals including achieving the best seizure control possible with the minimal amount of anticonvulsant drugs, improving the client's self-image, increasing social interaction, reducing intrauterine or neonatal exposure to anticonvulsant drugs, increasing the client's knowledge of seizure disorders and their treatment to enhance compliance, and preventing or detecting and treating toxic and adverse effects of anticonvulsant drugs.

INTERVENTION

Nursing measures may help reduce the number of seizure episodes. Many factors increase the risk of seizures by changing the biochemical environment in the CNS (Table 19-4). The nurse should strive to eliminate or control these factors in the acutely ill client and to teach clients who manage their own regimens about techniques for reducing their impact.

Table 19-4. Nursing Management of Factors Predisposing to Recurrent Seizure Activity

Factors	Intervention
Fever	Prompt and vigorous treatment of febrile illness
	Control of high temperatures with tepid baths, hypothermia blankets, cold applications, or antipyretic drugs
Hypoxia	Prevention of chronic respiratory disease by avoidance of smoking and air pollution
	Prompt and vigorous treatment of respiratory infections
	Careful attention to oxygen needs in sports such as scuba diving
Hypoglycemia	Discussion of regular, nutritious meals
	Avoidance of concentrated carbohydrates by clients subject to reactive hypoglycemia
	Avoidance of insulin reactions by diabetics
Calcium ion deficiency	Prevention of hyperventilation by good emotional hygiene and breathing into a paper bag at the beginning of an episode
	Encouragement of regular, moderate exercise to induce mild physiologic acidosis
Sodium imbalance	Avoidance of excessive sodium intake, especially by female clients during the premenstrual period and by those on oral contraceptives
	Avoidance of water intoxication and hyponatremia by adequate salt intake in environments conducive to excessive perspiration
Sympathoadrenal response	Teaching of stress management techniques and good emotional hygiene
	Avoidance of exhaustion
Alcohol	Avoidance of intoxication of any degree (mild intoxication depresses CNS inhibition, and severe intoxication is often complicated by dehydration and hypoglycemia)
Repetitive stimuli of specific frequencies (strobe lights, repetitive bells)	Avoidance of discotheques or other environments where such stimuli are pervasive
	Avoidance of looking at emergency strobe lights on ambulances and police vehicles

Acute intercurrent illnesses must be vigorously treated; fever and hypoxia must be controlled or eliminated. Maintaining fluid and electrolyte balance is crucial. Reducing stress and promoting good mental health help minimize the impact of endogenous biochemicals conducive to seizures. Good habits contribute not only to vigorous physical health but also to a feeling of general well-being. These benefits can enhance seizure control. Good nutrition, including ample intake of vitamin D and folic acid, is needed to maintain optimal health.

If the nurse finds that the client is pregnant or is planning to have children in the near future, the physician should be consulted. To protect the fetus, drug dosages should be reduced as much as possible before and during pregnancy. The client should inform the physician promptly if seizures occur, because seizures during pregnancy can be harmful to the fetus. Lactation is generally contraindicated for mothers on anticonvulsant drugs. Health measures to reduce the risk of seizures and the need for high drug doses are particularly beneficial to women of childbearing age.

Managing the Drug Regimen. Clients must be monitored closely for therapeutic, toxic, and side effects of anticonvulsant drugs, especially when drug therapy is initiated, when dosages or drug agents are changed, or when intercurrent illness complicates the response to treatment. When anticonvulsant therapy is initiated, side effects are common. To limit their severity, drug dosages are begun at a low level and are gradually increased until adequate control is achieved. Seizures should decrease as serum levels approach the therapeutic range.

Many anticonvulsants have common side effects. The nurse should appraise the client's mental and neurologic function and behavior carefully. Nursing measures to improve GI function are important in maintaining effective control. Administering the medications with meals reduces the incidence of gastric symptoms. The client needs considerable support during this period. Nursing measures to ameliorate side effects may encourage compliance by increasing comfort.

The nurse must be aware of the side effects unique to each drug and must monitor the client carefully for them. Preventive measures should be taken when possible. For example, gingival hypertrophy from phenytoin is less common and less pronounced when the client practices meticulous oral hygiene and gum massage.

Once an optimal regimen is established, the nurse must administer, or teach the client to administer, doses regularly, at consistent intervals in relation to diurnal patterns of rest or activity and in relation to meals. The drug regimen may change from time to time because of allergy, side effects, toxicity, or loss of seizure control. Most adverse reactions are dose-dependent and are alleviated by careful reduction of dosage.

Whenever drugs are added to or deleted from the treatment regimen, the client's response to all drugs is likely to be altered. Assessing the client's response to medication is key to evaluating the new drug regimen. Serum drug levels provide pertinent data but should never be the sole basis for evaluation. Careful, accurate clinical assessment of the client is essential.

Allergic reactions, such as liver impairment, blood dyscrasias, and skin eruptions, may progress to life-threatening problems and should be reported immediately to the physician. In most cases, the drug will be discontinued, and loading doses (higher-than-normal doses) of a different anticonvulsant drug may be ordered to prevent seizures during the transition period. Initially, side effects from loading doses are likely to be pronounced. Omitting doses may cause seizure activity to occur. Abrupt, complete withdrawal of anticonvulsants may precipitate status epilepticus.

Emergency Treatment of Status Epilepticus. Status epilepticus requires intensive medical and nursing care. For rapid effect, medications are commonly administered IV. Diazepam is the agent of choice. If response is inadequate, other drugs may be added. A general anesthetic may be administered in refractory cases. Treatment is best carried out in an intensive care unit where skilled nursing care is available. Vital signs must be closely monitored.

The rate of infusion must be controlled carefully. Infusion pumps are recommended. If IV phenytoin is ordered, normal saline solution or special solvent must be used as the vehicle, and no other drugs may be added to it. The infusion rate should not exceed 50 mg/min. Phenytoin precipitates out of solution easily; it is incompatible with glucose or acid solutions and most other drugs. Infusions should be monitored closely for particle formation. The client should be monitored for phlebitis and infiltration. In some cases of intermittent infusion, an in-line filter may be used. Because phenytoin can cause cardiac arrhythmias, clients receiving it IV (especially the elderly, those with heart disease, and those with unstable vital signs) should be monitored for cardiac arrhythmias.

Phenytoin solutions are very irritating to tissues. Should discoloration or edema develop distally to the IV site, the IV line should be removed immediately and the physician notified. Continued infusion can lead to ischemia and tissue necrosis, manifested by purple discoloration of the hand or foot, skin blisters, and sloughing of tissues (so-called "purple glove syndrome"). The limb should be elevated above the chest and warm compresses applied to the hand or foot. The nurse should monitor peripheral pulses, skin color and temperature, and capillary refill. Purple glove syndrome can lead to extensive tissue damage and subsequent amputation.

Status epilepticus is very disturbing to the client's family or friends who are present during such episodes. To allay anxiety, they should be offered emotional support and sufficient explanation of what is occurring.

Care should be taken to protect the privacy of clients brought to the medical facility by strangers or casual acquaintances. The nurse should ascertain the status of the persons accompanying the client and use judgment in discussing the client's condition with them.

After the acute episode resolves, clients are commonly lethargic and confused. The duration of this postictal state is proportional to the duration of the seizure. As mental alertness returns, clients need an explanation of what has happened and must be oriented to their surroundings. They may be disturbed by the recurrence of seizures. In addition to the usual emotional impact of sudden illness and institutionalization, disruption of seizure control may arouse embarrassment or shame. There may also be practical consequences, such as the loss of a driver's license. In many states, the right to drive is suspended until the person has again been free of seizures for at least 1 year. Clients need considerable emotional support and assistance in coping with such stressors.

Maintaining Self-Image. Control of seizures with a stable drug regimen is important to enhancing the client's self-image and social interaction. Nurses and other healthcare personnel should treat the client with respect and warm acceptance. The client should be encouraged to maintain existing social relationships and develop new ones. This can be facilitated by teaching the client ways to counter drug-related cosmetic changes and enhance his or her physical appearance.

Client Education. In the past, epilepsy was regarded as a sign of genetic inferiority, mental incapacity, and personal deficiency, and the traditional stigma attached to this condition has not entirely subsided. Consequently, the feelings connected with an epilepsy diagnosis may be so strong that neither clients nor their families are receptive to teaching until they can cope with their emotional response to the illness (see Critical Thinking Challenge).

Clients and their families need reassurance that seizure disorders have a physical cause and are not a form of mental illness. The attitude that the nurse conveys with regard to epilepsy will have a pronounced effect. If the nurse treats the client with respect and warm acceptance and discusses the disorder matter-of-factly, client and family acceptance of the diagnosis will be facilitated.

The nurse should provide a careful explanation of the seizure disorder and the treatment plan. A discussion of general health measures that decrease the risk of seizures should be included. Because so much information must be covered, several teaching sessions may be required; written materials should be given for reference.

If clients are unaware of seizure occurrences, someone close to them should monitor and keep a written record of the frequency of the seizures. This should be discussed openly with clients, and permission should be obtained before recruiting a family member or other

CRITICAL THINKING CHALLENGE
Case Analysis

Read about Donna, the 19-year-old secretarial school student, in the Example of Nursing Process for Changes in Anticonvulsant Drug Regimen. Then consider the following questions.

1. What teaching does Donna need regarding her medication regimen?
2. Donna asks, "Will these medications control my seizures?" How would you respond?
3. Donna is engaged to be married and is concerned about having children. She asks, "Will my medications interfere with pregnancy? Can I go off the medications when I'm pregnant? Will epilepsy pass on to my children?" How would you answer?
4. As you and Donna talk further, you learn that she frequently stays up all night studying, is very active in intramural basketball, diets quite strictly, avoiding foods high in fat and calories, and skips meals. What advice would you give her, and why?

person for this responsibility. The monitor should receive an explanation of the different types of seizure manifestations. This helps detect episodes that may differ from the client's usual pattern.

Many clients must learn new ways to maintain an acceptable appearance. The nurse can discuss side effects such as facial coarsening and hirsutism from phenytoin. These effects may be particularly disturbing to female clients, as may the unsightly gingival hypertrophy that some clients experience with phenytoin. Other anticonvulsants (valproic acid) can cause excessive but transient hair loss.

For women, the nurse can suggest bleaching undesirable facial hair; this is usually preferable to shaving, because the stubble that appears after shaving is more noticeable than light-colored hair. Electrolysis may destroy hair follicles, but this process is prolonged, uncomfortable, and expensive. Moreover, eliminating all hair follicles results in a shiny appearance, because the fine hairs that impart a downy appearance are gone. When alopecia is a problem, a wig or hairpiece may be used to disguise hair loss.

Clients should be taught how to perform meticulous skin care to minimize acne, which develops with some anticonvulsants. Facial features can be defined and enhanced with makeup. Careful oral hygiene, including flossing, helps minimize gingival hypertrophy.

Clients may inquire how long medication must be continued. In some cases of childhood and post-traumatic epilepsy, medication can eventually be discontinued after a suitable weaning period. However, this is usually not attempted until after 2 to 4 years of treatment. Most clients with idiopathic epilepsy need anticonvulsant therapy indefinitely. The nurse should prepare clients for the prolonged drug therapy and should never promise that the therapy will be temporary.

Clients should be cautioned to avoid abruptly discontinuing drug therapy and to consult the physician if conditions occur that interfere with medication. Women of childbearing age should be cautioned to consult the physician before conceiving, because anticonvulsant drugs tend to be teratogenic. During pregnancy, the drug regimen should provide the lowest dosage required for seizure control. Dosages must not be decreased or discontinued without medical advice, however, because seizures are also detrimental to the fetus.

Clients taking phenytoin should be cautioned to buy the same trade name preparation each time the prescription is filled to avoid variations in blood levels of the drug. These variations stem from the differing bioavailability among drug brands.

Clients should be urged to take anticonvulsant drugs with food to minimize GI side effects. They should be cautioned about missing doses, which can precipitate seizures.

OUTCOME EVALUATION

Data required for evaluation include absence or decreased incidence of seizures; changes (reductions) in drug dosage; statements by the client relating to self-image, self-confidence, and social interactions; absence of congenital anomalies or anticonvulsant drug effects in female clients' children; absence of toxic or side effects in clients; and ability of clients to relate information conveyed during teaching sessions.

❖ CHECKLIST OF NURSING ACTIONS

When Maintenance Anticonvulsant Therapy is Ordered

- ❑ Urge clients to avoid strobe lights, which may exacerbate seizure activity, and conditions that may cause hypoxia, hypoglycemia, exhaustion, and sodium and water retention (these may increase seizure frequency).
- ❑ Help clients develop effective stress management techniques to prevent sympathoadrenal reactions.
- ❑ Caution clients to avoid alcohol intoxication.
- ❑ Stress the importance of good seizure control, especially when absence seizures are the only evidence of epilepsy.
- ❑ Urge clients to take the drugs as ordered. Warn against abrupt discontinuation of medication.
- ❑ Encourage clients to take anticonvulsant drugs with food.
- ❑ Teach clients the toxic and side effects of their anticonvulsant drugs that indicate the need for medical reappraisal.
- ❑ Teach clients how to minimize side effects of medication.

- ❑ Monitor clients carefully for therapeutic response, toxic effects, and side effects, especially when combinations of drugs are ordered.
- ❑ Refer clients to the physician for adjustment of dosage if response to the drugs is inadequate or if toxic effects occur.
- ❑ Teach clients receiving phenytoin techniques of good oral hygiene and gum massage.
- ❑ Warn clients that anticonvulsant drugs can cause drowsiness and incoordination that make operating a motor vehicle or other power machinery dangerous.
- ❑ Advise clients to verify that the pharmacist consistently refills prescriptions for phenytoin with the same trade name drug.

When Anticonvulsants Are Given for Status Epilepticus

- ❑ Monitor clients closely for toxic signs of drugs given IV.
- ❑ Be prepared to assist with emergency treatment if cardiovascular shock or cardiac arrest occurs.
- ❑ Support family members or friends who accompany the client to the health care facility.
- ❑ Protect the client's privacy.

Bibliography

Blake GJ. (1991). Carbamazepine for trigeminal neuralgia and pain. *Neurology* 36, 594–595 (April).

Brodie MJ. (1993). Felbamate: A new antiepileptic drug. *Lancet, 341*(1), 445–446.

*Byers VL. (1993). Novel antiepileptic drugs. *J Neuroscience Nursing, 25*(6), 375–379.

(1990). Consult stat: Use caution when administering magnesium sulfate. *RN, 53*(11), 100–101.

Devinsky I. (1994). On seizure disorders. *Clinical Symposia, 46*(1), 2–34.

Dreifuss FE. (1991). Toxic effects of drugs used in the ICU: Anticonvulsant agents. *Crit Care Clin, 7*, 521–532.

Elives R. (1991). Management of epilepsy. *Practitioner, 235*, 563–668.

Fackelmann KA. (1991). Epilepsy and pregnancy: a drug dilemma. *Science News, 140*(7), 11.

Farwell JR, et al. (1990). Phenobarbital for febrile seizure: Effects on intelligence and on seizure recurrence. *N Engl J Med, 322*(6), 364.

Fisher RS. (1993). Emerging anti-epileptic drugs. *Neurology, 43*(suppl 5), 12–17.

*French F. (1994). The long-term management of epilepsy. *Ann Intern Med, 120*, 411.

(1994). Gabapentin (Neurontin): Added protection against seizures. *ASN, 94*(9), 53.

*Recommended for further reading.

Gannon SL. (1993). Epilepsy in the elderly. *J Neuroscience Nursing, 25*(5), 273.

Glenn MB. (1991). Anticonvulsants reconsidered. *J Head Trauma Rehab, 6*(3), 85–88.

Harden C. (1994). New antiepileptic drugs. *Neurology, 44,* 787–795.

Hardman JG, Linbird LE, Molinoff PB, et al. (eds). (1996). *Goodman and Gilman's Pharmacological basis of therapeutics,* 9th ed. New York: McGraw-Hill.

*Hopkins S. (1994). Epilepsy: Advances in anticonvulsant drugs. *Nursing Standard, 8*(15), 24–25.

Hussar DA. (1994). Antiepileptic: gabapentin. *Nursing '94, 24*(12), 55.

*Kupecz D. (1995). New drugs for the treatment of epilepsy. *Nurse Practitioner, 20*(5), 82–85.

Lannon SL. (1995). Controlling seizures in the elderly. *Nursing '95, 95*(3), 32.

Lannon SL. (1993). Epilepsy in the elderly. *J Neuroscience Nursing, 25*(5), 273–285.

Lazar RB. (1995). Felbamate: Is there a role in the prevention and management of posttraumatic epilepsy? *J Head Trauma Rehab, 10*(1), 87–89.

Legion V. (1991). Health education for self-management by people with epilepsy. *J Neuroscience Nursing, 23*(5), 300–305.

Mattson RH. (1994). Current challenges in the treatment of epilepsy. *Neurology, 44*(suppl), 54.

Anonymous. (1994). New anti-seizure medications you should know about. *Case Management Advisor, 5*(7), 99–100.

Anonymous. (1995). New drugs: Lamotrigine. *Am J Nurs, 95*(5), 61–64.

O'Brien K. (1991). Managing the seizure patient. *Nursing '91, 21*(1), 63–65.

Rose BA. (1993). Neurologic therapies in critical care. *Crit Care Nurs Clin North Am, 5*(2), 237–246.

Russell A. (1995). Epilepsy. *Nursing Standard, 10*(3), 33–39.

*So E. (1993). Update on epilepsy. *Med Clin North Am, 77,* 203–214.

Taylor CP. (1994). Emerging perspectives on the mechanism of action of gabapentin. *Neurology, 44*(suppl 5), 510–516.

*Wyler AR. (1993). Modern management of epilepsy. *Postgrad Med, 94*(3), 97.

Ziemba SK. (1995). Seizures. *Am J Nurs, 95*(2), 32–33.

*Recommended for further reading.

For more information and sample tests and activities, refer to Chapter 19 in the Student Workbook for Clinical Pharmacology and Nursing Management, 5th edition, available through your bookstore.

20

Drugs That Affect Emotional and Psychologic Functions

A wide range of psychoactive drugs is available, with various side effects and pharmacologic actions. Advances in psychopharmacology and nonpharmacologic therapeutic interventions have drastically improved the quality of life for many persons. Before the 20th century, the use of medications for mental illness remained largely undeveloped. People have experimented with mind-altering chemicals throughout history, but sociocultural beliefs and scientific developments have greatly influenced the therapeutic value and use of these medications. Not until the 18th century did clinicians begin to consider a possible link between psychiatric symptoms and anatomic abnormalities. Observations of poor care and often punitive treatments marked the 19th century, raising important ethical questions about traditional intervention. The need to find more humane and scientific therapies, including medications, became increasingly evident.

In the early 20th century, psychopharmacology was still in its infancy. The use of barbiturates for anxiety emerged, although interventions remained largely custodial. Treatments for refractory mental illness included the use of insulin, electroconvulsive therapy, hydrotherapy, and surgical lobotomies. These approaches often had little effect. Psychoanalysis was an alternative therapy for persons who could afford it. In the midst of the 20th century, pharmacologic developments rapidly emerged, beginning with the synthesis of antipsychotic medications. These advances radically changed treatment options for the mentally ill. Psychopharmacology has provided the means for relieving many debilitating symptoms, including depression, psychosis, anxiety, and mood swings. Use of mechanical restraints declined. Isolation decreased among persons suffering from schizophrenia. Because of pharmacologic developments, many persons can now live in the community rather than in institutional confinement.

Psychoactive drugs include antipsychotic, anxiolytic, antidepressant, and mood stabilizing agents. The choice of medications is influenced by several factors, including the type of disorder, the severity of symptoms, standard treatment approaches, previous treatment responses and experiences, perceptions of medication, and willingness to follow a medication regimen. Medication therapy is a single component of a multifaceted treatment plan. Although medication does not cure psychiatric disorders, pharmacologic advances during the 20th century have enhanced the well-being of countless persons.

General Considerations

The goal of psychopharmacologic intervention is to provide symptomatic relief, thus ideally contributing to improved functional status and quality of life. Although current medications do not cure psychiatric illness, they provide many persons with an opportunity to live a productive and rewarding life outside of an institution. Furthermore, medications may make it possible for the person to take part in other kinds of psychiatric treatments, such as psychotherapy. Depending on the type of disorder, many clients respond to less invasive nonpharmacologic interventions. Medication intervention is one component of a larger treatment plan.

Clients with psychiatric illnesses often exhibit a wide range of complex behaviors that may affect their capacity for therapeutic adherence. Thus, compliance is a key area of consideration and assessment. For example, severely depressed clients may need antidepressant medications, but they are at significant risk of using these medications to commit suicide by overdose. Clients exhibiting disorganized thinking or impulsive behavior may have difficulty adhering to a medication regimen. Therefore, the disorder itself can significantly confound a person's ability to adhere to the medication regimen, as can his or her values and perceptions of the medication. Psychiatric symptoms may alter the client's values. For instance, clients with paranoid schizophrenia may believe that medications are poison and that the healthcare provider is trying to harm them. Furthermore, unpleasant side effects commonly result from drugs used therapeutically, so that drug administration can be risky. Because specific knowledge regarding psychoactive drug mechanisms is limited, treatment responses are sometimes difficult to predict.

Pathophysiology of Psychiatric Illness

Clinical studies provide increasing evidence that biologic, as well as psychosocial, influences may contribute to the development, expression, and chronicity of psychiatric illnesses. Investigators are focusing on the role of neuronal signaling in the central nervous system (CNS) and the potential influence on emotions and behaviors. The neuroanatomic and neurophysiologic regulation of intellectual functions, sensory input, visual and auditory reflexes, and emotions continues to prompt research on underlying biobehavioral dynamics.

Neuronal signaling involves the transmission of signals from the presynaptic neuron to the postsynaptic neuron (Fig. 20-1). Chemicals called neurotransmitters relay signals from one cell to another (Box 20-1). The presynaptic neuron receives signals that elicit a cellular

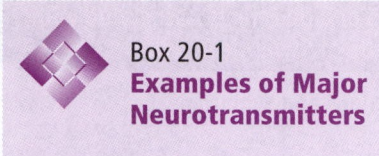

Box 20-1
Examples of Major Neurotransmitters

Acetylcholine

Dopamine

Gamma-aminobutyric acid (GABA)

Glutamate

Serotonin

Norepinephrine

response involving the release of neurotransmitters into the synaptic cleft. Following its release into the synaptic cleft, the neurotransmitter can interact with receptors on the cell membrane of the postsynaptic neuron, as well as with receptors (known as autoreceptors) on the presynaptic neuron. Once the neurotransmitter binds to a receptor site, subsequent physiologic responses indirectly influence behavior. Specific receptors are associated with the different neurotransmitters (Box 20-2). Other unidentified receptors may also exist. After release from the presynaptic neuron, neurotransmitters return to the presynaptic cell for storage and future release (reuptake). Alternatively, the neurotransmitter can break down into metabolites for excretion rather than interact with receptors or engage in presynaptic reuptake.

Researchers have focused on understanding the extent to which abnormal neurotransmission contributes to psychopathology. Abnormalities occurring with one particular type of neurotransmitter system do not appear to explain fully the etiology of psychiatric disorders. Mental illness is more likely to involve alterations among several neurotransmitters, as well as psychosocial factors. For example, excessive dopamine and norepinephrine and the ratio of dopamine to serotonin are thought to be involved in schizophrenia. Increased levels of the excitatory amino acid glutamate may contribute to hallucinations and other psychotic symptoms. Increased CNS levels of norepinephrine and decreased

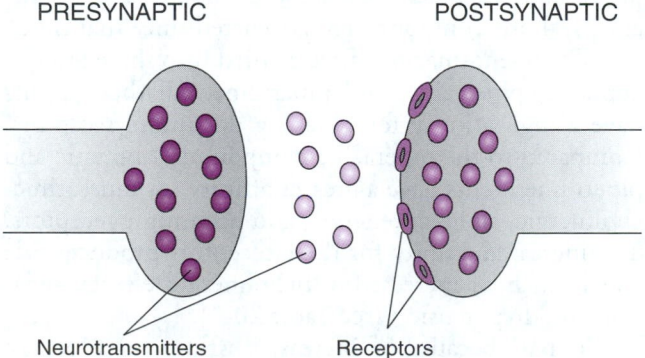

PRESYNAPTIC   POSTSYNAPTIC

Neurotransmitters   Receptors

Figure 20-1. Representation of neuronal signaling. Released from the neuron near the synapse (the presynaptic neuron), neurotransmitters relay impulses across the synapse to receptors on the nearby neuron (the postsynaptic neuron). After their release, the neurotransmitters may return to the nerve cell for storage (known as re-uptake) or they may break down into metabolites for excretion.

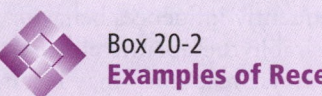

Box 20-2
Examples of Receptor Types

Adrenergic:	α_1, α_2, β_1, β_2
Cholinergic:	muscarinic (M_1–M_5), nicotinic
Dopaminergic:	D_1–D_5
Serotonergic:	5-HT$_{1A-F}$, 5-HT$_2$, 5-HT$_3$*

*5-HT = 5-hydroxytryptamine, the chemical name for serotonin

Table 20-1. Examples of Side Effects Associated with Pharmacologic Blockade of Synaptic Activity

Type of Side Effect	Signs and Symptoms
Adrenergic	
α_1	Postural hypotension, dizziness, sedation
α_2	Sexual disturbance
Cholinergic	Dry mouth, blurred vision, constipation, urinary retention
Dopaminergic	
D_2	Extrapyramidal symptoms
Histaminergic	
H_1	Sedation, postural hypotension, weight gain

gamma-aminobutyric acid (GABA) are associated with anxiety. Decreased CNS levels of norepinephrine and serotonin are linked to depression.

Altered neurotransmission may result from several possible synaptic mechanisms. For example, too much or too little neurotransmitter may be released from the presynaptic cell. The reuptake mechanism may be poorly regulated, leading to excessive or diminished amounts of the neurotransmitter left in the synaptic cleft. Changes in the sensitivity of presynaptic or postsynaptic receptors (hypersensitive or hyposensitive) may alter the receptor's ability to bind with neurotransmitters.

Psychopharmacology helps regulate altered neurotransmission in the CNS. Psychoactive drugs target mechanisms involved in neurotransmission to enhance or inhibit cellular responses. Some pharmacologic agents are associated with a particular neurotransmitter. For example, the selective serotonin reuptake inhibitors (SSRIs), often used in the treatment of depression, are selective in blocking the reuptake of serotonin into the presynaptic neuron. Thus, SSRIs increase the amount of serotonin available in the synaptic cleft for receptor binding. Psychoactive agents also have varied affinity for differing types of receptors. Such differences contribute to the diverse therapeutic effects, adverse reactions, and side effect profiles of medications (Table 20-1).

In summary, medications can modify CNS neurotransmission, which subsequently influences behavior. In addition to the drugs' desirable therapeutic effects, undesirable consequences (adverse reactions) may result.

Psychoactive Drug Classes

Psychoactive drugs are categorized according to their major uses. Some medications have therapeutic indications for several conditions. General categories of psychoactive drugs are antipsychotics, anxiolytics, antidepressants, and mood stabilizers. The following sections outline the major classes and the pharmacodynamics, pharmacokinetics,

therapeutic uses, adverse reactions, interactions, and precautions and contraindications associated with these agents. Key nursing management issues related to the psychoactive drug categories are also discussed.

Antipsychotic Agents

Antipsychotic medications, also referred to as major tranquilizers, are generally used for psychiatric conditions characterized by altered mental status and disturbed thought processes. Psychotic symptoms include paranoid thinking, disorganized speech, delusions, and hallucinations. Aggressive behavior and altered mood may also occur. Characteristically, persons with psychotic symptoms have distorted perceptions of reality that interfere with conducting activities of daily living. Psychotic symptoms may also jeopardize the person's safety. Antipsychotic agents help provide symptomatic relief from psychotic symptoms and may enhance the person's quality of life.

The major classes of antipsychotic agents are phenothiazines, thioxanthenes, butyrophenones, diphenylbutylpiperidine, dibenzoxazepines, and dihydroindolone (Table 20-2). Dibenzodiazepine and benzisoxazole (Table 20-3) are two additional classes labeled as atypical antipsychotic agents. In general, antipsychotic agents do not induce chemical dependency.

Phenothiazines

The use of phenothiazines in treating psychiatric illness resulted from efforts to find a drug to calm preoperative patients. In the early 1950s, the French surgeon Laborit observed ataraxia (calmness without sedation) in preoperative clients receiving chlorpromazine. These observations led Laborit to propose trying chlorpromazine to calm agitated psychotic persons. The use of chlorpromazine in the clinical setting increased rapidly when clinical experiments supported the calming effect of chlorpromazine in agitated clients. Development of additional antipsychotic compounds has occurred since that time.

The phenothiazines are classified into three groups: aliphatic, piperazine, and piperidine. All these agents have a high affinity for blocking dopamine receptors. Compared to the piperazine compounds, aliphatic and piperidine agents have a greater affinity for muscarinic-cholinergic, alpha-adrenergic, and histaminic receptors. The increased affinity for these receptors produces side effects such as increased anticholinergic effects, sedation, and hypotension (see Table 20-2).

In part because of increased affinity in blocking dopamine (D_2) receptors in the nigrostriatal region of the brain, piperazine agents are more likely to produce extrapyramidal symptoms (EPS) such as akathisia, dystonia, and parkinsonism (Box 20-3). Thus, an awareness of drug action allows clinicians to anticipate and assess for specific side effects and adverse reactions (see Table 20-1).

Table 20-2. Antipsychotic Agents

Drug	Dosage Form*	Potency	Range of Daily Adult Oral Dose† (mg/day)
Phenothiazines			
Aliphatic			
chlorpromazine (Thorazine)	PO, IM, SUP	low	200–800
Piperidine			
mesoridazine (Serentil)	PO, IM	moderate	30–400
thioridazine (Mellaril)	PO	low	150–800
Piperazine			
fluphenazine (Prolixin)	PO, IM	high	1–60
perphenazine (Trilafon)	PO, IM	high	12–32
trifluoperazine (Stelazine)	PO, IM	high	4–20
Thioxanthenes			
thiothixene (Navane)	PO, IM	high	6–60
Butyrophenones			
haloperidol (Haldol)	PO, IM	high	1–15
Diphenylbutylpiperidines			
pimozide (Orap)	PO	high	<0.2 mg/kg, or <10 mg/day
Dibenzoxazepine			
loxapine (Loxitane)	PO, IM	high	20–100
Dihydroindolone			
molindone (Moban)	PO	high	50–225

*PO = oral, IM = intramuscular, SUP = suppository
†Dose varies according to indicated use and severity of symptoms.

Box 20-3
Recognizing Extrapyramidal Symptoms

Several undesirable side effects associated with psychotropic drugs are known as extrapyramidal symptoms (EPS) because they affect the extrapyramidal tract. They include akathisia, dystonia, and parkinsonism. EPS are often responsive to treatment with anticholinergic and antiparkinson agents.

Akathisia

Extreme, uncontrollable restlessness

Compulsion to move around, pacing, difficulty sitting still

Dystonia

Rapid onset (within hours or days after antipsychotic medication begins or dosage changes); may be frightening for the client

Involuntary muscle contractions of the head, neck, and face; possible difficulty swallowing, opening the mouth, or moving the tongue or jaw

Spasms of the neck, causing hyperextension of head

Oculogyric crisis: fixed upward gaze resulting from extraocular muscle spasms

Parkinsonism

Onset within weeks or months after antipsychotic drug therapy begins

Muscular rigidity (often undetected)

Tremor (tremor + rigidity = cogwheeling)

Pill rolling (repetitive rubbing of the thumb against the index finger)

Akinesia (immobility): slowed movements and decreased ability to initiate movement, masklike facial expression, decreased eye blinking, drooling, shuffling gait

Table 20-3. Atypical and Novel Antipsychotic Agents

Drug	Dosage Form	Targeted Daily Adult Dose Range (mg/day)
Dibenzodiazepine		
clozapine (Clozaril)	Oral	300–450
Benzisoxazole		
risperidone (Risperdal)	Oral	4–6
Pirenzepine		
olanzapine (Zyprexa)	Oral	10–20

Thioxanthenes

Thioxanthenes are structurally similar to phenothiazines. Thiothixene (Navane) is one of the most potent thioxanthene agents. High-potency antipsychotic agents are associated with EPS.

Butyrophenones

Haloperidol (Haldol) is the only butyrophenone approved for use as an antipsychotic agent in the United States. Haloperidol is an extremely potent drug with high affinity for blocking dopamine (D_2) receptors. Thus, it is also associated with EPS.

Other Agents

Pimozide is the single diphenylbutylpiperidine available in the United States. Although approved only for use in Tourette syndrome in the United States, pimozide and other diphenylbutylpiperidine agents, including fluspirilene and penfluridol, are used as antipsychotics in other countries (Marder & Van Putten, 1995). Pimozide is associated with relatively high EPS effects and low anticholinergic, hypotensive, and sedative effects. Dibenzoxazepine and dihydroindolone compounds (loxapine and molindone, respectively) are likely to have high EPS effects.

Atypical and Novel Agents

The dibenzodiazepine compound clozapine (Clozaril) is often called an atypical antipsychotic (Box 20-4) because it has several differences from traditional antipsychotic agents. Clients receiving atypical antipsychotic drugs may experience a significant reduction of symptoms—and possibly symptom remission—even if they did not respond well to traditional antipsychotic agents. This level of improvement is markedly different from that observed following traditional antipsychotic therapy. Other novel antipsychotic agents include risperidone and olanzapine. Similar to clozapine, these agents appear to decrease negative symptoms of psychosis (eg, blunted affect) and positive symptoms (eg, hallucinations and delusions); traditional antipsychotic agents tend to reduce positive symptoms only.

Differing from traditional antipsychotics, atypical agents are associated with lower risk for EPS. Clozapine, for example, is generally not associated with tar-

dive dyskinesia (TD), although it may produce significant and life-threatening agranulocytosis. High-dose olanzapine and risperidone may induce EPS in some clients. Because atypical and novel antipsychotic agents may reduce the risk for EPS and TD, a trial of these drugs may be appropriate in clients who cannot tolerate traditional antipsychotic drugs. Atypical and novel antipsychotic agents may benefit clients who are unresponsive to traditional antipsychotic therapy.

Pharmacodynamics. Antipsychotic agents block dopamine receptors in the CNS; thus, they are dopamine receptor antagonists. Research suggests that antipsychotic agents exert their antipsychotic effect by blocking the dopamine receptors in the mesolimbic and mesocortical areas of the CNS. Traditional antipsychotic agents block several dopamine receptor subtypes, including D_2 (see Table 20-1). Atypical agents show a different affinity profile, having a lower capacity to bind to D_2 receptors. The decreased affinity for D_2 receptors may explain the decreased EPS symptoms with these agents (see Table 20-2). Additionally, clozapine and risperidone have a greater affinity for serotonin receptors ($5\text{-}HT_{2c}$). Both clozapine and traditional low-potency antipsychotic agents are muscarinic-cholinergic antagonists, resulting in associated side effects (see Box 20-2 and Table 20-1). Antipsychotic agents also block dopamine receptors in the medulla, resulting in an antiemetic effect. Differences in affinity for receptor subtypes may explain why some persons unresponsive to one drug will respond to another agent. Drug-induced behavioral effects (both therapeutic and undesirable) may reflect the CNS anatomic loci of drug action.

Pharmacokinetics. Antipsychotic medications are available in oral and parenteral preparations. Oral preparations include tablets, capsules, liquid concentrate, liquid suspension or elixir, and syrup. Parenteral preparations include those given by intramuscular (IM) injection. Chlorpromazine (Thorazine) is available as a

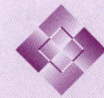

Box 20-4
Anticholinergic and Antiparkinson Agents for Drug-Induced EPS

Anticholinergic Aents

benztropine (Cogentin)
biperiden (Akineton)
procyclidine (Kemadrin)
trihexyphenidyl (Artane)

Antiparkinson Agents

amantadine (Symmetrel)
diphenhydramine (Benadryl)

suppository for antiemetic indications. Some agents are prepared in sustained-release form. Both oral and parenteral preparations are generally well absorbed. Food, antacids, cigarette smoking, and possibly coffee can decrease the absorption of oral preparations. Oral antipsychotic agents generally have peak effect within 1 to 4 hours after administration. Parenterally administered antipsychotic drugs have a rapid onset of action, with peak effect occurring 30 to 60 minutes after IM injection. These drugs are highly lipophilic, increasing access across the blood-brain barrier and entry into the CNS. Tables 20-2 and 20-3 provide general dosage information for the antipsychotic agents. Because of the many preparations and varying doses, the reader should consult the manufacturer's package insert before use.

Several factors, including the route of administration and the client's age, rate of metabolism, and concurrent medications, influence the half-life of antipsychotic agents. Therefore, the half-life of an antipsychotic medication varies widely from one person to another. Generally, the half-life of oral antipsychotic agents ranges from 10 to 40 hours. Treatment with these drugs often takes several weeks to achieve maximal effect. Some agents are prepared in slow-release form known as depot medications. Slow-release agents administered by IM injection have a much longer half-life and may take up to several months to reach a full effect. The long half-life of IM-administered antipsychotic drugs allows for intermittent dosing. For instance, IM fluphenazine can be administered every 2 weeks, making IM preparations particularly helpful for clients who have difficulty adhering to a daily medication regimen.

Because of the long half-life of antipsychotic agents administered IM, traces of medication can be found in the blood several months after the client discontinues drug therapy. Psychoactive agents accumulate in body tissues when administered over time. The tissues then slowly release the accumulated supply after discontinuation of the drug. Continual release is the reason traces of the drug can be found in urine several months after the medication has been stopped. The degree of accumulation is an important consideration when instituting a new drug regimen after discontinuing an antipsychotic agent. Knowledge of possible prolonged drug levels is also important for calculating necessary time intervals between incompatible drugs.

Orally administered antipsychotic agents undergo the metabolic process known as hepatic first-pass. Many metabolites of antipsychotic drugs are active and have significant physiologic effects. Some metabolites are more active than the parent drug, as with thioridazine (Mellaril). Most antipsychotic agents are highly bound to protein (greater than 90%); thus, extreme caution is warranted when they are used simultaneously with other highly protein-bound agents (eg, warfarin, digoxin). Because protein-bound agents compete with one another for protein binding, concurrent administration can result in drug displacement and lead to life-threatening toxicity. Excretion of antipsychotic drugs and their metabolites is largely through the kidneys.

Therapeutic Uses. Antipsychotic agents are most commonly used to treat psychotic disorders, including schizophrenia, schizoaffective disorder, depression with psychotic features, and psychotic symptoms observed in organic brain syndromes (eg, delirium, dementia). Some agents, including pimozide and haloperidol, are used to treat symptoms of Tourette syndrome. Antipsychotic drugs help manage severe agitation, acute manic episodes, and mania in clients refractory to treatment with standard mood stabilizers. Antipsychotic medications may provide symptomatic relief from chorea and agitation in Huntington's disease. Some antipsychotic agents are used to treat pervasive developmental disorders and mental retardation. Due to their antiemetic properties, antipsychotic agents are helpful in relieving nausea and vomiting.

Adverse Reactions. The development of EPS is a major concern with antipsychotic therapy (see Box 20-3). The symptoms usually are not identified until they are severe. Unfortunately, EPS are frequently misinterpreted as anxiety or agitation (Weiden et al., 1987). EPS can be extremely debilitating but are usually treatable. Ongoing assessment for EPS can lead to early identification and treatment. Clients generally develop EPS in the first few weeks of treatment; symptoms appear to be dose-dependent. An increase in antipsychotic drug dosage warrants particularly close assessment for EPS. With atypical antipsychotics, EPS appear to be less common. Because high-potency antipsychotics, such as haloperidol, have a greater risk for inducing acute dystonic reactions, the client needs close monitoring. Males and younger persons are more likely to develop acute dystonic reactions (Lavin & Rifkin, 1992).

Administration of antiparkinson medication quickly alleviates dystonic reactions (see Box 20-4). Anticholinergic and antiparkinson agents are cholinergic-blocking drugs thought to decrease EPS symptoms by altering the balance of acetylcholine and dopamine in the CNS. Anticholinergic and antiparkinson agents are sometimes administered prophylactically. Lower drug doses may help prevent EPS.

Tardive dyskinesia, an involuntary movement disorder induced by chronic antipsychotic therapy, may occur after several months or years of antipsychotic use. It is likely to affect up to 20% of persons who take these drugs for more than 1 year (Marder & Van Putten, 1995). Symptoms of TD include rhythmic, stereotyped movements such as chewing, puckering, lip smacking, protrusion of the tongue, facial grimacing, and choreiform (wormlike) motion involving the tongue, fingers, toes, and occasionally the trunk. Early symptoms include facial tics, oral movements, and rocking motions. Symptoms increase with excitement, subside after relaxation, and are not apparent during sleep. The onset of TD is sudden and can be frightening to clients, their families, and staff. Irreversible TD is associated with long-term antipsychotic use. Populations at risk for developing TD include the elderly, persons with concurrent affective illness, and clients receiving high doses of antipsychotic agents over an extended period (Kane & Lieberman, 1992).

Neuroleptic malignant syndrome (NMS) is a serious and potentially fatal adverse reaction to antipsychotic agents. Cardinal features include extreme muscle rigidity and fever. NMS symptoms usually occur within 1 month of initiation of drug therapy. Additional symptoms include increased sweating, pulse rate, and blood pressure, as well as confusion and leukocytosis. The severity of the reaction can vary; fatalities occur in up to 15% of cases. Treatment of NMS involves supportive care and immediate discontinuation of the antipsychotic agent. Symptoms usually subside within 1 month after discontinuation of the antipsychotic agent.

Other neurologic effects include seizures. Because antipsychotic drugs are associated with a lowered seizure threshold, extreme caution should be used in persons with a seizure history. Sedation and drowsiness may occur and are more frequent with the use of low-potency antipsychotic agents.

Anticholinergic effects are particularly associated with low-potency antipsychotic agents. These symptoms include dry mucous membranes, mydriasis, blurred vision, constipation, and urinary retention. Confusion and disorientation are associated with higher doses or concomitant administration of other anticholinergic agents.

Cardiovascular effects include postural hypotension, the result of alpha-adrenergic receptor blockade, which occurs more often with low-potency antipsychotic agents. Symptoms include dizziness and faintness and are prominent when rising from a lying or sitting position. Sometimes syncope occurs. The elderly and clients receiving parenteral agents are at greater risk for drug-induced postural hypotension. Tachycardia and changes in cardiac conduction are more common with low-potency antipsychotic agents. Electrocardiogram (ECG) changes, including prolonged Q-T and P-R intervals, usually remain within a normal range. Prolonged Q-T and P-R intervals in the normal range are generally not clinically significant unless the client has a history of a cardiac condition or the drug dosage exceeds that recommended. Several antipsychotic agents, including chlorpromazine, haloperidol, thioridazine, and pimozide, can have potentially serious cardiotoxic effects, including altered Q-T intervals.

Cutaneous effects involve allergic skin reactions, such as rashes or exfoliative dermatitis. Dermatologic reactions typically occur during the initial months of treatment. Low-potency antipsychotic agents cause photosensitivity or extreme sensitivity to sunlight. This effect may result in severe sunburn in unprotected persons. Although rare, exposure to the sun can change skin pigmentation, resulting in blue-gray spots. Cutaneous pigmentation changes are associated with low-potency medications.

Gastrointestinal (GI) effects, characterized by constipation and decreased intestinal motility, may be a consequence of acetylcholine blockade. Dyspepsia and diarrhea occur less commonly.

Neuroendocrine effects may occur as well. In general, traditional antipsychotic agents can block hypothalamic D_2 receptors. This limits dopamine's normal regulatory effect in inhibiting prolactin release from the pituitary. Thus, side effects resulting from hyperprolactinemia may be manifested. Gynecomastia, impotence, and rarely galactorrhea occur in men. Amenorrhea, menstrual irregularities, breast engorgement, lactation, and anorgasmia are possible drug-related effects in women. Weight gain and hyperthermia are additional symptoms possibly related to antipsychotic drug influences on hypothalamic functioning.

Hepatic effects, including cholestatic jaundice characterized by nausea, abdominal pain, elevated temperature, chills, pruritus, and abnormal liver function test results (eg, elevated alkaline phosphatase and bilirubin), are rare. Cholestatic jaundice typically occurs during the first few months of drug therapy. Treatment involves discontinuing the medication.

Ocular effects, such as pigmentation or discoloration of the lens, conjunctiva, cornea, and retina, are associated with low-potency antipsychotic agents. Unless severe, pigmentary changes generally do not alter vision. Irreversible visual impairment, including blindness, may occur with pigmentary retinopathy, an adverse effect associated with doses of thioridazine exceeding 800 mg daily (Hyman et al., 1995). Blurred vision may result from anticholinergic effects. Before the client starts low-potency antipsychotic therapy, the nurse must assess for a history of narrow-angle glaucoma.

Hematologic effects may include agranulocytosis, the depression of leukocyte production—a rare adverse reaction to antipsychotic agents. The onset of agranulocytosis is sudden and usually occurs in the first few months of drug therapy. This condition is serious and can result in death. Symptoms include sore throat, fever, weakness, and other signs of infection. The client with agranulocytosis must stop drug treatment at once, and appropriate isolation precautions must be initiated to prevent transmitting infection. Agranulocytosis affects about 2% of clients taking clozapine. Strict weekly white blood cell (WBC) monitoring is necessary throughout clozapine treatment, as well as for several weeks after drug therapy is discontinued.

Drug Interactions. Concurrent administration of antipsychotic agents with anticholinergic drugs, including antihistamines, antiparkinson agents, and antidepressants, may potentiate anticholinergic side effects. Antacids decrease absorption of antipsychotic agents; thus, it is better to separate administration of antacids and antipsychotic medications by about 2 hours. Taking epinephrine with antipsychotic drugs can result in a paradoxical decrease in blood pressure; therefore, epinephrine should not be used to counteract hypotensive side effects. Concomitant use of antipsychotic drugs and alcohol, barbiturates, narcotics, or benzodiazepines increases the CNS depressant effects, including increased sedation. Carbamazepine may suppress bone marrow and is avoided during clozapine therapy. Cigarette smoking can decrease antipsychotic plasma concentrations. Fluoxetine may increase antipsychotic blood levels. Other agents potentially influencing plasma levels of antipsychotic drugs include the beta blockers propranolol and pindolol, and amitriptyline. The therapeutic antihypertensive effect of guanethidine can be impaired by chlorpromazine, haloperidol, and thiothixene, thus necessitating close monitoring of blood pressure in persons receiving both agents. Antipsychotic drugs can block the effect of levodopa. Simultaneous administration of two or more antipsychotic agents does not appear to have any significant therapeutic value and may increase the risk for adverse effects.

Precautions and Contraindications. Although antipsychotic medications help many persons, they have serious physiologic effects and must be used cautiously. Few data are available on the efficacy of antipsychotic medications in children compared to efficacy in adults. Body weight, metabolism, and neurologic development are important factors. Elderly persons are more prone to adverse reactions, particularly anticholinergic effects and TD. Low-potency antipsychotic medications are contraindicated for persons with conditions sensitive to anticholinergic effects (eg, narrow-angle glaucoma, prostatic hypertrophy).

In general, pregnant women should avoid psychoactive drugs, particularly during the first trimester. The need for relieving severe psychiatric symptoms during pregnancy must be weighed carefully against potential teratogenic effects.

Because many psychoactive drugs and their active metabolites are biotransformed by the liver and excreted by the kidneys, psychoactive drugs must be used cautiously in clients with compromised renal or liver function. Agents with potentially severe cardiotoxicity following overdose (eg, thioridazine, mesoridazine, and pimozide) should be avoided in persons at risk for suicide. These agents are contraindicated in clients with a known hypersensitivity or allergic reaction to the drug.

Antipsychotic medications are contraindicated in comatose patients and in persons likely to experience a significant CNS depressant effect from other substances (eg, alcohol, barbiturates). Cautious use is warranted in clients with a history of respiratory distress, including asthma and emphysema, because of the antipsychotic agent's CNS depressant effect. Pimozide (Orap) is contraindicated in patients receiving macrolide antibiotic therapy (eg, erythromycin, clarithromycin).

■ SUMMARY

Antipsychotic drugs help relieve psychotic symptoms and are commonly used in the treatment of psychotic disorders. Drug properties, including

affinity for receptors and loci of action in the CNS, influence the therapeutic effect and side effect profile. High-potency drugs are generally associated with EPS; low-potency antipsychotic agents tend to be associated with anticholinergic effects. Although antipsychotic medications often provide beneficial effects, they are not curative. Rather, they provide some symptomatic relief and may improve individual functioning and quality of life.

❖ NURSING MANAGEMENT: CLIENT RECEIVING ANTIPSYCHOTIC AGENTS

Preparing antipsychotic medications for administration requires great care. For example, oral concentrates can be mixed with juice before administration, but not with beverages containing caffeine. Oral concentrates must be diluted soon before administration. Antipsychotic agents require careful handling, as direct contact with these agents can result in contact dermatitis. Several agents, such as haloperidol, must be stored in light-resistant containers. Because of the numerous potential adverse effects, varying individual responses, and drug interactions, thorough assessments and prompt interventions are critical.

NURSING PROCESS

ASSESSMENT

Before administering drug therapy, the nurse completes a comprehensive baseline nursing assessment, followed by subsequent assessments at regular intervals. A comprehensive assessment involves evaluating the client's functional health patterns, addressing such areas as activity and rest, circulation, ego integrity, elimination, foods and fluids, hygiene, neurosensory function, pain and discomfort, respiration, safety, sexuality, social interactions, teaching and learning needs, and discharge planning considerations (Doenges & Moorhouse, 1996).

Regular ongoing assessment is imperative. Routine collection of assessment data helps guide subsequent interventions and helps meet the client's needs. Careful and frequent assessments of signs and symptoms facilitates early identification and prompt intervention.

The nurse assesses and records the presence or absence of overt signs of emotional disturbances, including hallucinations, delusions, anxiety, depression, and suicidal and homicidal ideation, plan, and intent. Depressed clients are at greatest risk for committing suicide when they begin to feel slightly better and have enough energy to act on the suicidal thought. The client's mental status (eg, orientation to person, place, and time) must be thoroughly assessed at baseline and regularly during drug therapy. Vital signs, including pulse rate, orthostatic blood pressures, respiration, and body temperature, are important data to include in the baseline assessment.

The client's previous experience with, perceptions of, and attitudes about medications should be explored. It is important to obtain a history of previous medication use, efficacy, reason for discontinuation, and related experiences. Screening for risk factors and contraindicated conditions, including pregnancy, narrow-angle glaucoma, cardiac conditions, renal impairment, and hepatic dysfunction, is critical before initiating drug therapy.

NURSING DIAGNOSES

Possible nursing diagnoses specifically related to antipsychotic medications include:

- Impaired Verbal Communication, related to medication-induced EPS effects
- Acute Confusion, related to medication-induced TD or neurotoxicity
- Constipation, related to medication
- Fatigue, related to medication-induced sedation
- Fear, related to knowledge deficit about medications
- Risk for Fluid Volume Deficit, related to medication-induced NMS
- Risk for Infection, related to medication-induced agranulocytosis
- Risk for Injury, related to medication-induced orthostatic hypotension
- Knowledge Deficit, related to lack of exposure to medication information
- Altered Oral Mucous Membrane, related to medication
- Impaired Physical Mobility, related to effects of medication (eg, sedation, EPS, TD)
- Sexual Dysfunction, related to medication
- Risk for Impaired Skin Integrity, related to drug-induced photosensitivity
- Urinary Retention, related to medication

PLANNING

Planning efforts are directed at increasing the efficacy of drug therapy and decreasing the severity of side effects.

INTERVENTION

After beginning the antipsychotic medication, clients are monitored for signs and symptoms of therapeutic response, allergic reaction, and adverse effects. Because initial hypotension usually occurs, clients are encouraged to remain in a recumbent position for 1 hour after initial doses. Resuming a supine position typically manages and relieves symptoms. Clients gradually learn to make positional changes to accommodate this effect. The client must change position gradually, first sitting on the edge of the bed for a few minutes before standing. Side rails and assisted ambulation may be necessary early on.

In clients with severe hypotension, intravenous (IV) fluids are given, followed by pressor agents selective for alpha-adrenergic receptors if symptoms persist. Alpha-adrenergic pressor agents such as metaraminol (Aramine) and norepinephrine (Levophed) are used instead of drugs with mixed alpha- and beta-stimulating properties. Agents with mixed alpha- and beta-adrenergic properties may induce a paradoxical response, further jeopardizing blood pressure. Epinephrine is *not* used to treat antipsychotic-induced hypotension.

Signs and symptoms of EPS, TD, and NMS should be reported promptly to the prescribing clinician, who may order an anticholinergic or antiparkinson agent to help relieve these symptoms. The nurse can help calm clients experiencing EPS by reducing environmental stimulation. EPS may subside somewhat as environmental stimulation and stress decrease.

Early detection of TD increases the possibility of reversing the symptoms, although older persons are more susceptible to irreversible effects. Assessment for TD includes regular monitoring for abnormal movements. The Abnormal Involuntary Movement Scale (AIMS) from the U.S. Public Health Service is a useful assessment tool. It is particularly helpful to obtain a baseline AIMS rating before antipsychotic treatment begins. Periodic evaluations can then be made during each subsequent year of therapy. Because there is no known treatment for TD, early detection is crucial. The lowest effective dose of an antipsychotic agent is prescribed to minimize the risk of TD. Reducing the drug dose, discontinuing the agent, or using an alternative antipsychotic medication may be helpful and should be discussed with the prescribing clinician. If traditional antipsychotic agents induce TD, an atypical antipsychotic drug may be considered.

The prescriber must be informed promptly of increased irritability or agitation, urinary retention, jaundice, and abnormal WBC test results. With symptoms of infection, the client should have an immediate WBC count with differential. If the client has agranulocytosis, antipsychotic drug treatment is discontinued at once and appropriate isolation procedures are instituted to prevent infection. Because of the increased risk and rapid onset of agranulocytosis during clozapine therapy, strict weekly WBC monitoring is needed for the duration of drug therapy and for several weeks after its discontinuation. A WBC count less than $3,000/mm^3$ or a neutrophil count less than $1,500/mm^3$ warrants discontinuation of clozapine.

Measures to prevent constipation include adequate fluid intake, exercise, and a fiber-rich diet. Use of laxatives may be indicated. In clients with urinary retention, urine output is monitored.

Clients need opportunities to ask questions about their medication regimen. It usually helps to ask the client about how the medication affects all aspects of functioning. When clients are approached in a supportive manner, they may report side effects that may otherwise be embarrassing or difficult to share. This is particularly relevant to an adverse effect such as sexual dysfunction.

When administering antipsychotic medications, as with any other medications, the nurse must remain with the client until the client swallows the drug. The confusion and disorientation experienced by psychotic clients can interfere with their ability to follow instructions for taking medication. In clients with paranoia, fear of poisoning may impair their capacity to take medications, and they may attempt to hide them. Concealing drugs is a serious problem because it can endanger the client and others. Hiding medications increases the risk of an overdose by the client or others who may encourage or convince the client to give them the drug. Furthermore, relief from symptoms is compromised, and this may exacerbate the client's condition. As with any medication, drug doses should not be given if the nurse believes them to be prescribed in unsafe dosages, contraindicated due to use of another drug or medical condition, or responsible for serious adverse reactions.

Client Education. Educating the client early in the treatment course helps reduce anxiety about adverse reactions and promotes adherence to the treatment plan. Inform clients and their families that it may take several weeks (3–6) for a therapeutic response. Warning about the anticipated lag time helps support the client, who may otherwise be discouraged during the first few weeks of treatment. Advise clients and their families to follow directions for administering the drug carefully, and tell them what to do about taking or not taking a missed dose. Instruct clients to avoid contact with the medication if the drug can cause contact dermatitis. Caution clients against discontinuing medication before consulting the prescribing clinician, because sudden discontinuation can cause relapse or deterioration. If adverse drug reactions are severe or persistent, advise the client to consult the prescribing clinician regarding a change in the drug regimen.

Clients must learn about avoiding and managing adverse effects. Lightheadedness and dizziness may be reduced by rising slowly or making gradual positional changes. The nurse can demonstrate positional changes (eg, how to sit on the edge of the bed for a few minutes before standing, how to rise slowly to a standing position). Provide reassurance, and inform clients that many people who take the drug adjust to it within a few days. The client should also be advised to avoid driving an automobile, operating machinery, or performing tasks requiring mental alertness and motor coordination until his or her response to the drug is predictable.

Inform the client about drug interactions and synergistic effects. Clients should avoid alcohol because it has a depressant effect and lowers the seizure threshold. Instruct clients to wear protective clothing, sunglasses, and sun block preparations and to avoid direct sunlight if photosensitivity is a side effect of drug therapy. Encourage them to use sugarless hard candies or chewing gum, sip small amounts of fluid frequently, or rinse their mouths often if oral dryness develops. Stress the importance of regular eye examinations and of reporting any peculiar ocular discoloration, EPS, or other drug effects to the prescriber for further evaluation and possible dosage adjustment. Clients should be urged to report signs and symptoms of infection immediately.

OUTCOME EVALUATION
Data may reflect the client's emotional status, vital signs (including postural blood pressures), absence or presence of adverse effects (eg, orthostatic hypotension), and subsequent consequences of these effects (eg, falls), as well as the client's comfort level and ability to manage the drug regimen.

The following are examples of possible desirable outcomes: hemodynamic stability, sustained orientation to reality, reduced symptoms of psychosis, normal bowel functioning, participation in treatment program, self-performance of activities of daily living, maintained fluid volume, maintained skin integrity, identification and verbalization of signs and symptoms of infection, absence of injury, identification and verbalization of potential drug interaction, and identification and verbalization of management strategies for adverse reactions. The evaluation process helps determine the therapeutic benefit of the medication to the client.

❖ **CHECKLIST OF NURSING ACTIONS**

- ❑ During assessment, explore and record the client's reports of functional health patterns before drug therapy begins and observations of functional health patterns during drug therapy.
- ❑ Assess and reassess the client's suicidal thoughts and intent throughout therapy. Also assess risk factors associated with drug therapy.
- ❑ Administer antipsychotic drugs as prescribed. Watch the client take the medication. Monitor for therapeutic drug effects.
- ❑ Monitor laboratory test results, particularly the WBC count, for indications of agranulocytosis.
- ❑ Teach the client about drug therapy and identify possible adverse effects, such as EPS, TD, NMS, postural hypotension, and constipation.
- ❑ Teach the client about adverse reactions to report and strategies to manage unpleasant side effects, such as hypotension and constipation.

Anxiolytic Agents

Anxiolytics, also known as antianxiety agents or minor tranquilizers, are used primarily to alleviate psychiatric conditions in which anxiety is the prominent feature. Symptoms of anxiety include tension, restlessness, fear, and worry. Physiologic symptoms commonly related to anxious states include palpitations, increased perspiration, GI upset, and shortness of breath. Episodes of anxiety having a sudden onset are often described as an anxiety or panic attack, accompanied by extreme apprehension, feelings of impending doom, and a fear of losing control. Anxiolytic agents provide symptomatic relief of anxiety, although they do not cure the underlying pathology. Anxiolytic drug therapy is just one component of a comprehensive treatment plan.

Anxiolytic agents include the benzodiazepines and other nonbenzodiazepine agents such as buspirone, zolpidem, and hydroxyzine (Table 20-4). Several SSRIs are also used as antianxiety agents; they are discussed in the following section on antidepressant medications. Use of barbiturates and the propanediol agent meprobamate (Equanil, Miltown) has become fairly obsolete as safer agents, such as the benzodiazepines, have been developed. Tolerance and addiction may develop when taking the benzodiazepines for an extended time. Tolerance, dependency, and the risk of lethal overdose during benzodiazepine therapy are significantly lower than that previously observed with barbiturates.

Buspirone and zolpidem are nonbenzodiazepine drugs used primarily in treating generalized anxiety disorder and anxiety associated with psychoneurosis or organic illness, respectively. Hydroxyzine, an antihistamine, is used in treating short-term insomnia.

Table 20-4. Anxiolytic Agents

Drug	Dosage Form*	Range of Daily Adult Oral Dose† (mg/day)
Benzodiazepines		
alprazolam (Xanax)	PO	0.50–10
triazolam (Halcion)	PO	0.125–0.25
lorazepam (Ativan)	PO, IM	1–12
oxazepam (Serax)	PO	30–120
temazepam (Restoril)	PO	7.5–30
chlordiazepoxide (Librium)	PO, IM	15–100
clonazepam (Klonopin)	PO	0.5–20
clorazepate (Tranxene)	PO	7.5–60‡
diazepam (Valium)	PO, IM	2–40
flurazepam (Dalmane)	PO	15–30
Other Agents		
buspirone (BuSpar)	PO	15–60
zolpidem (Ambien)	PO	5–10
hydroxyzine (Atarax)	PO	200–400

*PO = oral, IM = intramuscular
†Dose must be individualized; doses vary according to indicated use and severity of symptoms.
‡Up to 90 mg daily for acute alcohol withdrawal.

Benzodiazepines

Because of their effectiveness, benzodiazepines are the most widely prescribed drugs for anxiety (Ballenger, 1995). Many different benzodiazepines are available, and the choice of an agent is largely related to the desired onset of effect and drug potency. Some conditions, including panic disorder, are more responsive to high-potency benzodiazepines.

Pharmacodynamics. Benzodiazepines exert a therapeutic effect by binding to $GABA_A$ receptors in the brain. They do not appear to have an effect on $GABA_B$ receptors. Benzodiazepines cause $GABA_A$ receptors to increase the opening of chloride channels along the cell membrane, leading to an inhibitory effect on cell firing. Thus, they act as $GABA_A$ agonists (Hsiao & Potter, 1990). To a lesser extent, zolpidem also exerts an effect on $GABA_A$ receptors. Other neurotransmitters (eg, serotonin, norepinephrine) may play a role in the therapeutic effect of benzodiazepines.

Benzodiazepines appear to raise the seizure threshold, and some of the agents, including clonazepam, are specifically used as anticonvulsants. The exact mechanisms of benzodiazepines in producing antianxiety and anticonvulsant effects are not fully understood, although they may involve receptor activity in the limbic system, hypothalamus, and cortical regions of the brain.

The nonbenzodiazepine agent buspirone, an azaspirone, is primarily a serotonergic presynaptic (5-$HT1_A$) agonist and a partial postsynaptic (5-$HT1_A$) receptor agonist. Buspirone does not appear to have an effect on GABA receptors. Both buspirone and zolpidem have less sedative, muscle relaxant, and anticonvulsant properties than benzodiazepines. Buspirone does not appear to induce dependency; this effect in zolpidem remains less understood. Hydroxyzine, an antihistamine, acts as an H_1-receptor antagonist; it does not appear to induce drug dependency.

Pharmacokinetics. Anxiolytics are available in varied preparations, including oral and parenteral forms. Some agents are available in sustained-release form. When given on an empty stomach, oral preparations are generally well absorbed in the GI tract. Absorption of IM preparations varies and can be erratic. Use of well-developed muscle allows better IM drug absorption. IV preparations are generally given only for preoperative use or for seizure treatment. The manufacturer's instructions should be consulted before preparing IV anxiolytics because this requires extreme care, particularly in preparing the diluent and rate of administration. Exceedingly rapid IV administration increases the risk for acute respiratory arrest. Benzodiazepines are lipophilic, so they readily enter the CNS.

General dosage information for anxiolytic agents is provided in Table 20-4. Because of the varied dosages and dosage forms, the reader should review the manufacturer's package insert before preparation or administration of the drug.

The half-life of anxiolytic agents ranges from several hours to several days. Similarly, peak plasma levels are diverse, occurring 30 minutes to several hours after administration. Agents with longer half-lives require less frequent dosing. The administration of long-acting doses at bedtime ensures full use of the sedative effect for sleep. However, extended effects may contribute to morning and midday drowsiness. High-potency anxiolytics carry a greater risk for inducing drug dependency than low-potency agents.

Benzodiazepines are highly protein bound, so caution must be used when they are given with other protein-bound agents. Benzodiazepine metabolic pathways vary. Several benzodiazepines have active metabolites. Although the parent drug may have a short distribution half-life (eg, oral diazepam), the elimination half-life may be prolonged due to active metabolites. Thus, active metabolites contribute to a cumulative drug effect with repeated administration. Traces of the benzodiazepine can be found in urine long after discontinuing drug therapy.

Therapeutic Uses. Benzodiazepines are used to treat anxiety disorders, including generalized anxiety disorder, social phobia, and panic disorder. They are also used to relieve performance and situational anxiety. Benzodiazepines are not intended for long-term use, nor for minor stresses of daily living. Some benzodiazepines, including chlordiazepoxide, are used to treat alcohol withdrawal. Their muscle relaxant, anticonvulsant, and sedative effects make benzodiazepines useful for treating alcohol withdrawal and controlling psychomotor excitability. Benzodiazepines are also used for treating antipsychotic drug-induced akathisia and, as an adjunct, for treating insomnia and acute mania. The nonbenzodiazepine buspirone is used primarily in treating generalized anxiety disorder; zolpidem and hydroxyzine are used for short-term insomnia.

Adverse Reactions. Adverse effects of benzodiazepines are generally observed at the beginning of drug treatment and are usually relieved with dosage reductions. Benzodiazepines commonly induce drowsiness and ataxia, which are more likely to occur in the elderly. Transient memory impairments, including anterograde amnesia, are associated with certain benzodiazepines, including triazolam and zolpidem. Reactions of rage, excitement, and hostility have been reported during chlordiazepoxide therapy, although this does not necessarily imply a causal relation. Increased depression, confusion, headache, vertigo, GI disturbances, menstrual irregularities, and changes in libido are less common. Urticaria may occur with drug hypersensitivity.

Drug Interactions. Antacids decrease the absorption of benzodiazepines. Cimetidine increases plasma levels of long-acting benzodiazepines. Other agents increasing plasma benzodiazepine levels include erythromycin, oral contraceptives, and some antidepressant agents. Carbamazepine decreases plasma benzodiazepine levels. Simultaneous use of most anxiolytic agents and antihistamines, barbiturates, monoamine oxidase inhibitors (MAOIs) and other cyclic antidepressants, and alcohol potentiates CNS depression. Therefore, the dosage of CNS depressants should be reduced when used with anxiolytic agents. By increasing the metabolism, cigarette smoking can decrease the effectiveness of some anxiolytic drugs.

Precautions and Contraindications. Clients taking benzodiazepines are at risk for tolerance and dependency, although these drugs are less addictive than alcohol, nicotine, cocaine, and previously used barbiturate-based antianxiety agents (Hyman et al., 1995). Gradual withdrawal is essential if dependence develops. Elderly clients are more vulnerable to drug-induced drowsiness, ataxia, and confusion. Because benzodiazepines are lipophilic, these agents may accumulate in fat tissues, placing obese clients at greater risk for increased drug levels. Cautious use is required in persons with impaired hepatic or renal functioning because anxiolytic agents rely on hepatic metabolism and renal clearance.

Because of the potential for addiction, use of benzodiazepines by clients with a history of substance abuse is usually contraindicated. Benzodiazepines are also avoided during pregnancy, particularly in the first trimester. Hydroxyzine is specifically contraindicated in early pregnancy. History of acute narrow-angle glaucoma is a contraindication for some benzodiazepines, including alprazolam, diazepam, and lorazepam. Use of anxiolytic agents in persons with a known hypersensitivity or allergic reaction to the drug is contraindicated.

■ SUMMARY

Anxiolytic agents are used to alleviate significant and debilitating levels of anxiety. Benzodiazepines are the most frequently used anxiolytics, although nonbenzodiazepine drugs are available. Both tolerance and dependence may develop when using benzodiazepines, and a withdrawal reaction can occur. The benzodiazepines are a safer alternative to treating anxiety than the previously used barbiturates.

❖ NURSING MANAGEMENT: CLIENT RECEIVING ANXIOLYTIC AGENTS

Extreme caution is required when giving parenteral doses of anxiolytic agents. The manufacturer's instructions should be consulted before preparing and administering the drug.

NURSING PROCESS

ASSESSMENT

After conducting a thorough baseline assessment of the client's functional health patterns and subsequently conducting reassessments at regular intervals, the nurse must consider additional factors, such as concurrent medications and other substances. These data are pertinent to potential drug interactions and the identification of clients in whom benzodiazepines are contraindicated. A drug history of prescribed, over-the-counter, and abused substances is obtained. Signs and symptoms of adverse effects, dependency, and abrupt withdrawal are additional areas requiring ongoing assessment. Signs of drug dependency include recurring requests for dose escalation, repeated requests for administration of medication before the prescribed time, and irritability if drug administration is delayed. Symptoms of withdrawal include insomnia, restlessness, extreme irritability, and nervousness.

NURSING DIAGNOSES

Possible nursing diagnoses related to anxiolytic medications include:

- Nonadherence, related to medication-induced dependence and the client's value system
- Acute Confusion, related to medication-induced sedation or drug sensitivity
- Ineffective Denial, related to medication-induced dependency
- Fatigue, related to medication-induced sedation
- Knowledge Deficit, related to lack of exposure to medication information
- Impaired Social Interaction, related to medication-induced sedation

PLANNING

The nursing care plan is based on outcome goals and interventions specific to the nursing diagnoses.

INTERVENTION

The client's response to medication therapy must be carefully monitored for efficacy and for hypersensitivity and other adverse effects. Interventions during anxiolytic therapy are largely supportive, providing reassurance and education. For clients affected by drowsiness and ataxia, ongoing assessment of gait is important, and use of side rails or assisted ambulation may be necessary, particularly for elderly clients. If the client experiences excessive drowsiness and ataxia, the prescribing clinician should be consulted, because a reduction in drug dosage may provide relief. Signs and symptoms of dependency and acute withdrawal must be reported promptly to the prescribing clinician and supportive measures instituted.

Client Education. The nurse must explain the effects of anxiolytic medications, including adverse effects, synergistic effects, and drug interactions. The nurse must caution the client not to discontinue drug therapy abruptly; rather, the client should consult the prescribing clinician regarding discontinuation and gradual withdrawal of medication. The client also needs information about how medication will affect coordination and skills, such as operating machinery (eg, motor vehicles, lawn mowers) requiring mental alertness and motor coordination. The client also must be warned to avoid alcohol because of the potentiating CNS depressant effect.

OUTCOME EVALUATION

Possible desirable outcomes include reduced symptoms of anxiety and tension, decreased anxiety verbalized by the client, absence of or decrease in medication-related adverse effects, identification and verbalization of adverse effects and potential drug interactions, and absence of signs and symptoms of dependency.

❖ CHECKLIST OF NURSING ACTIONS

- ❑ Before anxiolytic therapy begins, take a complete health and drug history and assess for possible hypersensitivity to the prescribed antianxiety agent.
- ❑ Monitor the client's response to medication. Observe for therapeutic drug effect and signs and symptoms of adverse effects, such as dependency and withdrawal.
- ❑ Teach the client alternative strategies to reduce stressors, cope with anxiety, and avoid dependency on medication.
- ❑ Advise the client not to stop taking the medication abruptly without consulting the prescribing clinician. Explain the signs and symptoms of withdrawal.
- ❑ Provide supportive care, such as encouragement and education. Stay with a highly anxious client until anxiety subsides.

Antidepressants and Mood Stabilizers

Antidepressant medications and mood stabilizers are used primarily to treat conditions involving mood disturbances. Antidepressants are helpful in relieving debilitating depressive symptoms. Depression can significantly disrupt activities of daily living and is characterized by low self-esteem, sadness, thoughts of death, psychomotor retardation or agitation, sleep disturbances, fatigue, and decreased energy. Clients with significant depression may be contemplating suicide and are at risk for self-inflicted injury.

Mood stabilizers target manic behavior or mood swings that fluctuate between mania and depression. Manic symptoms include euphoria, flights of ideas, grandiosity, excessive energy, psychomotor agitation, decreased need for sleep, poor judgment, and accelerated and pressured speech. Depressive and manic episodes may be accompanied by symptoms of anxiety and psychosis.

Major classes of antidepressant agents include the SSRIs, cyclic compounds, and MAOIs. Mood stabilizers are represented by lithium carbonate. Increasing evidence suggests that anticonvulsants and calcium channel blockers may have a role in treating clients who do not respond to lithium therapy.

Selective Serotonin Reuptake Inhibitors

The development of SSRIs has greatly changed the outcome of using antidepressant medication. Examples of SSRIs are fluoxetine (Prozac) and sertraline (Zoloft).

Pharmacodynamics. SSRIs block the reuptake of serotonin into the presynaptic cell, augmenting the levels of the neurotransmitter at the synapse. SSRIs are selective for blocking serotonin as opposed to other neurochemicals—hence their name. SSRIs also exert an effect on postsynaptic neurons. SSRIs have decreased affinity for anticholinergic and alpha-adrenergic receptors; therefore, they are likely to produce fewer side effects and adverse effects than other antidepressant agents.

Pharmacokinetics. SSRIs are available in oral preparations and are well absorbed in the GI tract. They are highly protein bound. Peak plasma levels range from 2 to 8 hours after oral administration. The half-life of parent SSRI compounds vary, with most averaging 20 to 25 hours. An exception to this is the half-life of fluoxetine, which may be as long as 72 hours. Many SSRIs have active metabolites with extended half-lives. Long half-lives contribute to the prolonged drug effect and necessitate extended time intervals before increasing dosage. Half-life must be considered when using other medications, particularly agents requiring similar metabolic pathways or other serotonin-potentiating agents. The hepatic metabolism of SSRIs depends on the cytochrome P450 enzyme system. The onset of a therapeutic antidepressant effect typically occurs 2 to 4 weeks after drug therapy begins. Dosage information for SSRIs is provided in Table 20-5.

Therapeutic Uses. SSRIs are used primarily in treating depression and obsessive-compulsive disorder. They may also be useful in treating bulimia nervosa. SSRIs are often the first-line antidepressant treatment unless contraindications, tolerance, or client experiences suggest otherwise.

Adverse Reactions. Serotonin syndrome is an adverse reaction resulting from SSRI interaction with MAOIs and other serotonergic agents, such as clomipramine or buspirone (Sternbach, 1991). This is a serious reaction that can result in seizures, coma, or death. Symptoms include fever, agitation, hypertension, hyperthermia,

Table 20-5. Antidepressant Agents

Drug	Dosage Form*	Range of Daily Adult Oral Dose (mg/day)†
Selective Serotonin Reuptake Inhibitors (SSRIs)		
fluoxetine (Prozac)	PO	20–80
fluvoxamine (Luvox)	PO	100–300
paroxetine (Paxil)	PO	20–50
sertraline (Zoloft)	PO	50–200
Tricyclics		
amitriptyline (Elavil)	PO, IM	50–300
clomipramine (Anafranil)	PO	25–250
desipramine (Norpramin)	PO	50–300
doxepin (Sinequan)	PO	50–300
imipramine (Tofranil)	PO, IM	50–300
nortriptyline (Aventyl, Pamelor)	PO	25–100
protriptyline (Vivactil)	PO	10–60
Tetracyclics		
maprotiline (Ludiomil)	PO	75–300
mirtazapine (Remeron)	PO	15–45
Monamine Oxidase Inhibitors (MAOIs)		
Irreversible		
phenelzine (Nardil)	PO	15–90
tranylcypromine (Parnate)	PO	10–30
isocarboxazid (Marplan)‡	PO	30–50
Reversible		
moclobemide (Manerix)‡	PO	150–600
Other Cyclic Antidepressants		
amoxapine (Asendin)	PO	150–300
buproprion (Wellbutrin)	PO	200–450
nefazodone (Serzone)	PO	200–600
trazodone (Desyrel)	PO	150–600
venlafaxine (Effexor)	PO	75–375

*PO = oral, IM = intramuscular
†Doses vary according to indicated use and severity of symptoms.
‡Not available in the United States

rigidity, and myoclonus. Symptoms vary depending on the severity of the syndrome.

Neurologic effects commonly include insomnia or somnolence. Drowsiness, fatigue, tremor, asthenia, myoclonus, and seizures may also occur. EPS are rarely observed with SSRI therapy. Cardiovascular effects include possible tachycardia and hypertension. GI effects, particularly nausea, may remit with time. Dyspepsia, diarrhea, and change in appetite and weight may also occur. Neuroendocrine effects are generally limited to sexual disturbances, such as delayed ejaculation and anorgasmia. Hematologic effects, such as elevated liver transaminase levels, may occur with fluvoxamine therapy. Respiratory effects include increased instances of sinusitis, rhinitis, and upper respiratory infections. Other effects include nervousness and anxiety and, occasionally, chills, malaise, edema, dry mouth, pruritus, and increased sweating. SSRI therapy may precipitate a manic reaction.

Drug Interactions. Concomitant use of SSRIs with MAOIs and other serotonergic agents (eg, clomipramine, buspirone) increases the risk of inducing a serotonin syndrome. In general, 5 weeks should elapse after discontinuing fluoxetine and before starting MAOI therapy. A 2-week "washout" period should follow discontinuation of other SSRIs before MAOI treatment begins.

Drugs highly bound to protein, including warfarin, coumadin, and digitoxin, are displaced with SSRI therapy. Increased plasma concentrations can have serious cardiovascular and toxic effects, thus requiring lower dosages with concomitant use of an SSRI.

Cimetidine may increase plasma SSRI concentrations. Other possible SSRI drug interactions include increases in plasma concentration of lithium, phenytoin, benzodiazepines, and theophylline. Terfenadine and astemizole are contraindicated during fluvoxamine therapy.

Precautions and Contraindications. In general, elderly clients can better tolerate the effects of SSRIs than the effects of other antidepressants. However, older clients are more likely to have coexisting medical conditions or to use other medications that may alter hepatic functioning. Decreased renal clearance is also a concern in older adults because renal and hepatic impairment increases the risk of adverse effects and drug toxicity. Reduced dosages are used in elderly clients to decrease the risk of adverse reactions. Cautious use of SSRIs in clients with hepatic or renal failure is imperative.

Use of SSRIs during pregnancy is usually avoided, particularly in the first trimester. However, extreme suicidality may necessitate intervention. In any case, the risks and benefits must be carefully considered. Although SSRIs are less dangerous in overdoses than other antidepressants, cautious use is needed with severely depressed and suicidal clients. Concurrent use of MAOIs is contraindicated with fluoxetine. Use of an SSRI in a client with a known hypersensitivity or allergic reaction to the drug is contraindicated.

Tricyclic and Other Cyclic Antidepressants

Examples of tricyclic agents are amitriptyline (Elavil) and imipramine (Tofranil). Examples of tetracyclic antidepressants are maprotiline (Ludiomil) and mirtazapine (Remeron). Examples of other heterocyclic agents are amoxapine (Ascendin) and buproprion (Wellbutrin).

Pharmacodynamics. Tricyclic agents block the reuptake of norepinephrine and serotonin, thereby increasing the amount of CNS neurotransmitter available for receptor binding. The increased action of these neuro-transmitters in the hypothalamus is thought to stimulate behavior and elevate mood. This antidepressant action conform to the idea that decreased serotonin and norepinephrine function in the CNS results in depression. This is also known as the monoamine hypothesis (Schildkraut, 1965). Recent studies suggest that other neurochemical systems may be involved in depression.

Because tricyclic antidepressants have varying affinities for muscarinic receptors, their use produces a range of anticholinergic effects among different tricyclic drugs. Tetracyclic agents appear to have pharmacologic mechanisms similar to those of the tricyclics. Other heterocyclic agents tend to have different pharmacologic properties than the tricyclic or tetracyclic agents. For example, amoxapine, buproprion, nefazodone, trazodone, and venlafaxine have varying affinities for dopamine, norepinephrine, and serotonin receptors. Buproprion, nefazodone, and venlafaxine have relatively little cholinergic, alpha-adrenergic, or histamine (H_1) receptor activity. Amoxapine has modest affinity for cholinergic, histamine (H_1), and alpha-adrenergic receptors. Similarly, trazodone has moderate alpha-adrenergic receptor activity, possibly contributing to the hypotensive effect observed with this drug.

Pharmacokinetics. Most tricyclic agents are available only as oral preparations. They are rapidly absorbed in the GI tract. Peak plasma levels vary, usually occurring in the first few hours after drug administration. The half-life of tricyclics varies. The average elimination half-life is 24 hours. Thus, a single daily dose given at bedtime is usually effective. Divided doses may be more beneficial for clients experiencing side effects. Tricyclic agents are lipophilic, increasing access into the CNS. They are highly bound to proteins. Hepatic metabolism of tricyclics depends on the cytochrome P450 enzyme system, yielding both active and inactive metabolites.

General dosage information for tricyclic agents is provided in Table 20-5. Onset of therapeutic effects usually occurs within the first 2 weeks. Therapeutic doses vary significantly among clients and are influenced by several factors, including metabolic rate. An initial tricyclic dosage is usually low, allowing for a gradual increase if necessary. Therapeutic blood levels have been identified for desipramine, imipramine, and nortriptyline (Rudorfer & Potter, 1987). The efficacy of tricyclics appears to occur within a narrow range: when levels fall below or rise above the serum window, therapeutic effect is less likely. Blood values are particularly informative if therapeutic adherence is a concern or if the rate and extent of metabolism are in question. Usually the drug is discontinued if no therapeutic behavioral response is observed after 4 to 8 weeks of dosage at a therapeutic range. When discontinuing tricyclic antidepressants, the dose is gradually tapered to prevent the rare occurrence of withdrawal symptoms. The substitution of another antidepressant and the addition of other agents to the regimen are options for clients who seem unresponsive to tricyclic agents.

Other cyclic agents (nontricyclic) are available in oral preparations. The pharmacokinetics of these agents vary. Some cyclic agents rely on P450 enzyme metabolism, making it important to assess drug compatibility when other agents are used concurrently. Buproprion has relatively few drug interactions, making it potentially advantageous in the presence of polypharmacy.

Therapeutic Uses. Tricyclic agents are used primarily for treating depression. Clomipramine is approved in the United States for managing obsessive-compulsive disorder only. In addition to depression, imipramine is used for treating enuresis (bedwetting) in children. Insomnia, bulimia nervosa (except for buproprion), chronic pain, migraine headaches, and panic disorder are additional suggested uses of cyclic antidepressants.

Adverse Reactions. The following adverse effects refer to reactions associated with the use of tricyclic agents unless otherwise noted.

Neurologic effects of tricyclic agents involve a slight CNS depressant effect. Confusion and drowsiness may occur, most notably in the elderly client. Less common effects include nightmares, insomnia, ataxia, paresthesias, tremor, and tinnitus. Buproprion is associated with an increased risk of seizures. Dizziness, nervousness, anxiety, somnolence, asthenia, and tremor are associated with venlafaxine. Somnolence also occurs with venlafaxine and nefazodone; about 25% of clients receiving venlafaxine experience somnolence.

Anticholinergic effects are the most commonly encountered reactions to tricyclic medications. Symptoms such as dry mouth, blurred vision, constipation, and urinary retention are common. Delirium, confusion, agitation, and restlessness are seen with anticholinergic toxicity. Paradoxically, the client may experience excessive sweating. Severe urinary retention may necessitate treatment with a cholinergic agent such as bethanechol (Urecholine).

Among the most common and potentially dangerous cardiovascular effects of tricyclic medications are postural hypotension and tachycardia. These symptoms usually result from the effect of tricyclic alpha-adrenergic receptor blockade. Hypotension is associated with trazodone. Postural hypotension symptoms, including dizziness and faintness, are most likely to be seen during positional changes. Tolerance to postural hypotension and tachycardia generally develops within the first week of drug therapy, although blood-pressure changes may persist. Older adults and clients with a history of cardiac disease are more vulnerable to the cardiovascular effects of antidepressant agents.

Changes in cardiac conduction can occur as well. They include arrhythmias, heart block, and prolonged Q-T, P-R, and QRS intervals on the ECG. Increased P-R and QRS intervals have been associated with toxic-

ity. Thus, cardiac functioning can be compromised with an overdose of these drugs. Clients with previous heart conditions are at greater risk for sudden death, which is rare.

Effects on the GI system include nausea, vomiting, diarrhea, constipation, and epigastric distress. Nausea is experienced by about 33% of clients receiving venlafaxine.

Ocular effects include blurred vision, which results from the anticholinergic properties of tricyclic agents. It tends to resolve within a few weeks of starting drug therapy.

Tricyclic agents tend to have few neuroendocrine effects. Libido may decrease, but it may be difficult to determine whether sexual disturbances are attributable to the drug or to depression. Sexual disturbances are dose-dependent with some cyclic agents such as venlafaxine. Discontinuation of trazodone is indicated after drug-induced priapism, which is rare. Compared to other agents, buproprion appears to have little effect on sexual functioning.

A rare hematologic effect, agranulocytosis, can occur during tricyclic treatment. The onset is sudden, and the condition may be life-threatening. Symptoms include fever, sore throat, general malaise, and other signs of infection.

Cutaneous effects include rash and occasional photosensitivity. Antihistamines or drug discontinuation may relieve the rash; photosensitivity can be managed by wearing protective clothing and sunscreens.

Weight change and allergic drug reactions are less common with tricyclic agents than with other antidepressants. Clients taking venlafaxine report increased sweating.

Drug Interactions. Simultaneous use of tricyclic agents with anticholinergic drugs, including antihistamines, antiparkinson agents, and low-potency antipsychotic agents, potentiates anticholinergic side effects. Drugs that increase tricyclic plasma levels include acetazolamide, acetylsalicylic acid, antipsychotic agents, dexamethasone, methylphenidate, MAOIs, thiazides, and thyroid hormones. Agents decreasing tricyclic plasma levels include alcohol, barbiturates, carbamazepine, oral contraceptives, phenobarbital, primidone, rifampin, and cigarette smoking. Because of the significant risk for serotonin syndrome, concomitant use of MAOIs and most cyclic agents is contraindicated.

Precautions and Contraindications. Elderly clients are more sensitive than others to the anticholinergic and alpha-adrenergic antagonist effects of cyclic agents. Because of this, they are at greater risk for adverse effects. Hypotensive drug effects may leave older clients more prone to falls. Older adults are also more likely to have concurrent pharmacotherapy for medical illnesses, increasing the risk for drug interactions. Serious adverse reactions, including tachycardia, urinary retention, hyperpyrexia, delirium, and coma, have occurred in children receiving a tricyclic agent to treat enuresis. Use of these agents during pregnancy is generally avoided, particularly during the first trimester. Although suicidality may warrant the need for antidepressant use during pregnancy, the risks and benefits must clearly be considered by both the client and prescriber. Tricyclics require cautious use in persons with compromised hepatic or renal function. Extreme caution is warranted in clients with a history of cardiac disease because of the potential for cardiovascular toxicity.

Tricyclic antidepressants are contraindicated for persons with conditions sensitive to anticholinergic effects (eg, narrow-angle glaucoma, prostatic hypertrophy). Buproprion is contraindicated in persons with a seizure history or a history of bulimia nervosa because of the increased risk of seizures in these clients. These agents must not be used in clients with a known hypersensitivity or allergy to them. Concurrent use of MAOIs and cyclic agents is also contraindicated for most cyclic agents.

Monoamine Oxidase Inhibitors

Monoamine oxidase is an enzyme responsible for breaking down certain body chemicals. There are two types of MAO enzymes: MAO-A and MAO-B. These enzymes are found throughout the body, including the brain. MAO enzymes are present in nonspecific neurons as well as neurons associated with a particular neurotransmitter. MAO-A enzyme is found in dopaminergic and noradrenergic neurons. MAO-B enzyme tends to be present in serotonin neurons. MAO inactivates unstored intracellular amines (eg, dopamine, norepinephrine, serotonin) by breaking them down. MAOIs block this process. Phenelzine (Nardil) is an example of an irreversible MAOI; moclobemide (Manerix) is an example of a reversible MAOI.

Pharmacodynamics. The action of MAOIs increases the availability of amines for synaptic release. Other intracellular compensatory mechanisms important to the efficacy of MAOIs are not fully understood. Because MAOIs inactivate MAO throughout the body, amine-containing foods normally catabolized by MAO in the gut are instead absorbed into the bloodstream. This effect increases the availability of amines in the CNS, contributing to further release of neurotransmitters. A serious reaction called hypertensive crisis can result from this combined increase in CNS neurotransmitters. Clients considered for MAOI therapy must be able to comply with dietary restrictions that limit the consumption of amine-containing foods, particularly those with tyramine (Box 20-5). Hypertensive crisis is associated with MAO-A and high-dose MAO-B inhibitors. Thus, clients on high doses of MAO-B inhibitors must adhere to dietary precautions as well.

MAOIs are classified as reversible or irreversible, based on the permanency with which MAOIs bind to

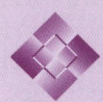

Box 20-5
Tyramine-Containing Foods to Avoid in MAOI Therapy

Tyramine and other pressor amines are broken down in the GI tract by MAO enzymes. The presence of MAOIs allows these substances to be absorbed in high concentrations, possibly resulting in hypertensive crisis. Foods to avoid include:

- Fruits and vegetables: avocados, bananas, fava beans, figs, raisins, sauerkraut
- Dairy products: cheeses (aged, bleu, Camembert, cheddar, mozzarella, Parmesan, Romano, Roquefort, Stilton), sour cream, yogurt
- Meats and fish: chicken livers, pickled herring and caviar, fermented sausages such as bologna, pepperoni, salami
- Beverages: beer; hot chocolate and cocoa drinks; colas and other caffeine-containing drinks; coffee and tea; red wines, particularly Chianti and sherry
- Other: chocolate, cocoa, licorice, soy sauce, yeast products

MAO molecules. Irreversible agents permanently bind to MAO molecules, making them forever inactive. MAO activity gradually resumes after discontinuation of irreversible MAOIs as new MAO molecules are synthesized. Thus, irreversible MAOI agents produce a long-lasting blockade. Reversible MAOIs are not permanent, allowing MAO function to return more quickly after drug discontinuation.

Pharmacokinetics. MAOIs are available in oral preparations and are well absorbed in the GI tract. Relatively little information is available on the pharmacokinetics of these agents, although inhibition of MAO activity is thought to peak within 1 week. Onset of therapeutic effects occurs 2 to 4 weeks after a maximal therapeutic dose. The initial dosage is usually low, allowing the dosage to be increased as necessary and as tolerated. General dosage information for MAOIs is provided in Table 20-5. MAOIs are generally discontinued gradually. The client must continue to comply with the drug-related dietary restrictions for about 2 weeks after discontinuing the drug because MAO levels do not immediately return to normal.

Therapeutic Uses. These agents are used to treat atypical and major depressive disorders, phobic anxiety, and panic disorder. Whether a client takes an MAOI or a tricyclic agent depends largely on the previous response to these agents and to the client's ability to comply with the dietary restrictions.

Adverse Reactions. Severe headache and high blood pressure are the cardinal features of a hypertensive crisis, which requires immediate treatment. Associated symptoms include stiffness of the neck, diaphoresis, nausea, and vomiting. Hypertensive crisis can lead to a stroke and can be fatal. If a hypertensive crisis occurs, the MAOI should be discontinued at once. Treatment of severe hypertensive crisis usually involves administering an antihypertensive agent, such as IV phentolamine mesylate, which blocks alpha-adrenergic receptors.

Serotonin syndrome, an adverse reaction caused by the interaction of an SSRI and other serotonergic agents, is serious because convulsions, coma, or death may result. Symptoms include elevated temperature, agitation, ocular oscillation, hypertension, hyperthermia, rigidity, and myoclonus and vary depending on the severity of the reaction.

Neurologic effects include sedation (associated with phenelzine), which most notably affects elderly clients. Severe insomnia can result from tranylcypromine. Less common neurologic effects include nightmares, paresthesia of extremities, myoclonic jerks, tinnitus, ataxia, and tremor. Episodes of hypomania, possibly from neurochemical overstimulation, may follow MAOI use.

Cardiovascular effects include postural hypotension and hypertension, as well as hypertensive crisis. GI effects such as nausea, diarrhea, constipation, and abdominal discomfort may occur. Sexual disturbances such as impotence, ejaculatory problems, and anorgasmia may occur. Weight gain and dry mouth are associated with phenelzine use.

Drug–Drug Interactions. Simultaneous use of MAOIs with SSRIs and other serotonergic agents increases the risk of inducing a potentially fatal serotonin syndrome; therefore, MAOIs are not used with SSRIs. A 5-week period should elapse between discontinuation of fluoxetine and the beginning of MAOI treatment. A 2-week period should elapse between discontinuation of other SSRIs and the beginning of MAOI treatment.

Hypertensive crisis may result from concurrent use of MAOIs and sympathomimetic drugs. Examples include amphetamines, dopamine, epinephrine, oxymetazoline, and pseudoephedrine. Because some of these agents are ingredients in over-the-counter medications, clients must be warned about the possibility of interactions with nonprescription agents. Buproprion and levodopa may induce a hypertensive crisis. MAOIs are contraindicated in persons taking guanethidine. Coadministration of MAOIs and oral hypoglycemic agents decreases serum glucose levels.

Drug–Food Interactions. These agents interact with foods and beverages that contain tyramine, and hypertensive crisis may result (see Box 20-5).

Precautions and Contraindications. The client must adopt a tyramine-free diet. A severe headache is usually the first warning of a hypertensive crisis, which requires discontinuation of the drug and immediate medical attention. Hypertensive crisis can also be precipitated by the combined use of MAOIs with other drugs as well as foods.

An overdose of MAOIs is severely toxic. Use in severely depressed clients necessitates extreme caution. Elderly clients are at greater risk for MAOI-induced adverse effects. Hypotensive episodes increase the risk for falls. Elderly clients generally require lower doses than younger adults. In additions, older adults are more likely to have coexisting medical conditions, to take other medications that may alter hepatic functioning, and to have decreased renal clearance. Extreme caution is warranted when using MAOIs in clients with altered renal or hepatic function, cardiovascular disease, epilepsy, a history of cerebrovascular accident (stroke), pheochromocytoma, and hyperexcitability or agitation. Other antidepressant agents is a consideration in these clients.

The use of MAOIs is avoided during pregnancy; alternate antidepressants should be used if symptoms require intervention. These agents are contraindicated in clients with a known hypersensitivity or allergic reaction to them.

Lithium

Mood stabilizers such as lithium carbonate are used to regulate severe fluctuations of mania, as in bipolar disorders.

Lithium, an element on the periodic chart, was first used to treat gout in the mid-1800s. It was later used as a salt substitute until hazardous toxicity was reported in the 1940s. During the mid-1900s, investigative efforts by Cade led to the discovery of lithium's antimanic properties. The Food and Drug Administration (FDA) approved the use of lithium for acute mania in 1970, although it was already widely used in other countries. Lithium provides symptomatic relief of acute hyperactivity. In contrast to antipsychotic agents, lithium does not produce sedative effects that may interfere with intellectual activity or daily functioning.

Pharmacodynamics. The specific mechanisms of lithium's action are not fully understood. It enhances serotonin, norepinephrine, GABA, and acetylcholine function in the CNS. It decreases central dopamine turnover and also influences second messenger systems (subsequent neurochemical signals following neurotransmission). The extent to which these actions contribute to an antimanic effect remains an area of intense investigation.

Pharmacokinetics. Lithium is available in oral preparations that are well absorbed in the GI tract. Chloride forms are associated with greater GI irritability than carbonate salt preparations. A peak serum lithium level occurs in 1 to 2 hours (4 hours with sustained-release preparations). Lithium's half-life is about 24 hours in healthy young adults. It is unbound to plasma proteins and is distributed throughout the body. Lithium is excreted almost exclusively by the kidneys. An inverse relation exists between sodium intake and lithium excretion: lower sodium intake decreases lithium excretion, potentially resulting in drug toxicity. Onset of therapeutic behavioral effects occurs within the first 2 weeks of drug therapy.

Lithium dosage is based on the client's medical history, concurrent medications, severity of illness, lean body mass, clinical response, and serum drug levels. Because a narrow margin exists between therapeutic and toxic blood levels, the serum lithium concentration must be monitored routinely. Levels of 1.0 to 1.2 mmol/L are the most therapeutic. Serum levels are generally higher during the acute phase of illness, as is the dosage. Toxicity usually occurs when the serum lithium level exceeds 1.5 mmol/L, making it necessary to discontinue the drug and to resume therapy at a lower dose. Blood samples are obtained more often during the initial phase of therapy (about twice a week) to help guide dosage adjustments. Weekly samples are obtained during the stabilization phase of therapy, followed by monthly collections during the initial maintenance phase. Serum levels are monitored up to every 3 months with long-term lithium use. Gradual tapering over several weeks is used when discontinuing lithium because rapid or abrupt discontinuation is associated with recurrence of manic or depressive symptoms. General dosage information for lithium is provided in Table 20-6.

Therapeutic Uses. Lithium is used primarily to treat acute mania and bipolar illness (alternating episodes of mania and depression). Manic symptoms include hyperactivity, pressured speech, flight of ideas, decreased need for sleep, poor judgment, and grandiosity. Lithium is sometimes used prophylactically to prevent relapse. It is particularly advantageous in treating bipolar disorders, given that antidepressant agents can induce manic episodes.

Adverse Reactions. The severity of adverse reactions is usually related to lithium blood levels. Neurologic effects—poor memory, drowsiness, and fatigue—affect about 33% of clients taking these agents. Tremors occur more frequently during the initial phase of treatment.

Incoordination and muscle weakness are early signs of possible drug toxicity. Confusion and EPS may develop with drug toxicity as well.

Cardiovascular effects include ECG changes, such as inverted or flattened T waves. Arrhythmias generally occur in clients with a preexisting cardiac condition. Hypotension and bradycardia may ensue. Neuroendocrine effects, such as thyroid disorders (goiter, hypothyroidism), occur in up to 5% of persons taking lithium, prompting treatment with small doses of thyroid medication (Lenox & Manji, 1995). GI effects, such as nausea, may occur during the first few days of treatment but usually subside thereafter. Diarrhea, nausea, and vomiting are possible early signs of drug toxicity.

Renal effects, including increased thirst and polyuria, are the most common side effects of lithium therapy. These symptoms are more prevalent during the initial treatment phase but may persist throughout therapy. An acute increase in the serum creatinine level requires discontinuation of the drug. Other effects include weight gain and transient edema, unrelated to alterations in renal function.

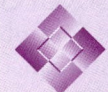

Toxicity Alert: Lithium

Incoordination and muscle weakness are early signs of possible drug toxicity, as are confusion, EPS, diarrhea, nausea, and vomiting. Neurotoxicity, a serious adverse effect that can result in seizures, coma, or death, is generally reversible within 5 to 10 days after discontinuation of lithium therapy. Major toxic effects necessitate immediate discontinuation of the drug.

Drug Interactions. Diuretics (eg, thiazides) and nonsteroidal antiinflammatory agents (eg, ibuprofen, naproxen) interfere with lithium clearance, thereby increasing the risk of toxicity. Angiotensin-converting enzyme inhibitors and antibiotics (eg, metronidazole, tetracycline) increase plasma lithium levels, similarly increasing the risk for toxicity. Concurrent use of calcium channel blockers and antipsychotic agents may result in neurotoxicity. Coadministration of lithium with antipsychotic agents may exacerbate EPS. Acetazolamide, theophylline, and osmotic diuretics decrease plasma lithium levels. Caffeine may induce a mild reduction in lithium blood levels. Dietary sodium restriction enhances the risk for lithium toxicity.

Precautions and Contraindications. To decrease the risk of toxicity, clients should maintain normal salt intake and adequate fluids. Elderly persons are at increased

Drug	Dosage Form	Usual Range of Adult Dose*
lithium carbonate (Eskalith)	Oral	900–1800 mg/day
valproic acid (Depakene)	Oral	15–60 mg/kg/day

Table 20-6. Mood Stabilizers

*Estimated dose range to achieve therapeutic serum lithium level

risk for drug toxicity due to decreased lean body mass and renal clearance. Lithium is not customarily used by clients with impaired renal or cardiovascular function or by clients on a sodium-restricted diet. Without alternate treatment, lithium is used with extreme caution in these clients and may require daily blood monitoring for toxicity.

Before beginning lithium therapy, the client needs baseline laboratory assessments of kidney function (routine urinalysis, urine specific gravity, serum creatinine level). Decreased renal concentration is associated with chronic lithium therapy, contributing to symptoms of nephrogenic diabetes insipidus. This effect is usually reversible on discontinuing drug therapy.

Lithium use during pregnancy is generally avoided; use in the first trimester is associated with Ebstein's anomaly. Lithium is used cautiously in clients with hypothyroidism. Because of the extent of potential drug toxicity, the suicide risk should be assessed routinely. Use of lithium in persons with a known hypersensitivity or allergic reaction to it is contraindicated.

Because of adverse reactions, fear of toxicity, denial of illness, and enjoyment of exhilaration during manic episodes, some clients refuse lithium therapy or stop taking it once they leave the treatment setting.

Anticonvulsants and Calcium Channel Blockers

Although there is increasing evidence that anticonvulsants and calcium channel blockers may be helpful in treating lithium-refractory mania, these agents are not approved by the FDA for treating mania. The exception is valproic acid (see Table 20-6).

❖ SUMMARY

Depression and mania are characterized by mood changes or swings. Antidepressant agents include the SSRIs, cyclic compounds, and MAOIs. Lithium is the usual first-line medication for treating mania-related conditions. Researchers are exploring the potential use of anticonvulsant agents and calcium channel blockers for clients who cannot tolerate lithium's adverse effects or who are refractory to lithium therapy.

❖ NURSING MANAGEMENT: CLIENT RECEIVING ANTIDEPRESSANTS AND MOOD STABILIZERS

Because both antidepressant agents and mood stabilizers are highly toxic and can be fatal in overdoses, close observation of clients for signs of suicidality is imperative, particularly during initial relief from depressive symptoms. This is when depressed clients may begin to have enough energy to act on their suicidal thoughts.

Manic clients usually exhibit poor judgment, excessive activity, and euphoria in the acute phase of illness;

thus, they may fail to adhere to medication regimens, particularly because they often find the euphoric mood desirable and know that the euphoria is counteracted by drug therapy. In addition, excessive activity may lead to changes in food and fluid intake, resulting in potentially dangerous electrolyte imbalances.

NURSING PROCESS

ASSESSMENT

A comprehensive baseline assessment of the client's functional health patterns is key. After initiation of drug therapy, regular assessment of functional health patterns helps determine the therapeutic value of the medication. The client's mental status (eg, orientation to person, place, and time) is thoroughly assessed at baseline and at regular intervals during drug therapy. Vital signs, including pulse rate, orthostatic blood pressures, respiratory rate, and body temperature, are additional data for the baseline assessment, as are assessments of renal function and fluid and electrolyte levels.

Emotional status and suicidal risk are assessed routinely and thoroughly. A history of the client's previous medication experiences and related perceptions and attitudes is compiled. The history should include details of previous medication use, efficacy, reason for discontinuation, related experiences, and use of over-the-counter medications, alcohol, cigarettes, caffeine, and illegal substances. Identification of potential drug interactions is key.

Before drug therapy begins, clients are screened for contraindications or conditions that present increased risk for adverse reactions. Assessment for pregnancy and cerebrovascular, cardiac, hepatic, and renal conditions helps to determine the necessary precautions or to identify contraindications of the proposed treatment agent. Similarly, the nurse assesses for drug sensitivities, a history of seizures, narrow-angle glaucoma, or pheochromocytoma, and the client's diet. Baseline and follow-up ECGs may be indicated, particularly in clients with preexisting cardiac problems.

NURSING DIAGNOSES

Possible nursing diagnoses related to antidepressant drug therapy include:

- Constipation, related to medication
- Diarrhea, related to medication
- Risk for Infection, related to medication-induced agranulocytosis
- Risk for Injury, related to medication-induced orthostatic hypotension
- Knowledge Deficit, related to lack of exposure to medication information
- Altered Oral Mucous Membrane, related to medication
- Risk for Poisoning, related to medication toxicity

- Sleep Pattern Disturbance, related to medication-induced somnolence or insomnia
- Ineffective Management of Therapeutic Regimen (Individual), related to MAOI-required dietary restrictions
- Urinary Retention, related to medication

Possible nursing diagnoses related to lithium therapy include:

- Fluid Volume Excess, related to medication
- Knowledge Deficit, related to lack of exposure to medication information
- Ineffective Management of Therapeutic Regimen (Individual), related to fear of drug-induced decrease in euphoria
- Risk for Poisoning, related to potential lithium toxicity

PLANNING

Interventions specific to nursing diagnoses and goals are identified. Goals may include increasing the efficacy of drug therapy and decreasing the severity of adverse effects. Client and family involvement in the planning process helps them feel valued, increases the client's self-determination as appropriate, increases his or her problem-solving skills, and helps in setting realistic objectives.

INTERVENTION

Because of the hypotensive and hypertensive reactions to antidepressant therapy, regular blood-pressure monitoring is essential. During the initial doses, and after an increase in dosage, orthostatic blood pressures are assessed 30 minutes after drug administration. Symptoms of hypotension include dizziness and faintness and are usually relieved by having the client lie down. With severe continuous hypotension, IV fluids may be indicated. Subsequent administration of a pressor agent specific for alpha-adrenergic receptors (eg, norepinephrine) is a possible intervention. Epinephrine is *not* used because it may further lower the blood pressure.

Elevated blood pressure and headaches are signs of hypertensive crisis. MAOI therapy is immediately discontinued if hypertensive crisis occurs. Treatment of a severe hypertensive event usually involves administering an antihypertensive agent such as IV phentolamine mesylate. The nurse should then investigate any precipitating events, as they may be related to a suicide attempt or failure to adhere to the dietary regimen. Difficulties with dietary restrictions should be taken seriously and reported to the prescribing clinician immediately.

Although agranulocytosis is a rare adverse effect of antidepressant medications, it is necessary to know how to manage it, particularly because it occurs suddenly and may be life-threatening. Symptoms of infection are warning signs that necessitate a WBC count with differential. Drug treatment is discontinued if agranulocytosis develops, and appropriate isolation procedures are instituted.

CRITICAL THINKING CHALLENGE
Case Analysis

Mrs. Turner, a 72-year-old woman, is hospitalized in the psychiatric unit for depression. She has been receiving an antidepressant medication for several days, but she will not get out of bed on her own in the morning without constant prompting and assistance from the nursing staff. What hypotheses would explain her behavior?

Early interventions directed at preventing or relieving discomfort from cutaneous, GI, and other symptoms is likely to increase adherence to the drug regimen. Adequate measures should be instituted to counteract photosensitivity. Constipation may be avoided by adequate exercise and intake of dietary fiber; in some cases, laxatives may be needed. To relieve dry mouth, the client may suck on ice chips or sugarless hard candies and gum (to prevent caries), sip liquids frequently, and rinse the mouth often. For clients affected by drowsiness, ongoing assessment of gait is important; the use of side rails or assisted ambulation may be necessary for safety's sake. Drug-induced dyspepsia may be alleviated by administering the agent with meals, although this may also decrease drug absorption. Insomnia is often relieved by administering the agent in the morning; conversely, sedation is frequently reduced when the drug is administered at bedtime.

Lithium levels require close monitoring. Transient symptoms of nausea, tremor, diarrhea, thirst, and polyuria may appear when lithium therapy is initiated, but they usually rapidly diminish or disappear. At this point, the client should be monitored closely to determine whether the symptoms are early signs of toxicity or are merely transient.

Blood samples to measure antidepressant and lithium levels should be collected at least 10 hours after the last oral dose, because this provides a more stable reflection of actual drug levels. Waiting several days after an increase in dosage allows a more accurate assessment of blood concentration. Blood samples are usually obtained first thing in the morning, before administering the morning medication dose.

Client Education. The client taking antidepressant or mood-stabilizing drugs needs thorough instructions about the drugs, their uses, and possible adverse effects. For example, the client taking an MAOI must clearly understand drug–diet interactions and related risks and adverse effects. The nurse can discuss this information and ask the client to restate it to assess how well the client understands it. Providing a written list of the restricted foods also may encourage therapeutic adherence (see Box 20-5); the client should tape the list to the refrigerator at home. Family members must understand the serious consequences of giving the client tyramine-rich foods during therapy and sooner than 2 weeks after drug discontinuation. Caution the client not to take cough medicine and cold preparations while on MAOIs.

The client must know about any anticipated lag time before a therapeutic response occurs. He or she should take the medication as prescribed because as-needed or erratic dosing is ineffective.

To prevent withdrawal and associated adverse effects, the nurse should caution the client against abrupt and unsupervised discontinuation of medication. The client should consult the prescribing clinician regarding discontinuation and gradual withdrawal of medication. If adverse effects persist, the possibility of adjusting the dosage or administering the drug in divided doses should be discussed with the prescribing clinician.

The client must learn to recognize any adverse reactions (eg, hypertensive crisis, signaled by the cardinal signs of headache and elevated blood pressure). These should be reported immediately to the prescriber, and the client should go to an emergency room immediately. Clients can be taught strategies to avoid or deal with various adverse effects, such as drowsiness, dizziness and lightheadedness from orthostatic hypotension, drug interactions, and synergistic effects. Although agranulocytosis is rare in clients taking antidepressants, they should learn to recognize signs and symptoms of infection and report them immediately to the nurse or prescribing clinician.

The client taking lithium must maintain a stable intake of dietary salt and fluids. Crash diets and fasting lead to sodium depletion, elevated lithium blood levels, and possible toxicity. Discuss with the client and family the symptoms of lithium toxicity (drowsiness, diarrhea, confusion, vomiting, muscle weakness, ataxia) and the need to discontinue the drug and notify the prescribing clinician immediately if they occur.

Stress the importance of regular testing of serum levels. Educate clients about drug interactions and the need to avoid concomitant use of diuretics. Caution clients against changing their drug therapy, and discuss the need to maintain the lithium level in the blood even after they feel better. Doses should not be increased by the client, because the margin between the toxic level and therapeutic level is very small. Increased sodium loss through increased sweating, or any condition where sodium depletion occurs, and strategies for dosage adjustments must be discussed with the prescriber.

Women taking tricyclics and lithium should avoid breast-feeding, because these drugs are secreted in breast milk and may be potentially harmful to the newborn.

OUTCOME EVALUATION

Some desirable outcomes related to antidepressant therapy include appropriate dietary choices by the client on an MAOI; client understanding of the need to follow a tyramine-free diet (with MAOI therapy); and increased eye contact and interpersonal interactions. Other desirable outcomes include absence of drug toxicity, improved sleep patterns, ability to cope with and relieve dry mouth, normal bowel functioning, hemodynamic stability, and recognition of signs and symptoms of infection. Ideally, the client remains injury-free, performs self-care activities, and demonstrates a measurable increase in activity level.

For clients taking lithium, desirable outcomes may include stable fluid volume, client understanding of sodium and fluid intake requirements, client understanding of blood monitoring to help maintain a therapeutic serum lithium level, improved sleep pattern, and involvement in problem-solving activities.

❖ **CHECKLIST OF NURSING ACTIONS**

❑ Perform baseline assessments for clients beginning therapy with antidepressant or mood-stabilizing drugs.

❑ Encourage client and family involvement in developing the nursing care plan and establishing goals and desired outcomes for drug therapy.

❑ Perform monitoring regularly, as often as required by the client's condition. For example, arrange for laboratory testing as needed to confirm therapeutic or toxic drug levels in the blood.

❑ Develop and carry out teaching programs about the client's medication and therapeutic regimen. Involve the client and family in educational sessions—for example, teaching about dietary recommendations and adverse reactions. Encourage the client to adhere to dietary restrictions and the family to support him or her in doing so.

❑ Promote safety by advising clients about drug effects. For example, advise against driving an automobile, operating machinery, or performing tasks requiring mental alertness and motor coordination until the response to drug therapy is known.

❑ Inform clients about drug interactions and synergistic effects, such as those associated with alcohol.

❑ Advise clients that orthostatic hypotension can be reduced if they rise slowly and change positions gradually, sitting on the edge of the bed for a few minutes before standing.

❑ For clients taking MAOIs, provide a written list of foods and beverages to be avoided.

❑ Reevaluate the nursing care plan as needed, providing follow-up care and referrals to community agencies as appropriate to achieve identified and desired outcomes.

References

Ballenger JC. (1995). Benzodiazepines. In Schatzberg AF, Nemeroff CB, eds. *Textbook of psychopharmacology*. Washington, DC: American Psychiatric Press, pp. 215–230.

Doenges ME, Moorhouse MF. (1996). *Nurse's pocket guide: Nursing diagnoses with interventions*, 5th ed. Philadelphia: FA Davis.

Hsiao JK, Potter WZ. (1990). Mechanisms of action of antipanic drugs. In JC Ballenger, ed. *Clinical aspects of panic disorder*. New York: Wiley-Liss, pp. 297–317.

Hyman SE, Arana GW, Rosenbaum JF. (1995). *Handbook of psychiatric drug therapy*, 3d ed. New York: Little, Brown.

Kane JM, Lieberman JA. (1992). Tardive dyskinesia. In Kane JM, Lieberman JA, eds. *Adverse effects of psychotropic drugs*. New York: Guilford Press, pp. 235–245.

Lavin MR, Rifkin A. (1992). Neuroleptic-induced parkinsonism. In Kane JM, Lieberman JA, eds. *Adverse effects of psychotropic drugs*. New York: Guilford Press, pp. 175–188.

Lenox RH, Manji HK. (1995). Lithium. In Schatzberg AF, Nemeroff CB, eds. *Textbook of psychopharmacology*. Washington, DC: American Psychiatric Press, pp. 303–349.

Marder SR, Van Putten T. (1995). Antipsychotic medications. In Schatzberg AF, Nemeroff CB, eds. *Textbook of psychopharmacology*. Washington, DC: American Psychiatric Press, pp. 247–261.

Rudorfer MV, Potter WZ. (1987). Pharmacokinetics of antidepressants. In Meltzer HY, ed. *Psychopharmacology: The third generation*. New York: Raven Press, pp. 1353–1364.

Schildkraut JJ. (1965). The catecholamine hypothesis of affective disorders: A review of supporting evidence. *Am J Psychiatry, 122*, 509–522.

Sternbach H. (1991). The serotonin syndrome. *Am J Psychiatry, 148*, 705–713.

Weiden PJ, Mann JJ, Haas G, et al. (1987). Clinical nonrecognition of neuroleptic-induced movement disorders: A cautionary study. *Am J Psychiatry, 144*, 1148–1153.

Gardos G, Casey DE, Cole JO, et al. (1994). Ten-year outcome of tardive dyskinesia. *Am J Psychiatry, 151,* 836–841.

Garvey CA, Gross D, Freeman L. (1991). Assessing psychotropic medication side effects among children. A reliability study. *J Child Adolesc Psychiatr Ment Health Nurs, 4(4)*, 127–131.

Glod CA. (1991). Psychopharmacology and clinical practice. *Nurs Clin North Am, 26*(2), 375–399.

Glod CA, Mathieu J. (1993). Expanding uses of anticonvulsants in the treatment of bipolar disorder. *J Psychosocial Nurse Ment Health Serv, 31*(5), 37–39.

Goff DC, Baldessarini RJ. (1993). Drug interactions with antipsychotic agents. *J Clin Psychopharmacol, 13*, 57–67.

Kane JM, Lieberman J, eds. (1992). *Adverse effects of psychotropic drugs*. New York: Guilford Press.

Roose SP, Glassman AH, Attia E, Woodring S. (1994). Comparative efficacy of selective serotonin reuptake inhibitors and tricyclics in the treatment of melancholia. *Am J Psychiatry, 151*, 1735–1739.

Siegel GJ, Agranoff BW, Albers RW, Molinoff PB, eds. (1993). *Basic neurochemistry*, 5th ed. New York: Raven Press.

Schatzberg AF, Nemeroff CB, eds. (1995). *Textbook of psychopharmacology*. Washington, DC: American Psychiatric Press.

Thapa PB, Gideon P, Fought RL, Ray WA. (1995). Psychotropic drugs and risk for recurrent falls in ambulatory nursing home residents. *Am J Epidemiol, 142*(2), 202–211.

This chapter supported in part by USPHS grant K07 MH00965 to Dr. B. E. Wolfe from the National Institute of Mental Health

Bibliography

Blair DT, Dauner A. (1993). Neuroleptic malignant syndrome: Liability in nursing practice. *J Psychosocial Nurse Ment Health Serv, 31*(2), 5–12.

Cooper JR, Bloom FE, Roth RH. (1996). *The biochemical basis of neuropharmacology*, 7th ed. New York: Oxford University Press.

For more information and sample tests and activities, refer to Chapter 20 in the Student Workbook for Clinical Pharmacology and Nursing Management, 5th edition, available through your bookstore.

VII

Drugs Affecting the Cardiovascular and Renal Systems

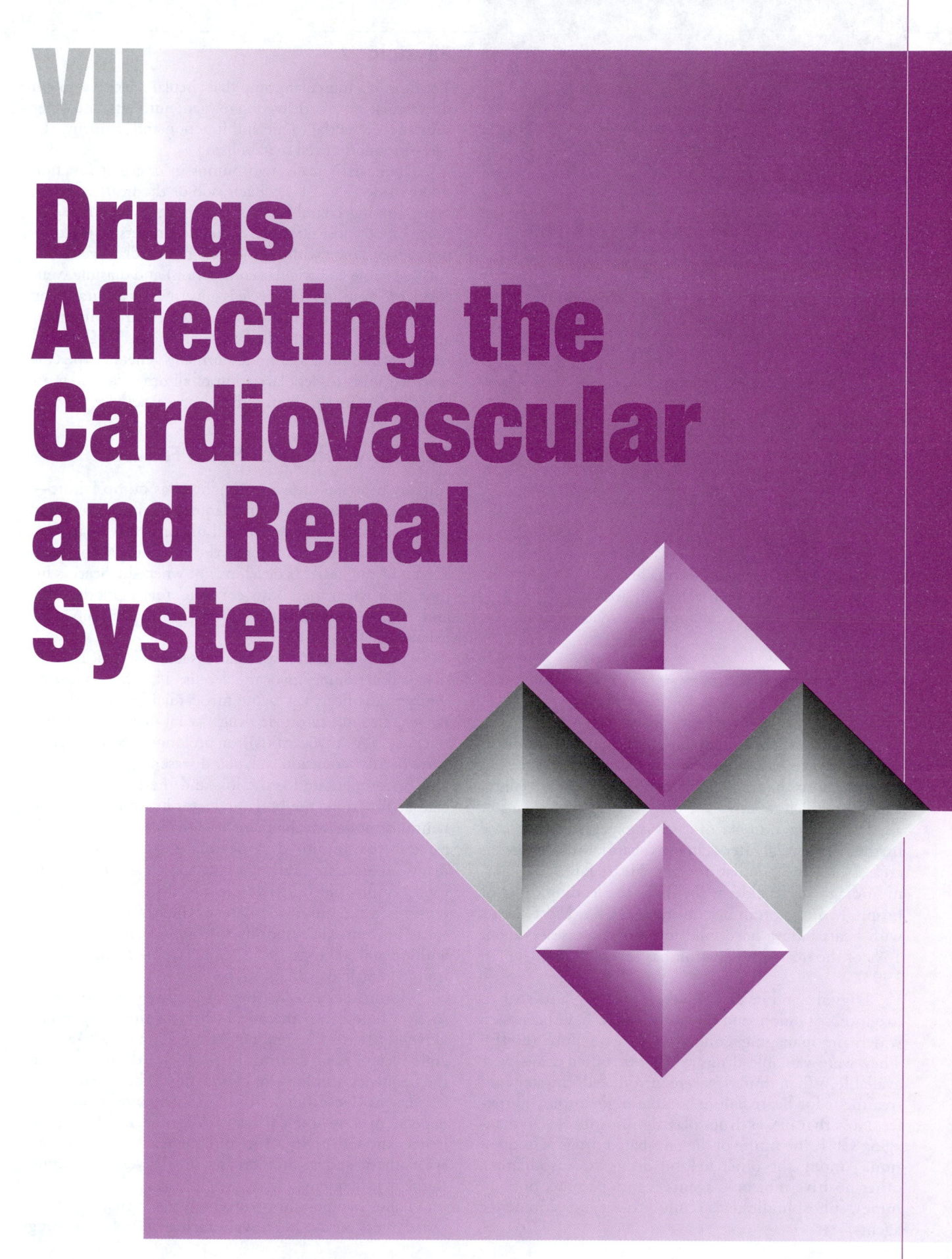

21

Drugs That Manage Heart Failure

Heart failure is a growing public health problem in the United States, where it is estimated that more than 3 million people have heart failure and 400,000 new cases are diagnosed yearly (Garg et al., 1993). The number of cases is expected to increase further as survival after acute myocardial infarction increases and the population ages. Heart failure, a common diagnosis in elderly clients, is the leading cause of hospital admission in persons over age 65. Most clients with heart failure have mild to moderate disease; about 15% of the treated population has severe failure (Rajfer, 1993).

Digitalis and its derivatives, found in plants such as foxglove, sea onion, and lily of the valley, have been used widely in managing congestive heart failure (CHF). They were valuable drugs when few other drugs were available. When diuretics were introduced, the standard treatment for heart failure became digoxin plus diuretics. Now that newer drugs play significant roles in managing CHF, the future of digitalis-based drugs is in question. Among the other helpful drugs are vasodilators, other positive inotropic agents (eg, dopamine, dobutamine), phosphodiesterase inhibitors, and adrenergic agents.

Physiology

The heart is a muscular pump that circulates blood through the vascular system, delivering oxygen, nutrients, and other substances essential to life and function and removing the waste products of cell metabolism.

The heart is really two pumps in one that function side by side (Fig. 21-1). Each side of the heart is, itself, two pumping chambers: an atrium and a ventricle. To move blood most effectively, these chambers must function out of phase with each other. The cardiac cycle consists of systole (ventricular contraction) and diastole (ventricular relaxation). The cycle is governed by a conducting system. In normal cardiac conduction, electrical impulses are generated and propelled through the heart. Depolarization of the sinoatrial node normally generates the current that leads to depolarization of all other cardiac muscle cells. Calcium facilitates this electrical activity.

Pathophysiology of Heart Failure

Initially heart failure was thought of as pump failure—failure of the heart to pump adequate quantities of blood to meet the needs of peripheral organs. Now heart failure is considered a disorder of the circulation, not just a disease of the heart. It develops not when the heart is injured, but when the body's compensatory hemodynamic and neurohormonal mechanisms are overwhelmed or exhausted (Packer, 1992).

The key event in heart failure is loss of a critical quantity of functioning myocardial cells. This can follow an injury to the heart (eg, acute myocardial infarction), toxins (eg, alcohol, cytotoxic drugs), viral or parasitic infection (eg, viral myocarditis), or prolonged cardiovascular stress (eg, hypertension, valvular disease).

To compensate for the loss and thereby to preserve cardiac function, the body activates hemodynamic and neurohormonal mechanisms to enhance the contractile force of the uninjured myocardial cells. These mechanisms incorporate Starling's law: a decrease in the ability to empty the ventricle during systole increases the tension on the uninjured parts of the heart during diastole; the ventricle responds to this increase in preload with enhanced contractions. The stronger contractions lead to ventricular dilation.

Meanwhile, a decrease in the ability of the ventricle to eject blood into the aorta activates the sympathetic nervous system. The resultant stimulation of beta-adrenergic receptors in the uninjured myocardium increases the frequency and force of contraction. These two mechanisms involve different but complementary calcium-dependent inotropic pathways. Ventricular dilation enhances the sensitivity of myofilaments to calcium, and sympathetic activation increases the delivery of calcium to the myofilaments.

These compensatory mechanisms increase the internal stress on the heart wall during diastole, resulting

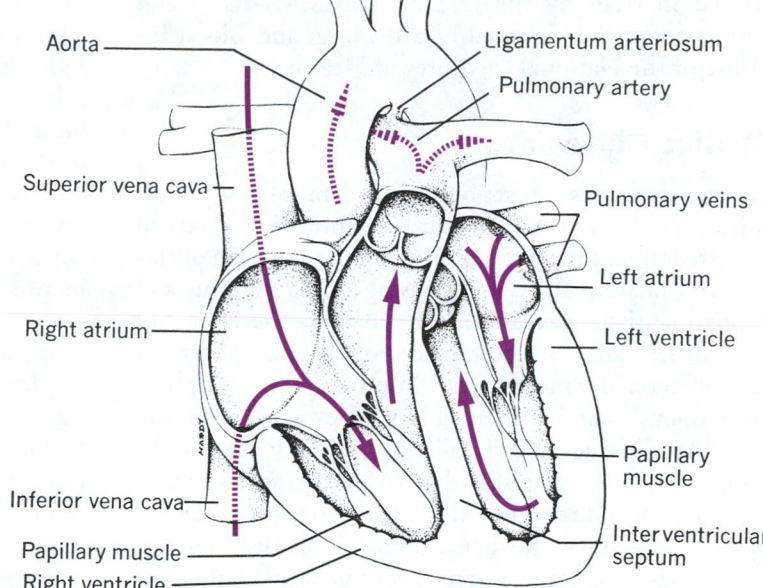

Figure 21-1. The heart pumps blood throughout the body (in the direction indicated by the arrows). The right side of the heart receives blood from the body and pumps it into the lungs where carbon dioxide is exchanged for oxygen. The oxygenated blood then enters the left side of the heart and is propelled through the peripheral vascular system to nourish the cells of the body.

in eventual structural distortion and accelerated energy expenditure. This induces the synthesis of certain myofibrillar proteins, which in turn promote ventricular wall thickening (ventricular hypertrophy). The thickened wall reduces ventricular strain. In addition, the proteins synthesized are bioenergetically more efficient than the ones initially present. So, initially, ventricular hypertrophy strengthens the heart and reduces its workload and energy expenditure.

At the same time, and related to increased diastolic wall stress in the atria, atrial stretch stimulates the atrial baroreceptors. These inhibit sympathetic outflow from the central nervous system, and atrial natriuretic peptide is secreted. This peptide inhibits the release of the neurotransmitter norepinephrine and its actions on peripheral blood vessels. The peptide also exerts direct vasodilatory and natriuretic effects that reduce the hemodynamic load on the heart.

When cardiac output drops, systemic perfusion pressure is maintained by peripheral vasoconstriction and sodium retention. The release of atrial natriuretic peptide becomes blunted after long-term atrial distention, and the released peptide can no longer suppress the release of renin or dilate peripheral blood vessels. In addition, the release of endothelium-derived relaxing factor is diminished in persons with heart failure. As a result, the actions of vasoconstrictors are unopposed.

Heart failure symptoms trigger the renin–angiotensin mechanism. The activation of the sympathetic nervous system increases the release of renin. Angiotensin exerts constrictor effects in the kidney, enhancing proximal tubular sodium reabsorption. Angiotensin also augments sodium reabsorption directly and indirectly by stimulating the release of aldosterone. Angiotensin stimulates the cerebral thirst center, which may lead to increased water intake and retention, and

enhances the release of pituitary vasopressin, which decreases water excretion. Water retention occurs from the increase in water intake (resulting from stimulation of the cerebral thirst center) and the decrease in water excretion (resulting from the enhanced release of pituitary vasopressin). These salt- and water-retaining effects are potentiated by the stimulation of renal sympathetic nerves in early heart failure and by a fall in renal blood flow in late heart failure. The development of peripheral vasoconstriction and sodium retention represents an important shift, with the cardiovascular system moving from a state of compensation to a state of decompensation.

Over time, the hemodynamic and neurohormonal mechanisms lose their ability to compensate; they then cause more deleterious than beneficial effects. For example, prolonged ventricular dilation leads to thinning and necrosis of the ventricular wall, destroying myocardial cells in previously uninjured segments of the heart. Progressive ventricular dilation may undermine mitral valve support, with subsequent mitral valve regurgitation. The hypertrophic response may actually increase energy demands. This happens because the number of energy-consuming myofibrils increases but the supply of energy decreases because the thickened wall impairs oxygen diffusion.

Prolonged activation of the sympathetic nervous system and the renin–angiotensin mechanism has adverse effects: high concentrations of norepinephrine and angiotensin exert direct toxic effects on myocardial cells. Alterations in intracellular cyclic adenosine monophosphate (c-AMP) and potassium levels result and may exert adverse electrophysiologic effects, provoking lethal arrhythmias.

The question of whether cardiac glycosides improve the survival rates of clients with heart failure is addressed in trials by the Digitalis Investigators Group sponsored by the National Heart, Lung, and Blood Institute of the National Institutes of Health.

Cardiac Glycosides

Cardiac glycosides can act on the mechanical component of heart failure (reduced myocardial contractility) and can also strengthen the force and prolong the duration of cardiac contraction, thereby increasing cardiac output and improving tissue perfusion. In addition, the effects of these drugs can promote recovery of the ailing heart by various secondary mechanisms. Improved blood supply to the kidneys increases their ability to excrete water and salts. This diuretic effect is enhanced by a reduction in the compensatory mechanisms that favor sodium and water retention. By reducing blood volume, diuresis reduces peripheral resistance, further improving cardiac output. Cardiac glycosides also improve coronary circulation, inhibit responsiveness to ectopic stimuli in the heart, and tend to eliminate premature contractions.

Despite current research and changes in thinking about the actions of some cardiac glycosides, these agents continue to play a role in managing cardiovascular disease. Digitalis-derived drugs (eg, digoxin) are reported to be among the ten most commonly prescribed drugs in the United States (Meissner & Gever, 1993).

Pharmacodynamics. Each of the cardiac glycosides has a chemical structure consisting of a sugar, a steroid, and a five- or six-member lactone ring. Although many glycosides have been produced, only a few are customarily used in clinical practice (Table 21-1).

Exactly how cardiac glycosides work is unknown. The current hypothesis is that they bind to and inhibit sodium/potassium-activated adenosine triphosphatase (Na,K-ATPase) in the myocardial cell membrane, inhibit the sodium pump, and thus bring about a rise in the intracellular sodium concentration. As a consequence, sodium–calcium exchange is stimulated and additional calcium entering the cell is taken up in the sarcoplasmic reticulum. With each heart beat, there is an increased release of calcium from the sarcoplasmic reticulum, thus increasing the strength of the heart contraction—a positive inotropic effect (Poole-Wilson, 1994).

In the client with heart failure, digoxin slows the cardiac conduction system and therefore the heart rate. It does this by increasing central parasympathetic output and decreasing central sympathetic outflow. The result is an enhanced vagal effect, which reduces conduction velocity (negative dromotropic effect) and lengthens action potential in the conducting tissues of the heart. Box 21-1 lists the types of chemical effects on the heart.

Pharmacokinetics. Gastrointestinal (GI) absorption of cardiac glycosides varies with the polarity of the drug, the drug product, and the manufacturer. Polar drugs are those having electrical charges on the molecule. Although the molecule as a whole is electrically neutral (because the number of negative and positive charges are equal), one or more sites on it exhibit a negative charge, and one or more others are positively charged. Relatively nonpolar compounds (eg, digitoxin) are completely absorbed. Digoxin, which is more polar than digitoxin, is less completely absorbed. Deslanoside

Table 21-1. Cardiac Glycosides

Drug Name	Loading Dose*	Maintenance Dose	Onset	Action Peak	Half-life
deslanoside (Cedilanid-D)	Adults: 1.6 mg, divided in 1 or 2 doses (maximum digitalizing dose: 2 mg)	not used for maintenance	IV: 10 min IM: 30 min	IV: 20 min–4 hr	33–36 hr
digoxin (Lanoxin, Lanoxicaps)	*Oral tablets and elixir:* Infants 1–24 mo: 35–60 µg/kg Children 5–10 yr: 20–35 µg/kg Adults and children older than 10 yr: 10–15 µg/kg *Liquid-filled oral capsules:* Adults and children older than 10 yr: 8–12 µg/kg *IV solutions:* Infants 1–24 mo: 30–50 µg/kg Adults and children older than 10 yr: 8–12 µg/kg	*Oral tablets and elixir:* 25–35% of oral loading dose	0.5–2 hr	6–8 hr	34–44 hr
digitoxin	Infants 2 wk–1 yr: 45 µg/kg Children 2–12 yr: 30 µg/kg or 750 µg/m² Adults and children 12 yr and up: 1.2–1.6 mg	10% of total digitalizing dose	30 min–2 hr	4–12 hr	5–7 days

*Total loading doses are divided and fractional doses administered q4–12 h during first 24 hr of treatment.

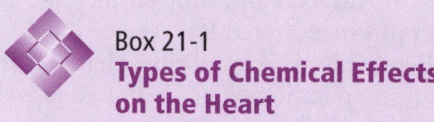

Box 21-1
Types of Chemical Effects on the Heart

Inotropic: affect the strength of contraction of cardiac muscle

Chronotropic: affect the rate of contraction of cardiac muscle

Dromotropic: affect the conductivity of cardiac tissue

is more polar than digoxin and is so poorly absorbed after oral administration that it is administered only parenterally. Binding by plasma proteins also varies with polarity: more polar compounds are less bound than nonpolar drugs. At therapeutic plasma concentrations, digitoxin is 97% protein bound, digoxin 20% to 30% protein bound.

Cardiac glycosides are widely distributed in body tissues. Concentrations are highest in the heart, kidneys, intestine, stomach, liver, and skeletal muscle. The lowest concentrations are in the plasma and brain. The drugs cross the placenta and are distributed in breast milk.

Metabolism varies with polarity. Highly polar glycosides (eg, digoxin, deslanoside) are not metabolized appreciably; less polar compounds (eg, digitoxin) are extensively metabolized by the liver. Excretion is primarily by the kidneys. Cardiac glycosides are not removed by dialysis.

Plasma concentrations of cardiac glycosides are helpful but not absolute indicators of therapeutic and toxic drug effects. Individual response to a given concentration is influenced by serum electrolytes (particularly potassium, calcium, and magnesium), acid–base balance, the type of cardiac disorder, thyroid status, autonomic nervous system activity, and other drugs administered concurrently. Hypokalemia increases the toxic potential of a given drug level; clients with supraventricular tachycardias (atrial fibrillation or atrial flutter) may require higher plasma concentrations than do clients with heart failure.

Digitalis is reputed to be a cumulative drug (one with a tendency to increase in concentration and cause toxicity). However, it is probably no more likely to accumulate in body tissues than many other substances with long half-lives.

Therapeutic Uses. Cardiac glycosides are used for treating heart failure and certain atrial arrhythmias, such as atrial fibrillation and atrial flutter. By inhibiting the conductivity of the heart, cardiac glycosides reduce the number of impulses that reach the ventricles and slow the rate of ventricular contraction. This prolongs diastole, improves ventricular filling, and increases cardiac output.

Dosage and Administration. Commonly, cardiac glycosides, such as digoxin and digitoxin, are initially administered in loading doses depending on the client's age, size, and medical condition (Box 21-2). Other dosing considerations include the particular drug and the administration route chosen. The loading dose is usually divided and administered over a period of 24 hours (usually every 6 hours).

Once the client is digitalized, maintenance doses are given once daily. They are usually proportional to the daily losses from metabolism or excretion. In addition, they are relatively high for the glycosides eliminated by the kidneys (if the client has normal renal function) because about one third of the drug is excreted in the urine daily.

Because digitoxin is metabolized more slowly in the liver, its maintenance dose is only about 10% of the loading dose. Renal or liver impairment slows elimination of certain drugs and requires reduction of the maintenance dose. Because it is not eliminated by the kidneys, digitoxin may be the drug of choice for clients with renal disease. On the other hand, agents excreted through the kidneys are preferable for persons with hepatic impairment.

Most children require proportionately higher doses of the cardiac glycosides—up to 50% more than adults according to weight. Premature and immature infants are very sensitive and require reduced dosages.

Adverse Reactions. Digitalis is an example of a drug with a narrow safety margin. Therapeutic doses are fully 50% to 60% of toxic doses.

Cardiac glycosides are irritating to tissue and are rarely injected intramuscularly because pain, muscle fasciculation, and necrosis can occur at the injection site.

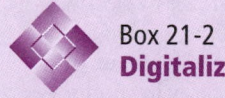

Box 21-2
Digitalization

To promote a desired and speedy response to cardiac glycosides, the initial doses must usually be several times the magnitude of those required for maintenance. Tissue depots (plasma proteins and other body tissues) must be saturated before therapeutic serum concentrations of the drugs are stabilized. Such accelerated dosage regimens are termed *digitalization*.

Rapid digitalization is best accomplished in a controlled environment (eg, coronary care unit) with facilities and monitoring equipment for continuous assessment of cardiac function and prompt treatment of any serious arrhythmias that might occur. Intravenous administration of a cardiac glycoside, which may be required, is a particularly hazardous undertaking.

Most adverse reactions to cardiac glycosides are symptoms of toxicity (see Toxicity Alert: Digitalis), indicating the need for a careful appraisal for overdose and possible dose reduction. Symptoms of toxicity include GI symptoms, vision disturbances, bradycardia (apical rate less than 60/min in adults), tachycardia (apical rate greater than 100/min in adults), and CNS symptoms.

Toxicity Alert: Digitalis

Because the margin between therapeutic and toxic levels of cardiac glycosides is so narrow, the nurse must be vigilant for signs and symptoms of digitalis toxicity.

Early Toxicity

- Anorexia (almost always the first sign)

Moderate Toxicity

- Nausea, vomiting, sometimes with abdominal pain and increased salivation (usually appears 1–3 days after anorexia)
- Fatigue (ranges from drowsiness to muscle weakness)
- Vision disturbances, such as misperceived colors, particularly green and red, or yellow or green halos around objects (usually occur a few days before cardiac signs)
- Mental disturbances, such as confusion, depression, even psychosis (common in elderly and in clients with atherosclerosis)

Severe Toxicity

- Diarrhea, weakness, headache, malaise, diplopia, scotomata
- Arrhythmia—may decrease heart rate by slowing conduction and increasing refractory period at atrioventricular node; may increase heart rate by creating abnormal pacemaker activity in conductive tissue; may cause two or more concurrent arrhythmias; may cause premature ventricular contractions, ventricular fibrillation, or cardiac arrest

Many symptoms of toxicity of the cardiac glycosides resemble those of the heart conditions for which they are prescribed, so differentiating the two requires careful assessment. Comparing the serum glycoside level with the usual therapeutic range is sometimes helpful but can be misleading because physiologic response to the drugs can be excessive even when serum levels are not. Perhaps the best diagnostic tool is the electrocardiogram (ECG). A therapeutic digitalis level tends to alter certain segments of the ECG by narrowing the QRS complex, depressing or inverting T waves, and slowing the heart rate (Fig. 21-2). Increasing drug effects prolong the P-R interval and shorten the Q-T interval. Large doses produce altered P waves.

When the client's physical condition changes, the response to digitalis preparations may be altered as well, particularly if any of the following occur:

- Vomiting, diarrhea, or other GI disorder (changes ability to absorb digitalis)
- Acid–base or electrolyte disturbances, such as hypokalemia, hypomagnesemia, or hypocalcemia (change the heart's sensitivity to digitalis)
- Hypothyroidism (alters the client's ability to metabolize digitalis)
- Liver or kidney disease (changes the ability to metabolize or excrete digitalis).

A client who undergoes electrical cardioversion to manage arrhythmia should be observed carefully for digitalis toxicity because this procedure increases the heart's sensitivity to digitalis.

When initial signs or symptoms of toxicity develop, one or more daily doses of the glycosides are omitted. Medication is not resumed until these indicators disappear.

Drug Interactions. Digoxin interacts with many drugs (Table 21-2). Antacids, antidiarrheals, and ion-exchange resins interact with digoxin to decrease digoxin absorption, which decreases digoxin effectiveness.

After administration of succinylcholine to fully digitalized clients, cardiac arrhythmias have developed. Succinylcholine appears to potentiate the cardiac conduction effects of digitalis preparations and may produce increased ventricular irritability. Depolarizing muscle relaxants may produce a sudden shift of potassium from inside the muscle cell to outside. In the digitalized myocardium, arrhythmias could result.

Some drugs increase the potential for toxicity by causing hypokalemia. These drugs include thiazide and loop diuretics that waste potassium, amphotericin B, and corticosteroids. Diuretics such as furosemide (Lasix), ethacrynic acid (Edecrin), bumetanide (Bumex), chlorthalidone (Hygroton), and metolazone (Zaroxolyn) have been implicated. The magnesium deficiency that can occur after diuretic therapy may also contribute to digoxin toxicity.

Other drugs that increase the potential for toxicity include quinidine, verapamil, and erythromycin. When quinidine is coadministered with digoxin, the serum digoxin concentration almost doubles (Abernethy & Andrawis, 1993). The client may experience cardiac arrhythmias and the other usual symptoms of digitalis toxicity.

About 10% of clients who take digoxin carry an intestinal organism, *Eubacterium lentum*, that inactivates 30% to 40% of the digoxin taken. In these clients, a therapeutic digoxin dose can be toxic if the intestinal flora are disturbed by an antibiotic such as erythromycin. Administering erythromycin to the client on

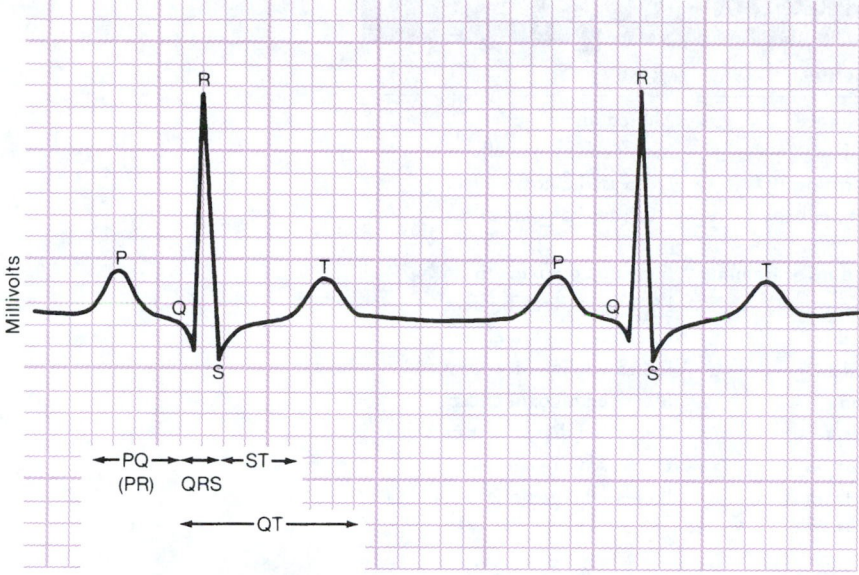

Millivolts

←PQ→ ←→ ←ST→
(PR)   QRS
←——QT——→

Key:

Each vertical square represents one tenth of a milli-
    volt of electrical charge

Each horizontal square equals 0.04 seconds of time.

Approximate values for normal intervals:

PQ(PR) interval—0.16 sec.
QT interval—0.3 sec.
QRS interval—0.08 sec.
P wave—0.08 sec.
ST interval—0.1 sec.

P wave = Electrical changes associated with atrial depolarization
QRS Complex = Electrical changes associated with ventricular depolarization
T wave = Electrical changes associated with ventricular repolarization
The electrical changes associated with atrial repolarization normally coincide with the QRS complex
    and are obscured by it.

Time (0.04 seconds per square)

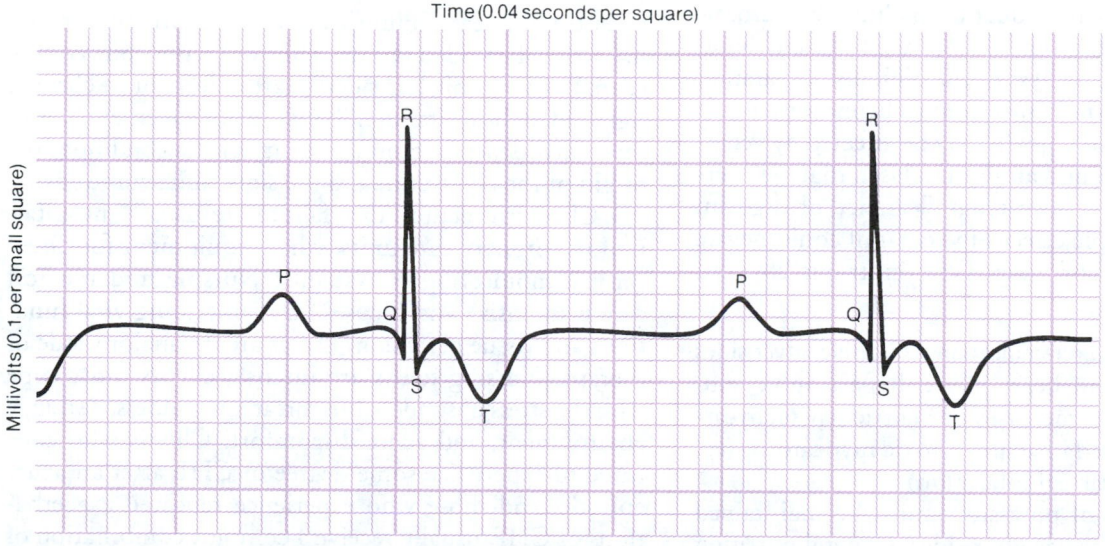

Millivolts (0.1 per small square)

Figure 21-2. A normal ECG tracing appears at top. Electrical changes associated with atrial repolarization normally coincide with the QRS complex and are obscured by it. The amplitude
and direction of tracings vary depending on placement of the electrodes for various leads. Compared with the normal ECG, the tracing below the top tracting illustrates the pattern normally
seen in therapeutic digitalization. It reflects a prolonged P-R interval, a shortened Q-T interval,
and T-wave inversion.

Table 21-2. Selected Drug Interactions Involving Digoxin

Agent	Mechanism of Action	Result
amiloride	Increase renal clearance	Altered digoxin effect
amphotericin B	Cause hypokalemia	Increased digoxin effect
antacids	Decrease GI absorption	Decreased digoxin effect
barbiturates	Enzyme induction, enhanced metabolism	Decreased digoxin effect
calcium	Calcium action on myocardium	Increased digoxin effect
cholestyramine	Decrease GI absorption	Decreased digoxin effect
corticosteroids	Cause hypokalemia	Increased digoxin effect
diuretics (thiazide & loop)	Cause hypokalemia	Increased digoxin effect
erythromycin	Enzyme inhibition	Increased digoxin effect
kaolin–pectin mixtures	Decrease GI absorption	Decreased digoxin effect
metoclopramide	Decrease GI absorption	Decreased digoxin effect
quinidine	Displace digoxin from tissue-binding sites, decrease renal clearance	Increased digoxin effect
spironolactone	Decrease renal clearance	Altered digoxin effect
thyroid preparations	Change renal clearance of digoxin	Increased or decreased digoxin effect
verapamil	Decrease renal clearance	Increased digoxin effect

digoxin may increase the active digoxin serum concentration up to 100%. Apparently, the erythromycin reduces the population of bacteria that inactivate the digoxin. The rise in the serum digoxin level increases the risk of toxicity.

Drugs that decrease the activity of digitalis preparations by hepatic enzyme induction include the barbiturates, phenytoin, rifampin, and possibly phenylbutazone. Thus, the effectiveness of the digitalis preparation is decreased and the dose may need to be increased.

Renal clearance of digoxin may be affected by verapamil, spironolactone, and amiloride. Used together, verapamil and digoxin reduce renal clearance of digoxin. The negative inotropic effect of verapamil could negate some of the benefits of the positive inotropic effect of digoxin.

Precautions and Contraindications. Cardiac glycosides are contraindicated in heart block, hypertrophic subaortic stenosis, and some cases of ventricular tachycardia. Caution is advised in acute or toxic myocarditis (eg, that following myocardial infarction).

Adequate levels of potassium must be maintained in clients receiving cardiac glycosides. General nutrition should be supported to ensure optimal levels of other electrolytes (eg, magnesium, calcium).

■ SUMMARY

Cardiac glycosides exert positive inotropic, negative chronotropic, and negative dromotropic effects on the heart. They have been widely used to treat clients with CHF. These drugs have a narrow margin of safety, and the nurse should assess each client for signs and symptoms of toxicity before each dose. Anorexia, nausea or vomiting, distur-

bances in vision, and a very slow or very rapid heart rate are some indicators of toxicity.

❖ NURSING MANAGEMENT: CLIENT RECEIVING A CARDIAC GLYCOSIDE

Clients with heart failure are usually identified as being in acute left-sided heart failure (acute pulmonary edema), in chronic left-sided heart failure, or in chronic right-sided heart failure. Nursing management varies somewhat depending on the acuity of the condition, the origin of the condition, and the signs and symptoms.

Clients in acute heart failure are usually hospitalized in coronary care units, where equipment for direct cardiac monitoring is available. Nursing and medical care is intensive and focuses on maintaining vital functions and tissue perfusion. Drugs are the major mode of therapy. Nursing needs are intense: clients must cope with the stress of sudden, life-threatening illness, a strange environment, and acute discomfort. Clients who continue to experience some degree of CHF after an acute episode, and those who experience repeated exacerbations of CHF, usually receive a complex combination of medications, which include cardiac glycosides. Dosages of all drugs must be carefully adjusted for optimal effect. All clients require help managing their medications.

NURSING PROCESS

ASSESSMENT

A detailed health history should be obtained in an interview with the client, if possible. A family member or another significant person may become the primary source of data, especially if the client's level of consciousness is impaired by poor oxygenation of the brain.

Most clients in acute heart failure feel fearful and anxious because they are aware of the life-threatening nature of the illness; anxiety is heightened if the client is admitted to the coronary care unit. Family members and others may be prone to fear, anxiety, and feelings of helplessness as well. If these feelings are evident, they may intensify similar feelings in the client.

A drug history must be obtained. Clients with more chronic failure often require several drugs, some of which may interact in a harmful manner. All drugs used by the client should be documented, including prescription, over-the-counter, and social drugs (caffeine, nicotine, and alcohol).

Risk factors predisposing to drug toxicity should be identified. These include hepatic or renal impairment, use of potassium-wasting diuretics, and hormone use. Hepatic or renal impairment causes drugs to accumulate; unusual stress contributes to depletion of potassium. Immobility may be accompanied by hypercalcemia associated with bone demineralization.

The nursing assessment should also involve a baseline physical examination, including vital signs, apical and radial pulse rates, cardiac rhythm and sounds, skin color, tissue turgor, degree and sites of edema, peripheral perfusion findings, level of consciousness, level of energy, and some measure of central venous pressure. Cyanosis, dyspnea, increased venous pressure, edema, delayed capillary refill, lack of energy, and altered level of consciousness are signs and symptoms of cardiac decompensation.

Nutritional status should be appraised, with particular attention to fluid, electrolyte, and acid–base balance. Hypokalemia, hypercalcemia, hypomagnesemia, and alkalosis predispose the client to digitalis toxicity. Bowel status is also important. Constipation causes vagal stimulation, which tends to slow the heart; diarrhea can cause rapid potassium depletion.

The nurse should appraise the client's current health practices. Adherence to the current drug regimen should be determined. The client's ability to incorporate self-care measures appropriate to the level of disability into his or her lifestyle must be evaluated.

The idea of chronic dependence on medication or other special treatment may be difficult for the client and family to accept and integrate into living patterns. The success of treatment is measured by quality of life, as well as by adherence to the therapeutic regimen.

NURSING DIAGNOSIS

Diagnoses related to the drug regimen may focus on potential toxic effects, such as:

- Altered Nutrition: Less than Body Requirements, related to drug-induced anorexia, nausea, or diarrhea
- Decreased Cardiac Output, related to drug-induced arrhythmias, impaired cardiac conductivity, and abbreviated diastole
- Visual Sensory/Perceptual Alterations: drug-induced disturbance in yellow and green color perception

- Ineffective Management of Therapeutic Regimen (Individuals), related to complex drug therapy
- Knowledge Deficit, related to heart failure and drug therapy

PLANNING

Goals of nursing care for clients with heart failure include administering therapy to increase cardiac output and tissue perfusion, decrease interstitial and blood fluid volumes, improve gas exchange in the lungs, alleviate or eliminate dyspnea, decrease the risk of skin breakdown, provide physical care needed by the client, increase tolerance for activity, and optimize amount of sleep. Additional goals are to provide clients and families with the information needed to cope with the illness, promptly detect and treat drug toxicity, and increase effective management of the treatment regimen (see the Critical Thinking Challenge).

INTERVENTION

Much of the nursing care administered depends on the therapeutic regimen. The nurse administers medications (including oxygen), monitors the client's response to treatment, and adjusts treatment in accord with this response and standard protocols when appropriate. A normal therapeutic response to cardiac glycosides is

CRITICAL THINKING CHALLENGE
Case Analysis

You are caring for two clients who have different medical diagnoses but who are both receiving a cardiac glycoside. Mrs. Anselm, a widow with no family, is 74 years old. She has long-standing congestive heart failure and mitral valve regurgitation. Mr. Mayfield, age 60, has heart failure and arrhythmias. He has been considering retirement from his job as a supermarket butcher.

You have conducted a nursing assessment of each client and have documented their subjective complaints and objective evidence gathered during the physical examination. Your data include individual medication histories. Mrs. Anselm also takes furosemide (Lasix) to promote diuresis. Mr. Mayfield also takes antacids and laxatives to manage GI complaints.

1. Consider which of your clients' subjective and objective complaints could be caused by the cardiac glycoside and which by some other medication they are receiving. Discuss how you came to this conclusion.
2. Propose and prioritize interventions you would perform to help each client prevent adverse reactions to the cardiac glycoside (and the other medications).
3. Identify the teaching–learning needs of each client. Develop a teaching plan specific to each client's needs. Explain the similarities and differences of these teaching plans.
4. With hindsight, what additional information would you have gathered during the assessment interviews?

characterized by a stronger and slower pulse rate, diuresis, and decreased dyspnea.

Administering digitalis preparations requires special care. Because of the drug's potency and narrow safety margin, medication errors of small magnitude may have serious consequences. Because an overdose as small as ⅛ mg could represent a doubling of the therapeutic maintenance dose, the nurse must clearly differentiate between maintenance and loading doses.

Dosage errors are particularly likely to occur in medication areas where many different digitalis preparations are stored. The names of digitalis preparations are similar enough to make differentiation difficult. Drug errors may be reduced by stocking only those preparations in common use. The unit-dose system of individual rather than stock drug supplies is also preferred for safety.

Oral cardiac glycosides should not be administered with meals that have a high fiber content. Studies have shown that it binds with the fiber, reducing the amount of medication available for absorption. Because cardiac glycosides are usually administered only once a day, they are customarily given after breakfast.

Close monitoring of the client's potassium level is necessary. Clients who have difficulty eating, who sustain abnormal fluid losses from diarrhea or fistula drainage, or who are on potassium-wasting diuretics are at risk for digitalis toxicity. Additionally, all clients subject to high stress levels lose potassium through the kidneys in response to high levels of the adrenocortical hormones (eg, aldosterone, cortisone).

Toxicity can also develop in clients who cannot detoxify and eliminate the drug at the normal rate (those with marginal liver or kidney function). Infants may be unable to handle the drug efficiently because their organs are immature; elderly persons are likely to have some degree of damage to these organs. If the client has adequate kidney function, the nurse should encourage consumption of foods rich in potassium to reduce the risk of digitalis toxicity.

Because cardiac glycosides have such narrow safety margins, monitoring must include careful attention to indications of therapeutic response and early signs of toxicity. Laboratory tests measuring drug concentrations must be considered carefully, but they are relative, not absolute, indicators of potential toxicity. Individual response to specific drug concentrations is altered by many factors, including electrolyte and hormone levels, acid–base balance, and the degree of cardiac pathology. Laboratory data must be interpreted in light of the total clinical picture.

Because many signs and symptoms of toxicity from the cardiac glycosides are identical to those of heart failure, they are only partially reliable as indicators of drug toxicity. The client with heart failure is likely to experience malaise, anorexia, nausea, vomiting, or alterations in levels of consciousness. Changes in vision are good evidence of toxicity, but they do not occur consistently. The timing and sequence of symptoms may be helpful.

Nausea early in the course of glycoside therapy may result from poor perfusion of the intestinal tract rather than drug toxicity. If a period of client improvement (indicating therapeutic response to medication) is followed by renewed GI problems, toxicity is much more likely to be the cause. An apical pulse rate below 60 or above 100 in adults suggests toxicity, as does an increase in pulse deficit (the difference between the apical and the radial pulse rates). Judgment in interpreting such data is necessary.

Assessment for toxicity should be performed before each scheduled dose of medication. The nurse must be particularly alert to early signs and symptoms of toxicity. Diagnosis at this stage allows for early correction. By the time late symptoms develop, when the diagnosis is obvious, the client is likely to be in serious difficulty (see Toxicity Alert: Digitalis).

If a diagnosis of toxicity seems likely, cardiac glycosides should be withheld and the prescribing clinician notified of the client's condition. The clinician may order potassium supplements if the client's levels are low. Usually, omission of one or more doses of the glycosides lowers the serum concentration below the toxic level. Nursing measures to support general physiologic function and maintain fluid and electrolyte balance are helpful not only to correct toxicity but also to delay or prevent it.

Nursing measures designed to eliminate stressors and help the client minimize the stress response allay toxicity by conserving body potassium stores. Both the family and client need emotional support.

The use of cardiac glycosides in treating acute heart failure often alleviates the symptoms of heart failure and restores homeostasis. Unless the underlying cause of cardiac impairment can be corrected, however, failure can recur. Although cardiac glycosides may be withdrawn after resolution of an acute episode, they are sometimes used for prolonged periods.

Client Education. Clients in acute heart failure cannot absorb large amounts of information at one time, nor can their families or significant others. The nurse should develop and implement a teaching plan appropriate to their status. Comprehensive teaching should be postponed until the client's physical condition appears to stabilize.

Clients who live at home and manage their own care need teaching designed to help them manage their drug regimen (see the Critical Thinking Challenge). Instructions should stress maintaining adequate potassium intake, techniques for self-monitoring for early signs and symptoms of digitalis toxicity, and actions to take if those signs appear.

When adherence is a problem, the nurse must identify and try to eliminate the underlying reasons. Sometimes clients omit drug dosages when they are feeling well, believing that medicines can be taken on an as-needed basis. Sometimes the client has too little money to cover both medication and essential living expenses. If the client must choose, for example, between paying for medicine or heat during cold weather, one should be not surprised if adherence to drug therapy takes second place.

If clients have difficulty remembering to take all their drugs, the nurse can help them develop a system to ensure regular dosage. Showing clients how to prepare all medications needed for the day, sorted according to administration time, is usually helpful. To maintain a therapeutic blood level, cardiac glycoside preparations should be given at about the same time each day. This is particularly important if digoxin is used, because more than a third of the drug is excreted normally in 24 hours, and blood levels can drop by half if the daily dose is delayed, for example, from morning to evening.

Clients should learn how to monitor the pulse for rate and rhythm for a full minute before taking a cardiac glycoside. The nurse can identify and explain the general normal range (60–100 beats/min). The client should call the prescriber if the pulse rate is outside a range set by the prescriber based on the client's condition or other medications. The prescriber should also be consulted if GI upset (anorexia, nausea, vomiting, or diarrhea) develops (see Home and Community Care: Mental Notes).

Clients need to know that digitalis preparations are potent poisons and, therefore, should be stored in a secure place away from children and pets.

OUTCOME EVALUATION

Data required for evaluation include vital signs (especially blood pressure, pulse, and respirations); descriptions of color perception, tissue turgor, and peripheral circulation; absence or presence of rales and rhonchi; serum potassium levels; serum digoxin levels; and statements by the client relating to difficulty or ease in breathing. The client's ability to repeat to the nurse information conveyed during teaching sessions also provides the nurse with an estimate of the client's learning progress. Additional data include statements by the client and family concerning their perceptions of stress.

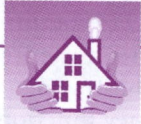

HOME AND COMMUNITY CARE

Mental Notes

The following notes are an example of how a nurse might think when constructing a teaching plan for a client and family about a discharge regimen involving a cardiac glycoside.

Preliminary Assessment

✔ **Client's knowledge:** Cardiac glycoside purpose and action, adverse effects, potential interactions, dosage schedule
✔ **Client's habits:** Nutrition, such as use of processed foods and potassium-rich foods; primary food purchaser and preparer; activity limitations and allowances
✔ **Client's circumstances and influencing factors**
  • Age
  • Self-care attitude and ability
  • Previous experience with cardiac glycosides and other prescribed or over-the-counter medications
  • Financial situation (ability to pay for and obtain medications)
  • Physical condition, such as visual deficits, manual dexterity, level of alertness
  • Psychologic effects of physical condition

Goals and Planning

✔ Reduce risk of adverse effects and drug interactions.
✔ Promptly detect and treat adverse reactions or drug interactions.
✔ Decrease knowledge deficit related to drug regimen.

Intervention

✔ **Provide anticipatory guidance**
  • Explain potential adverse reactions and interactions.
  • Set up drug administration schedule that incorporates client's lifestyle.
  • Urge client to use only one pharmacy for obtaining medications.
  • Have client post prescriber's telephone number in an easily accessible place.
✔ **Teach Skills**
  • Show client how to take and monitor pulse rate.
  • Reinforce pulse rate range parameters.
  • Encourage client to keep a pulse rate diary.
✔ **Facilitate learning**
  • Provide reinforcement materials, such as written instructions, especially for how to take a pulse.
✔ **Involve family**
  • Enlist aid of family members if client has difficulty taking his or her own pulse or adhering to medication schedule.
✔ **Schedule follow-up**
  • Reinforce need for follow-up laboratory tests.
  • Encourage client to schedule and keep follow-up appointments.
  • Arrange for transport as needed to promote follow-up.

❖ CHECKLIST OF NURSING ACTIONS

Acute Heart Failure

- ❏ Assess clients directly for cardiorespiratory status; supplement observations with ECG, blood pressure, and laboratory data.
- ❏ Assess the emotional reaction of clients and families to the life-threatening illness.
- ❏ Protect the client from exertion.
- ❏ Differentiate carefully between digitalizing and maintenance doses of cardiac glycosides.
- ❏ Monitor clients for therapeutic and toxic reactions to cardiac medication. Evaluate clients carefully before administering each dose of these drugs.
- ❏ Withhold cardiac glycosides when clients exhibit early signs and symptoms of toxicity.
- ❏ Unless otherwise contraindicated, encourage ingestion of foods and fluids rich in potassium.
- ❏ Eliminate unnecessary stressors and help the client reduce stress levels.
- ❏ Teach the client essential information about the treatment regimen; postpone detailed and comprehensive teaching until the client's condition stabilizes.

Chronic Heart Failure

- ❏ Periodically perform a general health assessment, with emphasis on cardiovascular function.
- ❏ Before giving each dose of cardiac glycosides, assess for evidence of drug toxicity.
- ❏ Administer cardiac glycosides daily at about the same time after a meal.
- ❏ Analyze the drug regimen for risk of adverse drug reactions and interactions.
- ❏ Monitor the client for signs and symptoms of adverse drug reactions and interactions.
- ❏ Encourage digitalized clients with good renal function to increase their intake of dietary potassium, especially when potassium-wasting diuretics are used concurrently.
- ❏ Help clients develop stress management skills.
- ❏ Discuss ways to avoid constipation; teach measures to promote fecal elimination.
- ❏ Inform clients about extracardiac and cardiac signs and symptoms of toxicity and signs and symptoms of interactions. Teach them (and family members) how to monitor pulse rates.
- ❏ When clients need financial aid to adhere to drug therapy, make referrals to appropriate agencies.
- ❏ Help the client devise a system that promotes accurate administration of all drugs.
- ❏ To prevent accidental poisoning, warn clients to store medicines in secure areas.

Digitalis Antidote: Digoxin Immune Fab

Acute digitalis toxicity carries a definite risk of cardiac arrest, and immediate medical attention is required. A parenteral antidote for digoxin toxicity, digitalis immune fab (Digibind), is available to treat severe toxicity.

Digoxin immune fab is the first biologic preparation to be approved as a specific antidote to a drug. The antigen-binding fragments (fab) are made from antidigoxin antibodies acquired from sheep.

Pharmacodynamics. Digoxin immune fab fragments bind molecules of digoxin, making them unavailable for binding at their site of action. The fab fragment/digoxin complex accumulates in the blood and is excreted by the kidneys. Ordinarily, improvement in signs and symptoms of digoxin intoxication begins in less than 30 minutes.

Pharmacokinetics. The onset of action is in less than 1 minute; the agent's half-life is 15 to 20 hours. While antigen-binding fragments are circulating in the blood, laboratory assays for digoxin may indicate an increase in serum levels; this is because the drug bound to the antigen-binding fragments is measured along with the free digoxin. Elimination from the body of the fragments and the digoxin they bind depends on kidney function. Several days may be required for elimination. During this interval, digoxin immune fab remaining in the blood is likely to render further doses of digoxin ineffective.

Therapeutic Uses. Use of digoxin immune fab is limited to life-threatening overdoses in clients who have severe cardiovascular disruption (shock, cardiac arrest, severe ventricular arrhythmias, progressive bradycardia) or serum potassium exceeding 5 mEq/L.

Dosage and Administration. The dose of digoxin immune fab is computed according to the amount of digoxin taken or drug serum levels. Usually a 40-mg dose of digoxin immune fab binds about 0.6 mg of digoxin or digitoxin. In clinical testing, average doses were in the range of 120 to 400 mg. The drug is marketed in vials containing 40 mg and costs about $245 per vial.

Digoxin immune fab is administered intravenously (IV) either by bolus or by infusion over a 30-minute period. It should be infused through a 0.22-μm membrane filter.

Adverse Reactions. Experience with this antidote is limited, and few adverse reactions have been reported. The use of this antidote is likely to withdraw all digoxin from the client's system and precipitate the cardiac malfunctions for which the cardiac glycoside was originally prescribed. For this reason, its use is likely to be followed by low cardiac output, CHF, and atrial tachycardia. Hypokalemia may also develop.

Precautions and Contraindications. Because it is an animal product, digoxin immune fab has the potential to cause allergic reactions. Clients at risk for allergic reaction to this drug (those with allergy to sheep protein or wool and those who have previously received digoxin immune fab) should undergo skin testing before receiving the drug. Skin testing is not recommended as a routine procedure for all clients, however, because it delays treatment.

If possible, serum digoxin concentrations should be measured before the antidote is given. Potassium levels should be monitored carefully for several hours after giving the drug.

■ SUMMARY

Digoxin immune fab is an antidote used for severe cardiac glycoside toxicity. The client requires careful monitoring throughout antidote therapy to prevent cardiac malfunction.

❖ NURSING MANAGEMENT: CLIENT RECEIVING DIGOXIN IMMUNE FAB

A client diagnosed with digitalis toxicity should be hospitalized for immediate treatment. The hospital setting is important because it has facilities for cardiac monitoring and emergency treatment. In addition, the digoxin immune fab must be given IV.

NURSING PROCESS

ASSESSMENT

Required assessment data include signs and symptoms of digitalis toxicity, a complete drug history, and laboratory data defining electrolyte values (see Example of Nursing Process for Digoxin Toxicity). Serum drug level measurements are also helpful. Plasma concentrations between 0.5 and 2.0 mg/mL for digoxin and between 10 and 35 mg/mL for digitoxin are considered therapeutic. A definitive diagnosis can be made from an ECG exhibiting a prolonged P-R interval, a short Q-T interval, and abnormal P waves.

NURSING DIAGNOSIS

Nursing diagnoses related to toxicity from cardiac glycosides include:

- Risk for Injury, related to digoxin toxicity
- Altered Nutrition: Less than Body Requirements, related to drug-induced anorexia, nausea, or diarrhea
- Fluid Volume Deficit, related to increased loss secondary to vomiting and diarrhea
- Visual Sensory/Perceptual Alterations: Drug-induced disturbance in yellow and green color perception
- Knowledge Deficit, related to antidote therapy

PLANNING

Goals of nursing care are to prevent cardiac arrest by controlling arrhythmias, to detect and treat cardiac arrest should it occur, to improve nutritional status, to correct fluid deficits, and to provide information about toxicity management.

INTERVENTION

The medical treatment of acute cardiac glycoside toxicity requires 1) immediate suspension of glycoside administration and 2) general supportive measures to promote metabolism or excretion of the drug, or both. Cardiac monitoring is necessary. Antiarrhythmic drugs and potassium may be required. Therapy carries a risk of serious complications because overmedication with antiarrhythmics and parenteral potassium may further disrupt heart function and cause cardiac arrest. Digoxin immune fab may be used in severe cases. Nurses may be responsible for administering IV bolus medication (in accordance with established protocols), as well as infusions.

Healthcare staff must be prepared to initiate cardiopulmonary resuscitation should cardiac arrest occur. Clients receiving digoxin immune fab should be monitored closely for allergic reactions to the antidote, hypokalemia, and recurring symptoms of cardiac failure.

Nursing measures to alleviate discomfort from GI disturbances (nausea, vomiting, and diarrhea) should be instituted. Food and fluids should be withheld if nausea is apparent. When tolerated, warm tea or ginger ale helps relieve nausea. Medications may be ordered to control nausea or diarrhea. As the client improves, juices and foods rich in potassium should be offered. IV potassium is relatively dangerous because it can rapidly raise blood potassium levels to toxic levels. However, it cannot be discontinued until the client can ingest adequate potassium, either in food or as a supplement. Because hypokalemia is usually accompanied by hypochloremia, potassium chloride is usually the supplement of choice. Potassium citrate, potassium bicarbonate, or potassium gluconate may be used, but only if the client's chloride level is normal. The nurse can help the client adhere to the potassium supplement regimen by determining the form most agreeable to the client. Preparations that must be diluted can be diluted in any beverage the client chooses, from water to coffee to juice, which should be sipped slowly during or after a meal. To avoid excess carbonation, effervescent preparations should be ingested only after bubbling subsides. The client taking a potassium supplement must be monitored for GI symptoms, as these supplements can cause GI irritation and ulceration.

If visual changes disturb the client, abnormal perceptions may be diminished or masked by manipulating environmental stimuli. If the client's color vision is disturbed, visual stimuli should be minimized and pleasant stimuli provided to the other senses. Backrubs provide tactile stimulation, and the client may enjoy listening to music.

Example of Nursing Process for Digoxin Toxicity

The client is a 62-year-old retired waitress who has been under treatment for chronic congestive heart failure for a year and a half. She has been admitted to an acute care facility with complaints of nausea, vomiting, and diarrhea since the previous day. She thinks she may have "picked up a stomach bug" but is concerned because her pulse is irregular and she has occasional periods of palpitations.

On admission, her vital signs are temperature 37.5°C (98°F), radial pulse 60/min, apical pulse 104/min, respirations 22/min, and BP 112/86. Tissue turgor is poor, as evidenced by tenting when skin is pinched. Mucous membranes appear dry. The client is being maintained at home with digoxin, and hydrochlorothiazide 50 mg/day.

The client is transferred to the coronary care unit, where a printout from her cardiac monitor shows a short Q-T interval and prolonged P wave. A diagnosis of digoxin toxicity is made.

Results of blood tests show a potassium level of 3.4 mEq/L and a plasma digoxin level of 2.4 ng/mL. An IV infusion of 1,000 mL of D_5W with 40 mEq potassium is ordered to run at a rate of 125 mL/hr.

Assessment Data

Nausea, vomiting, diarrhea

BP 112/86

Tenting of skin

Vomiting and diarrhea

Serum potassium 3.4 mEq/L

Plasma digoxin level 2.4 ng/mL

Client's lack of awareness of the nature of her illness

Nursing Diagnosis	Intervention	Goals and Outcomes
Fluid Volume Deficit, related to increased loss from the intestinal tract due to vomiting and diarrhea secondary to digoxin toxicity	**Administer** IV fluids as ordered; control the rate of flow with an infusion-control device.	Within 24 hours, tissue turgor will improve as shown by decreased or absent tenting on pinching of the skin.
	Keep an accurate record of fluid intake and output.	Systolic blood pressure will rise above 120 mm Hg.
Risk for Decreased Cardiac Output, related to cardiac arrhythmias secondary to digoxin toxicity	**Monitor** client for ECG changes characteristic of digitalis toxicity.	Ventricular flutter or fibrillation will not occur; if one does occur, circulation will be promptly restored by cardiopulmonary resuscitation.
	Initiate cardiopulmonary resuscitation if warranted.	
	Offer client clear fluids that help correct nausea, such as ginger ale or tea.	Serum potassium level will increase to normal range.
	When nausea subsides, **offer** the client foods rich in potassium.	The client will report that she no longer feels nauseated.
Knowledge Deficit concerning the drug regimen used to treat congestive heart failure	**Coach** client through procedures necessary for immediate care.	The client will actively collaborate in the treatment regimen.
	Prepare a teaching plan about cardiac failure and the drug regimen used to treat it; postpone teaching until current crisis is resolved.	The client will not experience a recurrence of serious digitalis toxicity.

Recovery is relatively rapid when the cardiac glycoside involved has a short half-life, provided renal function is adequate. Digitoxin, which is metabolized by the liver, is more slowly eliminated from the body.

When clients recover from the acute phase of illness, the source of the imbalance must be identified. The nurse should explore with clients their self-medication practices. Drug containers from the client's home can be examined to determine if the proper drugs and doses are available. If the client's prescription medications have changed, a review of current dosage instructions may help; the client may misunderstand the regimen or may be taking both old and new medications. A complete review of drug use—prescription and nonprescription—is necessary to identify drug interactions that may have contributed to the toxic reaction.

Factors that affect electrolyte balance must also be investigated. A potassium-poor diet, a temporary digestive upset, unusual stress, or acid–base imbalance may deplete body potassium. Hypercalcemia and hypomagnesemia potentiate the effects of digitalis and may precipitate toxicity (eg, the softening of drinking water reduces magnesium intake). Changes in electrolyte levels can cause toxicity despite a constant serum concentration of drug.

Client Education. Once the factors contributing to toxicity are identified and the medical emergency is resolved, the nurse can teach the client strategies to avoid recurrence. Preventive measures include careful attention to diet, correction of medication errors, and control or better management of stress. The client should be cautioned to seek early medical attention for changes in health status.

OUTCOME EVALUATION

Data required for evaluation include the absence of cardiac arrest, the correction of cardiac arrhythmias should they occur, laboratory data indicating normal potassium levels and drug serum levels below the toxic range, alleviation or elimination of signs of toxicity, and statements by clients that they feel better and that any visual disturbances have subsided (see Example of Nursing Process for Digoxin Toxicity).

Other Drugs for Managing Heart Failure

Mortality in heart failure remains high. Until recently, heart failure was considered a mechanical disorder, and treatment focused on achieving hemodynamic goals. Now we know that the development and progression of heart failure depend on the interrelation of hemodynamic and neurohormonal factors. Primary pathophysiologic features of heart failure include increased ventricular wall stress and increased neurohormonal activity. The three factors that contribute to increased ventricular wall stress are sodium retention (managed with diuretics), peripheral vasoconstriction (managed with direct-acting vasodilators), and reduced myocardial contractility (managed with positive inotropic agents) (Packer, 1992). Diuretics are discussed in detail in Chapter 27 and vasodilators in Chapter 24, but their role in CHF is outlined briefly here.

As research on heart failure continues, additional pharmacologic choices will become available. One example is flosequinan, a vasodilator that acts on arteries and veins and reduces sympathetic outflow to the heart. Another example is pimobendan, a phosphodiesterase inhibitor that enhances myocardial contractility by increasing the sensitivity of myofilaments to calcium. Vesnarinone is a phosphodiesterase inhibitor that increases the delivery of calcium to myofilaments by enhancing sodium influx into cells. It slows heart rate and has an antiarrhythmic effect. Bucindolol, a new beta blocker, dilates peripheral blood vessels directly; carvedilol, another beta blocker, dilates peripheral vessels by antagonistic action on alpha-adrenergic receptors (Parker, 1992). Drugs that interfere with the activity of renin (renin inhibitors) or with the interaction of angiotensin II and its receptor (angiotensin antagonists) are also being developed.

Drugs That Reduce Ventricular Wall Stress
Diuretics
The goals of diuretic therapy in heart failure are to relieve peripheral edema and pulmonary congestion, to reduce preload, and to normalize cardiac filling pressures (Wright, 1995). Diuretics alleviate the sodium retention characteristic of heart failure by inhibiting sodium and chloride reabsorption at specific sites in the renal tubules. Diuretics act on the distal tubules (thiazides and potassium-sparing diuretics) or on the loop of Henle (loop diuretics). Distal tubule diuretics modestly increase sodium excretion. However, they lose their effectiveness when renal function is impaired (eg, when the glomerular filtration rate falls below 30 mL/min). Loop diuretics increase sodium excretion to a greater degree. They retain their effectiveness until the glomerular filtration rate falls below 5 mL/min.

Loop diuretics have some vasodilating properties, enabling them to increase venous capacitance and reduce preload. Loop diuretics and thiazide diuretics may be combined. Potassium-sparing diuretics may be used when potassium conservation is desired.

Diuretics alone cannot maintain the stability of clients with heart failure. In addition, diuretic use is associated with a high risk of electrolyte depletion (potassium and magnesium) that may predispose the client to the development of dangerous arrhythmias. In time, other types of diuretics (eg, the experimental atriopeptidase inhibitors) may be available that have more favorable effects on the neurohormonal component of CHF.

Vasodilators
Vasodilators can alleviate peripheral vasoconstriction in heart failure by directly relaxing vascular smooth muscle at specific sites in the peripheral circulation. Three classes of direct-acting vasodilators have been developed: those that act mainly on peripheral veins (eg, nitrates, molsidomine), those that act mainly on peripheral arteries (eg, hydralazine, minoxidil, calcium channel blockers), and those with combined actions on both arteries and veins (eg, flosequinan) (Packer, 1992). The goals of vasodilator therapy are to relieve symptoms, improve cardiac filling pressures, and decrease arterial impedance (Wright, 1995).

Nitrates, such as isosorbide dinitrate, are venodilators; in high doses they dilate arterioles. They have been especially helpful in clients with heart failure related to ischemic heart disease. Although they exhibit favorable hemodynamic effects on a short-term basis, they seem to have limited long-term efficacy. The lack of efficacy has been attributed to tolerance to the vasodilator effects during long-term use.

Some direct-acting vasodilators (eg, calcium channel blockers) have negative inotropic effects. In controlled trials, clients treated with calcium channel blockers (verapamil, nifedipine, and diltiazem) were at higher risk of worsening heart failure with death than clients not using these drugs. Initially, the reduction in arterial resistance that occurs produces favorable hemodynamic effects, but these are usually negated over time by a reflex stimulation of the renin–angiotensin–aldosterone mechanism and the sympathetic nervous system.

New calcium antagonists that decrease rather than increase sympathetic nervous system activity (eg, amlodipine, felodipine) are being evaluated for long-term effects (Packer, 1992).

Hydralazine is an arterial smooth muscle relaxant that reduces systemic vascular resistance. Treatment with this agent reduces afterload and interrupts the vicious cycle of heart failure. However, study findings fail to demonstrate any long-term benefits with hydralazine alone. Some studies of therapy combining hydralazine and isosorbide dinitrate indicate that this combination may reduce mortality, but the use of the combination is limited by frequent side effects (Wright, 1995).

Other Positive Inotropic Agents

Positive inotropic drugs reduce wall stress by augmenting the contractility of the failing heart. Digitalis-type drugs have been the focus of this chapter's discussion, but other positive inotropic agents may be used.

In the myocardium, c-AMP is the second messenger that modifies intracellular calcium and the events of myocardial contraction. Intracellular levels of c-AMP are low in a failing heart. Drugs have been developed that enhance cardiac contractility by increasing the concentration of intracellular c-AMP. This can be done by augmenting its synthesis (using beta-adrenergic agonists) or by inhibiting its degradation (using phosphodiesterase inhibitors). The c-AMP–dependent agents dilate peripheral blood vessels as well as enhancing contractile force so that they produce a greater reduction in wall stress than digitalis-type drugs.

Dopamine and dobutamine are the most extensively studied beta-adrenergic agonists in heart failure. Short-term parenteral therapy with these agents in acute decompensatory heart failure has produced short-term improvement in symptoms and hemodynamic parameters. Again, however, long-term treatment with this type of drug is associated with increases in cardiovascular morbidity and mortality.

Phosphodiesterase inhibitors prevent the breakdown of c-AMP by inhibiting phosphodiesterase. The subsequent increase in c-AMP leads to increased myocardial contractility and peripheral vasodilatation. This action is similar to the action of methylxanthines (eg, theophylline), but the drugs being studied in relation to heart failure are more cardioselective. Two groups of drugs being studied are bipyridine derivatives (amrinone and milrinone) and imidazole derivatives (enoximone and piroximone).

Amrinone (Inocor) has both inotropic and vasodilator properties. Its full mechanism of action is unknown, but it reduces preload and afterload, increases myocardial contractility, and increases resting cardiac output. Amrinone therapy usually involves a dosage of 0.75 mg/kg given by slow IV injection over a period of 2 to 3 minutes. Amrinone cannot be diluted in any solution containing dextrose and cannot be infused into IV lines containing furosemide. Monitoring cardiac output, pulmonary capillary wedge pressure, and central venous pressure helps evaluate response. The initial dose is followed by a maintenance infusion of 5 to 10 g/kg/min with additional bolus injections after 30 minutes, if needed. The total dose should not exceed 10 mg/kg/day.

Amrinone has a half-life of 3.6 to 7.5 hours. It is metabolized by the liver and excreted by the kidneys (about 63%) and feces (about 18%). Amrinone is associated with a high incidence of adverse effects (eg, GI symptoms, arrhythmias, dose-dependent but asymptomatic thrombocytopenia, hypersensitivity reactions). It must not be administered concurrently with disopyramide because severe hypotension has occurred.

Milrinone (Primacor) is about 20 times as potent as amrinone and does not cause thrombocytopenia. Adverse reactions include arrhythmias and hypotension. Like amrinone, milrinone interacts with disopyramide. It is incompatible with furosemide and procainamide.

Some think that the reduction in c-AMP levels associated with heart failure may be an adaptive response for myocardial preservation. In addition, mortality statistics in various studies have led some to think that pharmacologically induced elevations of c-AMP may accelerate disease progression or induce ventricular arrhythmias (Wright, 1995).

Drugs That Reduce Neurohormonal Activity
Angiotensin-Converting Enzyme Inhibitors

Angiotensin-converting enzyme (ACE) inhibitors have favorable hemodynamic and neurohormonal effects in heart failure and after acute myocardial injury. In heart failure, ACE inhibitors, such as captopril (Capoten) and enalapril (Vasotec), are smooth muscle vasodilators that improve peripheral circulation and decrease afterload and, therefore, left ventricular filling pressure. They thereby increase cardiac output and exercise tolerance.

From a hemodynamic aspect, ACE inhibitors decrease the progressive left ventricular dysfunction that develops after acute myocardial injury. In some studies, ACE inhibitors were associated with a reduced incidence of recurrent myocardial infarction. From a neurohormonal aspect, they reduce the direct toxic effects of angiotensin on myocardial cells that may lead to cell necrosis and disease progression (Packer, 1992). For more information, see Chapter 25.

Beta-Adrenergic Antagonists

Because an elevated plasma norepinephrine level and impaired beta-receptor function are associated with heart failure, it has been proposed that beta-adrenergic antagonist therapy may improve response to circulating catecholamines and have other positive effects in clients with heart failure. Beta-adrenergic antagonists, such as metoprolol (Lopressor) and propranolol (Inderal), have indeed had favorable effects in clients with myocardial infarction complicated by heart failure. However, the negative effects of beta-adrenergic antagonists on myocardial contractility, heart rate, and conduction may exacerbate the symptoms of heart failure in certain clients.

◼ SUMMARY

Drugs can produce favorable hemodynamic effects by reducing ventricular wall stress, but benefits are not likely to be sustained if these agents activate endogenous neurohormonal systems. Similarly, drugs can exert beneficial neurohormonal actions by antagonizing the effects of either the sympathetic nervous system or the renin–angiotensin mechanism, but these drugs are unlikely to be well tolerated if they also depress cardiac function. Ideally, therapeutic management in CHF should produce favorable effects on both hemodynamic and neurohormonal systems.

References

Abernethy DR, Andrawis NS. (1993). Critical drug interactions: A guide to important examples. *Drug Ther, 10,* 15.

Garg R, Packer M, Pitt B, et al. (1993). Heart failure in the 1990s: Evolution of a major public health problem in cardiovascular medicine. *J Am Coll Cardiol, 22*(4), suppl. A, 3A–5A.

Meissner JE, Gever LN. (1993). Reducing the risks of digitalis toxicity. *Nursing '93, 7,* 47–51.

Packer M. (1992). Pathophysiology of chronic heart failure. *Lancet, 340*(July 11), 88–92.

Packer M. (1992). Treatment of chronic heart failure. *Lancet, 340*(July 11), 92–95.

Poole-Wilson P. (1994). Cardiac glycosides: Impact on mortality. In Singh BN, Dzau VJ, Vanhoutte PM, Woosley RL, eds. *Cardiovascular pharmacology and therapeutics.* New York: Churchill-Livingstone.

Rajfer SI. (1993). Perspective of the pharmaceutical industry on the development of new drugs for heart failure. *J Am Coll Cardiol, 22*(4), suppl. A, 198A–200A.

Wright JM. (1995). Pharmacologic management of congestive heart failure. *Crit Care Nurs Q, 18*(1), 32–44.

Bibliography

Banasik JL. (1994). Endothelins: New players in cardiovascular physiology and disease. *J Cardiovasc Nurs, 8*(3), 87–104.

Brandt RR, Wright S, Redfield MMet al. (1993). Atrial natriuretic peptide in heart failure. *J Am Coll Cardiol, 22,* suppl. A., 86A–92A.

Braunwald E, ed. (1992). *Heart disease: A textbook of cardiovascular medicine,* 4th ed. Philadelphia: WB Saunders.

Cohen AF, Kroon R, Schoemaker R, et al. (1991). Influence of gastric acidity on the bioavailability of digoxin. *Ann Intern Med, 115*(7), 540–545.

Dietz R, Waas W, Süsselbeck T, et al. (1993). Improvement of cardiac function by angiotensin-converting enzyme inhibition. *Circulation, 87,* suppl. IV, IV108–IV116.

Ferguson DW. (1993). Sympathetic mechanisms in heart failure: Pathophysiological and pharmacological implications. *Circulation, 87,* suppl. VII, VII68–VII75.

Hardman JG, Limbird LE, Molinoff PB, et al. (eds.) (1996). *Goodman and Gilman's The pharmacological basis of therapeutics,* 9th ed. New York: McGraw-Hill.

Kegel LM. (1995). Advanced practice nurses can refine the management of heart failure. *Clinical Nurse Specialist, 9*(2), 76–81.

Morton MR, Cooper JW. (1989). Erythromycin-induced digoxin toxicity. *DICP, Ann Pharmacother, 23*(9), 668–670.

Olin BR, ed. (1995). *Drug facts and comparisons,* 49th ed. St. Louis: Facts and Comparisons.

Pouleur H, Rousseau MF, Van Eyll C, et al. (1993). Cardiac mechanics during development of heart failure. *Circulation, 87,* suppl. IV, IV14–IV20.

Pratt NG. (1993). Neurohormonal response to ventricular failure: Pharmacologic management. *J Cardiovasc Nurs, 8*(1), 49–62.

Singh BN, Dzau VJ, Vanhoutte PM, Woosley RL, (eds.) (1994). *Cardiovascular pharmacology and therapeutics.* New York: Churchill- Livingstone.

Vander AJ, Sherman JH, Luciano DS. (1994). *Human physiology,* 6th ed. New York: McGraw-Hill.

Withering W. (1977). *An account of the foxglove and some of its uses: With practical remarks on dropsy and other diseases.* (Reprint of 1785 edition.) Wakefield, NH: Longwood Publishing Group.

For more information and sample tests and activities, refer to Chapter 21 in the Student Workbook for Clinical Pharmacology and Nursing Management, 5th edition, available through your bookstore.

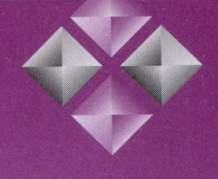

22

Drugs That Regulate Cardiac Rhythm

Cardiac arrhythmias, also known as cardiac dysrhythmias, are disturbances in the normal rhythm of the heartbeat. Such abnormalities of heart function disrupt normal cardiac output and predispose to congestive heart failure and sudden cardiac death. Sudden cardiac death accounts for more than 450,000 deaths each year in the United States (Dunnington, 1993). It represents the most extreme case of hemodynamic compromise resulting from a cardiac arrhythmia (Carrieri-Kohlman et al., 1993). Primary ventricular fibrillation is the most frequent arrhythmia underlying this event, although some deaths may be preceded by organized ventricular tachycardia.

Antiarrhythmic drugs were developed to help correct abnormal patterns of contraction or marked increases or decreases in the heart rate. Although positive chronotropic agents, such as atropine, epinephrine, and isoproterenol, are occasionally administered to correct bradycardia, drugs commonly used as antiarrhythmics are all myocardial depressants. They may be grouped into four classes according to their mechanism of action (Table 22-1). Within each class, individual drugs differ, as do their therapeutic effectiveness in any client. If a therapeutic response is not achieved with one drug, the client may respond to another in the same class.

All antiarrhythmic drugs have the potential to worsen arrhythmias or to cause new ones. Around-the-clock monitoring of the client's electrocardiogram (ECG) is usually needed when the client begins antiarrhythmic therapy or when the antiarrhythmic drug is changed.

Pathophysiology of Abnormal Cardiac Rhythms

A normal heartbeat is initiated in the sinoatrial node and follows a consistent pathway of depolarization through the atria, atrioventricular (AV) node, His-Purkinje system, and finally the ventricular myocardium. Electrical depolarization of the heart is normally followed by atrial and then ventricular contraction. Rhythm disturbances may be categorized in many ways: by origin (atrial, junctional, ventricular), by rate (tachyarrhythmias, bradyarrhythmias), and by chronicity (acute, chronic). Arrhythmias occur because of abnormalities in the initiation or conduction (or both) of the cardiac impulse. Disturbances in impulse formation include depressed sinus node automaticity, enhanced automaticity, abnormal automaticity, or triggered automaticity. Disturbances in impulse propagation include conduction blocks and reentry arrhythmia. There are also mixed disturbances of impulse propagation and conduction (Table 22-2).

Causes of arrhythmias include ischemic heart disease, congestive heart failure, infections, structural lesions of the heart, trauma, electrolyte imbalance, and drugs. Tachyarrhythmias (tachycardia associated with an irregular heart rhythm) may affect the atria or the ventricles, may be constant or paroxysmal, and may range from 100 beats per minute (bpm) to flutter or fibrillation that is too rapid to count. Moderate tachycardia can occur naturally as the result of fever or sympathetic nerve stimulation. Other causes include stimulant drugs (eg, caffeine, nicotine, amphetamines), myocardial inflammation (eg, after infarction), or myocardial irritability (eg, during ischemia).

Flutter and fibrillation are characterized by very rapid, uncoordinated contractions of the myocardium. The frequency of contraction in flutter is lower than in fibrillation. Atrial flutter or fibrillation reduces cardiac output but is generally not an emergency. Ventricular fibrillation is incompatible with life and requires immediate intervention to sustain perfusion of body tissues. When the AV node is bombarded by rapid impulses from the atria, it cannot respond to all the impulses, and ventricular response may be regular or irregular and usually occurs at a fractional rate (eg, the ventricles may respond to half of the stimuli).

Table 22-1. Classifying Disturbances in Cardiac Rhythm

Kind of Disturbance	Examples
Disturbances in Impulse Formation	
Depressed sinus node automaticity	Sinus bradycardia
	Sinus arrhythmia
	Wandering pacemaker
	Sinus pauses or arrest
Enhanced automaticity	Escape beats or rhythms (atrial, AV junctional, ventricular)
	Premature atrial, junctional, or ventricular beats
	Ectopic supraventricular tachycardias (paroxysmal or nonparoxysmal)
	Paroxysmal ventricular tachycardias
	Parasystolic rhythms
Abnormal automaticity	Late ischemic ectopy (postmyocardial infarction)
	Late ischemic tachyarrhythmias
Triggered automaticity	Early after-depolarizations, such as ventricular ectopy or torsades de pointes
	Delayed after-depolarizations; for example, digitalis-induced ventricular arrhythmias or exercise-induced ventricular arrhythmias
Disturbances in Impulse Propagation	
Conduction blocks	Sinoatrial block
	Intra-atrial blocks
	AV blocks, including first-degree, second-degree (Mobitz I, known as Wenkebach, and Mobitz II)
	High-degree or advanced AV block
	Third-degree or complete AV block
Reentry arrhythmias	Paroxysmal supraventricular tachycardias (AV nodal reentrant tachycardia; atypical AV nodal reentrant tachycardia; orthodromic AV reciprocating tachycardia; antidromic AV reciprocating tachycardia; nodoventricular bypass tract)
	Circus movement tachycardias (atrial flutter or fibrillation, ventricular flutter or fibrillation)
	Atrial, junctional, and ventricular extrasystoles
	Ventricular tachycardia
Mixed Disturbances of Impulse Conduction and Propagation	
	AV dissociation
	Wolff-Parkinson-White syndrome
	Electrical alterans
	Lown-Ganong-Levine syndrome

Table 22-2. Classification of Antiarrhythmic Drugs

Class	Mechanism of Action	Examples
I	Sodium channel blockade	
IA	Moderate depression of sodium influx during depolarization; prolonged repolarization	quinidine, procainamide, disopyramide
IB	Minimal depression of sodium influx during depolarization; shortened repolarization	lidocaine, mexiletine, phenytoin, tocainide
IC	Marked depression of sodium influx during depolarization; little effect on repolarization	flecainide, propafenone
Other		moricizine
II	Beta-adrenergic blockade	acebutol, esmolol, propranolol, sotalol
III	Prolonged repolarization	amiodarone, bretylium, sotalol
IV	Calcium channel blockade	verapamil
Other	Slow atrioventricular node conduction	adenosine

Ventricular arrhythmias such as tachycardia and fibrillation are life-threatening. Torsades de pointes (French for "twisting of the points") is polymorphic ventricular tachycardia that occurs in the setting of a lengthened Q-T interval, reflecting prolonged cardiac repolarization (Makkar et al., 1993). This arrhythmia may cause syncope or may even precipitate ventricular fibrillation and cardiac arrest. Although some persons may be prone to this arrhythmia because of a congenital abnormality of cardiac repolarization, the arrhythmia is more commonly an acquired disorder resulting from electrolyte abnormalities or administration of drugs that prolong the Q-T interval. Drugs discussed in this chapter that may cause torsades de pointes include quinidine, procainamide, disopyramide, amiodarone, and sotalol.

Bradyarrhythmias also may affect the atria or the ventricles. Except in athletes (whose stroke volume output is large), rates lower than 60 bpm are considered abnormal. Diseases characterized by bradycardia include carotid sinus syndrome, in which the carotid sinus is unusually sensitive to pressure (as a result of arteriosclerosis), and Stokes-Adams syndrome, in which the atrial impulse does not reach the ventricles, which then beat at their own, slower, intrinsic rhythm.

Irregular heartbeats may arise from irritable (ectopic) foci in the myocardium or blocks in impulse transmission. These foci produce extrasystoles, or premature atrial or ventricular beats. Sometimes ectopic foci generate impulses fast enough to capture control from the sinoatrial node and dictate the rhythm of cardiac contraction. At other times, they generate extra beats out of synchrony with the basic rhythm of the heart. Blocks in impulse conduction also cause rhythm irregularities. They may occur when part of the cardiac muscle is depressed by biochemical abnormalities or nonfunctional due to necrosis or scarring. Blocks tend to deflect impulses, causing them to follow abnormal pathways. Circuitous impulses are more likely to develop in enlarged hearts in which the conduction of impulses through the myocardium is prolonged.

Cardiac arrest is the cessation of all heart contraction. The underlying cause is usually hypoxia.

Some arrhythmias respond well to mechanical or physical treatment. Cardiac massage may be effective in maintaining circulation when heart function is inadequate to sustain life. Electric shock is used to abolish the chaotic impulses of fibrillation. After defibrillation (or cardioversion, as the procedure is termed when used to correct atrial fibrillation), the heart is temporarily refractory to all stimuli. On recovery, the heart usually resumes normal impulse conduction. Conduction deficiencies (heart block) may be controlled by pacemaker devices that deliver periodic electrical stimuli to the ventricles. Automatic internal cardiac defibrillators are needed in other situations. However, antiarrhythmic drugs are usually needed and are helpful for managing arrhythmias.

Class I Drugs: Sodium Channel Blocking Agents

Drugs of this class include several local anesthetic-type antiarrhythmic drugs (lidocaine, procainamide), an isomer of quinine (quinidine), and an anticonvulsant (phenytoin). These are called membrane-stabilizing agents. Class I antiarrhythmics are further categorized into four subclasses: IA, IB, IC, and others.

Class IA Drugs

Class IA drugs include quinidine, procainamide, and disopyramide (Table 22-3). An investigational agent in this class is cifenline (Cipralan).

Quinidine

Quinidine (Duraquin, Quinaglute), one of the first drugs observed to have antiarrhythmic activity, is structured much like quinine. In fact, the natural source of quinidine and quinine is the bark of the South American cinchona tree (cinchona alkaloids). Quinine is used for its antimalarial effects.

Pharmacodynamics. Quinidine depresses myocardial excitability, conduction velocity, and contractility. It blocks the fast sodium channel in the myocardial membrane, thereby slowing the rate of the rise of the action potential and prolonging the effective refractory period. In addition, it exerts an indirect anticholinergic effect (decreases vagal tone).

Pharmacokinetics. There are three quinidine salts: quinidine sulfate, quinidine gluconate, and quinidine polygalacturonate. They have differences in active drug content, quinidine absorption, and time to peak plasma level.

Quinidine is rapidly and well absorbed (70%–73%) from the gastrointestinal (GI) tract after oral administration. Peak plasma concentrations are achieved for quinidine gluconate in 3 to 5 hours and for quinidine sulfate in 1 to 3 hours. Quinidine is extensively bound to plasma proteins, with 10% to 20% of the dose free in the circulation. It is metabolized extensively in the body, primarily by the liver, with several metabolites. Whether these metabolites have antiarrhythmic activity remains controversial. In hepatic insufficiency, the unbound fraction may be significantly increased; in clients with cirrhosis, the elimination half-life may be prolonged. The effect of renal dysfunction on quinidine disposition remains controversial as well (Olin, 1995). Urinary acidification facilitates quinidine elimination and alkalinization retards it. Average therapeutic serum levels are reportedly 2 to 7 µg/mL, with toxic reactions occurring at 5 to 8 µg/mL or greater.

Therapeutic Uses. Quinidine is used to treat premature atrial, AV junctional, and ventricular contractions, paroxysmal atrial (supraventricular) tachycardia, paroxysmal AV junctional rhythm, atrial flutter, paroxysmal

Table 22-3. Antiarrhythmic Drugs: Class IA

Drug Name	Dosage Forms	Usual Dosage	Adverse Reactions
disopyramide (Norpace)	Oral capsules, extended-release capsules	Adults: conventional tablets: 150 mg q6h; extended-release capsules: 300 mg q12h PC: C	Blurred vision, dry mouth, nose, eyes, constipation, urinary hesitancy and retention, cardiogenic shock, heart block, torsades de pointes, respiratory difficulty/laryngospasm
procainamide (Procan SR, Pronestyl, Procanbid)	Oral capsules, tablets, sustained-release tablets; extended-release tablets; IM; IV	Adults: 50 mg/kg/day or 250–625 mg q3h (capsules/tablets) or 500 mg–1.25 g q6h (sustained-release tablets); IV by loading infusion of 1 g diluted to 50 mL at rate of 1 mL/min for 25–30 min or by direct injection at 50 mg/min to total of 500 mg PC: C	Lupus-like syndrome, ventricular fibrillation, torsades de pointes, agranulocytosis
quinidine sulfate (Quinora, Quinidex Extentabs)	Oral tablets, sustained-release tablets	Adults: 200–300 mg 3 or 4 times/day (tablets); 300–600 mg q8–12 h (sustained-release tablets); Children: 30 mg/kg/24 h in 5 divided doses PC: C	Nausea, vomiting, diarrhea, abnormal pain, widened QRS complex, heart block, ventricular flutter, ventricular fibrillation, torsades de pointes, acute hemolytic anemia, agranulocytosis, respiratory depression, vascular collapse, cinchonism

KEY: PC = pregnancy risk category (see Appendix A).

and chronic atrial fibrillation, and paroxysmal ventricular tachycardia not associated with complete heart block. It is used for maintenance therapy after electrical conversion of atrial fibrillation or flutter.

Dosage and Administration. The quinidine content varies depending on the form—sulfate, gluconate, or polygalacturonate. Therefore, these drug forms cannot be considered interchangeable, and dosage adjustment is likely if one form is substituted for another. The usual dosage depends on the particular quinidine preparation and its dosage form (extended-release form or regular). A typical dose for an extended-release form is 300 to 600 mg every 8 or 12 hours.

The effective dosage varies widely due to several factors, including the arrhythmia being treated. Clients with rapid elimination, often resulting from concomitant administration of metabolic inducers, may require a higher dosage. If the drugs that induce hepatic metabolism are discontinued, the quinidine dosage may need to be reduced.

Quinidine may be given parenterally if the client is being closely monitored to detect any change in cardiac rate or rhythm.

Before therapy to alleviate atrial flutter or fibrillation is initiated, anticoagulants may be administered to reduce the risk of thrombotic complications.

Adverse Reactions. The most common adverse effects associated with quinidine include nausea, vomiting, diarrhea, and abdominal pain. Life-threatening adverse reactions include widened QRS complex, heart block, ventricular flutter, ventricular fibrillation, torsades de pointes, acute hemolytic anemia, agranulocytosis, respiratory depression, and vascular collapse.

Cinchonism is an adverse effect characterized by tinnitus, hearing loss, headache, nausea, dizziness, vertigo, lightheadedness, and disturbed vision. This complex of side effects can occur after a single dose of quinidine.

The effect of quinidine is enhanced by potassium and reduced with hypokalemia. The risk of drug-induced torsades de pointes is increased by concomitant hypokalemia.

Drug–Drug Interactions. When quinidine is coadministered with digoxin, two different interaction mechanisms occur by which the serum digoxin concentration nearly doubles (Abernathy & Andrawis, 1993). Quinidine metabolism is inhibited by cimetidine and induced by phenytoin, phenobarbital, and rifampin; the latter agents lead to subtherapeutic quinidine concentrations. Potassium enhances the effect of quinidine. Other substances that interact with quinidine include amiodarone, antacids, nifedipine, sucralfate, verapamil, anticoagulants, beta blockers, disopyramide, procainamide, propafenone, and tricyclic antidepressants.

Drug–Laboratory Test Interactions. Triamterene interferes with the fluorescent measurement of quinidine serum levels.

Precautions and Contraindications. Quinidine often must be used cautiously in clients with renal disease, heart failure, or hepatic insufficiency. It is contraindicated during pregnancy and lactation and in clients with an allergy to the drug, second- or third-degree heart block, or myasthenia gravis.

Procainamide

Procainamide (Procan SR, Pronestyl) may be prescribed for several common arrhythmias.

Pharmacodynamics. Procainamide increases the effective refractory period of the atria and, to a lesser extent, the bundle of His-Purkinje system and ventricles of the heart. Procainamide depresses myocardial excitability. Its vagal blocking action is weaker than that of quinidine, and it has less of a depressant action on cardiac contractility.

Pharmacokinetics. After procainamide is administered orally, plasma levels reach about 50% of peak in 30 minutes, 90% of peak at 60 minutes, and peak at 90 to 120 minutes. Only 15% to 20% of the drug is bound to plasma proteins.

Procainamide is metabolized extensively in the liver by the enzyme *N*-acetyltransferase to *N*-acetylprocainamide (NAPA). Acetylation of procainamide may occur predominantly as a first-pass effect after oral administration. The rate of metabolism varies widely and is under genetic control. Rapid acetylators have higher plasma concentrations of NAPA and excrete larger amounts of NAPA in urine than slow acetylators. NAPA's actions are similar to those of procainamide, although it is less potent.

The elimination half-life of procainamide is 3 to 4 hours in clients with normal renal function, but reduced creatinine clearance and advancing age each prolong the elimination half-life. Half-life and renal clearance are also reduced in infants. Both procainamide and NAPA are eliminated by active tubular secretion as well as by glomerular filtration.

Therapeutic Uses. Procainamide may be prescribed to prevent recurrence of arrhythmias after cardioversion of atrial fibrillation. It is also used to treat atrial flutter, paroxysmal atrial tachycardia, and ventricular tachycardia.

Dosage and Administration. Tablets and capsules are formulated in 250-, 375-, and 500-mg strengths. An initial daily oral dose of up to 50 mg/kg may be given in divided doses every 3 hours. For clients over age 50 or for clients with renal, hepatic, or cardiac insufficiency, lesser amounts or longer intervals are usually advised to decrease dose-related adverse effects. Extended-release products are not recommended for initial therapy. Parenteral preparations are available. The extended-release preparations (250 mg–1 g) allow dosing every 6 to 8 hours. A typical maintenance dose would be 500 mg every 6 hours.

Adverse Reactions. Some think that the incidence of adverse effects associated with long-term procainamide therapy limits its usefulness. The most common adverse reaction to procainamide is a syndrome that resembles systemic lupus erythematosus. It affects possibly 50% of clients requiring large doses of procainamide for a year or more. If the syndrome is identified, treatment with procainamide is generally discontinued because of the possibility of pleural effusion and potentially lethal pericardial tamponade. Sometimes, however, a corticosteroid preparation is added to the drug regimen to permit continued use of procainamide. Clients who are rapid acetylators seem less likely to develop the syndrome.

Life-threatening adverse reactions include ventricular fibrillation, torsades de pointes, and agranulocytosis (with repeated use). Because evidence of bone marrow dysfunction usually occurs during the first 3 months of therapy, clients are advised to have complete blood counts (including white cell, differential, and platelet counts) performed weekly during the first 3 months and periodically thereafter. If the drug must be discontinued because of evidence of bone marrow dysfunction, blood counts usually return to normal within 1 month of discontinuing procainamide. Some clinicians consider the extended-release form to be particularly responsible for these problems.

Drug–Drug Interactions. Procainamide interacts with cimetidine and ranitidine; this blocks its tubular secretion and thus increases its bioavailability. Interactions have also been reported with beta blockers, ethanol, quinidine, trimethoprim, and lidocaine.

Drug–Laboratory Test Interactions. Lidocaine, meprobamate, and propranolol may interfere with fluorescent measurement of procainamide serum levels.

Precautions and Contraindications. Procainamide must be used cautiously in clients with impaired renal or hepatic function. It should be avoided by clients who are allergic to procainamide, procaine or similar drugs, and tartrazine, because some preparations (eg, Pronestyl) contain tartrazine. It is also contraindicated during pregnancy and lactation and in clients with heart block, systemic lupus erythematosus, or torsades de pointes.

Disopyramide

Disopyramide (Norpace) is a class IA drug that is pharmacologically but not chemically similar to procainamide and quinidine.

Pharmacodynamics. Disopyramide increases the action potential duration of normal cardiac cells and prolongs the refractory period. It also decreases the disparity in refractoriness between infarcted and adjacent normally perfused myocardium.

Pharmacokinetics. Disopyramide is rapidly and almost completely absorbed from the GI tract (about 90%) after oral administration. Peak plasma concentrations occur within 2 hours after an oral dose. It is bound to plasma proteins, but binding may range from 50% to 65%, depending on plasma concentration. The therapeutic plasma level of disopyramide ranges from 2 to 4 µg/mL.

The hepatic metabolism of disopyramide is not well understood. About 50% is excreted in the urine as unchanged drug and 30% as metabolites. The plasma half-life ranges from 4 to 10 hours, with a mean of 6.7 hours. When renal function is impaired, half-life values range from 8 to 18 hours, so the dose in clients with renal failure should be decreased to avoid drug accumulation.

Therapeutic Uses. Disopyramide is used in treating ventricular arrhythmias that are life-threatening.

Dosage and Administration. The usual dosage is 150 mg three or four times a day, with a maximal dose of 800 mg/d. Dosage reduction is necessary for clients with hypotension, possible cardiac decompensation, reduced left ventricular function, or cardiomyopathy. Extended-release preparations are available.

Adverse Reactions. The most common adverse reactions associated with disopyramide include anticholinergic side effects, such as blurred vision; dry mouth, nose, and eyes; constipation; and urinary hesitancy and retention. Life-threatening adverse reactions include cardiogenic shock, heart block, torsades de pointes, and respiratory difficulty, such as laryngospasm. Another serious adverse reaction is hypotension. Disopyramide may be ineffective in clients with hypokalemia, and its toxic effects may be enhanced with hyperkalemia.

Drug Interactions. Phenytoin and rifampin induce liver metabolism of disopyramide, thereby increasing its elimination and perhaps lowering its therapeutic effect. Procainamide and lidocaine may interact with disopyramide to cause widening of the QRS complex or QT prolongation. Erythromycin may increase disopyramide plasma levels and cause arrhythmias. Concurrent use of quinidine and disopyramide may result in increased disopyramide serum levels (disopyramide toxicity) or decreased quinidine levels (decreased response to quinidine).

Precautions and Contraindications. Because of its anticholinergic effects, disopyramide may be contraindicated in clients with glaucoma or obstructive uropathy. To manage anticholinergic effects, an acetylcholinesterase inhibitor, such as physostigmine or neostigmine, might be added to the drug regimen. Disopyramide tends to have negative inotropic properties, so it may cause or aggravate congestive heart failure and should not be used in clients with uncompensated or marginally compensated congestive heart failure.

Class IB Drugs

Class IB drugs include lidocaine, mexiletine, phenytoin, and tocainide (Table 22-4).

Lidocaine

Lidocaine (Xylocaine HCl) produces no change in myocardial contractility, but it does raise the ventricular fibrillation threshold.

Pharmacodynamics. Class IB drugs have less effect on sodium influx than class IA drugs. They shorten rather than prolong repolarization, and they depress ventricular automaticity. They decrease the action potential duration and the effective refractory period.

Pharmacokinetics. Lidocaine is ineffective orally because 60% to 70% is metabolized by the liver before reaching the systemic circulation. Two of its metabolites exhibit both antiarrhythmic and convulsant properties. Less than 10% of the drug is excreted unchanged in the urine, and renal elimination plays an important role in the elimination of the metabolites. Lidocaine exhibits a biphasic half-life; a half-life of about 10 minutes explains the short duration of action following intravenous (IV) bolus administration. If infusions are given for more than 24 hours, half-life may be 3 hours or more. Lidocaine is about 50% protein bound. Therapeutic serum levels are 1.5 to 6 µg/mL; levels of more than 6 to 10 µg/mL are usually toxic.

Therapeutic Uses. Lidocaine is the drug of choice for the short-term management of serious ventricular arrhythmias (eg, after myocardial infarction and during heart surgery or cardiac catheterization).

Dosage and Administration. The initial bolus dose is usually 50 to 100 mg IV, and it may be repeated in 5 minutes. Dosage should not exceed 200 to 300 mg in 1 hour. Continuous IV infusion may be necessary to maintain antiarrhythmic effects. The usual maintenance infusion rate is 1 to 4 mg/min (20–50 µg/kg/min). Clients should be switched to oral antiarrhythmic agents as soon as possible for maintenance therapy. When used in clients who are elderly or have heart failure, dosages may need adjustment. Changes in hepatic blood flow that may result from heart failure can alter lidocaine's pharmacokinetics.

Adverse Reactions. Common adverse effects of lidocaine include drowsiness, dizziness, transient paresthesias, and other central nervous system (CNS) symptoms. If the plasma concentration exceeds 8 µg/mL, more life-threatening reactions can occur: seizures, hypotension, respiratory depression, decreased cardiac output, and coma.

Drug Interactions. Use of lidocaine with beta blockers, cimetidine, procainamide, or tocainide increases the possibility of lidocaine-related adverse reactions.

Precautions and Contraindications. Lidocaine is used with caution in clients with hepatic or renal failure due to possible toxic accumulation of lidocaine or its metabolites. It is not given to clients who are allergic to it or who have any form of heart block or reduced cardiac output.

Mexiletine

Mexiletine (Mexitil) is an analog of lidocaine and is structurally similar to tocainide.

Table 22-4. Antiarrhythmic Drugs: Class IB

Drug Name	Dosage Forms	Usual Dosage	Adverse Reactions
lidocaine (Xylocaine)	IM; IV; *Note:* these must be marked "for cardiac arrhythmias"; preparations for local anesthesia that contain preservatives of vasopressors should not be used.	Adults: IV: *bolus:* 50–100 mg, dosage not to exceed 200–300 mg/h; *continuous infusion:* 1–4 mg/min or 20–50 µg/kg/min PC: B	Drowsiness, dizziness, transient paresthesias, seizures, hypotension, respiratory depression, decreased cardiac output, coma
mexiletine (Mexitil)	Oral capsules	Adults: 200–300 mg q8h PC: C	Dizziness, tremor, nervousness, incoordination, nausea, vomiting, heartburn, exacerbation of arrhythmias
phenytoin (Dilantin)	Oral chewable tablets, oral suspension, oral prompt capsules, oral extended-release capsules, IM, IV	Adults: IV: 50 mg q5min to total of 1,000 mg; Oral: 200–400 mg/day *Note:* consult further if using this for anticonvulsant therapy PC: D	Gingival hyperplasia, drowsiness, nystagmus, ataxia, dysarthria, slurred speech, mental confusion, insomnia, nervousness, diplopia, fatigue, irritability, depression, numbness, headache, cardiovascular collapse, agranulocytosis, toxic epidermal necrolysis
tocainide (Tonocard)	Oral tablets	Adults: 400–600 mg q8h PC: C	Tremors, dizziness, nausea, visual disturbances, exacerbation of arrhythmias, pulmonary complications, agranulocytosis

KEY: PC = pregnancy risk category (see Appendix A).

Pharmacodynamics. Mexiletine is a class IB drug whose mechanism of action is the same as lidocaine's.

Pharmacokinetics. Mexiletine is well absorbed after oral administration. Peak blood levels are reached in 2 to 3 hours. It is 50% to 60% bound to plasma proteins. Its elimination half-life ranges from 10 to 12 hours, but decreased hepatic function prolongs that to 25 hours. Mexiletine is extensively metabolized by the liver before elimination. Decreased renal function has not been noted to prolong elimination half-life significantly. Urinary acidification accelerates excretion; alkalinization retards it. Therapeutic plasma levels are 0.5 to 2 µg/mL.

Therapeutic Uses. Mexiletine is used for life-threatening ventricular arrhythmias, such as sustained ventricular tachycardia. It may reduce pain and paresthesias associated with diabetic neuropathy, but these are unlabeled uses.

Dosage and Administration. The usual dosage is 200 mg every 8 hours. Doses should be increased only every 2 to 3 days, and the daily dose should not exceed 1,200 mg. Clients with severe liver disease may require lower doses. Clients with severe right-sided heart failure can experience a reduction in hepatic metabolism of mexiletine; therefore, a reduction in dose may be needed. The drug may be given with food.

Adverse Reactions. The most common adverse effects associated with mexiletine include dizziness, tremor, nervousness, incoordination, nausea, vomiting, and heartburn. Life-threatening adverse reactions include exacerbation of arrhythmias.

Drug Interactions. Metoclopramide causes a faster gastric emptying time, which accelerates the rate of mexiletine absorption and possibly increases mexiletine's effects. Narcotics, atropine, and magnesium/aluminum hydroxide antacids may slow absorption. Phenytoin and rifampin induce liver metabolism of mexiletine, thereby increasing its elimination and perhaps lowering its therapeutic effect. Cimetidine may increase or decrease mexiletine plasma levels. Serum theophylline levels may be increased when it is taken concurrently with mexiletine.

Precautions and Contraindications. Mexiletine must be used with caution in clients with a seizure disorder, hypotension, or severe heart failure.

Phenytoin

Phenytoin, or diphenylhydantoin (Dilantin), is structurally related to barbiturates and was introduced in 1938 for use in treating seizure disorders. It was first used in 1950 for treatment of cardiac arrhythmias.

Pharmacodynamics. Phenytoin's electrophysiologic actions somewhat resemble those of lidocaine and the other class IB drugs. It decreases cardiac automaticity.

Pharmacokinetics. After oral administration, phenytoin is absorbed from the small intestine. Absorption rate and extent vary and depend on the specific preparation; therefore, brand interchange is not recommended. Dosage adjustments may be required when switching from extended-release to regular products. Regular products reach peak plasma levels in 1.5 to 3 hours.

Plasma protein binding ranges from 87% to 93%. Because phenytoin is poorly and erratically absorbed after intramuscular (IM) administration, it should not be administered by this route. Therapeutic plasma concentration is 10 to 20 μg/mL. Phenytoin is metabolized by hepatic microsomal enzymes, and metabolites are excreted in the urine. A genetically determined limitation in ability to metabolize phenytoin has been identified.

Therapeutic Uses. In relation to cardiac arrhythmias, phenytoin is most useful for treating supraventricular and ventricular arrhythmias associated with digitalis toxicity. Used prophylactically, phenytoin may prevent postcardioversion arrhythmias, especially in the client receiving a digitalis preparation. In addition, phenytoin has been used to treat ventricular arrhythmias that follow myocardial infarction, open-heart surgery, anesthesia, cardiac catheterization, cardioversion, and angiography. It is ineffective for atrial flutter or atrial fibrillation.

Dosage and Administration. Administered IV, doses of 50 mg can be given every 5 minutes until the arrhythmia stops or until a total of 1,000 mg has been given. Oral maintenance therapy can then commence (200–400 mg/day).

Adverse Reactions. The most common adverse reactions with phenytoin include gingival hyperplasia and drowsiness. Gingival hyperplasia may be reduced by good oral hygiene, including gum massage, frequent brushing, and appropriate dental care. Adverse CNS effects include nystagmus, ataxia, dysarthria, slurred speech, mental confusion, insomnia, transient nervousness, diplopia, fatigue, irritability, depression, numbness, and headache. Life-threatening adverse reactions include cardiovascular collapse, agranulocytosis, aplastic anemias, and toxic epidermal necrolysis.

Rapid IV administration (in excess of 50 mg/min) has been associated with serious toxicity, such as hypotension and respiratory arrest. The diluent supplied with phenytoin is not pharmacologically inert, and some of the adverse effects attributed to phenytoin may indeed be associated with the diluent, which has a high pH (11) and contains propylene glycol and ethyl alcohol. Because of the high pH, IV administration may cause local venous irritation. Each dose should be followed by normal saline solution to flush the vein.

Drug–Drug Interactions. Multiple drug interactions have been reported. Increased phenytoin effect may occur when any of these drugs are administered concurrently: allopurinol, amiodarone, benzodiazepines, chloramphenicol, cimetidine, disulfiram, fluconazole, isoniazid, metronidazole, miconazole, omeprazole, phenacemide, phenylbutazone, succinimides, sulfonamides, trimethoprim, valproic acid, salicylates, tricyclic antidepressants, chlorpheniramine, ibuprofen, and phenothiazines. In most cases, the increased effect results from inhibited phenytoin metabolism. Decreased phenytoin effect may occur when any of these drugs are administered concurrently: barbiturates, carbamazepine, diazoxide, rifampin, theophylline, antacids, charcoal, sucralfate, antineoplastics, folic acid, influenza virus vaccine, loxapine, nitrofurantoin, and pyridoxine. Phenytoin may decrease the effect of acetaminophen, amiodarone, carbamazepine, cardiac glycosides, corticosteroids, dicumarol, disopyramide, doxycycline, estrogens, haloperidol, methadone, mexiletine, oral contraceptives, quinidine, theophylline, valproic acid, cyclosporine, dopamine, furosemide, levodopa, levonorgestrel, mebendazole, phenothiazines, and sulfonylureas.

Drug–Food Interactions. Phenytoin interacts with enteral formulas. When the feeding tube empties directly into the small intestine and phenytoin is followed by continuous feedings, the GI residence time may be inadequate for total phenytoin dissolution. Overall phenytoin bioavailability, therefore, is compromised (Fleischer et al., 1990). In addition, a binding interaction may occur between phenytoin and one or more components of the enteral formula. Monitoring of plasma levels is important.

Evidence indicates that phenytoin may interfere with folic acid metabolism. Long-term phenytoin therapy may result in folate deficiency, possibly progressing to megaloblastic anemia. Folic acid therapy may be needed.

Drug–Laboratory Test Interactions. Phenytoin may interfere with the metyrapone and dexamethasone tests.

Precautions and Contraindications. Phenytoin should be used cautiously in clients with acute intermittent porphyria, hypotension, and severe myocardial insufficiency. It is contraindicated with certain bradycardias and in clients sensitive to hydantoins. Phenytoin may raise blood glucose levels in hyperglycemic persons, and clients with diabetes mellitus must monitor blood glucose levels regularly. Adjustment of dosage of the hypoglycemic drug may be needed.

Tocainide

Tocainide (Tonocard), a class IB drug, is a primary amine analog of lidocaine.

Pharmacodynamics. Tocainide's mechanism of action is the same as that of lidocaine. Most clients who respond to lidocaine also respond to tocainide.

Pharmacokinetics. The bioavailability of tocainide approaches 100% after oral administration. Peak serum concentrations are reached in 0.5 to 2 hours. Unlike lidocaine, tocainide undergoes negligible first-pass hepatic processing. From 10% to 20% is plasma protein bound. Tocainide appears to have no pharmacologically active metabolites. About 40% is eliminated via the kidneys unchanged; the rest of it undergoes glucuronidation before renal excretion. The average half-life, about 15 hours, is increased in severe renal dysfunction. The therapeutic range is 4 to 10 μg/mL.

Therapeutic Uses. Tocainide is used to suppress symptomatic ventricular arrhythmias associated with a prolonged Q-T interval. It has no appreciable effect on atrial arrhythmias. It has been used safely in clients with acute myocardial infarction and various degrees of heart failure. It exerts a small negative inotropic effect. It may be beneficial in treating myotonic dystrophy and trigeminal neuralgia.

Dosage and Administration. Variation in individual responsiveness to tocainide has been noted, so dosages may need adjustment based on client evaluation. The initial dose is usually 400 mg every 8 hours (range, 1,200 to 1,800 mg/day given in three divided doses). Dose-related adverse reactions tend to occur early in treatment, usually decreasing in severity and frequency with time. Some effects may be minimized by taking tocainide with food (the extent of its bioavailability seems unaffected by food).

Adverse Reactions. The most common adverse effects of tocainide include tremors, dizziness, nausea, and visual disturbances. Life-threatening adverse reactions include exacerbation of arrhythmias, pulmonary embolism, and agranulocytosis.

Agranulocytosis, bone marrow depression, leukopenia, neutropenia, aplastic/hypoplastic anemia, thrombocytopenia, and septicemia and septic shock have occurred. Because these problems are usually noted in the first 3 months of therapy, complete blood counts, including white blood cell, differential, and platelet counts, should be performed weekly during that period and periodically thereafter. If one of these problems necessitates drug discontinuation, blood counts usually return to normal within 1 month.

Pulmonary fibrosis, interstitial pneumonitis, fibrosing alveolitis, pulmonary edema, and pneumonia have occurred, often in seriously ill clients with fatalities. Clients should be instructed to report promptly any pulmonary symptoms, including exertional dyspnea, cough, and wheezing.

Drug Interactions. Cimetidine and rifampin appear to decrease tocainide's bioavailability. Metoprolol is also known to interact with tocainide.

Precautions and Contraindications. Cautious use is required for clients with heart failure, cardiac conduction abnormalities, hepatic or renal disease, potassium imbalance, or bone marrow failure of any type. Contraindications include allergy, pregnancy, and lactation.

Class IC Drugs

Class IC drugs include flecainide (Tambocor) and propafenone (Rhythmol) (Table 22-5).

Flecainide

Pharmacodynamics. Drugs in class IC have the greatest effect on sodium influx and do not appreciably affect repolarization. They depress cardiac conductivity, especially in the His-Purkinje system. Structurally, part of the flecainide molecule is similar to that of procainamide, except it lacks the section that is probably responsible for the lupus-like syndrome attributed to procainamide.

Pharmacokinetics. Flecainide is well absorbed after oral administration. Food or antacids do not affect absorption. Flecainide is not extensively bound by plasma proteins (about 40%). Peak plasma levels are attained at about 3 hours. About 30% of a dose is excreted unchanged in urine; the rest of the drug is biotransformed to two major metabolites that undergo renal excretion. The half-life ranges from 12 to 27 hours. If the client has renal impairment, the extent of unchanged drug in urine is reduced and the half-life is prolonged.

Therapeutic Uses. Flecainide is used for frequent premature ventricular contractions and sustained ventricular tachycardia. Flecainide is not recommended for clients with chronic atrial fibrillation. Increased premature ventricular contractions, ventricular tachycardia, and deaths have been reported when clients were treated with flecainide for atrial fibrillation or flutter (paradoxical effect).

Dosage and Administration. The recommended starting dose is 50 mg every 12 hours. Doses may be increased in increments of 50 mg twice daily every 4 days as necessary. The 4-day time interval between dosage adjustments is based on the fact that steady-state plasma levels in normal renal and hepatic function may not be achieved for 3 to 4 days after initiating therapy at a given dose.

Adverse Reactions. The most common adverse reactions with flecainide include dizziness, including lightheadedness, faintness, unsteadiness, and near syncope, dyspnea, headache, visual disturbances, and nausea. Life-threatening adverse reactions include new or worsened arrhythmias.

Flecainide increases the endocardial pacing threshold so that pacemaker-dependent clients may need their pacemakers reprogrammed. In fact, flecainide may be unsuitable for clients with pacemakers. New or worsening heart failure occurs in a small but significant percentage of those receiving flecainide.

Drug Interactions. Evidence suggests that amiodarone, cimetidine, disopyramide, propranolol, cigarette smoking, verapamil, and digoxin have the potential to cause clinically important drug interactions with flecainide. Amiodarone, cimetidine, and propranolol appear to increase flecainide plasma levels and bioavailability.

Precautions and Contraindications. Flecainide must be used with caution in clients who have pacemakers, potassium imbalance, or hepatic or renal disease. Cautious use is required in clients with cardiac conduction abnormalities because the drug has been shown to have

Table 22-5. Antiarrhythmic Drugs: Class IC

Drug Name	Dosage Forms	Usual Dosage	Adverse Reactions
flecainide (Tambocor)	Oral tablets	Adults: *initially* 50–100 mg q12h depending on arrhythmia; maximum dose is 300–400 mg/day depending on arrhythmia PC: C	Dizziness, lightheadedness, faintness, unsteadiness and near syncope, dyspnea, headache, visual disturbances, nausea, new or worsened arrhythmias
propafenone (Rythmol)	Oral tablets	Adults: 150 mg q8h, maximum of 900 mg/day PC: C	Dizziness, nausea and vomiting, alterations in taste, constipation, new or worsened arrhythmias

PC = pregnancy risk category (see Appendix A).

ventricular proarrhythmic effects in clients with atrial fibrillation or flutter. It has a negative inotropic effect and may cause or worsen heart failure. It is contraindicated in lactation.

Propafenone

Propafenone exhibits class IC properties in that it markedly depresses sodium influx during depolarization.

Pharmacodynamics. Propafenone slows conduction. It also exhibits a local anesthetic effect, limited beta-adrenergic blocking, and weak calcium channel blocking actions.

Pharmacokinetics. After oral administration, propafenone is absorbed almost completely, but its bioavailability is usually less than 20% due to extensive first-pass metabolism. There are two genetically determined patterns of metabolism. In nearly 90% of clients, the drug is rapidly and extensively metabolized with an elimination half-life of 2 to 10 hours. Some of the metabolites are active and have demonstrated antiarrhythmic activity. In less than 10% of clients, metabolism is slower because a certain metabolite is not formed or is minimally formed. The elimination half-life in these clients ranges from 10 to 32 hours.

There are significant differences in plasma concentrations of propafenone in slow and extensive metabolizers: the former achieve concentrations 1.5 to 2 times those of the extensive metabolizers. Because of these differences, clients should be watched closely for clinical (ECG) evidence of toxicity.

Therapeutic Uses. Propafenone is used for sustained suppression of ventricular tachycardia. It has been used also for certain supraventricular arrhythmias.

Dosage and Administration. The initial dose is 150 mg every 8 hours, increased at intervals of 3 to 4 days up to a maximum of 900 mg daily. Propafenone should be administered with food.

Adverse Reactions. The most common adverse effects of propafenone include dizziness, nausea and vomiting, alterations in taste sensation, and constipation. Life-

threatening adverse reactions include new or worsened arrhythmias.

Drug Interactions. Use with warfarin may cause plasma warfarin levels to rise. Concurrent use with cimetidine or quinidine can result in increased propafenone effects. Rifampin increases propafenone clearance and, therefore, leads to a loss of its therapeutic effect. Use with beta blockers or digoxin may increase the pharmacologic effects of those drugs.

Precautions and Contraindications. Propafenone must be used cautiously in clients with renal or hepatic dysfunction. Clients with impaired hepatic function should receive only 20% to 30% of the recommended dose. Propafenone, like flecainide, must be used cautiously with clients with cardiac conduction abnormalities or heart failure. In general, clients with chronic bronchitis or emphysema should not receive propafenone or other drugs with beta-adrenergic blocking activity. It should not be used during pregnancy (teratogenic effect) or lactation.

Other Class I Drugs
Moricizine

Moricizine (Ethmozine) is a class I drug that shares properties with other class I drugs but does not fit any of the existing subclasses precisely. Many of its antiarrhythmic effects are similar to those of class IA drugs, but its uses and adverse effects are more similar to those of class IC drugs.

Pharmacodynamics. Moricizine reduces the fast inward current action potential carried by sodium. It shortens repolarization, decreasing the duration of the action potential. The drug has minimal effect on the action potential amplitude and on normal automaticity. Moricizine prolongs the P-R interval, QRS interval, AV nodal conduction time, and His-Purkinje conduction time.

Pharmacokinetics. Moricizine is absorbed after oral administration and undergoes significant first-pass metabolism, resulting in a bioavailability of about 35%. Peak plasma concentrations are usually reached within

0.5 to 2 hours. Administration after a meal delays the rate of absorption but not the extent of absorption. It is 95% bound to plasma proteins. It undergoes extensive biotransformation in the liver, with less than 1% excreted unchanged in the urine. There are at least 26 metabolites, all found in very small amounts. The plasma half-life is about 2 hours. About 56% is excreted in the feces, 39% in the urine.

Therapeutic Uses. Moricizine is used for life-threatening ventricular arrhythmias, such as sustained ventricular tachycardia, that have not responded to other drugs.

Dosage and Administration. The usual dosage is 200 mg every 8 hours initially, then between 600 and 900 mg daily. The dose may be adjusted in increments of 150 mg/day at 3-day intervals.

Adverse Reactions. The most common adverse effects of moricizine include dizziness, lightheadedness, anxiety, headache, euphoria, and perioral numbness. The most serious adverse reaction has been arrhythmias.

Drug Interactions. Moricizine appears to decrease theophylline concentration, and it also interacts with cimetidine, digoxin, and propranolol. Concomitant administration of cimetidine results in decreased moricizine clearance, which would mandate dosage reduction of moricizine if the combination were used.

Precautions and Contraindications. Moricizine must be used cautiously in clients with hepatic or renal disorders. Like many other antiarrhythmic drugs, it can provoke new rhythm disturbances or worsen existing arrhythmias (proarrhythmic effects). It is contraindicated in heart block, cardiogenic shock, hypersensitivity to the drug, pregnancy, and lactation.

▪ SUMMARY

Class I antiarrhythmic drugs depress cardiac action by blocking the sodium channel in the myocardial membrane, generally exerting negative inotropic, chronotropic, and dromotropic effects. They are used to treat or prevent the recurrence of tachyarrhythmias. They can cause a variety of adverse reactions, including arrhythmias and decreased cardiac output.

Although maintenance therapy to prevent recurring arrhythmias is prescribed for nonhospitalized clients, therapy is usually initiated in critical care facilities in which cardiovascular function can be monitored closely and cardiopulmonary resuscitation can be initiated without delay, if necessary.

Class II Drugs: Beta-Adrenergic Blocking Agents

Beta-adrenergic blocking agents used as antiarrhythmics include acebutolol, esmolol, propranolol, and sotalol (Table 22-6). Beta-adrenergic blocking agents are not powerful antiarrhythmics, but some evidence indicates that they reduce the incidence of sudden death related to ventricular fibrillation after myocardial infarction. They do this by preventing development of that arrhythmia (Hampton, 1994). This positive feature is in contrast to the experience with some other antiarrhythmic drugs in persons who sustain myocardial infarction. Chapter 25 gives more information on beta-adrenergic blockers.

Propranolol

The beta-adrenergic blocking agent with the longest history of use, propranolol (Inderal), is discussed here. Until 1978, it was the only drug in this class approved by the Food and Drug Administration. Sotalol is a beta-adrenergic blocking agent that also has class III antiarrhythmic activity; it is discussed under class III drugs. Acebutolol and esmolol are other class II drugs but are cardioselective beta-adrenergic blocking agents rather than nonselective, as propranolol is.

Pharmacodynamics. Propranolol and other class II drugs block the effects of the adrenergic nervous system or adrenergic drugs (norepinephrine, epinephrine, isoproterenol, dopamine) on the heart. With the administration of propranolol, the adrenergic system can no longer initiate responses mediated by activation of beta-adrenergic receptors. These responses include increases in heart rate and cardiac contractile force in response to exercise, stress, excitement, and other factors; an increase in AV conduction velocity; relaxation of bronchial smooth muscle and a decrease in airway resistance; and release of insulin from beta cells in the islets of Langerhans.

The blockade's consequences on the overall regulation of the cardiovascular system must be considered when a beta-adrenergic blocking agent is used. Clients with normally functioning cardiovascular systems may be able to tolerate a blockade of adrenergic transmission to the heart; however, those with compensated heart failure are dependent on adrenergic tone to maintain adequate cardiac output. Removal of such tone may precipitate acute congestive heart failure.

Propranolol also has a membrane-stabilizing (local anesthetic) property that can contribute to its antiarrhythmic action. This property can account for propranolol's antiarrhythmic effect against the arrhythmias in which beta-receptor stimulation does not play a role.

As a result of the two properties, heart rate decreases and the cardiovascular system's potential for response to stressors diminishes. Impulse conduction through the sinoatrial and AV nodes is delayed and myocardial automaticity is reduced. Blood pressure also declines.

At low plasma propranolol concentrations (less than 100 ng/mL), the antiarrhythmic action is a result of beta-adrenergic blockade. However, plasma concentrations exceeding 100 ng/mL are needed to reduce the

Table 22-6. Antiarrhythmic Drugs: Class II

Drug Name	Dosage Forms	Usual Dosage	Adverse Reactions
acebutolol (Sectral)	Oral capsules	Adults: *initially* 200 mg twice daily, increased to maximum of 1,200 mg/day PC:B	Fatigue, bradycardia, diarrhea, constipation, agranulocytosis
esmolol (Brevibloc)	IV	500 μg/kg/min for 1 min; followed by 4-min maintenance infusion of 50 μg/kg/min; may need to be repeated PC: C	Dizziness, hypotension (dose-related), bronchospasm, infusion site inflammation
propranolol (Inderal)	Oral tablets, sustained-release capsules, solution, concentrated solution; IV	Adults: 10–30 mg tid or qid for arrhythmias PC: C	Bradycardia, hypotension, peripheral vascular insufficiency, heart block, congestive heart failure, confusion, fatigue, drowsiness, nausea, vomiting, diarrhea or constipation, flatulence, epigastric discomfort

KEY: PC = pregnancy risk category (see Appendix A).

ventricular rate in certain situations. At this plasma concentration, in addition to beta-adrenergic blockade, the direct depressant action of propranolol on AV transmission occurs.

Pharmacokinetics. Propranolol is almost completely absorbed from the GI tract after oral administration. Peak plasma concentrations are observed 2 hours after administration. First-pass metabolism significantly decreases bioavailability. About 93% of the drug is bound to plasma proteins. It is metabolized in the liver by four different pathways. Some of its metabolites can produce beta-adrenergic blockade. In clients with hepatic disease, propranolol metabolism is decreased, so bioavailability may increase. Hepatic disease also decreases the plasma protein-bound fraction and increases free propranolol. Hyperthyroidism may increase propranolol clearance by the liver. The half-life for propranolol is 3 to 5 hours. Its route of elimination is the kidney, although some fecal elimination occurs. After absorption, propranolol is widely distributed across the blood-brain barrier and the placenta. It is also secreted into breast milk.

Therapeutic Uses. Propranolol is usually used with another agent in treating arrhythmias. For example, propranolol with a cardiac glycoside can be used to manage the ventricular rate in clients with atrial flutter or fibrillation. Propranolol is also used in treating recurrent supraventricular tachyarrhythmias associated with the Wolff-Parkinson-White syndrome. Propranolol is highly effective in treating digitalis-induced arrhythmias. However, it is not the drug of choice in digitalis toxicity because of its additional effects on the cardiovascular system.

Combining propranolol with quinidine to prevent recurrence of atrial fibrillation after cardioversion may be more effective than administering quinidine alone. Combining propranolol and procainamide has been helpful in managing persistent ventricular fibrillation.

Intravenous administration of propranolol suppresses the arrhythmias associated with halothane or cyclopropane anesthesia. It also relieves ventricular outflow obstruction in hypertrophic obstructive cardiomyopathy and hypertrophic subaortic stenosis.

Propranolol is used prophylactically for clients who experience migraine headaches (it apparently inhibits cerebral vasodilation and arteriolar spasms), and it has been used to relieve acute panic symptoms (eg, stage fright).

Dosage and Administration. Propranolol may be administered orally or IV. The typical dose for supraventricular arrhythmias is 10 to 30 mg three or four times a day. The treatment of ventricular arrhythmias may require over 300 mg daily. When given IV for arrhythmias occurring under anesthesia, the usual dose ranges from 1 to 3 mg, with a rate of administration not exceeding 1 mL/min.

Adverse Reactions. Adverse effects include bradycardia, hypotension, peripheral vascular insufficiency, heart block, congestive heart failure, or cardiac arrest. CNS reactions include disorientation to time and place, short-term memory loss, emotional lability, and clouded sensorium. Perhaps the most common adverse effects include confusion, fatigue, and drowsiness. They are usually reversible once the drug is withdrawn. GI reactions include nausea, vomiting, diarrhea or constipation, epigastric discomfort, and flatulence. Other adverse reactions include allergic signs and symptoms.

Hypoglycemia has been reported in clients with diabetes mellitus on insulin, in children during recovery from anesthesia, and in clients after partial gastrectomy. The mechanism may be related to the fact that the beta-receptor blockade prevents adrenergic stimulation of glycogenolysis in skeletal muscle, which would normally result in an increase in plasma lactate. Lactate is subsequently converted by the liver to glucose. At the same time, insulin reactions are more difficult to detect in the client receiving propranolol because signs and symptoms relating to sympathoadrenal hyperactivity, which normally help the nurse identify hypoglycemia, are absent. On the other hand, hyperglycemia may be seen. This seems to be related to the blocking of insulin release from the pancreas.

Abrupt withdrawal of beta-adrenergic blocking agents may be followed by rebound sympathetic overactivity. A withdrawal syndrome of tremulousness, sweating, severe headache, malaise, palpitation, rebound hypertension, myocardial infarction, and arrhythmias has been identified.

Drug–Drug Interactions. Beta-adrenergic blocking agents interact with multiple drugs; the discussion here is representative rather than complete. Nonsteroidal antiinflammatory agents, barbiturates, cholestyramine and colestipol, aluminum and calcium salts, rifampin, and phenytoin may decrease bioavailability and plasma levels of certain beta-adrenergic blocking agents, resulting in decreased pharmacologic effect. Concurrent use of loop diuretics, phenothiazines, cimetidine, antithyroid drugs, and other antihypertensives may increase the effects of propranolol. When beta-adrenergic blocking agents and haloperidol are used together, the pharmacologic effects (hypotensive episodes) related to both drugs may be increased.

Concurrent use of beta-adrenergic blocking agents and prazosin may increase the postural hypotension produced by prazosin. Pharmacologic antagonism between nonselective beta-adrenergic blocking agents and theophylline can reduce the effects of one or both drugs. Propranolol may increase the anticoagulant effect of warfarin and the cardiac effects of calcium channel blockers, digitalis, and lidocaine. Hypoglycemic effects of sulfonylureas may be relieved by beta-adrenergic blocking agents.

Drug–Food Interactions. Food enhances the bioavailability of propranolol, although this effect is not noted with all beta-adrenergic blocking agents. Thus, the drug should be taken under the same conditions and at the same time each day.

Drug–Laboratory Test Interactions. Beta blockers may alter blood glucose levels and interfere with glucose or insulin tolerance test results. Propranolol may cause elevated blood urea nitrogen levels in clients with severe heart disease. It may also cause elevated serum transaminase, alkaline phosphatase, and lactic dehydrogenase values. Propranolol may interfere with glaucoma screening tests due to effects on intraocular pressure.

Precautions and Contraindications. Sinus bradycardia and greater than first-degree heart block are contraindications to using propranolol because it can further depress AV conduction. Chronic obstructive pulmonary disease is a contraindication to the use of propranolol because the resulting blockade would intensify the degree of airway obstruction.

Propranolol should always be decreased gradually when it is being discontinued, over a period of 1 to 2 weeks. Exacerbation of angina, myocardial infarction, ventricular arrhythmias, and death have occurred after abrupt withdrawal. The manufacturer recommends that it be withdrawn gradually 48 hours before major surgery in most cases, although some prescribers prefer to continue propranolol at lower doses.

■ SUMMARY

Propranolol is a nonselective beta-adrenergic blocking agent (blocks both beta-1 and beta-2 adrenoreceptors) that also has membrane-stabilizing properties. It is administered to control hypertension and certain arrhythmias and in various other situations. There are many potential adverse reactions, including bradycardia, hypotension, congestive heart failure, bronchospasm, and hyperglycemia or hypoglycemia.

Class III Drugs: Drugs That Prolong Repolarization

Class III antiarrhythmic drugs include amiodarone, bretylium, and sotalol (Table 22-7).

Amiodarone

Amiodarone (Cordarone) is a benzofuran derivative; much of the drug is iodine.

Pharmacodynamics. Amiodarone's antiarrhythmic effect may result from a prolongation of the myocardial cell action potential duration and refractory period and noncompetitive alpha- and beta-adrenergic inhibition.

Pharmacokinetics. Absorption after oral administration is slow and variable. Bioavailability is about 50%. Maximum plasma concentrations are attained 3 to 7 hours after a dose. Therapeutic effects on abnormal rhythms are not seen before 2 to 3 days and may take 1 to 3 weeks. The time to effect may be shorter when a loading-dose regimen is used. Amiodarone concentrates in the body in adipose tissue, liver, spleen, and lungs. A high percentage (96%) is bound to plasma proteins. It is metabolized in the liver, producing one metabolite. The main route of elimination is via hepatic excretion into bile. The mean half-life is 53 days, so antiarrhythmic effects may persist for weeks or months after the client discontinues the drug.

Therapeutic Uses. Amiodarone is approved for use only for life-threatening recurrent ventricular tachyarrhythmias that are resistant to control by other means. Unlabeled uses include refractory sustained or paroxysmal atrial fibrillation and paroxysmal supraventricular tachycardia.

Dosage and Administration. The dosing schedule for amiodarone relates to its unique pharmacokinetic prop-

Table 22-7. Antiarrhythmic Drugs: Class III

Drug Name	Dosage Forms	Usual Dosage	Adverse Reactions
amiodarone (Cordarone)	Oral tablets, IV	Adults: loading dose of 800–1,600 mg/day for 1–3 wk, then maintenance of 400 mg/day PC: C	Muscle weakness, fatigue, dizziness, corneal microdeposits, anorexia, nausea, vomiting, constipation, photosensitivity, cardiogenic shock, bradycardia, heart block, torsades de pointes, pulmonary toxicity
bretylium (Bretylol)	IV	Adults: *initially* 5–10 mg/kg over 8 min diluted; doses q1–2h as needed; or continuous infusion of 1–2 mg/min PC: C	Hypotension, nausea, vomiting, increased premature ventricular contractions
sotalol (Betapace)	Oral tablets, IV	Adults: *initially* 80 mg bid, maximum dose 640 mg/day; IV 0.2–1.0 mg/kg	Bradycardia, dyspnea, chest pain, palpitations, fatigue, dizziness, arrhythmias, torsades de pointes

KEY: PC = pregnancy risk category (see Appendix A).

erties and its adverse effects. A typical loading dose for life-threatening ventricular arrhythmias is 800 to 1,600 mg/day for 1 to 3 weeks until a therapeutic response is achieved. The dose is reduced to 600 to 800 mg/day after 1 month. The maintenance dose after that is about 400 mg/day.

Adverse Reactions. The most common adverse effects of amiodarone include muscle weakness, fatigue, dizziness, corneal microdeposits, anorexia, nausea, vomiting, constipation, and photosensitivity. Life-threatening adverse reactions include cardiogenic shock, marked sinus bradycardia, or sinus arrest and heart block. The arrhythmia torsades de pointes is associated with amiodarone.

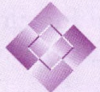

Toxicity Alert: Amiodarone

A potentially fatal toxicity associated with amiodarone is pulmonary toxicity characterized by cough and progressive dyspnea. The disorder is thought to result from indirect toxicity (hypersensitivity pneumonitis) or direct toxicity (interstitial alveolar pneumonitis). Hypersensitivity pneumonitis usually appears earlier in amiodarone therapy. Interstitial pneumonitis may result from phospholipidosis (foamy cells, foamy macrophages) due to inhibition of phospholipase.

Preexisting pulmonary disease does not appear to increase the risk of developing pulmonary toxicity; however, clients with pulmonary disease have a poorer prognosis if pulmonary toxicity does develop.

If there is dose reduction or withdrawal of amiodarone, reduced symptoms of toxicity are usually noted in the first week.

Drug–Drug Interactions. Amiodarone blocks the metabolism of many drugs. Because of its slow elimination, its potential for interaction with other drugs persists for months after its discontinuation. It interacts with beta blockers, digoxin, flecainide, phenytoin, procainamide, quinidine, theophylline, and warfarin, increasing the concentration of these drugs in each instance.

Drug–Laboratory Test Interactions. Elevated hepatic enzyme levels appear frequently. In most cases the client is asymptomatic. However, if the increase exceeds three times the normal value, dose reduction or drug discontinuation should be considered. Amiodarone also alters the results of thyroid function tests, because it affects peripheral conversion of thyroxine to triiodothyronine. It can cause hypothyroidism or hyperthyroidism.

Precautions and Contraindications. Any new respiratory symptom suggests pulmonary toxicity; therefore, physical examination, chest x-ray, and pulmonary function tests should be carried out. Asymptomatic corneal microdeposits appear in almost all adults treated with amiodarone for more than 6 months. They can interfere with vision and are reversible on discontinuation or reduction of the drug dose.

Sinus bradycardia and greater than first-degree heart block are contraindications to using amiodarone because this drug can exacerbate a serious arrhythmia.

Antiarrhythmics may be ineffective or arrhythmogenic in clients with hypokalemia. Any potassium or magnesium deficiency should be corrected before therapy with amiodarone begins. Contraindications also include pregnancy and lactation.

Bretylium

Pharmacodynamics. Initially taken up by sympathetic neurons, bretylium (Bretylol) causes a release of neuronal stores of epinephrine, which affects the myocardium (eg, tachycardia) and peripheral vascular resistance (eg, rise in blood pressure). These effects occur soon after administration, possibly temporarily worsening the client's cardiovascular condition. Subsequent therapeutic mechanisms are incompletely understood. Bretylium blocks the release of norepinephrine. By doing so, it delays repolarization and thereby prolongs both the action potential duration and the effective refractory period. In the peripheral vasculature, inhibited norepinephrine release causes hypotension, which is one of bretylium's more serious adverse reactions. The drug has a positive inotropic action on the myocardium, however, which is uncommon among antiarrhythmics.

Pharmacokinetics. Bretylium is administered by IV or IM injection; oral absorption is poor. Antifibrillatory effects occur within minutes of an IV injection, but suppression of ventricular tachycardia and other ventricular arrhythmias develops more slowly, from 20 minutes to 2 hours after administration.

Protein binding is negligible. Bretylium's half-life is 6 to 8 hours. More than 90% of the administered dose is excreted in the urine as the unchanged drug. Thus, the dose should be reduced in clients with impaired renal function.

Therapeutic Uses. Bretylium is not a first-line antiarrhythmic agent, but it is useful in treating life-threatening ventricular arrhythmias, principally recurrent ventricular tachycardia or fibrillation, especially when conventional agents have proved ineffective.

Dosage and Administration. When the drug is administered IM, it is given in undiluted form. Bretylium is diluted before IV administration. A dose of 5 to 10 mg/kg may be administered over 8 minutes. More rapid infusion may cause nausea and vomiting. Subsequent doses may be given at 1- to 2-hour intervals if the arrhythmia persists. Bretylium may be diluted and administered as a constant IV infusion at a rate of 1 to 2 mg/min.

Adverse Reactions. The most common adverse effects of bretylium include hypotension, nausea, and vomiting. Life-threatening adverse reactions include increased frequency of premature ventricular contractions.

Drug Interactions. If bretylium is used with antihypertensive agents and certain antiarrhythmics, hypotensive effects may be additive. It may worsen digitalis-induced arrhythmias, and concurrent use is not recommended.

Precautions and Contraindications. Bretylium must be used cautiously in clients with hypotension and shock or renal disease, and those who are lactating. Bretylium-induced hypotension (systolic blood pressure of 75 mmHg or less) must be treated and may be reversed by administering IV fluids to increase circulating blood volume and by cautiously administering IV norepinephrine.

Sotalol

Sotalol (Betapace) is a nonselective beta-adrenergic blocking agent (class II effect), having about one third the beta-blocking property of propranolol.

Pharmacodynamics. Sotalol prolongs the action potential duration in all cardiac tissues. It is this property that causes it also to be classified as a class III agent (Dunnington, 1993). It prolongs the absolute and relative refractory periods of the atria, ventricles, AV node, and accessory pathways. It slows the heart rate.

Pharmacokinetics. Sotalol is absorbed rapidly and almost completely after oral administration. However, absorption may be reduced by food. Bioavailability is close to 100%. Sotalol has minimal or no protein binding. No metabolites have been detected. The elimination half-life varies from 10 to 15 hours. Most of the drug is excreted unchanged in the urine by glomerular filtration. About 10% is excreted unchanged in the feces. The therapeutic plasma level ranges from 1 to 3 µg/mL.

Therapeutic Uses. Sotalol is approved for treating documented ventricular arrhythmias, such as sustained ventricular tachycardia, that are judged to be life-threatening. Sotalol is also as effective as quinidine in maintaining sinus rhythm after cardioversion of atrial fibrillation (Hampton, 1994). Additional data indicate it is likely to be effective in reducing the incidence of atrial flutter and fibrillation in clients who undergo coronary artery bypass surgery.

Dosage and Administration. Sotalol is available as oral and IV preparations. The recommended oral starting dose is 80 mg twice daily, with adjustments to 320 mg daily as necessary. Previous antiarrhythmic drugs should be withdrawn for at least two or three plasma half-lives before starting sotalol. Appropriate dose adjustments must be made for clients with impaired renal function (Dunnington, 1993). IV doses (0.2–1.0 mg/kg) have been used for acute arrhythmias.

Adverse Reactions. The most common adverse effects of sotalol include bradycardia, dyspnea, chest pain, palpitations, fatigue, dizziness, and GI effects. Life-threatening adverse reactions include arrhythmias. Sotalol prolongs the Q-T interval and, therefore, can induce torsades de pointes.

Drug–Drug Interactions. Concurrent use with verapamil may increase sotalol's effects. The antihypertensive effects of this drug may be increased or decreased by some interactant drugs.

Drug–Food Interactions. Potentially malignant arrhythmias can occur in clients with low potassium levels. Moreover, drug absorption may be reduced by food, especially milk and milk products, due to interaction between sotalol and calcium.

Drug–Laboratory Test Interactions. Sotalol can cause false results with glucose or insulin tolerance tests.

Precautions and Contraindications. Sotalol must be used cautiously in clients with diabetes. It is contraindicated in clients with sinus bradycardia, heart block, cardiogenic shock, heart failure, or chronic obstructive pulmonary disease, and in those who are pregnant or lactating.

■ SUMMARY

Class III drugs alter cardiac arrhythmias by slowing heart action by prolonging the action potential duration or prolonging repolarization in the myocardium. Individual effects of these drugs that supplement the antiarrhythmic action include sodium channel blockade, increased conduction time, reduced sinus node automaticity, adrenergic blockade, and increased refractory period in the heart. Adverse effects include impairment of cardiovascular, pulmonary, hepatic, and GI function, and exacerbation of cardiac arrhythmias. When therapy with these drugs is initiated, clients are usually under close observation in acute care facilities.

Class IV Drugs: Calcium Channel Blocking Agents

Class IV antiarrhythmics, calcium channel blocking agents, are discussed further in Chapter 25.

Verapamil

Verapamil (Calan, Verelan) is the only calcium channel blocking agent used to treat arrhythmias (Table 22-8).

Pharmacodynamics. Calcium ions, like the sodium ions affected by class I antiarrhythmics, contribute to depolarization and repolarization by moving back and forth across cardiac cell membranes. Blockade of cardiac calcium channels can reduce sinoatrial node automaticity, delay AV nodal conduction, and reduce myocardial contractility.

Verapamil slows AV conduction and prolongs the refractory period within the AV node. With this mechanism, it can reduce increased ventricular rate related to atrial flutter or atrial fibrillation. By interrupting reentry at the AV node, verapamil can restore normal sinus rhythm in clients with supraventricular tachycardias, including Wolff-Parkinson-White syndrome. The drug does not alter the normal atrial action potential.

Verapamil also produces peripheral vasodilation by a relaxant effect on vascular smooth muscle cells, which reduces systemic peripheral resistance and myocardial afterload. Thus, it reduces myocardial oxygen consumption, which probably explains its ability to improve exercise tolerance in clients with angina pectoris.

Pharmacokinetics. Verapamil may be administered orally or IV. Oral doses are well absorbed (90%), but absolute bioavailability ranges from 20% to 35% because of extensive first-pass hepatic metabolism. About 90% is bound to plasma proteins. After oral administration, verapamil reaches peak plasma concentration in 1 to 2 hours, but it shows wide individual variation. Half-life ranges from 3 to 7 hours. Steady-state plasma concentration is usually achieved within 48 hours. About 70% of the drug is eliminated as metabolites via the kidney. The therapeutic plasma concentration range is 80 to 300 ng/mL.

Therapeutic Uses. Verapamil is used in managing supraventricular tachyarrhythmias, angina pectoris, and hypertension. Treatment of migraine headaches is an unlabeled use.

Dosage and Administration. For arrhythmias, the oral dosage range of verapamil is usually 240 to 480 mg/day in divided doses 3 or 4 times a day. It may be administered without regard to meals. For supraventricular tachyarrhythmias, 5 to 10 mg may be given IV as a slow injection over at least 2 minutes. The dose may be repeated in 30 minutes if the initial response is inadequate. Continuous ECG and blood-pressure monitoring is required during parenteral administration because a few clients may have life-threatening adverse responses such as rapid ventricular rate, marked hypotension, or extreme bradycardia.

Adverse Reactions. The administration of verapamil is well tolerated by most clients. Most complaints are

Table 22-8. Antiarrhythmic Drugs: Class IV

Drug Name	Dosage Forms	Usual Dosage	Adverse Reactions
verapamil (Calan)	Oral tablets, sustained-release tablets, sustained-release capsules; IV	Adults: 240–480 mg/day in divided doses IV: bolus: 5–10 mg over 2 min; repeat in 30 min PC: C	Constipation, nausea, gastric discomfort, hypotension, dizziness, headache, atrioventricular block

KEY: PC = pregnancy risk category (see Appendix A).

about constipation, and perhaps nausea and gastric discomfort. Other adverse reactions include hypotension, dizziness, and headache. Life-threatening adverse reactions include AV block.

Drug–Drug Interactions. A major interaction has been with digoxin, whose clearance is reduced by verapamil. The negative inotropic effect of verapamil could negate some of the benefits from the positive inotropic action of digoxin. Digoxin dosage adjustments are required. Other interactions reported have been with barbiturates, calcium salts, dantrolene, histamine (H$_2$) antagonists, phenytoin, quinidine (hypotension), rifampin, sulfinpyrazone, vitamin D, beta blockers (hypotension, decreased cardiac output), carbamazepine, cyclosporine, lithium, prazosin, and theophylline.

Drug–Laboratory Test Interactions. Elevated transaminase levels, with or without concomitant elevated alkaline phosphatase and bilirubin levels, have occurred with verapamil. Some elevations are transient and disappear with continued verapamil treatment, but some cases of hepatocellular injury have been identified.

Precautions and Contraindications. Verapamil is generally contraindicated in clients with severe hypotension, cardiogenic shock, second- or third-degree AV block, severe congestive heart failure, or sick sinus syndrome, and in those who are pregnant or lactating. It must be used cautiously in clients with renal or hepatic dysfunction.

■ SUMMARY

Verapamil is the only calcium channel blocker used as an antiarrhythmic drug. It can be administered IV or orally in treating supraventricular tachycardias. Some adverse effects are constipation, hypotension, and bradycardia.

Other Antiarrhythmic Drugs

Adenosine

Adenosine (Adenocard) is an endogenous substance found in all body cells that is an important physiologic mediator in different organ systems. It is produced in myocardial cells by dephosphorylation of adenosine monophosphate and by degradation of *S*-adenosylhomocysteine (DiMarco, 1994).

Pharmacodynamics. Adenosine slows conduction through the AV node.

Pharmacokinetics. After administration, adenosine is taken up by erythrocytes and vascular endothelial cells. Its estimated half-life is less than 10 seconds. It is primarily metabolized to inosine and adenosine monophosphate.

Therapeutic Uses. Adenosine can be used for conversion of paroxysmal supraventricular tachycardia into sinus rhythm, including that associated with Wolff-Parkinson-White syndrome. It has been proposed as a diagnostic aid during myocardial perfusion imaging to assess clients with suspected coronary artery disease. It is an orphan drug and has been used in treating brain tumors in conjunction with carmustine (BCNU).

Dosage and Administration. Adenosine is given by rapid IV bolus. A dose of 6 mg is given as a rapid bolus over a 1- to 2-second period. If the first dose does not achieve therapeutic results within 1 to 2 minutes, a rapid IV bolus dose of 12 mg may be given. The 12-mg dose may be repeated one more time.

Adverse Reactions. The most common adverse effects include facial flushing, dyspnea, and chest pressure. First-, second-, or third-degree heart block may be produced, but because of the very short half-life the effect is generally self-limiting.

Drug Interactions. Theophylline appears to inhibit the effects of adenosine; carbamazepine and dipyridamole may increase its effects.

Precautions and Contraindications. Adenosine must be used with caution in clients with asthma (possibility of bronchospasm). It is contraindicated in clients who are hypersensitive to the drug and in clients with untreated heart block, sick sinus syndrome, atrial flutter, atrial fibrillation, or ventricular tachycardia.

■ SUMMARY

Adenosine acts as an antiarrhythmic by slowing conduction through the AV node. It is administered by IV bolus to convert paroxysmal supraventricular tachycardia into sinus rhythm.

❖ NURSING MANAGEMENT: CLIENT RECEIVING ANTIARRHYTHMIC DRUGS

The most dangerous adverse effect of antiarrhythmic drugs is the aggravation of preexisting arrhythmias or the provocation of new ones. Our limited knowledge about the mechanism of arrhythmias and the mode of action of antiarrhythmic drugs makes it difficult to predict the clinical response accurately. The use of antiarrhythmic drugs should be considered hazardous, particularly during the initial stages of therapy.

NURSING PROCESS

ASSESSMENT

Data required for assessment include a history of health problems related to cardiovascular disease and other systemic disorders, a complete drug history, and appraisal of current cardiovascular status, including an identification of the arrhythmia, an assessment of the client's attitudes and feelings toward the current illness, and evidence of the client's and family's knowledge of cardiac rhythm disorders and their treatment. Clients should be asked about specific risk factors for serious adverse effects associated with the drugs to be used. The degree of stress and specific stressors affecting the client should be determined.

NURSING DIAGNOSIS

Diagnoses stemming from the use of antiarrhythmic drugs include:

- Risk for Injury, related to drug effects
- Ineffective Management of Therapeutic Regimen (Individual), related to adverse effects of some antiarrhythmics or failure to understand the consequences of not adhering to prescribed drug regimen

Selected nursing diagnoses for clients affected by cardiac arrhythmias include:

- Decreased Cardiac Output, related to abnormal heart rate or rhythm
- Activity Intolerance, related to decreased energy from impaired tissue perfusion
- Anxiety, related to concerns about the impact of the illness or treatment on lifestyle
- Knowledge Deficit about cause and treatment of arrhythmia, related to lack of information
- Fear, related to risk of further cardiac malfunction secondary to arrhythmia or treatment

PLANNING

Goals related to drug therapy include maintenance of adequate systemic tissue perfusion, increased client safety, adherence to the therapeutic regimen, and increased knowledge of medication and its effects.

Overall desired outcomes resulting from general nursing care include maintained cardiac output, increased activity tolerance, reduced fear and anxiety, increased understanding of rhythm disorder, and prevention or prompt detection and management of adverse events.

INTERVENTION

For the acutely ill hospitalized client with cardiac arrhythmias, the nurse intervenes directly to achieve treatment goals (Box 22-1). In addition to general interventions, the nurse is responsible for various nursing measures specific to the antiarrhythmic drugs. Regular cardiovascular assessments must be carried out to evaluate drug effects.

Detecting Complications. The nurse must anticipate potential adverse drug reactions and interactions. When such effects are identified, measures must be taken to manage them. For example, because amiodarone potentiates the effect of digoxin, warfarin, and theophylline, among others, their serum levels should be monitored if they are used concurrently. The prescriber may act to prevent digoxin toxicity by halving the digoxin dose in a client starting amiodarone.

Antiarrhythmic drugs can accumulate in clients with hepatic or renal dysfunction, so clients should be observed carefully for signs and symptoms of increasing hepatic or renal impairment. Drug dosages may need to be changed based on these data.

For clients receiving tocainide or amiodarone, the nurse must monitor pulmonary status regularly, noting complaints of shortness of breath or cough. In these clients, baseline chest x-rays and pulmonary function tests are advisable, with follow-up chest x-rays every 3 to 6 months.

In clients also receiving procainamide, phenytoin, tocainide, or acebutolol, the nurse must monitor for signs of agranulocytosis. Leukopenia or thrombocytopenia may develop weeks after treatment begins, and the nurse should teach the client to recognize and report signs of infection or abnormal bruising or bleeding immediately.

Managing New Arrhythmias. As noted before, antiarrhythmic drugs can cause arrhythmias; this is referred to as their proarrhythmic effect. Thus, the nurse must be alert for new arrhythmias—for example, the

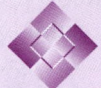

Box 22-1
Nursing Interventions for Clients Receiving Antiarrhythmics in Acute Care

The following are some key nursing interventions for hospitalized clients receiving treatment for cardiac arrhythmias.

- Assess cardiovascular status frequently.
- Report signs and symptoms of inadequate tissue perfusion.
- Monitor for signs and symptoms of arrhythmias (eg, complaints of palpitations or syncope, abnormal pulse rate or rhythm)
- Evaluate cardiac monitor information.
- Initiate appropriate protocols depending on the type of arrhythmia (eg, IV lidocaine for premature ventricular contractions).
- Administer supplemental oxygen as needed.
- Monitor tissue oxygen saturation via pulse oximetry and assess arterial blood gas values as necessary.
- Monitor serum electrolyte levels (eg, potassium, sodium, calcium, magnesium) regularly.
- Restrict client's activity based on tolerance and severity of arrhythmia.
- Prepare client for studies to diagnose the conduction problem or to evaluate the effectiveness of therapy.
- Implement measures to reduce fear and anxiety. Provide encouragement and support.
- Explain cause and treatment of arrhythmia in everyday language.
- Assess and monitor pacemaker or automatic implantable cardioverter defibrillator if appropriate.

development of torsades de pointes in clients taking quinidine, procainamide, disopyramide, amiodarone, or sotalol. Women are more at risk for this arrhythmia than men, particularly during administration of cardiovascular drugs that prolong cardiac repolarization (Makkar, 1993). Electrolyte disturbances such as hypokalemia or hypomagnesemia or a liquid protein diet may contribute to its development as well. Certain noncardiac drugs, such as phenothiazines, tricyclic antidepressants, certain antihypertensive drugs, antibiotics, diuretics, and antihistamines, may also set the stage for torsades de pointes by prolonging the Q-T interval (Schoenbaum, 1995). This arrhythmia may appear as an unexplained syncope. The drug protocol may direct the nurse to discontinue the drug if there is QRS widening and Q-T prolongation to a certain degree (eg, 50% of R-R interval). Magnesium sulfate or a pacemaker may be used to treat this arrhythmia. This, and other proarrhythmic events, often occur within days of starting therapy, but they may also occur unexpectedly later in the course of long-term treatment.

Managing Hypotension and Heart Failure.
Some antiarrhythmic agents (verapamil, esmolol, propranolol, bretylium, moricizine, sotalol) may cause hypotension or contribute to the development of heart failure. To promote client safety, the nurse must teach the client to avoid sudden changes in position to reduce the severity of any postural hypotension experienced. Blood pressure should be monitored frequently, especially in clients with known ventricular dysfunction or hypertrophy. Protocol may direct the nurse to discontinue the antiarrhythmic drug if severe hypotension occurs. The client's intake and output and weight should be monitored for any indications of heart failure (eg, edema, weight gain, output less than intake, fatigue, shortness of breath).

Managing Thyroid Abnormalities.
Because amiodarone contains iodine, which is ultimately released into the circulation, it inhibits the conversion of thyroxine to triiodothyronine. It can cause hypothyroidism or hyperthyroidism; the latter is a greater potential threat to cardiovascular status. Baseline thyroid function test values must be obtained and recorded, and the tests must be repeated periodically.

Avoiding Administration Errors.
Special care should be taken to prevent errors when using parenteral antiarrhythmics. The rate of flow of IV solutions containing antiarrhythmic drugs should be controlled by an infusion controller or pump to prevent inadvertent overdose, which could cause cardiac arrest.

Some drugs are incompatible with emergency drugs that may be needed by the client. The IV equipment must provide for separation of the incompatible substances. Brownish quinidine solutions must be discarded. Lidocaine solutions should be clearly marked "for cardiac arrhythmias," because lidocaine preparations used for local anesthesia contain preservatives and vasopressors that are contraindicated for the cardiac client.

Client Education.
To promote effective client management of the therapeutic regimen, the nurse must assess the client's ability to implement and adhere to the prescribed drug regimen. The nurse begins by explaining the arrhythmia in terms the client can understand, encourages questions, clarifies misconceptions, and provides verbal and written instructions about medication therapy. The nurse also helps the client discuss concerns regarding the medication therapy. Significant others should be included as appropriate in explanations and teaching sessions. The nurse should reinforce behaviors fostering adherence.

Although antiarrhythmic therapy is more risky than some other drug therapies, it can significantly improve cardiac function in many clients. Maintenance doses can be administered for long periods. These clients and their families should be aware that cardiac emergencies may arise. They should be taught the signs and symptoms of cardiac arrest, heart failure, and pulmonary and peripheral embolism. Family members and other responsible caregivers should be trained in cardiopulmonary resuscitation. The client and family should learn about available emergency services and how to use them, and post emergency telephone numbers near the phone.

The client on long-term antiarrhythmic therapy should be taught accurate dosing, proper drug storage, and monitoring of response. The nurse must describe the possible adverse effects of the drug and measures to take if they occur. Clients should learn to monitor their pulses and to recognize pulse alterations and signs and symptoms of heart dysfunction. Specific instructions should be given regarding normal parameters and the action required when abnormalities develop.

In clients receiving several other drugs (eg, anticoagulants, digitalis, diuretics), the nurse should stress the risks of multiple drug regimens, such as the potential for drug interactions, altered drug responses, and increased risk for adverse reactions (see Chap. 6 for a discussion of multidrug therapy).

The teaching plan should also include instructions for managing stress, diet, and fluid intake, techniques for minimizing the effects of postural hypotension (maintaining ample hydration, slowly rising from a prone or seated position), and measures to promote optimal elimination if urinary retention, diarrhea, or constipation develops (see the Critical Thinking Challenge).

OUTCOME EVALUATION
Data required for evaluating the success of the nursing care plan relate to cardiac output, activity tolerance, fear and anxiety, knowledge deficit, tissue perfusion status, incidence or absence of injury, adherence or lack of adherence to the therapeutic regimen, and incidence or absence of complications resulting from the antiarrhythmic agent.

CRITICAL THINKING CHALLENGE
Case Analysis

Acute Care

Mr. Smith, age 61, is admitted to the coronary care unit after sustaining a myocardial infarction. He is connected to a cardiac monitor and the initial cardiovascular assessment is done. At first the monitor shows he is experiencing occasional premature ventricular contractions (PVCs), but 2 hours later the monitor shows he is experiencing about six PVCs in 3 seconds, followed by a short run of ventricular tachycardia. Standing orders permit using lidocaine (Xylocaine) for treating six or more PVCs per minute.

1. After administering lidocaine, what adverse effects will you observe Mr. Smith for?
2. If Mr. Smith exhibits twitching and some tremors, establish his priority needs and propose effective nursing strategies.
3. Explain the rationales that support your actions.
4. If your interventions fail to control the PVCs, propose some other options. Detail the circumstances for these options and explain your rationale.

Home Care

Mr. Smith is being discharged after acute care management of a myocardial infarction complicated by arrhythmias. Since his admission, you have learned that 1 year ago he was treated for peptic ulcer disease and that he is planning to retire soon. He is being discharged on quinidine (Quinidex Extentabs) 300 mg q12h. He did not take this medication before his heart attack. You are preparing a discharge plan that includes a focus on arrhythmia and drug therapy.

1. Consider and prioritize the topics you need to explore with Mr. Smith before you begin your discharge teaching interventions.
2. Develop at least three broad nursing diagnoses and outcome goals to include in the teaching plan.
3. Propose at least six individualized nursing strategies to teach Mr. Smith about effective medication management and to provide anticipatory guidance.

❖ CHECKLIST OF NURSING ACTIONS

- Screen clients for risk factors for adverse drug reactions, and verify that the prescribing clinician is aware of these factors.
- Assess cardiovascular status frequently by assessing pulse rate and character, blood pressure, cardiac monitoring data and ECG tracings, tissue oxygenation, and electrolyte levels.
- Implement measures to promote rest or improve activity tolerance.
- Prevent errors in the administration of antiarrhythmics, especially IV preparations.

- Assess client for signs and symptoms of fear and anxiety.
- Minimize stressors on client and family, and teach stress management techniques.
- Assess for indications that the client may be unable to manage the therapeutic regimen.
- Encourage questions and clarify misconceptions from client and family to encourage adherence to the regimen.
- Observe for indications of drug interactions; verify that the prescribing clinician is aware of such indications.
- Watch for signs and symptoms of thromboemboli in clients who experienced atrial flutter or fibrillation.
- Carefully observe clients with decreased hepatic or renal function for signs of drug toxicity.
- Help clients ambulate; take safety measures to prevent falls.
- Institute nursing measures to reduce the risk of adverse reactions specific to the antiarrhythmic drugs used; monitor clients for signs and symptoms (especially for pulmonary toxicity, agranulocytosis, new arrhythmias, severe hypotension, and congestive heart failure).
- Be prepared to administer emergency care for life-threatening arrhythmias or cardiac arrest.
- Before discharge, help families prepare for managing medical emergencies for which the client is at high risk.
- Teach clients and families how to manage the drug regimen at home.
- Teach clients and families to avoid stressors that may increase the risk of arrhythmia.

References

Abernathy DR, Andrawis NS. (1993). Critical drug interactions: A guide to important examples. *Drug Therapy, 10,* 15.

Carrieri-Kohlman V, Lindsey AM, West CM. (1993). *Pathophysiological phenomena in nursing,* 2d ed. Philadelphia: WB Saunders.

DiMarco JP. (1994). Adenosine. *Cardiol Rev, 2*(1), 33–41.

Dunnington CS. (1993). Sotalol hydrochloride (Betapace): A new antiarrhythmic drug. *Am J Crit Care, 2*(5), 397–405.

Fleischer D, Sheth N, Kou JH. (1990). Phenytoin interaction with enteral feedings administered through nasogastric tubes. *J Parenteral Enteral Nutr, 14,* 513–516.

Hampton JR. (1994). Choosing the right beta-blocker. *Drugs, 48*(4), 549–568.

Makkar RR, Fromm BS, Steinman RT, et al. (1993). Female gender as a risk factor for torsades de pointes associated with cardiovascular drugs. *JAMA, 270* (21), 2590–2597.

Olin BR, ed. (1995). *Drug facts and comparisons,* 50th ed. St. Louis: Facts and Comparisons.

Schoenbaum M. (1995). Recognizing torsades de pointes, *AJN, 95*(2), 54.

Bibliography

Aronson RS, Ming Z. (1993). Cellular mechanisms of arrhythmias in hypertrophied and failing myocardium. *Circulation, 87,* suppl. VII, VII76–VII83.

Braunwald E, ed. (1992). *Heart disease: A textbook of cardiovascular medicine,* 4th ed. Philadelphia: WB Saunders.

Friedman PL. (1994). Subtleties of dosing oral antiarrhythmics. *CVRR, 10,* 45–53.

Hansten P, Horn J. (1993). *Drug interactions: updates,* 8th ed. Vancouver, WA: Applied Therapeutics.

Hardman J, Limbird LE, et al., (eds.). (1996). *Goodman and Gilman's The Pharmacological Basis of Therapeutics,* 9th ed. New York: McGraw-Hill.

Hohnloser SH, Woosley RL. (1994). Sotalol. *N Engl J Med, 331*(1), 31–38.

Nattel S. (1993). Comparative mechanisms of action of antiarrhythmic drugs. *Am J Cardiol, 72*(11), 13F–17F.

Singh BN. (1993). Choice and chance in drug therapy of cardiac arrhythmias: Technique versus drug-specific responses in evaluation of efficacy. *Am J Cardiol, 72*(11), 114F–124F.

Singh BN, Dzau VJ, Vanhoutte PM, Woosley RL, eds. (1994). *Cardiovascular pharmacology and therapeutics.* New York: Churchill-Livingstone.

Stahl L. (1995). How to manage common arrhythmias in medical patients. *AJN, 95*(3), 36–41.

Teo KK, Yusuf S, Furberg CD. (1993). Effects of prophylactic antiarrhythmic drug therapy in acute myocardial infarction. *JAMA, 270*(13), 1589–1595.

Yacone-Morton LA. (1995). Antiarrhythmics. *RN, 4,* 26–31.

For more information and sample tests and activities, refer to Chapter 22 in the Student Workbook for Clinical Pharmacology and Nursing Management, 5th edition, available through your bookstore.

23

Drugs That Regulate Lipid Levels

The circulatory system, a continuous, closed circuit of vessels, carries the blood pumped by the heart through the lungs and periphery of the body. The drugs discussed in this chapter regulate lipid levels, an important factor in vessel patency.

Vascular Physiology

The flow of fluid through the circulatory system depends on the patency of the vessels and pressure gradients, which propel liquids from the arteries to the veins and back to the heart. Maintenance of the pressure gradients requires adequate pumping action by the heart to establish high pressure in the vessels opening from the ventricles, elasticity of the arteries to moderate and prolong this pressure, and a degree of peripheral resistance sustained by partial constriction of the smaller vessels.

Vascular Pathophysiology

In addition to cardiac malfunction and changes in the volume of circulating blood, changes in the blood vessels can decrease blood flow through the circulatory system.

Circulation is reduced by processes that decrease the patency of the blood vessels, impair their elasticity, cause inappropriate vasoconstriction or vasodilatation, or interfere with venous return. Patency may be reduced by external pressure (the cause of decubitus), internal obstructions (thrombi, emboli, tumors), and atherosclerosis. Elasticity is reduced in arteriosclerosis, a process involving progressive fibrosis and calcification of the vascular wall.

This chapter focuses mainly on atherosclerosis as a cause of circulatory malfunction (Box 23-1) and on drugs used to retard atherosclerosis or to promote regression of existing plaque (atheromas). The drugs do not all have the same effects on cholesterol, triglycerides, and lipoproteins. The drugs discussed below should be used only in conjunction with a therapeutic diet and exercise.

Pathophysiology of Atherosclerosis

Atherosclerosis is a disease of the large and medium arteries (eg, coronary, cerebral, femoral, and aorta arteries). Most mortality associated with atherosclerosis is due to occluded coronary arteries (coronary artery disease), which are responsible for producing myocardial ischemia and infarction. Atherosclerosis can also cause cerebrovascular accidents (stroke), peripheral vascular

Box 23-1
Factors Contributing to Atherosclerosis*

Genetic predisposition

Smoking

Diet rich in fat and calories

Obesity

Blood cholesterol levels

Stress

Hormone status

Disease (eg, diabetes mellitus)

Hypertension

Aging

*Contributing factors are accelerated in developed countries with advanced technology.

disease, and renal failure, depending on the location of atheromatous lesions.

Primary pathologic processes of atherosclerosis appear to involve 1) a reaction to injury of the vessel wall, 2) a response to serum lipid levels, and 3) cellular transformation (Copstead, 1995).

Experts think that injury to the vessel wall, such as nonspecific damage to the endothelial surface of the arterial intima, produces a change in the permeability of the wall. Normal barrier features are lost. Sources of injury are associated particularly with smoking, hypertension, and high levels of circulating substances such as lipoproteins, catecholamines, angiotensin, or hormones. Serum constituents such as lipoproteins and platelets then enter the injured intimal lining.

In the second process—the response to serum lipid levels—high concentrations of cholesterol in the form of low-density lipoproteins (LDLs) are transported into the walls of the artery, where they produce irritation. It is thought that LDL is converted to oxidized LDL, which destroys the receptor needed for normal receptor-mediated clearance of LDL. The oxidized LDL induces monocyte attachment and endothelial dysfunction. Dysfunctional endothelial cells express cell adhesion molecules, which leads to further monocyte adhesion (attachment).

The third process involves monocytes in the vessel wall differentiating into macrophages, taking up lipids (oxidized LDL), and remaining locally as foam cells (Rang et al., 1995). These cells subsequently evolve into the fatty streaks that are the earliest atherosclerotic lesions (Copstead, 1995). An additional factor of current interest is lipoprotein (a) (Lp[a]), which is linked to apo B of LDL by a disulfide bridge to plasminogen. Numerous studies show a positive relation between Lp[a] concentration and coronary heart disease (Patsch & Gotto, 1995).

Dysfunctional endothelial cells may synthesize less nitric oxide synthase, which in turn may lead to a decrease in the release and activity of endothelial-derived relaxing factor. The loss of this factor interferes with normal vasodilation. Platelets, macrophages, and endothelial cells release chemotaxins and growth factors. As a result, smooth muscle cells proliferate and connective tissue components are deposited in the form of fibrous plaques known as atheromas, the lesions most characteristic of atherosclerosis.

Atheromas that then extrude from the intima alter blood flow in varying degrees. The most complicated or advanced lesion has a necrotic inner part because of the lack of blood supply. Dead tissue, cellular debris, hemorrhage, thrombus formation, and lipid calcification all contribute to the increasing rigidity of the lesion. The fibrous caps of the lesions may ulcerate or be lysed away by enzymes. Before signs and symptoms of atherosclerosis appear, the blood flow to a given organ is diminished by more than 50% (Copstead, 1995).

Role of Lipids and Lipoproteins

Because of their minimal solubility in water or plasma, lipids, except fatty acids, are packaged into structures called lipoproteins. The principal function of lipoproteins is to distribute lipids among their sites of synthesis, storage, use, and excretion.

The five kinds of lipoproteins are chylomicrons, very low-density lipoproteins (VLDLs), intermediate-density lipoproteins, low-density lipoproteins (LDLs), and high-density lipoproteins (HDLs). The degree to which elevated blood lipids contribute to heart disease is determined by their distribution among the various lipoprotein classes. High concentrations of all lipids except the HDLs are associated with an increased risk of atherosclerosis. High serum levels of triglycerides and LDLs (containing a high proportion of cholesterol) are associated with coronary artery disease.

High-density lipoproteins may exert a protective effect against atherosclerosis and may promote the mobilization and metabolism of cholesterol, thereby reducing its deposition in vessel walls.

In humans, lipoproteins are produced by the intestine and liver. Exogenous and endogenous lipid transport pathways have been distinguished according to lipid origin, but these pathways overlap.

In the exogenous pathway, cholesterol and triglycerides derived from the gastrointestinal (GI) tract are transported in the lymph and then in the plasma as chylomicrons to muscle and adipose tissue. On the vascular endothelial cells, triglycerides are hydrolyzed by a lipoprotein lipase, and the free fatty acids are taken up by the tissues. The chylomicron remnants pass to the liver, bind to receptors on hepatocytes, and undergo endocytosis. Cholesterol is liberated within the liver cell and may be stored, oxidized to bile acids, or secreted in the bile unaltered. It also may enter the endogenous pathway of lipid transport.

In the endogenous pathway, cholesterol and triglycerides are transported as VLDL to muscle and adipose tissue, where the triglycerides are hydrolyzed and the fatty acids enter the tissues as described above. During this process, the lipoprotein particles become smaller but still ultimately become LDL, the source of cholesterol for synthesis of steroids, plasma membranes, and bile acids. Cells requiring cholesterol for these purposes synthesize receptors that recognize LDL, enabling them to take up LDL (Rang et al., 1995).

Classification of Hyperlipoproteinemias

The normal processing of lipids and lipoproteins in the body has just been described. When abnormal processing of lipids occurs, the result may be a primary or secondary processing disorder. These disorders are called hyperlipoproteinemias.

The primary forms are genetically determined and can be divided into two groups: those caused by an in-

Table 23-1. Frederickson–WHO Classification of Hyperlipoproteinemia

Type and Incidence	Lipoprotein Elevated	CHOL	TG	Risk of Atherosclerosis
I, very rare	chylomicrons	+	+++	NE
IIa, common	LDL	++	NE	High
IIb, common	LDL + VLDL	++	++	High
III, somewhat uncommon	βVLDL	++	++	Moderate
IV, common	VLDL	+	++	Moderate
V, uncommon	chylomicrons VLDL	+	++	NE

CHOL = cholesterol; TG = triglycerides; LDL = low-density lipoprotein; VLDL = very low-density lipoprotein, βVLDL = abnormal form of VLDL, + = increased concentration, NE = not elevated

herited, single-gene defect and those that appear to be caused by a combination of several genetic factors that act together with various environmental insults (eg, diets high in saturated fats and cholesterol). Secondary hyperlipoproteinemias are complications of a more generalized metabolic disturbance, such as diabetes mellitus, hypothyroidism, alcoholism, nephrotic syndrome, chronic renal failure, liver disease, and administration of certain drugs. The hyperlipoproteinemias are classified according to which lipoprotein particle is increased (Table 23-1). The classification is known as the Frederickson–WHO (World Health Organization) classification. The greatest risk of coronary artery disease occurs from the hyperlipoproteinemia called familial hypercholesterolemia, type IIa.

Associated Factors

Based on recent, albeit short, trials, a 2% reduction in coronary heart disease results from each 1% reduction in serum cholesterol concentrations (Kramer, 1995). The reduction in coronary heart disease rates with long-term cholesterol lowering may be even greater. In 1993, the second report of the Expert Panel on Detection, Evaluation, and Treatment of High Blood Cholesterol in Adults presented the National Cholesterol Education Program's updated recommendations for cholesterol management (Expert Panel, 1993). The guidelines emphasize the importance of maximizing the benefits of nondrug therapies (eg, diet, weight loss, exercise) before adding pharmacologic therapy. According to the report, desirable blood cholesterol is about 200 mg/dL and high blood cholesterol exceeds 240 mg/dL. Borderline-high ranges from 200 to 239 mg/dL. HDL levels should be 35 mg/dL or more and LDL levels should be less than 130 mg/dL.

For diet therapy, the step I or step II diets of the American Heart Association can be used (Table 23-2). These are similar to the National Cholesterol Education Program's eating pattern recommendations (Kramer, 1995). These diets are intended to reduce the amount of saturated fat and cholesterol progressively and to

help achieve a desirable weight by eliminating excess calories. Total fat constitutes saturated fat, monounsaturated fat, and polyunsaturated fat, each having a different effect on serum cholesterol levels. All foods contain an assortment of the three in various combinations. Diet therapy is discussed in greater detail in the nursing management sections of this chapter.

Exercise has long been valued for its protective effect on the vascular system. It uses up calories, thereby reducing the substrate available for lipid synthesis. Exercise also tends to blunt the appetite and to increase the proportion of protective HDL in the blood.

Other protective effects are offered by the hormones estrogen and thyroxine, which tend to reduce atherosclerosis. Thyroxine lowers cholesterol and triglyceride levels. Part of this effect stems from thyroxine's diversion of calories for energy, which reduces the substrate available for the body's synthesis of cholesterol and fats.

Before menopause, women are at low risk for coronary heart disease, possibly because of their higher estrogen levels. After menopause, when estrogen levels drop, more postmenopausal women have high levels of plasma cholesterol than men of the same age (Arca et al., 1994). Many postmenopausal women have high-risk LDL cholesterol levels. It has been suggested that the decrease in estrogen secretion with cessation of ovarian function probably contributes to higher LDL

Table 23-2. Recommended Dietary Components

Component	Step I Diet	Step II Diet
Total fat	≤30%	≤30%
Saturated fat	8%–10%	<7%
Polyunsaturated	up to 10%	up to 10%
Monounsaturated	up to 15%	up to 15%
Carbohydrate	≥55%	≥55%
Protein	15%–20%	15%–20%
Cholesterol	≤300 mg%mg/d	≤200 mg%mg/d

cholesterol levels in postmenopausal women, and in women with a genetic propensity, loss of estrogens may have raised their LDL levels to the high-risk range (Arca et al., 1994). Some experts think that estrogen replacement therapy in postmenopausal women with high LDL levels may obviate the need for other drug therapy.

HMG-CoA Reductase Inhibitors

The introduction of a new class of drugs derived from fungi has been important to treatment for the hyperlipoproteinemias. The first such drug was mevasatin, isolated in Japan in 1976. The first drug widely used within the class was lovastatin. The drugs included in this class at this time are fluvastatin, lovastatin, pravastatin, and simvastatin (Table 23-3).

Fluvastatin

Approved for use in 1993, fluvastatin (Lescol) is the first entirely synthetic HMG-CoA reductase inhibitor and is structurally distinct from the fungus-derived agents. Its price is half that of the other HMG-CoA reductase inhibitors.

Pharmacodynamics. The agents is this group competitively inhibit 3-hydroxy-3-methylglutaryl-coenzyme A (HMG-CoA) reductase. This enzyme is associated with an early step in the hepatic biosynthesis of cholesterol in the conversion of HMG-CoA to mevalonate. Because the enzyme is not completely inhibited, mevalonate is available in amounts necessary to maintain homeostasis.

Pharmacokinetics. Following oral administration, fluvastatin is 98% absorbed. It may be taken without regard to meals because although its rate of absorption is affected, there are no apparent differences in lipid-lowering effect. It undergoes extensive first-pass hepatic extraction. Absolute bioavailability is 24%. It is 98% bound to plasma proteins. It undergoes biotransformation but does not seem to have any active circulating metabolites. It does not cross the blood-brain barrier. Only 5% is excreted in the urine; about 90% is

excreted in the feces. The drug has a half-life of about 1.2 hours.

Therapeutic Uses. Fluvastatin is used as an adjunct to diet for reducing elevated total and LDL cholesterol levels in clients with primary hyperlipoproteinemia (types IIa and IIb) when the response to diet and other cholesterol-lowering measures has been inadequate.

Dosage and Administration. Fluvastatin is given once a day with the evening meal or at bedtime, primarily because most cholesterol synthesis occurs at night. Starting dosage of 20 mg is increased to 40 mg if needed. Maximal reductions in the LDL should occur after 4 weeks at any given dose. It can be safely administered with cholestyramine or niacin, but it should be taken at least 2 hours after the cholestyramine to avoid drug interaction.

As with other drugs of this class, the client should also be on a therapeutic diet and an appropriate exercise regimen. The treatment will probably last several years, or it may be lifelong.

Adverse Reactions. Adverse reactions include headache, dyspepsia, back pain, and abdominal pain or cramps. Adverse reactions for the major classes of drugs used to combat atherosclerosis are summarized in Table 23-4.

Drug–Drug Interactions. Fluvastatin alters digoxin's pharmacokinetics, increasing the rate of its clearance. The histamine (H_2) antagonists appear to increase the bioavailability of fluvastatin and reduce its clearance. Fluvastatin decreases the bioavailability of rifampin and doubles its clearance.

Drug–Laboratory Test Interactions. Some clients on fluvastatin develop significant and sustained elevations in liver transaminase levels; this also occurs with some other drugs used in treating atherosclerosis.

Precautions and Contraindications. Fluvastatin must be used cautiously in clients with cataracts and impaired liver function. It is contraindicated during pregnancy and lactation and in clients allergic to fluvastatin. Be-

Table 23-3. Pharmacokinetic Profiles of HMG-CoA Reductase Inhibitors

	Fluvastatin	Lovastatin	Simvastatin	Pravastatin
Dose	20–40 mg	20–80 mg	10–40 mg	20–40 mg
Effect of food on absorption	no	yes	no	no
Active plasma metabolites	no	yes	yes	yes
Protein binding	98%	95%	95%	50%
Crosses blood-brain barrier	no	yes	yes	no
Excretion	5% urine 90% feces	10% urine 83% feces	13% urine 60% feces	20% urine 70% feces

Table 23-4. Primary Adverse Effects of Lipid-Lowering Drug Groups

Adverse Reactions	Bile Acid-Sequestering Resins	Nicotinic Acid	HMG-CoA Reductase Inhibitors	Fibric Acid Derivatives
GI				
Constipation	x		x	
Diarrhea	x		x	x
Abdominal pain	x	x	x	
Flatulence	x		x	
Nausea and vomiting	x	x	x	x
Ulcer		x		
CNS				
Headache	x	x	x	
Drowsiness	x			
Insomnia			x	
GU				
Dysuria	x			
Hematuria	x			
CV				
Flushing		x		
Warmth		x		
Urticaria		x		
MS				
Myalgia			x	
Myopathy			x	
Rhabdomyolysis			x	

cause of its possible effect on liver transaminases, liver function tests should be performed before fluvastatin treatment begins, at 6 and 12 weeks, and every 6 months thereafter.

Lovastatin

Pharmacodynamics. Lovastatin (Mevacor) has been the most extensively studied HMG-CoA reductase inhibitor. It was isolated from cultures of *Aspergillus terreus* and was approved for use in 1989. Its mechanism of action was discussed under fluvastatin.

Pharmacokinetics. Lovastatin is 35% absorbed after oral administration. It undergoes extensive first-pass hepatic extraction. Less than 5% of an oral dose reaches the general circulation as active inhibitor. It is 95% bound to plasma proteins. The drug is metabolized in the liver to active metabolites. Only 10% is excreted in the urine; about 83% is excreted in the feces. Peak plasma concentrations are obtained in 2 to 4 hours. It crosses the blood-brain and placental barriers.

Therapeutic Uses. Lovastatin is used as an adjunct to diet for reducing elevated total and LDL cholesterol levels in clients with primary hyperlipoproteinemia (types IIa and IIb) when the response to diet and other cholesterol-lowering measures has been inadequate. It may be useful in diabetic dyslipidemia and nephrotic hyperlipidemia.

Dosage and Administration. Lovastatin is available in 10-, 20-, and 40-mg tablets; the daily dosage is 20 to 80 mg in single or divided doses. Dosage adjustments may be made as necessary every 4 weeks. The maximum dose is 80 mg/day. Peak effect of the drug is achieved in 6 to 8 weeks. If a single daily dose is used, it should be administered with the evening meal because most cholesterol synthesis occurs at night. If lovastatin is taken without food, plasma concentrations of the drug are about two-thirds those reached when the drug is administered immediately after a meal.

As with other drugs of this class, the client should also be on a therapeutic diet and exercise regimen. Treatment will probably last several years, or it may be lifelong.

Adverse Reactions. This drug is generally well tolerated. Insomnia is one adverse reaction. Myalgia has occurred with lovastatin. Some clients have developed a myopathy (eg, myalgia or muscle weakness associated with markedly elevated CPK levels) or rhabdomyolysis. Renal failure can occur secondary to rhabdomyolysis. Most clients who developed myopathy while taking lovastatin were receiving concomitant therapy with cyclosporine, erythromycin, gemfibrozil, or niacin.

Drug–Drug Interactions. Drug interactions have been reported with warfarin, cyclosporine, erythromycin, gemfibrozil, and niacin.

Drug–Laboratory Test Interactions. Marked and persistent increases in aspartate amino transferase (AST, alanine aminotransferase [ALT]), alkaline phosphatase, and bilirubin levels have been noted in some clients taking lovastatin. When the drug was discontinued, transaminase levels usually fell slowly to pretreatment levels. Increases usually appeared 3 to 12 months after starting lovastatin therapy and were not associated with jaundice or other clinical signs or symptoms.

Transient elevated creatine kinase (CK) levels have occurred. As noted above, some clients have developed a myopathy with markedly elevated CPK levels.

Precautions and Contraindications. Lovastatin must be used cautiously in clients with impaired liver function and cataracts because cataracts developed in laboratory animals (not humans) given lovastatin. Because of the possible effect on liver enzymes, liver function tests should be performed before initiating therapy, every 4 to 6 weeks during the first 3 months of therapy, every 6 to 12 weeks during the next 12 months, and then at 6-month intervals. Lovastatin is contraindicated in pregnancy (skeletal malformations have occurred in animals given lovastatin) and lactation, and in clients with known allergy to lovastatin and fungal by-products.

Because of an apparent relation between increased plasma levels of active metabolites of the inhibitor and myopathy, the lovastatin dose should not exceed 20 mg/day in clients on immunosuppressants (Olin, 1995).

Pravastatin

Pharmacodynamics. Pravastatin (Pravachol) was approved for use in 1991. Its mechanism of action is the same as that of fluvastatin.

Pharmacokinetics. Pravastatin is absorbed after oral administration. The presence of food seems to reduce systemic bioavailability, but the lipid-lowering effects are similar whether taken with or before meals; thus, it may be taken without regard to meals. It undergoes extensive first-pass hepatic extraction. Absolute bioavailability is 17%. It is about 50% bound to plasma proteins. About 20% is excreted in the urine, 70% in the feces. The drug has a half-life of about 1.8 to 2.6 hours.

Therapeutic Uses. It is used as an adjunct to diet for reducing elevated total and LDL cholesterol levels in clients with primary hyperlipoproteinemia (types IIa and IIb) when the response to diet and other cholesterol-lowering measures has been inadequate.

Dosage and Administration. Pravastatin is available in 10-, 20-, and 40-mg tablets. The initial dose is 10 to 20 mg once daily at bedtime, with a maximum daily dose of 40 mg. As with other drugs of this class, the client should also be on a therapeutic diet and an appropriate

exercise regimen. The treatment will probably last several years, or it may be lifelong.

Adverse Reactions. This drug is generally well tolerated. Pravastatin does not appear to cause insomnia. Localized musculoskeletal pain, nausea and vomiting, headache, diarrhea, and abdominal pain or cramps have been reported. As with the other drugs in this class, the nurse should be alert to the possibility of myalgia and its related problems, as described above.

Drug Interactions. Warfarin, bile acid sequestrants, and gemfibrozil are interactants. With bile acid sequestrants, a 40% to 50% decrease in pravastatin bioavailability may occur. If the two must be taken concurrently, the pravastatin should be taken 1 hour before or 4 hours after the bile acid sequestrant.

Precautions and Contraindications. Precautions and contraindications are the same as for fluvastatin and lovastatin. Liver transaminase levels should be monitored.

Simvastatin

Pharmacodynamics. Simvastatin (Zocor) was approved for use in 1991. Its mechanism of action is the same as that of fluvastatin.

Pharmacokinetics. Simvastatin is 85% absorbed after oral administration. When simvastatin is given under fasting conditions, the plasma profile is similar to that obtained when it is administered with food, so it may be taken without regard to meals. Simvastatin undergoes extensive first-pass hepatic extraction. Less than 5% of an oral dose reaches the general circulation as active inhibitor. Only 13% is excreted in urine; 60% is excreted in the feces. It is 95% bound to plasma proteins.

Therapeutic Uses. This drug is used as an adjunct to diet for reducing elevated total and LDL cholesterol levels in clients with primary hyperlipoproteinemia (types IIa and IIb) when the response to diet and other cholesterol-lowering measures has been inadequate.

Dosage and Administration. Simvastatin is available as 5-, 10-, 20-, and 40-mg tablets. The initial dose is 5 to 10 mg once daily in the evening. Dose adjustments may be made at intervals of at least 4 weeks. The daily dose should not exceed 40 mg. As with the other drugs in this class, the client should also be on a therapeutic diet and an appropriate exercise regimen. Treatment may be long term or lifelong.

Adverse Reactions. This drug is generally well tolerated. Reported adverse effects include headache, insomnia, abdominal pain and cramps, and constipation. As with the other drugs in this class, the nurse should be alert to the possibility of myalgia and related problems.

Drug–Drug Interactions. Drug interactions have been reported with warfarin (increased bleeding effects) and gemfibrozil (possible myopathy or rhabdomyolysis).

Precautions and Contraindications. Precautions and contraindications are the same as for other drugs in this class.

Bile Acid-Sequestering Resins

Cholestyramine (Questran) and colestipol (Colestid) are anion-exchange resins, called bile acid sequestrants, used as antilipemics. Because these resins are not absorbed from the GI tract, they appear to be the safest antilipemics available.

Cholestyramine and Colestipol

Pharmacodynamics. Bile acid sequestrants bind bile acids in the intestine to form an insoluble complex that is excreted in the feces. The increased fecal loss of bile acids leads the body to try to compensate by increasing the rate of metabolism of cholesterol to bile acids. This leads to increased expression of LDL receptors on liver cells and, consequently, increased removal of LDL from the blood (Rang et al., 1995). The agents either have no effect on or increase triglyceride, VLDL, and HDL levels. The reduction of serum bile acid levels by cholestyramine reduces bile acid depots in the dermal tissues, with a resultant decrease in pruritus.

Pharmacokinetics. Anion-exchange resins are poorly absorbed systemically. They act locally in the GI tract and are excreted in the feces. The fall in LDL concentration is apparent in 4 to 7 days. Treatment with these resins may result in a 20% reduction in LDL. A decline in serum cholesterol is usually evident by 1 month. When the resins are discontinued, the serum cholesterol level usually returns to baseline within 1 month (Olin, 1995).

Therapeutic Uses. Both resins may be used to treat familial hyperlipoproteinemia type IIa or IIb. They are not helpful in clients with elevated concentrations of VLDL and HDL, and they are not used in types I, III, IV, or V hyperlipoproteinemia. Cholestyramine also may be used to relieve pruritus associated with biliary disease. Cholestyramine has been used to treat chlordecone (Kepone) pesticide poisoning. By binding chlordecone in the intestine, it inhibits its enterohepatic recirculation; it then increases its fecal excretion.

Dosage and Administration. Cholestyramine comes in a powder (Questran or Questran Light) or tablets. Colestipol comes in granules or tablets. The usual dosage is 4 to 24 g daily (cholestyramine) or 5 to 30 g daily (colestipol). Usually the total dosage is divided into two doses a day, taken with meals.

To avoid esophageal irritation or obstruction and intestinal obstruction, dry forms (powder or granules) must be mixed with fluids before administration. The preparations have a sandy or gritty quality and may be mixed in soups, cereals, pulpy fruits (eg, applesauce, crushed pineapple), or puréed foods. Colestipol will not dissolve. Colestipol tablets must not be cut, chewed, or crushed.

The lipid-lowering effect of 4 g cholestyramine is equivalent to that of 5 g colestipol.

Adverse Reactions. The most common adverse effects of cholestyramine and colestipol involve the GI tract: constipation, abdominal or rectal pain, distention or bloating, cramping, belching, flatulence, anorexia, nausea, vomiting, diarrhea, heartburn, and steatorrhea. Peptic ulceration, hemorrhoidal bleeding, dental bleeding, dysphagia, sour taste, hiccups, pancreatitis, cholecystitis or cholelithiasis, and diverticulitis have been reported.

Because it liberates chlorides in the GI tract, cholestyramine can cause hyperchloremic acidosis. This condition accelerates urinary calcium excretion and increases the risk of osteoporosis. Other body systems may also be affected. Symptoms of central nervous system involvement include headache, dizziness, anxiety, vertigo, drowsiness, insomnia, fatigue, and weakness. Rash, urticaria, musculoskeletal pain, dysuria, hematuria, and urine with a burnt odor may occur.

Drug–Drug Interactions. Anion-exchange resins are nondiscriminatory in their actions; they bind drugs administered concurrently and nutrients as well as bile acids, leading to decreased intestinal absorption of the drugs or nutrients (Box 23-2). Therefore, other drugs should be taken 1 hour before or 4 hours after the resin.

Drug–Laboratory Test Interactions. Transient and modest elevations of AST, ALT, and alkaline phosphatase levels have been observed. Some clients have an increase in serum phosphorus and chloride levels and a decrease in sodium and potassium levels. In addition, test values may reflect an increased prothrombin time.

Precautions and Contraindications. These drugs should be used with caution in clients with preexisting bowel disease or intractable constipation. Constipation occurs in 10% to 20% of recipients. Fecal impaction may occur as well, and hemorrhoids may be aggravated. Measures should be taken to prevent constipation, especially in clients with coronary artery disease. Clients may need vitamin A, D, K, and folic acid supplements with long-term drug therapy. These drugs are contraindi-

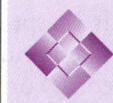

**Box 23-2
Drugs That Bind
With Bile-Sequestering Resins**

Antibiotics (including penicillin, tetracyclines, cephalexin, clindamycin, trimethoprim), anticoagulants, corticosteroids, fat-soluble vitamins (A, D, E, K), iron preparations, thiazide diuretics, chenodiol, digitalis preparations, folic acid, mefenamic acid, phenobarbital, phenylbutazone, thyroxine, thyroid hormone

cated in clients allergic to bile acid sequestrants or tartrazine, in pregnant or lactating clients, and in clients with complete biliary obstruction.

Nicotinic Acid

When administered in very large doses, nicotinic acid (niacin) can lower plasma cholesterol and triglyceride concentrations. Niacin, vitamin B_3, is the common name for nicotinic acid. Nicotinic acid functions in the body as a component of two coenzymes: NAD (nicotinamide adenine dinucleotide, coenzyme I) and NADP (nicotinamide adenine dinucleotide phosphate, coenzyme II), which play roles in the oxidation/reduction reactions essential for tissue respiration. Niacin is widely available as an over-the-counter (OTC) product and is one of the least expensive drugs for managing hyperlipoproteinemias.

Pharmacodynamics. The antilipemic effect of niacin is thought to be derived, in part, from a lowering of the plasma concentration of free fatty acid. Circulating free fatty acid is derived mostly from adipose tissue, and niacin inhibits lipolysis in adipose tissue. Circulating free fatty acid is a main source for synthesis of triglycerides in the liver. Thus, a reduction in free fatty acid can lead to a decrease in triglyceride synthesis.

Niacin decreases the hepatic production of VLDL, which is accompanied by a drop in its metabolic products, intermediate-density lipoproteins and LDL (Patsch & Gotto, 1995). Other actions that may decrease the risk of thrombosis are an increase in tissue plasminogen activator (and thus possibly increased thrombolysis) and a decrease in plasma fibrinogen (Rang et al., 1995). Niacin also reduces levels of Lp[a], whose concentration has a positive relation with coronary heart disease.

Pharmacokinetics. Niacin is a water-soluble vitamin readily absorbed after oral administration. It is metabolized to niacinamide, which is widely distributed in the body and in breast milk. Both unchanged niacin and its metabolites are excreted by the kidneys. About one third of an oral dose is excreted unchanged in the urine. Peak serum concentrations usually occur within 45 minutes, and plasma elimination half-life is about 45 minutes.

Therapeutic Uses. Niacin is considered effective in all types of hyperlipoproteinemia except type I. It is especially useful in type V with clients who do not respond to gemfibrozil (discussed below). It is also used to correct nicotinic acid deficiency and to prevent or treat pellagra.

Dosage and Administration. The recommended daily dietary allowance of niacin is 20 mg. For hyperlipoproteinemia, the dose is 1 to 2 g—three times the daily recommended dose—with a maximum daily dose of 6 g.

Niacin therapy may start with three 100- or 200-mg tablets a day. Over a 1- to 3-week period, additional tablets are added. This slow increase in dosage seems to help decrease difficulties with certain adverse reactions. LDL levels may fall in 5 to 7 days, and the maximal effect occurs in 3 to 5 weeks. The decrease in LDL is greater if niacin is used with a bile acid-sequestering resin.

Niacin is available in many dosage forms, including 25- to 500-mg tablets, sustained-release (SR) tablets and capsules, elixir, and injection. It is usually taken with meals or just after meals. Only two products, Niacor and Nicolar, have been approved by the Food and Drug Administration (FDA) for use in treating hyperlipoproteinemia. All other preparations in the various dosage forms are available as OTC drugs and are not regulated by the FDA.

Adverse Reactions. In the high dosages required for treating hyperlipoproteinemias, niacin has several disadvantages. It causes vasodilatory side effects in almost all clients, particularly when given in an immediate-release dosage form. In clinical trials, about 25% of clients had to stop using niacin because of these symptoms. Although SR forms were recommended to reduce the vasodilatory side effects, they produced GI effects. In addition, several instances of hepatotoxic effects associated with SR niacin were reported (McKenney et al., 1994).

Vasodilatory effects include flushing and a sensation of warmth, especially of the face and upper body. Itching or tingling with headache may also occur. Some experts think the flush response can be decreased by taking a dose of a prostaglandin inhibitor, such as aspirin, at a dose of 325 mg 30 minutes to 1 hour before or 30 minutes after the dose of niacin.

Gastrointestinal reactions include nausea, vomiting, abdominal pain, and diarrhea. Niacin causes histamine release, which increases hydrochloric acid secretion in the stomach. Peptic ulcers have been reported.

Drug–Drug Interactions. Niacin may interact with some antihypertensive drugs to increase postural hypotension. Drug interactions with HMG-CoA reductase inhibitors (myopathy) have been reported as well.

Drug–Laboratory Test Interactions. A substantial increase in liver aminotransferase (more than three times the upper limit of normal) and alkaline phosphatase levels have been noted in clients receiving SR niacin. Apparently these abnormal values return to normal within weeks of niacin discontinuation, although some cases of severe liver dysfunction and fulminant hepatitis have been reported. Decreased glucose tolerance has also been reported.

Precautions and Contraindications. Some niacin products contain tartrazine, which may cause acute asthma attacks in persons with aspirin allergy. Niacin therapy is contraindicated in pregnancy and lactation. Liver function tests should be monitored.

Fibric Acid Derivatives

Gemfibrozil

Fibric acid derivatives (fibrates) used to decrease plasma concentrations of triglycerides and cholesterol include gemfibrozil (Lopid) and clofibrate (Atromid S). Other fibric acid derivatives—fenofibrate, bezafibrate, and ciprofibrate—are used in Europe. The use of clofibrate itself is no longer recommended because of a low risk/benefit ratio (Patsch & Gotto, 1995) and because there is no evidence that it has a beneficial effect on cardiovascular mortality. Clofibrate users have twice the risk of developing cholelithiasis and cholecystitis requiring surgery as do nonusers. The drug increases the secretion of cholesterol into the bile and decreases the hepatic conversion of cholesterol into bile acids, thereby increasing the saturation, or lithogenicity, of bile (Patsch & Gotto, 1995). The increased incidence of gallstone formation and cholecystitis is not associated with gemfibrozil.

Pharmacodynamics. Gemfibrozil decreases serum triglyceride and VLDL levels and increases HDL levels. The mechanisms of action are not fully understood. Gemfibrozil stimulates lipoprotein lipase and thereby increases the hydrolysis of triglycerides in chylomicron and VLDL particles and liberates free fatty acid for storage in fat or metabolism. It also probably reduces hepatic VLDL production and increases hepatic LDL uptake (Rang et al., 1995). Unlike nicotinic acid, fibrates do not consistently lower plasma concentrations of Lp[a]. The desired effects are usually fully evident within 3 or 4 weeks.

Pharmacokinetics. Gemfibrozil is well absorbed from the GI tract. Peak plasma levels occur in 1 to 2 hours. The drug undergoes oxidation to form hydroxy-methyl and carboxyl metabolites. It has a plasma half-life of 1.5 hours. About 70% is excreted in the urine as metabolites, and 6% is excreted in the feces. Gemfibrozil is highly (95%) protein bound.

Therapeutic Uses. Gemfibrozil may be used for clients with types IIb, III, IV, and V hyperlipoproteinemia. Fibrates may be combined with nicotinic acid or bile acid sequestrants; these drugs appear to be additive in lowering LDL and triglyceride levels and in raising HDL levels. When the fibrate is given with the bile acid sequestrant, the administration of the two drugs must be separated by 2 hours to ensure full bioavailability of the fibrate (Patsch & Gotto, 1995).

Dosage and Administration. Gemfibrozil is available in capsule and tablet form. The usual adult dose is 1,200 mg/day in two divided doses, 30 minutes before the morning and evening meals.

Adverse Reactions. Gemfibrozil causes mild to moderate GI irritation, including nausea, vomiting, diarrhea, and dyspepsia, in up to 10% of clients, but these effects usually are transient and tend to decrease or terminate with continued therapy. Myositis may occur, however, particularly if gemfibrozil is combined with lovastatin (see below). Myositis begins as weakness and muscle and joint tenderness.

Drug–Drug Interactions. Combination treatment with fibrate and an HMG-CoA reductase inhibitor is effective in lowering both VLDL and LDL levels and in increasing the HDL level. Unfortunately, the drug combination of gemfibrozil and lovastatin was accompanied by myositis in 3% of clients in one study, enough to discontinue the combination (Glueck et al., 1992). No client had rhabdomyolysis, myoglobinuria, or renal failure, but these complications were reported in other studies. The drug combination must be used with extreme caution, if at all. Interactions have also been reported with oral anticoagulants (increased bleeding effects).

Drug–Laboratory Test Interactions. High CPK levels would be an indicator of the myositis referred to in the gemfibrozil–lovastatin interaction. Mild hemoglobin, hematocrit, and white blood cell decreases have been recorded, but these levels stabilized during long-term administration. Abnormally elevated liver function test values have been reported but usually reverse with drug discontinuation.

Precautions and Contraindications. Contraindications to gemfibrozil therapy include hepatic or renal dysfunction, primary biliary cirrhosis, gallbladder disease, pregnancy, and lactation. Periodic blood counts should be performed during the first 12 months of gemfibrozil administration. Blood glucose levels may fluctuate during long-term therapy and should be monitored.

Miscellaneous Drugs

Other substances known to affect lipid metabolism include neomycin, estrogens, beta-sitosterol, and omega-3 fish oils.

Neomycin

This aminoglycoside antibiotic is largely unabsorbed when taken orally. At a dose of about 1 to 3 g daily, neomycin lowers serum cholesterol by precipitating bile acids and preventing their resorption in the ileum. Hence, its mechanism of action seems to be similar to that of the bile acid-sequestering resins. It can reduce total serum cholesterol levels by 10% to 20%. The potential for nephrotoxicity and ototoxicity exists, however. Diarrhea and malabsorption of nutrients are other possible side effects.

Estrogens

The decrease in natural estrogens during menopause usually leads to increased levels of LDL cholesterol and a rise in cardiovascular risks for the client. As discussed earlier, estrogen replacement therapy in postmenopausal women with high LDL levels may eliminate the need for other drug therapy.

Beta-Sitosterol

Beta-sitosterol is a plant sterol with a structure similar to that of cholesterol. It is not absorbed and its mechanism of action is unknown, but it may inhibit the absorption of dietary cholesterol. It is used only for clients who have excessive LDL levels and who appear extremely sensitive to dietary cholesterol. Adverse effects include a mild laxative effect, nausea, and vomiting. The dose is 6 g (mixed with coffee, tea, fruit juice, or milk to increase palatability) administered 30 minutes before meals and at bedtime.

Omega-3 Fish Oils

The interest in fish oils stems from observations that the Greenland Eskimos, whose diet is rich in seafood, have low levels of plasma triglycerides and little heart disease. The mechanism of action in relation to plasma triglyceride concentration is uncertain, but inhibition of hepatic triglyceride secretion is a possibility.

Fish oils may be beneficial in types IV and V (and possibly III) hyperlipoproteinemia. Fish oil is contraindicated in clients with type IIa hyperlipoproteinemia because of the increase in LDL that it causes (Rang et al., 1995). Fish oil has been used in an attempt to reduce the incidence of pancreatitis (clients with high triglycerides are often labile and may quickly develop very high triglycerides, increasing the risk for pancreatitis).

Fish oils, which are rich in highly unsaturated fatty acids, including eicosapentenoic and docosahexenoic acids, have potentially useful effects, such as inhibition of platelet function, prolongation of bleeding time, antiinflammatory effects, and reduction of plasma fibrinogen. However, in some diabetic clients, carbohydrate metabolism may be further impaired (Patsch & Gotto, 1995).

Fish high in fish oils are mackerel, dogfish, Atlantic salmon, herring, lake trout, and tuna. OTC fish oil products provide the client with little information regarding the source of their contents. Some fish oil preparations are made from fish livers, which can be high in pesticides, heavy metals, and other environmental contaminants. They may contain potentially toxic amounts of the fat-soluble vitamins A and D and even quantities of cholesterol. The manufacture of fish oil capsules is not under FDA control. A dose of 3 g is equivalent to 8 ounces of salmon. A recommended safe dose of fish oil must be determined to prevent deleterious effects (Davis & Sherer, 1994).

■ SUMMARY

Initial treatment for hyperlipoproteinemia involves diet and exercise; drugs are used only when diet and exercise alone are ineffective. Commonly used agents are HMG-CoA reductase inhibitors, bile acid-sequestering resins, nicotinic acid, and fibric acid derivatives (Table 23-5).

❖ NURSING MANAGEMENT: CLIENT RECEIVING A LIPID-LOWERING DRUG

Prevention or management of elevated lipid levels requires a healthful lifestyle, in particular a sound diet and regular exercise. For most clients, the most effective approach is a prudent diet consisting of a variety of foods rich in essential nutrients, adequate in protein, low in cholesterol and saturated fats, and containing enough calories to maintain ideal body weight. Exercise should involve all body muscles without stressing joints or bones; swimming and walking are ideal. Exercise should last 20 to 30 minutes, occur at least three times weekly, and be vigorous enough to stimulate the heart and lungs.

The greater part of nursing management for clients receiving drug therapy for atherosclerosis and hyperlipoproteinemias consists of education about drugs, diet, exercise, and various appropriate lifestyle changes. Clients must understand that:

- Drug therapy is palliative, and certain risks accompany the pharmacologic reduction of lipid levels.
- Drug therapy seldom reverses the effects of poor health practices, nor is it a substitute for a prudent lifestyle that includes a moderate diet and regular exercise.
- Drug treatment for hyperlipoproteinemia may involve multiple agents; for example, clients with contributing illnesses, such as hormone imbalances, are likely to be taking several drugs concurrently, some of which may interact, complicating management of therapy.
- Drugs used to control or lower lipid levels do not correct the faulty metabolism that caused the abnormal blood lipid levels.

Table 23-5. Summarizing the Effects of Lipid-Lowering Drugs

Drug	CHOL	TG	VLDL	LDL	HDL
cholestyramine	↓	→↑	→↑	↓	→↑
colestipol	↓	→↑	↑	↓	→↑
fluvastatin	↓	↓	↓	↓	↑
gemfibrozil	↓	↓	↓	→↓	↑
lovastatin	↓	↓	↓	↓	↑
nicotinic acid	↓	↓	↓	↓	↑
pravastatin	↓	↓	↓	↓	↑
simvastatin	↓	↓	↓	↓	↑

CHOL = cholesterol level; TG = triglycerides; VLDL = very low-density lipoproteins; LDL = low-density lipoproteins; HDL = high-density lipoproteins

NURSING PROCESS

ASSESSMENT

All adults age 20 and older should have an initial serum cholesterol and HDL level baseline screening and a re-evaluation every 5 years thereafter. Clients with abnormal cholesterol and triglyceride values or hyperlipoproteinemia need further assessment to identify other cardiovascular risk factors (see the Critical Thinking Challenge, Part I). Some risk factors are lack of exercise, undue stress, obesity, and disorders such as hypertension, diabetes mellitus, and hypothyroidism. If endocrine disease is detected, serum glucose and thyroid function tests are pertinent.

A complete physical examination of current cardiovascular status is in order as well. The reproductive status of women of childbearing age should be determined.

The drug history should include specific data on the use of alcohol, tobacco, hormones, and cardiovascular drugs. The health history should describe diet and exercise patterns; these are important factors related to both disease and treatment. The interviewer usually explores food choices and methods of preparation, portion sizes, and frequency of consumption.

If drugs are indicated as part of the management plan, the nurse must assess the client's attitude toward their use and determine the impact that drug therapy will have on the client's emotional status and motivation for adherence. By the time drug treatment is considered, clients have usually failed to reduce their blood lipid levels sufficiently by diet and exercise programs, and they may feel discouraged. Some clients see drug therapy as their only hope for controlling a life-threatening condition; others may erroneously view drugs as an alternative to diet and exercise.

The client's knowledge (and that of significant others) about atherosclerosis and its treatment should be assessed.

NURSING DIAGNOSIS

Nursing diagnoses suited to clients for whom lipid-lowering drugs are prescribed include:

- Knowledge Deficit, related to drugs and the self-care regimen required for managing hyperlipoproteinemia
- Ineffective Management of Therapeutic Regimen (Individual), related to dietary restrictions and adverse drug effects
- Risk for Injury, related to possible adverse reactions and drug interactions

Nursing diagnoses vary depending on the medications prescribed. Additional nursing diagnoses that may be appropriate include:

 CRITICAL THINKING CHALLENGE
Case Analysis

Part I

Dr. Jones, age 29, is a faculty member in the Department of Psychology. He has a family history of early and severe cardiovascular disease. His father died of a myocardial infarction at age 39. His older brother is under treatment for hypercholesterolemia. He is married and has 2 sons. He is being treated in the Cardiac Fitness Clinic for hyperlipoproteinemia. The physician has prescribed lovastatin (Mevacor).

In talking with Dr. Jones, you learn that 2 years ago he was warned that his plasma cholesterol level was high. He was treated with nicotinic acid and cholestyramine but these regimens did not lower the level below 260 mg/dL. He tells you, "The men in my family tend to die young. I try to live each day to the fullest because my time may be limited."

1. To promote adherence with the new medication, propose some strategies for convincing Dr. Jones that this drug will work even though two other drugs seem to have failed. For example, how would you explain the differences in the mechanisms of action for lovastatin as compared with those of nicotinic acid and cholestyramine? Explain two more strategies.
2. Prioritize the laboratory data you would want available to study and monitor further. What would you expect the data to reveal, and how would you apply the information to a teaching plan for Dr. Jones?

3. Discuss some obstacles that you may have to overcome in teaching Dr. Jones about his condition and his medication.

Part II

Dr. Jones says he needs some counseling to maximize his use of self-care measures in terms of diet and exercise, because he cannot depend on drug therapy alone to manage his hyperlipoproteinemia. You are preparing a care plan. The chief nursing diagnosis is Knowledge Deficit, related to self-care regimen required for managing hyperlipoproteinemia.

1. Identify at least two broad goals for your nursing care plan.
2. Develop some individualized nursing strategies for the following broad categories of intervention to make your plan meaningful to Dr. Jones:
   - Anticipatory guidance: Propose some lifestyle areas to explore with Dr. Jones in preparing an exercise program. Identify three important areas to investigate. Explain why you think these areas are significant.
   - Learning facilitation: Construct a written exercise plan to provide as a sample reference for Dr. Jones.
   - Family involvement: Which family members would you include in teaching sessions with Dr. Jones? Analyze each family member's role in and potential contribution to Dr. Jones's exercise regimen.

- Constipation, related to adverse drug effects
- Altered Comfort: Cutaneous flush and pruritus related to drug-induced vasodilation
- Altered Nutrition: Less than Body Requirements, related to drug-induced impaired absorption of fat-soluble vitamins

PLANNING

The anticipated outcomes of nursing care include lower serum cholesterol levels, adherence to a prescribed diet and drug regimen, increased knowledge and understanding, and alleviation or elimination of adverse drug effects. In setting goals for dietary therapy, slow, gradual changes are usually more successful than abrupt, disruptive changes. This usually prevents the client from feeling overwhelmed, allows time for adaptation, and contributes to a sense of accomplishment rather than defeat.

INTERVENTION

A team approach to dietary counseling is best. Because of time constraints in most healthcare settings, diet instruction must be condensed. In some instances, follow-up referrals may be made to a dietitian or nutritionist and may be conducted by telephone or during office visits. After initial instruction, a period of at least 6 months of assistance and support from dietary counselor(s), family, and friends is usually needed to achieve the desired dietary changes.

There are two stages involved in motivating the client to take part in diet therapy: personalizing the benefits of change, and raising consciousness and opportunities for thinking about change efforts (Kramer, 1995). Emphasizing the gains to be achieved by changes, rather than the risks associated with not changing, is usually effective.

Because many clients are relatively young, dietary limitations and drug therapy may be poorly accepted if clients still have a great need to conform with their peers. On the other hand, because food preferences are less entrenched in youth, younger clients may adapt to dietary changes more easily than older people. The nurse can help clients integrate the dietary regimen into their daily activities, thereby minimizing its impact on their lifestyles. Both the client and the person who does the shopping and cooking should be involved in this process.

When drug therapy begins, the nurse should evaluate clients for adverse effects characteristic of the drugs prescribed. The client's laboratory data must be monitored as well.

To succeed, interventions must provide the client with encouragement and support, promote self-esteem and self-image, and reinforce the client's positive efforts to adhere to the treatment plan.

Client Education. The client needs materials such as pamphlets, audio cassettes, and videotapes to supplement teaching. These materials should include a record of suggested dietary changes, sample menus, snack suggestions, ideas for eating in restaurants, an exercise

log, and a phone number for a dietitian or nurse who can answer questions about lifestyle changes or drug therapy.

Because the client must reduce total fat, saturated fat, and cholesterol intake, he or she must learn which foods contain these elements (Box 23-3).

To promote exercise, the nurse should focus on convenient exercise alternatives that are accessible in all seasons and enjoyable. Swimming and brisk walking are generally suitable and popular choices (see the Critical Thinking Challenge, Part II).

If the client is taking cholestyramine or colestipol, careful instructions are needed on how to take the specific formulation. This client also must know how to

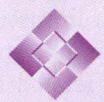

Box 23-3
Fat Facts

- Processed meats, such as bacon, sausage, and hot dogs, contain large amounts of saturated fats (and sodium).
- Ground beef should be extra-lean and drained or rinsed after cooking.
- Step I diets limit consumption of lean meat, poultry, and fish to 5 to 6 ounces daily.
- Step II diets focus on portion sizes. No portion of meat should be larger than a deck of playing cards (equivalent to 3 ounces).
- Healthful cooking methods allow fat to drip away from the meat (broiling, grilling, steaming, poaching). Microwaving and stir-frying in small amounts of oil are also appropriate.
- Saturated fats raise serum cholesterol and LDL levels. They are usually solid at room temperature (eg, lard or butter). They are composed of a chain of carbon atoms that carry the maximum number of hydrogen atoms possible.
- Some foods with high amounts of saturated fats are butter, cheese, cream, whole milk, and ice cream. Highly saturated vegetable oils are coconut, palm, and palm kernel oils, and cocoa butter (in solid chocolate).
- Reading food labels is a good way to identify the highly saturated fats commonly found in nondairy creamers, whipped toppings, processed foods, bakery items, and microwave popcorn.
- Corn, soybean, canola, sunflower, olive, peanut, safflower, and rice bran oils are primarily unsaturated vegetable oils.
- Monounsaturated fats (in olive oil, peanut oil, and canola oil) lower LDL levels but not HDL levels.
- Hydrogenation is the process of adding hydrogen atoms to an unsaturated fat, converting a liquid oil into a solid. Recent research indicates that hydrogenated fatty acids (called trans-fatty acids) raise LDL levels almost as much as cholesterol-raising saturated fatty acids do.

manage constipation by drinking fluids liberally and eating fiber-rich foods.

In addition to preparing and implementing a teaching plan emphasizing the facts and skills needed to achieve maximum effect from the diet, exercise, and drug regimens, the nurse must help clients correct any factors that limited their success with previous diet and exercise regimens. Clients should be referred to sources of additional help—for example, to the American Heart Association for literature and cookbooks featuring foods low in cholesterol and saturated fats.

Because adverse drug effects may impair therapeutic adherence, the client should be informed of the side effects most likely to occur and those that require medical attention. Many adverse effects are transient and tend to subside as treatment continues. In addition, because these drugs have a short history of use, the client should be urged to inform healthcare personnel of any unusual signs and symptoms that may represent an adverse reaction to a specific drug.

Finally, the nurse must convey the idea that the aim of treatment is control. In this respect, using drugs to combat atherosclerosis is similar to using insulin to control diabetes. Therapy is required for a long period, perhaps for life. The client must adjust to living with a chronic condition and incorporate the treatment regimen into a new lifestyle that can be maintained indefinitely.

OUTCOME EVALUATION

Data required for evaluation include client statements reflecting increased self-esteem, reporting the incidence or absence of adverse drug effects, and indicating the ability of the client and significant others to implement the self-care measures recommended.

Changes in total cholesterol and LDL concentrations are the indicators of drug response and effectiveness. A minimal goal is to reduce the LDL cholesterol level to 160 mg/dL or less and the serum cholesterol level to 200 mg/dL or less. Serum lipid and lipoprotein levels should be measured 4 to 6 weeks after treatment begins and every 3 to 6 months thereafter.

❖ CHECKLIST OF NURSING ACTIONS

For each client, assess the risk factors for cardiovascular disease.

❑ Encourage lifestyles that promote cardiovascular health by teaching clients to choose a prudent diet, exercise regularly, avoid smoking and excessive alcohol, and learn to manage stress.

❑ Give emotional support to clients for whom drugs to lower lipid levels are prescribed. Reassure them that the therapeutic regimen can lower plasma levels of harmful cholesterol and LDL.

❑ Refer clients to dietitians or to the American Heart Association for helpful literature and other assistance in adopting the prescribed therapeutic diet.

❑ Help clients integrate the therapeutic regimen into their lifestyles.

❑ Teach clients to recognize the therapeutic and adverse responses to drugs and when to consult the prescriber for modification of the regimen.

Drugs Used to Dissolve Cholesterol-Containing Gallstones

When cholesterol concentrates in bile in levels that exceed the capacity of bile acids and lecithin to dissolve it, crystals can precipitate and coalesce into gallstones. Stones that block bile flow cause severe pain and potential organ damage. Surgical removal by cholecystectomy is the most common and effective treatment for gallstones. Newer nonsurgical techniques, such as shock wave lithotripsy, are increasingly used. Occasionally, drugs may be used in an attempt to dissolve the gallstones if they are composed of cholesterol and not calcified. Two drugs are approved for this therapy: chenodiol (Chenix) and ursodiol (Actigall). Another drug, monoctanoin (Moctanin), is administered via a tube placed endoscopically in the bile duct at the time of surgery or later. The following discussion focuses on chenodiol therapy. Chapter 28 includes further discussion of other drugs that dissolve gallstones.

Chenodiol

Pharmacodynamics. Chenodiol is a naturally occurring bile acid. It blocks hepatic synthesis of cholesterol and cholic acid, thereby reducing biliary cholesterol levels and gradually dissolving gallstones composed of cholesterol.

Pharmacokinetics.
Chenodiol is well absorbed orally but undergoes extensive first-pass hepatic clearance. It is converted in the colon to lithocholic acid, which is largely excreted in the feces; the remainder is absorbed and metabolized in the liver.

Therapeutic Uses. Chenodiol is used for treating gallstones in clients who refuse surgery or whose age or health status makes them unsuitable for surgery.

Dosage and Administration. The usual dose is 250 mg twice a day for 2 weeks. Thereafter, the dose is increased by 250 mg/day each week until the recommended dose of 13 to 16 mg/kg/day or the maximally tolerated dose is reached.

Treatment may be discontinued if no response occurs after 15 to 18 months. In this time the drug should reduce the bile stones so that they are small enough to pass out of the bile ducts spontaneously. The likelihood of stone dissolution decreases as the size and number of stones increase. Up to 50% of clients develop new stones within 5 years of therapy discontinuation. Serial cholecystograms monitor for recurrence. The drug has no apparent effect on calcified gallstones.

Adverse Reactions. Adverse effects include nausea, vomiting, abdominal pain, and diarrhea. In clients unable to form hepatic sulfate conjugates of lithocholic acid, hepatotoxicity can occur.

Drug–Drug Interactions. Interactions have been reported with bile acid-sequestering resins (decreased chenodiol absorption). Aluminum-based antacids may reduce absorption of chenodiol. Estrogens and oral contraceptives may counteract the effectiveness of chenodiol by increasing hepatic secretion of cholesterol.

Drug–Laboratory Test Interactions. Elevated serum cholesterol and HDL levels may occur. Serum cholesterol levels are usually monitored at 4- to 6-month intervals. Elevated liver enzyme levels may also occur.

Precautions and Contraindications. Chenodiol is not used in clients allergic to the drug, those who are pregnant or lactating, or those with bile duct abnormalities. Elevated liver enzyme levels indicate hepatotoxicity. If ALT levels exceed three times the upper limit of normal, chenodiol is discontinued.

References

Arca M, Vega GL, Grundy SM. (1994). Hyperlipoproteinemia in postmenopausal women: Metabolic defects and response to low-dose lovastatin. *JAMA, 271*(6), 453–459.

Copstead LC. (1995). *Perspectives on pathophysiology.* Philadelphia: WB Saunders.

Davis JR, Sherer K. (1994). *Applied nutrition and diet therapy for nurses,* 2d ed. Philadelphia: WB Saunders.

Expert Panel on Detection, Evaluation and Treatment of High Blood Cholesterol in Adults. (1993). Summary of the second report of the National Cholesterol Education Program (NCEP) expert panel on detection, evaluation, and treatment of high blood cholesterol in adults (Adult Treatment Panel II). *JAMA, 269*(23), 3015–3023.

Glueck CJ, Oakes N, Speirs J, Tracy T, Lang J. (1992). Gemfibrozil-lovastatin therapy for primary hyperlipoproteinemias. *Am J Cardiol, 70*(1), 1–9.

Kramer LM. (1995). Implementing new dietary guidelines of the national cholesterol education program. *AACN Clinical Issues, 6*(3), 418–431.

McKenney JM, Proctor JD, Harris S, Chinchili VM. (1994). A comparison of the efficacy and toxic effects of sustained-vs immediate-release niacin in hypercholesterolemic patients. *JAMA, 271*(9), 672–677.

Olin BR (ed). (1995). *Drug facts and comparisons,* 50th ed. St. Louis: Facts and Comparisons.

Patsch W, Gotto AM Jr. (1995). High-density lipoprotein cholesterol, plasma triglyceride, and coronary heart disease: Pathophysiology and management. *Advances in Pharmacology, 32,* 375–426.

Rang HP, Dale MM, Ritter JM, Gardner P. (1995). *Pharmacology.* New York: Churchill-Livingstone.

Bibliography

Anonymous. (1995). Cholesterol screening for adults. *Nurse Practitioner, 20*(6), 66.

Berliner JA, Navab M, Fogelman AM, et al. (1995). Atherosclerosis: Basic mechanisms. *Circulation, 91*(9), 2488–2496.

Castelli WP. (1994). Blood pressure and lipids. *Cardiol Rev, 2*(2), 77–82.

Falk E, Shah PK, Fuster V. (1995). Coronary plaque dysfunction. *Circulation, 92*(3), 657–671.

Fuster V. (1994). Mechanisms leading to myocardial infarction: Insights from studies of vascular biology. *Circulation, 90*(4), 2126–2146.

Gotto AM Jr. (1993). Dyslipidemia and atherosclerosis: A forecast of pharmacological approaches. *Circulation, 87*(Suppl. III), III54–III59.

Hardman JG, Limbird LE, Molinoff PB, et al. (eds). (1996). *Goodman and Gilman's The pharmacological basis of therapeutics,* 9th ed. New York: McGraw-Hill.

Havel RJ, Rapaport E. (1995). Management of primary hyperlipidemia. *N Engl J Med, 332*(22), 1491–1498.

Levine GN, Keaney JF Jr, Vita JA. (1995). Cholesterol reduction in cardiovascular disease. *N Engl J Med, 332*(8), 512–521.

Levy RI, Troendle AJ, Fattu JM. (1993). A quarter-century of drug treatment of dyslipoproteinemia, with a focus on the new HMG-CoA reductase inhibitor fluvastatin. *Circulation, 87*(Suppl. III), III45–III53.

Reece SM. (1995). Toward the prevention of coronary heart disease: Screening of children and adolescents for high blood cholesterol. *Nurse Practitioner, 20*(2), 22.

Scarpa WJ Jr. (1994). New therapy update. *CVRR, 5,* 70.

Singh BN, Dzau VJ, Vanhoutte PM, Woosley RL (eds). *Cardiovascular pharmacology and therapeutics.* New York: Churchill-Livingstone.

For more information and sample tests and activities, refer to Chapter 23 in the Student Workbook for Clinical Pharmacology and Nursing Management, 5th edition, available through your bookstore.

24

Drugs That Affect Circulation

Physiology of the Coronary Vascular System

The blood supply to the heart is provided by the coronary arteries. The major coronary arteries give rise to several smaller branches. The right coronary artery (RCA) originates in the sinus of Valsalva near the aortic valve's anterior cusp. In most people, the RCA gives rise to a posterior descending vessel that supplies blood to the posterior heart. The RCA supplies blood to the right atrium, right ventricle, intraventricular septum, sinus node, atrioventricular node, and bundle of His.

The left coronary artery (LCA) arises near the aortic posterior cusp and soon divides into the anterior descending and circumflex branches. The left anterior descending branch moves blood to the right atrium, the anterior and apex of the left ventricle, the anterior papillary muscles, the right and left bundle branches, and the intraventricular septum. The left circumflex branch supplies the left atrium, the posterior and anterior of left ventricle, and the sinus node (Copstead, 1995). Branching off the major coronary arteries are smaller vessels that penetrate the myocardium and diverge into small arterioles and capillaries. Most of the heart's capillary beds drain into the coronary veins, which then empty into the right atrium through the coronary sinus.

Pathophysiology of Myocardial Ischemia

Ischemia refers to an inadequate supply of oxygen to an organ. Myocardial ischemia covers a group of clinical syndromes, with chronic stable angina at one end of the continuum and acute myocardial infarction (MI) at the other. All the syndromes share an imbalance between myocardial oxygen demand and coronary blood flow. The most frequently recognized primary cause of myocardial ischemia is atherosclerosis of the coronary arteries (see Chap. 23 for a discussion of atherosclerosis).

Fibrous plaques, or atheromas, are the lesions most characteristic of atherosclerosis. They extrude from the intima and are responsible for narrowing the arterial lumen and altering blood flow. When plaque causes the artery to narrow enough to limit blood flow and decrease coronary perfusion during times of increased myocardial workload (eg, physical exertion, emotional strain), ischemia results. Angina pectoris is a disorder characterized by chest pain associated with intermittent periods of myocardial ischemia. Acidosis and other chemical changes in the myocardium initiate impulses of pain that may be felt in the chest or referred to the left shoulder and arm, the throat and chin, or the epigastrium.

Atheromas may also rupture, leading to the formation of a thrombus, an aggregation of platelets, fibrin, and entrapped cellular elements. An occluding thrombus is one that occupies the entire lumen of a vessel and obstructs blood flow. The occlusive thrombosis that follows an atheromatous rupture may be responsible for the manifestations of acute coronary syndromes. They include unstable angina, acute MI, and sudden cardiac death. However, not all ruptured atheromas produce an acute coronary syndrome.

Changes in vasomotor tone in atherosclerotic coronary arteries can contribute to ischemic heart disease. Spasm of a coronary artery may disrupt or cause the rupture of a plaque. Platelet activation may lead to the release of vasoactive chemicals, which may contribute to vasospasm.

The vascular endothelium generates substances that play roles in modulating vasomotor tone. Acetylcholine, bradykinin, and histamine produce coronary vasodilation by binding endothelial receptors that then cause release of endogenous vasodilators. These vasodilators include prostacyclin (PGI_2) and endothelium-derived relaxing factor.

The endothelium also produces a potent vasoconstricting peptide called endothelin-1. A cholesterol-rich diet, thrombin, and other factors lead to increased release of endothelin-1. Under usual conditions, endothelium-derived relaxing factor appears to predominate over endothelin-1. However, in atherosclerosis, vasodilating endothelial functions are impaired and paradoxically become vasoconstricting, leukocyte-adhesive, and prothrombotic (Effat, 1995). Once a thrombus begins forming, platelet activation releases substances, such as thromboxane A_2 and serotonin, that induce further vasoconstriction and platelet aggregation.

Excessive vasodilatation causes neurogenic shock. Local vasospasm contributes to hypoxia in such conditions as transient ischemic attacks. Conversely, compensatory vasoconstriction in response to hypovolemic or cardiogenic shock seriously impairs peripheral circulation while preserving the perfusion of vital organs.

Vasodilators

Drug therapy is prescribed for ischemic heart disease to increase myocardial oxygen supply, decrease myocardial oxygen demand, or both. The major therapeutic drug categories include antiplatelet agents, anticoagulants, nitrates, beta-adrenergic receptor antagonists, calcium channel antagonists, angiotensin-converting enzyme inhibitors, and thrombolytic agents. This chapter is concerned primarily with the action of nitrates and thrombolytic agents, but a brief overview of the other agents is included.

Nitrites and Nitrates

Nitrogenous compounds used as vasodilators in treating angina pectoris include amyl nitrite, erythrityl tetranitrate, nitroglycerin (NTG), isosorbide dinitrate, and pentaerythritol tetranitrate (Tables 24-1 and 24-2). The discovery of NTG for treating angina pectoris dates from 1879. For medicinal use, organic nitrates are generally preferred to nitrites. They act as rapidly and are much more potent.

Pharmacodynamics. Nitrates exert their direct relaxant effect on smooth muscle cells of veins, arteries, and arterioles by first being converted to nitric oxide by metabolic enzymes. In producing nitric oxide, the nitrates interact with sulfhydryl groups. The resultant nitric oxide activates the enzyme guanylate cyclase, which initiates the conversion of guanosine triphosphate to cyclic guanosine monophosphate (cGMP), whose action leads to vasodilation and vessel relaxation (Rutherford, 1995). Few experts agree which enzyme or enzymes convert the nitrate to nitric oxide. Multiple enzymes may account for differences in the pharmacology of the various nitrates (Fung, 1993).

Increased venous capacitance and venodilation of the postcapillary vessels promote peripheral pooling of blood and decrease venous return to the heart. This in turn reduces left ventricular end-diastolic pressure (preload). Reduced preload leads to reduced myocardial oxygen demand. Then, arteriolar relaxation reduces systemic vascular resistance and arterial pressure (afterload). Myocardial oxygen consumption or demand is decreased by both arterial and venous effects of NTG and a more favorable supply/demand ratio is achieved.

When the need for oxygen is reduced below the level supplied by coronary circulation, ischemia is relieved and chest pain subsides.

In coronary circulation, the nitrates redistribute circulating blood along collateral channels, improving perfusion to the ischemic myocardium. Nitrates may also inhibit platelet activation and aggregation, which also may contribute to the antiischemic effects (Clem, 1995). The subendocardium is particularly vulnerable to ischemia, and nitrite and nitrate action favors subendocardial perfusion. Distended ventricles, without nitrate use, mechanically interfere with blood flow in the arteries supplying the subendocardial areas. The diminished preload resulting from nitrate use decreases left ventricular volume. The reduced volume relieves mechanical pressure and allows blood to flow more easily through the subendocardium.

Pharmacokinetics. Nitrites and nitrates are available for sublingual, buccal, oral, dermal, inhalant, and intravenous (IV) use. When given orally, the drugs undergo first-pass metabolism by the liver and are metabolized by nitrate reductase. Some of the metabolites are pharmacologically active, although their potency decreases with each successive loss of a nitrate group. These denitrated metabolites are eliminated more slowly than are their parent compounds. Therefore, they may accumulate sufficiently in the body to contribute to the drug action (Fung, 1993).

Nitroglycerin is readily absorbed through intact skin when applied topically, and ointments and transdermal systems provide a gradual release of the drug that reaches target organs before hepatic inactivation. Nitrites and nitrates are excreted by the kidneys.

Therapeutic Uses. Sublingual, transmucosal, or translingual spray forms of NTG, sublingual isosorbide dinitrate, and inhaled amyl nitrite are used for acute anginal episodes. Because of the more rapid relief of pain with sublingual NTG, sublingual isosorbide dinitrate should be reserved for clients who cannot tolerate or who do not respond to sublingual NTG.

For prophylaxis and long-term management of recurrent angina, topical, transdermal, translingual spray, transmucosal, and oral sustained-release forms of NTG may be used, as well as forms of isosorbide dinitrate, isosorbide mononitrate, erythrityl tetranitrate, pentaerythritol tetranitrate. IV NTG may be used to control blood pressure in perioperative hypertension associated with surgery, especially cardiovascular procedures. It also may be used for clients with congestive heart failure associated with acute MI and angina pectoris unresponsive to other agents. It may be used to produce controlled hypotension during surgical procedures.

Topical NTG (2%) ointment may be used to dilate peripheral veins to facilitate venous access (Griffith et al., 1994).

Table 24-1. Nitrites and Nitrates

Drug Name	Preparations	Usual Dosage	Onset	Duration
amyl nitrite (Amyl Nitrate Aspirols, Amyl Nitrate Vaporole)	Inhalant	0.18–0.3 mL as needed	30 sec	3–5 min
nitroglycerin	IV	5 mcg/min & increase by 5–10 mcg/min q5–10 min to desired response	1–2 min	3–5 min
	Sublingual	0.15–0.6 mg prn at 3- to 5-min intervals	1–3 min	30–60 min
	Translingual spray	0.4–0.8 mg metered spray; 1 or 2 sprays under tongue & repeat at 3- to 5-min intervals prn	2 min	30–60 min
	Transmucosal tablet	1 mg q3–5hr	1–2 min	3–5 hr
	Oral, sustained-release	1.3–9 mg PO bid or tid	20–45 min	3–8 hr
	Topical ointment	15–30 mg tid or bid	30–60 min	2–12 hr
	Transdermal	0.1–0.6 mg/hr	30–60 min	up to 24 hr
isosorbide dinitrate (Iso-Bid, Isordil, Isoket, Isosorb, Sorbitrate, Sorbitrate SA)	Sublingual	2.5–10 mg q2–3h prn	2–5 min	1–3 hr
	Chewable	5–10 mg q2–3hr		
	Oral	5–30 mg qid	20–40 min	4–6 hr
	Oral, sustained-release	40 mg q8–12hr	up to 4 hr	6–8 hr
isosorbide mononitrate (Monoket, ISMO, Imdur)	Oral	20 mg bid, 7 hr apart	30–60 min	no data
	Oral extended-release tablets	30–60 mg qd in morning		
erythrityl tetranitrate (Cardilate, Coronex, Dilatrate)	Sublingual	5–10 mg	5 min	3 hr
	Oral	10 mg tid ac with additional doses as needed up to 100 mg qd	15–30 min	6 hr
pentaerythritol tetranitrate (Desatrate, Myocardol, Naptrate, Neo-Corvas, Nitrin, Pentraspan, Peritrate SA, Vasolate)	Oral	10–40 mg qid	20–60 min	5 hr
	Oral extended-release tablets, capsules	30–80 mg q12hr	30 min	up to 12 hr

In addition to their use in the treatment of angina pectoris, nitrites and nitrates are also prescribed to relieve paroxysmal nocturnal dyspnea, esophageal spasm, and biliary colic. They may be helpful in ureteral colic and bronchial asthma. Amyl nitrate is used as an adjunct in the treatment of cyanide poisoning.

When administered IV concurrently with packed red blood cells, NTG reduces the risk of excessive preload and pulmonary edema secondary to the increased blood volume. This technique permits transfusions in clients with congestive heart failure.

Unlabeled uses of NTG ointment include adjunctive treatment of Raynaud's disease and other peripheral vascular diseases.

Dosage and Administration. Dosages are reviewed in Tables 24-1 and 24-2. With IV NTG, dosage typically starts at 5 µg/min and increases by 5 to 10 µg/min every 5 to 10 minutes until the desired response occurs.

Adverse Reactions. The adverse effects associated with nitrate preparations are predictable extensions of their pharmacologic effects. Dilation of cutaneous vessels causes flushing. Drug-induced dilation of cerebral blood vessels and vascular congestion there apparently is responsible for the throbbing headaches. Venous pooling can cause ankle edema.

A moderate but persistent vasodilation may reduce perfusion in some areas of the body or interfere with the normal compensatory vasoconstriction that maintains cerebral circulation in the upright position. This produces orthostatic or postural hypotension, which is characterized by weakness, dizziness, and fainting with sudden changes in position. Reduced blood pressure in the aortic and carotid sinuses may trigger reflex tachycardia.

Headache may be a transient effect, and the loss of headache may reflect nitrate tolerance (see p. 466). Acetaminophen may be used for relief. Headaches provoked by nitrates recur after a period of nitrate abstinence.

Sublingual NTG tablets may cause a local burning or tingling sensation in the oral cavity, and for years this was considered an indication of the drug's "freshness." This effect is not a reliable indicator of freshness, however, and some older clients may not experience this effect even with new NTG tablets.

Table 24-2. Nitroglycerin: Preparations and Dosages

Preparations	Usual Dosage
To Manage Chronic Angina Pectoris	
Sustained-release tablets (Nitrong)	2.6 mg tid or qid, titrated upward until side effects limit dose; maximum 26 mg qid
Sustained-release capsules (Nitro-Bid Plateau Caps, Nitrocine Timecaps, Nitroglyn)	2.5 mg tid or qid, titrated upward until side effects limit dose; maximum 26 mg qid
Controlled-release buccal tablets (Nitrogard)	1 mg q3–5h during waking hours
Transdermal systems (Minitran, Nitro-Dur, Transderm-Nitro, Nitroglycerin Transdermal, Nitrosdisc, Deponit)	0.2–0.4 mg/hr; patch-on period of 12–14 hr and patch-off period of 10–12 hr
Topical ointment (Nitro-Bid, Nitrol)	0.5 inch (12.5 mm/7.5 mg nitroglycerin) q8h; increase by 0.5 inch with each application to achieve desired effects
To Relieve Acute Attack or Prophylaxis Before Stressful Activity	
Sublingual tablets (Nitrostat)	0.15 mg/L/400 gr–0.6 mg/L/100 gr dissolved under tongue or in buccal pouch (between cheek and gum) at first sign of an acute attack; repeat q5 min until relief. Take no more than 3 tablets in 15 min; if pain continues, notify physician.
	May be used prophylactically before activities that may precipitate attack.
Translingual spray (Nitrolingual)	At onset of attack, spray 1 or 2 metered doses onto or under tongue, no more than 3 metered doses within 15 min. If pain continues, notify physician.
	May be used prophylactically before activities that may precipitate attack.
Emergency Relief of Acute Attack	
IV infusion (Tridil, Nitro-Bid IV, Nitroglycerin in 5% Dextrose)	5 mcg/min via an infusion pump. Titrate to situation in 5-mcg/min increments with increases q3–5 min until response is noted. If no response occurs at 20 mcg/min, use increments of 10–20 mcg/min; titrate carefully and monitor closely; no fixed optimal dose.

Other adverse effects include a rash (seen more with pentaerythritol tetranitrate and topical NTG). Contact dermatitis from transdermal NTG preparations may occur. The transdermal delivery system itself, not the NTG, may be responsible. NTG ointment may, however, cause topical allergic reactions.

Methemoglobinemia is rare. Formation of methemoglobin is dose-related. In genetic hemoglobin abnormalities that favor methemoglobin formation, even conventional doses of nitrates may produce harmful concentrations of methemoglobin. Tissue hypoxia due to methemoglobinemia can lead to cyanosis, metabolic acidosis, coma, convulsions, and death from cardiovascular collapse. Infants can be poisoned by relatively small amounts of nitrates. Poisoning may result from accidental ingestion, explosive powders, or well water with a high nitrate content. Use of water high in nitrates for home dialysis may cause toxic methemoglobinemia.

Intravenous NTG contains substantial amounts of ethanol as a diluent. When high doses are used, ethanol intoxication may develop.

Tolerance. Evidence indicates that partial or complete tolerance develops in clients treated with nitrates. Tolerance is the attenuation or loss of one or several of the effects of the nitrates. Industrial exposure to organic nitrates induces both tolerance and physical dependence, and withdrawal from contact with the substance has been reported to produce severe myocardial isch-

emia and pain, MI, or sudden death. It is not known what mechanisms are responsible for nitrate tolerance, but some experts suspect neurohormonal activation of plasma volume expansion and depletion of intracellular sulfhydryl cofactors (Fung, 1993). The occurrence of tolerance is somewhat variable and unpredictable and may be related to the size of dose, the dosing interval, and the duration of action of the preparation.

Strategies aimed at avoiding tolerance include using shorter-acting nitrates at the smallest effective doses (at lower doses, organic nitrates may not activate neurohormonal mechanisms), administering fewer daily doses, and allowing a nitrate-free interval (eg, a 10- to 12-hour nitrate-free interval during each 24-hour period), which may regenerate nitrate sensitivity the following day. The period may correspond to the time required for the regeneration of the sulfhydryl cofactor needed for the metabolic activation, or for neurohormonal compensatory mechanisms to dissipate. For example, a dosing regimen for isosorbide dinitrate of morning, noon, and mid-afternoon doses may be used, or a transdermal NTG regimen could feature a 12-hour patch-free interval (applied in the morning and removed in the evening). Throughout the nitrate-free interval, sublingual or buccal NTG may be administered if needed. See Focus On Nitrites and Nitrates: Similarities and Differences.

Drug Interactions. Drug interactions have been reported between nitrates and alcohol, aspirin, calcium channel blockers, and ergot derivatives (eg, dihydroergotamine) and between NTG and heparin. With the calcium channel blockers, marked symptomatic orthostatic hypotension may occur, and dosage adjustment of either of the agents is often necessary. With heparin, the pharmacologic effect of nitrates may be decreased.

Precautions and Contraindications. Nitrates are contraindicated in clients with allergy to nitrates, severe anemia, acute MI, cerebral hemorrhage or head trauma, or hypertrophic cardiomyopathy, and in pregnant or lactating clients. Nitrates must be used cautiously in

FOCUS ON

Focus on Nitrites and Nitrates: Similarities and Differences

Similarities	Differences
Pharmacodynamics	
These agents directly relax vascular smooth muscle. They produce vasodilation and reduce myocardial oxygen demand. Preload and afterload are reduced.	
Pharmacokinetics	
These agents are available for sublingual, buccal, oral, dermal, inhalant, and IV use. They are metabolized by the liver and excreted by the kidneys.	• The only inhalant is **amyl nitrate**. It has been abused for sexual stimulation. The effect of inhalation is almost instantaneous, causing lightheadedness, dizziness, and euphoria.
	• **Isosorbide dinitrate** comes in sublingual, chewable, oral tablets, sustained-release tablets, and sustained-release capsules.
	• **Isosorbide mononitrate** comes in tablets and extended-release tablets.
	• **Erythrityl tetranitrate** is available as oral or sublingual tablets.
	• **Pentaerythritol tetranitrate** is available as tablets, sustained-release tablets, and sustained-release capsules.
	• **Nitroglycerin** is available in these forms: IV, sublingual, translingual spray, transmucosal buccal controlled-release tablet, sustained-release tablet and capsule, topical ointment, and transdermal systems.
Therapeutic Uses	
These agents are used for acute anginal episodes and for prophylaxis and long-term management of recurrent angina.	• **IV nitroglycerin** may be used for control of blood pressure in certain situations. The topical ointment form may be used topically to dilate peripheral veins to facilitate venous access. It has been used as adjunctive treatment of Raynaud's disease and other peripheral vascular diseases.
	• **Amyl nitrate** is used as an adjunct in the treatment of cyanide poisoning.
Adverse Reactions	
These include flushing, throbbing headaches, ankle edema, orthostatic/postural hypotension characterized by weakness, dizziness, and fainting, reflex tachycardia.	• **IV nitroglycerin** may cause ethanol intoxication at high doses. Transdermal systems may cause contact dermatitis (the system, not the nitroglycerin). Topical ointment may cause topical allergic reactions. Sublingual nitroglycerin tablets may cause local burning or tingling in oral cavity.
Drug Interactions	
Drug interactions have been reported between nitrates and alcohol, aspirin, calcium channel blockers, ergot derivatives, and heparin.	
Precautions and Contraindications	
These include hypersensitivity to nitrates, severe anemia, closed-angle glaucoma.	• **Amyl nitrate** is contraindicated in pregnancy.
	• **IV nitroglycerin** is contraindicated in hypotension or uncorrected hypovolemia, increased intracranial pressure, constrictive pericarditis, and pericardial tamponade. Transdermal systems can be contraindicated with allergy to adhesives.

(continued)

FOCUS ON

Focus on Nitrites and Nitrates: Similarities and Differences (continued)

Similarities (continued)

Nursing Considerations

Assess cardiopulmonary status at baseline and regularly for evaluation of response to nitrate therapy. Assess complaints of chest pain and any factors associated with it, such as associated activities. Institute measures to relieve headaches, such as cool compresses, rest, and mild analgesics.

Instruct client in disease, drug therapy regimen, storage precautions, techniques for proper administration of specific drug form, and adverse effects. Instruct as to safety precautions associated with orthostatic/postural hypotension. Instruct client not to discontinue drug abruptly. Instruct client to avoid alcohol when taking drug.

Differences (continued)

• When using **IV nitroglycerin,** dilute as instructed and use special infusion sets. No other drug should be administered in the same solution or via the same tubing. Apply transdermal systems at same time each day after removal of old patch, and rotate sites of application, using clean, dry, hairless skin of chest or upper extremities free from cuts, scratches, or irritation. Avoid skin contact with topical ointment and wash hands thoroughly after administering.

---

clients with hypotension or hypovolemia, hepatic or renal dysfunction, and some types of heart disease (eg, constrictive pericarditis, pericardial tamponade).

▪▪ SUMMARY

Nitrites and nitrates are vasodilators used for treating angina pectoris. Their mechanisms of action reduce preload and afterload and lead to reduced myocardial oxygen demand. Adverse effects include headache, hypotension, and some degree of tolerance. Varying drug regimens are used to try to decrease the anticipated tolerance.

❖ NURSING MANAGEMENT: CLIENT RECEIVING NITRITES AND NITRATES

Clients receiving treatment for angina pectoris generally have coronary artery atherosclerosis, which reduces the blood flow to the myocardium below the level required for optimal function. Ischemia and chest pain develop when the myocardium's need for oxygen exceeds the capacity of the coronary circulation to deliver it. Pain occurs at first only with extreme exertion, but as the process progresses, less-strenuous activity precipitates discomfort. In the final stages of coronary artery disease, oxygen supplies to the myocardium are so low that even minimal work by the heart results in exhaustion and constant pain, even during rest.

Use of nitrate vasodilators may improve the client's quality of life by alleviating pain and increasing tolerance to exercise. Therapy is often initiated with sublingual NTG tablets to be taken as necessary to terminate a pain episode. Use of these tablets before exertion may prevent pain. Later, the drug regimen usually includes a transdermal preparation of nitrate or a sustained-release form of ni-

trate. Because nitrates may cause severe adverse effects and possibly tolerance, clients need considerable assistance in managing their medication regimens for optimal benefit.

NURSING PROCESS

ASSESSMENT

Data required for the initial assessment of clients receiving nitrates include a complete assessment of cardiovascular status. Specific information should reflect activities that cause anginal pain and whether rest relieves the pain. The nurse should determine the client's knowledge of coronary artery disease, attitude toward drug use, and goals for therapy.

NURSING DIAGNOSIS

Some nursing diagnoses related to drug therapy for coronary artery disease include:

• Pain: Headache related to vasodilation
• Altered Tissue Perfusion: Impaired cerebral perfusion related to postural hypotension secondary to use of NTG

Many clients have:

• Knowledge Deficit, related to lack of exposure to nitrate vasodilators and their use

Nursing diagnoses related to the disease process include:

• Activity Intolerance: Chest pain on exertion related to imbalance between oxygen supply and demand secondary to coronary artery disease

PLANNING

The goals and outcomes of nursing care are to alleviate or eliminate chest pain, increase activity tolerance, prevent or alleviate adverse drug effects (eg, headache, postural hypotension, tolerance), and reduce knowledge deficits (see the Critical Thinking Challenge).

INTERVENTION

The dosage and timing of NTG medication vary considerably, depending on the route of administration and the drug. Relatively small doses are required for sublingual administration. When administered by this route, NTG has an onset of action within 3 minutes and duration up to 60 minutes. If a single dose is ineffective, it may be repeated after 5 minutes. No more than three doses should be taken for any one episode, because pain not relieved by three doses may result from MI rather than ischemia. At such times, prompt medical treatment is vital.

Nitroglycerin is most effective in controlling angina when it is administered immediately after the onset of pain. For this reason, even in acute care settings, NTG is usually kept in the client's possession and is self-administered. For proper assessment of the client, the amount of drug used must be monitored and recorded. A record may be kept by the client, or the nurse may place a limited supply of the drug at the bedside, noting the number of tablets used and replacing them periodically.

Transdermal preparations include ointment and skin patches. Because clients usually must manage ointment or patch therapy at home by themselves, most of the information about their use is included in the section on client education. Each system has a different mechanism of drug delivery, and systems should not be considered interchangeable. For example, Nitrodisc contains NTG mixed in a solid polymer similar to silicone. The drug is absorbed through the skin from the polymer, which also contains a cosolvent to enhance skin penetration. On the other hand, in the Transderm-Nitro system, a semipermeable membrane between the drug and the skin is the controlling factor for drug delivery.

A transdermal drug penetrates the outer layers of the epidermis by passive diffusion at a constant rate; then it is absorbed into the circulation. The patches are regulated by a concentration gradient—in other words, a high concentration of drug in the patch forces the drug to the skin, where it is not as concentrated.

The old patch must always be removed immediately before applying the new one. Patches should be applied at the same time each day. The nurse should document the time of administration, drug, dose, and application site in the medication record. The date and time should also be written on the patch: if the patch falls off, checking the label will reveal whether the patch can be reapplied or replaced. This ensures that the client does not receive too much or too little drug.

Emergencies and Intravenous Drug Delivery. In an emergency, the nurse must remove any transdermal NTG applied to a client's chest because a cardioverter, or defibrillator, should not be discharged through a paddle electrode that overlies a transdermal NTG system. Aluminum on transdermal patches can cause smok-

CRITICAL THINKING CHALLENGE
Case Analysis

Dr. Jones, age 29, is the client you met in Chapter 23. He has a family history of early and severe cardiovascular disease. He has been receiving lovastatin (Mevacor) for a few months, and in the last month his cholesterol level has decreased. However, he has experienced episodes of chest pain on exertion, and the last episode led to hospital admission. The physician ruled out myocardial infarction but established a diagnosis of angina pectoris and prescribed both sublingual nitroglycerin prn and isosorbide dinitrate (Isordil Titradose) 10 mg tid.

1. What nursing diagnoses would you establish for Dr. Jones?
2. Develop at least two broad goals for each nursing diagnosis.
3. Clients taking nitrates on a regular basis can develop tolerance. How would you explain tolerance to this well-educated client?
4. How would you schedule the isosorbide dinitrate to promote a nitrate-free interval each day for Dr. Jones?

ing and electrical arcing during defibrillation, producing thermal burns.

Intravenous NTG may be used perioperatively or during critical care. It is diluted in 5% dextrose in water or in normal saline solution and not used for direct IV injection without dilution. No other drug should be administered in the same solution or through the same tubing. Glass bottles hold the NTG solution, and special infusion sets are used because NTG may be adsorbed by the polyvinyl chloride IV tubing in general use.

Some possible related problems include greater adsorption occurring with low flow rates, high concentrations, and long tubing. In addition, some filters in the administration sets absorb NTG; some infusion controllers may not work well with the special infusion set (ie, the special tubing tends to be less pliable than conventional tubing). Excessive flow at low infusion rate settings may result, causing alarms or unregulated gravity flow when the infusion pump is stopped. Infusion pumps should be pretested with the infusion set. During IV administration, the nurse monitors blood pressure and heart rate constantly, and often records other measurements such as pulmonary capillary wedge pressure. As the client responds, the dose can be reduced. The client then must be weaned from IV NTG by decreasing the IV dose 5 to 10 mcg every 15 minutes. Even with weaning, adverse reactions may occur up to an hour after drug discontinuation.

Management of Adverse Effects. The throbbing headache induced by nitrates tends to subside if the drug is used on a regular basis. Applying cold compresses to the head and helping the client rest in a quiet environment may help relieve discomfort. Mild analgesics (eg, acetaminophen) may be administered to reduce headache pain as well. The client should be encouraged to continue using the drug for an adequate trial period to see if tolerance (with reduced headache) develops.

Nitrates reduce blood pressure and can cause dizziness, fainting, and weakness. If these symptoms are troublesome, helping the client to rest in a recumbent position may provide relief. Vital signs should be monitored. To reduce the risk of falls, the client may need assistance when ambulating. If the client is susceptible to shock from some other medical condition, an alternative treatment for the angina (oxygen and rest) may be used in preference to the drug.

Client Education. The nurse must prepare and implement a teaching plan about nitrate drugs and must help the client manage the drug regimen effectively. Because clients usually control and manage NTG therapy themselves, they must receive complete information about the drug. Clients who experience adverse effects must know how to cope with them. For example, clients experiencing postural hypotension should be taught to move and change position slowly and to avoid alcohol, which tends to intensify the reaction. They also must report adverse effects to the healthcare provider.

Proper drug storage and administration techniques should be carefully explained. Because NTG is sensitive to air, light, heat, and moisture, it requires special handling and storage to preserve its effectiveness (see Home and Community Care: Guidelines for Nitroglycerin).

The client should be informed, as appropriate, that several transdermal NTG systems (patches) are available (eg, Transderm-Nitro, Nitro-Dur, Nitrodisc, Deponit, Minitran). Release rates vary from 0.1 to 0.6 mg/hour, and product differences include ease of application and removal, adhesiveness, comfort, size, and appearance. Each system has a different mechanism of drug delivery, so systems should not be considered interchangeable.

Because the drug and the patches are somewhat irritating, the client should rotate the sites of application and learn to recognize excessive skin irritation. Redness and itching at the old patch site are fairly common. Irritated skin should be exposed to air if possible, and the client should be urged to avoid scratching.

The client must know that the aluminum in skin patch medications can contribute to accidental burns. Exposed to microwaves, ultrasound, or electrical currents, metal becomes hot. Microwave ovens in good repair do not pose a significant hazard, but second-degree burns have resulted from exposure to a leaky unit.

The client should not stop using the drug abruptly. Weaning is recommended to prevent rebound symptoms.

The client should use sublingual NTG before beginning activities that precipitate anginal episodes. Helping the client plan regular activity may be desirable to keep him or her relatively active, a factor in developing collateral circulation in the myocardium. Of course, the kinds and frequency of activities must be appropriate to the severity of coronary artery disease. The client who cannot walk without chest pain will not be able to undertake strenuous activities simply by using NTG.

Transdermal or sustained-release products have very different onsets and durations of actions than sublingual NTG, and they cannot reliably stop or prevent an anginal attack. This limitation must be stressed to the client, who should always have available an immediate-acting (sublingual) dosage form.

OUTCOME EVALUATION

Data required for evaluation include statements by the client that physical activity has increased, that anginal pain has subsided or disappeared, and that headache and postural hypotension have decreased or disappeared. Another measure is evidence that the client is correctly managing the drug regimen, such as a decrease in blood pressure and pill counts indicating that all the prescribed medicine is taken. See Example of Nursing Process for Nitroglycerin Therapy. Physical data required for evaluation are based on the baseline blood pressure and heart rate assessed before NTG therapy and after the client has been at rest for 10 minutes. Vital signs should be taken again 1 hour after drug administration. An appropriate dosage produces a blood-pressure drop of 10 mmHg with the client in a resting position.

❖ CHECKLIST OF NURSING ACTIONS

When Nitroglycerin is Prescribed for Angina Pectoris

- ❏ Instruct clients to allow sublingual tablets to dissolve under the tongue.
- ❏ Monitor the number of sublingual tablets used and the client's response to them.
- ❏ Instruct clients in proper storage of the medication.
- ❏ Instruct clients to replace their supply of sublingual tablets every 3 months.
- ❏ Instruct clients to rotate the site used for transdermal preparations.
- ❏ Administer analgesics to relieve headache when it occurs.
- ❏ Instruct the client to rest quietly when headache or faintness occurs after medication administration.
- ❏ Encourage clients to continue the therapeutic regimen until tolerance to the drug's adverse effects develops.
- ❏ Help the client manage the drug regimen for optimal therapeutic effect, including maintenance of normal lifestyle.

Other Agents Used to Treat Ischemic Heart Disease

Other drug categories used in the pharmacotherapy of ischemic heart disease include antiplatelet agents, anticoagulants, beta-adrenergic blocking agents, calcium

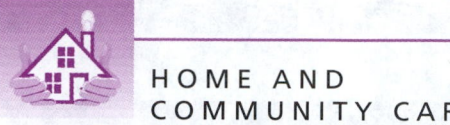

HOME AND COMMUNITY CARE

Guidelines for Nitroglycerin

Most clients self-manage their nitroglycerin regimen. Clients new to the medication may benefit from these guidelines for safe use and storage.

Sublingual Tablets

- Because moisture helps sublingual tablets dissolve, drink fluid before placing sublingual nitroglycerine under the tongue.
- If a single dose is ineffective, repeat the dose after 5 minutes.
- If a buccal tablet is used, hot drinks help dissolve it after placing it between the gum and cheek or upper lip.
- Do not take more than three doses for an episode of pain. If the pain continues after three doses, seek prompt medical care.
- Store tablets in their original container—a small brown glass bottle with metal screw cap. Do not transfer them to any other container because they may rapidly lose potency in metal, plastic, or cardboard boxes. Because the drug is volatile, remove any cotton, paper, or other material that could absorb the vapors.
- Protect nitroglycerin from body heat. Avoid carrying it in pockets of close-fitting garments.
- Keep the drug away from small children, who are highly susceptible to nitrate poisoning.
- Keep the medication in a dry, dark place—not a bathroom cabinet or a refrigerator.
- Despite these precautions, nitroglycerin deteriorates over time. Discard tablets 3 months after the container seal is broken.

Translingual Sprays

- Administer the translingual spray directly onto the oral mucosa; preparation is not to be inhaled. The spray delivers 0.4 mg/metered dose. At onset of attack spray one or two metered doses onto the oral mucosa. No more than 3 doses/15 min should be used. If pain persists, seek medical attention. The spray may be used prophylactically 5 to 10 minutes before activity that might precipitate an attack.
- Nitroglycerin sprays may have a 3-year storage life at room temperature, but they must be stored away from excessive heat.

Oral Tablets

- Take an oral nitrate tablet on an empty stomach with a glass of water.
- Do not crush or chew a sustained-release tablet, because doing so may produce an undesired effect.

Topical Preparations

- Apply ointment or patch to clean, dry, hairless skin of the chest or upper arm. The skin should not have scratches, cuts, or other irritations. If necessary, clip hair with scissors (not a razor, because shaving affects the skin and lets the drug penetrate too quickly).
- Before a new dose is applied, wash the old site with soap and water to remove any drug residues. Select a new site for the new dose. Rotating application sites prevents skin inflammation and irritation.
- Avoid applying the medication to skin folds or areas lower than the elbow. Also avoid areas that you move frequently, because frequent motion increases circulation and drug absorption.
- Always remove the old patch right before applying a new one.
- Apply patches at the same time each day.
- Protect the patch and check to be sure it is intact after showering, perspiring, or swimming.
- Discard old patches carefully because leftover nitroglycerin may be hazardous to children or pets. Fold the patch in half with sticky sides touching, and place in a foil pouch for disposal.
- If using ointment (Nitroglycerin, Nitro-Bid, Nitrol) from tubes, measure the prescribed amount onto the special dose-measuring paper. Fold the paper to spread the ointment evenly in a thin layer. Unfold the paper and place it on the skin. Tape the borders of the patch to the skin with paper tape. Do not rub in the ointment because rapid absorption will interfere with the desired action.
- Do not store ointment tubes near toothpaste or other medications in tubes. Nitroglycerin mistaken for and used as toothpaste or other dental products can cause problems.

channel antagonists, angiotensin-converting enzyme inhibitors, and thrombolytic agents.

Antiplatelet Agents

Major antiplatelet agents include aspirin (discussed in detail in Chap. 36) and ticlopidine. With ischemic heart disease, aspirin has been effective in reducing the mortal-ity associated with stable or unstable angina, acute MI, and coronary artery bypass grafting and angioplasty. Its antiplatelet effects result from its inhibitory effect in formation of thromboxane A_2, which causes platelet aggregation. The antiplatelet effects last for the life of the platelet (7–10 days). Because of the rapid turnover of platelets, platelet function returns to normal about 7

Example of Nursing Process for Nitroglycerin Therapy

The client is a 58-year-old man with a 3-year history of angina pectoris, which has been fairly well controlled until recently with sublingual nitroglycerin medication. Lately, because he has needed medication more often, he has returned to the physician for further assistance. The physician has prescribed Nitro-Dur, one patch worn for 12 hours daily.

Assessment Data
Nitro-Dur therapy

Nursing Diagnosis	Intervention	Goals and Outcome Criteria
Potential complication: Impaired Skin Integrity	**Advise** the client and family that medical identification bracelet should be worn to alert emergency personnel to use of Nitro-Dur (must be removed if defibrillation is necessary to avoid burn injury).	The client will not sustain burn injury related to the patch.
	Advise client to rotate sites of patch application.	The client will not develop evidence of skin disruption such as erythema and pruritus.
	Advise client to wash site of previous dose with soap and water to remove drug residues.	
Risk for Injury to others, related to contact with the patch	**Teach** the client to apply the patch to a clean, dry, hairless skin area of chest or upper extremities that is not subject to any friction that could dislodge the patch.	Others will not be medicated by the patch.
	Teach client to check that patch is intact after showering, heavy perspiration, or swimming.	
	Teach client to dispose of patch correctly when it is removed by folding it in half with the sticky sides touching and placing it in its foil pouch for disposal.	

days after aspirin therapy is discontinued. The recommended doses of aspirin for cardiovascular disorders range from 80 to 325 mg daily. The dosages of aspirin most frequently used in the United States are 81, 162, and 325 mg (Clem, 1995).

Ticlopidine (Ticlid) is another antiplatelet agent used. Dipyridamole (Persantine) was used in coronary artery disease in the past for antiplatelet purposes, but today it is used only in clients with prosthetic heart valves.

Ticlopidine inhibits platelet aggregation and release of platelet granule constituents. It interferes with platelet membrane function by inhibiting platelet–fibrinogen binding induced by adenosine diphosphate and subsequent platelet–platelet interactions. The effect on platelet function is irreversible for the life of the platelet. In clients who have a documented aspirin allergy, 250 mg ticlopidine twice daily is an alternative antiplatelet agent in selected situations.

Anticoagulants

The rationale for using anticoagulants in ischemic heart disease is based on coronary thrombosis and rethrombosis. Anticoagulants do not affect the rapidity of thrombolysis, but they prevent early rethrombosis after thrombolysis and prevent late thrombosis and reocclusion (Clem, 1995). The two major anticoagulants used are heparin and warfarin (discussed in detail in Chap. 26).

Heparin is used in unstable angina and acute MI, especially when using short-acting thrombolytics (ie, alteplase). The anticoagulation goal of heparin therapy in acute MI and unstable angina is to achieve an activated partial thromboplastin time of 1.5 to 2 times the control. Hemorrhage is the most common adverse effect of heparin therapy. Concomitant use of aspirin and heparin has increased the risk of bleeding, but this combination is used quite commonly with acute MI and unstable angina because the benefits of using the two agents together seem to outweigh the increased risk of bleeding.

The benefit of warfarin in ischemic heart disease is not as clear as it is with heparin. When used in MI, the therapeutic goal for warfarin therapy is an International Normalized Ratio (INR) of 2 to 3. It takes 5 to 7 days to reach a therapeutic INR with warfarin. Using aspirin and warfarin together for certain indications (including acute MI) improves efficacy without increasing bleeding complications.

Beta Blockers

Beta-adrenergic blocking agents are used for many different cardiovascular disorders and are discussed in detail in Chapter 25. The mechanism by which beta blockers are beneficial in ischemic heart disease is their reduction in myocardial oxygen demand by negative inotropic (decreased force of myocardial contraction) and negative chronotropic (decreased heart rate) effects. Studies of the benefits of beta blockers administered after MI show that in the acute MI phase, selected beta blockers reduce the infarct size and decrease mortality rate. Despite the benefits, the negative inotropic and chronotropic properties of beta blockers can precipitate congestive heart failure, heart block, or hypotension.

Calcium Channel Blockers

There are four categories of calcium channel blockers. In general, the dihydropyridine group (including nifedipine, isradipine, felodipine, amlodipine, and nicardipine) exerts its major effect through peripheral vasodilation. The calcium channel blockers exert their antianginal effects by coronary vasodilation (which increases myocardial oxygen demand) and by reducing myocardial oxygen demand through peripheral vasodilation and decreased myocardial contractility. Also, the slowing of conduction through the sinus and atrioventricular nodes attenuates the increase in heart rate with exertion, thereby reducing exertional angina symptoms.

Various adverse reactions are associated with calcium channel blockers. One effect of the dihydropyridine group is reflex tachycardia, which can complicate ischemic heart disease because it increases myocardial oxygen demand. Fortunately, this effect seems to occur less commonly with longer-acting and sustained-release forms of the dihydropyridines.

Angiotensin-Converting Enzyme Inhibitors

The use of angiotensin-converting enzyme (ACE) inhibitors in ischemic heart disease is relatively recent. Left ventricular remodeling after MI consists of a thinning of the ventricular muscle in the infarct area and left ventricular dilation. The ACE inhibitors seem to prevent this process, probably by reducing afterload.

Thrombolytics

In the late 1970s, it was observed that coronary thrombosis occurred very early in most acute MIs and that reperfusion of occluded coronary arteries may limit the size of the MI. Streptokinase was the thrombolytic agent used at that time. It was administered through an intracoronary catheter. Because a catheterization laboratory was needed to use thrombolytics, and this often presented difficulties, IV thrombolytics were developed (eg, anisoylated plasminogen streptokinase activator complex [APSAC] and recombinant tissue plasminogen activator (t-PA). In contrast to anticoagulants, which prevent the propagation of thrombi, the thrombolytic agents promote the lysis of thrombi by converting plasminogen to plasmin, causing the degradation of fibrin and fibrinogen and, ultimately, clot dissolution (Clem, 1995).

The fibrinolytic activity of t-PA may be more intense than the others because its plasminogen activation is more fibrin-selective. The thrombolytics have been underused, although there are some relative and absolute contraindications to their use (eg, cerebrovascular accident within 2 months, severe uncontrolled hypertension, major surgery in the past 10 days, subacute bacterial endocarditis, diabetic hemorrhagic retinopathy). In addition, streptokinase and APSAC are derived from streptococci, and recent administration of streptokinase or APSAC can cause the formation of streptokinase-neutralizing antibodies that inhibit streptokinase-induced thrombolysis, rendering it ineffective. Streptokinase products should not be readministered for 6 to 12 months after the client receives streptokinase.

More recent advances in agents used for treating ischemic heart disease include abciximab, a monoclonal antibody that binds to the glycoprotein IIb/IIIa receptor on platelets (see Chap. 26). By binding to this receptor, an antiplatelet effect is achieved. The use of this agent has been confined to selected clients undergoing percutaneous transluminal coronary angioplasty.

Vasoconstrictors

Vasoconstrictor (vasopressor) drugs (Table 24-3) are effective in reversing shock due to inappropriate dilation of the peripheral blood vessels. They are the treatment of choice in anaphylactic and neurogenic shock. They are sometimes used in treating orthostatic hypotension and when the drop in blood pressure is induced by spinal anesthesia. In other types of shock, vasoconstrictors are not used as frequently as they were in the past. Although their administration raises blood pressure, it may not improve blood flow. In cardiogenic and hypovolemic shock, significant reflex vasoconstriction is usually present. Intensification of this response by drugs may seriously compromise circulation. Only when these types of shock are associated with failure of the normal compensatory vasoconstriction are vasopressor agents helpful.

Table 24-3. Selected Vasoconstrictors

Drug Name	Routes of Administration	Usual Dosage	Uses	Mechanism of Action
epinephrine (Adrenalin chloride)	IV	5–10mL 1:10,000, repeat at 5-min intervals as required OR 1 mg in 250 mL 5% D/W to run at 1–4 mcg/min or 15–60 mL/hr	Cardiac arrest	Nonspecific activation of alpha- and beta-adrenergic receptor sites
	intracardiac	3–5 mL 1:10,000	Cardiac arrest	
	SC, IM	Adults: 0.3–0.5 mL 1:1,000, repeat q20 min	Bronchospasm (as in anaphylaxis)	
	SC	Child: 0.01 mg/kg 1:1,000, repeat q20 min	Bronchospasm (as in anaphylaxis)	
	topical	Nasal: 1–2 drops 0.1% solution q4–6h Topical: 1:1,000–1:10,000	Hemostasis	
	ophthalmic	1–2 gtt 0.25%–2% solution	Glaucoma	
		1–2 gtt 0.1% solution PC: C	Ocular mydriasis and hemostasis	
mephentermine sulfate (Wyamine)	IM IV	30–45 mg in single injection OR in 5% dextrose solution to run at rate of 1.0 mg/min PC: D	Hypotension secondary to spinal anesthesia, maintenance of BP in shock after hemorrhage while fluid replacement is accomplished	Activates alpha-adrenergic receptor sites on blood vessels and activates cardiac beta receptors
metaraminol (Aramine)	IM SC	2–10 mg	Acute hypotensive states associated with spinal anesthesia and treatment of drug-induced hypotension	Activates alpha-adrenergic receptor sites on blood vessels and activates cardiac beta receptors
	IV	0.5–5 mg followed by infusion of 15–100 mg in 500 mL 5% dextrose solution PC: D		
methoxamine (Vasoxyl)	IV IM	3–5 mg by slow injection 10–15 mg just before anesthesia, repeat if needed in 15 min PC: C	For supporting, restoring, or maintaining BP during anesthesia	Activates alpha-adrenergic receptors
phenylephrine (Neo-Synephrine)		2–5 mg of 1% solution	For supporting, restoring, or maintaining BP during anesthesia and treatment of drug-induced hypotension	Activates alpha-adrenergic receptors
	SC IM IV	0.1–0.5 mg of 0.1% solution, may repeat in 15 min or in IV solution		
norepinephrine (Levophed)	IV	4 mL/250–1,000 mL of 5% dextrose solution; average maintenance dose, 2–4 mcg/min or 0.5–1 mL/min PC: D	Acute hypotensive states	Activates alpha-adrenergic receptor sites on blood vessels and activates cardiac beta receptors

PC = pregnancy risk category (see Appendix A).

Local anesthetics are customarily mixed with vasoconstrictors to produce constriction of nearby blood vessels. This slows systemic absorption and prolongs the local effect of the anesthetic, allowing adequate anesthesia with minimal doses.

Vasoconstrictors are also active ingredients in nose drops and eye drops designed to reduce local congestion. Rebound hyperemia often occurs when the effect of a dose wears off. If the drug is repeated, physical dependency may develop; psychological dependency does not usually develop. Excessive use of such topical agents may cause systemic toxicity due to repeated absorption of the drug.

Pathophysiology of Peripheral Vascular Disease

Peripheral vascular disease can involve the arterial, venous, or lymphatic system. Occlusion of the arterial blood supply by atherosclerosis causes symptoms that vary in severity. Intermittent claudication is the pain, ache, or cramp that occurs in a muscle with an inadequate blood supply that is stressed by exercise. This is usually a segmental disease, with marked variation from person to person in its extent. Further occlusion results in severe ischemia in which the foot or leg is cold and skin changes occur. In this advanced stage, ulceration and gangrene of the toes are common.

Normal blood flow through the veins of the lower extremities and abdomen is often impaired by varicose veins. Tortuous, distended veins with incompetent valves develop most often in persons subject to increased hydrostatic pressure in the veins or obstruction of venous flow. Familial predisposition (apparently due to relatively weak vein structures) increases the risk. Factors associated with early onset of varicosities include obesity, pregnancy, abdominal tumors, long periods of sitting or standing in one place, and constrictive clothing.

When venous pressure rises for prolonged periods, the veins become overdistended. This weakens the wall and prevents the valves from closing completely, further reducing venous return and increasing congestion. Venous distention tends to progress, with eventual destruction of the valves and development of enlarged, tortuous vessels. Increased venous pressure is reflected by increased capillary pressure, and peripheral perfusion is reduced. Painful, weak muscles and edema ensue. Stasis ulcers or gangrene can develop.

When conservative measures for treating varicose veins prove inadequate, venous pooling can be reduced by eliminating some of the incompetent, overdistended vessels. Surgical removal of the varicosities is often preferred. When this is contraindicated or less than optimal, veins can be obliterated by the injection of irritating sclerosing drugs, which induce fibrosis of the vessels.

Drugs Used With Peripheral Vascular Disease

Peripheral vasodilators were used in the past to treat peripheral arterial disease, but their efficacy in relieving the ischemia is severely limited. They may increase blood flow to nonischemic areas. These peripheral vasodilators are briefly reviewed in Table 24-4. Some of these agents have also been used for treating cerebrovascular insufficiency in elderly clients. In that situation, these drugs can cause hypotension, which can actually result in reduced cerebral perfusion, negating any potential benefit from the cerebral vessel dilation. By different mechanisms, pentoxifylline may play a positive role in peripheral vascular disease of arterial origin.

Pentoxifylline

Pentoxifylline (Trental) is a xanthine derivative structurally related to the methylxanthines (caffeine, theophylline) and is categorized as a hemorrheologic agent.

Pharmacodynamics. Pentoxifylline produces hemorrheologic effects, lowering blood viscosity and improving erythrocyte flexibility. Thus, it increases blood flow to the affected microcirculation and enhances tissue oxygenation. It increases cellular adenosine triphosphate content via a membrane-stabilizing action, thus reducing red blood cell aggregation. It stimulates prostacyclin formation and release. It inhibits phosphodiesterase

Drug Name	Preparations	Usual Dosage	Adverse Reactions
Table 24-4. Peripheral Vasodilators			
cyclandelate (Cyclan, Cyclospasmol)	Tablets Capsules	Initial: 1.2–1.6 g/d in divided doses before meals & at bedtime; maintenance: 400–800 mg/d in 2–4 divided doses PC: C	GI distress, flushing, headache, weakness, sweating, dizziness, tachycardia
isoxsuprine (Vasodilan, Voxsuprine)	Tablets IM	10–20 mg tid or qid PC: C	Flushing, palpitations, nausea, dizziness, skin rash, tachycardia, abdominal stress, hypotension, nervousness
ethaverine (Ethaquin, Ethatab, Ethavex-100, Isovex)	Tablets Capsules	100 mg tid, may be increased to 200 mg tid PC: C	GI distress, dryness of throat, hypotension, malaise, vertigo, headache, lassitude, drowsiness, flushing, sweating
papaverine (Pavabid Plateau, Pavarine Spancaps, Pavased, Pavasule, Pavabid HP)	Tablets Timed-release capsules Timed-release tablets IM	100–300 mg 3–5 times qd PC: C	GI distress, flushing, sweating, headache, fatigue, rash, diarrhea, dizziness, tachycardia, anorexia
nylidrin (Adrin, Arlidin)	Tablets	3–12 mg tid or qid PC: C	Trembling, nervousness, weakness, dizziness, nausea, vomiting, postural hypotension, palpitations

PC = pregnancy risk category (see Appendix A).

degradation of platelet cAMP. The increase of cAMP levels decreases the synthesis of thromboxane A_2. The net result is reduced platelet aggregation. The drug also increases fibrinolytic activity and decreases fibrinogen concentration.

Pharmacokinetics. After oral administration, pentoxifylline is extensively absorbed. It undergoes hepatic first-pass effect. Plasma levels of the parent drug peak within 1 hour. Excretion is by the urine, although about 4% of the dose can be recovered in the feces.

Therapeutic Uses. Pentoxifylline is used to treat peripheral arterial disease. Unlabeled uses have included cerebrovascular insufficiency, transient ischemic attacks, sickle-cell thalassemias, strokes, eye circulation disorders, and Raynaud's disease.

Dosage and Administration. The dosage is 400 mg three times daily with meals. Therapeutic effects may be seen within 2 to 4 weeks, but therapy should continue for 8 weeks for full evaluation of its effect. The clearance of pentoxifylline is reduced in clients with renal impairment, so a lower dosage may be necessary.

Adverse Reactions. Frequent adverse reactions include dyspepsia, nausea, vomiting, dizziness, and headache.

Drug Interactions. A possible interaction between pentoxifylline and warfarin has been reported, in that the prothrombin time was prolonged and bleeding occurred. Pentoxifylline may interact with histamine (H_2) antagonists, causing increased effects from the antagonist.

Precautions and Contraindications. Pentoxifylline must be used cautiously in pregnancy. It is contraindicated in lactation and in clients with known allergy to the drug or to methylxanthines (eg, caffeine, theophylline).

Sclerosing Agents

Sclerosing agents currently used to treat varicose veins include ethanolamine oleate (Ethamolin), morrhuate sodium (Scleromate), and sodium tetradecyl sulfate (Sotradecol).

Pharmacodynamics. Sclerosing agents irritate the intimal endothelium of the vein, producing an inflammatory response. A blood clot develops that occludes the vein and leads to formation of fibrous tissue, resulting in obliteration of the vein.

Pharmacokinetics. Sclerosing agents are injected directly into the affected veins. They are not absorbed systemically but act locally at the injection site.

Therapeutic Uses. Morrhuate sodium and sodium tetradecyl sulfate can be used to treat small, uncomplicated varicose veins of the lower extremities or as a supplement to venous ligation to obliterate residual varicose veins or to reduce the risk of surgery. Morrhuate sodium has been used for internal hemorrhoids, but its effectiveness has not been conclusively established.

Ethanolamine oleate may be used to prevent rebleeding of esophageal varices that have recently bled. It is not indicated for nonbleeding varices, nor is it recommended for varicosities of the leg. When ethanolamine oleate is used for esophageal varices, sclerosis is a delayed rather than an immediate effect, occurring about 2.5 months after injection. Sclerotherapy with this agent has no beneficial effect on portal hypertension, the cause of esophageal varices, so recanalization and collateralization may occur, necessitating reinjection. Ethanolamine oleate is introduced to the target area through a flexible fiberoptic esophagoscope. Sclerosing agents are administered by the physician, usually in an outpatient or office procedure.

Dosage and Administration. The usual dose of morrhuate sodium for the obliteration of small or medium veins is 50 to 100 mg (1–2 mL); for large veins it is 150 to 250 mg. The drug may be given as multiple injections at one time or in single doses. Therapy may be repeated at 5- to 7-day intervals, depending on the client's response.

Adverse Reactions. With morrhuate sodium, the client may report burning or cramping sensations and urticaria. Tissue sloughing and necrosis with extravasation have occurred. With sodium tetradecyl, a permanent discoloration of skin along the path of the sclerosed vein segment may result. Anaphylactoid and allergic reactions have occurred. With ethanolamine oleate, the most common adverse reactions are pleural effusion, esophageal ulcer, esophageal stricture, and pneumonia.

Precautions and Contraindications. Injection therapy is contraindicated for clients with acute local or systemic infection, for those in whom there is significant valvular or deep venous incompetence, and for those with underlying arterial disease. Only a few vessels can be treated at one time. Excessive obliteration of venous vessels can compromise circulation and, in extreme cases, require amputation of a lower limb.

❖ NURSING MANAGEMENT: CLIENT RECEIVING AN AGENT FOR PERIPHERAL VASCULAR DISEASE

For a client receiving pentoxifylline, the nurse must observe for adverse reactions. Pentoxifylline may cause hypotension, so clients with coronary artery disease with angina or clients receiving concomitant antihypertensive therapy should be monitored closely for complaints of chest pain or signs of arrhythmias. Because dizziness may occur, clients should take precautions to prevent injury related to driving or operating hazardous machinery.

Nursing management of the client receiving a sclerosing agent focuses on relieving discomfort, detecting and treating potential allergic reaction, and educating the client to perform effective self-care after discharge.

NURSING PROCESS

ASSESSMENT

Initial assessment of the client seeking sclerotherapy should include a complete history of venous disease, including episodes of thrombophlebitis, vein surgery, and previous sclerotherapy. The client should be examined to determine the extent of superficial vein involvement. A phlebogram is usually performed to evaluate venous circulation.

The client's drug history should be reviewed to assess the potential for allergic reaction to the sclerosing drugs. A client with multiple allergies or a family history of allergy, particularly of reactions to sclerosing agents, is at increased risk for allergic reaction during treatment, especially if the client has been treated with these drugs in the past. To determine possible sensitivity, a small amount may be injected into a varicose vein 24 hours before administering a large dose.

NURSING DIAGNOSIS

Nursing diagnoses arising from sclerotherapy are:

- Pain (aching sensation, feeling of stiffness), related to inflammatory process secondary to sclerotherapy
- Risk for Injury, related to drug-induced anaphylaxis

PLANNING

Goals of nursing care include alleviating or eliminating pain and preventing or promptly detecting and managing allergic reaction to the prescribed drugs.

INTERVENTION

The nurse supports and assists the client as necessary during the treatment procedure. Equipment and supplies for the treatment of anaphylaxis should be at hand before the procedure is started. The nursing staff must be prepared to treat anaphylaxis should it occur. The nurse also prepares and implements a teaching plan to help the client manage self-care at home after the procedure.

Client Education. The nurse should encourage the client to use conservative measures to manage peripheral venous disease. Progression of venous degeneration can be delayed by such health measures as losing excess weight, periodically elevating the extremities, wearing elastic support hose, avoiding standing for long periods, and avoiding clothing that hampers circulation in the legs. Clients should be encouraged to continue such practices even if sclerotherapy is used.

When sclerotherapy is used, the client should be instructed that severe pain or local tissue sloughing, which indicates an adverse reaction to the drugs, must be reported promptly for follow-up care.

Warm compresses and a mild analgesic such as aspirin, ibuprofen, or acetaminophen can be used to relieve discomfort at the injection sites. Injection therapy is an adjunct to, not a substitute for, other methods of treating varicose veins.

OUTCOME EVALUATION

Data required for evaluation include the client's reports of absence or presence of pain and absence or presence of evidence of allergic reaction.

❖ CHECKLIST OF NURSING ACTIONS

- ❑ Monitor clients using agents for peripheral arterial disease for adverse reactions.
- ❑ Assess clients seeking injection therapy regarding previous treatment of varicosities.
- ❑ Be prepared to treat sensitivity reactions, including anaphylaxis, when sclerosing agents are used.
- ❑ Instruct clients to report to the physician severe pain or tissue sloughing at the sites of injection.
- ❑ Teach clients health measures to delay the progression of venous degeneration (reduction of excess weight, intermittent exercise, avoidance of restrictive clothing and long periods of standing or sitting).

References

Clem JR. (1995). Pharmacotherapy of ischemic heart disease. *AACN Clinical Issues, 6*(3), 404–417.

Copstead LC. (1995). *Perspectives on pathophysiology.* Philadelphia: WB Saunders.

Effat MA. (1995). Pathophysiology of ischemic heart disease. *AACN Clinical Issues, 6*(3), 369–374.

Fung H. (1993). Clinical pharmacology of organic nitrates. *Am J Cardiol, 72*(9), 9C–15C.

Griffith P, James B, Cropp A. (1994). Evaluation of the safety and efficacy of topical nitroglycerin ointment to facilitate venous cannulation. *Nursing Research, 43*(4), 203–206.

Rutherford JD. (1995). Nitrate tolerance in angina therapy: How to avoid it. *Drugs, 49*(2), 196.

Bibliography

Albert NM. (1995). High-risk unstable angina: Keeping pace with current research findings. *AACN Clinical Issues, 6*(1), 110–120.

Antonaccio M, ed. (1990). *Cardiovascular pharmacology,* 3d ed. New York: Raven Press.

Buttaro M. (1994). Staying on top of transdermal drug patches. *Nursing '94, 24,* 41–44.

Craig CR, Stitzel RE. (1990). *Modern pharmacology,* 3d ed. Boston: Little, Brown and Co.

Gleeson B. (1991). Loosening the grip of anginal pain. *Nursing '91, 21,* 33–39.

Gleeson B. (1991). Teaching your patient about his antianginal drugs. *Nursing '91, 21,* 65–72.

Hardman JG, Limbird LE, Molinoff PB, et al. (eds). (1996). *Goodman and Gilman's The pharmacological basis of therapeutics,* 9th ed. New York: McGraw-Hill.

Katz B, Rosenberg A, Frishman WH. (1995). Controlled-release drug delivery systems in cardiovascular medicine. *Am Heart J, 129*(2), 359–368.

Owen A. (1995). Tracking the rise and fall of cardiac enzymes. *Nursing '95, 25*, 35–38.

Parker JO. (1993). Nitrates and angina pectoris. *Am J Cardiol, 72*(9), 3C–8C.

Pearson T, Rapaport E, Criqui M, et al. (1994). Optimal risk factor management in the patient after coronary revascularization. *Circulation, 90*(6), 3125–3133.

Williams K, Morton PG. (1995). Diagnosis and treatment of acute myocardial infarction. *AACN Clinical Issues, 6*(3), 375–386.

Yacone-Morton LA. (1995). Inotropic agents and nitrates. *RN, 58*(3), 22–28.

For more information and sample tests and activities, refer to Chapter 24 in the Student Workbook for Clinical Pharmacology and Nursing Management, 5th edition, available through your bookstore.

25

Drugs That Regulate Blood Pressure

Physiology of Blood Pressure

The circulatory system is a continuous, closed circuit of vessels that carry the blood pumped by the heart through the lungs and periphery of the body. The flow of fluid through this system depends on the patency of the vessels and on pressure gradients, which propel liquids from the arteries to the veins and back to the heart.

Maintenance of the pressure gradients requires adequate pumping action by the heart to establish high pressure in the vessels opening from the ventricles, arterial elasticity to moderate and prolong this pressure, and a degree of peripheral resistance sustained by partial constriction of the smaller vessels.

Arterial blood pressure varies with the cardiac cycle. The systolic pressure corresponds to ejection of blood from the left ventricle into the arteries. This fluid volume distends the blood vessel, stretching the muscle fibers and raising the intraluminal pressure above that of the distal arterioles, capillaries, and venules. The pressure gradient established in this way causes blood to flow rapidly toward the capillary bed.

Arterial pressure falls to its lowest point (diastolic) just before the next ventricular ejection phase. The diastolic pressure is determined in part by the diameter of the arterioles, which is also the major determinant of systemic vascular resistance (SVR). Therefore, the diastolic value provides an estimate of SVR. Blood pressure is the product of cardiac output and vascular resistance and is affected by changes in both. Vasoconstriction, a narrowing of vessel diameter, increases SVR and diastolic blood pressure; vasodilation reduces SVR and diastolic blood pressure. The pulse pressure is the difference between systolic and diastolic pressures.

The aortic and carotid baroreceptors are important regulators of arterial blood pressure. A drop in arterial pressure results in activation of sympathetic nerves to the heart and vessels and inhibition of parasympathetic influence on the heart. Blood pressure returns toward normal as heart rate, cardiac output, and SVR increase.

Several chemical mediators influence arteriolar diameter and, therefore, blood pressure. Mediators that generally cause vasoconstriction and elevate blood pressure include angiotensin II, vasopressin, and some prostaglandins. Mediators that reduce blood pressure include histamine, nitric oxide, and some prostaglandins.

Pathophysiology of Hypertension

Circulation is reduced by processes that decrease the patency of the blood vessels, impair their elasticity, cause inappropriate vasoconstriction or vasodilation, or interfere with venous return. Patency may be reduced by external pressure (the cause of decubitus ulcers), internal obstructions (thrombi, emboli, tumors), and atherosclerosis. Elasticity is reduced in arteriosclerosis, a degenerative process involving progressive fibrosis and calcification of the vascular wall. Inappropriate vasodilation is seen in neurogenic shock and postural hypotension; excessive vasoconstriction is characteristic of hypertension.

Hypertension is defined as blood pressure persistently elevated above 140 mmHg systolic or 90 mmHg diastolic (Copstead, 1995). Hypertension increases the heart's workload and the risk of degenerative changes in the blood vessels as well as in other body organs (eg, kidneys, brain, heart, eyes). The degree and duration of hypertension determine the severity of organ damage.

Hypertension has a few forms: *essential hypertension* (also called primary or idiopathic high blood pressure), which has no identifiable cause, and *secondary hypertension*, which is attributable to an identifiable cause, such as renal, endocrine, vascular, or neurologic disorders, pregnancy, or the use of an exogenous substance (Box 25-1).

Certain risk factors contribute to hypertension, both physical and environmental. These include age (blood pressure rises consistently with age), race (hypertension occurs two to three times more often in African Americans than in European Americans), family history, obesity, excess sodium intake, and stress.

The phrase "silent killer" is commonly applied to hypertension and indicates that few signs and symptoms exist. When signs and symptoms do occur, such as headache, retinopathy, seizures, and coma, they may signify advanced hypertension. Hypertension can be classified into four stages (Table 25-1).

Box 25-1
Causes of Secondary Hypertension

Renal Hypertension

Renovascular disease

Preeclampsia and eclampsia

Renal parenchymal disease

Nephroblastoma

Glomerulopathic syndromes

Endocrine Hypertension

Primary aldosteronism secondary to bilateral adrenal hyperplasia

Severe Cushing's disease

Pheochromocytoma (tumor of adrenal medulla)

Acromegaly

Hyperparathyroidism

Cardiovascular Disease

Coarctation of aorta

Aortic aneurysm

Dissection of aorta

Malignant Hypertension/Hypertensive Encephalopathy (Exogenous Substances)

Estrogen-containing oral contraceptives

Sympathomimetics

Clonidine withdrawal

MAOIs with sympathomimetics

Tricyclic antidepressants with sympathomimetics

Corticosteroids

ACTH

Hypertension in Special Populations

The prevalence of hypertension in the United States is exceedingly high in persons over age 60, occurring in 60% of non-Hispanic whites, 61% of Mexican Americans, and 71% of non-Hispanic blacks (Hall, 1994). Other special populations in terms of hypertension are children and pregnant women.

Older Adults

Older hypertensive adults have a high occurrence of hypertension-related disease, including coronary artery disease, stroke, left ventricular hypertrophy, heart failure, and peripheral arterial disease. Diabetes is also more prevalent in the elderly. Effective treatment of hypertension reduces the risk of cardiovascular complications among older adults.

Several pathophysiologic changes associated with aging contribute to hypertension in older adults. Decreased arterial compliance results from increased stiffness of the arterial wall and is associated with an increase in peripheral arterial resistance. In younger people, the cardiac volume generated during each systole is absorbed to some degree by the elasticity of the arterial walls. With aging, arterial walls become stiffer and have less ability to distend and absorb this wave of pressure, which produces a widened pulse pressure (Chutka, 1995).

Decreased plasma volume and a decline in baroreceptor function increase the elderly person's risk for orthostatic hypotension. Older adults are less able to produce a compensatory tachycardia and vasoconstriction in response to an orthostatic posture. Orthostatic hypotension is often worsened when certain antihypertensive agents are used.

Other changes that occur in elderly adults include an increase in catecholamine levels and a decrease in plasma renin and aldosterone values. Alpha-adrenergic activity, which mediates vasoconstriction, remains intact with aging, but beta-adrenergic responsiveness, which mediates vasodilatation, declines with aging.

Older adults tend to demonstrate a decreased natriuretic capability and are susceptible to peripheral edema related to changes in sodium and fluid intake. Renal function, both glomerular filtration and renal plasma flow, generally declines with age. Creatinine clearance falls markedly after age 60. This can impair the removal of various drugs that depend on renal excretion (Hall, 1994). Often the total body potassium level is decreased significantly in older adults, which is related to their reduced lean body mass.

Children

Children are another special population in terms of hypertension. Kidney disease accounts for about 80% of cases of pediatric hypertension. With dosage adjustments, most of the same antihypertensive drugs used for adults can be used for children.

Table 25-1. Classification and Follow-Up of Blood Pressure for Adults Age 18 and Older

Category (Blood Pressure)	Systolic Pressure (mmHg)	Diastolic Pressure (mmHg)	Follow-Up
Normal	<130	<85	Recheck in 2 years
High normal	130–139	85–89	Recheck in 1 year
Hypertension			
Stage 1 (mild)	140–159	90–99	Confirm within 2 months
Stage 2 (moderate)	160–179	100–109	Evaluate or refer within 1 month
Stage 3 (severe)	180–209	110–119	Evaluate or refer within 1 week
Stage 4 (very severe)	≥210	≥120	Evaluate or refer immediately

These decisions should be based on the average of two or more readings taken at each of two or more visits after an initial screening. When systolic and diastolic pressures fall into different categories, the higher category should be selected to classify the blood-pressure status.

Adapted from: *The Fifth Report of the Joint National Committee on Detection, Evaluation, and Treatment of High Blood Pressure.* (1993). Bethesda, MD: National Institutes of Health, National Heart, Lung, and Blood Institute (NIH Publication No. 93-1088).

Pregnant Women

If drug therapy for hypertension is necessary in a pregnant woman (see Chap. 10), methyldopa, beta blockers, or hydralazine may be the treatment of choice. Diuretic therapy is controversial because these drugs may reduce maternal blood volume and underperfuse the placenta. Angiotensin-converting enzyme (ACE) inhibitors are avoided because they may have a negative effect on the fetus. Hypertensive emergencies may involve the use of hydralazine, diazoxide, or labetalol. Magnesium sulfate has been given for eclampsia and the hypertensive component because eclampsia is accompanied by excessively low serum magnesium levels. Although magnesium sulfate does not lower blood pressure, it is effective as an anticonvulsant.

Ethnicity

The genetic characteristics of some ethnic groups can alter the response to antihypertensive agents. The incidence of hypertension and the severity of associated problems are greater in certain racial groups. Diuretics and calcium channel blockers are more effective than beta blockers or the usually effective doses of ACE inhibitors in African Americans (*Medical Letter*, 1995). On average, these clients have lower plasma renin levels, which may explain why beta blockers, which lower renin secretion, may not work so well.

Antihypertensive Drug Therapy

Management of hypertension requires eliminating or modifying as many risk factors as possible. Sometimes weight reduction, stress management, sodium restriction, exercise, modification of dietary fats, and alcohol restriction are sufficient to return blood pressure to normal levels. However, drug regimens are commonly instituted to reduce excessive pressures and maintain them at the desired level.

In the 1970s and early 1980s, the Joint National Committee on Detection, Evaluation, and Treatment of High Blood Pressure (JNC) issued treatment recommendations known as the "stepped-care model" (Walz, 1994). This model recommended diuretics as the initial therapeutic agent; if blood pressure remained uncontrolled, other drugs were added in a stepwise fashion.

Studies using the stepped-care model demonstrate that hypertension can be lowered, that the risk of stroke can be reduced, and that mortality in clients with essential hypertension can be reduced with the prescribed approach. However, hypertension is also a risk factor in coronary artery disease, which may lead to myocardial infarction (MI) and sudden death. Controlling blood pressure with the stepped-care model did not result in a documented decrease in this cardiac-related morbidity and mortality. Because findings suggested that using diuretics and beta blockers does not the resolve all the problems associated with hypertension, some clinicians proposed increased individualization of hypertension management. They argued that drug selection should be based on the client's age, race, lifestyle, and current health status (presence or absence of left ventricular hypertrophy [LVH], hyperglycemia, and elevated serum lipoprotein levels). They pointed out that LVH and atherosclerosis, which may accompany hypertension, increase a client's risk of MI and death. These two disorders, however, respond selectively to antihypertensive agents. Research indicates that calcium channel blockers and ACE inhibitors may improve LVH and have little negative effect on lipid profiles, which influence

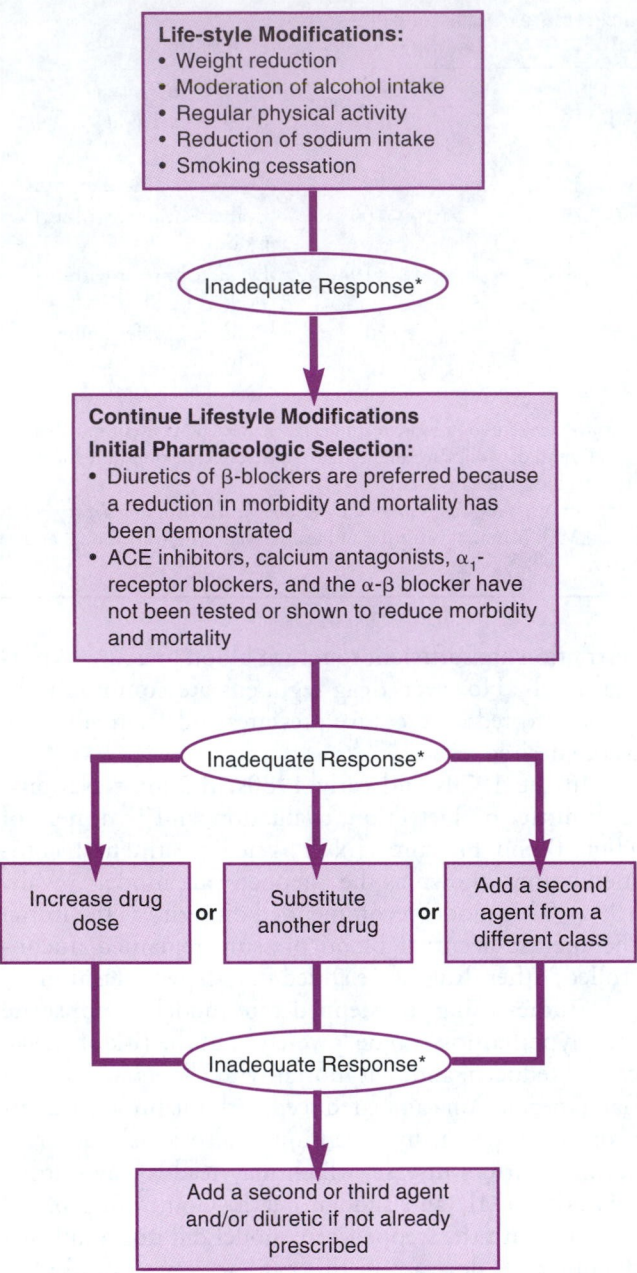

JNC-V Treatment Algorithm for Individualized Management of Hypertension

Life-style Modifications:
- Weight reduction
- Moderation of alcohol intake
- Regular physical activity
- Reduction of sodium intake
- Smoking cessation

Inadequate Response*

Continue Lifestyle Modifications
Initial Pharmacologic Selection:
- Diuretics of β-blockers are preferred because a reduction in morbidity and mortality has been demonstrated
- ACE inhibitors, calcium antagonists, α₁-receptor blockers, and the α-β blocker have not been tested or shown to reduce morbidity and mortality

Inadequate Response*

Increase drug dose **or** Substitute another drug **or** Add a second agent from a different class

Inadequate Response*

Add a second or third agent and/or diuretic if not already prescribed

*Response means achieved goal blood pressure, or patient is making considerable progress toward this goal.

Figure 25-1. Joint National Committee, V, treatment algorithm for individualized management of hypertension. (Adapted from: *The Fifth Report of the Joint National Committee on Detection, Evaluation, and Treatment of High Blood Pressure.* (1993). Bethesda, MD: National Institutes of Health, National Heart, Lung, and Blood Institute (NIH Publication No. 93-1088).

atherosclerosis, whereas the traditional initial stepped-care agents may be less effective in reversing LVH and have a more substantial negative effect on lipid profiles.

The shortcomings in the traditional approach contributed to changes in the 1988 and 1993 JNC rec-ommendations. In 1988, the JNC widened the scope of treatment to include diuretics, beta blockers, ACE inhibitors, and calcium antagonists (calcium channel blockers) as step I agents for the initial drug treatment of hypertension. In 1993, the JNC expanded the step I list further to include the selective alpha-1 adrenorecep-tor blockers and combined alpha- and beta-adrenergic blockers (National Institutes of Health, 1993). The modification of the stepped-care model, therefore, in-cluded individualization of client risk and status of dis-ease as criteria for choosing the initial antihypertensive agent or agents (Fig. 25-1).

In treatment to reduce elevated blood pressure, the target diastolic blood pressure is less than 90 mmHg, the goal recommended in the JNC guidelines (Farnett & Mulrow, 1994). A decrease in diastolic pressure to less than 85 mmHg may impair diastolic myocardial per-fusion pressure in susceptible clients (those with preex-isting cardiovascular disease). Newer data indicate that diastolic blood pressures under 85 mmHg may be asso-ciated with increased coronary heart disease mortality.

Current agents in use as antihypertensives include diuretics (see Chap. 27), sympathetic inhibitors, direct-acting vasodilators, ACE inhibitors, angiotensin-recep-tor antagonists, and calcium channel blocking agents.

Sympathetic Inhibitors

The sympathetic inhibitors include these drug subgroups: adrenergic blocking agents, central action inhibitors, blockers of neuroeffector transmission, and some mis-cellaneous agents. The adrenergic blocking agents can be separated into subcategories that produce combined al-pha-1 and alpha-2 adrenoreceptor blockade, selective al-pha-1 adrenoreceptor blockade, beta-adrenergic block-ade, and combined alpha- and beta-adrenergic blockade.

Adrenergic Blocking Agents
Combined Alpha-1 and Alpha-2 Adrenergic Blockers
Combined alpha-1 and alpha-2 adrenergic blocking agents (Table 25-2) include phenoxybenzamine (Dibenzyline), phentolamine (Regitine), and tolazoline (Priscoline). Phen-tolamine is discussed as representative of the group.

Pharmacodynamics. The combined alpha-1 and alpha-2 adrenergic blocker phentolamine reduces systemic and pulmonary resistance and, thus, lowers blood pressure. It prevents catecholamines from activating smooth muscle alpha-receptors, which normally cause vasoconstriction. Phentolamine prevents vasoconstriction in both arterial and venous beds.

Pharmacokinetics. When given intravenously (IV) during surgery, phentolamine reaches peak action in 2 minutes. Its duration of action is 10 to 15 minutes. Its half-life is 19 minutes. It is excreted in the urine.

Therapeutic Uses. The combined alpha-1 and alpha-2 adrenergic blockers, specifically phentolamine, are used

Table 25-2. Adrenergic Blocking Agents

Drug Name	Preparation	Usual Dosage	Adverse Reactions
Combined Alpha-1 and Alpha-2 Adrenergic Blocking Agents			
phenoxybenzamine (Dibenzyline)	Capsules	20–40 mg 2 or 3 times/d PC: C	Miosis, nasal congestion, vomiting, hypotension
phentolamine (Regitine)	IM IV	2–5 mg prn PC: C	Hypotension, tachycardia, arrhythmias, angina, abdominal pain, nausea, vomiting, diarrhea
tolazoline (Priscoline)	IV	1–2 mg/kg/hr via IV infusion PC: C	Hypotension, GI bleeding, acute renal failure, hypochloremic alkalosis, thrombocytopenia
Selective Alpha-1 Adrenergic Blocking Agents			
doxazosin mesylate (Cardura)	Tablets	2–16 mg/d in 1 dose PC: B	Similar to prazosin, but with less hypotension after first dose
prazosin (Minipress, Hypovasc)	Capsules	1 mg at bedtime, then 1 mg bid or tid; up to 20 mg/d PC: C	Syncope with first dose, dizziness and vertigo, palpitations, fluid retention, headache, drowsiness, weakness, anticholinergic effects
terazosin (Hytrin)	Tablets Capsules	1–5 mg qd PC: C	Similar to prazosin
Beta-Adrenergic Blocking Agents			
acebutolol (Sectral)	Capsules	200–1200 mg in 1 or 2 doses PC: B	See Table 25-3
atenolol (Tenormin)	Tablets IV	25–100 mg in 1 or 2 doses 5 mg over 5 min, repeat 10 min later PC: C	See Table 25-3
betaxolol (Kerlone)	Tablets Ophthalmic solution	5–40 mg in 1 dose 1 drop bid PC: C	See Table 25-3
bisoprolol fumarate (Zebeta)	Tablets	5–20 mg in 1 dose PC: C	See Table 25-3
carteolol (Cartrol)	Filmtab tablets	2.5–10 mg in 1 dose PC: C	See Table 25-3
esmolol (Brevibloc)	IV	50–200 mcg/kg/min PC: C	See Table 25-3
metoprolol tartrate (Lopressor)	Film-coated tablets	50–200 mg in 1 or 2 doses PC: B	See Table 25-3
metoprolol succinate (Toprol-XL)	Extended-release tablets	50–200 mg qd PC: B	See Table 25-3
nadolol (Corgard)	Tablets	20–240 mg in 1 dose PC: C	See Table 25-3
penbutolol (Levatol)	Tablets	20–80 mg in 1 dose PC: C	See Table 25-3
pindolol (Visken)	Tablets	10–60 mg in 2 doses PC: B	See Table 25-3
propranolol hydrochloride (Inderal, Inderide LA)	Tablets Extended-release capsules	40–240 mg in 2 doses 80–240 mg in 1 dose	See Table 25-3
Propranolol (Intensol)	Oral solution IV	4, 8, & 80 mg/mL: dosage based on indication 1–3 mg at 1 mg/min, may repeat once after 2 min PC: C	

PC = pregnancy risk category; see Appendix A.

(continued)

Table 25-2. (Continued)			
Drug Name	**Preparation**	**Usual Dosage**	**Adverse Reactions**
Beta-Adrenergic Blocking Agents (continued)			
sotalol (Betapace)	Tablets	160–320 mg/d in 2 doses PC: B	See Table 25-3
timolol maleate (Blocadren)	Tablets Ophthalmic solution	10–40 mg/d in 2 doses 1 gtt of 0.25%–0.5% bid PC: C	See Table 25-3
Combined Alpha- and Beta-Adrenergic Blocking Agents			
labetalol (Normodyne, Trandate)	Tablets IV	200–1200 mg in 2 doses 20 mg IV over 2 min, with additional doses as needed or 2 mg/min via IV infusion PC: C	Similar to other beta-adrenergic blocking agents, but has intrinsic sympathomimetic activity and more orthostatic hypotension; fever; hepatotoxicity
carvedilol (Coreg)	Tablets	6.25 mg bid PC: C	Dizziness, fatigue, back pain, rhinitis, bradycardia, diarrhea

PC = pregnancy risk category; see Appendix A.

to manage the hypertension and sweating of pheochromocytoma (tumor of the adrenal medulla). Phentolamine can be used to diagnose pheochromocytoma (phentolamine blocking test), but it is not the procedure of choice. Phentolamine can prevent or control hypertension during surgical removal of the pheochromocytoma. It does not produce the sustained antihypertensive effect needed to treat hypertension over the long term. Phentolamine is also used to prevent and treat dermal necrosis and sloughing following IV administration or extravasation of norepinephrine or dopamine.

Unlabeled uses include treating hypertensive crises secondary to interactions between monoamine oxidase inhibitors (MAOIs) and sympathomimetic amines, and rebound hypertension on withdrawal of clonidine, propranolol, or other antihypertensives.

Dosage and Administration. During surgery to remove a pheochromocytoma, 2 to 5 mg is given IV or intramuscularly (IM) to an adult as needed. To prevent necrosis related to IV administration of norepinephrine, 10 mg may be added to each liter of IV fluid containing the norepinephrine. To treat extravasation, it is injected directly into the affected area, intradermally (5–10 mg in 10 mL of 0.9% sodium chloride solution). This must be done within 12 hours of the extravasation.

Adverse Reactions. Reflex increases in heart rate, contractile force, and plasma renin activity are among the adverse effects. Others include acute and prolonged hypotensive episodes, cardiac arrhythmias, dizziness, flushing, orthostatic hypotension, nasal stuffiness, nausea, vomiting, and diarrhea.

Drug Interactions. The vasoconstrictive and hypertensive effects of epinephrine and ephedrine are antagonized by phentolamine.

Precautions and Contraindications. Phentolamine must be used with caution in pregnancy or lactation. It is contraindicated in coronary artery disease because MI has occurred, usually in association with marked hypotension, which may occur with phentolamine.

Selective Alpha-1 Adrenergic Blocking Agents
Prazosin (Minipress), terazosin, and doxazosin selectively block postsynaptic alpha-1 adrenergic receptors. Prazosin is discussed as the prototype of the group.

Pharmacodynamics. The selective alpha-1 adrenergic receptor blockers differ from combined alpha-1 and alpha-2 blockers in that the selective agents do not block alpha-2 presynaptic receptors, so they do not cause reflex tachycardia. Prazosin and other drugs in this group affect both supine and standing blood pressure; the effect is most pronounced on the diastolic pressure. The use of prazosin as a single antihypertensive agent is limited by its tendency to cause sodium and water retention and increased plasma volume.

Pharmacokinetics. Prazosin is extensively metabolized, and the metabolites are active. Peak plasma levels occur in 1 to 3 hours. Duration of antihypertensive effect is 10 hours. In chronic renal failure, elimination half-life may be prolonged, protein binding decreased, and peak plasma concentrations increased. About 90% of prazosin is eliminated in feces, about 10% in urine.

Therapeutic Uses. Prazosin's potency is comparable to that of propranolol, methyldopa, and clonidine as an antihypertensive. Prazosin is useful in managing clients with hypertension with hyperlipidemia. Some studies show that it decreased total cholesterol levels and levels of low-density lipoprotein (LDL) and increased levels of high-density lipoprotein (HDL) (*Medical Letter*, 1995).

An unlabeled use of prazosin (but a labeled use for terazosin and doxazosin) is treatment of benign prostatic hypertrophy and prostatism. In benign prostatic hypertrophy, the drug reduces symptoms and improves urine flow by relaxing smooth muscle, a result of blockade of alpha-1 adrenoreceptors in the bladder neck and prostate. Because the bladder body has relatively few alpha-1 receptors, the drug reduces the bladder outlet obstruction without affecting bladder contractility.

In another unlabeled use, prazosin was found to reduce clinical symptoms and increase exercise tolerance in short-term studies of subjects with refractory congestive heart failure (CHF) (Olin, 1995). It apparently decreases afterload and preload. It should be used with a diuretic because of its tendency to increase plasma volume.

Dosage and Administration. An adult should be started on 1 mg at bedtime, then 1 mg twice or three times daily; the dose of prazosin may be increased to 20 mg/day. Food may delay absorption but does not affect the extent of absorption.

Adverse Reactions. Prazosin is known for its first-dose effect: marked hypotension, especially orthostatic hypotension, and syncope with sudden loss of consciousness. This effect may be minimized by limiting the initial dose to 1 mg and giving it at bedtime. Dosage increases can be made every 2 weeks. A similar effect may occur if therapy is interrupted for more than a few doses, if dosage is increased rapidly, or if another antihypertensive agent is introduced. Occasionally, syncope is preceded by severe supraventricular tachycardia, with a heart rate of 120 to 160 beats per minute. Other common adverse effects include dizziness, lightheadedness, headache, and drowsiness. The incidence of orthostatic hypotension is higher in elderly clients.

Drug Interactions. Beta-adrenergic blocking agents may intensify the acute postural hypotensive reaction that follows the first dose of prazosin. The antihypertensive effect of clonidine may be decreased. Verapamil appears to increase the serum levels and effects of prazosin.

Drug–Laboratory Test Interactions. False-positive results may occur in screening tests for pheochromocytoma in clients being treated with prazosin. Prazosin should be discontinued and the client should be retested in 1 month if an elevated vanillylmandelic acid (VMA) level is recorded.

Precautions and Contraindications. Prazosin is contraindicated in clients who are allergic to the drug or who are pregnant or lactating. Nursing measures are needed to assist the client with possible postural hypotension or syncope.

Beta-Adrenergic Blocking Agents

Some experts categorize the beta-adrenergic blocking agents into nonselective, combined beta-1 and beta-2 adrenergic blocking agents and cardioselective (predominantly beta-1 adrenergic blockers) agents. Cardioselective beta blockers have a greater affinity for beta-1 receptors (in cardiac muscle) than beta-2 receptors (in bronchial and vascular musculature) and are preferred for clients with respiratory diseases such as asthma or chronic obstructive disease. However, cardioselectivity is lost when the medications are used in higher doses. Even with low doses of the cardioselective agents, bronchospasm may occur. Therefore, these agents are grouped together in this chapter, although Table 25-3 identifies the ones categorized as cardioselective. Also see Focus On Beta-Adrenergic Blocking Agents: Similarities and Differences on p. 487.

One group of beta-adrenergic blocking agents has intrinsic sympathomimetic activity (acebutolol, carteolol, penbutolol, pindolol), which means they produce less resting bradycardia and less reduction in cardiac output than do traditional beta blockers. This property is also indicated in Table 25-3. This drug group, unlike other beta blockers, apparently does not increase serum triglyceride concentrations or decrease HDL cholesterol levels (*Medical Letter*, 1995). In addition, they can lower blood pressure with less of a decrease in resting heart rate and may be preferred for clients who develop symptomatic bradycardia with other beta blockers.

Propranolol (Inderal), having neither cardioselective nor intrinsic sympathomimetic activity, was discussed as the prototype beta-adrenergic blocking agent in Chapter 22. Propranolol is used in hypertension management, but because it was discussed in detail earlier, betaxolol (Kerlone), metoprolol (Lopressor, Toprol XL), and pindolol (Visken) will be discussed as representative agents in this chapter. Table 25-4 outlines combination agents (those that combine a diuretic with a beta-adrenergic blocking agent or some other agent).

Pharmacodynamics. The physiologic responses mediated by activation of beta-adrenergic receptors include:

- Increases in heart rate and cardiac contractile force in response to exercise, stress, excitation, and other factors
- Increase in atrioventricular conduction velocity
- Relaxation of bronchial smooth muscle and decreased airway resistance
- Release of insulin from beta cells in the islets of Langerhans.

Beta-adrenergic blocking agents prevent or decrease the ability of the adrenergic system to initiate these responses.

Beta-adrenergic receptor blockade is useful in conditions in which sympathetic activity is detrimental, possibly because of pathologic or functional changes. Individual beta-adrenergic blocking agents may be more appropriate for one pathophysiologic situation than for another, depending on their cardioselectivity or intrinsic sympathomimetic activity. Beta blockers are effective antihypertensives used alone or with other antihypertensives. They reduce systolic and diastolic blood pressure at rest and on exercise and decrease standing

Text continues on page 489.

Table 25-3. Beta-Adrenergic Blocking Agents

Drug Name	Cardio-selective	ISA	Preparation	Usual Dosage	Adverse Reactions
acebutolol (Sectral)	Yes	Yes	Capsules	200–1200 mg in 1 or 2 doses PC: B	Causes less bradycardia than other beta blockers (see atenolol)
atenolol (Tenormin)	Yes	No	Tablets	25–100 mg in 1 or 2 doses	Bradycardia, heart block, aggravation of peripheral vascular insufficiency, fatigue, weakness, decreased libido, reduced exercise tolerance, may mask symptoms of and delay recovery from hypoglycemia, depression, insomnia, vivid dreams, bronchospasm, aggravation of allergic reactions, increased serum triglycerides, decreased HDL cholesterol
			IV	5 mg over 5 min, repeat 10 min later PC: C	
betaxolol (Kerlone)	Yes	No	Tablets	5–40 mg in 1 dose	See atenolol
			Ophthalmic solution	1 drop bid PC: C	
bisoprolol fumarate (Zebeta)	Yes	No	Tablets	5–20 mg in 1 dose PC: C	See atenolol
carteolol (Cartrol)	No	Yes	Filmtab tablets	2.5–10 mg in 1 dose PC: C	No clear advantage except when clients have bradycardia and must receive beta blocker because it causes less bradycardia than the others; otherwise see atenolol
esmolol (Brevibloc)	Yes	No	IV	50–200 mcg/kg/min PC: C	See atenolol
metoprolol tartrate (Lopressor)	Yes	No	Film-coated tablets	50–200 mg in 1 or 2 doses PC: B	See atenolol
metoprolol succinate (Toprol-XL)	Yes	No	SR tablets	50–200 mg qd PC: B	See atenolol
nadolol (Corgard)	No	No	Tablets	20–240 mg in 1 dose PC: C	See atenolol
penbutolol (Levatol)	No	Yes	Tablets	20–80 mg in 1 dose PC: C	Causes less bradycardia than other beta blockers (see atenolol)
pindolol (Visken)	No	Yes	Tablets	10–60 mg/d in 2 doses PC: B	Causes less bradycardia than other beta blockers (see atenolol)
celiprolol* (Selecor)	Yes	Yes	Oral	200–600 mg in 1 dose	GI symptoms, heart block, bradycardia
propranolol hydrochloride (Inderal)	No	No	Tablets	40–240 mg/d in 2 doses	See atenolol
			SR capsules, Oral solution	80–240 mg in 1 dose	
			IV	1–3 mg at 1 mg/min, may repeat once after 2 min PC: C	See atenolol
sotalol (Betapace)	No	No	Tablets	160–320 mg/d in 2 doses PC: B	See atenolol
timolol maleate (Blocadren)	No	No	Tablets	10–40 mg/d in 2 doses	
			Ophthalmic solution	1 drop of 0.25%–0.5% bid PC: C	

ISA = intrinsic sympathomimetic activity; SR = sustained-release product.
*investigational
PC = pregnancy risk category

FOCUS ON

Focus on Beta-Adrenergic Blocking Agents: Similarities and Differences

Similarities

Pharmacodynamics

Beta blockers compete with norepinephrine and epinephrine for available peripheral beta-receptor sites; they block the agonistic effect of these sympathetic neurotransmitters. They function as antihypertensives, they depress the automaticity of the sinus node, they decrease AV and intraventricular conduction velocity, and they reduce myocardial oxygen demand.

Pharmacokinetics

These agents are adequately absorbed by the GI tract, metabolized by the liver, and excreted by the kidneys.

Therapeutic Uses

These agents are used in hypertension, angina pectoris, after MI, migraine prophylaxis, and certain arrhythmias.

Adverse Reactions

These include bradycardia, heart block, aggravation of peripheral vascular insufficiency, fatigue, weakness, decreased libido, reduced exercise tolerance, hypoglycemia/hyperglycemia, depression, insomnia, vivid dreams, bronchospasm, aggravation of allergic reactions, increased serum triglycerides, and decreased HDL cholesterol.

Drug Interactions

Most beta blockers interact with aluminum and calcium salts, barbiturates, cholestyramine and colestipol, NSAIDs, ampicillin, rifampin, calcium channel blocking agents, haloperidol, histamine (H2) antagonists, hydralazine, loop diuretics, MAOIs, phenothiazines, propafenone, quinidine, ciprofloxacin, thyroid drugs, anticoagulants, benzodiazepines, clonidine, disopyramide, epinephrine, lidocaine, prazosin, sulfonylureas, and theophylline.

Differences

- Cardioselective beta blockers have greater affinity for beta-1 receptors in cardiac muscle than beta-2 receptors in bronchial and vascular musculature. Cardioselective agents are **acebutolol, atenolol, betaxolol, bisoprolol, esmolol,** and **metoprolol**.
- Some beta blockers have intrinsic sympathomimetic activity, which means they produce less resting bradycardia and less reduction in cardiac output than other beta blockers: **acebutolol, carteolol, penbutolol,** and **pindolol**.

- A significant percentage of **acebutolol** and **atenolol** are excreted in the feces. The lipid solubility of **acebutolol, atenolol, betaxolol, bisoprolol, esmolol, carteolol, nadolol,** and **sotalol** is low. The lipid solubility of **metoprolol, penbutolol,** and **propranolol** is higher. Drugs with higher lipid solubility can cross the blood-brain barrier.
- Most of the agents have an elimination half-life of less than 12 hours, but the half-life for **betaxolol** and **nadolol** is 14–22 hours and 20–24 hours respectively.
- **Atenolol, esmolol,** and **propranolol** have IV preparations.

- **Esmolol** and **sotalol** are not used to treat hypertension.
- **Atenolol, metoprolol, nadolol,** and **propranolol** are used with angina pectoris.
- **Atenolol, esmolol, metoprolol, nadolol, propranolol,** and **timolol** are given after MI.
- **Propranolol, timolol, atenolol, metoprolol,** and **nadolol** are used for migraine prophylaxis.
- **Betaxolol** and **timolol** are used for eye diseases.

- **Acebutolol, carteolol, penbutolol,** and **pindolol** cause less bradycardia than the others.
- **Carteolol, nadolol, penbutolol, pindolol, propranolol, sotalol,** and **timolol** are apt to cause more difficulties with bronchospasm and allergic symptoms.

- There are more similarities than differences. **Metoprolol** can be used as an example. There are increased effects of metoprolol with verapamil, cimetidine, and thyroid drugs. There are increased effects of both drugs if metoprolol is taken with hydralazine. There are increased serum levels and toxicity of IV lidocaine, if given concurrently. There is increased risk of postural hypotension with prazosin. There are decreased antihypertensive effects if taken with NSAIDs, clonidine, or rifampin. There are decreased therapeutic effects with barbiturates. Hypertension occurs and is followed by severe bradycardia if it is given concurrently with epinephrine.

(continued)

FOCUS ON

Focus on Beta-Adrenergic Blocking Agents: Similarities and Differences (continued)

Similarities (continued)

Precautions and Contraindications

Care must be taken if these agents are used with CHF, bradycardia, chronic obstructive pulmonary disease, or diabetes mellitus.

Nursing Considerations

Assess cardiopulmonary status at baseline and ongoing for changes. Assess blood pressure (lying, sitting, and standing) for changes. Assess pulse rate and rhythm. Instruct client about disease, adverse reactions, and how to integrate agent into lifestyle.

Differences (continued)

- **Esmolol** is used for supraventricular tachycardia in emergency situations, but generally is not used for longer than 24 hours.
- **Sotalol** is used for ventricular arrhythmias, but it can be proarrhythmic, and hypokalemia or hypomagnesemia seem to increase the risk of new or worsened arrhythmias.

- Food may enhance the bioavailability of **propranolol** and **metoprolol,** so these drugs should be administered at a consistent time each day in relation to meals.
- **Sotalol** absorption may be reduced by food, so it should be given on an empty stomach.

Table 25-4. Representative Combination Antihypertensive Agents

Beta-Adrenergic Blocking Agent and Diuretic

Trade Name	Blocking Agent	Diuretic
Corzide 40/5 or Corzide 80/5	nadolol 40 or 80 mg	bendroflumethiazide 5 mg
Inderide	propranolol 40 or 80 mg	hydrochlorothiazide 25 or 50 mg
Inderide LA	propranolol 80, 120, or 160 mg	hydrochlorothiazide 50 mg
Lopressor HCT	metoprolol 50 or 100 mg	hydrochlorothiazide 25 or 50 mg
Tenoretic	atenolol 50 or 100 mg	chlorthalidone 25 mg
Timolide	timolol 10 mg	hydrochlorothiazide 25 mg
Ziac	bisoprolol 2.5, 5, or 10 mg	hydrochlorothiazide 6.25 mg

ACE Inhibitor and Diuretic

Trade Name	ACE Inhibitor	Diuretic
Capozide 25/15 or Capozide 50/25	captopril 25 or 50 mg	hydrochlorothiazide 15 or 25 mg
Lotensin HCT	benazepril 5, 10, 20 mg	hydrochlorothiazide 6.25, 12.5, or 25 mg
Prinzide	lisinopril 10 or 20 mg	hydrochlorothiazide 12.5 or 25 mg
Vaseretic	enalapril 10 mg	hydrochlorothiazide 25 mg
Zestoretic	lisinopril 20 mg	hydrochlorothiazide 12.5 or 25 mg

Other Combinations

Trade Name	Component #1	Component #2
Aldoclor 250	methyldopa 250 mg	chlorothiazide 250 mg
Aldoril-15 or Aldoril-25; Aldoril D30 or Aldoril D50	methyldopa 250 or 500 mg	hydrochlorothiazide 15, 25, 30, or 50 mg
Apresazide 25/25	hydralazine 25 mg	hydrochlorothiazide 25 mg
Combipres 0.1	clonidine 0.1 mg	chlorthalidone 15 mg
Enduronyl	deserpidine 0.25 mg	methyclothiazide 5 mg
Esimil	guanethidine 10 mg	hydrochlorothiazide 25 mg
Hydropres	reserpine 0.125 mg	hydrochlorothiazide 25 or 50 mg
Hyzaar	losartan 50 mg	hydrochlorothiazide 12.5 mg
Minizide 1	prazosin 1 mg	polythiazide 0.5 mg

and supine blood pressure. Several mechanisms have been proposed to explain the antihypertensive action of beta blockers:

- Their effect on the central nervous system (CNS) leads to reduced sympathetic outflow to the periphery.
- They promote competitive antagonism of beta-adrenergic agonists for available peripheral beta-receptor sites (including those responsible for renin release from the kidneys).
- They initiate a presynaptic action inhibiting neurotransmitter release.

No single mechanism seems to offer a complete explanation. For example, because beta blockers can lower blood pressure irrespective of their capacity to enter the brain, the CNS effect theory provides only a partial explanation (Robertson & Ball, 1994).

Most beta blockers have an inhibitory effect on renin release, consequently reducing plasma angiotensin II levels. Peripheral concentrations of plasma angiotensin II have an effect on arterial pressure, so inhibition of renin secretion must contribute to the fall in blood pressure. However, this theory does not fully explain the antihypertensive effect—for example, pindolol is a beta blocker that lowers pressure but has an inconsistent effect on renin release.

Beta blockers compete with norepinephrine and epinephrine for available peripheral beta-receptor sites, leading to depressed automaticity of the sinus node and ectopic pacemaker and decreased atrioventricular and intraventricular conduction velocity. They reduce myocardial oxygen demand by negative inotropic (decreased force of myocardial contraction) and negative chronotropic (decreased heart rate) effects. The reduction in myocardial oxygen demand induced by beta blockers in long-term use can prevent symptoms associated with angina (eg, delay the onset of pain during exercise) and increase work capacity.

The mechanism by which beta-adrenergic blockade helps manage migraine headache has not been established. The headache pain is thought to be related to vasodilation. Blocking craniovascular beta receptors may decrease cerebral vasodilation and arteriolar spasms, therefore decreasing pain. Beta blockers approved by the Food and Drug Administration for treating migraines include propranolol and timolol. Atenolol, metoprolol, and nadolol also have unlabeled use for migraines.

Pharmacokinetics. Systemic bioavailability following oral administration of propranolol or timolol is low because of significant first-pass hepatic metabolism. Ingestion with food enhances the bioavailability of propranolol and metoprolol, but this effect is not noted with betaxolol or pindolol. Propranolol and metoprolol readily enter the CNS; other beta blockers, because of their high water solubility, do not cross the blood-brain barrier. These latter drugs may have a lower incidence of CNS side effects.

The bioavailability of betaxolol is 89%, half-life is 14 to 22 hours, and protein-bound status is 50%. The bioavailability of non–long-acting metoprolol is 40% to 50% (long-acting metoprolol, 77%), half-life is 3 to 7 hours, and protein-bound status is 12%. The bioavailability of pindolol is about 100%, half-life is 3 to 4 hours, and protein-bound status is 40%. All three drugs are metabolized by the liver and excreted in the urine, but the amount excreted unchanged in the urine ranges from 5% (metoprolol) to 40% (pindolol).

Therapeutic Uses. Labeled uses of betaxolol include hypertension, intraocular hypertension, and chronic open-angle glaucoma (see Chap. 39). Labeled uses of metoprolol include hypertension, angina pectoris, MI. Unlabeled uses of metoprolol include ventricular arrhythmias or tachycardias, atrial ectopy, migraine prophylaxis, essential tremors, aggressive behavior, antipsychotic-induced akathisia, enhanced cognitive performance, and CHF. Labeled uses of pindolol include hypertension. Unlabeled uses of pindolol include ventricular arrhythmias or tachycardias, antipsychotic-induced akathisia, and anxiety.

Dosage and Administration. Dosages of the same drug vary depending on the client and the client's condition. When betaxolol is used to manage hypertension, the initial dose is 10 mg once daily, alone or added to diuretic therapy (for older adults, the recommended starting dose is 5 mg). The drug is available in 10- and 20-mg tablets. The full antihypertensive effect is usually realized within 7 to 14 days; if the desired response is not achieved, the dose can be doubled. Increasing the dose over 20 mg does not produce a statistically significant additional antihypertensive effect. Reduced heart rate can be anticipated with increasing dosage. In discontinuing treatment, betaxolol should be gradually decreased and withdrawn over 2 weeks.

When metoprolol is used to manage hypertension, the initial dose is 100 mg/day in single or divided doses, alone or added to diuretic therapy. The drug is available in 50- and 100-mg tablets and as an injection (1 mg/mL). The dose may be increased at weekly (or longer) intervals until optimal blood-pressure reduction is achieved. In general, the maximal effect of any given dosage level will be apparent after 1 week of therapy. The maintenance dose is 100 to 450 mg/day. For angina, the initial dosage is 100 mg/day in two divided doses; the effective dosage range is 100 to 400 mg/day.

In clients with MI, treatment should begin as soon as possible after the client is hemodynamically stable. Three IV bolus injections of 5 mg each are administered at about 2-minute intervals. During IV administration, the blood pressure, heart rate, and electrocardiogram should be monitored carefully. If clients tolerate the full IV dose, they are given 50 mg orally every 6 hours beginning 15 minutes after the last IV dose; that dosage continues for 48 hours. Subsequently, a maintenance dose of 100 mg twice daily is used. Data suggest that treatment should continue for 1 to 3 years. Extended-release tablets of metoprolol are available in 50-, 100-, and 200-mg strengths.

The initial pindolol dose for hypertension is 5 mg twice daily, alone or added to diuretic therapy. The drug is available in 5- and 10-mg tablets. The antihypertensive response usually occurs within the first week of treatment, but maximal response may take 2 weeks or longer. If blood pressure does not decrease satisfactorily in 3 to 4 weeks, the dose is increased in increments of 10 mg/day at 3- to 4-week intervals, to a maximum of 60 mg/day.

Adverse Reactions. Consequences of beta-adrenergic blockade on overall regulation of the cardiovascular system must be considered when a beta-adrenergic blocker is used. Clients with normally functioning cardiovascular systems may be able to tolerate a blockade of adrenergic transmission to the heart. However, those with compensated heart failure depend on adrenergic tone to maintain adequate cardiac output, and removal of such tone may precipitate acute CHF. Additionally, because of their negative inotropic and chronotropic properties, beta blockers can precipitate CHF, heart block, or hypotension. Metoprolol, for example, decreases sinus heart rate in most clients. This decrease is greatest in clients with high initial heart rates and lowest in clients with low initial heart rates. Metoprolol slows atrioventricular conduction and may produce significant first-, second-, or third-degree heart block. If the rate decreases to below 40 beats per minute or heart block occurs, metoprolol may be discontinued and additional therapies—including IV atropine—initiated.

Beta-2 adrenergic blockade results in passive bronchial constriction by interfering with endogenous adrenergic bronchodilator activity.

Hypoglycemia has been associated with the use of beta blockers in clients with diabetes mellitus who use insulin. Hypoglycemia may be related to drug-induced inhibited glycogenolysis in skeletal muscle, which would normally result in an increase in plasma lactate. Lactate is subsequently converted by the liver to glucose. At the same time, insulin reactions are more difficult to detect in the client receiving a beta blocker because signs and symptoms relating to sympathoadrenal hyperactivity, which normally help the nurse identify hypoglycemia, are absent. On the other hand, hyperglycemia may occur, and this seems to be related to the blocking of insulin release from the pancreas. The cardioselective beta blockers are less likely to delay recovery from hypoglycemia or cause severe hypertension when hypoglycemia leads to an increase in circulating epinephrine (*Medical Letter*, 1995).

Abrupt withdrawal of beta-adrenergic blocking agents may be followed by rebound sympathetic overactivity. A withdrawal syndrome of tremulousness, sweating, severe headache, malaise, palpitation, rebound hypertension, MI, and arrhythmias has been identified. When discontinuing chronically administered beta-adrenergic blocking agents, the dosage should be reduced gradually over 1 to 2 weeks. If therapy with an alternative beta-adrenergic blocking agent is desired, the client may be transferred directly to comparable doses of another agent without interrupting therapy.

Drug–Drug Interactions. The widespread use of beta-adrenergic blockers in various situations is reflected in the multiple drug interactions identified between beta blockers and other drugs, including aluminum salts, barbiturates, calcium salts, cholestyramine, colestipol, nonsteroidal antiinflammatory agents (NSAIDs), ampicillin, rifampin, calcium channel blocking agents, haloperidol, histamine (H_2) antagonists, hydralazine, loop diuretics, MAOIs, phenothiazines, propafenone, quinidine, ciprofloxacin, thyroid drugs, anticoagulants, benzodiazepines, clonidine, disopyramide, epinephrine, lidocaine, prazosin, sulfonylureas, and theophylline. Metoprolol specifically is implicated with histamine (H_2) antagonists, hydralazine, MAOIs, propafenone, thyroid drugs, and benzodiazepines.

Drug–Laboratory Test Interactions. Beta-adrenergic blockers may produce hypoglycemia, interfering with glucose or insulin tolerance test results. Propranolol and metoprolol may cause elevated serum transaminase, alkaline phosphatase, and lactic acid dehydrogenase (LDH) levels. Minor but persistent elevations in AST and alanine aminotransferase (ALT) levels have occurred in clients treated with pindolol, but progressive elevations were not observed and liver injury has not been reported. Alkaline phosphatase, LDH, and uric acid levels are also elevated rarely, but the significance is unknown. Beta blockers may adversely affect the lipid profile by elevating triglyceride and reducing HDL cholesterol levels (Chutka, 1995).

Precautions and Contraindications. It is contraindicated to administer metoprolol to a client with MI if the client also has severe bradycardia, significant heart block, or severe hypotension. In general, chronic obstructive pulmonary disease is a contraindication to the use of beta blockers because the resulting blockade would intensify the degree of bronchospasm or airway obstruction. Because of their relative cardioselectivity, however, low doses of acebutolol, atenolol, metoprolol, and bisoprolol may be used with caution with clients with bronchospastic disease who do not respond to, or cannot tolerate, other antihypertensive treatment.

The necessity or desirability of withdrawing beta blockers before major surgery is controversial. The risk of excessive myocardial depression during general anesthesia may be enhanced. If the beta blockers are withdrawn, a 48-hour interval should occur between the last dose and anesthesia. If beta blockers are not withdrawn, care should be taken with anesthetic agents known to depress the myocardium. In emergency surgery, the effects of beta-adrenergic blocking agents may be reversed by administering beta-receptor agonists (dopamine, norepinephrine).

Combined Alpha- and Beta-Adrenergic Blockers

Labetalol (Normodyne, Trandate), the first drug in this category, is a nonselective combined beta-1 and beta-2 adrenergic blocker and a selective alpha-1 adrenergic blocker; it is more potent as the former than the latter. A similar agent, carvedilol (Coreg), was approved in 1995.

Pharmacodynamics. The alpha- and beta-blocking actions decrease blood pressure. Alpha blockade results in vasodilation, decreased peripheral resistance, and orthostatic hypotension but only slightly affects cardiac output and coronary artery blood flow. Due to alpha-1 receptor blocking activity, standing blood pressure is lowered more than supine. Renal blood flow and the glomerular filtration rate are relatively unchanged.

Pharmacokinetics. Oral labetalol is completely absorbed, and peak plasma levels occur in 2 to 4 hours. The duration of effect lasts from 8 to 12 hours, depending on dose. The maximal effect from an IV dose occurs in 5 minutes. There is extensive first-pass effect, so absolute bioavailability is 25%, but this is increased by food. In older adults, labetalol is about 50% protein bound. About 55% to 60% of a dose appears in urine as metabolites or as unchanged drug in the first 24 hours. Neither hemodialysis nor peritoneal dialysis removes a significant amount of drug. In decreased hepatic or renal function, elimination half-life is not altered.

Therapeutic Uses. Labetalol seems to decrease blood pressure more promptly than beta-adrenergic blockers, and it does not affect serum lipid levels. It is often used with thiazide and loop diuretics to counteract the volume expansion that occurs with its use. It has been used parenterally in severe hypertension, such as that associated with pheochromocytoma.

Dosage and Administration. An initial oral dose of labetalol is about 100 mg twice daily, alone or added to a diuretic. Dosage adjustments may be made every 2 to 3 days, in increments of 100 mg twice daily, based on standing blood pressure. A typical maintenance dose is 200 to 400 mg twice daily, but clients may require 1,200 to 2,400 mg daily.

In severe hypertension or hypertensive emergencies, 20 mg may be injected over 2 minutes, followed by additional injections of 40 to 80 mg every 10 minutes until the desired supine blood pressure is attained or a total of 300 mg is given. Another option is to administer 2 mg/min IV, with the client supine during the infusion. Symptomatic orthostatic hypotension is likely to occur if clients are allowed to be upright within 3 hours of receiving the drug.

Adverse Reactions. Labetalol is usually well tolerated. Adverse effects include nausea, dizziness, and orthostatic hypotension (which may be more frequent than with beta-adrenergic blockers). Transient scalp tingling may occur, especially with initial treatment. As discussed under beta-adrenergic blocking agents, beta-adrenergic blockade has a negative effect on clients who have compensated heart failure and who depend on adrenergic tone to maintain adequate cardiac output.

Drug–Drug Interactions. Drug interactions have been reported with cimetidine, glutethimide, halothane, and nitroglycerin. Labetalol can blunt the bronchodilator effect of beta-adrenergic agonists, such as albuterol, in clients with bronchospasm, so greater than normal doses of the agonist are needed. Cimetidine increases the bioavailability of oral labetalol. Glutethimide may decrease the effects of labetalol by inducing liver enzymes that metabolize labetalol. Synergistic adverse effects on cardiovascular hemodynamics may occur with concurrent administration of halothane and IV labetalol. Labetalol blunts the reflex tachycardia that may be produced by nitroglycerin; it does not prevent the hypotensive effect of nitroglycerin.

Drug–Laboratory Test Interactions. The labetalol metabolite in urine may falsely increase urinary catecholamine levels measured by a certain method. Reversible increases of serum transaminase levels occur in about 4% of clients; more rarely, reversible increases in blood urea levels occur.

Precautions and Contraindications. Oral labetalol must be used cautiously in clients with diabetes or hypoglycemia (it can mask cardiac signs of hypoglycemia) and in clients with chronic obstructive pulmonary disease. The drug is contraindicated in clients with sinus bradycardia, second- or third-degree heart block, cardiogenic shock, heart failure, or asthma, and in those who are pregnant or lactating.

Agents With Central Antihypertensive Action

The second major subgrouping of sympathetic inhibitors includes the agents that have a central antihypertensive action (Table 25-5). This drug group includes clonidine, guanabenz, guanfacine, and methyldopa. Methyldopa (Aldomet) and clonidine (Catapres) are representative drugs.

Pharmacodynamics. Methyldopa and clonidine have comparable antihypertensive potency. The mechanism by which methyldopa lowers arterial pressure is not completely understood, although several mechanisms have been proposed. For example, methyldopa may inhibit the enzyme dopa-decarboxylase, thereby limiting the generation of catecholamines. Another possible mechanism is that one of its metabolites, alpha-methylnorepinephrine, may activate alpha-2 receptors in the cardiovascular regulatory centers, which leads in turn to decreased sympathetic outflow from the CNS of vasoconstrictor and cardioaccelerator impulses. This produces vasodilation and lower arterial pressure. Cardiac output is usually unchanged or somewhat reduced. Renal blood flow and glomerular filtration rate are maintained, and myocardial and cerebral blood flows are

Table 25-5. Other Classes of Antihypertensive Agents

Drug Name	Preparation	Usual Dosage	Adverse Reactions
Centrally Acting Adrenergic Inhibitors			
clonidine (Catapres, Catapres TTS)	Tablets Transdermal system	0.1–0.6 mg in 2 doses one patch weekly PC: C	Dry mouth, drowsiness, dizziness, sedation, constipation, fatigue, headache, rebound hypertension; contact dermatitis with patches
guanabenz (Wytensin)	Tablets	4–64 mg in 2 doses PC: C	Similar to clonidine
guanfacine (Tenex)	Tablets	1–3 mg in 1 dose PC: B	Similar to clonidine, but milder
methyldopa (Aldomet, Presinol, Sembrina)	Tablets Oral suspension IV	250 mg–2g in 2 doses PC: C	Sedation, headache, weakness, dry mouth, nasal stuffiness, diarrhea, rash
Blockade of Neuroeffector Transmission			
guanadrel (Hylorel)	Tablets	10–75 mg in 2 doses PC: B	Similar to guanethidine, but less diarrhea
guanethidine (Ismelin)	Tablets	10–100 mg in 1 dose PC: C	Orthostatic hypotension, diarrhea, bradycardia, sodium and water retention
reserpine (Novoserpine, Reserpoid, Sandril, Serfin, Serpalen, Serpasil, Ser-Ap-Es)	Tablets	0.05–0.1 mg in 1 dose PC: C	Depression; nightmares; nasal stuffiness; drowsiness; GI disturbances; bradycardia
Miscellaneous Agents: Ganglionic Blocking Agents			
mecamylamine (Inversine)	Tablets	2.5 mg bid adjusted upwards to an average dose of 25 mg/d PC: C	Orthostatic hypotension, blurred vision, dry mouth, anorexia, nausea, vomiting, diarrhea, constipation, paralytic ileus, urinary retention
Miscellaneous Agents: Monamine Oxidase Inhibitors (MAOIs)			
pargyline (Eutonyl)	Tablets	25–50 mg qd	Orthostatic hypotension, dry mouth, headache, nightmares
Direct-Acting Vasodilators			
hydralazine (Apresoline)	Tablets IM IV	40–200 mg in 2–4 doses PC: C	Headache, palpitations, reflex tachycardia, anorexia, nausea, vomiting, diarrhea, paresthesias, numbness, tingling
minoxidil (Loniten)	Tablets	2.5–4.0 mg in 1 or 2 doses PC: C	Tachycardia, sodium and water retention, hypertrichosis, hypersensitivity skin reactions
Angiotensin II Receptor Antagonist			
losartan (Cozaar)	Tablets	50 mg qd PC: D (in second and third trimesters) PC: D	Dizziness, insomnia, muscle cramps, leg pain, GI upset

PC = pregnancy risk category; see Appendix A.

reportedly increased. Methyldopa causes plasma volume expansion and possibly fluid retention; a diuretic is usually administered concurrently. The coadministration of a diuretic enhances the antihypertensive efficacy of methyldopa (and clonidine).

Clonidine is an imidazoline derivative whose action also involves cardiovascular regulatory centers. Whereas clonidine acts directly, methyldopa must first be converted to alpha-methylnorepinephrine.

Pharmacokinetics. Oral absorption of methyldopa varies, with an average of 25%. Peak plasma levels are achieved in 2 to 4 hours. A period of about 2 days is required to establish maximal antihypertensive effects. Effective IV doses cause a decline in blood pressure that may begin in 4 to 6 hours. Metabolism is complex and not completely understood. The main metabolite is formed in intestinal cells. About 70% of the absorbed drug is excreted in the urine.

Blood pressure declines within 30 to 60 minutes of an oral dose of clonidine. The peak plasma level occurs in about 3 to 5 hours, with a plasma half-life of 12 to 16 hours. About 50% of the absorbed dose is metabolized in the liver. Half-life is increased to 30 to 40 hours in clients with impaired renal function. Clonidine and its metabolites are excreted mainly in the urine.

Therapeutic Uses. Methyldopa is used for mild to moderate primary hypertension. Because it lowers blood pressure without compromising renal blood flow or glomerular filtration rate, it is particularly useful in treating hypertension complicated by renal disease. However, it is usually ineffective in end-stage renal disease and the accompanying severe hypertension.

Clonidine is also used for mild to moderate hypertension. It may be combined with a diuretic, vasodilator, and beta blocker. It also is especially useful in clients with renal disease. Unlabeled treatment uses include alcohol withdrawal, smoking cessation facilitation, methadone/opiate detoxification, Tourette syndrome, menopausal flushing, postherpetic neuralgia, and ulcerative colitis. It is also used to diagnose pheochromocytoma.

Dosage and Administration. Initial therapy with methyldopa is 250 mg two or three times a day for 48 hours. Dosage adjustments may be made at intervals of not less than 2 days. The drug may cause sedation, so dosage increases should be provided in the evening. Maintenance therapy is usually 500 mg to 3 g daily in 2 to 4 doses. Tolerance may occur, usually between the second and third month of therapy. Adding a diuretic or increasing the dosage of methyldopa often restores blood-pressure control. When given IV, the dose is added to 100 mL of 5% dextrose in water and administered over 30 to 60 minutes. IV therapy is generally used only until control is obtained; then oral therapy continues.

The initial dose of clonidine is 0.1 mg twice daily. Dosage increases may be made each day until the desired response is achieved. The maximal dose is 2.4 mg/day. The drug may cause sedation, so dosage increases should be slow and most of the daily dose should be given at bedtime. Tolerance may occur.

Clonidine is available in a transdermal system (Catapres-TTS). This should be applied once a week to a hairless area of intact skin on the upper arm or torso. Sites should be rotated. The antihypertensive effect of the system may not begin until 2 or 3 days after application. Therapeutic plasma levels are lower than those occurring during oral therapy with equipotent doses. Thus, when substituting this system for another antihypertensive agent, a gradual reduction of the prior dosage is advised.

Adverse Reactions. The most common adverse effects of methyldopa are sedation, headache, weakness, dry mouth, nasal stuffiness, rash, and diarrhea. Urine discoloration may occur when urine is exposed to air (it may darken, because methyldopa breaks down into its metabolites). Some methyldopa products contain sulfites that may trigger allergic reactions in susceptible persons.

The most common adverse effects of clonidine include dry mouth, drowsiness, dizziness, sedation, and constipation. Constipation, dizziness, headache, and fatigue tend to diminish within 4 to 6 weeks. Orthostatic hypotension is mild because supine pressure is reduced to essentially the same extent as standing pressure (and seems less a factor than it is with methyldopa). The drug reduces heart rate but does not alter normal hemodynamic responses to exercise.

Transient localized skin reactions have been reported with the transdermal system. Reactions include pruritus, erythema, localized vesiculation, hyperpigmentation, and excoriation. If oral clonidine is substituted for transdermal clonidine, a generalized skin rash may develop.

Drug–Drug Interactions. Drug interactions have been reported between methyldopa and haloperidol (dementia, high incidence of sedation), levodopa (additive hypotensive effects), lithium (symptoms of lithium toxicity), propranolol (paradoxical hypertension), sympathomimetics, and tolbutamide (enhanced hypoglycemic effects).

Tricyclic antidepressants may block the antihypertensive effects of clonidine. Withdrawal hypertension caused by abrupt discontinuation of clonidine may be more severe in clients also taking beta-adrenergic blockers.

Drug–Laboratory Test Interactions. Methyldopa may interfere with test results measuring urinary uric acid, serum creatinine, and AST levels. Falsely high levels of urinary catecholamines may occur in urine samples when the client is receiving methyldopa; this interferes with diagnosing pheochromocytoma. Methyldopa does not interfere with VMA measurement.

With prolonged therapy, a positive direct Coombs' test result occurs in 10% to 20% of clients, usually between 6 and 12 months of therapy. The lowest reported incidence was at a dosage of 1 g/day or less. These test results are associated rarely with hemolytic anemia. In addition, a positive indirect Coombs' test result may occur less often. It may interfere with crossmatching of blood. If Coombs'-positive hemolytic anemia occurs, anemia usually resolves promptly after discontinuation of methyldopa. It may take weeks to months, however, before the positive Coombs' test result reverts to normal after methyldopa discontinuation. Rarely, a reduction of the white blood cell count has been documented, but the count returns to normal on discontinuation of the drug.

With clonidine, there may be decreased urinary excretion of catecholamines.

Precautions and Contraindications. If clonidine therapy is stopped suddenly, marked rebound hypertension related to excessive sympathetic discharge may occur. This significant effect is more a feature of clonidine therapy than methyldopa therapy. When clonidine is discontinued, the dose should be reduced gradually over 2 to 4 days to avoid this effect. Hypertensive encephalopathy and death have been reported after abrupt cessation of therapy.

In clients with uremia, the active metabolites of methyldopa accumulate, so the drug must be used with caution in clients with renal failure. The drug is removed by hemodialysis, which affects the timing of administration. Because methyldopa has been known to cause a fatal hepatic necrosis, liver function should be monitored. If addressed promptly, abnormalities in liver function revert to normal when the drug is discontinued. Blood counts should be monitored because white cell and platelet counts may change; hemolytic anemia has occurred.

Agents Causing Blockade of Neuroeffector Transmission

These agents are also referred to as peripheral antiadrenergics or peripherally acting adrenergic antagonists. Drugs in this group include guanadrel, guanethidine, and reserpine derivatives. Guanethidine (Ismelin) is considered a prototype of the group (see Table 25-5). *Rauwolfia serpentina* (snakeroot), found in India, Sri Lanka, Burma, and Java, contains 20 antihypertensive alkaloids; one of them is reserpine. Although the net result is similar, reserpine does not interfere with norepinephrine in the same way that guanethidine does. The rauwolfia alkaloids are infrequently used today, largely because they have the potential to elicit a wide range of adverse reactions and because other agents are just as effective.

Pharmacodynamics. The accumulation of guanethidine in adrenergic neurons disrupts the process by which action potentials trigger the release of stored norepinephrine. With norepinephrine release prevented, vascular smooth muscle contraction is reduced (because sympathetic nerve stimulation is reduced), and blood pressure decreases. A gradual depletion of norepinephrine stores in the nerve endings follows. The result is a prolonged reduction in heart rate and peripheral vascular resistance.

Guanethidine exemplifies the concept that the initial physiologic changes occurring in early treatment may change with chronic treatment. During early treatment, cardiac output decreases and a proportional decrease in renal, splanchnic, and cerebral blood flow occurs. With long-term therapy, however, hemodynamic adjustments occur and cardiac output gradually increases to pretreatment levels. A reduction in renal blood flow and glomerular filtration rate occurs in the early treatment period, but no significant changes appear to occur in renal function with long-term therapy.

Pharmacokinetics. Guanethidine is incompletely absorbed (3%–50%) after oral administration. It is partially metabolized by the liver to three metabolites. Guanethidine and its metabolites are excreted primarily in the urine. The drug is eliminated slowly because of extensive tissue binding (half-life 4–8 days).

Therapeutic Uses. Guanethidine is an extremely potent antihypertensive agent, but it is not widely used because of its associated adverse effects and prolonged half-life. When it is used, the indications are moderate and severe hypertension and renal hypertension (eg, that secondary to pyelonephritis, renal amyloidosis, and renal artery stenosis). It is always used with a diuretic.

Dosage and Administration. The initial dose is usually 25 to 50 mg. Dosage may be increased by 25 to 50 mg each day or every other day as indicated. The client should not be discharged from the hospital until the effect of the drug on the standing blood pressure is known.

Adverse Reactions. Reflex sympathetic nervous activity normally causes vasoconstriction when the client assumes an upright position. Because the sympathetic venoconstrictive mechanisms are inhibited by the guanethidine, orthostatic effects are common. Fainting may occur unless the client is warned to sit or lie down with the onset of dizziness or weakness. Orthostatic hypotension is marked in the morning and is accentuated by prolonged standing, hot weather, alcohol, or exercise. Orthostatic effects may be particularly bothersome during the initial dosage adjustment period.

Bradycardia, sodium and water retention, and diarrhea are common adverse effects. Diarrhea may be severe, necessitating discontinuation of the medication.

Drug Interactions. Drug interactions have been reported between guanethidine and anorexiants, haloperidol (hypotensive effect antagonized), minoxidil (profound orthostatic effects), MAOIs, phenothiazines (hypotensive effect inhibited), sympathomimetics, and tricyclic antidepressants (hypotensive effect inhibited).

Precautions and Contraindications. Guanethidine must be given with caution to clients with coronary artery disease, recent MI, cerebrovascular disease, bronchial asthma, active peptic ulcer or ulcerative colitis (may be aggravated by an increase in parasympathetic tone), and renal dysfunction. It is contraindicated in those who are allergic to it and in pregnancy and lactation.

Miscellaneous Agents

Miscellaneous agents (see Table 25-5) include ganglionic blocking agents and an MAOI. Synaptic transmission in the ganglia of the autonomic nervous system is mediated by acetylcholine. The transmission can be reduced by preventing the attachment of acetylcholine to the receptor sites of the autonomic ganglia. Mecamylamine (Inversine) does this.

Mecamylamine is nonselective in its blocking action, so it reduces neurotransmission in both sympathetic and parasympathetic ganglia. Blockage of impulse transmission in the sympathetic system decreases vascular tone, producing vasodilation and hypotension and decreasing venous return to the heart (and, consequently, cardiac output). Blockage of impulse transmission in the parasympathetic system produces significant adverse reactions. Mecamylamine is an extremely potent antihypertensive agent, but it is not used frequently because of the extensive adverse reactions. It is indicated for moderately severe to severe essential hypertension and uncomplicated malignant hypertension.

The miscellaneous grouping also includes one MAOI approved for treating hypertension. Pargyline (Eutonyl) lowers blood pressure by blocking the release of norepinephrine at the sympathetic neuroeffector junctions, thereby interfering with vasoconstriction. However, because of difficulties involving interactions with MAOIs, pargyline is rarely used.

Direct-Acting Vasodilators

This class of drugs, widely used in managing high blood pressure, includes hydralazine (Apresoline) and minoxidil (Loniten), both of which are representative (see Table 25-5).

Pharmacodynamics. Direct-acting vasodilators produce peripheral vasodilation by direct relaxation of vascular smooth muscle. Hydralazine alters cellular calcium metabolism, thus interfering with the calcium movements in the vascular smooth muscle that are responsible for initiating or maintaining the contractile state. The peripheral vasodilating effect results in decreased arterial blood pressure (diastolic more than systolic) and decreased peripheral vascular resistance. The dilation of arterioles instead of veins minimizes orthostatic hypotension and promotes increased cardiac output. There is a reflex increase in sympathetic stimulation of the heart (increased heart rate). An increase in plasma renin level—in response to reflex sympathetic discharge—leads to production of angiotensin II, which stimulates aldosterone reabsorption and thereby sodium reabsorption and water retention. Because of the reflex sympathetic stimulation of the heart, these agents often are administered along with a drug that inhibits sympathetic activity (ie, a beta-adrenergic blocker).

Minoxidil, a piperidino-pyrimidine derivative, is not related chemically to hydralazine, but it is a direct-acting peripheral vasodilator and appears to block calcium uptake through the cell membrane. It reduces elevated systolic and diastolic blood pressure by decreasing peripheral vascular resistance. In studies, it reduced supine diastolic blood pressure by 20 mmHg in 75% of persons evaluated. Like hydralazine, it increases heart rate, cardiac output, renin secretion, sodium reabsorption, and water retention.

Pharmacokinetics. Hydralazine is rapidly absorbed after oral administration. Bioavailability is 30% to 50%. Protein binding is 87% and half-life is 3 to 7 hours. Peak plasma concentrations occur 1 to 2 hours after ingestion; duration of action is 6 to 12 hours. Hydralazine undergoes extensive hepatic metabolism. It is excreted in the urine as active drug and metabolites.

Minoxidil is 90% absorbed after oral administration. It is not protein bound and concentrates in arteriolar smooth muscle. After a single oral dose, blood pressure usually starts to decline within 30 minutes and reaches a minimum value in 2 or 3 hours. About 90% of minoxidil is metabolized, predominantly by conjugation with glucuronic acid. Metabolites exert much less pharmacologic effect than minoxidil itself, and all are excreted principally in the urine.

Therapeutic Uses. Hydralazine is used for clients with moderately severe essential hypertension. Because it reduces vascular resistance, hydralazine also reduces afterload and could potentially assist in managing CHF; however, studies have failed to demonstrate any long-term benefits of using hydralazine alone for CHF.

Minoxidil can produce a greater drop in blood pressure than hydralazine and is used for hypertension resistant to other forms of therapy and for severe hypertension that may be life-threatening. It is especially used for hypertension in clients with renal failure because it produces no significant changes in renal blood flow or glomerular filtration rate. In hypertension management, both vasodilators are usually used in combination with a beta blocker (to minimize the reflex increase in heart rate) and a diuretic (to avoid sodium and water retention).

Topical minoxidil (Rogaine) is used for treating androgenetic alopecia, expressed in males as baldness of the vertex of the scalp and in females as diffuse hair loss or thinning. At least 4 months of twice-daily applications are required before hair regrowth can be expected. Accidental ingestion of the topical agent may produce adverse systemic effects. Increased systemic absorption may occur if more frequent or larger-than-directed doses of the topical form are used or if the drug is applied to skin surfaces other than the scalp. Use of the oral preparation to promote hair growth is not approved.

Dosage and Administration. Treatment with hydralazine should begin with 10 mg four times daily for the first 2 to 4 days and then increase to 25 mg four times daily. It is available as 10- to 100-mg tablets and in 20-mg/mL injection form. For maintenance, the daily dosage should be limited to 200 mg daily to decrease the possibility of a reaction resembling systemic lupus erythematosus. The bioavailability of hydralazine is enhanced by the concurrent ingestion of food. Hydralazine can be administered parenterally when it cannot be given orally.

Minoxidil's initial dosage is 5 mg/day as a single dose. The daily dosage can be increased to 100 mg, but the typical dosage is 10 to 40 mg daily. It should be given with a beta blocker and a loop diuretic because of associated fluid retention and reflex tachycardia.

Adverse Reactions. Adverse effects from hydralazine include headache, palpitations, reflex tachycardia, anorexia, nausea, vomiting, and diarrhea. Peripheral neuritis, manifested by paresthesias, numbness, and tingling, has been observed; it may be due to an antipyridoxine effect. If neuritis symptoms develop, pyridoxine (vitamin B_6) may be added to the drug regimen. Exacerbation of anginal symptoms may occur, and the drug has been implicated in MI.

Hydralazine may produce a lupuslike syndrome, including arthralgia, dermatoses, fever, splenomegaly, and glomerulonephritis. Generally this happens after 6 months of continuous therapy in clients who are slow acetylators and with doses in excess of 200 mg/day. Slow acetylators generally have higher plasma hydralazine levels and require lower doses to maintain control of blood pressure. The lupuslike syndrome usually regresses with drug discontinuation, but steroidal therapy may be necessary and residual effects may remain for years. Some hydralazine preparations contain tartrazine, which may cause allergic reactions in susceptible clients.

Minoxidil's adverse effects include tachycardia, electrocardiogram changes, edema, sodium and water retention, and hypertrichosis. Hypertrichosis—the elongation, thickening, and enhanced pigmentation of fine body hair—develops in 80% of clients within 3 to 6 weeks of therapy. Hypersensitivity skin reactions and Stevens-Johnson syndrome have occurred. Serious adverse reactions include pericardial effusion, occasionally progressing to tamponade, and exacerbation of anginal symptoms.

Drug–Drug Interactions. Drug interactions with hydralazine have involved beta-adrenergic blocking agents (serum levels of either drug may be increased when they are used concurrently) and NSAIDs (decreased effect of hydralazine). Guanethidine interacts with minoxidil, causing profound orthostatic effects.

Drug–Laboratory Test Interactions. Hydralazine may cause some decrease in total cholesterol levels. Blood dyscrasias have been reported. Hydralazine interferes with one method of determining urinary 17-hydroxycorticosteroids.

Early in minoxidil therapy, hematocrit, hemoglobin, and red blood cell count usually decrease; serum alkaline phosphatase, blood urea nitrogen (BUN), and creatinine levels may increase.

Precautions and Contraindications. Clients receiving hydralazine should have complete blood counts and antinuclear antibody (ANA) titer determinations made before and during prolonged therapy because of the possibility of blood dyscrasias or lupuslike syndrome. Hydralazine is contraindicated in mitral valve disease and coronary artery disease. It must be used cautiously in clients with increased intracranial pressure or severe hypertension with advanced renal damage, and in lactation.

Minoxidil is contraindicated in pheochromocytoma. It must be used cautiously after MI and in CHF. It is not recommended during pregnancy or lactation.

Angiotensin-Converting Enzyme Inhibitors

Angiotensin-converting enzyme inhibitors were formerly used to treat severe hypertension that did not respond to other medications. Currently, ACE inhibitors are used for early hypertension control in clients with normal renal function. Typical agents in this category are benazepril, captopril, enalapril, fosinopril, lisinopril, moexipril, quinapril, and ramipril (Table 25-6). Captopril, the oldest in the category, is discussed as a prototype. See Focus On ACE Inhibitors: Similarities and Differences on page 498.

Pharmacodynamics. Renin is synthesized by the kidneys and released into the circulation, where it acts on a substrate to produce angiotensin I. Angiotensin I is then converted by ACE to angiotensin II, a potent vasoconstrictor that also stimulates aldosterone secretion from the adrenal cortex. ACE inhibitors prevent the conversion of angiotensin I to angiotensin II. Inhibiting the enzyme results in reduction of peripheral arterial resistance and blood pressure. Standing and supine blood pressures are lowered to about the same extent.

Inhibition of ACE also appears to decrease the inactivation of bradykinin (normally ACE degrades bradykinin), an endogenous vasodilator, and this accumulation of kinins in various tissues may contribute to the pressure-lowering effect and certain adverse reactions.

Increased prostaglandin synthesis may also play a role in the peripheral vasodilating and antihypertensive action of captopril. Single doses of captopril increase urinary excretion of prostaglandin E_2 and plasma levels of its metabolites. Captopril's antihypertensive effects persist longer than does demonstrable inhibition of circulating ACE.

Pharmacokinetics. About 75% of captopril is absorbed after oral administration, but absorption is reduced significantly by food. With other ACE inhibitors, the *rate* of absorption may be more affected by food than the *extent* of absorption, and with others food may not affect absorption. Captopril's onset of action is 15 minutes and the duration of action is dose-related. Peak serum levels are reached in 30 to 90 minutes, and blood-pressure reduction peaks within about 60 to 90 minutes after oral administration. Captopril is 25% to 30% protein bound. Plasma half-life when renal function is normal is less than 2 hours; however, as with all ACE inhibitors, impaired renal function prolongs half-life (in this case, from 3.5 to 32 hours). About 40% to 50% of captopril is eliminated unchanged in the urine.

Therapeutic Uses. These agents are effective and well tolerated for treating hypertension. They are less effec-

Table 25-6. ACE Inhibitors

Drug Name	Preparations	Usual Dosage	Adverse Reactions
benazepril (Lotensin)	Tablets	10–40 mg in 1–2 doses PC: (see below)	Headache, cough, rash
captopril (Capoten)	Tablets	12.5–150 mg in 2 or 3 doses	Neutropenia/agranulocytosis, maculopapular rash, angioedema, hyperkalemia, cough
enalapril (Vasotec)	Tablets IV	2.5–40 mg in 1 or 2 doses 1.25 mg q6h over 5 min	Headache, dizziness, hypotension including orthostatic hypotension, acute renal failure, hyperkalemia, cough
fosinopril (Monopril)	Tablets	10–40 mg in 1 or 2 doses	Headache, hyperkalemia, cough
lisinopril (Prinivil, Zestril)	Tablets	5–40 mg in 1 dose	Headache, hyperkalemia, cough
moexipril (Univasc)	Tablets	7.5–30 mg in 1 or 2 doses	Cough, dizziness, diarrhea, flu syndrome, pharyngitis, blushing, rash, myalgia
quinapril (Accupril)	Tablets	5–80 mg in 1 or 2 doses	Angioedema, hyperkalemia, cough, agranulocytosis
ramipril (Altace)	Capsules	1.25–20 mg in 1 or 2 doses	Angioedema, hyperkalemia, cough, rash
trandolapril (Mavik)	Tablets	1 mg qd in nonblack clients, 2 mg qd in black	Cough, dizziness, diarrhea

ACE inhibitors are contraindicated in pregnancy during the second and third trimesters (PC: D). PC: C in first trimester. When used in pregnancy during the second and third trimesters, ACE inhibitors can cause injury, including hypotension, neonatal skull hypoplasia, anuria, reversible or irreversible renal failure, and death.

tive, but not ineffective, in African Americans. They have favorable hemodynamic and neurohormonal effects in clients with heart failure and after acute MI. They decrease afterload and left ventricular filling pressure, thereby increasing cardiac output and exercise tolerance. When captopril is used in CHF, it is usually combined with diuretics and digitalis (unless digitalis is poorly tolerated). From a neurohormonal aspect, they reduce the direct toxic effects of angiotensin on myocardial cells that may lead to cell necrosis and disease progression (Packer, 1992).

Captopril has a protective effect on the kidneys in clients who have insulin-dependent diabetes mellitus with established diabetic nephropathy. It decreases urinary protein excretion and retards the progression of the renal disease, lowering the risk for death, dialysis, or transplantation. Captopril's effects in this situation seem to be independent of its function as an antihypertensive agent.

Unlabeled uses for captopril include managing hypertensive crises, neonatal and childhood hypertension, rheumatoid arthritis, hypertension related to scleroderma, renal crisis, Bartter's syndrome, Raynaud's syndrome, and hypertension of Takayasu's disease.

Dosage and Administration. Captopril is available in 12.5- to 100-mg tablets. It should be administered 1 hour before meals. If possible, any previous antihypertensive drugs should be discontinued 1 week before captopril therapy begins. Initial treatment for hypertension is 25 mg two or three times a day. Dosage may be increased to 50 mg two or three times a day after 1 to 2 weeks and further increased to 150 mg two or three times a day as needed. The maximal daily dose is 450 mg.

With CHF, the usual initial dosage is 25 mg three times a day; dosage increases should generally be de-

layed for 2 weeks. Again, the maximal daily dose is 450 mg.

The target maintenance dose after MI is 50 mg three times daily. Therapy may be initiated as early as 3 days after MI. With diabetic nephropathy, the recommended dose for long-term use is 25 mg three times daily.

Adverse Reactions. Cough occurs commonly in clients treated with ACE inhibitors (incidence 5%–39%). Some reports indicate that inhaling cromolyn (Intal) may relieve the cough. ACE inhibitors may cause a profound drop in blood pressure (exaggerated hypotensive response) within 1 to 3 hours of the first dose. Clients with high levels of plasma renin activity (including those who are volume-depleted or taking diuretics and those with renovascular hypertension or CHF) may be those who have excessive hypotensive responses to ACE inhibitors. Clients with bilateral renovascular disease whose renal perfusion is maintained by high levels of angiotensin II may develop acute renal failure when using an ACE inhibitor.

Rashes are fairly common with captopril, and allergic reactions (anaphylaxis, angioedema) also may occur. Rarely, ACE inhibitors have been associated with a syndrome that starts with jaundice and progresses to fulminant hepatic necrosis and, sometimes, death. The mechanism for this syndrome is not understood. Captopril-specific side effects, which may be due to a sulfhydryl group in the molecule, include taste loss or disturbance and neutropenia.

Drug–Drug Interactions. The antihypertensive effects of ACE inhibitors may be increased by diuretics and adrenergic blocking agents and other antihypertensive

FOCUS ON

Focus on ACE Inhibitors: Similarities and Differences

Similarities

Pharmacodynamics

Renin is synthesized by the kidneys and released into the circulation, where it acts on a substrate to produce angiotensin I. Angiotensin I is then converted by ACE to angiotensin II, a potent vasoconstrictor that also stimulates aldosterone secretion from the adrenal cortex. ACE inhibitors prevent the conversion of angiotensin I to angiotensin II. Inhibiting the enzyme results in decreased vasoconstriction and reduced peripheral vascular resistance.

Hypertension is often characterized by insulin resistance, and ACE inhibitors have been found to improve insulin sensitivity.

Pharmacokinetics

ACE inhibitors differ in terms of chemical structure, prodrug/active drug status, and lipid solubility, but the impact on clinical use is not clear.

They differ in duration of a clinically significant antihypertensive effect, and this can affect the number of daily doses needed.

ACE inhibitors are eliminated predominantly through the kidneys.

Therapeutic Uses

These agents are used in hypertension, following myocardial infarction to attenuate left ventricular dysfunction, and in congestive heart failure.

Adverse Reactions

Cough, headache, rash, angioedema, hyperkalemia, hypotension

Drug Interactions

Diuretics and adrenergic blocking agents may increase antihypertensive drug effects of ACE inhibitors. Nitrates may be potentiated. Potassium-sparing diuretics and potassium supplements can contribute to hyperkalemia when used with ACE inhibitors.

Precautions and Contraindications

Some clients are at risk of developing renal failure when an ACE inhibitor is used

ACE inhibitors may be contraindicated in clients receiving immunosupressants. They are contraindicated in clients allergic to sulfonamides and in the second and third trimesters of pregnancy.

Nursing Considerations

Assess cardiopulmonary status at baseline and ongoing for changes. Assess blood pressure (lying, sitting, and standing) for changes. Instruct client about disease, adverse reactions, and how to integrate agent into lifestyle.

Differences

- Increased prostaglandin synthesis may also play a role in the action of **captopril.**

- **Lisinopril** has been shown to improve insulin sensitivity to a greater degree than other ACE inhibitors.

- Because the liver has no real role with **lisinopril,** it could be the best choice with clients with hepatic insufficiency.

- **Lisinopril, enalapril,** and **trandolapril** seem to guarantee better control of 24-hour blood pressure with once-daily administration.

- **Fosinopril, ramipril, spirapril,** and **trandolapril** are eliminated by the liver as well as the kidney. When one route of elimination is reduced, there is a compensatory rise in excretion by the alternative route. These agents can be administered to clients with renal failure without changing the dose.

- **Captopril, enalapril, lisinopril,** and **quinapril** are used in CHF.

- Adverse reactions specific to **captopril** include taste loss or disturbance.

- The antihypertensive effect of **captopril** can be reduced by concurrent use of indomethacin, aspirin, and other NSAIDs.

- Neutropenia with myeloid hypoplasia has resulted from use of **captopril**; its incidence is higher with renal failure and collagen disease (such as scleroderma or systemic lupus erythematosus) with impaired renal function. Some fatalities have occurred.

- Administer **captopril** 1 hour before meals.

drugs, and by severe sodium and fluid restriction. Drug interactions occur between ACE inhibitors and potassium-sparing diuretics and potassium supplements. The antihypertensive efficacy of captopril can be reduced by NSAIDs. This interaction appears due to inhibition by NSAIDs of prostaglandin synthesis; prostaglandins seem to play a positive role in the antihypertensive effect of ACE inhibitors. Vasodilators (nitrates) may be potentiated by ACE inhibitors.

Drug–Laboratory Test Interactions. Neutropenia with myeloid hypoplasia has resulted from captopril. Its incidence is higher with renal failure and collagen disease with impaired renal function. In general, the neutrophil level returned to normal in 2 weeks after captopril was discontinued, but some cases were fatal in association with infection and concurrent serious illness. Hyperkalemia has been observed in some clients receiving ACE inhibitors. Serum potassium may rise due to the absence of aldosterone activity. The reduced circulating aldosterone is associated with a potassium-sparing effect. Additional risk factors for development of hyperkalemia may include use of potassium-sparing diuretics, potassium supplements, renal insufficiency, and diabetes mellitus.

Captopril may decrease fasting blood sugar in the nondiabetic client and may cause hypoglycemia in the diabetic controlled with antidiabetic drug therapy.

Precautions and Contraindications. Clients who have poor renal function but who are not diabetics when ACE inhibitor therapy is being considered may need to try other classes of antihypertensives first. The drug may be contraindicated in clients receiving immunosuppressants or other drugs that normally cause leukopenia or agranulocytosis. White blood cell and differential counts are recommended before therapy begins and at approximately 2-week intervals during early therapy with ACE inhibitors. The drugs are contraindicated in clients allergic to sulfonamides and in the second and third trimesters of pregnancy.

Angiotensin Receptor Antagonist

Approved for use in 1995, losartan (Cozaar) is the first of a new class of antihypertensives, angiotensin II receptor antagonists.

Pharmacodynamics. Losartan blocks the vasoconstrictor and aldosterone-secreting effects of angiotensin II by selectively blocking the binding of angiotensin II to the AT_1 receptor found in vascular smooth muscle and the adrenal gland. Losartan is a reversible, competitive inhibitor of the AT_1 receptor.

Pharmacokinetics. After oral administration, it is well absorbed, and bioavailability is 33%. Peak concentrations of losartan and its active metabolite are reached in

1 hour and in 3 to 4 hours, respectively. Losartan and its active metabolite are highly bound to plasma proteins. Losartan crosses the blood-brain barrier poorly, if at all. It undergoes substantial first-pass metabolism in the liver. About 14% of losartan is converted to an active metabolite that is 10 to 40 times more potent than losartan and appears responsible for much of the angiotensin II receptor antagonism. After an oral dose, about 35% is recovered in the urine and 50% in the feces.

Therapeutic Uses. Losartan is approved for the treatment of hypertension, alone or in combination with other antihypertensive agents. It is less effective in African Americans.

Dosage and Administration. The usual starting dose is 50 mg once daily (25 mg if the client is on a diuretic or has a history of hepatic impairment). Dosage increases to a higher once-daily dose or a twice-daily regimen may be made. Losartan may be administered with or without food.

Adverse Reactions. To date, losartan is well tolerated. Reported adverse effects include diarrhea, dyspepsia, muscle cramps and myalgia, back and leg pain, dizziness, insomnia, nasal congestion, cough, and sinus disorder or sinusitis. The most common effects are dizziness and diarrhea.

Drug–Drug Interactions. Drug interactions have been reported with cimetidine (increased losartan effect) and phenobarbital (decreased losartan effect).

Drug–Laboratory Test Interactions. Despite the effect of losartan on aldosterone secretion, very little effect on serum potassium level has been observed in blood tests.

Minor increases in BUN or serum creatinine levels were observed in some clients treated with losartan alone. Small decreases in hemoglobin and hematocrit values occurred in clients treated with losartan alone. Occasional elevations of liver enzyme or serum bilirubin levels have occurred.

Precautions and Contraindications. In clients with hepatic dysfunction, the bioavailability of losartan is two times higher and the clearance about 50% lower, so these clients need smaller doses. Losartan must be used cautiously in clients with severe CHF or renal artery stenosis. It is contraindicated in the second and third trimesters of pregnancy.

Calcium Channel Blocking Agents

The calcium channel blockers are classified by structure: diphenylalkylamines (verapamil), benzothiazepines (diltiazem), and dihydropyridines (amlodipine, felodipine, isradipine, nicardipine, nifedipine, nimodipine, nisoldipine). Verapamil, the diphenylalkylamine, was discussed in Chapter 22 because it is used to treat arrhythmias. In this chapter, one benzothiazepine, diltiazem

(Cardizem), and one dihydropyridine, nifedipine (Procardia, Adalat), will be discussed as prototypes of these two classes.

Pharmacodynamics. The calcium channel blocking agents are a very important group of drugs (Table 25-7). In contractile cells of the myocardium, calcium links excitation to contraction (excitation/contraction coupling). Contractile processes of myocardial and vascular smooth muscle depend on the movement of extracellular calcium ions into certain myocardial and vascular cells through specific ion channels. Calcium channel blocking agents lower the intracellular calcium concentration by reducing the transmembranous slow calcium influx, which normally occurs during membrane depolarization. The inhibition of calcium influx into cells prevents the rise in calcium levels and results in diminished vascular tone, vascular smooth muscle relaxation,

Table 25-7. Calcium Channel Blocking Agents

Drug Name	Preparation	Usual Dosage	Adverse Reactions
verapamil (Calan, Isoptin, Calan SR, Isoptin SR, Verelan, Covera-HS)	Tablets Sustained-release tablets Sustained-release capsules Injection Controlled onset extended release	80 mg tid (hypertension) PC: C	Dizziness, lightheadedness, constipation, hypotension, peripheral edema
diltiazem (Cardizem, Cardizem SR, Cardizem CD, Dilacor XR, Tiazac)	Tablets Sustained-release capsules	240–360 mg qd PC: C	Dizziness, lightheadedness, headache, asthenia, peripheral edema, AV block, bradycardia, flushing
nifedipine (Adalat, Procardia, Procardia XL, Adalat CC)	Capsules Sustained-release tablets	30–90 mg qd PC: C	Dizziness, lightheadedness, nervousness, headache, weakness, shakiness, paresthesias, somnolence, asthenia, insomnia, nausea, diarrhea, constipation, abdominal discomfort, dry mouth, flatulence, peripheral edema, hypotension, palpitations, CHF, MI, pulmonary edema, rash, flushing, nasal congestion, micturition disorder, sexual disorders, shortness of breath, muscle cramps, joint stiffness, cough
amlodipine (Norvasc)	Tablets	5–10 mg qd PC: C	Dizziness, lightheadedness, headache, fatigue, peripheral edema, palpitations, flushing
felodipine (Plendil)	Extended-release tablets	2.5–10 mg qd PC: C	Same as amlodipine
isradipine (DynaCirc)	Capsules	2.5–10 mg qd PC: C	Same as amlodipine
nicardipine (Cardene, Cardene SR)	Capsules Sustained-release capsules IV	20–40 mg tid 30 mg bid titrate at 5–15 mg/hr PC: C	Same as amlodipine
nimodipine (Nimotop)	Capsules Liquid	60 mg q4h PC: C	Headache, diarrhea, hypotension
bepridil (Vascor)	Tablets	200 mg/d PC: C	Dizziness, lightheadedness, drowsiness, nervousness, headache, asthenia, tinnitus, tremor, nausea, diarrhea, abdominal discomfort, dry mouth, palpitations, shortness of breath, anorexia
nisoldipine (Nisocor, Sular)		20 mg/d PC: C	Dizziness, lightheadedness, headache, fatigue, lethargy, nausea, peripheral edema, flushing
nitrendipine* (Baypress)		10–80 mg/d in single dose or 2 or 3 divided doses PC: C	Headache, fatigue, peripheral edema, flushing, palpitations, dizziness

*Investigational
PC = pregnancy risk category (see Appendix A).

and, consequently, vasodilation and lowered blood pressure. Calcium channel blockers dilate the coronary arteries and arterioles, both in normal and ischemic regions. This increases myocardial oxygen delivery.

These agents also reduce arterial blood pressure at rest and with exercise by dilating peripheral arterioles and reducing total peripheral resistance (afterload) against which the heart works. This reduces myocardial energy consumption and oxygen requirements, which probably explains their effectiveness in chronic angina pectoris.

Although these agents are similar in that they all act on the slow (calcium) channels, they have different degrees of selectivity in their effects on vascular smooth muscle, myocardium, or specialized conduction and pacemaker tissues. This heterogeneity of the calcium blockers partly determines their clinical application and the different adverse reactions produced by each agent. See Focus On Calcium Channel Blockers: Similarities and Differences.

Pharmacokinetics. Nifedipine is 90% absorbed after oral administration, and bioavailability is 45% to 86%. Onset of action is 20 minutes, with peak plasma levels recorded in 0.5 to 6 hours. It is 92% to 98% protein bound. Diltiazem is 80% to 90% absorbed after oral administration, and bioavailability is 40% to 67%. Onset of action is 30 to 60 minutes, with peak plasma levels in 2 to 11 hours. It is 70% to 80% protein bound.

Therapeutic Uses. Nifedipine and diltiazem are approved for treating hypertension and angina.

Dosage and Administration. Nifedipine is available in 10- and 20-mg capsules and 30- and 90-mg sustained-release (SR) tablets. Clients with hypertension may receive the SR dosage form (Procardia XL), administered once daily. The SR tablets must be swallowed whole, not chewed or divided. Debate exists over the sublingual bioavailability of nifedipine. The capsules have been punctured and administered sublingually (contents squeezed under the tongue) as needed when blood pressure is high. Some studies report sublingual absorption and therapeutic blood-pressure reduction, and others do not (Robertson & Ball, 1994).

Diltiazem is available in 30- to 120-mg tablets and 60- to 300-mg SR capsules. Again, the SR forms (Cardizem SR, Cardizem CD) are the ones used for hypertension management. Cardizem SR is started at 60 to 120 mg twice daily. The optimal dosage range is 240 to 360 mg/day. Cardizem CD is started at 180 to 240 mg once daily, with a range of 240 to 360 mg once daily. It may take 14 days for maximal antihypertensive effect. Cardizem CD may also be used for angina.

Diltiazem is available in parenteral form for use with paroxysmal supraventricular tachycardia. The initial bolus dose, 0.25 mg/kg, is administered over 2 minutes (20 mg is an average dose). If response is inadequate, a second dose may be administered after 15 minutes. A continuous IV infusion may be administered in clients with atrial fibrillation or atrial flutter at 10 to 15 mg/hour, but it is not recommended for infusion exceeding 24 hours.

Adverse Reactions. Adverse effects include headache, dizziness, edema, changes in heart rate (tachycardia), nausea, rash, and constipation. Calcium channel blockers do not have deleterious effects on serum lipid levels or glucose metabolism (as do beta blockers).

Nifedipine has its greatest effect on vascular smooth muscle, so the incidence of adverse effects resulting from vasodilation (eg, headache, flushing) is greater.

Cardiovascular effects, including ankle edema, CHF, MI, and pulmonary edema, are more prominent with nifedipine. The edema may be due to arterial vasodilation.

Drug–Drug Interactions. Drug interactions have been reported between nifedipine, felodipine, and histamine (H_2) antagonists, quinidine, anticoagulants, beta blockers, digitalis, parenteral magnesium sulfate, and theophyllines. Drug interactions have been reported between diltiazem and histamine (H_2) antagonists, beta blockers, carbamazepine, cyclosporine, digitalis, encainide, lithium, and theophyllines. Beta blockers can increase bradycardia when used with diltiazem.

Drug–Food Interactions. Nifedipine interacts with grapefruit juice (see Chap. 6).

Drug–Laboratory Test Interactions. Rare and usually transient, but occasionally significant, elevations of enzymes (eg, alkaline phosphatase, CPK, LDH, AST, ALT) have occurred with diltiazem and nifedipine. These changes reverse after drug discontinuation. The laboratory abnormalities have rarely been associated with clinical symptoms; however, cholestasis with or without jaundice and allergic hepatitis have occurred with nifedipine. Positive direct Coombs' test findings with or without hemolytic anemia have been recorded with nifedipine.

Precautions and Contraindications. Because diltiazem can affect atrioventricular conduction, it must be used with caution in clients also taking a beta blocker. Diltiazem and nifedipine are contraindicated in clients who are allergic to the drugs, pregnant, or lactating. Diltiazem is also contraindicated in second- or third-degree heart block and hepatic or renal dysfunction.

Abrupt withdrawal of calcium channel blockers may cause rebound angina, probably the result of increased flow of calcium into cells, causing coronary arteries to spasm. When discontinuing drug therapy, the client should have a gradually tapered dosage under medical supervision.

■ SUMMARY

Hypertension is an all-too-common cardiovascular health problem. In some clients, hypertension can be managed without drugs, but many require a drug regimen. The many types of antihypertensives include diuretics, sympathetic inhibitors (adrener-

FOCUS ON

Focus on Calcium Channel Blockers: Similarities and Differences

| Similarities | Differences |

Similarities

Pharmacodynamics

Contractile processes of myocardial and vascular smooth muscle depend on movement of extracellular calcium ions into certain myocardial and vascular cells. Calcium channel blockers lower the intracellular calcium concentration by reducing transmembranous calcium influx, and this results in diminished vascular tone, vascular smooth muscle relaxation, and, consequently, vasodilation and lowering of blood pressure.

Pharmacokinetics

These agents are well absorbed from the GI tract and are extensively metabolized by the liver.

Therapeutic Uses

These agents are used for hypertension and angina pectoris.

Adverse Reactions

Headache, dizziness, edema, changes in heart rate (tachycardia), nausea, rash, and constipation. Some have been associated with a decrease in platelet aggregation and an increase in bleeding time (thought to be a function of inhibition of calcium transport across the platelet membrane). Abrupt withdrawal may cause rebound angina.

Drug Interactions

Histamine (H_2) antagonists, beta blockers, digitalis preparations, and theophylline generally interact with calcium channel blocking agents. Antihypertensives are potentiated.

Precautions and Contraindications

All must be used cautiously in clients with CHF and impaired liver function. Although possibly advantageous in some clients, coadministration of calcium channel blockers and beta blockers may result in increased adverse effects on myocardial contractility or AV conduction.

Nursing Considerations

Assess cardiopulmonary status at baseline and ongoing for changes. Assess blood pressure (lying, sitting, and standing) for changes. Instruct client about disease, adverse reactions, and how to integrate agent into lifestyle.

Differences

- The calcium channel blockers are classified by structure: diphenylalkylamines (**verapamil**), benzothiazepines (**diltiazem**), dihydropyridines (**amlodipine, felodipine, isradipine, nicardipine, nifedipine, nisoldipine,** and **nimodipine**). The structural differences determine the tissues where they have the greatest impact.

- The agents with IV preparations include **nicardipine, diltiazem,** and **verapamil.**

- **Amlodipine, bepridil, diltiazem, nicardipine, nifedipine,** and **verapamil** are indicated for angina pectoris.
- **Amlodipine, diltiazem SR, felodipine, isradipine, nicardipine, nifedipine SR, verapamil,** and **verapamil SR** are indicated for essential hypertension.
- **Verapamil** is used for supraventricular tachyarrhythmias.

- **Nifedipine** has prominent cardiovascular effects, including ankle edema, CHF, MI, and pulmonary edema.
- **Verapamil, nifedipine,** and **felodipine** may have a greater hypotensive effect in the elderly than in younger clients.

- Drug interactions have been reported between **nifedipine** and quinidine, anticoagulants, and magnesium sulfate.
- Drug interactions have been reported between **diltiazem** and carbamazepine, cyclosporine, and lithium.

- Adverse effects have occurred when **verapamil** is used with ventricular tachycardia without a supraventricular origin.

- If nausea occurs with **bepridil,** it may be taken with meals or at bedtime.
- Sustained-release preparations, as **nifedipine** and **diltiazem,** should be swallowed whole and not crushed or chewed.
- **Nifedipine** and **felodipine** interact with grapefruit juice.

gic blocking agents, central action inhibitors, blockers of neuroeffector transmission, miscellaneous agents), direct-acting vasodilators, ACE inhibitors, and calcium channel blocking agents. Clients experience adverse reactions related to the medications because the agents influence various body processes and because other drugs are added to the regimen to manage unwanted effects of the antihypertensive agent.

❖ NURSING MANAGEMENT: CLIENT RECEIVING ANTIHYPERTENSIVE DRUG THERAPY

Early and vigorous treatment of hypertension is important: adequate control of blood pressure reduces the risk of stroke and decreases mortality in clients with essential hypertension. For example, studies indicate that a reduction in diastolic blood pressure of about 5 to 6 mmHg is associated with a relative reduction in the risk of stroke of 35% to 40% (McVeigh et al., 1995). The same study estimated that 15% to 25% of adults in the United States have blood pressures above normal, and at least half are unaware of the problem. Only half of those diagnosed are treated; of these, only half are adequately controlled. The figures imply that only one person in eight who is at risk is receiving adequate treatment. Case finding and referral are important nursing responsibilities.

Commonly, clients with hypertension receive more than one medication. For example, some antihypertensive agents encourage sodium and fluid retention (minoxidil, methyldopa) or reflex tachycardia (hydralazine, phentolamine). Thus, the effects of these agents may require treatment with additional drugs; for example, a beta blocker is usually given with hydralazine, and a potent loop diuretic is often required with minoxidil therapy.

Adherence rates for antihypertensive therapy are reportedly 45% to 65% (Rudd, 1994). Some of the rest adhere partially to the regimen; consequences of partial adherence with antihypertensive therapy include submaximal benefit, increased hospitalization, and increased cardiovascular morbidity. Partial compliers are more likely to respond to adherence-enhancing interventions than are noncompliers. Many factors are involved in adherence and nonadherence. It is difficult for clients to appreciate the importance of therapy when the condition is asymptomatic, as hypertension usually is. Treatment is long term and may be lifelong. Buying medication is a financial drain. Adverse effects of the drug regimen can be uncomfortable or otherwise distressing.

One strategy to promote adherence is to simplify a complex regimen. Several drugs are available in SR forms. The simplest possible regimen is one pill once a day. One antihypertensive agent comes in a transdermal patch that has to be changed only once a week. The nurse can improve adherence by exploring the factors associated with nonadherence and working with the client to reduce their impact.

NURSING PROCESS

ASSESSMENT

Nurses are in a position to refer many clients with previously undetected hypertension for definitive diagnosis. Hypertension screening clinics are often initiated and managed by nurses. Persons with blood pressures exceeding 140 mmHg systolic or 90 mmHg diastolic should be referred to a physician for evaluation.

Initial assessment of clients with hypertension should include a complete history (and family history) and physical examination. Identification of the patient's cardiovascular risk profile is essential for subsequent nursing management. Care should be taken to follow the correct principles of blood-pressure assessment during the physical examination (eg, correct size of cuff for the size of the client's arm; blood-pressure readings taken in three positions in the right sequence).

All clients should have a urinalysis to detect blood, protein, and glucose. Blood specimens must be analyzed for glucose, potassium, creatinine, total and HDL cholesterol, and uric acid levels. Elevated fasting blood glucose levels, elevated plasma cholesterol levels, and low HDL cholesterol levels all markedly increase cardiovascular risk associated with high blood pressure.

Clients' knowledge of hypertension and cardiovascular disease and their treatment should be assessed. Clients should be screened for contraindications to antihypertensive agents and for risk factors for adverse reactions to these agents. For clients already receiving an antihypertensive agent, the nurse must know the name of the drug, the length of time on the drug, the client's attitude toward drug use, any adverse reactions, and current use of over-the-counter drugs.

NURSING DIAGNOSIS

Clients receiving medication for hypertension are likely to be affected by:

- Altered Tissue Perfusion, related to diminished peripheral blood flow secondary to increased peripheral vascular resistance
- Ineffective Management of the Therapeutic Regimen (Individual), related to difficulty in making lifestyle changes, adverse reactions to the prescribed antihypertensive agent, lack of understanding of implications of not following treatment plan, or insufficient financial resources
- Fluid Volume Excess: Edema, related to excessive sodium intake or sodium retention secondary to antihypertensive agent therapy
- Risk for Injury, related to dizziness, lightheadedness, and syncope secondary to drug-induced orthostatic hypotension

Most clients for whom drugs are prescribed have been under nonpharmacologic treatment for hypertension. Therefore, they should have some knowledge about the disease and its complications, but many clients have:

- Knowledge Deficit: Antihypertensives and their use related to unfamiliarity with their action and adverse reactions

PLANNING

Goals of nursing care include reduced blood pressure, adherence to therapeutic regimen (for the obese client, weight loss; for tobacco users, reduction or elimination of tobacco use; for clients using alcohol, reduction of alcohol use; improved management of stress; verbalized adherence with self-administration of medications), reduced risk of hypervolemia and edema, reduced incidence and severity of orthostatic hypotension, increased knowledge, and pre-vention of potential complications. See the Example of Nursing Process for Nifedipine Therapy.

INTERVENTION

Nursing care of clients with chronic hypertension in-cludes helping the client adopt a lifestyle conducive to cardiovascular health and helping the client manage the drug regimen for maximal benefit. Response to therapy for hypertension can be greatly enhanced by nursing measures to reduce contributing factors such as obesity, excessive intake of sodium, lack of exercise, and stress.

Useful strategies for promoting adherence include increased attention and supervision and continuous positive reinforcement. Friends and family members may help in providing attention and positive reinforce-ment. The explicit treatment goal should be stated and reinforced, and there should be realistic short-term ob-jectives about salt restriction, weight loss, moderation

---

Example of Nursing Process for Nifedipine Therapy

The client is a 40-year-old black man with a 6-month history of hypertension. He has been treated with hydrochlorothiazide and a beta-adrenergic blocking agent with good response. However, he has been experiencing fatigue and sleepiness, which he feels are interfering with his job performance. The physician is planning to phase out the beta-adrenergic blocking agent and replace it with a calcium channel blocking agent, nifedipine (sustained-release preparation).

Assessment Data

Complaint of fatigue and sleepiness associated with antihypertensive therapy; change in antihyperten-sive medication

Beginning therapy with nifedipine

Nursing Diagnosis	Intervention	Goals and Outcomes
Potential Noncompliance, related to adverse reactions of prescribed antihy-pertensive agent	**Reinforce** the client's positive action of reporting adverse reactions to his healthcare provider promptly. **Reinforce** that treatment goals for client are reduced blood pressure, adherence to therapeutic regimen, and avoidance of adverse reactions.	The client will report that fatigue and sleepiness are decreased or absent once the beta-adrenergic blocking agent has been discontinued. The client will keep appointments with the healthcare provider. The client will promptly report any difficulties he attributes to nifedipine therapy.
Knowledge Deficit: nifedipine use	**Teach** client how nifedipine works and how it differs from former drug. **Teach** proper use of sustained-release (SR) preparation.	The client will state that his diet does not include grapefruit juice or grape-fruit. The client will report regularly for of-fice appointments and laboratory tests.
Pain: Headache related to antihyper-tensive therapy; potential for chest pain, edema, and/or dyspnea related to drug therapy	**Explain** the interaction between nifedipine and such substances as grapefruit juice. **Reinforce** the impor-tance of regular medical supervision. **Identify** adverse reactions that are likely to occur and explain measures that can be taken (headache: use of acetamino-phen; cardiovascular symptoms: report to the healthcare provider).	If headache develops, the client will be able to implement methods to relieve discomfort.

of alcohol use, exercise, and smoking cessation. Antihypertensive agents and lifestyle modifications must be integrated into the client's daily routine (eg, considering work, sleep, and eating habits). Emphasis should be on modifications of lifestyle rather than complete change. Consistent dosage may be difficult for clients with memory deficits. The nurse should help clients devise a system for taking medication that will help prevent dose omissions; this may include special medication dispensers, with or without alarms.

Client Education. Public education and case finding are vitally important to identify adults with undiagnosed hypertension. Laypeople may still be unaware of the importance of early and continuing treatment of this condition, although information campaigns through the media do convey this message. Screening clinics held at fairs, shopping malls, hospitals, and other community sites are proliferating. Nurses play an active role in informing people of the risks of hypertension and in identifying persons with the disease.

Clients need help in carrying out health measures designed to enhance the medical treatment of hypertension. Counseling and instruction are required in the areas of diet, exercise, emotional health, smoking cessation, and moderation or elimination of alcohol consumption. Caffeine intake should be discouraged because it stimulates the sympathetic nervous system and may contribute to raising blood pressure. Losing excess weight often lowers blood pressure, sometimes to normal. Sodium intake must be limited to prevent hypervolemia. The client may need to learn new techniques for managing stress to minimize psychologic and physiologic reactions to stressors. Some people benefit from biofeedback training or hypnosis to promote vasodilation. Moderate exercise is helpful, not only to accelerate weight loss but also to promote sleep and reduce emotional stress. See the Critical Thinking Challenge, Part I.

Clients at risk for injury because of dizziness, lightheadedness, or syncope from an antihypertensive should be taught how to compensate for these difficulties. The client should rise from a lying to standing position by sitting up slowly, sitting quietly for a few minutes to allow time for the body to adjust to the change in position, and then standing slowly. The client should be taught to avoid activities that contribute significantly to vasodilation, which might worsen orthostatic hypotension (eg, hot baths and showers, steam rooms, saunas). Information should be provided about community resources and support groups that can help the client make any needed lifestyle changes (eg, American Heart Association, smoking cessation programs, weight loss programs, stress management classes).

Regular medical supervision is as important for clients on long-term therapy for hypertension as it is for clients with other chronic conditions. The number of visits to healthcare providers can be reduced, however, if clients learn to monitor their own progress. Most

CRITICAL THINKING CHALLENGE
Case Analysis

Part I

Jacob Andrews, age 76, has a history of non–insulin-dependent diabetes mellitus, hypertension, and one episode of mild congestive heart failure. His diabetes is controlled by diet (1,800 calories daily). Antihypertensive medication has been limited to hydrochlorothiazide 50 mg/day. Until recently, his blood pressure was 130–160/80–86. However, in the last month, it was consistently higher, at 170–180/90–100. The physician is considering adding a beta-adrenergic blocking agent to Mr. Andrews' drug regimen.

1. This is the first time you have met Mr. Andrews, and part of his medical record appears to be missing. What assessment data do you need to obtain to develop a comprehensive nursing care plan for him? Why are these data essential?

2. You learn that Mr. Andrews will continue to take hydrochlorothiazide. Identify what you need to know about his past use of hydrochlorothiazide for best planning. Because he has been receiving this drug for a while, what should he be able to tell you about it? Explain why hydrochlorothiazide (or any diuretic) is usually the first medication prescribed for hypertension control.

3. Compare and contrast the advantages and disadvantages of Mr. Andrews' use of a beta-adrenergic blocking agent.

Part II

You are visiting Mr. Andrews at home for the first time since he was discharged from the hospital. You have reviewed his medical record and discharge summary and have developed a general care plan for Knowledge Deficit, related to drug therapy and adverse reactions. Mr. Andrews is a widower, his only nearby relative is a newly married granddaughter who helps him with grocery shopping. His income is limited to his social security pension and his retirement pension.

1. List and prioritize some goals you have for your visit that relate to your care plans.

2. Explain how you would individualize the following broad categories of nursing intervention to make your work with Mr. Andrews productive:

   • Teaching: Mr. Andrews' pulse rate is 20 points below that recorded in the discharge summary. Discuss the implications of this finding. What kinds of instruction and reference (teaching) materials can you give Mr. Andrews to help him carry out effective self-care?

   • Self-responsibility: Develop a method for helping Mr. Andrews keep a record of his blood pressure until you visit him again.

   • Family involvement: How can you best involve Mr. Andrews' family in helping him adjust to his new medication regimen?

   • Community referrals: Identify at least three community resources or agencies that, in an ideal world, would be available to help Mr. Andrews adhere to his therapeutic regimen. Support your choices and assign specific functions to these groups or individuals.

clients or a family member can learn to use a sphygmomanometer to measure blood pressure. This provides clients with a sense of control and the ability to know when to seek prompt medical attention. Clients need help choosing a reliable instrument and in developing skill in the procedure. Readings should be taken regularly, at the same time of day and under similar conditions. Morning pressures are apt to be lower than those taken in the afternoon. Activity, emotional stress, eating, and sleep all affect readings. Clients should be advised how to record the values, and they should be encouraged to bring the records to follow-up appointments with the healthcare provider. The records can help the provider assess the effects of the drug regimen and adjust it if necessary.

The nurse should prepare and implement a teaching program to inform the client about the specific antihypertensive drug regimen. The teaching plan should be implemented in stages, based on client and family readiness. Printed materials should accompany verbal instruction. Questions should be encouraged and misconceptions clarified. Clients should be told what specific signs and symptoms to report to the healthcare provider (eg, chest pain, edema, weight gain, frequent or uncontrollable nose bleeds, persistent headache or headache present on awakening, continued or severe dizziness, changes in vision). Clients should be advised that the medication should not be stopped abruptly, due to the potential for adverse reactions (eg, rebound hypertension, anginal attacks).

The nurse should stress that hypertension is a chronic condition and that adherence to the treatment plan is necessary to delay or prevent complications. The client needs to continue taking the medication, even if he or she feels better. The client should be told that some adverse reactions experienced early in therapy will subside with continued therapy. If the client forgets a dose, he or she should not take the forgotten dose and should not try to catch up by taking two doses next time.

OUTCOME EVALUATION

The client should be monitored carefully for both therapeutic and adverse reactions to the antihypertensive agent and for adherence to the therapeutic regimen. Because doses are tailored to individual needs and minimally effective dosages are desirable, evaluation of response is critical for proper adjustment of the regimen. Data required for evaluation include serial measures of vital signs, mental status, peripheral circulation, capillary refill, and intake and output. Additional data from the client include reports about use of tobacco and alcohol, food consumption in relation to the recommended diet, serial measurements of blood pressure taken at home, subjective assessment of stress levels, statements reflecting an understanding of the implications of following or not following the treatment plan, statements about incidence or absence of signs and symptoms of complications of hypertension, and statements about incidence or absence of adverse reactions to the drug. See the Critical Thinking Challenge, Part II.

❖ CHECKLIST OF NURSING ACTIONS

- ❏ Play an active part in identifying persons with hypertension.
- ❏ Help clients improve their self-care practices designed to enhance the medical regimen (eg, stress reduction, increased exercise, diet modification).
- ❏ Help the client follow the prescribed regimen. Help integrate the treatment plan into the client's lifestyle.
- ❏ Monitor regularly the status of clients being treated for hypertension (eg, vital signs, weight, specified laboratory tests) for reactions to therapy.
- ❏ Assess clients for risk factors for adverse reactions to prescribed drugs.
- ❏ Monitor regularly for adverse reactions to the drugs and for changes in health status that may indicate previously unrecognized adverse reactions.
- ❏ Reassure clients that some adverse reactions are transient and are likely to subside with continued therapy.
- ❏ Teach appropriate coping strategies for drug-induced adverse reactions (eg, orthostatic hypotension).
- ❏ Advise clients of signs and symptoms that should be reported promptly to the healthcare provider; they may require adjustment of the therapeutic regimen.

Agents Used for Hypertensive Emergencies

Acute hypertensive crises are uncommon but life-threatening. The blood pressure rises rapidly to very high levels—usually the diastolic pressure exceeds 120 mmHg. There is a risk of cerebrovascular hemorrhage or seizure. Vigorous treatment is essential to lower the blood pressure. The etiology of hypertensive crisis varies. It may be a complication of pregnancy, cerebrovascular accident, or perioperative hypertension. Treatment is influenced by the underlying condition. Thus, magnesium sulfate would be used to prevent or control seizures in preeclampsia or eclampsia of pregnancy. Episodes resulting from excessive catecholamine secretion in pheochromocytoma may respond well to a combined alpha-1 and alpha-2 adrenoreceptor blocker. A parenteral form of an agent discussed earlier in this chapter (methyldopa, hydralazine, labetalol) or an agent reserved for such a situation (diazoxide, nitroprusside) may be used. The latter drugs will be discussed briefly.

Pharmacodynamics. Diazoxide is a nondiuretic antihypertensive that is structurally related to the thiazides.

It promptly reduces blood pressure by relaxing smooth muscle in the peripheral arterioles. Increases in heart rate and in cardiac output occur as blood pressure is reduced. Coronary blood flow is maintained. Renal blood flow is increased after an initial decrease.

Nitroprusside relaxes vascular smooth muscle and consequently dilates peripheral arteries and veins. It is more active on veins than on arteries. Dilation of veins promotes peripheral pooling of blood and decreases venous return to the heart, thereby reducing preload. Arteriolar relaxation reduces systemic vascular resistance, systolic arterial pressure, and afterload. Dilation of the coronary arteries also occurs. The heart rate increases slightly, and the drug has a variable effect on cardiac output. Renal vasodilation occurs.

Pharmacokinetics. Diazoxide is extensively bound to serum protein and may therefore displace other highly protein-bound agents. The plasma half-life is 20 to 36 hours. The duration of antihypertensive effect varies but is generally less than 12 hours. Generally, hypotensive effects begin within 1 minute and peak within 2 to 5 minutes. Blood pressure increases gradually over the next 20 minutes and then more slowly over the next 3 to 15 hours.

The hypotensive effect of nitroprusside is seen within 1 to 2 minutes after the start of an adequate infusion, and it dissipates almost as rapidly after an infusion is discontinued. The drug is cleared by intraerythrocytic reaction with hemoglobin; the products of the reaction are cyanmethemoglobin and cyanide ion. Safe use of nitroprusside must be guided by knowledge of the further metabolism of these products.

Therapeutic Uses. Diazoxide is indicated for short-term use in severe, nonmalignant and malignant hypertension. This drug increases the blood glucose level by decreasing insulin release and increasing glucose. Thus, it is also occasionally used in hyperinsulinism in infants and children and in inoperable pancreatic islet cell cancers.

Nitroprusside is indicated for immediate reduction of blood pressure in clients in hypertensive crisis and for production of controlled hypotension to reduce bleeding during surgery in selected clients.

Dosage and Administration. During and immediately after injection of diazoxide, the client should remain supine. The drug is administered undiluted and rapidly, in 30 seconds or less, by IV injection in doses of 1 to 3 mg/kg. Extravasation must be avoided because the agent is irritating to tissue. The dose may be repeated in 5 to 15 minutes as needed. The drug may be used again over 4 to 5 days, but it should not be used for longer than 10 days.

The contents of a 50-mg vial of nitroprusside are dissolved in 2 to 3 mL dextrose in water. The initially reconstituted solution is further diluted in 250 to 1,000 mL sterile 5% dextrose injection. The drug is sensitive to light and becomes less active when exposed to light.

Therefore, the diluted solution must be wrapped with opaque material; it is unnecessary to cover the infusion drip chamber or the tubing. No other drug may be incorporated into the infusion. The infusion should be started at a very low rate (0.3 µg/kg/min) with gradual upward titration as needed; the maximal recommended infusion rate is 10 µg/kg/min. Diluted solution must be discarded after 24 hours.

Adverse Reactions. The most common adverse reactions with diazoxide include hypotension, nausea and vomiting, dizziness, and weakness. Organ ischemia can be caused by hypotension or by a very rapid drop in pressure. Beta blockers may be needed during diazoxide therapy to control cardiac responses. Diazoxide also causes hyperglycemia, and because diabetes will develop, diazoxide is not used on a chronic basis.

Adverse reactions to nitroprusside include abdominal pain, apprehension, diaphoresis, dizziness, and headache when the blood pressure falls too rapidly. Reflex tachycardia is common and can be dangerous to clients with ischemic heart disease. Beta blocker therapy may be a necessary adjunct in selected situations. Organ ischemia can occur if the blood pressure falls too much or too quickly. With nitroprusside, the blood pressure is usually stabilized at only 30% or 40% below predrug levels because of the danger of organ ischemia. Fatal cyanide poisoning can occur when the maximal dose is infused for longer than 10 minutes. Signs and symptoms of cyanide poisoning include metabolic acidosis, dizziness, headache, ataxia, coma, thready pulse, impaired reflexes, and cherry-red coloration of the blood and skin.

Drug Interactions. Drug interactions have been reported between diazoxide and phenytoin (reduced seizure control). No specific drug interactions have been reported between nitroprusside and other agents.

Precautions and Contraindications. Diazoxide is contraindicated in clients with allergy to thiazides or other sulfonamide derivatives and in pregnancy or lactation. In general, it must be used with extreme caution in any client.

Nitroprusside should be used cautiously in hepatic and renal insufficiency, hypothyroidism, and pregnancy and lactation. It should not be used to produce controlled hypotension during surgery in clients with known inadequate cerebral circulation. Materials should be readily available in case of cyanide toxicity whenever nitroprusside is used.

❖ NURSING MANAGEMENT: CLIENT RECEIVING DRUG THERAPY FOR HYPERTENSIVE CRISIS

Hypertensive crisis is best treated in special care units where the client can be closely monitored and emergency measures can be instituted quickly and easily should the need arise. Constant and close supervision is required to prevent dangerous complications. Although rapid reduction of blood pressure is desired, abrupt or excessive drops can compromise circulation to vital organs. IV antihypertensives act very quickly, and the use of these drugs can be dangerous.

NURSING PROCESS

ASSESSMENT

The client treated for hypertensive crisis is acutely ill and is likely to be anxious and fearful. Evaluation should include assessment of emotional reaction to the life-threatening situation, vital signs, and signs and symptoms of specific end-organ damage. For example, in observing for complications such as impaired renal function, the nurse should assess hourly urine output, urine specific gravity, BUN, serum creatinine, serum potassium, calcium, and phosphorus levels, and creatinine clearance. In observing for cerebrovascular accident or hypertensive encephalopathy, the nurse should assess for dizziness, syncope, visual disturbances (blurred vision), headache, vomiting, mental status (change in alertness and orientation, memory impairment, impaired judgment, agitation, impaired thought process), pupillary reactions, and sensory and motor function (focal motor weakness).

NURSING DIAGNOSIS

Diagnoses for these clients include:

- Anxiety, related to perception of threat to life

Administration of antihypertensive drugs may cause:

- Risk for Injury, related to complications of nitroprusside (or other antihypertensive agent) therapy

PLANNING

Goals of nursing care include reducing anxiety and fear, reducing blood pressure to more normal levels, preventing or promptly detecting and correcting injury related to the antihypertensive agent, and reducing the risk of complications.

INTERVENTION

To protect the anxious or fearful client, the nurse should establish a therapeutic relationship as soon as possible, characterized by the nurse's genuine concern for the client's welfare and the client's trust in the nurse. Once the client's trust is earned, the nurse will be effective when offering reassurance. Clients should not be told that "everything will be all right." Instead, the nurse should remind clients that the staff is skilled and will use every means possible to improve the medical condition and resolve the crisis.

The administration of IV infusions is a nursing responsibility. The nurse should maintain infusions at the proper rate, using an automatic control device such as an infusion pump or controller. The nurse should follow directions for protecting sensitive drugs from conditions conducive to deterioration (eg, nitroprusside must not be exposed to light).

The client should be observed closely for response to treatment. Blood pressure should decline steadily but gradually (drastic changes in blood pressure can occur within 2 to 5 minutes, but this is undesirable). If hypotension occurs, the IV infusion should be stopped and the client placed in the Trendelenburg position to increase venous return.

A strict accounting of fluid intake and output is required. Fluid intake should err on the low side, because hypervolemia further increases blood pressure. Clients should be monitored closely for peripheral edema or respiratory difficulties signifying pulmonary edema.

Client Education. The client treated for hypertensive crisis is acutely ill. Teaching is confined to explanations of the treatment regimen, designed to allay apprehension and to secure the client's cooperation. Health teaching should be deferred until the acute phase of illness has been resolved.

OUTCOME EVALUATION

Data required for evaluation include serial measurements of vital signs, especially blood pressure, incidence or absence of signs and symptoms of potential complications (eg, stroke, renal failure), and reports from clients concerning physical and emotional comfort.

❖ CHECKLIST OF NURSING ACTIONS

- ❑ Establish a nurse–client relationship characterized by concern (nurse) and trust (client).
- ❑ Offer the client reassurance and emotional support.
- ❑ Use an infusion control device to maintain a steady infusion rate.
- ❑ Monitor the client closely for response to treatment; take frequent vital signs, especially blood pressure.
- ❑ Monitor the client closely for adverse drug reactions, including abrupt drops in blood pressure, infiltration, respiratory impairment, and hypervolemia.
- ❑ Maintain a strict accounting of fluid intake and output; maintain a minimal intake to avoid hypervolemia.

References

Chutka DS. (1995). Selection of antihypertensive medications for the elderly. *Hosp Formul, 30*(3), 148–160.

Copstead LC. (1995). *Perspectives on pathophysiology.* Philadelphia: WB Saunders Co.

———. (1995). Drugs for hypertension. *The Medical Letter, 37*(949), 45–50.

Farnett LE, Mulrow CD. (1994). Anti-hypertensive therapy and the J-curve. *Cardiol Rev, 2*(4), 174–182.

Hall WD. (1994). Hypertension in the elderly. *Cardiol Rev, 2*(3), 157–164.

McVeigh GE, Flack J, Grimm R. (1995). Goals of antihypertensive therapy. *Drugs, 49*(2), 162–175.

National Institutes of Health. (1993). The fifth report of the Joint National Committee on Detection, Evaluation and Treatment of High Blood Pressure (NIH Publication No. 93-1088).

Olin BR, ed. (1995). *Drug facts and comparisons,* 49th ed. St. Louis: Facts and Comparisons.

Packer JO. (1992). The neurohormonal hypothesis: A theory to explain the mechanism of disease progression in heart failure. *J Am Coll Cardiol, 20*(1), 248–253.

Robertson JI, Ball SG. (1994). *Hypertension for the clinician.* London: WB Saunders Co.

Rudd P. (1994). Compliance with antihypertensive therapy: A shifting paradigm. *Cardiol Rev, 2*(5), 230–240.

Walz DW. (1994). Hypertension management: The case for individualized therapy. *Clinical Reviews,* (4), 53–74.

Leonetti G, Cesare C. (1995). Choosing the right ACE inhibitor. *Drugs, 49*(4), 516–535.

Lewis EJ, Hunsicker LG, Bain RP, et al. (1993). The effect of angiotensin-converting-enzyme inhibition on diabetic nephropathy. *N Engl J Med, 329*(20), 1456–1462.

Reisin E. (1994). Obesity-related hypertension: Antihypertensive drug approaches. *CVRR,* (3), 13–18.

St. John Hammond PG. (1994). Once-a-day antihypertensive therapy: Comparison of extended-release diltiazem HCl and extended-release nifedipine. *CVRR,* (7), 46.

Wright JM. (1995). Pharmacologic management of congestive heart failure. *Crit Care Nurs Q, 18*(1), 32–44.

Bibliography

Clem JR. (1995). Pharmacotherapy of ischemic heart disease. *AACN Clinical Issues, 6*(3), 404–417.

Cuddy RP. (1995). Hypertension: Keeping dangerous blood pressure down. *Nursing '95,* (8), 35–41.

Cuddy RP. (1993). Hypertension update. *Advance for Nurse Practitioners, 1* (8):22–23, 26.

Hardman JG, Limbird LE, Molinoff PB, et al. (eds). (1996). *Goodman and Gilman's The pharmacological basis of therapeutics,* 9th ed. New York: McGraw-Hill.

For more information and sample tests and activities, refer to Chapter 25 in the Student Workbook for Clinical Pharmacology and Nursing Management, 5th edition, available through your bookstore.

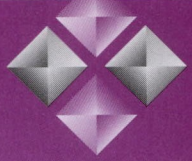

26

Drugs That Affect Hemostasis

Blood is a delicately balanced chemical mixture that remains fluid while circulating in an undamaged vascular system. Hemostasis, the arrest of blood loss from damaged blood vessels, is a very complex process that involves vasospasm, formation of a platelet plug, and fibrin formation (Rang et al., 1995).

Hemostasis

Platelets are the smallest of the formed elements in the blood. Normally there are 150,000 to 350,000 platelets per cubic millimeter of blood. Platelets have an important role in the response of blood vessels to injury.

In a normal, undamaged blood vessel, the endothelium plays an active part in preventing thrombus formation. It generates and releases prostacyclin and nitric oxide, which inhibit platelet aggregation, and also plasminogen activator and the anticoagulant substances heparin and heparin sulfate. The endothelium also expresses thrombomodulin, a receptor/cofactor involved in activating coagulation inhibitor, protein C.

When the endothelium is damaged—for example, when an atherosclerotic plaque is ruptured or a vessel is cut or injured—the vessel immediately constricts. The platelets that adhere to components of the subendothelium are activated and join together into aggregates to plug the injured, leaking vessel.

Adhesion involves the linking of subendothelial components to glycoprotein (GP) IIb receptors on the platelet membrane by von Willebrand factor. *Activation* involves shape changes, followed by the release of biologically active substances, some from storage granules (adeno-

Box 26-1
Clotting Factors

   I. Fibrinogen—a high-molecular-weight plasma protein produced by the liver

  II. Prothrombin—a plasma glycoprotein produced in the liver from vitamin K

 III. Tissue thromboplastin—produced by a number of body tissues

 IV. Calcium—a serum electrolyte, active only in ionized form

  V. Proaccelerin, labile factor—a plasma protein

 VI. This number was assigned to a factor thought to be an intermediate product of prothrombin conversion. This substance is not believed to play a role in coagulation.

 VII. Stable factor, serum prothrombin conversion accelerator

VIII. Antihemophilic factor—a plasma protein

 IX. Christmas factor—a serum component produced in the liver from vitamin K

  X. Stuart factor—a serum component produced in the liver from vitamin K

 XI. Plasma thromboplastic antecedent—a component of both serum and plasma

 XII. Hageman factor—a component of both serum and plasma

XIII. Fibrin-stabilizing factor

sine diphosphate [ADP] and fibrinogen) and some synthesized (platelet-activating factor and thromboxane [TXA_2]). These substances enhance vasoconstriction and aggregation. They also contribute to vessel repair. *Aggregation* involves links formed by fibrinogen binding to the GPIIb/IIIa receptors on adjacent platelets.

A mass of aggregated platelets forms a plug. Together with vessel constriction, it maintains hemostasis in small vessels until the platelet plug is reinforced by fibrin. The platelet plug is usually completely formed within 3 to 7 minutes.

Blood coagulation involves the conversion of fluid blood to a solid gel or clot. Blood coagulation factors, except for tissue factor (factor III, tissue thromboplastin) and calcium, circulate in the bloodstream in an inactive state (Box 26-1). The liver is responsible for synthesizing coagulation factors, except for part of factor III. Factors II, VII, IX, and X depend on vitamin K for synthesis and normal activity (Copstead, 1995).

The clotting system consists of a cascade of enzymes and the blood coagulation factors I through XIII. At each step in the cascade, a circulating protein, or inactive clotting factor, undergoes proteolysis, transforming it into an active form that then triggers the next clotting factor. The last enzyme, thrombin, derived from prothrombin (factor II), converts soluble fibrinogen (enzymatic cleavage) to an insoluble meshwork of fibrin in which blood cells are trapped, forming the clot. This conversion is the last step and the main event, although fibrin itself forms only 0.15% of a total blood clot.

The cascade follows two pathways: extrinsic and intrinsic (Fig. 26-1). The intrinsic pathway requires several minutes for fibrin formation; the extrinsic pathway forms fibrin in seconds by bypassing the initial cascade steps. Intrinsic pathway function is measured by activated partial thromboplastin time (APTT), the extrinsic pathway by prothrombin time (PT) (Raimer & Thomas, 1995). Both pathways result in the conversion

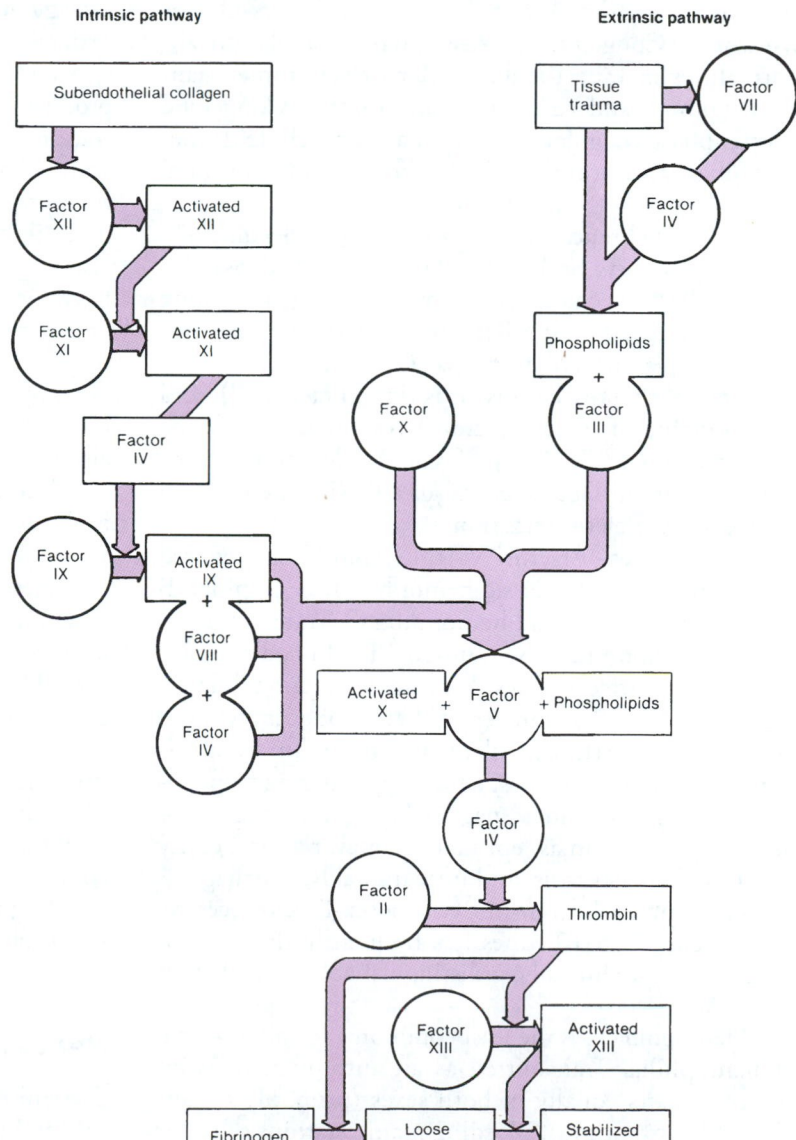

Figure 26-1. The mechanism of coagulation.

of prothrombin to thrombin. Calcium and a negatively charged phospholipid are essential for three of the steps—action of factor IX on X, factor VII on X, and factor X on II. The negatively charged phospholipid is provided by activated platelets that have adhered to the damage site.

In the final stage of clot formation (clot retraction), the components of the fibrin clot—the platelet plug, fibrin strands, and trapped red blood cells—are compressed into a firm clot. This stage takes about 1 hour. As the fibrin clot is forming, fibrinolysis or clot dissolution begins. This process prevents excessive clotting and vessel occlusion.

Defects of Hemostasis

Abnormalities of hemostasis include vessel wall abnormalities, platelet hemostatic mechanism abnormalities, and plasma or fluid phase disorders. Congenital coagulopathies due to abnormal structure or function of blood vessels include hereditary hemorrhagic telangiectasia (Rendu-Osler-Weber disease) and Ehlers-Danlos syndrome. Congenital platelet phase coagulation abnormalities include Kasabach-Merritt syndrome (giant hemangioma) and von Willebrand disease. Congenital plasma phase coagulation abnormalities include the hemophilias, antithrombin III deficiency, and congenital afibrinogenemia (Srnec, 1993).

Von Willebrand disease is an inherited bleeding disorder that affects both sexes. Formerly called pseudohemophilia, it is characterized by a prolonged bleeding time, decreased factor VIII activity in the plasma, and decreased platelet adhesiveness. Cryoprecipitate is the mainstay of therapy because it is rich in factor VIII and von Willebrand factor (factor VIII concentrates lack the large molecular form of von Willebrand factor). Von Willebrand factor acts as an adhesive mediator in platelet-to-platelet interaction.

Deficiencies of factors VIII, IX, and XI are referred to as hemophilia A (classic hemophilia), hemophilia B (Christmas disease), and hemophilia C. Transmitted by females, hemophilia A is an inherited X-linked recessive disorder that affects males. It causes a functional defect in the factor VIII molecule that produces reduced plasma factor VIII coagulant activity. Clinical manifestations include soft-tissue bleeding, ranging from relatively harmless hematomas to life-threatening retroperitoneal hematomas, epistaxis, hematuria, oral cavity bleeding, hemarthrosis, and intracranial hemorrhage.

Hemophilia B, transmitted as a sex-linked recessive trait, occurs 7 to 10 times less frequently than hemophilia A. It is clinically indistinguishable from hemophilia A.

Hemophilia C is the least common and mildest form of hemophilia. Transmitted as an autosomal recessive trait, it occurs equally in both sexes (primarily in persons of Jewish origin). Bleeding manifestations of factor XI deficiency include nose bleeds, menorrhagia, and bleeding after dental extraction and surgical procedures.

Disorders Affecting Hemostasis

Hemorrhagic disease of the newborn is a coagulation disorder that may occur 48 to 72 hours after birth. It is rare in Western countries because newborns routinely receive vitamin K. Acquired vitamin K deficiency may result in bleeding due to a coagulation defect and may occur with malnutrition, malabsorption, chronic hepatic disease, antibiotic therapy, and oral anticoagulant therapy.

Disseminated intravascular coagulation (DIC) is an acquired hemorrhagic syndrome that occurs secondary to factors such as cancer, sepsis, snakebite, abruptio placentae, traumatic and crushing injuries, transfusions of incompatible blood, burns, and shock. Accelerated intravascular clotting, which begins in small vessels, rapidly consumes coagulation factors. At the same time, the fibrinolytic system is activated to break down the clots. The paradoxical combination of coagulation, anticoagulation, and fibrinolysis ultimately leads to hemorrhage.

Thrombocytopenia is a result of decreased platelet production, increased destruction of platelets, or sequestration of platelets in the liver or spleen. Chemotherapy and radiation therapy produce thrombocytopenia by temporarily destroying platelet-producing megakaryocytes in the bone marrow. Bone marrow malignancy also interferes with normal cell production. Clients may have normal bone marrow function with increased destruction or consumption of platelets, as in splenomegaly and DIC. Some drugs, such as heparin, quinidine, hydrochlorothiazide, and others, can cause thrombocytopenia when antibodies formed against the drug also destroy platelets.

A common complication of many hepatic disorders is abnormal hemostasis. Liver disease alters the synthesis and transport of bile, which is necessary for normal fat digestion and absorption. Impaired absorption and metabolism of vitamin K, which is fat-soluble, result in decreased hepatic synthesis of certain coagulation factors. The liver also plays a role in removing activated coagulation/fibrinolytic proteins. Failure to do so adequately may lead to an imbalance between clot formation and clot dissolution, manifested clinically by DIC. Liver disease may alter normal production of coagulation inhibitors and contribute to the hypercoagulable component of DIC. Another factor contributing to bleeding associated with liver disease is thrombocytopenia, probably related to sequestration of platelets in the enlarged spleen.

Hemostatics

Systemic and topical hemostatics (Table 26-1) function to stop bleeding.

Table 26-1. Systemic Hemostatics

Drug Name	Preparation	Usual Dosage	Additional Information
Whole blood	Fresh whole blood or citrated blood IV	1–2 pints	Fresh whole blood contains all factors necessary for clotting; citrated blood supplies all factors except calcium.
Plasma	Fresh plasma or fresh-frozen plasma IV		Fresh-frozen plasma is the only agent available to treat bleeding related to deficiencies of factor V, XI, XIII; might give diuretics or diphenhydramine hydrochloride concomitantly.
Platelets	IV	units	Indicated for treating certain types of thrombocytopenia; each unit of platelets can increase platelet count by 5,000–10,000/μL.
Cryoprecipitate	Removed precipitate from thawed fresh-frozen plasma IV	Initially 1 U/2 kg, followed by 1 U/15 kg/d (fibrinogen levels are used to monitor transfusion needs)	This is the only form of concentrated fibrinogen available.
Antithrombin III	Prepared from human plasma IV	1 IU/kg will increase antithrombin III level 1%–2%	Use heparin concomitantly.
Preparations of Specific Factors			
Antihemophilic factor	IV	Moderate hemorrhage: 15–25 U/kg initially, followed by 10–15 U/kg q8–12h as needed	Administer for hemophilia A.
Antiinhibitor coagulant complex (Autoplex T, Feiba VH Immuno)	IV	25–100 factor VIII correctional units/kg depending on severity of bleeding; repeat in 6 hr as needed	Give at 2–10 mL/min; more rapid rates increase incidence of adverse reactions.
Prothrombin complex (contains factor IX, prothrombin, factor X, factor VII, protein C)	IV	Example: 70-kg client with factor IX level of 0% must be elevated to 25%; give 1 U/kg ×70 kg ×25 = 1,750 U	Administer for hemophilia B.
Vitamin K₁, phytonadione (Mephyton, AquaMEPHYTON, Konakion)	Oral IM	Prophylaxis to newborn: 0.5–1.0 mg within 1 hr after birth Anticoagulant-induced prothrombin deficiency: 2.5–10 mg; repeat in 6–8 hr (parenteral) or 12–48 hr (oral) depending on PT	Preparation is not helpful for bleeding associated with use of heparin.
aminocaproic acid (Amicar)	Oral IV	5 g, followed by 1–1.25 g hourly	Administer no more than 30 g/24 hr.
tranexamic acid (Cyklokapron)	Oral tablets IV	Example: for dental extraction in hemophilia, give 10 mg/kg IV before surgery, and after surgery give 25 mg/kg orally 3 or 4 times/day for 2–8 days.	Product is 10 times more potent than aminocaproic acid.
desmopressin acetate (DDAVP)	IV	0.3 mcg/kg diluted in 10–50 mL saline; infused over 15–30 min	Monitor for water overload due to antidiuretic properties.
aprotinin (Trasylol)	IV through central line	Include test dose, loading dose, pump prime dose (dose to be added to priming fluid of cardiopulmonary bypass circuit), and constant infusion dose	Use with coronary artery bypass graft surgery.

Systemic Hemostatics

Systemic hemostatics include blood and blood products that include specific factors (Table 26-2). They also include vitamin K, antifibrinolytic agents, desmopressin acetate, and aprotinin.

Blood and Blood Products

Blood is composed of erythrocytes, leukocytes, and plasma and by volume is about 45% cells and 55% plasma. The average adult has 4 to 5 L of blood. Fresh whole blood provides all the factors necessary for clotting; citrated

Table 26-2. Preparations of Specific Factors

Drug Name	Preparation	Additional Information
Antihemophilic Factor		
antihemophilic factor (porcine) Hyate: C	Freeze-dried concentrate of AHF	Porcine derivative
Bioclate	Concentrated recombinant AHF	After reconstitution, also contains albumin (human), PEG, sodium, histidine, polysorbate 80, calcium
Helixate	Recombinant stable dried concentration of AHF	After reconstitution, also contains glycine, imidazole, polysorbate 80, calcium chloride, sodium, chloride, human albumin
Humate-P	Pasteurized purified lyophilized concentrate of AHF (human)	
Koate-HP	Stable dried concentrate of AHF, lyophilized	After reconstitution, contains heparin, PEG, glycine, polysorbate 80, TNBP, calcium chloride, aluminum, histidine, albumin (human)
Monoclate-P	Stable concentrate of AHF	After reconstitution, contains sodium, calcium chloride, albumin (human), mannitol, histidine
Profilate HP	Stable freeze-dried concentrate of AHF (human) suspended in heptane and heated	now
KoGENate	Recombinant AHF	
Recombinate	Concentrated recombinant AHF	After reconstitution, contains albumin (human), polyethylene glycol, sodium, histidine, polysorbate 80, calcium
Factor IX		
AlphaNine	Purified heat-treated/solvent preparation of factor IX derived from human plasma	Contains ≥50 U factor IX/mg protein.
AlphaNine SD	Purified, solvent detergent-treated preparation of factor IX derived from human plasma	Same as above
Konyne 80	Formerly called Konyne HT	Contains 100 IU factor IX/mL with histidine, mannitol, and mouse protein
Mononine	Lyophilized monoclonal antibody	

blood supplies all factors except calcium. If whole blood is administered, all blood components will also be administered. Separating whole blood into components and transfusing a client with a component permits replacement of specific deficiencies without giving the client unnecessary components or excessive volume. Rarely used for hemostasis purposes, whole blood is used mostly to replace acute blood loss or blood volume deficit and reduced oxygen-carrying capacity (see Chap. 48).

Plasma

Blood plasma is the liquid remaining after removal of the cellular components of the blood. Retrieval of plasma by centrifuging 1 unit of whole blood yields an average volume of 200 mL. Single-donor plasma is obtained from 1 unit of randomly donated whole blood. If a single-donor unit is immediately transfused, it is termed fresh plasma. Fresh plasma contains all the coagulation factors. Fresh-frozen plasma is the same plasma frozen within 6 hours of collection. The coagulation factors in fresh plasma remain stable for at least a year if the plasma is immediately frozen and stored at $-30°C$.

Plasma or fresh-frozen plasma may be indicated for replacing deficient plasma clotting factors. In hemophilia A, the use of plasma has been replaced largely by either cryoprecipitated or lyophilized concentrates of antihemophilic factor. Fresh-frozen plasma is the only agent currently available to treat bleeding episodes in clients with hereditary or acquired deficiencies of factors V, XI, or XIII. Plasma helps control bleeding during oral anticoagulant therapy until the action of administered vitamin K_1 is apparent. Fresh-frozen plasma has been recommended as a source of antithrombin III in clients deficient in this agent who are undergoing surgery or who are under treatment with heparin for thrombosis. Fresh-frozen plasma may halt the massive intravascular coagulation that may occur in newborns with homozygous protein C deficiency (Colman et al., 1994).

Platelets

Platelets for transfusion are obtained by centrifuging whole blood from several random donors or are available as a concentrate obtained by hemapheresis from a single donor. Both preparations are suspended in plasma to help maintain a pH of 6.0 or higher during storage.

Multiple-donor platelets are more readily available and can be less expensive. Platelet preparations may contain leukocytes and may cause nonhemolytic febrile reactions in some clients. Platelets also have antigens known as human leukocyte antigens (HLA). Some clients receiving multiple platelet transfusions become alloimmunized to HLA antigens. The antibodies thus formed destroy transfused platelets. However, screening tests can detect the antibodies. If they are present, HLA-matched platelets can be obtained by hemapheresis.

Platelet transfusion is indicated for the client with thrombocytopenia who is actively bleeding, if the platelet deficiency is causing or contributing to the bleeding. The goal is to maintain a platelet count greater than 50,000/mm³. The goal in treating DIC is to remove the underlying cause; however, thrombocytopenia may be severe enough to require platelet transfusion. Clients with thrombocytopenia related to chemotherapy, radiation therapy, or bone marrow malignancy can benefit from platelet transfusion as well.

A client receiving multiple-donor platelets can expect the platelet count to increase 5,000 to 10,000/µL. The platelets can be administered as rapidly as tolerated, but infusion should take no longer than 4 hours (Coffland & Shelton, 1993). The platelet life span is only about 7 days, so repeated platelet administration may be needed to control bleeding or to increase the platelet count significantly.

A client with rapid peripheral destruction of platelets does not benefit from platelet transfusion, because the transfused platelets are destroyed in the same way as the client's own platelets. This would be the case in idiopathic thrombocytopenic purpura. Clients with drug-induced thrombocytopenia do not benefit from platelet transfusion, either. Platelet dysfunction associated with uremia also does not respond well to transfused platelets.

Cryoprecipitate

When fresh-frozen plasma is thawed at 4°C, a thick white precipitate forms and can be removed by centrifugation. The removed precipitate is resuspended in plasma and frozen, and it can be stored for up to a year (Coffland & Shelton, 1993). Called cryoprecipitate, it is the only form of concentrated fibrinogen available, and each bag contains about 200 to 250 mg of fibrinogen. In addition to fibrinogen, it contains 46% of the factor VIII found in plasma, fibronectin, immunoglobulins, albumin, and von Willebrand factor. Indications for administering cryoprecipitate include von Willebrand disease, acute liver failure, DIC, acute hypofibrinogenemia, dysfibrinogenemia, afibrinogenemia, and mild hemophilia. It may also be used for fibronectin deficiency.

Antithrombin III

Antithrombin III is a plasma protein that inhibits plasma serine proteases, among them activated Stuart factor (factor Xa), thrombin, and plasmin. Hereditary antithrombin III deficiency is a relatively common cause of familial recurrent thrombosis. The therapy for thrombotic episodes might involve heparin, but it is difficult because the action of heparin is mediated through its binding to antithrombin III. Purified preparations of antithrombin III derived from human plasma are available. Infusions of antithrombin III, with or without concomitant heparin therapy, have been used, but to date therapy has been difficult to evaluate. In clients with DIC, the titer of antithrombin III may be reduced, suggesting the antithrombin III preparation may be helpful in this disorder also.

Preparations of Specific Factors

Antihemophilic Factor

Pharmacodynamics. Lyophilized preparations of factor VIII or antihemophilic factor (Hemofil M, Koate-HS, Koate-HP, Monoclate) are prepared from human plasma.

Pharmacokinetics. Coagulant levels rise rapidly after administration, then quickly decrease. Plasma half-life after the initial dose is 9 to 15 hours and increases with subsequent doses.

Therapeutic Uses. These preparations arrest moderate or severe bleeding in clients with hemophilia A and prevent hemorrhage that may occur with planned dental procedures or surgery. Adequate factor must be given to achieve clot formation and allow regrowth of fibroblasts for adequate healing.

Dosage and Administration. The concentrate and diluent are warmed to room temperature before mixing. The preparation must be administered intravenously (IV) within 3 hours of reconstitution. It should not be refrigerated after reconstitution because precipitation can occur.

Dosage is expressed in AHF units: one AHF unit equals the activity present in 1 mL of normal pooled human plasma. The dose is adjusted according to the client's weight, severity of bleeding, evidence of factor VIII inhibitor, and the desired level of factor VIII. The goal is usually to obtain a factor VIII level of at least 30% of normal, as this usually provides effective hemostasis. There is a linear dose-response relation, with a rise of about 2% in factor VIII activity for each unit of factor VIII/kg transfused.

The dose for moderate hemorrhage may be 15 to 25 U/kg initially, followed by 10 to 15 U/kg every 8 to 12 hours as needed. Doses less than 34 U/mL may be given at a rate of 10 to 20 mL over 3 minutes; doses greater than 34 U/mL should be given at a maximal rate of 2 mL/min.

About 6% to 10% of clients with hemophilia develop factor VIII inhibitor, an immunoglobulin G (IgG) antibody. Appearance of an inhibitor is usually associated with markedly reduced or absent response to factor VIII. The etiology of this inhibitor is unknown. It is believed that persons predisposed to the development of an inhibitor will do so by the time they have received 100 treatment-days of exposure to factor VIII (Srnec, 1993). Clients with inhibitors do not bleed more often than do other hemophiliac persons, but the bleeding episodes are difficult or impossible to control with factor VIII replacement.

Adverse Reactions. Mild reactions include headache, flushing, and abdominal pain. Stinging sensations may be reported at the venipuncture site. Rapid administration of antihemophilic factor tends to cause tachycardia. Acute anaphylactoid reactions may occur. Massive doses have resulted in acute hemolytic anemia, apparently related to contamination by isohemagglutinins.

Like other blood products, this preparation can convey viral hepatitis and the human immunodeficiency virus (HIV). Several methods have been used in an attempt to eliminate the risk of disease transmission.

Precautions and Contraindications. To prevent problems related to too-rapid transfusion, the pulse rate should be monitored during treatment and the infusion should be slowed if the pulse rate increases substantially.

Antiinhibitor Coagulant Complex
Pharmacodynamics. Antiinhibitor coagulant complex (Autoplex T, Feiba VH Immuno) is prepared from pooled human plasma.

Pharmacokinetics. It contains activated and precursor clotting factors. Kinin-generating system factors are also present.

Therapeutic Uses. It is indicated for clients with hemophilia A who have developed factor VIII inhibitor and who are bleeding or are to undergo surgery.

Dosage and Administration. The dose is 25 to 100 factor VIII correctional units/kg, depending on the severity of bleeding. It is given IV at 2 to 10 mL infusion solution/min. Faster infusion rates should be avoided because the incidence of adverse reactions rises with rapid infusion rates. The infusion may be repeated in 6 hours if needed. One unit of factor VIII correctional activity is defined as that amount of the substance that when added to an equal amount of factor VIII-deficient plasma corrects the clotting time to 35 seconds.

Adverse Reactions. Adverse reactions include fever, chills (hypersensitivity reactions), headache, flushing, and tachycardia. The client should be observed for indications of hypercoagulability and intravascular coagulation (dyspnea, coughing, chest or leg pain); the infusion should be terminated if such symptoms occur. Like other blood products, this preparation can convey viral hepatitis and HIV.

Drug Interactions. The possibility of hypercoagulation states increases with the concomitant use of an antiinhibitor coagulant complex and aminocaproic acid or tranexamic acid.

Concentrates of Vitamin K-Dependent Clotting Factors
Concentrates of the vitamin K-dependent clotting factors (prothrombin complex preparations) include Konyne-HT (heat-treated), Profilnine-HT, Proplex T, and Proplex SX-T.

Pharmacodynamics. These products are prepared from plasma that has been depleted of factor VIII and fibrinogen. The preparations, furnished in lyophilized form, predominantly contain factors VII, IX, and X, prothrombin, and protein C.

Pharmacokinetics. These preparations are administered IV. Reported half-lives are 12 to 40 hours, depending on the product.

Therapeutic Uses. These concentrates prevent or control hemorrhage caused by hemophilia B. Fresh-frozen plasma is also a choice in mild factor IX deficiency and may be used before these products. Some have suggested using these concentrates instead of plasma to treat acute bleeding resulting from overdose of oral anticoagulants. Proplex T (only) may be used to prevent or control bleeding episodes in persons with factor VII deficiency.

Dosage and Administration. Dosage, expressed in units, depends on the degree of deficiency and the desired hemostatic level of the deficient factor. For example, a 70-kg client with a factor IX level of 0%, which must be elevated to 25%, would receive 1 U/kg × 70 kg × 25, or a total of 1,750 U. These preparations are for IV use only. The infusion should be administered within 3 hours after reconstitution at a rate not exceeding 3 mL/min. The preparation should not be refrigerated after reconstitution because precipitation may occur.

Prophylaxis is the ideal treatment for proven congenital deficiency. A dosage of 10 to 20 IU/kg once or twice a week may prevent spontaneous bleeding in clients with hemophilia B.

Adverse Reactions. Rapid injection of these concentrates can cause headache, flushing, changes in blood pressure, transient fever, chills, tingling, urticaria, nausea, and vomiting. Discontinuing the infusion resolves symptoms. Some clients treated with these concentrates have sustained thromboembolic episodes, myocardial infarction (MI), or DIC. To prevent DIC, the blood level of factor IX should usually not be raised above 50% of normal. When large doses of the drug are required, prophylactic anticoagulation should be considered.

Like other blood products, these preparations may rarely convey viral hepatitis and HIV.

Vitamin K
Vitamin K is a fat-soluble agent crucial to the production of many proteins involved in coagulation. It is a cofactor for the hepatic insertion of carbon dioxide into the gamma-carbon of glutamic acid residues in the protein precursors of the vitamin K-dependent clotting factors (factors II, VII, IX, and X). Vitamin K is also needed to complete the synthesis of many other proteins.

Deficiency of vitamin K can result from inadequate intake or absorption or poor utilization, or as a consequence of vitamin K antagonist activity. Although the healthy liver has a 30-day store of vitamin K, deficiency can occur in 7 to 10 days in acutely ill clients. Deficiency of vitamin K from inadequate intake is uncommon in healthy persons but can occur in clients with restricted food intake or clients receiving total parenteral nutrition and antibiotics. Situations that could result in inadequate absorption of vitamin K include biliary obstruction, celiac disease and sprue, regional enteritis and ulcerative colitis (characterized by diarrhea), and extensive bowel resection. Hepatocellular disease may result in the inability of liver cells to use vitamin K to produce clotting factors. Antibiotic therapy inhibits vitamin K-producing intestinal microflora as well and may be a factor in some cases of vitamin K deficiency.

Bacterial flora in the jejunum and ileum synthesize vitamin K and provide about half the body's requirement. Newborns may develop hemorrhagic disease secondary to vitamin K deficiency because the intestine is sterile for a few days after birth. The safety and efficacy of giving vitamin K at birth to prevent hemorrhagic disease in the newborn are well documented in the literature; the practice is recommended by the American Academy of Pediatrics and the American College of Obstetrics and Gynecology. However, vitamin K is not administered universally.

Two naturally occurring forms of vitamin K are phylloquinone (vitamin K_1) and menaquinone (vitamin K_2). Phylloquinone, found in various green plants such as brussels sprouts, spinach, and cabbage, is the major dietary source of vitamin K. Menaquinone is synthesized, primarily by intestinal bacteria.

Phytonadione and Menadiol Sodium Diphosphate
Known also as vitamin K_1, phytonadione (Mephyton, AquaMEPHYTON, Konakion) is a fat-soluble synthetic compound identical to naturally occurring vitamin K_1. Menadiol sodium diphosphate (Synkayvite), or vitamin K_4, is a water-soluble synthetic analog of vitamin K. It is converted in the body to menadione (K_3), which is very potent.

Pharmacodynamics. These agents act in the body as naturally occurring vitamin K does.

Pharmacokinetics. Phytonadione may be administered orally or by injection. Bile salts must be present in the gastrointestinal (GI) tract for absorption to occur after oral administration. Oral phytonadione exerts its effect in 6 to 10 hours. Parenteral phytonadione usually controls hemorrhage within 3 to 6 hours. A normal prothrombin level may be obtained in 12 to 14 hours.

Although initially concentrated in the liver, vitamin K is rapidly metabolized and little tissue accumulation occurs. The drug crosses the placenta. Little is known about the metabolic fate or excretion of vitamin K preparations.

Therapeutic Uses. Phytonadione is the preferred drug for treating hypoprothrombinemia. However, adequate absorption of phytonadione occurs only in the presence of bile salts, whereas menadiol sodium diphosphate can be adequately absorbed without bile salts. Only phytonadione is used for prophylaxis and treatment of hemorrhagic disease of the newborn and for treatment of oral anticoagulant-induced prothrombin deficiency.

Vitamin K preparations are not helpful with bleeding caused by heparin.

Dosage and Administration. The prophylactic dose given to newborns is a single intramuscular (IM) dose of 0.5 to 1 mg within 1 hour after birth. For anticoagulant-induced prothrombin deficiency, a typical dose of phytonadione is 2.5 to 10 mg, or up to 25 mg initially. Subsequent doses are determined by PT response or clinical condition. If, in 6 to 8 hours after parenteral administration (or 12 to 48 hours after oral administration), the PT has not decreased sufficiently, the dose may be repeated.

Adverse Reactions. Reactions resembling allergy or anaphylaxis can occur after injection. The reactions may occur in persons receiving the drug for the first time; they tend to be most severe when the drug is administered IV. Local inflammation at the injection site may develop. Correct dosage of vitamin K for infants is critical because an overdose may cause irreversible negative effects. Menadiol sodium diphosphate may induce hemolysis of erythrocytes in clients deficient in glucose-6-phosphate dehydrogenase.

Drug Interactions. Mineral oil may decrease GI absorption of phytonadione with concurrent oral administration.

Antifibrinolytic Agents
Aminocaproic Acid
Aminocaproic acid (Amicar) is the prototype of a group of compounds that impede fibrinolysis.

Pharmacodynamics. Aminocaproic acid inhibits both plasmin (fibrinolysin) activity and the activation of plasminogen.

Pharmacokinetics. Aminocaproic acid is administered orally or IV. The drug is absorbed rapidly after oral administration and peak plasma levels occur within 2 hours. A single IV dose has a duration of action less than 3 hours. It penetrates body cells, including red blood cells. It does not appear to bind to plasma proteins. A major portion of the agent is excreted unmetabolized in the urine.

Therapeutic Uses. Aminocaproic acid is useful in limited situations. It has helped control hemorrhage after prostatectomy. It helps prevent repeated bleeding after dental extraction in clients with hereditary bleeding disorders and, possibly, additional bleeding after subarachnoid hemorrhage. It is indicated in a rare condition called primary fibrinolytic purpura.

Fibrinolysis, the desired objective with such agents as streptokinase, urokinase, or tissue plasminogen activator, may create a bleeding problem. In such cases, aminocaproic acid may be the antidote.

Dosage and Administration. An initial dose of 5 g orally or IV, followed by 1 to 1.25 g hourly, should achieve and sustain drug plasma levels at 0.13 mg/mL, the concentration apparently necessary for inhibiting fibrinolysis. Administration of more than 30 g/24 hours is not recommended. Studies in prostatectomy clients indicate that aminocaproic acid administered IV at 1 g/hour for 4 hours and then at 0.5 g/hour for an additional 8 hours reduces blood loss dramatically (Colman et al., 1994).

Adverse Reactions. The effects of aminocaproic acid are usually mild and abate when the drug is discontinued. Signs and symptoms include nausea, cramps, diarrhea, dizziness, tinnitus, hypotension, malaise, headache, nasal stuffiness, and conjunctival suffusion.

Drug–Drug Interactions. An increase in clotting factors, leading to a hypercoagulable state, may be produced by coadministration of aminocaproic acid and oral contraceptives or estrogens.

Drug–Laboratory Test Interactions. Serum potassium levels may be elevated by aminocaproic acid, especially in a client with impaired renal function.

Precautions and Contraindications. If aminocaproic acid is administered to a client with intravascular clots, the clots may not undergo lysis as they do normally. Fibrinolysis is a normal process, presumably active at all times to ensure the fluidity of blood. Theoretically, therefore, inhibition of fibrinolysis by aminocaproic acid may result in clotting or thrombosis. Thus, the drug is contraindicated in clients with fibrinolysis secondary to DIC because the compound may prevent the dissolution of clots in small blood vessels (eg, those of the glomeruli). It also may be inappropriate in bleeding that may complicate thrombotic thrombocytopenic purpura.

Tranexamic Acid

Tranexamic acid (Cyklokapron) is an antifibrinolytic whose actions are similar to those of aminocaproic acid but are about 10 times more potent. It diffuses rapidly into joint fluid and the synovial membrane; the same concentration is achieved in the joint fluid as in the serum. It is indicated for short-term use in hemophiliac clients to reduce or prevent hemorrhage. It is administered orally or IV. Adverse reactions include nausea, vomiting, and diarrhea.

Desmopressin Acetate

Desmopressin acetate is a posterior pituitary hormone that increases the titers of factor VIII and von Willebrand factor, presumably as a result of induced release from storage sites in vascular endothelial cells. Its hormonal aspects are discussed in detail in Chapter 33. It has helped clients with classic hemophilia or von Willebrand disease with a baseline factor VIII titer 5% to 10% of normal. It is useful for raising the factor VIII concentration to hemostatic levels sufficient to allow minor surgery and to control minor bleeding. Due to its antidiuretic properties, clients must be monitored to avoid water overload.

Aprotinin

Aprotinin, obtained from bovine lung, inhibits proteolytic enzymes with a variety of effects on the coagulation system. It inhibits plasmin and kallikrein actions. It preserves the adhesive glycoproteins in the platelet membrane, making them resistant to damage from mechanical injury that occurs during cardiopulmonary bypass. The net effect is to inhibit both fibrinolysis and the turnover of coagulation factors and to decrease bleeding.

In clients undergoing cardiac surgery requiring extracorporeal circulation by a heart-lung machine, adverse changes develop in the blood components, blood cells, and specific coagulation proteins. These changes cause a transient homeostatic defect during the intraoperative and immediate postoperative period that may result in diffuse bleeding despite correct surgical technique. Thus, aprotinin is used to reduce perioperative blood loss or the need for transfusion in clients who are having primary or repeated coronary artery bypass graft surgery, who face a high risk for bleeding, or who cannot receive a transfusion. The risk of hypersensitivity is high, and all clients treated with aprotinin should first receive a test dose to assess the potential for allergic reactions.

Topical Hemostatics

Over the years, many agents have been used to control bleeding at accessible sites. In ancient times, twigs and barks were applied to wounds; their benefit probably derived from their content of oxidation products of tannin that activate Hageman factor (factor XII), initiating clotting by means of the intrinsic pathway of thrombin formation. A modern equivalent is the application of a moistened tea bag, rich in tannins, to a bleeding dental socket. Spiderwebs, a folk remedy for bleeding, perhaps also activated Hageman factor. Styptic pencils, usually composed of alum, have long been used to control bleeding from minor cuts, such as those from shaving (Colman et al., 1994).

Several topical hemostatic substances are used to retard blood loss or promote coagulation, including epinephrine, oxidized cellulose, preparations of gelatin, and thrombin.

Epinephrine

Epinephrine stimulates vasoconstriction, slowing blood flow and allowing normal clotting to occur. It is particularly useful in controlling bleeding from tissues to which pressure cannot be applied. Some of the drug may be absorbed systemically, especially if applied to large areas.

Oxidized Cellulose

Oxidized cellulose (Oxycel, Surgicel) is available in pads, pledgets, and strips. When saturated with blood, the product swells into an adhesive mass that adheres to the bleeding surface. After 24 to 48 hours, it becomes gelatinous and can be removed, usually without causing additional bleeding, by irrigation with sterile water or saline solution. It does not alter normal blood clotting mechanisms. It is used in surgical procedures when ligation is inappropriate. It should not be packed into the affected area, nor wrapped too tightly around a body part, because swelling may cause obstruction and may interfere with the function of surrounding structures.

Gelatin Products

Available as a powder, sponge (Gelfoam), or film (Gelfilm, Gelfilm Ophthalmic), gelatin absorbs blood and water. A sponge implanted in tissue is absorbed completely within 4 to 6 weeks without inducing excessive scar tissue formation. The addition of thrombin solution to a gelatin sponge may be beneficial. The film is similar to the sponge but has a cellophane-like appearance in the dry state and a soft, elastic consistency when moistened. The film can be used, for example, to repair a pleural defect in connection with a thoracotomy; there would be subsequent ingrowth of regenerating pleural and fibrous tissue across the gradually resorbed implant. The film has several indications related to neurosurgery and ophthalmic surgery.

Because gelatin is an animal protein, allergic hypersensitivity may develop. Gelatin products are not recommended in the presence of infection; indeed, they could act as a bed for infection and abscess formation.

Thrombin

Powdered bovine thrombin (Thrombinar) may be used to help control localized, accessible bleeding from lacerated tissues or after dental extraction. Thrombin directly converts fibrinogen to fibrin. The contents of a 5,000-U vial dissolved in 5 mL of saline diluent can clot an equal volume of blood in less than a second. Blood at the traumatized site should be gently sponged away, and thrombin should then be applied directly to the bleeding site. The surface may be flooded using a sterile syringe and a small-gauge needle. Application of the powder itself may be more effective in the client known to have a hemostatic defect. Because thrombin is an animal derivative, it can induce allergic hypersensitivity.

■ SUMMARY

Various clotting disorders are characterized by excessive or prolonged bleeding. Some are associated with hereditary deficiencies of one or more clotting factors; others are associated with the inability to produce certain factors because of disease or iatrogenic conditions. The underlying problem is eliminated whenever possible, but replacement of the deficient clotting factor or factors often is necessary.

Systemic hemostatics include whole blood, plasma, platelets, cryoprecipitate, antithrombin III, preparations of certain specific factors, vitamin K, antifibrinolytic agents, desmopressin acetate, and aprotinin. Topical hemostatics include epinephrine, oxidized cellulose, gelatin products, and thrombin.

❖ NURSING MANAGEMENT: CLIENT RECEIVING A HEMOSTATIC AGENT

Whenever systemic hemostatics are administered, there is a chance of overcorrecting the clotting deficiency and producing a state of hypercoagulation. Such a condition is actually more dangerous than bleeding; lost blood can be replaced, but intravascular clots are difficult to remove or dissolve. The stressed client is particularly vulnerable to this complication because stress hormones induce an underlying hypercoagulability that is manifested once the coagulation defect is remedied. For this reason, treatment usually aims at restoring clotting factors to a minimally effective level. A gradual correction of the coagulation defect is desirable. Clients, who often feel desperate, may become impatient if treatment does not produce prompt improvement. They must be reassured that the blood loss can be replaced if necessary, and that a conservative approach is preferable in these situations.

When blood or blood products are administered, there is always a danger of incompatibility reactions. These are most common and most serious with whole blood, but they occasionally occur with fractional components, such as antihemophilic factor. (See Chap. 48 for precautions required during the administration of blood.) Infectious agents such as the hepatitis viruses and HIV also can be transmitted by blood and blood products. Clients who have received human blood products should be monitored for signs and symptoms of infection.

Blood and its derivatives are easily damaged by temperature extremes and rough handling. The nurse must understand the particular requirements of the preparation being used and adjust the procedures for its preparation and administration accordingly. For example, solutions (blood, plasma, reconstituted antihemophilic factor) are refrigerated until they are administered, but they must be protected from freezing. Both red blood cells and protein molecules are damaged by vigorous agitation or rough handling.

NURSING PROCESS
ASSESSMENT

Data required for assessment include the history of the bleeding disorder (onset, duration, and severity of bleeding), the current rate of blood loss, vital signs, color, warmth of skin and circulatory return to peripheral tissues, and results of laboratory tests for red blood cells, hemoglobin, hematocrit, platelets, PT, partial thromboplastin time (PTT), and blood type. Previous exposure and reaction to hemostatic agents should be determined.

NURSING DIAGNOSIS

Clients with prolonged or excessive bleeding will experience:

- Anxiety, related to potential death or infection
- Pain, related to multiple venipunctures and injections used with agents to control bleeding
- Risk for Injury, related to possible viruses in or allergic reaction to hemostatic agent

Clients and families may also have:

- Knowledge Deficit, related to coagulation deficiencies and their treatment

PLANNING

Goals of nursing care include alleviating anxiety, minimizing discomfort and pain, increasing coagulability to a minimally effective level, improving tissue perfusion and circulation, reducing the risk of adverse effects such as infection, promptly detecting and treating adverse reactions that develop, and increasing the client's knowledge about coagulation and hemostatic agents.

INTERVENTION

Nursing interventions to alleviate anxiety include promoting the client's trust in healthcare personnel by demonstrating competent nursing skills and conveying genuine concern for the client's welfare. Both clients and family should be encouraged to express their concerns, and the gravity of the client's situation should be acknowledged. Too often the clinical situation is characterized by an atmosphere of worry and hurry. This should be minimized as much as possible. Unnecessary stressors, such as prolonged fasting, noise, and glaring lights, should be eliminated. The family should be advised to maintain as healthful a routine as possible, eating, sleeping, and resting regularly.

Nursing measures to minimize pain include preventing multiple needle sticks when possible. Blood samples can sometimes be taken from existing IV lines.

Intravenous infusions of hemostatic agents should be given relatively slowly, and the total volume should be limited to prevent circulatory overload. An infusion pump or other device is required to control the flow rate. Concomitant administration of diuretics, such as furosemide, may reduce the danger of overload when large volumes are infused. Clients should be monitored for adverse effects specific to the prescribed agents. Clients receiving hemostatics of animal origin should be assessed regularly for an allergic reaction (urticaria, fever, nausea, or headache). Reactions may be treated with the antihistamine diphenhydramine hydrochloride (Bena-

dryl), or this agent may be given about 30 minutes before the hemostatic agent.

Safe administration of blood requires precautions to prevent administering mismatched blood. Even after following precautions, the nurse must closely observe clients receiving blood, especially during the infusion of the first 50 mL. Early signs and symptoms of a blood reaction include headache, flushing, tachycardia, back pain, hypotension, fever, chills, and neurologic changes. If these develop, the transfusion must be stopped immediately.

Topical hemostatics are often left in place to be absorbed by the body. When materials applied to bleeding sites must be removed, it is important to moisten them thoroughly with a sterile liquid such as normal saline solution. Removal of dry adherent substances can injure blood vessels, causing further bleeding. This principle also applies to the removal of nasal, vaginal, or other packing.

Client Education. Clotting deficiencies can be chronic health problems. Most clients and their families eventually learn a great deal about the specific disorder, but they may still need further education. Under the stress of an acute bleeding episode, they may be unable to recall facts or think rationally. The nurse should offer clients information necessary for coping with the treatment procedures without conveying an assumption that this knowledge is new. If time allows, the nurse should question clients to determine how sophisticated they are about their condition. However, even clients who are very knowledgeable should continue to receive coaching instructions that help them participate in treatment procedures. The nurse must also help the client recognize signs and symptoms of serious adverse effects and stress the importance of notifying the healthcare provider at once if they occur.

Clients deficient in vitamin K because of alterations in intestinal flora may benefit from learning about foods, such as buttermilk or yogurt, that contain *Lactobacillus* cultures. These foods help restore the normal flora, thereby increasing the production of vitamin K in the GI tract.

OUTCOME EVALUATION

Data required for evaluation include statements by the client indicating decreased fear, anxiety, and pain. The presence or absence of bleeding and the results of laboratory tests that measure coagulability will identify progress or lack of it, replacement of blood losses, and contained blood loss. Color, tests for peripheral circulation, and vital signs indicate changes in tissue perfusion. The presence or absence of adverse drug effects and their severity are needed to evaluate their prevention, detection, and treatment. Client education is measured by the client's ability to cooperate with treatment procedures and to recall information from teaching sessions.

- Eliminate or ameliorate stressors when possible.
- Reassure the client that blood loss can be replaced and that a conservative approach is desirable.
- Minimize the number of needle sticks.
- Use proper procedures when handling, storing, and preparing blood and its derivatives.
- Avoid rapid administration of IV preparations.
- Observe clients closely for adverse drug reactions. If possible, use nursing measures to reduce the risk and the severity of these reactions. Report reactions requiring further medical attention to the prescriber.
- Instruct clients receiving blood or blood products about the signs and symptoms of potential infection. Warn them to seek immediate medical attention if such reactions develop.
- Advise clients to include foods rich in vitamin K in the diet.

Anticoagulants

Drugs that inhibit clotting may be used either to prevent or treat thromboembolic disorders. Anticoagulant drugs do not dissolve existing clots but do interrupt the extension of these clots, which tend to enlarge because of the autocatalytic nature of coagulation. Table 26-3 compares various anticoagulants.

Heparin

Heparin is not really a single substance but a group of substances with molecular weights from 3,000 to 40,000. In the tissues, heparin is found in mast cells. It is also in the plasma and in the endothelial cell layer of blood vessels. It is an acidic mucopolysaccharide that carries an electronegative charge, which seems to account for many of its actions. For clinical use, it is extracted from beef lung or the intestinal mucosa of hogs.

Fragments of heparin with slightly different anticoagulant activity from the parent molecule are also available. The molecular weights vary from 4,000 to 15,000. These preparations, referred to as "low-molecular-weight heparins," are discussed below.

Pharmacodynamics. Small amounts of heparin with antithrombin III inhibit thrombosis by inactivating factor Xa and inhibiting the conversion of prothrombin to thrombin. Once active thrombosis develops, larger amounts of heparin, with antithrombin III, inactivate factors IX, X, Xa, XI, and XII and thrombin, inhibiting the conversion of fibrinogen to fibrin. The heparin/ antithrombin III complex is 100 to 1,000 times more potent as an anticoagulant than antithrombin III alone.

Heparin also prevents the formation of a stable fibrin clot by inhibiting the activation of factor XIII (fibrin-stabilizing factor). Other effects include the inhibition of thrombin-induced activation of factors V and VIII.

Pharmacokinetics. Heparin must be administered parenterally because it is broken down by digestion. It is readily absorbed when administered subcutaneously (SC) or IV. It should not be given IM because it is absorbed erratically and can cause bleeding at the injection site (hematoma). When given IV, the peak effect is in 5 to 10 minutes, with a duration of 2 to 6 hours. It is gradually absorbed SC with an onset of action of 30 to 60 minutes and a duration of 8 to 12 hours. It is highly bound to plasma proteins. Some heparin is metabolized by the liver enzyme heparinase, and the rest is excreted unchanged by the kidney.

After administration, heparin is widely distributed in the body; much of it is trapped in the interstitial fluid and reticuloendothelial cells. It does not cross the

Table 26-3. Comparison of Heparin, Enoxaparin, and Warfarin Sodium

	Heparin	Enoxaparin	Warfarin Sodium
Route(s) of administration	IV, SC	SC	PO, IV
Unit of measurement of doses	units	mg	mg
Frequency of dosage	twice a day SC, continuous IV infusion	twice a day SC	once daily
Onset of action	IV peak 5–10 min, SC 30–60 min	peak 3–5 hr after SC	peak 1.5–3 days
Antidote(s)	protamine sulfate	protamine sulfate	vitamin K
Laboratory test(s) for monitoring	APTT	no need for daily monitoring	PT, INR
Adverse reactions	hemorrhage, allergic reactions, thrombocytopenia	bleeding, fever, nausea, edema, confusion, skin reactions	hemorrhage, purple toe syndrome, alopecia
Pregnancy category	C	B	D
Source	bovine lung or porcine intestinal mucosa	porcine heparin	plant

placenta and is not distributed into breast milk. Although heparin is eliminated through the kidneys, it is not removed by hemodialysis.

Therapeutic Uses. Heparin is the anticoagulant of choice when an immediate effect is required. Heparin is approved for preventing and treating venous thrombosis, pulmonary embolism, and embolism caused by atrial fibrillation. It is also used in preventing cerebral thrombosis in evolving stroke and preventing and treating peripheral arterial embolism, and as an adjunct in treating coronary occlusion.

Heparin is also used to prevent clotting in equipment used for extracorporeal circulation and in blood samples when laboratory tests require unclotted blood.

In some situations, arterial catheters may be in place for hemodynamic monitoring and central venous lines may be used. When large volumes of IV fluids are contraindicated, intermittent IV therapy may be ordered. In such cases a heparin lock, which is an IV needle with a small well covered by a rubber diaphragm, may be in place. Heparin locks and central lines are flushed with saline solution or heparin in accord with institutional policy. Heparin in the needle inhibits clot formation in the lumen, thereby maintaining patency despite the absence of fluid flow for long periods. To prevent damage to the diaphragm and subsequent leakage, a small-gauge (25 or 26) needle is used. Injection should be slow, as with all IV medications delivered by the push technique.

Subanticoagulant doses of heparin (low-dose heparin) have been used to prevent thrombi in hospitalized clients at high risk (eg, postpartum mothers, older clients undergoing hip or abdominal surgery, clients with long bone fractures).

Heparin was once used to treat DIC, but this use is now controversial. Heparin may be helpful when ischemic organ dysfunction or failure or potential loss of life or limb exists because of the degree of microvascular thrombi. Heparin can prevent further microvascular obstruction by thrombi and minimize platelet aggregation. Heparin in low doses is a good antithrombin agent. Because excessive amounts of thrombin can theoretically stimulate the pathophysiologic coagulation and fibrinolysis processes in DIC, heparin should interrupt the repetitive nature of this cycle. Antithrombin III activity is greatly enhanced with heparin, as previously described. On the other hand, when DIC and septic shock occur concurrently, heparin is not thought to be beneficial (Bell, 1993). Because of the risk of bleeding, heparin is usually contraindicated for clients with active bleeding of any kind.

Dosage and Administration. The potency of commercial preparations of heparin is expressed in terms of units of heparin activity. There is heparin calcium (Calciparine) and heparin sodium (Liquaemin Sodium).

In acute situations requiring full anticoagulation, the drug is usually given IV, by continuous drip, at a dose of 20,000 to 40,000 U/day. Heparin can be added to IV solution from a multiple-dose vial or, preferably, a premixed preparation of a designated number of units in 250 to 500 mL of 0.45% to 0.9% sodium chloride solution is used. The infusion may be started after an IV bolus of 5,000 units. An infusion controller must be used. The infusion dosage is usually adjusted according to the results of coagulation tests. The best indicator is the APTT, which measures how heparin is inhibiting thrombin, factor Xa, and factor IXa. The recommended APTT range for most conditions requiring heparin therapy is 1.5 to 2 times the client's baseline time, normally 24 to 36 seconds. At times, however, a higher APTT may be required.

Low-dose heparin prophylaxis, before and after surgery, may reduce the incidence of postoperative deep vein thrombosis (DVT) in the legs. Dosage for this purpose might be 5,000 U SC 2 hours before surgery and 5,000 units every 8 to 12 hours for 7 days after surgery, or until the client is fully ambulatory. A small-gauge (25 or 26), ½″ to ⅝″ needle should be used to minimize tissue trauma. The SC sites are above the iliac crest and the abdominal fat layer.

When used to clear heparin locks, a dose of 10 to 100 U/mL of Heparin Sodium Lock Flush Solution may be given via the injection hub to prevent clot formation.

Adverse Reactions. Heparin is well tolerated by most clients. High-dose heparin therapy is used only in institutional settings where the recipient is under close medical supervision. The greatest risk is excessive bleeding; when this occurs, discontinuing the medication usually eliminates the symptoms. In severe cases, protamine sulfate is administered as an antidote (see below).

Allergic reactions or hypersensitivity may occur because heparin is derived from animal tissue. It should be used with caution in clients with a history of allergy. Before a therapeutic dose is given, a trial dose may be advisable. Have epinephrine 1:1,000 available.

Thrombocytopenia has occurred in clients receiving heparin. Other causes of thrombocytopenia should be ruled out before determining that thrombocytopenia relates to heparin administration. The incidence of heparin-associated thrombocytopenia is higher with bovine than with porcine heparin. The severity also appears to be dose-related. Early thrombocytopenia, which develops 2 to 3 days after starting heparin, tends to be mild and is due to the direct action of heparin on platelets.

Rarely clients develop new thrombus formation in association with thrombocytopenia resulting from irreversible, heparin-induced platelet aggregation. This is called heparin-induced thrombocytopenia and thrombosis (HITT) and is potentially fatal. Also called white clot syndrome, it occurs between days 3 and 12 of therapy, most often around day 6. Signs and symptoms include a platelet count below 100,000/mm³, thromboembolus or hemorrhage, and a positive platelet aggregation test. The process may lead to severe thromboembolic complications (eg, skin necrosis, gangrene of the extremities [possibly leading to amputation], MI, pulmonary embolism, or stroke). It is not known what causes HITT, but it may be an immune-mediated response. If HITT is suspected, heparin should be stopped and the prescriber notified. Protamine sulfate and plasmapheresis are used to treat HITT.

A toxic effect of heparin, reported with long-term treatment of 6 months or more, is osteoporosis with resultant spontaneous fractures. The reason for this is unknown.

Drug–Drug Interactions. Aspirin and nonsteroidal antiinflammatory agents (NSAIDs), cephalosporins, and penicillins may increase the risk of bleeding. Some sources say that IV nitroglycerin may decrease heparin's anticoagulant activity.

Drug–Laboratory Test Interactions. Heparin may prolong the PT, which may be the standard used for monitoring concurrent therapy with oral anticoagulants. Significant elevations of serum transaminase levels (AST and ALT) have been noted. Transaminase determinations are important in the differential diagnosis of some disorders, such as MI, so elevations must be interpreted carefully.

Precautions and Contraindications. These include hypersensitivity to heparin, severe thrombocytopenia, and any uncontrolled bleeding (ie, during labor and the immediate postpartum period). In addition, drugs that interact with heparin to increase the risk of bleeding are generally contraindicated for clients receiving heparin.

Enoxaparin

Enoxaparin (Lovenox) was introduced in 1993 as the first low-molecular-weight heparin derivative. A similar product is dalteparin sodium (Fragmin).

Pharmacodynamics. Enoxaparin appears to have two mechanisms of action: direct inhibition of thrombin by binding and enhancement of antithrombin III and inhibition of prothrombinase-mediated thrombin generation. However, the relative importance of these two mechanisms and other activities is unclear. Evidence suggests it is less likely than heparin to cause bleeding difficulties and more likely to prevent fatal pulmonary embolism.

Pharmacokinetics. Maximal effect of enoxaparin occurs 3 to 5 hours after SC injection. Elimination is believed to be through renal mechanisms. Enoxaparin does not appear to cross the placenta to any significant extent.

Therapeutic Uses. Clients who undergo orthopedic surgery, such as knee or hip replacement, have a high risk (40% to 80%) of developing venous thromboembolism, which precipitates fatal pulmonary embolism in about 2% of these clients (Noble et al., 1995). Prophylaxis for DVT is the principal indication for the use of enoxaparin.

Using enoxaparin to treat existing DVT and to prevent clotting in hemodialysis circuits has been studied. Clients undergoing general, urologic, or gynecologic surgery may also benefit from this drug.

Dosage and Administration. In clients undergoing hip replacement, one recommended dose is 30 mg twice daily by SC injection, with the initial dose given as soon as possible after surgery, but not more than 24 hours after surgery. The duration of administration ranges from 7 to 14 days. A second approach has been to use 40 mg once daily, initiated preoperatively. The drug is administered using the left and right anterolateral and left and right posterolateral abdominal wall, inserting the whole length of the needle into the skin fold (prefilled syringes with 26-gauge, 1/2 ″ needle) and holding the skin fold throughout the injection. Enoxaparin has little effect on PTT or PT. Daily monitoring is not usually needed.

Adverse Reactions. The incidence of bleeding related to enoxaparin use has been low. Other reported adverse effects include fever, nausea, peripheral edema, confusion, and skin reactions.

Drug–Drug Interactions. Enoxaparin may interact with oral anticoagulants and platelet inhibitors. Combined use of low-molecular-weight heparin preparations and the NSAID ketorolac (Toradol) may potentiate hemostatic effects; caution is advised.

Drug–Laboratory Test Interactions. Significant elevations of serum transaminase levels (AST and ALT) have been noted. Transaminase determinations are important in the differential diagnosis of some pathologies, such as MI, so elevations must be interpreted carefully. Some clients have exhibited thrombocytopenia.

Precautions and Contraindications. The contraindications to heparin use also apply to enoxaparin.

Antithrombin III-Independent Anticoagulants

Several antithrombin III-independent inhibitors of thrombin have recently become available: hirudin, hirugen, argatroban, and the peptide chloromethyl ketone inhibitor/PPACK.

Hirudin, the anticoagulant substance from the medicinal leech and the most potent known naturally occurring inhibitor of thrombin, has been synthesized by recombinant DNA techniques and is available for clinical use. It binds to the active catalytic site and the fibrinogen recognition site on thrombin. It has proved effective at inhibiting experimentally produced arterial and venous thrombosis. Unlike heparin, it causes little or no bleeding at clinically effective antithrombotic doses. Given IV, its half-life is 1 to 2 hours. It is excreted unchanged, mainly through the kidney.

Hirugen is a synthetic dodecapeptide derived from hirudin that binds directly to thrombin. Argatroban is a weak competitive inhibitor of thrombin with a half-life of only a few minutes. PPACK alkylates the active site in thrombin, inhibiting it irreversibly. These three compounds can reach and inactivate thrombin that is bound to fibrin (Rang et al., 1995).

Protamine Sulfate

Pharmacodynamics. Protamines are strongly basic proteins of low molecular weight, rich in arginine. They occur in the sperm of salmon and certain other fish. When administered to normal persons, protamine acts as a weak anticoagulant. However, when administered to clients who have been treated with heparin, protamine combines chemically with the acidic heparin to form a stable salt that has no anticoagulant properties.

Pharmacokinetics. Protamine sulfate has a rapid onset of action that persists about 2 hours. Heparin is neutralized within 5 minutes after IV injection of protamine sulfate. The metabolic fate of the heparin/protamine complex is unknown. One theory is that the heparin/protamine complex may be affected by fibrinolysin, thus freeing heparin.

Therapeutic Uses. Protamine is used IV for treating severe heparin overdosage. It is also used to terminate heparin anticoagulation after extracorporeal circulation or dialysis.

Dosage and Administration. Protamine sulfate 1 mg neutralizes about 90 USP units of heparin (bovine) or about 115 USP units (porcine). No more than 50 mg of protamine should be administered in any 10-minute period; it is given slowly IV over the 10 minutes. Dosage is calculated in relation to the dose of heparin, its route of administration, and the time elapsed since it was given. Coagulation tests should be performed 5 to 15 minutes after protamine is administered and again in 2 to 8 hours as the client is monitored for heparin rebound.

Adverse Reactions. Allergic reactions to protamine sulfate have been reported and are most likely in persons allergic to fish. Rapid injection of protamine causes an abrupt drop in blood pressure and bradycardia. A heparin rebound or rebound anticoagulation may be encountered as a complication 30 minutes to 18 hours after reversing the effects of heparin with protamine. No significant drug interactions have been reported.

Precautions and Contraindications. These include pregnancy, lactation, and allergy to the drug or to fish products.

Coumarin and Indandione Derivatives

The most commonly prescribed oral anticoagulant is the coumarin derivative warfarin sodium (Coumadin). The indandione anticoagulant anisindione (Miradon) is similar to the coumarin derivatives in action and adverse reactions. It has a greater incidence of severe adverse reactions, including cutaneous, hepatic, and hematologic effects, and is used primarily to treat clients who do not tolerate coumarin derivatives.

Pharmacodynamics. Warfarin sodium's chemical structure resembles that of vitamin K. It is thought to act mainly by competitively inhibiting this nutrient. The drug molecule is accepted by the liver in place of vitamin K. Normal vitamin K is not reduced as usual, thereby decreasing its role in the production of clotting factors II, VII, IX, and X.

The reduction in the synthesis of the clotting factors affects the coagulation processes. Anticoagulant effects depend on the half-lives of clotting factors. When warfarin sodium is administered, factor VII is affected first (half-life of 6 hours), then factors IX, X, and II, with half-lives of 24, 40, and 60 hours, respectively. Thus, an initial prolongation of PT is seen in 8 to 12 hours, but maximal anticoagulation is not reached for 3 to 5 days.

Oral anticoagulants have no direct effect on an established thrombus, nor do they reverse ischemic tissue damage caused by a thrombus. However, once thrombosis has occurred, anticoagulant treatment may prevent extension of the formed clot and secondary thromboembolic complications that may result in serious, possibly fatal, consequences.

Pharmacokinetics. Coumarin derivatives may be given orally. The preparations available vary in the degree to which they are absorbed in the GI tract. Dicumarol is poorly absorbed; warfarin sodium is rapidly absorbed. Large amounts of the drug are bound to plasma proteins (97% to more than 99%); it also accumulates in the lungs, liver, spleen, and kidneys.

Warfarin sodium has a half-life of about 48 hours, reaches its peak activity in 1.5 to 3 days, and has a duration of action of 2 to 5 days. It is metabolized by the hepatic microsomal enzyme system and excreted in the urine and feces as inactive metabolites. The coumarin derivatives can cross the placental barrier and are secreted in breast milk. The latter could be important because the newborn is already at risk for inadequate synthesis of vitamin K in the bowel.

Therapeutic Uses. Coumarin derivatives are approved for preventing and treating venous thrombosis and its extension, preventing embolism caused by atrial fibrillation, and as an adjunct in the prophylaxis of systemic embolism after MI. They have been used to prevent recurrent transient ischemic attacks (with unclear results). They should not be used in treating acute completed strokes due to the risk of fatal cerebral hemorrhage. Long-term oral anticoagulant therapy is used to prevent thromboembolic disorders in clients considered at high risk, including those with rheumatic heart disease (especially if atria are enlarged or fibrillating), prosthetic heart valves, or a history of MI.

Several factors may result in an increased response to the oral anticoagulants: carcinoma; hepatic disorders; biliary fistula; infection with concomitant antibiotic therapy, which may alter intestinal flora; renal insufficiency; recent surgery; radiation therapy; vitamin K deficiency; diarrhea; and poor nutritional state. Female and elderly clients appear more sensitive to these agents. Other factors appear to result in a decreased response: hyperlipidemia, diabetes, hypothyroidism, and hereditary resistance to oral anticoagulants.

Dosage and Administration. Warfarin sodium is usually administered once a day. While the client is in the hospital, doses are adjusted daily in accord with coagulation tests. The desired PT and international normalized ratio (INR) depend on the condition being managed. The usual aim of therapy is to adjust the dose to maintain the PT at 1.5 to 2.5 times a control value. A target INR range of 2.0 to 3.0 is recommended in most cases (3–4.5 recommended for clients with mechanical prosthetic heart valves). An injectable form of warfarin was recently approved for marketing.

Oral anticoagulants are sometimes prescribed with heparin use and are often used when long-term anticoagulant therapy is indicated. If warfarin sodium is administered over a long time on an outpatient basis, the client must first be stabilized with a maintenance dose. Periodic (usually monthly) coagulation tests are necessary to monitor the client's response to the drug.

The client should stay on a steady, well-balanced diet. Vitamin K affects how the body reacts to warfarin sodium, so the client should not increase or decrease significantly the consumption of foods rich in this vitamin, such as broccoli, cabbage, asparagus, spinach, brussels sprouts, turnip greens, kale, and liver.

Adverse Reactions. Warfarin sodium has a narrow therapeutic index, so the chances of adverse reactions are greater. Over time, the problems associated with warfarin sodium have been related mainly to bleeding. Because of the narrow therapeutic index, reliable and accurate monitoring of anticoagulant intensity is necessary to ensure that the dosage is optimally therapeutic. The traditional method of determining the efficacy of anticoagulant therapy with warfarin sodium has been the PT, but inconsistency in PT results is a problem (Bussey et al., 1992). Several variables may affect the results of the PT test, including equipment; sample collection methods, handling, and storage; and the sensitivity of the thromboplastin reagent (Oertel, 1995). To resolve the problem of variable PTs, the INR, which corrects for the variability in PT results, is recommended for use in monitoring oral anticoagulant therapy.

When abnormal bleeding occurs, anticoagulation should be partially or completely reversed. Treatment may require using phytonadione (vitamin K_1). In addition, all possible causes other than anticoagulant toxicity should be ruled out, especially if the bleeding is not affected by restoration of normal coagulation.

Anticoagulant therapy may promote the release of vascular plaque emboli and thereby increase the risk of complications, such as "purple toe syndrome." Discontinuation of therapy is recommended when such phenomena are observed. Other adverse reactions include nausea, diarrhea, pyrexia, dermatitis, urticaria, alopecia, mouth ulcers, paralytic ileus, and intestinal obstruction from submucosal hemorrhage.

Drug–Drug Interactions. Warfarin sodium is an example of a drug that, through its metabolism in the liver, is affected by enzyme inhibitors and enzyme inducers (see Chap. 6). Taken with an enzyme inhibitor, warfarin breakdown may be decreased and its plasma concentration increased; taken with enzyme inducers, its plasma concentration decreases. So many drugs affect the body's response to coumarin anticoagulants that the interactions are considered a prototype for the study of drug interactions (Table 26-4).

Table 26-4. Highly Probable Drug–Food Interactions With Warfarin Sodium

Substances That Potentiate Warfarin's Effect	Substances That Diminish Warfarin's Effect
acetaminophen	alcohol (chronic use/abuse)
aminoglycosides	barbiturates
amiodarone	carbamazepine
androgens	cholestyramine
aspirin and other salicylates	dicloxacillin
cephalosporins	ethchlorvynol
chloral hydrate	estrogens
cimetidine & other histamine (H_2) antagonists	glutethimide
clofibrate	griseofulvin
dextropropoxyphene	nafcillin
disulfiram	oral contraceptives
erythromycin	rifampin
influenza vaccine	spironolactone
loop diuretics	sucralfate
metronidazole	thiazide diuretics
miconazole	trazodone
NSAIDs	vitamin K
phenylbutazone	
propafenone	
propranolol	
quinidine	
quinolones	
sulfonamides	
tamoxifen	
tetracyclines	
thyroid drugs	
vitamin E	

Drug–Laboratory Test Interactions. Oral anticoagulants may color alkaline urine red-orange, and this may interfere with some laboratory tests.

■ SUMMARY

Anticoagulants may be used for preventing or treating such conditions as venous thrombosis, pulmonary embolism, and coronary thrombosis. These drugs do not dissolve existing clots, but they interrupt the extension of these clots. The most serious risk with heparin and warfarin therapy is excessive bleeding. Many drugs affect responses to the oral anticoagulants.

Antiplatelet Drugs

Whereas anticoagulants inhibit blood clotting, antiplatelet drugs interfere with the aggregation of platelets needed for clotting. These drugs include aspirin, dextran, sulfinpyrazone (Anturane), dipyridamole (Persantine), ticlopidine (Ticlid), and abciximab. Dipyridamole was discussed in Chapter 24. Aspirin is the most widely used antiplatelet agent.

Aspirin

Aspirin, discussed more fully in Chapter 36, alters the balance between thromboxane A_2, which promotes aggregation, and prostacyclin (PGI_2), which inhibits it. Aspirin inactivates prostaglandin synthetase irreversibly. This reduces both thromboxane A_2 synthesis in platelets and prostacyclin synthesis in endothelium. Vascular endothelial cells can synthesize new enzyme, whereas platelets cannot.

After administration of aspirin, thromboxane A_2 synthesis does not recover until the affected group of platelets is replaced; this usually takes 7 to 10 days. Furthermore, inhibition of the prostaglandin synthetase of the vascular endothelium requires higher amounts of aspirin than does inhibition of the prostaglandin synthetase of the platelet. Thus, low doses of aspirin given intermittently decrease the synthesis of thromboxane A_2 without drastically reducing prostacyclin synthesis (Rang et al., 1995).

Research has shown that aspirin reduces the risk of fatal or nonfatal MI in clients with unstable angina pectoris or previous heart attack. In studies, clients admitted for unstable angina or acute MI usually received heparin, but aspirin was also started with a loading dose of 160 mg, followed by 80 mg/day. Clients who met certain criteria would usually have the heparin converted to warfarin sodium and continue with warfarin sodium and aspirin for 3 months after discharge (Chesebro et al., 1994). After that, aspirin therapy may continue for life.

Clients with stable coronary artery disease may benefit from either aspirin (80–325 mg/day) or anticoagulant therapy. Clients at lower risk, with no overt coronary artery disease and no symptoms but with more than one risk factor for coronary artery disease, especially clients over age 60, may also benefit from low-dose aspirin therapy.

Clients with nonvalvular atrial fibrillation without clinical or echocardiographic risk factors for thromboembolism have a reduced risk of thromboembolism if they take 325 mg of enteric-coated aspirin daily. In clients with mechanical or bioprosthetic heart valves, the risk of thromboembolism is highest in the first 3 months after valve replacement. An anticoagulant and a platelet inhibitor (aspirin, 80–100 mg/day, or dipyridamole, 5–6 mg/kg/day) may be used. Clients who undergo aortocoronary artery bypass grafts should receive aspirin (80–325 mg/day), starting within 6 hours after the operation, with the first loading dose (160–325 mg) administered by nasogastric tube or rectal suppository.

Dipyridamole

Pharmacodynamics. Dipyridamole has vasodilator action. Its predominant action is on small resistance vessels. Dipyridamole is also thought to inhibit platelet aggregation to some degree.

Pharmacokinetics. After an oral dose, the average time to peak concentration is about 75 minutes. Dipyridamole is highly bound to plasma proteins. It is metabolized by the liver. The drug and its metabolites enter the enterohepatic cycle via secretion in bile and eventually are eliminated in the feces.

Therapeutic Uses. Dipyridamole has better antithrombotic effects against prosthetic materials (eg, artificial heart valves, arteriovenous shunts) than against biologic surfaces. Against biologic surfaces, aspirin has been as effective as combined aspirin and dipyridamole. Thus, dipyridamole is used for high-risk clients with mechanical prosthetic heart valves. It is believed that platelet reactivity and interaction with prosthetic cardiac valve surfaces is a significant factor in thromboembolic complications occurring in connection with prosthetic heart valve replacement.

Dosage and Administration. Dipyridamole is marketed as oral tablets of 25 to 75 mg. The usual adult dosage is 75 to 100 mg, four times daily.

Adverse Reactions. Adverse effects of dipyridamole are generally transient and minimal. They include dizziness, abdominal distress, headache, rash, diarrhea, vomiting, flushing, and pruritus. Worsening of angina has been reported.

Drug Interactions. The use of IV dipyridamole has decreased coronary vasodilation effects if used concurrently with theophylline.

Precautions and Contraindications. Dipyridamole must be used cautiously in clients with hypotension because peripheral vasodilation, an effect of the drug, may exacerbate hypotension. It is contraindicated in allergy to the drug and in pregnancy and lactation.

Ticlopidine

Ticlopidine is a thienopyridine derivative antiplatelet drug approved in 1991.

Pharmacodynamics. Ticlopidine appears to interfere with platelet membrane function by inhibiting ADP-induced platelet/fibrinogen binding and subsequent platelet/platelet interactions (Olin, 1995). The effect on platelet function is irreversible for the life of the platelet.

Pharmacokinetics. Maximal antithrombotic effects occur after 3 to 7 days of therapy. After ticlopidine therapy stops, bleeding time and other platelet function tests return to normal within 2 weeks in most clients. Ticlopidine is rapidly absorbed. Peak plasma levels occur about 2 hours after dosing. The drug is extensively metabolized by the liver and excreted in the urine (60%) and the feces (23%). Ticlopidine binds reversibly to plasma proteins.

Therapeutic Uses. In studies, ticlopidine has halved the incidence of MI, vascular mortality, and total coronary events. It also reduced the incidence of abrupt thrombotic occlusion and ischemic complications in clients undergoing percutaneous transluminal coronary angioplasty (PTCA), but not the incidence of restenosis (Chesebro et al., 1994). Ticlopidine has also been used in clients with transient ischemic attacks, intermittent claudication, chronic arterial occlusion, subarachnoid hemorrhage, coronary artery bypass graft surgery, arteriovenous shunts or fistulas for hemodialysis, open-heart surgery, glomerulonephritis, and sickle-cell disease.

Dosage and Administration. Maximal effect is reached at a dose of 500 mg/day. Ticlopidine tablets (250 mg) are taken twice daily with food to minimize GI adverse reactions.

Adverse Reactions. Adverse effects include diarrhea, nausea, dyspepsia, and rash. Neutropenia and thrombocytopenia have occurred and have limited the use of this drug.

Drug–Drug Interactions. Drug interactions have been reported with antacids (decreased ticlopidine plasma levels), digoxin (decreased digoxin levels), cimetidine (reduced ticlopidine clearance), aspirin, and theophylline (prolonged theophylline half-life).

Drug–Food Interactions. The oral bioavailability of ticlopidine increases when the drug is taken after a meal.

Drug–Laboratory Test Interactions. Neutropenia has occurred. When the drug was discontinued, the neutrophil counts returned to normal over 1 to 2 weeks. Neutropenia occurred 3 weeks to 3 months after the start of therapy. Thrombocytopenia may occur alone or with neutropenia. Ticlopidine therapy causes increased serum cholesterol and triglyceride levels. Elevations of alkaline phosphatase and transaminase levels have occurred.

Precautions and Contraindications. A complete blood count with white blood cell differential should be performed every 2 weeks, from the second week through the third month of therapy, because of the potential for blood abnormalities.

Abciximab

Abciximab (ReoPro) is the fab (antigen-binding fragment) of monoclonal antibody 7E3. The drug was approved by the Food and Drug Administration (FDA) in 1994.

Pharmacodynamics. Abciximab binds to the intact GPIIb/IIIa receptor of human platelets, which is the major platelet surface receptor involved in platelet aggregation. The drug inhibits platelet aggregation by preventing the binding of fibrinogen, von Willebrand factor, and other adhesive molecules to the receptor sites.

Pharmacokinetics. After bolus administration, plasma concentrations of abciximab decrease rapidly. The initial half-life is less than 10 minutes; the second phase half-life is about 30 minutes. Bleeding time returns to less than 12 minutes within 12 hours after the infusion ends in most clients and within 24 hours in 90% of clients. Platelet function generally recovers over 48 hours, although abciximab remains in the circulation in a platelet-bound state for up to 10 days.

Therapeutic Uses. Abciximab is used as an adjunct to PTCA or atherectomy for preventing acute cardiac ischemic complications in clients at high risk for abrupt closure of the treated coronary vessel. It is intended for use with aspirin and heparin.

Dosage and Administration. The recommended dosage is an IV bolus of 0.25 mg/kg administered 10 to 60 minutes before the start of PTCA, followed by a continuous IV infusion of 10 µg/min for 12 hours.

Adverse Reactions. Adverse effects include hypotension, bradycardia, nausea, vomiting, pain, and bleeding. Hypersensitivity reactions may occur; if symptoms of allergic reaction or anaphylaxis occur, the infusion should be stopped and appropriate treatment given. No drug interactions have been reported to date.

Precautions and Contraindications. Because it increases the risk of bleeding, abciximab is contraindicated with recent GI or genitourinary bleeding of clinical significance, history of stroke within 2 years or with a significant residual neurologic deficit, administration of oral anticoagulants within 7 days (in most cases), thrombocytopenia, recent major surgery or trauma, arteriovenous malformation or aneurysm, severe uncontrolled hypertension, and use of IV dextran.

Dextran

Low-molecular-weight dextran prolongs the bleeding time. Administration of 500–1000 mL IV on 1 day, followed by 500 mL per day for an additional 2 to 3 days would typically be used. The mechanism of action is unclear but may involve an alteration of platelet membrane function or inhibition of the factor VIII/von Willebrand factor complex. Dextran is associated with a low but dangerous incidence of anaphylactic reactions. Dextran has been used in clients undergoing angioplasty or placement of intravascular stents for prevention of acute thrombotic occlusion, but studies showing clear-cut benefits have not been done (Chesebro et al., 1994).

Sulfinpyrazone

Sulfinpyrazone competitively inhibits platelet prostaglandin synthetase. It reduces thrombus formation on subendothelium, inhibits platelet adhesion to collagen, and may protect endothelium from chemical injury. The most beneficial effects of sulfinpyrazone appear to be on prosthetic rather than biologic surfaces. The clinical benefits in clients with coronary artery disease vary, with questionable benefit after MI, no benefit with unstable angina, no benefit in preventing stroke, and probably some benefit in preventing aortocoronary vein graft occlusion (Chesebro et al., 1994).

■ SUMMARY

Platelet activation and aggregation are important components of hemostasis, and antiplatelet drugs can have a therapeutic affect on unwanted coagulation. Nursing management for clients receiving antiplatelet drugs is much the same as for anticoagulants.

❖ Nursing Management: Client Receiving an Anticoagulant or Antiplatelet Drug

Anticoagulant therapy is often used to treat acute, life-threatening conditions such as pulmonary embolism and MI.

Nursing Process

Assessment

The initial assessment of clients receiving anticoagulants includes a review of risk factors (Box 26-2), signs and symptoms of thrombi or emboli, previous exposure to anticoagulants, level of knowledge about thromboembolic disease and its treatment, emotional response to the life-threatening condition, and general stress level. Baseline data should include skin color, vital signs, peripheral pulses, warmth of peripheral tissues, and results of laboratory tests such as platelet count, bleeding time, APPT, PT, urinalysis, and stool examination for occult blood. A complete drug history should be taken.

Before any anticoagulant is administered, it must be determined whether the client is at risk for adverse reactions to the drug. A careful history must be taken to rule out contraindications to anticoagulants. A history of peptic ulcers or abnormal bleeding tendencies is particularly important. If heparin is to be used, the client should be questioned about any previous heparin therapy. Because heparin is an extract from animal tissues, initial exposure may induce hypersensitivity. If warfarin therapy is planned, pregnancy should be ruled out in women of childbearing age. A careful drug history is crucial to identify risks of complications from drug interactions.

Nursing Diagnosis

Nursing diagnoses related to anticoagulant therapy include:

- Risk for Injury, related to drug-induced hemorrhage or anaphylaxis
- Risk for Injury, related to potentially impaired gas exchange from drug-induced dislodgment of thrombus
- Altered Tissue Perfusion, related to hypercoagulability and venous stasis (associated with DVT)
- Body Image Disturbance, related to ecchymoses and petechiae (associated with subcutaneous heparin)
- Risk for Impaired Skin Integrity, related to venous stasis associated with decreased activity
- Fear, of death, related to potential complications of drug-related hemorrhage
- Knowledge Deficit concerning thromboembolic disorders and their treatment with medication

Planning

Goals of nursing management include improved tissue perfusion, reduced risk of adverse drug reactions, prompt detection and treatment of possible adverse drug effects,

Box 26-2
Client Characteristics That Increase Bleeding Risk With Anticoagulants

- Age over 60
- Liver dysfunction during therapy (heparin)
- Preexisting condition that increases risk of hemorrhage, such as cerebral aneurysm, recent intracranial bleeding (eg, subdural and subarachnoid bleeding)
- Recent neurosurgery or cerebrospinal surgery
- Serious cardiovascular disease (eg, subacute bacterial endocarditis, dissecting abdominal aortic aneurysm, severe hypertension)
- Underlying blood dyscrasias or hemostatic defects
- Peptic ulcer disease with active or recent bleeding
- Concurrent administration of NSAIDs or diuretics (warfarin)
- Alcoholism
- Macular degeneration (intraocular bleeding may occur), severe proliferative diabetic retinopathy or recent or anticipated ophthalmologic surgery
- Pregnancy (warfarin)

maintenance of skin integrity, adaptation to temporary changes in skin appearance, and increased knowledge related to thromboembolism and its treatment. See the Example of Nursing Process for Anticoagulant Therapy.

INTERVENTION

If the client is being treated for DVT, recommended activity restrictions must be observed. Some recommend elevating the legs; others oppose this. Positions that compromise venous blood flow (eg, crossing the legs, putting pillows under the knees, and sitting for long periods) should be avoided. A minimum fluid intake of 2500 mL/day should be maintained unless contraindi-cated to prevent increased blood viscosity, which leads to venous stasis.

During therapy, the client receiving an anticoagulant must be monitored carefully for adverse reactions. Heparin therapy is normally given for periods of 7 to 10 days, but warfarin may be used over periods of months or years. The degree of anticoagulation is monitored by bleeding time or APTT (for heparin) and PT and INR (for warfarin). Platelets are monitored when heparin and enoxaparin are used. Unlike the others, enoxaparin does not require routine laboratory monitoring of APTT or PT (of course, baseline coagulation values should be determined before therapy).

Example of Nursing Process for Anticoagulant Therapy

Your client, Joseph Macone, age 65, recently had orthopedic surgery. He felt somewhat discouraged at the amount of disability he was experiencing after surgery and resisted some of the physical therapy exercises. In the perioperative period, appropriate therapy was used in an attempt to prevent deep vein thrombosis (DVT). However, 14 days after surgery Mr. Macone was readmitted with DVT of the right leg. The care plan, developed during his hospitalization, anticipates that therapy will help restore circulation and perfusion and that the client will be discharged on an oral anticoagulant.

Assessment Data

Recent orthopedic surgery
Diagnosis of DVT
Restricted activity and mobility
Anticoagulant therapy
Need for discharge on oral anticoagulant

Nursing Diagnosis

Altered Peripheral Tissue Perfusion, related to obstructed venous blood flow in affected extremity associated with thrombus and inflammation of vessel and venous stasis

Potential complication: Pulmonary embolism related to dislodgement of thrombus

Intervention

Assess for impaired venous blood flow in the affected extremity.

Administer anticoagulants as ordered.

Assess for signs and symptoms of pulmonary embolus (eg, sudden intense chest pain, dyspnea, tachypnea, decreased PaO$_2$).

Auscultate breath sounds every 4 hours.

Avoid massaging affected extremity and caution client not to do so. Explain rationale.

Do not exercise affected extremity during acute phase of DVT.

If embolus is suspected, **prepare** client for diagnostic tests (eg, ventilation/perfusion lung scan, arterial blood gases) and place client in semi- to high Fowler's position.

Provide oxygen therapy as ordered.

Goals and Outcomes

The client will have improved venous blood flow in affected extremity as evidenced by diminished pain, tenderness, feeling of heaviness, and swelling.

The client will not experience a pulmonary embolism as evidenced by absence of sudden chest pain, unlabored respirations within normal rate range, usual mental status, and blood gas values within normal range.

(continued)

Example of Nursing Process for Anticoagulant Therapy (continued)

Nursing Diagnosis (continued)	Intervention (continued)	Goals and Outcomes (continued)
Risk for Injury: Bleeding related to drug therapy	**Assess** for internal bleeding (observe urine, stool, emesis, sputum). **Report** positive results. **Assess** for petechiae, purpura, ecchymoses. **Monitor** coagulant test results and discuss them with prescriber. **Assess** all venipuncture sites for bleeding. **Apply** gentle, prolonged pressure after venous/arterial punctures. **Include** significant others in teaching sessions, if possible, and provide written instructions as well. *Instruct client to:* -Avoid or adapt activities to decrease the risk for injury. -Take medication at the same time each day; avoid stopping medication abruptly; avoid making up for a missed dose. -Schedule and keep follow-up appointments for care and periodic blood tests. -Avoid taking OTC products containing aspirin and other salicylates. -Avoid regular or excessive intake of alcohol. -Maintain balanced intake of green, leafy vegetables or other vitamin K-rich foods. -Wear medical identification.	The client will not experience bleeding, or bleeding that occurs will be controlled.

Hospitalized clients receiving anticoagulants undergo daily venipunctures to collect blood for the necessary monitoring. Bleeding may not stop readily from these sites, and in some cases the nurse must apply a pressure dressing to the site.

Despite all precautions, large ecchymoses may occur; a common site is the antecubital space. Discomfort in the area may be diminished by applying warm packs intermittently. To relieve distress caused by the appearance of unsightly bruises, clients need reassurance that the change is temporary and that the ecchymoses are not dangerous.

Multiple needle sticks, such as those associated with twice-daily administration of subcutaneous heparin, contribute to both pain and ecchymoses. Nursing measures to enhance the client's body image and promote a decrease in any discomfort are important.

Accidental injury likely to produce further ecchymoses should be avoided. Hazards in the environment that increase the risk of falls, cuts, or other injury must be eliminated. Men should be shaved daily, using an electric shaver rather than razor blades.

The use of attractive garments and grooming aids should be encouraged. Women should be encouraged to continue using cosmetics if they normally do so. Clothing should cover ecchymoses.

Because the risk for GI hemorrhage is serious in clients receiving anticoagulants, measures to reduce gastric irritation should be taken. Acetaminophen, which does not have the antiplatelet properties of aspirin, is well tolerated by most people and can be recommended as an analgesic and antipyretic substitute for aspirin (which is contraindicated in anticoagulant therapy). Most antiinflammatory drugs that might be used in place of aspirin are themselves ulcerogenic and may need to be discontinued or avoided during anticoagulant therapy. For this reason, clients with severe arthritis have particular problems with heparin or warfarin anticoagulant therapy. Nursing measures to ameliorate the arthritic symptoms include reducing stress, preventing chilling (which increases muscle tone), applying warmth, and promoting adequate sleep.

Careful attention must be paid to signs of excessive bleeding, such as red, rust-colored, or smoky urine, bloody or tarry stools, petechiae, bleeding gums, epistaxis, blood in vomit or sputum, prolonged or excessive menses, severe or prolonged headache, excessive or unexplained bruising, and sudden abdominal or back pain. Back pain may indicate retroperitoneal hemorrhage. Hemarthrosis may cause painful, enlarged joints. Chemical tests of stools and urine for occult blood should be performed regularly. Any frank bleeding should be reported immediately. Equipment and appropriate personnel must be readily available for treatment, including transfusion. Vitamin K may be required for the treatment of warfarin toxicity; protamine is the antidote for heparin.

If the client is being treated for DVT, measures to maintain skin integrity are needed. Inspect the skin (especially bony prominences, dependent areas, and affected extremities) for pallor, redness, and breakdown. For the affected arm or leg, perform actions to protect it from excessive pressure. For example, keep the heel off the bed by using heel protectors or by elevating the ankle on a foam block or pillows.

Any anxiety and fear must be dealt with during the initial treatment stages. Most clients experience fear of sudden death from embolism, stroke, or other catastrophic complications of the disease. Also, clients may equate anticoagulation with bleeding disorders and believe that they can bleed to death from a scratch. The nurse must listen to and acknowledge such concerns. Correcting misconceptions about anticoagulant therapy reduces fear. The nurse should reassure clients that the drugs do not eliminate clotting but only delay it.

Controlling client fear is particularly important because the normal hormone response to fear (increased adrenaline and cortisone secretion) increases coagulation, thereby potentially requiring larger doses of medication. Fluctuations of emotional status contribute to an uneven response to anticoagulant drugs. For these reasons, the nurse should be particularly diligent in reducing all factors that contribute to stress. Prompt attention to call bells makes the client feel confident that treatment will be immediate should complications develop. A calm, confident demeanor on the nurse's part that conveys a concern for the client's well-being is reassuring.

Specific Interventions for Clients Receiving Heparin. When heparin is used to control clotting in extracorporeal circulation (hemodialysis, heart-lung machines), it is introduced into the blood as it leaves the client to enter the machine; protamine is added to the blood as it reenters the client. If the doses of the two drugs are carefully controlled, clients will not experience a significant change of coagulation in the body. However, these clients must be watched carefully for complications because any imbalance in the proportions of heparin and protamine can cause clotting problems.

Heparin is still available in multiple-dose vials, and special care must be taken when measuring doses from such vials because overdoses can be disastrous. Many hospitals require that every heparin dose be verified by a second nurse. This is always a wise precaution (see Table 26-3). Continuous IV drip administration is usually accomplished by using premixed heparin sodium and sodium chloride solutions. An infusion regulator is needed for all IV lines containing heparin. Special care is taken to minimize movement of the needle or catheter to prevent infiltration or irritation of the vein. The client receiving anticoagulants is particularly vulnerable to trauma.

Heparin should not be given IM because hematomas result. Usually, SC administration is ordered for small doses of heparin. Whenever a needle is inserted into tissue, small blood vessels may be penetrated and damaged. If an anticoagulant is then injected into the tissue or if the client has already been medicated, these blood vessels may not close off but continue to bleed slowly, causing large ecchymoses. For this reason, special care must be taken to minimize vascular damage while injecting heparin. The abdominal subcutaneous fat is preferred as an injection site because it contains fewer blood vessels.

Heparin injections should be positioned at least 2″ from any scar and from the umbilicus. The nursing care plan should specify a schedule of site rotation to minimize trauma. When administering heparin SC, omit aspiration and postinjection massage to minimize blood vessel damage. SC injection is inappropriate for very thin or cachexic clients because their fat deposits are inadequate to protect them from inadvertent IM injection.

Heparin also retards healing. Nurses should be alert to any indications of dehiscence in surgical wounds. Removal of stitches may need to be delayed.

Specific Interventions for Clients Receiving Warfarin Sodium. When warfarin is prescribed, the coagulability of blood is more stable when doses are given regularly; a specific hour should be established for medication. The same applies to outpatients. The periodic blood tests are likely to be scheduled for the morning hours, and the usual afternoon administration of the drug is continued. This provides stability and continuity in the medication regimen.

If a female client suspects pregnancy, the physician should be informed immediately if the client is receiving coumarin derivatives, because they cross the placenta.

Body levels of vitamin K depend not only on diet but on the maintenance of normal intestinal flora. Intestinal organisms, which synthesize vitamin K, play an important role in maintaining adequate levels. Adding an antibiotic to the regimen of a client receiving warfarin may reduce the intestinal flora and deplete body levels of vitamin K. This will increase the effect of warfarin and may lead to spontaneous bleeding. If antibiotics are necessary, close medical supervision is required. The ingestion of buttermilk, yogurt, or another dairy product containing live lactobacilli helps restore normal intestinal flora and may help ameliorate these effects.

Diet can affect the body's response to warfarin. Vitamin K inhibits the effect of the anticoagulant. Some literature advises clients receiving warfarin to avoid foods rich in vitamin K, but this advice is potentially dangerous because long-term avoidance of whole groups of foods increases the risk of malnutrition. The goal is consistency and regularity of intake. Clients should be advised to eat a diet consistent in this nutrient as long as warfarin is used.

Throughout therapy, the response to warfarin and other drugs used concurrently should be monitored carefully for adverse reactions caused by drug interactions. Dosages of both warfarin and other drugs may need to be manipulated to compensate for these effects. When warfarin or other drugs are discontinued, further dosage adjustments may be needed. The nurse or client may need to remind the physician of the total drug regimen so that appropriate adjustments can be made.

Client Education. Initial education is directed at helping the client cope with the impact of the disorder and treatment, dependence, and anxiety. Demonstration of technical competence and a warm concern for the client promotes trust and learning readiness. The nurse can then provide information about the drug and treatment regimen. This promotes client cooperation.

For clients receiving heparin, teaching topics include the procedures to be performed, the effects of the drugs, and safety precautions. A common source of concern to the client receiving heparin is injection into the subcutaneous tissue of the abdomen. The client should be informed that the needle does not penetrate abdominal organs, that medication is deposited into the pocket below the subcutaneous tissue, and that medication administration is actually safer and more comfortable in the abdomen because there are fewer blood vessels and bleeding at the site is minimal. Before discharge from the hospital, the client should be informed that some clients experience transient alopecia 4 to 12 weeks after heparin therapy. This condition is self-limiting, and no permanent effects occur.

For clients receiving warfarin, teaching includes instructions for self-managing the drug regimen successfully. Continued medical supervision is necessary, including regular visits to the healthcare provider and periodic blood tests. The client should be provided with written instructions for scheduling laboratory tests and future appointments. Clients should be told to take the medication at the same time each day and not to stop

taking medication abruptly. If a dose is forgotten, it may be taken within 8 hours of the time it is normally taken. If it is longer than 8 hours, the dose should not be taken, and the client should call the prescriber for further instructions (Catania, 1994).

The prescribed warfarin dose is established under a set of controlled circumstances in the hospital. If these conditions are altered, serious complications may develop. The healthcare provider must be consulted if the client wishes to discontinue or add any medications. Adding medications may increase or decrease the effect of the anticoagulant. Changes often require adjustment of warfarin dosage. Over-the-counter (OTC) and illegal drugs can alter the client's response to warfarin. OTC preparations may contain aspirin or other salicylates, phenobarbital, or vitamins, all of which affect the therapeutic action of the warfarin and other anticoagulants. The client should avoid regular or excessive intake of alcohol, which may alter drug effect.

All outpatient clients on warfarin sodium should wear or carry medical identification that lists the drug dosage and the names, addresses, and telephone numbers of the client and physician. Clients should be told to notify the dentist, any new physician or pharmacist, and other healthcare providers that they are using warfarin sodium.

Clients on prolonged anticoagulant therapy must learn strategies for promoting safety and minimizing the risk of bleeding (see Home and Community Care: Minimizing Bleeding Risks). Clients should be reassured that clotting is not abolished, only delayed. Although bleed-

HOME AND COMMUNITY CARE

Minimizing Bleeding Risks

- Use an electric razor rather than a razor with blade.
- Floss and brush teeth gently; use soft-bristled toothbrush and waxed floss.
- Avoid putting sharp objects (even toothpicks) in mouth.
- Wear gloves when gardening.
- Put nonslip mats in the bathtub and shower.
- Arrange furniture and area rugs to reduce chances of tripping and bumping.
- Do not walk barefoot.
- Cut nails carefully; consider podiatrist assistance for toenails.
- Avoid situations that could easily result in injury (eg, contact sports or skiing).
- Avoid blowing nose forcefully.
- Avoid straining to have a bowel movement.

ing will be more persistent than usual and can be troublesome, the client will not exsanguinate rapidly if minor injury occurs. Should the client experience serious injury, bleeding will be persistent. If emergency care personnel are aware of the drug regimen, corrective measures to control the bleeding can be instituted. Accidental injuries likely to produce further bleeding should be avoided. Hazards in the environment that increase the risk of injury must be eliminated.

For clients receiving aspirin as an antiplatelet agent, teaching must focus on the medicinal quality of the drug. Some clients may not regard aspirin as real medicine. They may have taken aspirin for years on their own for minor symptoms. Because clients may be conditioned to taking aspirin only as needed, they should be reminded that it is necessary to take prescribed doses regularly. The nurse should emphasize that because aspirin alters hemostasis, it deserves the respect given to any effective medicine. The nurse may also need to teach the client about aspirin's potential risks and adverse reactions. The nurse should also determine whether the client normally takes aspirin for other symptoms, such as pain or fever. If so, the client should be advised to substitute acetaminophen for aspirin.

OUTCOME EVALUATION

Data required for evaluation include vital signs and peripheral pulses (rate, strength, character), degree of pain or tenderness, feeling of heaviness or swelling of affected extremity (if the client has DVT), color and warmth of skin, presence or absence of unusual bleeding, and client reports indicating decreased fear and increased acceptance of the condition and therapy. The success of the teaching plan is judged by client comments indicating that information has been helpful in adapting to the treatment regimen, by the client's increased adherence to the regimen, and by the client's ability to repeat information conveyed during teaching sessions.

❖ CHECKLIST OF NURSING ACTIONS

- ❏ Screen client for risk factors for adverse drug reactions and drug interactions.
- ❏ Assess client for anxiety and fear.
- ❏ Assess client for knowledge about thromboembolic illness and its treatment.
- ❏ Monitor client carefully for adverse drug reactions and drug interactions.
- ❏ Eliminate unnecessary stressors and help client reduce stress levels through stress management techniques.
- ❏ Promote a positive self-image in clients affected by large or numerous ecchymoses.

- ❏ Before administering the first dose of heparin, ascertain whether the client has been previously exposed to the drug; assess his or her reaction to it and whether the client has a history of allergies.
- ❏ Ensure accuracy of heparin dosage; when possible, have another nurse verify the prepared dose.
- ❏ When heparin is administered by continuous IV infusion, use an IV infusion controller.
- ❏ Administer SC injections of heparin in the subcutaneous space of the abdomen; do not aspirate before injection or massage the site afterward.
- ❏ Administer daily doses of warfarin at the same time each day, preferably in the afternoon.
- ❏ Monitor the client for signs and symptoms of abnormal or excessive bleeding.
- ❏ Protect the client from trauma.
- ❏ Monitor results of coagulation tests and carry out related interventions.

CRITICAL THINKING CHALLENGE
Case Analysis

Part I

Bettina Tripp, age 43, is admitted to the emergency room with a diagnosis of acute deep vein thrombosis of the right leg.

1. What medication do you think the healthcare provider in charge will administer to this client?
2. What assessment data would support this drug choice?
3. As the nurse caring for Ms. Tripp until a hospital bed is ready, what signs or symptoms (relative to the drug) would concern you? Explain why they concern you.
4. What interventions would you implement should they occur?

Part II

Ms. Tripp was discharged after treatment for DVT. She has been referred to your home care agency for follow-up nursing care. You are the nurse assigned to visit her at home. The referral records indicate that her medication on discharge was warfarin sodium (Coumadin). In your initial meeting, you talk with Ms. Tripp about her health and lifestyle concerns.

1. In developing a helpful and realistic care plan, what would you assess with Ms. Tripp relative to warfarin therapy before you begin any teaching interventions? What data should the drug history include? How will you individualize intervention categories?
2. Ms. Tripp tells you, "I'm afraid of this medicine. My brother took Coumadin when he had a bad leg. But then he died. He had an embolism." How would you implement active listening techniques?

Fibrinolysis

Clots that form in the circulatory system obstruct blood flow. Deprived of blood, tissues beyond the clot sustain serious damage. Almost as soon as a blood (fibrin) clot forms, fibrinolysis or clot dissolution begins (Fig. 26-2). The body initiates this action to prevent excessive clotting and vascular occlusion. Fibrinolysis involves the action of two endogenous plasminogen activators: tissue-type plasminogen activator (t-PA) and urokinase-type plasminogen activator (u-PA). The principal role of t-PA is in fibrinolysis, whereas that of u-PA is mainly in cell migration and tissue remodeling (Rang et al., 1995).

Plasminogen, a serum beta-globulin, is deposited on the fibrin strands within a thrombus. Plasminogen activators are proteases that diffuse into the thrombus and cleave a particular bond in plasminogen to release the enzyme plasmin, also known as fibrinolysin. Plasmin acts on the fibrin meshwork, generating fibrin degradation products and lysing (disintegrating) the clot. Plasmin can digest not only fibrin but also fibrinogen, factors II, V, and VIII, and many other proteins. Its action is localized to the clot. Any plasmin that escapes into the circulation is inactivated by various plasmin inhibitors. In large clots, some of the fibrin remains unaffected; this clot residue produces a fibrotic scar.

Fibrinolytic Agents

Drugs may affect the fibrinolytic system by increasing the normal fibrinolytic process (fibrinolytic agents). Accelerated fibrinolysis restores circulation, prevents ischemia and tissue necrosis, and reduces fibrous scarring. This, in turn, reduces the permanent damage caused by such conditions as MI, cerebral thrombi, and peripheral arterial emboli.

Popularly called "clot-busters," fibrinolytic agents have been studied in clinical trials that attempt to answer questions about the value of early and sustained vascular patency, risk versus benefit for immediate intervention, bleeding rates associated with different agents, the roles of adjunctive and conjunctive therapy, and effects on mortality. Remaining questions relate to agent superiority, the need for adjunctive therapy, and risk versus benefit for high-risk clients. Current trials, such as Global Utilization of Streptokinase and t-PA for Occluded Coronary Arteries (GUSTO) and Thrombolysis in Myocardial Infarction (TIMI 4) may provide insight into such issues.

Streptokinase, anisoylated plasminogen streptokinase activator complex (APSAC), t-PA, and u-PA are some available fibrinolytic agents (Table 26-5). Box 26-3 lists contraindications to the use of fibrinolytic agents.

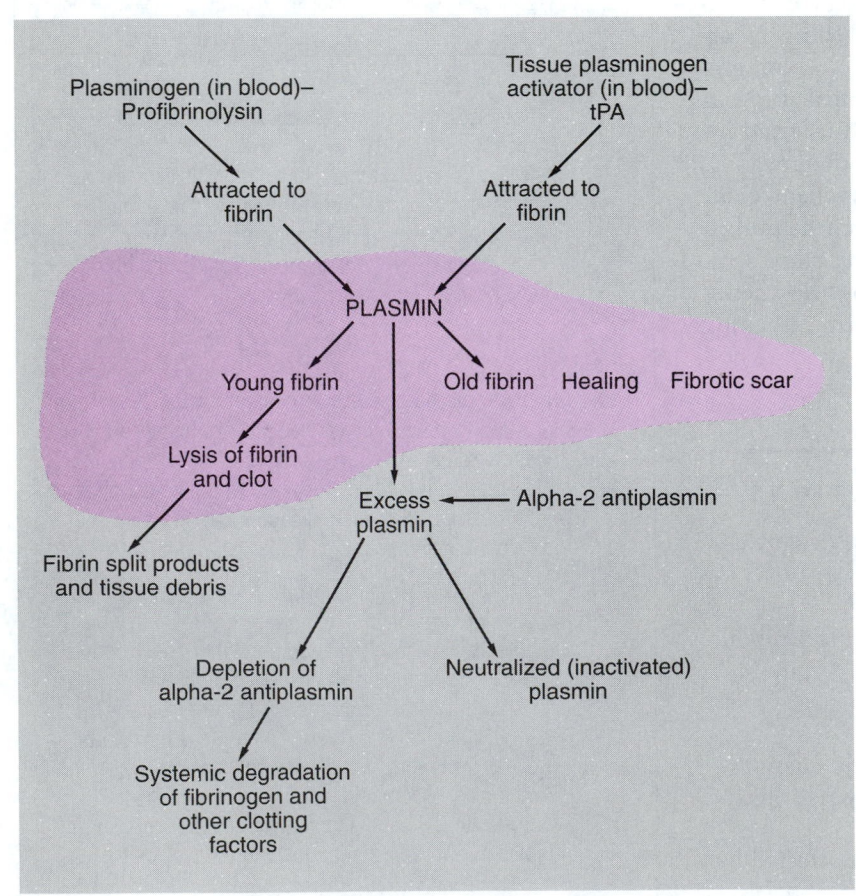

Figure 26-2. Physiologic mechanism of clot dissolution.

Table 26-5. Fibrinolytic Drugs*

Drug Name	Frequency of Reocclusion (%)	Half-life (min)	Usual Dosage	Adverse Reactions
streptokinase (Kabikinase, Streptase)	15	23	IV infusion: loading dose for 60 min, ±maintenance infusion for up to 72 hr	Serious bleeding, allergic reactions, hypotension, reperfusion arrhythmias
anisoylated plasminogen streptokinase activator complex (APSAC, anistreplace) (Eminase)	10	90	IV injection over 2–5 min	Serious bleeding, fewer allergic reactions than streptokinase
urokinase (u-PA) (Abbokinase)	10	16	IV infusion: loading dose for 5–10 min, maintenance infusion	Serious bleeding, reperfusion arrhythmias
tissue plasminogen activator (tPA, alteplase) (Activase)	20	5–8	IV injection over 2 min, then IV infusion over 3 hr	Serious bleeding, reperfusion arrhythmias

*Data on frequency of reocclusion and dosage and administration vary depending on source. These data reflect fibrinolytics used in MI.

Streptokinase

Streptokinase (Kabikinase, Streptase) is nonenzymatic protein produced by group C beta-hemolytic streptococci. The ability of streptokinase to break down fibrin clots was discovered in 1933, but not until 1980 did studies begin to show the benefits that could be obtained with early use of the drug in the client with MI.

Box 26-3
Contraindications to Using Fibrinolytic Agents

Absolute Contraindications

Recent (within 10 days) internal bleeding

Known predisposition to bleeding

History of cerebrovascular accident

Recent intracranial, intraspinal, or intraocular trauma or surgery

Intracranial atrioventricular malformations

Neoplasms or aneurysms

Severe uncontrolled hypertension

Recent (within 10 days) trauma (including cardiopulmonary resuscitation)

Relative Contraindications

Minor trauma

Diabetic retinopathy or hemorrhagic ophthalmic conditions

Pregnancy

Concurrent anticoagulation

Pharmacodynamics. Streptokinase first combines with circulating plasminogen, forming an activator complex. This activator complex converts plasminogen, confined both in the systemic circulation and in the thrombus, into plasmin (Weiner, 1993). Streptokinase has a systemic effect. The high levels of plasmin resulting from its use lead to a depletion in circulating fibrinogen (60%–80% drop) and factors V and VIII.

Pharmacokinetics. The half-life of streptokinase is about 18 minutes (which prolongs the plasmin production). Systemic low coagulability lasts for 24 to 36 hours.

Therapeutic Uses. Streptokinase is used in the treatment of MI, pulmonary embolism, DVT, arterial thrombosis, and occlusions in arteriovenous cannulas.

Dosage and Administration. For MI therapy, streptokinase is administered as soon as possible after the infarction. Best results are obtained when the drug is administered within the so-called "6-hour window of opportunity." In powder form, the preparation can be reconstituted with 5 mL of 5% dextrose in water injection or 0.9% sodium chloride injection. This diluent should be added slowly to the vial, directing it to the side of the vial, which is then gently rolled and tilted. Shaking the vial is avoided because foaming or increased flocculation can occur. Once reconstituted, the solution should be further diluted to a final volume of 45 to 100 mL (Weiner, 1993). The 1-hour IV infusion delivers about 1.5 million U (Dunn & Senerchia, 1993).

Intracoronary streptokinase has been used by administering a bolus dose of 10,000 to 30,000 U in a small volume of diluent. This is injected selectively into the occluded coronary artery over 15 seconds to 2 minutes. A maintenance infusion of 2,000 to 4,000 U/min follows. When streptokinase is used for severe venous thrombosis or pulmonary embolism, longer infusions, up to 72 hours, are given.

Adverse Reactions. Primary adverse effects include hypotension, allergic reaction, and serious bleeding. An adverse effect related to reperfusion that occurs as a result of using streptokinase is cardiac arrhythmia. A drawback of streptokinase use is its tendency to promote a burst of plasmin formation, which generates kinins; this causes hypotension.

Because it is extracted from cultures of streptococci, streptokinase must be biologically assayed and standardized. Nevertheless, it is still considered highly antigenic. It may produce allergic reactions characterized by rash, fever, urticaria, tachycardia, hypotension, and bronchospasm in mild to fatal degrees. When the recipient produces antibodies, he or she becomes refractory (unresponsive) to the drug for several months.

The main hazard of all fibrinolytics is bleeding, internal or superficial. Internal bleeding involves the GI tract, genitourinary tract, or retroperitoneal, ocular, or intracranial sites. Superficial bleeding is observed mainly at the introduction sites (eg, venous cutdowns, arterial punctures) or at surgical incision sites. IM injections should be avoided during treatment with fibrinolytic agents. Venipunctures should be performed carefully and only as required. Should arterial puncture be necessary, an upper extremity vessel should be used because it is more accessible for manual compression. A pressure dressing should be applied and the site checked frequently. Bleeding may be treated by giving an antifibrinolytic agent such as tranexamic acid, fresh plasma, or coagulation factors (Olin, 1995).

When ischemic cardiac tissue is reperfused, arrhythmias are likely to develop. The most common reperfusion arrhythmias are sinus bradycardia, accelerated idioventricular rhythm, ventricular extrasystoles, and ventricular tachycardia. Lidocaine may be infused prophylactically to reduce the risk of reperfusion arrhythmias.

Drug Interactions. Antiplatelet drugs and anticoagulants increase the risk of bleeding. No laboratory test interactions have been identified.

Precautions and Contraindications. Because streptokinase can cause an antigenic response, some institutions have policies that recommend concomitant use of diphenhydramine (Benadryl) or corticosteroids to counter the antigenic response.

Anisoylated Plasminogen Streptokinase Activator Complex

Anisoylated plasminogen streptokinase activator complex (APSAC, anistreplase) (Eminase) is a chemically engineered molecule comprising streptokinase bound to human lysine plasminogen, derived from pooled human blood. This complex is stabilized by the addition of an anisoyl group that sustains drug activity (Majoros, 1993).

Pharmacodynamics. This molecule remains inactive until it reaches the plasma, where it is broken down. Once induced, anistreplase acts primarily on the thrombus, but it also has systemic effects.

Pharmacokinetics. The main difference between streptokinase and this drug is its longer duration of action. Anistreplase breaks down or is released slowly. It remains stable and active for a long time. The half-life is longer than that of any other fibrinolytic (90–120 minutes), making it possible to administer this drug as a single bolus injection.

Therapeutic Uses. Anistreplase is used for managing acute MI in adults, for lysing thrombi obstructing coronary arteries, reducing the infarct size, improving ventricular function after MI, and reducing associated mortality.

Dosage and Administration. A potential advantage of anistreplase is the simple administration method of a 30-U IV bolus given over 2 to 5 minutes. Its fibrinolytic activity is sustained for 4 to 6 hours. Like t-PA, anistreplase is very costly.

Adverse Reactions. Anistreplase is thought to be less antigenic than streptokinase. The main hazard for all fibrinolytic agents is potentially serious bleeding; this was discussed in detail in the section on streptokinase.

Drug Interactions. These are the same as for streptokinase.

Precautions and Contraindications. Absolute contraindications include active internal bleeding and cerebrovascular disease. Relative contraindications include bleeding diatheses, pregnancy, and uncontrolled hypertension.

Urokinase

Urokinase (u-PA) (Abbokinase) is an endogenous substance involved in many physiologic processes. A urokinase receptor is found on the surface of monocytes and many other cell types. The urokinase used clinically is prepared from cultures of human embryonic kidney cells and must be biologically assayed and standardized. Recombinant single-chain urokinase plasminogen activator (r-scuPA) is available. It is converted to urokinase when it binds to fibrin.

Pharmacodynamics. Endogenously, urokinase is secreted from kidney cells as a pro-enzyme (scu-PA), from which the active enzyme plasminogen activator (tcu-PA) is derived by proteolysis. The tcu-PA activates plasminogen, causing an increase in plasmin levels throughout the body. When used therapeutically, urokinase is not specific for fibrin-bound thrombi, but, like streptokinase, has a systemic effect.

Pharmacokinetics. Urokinase has a half-life of about 15 minutes. After absorption, the drug concentrates in the liver and bladder. It has a duration of action of 12 to 24 hours. It is excreted in small amounts in bile and urine.

Therapeutic Uses. Urokinase is used in treating MI, pulmonary embolism, DVT, peripheral arterial thrombosis, and occlusion of central venous catheters. It is particularly useful for clients refractory to streptokinase due to previous exposure and antibody formation.

Dosage and Administration. Urokinase is not approved by the FDA for use in MI, but when used in that situation, a dose of 2 to 3 million U has been administered over 45 to 90 minutes, with half the dose given as an initial injection over 5 minutes and the rest given as a continuous infusion. The vial of powder is reconstituted with sterile water. It is important to reconstitute only with Sterile Water for Injection without preservatives (not Bacteriostatic Water for Injection). The resultant solution should be slightly straw-colored. The vial should be rolled and tilted to enhance reconstitution. The reconstituted urokinase should be diluted further with 0.9% sodium chloride solution or 5% dextrose in water. No other medication should be added to this solution. Because urokinase does not contain preservatives, it should be reconstituted immediately before use.

Urokinase has been given by intracoronary administration with doses of 6,000 U/min for periods of up to 2 hours. For peripheral arterial thrombosis, the tip of the infusion catheter is positioned in the proximal few centimeters of the clot.

Typically, heparin is administered concomitantly.

Adverse Reactions. Urokinase is not antigenic, so it does not result in drug resistance or allergic reactions. The main hazard for all fibrinolytic agents is potentially serious bleeding; this was discussed in detail in the section on streptokinase. As with streptokinase, when ischemic cardiac tissue is reperfused, arrhythmias are likely to develop.

Drug Interactions. Interactions are the same as with streptokinase.

Precautions and Contraindications. Urokinase is contraindicated in hypersensitivity to the drug, active internal bleeding, cerebrovascular accident within 2 months, intracranial or intraspinal surgery, and intracranial neoplasm. It must be used cautiously in clients with recent major surgery, pregnancy or recent delivery, lactation, known hemostatic defects, recent internal bleeding or trauma, severe hypertension, cerebrovascular disease, and diabetic hemorrhagic retinopathy.

Tissue Plasminogen Activator

Tissue plasminogen activator (t-PA, alteplase) (Activase) is a naturally occurring protein enzyme in endothelium, circulating blood, and tissues. Using recombinant DNA technology, large-scale production of recombinant t-PA is possible.

Pharmacodynamics. Endogenous t-PA is responsible for converting plasminogen into plasmin. What differentiates t-PA from other fibrinolytic agents is its ability to bind to fibrin in a thrombus and convert the trapped plasminogen to plasmin (local fibrinolysis). It has limited systemic effect—thus, it is clot-selective.

Pharmacokinetics. The liver clears t-PA rapidly from circulating plasma. More than 50% of t-PA in plasma is cleared within 5 minutes after the infusion ends.

Therapeutic Uses. Approved for treating MI and pulmonary embolism, t-PA is also used for treating peripheral arterial occlusions. One major disadvantage of t-PA is its cost (about $2,200 per dose).

Dosage and Administration. The standard dosage of t-PA for treating MI is 100 mg administered IV over 3 hours. Typically, a bolus of 6 to 10 mg is administered over 2 minutes, with an additional 50 to 54 mg administered over the remaining first hour. Then 20-mg increments are administered hourly over the next 2 hours, for a total dose of about 100 mg. Some clinicians recommend a weight-adjusted dose of 1.25 mg/kg (Weiner, 1993).

Each vacuum-packed vial of t-PA, supplied as sterile lyophilized powder containing 10, 20, or 50 mg, should be reconstituted using aseptic technique with the accompanying diluent of nonbacteriostatic sterile water for injection. Once reconstituted, the t-PA should be used within 8 hours. It can be diluted further to a concentration of 0.5 mg/mL using either 0.9% sodium chloride solution for injection or 5% dextrose in water solution for injection. After dilution, the drug should be administered IV by an infusion control device. In-line filters should not be used because t-PA may be absorbed onto the filter, resulting in incomplete administration of the medication.

Clients selected for t-PA treatment must receive the drug as soon as possible after acute chest pain begins. The quality of therapeutic response seems inversely related to the delay in treatment. Fibrinolytics should be given within 6 hours of onset of signs and symptoms of MI.

Due to the short-half life, treatment regimens have often included adjunctive IV heparin to reduce reocclusion rates.

Adverse Reactions. Again, the main hazard for all fibrinolytic agents is potentially serious bleeding (see the streptokinase discussion). t-PA appears to be nonantigenic and can be used in clients likely to have antibodies to streptokinase, such as those with recent streptococcal infections or those treated with streptokinase. As with streptokinase, arrhythmias are likely when ischemic cardiac tissue is reperfused.

Drug–Drug Interactions. Concomitant use of antiplatelet drugs and anticoagulants may increase the risk of bleeding.

Drug–Laboratory Test Interactions. During therapy, results of coagulation tests or measures of fibrinolytic activity may be unreliable. For example, t-PA in blood samples removed for analysis can degrade the fibrinogen in the sample.

■ SUMMARY

Four drugs capable of stimulating or accelerating the natural fibrinolytic process are streptokinase, anisoylated plasminogen streptokinase activator complex, urokinase, and t-PA. They are useful as treatment agents to dissolve dangerous intervascular clots (eg, coronary thrombosis, pulmonary emboli) and in certain other situations. Many large clinical trials continue to study which agent or combination regimen is best. Adverse reactions to these drugs include systemic anticoagulation (apparently least with t-PA), allergic hypersensitivity and subsequent refractoriness to treatment (streptokinase), and excessive bleeding.

❖ NURSING MANAGEMENT: CLIENT ON FIBRINOLYTIC THERAPY

Clients selected for fibrinolytic therapy are the victims of sudden onset of illness. They come to the healthcare setting anxious and in pain.

NURSING PROCESS

ASSESSMENT

As much information as possible should be obtained from the client's family or others. It is helpful if prescription drugs taken by the client are brought to the healthcare facility in their original containers. A complete drug history is needed.

It is important to determine when the symptoms began, because the time elapsed between the onset of symptoms and the initiation of fibrinolytic therapy critically affects the prognosis. The sooner treatment is begun, the greater the likelihood that tissue damage will be less permanent.

Determining risk factors for fibrinolytic therapy is primarily the physician's responsibility. However, the nurse can gather important information from the family while the physician is examining the client. Information about any contraindications for fibrinolytic therapy should be sought.

A total body assessment to identify any preexisting ecchymotic areas or open wounds is beneficial. Documentation of abnormal findings is necessary.

Necessary baseline and serial laboratory values include hematocrit and hemoglobin and creatine phosphokinase (CPK) with isoenzymes, plasma fibrinogen, fibrin degradation products, thrombin time, PT, bleeding time, and PTT. Blood must be typed and screened. A heparin lock can be inserted for drawing additional blood or delivering IV medication.

A knowledge assessment may be compiled relative to the client's and the family's understanding of the condition and treatment.

NURSING DIAGNOSIS

Nursing diagnoses arising from MI and related drug therapy include:

- Pain, related to tissue ischemia secondary to thrombi or emboli
- Anxiety, related to bleeding from drug therapy or possible death from infarction
- Risk for Injury: Drug-induced bleeding
- Decreased Cardiac Output, related to drug-induced arrhythmia after reperfusion

Most clients and their families exhibit:

- Knowledge Deficit, related to thrombolic disease and its treatment

PLANNING

Goals are to eliminate pain, restore circulation, alleviate or eliminate anxiety and fear, prevent or control hemorrhage, correct reperfusion arrhythmias, and reduce knowledge deficits of clients and their families about thrombolic disease and the use of fibrinolytic agents.

INTERVENTION

Nursing interventions should be directed at limiting the number and severity of potentially preventable bleeding events. All venipunctures should be completed before administration of the fibrinolytic agent. Blood drawing should be performed only by staff highly skilled in venipuncture. After venipuncture is performed, manual pressure should be applied to the site for several minutes before applying a pressure dressing. Usually at least two intravascular infusion lines are needed: an IV line for administering fibrinolytic drugs and a separate IV line for administering other drugs (eg, lidocaine). Each line should include an infusion controller.

Automatic blood-pressure cuffs should be used with caution in these clients. If used, the area under the cuff should be assessed frequently for ecchymosis. The cuff should not be inflated more often than necessary and the arm used should be changed frequently (Dunn & Senerchia, 1993).

After the fibrinolytic drug is administered, the nurse must monitor for potential bleeding. Regular assessment for oozing from IV access sites is needed. If a cardiac catheterization was performed and a hematoma forms at the site, the area should be marked clearly so that any increase in size can be noted.

A client with a femoral sheath in place will benefit from the use of leg immobilizers. With limited extraneous movement, the client may experience less bleeding from the intravascular insertion site. The client also requires continual hemodynamic monitoring and frequent hematocrit checks. If the hematocrit value drops significantly, the physician should be notified. If the client experiences hemodynamic compromise, blood products may need to be administered.

The nurse must also assess for subtle signs of retroperitoneal bleeding, such as back and flank pain, hematoma formation, a decrease in hematocrit value, hematuria, and hemodynamic compromise. Management of retroperitoneal bleeding must be quick and accurate because the vessels in the femoral area are large and carry high volumes of blood. Damage to femoral vessels results in extremely rapid blood loss. If the fibrinolytic agent is still being infused, it should be stopped immediately (as should any anticoagulant). Fresh-frozen plasma may be ordered, as well as packed red blood cells, to keep the hematocrit within an acceptable range. IV fluids can be given to maintain or replace volume. At the same time, an abdominal computed tomography (CT) scan should be performed and a surgeon consulted, because the client may need vascular surgery to repair the bleeding vessel.

The nurse must facilitate the client's trust in the healthcare staff. Competent and rapid response to the client's needs and an attitude of warm concern for the client and family promote this therapeutic relationship. Until the emergency resolves, the client cannot be counseled at length. However, the client may be assured that the staff's skill will ensure the best possible care. Crisis intervention techniques may be useful in helping the family cope, and family members should be kept informed in detail about treatment and the client's progress.

Clients with coronary thrombosis must be closely monitored for changes in cardiac rhythm. Arrhythmias are likely to develop when the clot is dissolved and perfusion is restored. Cardiac antiarrhythmic drugs, such as lidocaine, should be administered in accordance with established protocols.

Throughout the client's hospital stay, the nurse monitors pertinent diagnostic findings and intervenes to decrease the risk of infection. Strict aseptic technique is used with all procedures. To support general resistance to infection, the client should have a nourishing diet, adequate fluids, and ample rest and sleep. High stress levels suppress the immune response, so the nurse should eliminate unnecessary stressors and help the client control stress levels.

Client Education. Until the client is stabilized and the clot dissolved, he or she can cope only with essential information. The staff should explain to the client what is about to happen in terms of the client's perceptions of the experience—in other words, what the client is likely to feel. Information about invasive procedures such as arterial or venous punctures should be given immediately before the procedure. The longer the client anticipates such procedures, the higher the level of fear and stress.

During convalescence, both client and family should be taught (or retaught) about the disease, the treatment provided in the hospital, and the home treatment likely to be prescribed. Self-care measures to ameliorate the underlying condition (eg, exercise, diet, stress management) should be emphasized. If long-term anticoagulant or antiplatelet medication is prescribed, clients need instruction in proper administration of the drug, signs and symptoms of adverse reactions, and the signs and symptoms that should be reported to the healthcare provider. The client should be taught about the potential risks and adverse reactions associated with drug interactions, such as those that may occur with aspirin. The nurse should determine whether the client normally takes aspirin for other symptoms, such as pain or fever. If so, the client should be advised to substitute acetaminophen for aspirin because aspirin may interact with anticoagulant or antiplatelet therapies.

OUTCOME EVALUATION

Data required for evaluation include statements by the client indicating that fear and anxiety have decreased and that symptoms such as pain have decreased or abated. Surface bleeding, restlessness, pallor, change in vital signs, decrease in urine output, or evidence of blood in emesis, urine, sputum, or stools would be indicators of excessive bleeding in response to the drug. Confusion, speech or visual disturbances, or headache would indicate that intracranial hemorrhage may have occurred as an adverse reaction. Rapid or slow pulse, dizziness or lightheadedness, or information from electrocardiogram printouts could indicate the adverse reaction of arrhythmias. Teaching is evaluated by the client's ability to cooperate with treatment procedures and to repeat information conveyed during teaching. (See Example of Nursing Process for Fibrinolytic Therapy.)

❖ CHECKLIST OF NURSING ACTIONS

- ❑ Establish a therapeutic relationship characterized by trust in the nursing staff by the client.
- ❑ Explain to the client procedures to be done in terms of what he or she will experience.
- ❑ Keep the family informed of the client's condition and the progress of treatment.
- ❑ Assess the client for pain and anxiety.
- ❑ Evaluate the client for decreased tissue perfusion, excessive bleeding, or intracranial hemorrhage in response to the drug.
- ❑ Monitor clients with coronary artery thrombosis for cardiac arrhythmias, especially when coronary circulation is restored.
- ❑ Assist with emergency procedures, including parenteral administration of drugs.
- ❑ Handle enzyme drugs gently to prevent denaturation.
- ❑ Observe and record reactions to fibrinolytic therapy.
- ❑ Maintain strict aseptic techniques for surgical procedures.
- ❑ Teach the client and family self-care measures to promote cardiovascular function and to delay the progression of cardiovascular disease.

Example of Nursing Process for Fibrinolytic Therapy

The client is a 54-year-old man admitted to the emergency department with a tentative diagnosis of acute myocardial infarction. He has a history of diabetes and cardiovascular disease, having been treated for deep venous thrombosis about 6 months ago. He has had irregularities in cardiac rate and rhythm in the past, although none required hospital treatment. He takes some cardiovascular and diabetic medications. The client appears tense and anxious. He asks you, "I'm not going to die, am I?"

Assessment Data

Fibrinolytic therapy

History of anticoagulant therapy

Undergoing assessment procedures for myocardial infarction and fibrinolytic therapy

History of some cardiac irregularities of rate and rhythm and use of some cardiovascular medications

Nursing Diagnosis*	Intervention	Goals and Outcome Criteria
Risk for Injury: Bleeding	**Complete** venipunctures before administering agent.	The client will not experience bleeding, or bleeding that occurs will be controlled.
	Establish two IV sites.	
	Use smallest-gauge needle possible.	
	Assess vascular access sites for bleeding. Apply gentle, prolonged pressure after venipunctures.	
	Assess for internal bleeding (observe urine, stool, emesis, sputum). Report positive results.	
	Assess for signs of retroperitoneal bleeding, such as back and flank pain.	
	Assess for intracranial bleeding.	
	Assess vital signs. Follow institution's protocol for use of automatic blood-pressure cuffs.	
	Assess hemoglobin and hematocrit values and any coagulation study results; report abnormal results.	
	Instruct client about activities to avoid or adapt to decrease risk for injury.	
Potential Decreased Cardiac Output, related to reperfusion arrhythmias	**Assess** for abnormal rate, rhythm, or configurations on electrocardiogram. Report changes promptly. Assess for signs and symptoms of cardiac arrhythmias (eg, irregular apical pulse, pulse rate change, apical/radial pulse deficit, palpitations).	The client will not experience arrhythmias, or arrhythmias that occur will be corrected.
	Assess for signs of reduced cardiac output or inadequate tissue perfusion that may accompany arrhythmias (eg, decreased blood pressure, diminished peripheral pulses, dizziness/syncope, changes in mental state, pallor/cyanosis, weakness, shortness of breath).	

(continued)

Example of Nursing Process for Fibrinolytic Therapy (continued)

Nursing Diagnosis* (continued)

Potential Decreased Cardiac Output, related to reperfusion arrhythmias (continued)

Intervention (continued)

Administer prophylactic lidocaine before initiation of fibrinolytic therapy if ordered.

Keep atropine sulfate at bedside for bradyarrhythmias (especially if inferior wall MI is suspected).

Have emergency equipment and medications readily available for defibrillation or cardiopulmonary resuscitation.

Perform actions to reduce cardiac workload (eg, maintain activity restrictions, avoid activities that create Valsalva response, implement measures to promote rest and conserve energy, implement measures to prevent fluid volume excess).

Administer oxygen therapy as ordered.

Goals and Outcome Criteria (continued)

The client will not experience arrhythmias, or arrhythmias that occur will be corrected (continued)

*These nursing diagnoses are focused on fibrinolytic therapy. Other nursing diagnoses are critical when MI has occurred (eg, Pain, related to tissue ischemia; Anxiety, related to potential death) but are not discussed here.

References

Bell TN. (1993). Disseminated intravascular coagulation. *Crit Care Nurs Clin North Am, 5*(3), 389–410.

Bussey HI, Force RW, Bianco TM, Leonard AD. (1992). Reliance on prothrombin time ratios causes significant errors in anticoagulation therapy. *Arch Intern Med, 152,* 278–282.

Catania U-M. (1994). Monitoring coumadin therapy. *RN,* (2), 9–34.

Chesebro JH, Badimon JJ, Stein B, Fuster V. (1994). Platelet-active drugs. In Singh BN, Dzau VJ, Vanhoutte PM, Woosley RL, eds. *Cardiovascular pharmacology and therapeutics.* New York: Churchill-Livingstone.

Coffland FI, Shelton DM. (1993). Blood component replacement therapy. *Crit Care Nurs Clin North Am, 5*(3), 543–556.

Colman RW, Hirsh J, Marder VJ, et al., eds. (1994). *Hemostasis and thrombosis: Basic principles and clinical practice,* 3d ed. Philadelphia: JB Lippincott.

Copstead LC. (1995). *Perspectives on pathophysiology.* Philadelphia: WB Saunders.

Dunn S, Senerchia C. (1993). Bleeding complications in the patient with cardiac disease following thrombolytic and anticoagulant therapies. *Crit Care Nurs Clin North Am, 5*(3), 511–523.

Majoros K. (1993). Comparisons and controversies in clot buster drugs. *Crit Care Nursing Quarterly, 16*(2), 46–69.

Noble S, Peters DH, Goa KL. (1995). Enoxaparin. *Drugs, 49*(3), 388–410.

Oertel LB. (1995). International normalized ratio (INR): An improved way to monitor oral anticoagulant therapy. *Nurse Practitioner, 20*(9), 15–22.

Olin BR, ed. (1995). *Drug facts and comparisons.* St. Louis: Facts and Comparisons.

Raimer F, Thomas M. (1995). Clot stoppers: Using anticoagulants safely and effectively. *Nursing '95, 25*(3), 34–43.

Rang HP, Dale MM, Ritter JM, Gardner P. (1995). *Pharmacology.* New York: Churchill-Livingstone.

Srnec P. (1993). Congenital coagulopathies in the pediatric population. *Crit Care Nurs Clin North Am, 5*(3), 445–452.

Weiner B. (1993). Thrombolytic agents in critical care. *Crit Care Nurs Clin North Am, 5*(3), 355.

Bibliography

Brigden ML. (1995). When bleeding complicates oral anticoagulant therapy. *Postgrad Med, 98*(3), 153–168.

Burns D. (1993). Review of thrombolytic use in acute myocardial infarction, pulmonary embolism, and cerebral thrombosis. *Crit Care Nursing Quarterly, 15*(4), 1.

GUSTO Investigators. (1993). The effects of tissue plasminogen activator, streptokinase, or both on coronary-artery patency, ventricular function, and survival after acute myocardial infarction. *N Engl J Med, 329*(22), 1615–1622.

Hardman JG, Limbird LE, Molinoff PB, et al. (eds). (1996). *Goodman and Gilman's The pharmacological basis of therapeutics,* 9th ed. New York: McGraw-Hill.

Hickey A. (1994). Catching deep vein thrombosis in time. *Nursing '94, 24*(10), 34–41.

Hull R, Raskob G, Pineo G, et al. (1993). A comparison of subcutaneous low-molecular-weight heparin with warfarin sodium for prophylaxis against deep-vein thrombosis after hip or knee implantation. *N Engl J Med, 329*(14), 1370–1376.

Le DT, Weibert RT, Sevilla BK, et al. (1994). The international normalized ration (INR) for monitoring warfarin therapy: Reliability and relation to other monitoring methods. *Ann Intern Med, 120*(7), 552–558.

Mehta P, Mehta JL. (1994). Anticoagulants. In Singh BN, Dzau VJ, Vanhoutte PM, Woosley RL, eds. *Cardiovascular pharmacology and therapeutics.* New York: Churchill-Livingstone.

Thorp JA, Gaston L, Caspers DR, Pal ML. (1995). Current concepts and controversies in the use of Vitamin K. *Drugs, 49*(3), 376–387.

Weitz J. (1994). New anticoagulant strategies: Current status and future potential. *Drugs, 48*(4), 485–497.

For more information and sample tests and activities, refer to Chapter 26 in the Student Workbook for Clinical Pharmacology and Nursing Management, 5th edition, available through your bookstore.

27

Drugs That Affect the Kidneys

Diuretics are drugs that induce loss of body fluid by increasing the production of urine by the kidneys. Because the body's fluid balance is affected significantly by sodium ions, losing fluid usually involves increasing the kidney's excretion of sodium; thus, sodium loss is the primary mechanism by which many diuretics act. Although diuretics have a long history of effectively treating edema, many of the drugs currently used were unknown a generation ago.

Physiology of the Kidneys

The renal system comprises the kidneys, ureters, bladder, and urethra. Urine is formed by the kidneys and flows through the other structures to be excreted from the body. The regulation of body fluid and solutes is governed by processes known as filtration, reabsorption, and secretion.

The basic structural and functional unit of the kidney is the nephron, of which each kidney has about 1 million. The two types of nephrons are the cortical nephron (85%) and the juxtamedullary nephron (15%). They are named for their location.

The kidneys are highly vascular. Blood flows to their many parts through the renal artery, which branches into many small vessels, the smallest of which are the capillaries. Blood enters the glomerulus (the capillary bundle). The capillary bundle is encased in a sac called Bowman's capsule. Fluid and particles from the blood are filtered through three layers into Bowman's space: the capillary endothelial layer, the basement membrane, and the capsular epithelial layer. The process of glomerular filtration occurs here.

The product of filtration is the filtrate. It contains no red blood cells, a small amount of albumin, and essentially the same concentration of electrolytes and other small molecules as the plasma. This filtrate undergoes many further changes. At a glomerular filtration rate (GFR) of 125 mL/min, the kidneys produce 180 L of filtrate daily, but the average urine output is only 1,000 to 1,500 mL. Glomerular filtration is controlled by four pressures: glomerular capillary hydrostatic pressure, glomerular capillary colloid osmotic pressure, Bowman's space hydrostatic pressure, and Bowman's space colloid osmotic pressure.

Important roles in renal hemodynamics are played by the sympathetic nervous system, angiotensin II, antidiuretic hormone, dopamine, histamine, endothelin, endothelium-derived relaxing factor, and atrial natriuretic peptide. They work in concert to sustain glomerular filtration despite wide variations in systemic pressures (Holechek, 1992).

Although filtration occurs in the glomerulus, it is the tubular structures that transform filtered fluid into urine. The nephron tubule is divided into four segments: the proximal tubule, the loop of Henle, the distal tubule, and the collecting tubule.

The filtrate first enters the proximal tubules (Table 27-1). Tubular processes of reabsorption and secretion selectively alter and reduce the filtrate and form urine. Through tubular reabsorption, most of the filtrate moves into the peritubular capillaries or vasa recta capillaries and then returns to the bloodstream. The proximal tubule is the major site of reabsorption, although reabsorption occurs throughout the nephron. Reabsorption involves both passive (osmosis and diffusion) and active (carrier-mediated) transport mechanisms. The body secretes (removes) unwanted or excess substances by tubular secretion, which is the movement of solutes from the peritubular capillaries into the tubular system. Again, both passive and active transport mechanisms assist tubular secretion.

Excretion is the process by which unwanted substances are eliminated from the body through urine. These substances include the end products of metabolism such as urea, creatinine, uric acid, drugs, foreign chemicals, and unwanted amounts of such substances as sodium, potassium, and phosphate (Chmielewski, 1992).

Table 27-1. Characteristics of the Renal Tubule

Segment	Characteristics	Effects on Filtrate
Proximal tubule (from the glomerular membrane to the thin portion of the loop of Henle)	Capable of active transport of many substances (reabsorption of nutrients and electrolytes and secretion of hydrogen ions and drugs) Freely permeable to water	Reabsorbs virtually all glucose, protein, amino acids, acetoacetate ions, and vitamins Reabsorbs part of the sodium and potassium, with subsequent reabsorption of chloride ions by passive diffusion Reabsorbs some urea Actively secretes hydrogen ions and common drugs Reabsorbs about 65% of the water from the filtrate Maintains isotonicity between filtrate and blood
Descending portion of the thin segment of the loop of Henle	Highly permeable to water Moderately permeable to ions such as sodium and urea	Produces a hypertonic filtrate due to passive diffusion of fluid into the hypertonic interstitial fluid of the kidney medulla
Ascending portion of the thin segment of the loop of Henle	Less permeable to water and urea than descending portion	Maintains hypertonicity of filtrate
Early distal tubule (from the thick portion of the ascending loop of Henle to about the midpoint of the distal convoluted tubule)	Capable of active transport of chloride ions Relatively impermeable to water	Transports and reabsorbs solutes Renders the filtrate hypotonic
Late distal tubule (from the midpoint of the distal convoluted tubule to the collecting tubule)	Capable of actively reabsorbing sodium and secreting potassium in response to the hormone aldosterone	Adjusts concentration of sodium and potassium ions in the filtrate
Collecting tubule	Variably permeable to water, depending on the presence of antidiuretic hormone (ADH)	Concentrates urine

Pathophysiology

Throughout the body, transcapillary exchange of materials, through the interstitial space, to or from the cells, is another continuous process. The process is essential for exchange of gases and nutrients. As fluid moves through the interstitial space, most of it returns to the capillary bed. Increased fluid accumulation in the interstitial space can occur from more than one mechanism.

Edema is the excess accumulation of fluid in the interstitial component of the extracellular fluid compartment (Skov & Muwaswes, 1993). If the volume of fluid flowing through the capillaries exceeds the body's ability to return it to the venous circulation, the tissues swell and the fluid may overflow from the interstitium into spaces such as the peritoneal cavity (known as ascites), intestinal lumen, and thoracic cavity.

Progression of existing disorders can overwhelm reserve mechanisms that defend against edema. For example, a client with compromised cardiac function may experience additional compromise if a myocardial infarction occurs. In turn, pulmonary blood volume may increase and transcapillary fluid flux may exceed the body's compensatory ability to remove it. The fluid collected in the lung, as a result, is called pulmonary edema. Pulmonary edema limits ventilation and can lead to a life-threatening spiral of decreasing oxygenation and cardiac output.

Edema is described in terms of where the fluid accumulates (interstitial, intracavitary, or intracellular) and in terms of the initiating mechanism (eg, vasogenic, cellular, lymph). Some conditions result in edema from more than one mechanism (eg, the vasogenic and cellular mechanisms in cirrhosis). No matter what its cause, fluid overload that occurs as part of edema increases the workload of the heart, decreases tissue perfusion, and promotes decline in other organ systems.

Diuretics and Cardiovascular Disease

Heart failure is a potential consequence of most cardiac disorders and occurs when the heart cannot provide sufficient output to maintain body functions. Both acute and chronic congestive heart failure (CHF) involve fluid retention and edema.

Using diuretics to treat CHF can reduce preload and can promote the state of *compensated* CHF. Reversing fluid retention and reducing edema relieve symptoms and reduce some of the heart's workload. However, a reduction in preload must be attempted cautiously. Because the failing heart has a decreased capacity to regulate its contractility in response to changes in venous return, diuretic therapy that is too abrupt or severe may subject clients to the complications of decreased blood volume. Complications of decreased blood volume include decreased cardiac output and blood pressure. Therefore, diuretic drug therapy requires continuous evaluation, adjustment, and use of other measures to maximize cardiac performance.

Afterload reduction may be achieved in CHF management by promoting vasodilation with angiotensin-converting enzyme (ACE) inhibitors, calcium channel blockers, and direct vasodilators. ACE inhibitors lead to a disruption of angiotensin II function, which normally is an endogenous vasoconstrictor. Calcium channel blockers cause arteriolar dilation by inducing vascular smooth muscle to relax by decreasing calcium ions in smooth muscle cytoplasm. Again, excessive reduction in blood pressure must be avoided when using these agents.

Mild CHF often responds to dietary salt restriction and low doses of a thiazide diuretic. As CHF progresses, clients become refractory to thiazide diuretics, which are generally ineffective as single agents when the GFR falls below 20 to 30 mL/min. Under these conditions, loop diuretics and a tighter control of dietary salt are needed. Nevertheless, as clients move through the treatment strategies, the risks of volume depletion, azotemia, and electrolyte abnormalities increase sharply.

Renal sodium and fluid retention in clients with *decompensated* CHF lead to pulmonary edema. In this situation, diuretics may be life-saving, but decompensated CHF also predisposes clients to dangerous electrolyte imbalances (hypokalemia, hypomagnesemia, and hyponatremia). This risk further necessitates continuous re-evaluation of diuretic therapy.

Diuretics and Liver or Renal Disease

Cirrhosis of the liver incorporates multiple signs and symptoms, including ascites and peripheral edema. At later stages of cirrhosis, renal sodium excretion is often low due to reduced GFR and increased renal sodium reabsorption. Ideally, diuretics should help. Indeed, some clients experience increased plasma volume and enhanced sodium reabsorption related to aldosterone levels; diuretics may then be helpful. However, some clients appear to have a reduced effective blood volume, which leads to increased levels of hormones (renin, aldosterone, vasopressin, and norephinephrine) associated with volume depletion. These clients would have an adverse response to further volume depletion from diuretics.

Clients with acute and chronic renal failure commonly receive diuretic therapy. The nephrotic syndrome leads to renal losses of albumin that eventually lead to severe hypoalbuminemia and a drop in plasma oncotic pressure. This increases the movement of fluid into the interstitial spaces. Loop diuretics are often helpful, but aldosterone antagonists have proved less helpful.

Diuretics and Other Conditions

Other conditions in which diuretic therapy may be helpful include hypertension, diabetes insipidus, renal tubular acidosis, increased intracranial pressure, hypercalcemia, and increased intraocular pressure.

Drugs Used as Diuretics

As described above, factors that influence urine production include glomerular filtration, tubular reabsorption, and tubular secretion. Many substances increase urine production by the normal kidney, including dietary components such as water, osmotically active salts and sugars, and xanthines. Diuretics are drugs that cause a net loss of sodium and water from the body. Most diuretics act at the proximal tubule, loop of Henle, or distal tubule (Fig. 27-1). Most diuretics decrease reabsorption in the tubules. A resultant increase in the tubular

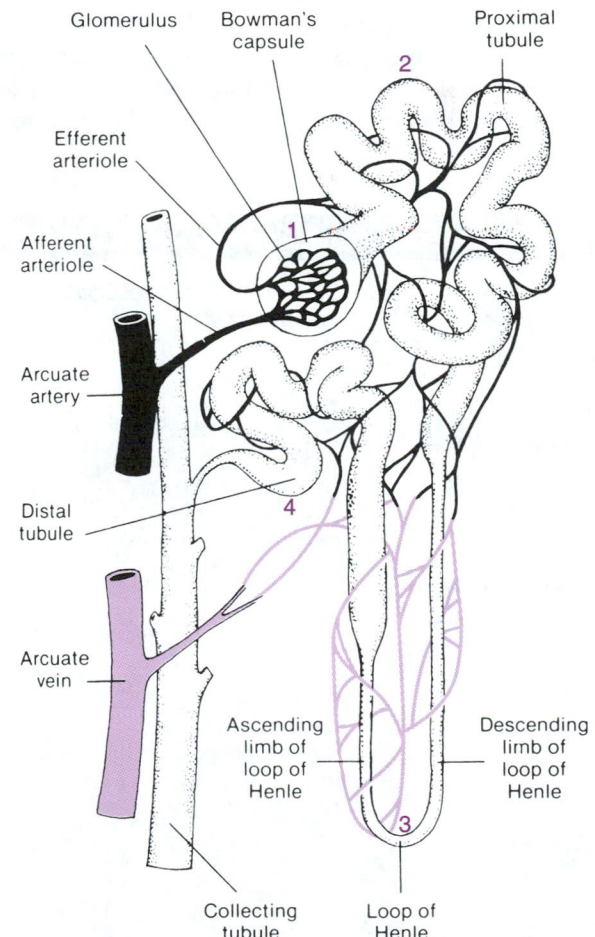

Figure 27-1. Sites of diuretic action. (*Site 1*) Renal vasculature. Agents that increase renal blood flow or renal artery hydrostatic pressure also increase glomerular filtration rate. (*Site 2*) Proximal tubule. Agents that decrease electrolyte reabsorption in the proximal tubule allow a large volume of filtrate to pass through to the distal tubule. (*Site 3*) Loop of Henle. High-ceiling diuretics reduce electrolyte reabsorption in the ascending loop of Henle. (*Site 4*) Distal tubule. Drugs may interfere with sodium reabsorption or may block the effects of aldosterone at this site.

fluid flow rate further interferes with reabsorption by reducing tubular transit time. Diuretics may cause natriuresis (excretion of abnormal amounts of sodium in the urine) or chloruresis (excretion of abnormal amounts of chloride in the urine).

The diuretic drugs include loop diuretics, thiazides, indolines, quinazolines, potassium-sparing agents, osmotic diuretics, and carbonic anhydrase inhibitors (Table 27-2). The diuretics used before 1920 were xanthines (caffeine, theophylline) and osmotic diuretics (eg, urea). The next agents introduced were the carbonic anhydrase inhibitors, which were developed from the sulfonamides, following the observation that sulfanilamide caused mild diuresis as a side effect. Modifications of the original structure led first to acetazolamide and later to a group of diuretics called the thiazides.

Further modifications led to the compounds furosemide and bumetanide (loop diuretics). These drugs are sulfonamide derivatives, but have few chemical features in common with the thiazides. Their mechanism of action is also different.

All these compounds effectively promoted sodium excretion, but they also caused potassium loss. This led to a search for potassium-sparing diuretics. Aldosterone antagonists, such as spironolactone, were introduced in 1962. Further work led to the development of amiloride and triamterene. Recent efforts involve the development of uricosuric diuretics to overcome the problem of increased plasma uric acid concentration resulting from diuretic use.

Adaptation to Diuretics

The first dose of a diuretic usually produces diuresis as anticipated. However, a new equilibrium or steady state is attained within 2 to 6 days, and postdiuretic sodium retention and tolerance to the diuretic occur. This is called the "braking phenomenon" (Brenner, 1996).

Clinicians think that diuretics may induce adaptations in the nephron in response to the increased rate at which sodium chloride is delivered to the kidney. The increased delivery rate stems from the use of a diuretic. In response, clinicians have developed a regimen to accompany drug therapy:

1. Dietary salt is restricted, even in clients receiving powerful diuretics. The goal is to maintain initial volume loss and avoid any weight gain (every 1 kg of body weight gained or lost represents 1 L of fluid).

Table 27-2. Electrolyte Imbalances That Diuretics May Induce

Imbalance Associated With Diuresis	Types of Diuretics Associated With Imbalance	Signs and Symptoms Caused by Imbalance
Potassium		
hypokalemia	osmotic carbonic anhydrase inhibitors loop thiazide	hypotension, tachyarrhythmias, muscle weakness, abdominal pain, diminished bowel sounds, paralytic ileus
hyperkalemia	potassium-sparing osmotic (in the elderly)	bradycardia, heart block, heaviness of limbs, nervousness, diarrhea, GI distress
Magnesium		
hypomagnesemia	loop	muscle weakness, vertigo, irritability, confusion, anorexia, nausea, generalized muscle spasticity
Sodium		
hyponatremia	osmotic (rare) carbonic anhydrase inhibitors loop thiazide	inability to concentrate, drowsiness, lethargy, confusion, stupor, coma; occasionally, agitation, psychosis, seizures
hypernatremia	osmotic	confusion, neuromuscular excitability, muscle weakness, seizures, thirst, dry skin, flushing, fever, agitation, oliguria or anuria
Calcium		
hypocalcemia	osmotic carbonic anhydrase inhibitors loop (in some situations) potassium-sparing	numbness and tingling of the extremities, muscle cramps, hyperreflexia, tetany, laryngeal stridor
hypercalcemia	loop (with chronic use) thiazide	deep bone and flank pain, anorexia, nausea, extreme thirst, weakness, confusion

Adapted from Byers JF, Goshorn J. (1995). How to manage diuretic therapy. *Am J Nurs*, 95(2), 42.

2. Clients who seem to become tolerant to one diuretic may respond to another type that acts on a different nephron segment.

3. Prolonged diuretic therapy should not be stopped abruptly, because the adaptations may persist for 2 weeks. Dietary salt restriction should be in place and diuretics should be withdrawn gradually if they need to be discontinued.

4. Selecting a diuretic with a prolonged action or giving the diuretic more frequently may enhance sodium chloride loss by limiting the time available for postdiuretic sodium retention.

Agents That Increase Glomerular Filtration

Fluids and xanthines are agents that may increase glomerular filtration.

Fluids

When kidney function is impaired due to hypovolemic shock, fluid administration may help. Administering fluids may raise the hydrostatic pressure in the glomerulus and restore function by promoting glomerular filtration. The subsequent dilution of urine in the tubule also helps protect the renal tissues from the chemical damage sometimes caused by very concentrated urine. The specific fluids used are selected to correct the electrolyte imbalances present.

Xanthines

Xanthines (theophylline, theobromine, caffeine) induce diuresis by several mechanisms. Their cardiotonic and vasopressor effects increase blood flow and glomerular filtration. They also reduce sodium and chloride reabsorption in the proximal tubule. The diuretic effect of xanthines is not pronounced, and their usefulness is limited because of their stimulant actions on the central nervous system (CNS). The diuretic effect of xanthines, although weak, may be additive with that of other diuretics.

Diuretics That Act Directly on the Nephron
Loop Diuretics

Diuretics that act in the loop of Henle are called the loop diuretics (Table 27-3). There are two subclasses: one includes furosemide (Lasix) and bumetanide (Bumex), and the other includes ethacrynic acid (Edecrin). Another diuretic in this group is torsemide (Demadex).

Pharmacodynamics. Loop diuretics are the most powerful of all diuretics, capable of causing 15% to 25% of the sodium in the filtrate to be excreted. This led to the term "high ceiling" diuretics, in a comparison with thiazide diuretics (Rang et al., 1995). Loop diuretics inhibit reabsorption of sodium and chloride in the thick ascending limb of the loop of Henle, although actions at other segments of the nephron also contribute to diuresis (see Fig. 27-1, site 3). The transport of sodium chloride out of the tubule into the interstitial tissue is inhibited by inhibiting the sodium/potassium/chloride ($Na^+/K^+/Cl^{--}$) carrier in the luminal membrane. Normally, sodium and chloride reabsorption is mediated by a $Na^+/K^+/Cl^{--}$ cotransport system. This system is reversibly blocked by loop diuretics, which bind to one of the chloride binding sites of the carrier. Inhibiting the outward transport of sodium and chloride means that the solute remains in the tubular fluid and holds water with it. As much as 25% of the glomerular filtrate may thus pass out of the nephron, a profuse diuresis.

Loop diuretics appear to have venodilating action. After intravenous (IV) administration of loop diuretics

Table 27-3. Loop Diuretics

Drug Name	Preparation	Usual Dosage	Adverse Reactions
bumetanide (Bumex)	Tablets	*Tablets:* 0.5–2 mg/day; maximum daily dose, 10 mg	Asterixis, encephalopathy with preexisting liver disease, ototoxicity, GI effects, difficulties with erection
	IV or IM	*IV:* 0.5–1 mg over 1–2 min	
		PC: C	
ethacrynic acid (Edecrin, Sodium Edecrin)	Tablets	*Tablets:* 50–200 mg qd	Most likely of four to cause GI upset and ototoxicity, neutropenia in critically ill clients, thrombocytopenia
	IV	*IV:* 0.5–1 mg/kg via a running infusion or directly IV over several min	
		PC: B	
furosemide (Lasix)	Tablets Oral solution	*Oral:* 20–80 mg qd; up to 600 mg/day	Ototoxicity, GI effects, interstitial nephritis with rash
	IV	*IV:* 40 mg over 1–2 min, may repeat	
		PC: C	
torsemide (Demadex)	Tablets	*Tablets:* 10–20 mg qd	Headache, dizziness, insomnia, syncope, GI effects, chest pain, arrhythmias, hypotension, cough, arthralgia, myalgia
	IV	*IV:* 10–20 mg qd over 2 min	
		PC: B	

PC = pregnancy risk category; see Appendix A.

to clients with acute CHF, a therapeutically useful vascular effect is seen *before* the onset of the diuretic effect.

These drugs cause significant potassium loss. The high flow rate of filtrate produced by these diuretics also favors potassium excretion by continually flushing it away, increasing the gradient from cell to lumen. Loop diuretics may also produce metabolic alkalosis because the loss of sodium and chloride (with the resultant volume depletion), along with potassium depletion, stimulates hydrogen ion secretion and bicarbonate generation. Loop diuretics significantly increase the excretion of calcium and magnesium. They increase urate excretion on a short-term basis but later reduce excretion (provided volume losses are not replaced).

Pharmacokinetics. Loop diuretics are administered orally or parenterally. They are well absorbed; their bioavailability ranges from 60% to 100% (see Focus On Loop Diuretics: Similarities and Differences). After oral administration, these drugs act within 30 minutes to 1 hour, peak in about 2 hours, and have a duration of action of 6 to 8 hours. After parenteral administration, they have an onset of action of 5 to 10 minutes, a peak effect in 15 to 60 minutes, and a duration of action of 30 minutes to 8 hours. Bumetanide has the shortest duration of action.

Torsemide has the longest duration of action and is considered a long-acting diuretic. Parenteral administration is indicated when a rapid onset of diuresis is desired or when gastrointestinal (GI) absorption is impaired.

Bumetanide is considered the most potent of the four agents, about 40 times more potent than furosemide. It tends to be more chloruretic than natriuretic. These drugs are excreted mostly by the kidneys.

Therapeutic Uses. Loop diuretics can relieve edema associated with CHF, especially severe left ventricular failure. They are used for acute pulmonary edema and also for edema associated with nephrotic syndrome or cirrhosis. Furosemide or torsemide may be used alone or with other antihypertensive drugs in managing hypertension. Ethacrynic acid may be used for short-term management of ascites related to cancer. Furosemide and ethacrynic acid have been also used to treat hypercalcemia.

Dosage and Administration. The oral dosage of furosemide is 20 to 80 mg/day for edema and hypertension. Dosages vary widely with CHF and renal disease; doses as high as 2 g have been used. When given parenterally for acute pulmonary edema, the usual initial dose is 40 mg over 1 to 2 minutes. If the response is not satisfac-

---

FOCUS ON

Focus on Loop Diuretics: Similarities and Differences

Similarities

Pharmacodynamics

Prime inhibition of reabsorption of sodium and chloride by loop diuretics occurs in thick ascending limb of the loop of Henle. Normally NaCl reabsorption is mediated there by the $Na^+/2Cl^-K^+$ cotransport system. This cotransport system is reversibly blocked by loop diuretics, which bind to one of the Cl^- binding sites of the carrier; this leads to reduced water reabsorption.

These drugs cause significant potassium loss. Decreased sodium absorption in the early parts of the nephron therefore results in increased delivery of sodium to the collecting ducts. The high flow rate of filtrate will favor potassium excretion by continually flushing it away.

Loop diuretics increase the excretion of calcium and magnesium. They increase urate excretion on a short-term basis, but later reduce excretion.

Pharmacokinetics

Protein binding of these agents exceeds 90%. When given orally, the loop diuretics have a duration of action of 6 to 8 hours. Their onset of action is within 30 to 60 minutes.

Differences

- **Bumetanide** may have additional action in the proximal tubule; it does not appear to act on the distal tubule.
- **Ethacrynic acid** forms a complex with cysteine; the complex is the active form of the drug.

- Loop diuretics are chemically diverse. Their bioavailability ranges from 60% to 100%, with **furosemide** the least bioavailable and **ethacrynic acid** the most.
- **Bumetanide** is more extensively metabolized than **furosemide.** Thus, it is less cumulative in renal failure; this may reduce the frequency of ototoxic effects.

(continued)

FOCUS ON

Focus on Loop Diuretics: Similarities and Differences (continued)

Similarities (continued)

Therapeutic Uses

Loop diuretics are used to treat moderate or severe edema due to CHF, cirrhosis of the liver, or nephrotic syndrome when these clients are refractory to more conservative measures (eg, salt restriction and thiazides). They are also used in clients with renal functional impairment, who are often unresponsive to thiazides alone.

Adverse Reactions

Azotemia can develop if diuresis is excessive or the fall in BP is too great. Loop diuretics can cause hyponatremia, hypokalemia, hypocalcemia, hypomagnesemia, and metabolic alkalosis. They can impair CHO tolerance. A drug allergy (or interstitial nephritis) develops in occasional clients. The danger of ototoxic injury is present, especially when high doses are given, especially to clients with impaired renal function.

Drug Interactions

Loop diuretics may interact with anticoagulants, chloral hydrate, digitalis preparations, lithium, theophyllines, cisplatin, aminoglycosides, NSAIDs, probenecid, and salicylates.

Precautions and Contraindications

Hypokalemia must be avoided.

Loop diuretics are used cautiously in clients with diabetes; increased dosage of antidiabetic agents may be needed. Loop diuretics are used cautiously in renal and liver disease, SLE, and pregnancy and lactation.

Loop diuretics are contraindicated in clients with known allergies to them or to sulfonamides.

Nursing Considerations

Instruct client in pathophysiology involved, drug therapy regimen, adverse reactions and interactions. Instruct in appropriate diet, such as including low-sodium and high-potassium foods. Instruct client to use sun block. Monitor blood sugars. Assess cardiopulmonary status and vital signs for changes. Monitor electrolytes frequently for changes. Assess for signs and symptoms of hypokalemia. Check daily weights for significant increases or decreases. Assess extremities and abdomen (such as measuring circumference) for presence and amount of edema.

Differences (continued)

- **Ethacrynic acid** is being studied for the possibility it will reduce intraocular pressure in glaucoma.
- **Bumetanide** may be beneficial in the treatment of adult nocturia (but not effective in prostatic hypertrophy).

- In some clients, **ethacrynic acid** has produced severe, watery diarrhea; this is a criterion for drug discontinuation.
- Because of the amount of sorbitol in **furosemide** solution vehicle, diarrhea, especially in children, may occur when higher doses are given.
- Clients with known sulfonamide sensitivity may show allergic reactions to **furosemide, torsemide,** or **bumetanide.**
- There have been occasional spontaneous reports of thrombocytopenia with **bumetanide.**

- An exaggerated adverse clofibrate reaction may occur when **furosemide** is used concurrently with clofibrate. Phenytoin may reduce diuretic effect of furosemide.

tory within 1 hour, another dose of 80 mg may be given. Furosemide as a parenteral solution is a mildly buffered alkaline solution and should not be mixed with highly acidic solutions. It also has formed a precipitate when mixed with certain antibiotics. Dosages for the other agents in the class appear in Table 27-3.

Adverse Reactions. Ototoxic reactions, including tinnitus, reversible and irreversible hearing impairment, deafness, and vertigo with a sense of fullness in the ears, have been reported. Deafness is usually reversible and of short duration (1–14 hours), but irreversible hearing impairment has occurred. Usually, ototoxicity is associated with rapid IV injection, with severe renal impairment, with doses several times the usual dose, and with concurrent use of other ototoxic drugs. Some argue that ototoxicity is more common with furosemide than with bumetanide.

Photosensitivity dermatitis occurs rarely with furosemide; it is reversed after drug withdrawal. Acute interstitial nephritis with fever, rash, and eosinophilia is an uncommon complication that may develop abruptly or some months after therapy is started with furosemide.

Severe diuretic-induced hyponatremia is an uncommon but serious complication of diuretic therapy. It may be complicated by seizures and must be handled as an emergency with intensive treatment. The management of severe hyponatremia remains controversial because some think that rapid correction may be very dangerous. Mild hyponatremia can be treated by withdrawing diuretics and restricting daily intake of free water to 1 L or less.

Loop diuretics inhibit potassium reabsorption by the loop of Henle, but the main mechanism of kaliuresis is increased distal potassium secretion. Metabolic alkalosis, which may complicate therapy with loop diuretics, increases distal potassium secretion. Diuretics stimulate the secretion of aldosterone and antidiuretic hormone, both of which promote distal potassium secretion. Hypokalemia may be mild or severe; severe hypokalemia clearly requires treatment, but the importance and management of mild hypokalemia remain controversial.

Loop diuretics also inhibit magnesium reabsorption in the loop of Henle. Prolonged therapy with loop diuretics reduces the plasma magnesium level by an average of 5% to 10%, and an occasional client has severe hypomagnesemia. Hypomagnesemia is associated with depression, muscle weakness, and atrial fibrillation. It may be treated with magnesium oxide or magnesium sulfate. Any existing magnesium deficit must be treated to manage hypokalemia successfully.

Loop diuretics usually do not change plasma calcium concentrations, although they cause a prompt decrease in serum calcium when they are given with saline infusion to clients with hypercalcemia.

Loop diuretics regularly cause a metabolic alkalosis. This effect is of special significance in clients with liver disease and ascites, in whom the alkalosis may provoke hepatic coma, and in those with underlying pulmonary insufficiency, in whom the alkalosis may diminish ventilation. Diuretic-induced metabolic alkalosis is best managed by administering chloride, a potassium-sparing diuretic, or a carbonic anhydrase inhibitor. Metabolic alkalosis impairs the natriuretic response to loop diuretics and therefore may contribute to diuretic resistance (Brenner, 1996).

Drug–Drug Interactions. Many drug interactions have been reported with loop diuretics. The effect has been to increase some therapeutic effect or adverse reaction of the interactant drug in the case of anticoagulants, chloral hydrate, lithium, and digitalis glycosides.

The actions of theophyllines may be enhanced or inhibited. With cisplatin or aminoglycosides, additive ototoxicity related to the diuretic occurs. Nonsteroidal antiinflammatory agents (NSAIDs), probenecid, and salicylates may reduce the diuretic's effect.

Clofibrate can cause myopathy in hyperlipidemic clients with the nephrotic syndrome; furosemide can potentiate this toxic response by displacing clofibrate from the depleted plasma protein-binding sites (Brenner, 1996).

Drug–Laboratory Test Interactions. Loop diuretics may decrease glucose tolerance, resulting in hyperglycemia in clients previously well controlled on sulfonylureas. Hyperglycemia is seen with all loop diuretics, but perhaps to a lesser degree than with thiazide diuretics. Acute symptomatic hypoglycemia with convulsions occurred in uremic clients who received doses of ethacrynic acid above those recommended.

Short-term administration of loop diuretics increases plasma cholesterol concentrations and raises the levels of low-density and very-low-density lipoproteins and triglycerides. These effects are probably due to extracellular volume depletion.

A rise in the ratio of blood urea to creatinine suggests extracellular fluid volume depletion. (Renal failure can be precipitated by overly vigorous diuresis.)

Precautions and Contraindications. Hypokalemia induced by loop diuretics is dangerous in clients at high risk for arrhythmia (eg, those taking digitalis glycosides, those with left ventricular hypertrophy, myocardial ischemia, cardiac failure, previous arrhythmias, or prolonged Q-T intervals). The serum potassium level should be maintained at 3.5 mEq. Diuretic-induced hypokalemia can be diminished by concurrent use of potassium chloride supplements.

Plasma lithium levels must be monitored closely when lithium is used concurrently with diuretics. Some diuretics may increase lithium's plasma concentration, and some may increase its clearance.

Prolonged diuretic therapy impairs glucose tolerance and may occasionally precipitate overt diabetes mellitus. Loop diuretics must be used cautiously in clients with diabetes, and increased dosage of antidiabetic agents may be needed.

Loop diuretics are used cautiously in renal and liver disease, in systemic lupus erythematosus (SLE), and in pregnancy and lactation. They are contraindicated in clients with known allergies to them or to sulfonamides.

Diuretics That Act on the Early Distal Tubule
Thiazide Diuretics

Pharmacodynamics. Thiazide diuretics act by decreasing the reabsorption of sodium and chloride in approximately equal amounts in the early distal convoluted tubules (see Fig. 27-1, site 4). It appears there is competition between chloride and thiazides for binding to one of the chloride-binding sites of the $Na^+/K^+/Cl^{--}$ cotransport system. They have no action on the thick ascending loop of Henle. Thiazides also increase the excretion of potassium, magnesium, and bicarbonate (Table 27-4).

Pharmacokinetics. Thiazides are absorbed rapidly from the GI tract; chlorothiazide can also be administered IV. They are extensively bound to plasma proteins. Some of these agents are more lipid-soluble (eg, bendroflumethiazide, polythiazide), have more pro-

longed action, and are more extensively metabolized. Onset of action is 1 to 3 hours and peak action occurs at 2 to 6 hours. The duration of action ranges from 6 to 72 hours, typically 6 to 12 hours. They are actively secreted by the proximal tubule of the kidney and are excreted in urine. See Focus On Thiazide Diuretics: Similarities and Differences.

Therapeutic Uses. Thiazides are among the drugs of choice for the treatment of hypertension in clients with well-preserved renal function. They are useful in treating edema associated with chronic CHF and chronic renal or hepatic disease. They become less effective if used alone in clients whose creatinine clearance is decreased (these clients usually require a loop diuretic instead of or along with the thiazide).

Dosage and Administration. All thiazides come in tablet form. Hydrochlorothiazide and chlorothiazide are also available as an oral solution and an oral suspension, respectively. Chlorothiazide is available for parenteral injection. Several other diuretic drugs are marketed in a

Table 27-4. Thiazide Diuretics

Drug Name	Preparation	Usual Dosage	Adverse Reactions
bendroflumethiazide (Naturetin)	Tablets	2.5–5 mg qd PC: C	Hyponatremia (mild to severe), hypokalemia, hypomagnesemia, blood dyscrasias, interstitial nephritis, pancreatitis, cholecystitis, sexual difficulties, photosensitivity
benzthiazide (Exna)	Tablets	50–150 mg qd divided into 2 doses PC: C	See above
chlorothiazide (Diuril, Diurigen, Diuril Sodium)	Tablets Oral suspension Powder for injection	*Oral:* 500 mg–1 g once or twice a day *Injection:* 250 mg/5 mL (for emergency use) PC: C	See above IV form: hematuria, alopecia
chlorthalidone (Thalitone, Hygroton)	Tablets	50 mg qd PC: C	See above
hydrochlorothiazide (Esidrix, HydroDiuril, Hydro-Par, Oretic)	Tablets Solution Intensol solution	*Tablets:* 25–100 mg *Solution:* 50 mg/5 mL *Intensol:* 100 mg/mL PC: B	See above
hydroflumethiazide (Diucardin, Saluron)	Tablets	25–200 mg qd (in divided doses when dosage exceeds 100 mg qd) PC: C	See above
methyclothiazide (Enduron, Aquatensen)	Tablets	2.5–10 mg qd PC: C	See above
polythiazide (Renese)	Tablets	1–4 mg qd PC: C	See above
quinethazone (Hydromox)	Tablets	50–100 mg qd PC: C	See above
trichlormethiazide (Naqua, Metahydrin, Diurese)	Tablets	2–4 mg qd PC: C	See above

*Usual adult maintenance dose for edema
PC = pregnancy risk category; see Appendix A.

Focus on Thiazide Diuretics: Similarities and Differences

Similarities

Pharmacodynamics

Thiazide diuretics increase the urinary excretion of sodium and chloride in approximately equivalent amounts. The major site of action is the early distal convoluted tubule, where they block sodium/chloride reabsorption. Thiazides also inhibit sodium chloride and fluid reabsorption from the medullary collecting duct. Thus, thiazides impair maximal urine dilution; the increase in sodium chloride excretion with impaired urine dilution (but intact concentration) predisposes clients to the development of hyponatremia during therapy (Brenner, 1996).

Other common actions include increased potassium and bicarbonate excretion, decreased calcium excretion, increased magnesium excretion, and uric acid retention. They also decrease extracellular fluid volume. With chronic therapy, peripheral vascular resistance falls (arteriolar dilation increases).

Pharmacokinetics

Thiazides are readily absorbed from the GI tract. They are extensively bound to plasma proteins.

Therapeutic Indications

Thiazides are among the drugs of choice for the treatment of hypertension, particularly if the client has well-preserved renal function. They are used in the management of many conditions involving edema (eg, CHF, cirrhosis, CRF) and are used in hypercalciuria, calcium nephrolithiasis, and diabetes insipidus.

Adverse Reactions

Thiazides have many adverse reactions in common (orthostatic hypotension, anorexia, epigastric distress, nausea, vomiting, abdominal pain, diarrhea, constipation, pancreatitis, impotence/reduced libido, leukopenia, thrombocytopenia, agranulocytosis, aplastic anemia, photosensitivity, rash, urticaria, cutaneous vasculitis, muscle cramp/spasm, hyperglycemia, hyperuricemia, and electrolyte imbalances).

Drug Interactions

Thiazides may interact with lithium, allopurinol, antineoplastics, NSAIDs, bile acid sequestrants, corticosteroids, and anticoagulants.

Differences

- The water-soluble thiazides (**chlorothiazide** and **hydrochlorothiazide**) inhibit carbonic anhydrase and at high doses increase sodium and bicarbonate excretion by a proximal mechanism.

- Absorption percentages vary from 50% (**hydrochlorothiazide**) to 100% (**bendroflumethiazide**). Half-lives vary from 2 to 3 hours (**bendroflumethiazide, chlorothiazide, trichlormethiazide**) to 25 hours (**polythiazide**).
- The more lipid-soluble drugs, like **polythiazide,** have a more prolonged action. **Polythiazide** has a duration of action of 24 to 48 hours, but **hydrochlorothiazide** has a duration of action of 6 to 12 hours.

- Some of these products (**benzthiazide, trichlormethiazide**) contain tartrazine, which may cause allergic-type reactions, including bronchial asthma, in certain clients.
- **Bendroflumethiazide, chlorothiazide, hydrochlorothiazide, hydroflumethiazide,** and **methyclothiazide** may cause respiratory distress, including pulmonary edema and pneumonitis.
- IV **chlorothiazide** can cause hematuria.

(continued)

Focus on Thiazide Diuretics: Similarities and Differences (continued)

Similarities (continued)	Differences (continued)
Precautions and Contraindications Thiazides are used cautiously in clients with fluid and electrolyte imbalances, renal and liver disease, gout, SLE, hyperparathyroidism, and pregnancy and lactation. They are contraindicated in clients with known allergies to them or to sulfonamides. **Nursing Considerations** Instruct client in pathophysiology involved, drug therapy regimen, adverse reactions and interactions. Instruct in appropriate diet, such as including low-sodium and high-potassium foods. Monitor blood sugars. Instruct client to use sun block. Caution client to change position slowly and dangle feet before getting out of bed. Assess cardiopulmonary status and vital signs for changes. Monitor electrolytes frequently for changes. Check daily weights for significant increases or decreases. Assess extremities and abdomen (such as measuring circumference) for presence and amount of edema.	• **Benzthiazide** and **trichlormethiazide** contain tartrazine, which may cause allergic-type reactions in susceptible clients.

combined dosage form with thiazide diuretics such as hydrochlorothiazide (Box 27-1).

Adverse Reactions. Fluid and electrolyte abnormalities with diuretics were discussed under loop diuretics. Thiazides may cause a mild chronic hyponatremia that is asymptomatic, but they can also cause a severe hyponatremia that develops rapidly; the latter requires therapy. Severe hyponatremia may be more likely to occur with elderly women with well-preserved renal function. Neurologic manifestations may accompany severe hyponatremia and may or may not be reversed after treatment for the hyponatremia. The management of severe hyponatremia remains controversial because it is thought that too-rapid correction may also be very dangerous. Mild hyponatremia thought to need treatment can be managed by withdrawing diuretics and restricting daily intake of free water to 1 L or less.

Diuretic-induced hypokalemia and hypomagnesemia are especially dangerous in clients with CHF (especially those who are receiving digitalis preparations or have a prolonged Q-T interval), cirrhosis of the liver, or myocardial ischemia or arrhythmias.

Thiazides can also cause a number of rare complications, such as interstitial nephritis, pancreatitis, cholecystitis and jaundice, and blood dyscrasias. Thiazide diuretics have been associated with impotence, decreased libido, difficulty in gaining or sustaining an erection, and difficulty in ejaculating. Although uncommon,

photosensitivity occurs with thiazides and appears more likely to occur with hydrochlorothiazide than with other thiazides. It is reversed after drug withdrawal.

Drug Interactions. Plasma lithium concentrations can increase with thiazide therapy because of increased reabsorption of fluid and lithium in the proximal tubule and decreased excretion.

Concurrent use of thiazides with allopurinol may increase the incidence of hypersensitivity reactions to

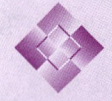

Box 27-1
Diuretic Combination Agents

Aldactazide: 25 or 50 mg spironolactone, 25 or 50 mg hydrochlorothiazide

Dyazide: 50 mg triamterene, 25 mg hydrochlorothiazide

Maxzide: 75 mg triamterene, 50 mg hydrochlorothiazide

Moduretic: 5 mg amiloride, 50 mg hydrochlorothiazide

See Chapter 25 for a discussion of other combination diuretic agents used in treating hypertension.

allopurinol. With antineoplastics, the antineoplastic-induced leukopenia may be prolonged.

Some NSAIDs (especially indomethacin) may reduce the diuretic and antihypertensive effects of thiazide diuretics. Bile acid sequestrants bind thiazides and reduce their absorption from the GI tract by up to 85%. Thiazides should be given 2 hours before the resin.

Corticosteroids may intensify electrolyte depletion, particularly hypokalemia, when given with thiazides. Anticoagulant effects may be diminished when thiazides and anticoagulants are used concurrently.

Drug–Laboratory Test Interactions. Thiazide diuretics cause hyperglycemia, which may be due to decreased hepatic glucose use. One study of thiazide-treated hypertensive clients found that magnesium administration that corrected hypomagnesemia improved glucose uptake, clearance, and metabolism. Possibly the combination of a potassium-sparing diuretic and the thiazide diuretic may prevent thiazide effects on serum glucose concentration (Brenner, 1996).

Like the loop diuretics, thiazides increase plasma cholesterol concentrations.

Prolonged thiazide therapy for hypertension increases the serum urate concentrations by one third. Because renal urate excretion is unchanged, urate clearance falls. The fall in clearance may be related to increased reabsorption secondary to extracellular volume depletion. Hyperuricemia is dose-related and does not normally cause problems unless the client is susceptible to gout or the serum urate level exceeds 12 to 14 mg/dL (Brenner, 1996).

Thiazides reduce renal calcium excretion, and this is accompanied by a small rise in serum calcium. This may have favorable long-term effects in counteracting osteoporosis.

Precautions and Contraindications. Some thiazide products contain tartrazine (eg, benzthiazide, trichlormethiazide), which may cause allergic-type reactions (including bronchial asthma) in certain susceptible clients. Thiazide diuretics must be used cautiously in clients with fluid and electrolyte imbalances, kidney and liver disease, gout, SLE, hyperparathyroidism, and pregnancy and lactation. They are contraindicated in clients with known allergies to them or to sulfonamides.

Indolines

The first in a new class of diuretics known as indolines is indapamide (Lozol). Some sources include the drug under the thiazide grouping because its pharmacologic effects and clinical uses are similar to those of hydrochlorothiazide.

Pharmacodynamics. Indapamide exerts a diuretic action similar to that of the thiazide diuretics. It enhances excretion of sodium, chloride, and water by interfering with the transport of sodium ions across the epithelium of the diluting segment of the renal tubules. In addition, it exerts a direct vascular effect that lowers blood pressure.

Pharmacokinetics. Indapamide is lipophilic and well absorbed when administered orally, in both the fasting and nonfasting state. It reaches its peak in 2 to 2.5 hours and has a duration of about 36 hours. It is metabolized in the liver and excreted in urine (60%). It is also excreted in feces (16%–23%). Elimination half-life is 14 hours.

Therapeutic Uses. Indapamide is used in managing edema caused by CHF and renal or hepatic disease. It may be used also in initial hypertension treatment.

Dosage and Administration. For edema, the adult dose is 2.5 mg as a single daily dose (in tablet form) in the morning. If the response is unsatisfactory after 1 week, the dose is increased to 5 mg/day.

For hypertension, the adult dose is 1.25 mg/day. If the response is unsatisfactory, this dosage can be increased every 4 weeks to a maximal daily dose of 5 mg. If it then seems necessary to combine this drug with another antihypertensive, the dose of the other agent should be reduced during the early treatment period.

Adverse Reactions. Indapamide reportedly has a lower incidence of causing major changes in serum electrolytes, uric acid, and glucose levels. However, the hypokalemia appears to be dose-dependent, so that hypokalemia is more likely to occur if higher doses of indapamide are used. Likewise, hyponatremia may be more common in elderly women (see thiazide discussion). Indapamide does not appear to increase serum cholesterol levels. Other adverse reactions include CNS effects (headache, nervousness, blurred vision), GI disturbances, dizziness and orthostatic hypotension, fatigue, cough, and muscle cramps.

Drug–Drug Interactions. Decreased lithium clearance may increase the risk of lithium toxicity. Drug-induced hypokalemia is dangerous for clients receiving digitalis preparations.

Drug–Laboratory Test Interactions. Because indapamide, like thiazide diuretics, may cause hypercalcemia and hypophosphatemia, it may need to be withheld before parathyroid testing.

Precautions and Contraindications. The indolines must be used cautiously in clients with fluid and electrolyte imbalances, renal and liver disease, gout, SLE, hyperparathyroidism, and pregnancy and lactation. They are contraindicated in clients with known allergies to them or to sulfonamides.

Quinazolines

Metolazone (Mykrox, Zaroxolyn) is an example of the quinazoline class.

Pharmacodynamics. This diuretic is structurally and pharmacologically similar to hydrochlorothiazide.

Pharmacokinetics. Metolazone is incompletely absorbed. The onset of action is in 1 hour, the peak in 2 to 8 hours. Its duration of action is 12 to 24 hours. It does not appear to be metabolized, and it is eliminated in the urine.

Therapeutic Uses. Metolazone appears to be more effective as a diuretic than thiazides in clients with severe renal failure. It is used in managing edema caused by CHF and renal or hepatic disease. It is also used for treating hypertension as the sole agent or to enhance the effectiveness of other antihypertensives. Antihypertensive effects may be observed in 3 to 4 days, but 3 to 4 weeks may be required for maximal effect.

Dosage and Administration. The typical dose is 5 to 20 mg/day for edema and 2.5 to 5 mg/day for hypertension. The metolazone formulations are not bioequivalent or therapeutically equivalent at the same doses— Mykrox is more rapidly and completely bioavailable— so brands should not be interchanged.

Adverse Reactions. Adverse reactions include dizziness, headache, GI symptoms, cardiac arrhythmias, chest pain, blood dyscrasias, rashes, and pruritus.

Drug–Drug Interactions. Decreased lithium clearance may increase the risk of lithium toxicity. Drug-induced hypokalemia is dangerous for clients receiving digitalis preparations.

Drug–Laboratory Test Interactions. The laboratory test implications and interactions are similar to those of other diuretics discussed above.

Precautions and Contraindications. Metolazone is not given to clients allergic to thiazides. Other precautions are the same as those for other diuretics.

Potassium-Sparing Diuretics

A few diuretics conserve potassium in the body while increasing sodium excretion (Table 27-5). Potassium-sparing diuretics can be divided into two general classes: those that do not interact with aldosterone receptors (eg, amiloride [Midamor], triamterene [Dyrenium]) and competitive antagonists of aldosterone (eg, spironolactone [Aldactone]).

Pharmacodynamics. In the kidney, potassium is filtered at the glomerulus and then absorbed parallel to sodium throughout the proximal tubule and thick ascending limb of the loop of Henle, so only minor amounts of potassium normally reach the distal convoluted tubule. As a result, potassium appearing in urine is secreted at the distal tubule and collecting duct. The potassium-sparing diuretics interfere with sodium reabsorption at the distal tubule (see Fig. 27-1, site 4), thus decreasing potassium secretion.

Spironolactone acts by competing for intracellular aldosterone receptors in the cells of the distal tubule. The result is an inhibition of the sodium-retaining action of aldosterone and a concomitant decrease in its potassium-secreting effect.

Triamterene and amiloride not only inhibit sodium reabsorption induced by aldosterone, but they also inhibit basal sodium reabsorption. They are not aldosterone antagonists. They act on the collecting tubules and collecting ducts, inhibiting sodium reabsorption and decreasing potassium excretion. Amiloride blocks the luminal sodium channels by which aldosterone produces its main effect, making less sodium available for transport across the basolateral membrane. It may inhibit Na^+,K^+-ATPase. Triamterene probably has a similar action. By preventing sodium entry, they also reduce sodium/hydrogen exchange and thus inhibit hydrogen excretion, resulting in some degree of alkalinization of the urine. Alkalinization is less marked with amiloride (Rang et al., 1995).

Table 27-5. Potassium-Sparing Diuretics

Drug Name	Preparation	Usual Dosage	Adverse Reactions
amiloride (Midamor)	Tablets	5–10 mg qd; doses >10 mg/day usually not needed PC: B	Headache, dizziness, paresthesia, tremors, nervousness, confusion, insomnia, depression, GI effects, weakness, fatigue, muscle cramps, extremity pain, cough, orthostatic hypotension, skin rash, pruritus, visual disturbances, tinnitus, neutropenia
spironolactone (Aldactone)	Tablets	25–200 mg/day PC: D	GI effects, lethargy, drowsiness, headache, confusion, ataxia, antiandrogenic effects, rash, pruritus
triamterene (Dyrenium)	Capsules	100 mg bid after meals; do not exceed 300 mg/day PC: B	GI effects, interstitial nephritis (when hydrochlorothiazide/triamterene combination used), thrombocytopenia, photosensitivity rash

PC = pregnancy risk category; see Appendix A.

Spironolactone decreases uric acid excretion. Triamterene and amiloride promote the excretion of uric acid. Amiloride decreases calcium excretion and is less likely than other diuretics to enhance magnesium excretion.

These three diuretics are important not because of their diuretic efficacy, which is less than that of other diuretics, but because of their potassium-sparing ability. They can be given with potassium-losing diuretics such as the thiazides to maintain potassium balance.

Pharmacokinetics. Potassium-sparing diuretics are administered orally.

Spironolactone is metabolized to active compounds (canrenones), is readily absorbed (over 90% bioavailable), and is more than 95% bound to plasma proteins. Its plasma half-life is only 10 minutes, but its active metabolite, canrenone, has a plasma half-life of 16 hours. Experts think its action is largely due to canrenone. The onset of action is very slow (24–48 hours); it takes 48 to 72 hours to reach peak effect.

Triamterene is well absorbed in the GI tract (30%–70% bioavailability). Its onset of action is 2 to 4 hours, with a peak action at 6 and 8 hours. Duration of action is 12 to 16 hours. Triamterene is rapidly hydroxylated to metabolites that retain diuretic action. Both the drug and its metabolites are excreted by the kidney, with half-lives of about 3 to 5 hours. It accumulates in clients with cirrhosis because of a decrease in hydroxylation and biliary secretion. It also accumulates in clients with renal disease because of a decrease in renal excretion.

Amiloride is incompletely absorbed (15%–25% bioavailability). It may have a slower onset of action, with a peak action at 6 to 10 hours and a duration of action of about 24 hours. It is secreted in active form into the tubule fluid.

Therapeutic Uses. Potassium-sparing diuretics are frequently used as adjuncts with potassium-wasting diuretics to prevent potassium loss. They are used also in primary hyperaldosteronism (Conn's syndrome), which is rare. They are used in secondary hyperaldosteronism due to hepatic cirrhosis complicated by ascites.

In an unlabeled use, amiloride may be useful in reducing lithium-induced polyuria without increasing lithium levels (as occurs with thiazides). Aerosolized amiloride (via nebulizer) appears to slow the progression of pulmonary function reduction in adults with cystic fibrosis.

Dosage and Administration. Amiloride and triamterene should be taken with meals because they can cause adverse GI effects. The administration of spironolactone with food appears to increase its absorption.

Adverse Reactions. The most serious adverse effect of these drugs is hyperkalemia, which is most likely to occur when the drugs are used alone without concurrent administration of potassium-wasting diuretics. The incidence of hyperkalemia is greater in clients with renal impairment or diabetes (with or without recognized renal insufficiency) and in the elderly. To treat hyperkalemia, the drug must be discontinued. Measures that could be used to reduce the hyperkalemia include administration of IV glucose (20%–50%) and regular insulin (using 0.25 and 0.5 U insulin/gram of glucose). If the client is acidotic or has a tachyarrhythmia, 44 mEq of sodium bicarbonate or 10 mL of 10% calcium gluconate or calcium chloride would be infused over several minutes. For atrioventricular block, transvenous pacing might be needed. If necessary, sodium polystyrene sulfate may be given orally or by enema. Persistent hyperkalemia could require dialysis.

Spironolactone can also cause GI upset (anorexia, nausea, vomiting, diarrhea, peptic ulceration) and antiandrogenic effects (eg, impotence, gynecomastia, testicular atrophy, postmenopausal bleeding). Skin rashes can occur.

Rarely, triamterene precipitates in the urine collecting system and causes renal stone disease. Triamterene may impart a harmless pale-blue fluorescence to the urine.

Drug–Drug Interactions. Triamterene can cause acute renal failure when given with indomethacin, even in normal clients.

The hyperkalemia these drugs cause is potentiated by other drugs that impair potassium excretion or raise the plasma potassium level (eg, ACE inhibitors, NSAIDs). Interaction with heparin can also potentiate the hyperkalemia because heparin limits aldosterone synthesis. If the client needs a blood transfusion, each liter of blood could contain 30 to 65 mEq of potassium, which would compound hyperkalemia. Low-salt milk or salt substitutes sometimes used by clients with renal disease can worsen hyperkalemia: low-salt milk can contain 60 mEq of potassium/L. Certain potassium-containing medications, such as parenteral penicillin G potassium, can also worsen hyperkalemia.

Interactions have also been reported between amilride and digoxin, triamterene and amantadine and cimetidine, and spironolactone and anticoagulants, digitalis preparations, mitotane, and salicylates.

Drug–Laboratory Test Interactions. Spironolactone and its metabolites can interfere with blood tests for digoxin, resulting in falsely elevated levels. Triamterene interferes with the evaluation of serum quinidine levels.

Precautions and Contraindications. Potassium-sparing diuretics are contraindicated in clients with limited renal reserve who cannot easily correct high potassium levels in the blood. These diuretics are not prescribed for clients with elevated blood urea nitrogen levels or those in acute renal failure. Amiloride and triamterene accumulate in clients with renal failure. Triamterene should be used very carefully in clients with cirrhosis of the liver because it can accumulate.

Diuretics That Modify Filtrate Content
Osmotic Diuretics

Diuretics that modify the filtrate content act indirectly by increasing either the osmolarity of the filtrate or the sodium load. There are four osmotic diuretics: glycerin/glycerol (Osmoglyn), isosorbide (Ismotic), mannitol (Osmitrol), and urea (Ureaphil).

Pharmacodynamics. Osmotic diuretics are pharmacologically inert substances that are filtered freely at the glomerulus but incompletely reabsorbed or not reabsorbed at all. Within the nephron, their main effect is exerted on the parts of the nephron that are freely permeable to water—the proximal tubule, the descending limb of the loop of Henle, and the collecting tubules. A high concentration of nonreabsorbable solute in the renal tubule increases osmotic pressure within the tubule, inhibiting diffusion of water from the tubule to the blood vessels of the nephron. This action increases the volume of fluid in the tubule and accelerates fluid flow, leading to increased fluid excretion. This has the secondary effect of reducing sodium reabsorption: the sodium concentration within the proximal tubule is now lower than it otherwise would be, and this alters the electrochemical gradient for reabsorption. However, the increase in sodium excretion is relatively smaller than the increase in water excretion, so these diuretics are not considered useful in treating conditions associated with sodium retention.

Pharmacokinetics. Osmotic diuretics (Table 27-6) may be administered orally or IV. The onset of action with oral glycerin or isosorbide occurs in 10 to 30 minutes; the onset of action with IV mannitol or urea is 30 to 45 minutes. All reach a peak action in 1 to 1.5 hours, with a duration of action of 4 to 8 hours. Mannitol is slightly metabolized, but for the most part osmotic diuretics are excreted intact in urine.

Therapeutic Uses. Osmotic diuretics are used to prevent acute renal failure during prolonged surgery or trauma; to prevent increased intracranial, cerebrospinal, or intra-ocular pressures during surgery, trauma, or disease; and to reduce intraocular pressure rapidly in acute glaucoma.

If given soon after the development of acute renal failure, mannitol and loop diuretics may convert oliguric to nonoliguric renal failure. Mannitol may also be successful in combating the symptoms of the dialysis disequilibrium syndrome.

Mannitol might be given to reduce brain mass before or after neurosurgery. It attracts water from the brain cells. Reduced cerebrospinal fluid pressure may be observed within 15 minutes after starting a mannitol infusion. It may be used to reduce intraocular pressure. When used preoperatively, it is administered 60 to 90 minutes before surgery to achieve maximal effect.

A 2.5% mannitol solution is used for urologic irrigation in transurethral prostatic resection or other transurethral surgical procedures. This minimizes the hemolytic effect of water alone, the entrance of hemolyzed blood into the circulation, and the resulting hemoglobinemia, considered a major factor in producing serious renal complications.

To prevent the toxic effects of cisplatin, mannitol may be useful added to saline solution to promote diuresis.

A 30% solution of urea is used to reduce intracranial pressure from cerebral edema. An unlabeled use is intra-amniotic injection to induce abortion.

Glycerin is used to interrupt acute attacks of glaucoma. It is administered before and after ocular surgery when reduction of intraocular pressure is indicated. In the blood vessels, glycerol's osmotic holding power promotes water movement into the intravascular space. By this mechanism, water is removed from the vitreous fluid of the eye. Although part of the glycerol is metabolized as calories, some is excreted, carrying water with it.

Dosage and Administration. Mannitol is administered by IV infusion only. The usual adult dose is 20 to 200 g/24 hours. The administration rate is adjusted to maintain a urine flow of at least 30 to 50 mL/hour. The contents of a vial are further diluted in sterile water for injection. When exposed to cool temperatures, mannitol

Table 27-6. Osmotic Diuretics

Drug Name	Preparation	Usual Dosage	Adverse Reactions
glycerin/glycerol (Osmoglyn)	Solution for oral use only	1–2 g/kg 1–1.5 hr before surgery PC: C	Nausea, vomiting, headache, confusion, disorientation
isosorbide (Ismotic)	Solution for oral use only	1.5 g/kg 2–4 times a day as needed PC: C	Nausea, vomiting, hiccups, CNS effects, headache
mannitol (Osmitrol)	IV	20–200 g/24 hr (depending on indication) PC: C	As above; also variations of circulatory overload, hyponatremia, hyperkalemia, metabolic acidosis
urea (Ureaphil)	IV	1–1.5 g/kg; do not exceed 120 g qd PC: C	As above; also chemical phlebitis to tissue necrosis near injection site

PC = pregnancy risk category; see Appendix A.

solution may crystallize; in such cases, the container of mannitol solution may be warmed in a hot water bath and then cooled to body temperature for administration. The administration set should include a filter.

Administration of mannitol may be preceded by a test dose for oliguric clients to determine whether the kidney can respond to the drug. The test dose should raise the urinary output to about 30 mL/hour.

When urea is administered, rapid IV administration should be avoided because it may be associated with hemolysis and increased capillary bleeding. The infusion rate should not exceed 4 mL/minute. The maximum daily dose is 120 g; a typical adult dose is 1 to 1.5 g/kg. The contents of a 40-g vial are mixed with 105 mL of 5% or 10% dextrose injection or invert sugar.

Glycerin is administered orally (lime-flavored solution) at a dose of 1 to 2 g/kg. Maximal reduction of intraocular pressure occurs 1 hour after glycerin administration, and the effect lasts about 5 hours.

Isosorbide is administered orally (vanilla/mint-flavored solution) at a dose of 1.5 g/kg. Palatability may be improved if the medication is poured over ice and sipped.

Adverse Reactions. Osmotic diuretics tend to induce nausea and vomiting and produce headache. Excessive loss of water and electrolytes may lead to serious imbalances, and the effects on electrolytes are complicated.

When administered IV, urea may cause phlebitis because it is irritating. Extravasation causes reactions ranging from mild irritation to pronounced tissue edema to sloughing and tissue necrosis.

Drug Interactions. Few drug interactions have been clearly identified, but urea may reduce the effectiveness of lithium by increasing its excretion and may potentiate the action of anticoagulants.

Precautions and Contraindications. Osmotic diuretics must be used cautiously in clients with renal disease. Expansion of extracellular fluid volume and hemodilution are predictable effects of mannitol infusion in clients with renal failure who cannot eliminate the drug. Circulatory overload, CHF, pulmonary edema, CNS depression, and severe hyponatremia can develop. Movement of potassium ions from the intracellular space to the extracellular space may cause hyperkalemia, and hyperkalemic metabolic acidosis may develop. Occasionally, urgent hemodialysis is needed to remove the drug. Osmotic diuretics are contraindicated in pregnancy and lactation.

Agents That Act on the Proximal Tubule

Diuretics that act primarily on electrolyte reabsorption in the proximal tubule (see Fig. 27-1, site 2) include xanthines and carbonic anhydrase (CAH) inhibitors (Table 27-7).

Carbonic Anhydrase Inhibitors

Carbonic anhydrase inhibitors are sulfonamide derivatives that increase the flow of alkaline urine. They include acetazolamide (Diamox), dichlorphenamide (Daranide), and methazolamide (Neptazane).

Pharmacodynamics. In the cells of the proximal tubule, the enzyme CAH catalyzes the formation of carbonic acid from carbon dioxide and water. Carbonic acid then dissociates to form hydrogen and bicarbonate ions, and the bicarbonate ion passes into the plasma. The hydrogen ion is secreted into the lumen of the proximal tubule, the secretion being balanced electrically by the opposite transport of sodium. In the lumen, the hydrogen ions combine with filtered bicarbonate ions to form carbonic acid, which dissociates to form water and carbon dioxide, which again is catalyzed by CAH. The carbon dioxide diffuses back into cells. The net effect of these processes is that much of the filtered bicarbonate is reabsorbed by the proximal tubule.

Drugs that inhibit CAH increase the volume of urine flow by preventing bicarbonate reabsorption. They also deplete extracellular bicarbonate. There is enhanced excretion of bicarbonate, sodium, potassium, and water, resulting in an increased flow of an alkaline urine (and a mild metabolic acidosis).

Table 27-7. Carbonic Anhydrase Inhibitors

Drug Name	Preparation	Usual Dosage	Adverse Reactions
acetazolamide (Diamox, Dazamide, Diamox Sequels)	Tablets Sustained-release capsules IV	*Glaucoma or preoperative treatment of glaucoma:* variable doses, possibly 250 mg qid *Diuresis:* 5 mg/kg qd *Acute mountain sickness:* 500–1,000 mg qd in divided doses or SR PC: C	Sulfonamide-type adverse reactions, GI effects, CNS effects, bone marrow depression, photophobia, metabolic acidosis
dichlorphenamide (Daranide)	Tablets	25–50 mg 1–3 times daily PC: C	See above
methazolamide (Neptazane)	Tablets	50–100 mg 2 or 3 times daily PC: C	See above

PC = pregnancy risk category; see Appendix A.

Inhibition of CAH is not limited to the renal tissues. In the eyes, it slows aqueous humor formation, thereby decreasing intraocular pressure.

Pharmacokinetics. The onset of action after oral administration of these diuretics is 1 to 4 hours (longest with methazolamide). Peak effect occurs in 1 to 8 hours (longest with methazolamide). Duration of action is 6 to 18 hours. These drugs are largely excreted within 24 hours, either as unchanged drug or as active metabolites.

Therapeutic Uses. Carbonic anhydrase inhibitors have been used in the past for managing edema associated with CHF, but this use is uncommon today. CAH inhibitors have proved useful in treating chronic simple (open-angle) glaucoma and secondary glaucoma. They may be used preoperatively in acute narrow-angle glaucoma to lower intraocular pressure when a delay of surgery is desired.

Acetazolamide has been used for preventing or ameliorating symptoms associated with acute mountain sickness (nausea, weakness, dizziness) in climbers attempting rapid ascent and in those who are susceptible to acute mountain sickness despite gradual ascent.

These agents may be useful as an adjunct in treating certain dysfunctions of the CNS (epilepsy). Inhibition of CAH in this area appears to retard abnormal, paroxysmal, excessive discharge from CNS neurons. The mechanism may be the lowered pH of the brain tissue.

Dosage and Administration. Acetazolamide is available as tablets, sustained-release capsules, and a powder for reconstitution for parenteral administration. If acetazolamide is given parenterally, it should be administered IV because the drug solution is alkaline and intramuscular injection is painful. The tablets may be crushed and suspended in a sweet syrup as an oral liquid dose form. In glaucoma, a typical dose is 250 mg orally one to four times daily, depending on response. For epilepsy, the usual dosage is 8 to 30 mg/kg/day in divided doses. In acute mountain sickness, a total of 500 to 1,000 mg/day is given in divided doses; treatment should be initiated 24 to 48 hours before ascent and should be continued as long as needed to control symptoms. The dosage for dichlorphenamide is 100 to 200 mg initially, followed by 100 mg/12 hours until the desired response is achieved; the maintenance dosage is 25 to 50 mg one to three times daily. The dosage for methazolamide is 50 to 100 mg two or three times daily.

Adverse Reactions. Inhibition of CAH reduces the kidneys' ability to excrete hydrogen ions. An inevitable side effect is some degree of metabolic acidosis. Other adverse reactions affect the GI system, the CNS (drowsiness, paresthesias, muscle weakness, flaccid paralysis), the hematopoietic system (agranulocytosis, aplastic anemia, other signs of bone marrow depression), and the renal system. Photophobia may occur.

Drug–Drug Interactions. Many drug interactions are possible. CAH inhibitors make the urine alkaline and thus may enhance or prolong the action of amphetamines, catecholamines, procainamide, quinidine, tricyclic antidepressants, and other basic drugs by decreasing their renal excretion. Renal excretion of lithium, barbiturates, nitrofurantoin, salicylates, and other acidic preparations may be increased and their effects decreased. Increased hypokalemia can result with combinations of CAH inhibitors and amphotericin B or corticosteroids. CAH-induced hypokalemia may cause toxicity from digitalis preparations if taken concurrently. Metabolic acidosis can occur if CAH inhibitors are given with salicylates. A reduced response to insulin and oral hypoglycemics has been noted.

Drug–Laboratory Test Interactions. Uric acid values may be increased. False-positive urinary protein determinations, falsely elevated values for urine urobilinogen, and depressed iodine uptake values may occur.

Precautions and Contraindications. These drugs should be used with caution in clients with chronic obstructive pulmonary disease when alveolar ventilation may be impaired because respiratory acidosis might be precipitated or aggravated. Uric acid excretion may be reduced, so gout may be exacerbated. Allergic reactions may occur.

▪ SUMMARY

Diuretics are drugs that promote urine production. Most act by interfering with electrolyte reabsorption in the kidney. They are prescribed to reduce edema caused by heart disease, renal disease, cirrhosis, and other conditions that involve sodium and water retention, such as hypertension. Drugs used as diuretics include loop diuretics, thiazides and indolines, quinazolines, potassium-sparing diuretics, osmotic diuretics, and CAH inhibitors.

❖ NURSING MANAGEMENT: CLIENT RECEIVING A DIURETIC

The adverse effects of diuretics include excessive diuresis, increased blood uric acid levels, and increased blood glucose concentrations. Fluid and electrolyte imbalances are likely to develop, and gout and diabetes mellitus may worsen.

NURSING PROCESS

ASSESSMENT

Before diuretic therapy is initiated, baseline data are needed for parameters likely to change with diuresis: body weight, skin turgor, vital signs, heart sounds, serum levels of electrolytes, liver and kidney function, and glucose and uric acid levels. Peripheral edema should be assessed and ankle circumference measured. With ascites, the circumference of the abdomen should be measured. Hearing should be assessed when loop diuretic use is anticipated. Intake and output patterns should be assessed, as should the need for an indwelling catheter. A drug history must be compiled in anticipation of possible drug interactions.

NURSING DIAGNOSIS

Nursing diagnoses likely to be made when clients receive diuretics include:

- Fluid Volume Excess, related to sodium and water retention secondary to CHF (or renal failure, hepatic impairment, hypertension)
- Fluid Volume Deficit, related to increased volume and frequency of urination
- Risk for Injury, related to electrolyte imbalances (hypokalemia, hyperkalemia)
- Knowledge Deficit, related to edema and diuretics used in its treatment
- Ineffective Management of Therapeutic Regimen (Individual), related to knowledge deficit, powerlessness, or lack of perceived benefits

PLANNING

Nursing goals include promoting sodium and water excretion, preventing fluid deficit, increasing knowledge, encouraging the client to adhere to the therapeutic regimen, and promoting normal electrolyte balance.

INTERVENTION

Whenever possible, diuretics should be administered early in the day so that the drug can be dissipated before bedtime, when the client's sleep would be interrupted by the need to urinate. If clients who receive diuretics are acutely ill or debilitated, the nurse should be available to help them to the bathroom without delay. Clients who cannot ambulate need a bedpan or urinal readily available or may temporarily require an indwelling catheter.

Clients who receive diuretics are on sodium-restricted diets. The degree of restriction varies with the severity of the edema, the type of diuretic used, and the prescriber's preference. Usually 500 to 2,000 mg of sodium are allowed. The nurse should be thoroughly familiar with the diet ordered. To help the client adhere to dietary salt restrictions, the nurse may suggest using herbs and flavorings to improve the taste of food. Seasonings that contain sodium, such as garlic salt, are not allowed, although the pure herb would be permitted. A nutritionist should be consulted if there is any doubt about the suitability of specific foods.

Daily body weights are the most sensitive measure of diuresis. To be reliable, weight must be measured at the same time each day, under standard conditions, using the same scale. Commonly, in the hospital, weights are recorded before breakfast, after the client has voided. The client should wear the same clothing at each weighing. If clients cannot stand alone, they may be weighed on a bed scale. A loss of 1 kg (2.2 lb) of body weight represents a loss of 1 L of fluid.

Clients on intensive diuretic therapy in the healthcare setting require close monitoring to detect early adverse reactions and toxicity. Diuretic therapy sometimes is continued for long periods. Nurses should be alert to adverse reactions characteristic of the specific diuretic ordered. Signs and symptoms should be listed in the client's nursing care plan. All diuretics can cause confusion due to electrolyte imbalance, and all can cause allergic reactions, including skin rash.

An accurate record of intake and output is essential. Measurements that are often ignored in monitoring fluid balance must be included in the record. For example, if the client is taking ice chips, the amount of fluid ingested in this way should be recorded accurately.

A client at risk for injury because of dizziness or lightheadedness while on a diuretic should be taught or helped to perform actions to compensate for these difficulties. The client should rise from a lying to standing position by sitting up slowly, sitting quietly for a few minutes to allow time for the body to adjust to the change in position, and then standing slowly. The client should be taught to avoid activities that contribute significantly to vasodilatation and might worsen orthostatic hypotension, such as hot baths and showers, steam rooms, and saunas. (See the Critical Thinking Challenge.)

Nurses can do much to prevent potassium deficiency. The prescriber may be asked if a potassium supplement should be ordered for the client who is receiving potassium-wasting diuretics. Foods rich in potassium should be offered to the client. Common sense and individual preference should influence the selection—for instance, a seriously ill client may prefer orange juice to a banana or dried apricot. Tea and coffee, if allowed, are significant sources of potassium.

If potassium deficiency develops despite all precautions, it must be detected as early as possible. The signs and symptoms of hypokalemia are described in Table

CRITICAL THINKING CHALLENGE
Case Analysis

Hugh Owen, age 77, was discharged 4 days ago from the hospital, where he was treated for acute congestive heart failure. Medication in the hospital included digoxin, 0.25 mg; furosemide, 20 mg bid; and spironolactone, 25 mg bid. Mr. Owen lives alone. He has no family, but a good friend lives a few houses away. You are visiting Mr. Owen for the first time tomorrow and are developing a potential care and teaching plan. You have a fair idea of what you want to cover in assessing Mr. Owen's adjustment and adherence to the therapeutic regimen.

Imagine your initial meeting with Mr. Owen. Compose a script of your conversation that focuses on diuretic therapy. Include elements that illustrate active listening, mutual goal setting, and learning facilitation.

27-2. The nurse should assess the client regularly for early signs and symptoms of hypokalemia, which may appear before serum potassium values are available. The laboratory data only confirm what should have been detected earlier by the nursing staff.

If parenteral infusion of potassium is ordered, the solution must be administered slowly. High concentrations of this electrolyte in body fluids can cause smooth muscle spasm and a weak heart action. IV infusions that contain potassium can cause vasospasm that compromises the IV line. More seriously, rapid IV administration can precipitate ventricular fibrillation.

Hypokalemia poses a particular risk for clients who receive digitalis because adequate levels of potassium are necessary to prevent digitalis toxicity. Common symptoms of early digitalis toxicity are anorexia and nausea. Food intake, the chief source of potassium, is interrupted. Potassium levels drop more rapidly, accentuating the toxic symptoms.

An important influence on potassium levels is the amount of stress imposed on the client, because stress stimulates cortisone secretion. Two effects of cortisone on the kidneys are increased potassium excretion and sodium retention. Stress, therefore, not only increases the risk of hypokalemia but reduces the therapeutic effect of the prescribed diuretics. Nursing measures to reduce stress are critical to treatment. Noxious stimuli, including noise and glaring lights, should be minimized.

Although less common, hyperkalemia also poses a danger for the client receiving a potassium-sparing diuretic, particularly if this is the only diuretic prescribed. Foods rich in this mineral (eg, orange juice, bananas, apricots, water in which vegetables are cooked, foods of animal origin) should be taken in moderate amounts only. Coffee, tea, and chocolate also contain significant amounts of potassium and should be limited. Hyperkalemia, which may develop quickly, predisposes the client to fatal cardiac arrhythmias, and the electrolyte imbalance requires early diagnosis and prompt corrective action.

Intensive diuresis may precipitate sodium and water depletion, a syndrome that resembles heat exhaustion. The signs and symptoms of this condition depend on the relative proportions of the two substances lost. If water and sodium are excreted in equal proportions, isotonic dehydration develops; if more sodium than water is lost, hypotonic dehydration occurs. These conditions are more apt to occur in hot, humid weather when large amounts of salt and water are lost through perspiration.

Diuretic therapy can affect intercurrent chronic disease. Diabetic clients should be monitored closely to facilitate control of hyperglycemia, which can increase when diuretics are used. Clients may need an increased dose of hypoglycemic drugs or an adjustment in diet. If the diuretic is reduced in dose or discontinued without adjusting the diabetic regimen, the client may experience hypoglycemic reactions. A history of gout should alert the nurse to take measures to prevent this complication.

Foods rich in purine, which tends to elevate further the body's production of uric acid, should be eliminated from the diet. Foods rich in purine include meat extracts (gravies, bouillon), organ meats, and legumes. Diabetes or gout could appear in clients who have previously not had these diagnoses. Every client who receives long-term diuretic therapy should be reviewed periodically for indications of drug-induced complications, and the nursing staff should work closely with the prescriber to develop an individualized drug regimen for optimal effect.

Client Education. The nurse should prepare and implement a teaching program about the specific diuretic regimen. Printed materials should accompany verbal instruction. Questions should be encouraged and misconceptions clarified. Clients should learn which signs and symptoms should be reported to the healthcare provider.

Clients should be advised that medication should not be stopped abruptly. They should be urged to take the drug regularly as directed; some clients tend to reduce the dose, taking the "water pill" only when they notice visible edema.

Diabetic clients should be advised to report signs or symptoms indicating altered blood glucose levels. They should be urged to monitor their blood glucose levels regularly and report significant deviations to the healthcare provider.

Clients who receive diuretics for the first time should be warned that they will urinate in amounts greater than normal. They should be urged to take the diuretic early in the day to minimize interruption of daytime activities and sleep from increased urine output and possible urgency.

Clients who may experience photosensitivity while taking certain diuretics should be advised to use a broad-spectrum sun block when outdoors.

Clients who take diuretics on a prolonged basis at home must be taught to assess their response to the medication. They should weigh themselves regularly, using the same scale and at the same time of day (preferably as soon as rising, after voiding but before eating).

Clients should be encouraged to purchase all medications from one pharmacy. Clients who receive diuretics on a continuing basis often receive several other drugs also, and many pharmacists maintain complete drug profiles and monitor drug regimens for incompatibilities, drug interactions, and other drug-related problems. These services can help the client avoid complications of therapy. Clients must also inform all their healthcare providers about their use of medications.

Clients should be advised against self-medication with over-the-counter drugs, such as laxatives or cathartics that enhance potassium loss or antacids that contain sodium, unless advised by the healthcare provider.

OUTCOME EVALUATION

The therapeutic response is evaluated by comparing urinary output to fluid intake, measuring serial weights, and observing reduction of edema (as measured by serial ankle or abdominal circumferences). Other data required for evaluation include laboratory data and physical evidence relating to electrolyte balance. (See Example of Nursing Process for Furosemide.)

❖ CHECKLIST OF NURSING ACTIONS

- ❑ Question the client about previous experience with drugs of this type.
- ❑ Carefully assess the client's fluid and electrolyte status.
- ❑ Whenever possible, administer diuretics early in the day to minimize their effects during sleeping hours.
- ❑ Advise the client that urine output will increase noticeably after diuretic therapy is begun.
- ❑ Monitor fluid status of acutely ill clients by keeping accurate intake and output records and daily weight charts.
- ❑ Unless clients are receiving potassium-sparing diuretics, encourage them to eat potassium-rich foods to prevent hypokalemia.
- ❑ Monitor clients closely for signs and symptoms of electrolyte imbalance and other adverse reactions specific to the drugs given.
- ❑ If signs and symptoms of hypokalemia develop, consult the prescriber about using potassium supplements or reducing the diuretic dosage.
- ❑ If signs and symptoms of hyperkalemia develop, consult the prescriber.
- ❑ Make sure the client's diet conforms to the prescribed sodium restrictions. Consult the dietitian about client preferences in food selection.
- ❑ Monitor diabetic clients who receive thiazide diuretics for glucose imbalance.
- ❑ Encourage clients receiving thiazide diuretics who have a history of gout to reduce dietary intake of purine.

Example of Nursing Process for Furosemide Therapy

The client, a 77-year-old retired railroad engineer, was admitted to the hospital a week ago for acute congestive heart failure. He has improved with a regimen of low-sodium diet, digoxin, and furosemide. For the last 2 days his vital signs have been normal. There is no visible edema except for swollen ankles in the evening. He is on maintenance doses of digoxin and furosemide.

When the client's medications are brought to him this morning, he complains of weakness and dizziness on arising. He moves listlessly and his abdomen appears somewhat distended. The client states he could not eat all his breakfast because he "just didn't have any appetite." His blood pressure is 110/84. Serum electrolyte values from 2 days ago show low-normal sodium and potassium.

Assessment Data

Low blood pressure

Weakness

Anorexia

Abdominal distension

Low–normal sodium and potassium

Dizziness on arising

Receives digoxin and furosemide

Nursing Diagnosis	Intervention	Goals and Outcomes
Potential Complication: Electrolyte imbalance (hypokalemia)	**Withhold** digoxin and furosemide for the moment. **Review** client's weight records and input and output records. **Consult** the prescriber for order for update on serum electrolytes. **Assess** further: monitor client's pulse for rate and rhythm, measure abdominal girth. **Offer** the client a glass of orange juice or a banana, a palatable source of potassium. **Evaluate** the client for stress. Reduce obvious stressors.	The client will state that he feels less weak and dizzy and is more interested in eating. The client's serum electrolytes will rise gradually. The client's abdominal girth will decrease.

- Teach clients how to assess their responses to medication.
- Teach clients the signs and symptoms to report to the prescriber.
- Stress the importance of taking diuretics regularly as ordered.

Resin Exchange Agents

Resin exchange agents, although they work via the GI tract, are discussed here because they may be used in treating clients with hyperkalemia. The only commercially available one for use with hyperkalemia is sodium polystyrene sulfonate (Kayexalate).

Pharmacodynamics. As sodium polystyrene sulfonate passes along the intestine, or is retained in the colon after administration by enema, the sodium ions are partially released and are replaced by potassium ions. This action occurs primarily in the large intestine.

Pharmacokinetics. The efficiency of this preparation is limited and unpredictable. Although the exchange capacity is predicted to be 3.1 mEq potassium/g, in reality it is about 1 mEq potassium/g. Because this is a wide range, electrolyte balance must be closely monitored. Onset of action after oral administration ranges from 2 to 12 hours and is longer after rectal administration.

Therapeutic Uses. This agent is used for treating hyperkalemia.

Dosage and Administration. The average adult oral dose is 15 to 60 g, best provided by administering 15 g one to four times daily. Sodium polystyrene sulfonate is a suspension of 15 g/60 mL, with a sodium content of 1.5 g/65 mEq. The suspension contains sorbitol solution, alcohol, propylene glycol, sodium saccharin, and methyl- and propylparabens; it is cherry-flavored (the sorbitol is used to combat any constipation the product might cause). Kayexalate is a powder that may be made into a suspension. Palatability can be increased by using low-potassium fruit juice, syrup, or soda.

The resin may be given as an enema, about 30 to 50 g every 6 hours. Because effective lowering of serum potassium with this agent may take hours, even days, this agent may not be sufficient to manage hyperkalemia that is considered life-threatening.

Adverse Reactions. This agent may absorb calcium or magnesium, causing imbalances such as hypocalcemia, hypomagnesemia, or even hypokalemia. It also may release sufficient sodium to cause problems for a client who cannot tolerate a high sodium load. The most common adverse reactions involve GI disturbances such as nausea, vomiting, anorexia, and constipation. Because the drug tends to solidify in the GI tract, it could cause fecal impaction.

Drug Interactions. Systemic alkalosis has occurred after cation exchange resins were administered orally in combination with nonabsorbable cation-donating antacids and laxatives (eg, magnesium hydroxide, aluminum carbonate).

References

Brenner BM. (1996). *Brenner & Rector's The kidney, Volume II*, 5th ed. Philadelphia: WB Saunders.

Chmielewski C. (1992). Renal anatomy and overview of nephron function. *ANNA J, 19*(1), 34–38.

Holechek MJ. (1992). Glomerular filtration and renal hemodynamics. *ANNA J, 19*(3), 237–248.

Rang HP, Dale MM, Ritter JM, Gardner P. (1995). *Pharmacology.* New York: Churchill-Livingstone.

Skov P, Muwaswes M. (1993). Edema. In Carrieri-Kohlman V, Lindsey AM, West CM, eds. *Pathophysiological phenomena in nursing*, 2d ed. Philadelphia: WB Saunders.

Bibliography

Byers JF, Goshorn J. (1995). How to manage diuretic therapy. *AJN, 95*(2), 38–43.

Copstead LC. (1995). *Perspectives on pathophysiology.* Philadelphia: WB Saunders.

Hardman JG, Limbird LE, Molinoff PB, et al. (eds). (1996). *Goodman and Gilman's The pharmacological basis of therapeutics*, 9th ed. New York: McGraw-Hill.

Hoes AW, Grobbee DE, Peet TM, Lubsen J. (1994). Do non-potassium-sparing diuretics increase the risk of sudden cardiac death in hypertensive patients? *Drugs, 47*(5), 711–733.

Olin BR, ed. (1995) *Drug facts and comparisons,* 50th ed. St. Louis: Facts and Comparisons.

Preisig P. (1992). Urinary concentration and dilution. *ANNA J, 19*(4), 351–355.

Radke KJ. (1994). The aging kidney: Structure, function, and nursing practice implications. *ANNA J, 21*(4), 181–192.

Solomon R, Werner C, Mann D, et al. (1994). Effects of saline, mannitol, and furosemide on acute decreases in renal function induced by radiocontrast agents. *N Engl J Med, 331*, 1416–1420.

For more information and sample tests and activities, refer to Chapter 27 in the Student Workbook for Clinical Pharmacology and Nursing Management, 5th edition, available through your bookstore.

VIII

Drugs Affecting the Gastrointestinal System

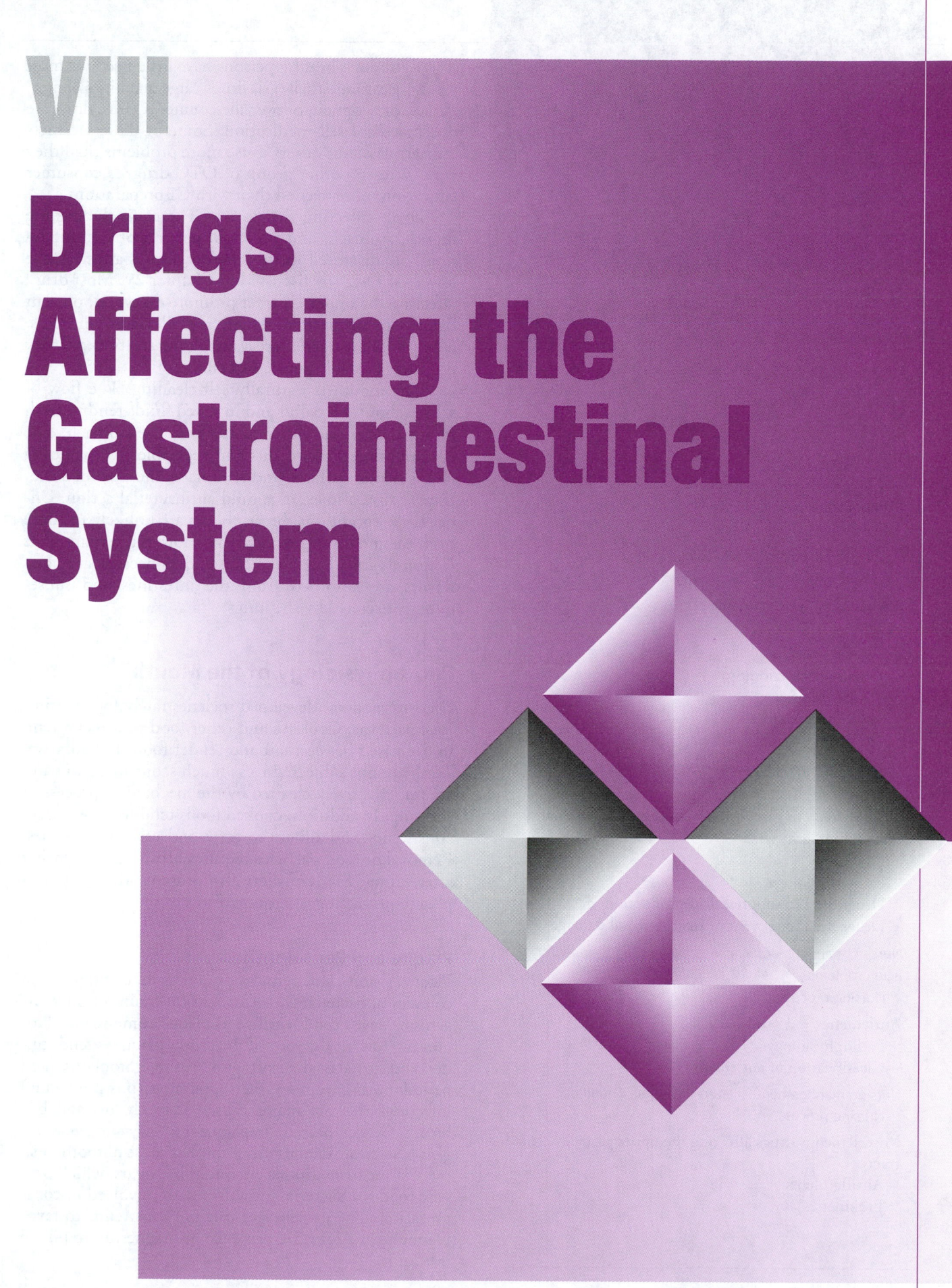

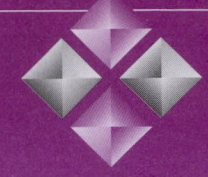

28

Drugs That Affect the Upper Gastrointestinal Tract

Although healthy persons have little need for most gastrointestinal (GI) drugs, large quantities of non-prescription, or over-the-counter (OTC), drugs are purchased for self-medication. Some of these products are harmless, but others cause more problems than they cure. With no other group of OTC drugs is consumer education more needed than with GI preparations.

Drugs affecting the upper GI tract (including the mouth, stomach, and proximal portion of the duodenum) are discussed in this chapter. Drugs affecting the lower GI tract are discussed in Chapter 29. Most drugs affecting the upper GI tract promote digestion, prevent damage to susceptible tissues, and alleviate symptoms. Some of these agents are valuable in treating primary disorders (notably peptic ulcers).

The mouth is naturally self-cleaning. The flow of saliva (about 1 L daily) and ingested fluids tend to wash food particles and other matter into the stomach. The consumption of raw fruits and vegetables mechanically cleans dental surfaces and stimulates the flow of secretions. Saliva also exerts a mild antibacterial action. Under these conditions, breath odors are unlikely to come from the mouth or nasopharynx. However, certain foods (onions, garlic, leeks) can cause odors because aromatic flavors are absorbed from the intestines and subsequently excreted by the lungs.

Pathophysiology of the Mouth

Diets in modern, developed societies rarely follow primitive patterns. Cooking and other food processing tend to decrease fiber content and render foods less abrasive. Teeth are not subjected to as much scouring action and are not effectively cleaned by the mechanical process of chewing. In addition, cooked foods tend to have a pasty consistency and adhere to teeth and other oral tissues. Removal of food particles requires brushing and rinsing after eating. Modern diets also promote the growth of plaque-producing microorganisms in the mouth.

Plaque and Periodontitis

Plaque, a stony, adherent deposit on teeth, is composed of colonies of bacteria. More than 1,000 strains of microorganisms have been identified as plaque components. Progressing toward the root of the tooth, plaque extends under and irritates the soft gum tissues. Stomatitis and periodontitis are among the suppurative (pus-producing) infections that are major causes of tooth loss and bad breath. Certain bacteria in plaque (eg, *Streptococcus mutagens*) also create dental caries, another cause of tooth loss.

Plaque formation is enhanced by sugars, which provide food for bacterial growth and are involved in coaggregation. The presence of calcium ions tends to favor plaque formation; the presence of magnesium tends to inhibit it.

Halitosis

Although some breath odors stem from retained secretions, crusts, and exudates in the mouth, these are temporary and can be controlled by basic oral hygiene. Other odors are excreted by the lungs. Oral hygiene does not affect halitosis caused by ingesting or inhaling substances that are excreted by the lungs (eg, tobacco smoke, alcohol, onions, garlic). Halitosis unrelieved by avoiding offending substances and conscientious hygiene may result from a medical problem. Vincent's angina, stomatitis, and oropharyngeal or lung abscesses cause bad breath of relatively short duration. Long-term bad breath may arise from catabolic metabolism (eg, weight reduction that produces ketosis) or from carcinoma in the mouth or respiratory tract.

Intermittent halitosis can be caused by gingivitis, oropharyngeal diverticulum (it traps food particles, which then decompose), nasal discharge, rhinitis, foreign body in the nose, sinusitis with postnasal drip, infection (in the throat, tonsils, adenoids, or lungs), or lung cancer. Other disorders that cause breath odors include respiratory infections (pharyngitis, tonsillitis), ketoacidosis (uncontrolled diabetes), liver failure, and uremia.

Agents Used to Treat the Mouth

Various agents are used to control and treat dental caries and plaque, gingivitis, mouth odors, and the oral mucous membranes (Table 28-1). Most preparations contain multiple ingredients; some contain alcohol.

❖ NURSING MANAGEMENT: CLIENT USING DENTAL PRODUCTS

The purpose of oral hygiene pharmaceuticals is to remove bacteria and bacteria-promoting matter from the teeth and mouth. Secretions may form crusts during the

Table 28-1. Agents Used to Treat the Mouth

Product	Preparations and Uses	Nursing Implications
Dentifrices	Cleaning agents formulated of abrasives (pumice, calcium carbonate, magnesium), flavorings, and other substances (glycerin, propylene glycol, dyes, fluoride)	Regular oral hygiene promotes client comfort.
Fluoride	Mechanism of action that prevents tooth decay and increases resistance of tooth enamel to acid and to caries is not fully understood. Fluoride inhibits microbes and desensitizes exposed root surfaces. Systemically absorbed fluorides are incorporated into crystalline structure of bone and growing teeth. Fluoride may be in drinking water, toothpaste, and oral rinses.	Excess use may mottle tooth enamel. Prolonged fluorosis may cause osteosclerosis; clients at risk are diabetics, kidney stone formers, women with recurring cystitis, and others who must maintain a high fluid intake. Signs and symptoms of fluoride allergy include rash, stomatitis, and GI or respiratory dysfunction.
Antiplaque rinses	Antimicrobial rinse used for about 30 seconds twice daily (AM and PM) after brushing teeth; treats gingivitis. Contains alcohol. About 30% remains in mouth after expectoration; poorly absorbed by GI tract.	Product may stain oral surfaces (teeth, tongue, restorations). Stain may be removed by professional prophylaxis. Product may alter sense of taste during treatment. Pregnancy category B
Mouthwashes	These oxidizing agents (containing sodium perborate, potassium permanganate, hydrogen peroxide, or carbamide peroxide) clean mouth, reduce bacterial flora, soothe mucous membranes, and stimulate secretion of saliva. Concentration strength varies; product must be expectorated.	Prolonged peroxide use may cause hairy tongue; prolonged potassium permanganate use can discolor mucous membranes purple. Ingestion may cause toxicity. Oxidation may cause bleeding in fresh wounds.
Saliva substitutes	These electrolyte solutions are moderately viscous and are applied topically.	Saliva substitutes are used to treat dry mouth resulting from radiation therapy, surgery involving the parotid gland, anticholinergic drug use, Sjögren's syndrome, or Bell's palsy.
Other (surfactants, aromatic oils, flavorings, antiseptics)	These rinses or lozenges clean or deodorize the mouth by reducing the surface tension of oral fluids, stimulate salivary glands, mask odors, and reduce bacterial flora, respectively.	Ingestion of excessive amounts may be toxic. Some products contain alcohol, which dries the mouth and inhibits salivation. Some products may cause painless mouth ulcers.

night, when the saliva flow decreases and bacterial growth accelerates, especially in mouth breathers. Food, especially sugars and starches, promotes the growth of microorganisms and the formation of plaque. Bacteria produce acids that dissolve tooth enamel, causing cavities and promoting decay. A program of careful and frequent oral hygiene can significantly decrease the incidence and severity of dental disorders as well as freshen the mouth and breath.

Fluoridated toothpastes and topical rinses are valuable adjuncts in preventing tooth decay. Brushing should loosen material from the surface of the teeth, gums, and tongue. Rinsing should rid the mouth of the free debris. Although oral hygiene retards the development of plaque, it cannot remove already developed plaque from teeth. This requires scraping and scaling by a dentist or dental hygienist, a procedure that should be performed at least every 6 months. Plaque is accelerated by carbohydrates, especially sugars, and the calcium ion. It is inhibited by magnesium.

For clients with active disease (periodontitis or caries), antiseptic mouthwashes (those containing sodium benzoate or benzoic acid) help reduce the oral microscopic flora. A hydrogen peroxide mouthwash is also antibacterial, but prolonged use can foster the development of an unsightly fungus called hairy tongue. (See Chap. 40 for more information on hydrogen peroxide.)

Recommended solution strengths for oxidizing agents used as mouthwashes vary. Sodium perborate, a white, odorless powder, is prepared as a 2% solution (0.5 tsp per 100 mL solution). Hydrogen peroxide should be prepared as a 1.5% solution. A solution is marketed in this strength specifically for use as mouthwash. The more usual hydrogen peroxide preparation, 3%, should be diluted 1:1 with water for oral use.

Because they are medicinal agents, these substances must be treated with the respect accorded any drug substance. Medicated solutions and those containing alcohol should be stored securely to prevent accidental ingestion and poisoning. Commercial mouthwashes often contain a considerable amount of alcohol; preparations with low concentrations (less than 27%) are preferred to those with higher alcohol content.

NURSING PROCESS

ASSESSMENT

Risk factors for dental plaque and caries include inadequate fluoride intake, impaired manual dexterity (interferes with good oral hygiene), high intake of carbohydrates (especially sugars), and high calcium intake (dietary or medicinal). Clients should be questioned specifically about use of fluoridated water, fluoride tablets, fluoridated toothpaste, and calcium supplements. Assessment of the mouth may disclose cavities, crusts, or discolored plaque. Colorless plaque may be revealed by chewing a tablet that stains plaque a bright color.

Assessment data include the kinds of preparations used by the client, the frequency of application, and the purposes for which they are used. If the client experiences persistent breath odors, the nurse should inquire about smoking, use of alcohol, and weight reduction regimens. Assessment for signs and symptoms indicative of diseases likely to produce such odors should be comprehensive. The nurse should also determine where substances used for oral hygiene are stored.

NURSING DIAGNOSIS

Nursing diagnoses related to the use of fluoride supplements or other drugs for dental disease may include:

- Impaired Tissue Integrity: Rough, discolored tooth enamel related to fluorosis secondary to excessive use or ingestion of toothpaste, rinsing solutions, or dietary supplements containing fluoride
- Risk for Impaired Skin Integrity: Rash related to allergic reaction secondary to exposure to fluoride
- Knowledge Deficit, related to proper preparation and use of dental drug products

PLANNING

Goals of treatment include improving oral hygiene, preventing dental caries and periodontitis, increasing or decreasing fluorine intake, and educating the client about good oral hygiene and dental drug products.

Nursing goals and outcomes may include the detection of diseases contributing to breath odors and referral of affected clients for definitive medical diagnosis and treatment. Goals also include reducing or eliminating smoking and alcohol consumption, reducing the risk of poisoning by accidental ingestion of mouthwashes and gargles, reducing breath odors by improving oral hygiene, and educating the client about oral hygiene

INTERVENTION

The nurse may refer the client to a dentist or dental hygienist for oral hygiene instruction, or the nurse may demonstrate these techniques and instruct the client directly. Clients who cannot perform oral hygiene because of impaired manual dexterity may want to learn about such aids as a jet spray (WaterPik) appliance, an interdigital stimulator (StimUdent), or a dental floss holder.

When the client cannot perform oral care, the nursing staff does so, using various aids available for this purpose. The removal of crusts and other debris requires other approaches. Papaya juice, which contains a proteolytic enzyme, is effective in breaking down crusts. Debris may be removed mechanically by irrigation with water, normal saline solution alone or with sodium bicarbonate, or a 1:6 solution of hydrogen peroxide and water.

Client Education. A basic teaching plan focused on dental products and oral hygiene should include instructions for brushing and flossing teeth after meals and snacks and scheduling regular professional cleaning by a dentist or dental hygienist twice a year. Clients with conditions requiring sodium-restricted diets (eg, hypertension, congestive heart failure) should be advised not to use salt and soda tooth powder, because some of it may be swallowed during use. Clients receiving calcium supplements for the control of osteoporosis should be warned that plaque may form more rapidly because of increased calcium ions in the saliva.

Dietary fluoride supplements may be recommended for clients in areas where water is low in fluoride. These supplements should not be used if the drinking water is fluoridated: such combinations can result in excessive fluoride intake, with subsequent damage to teeth and bones.

There is little need for the healthy person to use special agents for cleansing the mouth or throat. Commercial solutions are formulated to enhance flavor and eye appeal. Except when prescribed by a physician, they should be regarded as cosmetics rather than medicine and used sparingly because of their potential for adverse reactions. When ordered as part of a medical regimen, the client should be encouraged to use them as prescribed.

OUTCOME EVALUATION

Data required for evaluation include cleanliness of the mouth after oral hygiene and the incidence or absence of dental caries, plaque, gingivitis, and periodontitis. Other data required for evaluation include client reports of alcohol and cigarette use and breath odors, the incidence or absence of accidental poisoning involving mouthwashes, and frequency of referral for medical care of conditions underlying halitosis.

Digestants

Digestants are endogenous chemicals that promote the breakdown of food into absorbable particles. They include hydrochloric acid (HCl), enzymes (proteases, saccharases, lipases), and bile.

Normal Processes

In normal persons, digestants are secreted by the pancreas and liver and by the cells in the mucous membranes of the intestinal tract. HCl and pepsin are produced in the stomach, amylase, trypsin, and lipase by the pancreas, and bile by the liver. HCl promotes and activates pepsin and accelerates protein hydrolysis. Pepsin and other enzymes catalyze the breakdown of calorie nutrients in chyme. Bile acts as a surfactant to emulsify fat.

Abnormal Functioning

Several conditions can interfere with the body's production of digestants. Stomach cancer, for example, destroys secretory gastric cells. Pancreatitis interferes with pancreatic secretion, either temporarily by cell inhibition or permanently by cell destruction. Liver disease or biliary obstruction may decrease the secretion of bile

into the duodenum. Cystic fibrosis is characterized by the production of thick secretions that obstruct ducts and inhibit the secretion of several digestants. Surgical removal of secretory tissue (eg, gastrectomy) also reduces endogenous production of digestants.

Gastric Acidifiers

Hydrochloric acid and glutamic acid hydrochloride are used to lower gastric pH (Table 28-2).

Pharmacodynamics. Hydrochloric acid and glutamic acid hydrochloride restore the normal acidic environment of the stomach, thereby increasing the precipitation of caseinogen, converting pepsinogen into pepsin, and stimulating secretion by the duodenum. They also inhibit the multiplication of bacteria and stop the action of ptyalin.

Pharmacokinetics. Administered orally, gastric acidifiers enter the stomach, their site of action. They are handled by the body the same as endogenous HCl. When the food mass containing these acids reaches the duodenum, pancreatic juice (which has a basic pH) neutralizes the acid. In the small intestine, the salts produced by this reaction are absorbed into the bloodstream and used as are any other salts in food.

Therapeutic Uses. Gastric acidifiers are administered orally for replacing stomach acid in clients with an HCl deficiency (achlorhydria or hypochlorhydria).

Adverse Reactions. In the mouth, HCl reacts with tooth enamel, breaking down and eroding the enamel and forming cavities. In the esophagus, it can irritate tissue and promote ulcer formation. Carelessly handled acid may contact the skin, producing chemical burns. In large doses, gastric acidifiers can cause metabolic acidosis.

Precautions and Contraindications. Hydrochloric acid should be diluted and administered through a glass straw placed near the back of the mouth. Gastric acidifiers are contraindicated for persons with peptic ulcers or gastric hyperacidity. These agents should be stored in a secure place to prevent accidental ingestion.

Pancreatic Enzymes

Pancreatic enzymes contain lipases, proteases (trypsin and chymotrypsin), and saccharases (amylases). Pancreatin is a powder prepared from hog pancreas. For medicinal use, it is formulated as an enteric-coated tablet to prevent the active ingredients from disintegrating in the stomach.

Pharmacodynamics. In the duodenum, pancreatic enzymes perform the chemical functions of digestion normally performed by endogenous enzymes.

Pharmacokinetics. After the breakdown of nutrients in the small intestine, pancreatic enzymes are digested

Table 28-2. Digestants

Drug Name	Preparation	Usual Adult Dosage	Therapeutic Uses
Gastric Acidifiers			
hydrochloric acid	10% diluted solution for oral use	4–8 mL, tid, with meals.	Dyspeptic symptoms
glutamic acid hydrochloride	Capsules	340–680 mg with meals (340 mg contains 1.8 mEq HCl)	Absence of free HCl in stomach Achlorhydria Hypochlorhydria
Pancreatic Enzymes			
pancreatin (Digepepsin, Donnazyme)	Enteric-coated tablets Plain tablets Powder	8,000–24,000 U of lipase activity with each meal and snack PC: C	Replacement therapy for pancreatic insufficiency
pancrelipase (Cotazym, Zymase, Pancrease, Ilozyme; *Can:* Viokase)	Capsules Tablets Powders Packets	8,000–24,000 U of lipase activity/17 g of dietary fat with each meal and snack PC: C	Replacement therapy for pancreatic insufficiency; treats conditions of cystic fibrosis, pancreatitis, malabsorption syndrome
Bile Drugs			
dehydrocholic acid (Decholin)	Tablets	250–500 mg, tid, with meals or immediately after meals	Replacement therapy with deficiency or biliary stasis After surgery of the biliary system Cholangitis Cholecystitis
chenodiol (Chenix)	Oral tablets	250 mg AM and hs, or 500 mg hs PC: X	Dissolution of gallstones in clients at high risk for surgery
monoctanoin (Moctanin)	Liquid for infusion into biliary tract	Continuous perfusion into biliary tract: 3–5 mL/hr for 2–10 days PC: C	Dissolution of cholesterol (translucent) gallstones after cholecystectomy
ursodiol (Actigall) capsules		8–10 mg/kg/day in 2 or 3 divided doses PC:B	Dissolution of radiolucent, noncalcified gallstones

KEY: PC = Pregnancy risk category; see Appendix A.
Can: Canadian trade name.

and absorbed along with components of food and other digestant substances. Pancreatic lipase is irreversibly inactivated at a pH of 4.0 or less.

Therapeutic Uses. Pancreatic enzymes are used for replacement therapy in treating malabsorption caused by exocrine pancreatic insufficiency. Conditions causing this deficiency include cystic fibrosis, chronic pancreatitis, and pancreatectomy. Pancreatin is available in plain or enteric-coated oral tablets. Pancrelipase (Cotazym, Festal II, Ilozyme, Pancrease), a more concentrated preparation, is marketed as capsules (prompt or delayed-release), powder, and tablets (prompt or delayed-release). Dosages range from 8,000 to 36,000 U of lipase activity. These agents should be administered with food.

Adverse Reactions. Excessive doses of pancreatic enzymes can cause nausea, vomiting, or diarrhea. Extremely high doses are associated with hyperuricemia and uricosuria. Allergic reactions (most likely in persons allergic to pork) are characterized by sneezing, lacrimation, or rash. Inhalation of powdered pancreatic enzymes causes irritation of the mucosa and can precipitate bronchospasm in persons with allergic sensitivity to the substance.

Precautions and Contraindications. Initial doses of pancreatic enzymes are relatively low and are increased as necessary until steatorrhea abates. The preparation is contraindicated in persons with allergic hypersensitivity to it or to hog protein.

Bile Drugs

Chenodiol (Chenix), ursodiol (Actigall), and dehydrocholic acid (Decholin) are three bile salts available in drug formulations. Monoctanoin (Moctanin) is a semisynthetic glycerol given via the common bile duct to dissolve cholesterol gallstones. See Chapter 23 for a discussion of chenodiol.

Pharmacodynamics. Bile acids dissolve cholesterol in bile and facilitate bile drainage. In the intestines, bile acids emulsify fat, facilitating its enzymatic breakdown into absorbable fatty acids. Bile acids also act as choleretics—in other words, they stimulate hepatic production of a dilute bile. Monoctanoin and ursodiol dissolve gallstones.

Pharmacokinetics. Bile acids are administered orally and traverse the intestinal tract. They are subsequently digested like natural bile acids, with most entering the enterohepatic circulation and a small fraction excreted in feces. Monoctanoin is given directly into the biliary tract only; it is not given orally or parenterally.

Therapeutic Uses. Ursodiol is indicated for treating small noncalcified gallstones. Dehydrocholic acid is used as a laxative and is sometimes administered after gallbladder surgery to promote T-tube drainage. Monoctanoin is used to dissolve cholesterol (translucent) stones remaining after cholecystectomy.

Adverse Reactions. Bile acids may cause diarrhea and liver impairment. Both are reversible on withdrawal of the drugs. Treatment with monoctanoin should be stopped if chills, fever, leukocytosis, or severe right upper gastric pain occurs.

Precautions and Contraindications. Caution should be used when giving bile acids to clients with impaired liver function.

■ SUMMARY

Digestants are pharmaceutical preparations of chemicals essential for digestion. They include HCl, pancreatic enzymes, and bile acids. They are used in replacement therapy for clients with deficiencies of autogenous digestant compounds. In addition, bile acids are used for their laxative and choleretic effects; monoctanoin and ursodiol dissolve gallstones. Digestants are well tolerated by most clients but can cause adverse reactions, including damage to the teeth, allergic hypersensitivity, diarrhea, and liver impairment.

❖ NURSING MANAGEMENT: CLIENT RECEIVING A DIGESTANT

Whether the client is receiving a gastric acidifier, a pancreatic enzyme, or an agent that affects bile flow, nursing management concentrates on promoting therapeutic effect and preventing or minimizing adverse reactions.

NURSING PROCESS

ASSESSMENT

Before digestant therapy begins, clients should be evaluated for risk of adverse reaction. Clients with a history of peptic ulcer disease are likely to experience recurrent ulcer problems if they receive HCl. Clients with jaundice should not receive bile acids. When pancreatic enzymes are prescribed, clients should be assessed specifically for allergy to pork. A complete nutritional assessment should be done as well, with emphasis on signs and symptoms of malabsorption.

NURSING DIAGNOSIS

Clients receiving digestant medication may experience:

- Impaired Tissue Integrity: Erosion of tooth enamel related to hydrochloride ingestion secondary to achlorhydria
- Pain (in the joints), related to hyperuricemia secondary to pancreatic enzyme medication
- Diarrhea, related to stimulation of peristalsis by bile or bile acids
- Knowledge Deficit, related to digestant deficiencies and drug treatment
- Risk for Injury, related to potential drug-induced allergic hypersensitivity to pork protein in digestive enzymes or to possible hepatotoxicity

PLANNING

Goals of nursing care include preventing tooth damage by HCl, preventing or promptly detecting and treating hyperacidity in clients receiving HCl, preventing or promptly detecting and treating allergic reactions to digestant enzymes by clients allergic to pork protein, maintaining normal fecal elimination, promptly detecting and treating other adverse reactions to digestant medications, and educating the client about digestant deficiencies and their treatment.

INTERVENTION

Digestants are given with food to increase their efficacy in promoting digestion and (with pancreatic enzymes) to protect them from degradation by stomach acid. They should be administered with ample fluids to propel them into the stomach.

Hydrochloric acid solutions, usually 10% strength, must be further diluted 15 to 20 times before administration. Even at these dilutions, the acid is strong enough to injure tooth enamel and should not be allowed to touch the teeth. The solutions are administered through a glass straw placed in the back of the mouth. Each dose should be followed by water or other liquid to ensure that it washes from the esophagus into the stomach.

During digestant therapy, clients should be assessed to determine the therapeutic response to the medications and should also be monitored for adverse reactions. The teeth of clients receiving HCl should be examined regularly for erosion and cavities.

Clients receiving digestive enzymes may develop signs and symptoms of allergic reaction (sneezing, lacrimation, rash, wheezing) that require treatment with antihistamines or decongestants. When bile acids are prescribed, clients should be monitored for hepatotoxicity and diarrhea. Clients being treated with acids (hydrochloric or bile) should be watched for signs and symptoms of peptic ulcer disease.

Client Education. Clients taking HCl should be taught preventive measures to protect the teeth. After taking medication, they should neutralize any residual acid in the mouth by rinsing with a dilute sodium bicarbonate solution. Other digestants should be taken with 8 to

12 oz of water to ensure delivery into the stomach. All digestants should be taken with food. Fluids taken with pancreatic enzymes must not be hot, because enzymes may degrade at high temperatures.

Clients taking bile acids should be taught to recognize the signs and symptoms of toxicity. They should know the signs and symptoms that warrant consulting the prescriber to adjust the drug regimen.

Some OTC preparations contain digestants and claim to relieve digestive symptoms. The doses in these medicines are too low to correct medical conditions for which digestants are prescribed, so clients should not use these drugs as a substitute.

OUTCOME EVALUATION

Outcome criteria include intact tissues, particularly those of the mouth and teeth; reports of reduced pain or absence of discomfort related to bile drugs; absence of diarrhea related to drug-induced bile acid stimulation; absence of allergic reaction; and increased client knowledge about the therapeutic regimen.

❖ CHECKLIST OF NURSING ACTIONS

- ❑ Before initiating digestant medication, assess clients for factors that increase the risk of adverse reaction to these drugs.
- ❑ Administer digestants with or after meals so that they mix with the food mass in the digestive tract.
- ❑ Follow digestant medications with ample fluids to deliver them to the stomach.
- ❑ Dilute HCl solutions 15 to 20 times before administration.
- ❑ Administer HCl via a glass straw placed in the back of the mouth.
- ❑ Have clients rinse their mouths with dilute sodium bicarbonate solution after ingesting HCl.
- ❑ Monitor clients receiving digestants for adverse drug reactions.
- ❑ Teach clients receiving digestants how to administer the drugs and how to monitor themselves for adverse reactions.
- ❑ Caution clients taking digestants not to substitute OTC preparations for the prescription drugs.

Drug Therapy in Gastric Acidity and Gastrointestinal Mucosal Integrity

Physiology

The HCl produced by the stomach plays an essential role in digesting food. Protein digestion is initiated in the stomach by pepsin and a low pH. The combination promotes the hydrolysis of proteins to amino acids. Not only is acidity favorable to proteolysis, it is essential for the formation of pepsin.

The conversion of pepsinogen to active pepsin proceeds most rapidly in a medium with a pH of 2 or less, which is highly acidic. The conversion virtually ceases when the pH rises to 5 or more. The HCl produced by parietal cells in the gastric mucosa normally maintains a pH of 2 to 5, depending on the presence of food and other chemicals taken orally.

The secretion of HCl is increased by endogenous substances (acetylcholine, gastrin, and histamine). A proton pump is necessary to assist in the secretion of HCl.

Although a high degree of acidity is optimal for digestion, it is highly corrosive and potentially traumatic to tissue. Any cells damaged by the acid are also vulnerable to the action of pepsin. The normal GI tract has defenses against this threat.

Gastric mucosa secretes two kinds of mucus. One type is a thin lubricant similar to that produced by other parts of the tract to promote digestion and to propel the food mass. The second is a thick, viscid substance that forms a barrier between the gastric mucosa and its corrosive secretions. This type of mucus is unique to the stomach and protects the gastric mucosa from chemical damage by its own secretions.

Normal gastric mucosa appears to resist penetration by acid to a degree not shared by the mucosa of persons susceptible to peptic ulcer disease. The mucosa is also protected by the mucosal blood flow, which removes acids that may have damaged the epithelium, and by restitution, the creation of a fibrin cap over an injured area. Prostaglandins produced in the GI tract also prevent injury to the mucosa.

Mechanical barriers prevent the spread of undue amounts of acid to unprotected tissues outside the stomach. The lower esophageal sphincter prevents reflux of acid upward into the esophagus; the pyloric sphincter prevents leakage of acid into the duodenum. Stomach contents do enter the duodenum periodically during digestion, but normally, by the time this material leaves the stomach, some of the acid has been neutralized by buffer substances in the food. Moreover, only small volumes enter the duodenum at any one time, and they are quickly mixed with pancreatic secretions, which raise the pH to an alkaline level.

Pathophysiology

Discomfort and tissue damage can develop when the delicately balanced processes of digestion are disrupted. Excess acid production, inadequate mucus secretion, impaired mucosal resistance to acid penetration, inadequacy of the cardiac sphincter, hypermotility of the stomach, and inadequate pancreatic secretion are among the factors that predispose persons to problems attributed to hyperacidity. These are secondary to both genetic and environmental influences (Box 28-1).

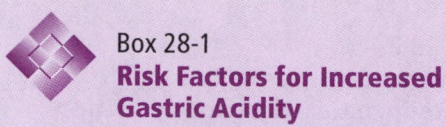

Box 28-1
Risk Factors for Increased Gastric Acidity

Disrupted Digestion

Excess acid production

Inadequate mucous secretion

Impaired mucosal resistance to acid penetration

Inadequacy of the lower esophageal sphincter

Hypermotility of the stomach

Inadequate pancreatic secretion

Genetic Factors*

Excess number of acid-secreting parietal cells

Inadequate mucous production

Mucosa susceptible to acid penetration

Metabolism that favors high levels of substances such as histamine

Diaphragm susceptible to hiatal hernia formation

Stress response patterns of parasympathetic activity

Undue sensitivity to external stimuli to acid production

Environmental Factors

Smoking

Overeating

Ingestion of gastric irritants

Undue stress

Excessive abdominal pressure (pregnancy, tight clothing, obesity)

Deficiency of the lower esophageal sphincter

Intermittent pressure on the stomach by the diaphragm

Abnormal passages in the tract

Infection with *Helicobacter pylori*

Drug therapy with NSAIDs

*Genetic factors are not completely understood but may include those listed here.

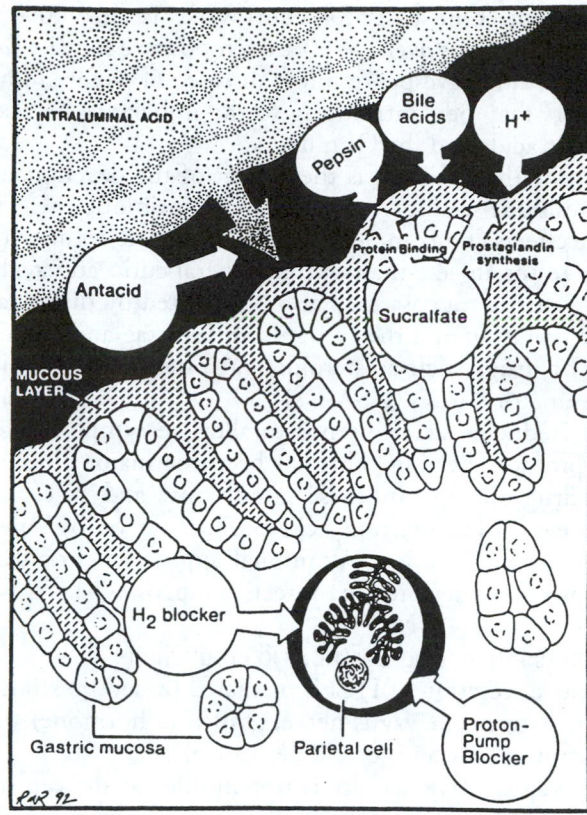

Figure 28-1. Mechanism of gastric mucosa injury and site of action for compounds used to manage peptic ulcer disease. The caustic action of stomach acid, pepsin, and bile salts can break down the intrinsic protective barrier to ulceration of the stomach. Alteration in regional blood flow also contributes to ulceration. Antacids directly neutralize intraluminal acid. Sucralfate stimulates prostaglandin synthesis which enhances the protective mucosal branch and can bind to pepsin, bile salts, and the ulcer surface. H_2 receptor antagonists and proton pump blockers have their effect directly on the parietal cell to inhibit acid production. H_2 receptor antagonists work at the histamine receptor and proton-pump blockers at the final site of acid production. Reproduced with permission from Manuel JJ. (1993). Clinical pharmacology of commonly used drugs in GI practice, part II. *Gastroenterology Nursing, 15*(4), 156–162.

Infection with a gram-negative spiral microorganism, *Helicobacter pylori*, is implicated in peptic ulcer disease. Its discovery in clients with peptic ulcer disease led to a new treatment approach. Treatment regimens include various combinations of bismuth, H2 blockers, and one or more anti-infective drugs (eg, tetracycline, metronidazole or clarithromycin, or amoxicillin).

Definitive diagnosis follows an endoscopic gastric biopsy. Other tests include serum tests for antibodies to *H pylori* and the urea breath test. A vaccine against *H pylori* infection is under development.

Helicobacter pylori can survive in the extreme acid environment of the stomach because it produces urease, an enzyme that catalyzes the formation of a substance that neutralizes gastric acid. *H pylori*'s spiral shape allows it to penetrate the mucosal lining; it then weakens the mucous protective barrier.

More than 90% of clients with peptic ulcer disease and more than 70% with gastric ulcers have *H pylori* in the stomach (National Institutes of Health, 1994). Despite a National Institutes of Health Consensus Statement (National Institutes of Health Consensus Panel, 1994) indicating that clients with peptic ulcer and *H pylori* infection should be treated with an anti-infective regimen, controversy continues over the preferred treatment. One basis for controversy is that 40% to 60% of persons over age 60 are seropositive for *H pylori* and do not have peptic ulcer disease. Therefore, other factors may be contributing to the imbalance between gastric acids and the GI mucosa.

Another concern is the danger of the development of resistant strains from widespread antibiotic use. The side effects and complexity of the antibiotic regimen often result in less-than-optimal therapeutic adherence. The gastric mucosa may also be affected by direct gastric irritation and the systemic antiprostaglandin activity of drugs such as steroids and nonsteroidal antiinflammatory drugs (NSAIDs).

Reducing acidity tends to alleviate symptoms and to promote healing. This has been the major objective of drug therapy in these conditions, and it can be achieved by inhibiting acid production or by subsequent neutralization. Additional approaches are drugs to protect or restore the protective mucosa.

Factors Influencing Gastric Acid Production

Gastric secretion of HCl is mediated by several stimuli: signals from the vagus nerve, gastrin (a hormone), and histamine (the amino acid derivative).

Vagus nerve activity is responsible for the cephalic phase of secretion, which is stimulated by the sight, sound, odor, and even thought of food. The parasympathetic system, of which the vagus nerve is a part, is one pathway by which emotional stress stimulates acid production.

Gastrin is produced by the antrum of the stomach in response to such stimuli as mechanical distention, extreme temperatures, and chemical irritants. The specific elements of the diet that act as irritants vary from person to person, but rich foods with high sugar and fat content, caffeine, alcohol, and strong flavoring agents, such as spices, are frequent offenders. Smoking is also believed to stimulate the parietal cells.

A negative feedback mechanism helps control the activity of the parietal cells. As the pH in the stomach drops, secretion declines, becoming totally blocked at a pH of 2. When food is ingested, it reacts with the acid secretions, raising the pH and stimulating further acid production.

Histamine stimulates acid secretion in much the same way as gastrin. Body levels of this chemical are increased in allergic reactions and any condition characterized by extensive tissue damage. Histamine stimulation of parietal cells may be the primary mechanism by which peptic ulcers develop. Stimuli that increase acid production also tend to relax the lower esophageal sphincter.

These mechanisms evoke potential interventions for reducing acid production: prevention of secretion of gastric acid, neutralization of gastric acid, and protection or restoration of mucosal damage. Therapeutic approaches are listed in Box 28-2. Anti-infectives may be given to eliminate infection with *H pylori*.

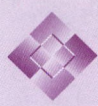

Box 28-2
Therapeutic Approaches to Reduce Gastric Acid Production

Reduce sensory stimuli related to food.

Modify the diet to include small, bland meals at moderate temperatures.

Avoid ingesting highly alkaline compounds.

Institute drug therapy with agents that reduce vagal nerve activity, suppress production of gastrin or histamine, inactivate gastrin or histamine, and block the stimulating effects of gastrin and histamine on the parietal cell.

Drugs Used to Suppress Acid Production

Medications to reduce acid production include anticholinergics, tranquilizers, histamine (H_2) receptor antagonists, and proton pump inhibitors.

Anticholinergics

Anticholinergics prescribed to inhibit vagal stimulation of the stomach include belladonna (as a tincture) and propantheline bromide. The use of these agents appears to be declining since the introduction of histamine (H_2) receptor antagonists. Both tranquilizers and anticholinergics are administered before meals. They may be combined in one preparation, as in the product Librax, which contains chlordiazepoxide hydrochloride and clidinium bromide (Quarzan). Anticholinergics and tranquilizers are discussed in detail in Chapters 16 and 20, respectively.

Histamine (H_2) Receptor Antagonists

In recent decades, drugs capable of inhibiting histamine (H_2) receptors have been developed. Four of these—cimetidine (Tagamet), famotidine (Pepcid), ranitidine (Zantac), and nizatidine (Axid)—have been approved by the Food and Drug Administration (FDA) for use in treating duodenal and gastric ulcers and conditions characterized by pathologic hypersecretion of gastric HCl (eg, Zollinger-Ellison syndrome). Cimetidine is also approved for the short-term treatment of active benign gastric ulcers. All are now available as nonprescription drugs. Table 28-3 summarizes the histamine (H_2) receptor antagonists.

Pharmacodynamics. Histamine (H_2) receptor antagonists competitively inhibit the action of histamine on the H_2 receptors that triggers parietal cell response to chemical stimulation. These receptors differ from the histamine (H_1) receptors, which mediate the local tissue effects of histamine in allergic and anaphylactic reactions. The latter are blocked by the classic antihistamines, which have no effect on secretory functions stimulated by H_2 receptors. The fact that they reduce acid secretion attributable not only to histamine but also to gastrin

Table 28-3. Histamine (H$_2$) Receptor Antagonists

Drug Name	Preparation	Usual Adult Dosage	Specific Adverse Reactions	Selected Drug Interactions
cimetidine (Tagamet, *Can:* Nu-Cimet, Peptol)	Tablets and liquid for oral administration Solution for IM or IV injection	300 mg q6–8h or 400 mg q12h Maximum daily dosage: 2.4 g PC: B	Nephrotoxicity greater than that of ranitidine Diarrhea Mania Inhibition of parathormone production Fever	Because cimetidine inhibits liver microsomal enzymes, it can cause higher than usual serum levels of the drugs usually metabolized by these enzymes. Antacids inhibit the absorption of cimetidine.
famotidine (Pepcid)	Oral Solution for IV injection	40 mg/d, given as a single dose; maintenance dose 20 mg/d Maximum daily dosage (for pathologic hypersecretion states): 640 mg PC: B	Diarrhea Reversible alopecia Diarrhea Transient irritation at injection site	No significant drug interactions have been reported to date.
ranitidine (Zantac)	Oral tablets Solution for IM or IV injection	150 mg q12h Maximum daily dosage: 400 mg PC: B	Nausea and vomiting, constipation, abdominal pain Hepatotoxicity greater than that of cimetidine Increased intraocular pressure Anaphylaxis	Ranitidine inhibits the metabolism of theophylline. Antacids inhibit the absorption of ranitidine.
nizatidine (Axid)	Pulvules for oral administration	300 mg hs PC: C	Diaphoresis Urticaria Somnolence	Nizatidine increases serum levels of aspirin.

KEY: PC = pregnancy risk category; see Appendix A.
Can: Canadian trade name

and vagal activity indicates that all three mechanisms may share, to some degree, a common pathway, possibly the H$_2$ receptor itself.

Reduced H$_2$ receptor activity results in reduced gastric acid output and concentration, with basal secretion affected to a greater degree than secretion in response to stimuli (food, insulin, histamine, pentagastrin, and caffeine). Pepsin levels are reduced indirectly as a result of the rise in gastric pH.

Pharmacokinetics. All four histamine (H$_2$) receptor antagonists are rapidly absorbed from the GI tract. Cimetidine, famotidine, and ranitidine undergo extensive first-pass metabolism, with bioavailability 50% to 88%. Nizatidine has 98% bioavailability and is the only one currently unavailable for intravenous (IV) use. All four drugs are widely distributed to most body tissues and fluids; except in liver disease, they do not cross the blood-brain barrier readily. Protein binding is relatively low, 10% to 19% for ranitidine, 15% to 20% for cimetidine and famotidine, and 35% for nizatidine. These drugs are distributed in breast milk; animal studies indicate that cimetidine crosses the placenta.

Histamine (H$_2$) receptor antagonists are metabolized by the liver. Hepatic metabolism is the major pathway for elimination of cimetidine and ranitidine; famotidine and nizatidine are excreted primarily by the kidneys. Cimetidine and ranitidine are removed by hemodialysis; famotidine is not. Elimination half-lives are about 2 hours and are prolonged in persons with impaired renal function.

Therapeutic Uses. Histamine (H$_2$) receptor antagonists are used for preventing and treating peptic ulcers and pathologic GI hypersecretory conditions (eg, Zollinger-Ellison syndrome, systemic mastocytosis, multiple endocrine adenomatosis, gastroesophageal reflux). Although not approved by the FDA for these purposes, histamine (H$_2$) receptor antagonists have also been used for treating other acid-related problems, such as hiatal hernia, esophagitis, acute GI bleeding, and gastritis, as well as for preventing stress ulcers.

Adverse Reactions. Histamine (H$_2$) receptor antagonists are generally well tolerated. The central nervous, cardiovascular, and musculoskeletal systems are affected most often. Signs and symptoms of central nervous system

(CNS) reactions include stupor, depression, headaches, dizziness, confusion, fatigue, and somnolence. In addition, histamine (H_2) receptor antagonists have been associated with rash, liver and kidney impairment, antiandrogen effects, and bone marrow depression.

Cimetidine sometimes causes feminization in males (gynecomastia, impaired sexual function). IV administration of cimetidine has resulted in disorientation, hallucinations, psychosis, and agitation, especially in clients over age 70. Bradycardia, hypotension, and cardiac arrest have been reported. Musculoskeletal pain (arthralgia, myalgia) may also occur. The use of cimetidine to treat clients who have had a gastrectomy or vagotomy or to treat those who have difficulty chewing has been associated with the development of phytobezoars (masses of undigested vegetable in the stomach). Other adverse effects include leukocytosis, blurred vision, bone marrow depression, liver abnormalities, and allergic reaction. Cimetidine may mask the signs and symptoms of pheochromocytoma, which then recur in exaggerated form when the histamine (H_2) blocker is discontinued .

Ranitidine can cause chronic headaches. IV ranitidine may cause bradycardia, tachycardia, and premature ventricular beats. The most common adverse reactions to nizatidine are diaphoresis and urticaria. Adverse effects of famotidine resemble those of ranitidine.

Drug–Drug Interactions. Cimetidine inhibits liver metabolism of many drugs that are administered concurrently. Drugs whose serum levels are increased when cimetidine is added to the treatment regimen include coumarin anticoagulants, tricyclic antidepressants, benzodiazepines, phenytoin, beta-adrenergic blocking agents, lidocaine, triamterene, and theophylline. When administered with morphine, cimetidine has caused apnea. The other agents appear to have minimal effects on liver metabolism of other drugs.

Drug–Laboratory Test Interactions. Ranitidine causes false-positive results in urine protein determinations using Multistix. Therefore, a sulfosalicylic acid reagent should be used for determining urinary protein during ranitidine therapy.

Precautions and Contraindications. Histamine (H_2) receptor antagonists should be used with caution in clients with renal or hepatic impairment; dosages must be reduced in renal failure. Cimetidine is contraindicated in clients with liver disease because liver impairment increases the permeability of the blood-brain barrier, increasing the risk of cimetidine-induced mental confusion. Symptomatic response to the drugs should not be interpreted as ruling out a gastric malignancy; it has been suggested (but not established) that cimetidine therapy may predispose clients to gastric carcinoma.

Cimetidine, famotidine, and ranitidine are in pregnancy category B, ranitidine in C. The drugs are not recommended for use in children or during lactation. They are contraindicated in persons with allergic hyper-

sensitivity to them. See Focus On Histamine (H_2) Receptor Antagonists: Similarities and Differences.

Proton Pump Inhibitors

Proton pump inhibitors block a step in the formation of HCl in the stomach. The two proton pump inhibitors available are omeprazole (Prilosec) and lansoprazole (Prevacid).

Pharmacodynamics. Proton pump inhibitors act by inhibiting the gastric enzyme $H^+,K^+,ATPase$, which catalyzes the final step of acid production at the secretory surface of the gastric parietal cell. They therefore block the final common pathway by which multiple stimuli act to stimulate gastric acid secretion.

Pharmacokinetics. Proton pump inhibitors are administered orally and are absorbed rapidly. They undergo extensive first-pass metabolism by the liver microsomal enzymes. Antisecretory effects last longer (as much as 72 hours) than suggested by their relatively shorter plasma half-life (less than 2 hours). Lansaprazole produces a more rapid increase in gastric pH. They are excreted via urine and feces.

Therapeutic Uses. Proton pump inhibitors are used in treating conditions requiring a reduction in stomach acid concentration (peptic ulcer, gastroesophageal reflux disease, Zollinger-Ellison syndrome).

Dosage and Administration. Adult dosages of omeprazole are 20 to 40 mg daily, given in one or two doses. The dose of lansoprazole is 15 or 30 mg daily before eating.

Adverse Reactions. Only mild adverse effects have been reported, and their incidence is low. They include headache, nausea and vomiting, abdominal pain, dyspepsia, flatulence, and diarrhea or constipation.

Drug–Drug Interactions. Because of the long-lasting and profound effect of proton pump inhibitors on gastric pH, the absorption of other drugs affected by gastric pH may be altered (eg, ampicillin, digoxin, iron salts, ketoconazole). Since they are metabolized by pathways regulated by the liver microsomal enzymes, there may be interactions with other drugs also metabolized by this pathway. Omeprazole inhibits the metabolism of warfarin, diazepam, and phenytoin, thereby increasing blood level of these drugs. The dosage of these drugs may need to be reduced if omeprazole is added to the drug regimen.

Drug–Food Interactions. Absorption of lansoprazole is diminished if given after food.

Precautions and Contraindications. Short-term use is recommended in light of increased carcinogenicity in rats receiving it in long-term therapy (24 months). Omeprazole is Pregnancy Category C and lansoprazole is Pregnancy Category B. The dosage of lansoprazole may need to be reduced in patients with impaired liver function.

FOCUS ON

Histamine (H$_2$) Receptor Antagonists: Similarities and Differences

Similarities

Pharmacodynamics

These agents inhibit the action of histamine on H$_2$ receptors of the parietal cells, decreasing gastric acid output and concentration regardless of the stimulating agent or basal condition.

Pharmacokinetics

These agents are rapidly absorbed from the GI tract and are metabolized by the liver. They are primarily excreted by the kidneys. Their elimination half-life ranges from 1 to 2.5 hours, peaking in 1 to 3 hours. They are widely distributed.

Therapeutic Uses

These agents are used to treat acute duodenal ulcers. They are also used to treat GI hypersecretory conditions such as Zollinger-Ellison syndrome, systemic mastocytosis, postoperative hypersecretion, and gastroesophageal reflux disease. They are also used in the treatment of short-term gastric ulcers and other acid-related problems such as hiatal hernia, gastritis, acute GI bleeding, and prevention of stress ulcers.

Adverse Reactions

These include: (CNS) depression, stupor, headache, dizziness, confusion, fatigue, somnolence; (CV) bradycardia, hypotension, cardiac arrest; (EENT) blurred vision; (GI) kidney impairment; (MS) musculoskeletal pain, arthralgia, myalgia; (SKIN) rash, allergic reaction; (HEMA) bone marrow depression, leukocytosis; (REPRO) bilateral gynecomastia, breast soreness.

Drug Interactions

Absorption of histamine (H$_2$) blockers is decreased by antacids.

Differences

- **Cimetidine** indirectly decreases pepsin secretion by decreasing the volume of gastric juice; it has a weak antiandrogenic effect.
- **Famotidine, nizatidine,** and **ranitidine** produce a dose-related reduction in pepsin secretion.

- Absorption of **cimetidine** and **ranitidine** may be impaired by the simultaneous administration of antacids.
- **Ranitidine** and **cimetidine** are distributed into breast milk, removed by hemodialysis, and undergo extensive first-pass metabolism. The half-life of parenteral **cimetidine** is 1.6 to 2.1 hours; parenteral **ranitidine** has a half-life of 2 to 2.5 hours; parenteral and oral **famotidine** has a half-life of 2.5 to 3.5 hours. The distribution of **famotidine** is unknown. The duration of **famotidine** is 10 to 12 hours; **cimetidine** is 6 to 8 hours; **nizatidine** is up to 12 hours; and **ranitidine** is 6 to 10 hours.
- **Cimetidine** is also excreted in breast milk. **Nizatidine** and **ranitidine** are also excreted in feces.

- **Cimetidine** has been used in treatment of acetaminophen overdose.
- **Ranitidine** is used in the treatment of theophylline toxicity and also has been used in prophylaxis of gastric damage caused by NSAIDs.

- IV **ranitidine** may cause cardiac arrhythmias.
- IV **cimetidine** may cause disorientation, hallucinations, agitation, psychosis, and cardiac arrhythmia.
- **Ranitidine** and **cimetidine** may cause itching, burning, and pain at the injection site.
- **Famotidine** may cause transient irritation at the IV site.
- **Famotidine** and **ranitidine** may cause constipation and diarrhea.
- **Famotidine** may cause flushing, palpitations, hypertension, and tinnitus.
- **Ranitidine** may cause vomiting and abdominal discomfort.
- **Nizatidine** may cause hyperuricemia and hepatocellular injury.

- The absorption of **ranitidine** and **famotidine** may be decreased by ketoconazole.
- **Cimetidine** inhibits liver metabolism of some drugs; it may cause increased serum levels/toxicity of lidocaine, metoprolol, procainamide, quinidine, oral anticoagulants, tricyclic antidepressants, benzodiazepines, phenytoin, and theophylline.
- **Cimetidine** may decrease the absorption of iron salts, tetracyclines, and tocainamide.
- **Ranitidine** and **cimetidine** can cause false-positive test results indicating gastric bleeding.

(continued)

Histamine (H₂) Receptor Antagonists: Similarities and Differences (continued)

Similarities (continued)

Precautions and Contraindications

These agents should be used cautiously in people with cirrhosis and impaired renal and hepatic function. These agents are contraindicated for clients with hypersensitivity to histamine (H₂) receptor antagonists.

Nursing Considerations

Instruct client in disease, treatment, drug therapy, regimen, adverse effects, and adherence; administer as a daily dose, preferably at bedtime; instruct client to take with food if necessary; separate doses of antacids by 1 to 2 hours; encourage client to avoid cigarette smoking; monitor blood studies for changes.

Differences (continued)

- **Cimetidine,** in large doses, should be used cautiously in clients with asthma. Cimetidine can decrease hepatic metabolism of drugs metabolized by the cytochrome P-450 pathway, resulting in potential increased serum levels of these drugs.
- **Cimetidine** is contraindicated in clients with liver disease.

- Administer IV **ranitidine** over 5 minutes or as an infusion over 15 to 20 minutes; do not dilute for IM injection.
- Administer **famotidine** IV push over 2 minutes or more and as an IV infusion over 15 to 30 minutes.
- Infuse IV **cimetidine** slowly over 30 minutes and warn client that IM injection of **cimetidine** may be painful; do not dilute **cimetidine** with sterile water for injection.
- Administer **famotidine** for best results at bedtime; instruct client that it may be taken with a snack and it may be taken concomitantly with antacids.
- **Nizatidine** cannot be given IV.

■ SUMMARY

Several drugs that inhibit acid production by the gastric mucosa are effective agents for treating peptic ulcers. They are often used to prevent stress ulcers as well. Adverse reactions to this group of drugs occur infrequently but are variable and affect many body systems. Because these drugs are relatively new, the nurse must monitor clients for signs and symptoms of long-term adverse effects that may not be documented. The recent availability of some of these drugs without a prescription points to the need to teach clients about their appropriate use. For example, because cimetidine inhibits microsomal enzymes, clients must be aware of potential interactions with other drugs and possible toxicity.

Drugs Used to Prevent or Treat Mucosal Damage

Antacids

Antacids are alkaline chemicals administered orally to neutralize HCl secreted by the stomach mucosa. They are used to relieve discomfort and reduce trauma caused by the corrosive effect of acid on exposed GI tissues. They usually act within 5 to 15 minutes, but their effects usually last only 2 hours. Antacids are also believed to have a restorative and protective effect on the gastric mucosa. Antacids can be purchased without a prescription and are widely used for self-medication without

supervision by healthcare professionals. Although generally safe, these drugs are not without adverse and toxic effects.

When prescribing antacids, the clinician must consider their therapeutic efficacy, their acceptability to the client, adverse reactions, and cost. Although the prescription may require adjustment to achieve optimal results, neither client nor nurse should substitute one antacid for another without consulting the prescriber.

Pharmacodynamics. Most antacids are alkaline salts or hydroxides of calcium, magnesium, or aluminum. They react chemically with HCl to form neutral or weak acid salts, thereby increasing gastric pH.

Among antacid preparations, the acid-neutralizing capacity (ANC) varies considerably. ANC is the mEq of HCl required to keep an antacid suspension at pH 3.5 for 10 minutes in vitro. A specific preparation may also vary over time, because drug manufacturers continuously reformulate antacid preparations. Liquid formulations are generally more effective than tablets (Table 28-4).

Pharmacokinetics. The salts resulting from the chemical neutralization occurring in the stomach mix with other materials in the GI tract and are subjected to the normal digestive process. If the chemical complex is broken down and absorbed, the body gains base reserve. If it is not, acidic material is carried out of the body in the feces.

Table 28-4. Properties of Selected Antacids

Drug Name	Ingredients*	Acid-Neutralizing Capacity Dose	Sodium Content/Dose
Alka-Seltzer Effervescent Antacid	Sodium bicarbonate, citric acid, potassium bicarbonate	21.2 mEq/2 tablets	592 mg/2 tablets
Amphojel	Aluminum hydroxide	13 mEq/2 tsp	14 mg/2 tsp
Basaljel Extra-Strength	Aluminum carbonate	29 mEq/2 tsp	46 mg/2 tsp
Maalox TC	Aluminum hydroxide, magnesium hydroxide	42 mEq/2 tsp	2.4 mg/2 tsp
Maalox Plus	Aluminum hydroxide, magnesium hydroxide, simethicone	11.4 mEq/2 tablets	2.8 mg/2 tablets
Mylanta II	Aluminum hydroxide, magnesium hydroxide, simethicone	36 mEq/2 tsp	2.2 mg/2 tsp
Di-Gel	Aluminum hydroxide, magnesium carbonate, magnesium hydroxide, simethicone	9.4 mEq/2 tablets	10 mg/2 tablets
Gelusil	Aluminum hydroxide, magnesium hydroxide, simethicone	22 mEq/2 tsp	1.4 mg/2 tsp
Milk of Magnesia	Magnesium hydroxide	80 mEq/30 mL	0
Riopan	Magaldrate†	8.8 mEq/5 mL	0.7 mg/5 mL
Titralac	Calcium carbonate, glycine	21 mEq/1 tsp	11 mg/1 tsp
	Calcium carbonate, glycine	19 mEq/2 tablets	0.6 mg/2 tablets
Tums	Calcium carbonate	21 mEq/2 tablets	5.4 mg/2 tablets

*Commercial preparations are frequently reformulated.
†A complex hydroxy-magnesium aluminate.

Therapeutic Uses. Antacids are used for treating peptic ulcers and other HCl-related conditions. Although antacids can produce healing of peptic ulcers, the need for frequent administration makes them inconvenient. Since they relieve pain from hyperacidity, they often are used in conjunction with other drug therapy.

Adverse Reactions. Although antacids have the potential for causing serious physiologic problems, they have a fairly wide safety margin. Clinical problems occur mainly when large doses are prescribed or OTC preparations are seriously abused. An appreciation of the risks of antacid therapy has been slow to develop, and adverse reactions may still be underdiagnosed.

Antacids tend to increase body fluid pH and can cause metabolic alkalosis. Systemic antacids such as sodium bicarbonate are readily absorbed and can cause systemic alkalosis. Nonsystemic antacids are not absorbed systemically to any great extent, except when given in high doses, on a long-term basis, or in clients with certain conditions. Nonsystemic antacids can, however, alter urinary pH and therefore could affect the elimination of other drugs.

The increase in gastric pH stimulates renewed secretion of acid, causing acid rebound, which may be severe. When antacids are the sole treatment agent, they must be administered repeatedly to maintain the lowered acidity. When administration is interrupted during the night, a very low pH may develop in the stomach, reversing the beneficial effects of daytime treatment.

Some adverse effects are specific to the metallic cations present in antacids (Table 28-5). Sodium increases the risk of overhydration and hypervolemia. Aluminum binds with dietary phosphate, forming an undigestable precipitate that is excreted in feces. This is the basis for the use of aluminum-based antacids in treating clients with significant chronic renal failure who have hyperphosphatemia. Aluminum ions inhibit smooth muscle contraction, thereby delaying gastric emptying. Aluminum antacids should be used cautiously in clients with gastric outlet obstruction.

Hypermagnesemia reduces impulse transmission, causing sedation and weakness. Myocardial rhythm is affected by magnesium and calcium. Aluminum and magnesium, which are both neurotoxic, are associated with encephalopathies. High serum levels of metallic ions during pregnancy can affect the fetus. Magnesium-containing antacids should be avoided in clients with significant renal failure.

The heavier metals (calcium, magnesium, and aluminum) form compounds with characteristically poor solubility. They predispose the client to calculi formations in both the GI tract and the renal system.

Aluminum and calcium compounds cause constipation; sodium and magnesium have a laxative effect. Both disturbances are common problems in antacid therapy. Drug manufacturers produce multiple preparations with varying combinations of antacids to try to balance the effects on bowel function and to minimize

Table 28-5. Adverse Reactions to Metallic Elements of Antacids

Ion	Adverse Reactions
Sodium	Water retention (increased risk of edema, over-hydration, hypervolemia, ascites, effusion, hypertension, premenstrual tension, heart failure)
	Reduced iron absorption
Calcium	Constipation
	Milk-alkali syndrome (including pronounced alkalosis)
	Rebound hyperacidity
	Potentiation of digitalis
	Renal calculi
	Impaired absorption of such drugs as tetracycline and iron
Magnesium	Diarrhea (increased risk of hypokalemia)
	Iron deficiency due to complexation of iron
	Hypermagnesemia (causing sedation, weakness, cardiac arrhythmias, and encephalopathy), especially in persons with renal impairment
	Impaired absorption of such drugs as tetracycline and iron
Aluminum	Constipation
	Binds with dietary phosphate, leading to phosphate depletion and osteomalacia
	Delayed gastric emptying
	Intestinal concretions (increased risk of colonic perforation and peritonitis)
	Encephalopathy
	Impairment of absorption of such drugs as tetracycline, digitalis, and isoniazid

these problems. Individual responses to the formulas vary. It is often necessary to try several products to determine the best one.

Milk-alkali syndrome, which can result in hypercalcemia and renal failure, may result from a high intake of calcium in antacids (or in milk or calcium supplements). An estimated 4 to 60 g of calcium carbonate can precipitate the syndrome (Newmark & Nugent, 1993).

Some antacid preparations contain sugar, which could lead to hyperglycemia in diabetic clients.

Drug Interactions. Antacids interact with many other drug agents. Within the GI tract, they combine chemically with some drugs, notably tetracycline antibiotics, forming complexes that resist digestion and pass unchanged out of the system. When administered with enteric-coated drugs, they may disintegrate the coating, releasing these drugs prematurely in the stomach. Elevations of pH also alter membrane transport of alkaline and acidic compounds, promoting passive diffusion of acidic chemicals and lipid membrane transport of alkaline chemicals. Passive diffusion of alkaline substances and lipid membrane transport of acidic substances are

inhibited. These effects can alter both absorption and excretion of many systemic drugs.

Digitalis is potentiated by hypercalcemia; calcium directly augments the ionic stimulation of cardiac contractility, thereby mimicking the action of digitalis. Magnesium may also potentiate digitalis by depleting potassium stores (causing hypokalemia) secondary to diarrhea.

Precautions and Contraindications. A certain percentage of most antacids is absorbed, altering blood chemistry and elevating the serum levels of individual metals. Sodium is contraindicated in many persons for whom water retention is harmful. Even healthy persons should avoid excessive sodium intake, which is associated with hypertension.

Magnesium and aluminum compounds should be used with caution by persons with impaired kidney function.

Antacid regimens should be tailored to the individual needs of clients. For example, combinations of both laxative and constipating agents may be needed to maintain normal fecal elimination.

■ SUMMARY

Antacids are basic compounds that act locally in the stomach to neutralize HCl and to protect the gastric mucosa. They are comparable to histamine (H$_2$) receptor antagonists in cost and effectiveness as antiulcer drugs. However, they must be administered more often than histamine (H$_2$) receptor antagonists. Antacids may alter the absorption of other drugs administered at the same time. They can also cause adverse reactions due to the local and systemic actions of the cation (metallic) portion of the molecules.

Sucralfate

Sucralfate is an anionic sulfated disaccharide structurally related to heparin.

Pharmacodynamics. Sucralfate's therapeutic effects appear to be local (ie, at ulcer sites in the upper GI tract) rather than systemic. Sucralfate reacts with HCl in the stomach to form a pastelike substance that is highly viscous and adhesive. This material binds to the surface of the GI mucosa, exhibiting a pronounced affinity for ulcer sites. Sucralfate does not reduce gastric acid output or concentration. The combination of a mechanical barrier and local acid neutralization may be important for protecting the ulcer site from the actions of pepsin, acid, and bile.

Pharmacokinetics. After oral administration, sucralfate is minimally absorbed from the GI tract. Only 3% to 5% of an oral dose reaches the systemic circulation as sucrose sulfate. Distribution has not been determined, and it is unknown whether sucralfate crosses the placenta or is distributed in breast milk. Most of the drug administered orally remains in the GI tract and is eliminated in feces. The small amount absorbed is excreted unchanged by the kidneys.

Therapeutic Uses. Sucralfate is approved for short-term treatment of duodenal ulcers. It has also been used for treating oral ulcers and gastric ulcers, as well as for preventing aspirin-induced gastric erosions. It also is used for preventing stress ulcers and GI bleeding in critically ill clients. The usual adult dosage is a 1-g tablet orally four times daily for 4 to 8 weeks.

Adverse Reactions. Sucralfate is generally well tolerated. Constipation affects about 2% of recipients; nausea, diarrhea, gastric discomfort, indigestion, dry mouth, rash, pruritus, back pain, dizziness, sleepiness, and vertigo have also been reported.

Drug Interactions. Sucralfate may bind to other oral drugs (cimetidine, phenytoin, tetracycline), reducing their bioavailability. Antacids should not be given within 30 minutes of sucralfate.

Precautions and Contraindications. Safety and efficacy in children have not been established. Evidence concerning mutagenicity, carcinogenicity, and teratogenicity of the drug is incomplete. Safe use during pregnancy and lactation has not been established. Because a small amount of aluminum is absorbed systemically during sucralfate therapy, the use of aluminum-containing antacids should be avoided in clients with chronic renal failure.

■ SUMMARY

Sucralfate is an antiulcer drug that acts mechanically by forming a protective coating over the ulcer site. It appears to be comparable in efficacy to antacids and histamine (H_2) receptor antagonists. Adverse reactions are relatively minor, affecting mainly the GI tract.

Misoprostol

Misoprostol (Cytotec) is a synthetic analog of prostaglandin E_1 (alprostadil).

Pharmacodynamics. It acts as a gastric antisecretory agent that reduces gastric acid secretion and also protects the mucosa from the irritant effects of drugs such as NSAID antirheumatics. It is believed that misoprostol exerts the same protective effects as does alprostadil, a prostaglandin that is antagonized by NSAIDs. The effects of misoprostol appear to be local rather than systemic.

Pharmacokinetics. Misoprostol is rapidly and completely absorbed from the GI tract. It is rapidly metabolized to an active metabolite, misoprostol acid, and two inactive metabolites. Food and antacids decrease the extent and delay the rate of systemic absorption. Although its action is local, the effects of misoprostol may be prolonged due to secretion of its active metabolite

into the GI tract from the blood. Misoprostol is widely distributed in test animals.

Onset of action occurs within minutes; action peaks at 60 to 90 minutes and lasts about 3 hours. Misoprostol acid (the active metabolite of misoprostol) is 80% to 90% protein bound. Distribution across the placenta or into milk is unknown.

Misoprostol and its metabolites are excreted primarily by the kidneys. Small amounts appear in the feces, probably via biliary elimination. Accumulation does not appear to occur with chronic administration. Serum half-life of the misoprostol acid is biphasic: 1.5 hours during the distribution phase and 20 to 40 minutes during the elimination phase. The drug is not removed by hemodialysis.

Therapeutic Uses. Misoprostol is used for preventing and treating NSAID-induced gastric ulcers in persons at high risk of developing complications from these ulcers, and for treating duodenal ulcers.

Dosage and Administration. Misoprostol is marketed as tablets containing 100 or 200 µg each. It is administered four times a day (after meals and at bedtime) in doses of 100 to 200 µg for up to 8 weeks. Dosage may be reduced for clients with renal impairment.

Adverse Reactions. Adverse effects involving the GI tract (diarrhea, nausea, abdominal pain) occur in up to 40% of recipients. Diarrhea is dose-related and usually self-limiting, lasting about 1 week.

Other adverse effects are less common. Reported CNS effects include headache, fatigue, dizziness, and anxiety. Other reactions involve the following systems: genitourinary and renal (menstrual irregularities, polyuria, dysuria, hematuria, urinary tract infection), hematologic (anemia, thrombocytopenia, increased sedimentation rate), sensory (visual abnormalities, conjunctivitis, earache, tinnitus, deafness), dermatologic (rash, dermatitis, alopecia, purpura), cardiovascular (blood-pressure changes, cardiac arrhythmias, phlebitis, angina, chest pain, edema), hepatic (altered liver function tests), and respiratory (infection, bronchospasm, epistaxis). Misoprostol can also cause abortion, fever, thirst, breast pain, impotence, arthralgia, myalgia, stiffness, back pain, and weight changes.

Drug Interactions. Misoprostol should not be used concurrently with magnesium antacids or other laxative preparations. To date, misoprostol appears to interact with few drugs. It has been effective in reversing cyclosporine toxicity in animals.

Precautions and Contraindications. Misoprostol is contraindicated in pregnant women (it causes uterine contractions) and clients with allergic hypersensitivity to prostaglandins. It is not recommended during lactation.

As a relatively new drug, misoprostol may produce other adverse effects not noted or reported to date.

Package inserts should be read each time a new supply is obtained because the information may be updated.

Caution should be used when the drug is prescribed for clients with inflammatory bowel disease or those prone to dehydration. Safety and efficacy in clients younger than age 18 have not been established.

■ SUMMARY

Several drugs act to inhibit acid production by the gastric mucosa or to protect the gastric mucosa. They are effective agents for treating peptic ulcers and are often used to prevent stress ulcers. Adverse reactions to this group of drugs are uncommon but are variable and affect many body systems. The nurse must monitor for and educate clients about signs and symptoms of adverse effects. The recent OTC availability of some of these drugs indicates the need to teach clients about appropriate use.

❖ NURSING MANAGEMENT: CLIENT RECEIVING DRUG THERAPY FOR GASTRIC ACID PROBLEMS

Treatment for acid-related problems is required in various conditions. Prescription of the drugs discussed above is an indication that the recipient is at risk; therefore, nursing measures to minimize acid secretion and enhance protection of the gastric mucosa are appropriate.

Because stress is believed to contribute to gastric acid production (by parasympathetic activity and secretion of adrenergic and glucocorticoid hormones), nursing measures to reduce stress along with drug therapy are therapeutic for the client suffering from hyperacidity. The nurse can help clients develop strategies for managing unavoidable stress. Periodic diversion is helpful when situational stress cannot be eliminated.

Smoking and alcohol consumption should be discouraged. So-called ulcer diets are no longer in common use, but adaptation of food intake is important. Any food that the client recognizes as contributing to symptoms of hyperacidity should be omitted. Coffee, chocolate, and foods rich in carbohydrates, fats, and spices may increase symptoms. The client should be urged to eliminate these items temporarily from the diet, then to test them individually for tolerance before resuming consumption.

Drug-induced ulcerations and bleeding are associated with certain antiinflammatory drugs such as steroids and NSAIDs. These potentially serious adverse effects are believed to result from the antiprostaglandin effect of these drugs, which weakens the gastric mucosa. NSAIDs also have a local irritant effect on the stomach. Bleeding from NSAID-induced ulcerations can be life-threatening and can occur without warning ulcer pain, especially in older adults. Clients must be taught to take NSAIDs with food and only as necessary. Because many NSAIDs are available without a prescription, education is needed.

Drug Therapy for Peptic Ulcers. Peptic ulcer disease is characterized by remissions and exacerbations. Multiple drugs, a modified diet, and rest are usually prescribed. Adherence to the medical regimen, although likely to fluctuate with the severity of symptoms, is vital to recovery. Continuous therapy is usually necessary for long periods. Research findings on antibiotic therapy for eradicating *H pylori* infection indicate remissions in up to 90% of clients who successfully complete therapy.

Drug Therapy for Gastroesophageal Reflux. In this disorder, the stomach contents reflux (back up) into the esophagus, irritating and damaging the esophageal mucosa. This can result in aspiration, strictures, hemorrhage, and perforation. The damage mechanisms are similar to those of peptic ulcer—an imbalance between hyperacidity and mucosal integrity. Treatment agents, therefore, include those used to treat peptic ulcer disease (histamine [H$_2$] receptor antagonists and proton pump inhibitors). An additional mechanism contributing to reflux is relaxation of the lower esophageal sphincter; drugs to stimulate gastric propulsion also may be used, such as bethanechol (Urecholine), metoclopramide (Reglan), and cisapride (Propulsid).

Besides encouraging adherence to the drug regimen, the nurse must also encourage measures to decrease reflux—for example, dietary adaptations (avoiding fatty meals, chocolate, alcohol, spearmint or peppermint, citric juices, cola, and milk), losing weight and wearing loose clothing, quitting smoking (smoking decreases lower esophageal sphincter pressure), and elevating the head of the bed 6" to 8".

Adherence to Drug Therapy. The critical nature of complications makes adherence to the therapeutic regimen especially important. Assessing compliance and intervening to encourage it are important nursing functions. Many clients omit doses of medications because the preparation is unpalatable, expensive, or inconvenient to carry (especially the liquid antacids).

Although the overall cost of histamine (H$_2$) receptor inhibitors and antacids is comparable, only prescription drugs are covered by most insurance plans. Hence, the client usually must bear all the cost of antacid treatment or OTC preparations of histamine (H$_2$) receptor antagonists.

Distressing adverse reactions can also reduce clients' motivation to adhere to the dosage schedule. Identifying and eliminating specific impediments to acceptance of the drug regimen are critical in improving adherence.

NURSING PROCESS

ASSESSMENT

Clients being treated for hyperacidity should be evaluated to determine their general health and nutritional status. If peptic ulcer disease has been diagnosed, the nurse should look for signs and symptoms of anemia, which can develop when ulcers bleed. The nature, severity, and chronology of pain associated with hyperacidity should be delineated. Stress levels and stress reduction skills should be evaluated. A complete drug history should be taken, with particular attention to NSAIDs and other medications likely to stimulate acid production.

NURSING DIAGNOSIS

Clients for whom medication is prescribed to relieve problems of hyperacidity and GI mucosal integrity may have:

- Knowledge Deficit, related to hyperacidity and drugs used for its treatment

Clients for whom histamine (H_2) receptor antagonists are prescribed may develop:

- Pain: Headache, muscle pains, bone and joint pain related to use of histamine (H_2) receptor antagonists
- Sexual Dysfunction: Decreased libido and potency secondary to cimetidine therapy

Common collaborative problems that should be differentiated from the nursing diagnoses include:

- Potential Complication: Hypovolemic shock related to hemorrhage, CNS effects, hepatotoxicity, or renal toxicity

Clients receiving misoprostol or proton pump inhibitors may develop:

- Pain, related to intestinal upset, nausea, vomiting, or abdominal discomfort
- Diarrhea

Clients receiving antacids are likely to develop:

- Constipation, related to use of aluminum or calcium antacids
- Diarrhea, related to the use of magnesium antacids

Clients receiving sucralfate may develop:

- Constipation or Diarrhea, related to adverse reaction to medication

A common collaborative problem related to antacid therapy that should be differentiated from the nursing diagnosis is:

Potential Complication: Phosphate deficiency or milk–alkali syndrome

PLANNING

Goals for nursing care and treatment include increased gastric pH, decreased pain, prompt detection and treatment of upper GI bleeding (if it develops), maintenance of normal fecal elimination, prompt detection and treatment of other adverse reactions to antihyperacidity medications, prevention of adverse drug interactions, and client education about hyperacidity and its prevention and treatment.

INTERVENTION

The nurse should regularly assess clients receiving antihyperacidity drugs for therapeutic response, gastric bleeding, known adverse reactions to prescribed drugs, changes indicative of previously unidentified adverse reactions, and adherence to the drug regimen. Reports of epigastric discomfort and tenderness or heartburn are significant indicators of continued tissue damage from excess acid. Symptoms attributable to hyperacidity should decline with treatment. Gastric bleeding may be detected by testing stools for occult blood, or by the presence of tarry stools or coffee-ground emesis.

Particular attention should be paid to signs and symptoms of alkalosis, changes in bowel function, and specific effects of the metallic ions contained in some of the drugs. Fecal elimination should be monitored; nursing measures may be used to alleviate mild constipation or diarrhea.

Clients receiving sucralfate, misoprostol, proton pump inhibitors, or histamine (H_2) receptor antagonists must be carefully evaluated for side effects and adverse reactions. Although they appear to have wide margins of safety, they are relatively new drugs and may have unrecognized potential for toxic effects.

The prescriber should be informed of the therapeutic response to the drug regimen and any complications (eg, gastric bleeding). The nurse should also consult the prescriber for possible changes in the drug regimen if the client develops adverse drug reactions (eg, persistent or severe constipation or diarrhea, impaired kidney or liver function, discomfiting CNS changes, susceptibility to infection, pain).

When oral antacids are administered, tablets should be chewed or sucked to dissolve the medication before being swallowed. The drugs will not combine efficiently with acid unless they reach the stomach in a solution or a finely divided form. When liquid antacids are administered, each dose should have sufficient volume and neutralizing capacity to reach the stomach. Small amounts of water may be given with antacids, but large amounts (more than 4 oz) stimulate gastric emptying and may propel the medication promptly into the small bowel.

Palatability is an important consideration. Plain compounds tend to taste chalky. Flavored preparations are available for many formulations.

Client Education. Clients requiring antacid prescriptions tend to take inadequate amounts, but the lay public generally overuses self-prescribed agents. The public has been conditioned to regard antacids as convenient home remedies for relieving minor symptoms, rather than as drugs for treating illness. Family traditions of dosing with antacids, advertisements extolling the virtues of fast relief for overindulgence, and the reluctance of medical insurance plans to pay for antacid therapy are some of the reasons antacids have been traditionally accepted as casual remedies. Their value as an effective treatment, with risks of adverse reactions and toxicity, is not appreciated. See the Critical Thinking Challenge.

Nurses who educate the public about self-medication should discourage the use of antacids and OTC histamine (H_2) receptor antagonists (cimetidine, famotidine, ranitidine) except in isolated incidents clearly related to unusual circumstances. Occasional self-medication to relieve distressing symptoms of overindulgence will probably cause no serious problems. More frequent use and the need for unusual doses are warning signals, and clients should be urged to seek medical attention to determine the underlying problem. A peptic ulcer, hiatal hernia, or other disorder may need treatment. Such treatment may well include continued use of antacids and histamine (H_2) antagonists, but in a more definitive fashion, with careful selection of the proper agent, a regular schedule of specific doses, and medical supervision.

Clients should be cautioned particularly against using sodium bicarbonate (baking soda) as an antacid. Although temporarily effective in relieving hyperacidity, sodium bicarbonate reacts with acid to generate a considerable amount of carbon dioxide gas, causing dangerous stomach distention. If part of the stomach wall is weakened, as in gastric ulcer disease, perforation can occur. This is a potentially fatal condition requiring immediate medical attention. Other problems related to using sodium bicarbonate are pronounced acid rebound and significant alkalosis (the chemical is easily and completely absorbed). Sodium bicarbonate's high sodium content can seriously disturb electrolyte balance and is particularly detrimental to persons who should restrict their sodium intake. Abdominal pain or heartburn is sometimes experienced during cardiac ischemia or infarction. Self-treatment with sodium bicarbonate can be detrimental if it causes a delay in seeking medical attention. Moreover, large doses of sodium in such situations predispose the client to congestive heart failure.

Clients taking NSAIDs (including aspirin) must learn about the danger of peptic ulceration and GI bleeding.

Nurses must stress that adherence to the prescribed regimen is critical to aid healing and to prevent complications, even when hyperacidity is in remission.

OUTCOME EVALUATION

Data needed for evaluation include gastric pH values, the client's report of increased comfort and decreased constipation or diarrhea, and evidence of the duration and severity of adverse drug reactions. (See Example of Nursing Process for Ranitidine and Antacid Therapy.)

❖ CHECKLIST OF NURSING ACTIONS

- ❏ Urge clients who frequently self-administer antacids to seek medical care to determine the cause of their symptoms.
- ❏ When drugs are prescribed to combat hyperacidity, help the client reduce stress levels and manage unavoidable stress effectively.
- ❏ Discourage smoking and alcohol consumption by clients with hyperacidity.
- ❏ Help clients identify and eliminate from their diets foods that stimulate acid secretion.
- ❏ Monitor clients receiving drugs to combat hyperacidity for therapeutic and adverse effects of the drugs.
- ❏ Instruct clients to chew antacid tablets thoroughly before swallowing.
- ❏ Supervise clients' use of antacids when these drugs are left at the bedside in institutional settings.
- ❏ Stress the importance of adherence to the medication regimen for preventing disease progression.
- ❏ Warn clients not to use baking soda as an antacid.
- ❏ Urge clients receiving new drugs, such as misoprostol or omeprazole, to report unusual signs and symptoms.

CRITICAL THINKING CHALLENGE
Issues Analysis

Many persons assign too much or too little value to advertising—especially advertising of drug products. As more and more drugs are available without a prescription, it becomes important for healthcare personnel to scrutinize and then educate clients about advertisers' claims.

Select an advertisement for an antacid or OTC histamine (H_2) receptor antagonist appearing in print or on TV or radio. Analyze the advertisement in terms of the stated message, the implied message, and the accuracy and adequacy of the information provided to the consumer.

1. What is the direct message?
2. Identify the intended audience. What persons of what age or condition are targeted?
3. Analyze the elements in the ad (color, design, pictures, symbols, action or gestures, dialogue). What do the elements imply?
4. Does the ad truthfully portray the approved indications of the advertised drug? Why or why not?

Antiemetics

Nausea and vomiting are common problems that require skilled nursing care. They herald the onset of many acute illnesses and accompany chronic illnesses, drug reactions, emotional disturbances, and pregnancy. Few symptoms are more distressing.

Pathophysiology

The vomiting reflex is complex and not well understood. Impulses from the cerebral cortex, the aural vestibular apparatus, and all parts of the GI tract stimu-

Example of Nursing Process for Ranitidine and Antacid Therapy

The client is a 65-year-old machinist with a long-standing history of peptic ulcer disease. He has been treated with antacids (Mylanta II, 15 mL q2h PRN), which he takes regularly after meals and at bedtime and at other times when heartburn occurs. Until recently, he has had no pronounced signs or symptoms of recurrent ulcers for over 5 years. Six months ago, he retired from his job. He consulted the physician because he has had increased heartburn and epigastric pain for several days, which the antacids do not control. An upper GI x-ray series reveals a small duodenal ulcer. The physician has prescribed ranitidine 150 mg bid and continued use of antacids PRN.

Assessment Data

The client complains of heartburn and epigastric pain that persists despite antacid medication

Medical diagnosis of duodenal peptic ulcer

Recent retirement

New prescription for ranitidine

Nursing Diagnosis	Intervention	Goals and Outcomes
Pain: Epigastric pain and heartburn related to inflammation and irritation secondary to hyperacidity and peptic ulcer; possible contributing factor, the stress of retirement	**Recommend** that the client continue to take a dose of antacid after meals and at bedtime until he is pain-free. **Instruct** the client to take ranitidine at 12-hour intervals, to maximize its inhibitory effect on stomach secretion of HCl. **Explore** with the client stressors affecting him since his retirement; help him decrease them. Review with the client stress management techniques he has used in the past; teach new techniques as appropriate.	Within a week the client will report that he is having little or no heartburn or epigastric pain.
Knowledge Deficit, relating to ranitidine and histamine (H_2) receptor antagonists	**Inform** the client that a few people who take ranitidine experience adverse reactions. Instruct him to report to his primary healthcare provider if he develops persistent, severe headaches, muscle or joint pains, or signs and symptoms of CNS disturbance. Inform the client that ranitidine is a fairly new drug and that it may have some adverse effects that remained unreported; advise the client to inform his primary healthcare provider of any unusual changes that coincide with the use of ranitidine.	The client will report significant signs and symptoms to the nurse or prescriber.

late the medullary centers that mediate the reflex. Many impulses are transmitted to the chemoreceptor trigger zone (CTZ) before the vomiting center goes into action. Impulses from the vomiting center stimulate a sequence of motor actions in the upper GI tract, which result in rapid emptying of the stomach. Closely associated with the vomiting center is an area whose excitation produces the sensation of nausea. Nausea is often accompanied by symptoms of autonomic (mainly parasympathetic) stimulation: increased perspiration, salivation, pallor, bradycardia, and hypotension.

Some reports of vomiting are actually regurgitation, not true vomiting. The nurse must be able to assess the phenomenon described to determine the appropriate nursing response (Table 28-6). Regurgitation is a relatively passive emission of material from the upper GI tract due to various mechanical factors, such as incomplete swallowing, eructation, or aspiration. Vomiting is characterized by reverse peristalsis, which forcibly empties the stomach.

Causes of vomiting are many, ranging from pregnancy to serious pathology. A complete assessment must be performed to determine the reason for the problem. The best approach is to eliminate the cause, but if it is impossible to correct the underlying pathology, measures are required to control nausea and reduce vomiting.

Table 28-6. Causes of Regurgitation and Vomiting

Patterns of Regurgitation or Vomiting	Associated Causative Conditions
Regurgitation	
Nonforcible regurgitation of undigested food or fluids, often during coughing episodes	Esophageal diverticula
	Insufficiency of gag reflex, leading to aspiration
Spitting up of small amounts of formula by infants	Propulsion of formula upward by gas bubbles during burping
Vomiting	
Vomiting after eating	Gastric irritability
	Presence of potent irritants in food
Deliberate or self-induced	Bulimia
Early-morning vomiting	Postnasal drip
	Pregnancy
	Uremia
	Chronic alcoholism
Forceful (projectile) vomiting, often without nausea	Pyloric stenosis
	Increased intracranial pressure
Bloody or coffee-ground emesis	Gastric bleeding
Vomitus of digested food 12 or more hours after eating	Duodenal obstruction
Vomitus of food with bile	Obstruction below the ampulla of Vater
Fecal vomiting	Obstruction low in the digestive tract
	Peritonitis
	Gastrocolonic fistula

Classification of Antiemetics

Antiemetic drugs are helpful adjuncts in controlling nausea and reducing vomiting. Selected antiemetics are listed in Table 28-7. The vomiting reflex can be interrupted at any point on its pathway. If vomiting is caused by GI irritation or pain, drugs given to reduce these problems may exert an antiemetic effect. Some general CNS depressants, such as phenobarbital, also suppress vomiting. The drugs generally classified as antiemetics act on the vomiting center, the CTZ, or the aural vestibular apparatus. Most of these drugs are anticholinergics, antihistamines, or phenothiazines (see Chaps. 16, 34, and 20, respectively).

The *anticholinergics* depress excitatory labyrinthine impulses in the vestibular nuclei. Their GI effects (decreased motility, secretion, and spasm) also tend to reduce enteric stimulation of the vomiting center. Of this group of drugs, scopolamine is most commonly used for antiemetic effect. It has a high incidence of anticholinergic side effects, such as tachycardia, palpitations, dry mouth, constipation, urinary hesitancy, urinary retention, impotence, dizziness, nervousness, and blurred vision. Because of its mydriatic effect, scopolamine is contraindicated in glaucoma.

The *antihistamines* depress selected portions of the CNS, but their antiemetic effects appear to be due in large part to their anticholinergic properties. Hydroxyzine (Vistaril) and dimenhydrate (Dramamine) are common antihistamine antiemetics. Dimenhydrate is often used to prevent motion sickness. In addition to anticholinergic side effects, antihistamines frequently cause drowsiness. See Chapter 34 for a detailed discussion of antihistamines.

Like antihistamines, *phenothiazines* are CNS depressants. Major antipsychotics, they are often prescribed to promote tranquility. They have antidopaminergic effects and are effective antiemetics, especially for drug-induced nausea and vomiting, but they carry a high risk of side effects. They are ineffective in the control of motion sickness. To avoid serious adverse reactions, prolonged use and high doses should be avoided. See Chapter 20 for a detailed discussion of phenothiazines.

Serotonin inhibitors are a relatively new type of antiemetic used in treating nausea and vomiting caused by cancer chemotherapy. They are believed to act by blocking 5-hydroxytryptamine (5-HT3) serotonin receptors in the chemoreceptor zone and on vagal nerve endings.

Many antiemetic drugs pose a risk of fetal damage, so their use should be avoided during pregnancy. Careful consideration of risks and benefits to both the mother and fetus must be weighed before prescribing antiemetics to pregnant women.

Benzquinamide

Benzquinamide (Emete-Con) is a benzoquinolizine derivative chemically unrelated to phenothiazine or antihistamine antiemetics.

Pharmacodynamics. The antiemetic effect of benzquinamide is thought to be due to its depressant action on the CTZ for emesis.

Pharmacokinetics. Benzquinamide is rapidly absorbed after oral, intramuscular (IM), or rectal administration. After absorption, it is distributed throughout body tissues. Protein binding is about 55% to 60%. It is unknown whether the drug enters the cerebrospinal fluid, crosses the placenta, or appears in breast milk. Benzquinamide is rapidly metabolized by the liver and excreted in the urine and the bile. Half-life is about 30 to 40 minutes.

Therapeutic Uses. Benzquinamide is used for preventing and treating nausea and vomiting associated with anesthesia and surgery.

Adverse Reactions. The most common adverse reaction to benzquinamide is drowsiness. CNS stimulation can also occur, as manifested by tremor, insomnia, restlessness, headache, excitement, and nervousness. GI

Text continues on page 589.

Table 28-7. Selected Antiemetic Drugs

Drug Name	Preparation	Mode of Action	Usual Dosage	Additional Information
Anticholinergics				
scopolamine (Transderm-Scop; *Can:* Transderm V)	Transdermal patch for topical application	Depression of labyrinthine impulses in the vestibular nucleus	Adults: one system programmed to deliver 0.5 mg of scopolamine over 72 hr PC: C	Scopolamine is considered one of the most effective drugs for the treatment of motion sickness, but it causes a high incidence of anticholinergic side effects.
Antihistamines				
buclizine (Bucladin-S)	Oral tablets	Depression of labyrinthine excitability and conduction in vestibular-cerebellar pathways	Adults: 50 mg 30 min before exposure to motion, repeated in 4–6 hr if required PC: C	Antihistamines possess CNS depressant, anticholinergic, anti-spasmodic, and local anesthetic activity. They are used to control motion sickness.
cyclizine (Marezine)	Oral tablets Solution for IM injection	Depression of labyrinthine excitability and conduction in vestibular-cerebellar pathways	Adults: 50 mg 30 min before exposure to motion, repeated in 4–6 hr if required Children: 25 mg 30 min before exposure to motion, repeated in 4–6 hr if required PC: C	
dimenhydrinate (Dramamine, *Can:* Gravol)	Oral tablets and solution Solution for IM or IV injection	Inhibition of vestibular stimulation, probably by inhibition of acetylcholine in the otolith system and the semicircular canals	Adults: 50–100 mg q4h PRN Children 2–5 yr: 12.5–25 mg PO up to tid Children 6–12 yr: 25–50 mg PO up to tid PC: B	
hydroxyzine (Anxanil, Atarax, Hyzine, Orgatrex, Vistacon, Vistaject, Vistaquel, Vistaril, Vistazine; *Can:* Multipax)	Oral tablets, capsules, solution, suspension Solution for IM injection	Possibly CNS inhibition of acetylcholine	Adults: *Oral:* 25–100 mg tid or qid PRN; *IM:* 50–100 mg q4–6h PRN Children: 1.1 mg/kg PC: C	Hydroxyzine is used to control nausea caused by radiation therapy, drug reactions, and surgery, as well as motion sickness.
meclizine (Antivert, Antrizene, Bonine, Dizmiss, Motion Cure, Ru-Vert M; *Can:* Bonamine)	Oral tablets, chewable tablets, chewable capsules	Depression of labyrinthine excitability and conduction in vestibular-cerebellar pathways	Adults: *For prevention of motion sickness:* 25–50 mg 1 hr before exposure to motion, repeated q24h PRN; *for control of vertigo:* 25–100 mg/day, in divided doses PC: B	Safety and efficacy of meclizine in children younger than 12 yr have not been established.
Phenothiazines				
chlorpromazine (Thorazine, Ormazine; *Can:* Largactil)	Oral tablets, solution, extended-release capsules Rectal suppositories Solutions for IM or IV injection	Possibly depression of the medullary CTZ by blockade of dopamine receptors	Adults: *Oral:* 10–25 mg q4–6h PRN; *rectal:* 100 mg q6–8h PRN; *IM:* initially 25 mg, then 25–50 mg q3–4h PRN as tolerated Children 6 mo or older: *Oral:* 0.55 mg/kg q4–6h PRN; *rectal:* 1.1 mg/kg q6–8h PRN; *IM:* initially 0.55 mg/kg q6–8h PRN PC: C	Phenothiazines are not effective in the control of motion sickness; they are used to control nausea caused by uremia, gastroenteritis, radiation sickness, carcinoma, and drug reactions.

KEY: PC = Pregnancy risk category; see Appendix A.
Can: Canadian trade name.

(continued)

Table 28-7. (Continued)

Drug Name	Preparation	Mode of Action	Usual Dosage	Additional Information
perphenazine (Trilafon)	Oral tablets and liquid Solution for injection	Antidopaminergic	Adults: *Oral:* 8–16 mg daily in divided doses; *IM:* 5 mg q6h PRN; *IV:* 5 mg Children 12 yrs or older: *IM:* 5 mg	When given IV, client must be in recumbent position.
prochlorperazine (Compazine; Ultrazine; *Can:* Provacin, Stemetil)	Oral tablets, solution, extended-release capsules Rectal suppositories Solutions for IV or deep IM injection	Possibly depression of medullary CTZ by blockade of dopamine receptors	Adults: *Oral:* (prompt) 5–10 mg tid or qid PRN; (extended-release) 15 mg once daily on arising PRN; or 10 mg q12h PRN; *rectal:* 25 mg bid PRN; *IM:* 5–10 mg, q3–4h PRN (maximum daily IM dosage: 40 mg) Children: *Oral:* (depending on weight) 2.5–10 mg/day, in divided doses; *IM:* 130 µg/kg/day, divided in 3 or 4 equal doses PC: C	
promethazine (Anergan, Phenazine, Phenergan, Prorex, Prothazine, Remsed, V-Gan; *Can:* Histanil)	Oral tablets and solutions Rectal suppositories Solutions for IM or IV injection	Depression of the CNS and inhibition of acetylcholine	Adults: 12.5–25 mg q4h PRN Children: 0.25–0.5 mg/kg, 4–6 times daily PRN Maximum rate of IV administration: 25 mg/min; maximum solution concentration for IV administration: 25 mg/mL PC: C	Also used as antihistamine and as adjunct to anesthesia.
Benzoquinolizine				
benzquinamide (Emete-Con)	Solution for IM or IV injection	Depression of the medullary CTZ	Adults: 0.5–1.0 mg/kg administered 15 min before emergence from anesthesia and repeated in 1 hr if required; subsequent doses q3–4h PRN	Benzquinamide is used for the prevention of postoperative nausea and vomiting when vomiting endangers the client or the results of surgery. Claims of freedom from hypotensive or autonomic effects are unproven. IV injection may cause sudden increase in blood pressure and cardiac arrhythmias; IV doses must be administered slowly.
Serotonin Receptor Inhibitors				
granisetron (Kytril)	Solution for IV infusion	Selective 5-HT3 serotonin receptor antagonism	Adults and children 2–16 yr: *IV:* 10 mcg/kg given within 30 min before initiation of chemotherapy PC: B	

KEY: PC = Pregnancy risk category; see Appendix A.
Can: Canadian trade name.

(continued)

Table 28-7. (Continued)

Drug Name	Preparation	Mode of Action	Usual Dosage	Additional Information
Serotonin Receptor Inhibitors (continued)				
ondanestron (Zofran)	Tablets or solution for IV infusion	Selective 5-HT3 serotonin receptor antagonism	Adults and children 12 yr or older: *Oral:* 8 mg q8h Children 4–12 yr: *Oral:* 4 mg q8h Adults and children 4–18 yrs: *IV:* three 0.15-mg/kg doses beginning 30 min before start of chemotherapy and then 4 and 8 hr after first dose	
Cannabis Derivative				
dronabinol (Marinol)	Liquid-filled oral capsules	Unknown	5 mg/m² 1–3 hr before antineoplastic chemotherapy treatment PC: B	CNS phenomena associated with marijuana use (hallucinations) may occur.
Unclassified				
metoclopramide (Clora, Reglan, Maxolon, Octamide, Reclomide; *Can:* Emex, Maxeran)	Oral tablets and solution Solution for IM or IV injection	Blockade of dopamine receptors in the medullary CTZ	Adults: *Oral:* 10 mg qid, ac and hs *IV:* (in antineoplastic therapy) 1–2 mg/kg 30 min before administration of an emetogenic drug, repeated q2–3h PRN PC: B	Metoclopramide is used to control emesis caused by antineoplastic chemotherapy. Metoclopramide is contraindicated in persons with pheochromocytoma or in whom increased GI motility might be dangerous.
trimethobenzamide (T-Gen, Tegamide, Ticon, Tigan, Arrestin, Benzacot, Brogan)	Oral capsules Rectal suppositories Solution for IM injection	Possibly inhibition of stimuli at the medullary CTZ	Adults: *Oral:* 250 mg tid or qid PRN; *IM or rectal:* 200 mg tid or qid Children: *Oral and rectal:* 15–20 mg/kg/day divided in 3 or 4 doses PC: C	Trimethobenzamide exhibits a weak antihistaminic activity.

KEY: PC = Pregnancy risk category; see Appendix A.
Can: Canadian trade name.

side effects include dry mouth, hiccups, anorexia, nausea, vomiting, abdominal cramps, and salivation. Shivering, sweating, flushing, weakness, and fatigue have been reported. Cardiovascular effects, which include alterations in blood pressure, atrial fibrillation, and premature atrial and ventricular contractions are associated with IV administration.

Precautions and Contraindications. Whenever possible, IV administration of benzquinamide should be avoided. This route is contraindicated for clients with cardiovascular disease or those who have received drugs that alter blood pressure or cause arrhythmias. Benzquinamide is also contraindicated for persons allergic to it.

Use of benzquinamide may mask the signs and symptoms of conditions such as intestinal obstruction, brain tumor, or drug overdose, so these conditions should be ruled out before the drug is administered.

Diphenidol

Pharmacodynamics. The mode of action of diphenidol (Vontrol) has not been explained, but it is believed to inhibit the medullary CTZ and conduction in vestibular-cerebellar pathways.

Pharmacokinetics. Diphenidol is well absorbed when administered orally or IM. Distribution is unknown. The drug is metabolized to inactive compounds; excretion is mainly in urine, with small amounts eliminated in feces. Biologic half-life has been reported as about 4 hours.

Therapeutic Uses. Diphenidol is used to control nausea and vomiting associated with surgery, malignant tumors, antineoplastic chemotherapy, radiation sickness, infectious disease, and labyrinthine disturbances, including those associated with Meniere's disease (hearing loss, tinnitus, vertigo) and surgery of the middle and inner ear.

Adverse Reactions. Diphenidol can produce CNS effects, including drowsiness, mental depression, sleep disturbances, blurred vision, dizziness, headache, visual and auditory hallucinations, disorientation, and confusion. Although they affect less than 1% of clients receiving the drug, acute reactions can be disturbing. Other signs and symptoms of adverse reactions to diphenidol include dry mouth, nausea, indigestion, rash, malaise, palpitation, and heartburn. Injection may cause transient decreases in blood pressure. Jaundice has also been reported.

Precautions and Contraindications. The use of diphenidol is limited to settings in which the recipient is under close, continuous supervision by healthcare professionals. If hallucinations, disorientation, or confusion occurs, the drug should be discontinued immediately. Diphenidol should be used with caution in clients with glaucoma or obstructive lesions of the GI or genitourinary tract. This drug is not recommended for treating persons with a history of sinus tachycardia. It is contraindicated in clients with anuria or a known allergic hypersensitivity to the drug. The oral tablets are contraindicated for clients with a known allergy to tartrazine, a coloring agent used in this formulation.

Trimethobenzamide

Trimethobenzamide (Tigan) is structurally related to the substituted ethanolamine antihistamines but exhibits only weak antihistaminic activity.

Pharmacodynamics. Although the precise mode of action of trimethobenzamide is unknown, it appears to inhibit stimuli at the medullary CTZ.

Pharmacokinetics. Trimethobenzamide is well absorbed when administered orally or IM. Distribution into human body tissues and fluids is unknown; in animals, the drug is distributed mainly into the liver, kidneys, and lungs. In animals, trimethobenzamide is metabolized by the liver, but its metabolism in humans has not been determined. The drug is excreted in the urine of both animals and humans and is found in the feces of animals.

Therapeutic Uses. Trimethobenzamide is used for controlling nausea and vomiting, especially when long-term therapy is anticipated. It is less effective than phenothiazines for controlling severe and potentially hazardous vomiting but causes fewer adverse effects than those drugs.

Adverse Reactions. Adverse effects of trimethobenzamide may involve the CNS (blurred vision, seizures, coma, depression, disorientation, vertigo, dizziness, drowsiness, and headache), the GI tract (diarrhea, jaundice, and exaggeration of preexisting nausea), and the bone marrow

(blood dyscrasias). Hypotension has been reported after IM injection. Pain, stinging, burning, and inflammation may also occur at injection sites. Adverse reactions are uncommon in clients receiving usual dosages of trimethobenzamide and very rarely require discontinuation of the drug.

Precautions and Contraindications. Trimethobenzamide should be administered with caution to clients with acute febrile illness, encephalitis, gastroenteritis, dehydration, and electrolyte imbalance. Children and elderly or debilitated persons are especially at risk for adverse reactions to trimethobenzamide. The drug should be discontinued if signs and symptoms of allergic hypersensitivity develop. Trimethobenzamide suppositories are contraindicated for clients allergic to benzocaine or similar local anesthetics. Safety during pregnancy and lactation has not been established.

Marijuana Derivative: Dronabinol

Dronabinol (Marinol) is a derivative of the hallucinogen marijuana, which is used medicinally to control nausea and vomiting caused by chemotherapy.

Pharmacodynamics. The active ingredient of dronabinol is delta-9-tetrahydrocannabinol (delta-9-THC, or THC), the principal psychoactive substance in *Cannabis sativa*. Its mechanism of action as an antiemetic is unknown. Tetrahydrocannabinol acts primarily on the CNS, and its antiemetic effect is probably central also.

Pharmacokinetics. Due to first-pass metabolism in the liver, only 10% to 20% of an oral dose is available systemically. Plasma levels peak 2 to 3 hours after ingestion. Tetrahydrocannabinol has a predilection for fatty tissues and is believed to be stored in fatty tissues for long periods. It is about 97% protein bound. The drug crosses the placenta and is concentrated and secreted in breast milk.

Therapeutic Uses. Dronabinol's medicinal use is limited to preventing or treating nausea and vomiting caused by chemotherapy. It is also used to stimulate the appetite of clients with AIDS. Dronabinol is supplied as liquid capsules. Initial dosage for adults is 5 mg/m² body surface area, taken 1 to 3 hours before administration of antineoplastic drugs. Subsequent doses are administered 2 to 4 hours apart for a total of four to six doses per day. If necessary, dosage may be increased in increments of 2.5 mg/m², but no dose should exceed 15 mg/m².

Adverse Reactions. Dronabinol exerts all the effects of marijuana and other centrally active cannabinols, including impairment of cognitive performance and memory, loss of inhibitions, and altered perceptions of reality (hallucinations, altered time perception). It can cause psychosis. Systemic physical effects include dry mouth, conjunctival injection, increased blood pressure, diarrhea, and musculoskeletal pain. Tetrahydrocannabinol also produces sexual changes (decreased rate of pregnancy in women, sexual impairment in men).

Precautions and Contraindications. Dronabinol is highly abusable. The use of dronabinol, especially for clients who have not used tetrahydrocannabinol previously, is limited to institutional settings where the recipient can be closely observed and where adverse reactions can be treated promptly. Prescriptions are limited to a few days' supply. Clients should avoid using alcohol or barbiturates when using the drug. They should also avoid hazardous tasks, such as operating power machinery. Dronabinol is contraindicated in clients with allergic hypersensitivity to tetrahydrocannabinol or sesame oil.

Serotonin Antagonists

Serotonin antagonists (granisetron and ondansetron) are used to treat nausea and vomiting induced by cancer chemotherapy. Cancer chemotherapeutic agents produce nausea and vomiting that results in the release of serotonin, which then causes more episodes of nausea and vomiting. These drugs are believed to block 5-HT3 serotonin receptors in the CTZ and on vagal nerve endings.

Pharmacodynamics. Granisetron and ondansetron are selective 5-HT3 receptor antagonists and block further nausea and vomiting caused by chemotherapeutic agents.

Pharmacokinetics. Oral doses of ondansetron are well absorbed and peak levels are achieved in 1.7 hours. Women may have higher plasma levels due to a greater extent and rate of absorption, slower clearance, and higher absolute bioavailability. Granisetron does not appear to have these gender differences. Ondansetron and granisetron are metabolized by the hepatic microsomal enzymes and therefore may be affected by other drugs affecting these enzymes. About 70% of ondansetron and 65% of granisetron is protein bound. Granisetron is excreted via feces and urine.

Therapeutic Uses. These drugs are used for treating chemotherapy-induced nausea and vomiting and preventing postoperative nausea and vomiting. Oral dosage of ondansetron is 8 mg three times a day for adults and children over age 12 years. The IV dosage for adults and children 4 to 18 years is three 15-mg/kg doses. Granisetron is administered IV at 10 µg/kg infused over 5 minutes, beginning 30 minutes before chemotherapy is initiated.

Adverse Reactions. Ondansetron and granisetron cause headaches, weakness, drowsiness or somnolence, and constipation. Side effects of ondansetron include dizziness, abdominal pain, musculoskeletal pain, and shivering. Granisetron may cause diarrhea, fever, taste disorders, and hypertension.

Precautions and Contraindications. Both drugs are classified as pregnancy category B drugs; their use by lactating clients should be avoided.

Glucocorticoids

Glucocorticoids also act as antiemetics and are sometimes used to prevent nausea and vomiting during antineoplastic chemotherapy. These drugs are discussed in detail in Chapter 30.

■ SUMMARY

Drugs from several chemical groups effectively reduce nausea and vomiting. Because they may mask the symptoms of underlying disease, care should be taken to evaluate the client thoroughly so that effective treatment may be prescribed for the underlying condition. Pregnancy should be ruled out, because many antiemetics are teratogenic. Nausea and vomiting can be reduced by the judicious use of anticholinergics, antihistamines, or phenothiazine tranquilizers, as well as individual drugs developed for their antiemetic effects.

❖ NURSING MANAGEMENT: CLIENT RECEIVING AN ANTIEMETIC

If allowed to persist, vomiting can undermine nutritional integrity and impair recuperative powers. Control of these symptoms is essential to the client's well-being. Pathologic conditions contributing to the problem must be treated to minimize their impact. Until a definitive diagnosis is made, the use of antiemetics should be avoided to prevent the masking of symptoms. The client must depend on nursing measures to ameliorate the symptoms.

Nausea and vomiting decrease when stimuli affecting the vomiting reflex are reduced. A decrease of all types of stimuli can be helpful. Noxious stimuli to all sensory modalities should be eliminated. Noise, offensive odors, distressing sights, emotional tension, pain, and similar stressors augment nausea. Even usually pleasant stimuli can add to reflex excitation. Body motion, which disturbs the vestibular apparatus in the inner ear, is particularly distressing. When nausea is acute, a quiet environment with subdued lighting is required; the client should be protected from the sights, sounds, and odors associated with food.

To minimize gastric irritation, offering frequent, small, bland meals may help. Foods that increase nausea should be eliminated. After episodes of vomiting, warm tea, ginger ale, or cola drinks may help reduce nausea. Effervescent beverages should be exposed to air until the gas bubbles dissipate and the liquid approaches room temperature, because carbonation contributes to gastric distention and increases discomfort. Large amounts of water, which stimulate nausea, should be avoided. Allow clients to choose the foods and beverages they prefer. Conditioning greatly influences response: a dish associated with a loving parent's care during childhood illness may be far better tolerated than foods believed to act pharmacologically to control nausea.

After a medical diagnosis is made, antiemetic drugs may be prescribed. In acute conditions, they are usually required for limited periods of time, the need declining as the underlying condition subsides. Clients with chronic conditions associated with nausea and vomiting receive antiemetics for longer periods of time.

Nursing Measures for Pregnant Clients. Antiemetics are not recommended during pregnancy because the safety of these drugs in pregnancy is not established. Some related compounds, such as thalidomide, are highly teratogenic. Vomiting in pregnancy is often relieved by the general measures outlined previously. Eating dry crackers before rising helps prevent or ameliorate morning sickness. The extra carbohydrates are thought to reduce the hypoglycemia caused by the energy requirements of the rapidly growing fetus. (Hypoglycemia is often associated with nausea.) In most cases, nausea and vomiting subside before the second trimester and do not seriously interfere with maternal nutrition.

NURSING PROCESS

ASSESSMENT

Determining and correcting the cause of nausea and vomiting are of primary importance. Complete assessment is vital to diagnosis and treatment. Exactly what the client means by nausea or vomiting must be determined—vomiting should be clearly differentiated from regurgitation and retching. The amount and character of emesis should be determined. The onset, frequency, duration, and associated circumstances of the symptoms provide important clues to etiology. Factors that either increase or alleviate the symptoms must be identified.

Physical assessment should include general appearance, vital signs, and an examination of the abdomen. When vomiting persists, nutritional status must be evaluated, with special attention to signs of fluid and electrolyte disturbances. Women of childbearing age should be questioned closely about the possibility of pregnancy.

A drug history should be taken before antiemetic therapy begins. Particular attention should be paid to the client's previous response to anticholinergics, antihistamines, and phenothiazines. Drugs in current use and those taken recently (2 weeks for most but longer for clients with liver or renal impairment) should be listed. This information must be evaluated to determine how likely it is that the nausea and vomiting might be an adverse reaction to a drug, how great a risk there is of interactions with antiemetic agents, and what the indications are of concomitant medical conditions.

The client should be questioned specifically about glaucoma, because antiemetics with anticholinergic properties are contraindicated in this condition. A family history of glaucoma indicates an increased risk of this problem in middle-aged or elderly clients.

NURSING DIAGNOSIS

Because most antiemetic drugs are CNS depressants, clients receiving them are likely to develop:

- Risk for Injury, related to drug-induced drowsiness secondary to CNS depression
- Pain: Fatigue, weakness, dizziness, disorientation, hallucinations, confusion, or depression related to CNS changes secondary to antiemetic medication
- Altered Tissue Perfusion: Hypotension related to vasodilation secondary to antiemetic medication
- Sensory/Perceptual Alterations: Blurred vision or hallucinations related to antiemetic medication
- Knowledge Deficit, related to drug therapy for nausea and vomiting

PLANNING

Goals of treatment and nursing care include alleviating or eliminating nausea and vomiting, improving nutrition, reducing discomfort, maintaining adequate blood pressure, restoring normal sensory perception, maintaining normal elimination, and educating the client or family about self-care measures to prevent or minimize nausea and vomiting.

INTERVENTION

The nurse's responsibilities in antiemetic therapy include administering medications, evaluating therapeutic responses, identifying adverse reactions, and teaching the client.

Careful drug administration enhances beneficial effects while minimizing adverse effects. For optimal results, nursing measures to control the symptoms are continued even when drugs are used.

Antiemetics are usually administered as needed (PRN). With active vomiting, the parenteral or rectal route is used because oral doses may not be retained. Preventive doses may be given by mouth. The client must be monitored carefully for adverse reactions. Safety precautions to prevent injury are important because the client may experience postural hypotension and drowsiness.

If phenothiazines are used, the drug must be discontinued at the earliest sign of akathisia. Paradoxically, nausea and vomiting can be increased by antiemetic drugs. If the client either fails to improve or develops other adverse reactions, a change in prescription or discontinuation of treatment may be required.

Chronically or Terminally Ill Clients. Chronically or terminally ill clients often experience nausea over long periods. Antiemetic medication should be timed to precede events known to precipitate symptoms. If nutrition is inadequate, medication may be needed before meals. Preventive use of the drugs allows oral administration of medication and controls nausea more effectively than treatment after the vomiting reflex activity is well established. Establishing a medication schedule designed to meet individual needs usually increases the client's response. A PRN order does not imply that the medication is restricted to use only after full-blown symptoms develop; the client may need preventive medication.

Nausea and vomiting can persist despite vigorous treatment by conventional means. Such refractory problems often develop in clients with malignant neoplasms. Whether the underlying disease itself or the radiation and antineoplastic drugs used for treatment cause this problem is unknown; perhaps both contribute. Cancer clients are poorly nourished at best, and an inability to eat further erodes their nutritional status. The problem is a serious one.

Client Education. Clients subject to motion sickness should be advised to take antiemetic medication at least 30 minutes before beginning a trip or activity that normally causes nausea and vomiting. If traveling in an automobile or bus, clients should sit near the front of the vehicle because they will be subject to fewer stimuli that result from the sway or bouncing of the vehicle. Such a position also facilitates focusing on objects directly ahead, a strategy that decreases the nausea-causing impact of peripheral visual stimuli.

Clients seeking advice about treating nausea and vomiting should be referred for medical assessment of the underlying condition. Habitual use of antiemetics is not advisable as a substitute for definitive medical care.

Clients with chronic or terminal conditions accompanied by nausea and vomiting should be taught how to decrease the stimuli accentuating these symptoms. Antiemetics should be taken regularly in such situations for their preventive effect.

Whenever antiemetic medication is required, clients should be warned not to operate power machinery, including automobiles, because the drugs can cause drowsiness.

OUTCOME EVALUATION

Data required for outcome evaluation include the absence or presence and severity of vomiting, the client's report about the absence or presence and severity of nausea, absence of signs and symptoms of undernutrition (including changes in weight), the client's reports about sensation and perception, frequency and consistency of bowel movements, absence or presence of rash and its severity, and ability of the client or family to perform self-care measures discussed in teaching sessions.

❖ CHECKLIST OF NURSING ACTIONS

- Assess clients subject to nausea and vomiting to determine the nature of their symptoms.
- Refer clients for definitive diagnosis and treatment.
- Decrease stimuli, especially noxious stimuli, to reduce the level of nausea and vomiting.
- Give careful mouth care after emesis.
- Recommend small, frequent bland feedings to minimize gastric irritation. Offer warm tea or flat ginger ale or cola drinks instead of water.
- Rule out pregnancy before administering antiemetic drugs.
- Administer preventive doses of antiemetics orally; medication during active nausea should be given rectally or parenterally.
- Monitor clients receiving antiemetics for drowsiness, postural hypotension, and (with phenothiazines) extrapyramidal effects.
- Teach clients subject to motion sickness to take antiemetic medication 30 minutes before undertaking the activity that causes nausea.
- For clients subject to chronic nausea, teach techniques to reduce the symptoms.

Miscellaneous Drugs Affecting the Upper Gastrointestinal Tract

Antiflatulents

Flatulence is a natural body process; it can increase with increased dietary bulk, neutralization of gastric acids, air swallowing, or the ingestion of gas-producing foods, such as cabbage. It can be excessive in clients with peptic ulcer disease, irritable or spastic colon, or diverticulosis.

Simethicone

An ingredient in some antacids and also available as tablets, capsules, or drops, simethicone (Gas-X, Mylanta Gas) disperses and prevents the formation of mucus-surrounded gas pockets in the GI tract. By lowering the surface tension of gas bubbles in the stomach and intestines, it allows the elimination of the gas more easily by belching or passing flatulence.

Prokinetics

Prokinetic drugs stimulate the upper GI tract. They are believed to act by increasing the effects of acetylcholine. They are used to treat esophageal reflux disorder and diabetic gastroparesis and to prevent nausea and vomiting. They should not be used in clients with intestinal obstruction, perforation, or GI bleeding.

Metoclopramide

Metoclopramide stimulates GI motility in the upper GI tract.

Pharmacodynamics. Metoclopramide's mode of action is unclear, but it appears to sensitize tissues to the effects of acetylcholine. It increases gastric contraction, relaxes the pyloric sphincter, and increases peristalsis in the duodenum and jejunum. It also increases the lower esophageal sphincter pressure. In the CNS, metoclopramide blocks dopamine receptors in the CTZ. It increases the CTZ threshold and decreases the sensitivity of visceral nerves that transmit afferent impulses from the GI tract to the vomiting center.

Pharmacokinetics. Metoclopramide is rapidly and well absorbed, with onset of action 30 to 60 minute after an oral dose and 1 to 3 minutes after an IV dose. It is not extensively bound to plasma proteins, and most (over 85%) of an oral dose is excreted in the urine within 72 hours. Distribution is not fully understood. In animals, the drug crosses the blood-brain barrier and is found in high concentrations in the area of the brain where the CTZ is located. Metoclopramide binds weakly to plasma proteins, principally to albumin. The drug crosses the placenta and is distributed in breast milk. Metoclopramide is not extensively metabolized. Both metabolites and unchanged drug are excreted in the urine and bile. The drug is only minimally removed by dialysis.

Therapeutic Uses. Metoclopramide is used to prevent nausea and vomiting in postoperative clients or in clients receiving cancer chemotherapy. It is used also to treat diabetic gastroparesis and gastroesophageal reflux disorder. It has also been used to improve lactation; elevated prolactin levels occur with chronic administration. The usual adult oral dosage is 10 to 15 mg up to four times a day (30 minutes before each meal and at bedtime). The usual IM dose is 10 mg. It is given IV slowly over at least 15 minutes; the initial dose is 1 to 2 mg/kg. If extrapyramidal symptoms occur, diphenhydramine (Benadryl) may be given IM.

Adverse Reactions. Adverse effects include depression, tardive dyskinesia, extrapyramidal symptoms (primarily dystonias), and parkinsonian symptoms. GI effects include nausea and bowel disturbances, especially diarrhea. Blood dyscrasias, including methemoglobinemia with overdosage in neonates, may occur. Tachycardia or bradycardia may occur. Rash, urticaria, or bronchospasm, especially in clients with asthma, have been reported. Endocrine effects include galactorrhea, gynecomastia, and impotence secondary to hyperprolactinemia.

Drug Interactions. Interaction between metoclopramide and digoxin results in decreased digoxin absorption. Concurrent use of cyclosporine and metoclopramide increases the toxic and immunosuppressant effects of cyclosporine.

Precautions and Contraindications. Sedation may occur, and clients should be warned about this effect and advised to avoid driving or other activities requiring alertness. Metoclopramide should be used cautiously in patients with hypertension because of possible release of catecholamines. Metoclopramide is contraindicated in persons with a history of seizures and in those in whom stimulation of GI motility might be dangerous (eg, mechanical obstruction or perforation). It is also contraindicated in clients with a history of sensitivity or intolerance to the drug. Caution should be used when the drug is administered to persons allergic to procainamide, because the two drugs are structurally similar.

Cisapride

Pharmacodynamics. Cisapride is believed to stimulate the release of acetylcholine at the mesenteric plexus. It increases the lower esophageal sphincter pressure and accelerates gastric emptying.

Pharmacokinetics. After oral administration, cisapride is rapidly absorbed and reaches peak plasma concentrations in 60 to 90 minutes. The amount and rate of absorption may be decreased by histamine (H_2) receptor antagonists. It is highly protein bound (about 95%). It is widely distributed and is excreted in the feces and urine.

Therapeutic Uses. It is used primarily in treating gastroesophageal reflux disorder. The adult dosage is 10 mg four times a day (at least 15 minutes before meals and at bedtime).

Adverse Reactions. Effects on the GI system include diarrhea, abdominal pain, nausea, constipation, flatulence, and dyspepsia. Other side effects include headache, urinary tract infection and frequent urination, rhinitis, sinusitis, pain, and fever.

Drug Interactions. The sedative effects of benzodiazepines and alcohol may be accelerated by cisapride. Coagulation times increase if cisapride is taken with oral anticoagulants, and the risk of serious ventricular arrhythmias exists with concurrent use of ketoconazole and similar antifungals.

Precautions and Contraindications. Cisapride is a pregnancy category C agent. Safety and efficacy in children have not been established.

Dexpanthenol

Dexpanthenol (Ilopan) is the alcohol analog of D-pantothenic acid, which plays a role in the synthesis of acetylcholine. Its exact mechanism of action is unknown. It is used to enhance peristalsis after surgery or in intestinal atony or paralytic ileus. It should not be used in the presence of intestinal obstruction or in clients with hemophilia. Adverse effects include itching, urticaria, intestinal colic, vomiting, and diarrhea.

Other drugs usually used for other conditions also have prokinetic effects: bethanechol, erythromycin, and the somatostatin analog octreotide acetate (Sandostatin), a drug used to treat endocrine tumors (Raiha & Sourander, 1993).

■ SUMMARY

Prokinetics help stimulate upper GI tract function in clients with decreased GI function. They should not be used in clients with obstruction, perforation, or GI bleeding.

References

National Institutes of Health. (1994). *Helicobacter pylori* in peptic ulcer disease. *JAMA, 272,* 65.

National Institutes of Health Consensus Development Panel on *Helicobacter pylori* in Peptic Ulcer Disease. (1994). *Helicobacter pylori* in peptic ulcer disease. *JAMA, 272,* 65–69.

Newmark K, Nugent P. (1993). Milk-alkali syndrome. A consequence of chronic antacid abuse. *Postgrad Med, 93*(1), 149–150.

Raiha I, Sourander L. (1993). GI motility disorders: Diagnostic workup and use of prokinetic therapy. *Geriatrics, 48*(11), 57–66.

Bibliography

Barker LR, Burton JR, Zieve PD, eds. (1995). *Principles of ambulatory medicine*, 4th ed. Baltimore: Williams & Wilkins.

Barthel JS. (1993). Eradication of *Helicobacter pylori* and recurrence of duodenal ulcer. *Ann Intern Med, 118*(Suppl 3), 69.

Bezzaro E. (1993). Changing perspectives of H_2 antagonists for stress ulcer prophylaxis. *Crit Care Nurs Clin North Am, 5*(2), 325.

Blaser MJ. (1992). Hypotheses on the pathogenesis and natural history of *Helicobacter pylori*-induced inflammation. *Gastroenterology, 102*(2), 720–727.

Clearfield HR. (1991). *Helicobacter pylori*: Aggressor or innocent bystander? *Med Clin North Am, 75*(4), 815–829.

Cotton P. (1994). NIH Consensus panel urges microbials for ulcer patients. Skeptics concur with caveats. *JAMA, 271*, 808–809.

Distasio S. (1993). Zofran makes chemo bearable. *RN, 56*(5), 56.

Fedotin MS. (1993). *Helicobacter pylori* and peptic ulcer disease: Reexamining the therapeutic approach. *Postgrad Med, 94*(3), 38–40.

Forbes GM, Glaser ME, Cullen DJ et al. (1994). Duodenal ulcer treated with *Helicobacter pylori* eradication: Seven-year follow-up. *Lancet, 343*, 258–260.

Gerchufsky M. (1995). Understanding peptic ulcer disease. *Advance for Nurse Practitioners, 3*(7), 11–15.

Hunt RH. (1991). Treatment of peptic ulcer disease with sucralfate: A review. *Am J Med, 91*(2A), 102S–106S.

Knapman J. (1993). Controlling emesis after chemotherapy. *Nursing Standard, 7*(15), 38.

Lewis M, Fishman D. (1994). Ondansetron for postoperative nausea and vomiting: in the absence of comparative trials. *Am J Hosp Pharm, 51*, 98.

Lichter I. (1993). Which emetic? *J Palliative Care, 9*(1), 42.

Locke GR, Talley NJ. (1993). Management of non-ulcer dyspepsia. *J Gastroenterol Hepatol, 8*(3), 279–286.

Mamel JJ. (1993). Clinical pharmacology of commonly used drugs in GI practice, part II. *Gastroenterol Nursing, 15*(4), 156–162.

Nachman JA. (1993). Postoperative nausea and vomiting. *Curr Rev Anesth, 15*(19), 159–164.

Peine CJ. (1992). Gallstone-dissolving agents. *Gastroent Clin North Am, 21*(3), 715.

Rhodes VA, McDaniel RW, Simms SG, Johnson M. (1995). Nurses' perceptions of antiemetic effectiveness. *Oncology Nursing Forum, 22*(8), 1243–1252.

Weber MS. (1995). Chemotherapy-induced nausea and vomiting. *Am J Nurs, 95*(4), 34.

Williams SG, DiPalma JA. (1992). Medication-induced digestive system injury in the elderly. *Geriatric Nursing, 13*(1), 39–42.

Young LY, Koda-Kimble MA, eds. (1995). *Applied therapeutics: The clinical use of drugs*, 6th ed. Vancouver, WA: Applied Therapeutics.

For more information and sample tests and activities, refer to Chapter 28 in the Student Workbook for Clinical Pharmacology and Nursing Management, 5th edition, available through your bookstore.

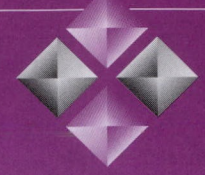

29

Drugs That Affect the Lower Gastrointestinal Tract

The lower gastrointestinal (GI) tract extends from the papilla of Vater to the anus. Drugs affecting this portion of the GI tract include antiflatulents, laxatives, antidiarrheals, and antiinflammatory drugs used to treat inflammatory bowel diseases.

Physiology of Flatulence

Gases are among the normal components of GI contents. Within the lower GI tract, excessive gas can be caused by compulsive air swallowing, by ingestion of antacids that produce carbon dioxide as a by-product of the neutralization reaction, or by increased fermentation in the GI tract.

Conditions promoting fermentation include the presence of large amounts of sugar, infection caused by organisms capable of fermentation, and prolonged passage time from increased dietary bulk, hypomotility, or material entrapped in the diverticuli. Certain foods, such as dried beans, notorious for causing flatulence, contain undigestible sugars that remain in the tract, promoting the growth of fermenting bacteria. The ability of the tract to expel gas can be impaired by immaturity (as in colicky babies), immobility, inadequate dietary fiber, depression, or neuropathy. All of these reduce intestinal motility.

When flatulence develops, it is important to treat the underlying causes whenever possible. Until this is accomplished and as long as chronic problems persist, antiflatulents can provide a measure of symptomatic relief.

Antiflatulents

Gas (flatus) that results from swallowed air or fermentation in the bowel is usually expelled from the stomach and colon promptly, causing no problems. Distention, discomfort, and pain can develop with unusual amounts of gas or gases that cannot be expelled.

Antiflatulent drugs promote the expulsion of gases by two mechanisms: mild irritation of the mucosa, which stimulates peristalsis, and defoaming, which causes small bubbles to coalesce into larger ones that are more easily eliminated. Antiflatulents also increase eructation and passage of gas from the rectum, which can be socially embarrassing.

Carminatives

Most irritant antiflatulents (carminatives) are aromatic oils, which stimulate intestinal motility by mild irritation. They are rarely prescribed as medical treatment but are frequently used as home remedies. Alcohol (in the form of whiskey or brandy) and peppermint (oil of peppermint or peppermint water) are popular. Small amounts of an alcoholic beverage or a few drops of peppermint are mixed with hot water for oral ingestion.

Simethicone

Simethicone (Mylicon, Silain) is a greasy, translucent liquid containing a mixture of liquid dimethylpolysiloxanes. Its antifoaming and water-repellent properties are derived from its ability to reduce surface tension. Simethicone decreases flatulence by causing gas bubbles in the GI tract to coalesce, forming larger masses, which are more easily expelled. Believed to be physiologically inactive, simethicone is considered nontoxic, but it is not recommended for treating infant colic because safety in infants and children is unproven. The drug is frequently combined with antacids (see Chap. 28), antispasmodics, and digestants in proprietary remedies.

Charcoal

Charcoal (Charcocaps) functions as an adsorbent for many substances. It eases flatulence by reducing the volume of intestinal gas and also helps control accompanying odor. Its use as an antidote in poisonings is discussed in Chapter 15. Because charcoal can adsorb drugs in the GI tract, it should be taken 2 hours before or 1 hour after other drugs.

❖ NURSING MANAGEMENT: CLIENT RECEIVING AN ANTIFLATULENT

When flatulence is a problem, the nurse should attempt to determine the cause.

NURSING PROCESS

ASSESSMENT

While taking the client's history, the nurse should ask about exercise and physical activity, diet (eg, foods that intensify flatulence, amount of fiber normally consumed), events occurring when flatulence first became a problem, and general health status. If a stroke or serious glucose imbalance preceded the onset of symptoms, neuropathy may be a contributing factor. A history of diabetes mellitus, multiple sclerosis, or other disease associated with nerve damage also may signify neuropathy. A long intestinal transit time and diverticulosis favor GI fermentation and increased gas production.

During the drug history, the nurse should ask about use of narcotic analgesics (eg, morphine, codeine) that tend to reduce propulsive peristalsis.

A complete physical examination of the abdomen should be performed to determine the degree of distention, tympany indicative of gas accumulations, and tenderness. The client should be observed to determine whether air swallowing is occurring.

NURSING DIAGNOSIS

Diagnoses appropriate for the client taking antiflatulent medication may include:

- Impaired Social Interaction, related to embarrassment secondary to frequent (or uncontrolled) eructation (or rectal expulsion of gas)

PLANNING

Goals of drug therapy include reducing intestinal gas production, reducing the volume of gas in the GI tract, or promoting gas expulsion.

INTERVENTION

In hospitalized clients, flatus often develops because of temporary immobility, lingering effects of general anesthetics, or the use of narcotic analgesics. The nurse should encourage ambulation as one means of stimulating peristalsis. If possible, nonnarcotic analgesics should be used to control pain. Warmth (eg, a hot-water bottle) applied to the abdomen is often helpful. If a rectal tube is used, it should be left in place for about 15 or 20 minutes at a time. As soon as the client can tolerate it, a normal diet with adequate fiber should be resumed gradually.

Nursing home residents are likely to develop flatus from neuropathy and limited mobility. Inadequate innervation of the intestinal tract is usually irreversible. These clients are usually affected by constipation and need a bowel regimen to promote normal fecal elimination. Stimulant laxatives may be prescribed as a part of the regimen. If the regimen does not control flatus adequately, the prescriber should be consulted, and an antiflatulent (eg, simethicone) may be prescribed. Foods that cause increased flatus should be eliminated from the diet.

Client Education. The nurse should help the client determine the cause of flatulence. The client should be informed about foods (eg, beans, cabbage, concentrated carbohydrates) that increase gas production in the GI tract. Beans may be tolerated if the client parboils and drains them before adding them to other ingredients. Exercise and ingestion of dietary fiber should be encouraged.

Clients affected by neuropathy or diverticulosis will have a chronic problem. For them and for colicky babies, peppermint may be recommended because it is inexpensive and readily available. The nurse can teach other clients about preparations containing simethicone. Over-the-counter (OTC) medications containing simethicone include Gas-X, Tempo, Di-Gel, Riopan Plus, Gelusil II, Gelusil M, and Mylanta II. Both peppermint and simethicone are relatively innocuous; alcohol should be discouraged because of its potential for toxicity.

OUTCOME EVALUATION

Data required for evaluation are reports by clients that they are more comfortable and that flatus has diminished. For clients whose social interaction had been impaired, an increase in social contacts and interaction would be significant.

Physiology of Fecal Elimination

After leaving the stomach, chyme enters the small intestine and is mixed with digestive enzymes, bile, and other secretions (Fig. 29-1). Nutrients are absorbed in this section of the GI tract, leaving a residue with the

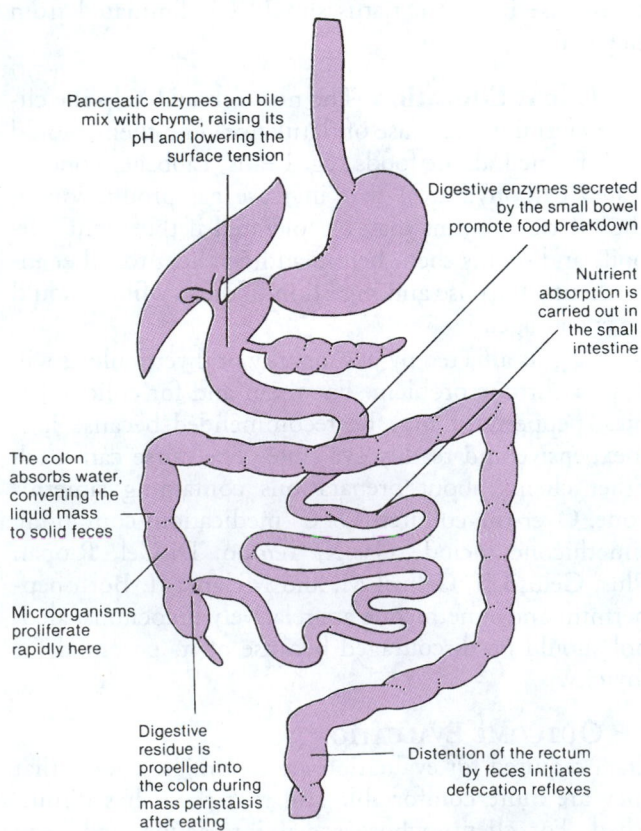

Pancreatic enzymes and bile mix with chyme, raising its pH and lowering the surface tension

Digestive enzymes secreted by the small bowel promote food breakdown

Nutrient absorption is carried out in the small intestine

The colon absorbs water, converting the liquid mass to solid feces

Microorganisms proliferate rapidly here

Digestive residue is propelled into the colon during mass peristalsis after eating

Distention of the rectum by feces initiates defecation reflexes

Figure 29-1. Lower part of the digestive tract.

consistency of watery gruel made up of undigestible fiber, water, electrolytes, bile pigments, digestive enzymes, mucus, and microorganisms. Several times a day, most notably after a meal, the ileocecal valve opens, and peristalsis propels part of this mass into the colon.

The colon reabsorbs fluids, electrolytes, and other substances, concentrating the residue into a smaller volume of soft to solid feces, stores this material for a time, and expels it from the body during defecation. Normal feces contain about three times more water than solids. In the moist, warm environment of the colon, microorganisms proliferate rapidly. About half the solid material in normal feces is composed of bacteria and other one-celled organisms.

Intestinal motility is regulated by local innervation, autonomic controls, nervous reflexes, and central nervous system (CNS) activity. Peristaltic waves are mediated by Auerbach's plexus, which lies between the circular and longitudinal muscular coats of the intestines. Sensory receptors in the mucous membrane transmit impulses to this myenteric plexus, which in turn stimulates smooth muscle contraction, producing pendulum and segmentation movements. These activities and intestinal tone may be influenced by acetylcholine in the intestinal wall.

Both the sympathetic and parasympathetic nervous systems (PNS) alter intestinal function. Sympathetic innervation is inhibitory, decreasing peristalsis and relaxing the smooth muscle. Sphincters constrict and secretion decreases. Parasympathetic activity stimulates secretion and motility and relaxes sphincters. Strong stimulation of the PNS can cause colic by inducing simultaneous contraction of large segments of intestine.

Reflexes coordinate functions of the GI tract. Gastrocolo-reflexes and duodenocolo-reflexes stimulate mass movements and propulsion of intestinal contents toward the anus. When feces enter the rectum, distention of the wall stimulates the myenteric plexus to initiate defecation. This weak reflex is fortified by spinal cord reflexes that increase PNS activity, augmenting peristaltic waves and initiating Valsalva's maneuver. This behavior (also called straining) involves taking a deep breath, closing the glottis, and contracting the abdominal muscles to increase intra-abdominal pressure. Straining, which facilitates defecation, also has pronounced effects on the cardiovascular system and can stress the heart.

Disturbances of Fecal Elimination

Minor disturbances in fecal elimination often occur in everyday life. Changes in diet, exercise, hydration, body rhythms, and emotions alter colonic function. Disease and medical regimens, such as bed rest and drug therapy, also disrupt normal patterns. A slowing of intestinal passage fosters excessive reabsorption of water and the formation of a hard, dry stool. Rapid passage allows too little time for reabsorption; stools tend to be watery and fluid, and electrolyte loss can be great.

The passage of infrequent, hard stools is termed constipation. The passage of frequent, semiliquid or liquid stools is termed diarrhea. These are relative terms with no precise meanings; the norms for fecal elimination vary from culture to culture, family to family, and person to person.

Laxatives

Before the development of modern medicine, laxatives were among the few truly effective remedies available to the medical practitioner. As a consequence, physicians tended to overprescribe them, a practice that fostered undue reliance on them by the lay public. Laxatives and antidiarrheals are valuable agents for treating many conditions, but their rational use requires a careful assessment of the factors associated with abnormal function and good judgment in determining their appropriate use.

Drug agents that stimulate defecation are called laxatives. Laxatives should not be used in undiagnosed abdominal pain, fecal impaction, or actual or suspected bowel obstruction or perforation. Use during the last trimester of pregnancy could stimulate premature labor.

A cathartic is a strong laxative that produces watery stools. Purgatives are even stronger agents that empty the bowel. When classified according to their mode of action, laxatives fall into five classes: irritant, hyperosmotic, bulk-forming, lubricant, and stool-softening (Table 29-1).

Irritant (and Vegetable) Laxatives

Irritant laxatives stimulate the intestinal mucosa, increasing motility and secretion. They may affect the small intestine and the colon. Stools tend to be watery and profuse, and intestinal pain and cramps may occur. Ideally, irritant laxatives should not affect the stomach or cause vomiting. They should be mild to prevent undue discomfort, and they should not induce systemic effects if absorbed.

Certain foods contain organic acids that act as mild laxatives: figs, prunes, pears, raisins, and rhubarb are known for their laxative effect.

Pharmacodynamics. The organic acids contained in laxative foods irritate the intestinal mucosa, stimulating reflex peristalsis. This action is supplemented by the food's cellulose content, which adds bulk to the stool, a further colonic stimulant.

Pharmacokinetics. Laxative foods pass through the GI tract fairly rapidly, a factor that decreases the absorption of the active ingredients. However, the potential for absorption of toxic amounts of the laxative compounds is present. The active ingredient of rhubarb, oxalic acid, is sufficiently concentrated in the plant's leaves to pose a serious threat of poisoning if the leaves are eaten.

Therapeutic Uses. Laxative foods should be incorporated in the diet in moderate amounts as part of a varied, balanced diet. Rhubarb is sometimes used by older adults as a home remedy for constipation. Prunes are frequently included in the diet to prevent constipation in such institutions as summer camps and nursing homes.

Adverse Reactions. Excessive use of laxative foods causes abdominal cramps, frequent stools, and fluid and electrolyte loss. Evacuation may be followed by a period of apparent or actual constipation. If the colon has been completely emptied, some time must elapse before feces accumulate sufficiently to produce another evacuation. Some foods (notably rhubarb) contain tannin, an astringent that produces constipation as an after-effect.

Precautions and Contraindications. Irritant laxatives, including those found in foods, are contraindicated in persons with a tendency toward colonic spasticity or those with chronic inflammatory bowel diseases (eg, ulcerative colitis, Crohn's disease).

Castor Oil

A product of the castor bean, castor oil is a bland, nonirritant oil used as a high-grade industrial lubricant and topical emollient.

Pharmacodynamics. Administered orally, castor oil has no effect on the stomach. During digestion, bile and pancreatic enzymes in the small intestine convert part of the oil to ricinoleic acid, a powerful irritant. Both the small and large intestines respond with increased motility and rapid passage of their contents; soft to watery stools are produced within 2 to 3 hours.

Pharmacokinetics. The extent of castor oil's absorption is unknown. Its active ingredient, ricinoleic acid, is absorbed slightly and subsequently metabolized like other fatty acids.

Therapeutic Uses. Castor oil is used to empty the bowel before such procedures as abdominal x-ray studies.

Adverse Reactions. Castor oil has a wide margin of safety. Large doses have little more effect than standard doses because the drug is rapidly eliminated by the purgative action it induces. Some people find the taste of castor oil disagreeable.

Precautions and Contraindications. Castor oil is contraindicated in persons in whom increased intestinal motility would be hazardous (eg, those with obstructive disease of the GI tract) and in persons with obstructive jaundice and pancreatic disease who lack the bile and pancreatic enzymes required for activation of the drug.

Anthraquinones

Anthraquinone (anthracene, emodin) cathartics include senna, aloes, and cascara sagrada.

Text continues on page 602.

Table 29-1. Drugs Used to Promote Fecal Elimination

Drug Name	Preparation	Usual Dosage	Additional Information
Irritant (Stimulant) Laxatives			
Vegetable Laxatives	Food (figs, prunes, pears, raisins, rhubarb)	One serving	Foods should be those preferred by the client.
castor oil (Alphamul, Emulsoil)	Oral capsules, suspension, and oil	Adults: 15–60 mL Children 2–12 yr: 5–15 mL Children younger than 2 yr: 1–5 mL A single dose is administered about 16 hr before surgery or procedure. PC: X	Castor oil is ineffective in the absence of bile or pancreatic enzymes. Unless the taste is disguised, the oil may cause nausea and vomiting.
Anthraquinones			
Aloin	Powder	Adults: 15 mg (herbal remedy)	Aloin is incorporated into the proprietary preparations Carter's Little Pills and Nature's Remedy. Although unreliable abortifacients, aloe and aloin are contraindicated in pregnant women.
cascara sagrada	Oral powder, suspension, tablets, fluid extract	Adults: 325 mg PC: C	Cascara sagrada is considered the mildest of the anthraquinone laxatives. A mixture of liquid cascara and milk of magnesia sometimes ordered for hospitalized persons is commonly termed (because of the color contrast between the two drugs) a "black and white."
senna (Black Draught, Casafru, Dr. Caldwell's Senna Laxative, Fletcher's Castoria, Gentlax, Senolax, Senexon, Senokot *Can:* Senokot)	Oral tablets, powder, capsules, and solution Rectal suppositories	Varies with the preparation PC: C	Senna is obtained from dried leaflets of cassia.
Diphenylmethane Cathartics			
bisacodyl (Bisco-Lax, Dulcagen, Dulcolax, Fleet Laxative, Theralax)	Enteric-coated oral tablets Rectal suppositories	*Oral:* Adults: 5–15 mg; children older than 3 yr: 5–10 mg or 0.3 mg/kg *Rectal:* Adults and children older than 2 yr: 10 mg; children 2 yr or younger: 5 mg PC: C	Repeated use of bisacodyl suppositories can cause inflammation of the rectal mucosa.
phenolphthalein (Alophen, Evac-U-Gen, Evac-U-Lax, Ex-Lax, Feen-A-Mint, Modane, Phenolax, Prulet)	Oral tablets, chewable tablets, wafers, and chewing gum	Adults: 60–194 mg	Phenolphthalein can discolor urine; alkaline urine will appear pink. Stools containing phenolphthalein turn pink if SSE are employed.
Hyperosmotic Laxatives			
glycerin, glycerol (Fleet Babylax, Sani-Supp)	Solution for enemas Rectal suppositories	Adults and children 6 yr or older: 5–15 mL Children younger than 6 yr: 2–5 mL *Rectal:* Adults and children 6 yr or older: 3 g Children younger than 6 yr: 1–1.5 g PC: C	Glycerin suppositories should be refrigerated for storage.

KEY: PC = pregnancy risk category; see Appendix A. *Can:* Canadian trade name.

(continued)

Table 29-1. (Continued)

Drug Name	Preparation	Usual Dosage	Additional Information
Hyperosmotic Laxatives (continued)			
lactulose (Cephulac, Cholac, Chronulac, Constilac, Constulose, Duphalac, Enulose; *Can:* Lactulax)	Oral syrup containing 10 g/15 mL	Adults: 15–60 mL daily as required PC: B	Lactulose is a synthetic dissaccharide analog lactose containing galactose and fructose.
Sorbitol, D-glucitol	Oral solution Rectal solution	*Oral:* Adults: 15 mL of a 70% solution *Rectal:* Adults: 120 mL of a 25%–30% solution; children 2 yr or younger: 30–60 mL of a 25%–30% solution	Sorbitol is sometimes used as an adjunct in therapeutic regimens employing sodium polystyrene sulfonate. It is also used in many low-calorie candy and diet foods; excess use can cause diarrhea and gas (diet food syndrome).
Saline Laxatives			
magnesium citrate (Citro-Nesia)	Oral solution	Adults: 100–200 mL Children 6–12 yr: 50–100 mL; children 2–5 yr: 4–12 mL PC: B	Compounds containing magnesium are relatively contraindicated for persons with impaired renal function.
magnesium hydroxide (Milk of Magnesia)	Oral suspension	Adults: 30–60 mL Children 6–12 yr: 15–30 mL; children 2–5 yr: 5–15 mL PC: B	Also used in lower doses as an antacid.
magnesium sulfate (Epsom salt)	Oral crystals and powder	Adults: 10–15 g Children 6–12 yr: 5–10 g; children 2–5 yr: 2.5–5 g PC: B	
polyethylene glycol-electrolyte solution (PEG-ES) (Colovage, Col-Lav, CoLyte, GoLYTELY, Go-Evac, NuLytely, OCL)	Oral solution	Adults: 250 mL q10 min up to 4 L PC: C	Solution is isotonic. No flavoring or other ingredients should be added to the solution.
potassium phosphate	Oral crystals and powder	Dosage depends on the preparation and combination of drugs used.	
sodium phosphate	Oral powder	Dosage depends on the preparation and combination of drugs used. PC: C	
Bulk-Forming Laxatives			
Bran	Food supplement, cereals	Adults: 1–4 oz	Bran is the outer husk of grain seeds, which is normally separated from the starch and germ during refinement of cereal products. Whole bran is somewhat irritating to the intestine and can aggravate spasticity of the bowel. It is contraindicated in intestinal obstruction, ulceration, stenosis, or adhesions. Bulk-forming laxatives must be given with ample fluids, and recipients must be kept well hydrated to produce a laxative effect.

KEY: PC = pregnancy risk category; see Appendix A. *Can:* Canadian trade name.

(continued)

Table 29-1. (Continued)			
Drug Name	**Preparation**	**Usual Dosage**	**Additional Information**
Bulk-Forming Laxatives (continued)			
calcium polycar-bophil (Equalactin, Fiberall, FiberCon, Fiber-Lax, Fiber-Norm, Mitrolan)	Oral tablets and chew-able tablets	Varies with the preparation PC: C	
karaya	Oral powder	Adults: 5–10 g	
Malt soup extract (Maltsupex)	Oral tablets, powder, and solutions	Adults: Tablet: 12–64 g Powder: Up to 32 g bid Children 6–12 yr: half of adult dose Infants 1 mo–2 yr: 6–16 g	
methylcellulose (Citrucel)	Oral tablets and solution	Adults: 4–6 g Children 6–12 yr: half of adult dose PC: C	
psyllium hydrophilic mucilloid (Effer-Syl-lum, Fiberall, Konsyl, Metamucil, Modane Bulk, Mucilose, Perdiem Fiber, Regu-loid, Serutan, Siblin, Syllact, V-Lax) *Can:* Karacil, Prodiem	Oral powder and chew-able pieces	Adults: 2.5–30 g Should be followed by a full glass of fluid to prevent esophageal obstruc-tion. Children 6–12 yr: 1.25–15 g PC: C	
Lubricant Laxatives			Plain mineral oil administered orally should be given only on an empty stomach to reduce the loss of fat-solu-ble vitamins; administer at least 2 hr before bedtime to reduce risk of regur-gitation and aspiration.
mineral oil (Agoral, Kondremul, Milki-nol, Neo-Cultol, Nu-jol, Zymenol) *Can:* Kondremul, Lansoyl	Oral liquid Oil enema	*Oral:* Adults: 15–45 mL; children older than 6 yr: 10–15 mL *Rectal:* Adults: 60–150 mL; children older than 6 yr: 60 mL PC: C	
Stool Softeners			Docusate may be administered as a single bedtime dose or in divided doses.
docusate (Colace, Doxidan, Doxate-C, Doxate-S, Doxinate, Kasof, Modane, Regulax, Regutol, Surfak)	Oral capsules and solu-tion	Adults and children older than 12 yr: 50–500 mg/day Children 2–12 yr: 40–120 mg/day; children younger than 3 yr: 10–40 mg/day PC: C	

KEY: PC = pregnancy risk category; see Appendix A. *Can:* Canadian trade name.

Pharmacodynamics. Anthraquinones act by irritating the intestinal mucosa and stimulating reflex peristalsis. Evacuation usually occurs within 6 to 12 hours but may be delayed for up to 24 hours.

Pharmacokinetics. Anthraquinone laxatives are only slightly absorbed from the small intestine. In the colon, enzymatic hydrolysis of glycosides in the drugs frees the pharmacologically active anthraquinones. Absorbed an-thraquinones are metabolized in the liver. The drugs and their metabolites are eliminated in feces by bile and in urine. Unabsorbed drug is eliminated directly in feces.

Therapeutic Uses. Proprietary preparations of anthra-quinone laxatives are widely used and sometimes abused. When laxatives are required medically, anthraquinones

(senna or cascara derivatives) are preferred over other stimulant drugs by many prescribers. They are pre-scribed for the relief of simple constipation and to pre-pare the bowel for diagnostic procedures such as x-ray examination of the GI tract with contrast media (Box 29-1). Aloe is not used medically as a laxative but is an ingredient in some herbal remedies.

Adverse Reactions. Stimulant (irritant) laxatives are habit-forming; prolonged use may result in dependency and loss of normal bowel function. Stimulant laxatives may produce abdominal discomfort, nausea, cramping, griping, and faintness. Among the anthraquinones, cas-cara sagrada is relatively mild, whereas aloe (aloin) is the most irritating. Irritant laxatives can also cause elec-trolyte disturbances (hypokalemia, hypocalcemia, acid–

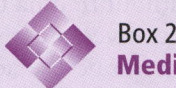
base imbalance), malabsorption, weight loss, and protein-losing enteropathy. Pathologic changes include structural damage to the myenteric plexus, severe and permanent loss of colonic motility, and hypertrophy of the muscularis mucosae. Atony and dilation of the colon sometimes resemble those seen in ulcerative colitis.

Anthraquinones may discolor the urine (from pink to red or brown to black). These drugs also discolor colonic mucosa (melanosis), an effect that appears to be innocuous.

Precautions and Contraindications. Anthraquinones are contraindicated in persons with symptoms suggestive of abdominal pathology (nausea, vomiting, acute abdominal pain) and those with intestinal obstruction.

Diphenylmethane Cathartics
Diphenylmethane cathartics include phenolphthalein and bisacodyl.

Pharmacodynamics. Diphenylmethane cathartics have their greatest effect on the colon. They act as irritants that stimulate reflex peristalsis. They require 6 or more hours to act and can be given at bedtime for results in the early morning.

Pharmacokinetics. Bisacodyl is not significantly absorbed from the GI tract. Up to 15% of orally administered phenolphthalein may be absorbed; some of the absorbed drug enters the enterohepatic circulation. After absorption into the bloodstream, diphenylmethanes are metabolized in the liver and excreted in the urine. They are distributed into breast milk.

Therapeutic Uses. Proprietary preparations containing diphenylmethanes are popular OTC laxatives. They have also been used medically to relieve constipation secondary to neurologic disease, idiopathic slowing of transit time, or constipating drugs, as well as to clean the bowel before GI surgery or diagnostic procedures.

Adverse Reactions. Side effects of diphenylmethanes include nausea, cramping, and faintness. Prolonged use may lead to laxative dependency, loss of normal bowel function, fluid and electrolyte imbalance, impaired nutrition, and weight loss. Rectal suppositories containing bisacodyl may cause irritation, inflammation, and a burning sensation of the rectal mucosa.

Allergic reactions to diphenylmethane laxatives include skin manifestations, renal irritation, encephalitis, respiratory disturbances, cardiac arrest, and (rarely) death. Skin problems include polychromatic skin eruptions, which may last several months. These drugs have been associated with Stevens-Johnson syndrome and systemic lupus erythematosus.

Precautions and Contraindications. Stimulant laxatives, including diphenylmethanes, are contraindicated in persons exhibiting signs and symptoms of abdominal pathology (nausea, vomiting, acute abdominal pain). They are not recommended for persons with abdominal cramps, anal or rectal fissures, or ulcerated hemorrhoids. Stimulant laxatives should not be prescribed for children younger than age 6. Safe use of bisacodyl during pregnancy has not been established. Diphenylmethane laxatives are contraindicated in persons with allergic sensitivity to them.

Hyperosmotic Laxatives
Hyperosmotic laxatives include glycerin, sorbitol, lactulose, and saline laxatives (magnesium cations and phosphate anions).

Pharmacodynamics. Hyperosmotic laxatives are thought to increase colonic fluid retention. The increased osmotic pressure in the bowel lumen may also promote movement of fluid across the intestinal mucosa from the extracellular fluid compartment. As a result, feces become more liquid, and the increased volume in the bowel stimulates stretch receptors, increasing peristalsis. Magnesium salts may also stimulate cholecystokinin release or reduce transit time.

Hyperosmotic laxatives tend to dehydrate the client. They may be the agent of choice in clients for whom a negative fluid balance is desired.

Besides its laxative effect, lactulose promotes reduction of blood ammonia levels in portal-system encephalopathy. It acidifies the contents of the bowel, promotes the outward diffusion and elimination of ammonia in the GI tract, and inhibits absorption of amines.

Pharmacokinetics. Rectally administered hyperosmotic laxatives are poorly absorbed. Preparations administered orally may be absorbed systemically, particularly magnesium-containing agents. The absorbed drugs are subsequently eliminated by the kidneys, whereas unabsorbed drugs are eliminated in feces.

Therapeutic Uses. Hyperosmotic laxatives, especially saline laxatives, are used to correct temporary constipation and to empty the bowel before surgery or procedures involving bowel examination. Saline laxatives are also used as adjuncts in treating poisoning because they hasten removal of some poisons from the GI tract. Sorbitol is frequently used with sodium polystyrene sulfonate to prevent constipation caused by that resin. In addition to its functions as a laxative, lactulose is used to treat portal system encephalopathy associated with high blood ammonia levels.

Adverse Reactions. Unless administered with sufficient fluid to produce an isotonic solution, saline cathartics tend to dehydrate the body and may cause electrolyte disturbances. Hypertonic preparations draw fluid into the lumen from the tissues. This fluid is excreted when the stool is evacuated. Dehydration is enhanced by the diuretic effect of these salts when the absorbed portion of the drugs is excreted in urine.

Glycerin may produce rectal discomfort, irritation, burning or griping, cramping, and tenesmus. The bitter taste of magnesium sulfate may cause nausea.

Saline laxatives are absorbed to some degree, increasing body levels of the particular metallic ion involved. These electrolyte changes are transient in clients with good renal function, who promptly excrete the salts in urine. If renal function is impaired, however, plasma content rises, and symptoms of excess may occur. Hypermagnesemia causes weakness, confusion, and sedation (about 20% of magnesium salts may be absorbed). Phosphates tend to reduce plasma levels of ionic calcium. Potassium toxicity arising from renal failure is heightened by the administration of a potassium-containing laxative. Sodium salts increase water retention and are contraindicated in congestive states, such as heart failure.

Lactulose may cause flatulence and abdominal cramping, especially when treatment begins. High dosages can cause diarrhea. Nausea and vomiting have also been reported. The fermentation of lactulose in the bowel may produce large accumulations of hydrogen gas.

Precautions and Contraindications. Hyperosmotic laxatives are contraindicated in clients with signs and symptoms of acute abdominal pathology (nausea, vomiting, acute abdominal pain). Magnesium compounds are contraindicated in clients with renal impairment, and sodium compounds should not be used by clients advised to restrict sodium intake.

If lactulose is used regularly, clients should be monitored for electrolyte disturbances (particularly hypokalemia) secondary to excessive loss of intestinal contents. This drug can cause high concentrations of gas in the bowel.

Bulk-Forming Laxatives

Bulk-forming laxatives are composed of polysaccharides and cellulose derivatives that are both hydrophilic and undigestible.

Pharmacodynamics. Within the digestive tract, bulk-forming laxatives swell in water to form gels or viscous solutions that soften the stool and increase its bulk. Peristalsis is stimulated, and transit time is reduced. Because the stool is soft, it passes easily without trauma to rectal or anal tissues. Bulk-forming laxatives are the most physiologic of the laxatives—they mimic the action of dietary fiber in the digestive tract.

Pharmacokinetics. Bulk-forming laxatives are not absorbed and are carried out of the body in feces.

Therapeutic Uses. Bulk-forming laxatives are often the treatment of choice in chronic constipation or laxative dependency not complicated by impaired intestinal motility caused by neural problems.

Adverse Reactions. Powdery formulations of bulk laxatives can cause suffocation or serious lung pathology if inhaled. When the drugs are taken with insufficient amounts of fluid, they may lodge in the esophagus, causing impaction and obstruction. This is most likely to occur in clients with swallowing problems.

Precautions and Contraindications. Bulk-forming laxatives should never be administered in dry form; they must be given with ample fluids (at least 8 oz for adults) to ensure propulsion of the dose beyond the cardiac sphincter into the stomach. In addition, without sufficient fluid, no bulk can be formed in the colon. Bulk-forming laxatives are contraindicated in persons with marked dysphagia.

Lubricant Laxatives

Lubricant laxatives include various oils, such as digestible vegetable oils and undigestible liquid petrolatum (mineral oil). Because lubricant laxatives must be used in quantity to ensure that a portion reaches the colon undigested, vegetable oils are not recommended for their laxative effect.

Pharmacodynamics. Oils retard the reabsorption of water from the fecal mass in the colon, preventing hardening of the stools. Oils also act as lubricants, facilitating stool passage.

Therapeutic Uses. Mineral oil is used by the lay public, and in selected cases by physicians, to control chronic constipation. Oils are used medically as retention enemas to soften stools in treating constipation or obstipation.

Adverse Reactions. Digestible oils are not used orally to treat constipation because they retard gastric motility and secretion and increase caloric intake.

Mineral oil is undigestible and poorly absorbed. However, the small amounts that are absorbed can cause a foreign body reaction in the mesenteric lymph nodes, intestinal mucosa, liver, and spleen. Although these reactions seem benign, the long-range safety of the drug is questionable. Mineral oil can leak past the anal sphincter, soiling undergarments, causing itching, and interfering with the healing of rectal lesions. As a lipid solvent, the drug interferes with the absorption of fat-soluble nutrients: vitamins A, D, and K dissolved in the unabsorbed portion of the oil are carried through the tract and excreted in feces.

Precautions and Contraindications. Mineral oil is usually administered between the last meal of the day and bedtime to minimize the risk of aspiration and the loss of fat-soluble vitamins. Because mineral oil taken at bedtime may be aspirated during sleep, causing lipid pneumonitis, there is no truly safe time to administer the drug. Persons receiving the drug over a long period should be monitored for signs and symptoms of fat-soluble vitamin deficiencies. Supplemental vitamins may be needed.

Stool Softeners

Stool softeners are moistening agents. They include sodium salts of docusate.

Pharmacodynamics. Stool softeners act by reducing surface tension in the bowel, promoting emulsification of the stool. They facilitate the incorporation of water into the fecal mass, thereby softening the stool. They may also affect motor and secretory functions of the digestive tract. The pharmacology of these compounds is not completely understood.

Pharmacokinetics. Stool softeners appear to be minimally absorbed; the portion that is absorbed is excreted in bile.

Adverse Reactions. Docusate compounds are toxic to human hepatic tissue cell cultures and theoretically could cause adverse reactions in the liver. However, in more than two decades of clinical practice, these drugs have been well tolerated, even when prescribed over long periods. Occasionally, GI pain, cramping, and skin rash may occur.

Precautions and Contraindications. Stool softeners should be administered with ample fluids to promote softening action in the bowel.

■ SUMMARY

Laxatives are drugs that stimulate fecal elimination. They are classified as irritant, hyperosmotic, bulk-forming, lubricant, or stool-softening. Irritant laxatives stimulate intestinal motility and secretion. Hyperosmotic laxatives draw water into the intestinal lumen, preventing dehydration and hardening of the stool. Bulk-forming laxatives stimulate the bowel by distention and also soften the stool. Lubricants and stool softeners promote the production of a soft stool.

In normal persons, constipation is best prevented by dietary management, hydration, exercise, and the promotion of habit. Laxatives may be needed to relieve temporary dysfunction or to compensate for permanent impairment of fecal elimination. Except for lubricants, laxatives should be taken with ample amounts of fluid. Excessive use of laxatives may cause dehydration, potassium loss or other electrolyte imbalances, steatorrhea, osteomalacia, vitamin and mineral deficiencies, or toxicity from absorption of chemical components.

❖ NURSING MANAGEMENT: CLIENT RECEIVING A LAXATIVE

The many and varied OTC laxative products indicate that the public frequently, even habitually, uses these agents. Nurses who have the greatest contact with clients are among the healthcare professionals who assess laxative use, administer various agents, and monitor their effects.

In long-term healthcare settings, nurses must be alert to situations that increase the risk of constipation—particularly relative inactivity, changes in diet, use of depressant drugs, inability to assume a normal posture for defecation, lack of privacy, and lack of opportunity to defecate at the normal time. Fasting required for diagnostic tests, anorexia, fluid and electrolyte imbalances, and increased stress levels tend to increase the risk of constipation.

Moreover, many drug regimens and various treatments disrupt normal bowel function: some reduce fluid and food intake, and some cause intestinal atony, leading to constipation. Laxatives are often helpful in ameliorating or controlling such conditions (see the Critical Thinking Challenge).

The client's disease may also cause constipation, especially when nerve function in the intestine is impaired. Neurologic diseases, such as stroke, multiple sclerosis, and diabetic gastroparesis, and cord injuries damage the nerves involved in stimulating motility, thus reducing peristalsis. Complete atony is not amenable to laxative therapy, but reduced motility often is.

CRITICAL THINKING CHALLENGE
Case Analysis

Mrs. Torrance, age 70, had coronary artery bypass surgery 5 days ago. She is complaining of abdominal distention, gas, and constipation. She has a history of peptic ulcer, irritable bowel, and diverticulosis. Her current medications are digoxin, atenolol, sucralfate, ranitidine, docusate, and warfarin. She also receives acetaminophen with codeine as needed for pain.

1. What additional data are needed to evaluate her problems?
2. What drugs may be affecting her situation?
3. What nondrug factors may be affecting her situation?
4. What nursing actions would you take, and what advice would you give Mrs. Torrance?

NURSING PROCESS

ASSESSMENT

When clients complain of constipation, it is necessary to ascertain exactly what they mean. Some clients think that constipation is failure to have a bowel movement every day. Depending on food and fiber intake, a person may or may not have a bowel movement that frequently. When stools are dry and hard, passed with difficulty or pain, and the client feels distended, a diagnosis of constipation can be made. A person who has soft stools at intervals greater than 24 hours may have prolonged intestinal transit time but not true constipation.

Additional data required for assessment include the frequency and consistency of stools, the ease or difficulty of passage, and prolonged sensations of fullness and distention in the distal bowel. The client's usual bowel functions in the absence of laxatives should be determined. The nurse then must assess the client's diet, hydration, activity level, and bowel habits to determine whether faulty habits cause or contribute to the problem.

Because changes in bowel habits may herald serious, underlying conditions (ranging from depression to malignant neoplasms), clients with constipation that does not respond to hygienic measures should be referred for a diagnostic evaluation to determine the cause of the condition.

Clients with abdominal pain or other symptoms of appendicitis must not receive laxatives until appendicitis is ruled out. The risk of perforation is sharply increased in victims of appendicitis who have been given a laxative. These drugs are also contraindicated in intestinal obstruction, inflammations (typhoid fever, ulcerative colitis), hemorrhage, and intussusception.

NURSING DIAGNOSIS

Clients receiving laxatives may have some of the following nursing diagnoses:

- Diarrhea, related to overstimulation of peristalsis secondary to laxative use
- Fluid Volume Deficit, related to excessive loss of water from the lower intestinal tract secondary to laxative-induced diarrhea
- Pain: Abdominal cramping, altered comfort, and nausea related to flatulence or overstimulation of the lower bowel secondary to laxative use
- Risk for Constipation, related to dehydration and hypokalemia secondary to laxative use
- Risk for Injury: Skin irritation or breakdown, fluid and electrolyte imbalances related to laxative use

Many clients have:

- Knowledge Deficit, related to normal fecal elimination, constipation, and appropriate use of laxatives

PLANNING

Goals of nursing care include restoring normal fecal elimination and preventing or promptly detecting and treating nausea, abdominal cramps and discomfort, dehydration, hypokalemia, acidosis, skin rash, or other adverse effects of laxative use. Alleviating fear is the goal for clients receiving anthraquinone laxatives. When client teaching is needed, increased knowledge about constipation, its prevention, and its treatment is a major goal.

INTERVENTION

In addition to needing laxatives, clients who are at high risk for constipation need nursing interventions to help prevent the condition. Emphasis should be on education, increasing the intake of fluids, fiber, and potassium, increasing physical activity, and establishing regular bowel habits.

Laxative foods may be offered, if allowed, in the diet. Choice of food should be dictated by client preference. For example, children who often refuse cooked prunes may accept dry prunes as snack foods. Pears and raisins exert laxative effects and are well liked by most people. Clients who refuse these foods may enjoy prune juice popsicles.

The timing of laxative administration in relation to the expected onset of action is important to prevent disrupting daily activities or sleep (Table 29-2).

Constipation secondary to medical treatments or illnesses can usually be prevented with a bulk laxative or stool softener. These types of laxatives must be given before the stool becomes hard and dry, 2 to 3 days before constipation is expected to develop.

Single episodes of temporary constipation are amenable to saline or irritant cathartics, or enemas. Temporary use of these agents is also appropriate when bulk laxatives or stool softeners with delayed onset of action are first administered, if the client has already become constipated. The choice of agent is determined by the client's general condition, associated pathology, and the preference of the client, nurse, or prescriber (Box 29-2).

Clients who cannot take oral preparations may need enemas or rectal suppositories. These are administered also when immediate evacuation is desired. Traditional enema solutions include tap water, soapsuds solution, and normal saline. Tap water is hypotonic and can be absorbed in large amounts. Soapsuds solutions, which are very irritating, are seldom prescribed today. Normal saline solution, which is isotonic, disturbs fluid and electrolyte balance the least. It is essentially nonirritating and is the solution of choice in most situations. Small hypertonic enemas, such as Fleet Phospho-Soda, may be prescribed when fluid loss is considered beneficial.

Table 29-2. Timing of Laxative Effect	
Type of Laxative	**Usual Time of Action**
Irritant	6–24 hr
Hyperosmotic	30 min–3 hr
Bulk-forming	12–72 hr
Lubricant	6–8 hr

Repeated enemas may be prescribed to clean the colon completely, but their use can remove nutrients from the intestine. Colonic hypermotility is reflected by increased motility of the small intestine. Chyme is propelled into the colon prematurely and removed by succeeding enemas. Clients may become weak and exhibit signs of stress, such as diaphoresis. These clients should be allowed to rest. Administering electrolyte-containing fluids (eg, coffee or tea) helps correct fluid and potassium depletion and often reverses the symptoms. The prescriber should be informed of the client's reaction before enemas are resumed.

Oral laxatives should be administered in the most palatable form possible. Some clients prefer milk of magnesia diluted with milk. The flavor of magnesium sulfate can be disguised in chilled grape juice. Laxatives marketed in enteric-coated form are virtually tasteless but should not be chewed, crushed, or administered concurrently with antacids because premature release of the agent in the stomach could cause irritation. The flavor of the drug would be evident as well.

Castor oil is more palatable if emulsified. Some clients prefer it with orange juice. This mixture can be emulsified and effervesced by adding a small quantity (0.5 tsp) of bicarbonate of soda immediately before ingestion. Caution should be exercised when disguising drug flavors with foods, however. Unless the drug flavor is well masked, the client could begin to dislike the food.

An alternative to disguising an unpalatable drug in food is chilling the tongue before administering the laxative. Chilling anesthetizes taste buds. The nurse can offer the client an ice cube or a popsicle to suck just before taking the drug. Bulk laxatives must be mixed with fluid immediately before ingestion, as they form a gel quickly after mixing. Ample fluids (for adults, one or two glasses) should be administered with all laxatives.

Box 29-2
Teaching Clients to Correct Constipation

Teaching clients to treat constipation by preventing it rather than relying on laxative agents is a key nursing intervention. Basic teaching focuses on diet, physical activity, bowel habits, and stress reduction.

Dietary Measures

- Encourage eating foods high in fiber, such as whole-grain cereals and breads, fruits, and vegetables. Some fruits and vegetables should be eaten raw because cooking tends to break down cellulose, the main source of dietary fiber. Other foods need to be cooked. Current cookbooks and magazines feature recipes for vegetarian and natural food products, such as granola, whole-grain breads, and vegetable casseroles.
- Point out that foods containing natural laxatives, such as prunes and rhubarb, are not necessarily helpful because dependence may merely shift from commercial to natural laxatives. Astringent foods (tea, blackberries, blueberries, elderberries) are best avoided.
- Advise clients about hydration. Ample hydration helps prevent excessive reabsorption of water from the stools. Adults need at least 8 glasses of fluid (1,500 mL) daily.
- Explain ways to maintain adequate dietary potassium intake, because hypokalemia reduces smooth muscle motility and can cause intestinal atony and constipation.

Physical Activity

- Outline a graduated program for increasing physical activity and exercise. Such a program helps tone all the body's muscles, including the smooth muscle of the intestine. Immobility and lack of exercise are causes of constipation.

- Advise clients to engage in regular exercise. Suggest 20-minute workouts at least three times weekly. Recommend activities that reflect the client's interests, that are feasible during bad weather, and that are suitable for one or two participants. If exercise is fun and available no matter what the season or number of people, it is more likely to become a habit. Suitable activity may including walking, cycling, swimming, dancing, golf, or tennis, depending on the client's age, physical condition, and lifestyle.

Bowel Routine

- Urge clients to establish a toileting routine to promote regularity. An initial defecation urge that is ignored will subside within 1 or 2 minutes. Habitual suppression weakens the reflex. Advise clients to choose a time of day when leisurely attention can be paid to bowel function. Because gastrocolic reflex appears strongest after the first meal of the day, the period after breakfast may be most suitable. Clients may need to adjust their sleeping habits to allow 15 to 20 minutes of extra time between breakfast and the rest of the day.

Stress Reduction

- Explain that for some people, constipation is initiated or increased by unusual stress. These people respond to stress with autonomic stimulation, characterized by a predominance of sympathetic over parasympathetic activity. (Other people, in whom parasympathetic activity predominates, may pass frequent, loose stools when under stress.) Help clients find ways to reduce or better manage stress in their lives.

When preparing doses of dry bulk laxatives, care should be taken to minimize their dispersion into the environment. Inhalation of bulk laxative dust can cause respiratory distress and allergic reactions.

Mineral oil should be administered on an empty stomach, a minimum of 2 hours before bedtime. Clients receiving mineral oil over an extended period should be monitored for deficiencies of fat-soluble vitamins.

Usually, laxatives are avoided in debilitated clients because laxatives increase fluid and electrolyte loss from the lower intestine. Therefore, their excessive use predisposes the client to dehydration, hypokalemia, nutritional depletion, and malnutrition. Repeated passage of watery stools, which sometimes contain digestive enzymes, can cause anal excoriation.

Client Education. The client with simple, primary constipation requires considerable teaching to acquire a healthy attitude toward bowel function and to reform bowel habits.

The nurse must inform clients that laxative use may become habitual and that undue reliance on these agents in preference to hygienic measures fosters psychologic dependence. Cathartics and purgatives, which empty the lower GI tract, retard stool production. This then may be misinterpreted as continued constipation, and repetition of the laxative dosage establishes physiologic dependency.

In clients who develop a pattern of alternate laxative and antidiarrheal use, the nurse must point out that the body needs time to reestablish normal and natural patterns. The habitual use of laxatives by persons with normally functioning intestinal tracts is not a healthy practice. Chronic use can lead to fluid and electrolyte imbalances, steatorrhea, osteomalacia, and vitamin and mineral deficiencies.

The nurse must also inform clients that laxatives may be abused by persons seeking to lose weight or by persons suffering from eating disorders such as bulimia. Excessive dosages may be consumed in these situations. Frequent or excessive laxative treatment is also a form of child abuse.

Incorporating instruction about diet and exercise is one strategy that may help prevent constipation. Modern diets of highly processed, fiber-deficient foods, decreased physical labor, sedentary lifestyles, and increasing life expectancy (many elderly adults experience decreased intestinal secretion and motility) contribute to irregular bowel function.

Instruction about laxative abuse is important. Adding prunes or pears to the diet may correct occasional problems. The rare use of saline or irritant laxatives to treat temporary constipation is probably not harmful if the cause of the disruption is minor and not likely to recur. Milk of magnesia or bisacodyl is relatively benign for such use.

The nurse must explain that recurrent problems must be investigated to identify the underlying cause and determine the corrective measures needed. Excessive use of laxatives can cause fluid and electrolyte de-

CRITICAL THINKING CHALLENGE
Case Analysis

Mr. Workman, age 80, recently moved to the city home of his daughter and son-in-law and their four children, ages 4 to 17 years. Mr. Workman lived in his own home in the suburbs until his wife died. He has his own bedroom but shares a bathroom with three of the children. He no longer takes his usual daily walks because he fears walking in the urban area. He is in generally good health. He has diabetes mellitus, treated with oral hypoglycemic agents and diet. His hypertension is controlled with a thiazide diuretic and a beta blocker. When his wife was alive, she prepared his meals. Currently, meals are prepared by Mr. Workman's daughter, but he is often left to reheat casseroles or leftovers. Because of the hectic schedule of the household members, rarely do all of them eat together.

Mr. Workman has recently developed constipation.

1. What factors related to his drug therapy may contribute to this problem?
2. What nondrug factors may be contributing to the problem?
3. Prepare a teaching plan for Mr. Workman addressing ways to solve his current problem and prevent recurrence.

pletion. Some clients, who are unable or unwilling to change their lifestyles, continue to have problems. For them, regular use of a bulk-forming laxative may be necessary. Bulk-forming laxatives must be taken prophylactically because they are not immediately effective. Peristalsis may be stimulated within 12 to 24 hours, but the appearance of soft stools requires 2 to 3 days. Chronic use of other laxatives should be discouraged unless prescribed for a chronic medical condition.

When prolonged laxative use is necessary, clients should be taught the proper techniques for administering the drugs, the adverse reactions that can occur, and precautions necessary to prevent complications. Clients taking phenolphthalein preparations need reassurance that the pink color imparted to alkaline urine and feces is harmless.

Specific parameters should be established for bowel function and signs and symptoms of adverse reactions. This gives the client a clear understanding of the circumstances requiring renewed evaluation by a healthcare professional.

Clients using herbal preparations should be cautioned about potential problems (see Home and Community Care: Hazards of Herbal Preparations).

OUTCOME EVALUATION

Evaluation depends on accurate and comprehensive monitoring of fecal elimination. The amount, consistency, and frequency of stools should be recorded. Clients should report that defecation is comfortable, without cramping, distention, or pain.

HOME AND COMMUNITY CARE

Hazards of Herbal Preparations

Clients who are advocates of herbal medicines should be cautioned about certain laxative preparations.

Aloin is not recommended for laxative use or any other purpose requiring internal consumption. This drug is considered too toxic for systemic use. Although it is contraindicated during pregnancy, aloin is not a reliable or safe abortifacient.

Psyllium preparations containing the whole seed are unsuitable for ingestion. The outer seed coat acts as a harsh irritant. When digested, a pigment is released that is absorbed and subsequently deposited as small granules in the renal tubules. The significance of these deposits is unknown. Manufacturers claim that refined psyllium preparations from which the seed coat has been eliminated do not cause renal pigmentation.

Mineral waters are reputed to enhance health. Although they do contain salts such as magnesium or sodium sulfates, they are not reliable laxatives. Commercial mineral waters are artificially prepared, factory-made solutions that are not formulated for medicinal purposes and should not be used for treating constipation.

❖ **CHECKLIST OF NURSING ACTIONS**

❏ Promote fecal elimination by teaching clients to exercise regularly, to include ample fluids, potassium, and fiber in the diet, and to develop a regular toileting routine.

❏ Identify clients at risk for constipation from pathology or medical regimens; recommend regular use of bulk laxatives or stool softeners to prevent alteration in fecal elimination.

❏ Monitor clients at risk for constipation; recommend a saline or stimulant laxative for temporary relief should constipation develop.

❏ Monitor clients receiving laxatives for adverse reactions to these drugs.

❏ Discourage repeated use of stimulant, saline, or lubricant laxatives.

❏ Avoid inhaling dry bulk laxative powders by minimizing their dispersion in the environment.

❏ Monitor clients using mineral oil for deficiency of fat-soluble vitamins.

❏ Warn clients against using aloe as an herbal laxative.

❏ Warn clients not to use laxatives when abdominal pain or other signs and symptoms of appendicitis, intestinal obstruction, or peritonitis are present.

Physiology of Diarrhea

Rapid passage of intestinal contents, which results in frequent, watery stools, may result from parasympathetic overactivity or local irritation of the bowel mucosa. These stimuli cause increased secretion and hypermotility of the bowel. The fecal mass, moistened and lubricated by large amounts of mucus, is rapidly propelled from the tract through the anus. Increased peristalsis in the large bowel is reflected in the small intestine, and chyme is carried prematurely into the colon, shortly to be eliminated by succeeding waves of peristalsis.

Because absorption of nutrients, bile, and digestive enzymes is not allowed to proceed to completion, dehydration, electrolyte depletion, and nutritional deficits may develop. The stool may be green due to undigested bile; its odor is abnormal and may be foul. The stool, which may contain active digestive enzymes, is irritating and may macerate perianal tissues.

The affected client experiences weakness, spasms and abdominal pain, and anal soreness. Weight loss with diarrhea is primarily caused by dehydration, although some lean body mass and fat may be broken down if caloric intake is inadequate.

Causes of Diarrhea

Many factors are associated with diarrhea (Table 29-3). Excessive PNS activity can occur when cholinergic drugs are used, in hyperthyroidism, during withdrawal from narcotics, and as a response to stress in susceptible persons. PNS stimulation is probably the mechanism by which emotions contribute to the incidence and severity of diarrhea. Some people respond to stress by autonomic stimulation characterized by a preponderance of PNS over sympathetic nervous system activity.

Colonic irritation may be caused by mechanical or chemical factors. Mechanical irritants are usually poorly masticated foods containing fibers and seeds. These are particularly troublesome in clients with diverticulosis. Impacted feces and bowel tumors can also stimulate hypersecretion or hypermotility of the bowel. Chemical irritants include bacterial toxins, drugs, poisons, stimulant laxatives, and toxic components of foods. Salmonella, cholera, and amebic dysentery are some infectious causes of diarrhea. These illnesses may be transmitted by personal contact or in food or water. They are associated with substandard sanitation.

Diarrhea is also an adverse reaction to many drugs. Antibiotics alter the microbial flora and environment and predispose to intestinal superinfections. Broad-spectrum

Table 29-3. Common Causative Factors in Diarrhea

Mechanism Involved	Examples	Corrective Measures
Excessive parasympathetic activity	Use of cholinergic drugs Narcotic withdrawal Stress-induced diarrhea Hyperthyroidism	Anticholinergic agents may be used for treatment.
Mechanical irritation	Poorly masticated foods containing fiber and seeds Bowel tumors Fecal impaction	Removal of the source of irritation is necessary for definitive treatment.
Chemical irritation	Bacterial toxins (echovirus, coxsackievirus, *Escherichia coli*, salmonella species, shigella species, *Entamoeba histolytica, Giardia lamblia,* and so on)	Some conditions are self-limiting and will resolve with supportive treatment designed to maintain fluid and electrolyte balance.
	Superinfection secondary to use of broad-spectrum antibiotics (eg, *Clostridium difficile*)	An antimycotic or other anti-infective may be needed to treat the superinfection, or the antibiotic prescription may need to be changed.
	Reaction to drugs (iron supplements, antacids, colchicine)	A change in the drug order may resolve the problem.
Increased osmotic pressure in the intestinal lumen	Malabsorption syndrome Excessive intake of salt or sugar	Definitive treatment of the underlying syndrome or a change in diet is needed.
Inflammation of the bowel	Ulcerative colitis Crohn's disease	Definitive treatment of the underlying condition is required.
Laxative abuse	Regular use of laxatives with inability to defecate without laxatives	Reeducation and assistance in establishing regular bowel habits are needed.

antibiotics are particular offenders. By suppressing the immune response, some anticancer agents and other immunosuppressants may allow microorganisms to grow in the GI tract. Barbiturates, especially in large doses, stimulate peristalsis. In some cases, suicide attempts with barbiturates have failed because the large doses ingested precipitated prompt evacuation of the drug in diarrheal stools. The body reacts to many drugs and poisons with a similar protective catharsis.

Antidiarrheal Agents

Fluid and Electrolyte Solutions

Correcting fluid and electrolyte imbalances is an important part of diarrhea treatment. Solutions are administered orally when possible. Diet is limited to clear fluids to rest the bowel. If the client cannot ingest enough fluid to replace losses, or if the imbalance is pronounced, parenteral solutions are administered. Dextrose in water is usually given first to establish optimal renal function. Mixtures of electrolytes in succeeding bottles replace body deficits; excesses are excreted by the kidney. Additional potassium may be ordered because losses of this electrolyte tend to be severe. Bicarbonate is often required to correct acidosis. Common antidiarrheal medications are reviewed in Table 29-4.

Lactobacillus acidophilus

Lactobacillus acidophilus (Bacid) is an acid-producing bacterium prepared in a concentrated, dried, and viable culture for oral administration. Its presence in yogurt preparations indicates that yogurt contains live acidophilus.

Pharmacodynamics. The *L acidophilus* bacterium helps restore the normal flora of the GI tract by inoculating the tract with a fresh culture of viable organisms. The acid produced by this bacterial growth creates an environment favorable to beneficial flora and unfavorable to fungi and bacteria that can cause diarrhea.

Therapeutic Uses. The *L acidophilus* bacterium is used to treat diarrhea arising from the modification of intestinal flora by antibiotics. It is also used for infectious diarrhea, ulcerative colitis, irritable colon, diverticulitis, colostomies, functional constipation, mucous or spastic diarrhea, and diarrhea following amebiasis.

Adverse Reactions. When treatment is initiated, intestinal flatus may increase temporarily.

Precautions and Contraindications. Use of *L acidophilus* is not recommended for infants and children under age 3, unless treatment is ordered and supervised by the prescriber. It is contraindicated for those who are sensitive to or intolerant of milk products (ie, lactase-deficient persons).

Bismuth Subsalicylate

Bismuth subsalicylate is believed to have antisecretory, antimicrobial, and antiinflammatory effects. It is used to treat indigestion, prevent traveler's diarrhea, and treat

Table 29-4. Antidiarrheal Medications

Drug Name	Preparation	Usual Dosage	Additional Information
Demulcents and Protectives			
bismuth subsalicylate (Pepto-Bismol, Bismatrol)	Chewable tablets, liquids	As recommended on package labels PC: C (D in the third trimester)	Tongue and stools may become black. Avoid taking aspirin with bismuth subsalicylate. This product is also used to treat *Helicobacter pylori* infection in pepticulcer disease and to prevent traveler's diarrhea.
Adsorbents			
charcoal	Tablets for oral use	600 mg–5 g PRN PC: C	Burned toast remains a traditional preparation used for "indigestion."
kaolin } ingredients pectin } in OTC preparations (Donnagel-MB, Kaodene, K-C, Kaopectate, Kaopectolin, K-P)	Liquid for oral use	15–30 mL of kaolin with pectin (an official mixture) after each unformed stool PC: C	Kaopectate is contraindicated in the presence of fever.
Opiates			
difenoxin (Motofen)	With atropine, oral tablets	Adults: 2 tablets initially; then 1 tablet q3–4h as needed up to 8 tablets in 24 hr PC: C	Avoid giving difenoxin with monoamine oxidase inhibitors to avoid serious hypertension. Use with caution in hepatic disease.
diphenoxylate (Logen, Lomanate, Lomotil, Lonox)	With atropine, oral tablets and solution	Adults: 2 tablets (containing 5 mg of diphenoxylate) tid or qid Children 2–12 yr: (liquid only): 0.3–0.4 mg/kg daily in 4 divided doses PC: C	Diphenoxylate is frequently used to treat traveler's diarrhea. This drug can trigger pancreatitis due to spasm of the sphincter of Oddi.
loperamide hydrochloride (Imodium, Kaopectate II, Pepto Diarrheal Control, Maalox Anti-Diarrheal Caplets, Imodium A-D)	Oral capsules	Adults: *Initially:* 4 mg; *thereafter:* 2 mg after each unformed stool (maximum daily dosage 16 mg) Children 2–5 yr: *Initially:* 1 mg tid; 6–12 yr: 2 mg tid; *thereafter:* 1 mg/10 kg only after each loose stool (not to exceed initial daily dose) PC: B	Loperamide acts directly on the nerve endings or intramural ganglia of the intestinal wall; it may also increase segmentation and retard forward motion through the intestine by enhancing contractions of intestinal circular musculature.
Opium			
camphorated tincture of opium (paregoric)	Oral liquid (2 mg morphine per 5 mL)	Adults: 5–19 mL 1–4 times daily Children: 0.25–9.5 mL/kg 1–4 times daily PC: B (D for prolonged use or use of high doses at term)	Camphorated tincture of opium is subject to Schedule III controls under the Federal Controlled Substance Act of 1970. Do not confuse with tincture of opium deodorized, which is 25 times stronger.
tincture of opium (laudanum, deodorized opium tincture)	Oral liquid (50 mg morphine per 5 mL)	Adults: 0.3–1 mL 1–4 times daily Children: Dilute tincture of opium 1:25 and give 0.2–0.7 mL, depending on weight PC: B (D for prolonged use or use of high doses at term)	Tincture of opium is subject to Schedule II controls under the Federal Controlled Substance Act of 1970.
Inoculants			
Lactobacillus acidophilus (Bacid, Intestinex, Lactinex)	Oral capsules, granules, and tablets	Adults: 2 capsules, 4 tablets, or 1 pkt of granules, tid or qid	*Lactobacillus acidophilus* may be administered with food or fluids. Fermented milk products, buttermilk, and yogurt also contain *L. acidophilus.*

KEY: PC = pregnancy risk category; see Appendix A.

Helicobacter pylori infection in peptic ulcer disease. Because it contains salicylate, clients also taking aspirin could develop aspirin toxicity (eg, ringing of ears). It should be avoided in clients taking anticoagulants. Clients should be told that their stools and possibly their tongue may be discolored black.

Anticholinergics

Drugs that reduce PNS activity alleviate intestinal hypermotility and hypersecretion. They are rarely used alone in treating diarrhea but may be used as adjuncts with adsorbent medications. Anticholinergics are particularly effective in relieving spasms and tenesmus because they inhibit smooth muscle spasm. The anticholinergic effects are not confined to the bowel but affect all body systems, producing the side effects characteristic of these drugs. Overuse of anticholinergics causes subsequent constipation, which can be severe. For a detailed discussion of anticholinergics, see Chapter 16.

Demulcents and Protectives

Certain salts of polyvalent metals are believed to soothe and coat the intestine, reducing irritation and overstimulation. Their effects seem to be limited and their efficacy has yet to be proven. Salts of bismuth, calcium carbonate, and magnesium oxide are commonly used for this purpose. They are ingredients in OTC remedies such as Pepto-Bismol.

Adsorbents

Adsorbent antidiarrheals include charcoal, chalk, kaolin, and pectin.

Pharmacodynamics. Adsorbents attract and hold other chemicals on the surface of their molecules. Their value in diarrhea is attributed to the immobilization and removal of toxins and irritants. Their actions are general rather than specific.

Pharmacokinetics. Adsorbent antidiarrheals appear not to be absorbed systemically in significant amounts.

Therapeutic Uses. They are used to alleviate the symptoms of acute, short-term episodes of diarrhea.

Adverse Reactions. Adsorbents affect beneficial substances as well as harmful ones. They inhibit intestinal absorption of water, electrolytes, nutrients, and drugs, preventing even local action by the latter. Kaolin and pectin may cause constipation, especially if fever, which can cause dehydration, is present.

Precautions and Contraindications. Kaolin and pectin preparations should not be used when fever is present. They should not be used in young children (under 3 years old) and debilitated, elderly clients without the supervision of a healthcare professional. When self-administered, adsorbents should not be used for longer than 48 hours before consulting a healthcare professional.

Astringents

Astringents used for controlling diarrhea include many folk remedies and some beverages.

Pharmacodynamics. Astringents are believed to reduce diarrhea by inhibiting secretion and forming a protective layer on the mucous membrane surface through the precipitation of protein in the tissues. The latter mechanism is not scientifically substantiated.

Pharmacokinetics. Astringent foods include tea, blueberries, blackberries, and elderberries. They are absorbed by the GI tract and metabolized as nutrients. The potassium they provide helps replace the losses that occur with excessive depletion of lower GI tract contents. Elderberry wine and blackberry cordial, prized as diarrhea remedies, also provide alcohol, whose tranquilizing properties may help relieve the subjective distress caused by the ailment. The alcohol is absorbed in the upper digestive tract and does not reach the colon.

Therapeutic Uses. Preparations made from berries are long-standing folk remedies for diarrhea. Tea is also a traditional remedy. It is sometimes prescribed for use in self-limiting acute diarrhea, even in children.

Adverse Reactions. Excessive use of astringents can cause constipation. Xanthines in tea can provoke restlessness or insomnia in inexperienced users, such as children. The alcoholic content of wines and cordials can also cause toxicity if consumed in appreciable quantities.

Precautions and Contraindications. Astringent preparations should be sipped or taken in small amounts at frequent intervals. As diarrhea subsides, the amount taken should be reduced gradually until the medication can be discontinued.

Opioids

Constipation is a side effect of all opioid analgesics. Opium is a well-known antidiarrheal. A common opioid preparation used to treat diarrhea is diphenoxylate and atropine (Lomotil).

Pharmacodynamics. Opium depresses the nervous system, thereby slowing the propulsive movement of the small and large intestines.

Pharmacokinetics. Opium preparations taken for the relief of diarrhea are absorbed, metabolized, and excreted like all opioid drugs (see Chap. 18).

Therapeutic Uses. Opiates are used to prevent or relieve acute diarrhea caused by chronic conditions such as diverticulosis or diverticulitis.

Adverse Reactions. In addition to the usual adverse reactions caused by opioid drugs, antidiarrheal preparations can slow the passage and excretion of toxins from the digestive tract.

Precautions and Contraindications. Opiates should not be used in infectious diarrhea or other conditions associated with toxins in the digestive tract because they slow the excretion of these irritants and prolong the pathologic condition.

The usual precautions and contraindications for opioid drugs apply to the preparations used to treat diarrhea. As narcotics, all are subject to the Controlled Substances Act.

Caution should be taken not to confuse camphorated tincture of opium with tincture of opium deodorized: the latter has 25 times more morphine than the latter.

■ SUMMARY

Whenever possible, the underlying cause of diarrhea should be eliminated. During acute nonfebrile episodes, an adsorbent such as kaopectate is often effective. Lomotil, a combination of an anticholinergic and an opioid (diphenoxylate and atropine), is frequently prescribed for traveler's diarrhea and chronic diarrhea in elderly clients. Overuse of astringent foods, which are common folk remedies for diarrhea, can cause subsequent constipation.

❖ NURSING MANAGEMENT: CLIENT RECEIVING AN ANTIDIARRHEAL

It may be unwise to suppress diarrhea until the cause is identified, because purging is a physiologic defense mechanism. Once the underlying problem is identified, the prescriber can decide how safe it is to suppress the diarrhea by palliative agents. The cause of the bowel disorder should be determined as soon as possible and definitive corrective treatment begun. Treatment often involves the use of drugs. Antibiotics are corrective in many enteric infections. The judicious use of cathartics to relieve impactions or to purge the intestine of chemical toxins may eliminate the sources of irritation.

NURSING PROCESS

ASSESSMENT

Assessment of the client with diarrhea requires a careful history and physical examination. The nature and timing of symptoms must be thoroughly explored. Data to be collected include the time of onset, duration, frequency, periodicity, quality, severity, location, and radiation of symptoms. The nature, volume, and frequency of stools must be delineated and the presence of blood, mucus, and fiber noted. Associated symptoms, such as fever, chills, cramping, pain, nausea, vomiting, and malaise, are clues to the underlying problem. Associated events (eg, dietary changes, travel, wilderness outings) and exposure to animals, inadequate sanitation, or people with similar symptoms may help clarify the cause.

During the physical examination, a careful evaluation of the client's fluid, electrolyte, and nutritional status must be made. Although fever develops in dehydration, it often suggests infection as well. Hyperpnea suggests acidosis; tachycardia suggests hypovolemia. A complete examination of the abdomen is particularly important. Excessive bowel sounds, tenderness, and hypermotility may be readily apparent. A palpable mass in the transverse or descending colon suggests a high fecal impaction or intestinal tumor.

Clients receiving broad-spectrum antibiotics are at risk for developing diarrhea secondary to overgrowth of opportunistic organisms such as fungi.

NURSING DIAGNOSIS

Diagnoses related to clients receiving antidiarrheal drugs may include:

- Constipation, related to parasympathetic inhibition secondary to anticholinergic antidiarrheal medication
- Pain: Flatulence related to increased intestinal fermentation secondary to administration of *L acidophilus*
- Risk for Injury, related to CNS depression secondary to ingestion of antidiarrheal medication containing alcohol

PLANNING

The first desired outcome in treating diarrhea is to prevent or detect and promptly correct fluid and electrolyte imbalances. Such complications are the most serious threat to the client's life and well-being. In many instances, achieving this goal allows the body to recuperate and eliminate the cause of diarrhea. The underlying cause must be treated if it is not a self-limiting condition.

Other goals of drug therapy include increased client comfort by reducing cramping and preventing anal excoriation. Stools must be reduced in number and in fluid content. If the condition is severe or chronic, it is important to promote nutrition and to conserve the client's strength. Adverse reactions to antidiarrheal medication should be promptly detected and treated.

INTERVENTION

Fluids and electrolytes administered orally can be lifesaving. These may be prepared by dissolving Gastrolyte (a commercial preparation containing salts) as directed. Ready-to-use oral electrolyte maintenance solutions include Pedialyte, Rapolyte, and Rehydralyte. Parenteral fluids are administered when oral fluids are not tolerated or when rapid correction of fluid and electrolyte imbalance is required.

Diet should be limited to clear liquids. Tea, gelatin, water, cola drinks, and commercial products such as Gatorade help replenish fluids and electrolytes without further irritating the GI tract. A glucose and electrolyte solution (prepared by dissolving 3.5 g of sodium chloride, 2.5 g of sodium bicarbonate, 1.5 g of potassium chloride, and 20 g of glucose in sufficient water to make 1 L of solution) may be offered in unlimited quantities. Artificial sweeteners, some of which can irritate the colon, should be avoided.

Clients at risk for diarrhea caused by overgrowth of microorganisms may be given foods containing *L acidophilus* (buttermilk, yogurt, cottage cheese). To maintain a relatively normal intestinal flora, these foods should be taken three or four times a day, at least 1 hour after or 2 hours before oral antibiotic medication. The client with acute diarrhea should be encouraged to rest. Narcotic analgesics may be ordered for sedation and for their antidiarrheal effect.

As the client responds to treatment, the diet may be advanced to solids with the omission of milk products. Because diarrhea temporarily depletes the GI disaccharidases required for the digestion of lactose, milk should be avoided for a few days. When it is again tolerated, yogurt or buttermilk helps restore normal intestinal flora.

Progression of ambulation depends on the client's strength and the degree to which activity stimulates intestinal motility. Activity may be allowed in the absence of fatigue, dizziness, or increased diarrhea. Antidiarrheal drugs are usually given orally. Lomotil may be administered at specific hours, but adsorbents and paregoric are often ordered after each stool. A maximum daily dose should be established to avoid overmedication, a frequent cause of subsequent constipation.

To avoid excoriation, the perianal area should be cleansed carefully after each evacuation. An emollient barrier such as white petrolatum or A and D Ointment may be applied. Prevention of skin breakdown is especially important in clients who are debilitated, immobile, or incontinent.

Antidiarrheal medications should be decreased as the client's condition improves. They should be discontinued altogether when stools become soft and the daily frequency of bowel movements drops to two.

Client Education. The client should be informed that mild or temporary diarrhea is not uncommon and is often amenable to simple home treatment. Rest and a clear liquid diet are usually effective. A healthcare professional should be consulted, however, if severe fluid losses develop or the client cannot take fluids orally.

The nurse must explain that dizziness and weakness are danger signs. If the loose stools persist beyond 48 hours (depending on severity), medical attention is also required. These recommendations apply to adults only. Infants and small children can quickly become seriously ill, developing fluid and electrolyte imbalances, and should always be seen by a physician very early in the illness.

In teaching strategies to prevent potentially chronic diarrhea, the nurse should urge the client to avoid gas-forming foods, such as cabbage and beans. Milk products should be eliminated for a trial period if lactase de-ficiency is suspected. Artificial sweeteners, laxative foods, and laxative drugs should be avoided as well. Assistance in reducing or managing stress is helpful to some clients. The nurse should point out that if the condition fails to respond to these measures, the client should seek a diagnostic workup to determine the cause of diarrhea.

Clients planning trips to locations where diarrhea is endemic may be advised to take along bismuth subsalicylate (Pepto-Bismol). This may be taken in a dosage of 60 mL (or four tablets) four times a day to control diarrhea. Prolonged use (longer than 3 weeks) can cause CNS toxicity, however.

OUTCOME EVALUATION

Fluid balance must be closely monitored. An accurate record of intake should be kept. The volume of liquid stools must be measured and included in output totals. The client should be carefully observed for signs and symptoms of dehydration, hyponatremia, hypokalemia, and acidosis. A careful record of the number, frequency, and characteristics of stools is essential. If progress is normal, stools will decrease in frequency and become less liquid. Other data required for evaluation include client reports regarding comfort and energy levels, signs and symptoms of nutritional deficiency, and presence or absence of anal excoriation.

❖ CHECKLIST OF NURSING ACTIONS

- ❑ Carefully assess the client presenting with diarrhea to determine the nature of the underlying condition. Evaluate the presence of weakness, pain, or discomfort, fluid and electrolyte imbalance, malnutrition, perianal skin breakdown, and emotional effect.
- ❑ Administer solutions to correct fluid and electrolyte imbalances.
- ❑ Promote rest in the client with diarrhea.
- ❑ During the acute phase of illness, limit diet to clear fluids, progressing to a milk-free full diet as tolerated. Delay milk products until the normal intestinal flora are restored.
- ❑ Clean the perianal area carefully after each defecation; apply emollients to prevent irritation.
- ❑ Monitor fluid balance, electrolyte balance, and number, frequency, and characteristics of stools in clients with diarrhea.
- ❑ Use antidiarrheal medications in moderation to avoid the development of subsequent constipation.
- ❑ Advise clients to seek medical attention early in the course of an illness characterized by diarrhea; this is critical in children, who become dehydrated very quickly.
- ❑ Advise clients about measures to prevent food-related diarrhea.

Antiinflammatory Drugs for Gastrointestinal Disease

Drug therapy for inflammatory bowel diseases such as ulcerative colitis includes the use of many types of drugs to suppress the inflammatory process. These drugs include sulfasalazine (Chaps. 41 and 42), immunosuppressants (Chaps. 46 and 47), corticosteroids (Chap. 30), and 5-aminosalicylic acid derivatives.

Mesalamine (Asacol, Rowasa) is 5-aminosalicylic acid, which results from the biodegradation of sulfasalazine. It is believed to be the active ingredient responsible for the antiinflammatory effect. Although the mechanism is unknown, the antiinflammatory effect in the colon is believed to be local rather than systemic. Olsalazine (Dipentum) is biotransformed to mesalamine.

These agents are generally well tolerated; the more common adverse effects include nausea, diarrhea, and headache. Salicylate toxicity may occur because mesalamine is an aminosalicylate. Mesalamine and olsalazine may be administered orally or rectally.

Bibliography

Beverly L. (1992). Constipation: Proposed natural laxative mixtures. *J Gerontologic Nurs, 18*(10), 5.

Carpenter D, Zielinski, DA, et al. (1992). How do you treat and control *C difficile* infection? *Am J Nurs, 92*(9), 22.

Ericsson CD, DuPont HL, et al. (1993). Traveler's diarrhea: Approaches to prevention and treatment. *Clin Infect Dis, 6,* 616.

Gorbach SL. (1990). Bismuth therapy in gastrointestinal diseases. *Gastroenterology, 99,* 863.

Hanauer SB, Baert F. (1994). Medical therapy of inflammatory bowel disease. *Med Clin North Am, 78*(6), 1413–1426.

Hanauer SB, Peppercorn MD, Present DH. (1992). Current concepts: New therapies in IBD. *Patient Care, 26*(13), 79–102.

Harari D, Gurwitz JH, Avorn J, Choodnovsky I, Minaker KL. (1994). Constipation: Assessment and management in an institutionalized elderly population. *J Am Geriatrics Soc, 42,* 947–952.

Hirschfeld S, Clearfield HR. (1995). Pharmacological therapy for inflammatory bowel disease. *Am Fam Physician, 51*(8), 1971–1975.

Neims DM, McNeill J, Giles TR, Todd F. (1995). Incidence of laxative abuse in community bulimic population: A descriptive review. *Int J Eat Disord, 17*(3), 211–228.

Sachar DB. (1995). Maintenance therapy in ulcerative colitis and Crohn's disease. *J Gastroenterol, 20*(2), 117–122.

Shafik A. (1993). Constipation: Pathogenesis and management. *Drugs, 45*(4), 528–540.

Travis SP, Jewell DP. (1994). Salicylates for ulcerative colitis—their mode of action. *Pharmacol Ther, 63*(2), 135–161.

For more information and sample tests and activities, refer to Chapter 29 in the Student Workbook for Clinical Pharmacology and Nursing Management, 5th edition, available through your bookstore.

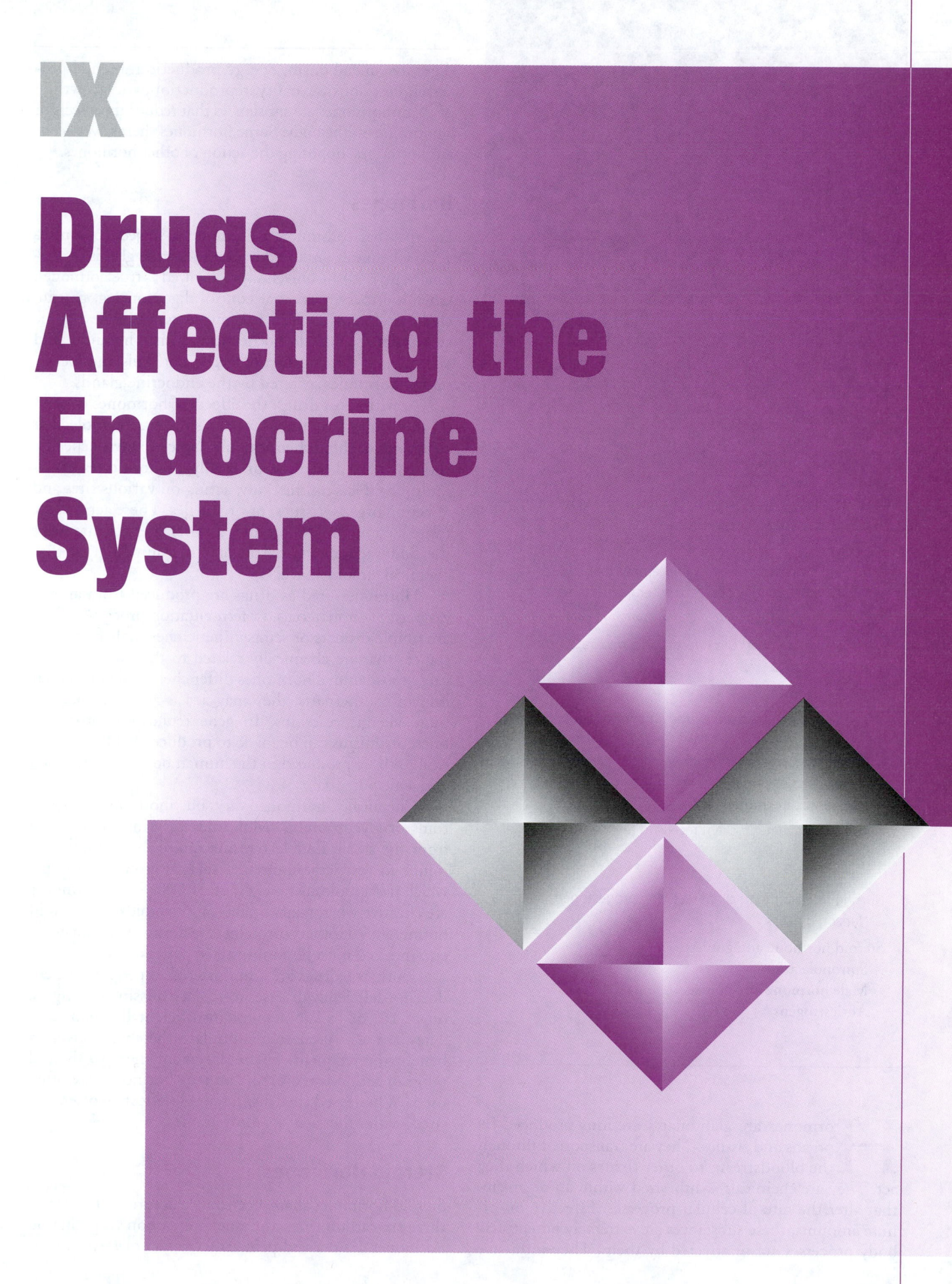

IX

Drugs Affecting the Endocrine System

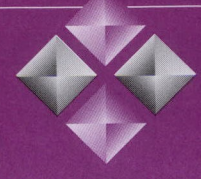

30

Drugs That Regulate Steroidal Hormone Levels

Hormones are glandular secretions produced by organs and tissues. They are transported through the bloodstream to other tissues on which they act. They are chemicals, synthesized within an organism, that alter the rate of cellular processes. Effective in minute amounts, these substances are extremely potent; few body processes are unaffected by them. They influence digestion, metabolism, energy production, mental processes, emotions, sexuality, reproduction, and growth.

Antihormones are substances that reduce the effects of a hormone on the body. Some hormones themselves act as antihormones, opposing the action of other hormones.

Hormones

Exactly what constitutes a hormone is subject to controversy. Chemicals produced by the endocrine glands (eg, pituitary, thyroid) are universally recognized as true hormones. Chemical messengers that control digestion (eg, gastrin, cholecystokinin) are also recognized as hormones. Some authorities also include biochemicals, such as histamine and serotonin, in this category; others do not. This unit focuses on the hormones secreted by the endocrine glands.

As with most drugs, the effects of hormones depend on molecular structure. Certain subunits or molecular structures of these chemicals are associated with specific actions. Each hormone or family of hormones exerts multiple effects on the body, acting on various sites and affecting organs, tissues, or organelles. These actions are related, combining to produce an overall effect that helps the body adapt to a particular environmental or biochemical circumstance.

Hormones used as drugs are produced from animal extracts, plant materials, or fermentation processes. They are simple extracts or semisynthetic chemicals from substances that are chemically related to the hormone. Because most animal hormones differ chemically from their human counterparts, they may act as antigens that can cause allergic reactions. In gene replication processes, microorganisms can be made to produce hormones identical to those produced in the human body, with reduced antigenic potential.

Chemically, hormones vary, but most are either steroids or glycoproteins. Molecules vary in size, ranging from the small, double tyrosine molecule of triiodothyronine to very large molecules such as growth hormone, which has a molecular weight of 21,500. Some hormones are effective when taken orally (most steroids and thyroid hormone), but others (proteins) are destroyed by digestive enzymes and must be administered parenterally.

Hormone drugs are administered to people with endocrine deficiency diseases to replace missing (see figure on p. 16) or to supplement insufficient biochemicals. They are also used to manipulate the metabolism to benefit the recipient. For replacement therapy, the full range of action is required, and true hormones are often used. When used as drugs, a single effect is often desired, with other actions undesirable.

Steroid Hormones

Steroid hormones share a central structure that contains three six-carbon rings and one five-carbon ring. Steroid hormones are derived primarily from cholesterol in the body, differing from each other in the number and nature of side groups or chains attached to the various rings (see page 16). The hormones produced by the adrenal cortex and the gonads—glucocorticoids, mineralocorticoids, and sex hormones—are all steroids. Certain hormones are precursors of others with markedly differing characteristics. For example, progesterone is converted to both mineralocorticoids and glucocorticoids. Androstenedione, an androgenic hormone, can be converted to either estrogens or another androgen, 11-beta-hydroxyandrostenedione.

Steroidal Functions

Steroid hormones perform many important functions in the body. Estrogens and androgens are responsible for sexual characteristics; their rhythmic secretion and relative concentrations determine sexual development and function. The glucocorticoids are vital to life, providing the responses necessary for physiologic adaptation to stress. The mineralocorticoids maintain blood volume necessary for proper circulation. All these hormones are available for use as pharmacologic agents.

Steroidal Actions

Steroid hormones react with receptor proteins in the cytoplasm of target cells to form complexes that then enter the nucleus (Fig. 30-1). There they bind with chromatin and influence the rate of protein and enzyme synthesis by stimulating the production of messenger ribonucleic acid (RNA). The protein or enzyme so produced determines the specific effects. For the most part, steroids are degraded by the liver and excreted in urine. Levels may be measured by either blood or urine assay.

Kinds of Steroids

The cortex of the adrenal glands produces several steroid hormones: mineralocorticoids, glucocorticoids, and sex hormones.

Corticosteroids are categorized as mineralocorticoids and glucocorticoids. Although both sexes produce both male and female sex hormones in the adrenal glands, the amounts are usually insignificant compared to the amounts secreted by the gonads. Mineralocorticoids and glucocorticoids share many functions, but glucocorticoids are characterized by widespread effects on body metabolism, inflammation, and immune response, with less pronounced effects on fluids and electrolytes. Mineralocorticoids exert greater effects on fluid and electrolyte balance.

Glucocorticoid secretion is triggered by pituitary secretion of adrenocorticotropin in response to stress. These corticoids alter metabolism to maintain or increase the blood glucose level. This action maintains brain and other vital functions when increased energy is required by the organism. These chemicals contribute to stress resistance by stimulating the central nervous system (CNS), inhibiting inflammation, and increasing

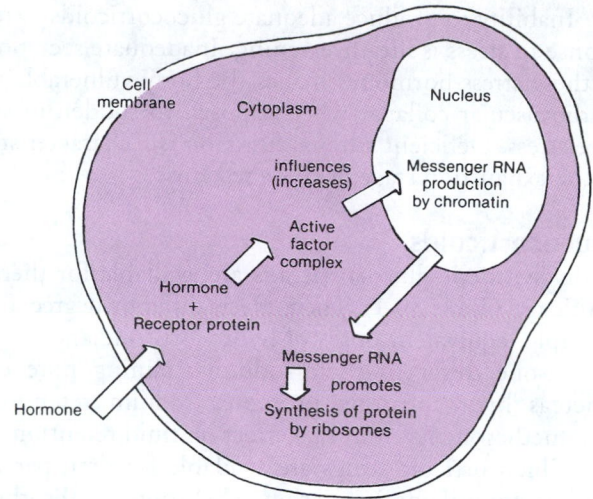

Figure 30-1. The mechanism of action of steroid hormones involves effects in cell nuclei.

coagulability of the blood. The increase in sodium and water retention provides additional blood volume. The glucocorticoids also suppress immune responses and inhibit growth.

The two main naturally occurring mineralocorticoids, desoxycorticosterone and aldosterone, act on the renal tubule to promote sodium reabsorption and potassium and hydrogen excretion. Water reabsorption increases secondary to sodium retention. As a result, blood volume and blood pressure are maintained at levels adequate for circulation.

Production of the mineralocorticoid hormones by the zona glomerulosa of the adrenal is independent of that of the other cortical steroids. Factors that affect mineralocorticoid secretion include potassium ion concentration in the extracellular fluid, volume of extracellular fluid, and sodium concentration in the extracellular fluid. Hormone secretion is stimulated by high potassium concentration, low blood volumes, and low sodium concentration.

Pathophysiology of Significant Hormone Deficiencies

A primary deficiency of adrenal corticosteroids in which production of glucocorticoids and mineralocorticoids is inadequate is Addison's disease, which results from destruction of the adrenal cortex by infection or hemorrhage.

Salt-losing adrenogenital syndrome is a congenital condition characterized by an inherited enzymatic interference with the synthesis of glucocorticoids and mineralocorticoids. When body levels of these corticosteroids are low, the pituitary is stimulated to produce large amounts of corticotropin. Although the adrenals cannot increase glucocorticoid or mineralocorticoid production, they do respond to corticotropin by increasing production of adrenal androgens, causing abnormally high testosterone levels and masculinization.

Inability to produce adequate glucocorticoids in response to stress is life-threatening. Inadequate secretion of these stress hormones makes the body vulnerable to cardiovascular collapse when exposed to sudden or severe stress. Deficient adrenal function is a characteristic of the exhaustion stage of stress response.

Glucocorticoids

Many synthetic glucocorticoids are available for therapeutic use (Table 30-1). Their effects differ by degree. For example, equivalent doses of hydrocortisone and dexamethasone differ in their sodium-retaining potency: whereas hydrocortisone promotes sodium retention, dexamethasone has minimal effect on fluid retention.

Glucocorticoid drugs are available for oral, parenteral, or topical administration. The drugs are absorbed by all routes. Aerosol and parenteral administration can produce rapid increases in blood levels. When it can be used, the oral route is preferred for systemic effect. Topical use always results in some systemic absorption and may produce systemic side effects. Whereas most glucocorticoid medications are limited to prescription use, many ointments and creams containing these drugs are available without a prescription.

Pharmacodynamics. Glucocorticoids function within the cell to influence protein production. They have the potential for producing a full range of hormone effects, including a rise in blood glucose level, sodium and water retention, increased potassium excretion, immunosuppression, CNS stimulation, mood elevation, inhibition of cell division, increased coagulability of blood, suppression of inflammation, and inhibition of corticotropin secretion. These drugs also blunt the senses, including that of pain. A few drug preparations are more specific in action in that they produce minimal sodium and water retention.

Pharmacokinetics. Glucocorticoids are effective by all routes. They are absorbed through the skin and mucous membranes as well as from the gastrointestinal (GI) tract. After absorption, they are distributed to all tissues through the bloodstream. They are metabolized by the liver and excreted by the kidneys.

Therapeutic Uses. Glucocorticoids are used as replacement therapy to maintain appropriate physiologic stress responses in clients with deficient adrenal function. Glucocorticoids are used also to treat various diseases because they have broad effects on basic physiologic processes (Table 30-2). Their uses include treating inflammatory diseases, allergic conditions, autoimmune diseases, organ rejection, cancers, and edema resulting from traumatic injury or surgery.

Although palliative rather than curative, the glucocorticoids are often the drugs of choice in the absence of better therapies. In combination with other drugs, glucocorticoids are used to suppress the immune response in recipients of organ transplants.

Dosage and Administration. The drug, route, dosage, and schedule of administration vary according to the condition being treated. In replacement therapy, the goal is to replicate the physiologic effects of the hormone being replaced, to achieve hormone balance, and to avoid symptoms of deficiency or excess. The drug is administered so as to mimic the normal diurnal pattern of hormone secretion (Fig. 30-2 on p. 624). Doses are given once or twice a day, on arising and if needed about 6 hours later. The basal dose is increased according to the degree of additional stress expected. Usually, double doses are taken for a mild increase in stress, such as a cold. Three or more times the basal dose may be needed to compensate for severe stress.

Relatively large doses are needed in acute addisonian crisis (circulatory shock resulting from a sudden inadequacy of the adrenal stress response). In clients with permanent deficiency, drug therapy must continue indefinitely. Temporary hyposecretion may respond to a course of glucocorticoid therapy to provide a period of rest, followed by gradual reduction of the dose to zero. Pituitary corticotropin production is suppressed by therapeutic use of the glucocorticoids, but serious deficiency states can be avoided by gradual withdrawal of the drugs.

Dexamethasone is the drug of choice for preventing cerebral edema because of its antiinflammatory effect, with minimal sodium and water retention. The drug is administered orally several times a day at equal intervals (eg, every 6 hours). A relatively stable blood level is desirable to maintain a constant effect. The drug is withdrawn gradually once the danger of cerebral edema subsides.

Prednisone, an oral glucocorticoid, is commonly used for other conditions that require a systemic drug effect. In short-term therapy, the drug is administered regularly, at frequent intervals, to maintain a constant blood level. In long-term therapy, larger doses are given every other day. This timing significantly reduces the incidence of side effects without impairing the therapeutic response. Alternate-day doses should be administered as soon as possible after waking in the morning.

Topical preparations are normally restricted to short-term use. Therefore, they tend to be administered regularly, several times a day.

Adverse Reactions. The glucocorticoids are potent medicines. When used in high doses or over a long period of time, toxic effects are common. In extreme cases, full-blown Cushing's syndrome develops. In this condition, many if not all of the toxic effects listed in Table 30-2 develop. Other side effects include leukocytosis, hiccups, abnormal hirsutism, menstrual disturbances, infertility, muscle weakening, thinning of the skin, ruddiness of complexion, and striae (stretch marks) on the torso and extremities. Glucocorticoids may double the incidence of peptic ulcers.

Text continues on page 624.

Table 30-1. Drug Preparations That Contain Glucocorticoid Hormones

Drug Name	Preparation	Usual Dosage
alclometasone dipropionate (Aclovate)	Topical cream and ointment (0.05%)	Apply a thin film to affected area bid or tid.
amcinonide (Cyclocort; *Can:* Mycoderm)	Topical cream and ointment	Apply a thin film to affected area bid or tid.
beclomethasone dipropionate (Beclovent, Propaderm, Vanceril; *Can:* Beclodisk, Beconase)	Oral aerosol inhaler	Adults: *Initial:* 84 µg (2 sprays) tid or qid (*maximum daily dosage:* 840 µg or 20 sprays) Children 6–12 yr: *Initial:* 42–84 µg (1 or 2 sprays), tid or qid (*maximum daily dosage:* 420 µg or 10 sprays) Not recommended for children younger than 6 yr of age
betamethasone (Celestone, Cel-U-Jec, Selestoject)	Oral tablets and solution (0.6 mg/5 mL) Solutions and suspension for injection	Adults: *Initial:* 2.4–4.8 mg/day, divided in 2–4 doses (*maximum daily dosage:* 7.2 mg) Children: 0.0175–0.25 mg/kg or 0.5–7.5 mg/m², divided in 3 or 4 doses *IM:* 0.5–9 mg or more/day (varying with the condition being treated)
betamethasone benzoate (Baben, Uticort)	Topical cream, gel, lotion, and ointment (0.025%)	Apply sparingly and rub gently into affected area 1–4 times daily.
betamethasone dipropionate (Alphatrex; *Can:* Diprosalic)	Topical cream, lotion, and ointment (0.05%) Topical aerosol spray	Apply sparingly and rub gently into affected area 1–4 times daily. *Maximum weekly dosage:* 45 g; *maximum course of treatment:* 14 days Spray an area the size of the client's hand not more than 3 sec from a distance of 15 cm tid–qid.
betamethasone valerate (Betacort, Valisone; *Can:* Celestoderm, Betacort, Betnovate, Rholosone)	Topical lotion, cream, and ointment (0.1%)	Apply sparingly and rub gently into affected area 1–4 times daily.
(Valisone Reduced Strength)	Topical lotion (0.01%)	Apply sparingly and rub gently into affected area 1–4 times daily.
clobetasol (Temovate; *Can:* Dermovate)	Topical cream and ointment (0.05%)	Apply sparingly and rub gently into affected area bid.
clocortolone (Cloderm)	Topical cream (0.1%)	Apply sparingly and rub gently into affected area 1–4 times daily.
cortisone (Cortone)	Powder and solution Oral tablets Suspension for IM injection	Dosage varies with the condition being treated and the response of the client; high doses are given initially, then decreased to the lowest effective maintenance dose. Daily dosage may be divided in 1 or 2 doses. Adults: *Initial:* Oral: 25–300 mg/day; *IM:* 20–300 mg/day Children: *Initial:* Oral: 0.7–10 mg/kg/day or 20–300 mg/m²/day; *IM:* 0.2–1.25 mg/kg/day or 7–37.5 mg/m²/day
desonide (DesOwen, Tridesilon)	Topical cream and ointment (0.05%–0.25%)	Apply sparingly and rub gently into affected area bid–qid.
desoximetasone (Esperson, Topicort)	Topical cream, gel, and ointment (0.05%–0.25%)	Apply sparingly and rub gently into affected area bid.
dexamethasone (AK-Dex, Decadron, Hexadrol, Maxidex, Mymethasone)	Oral elixir, tablets, solution and solution concentrate	Adults: 0.75–9 mg/day, divided in 2–4 doses Children: 0.024–0.34 mg/kg or 0.66–10 mg/m²/day, divided in 4 doses
(Aeroseb-Dex, Decaderm, Decaspray)	Topical aerosol spray (0.01%–0.1%)	Apply sparingly and rub gently into affected area tid or qid.
dexamethasone acetate (Decadron-LA, Dekasol-LA, Dexasone-L.A., Solurex L.A.)	Suspension for injection	Adults: *Initial:* 8–16 mg, q1–3wk Children younger than 12 yr: dosage has not been established
dexamethasone sodium phosphate (Decadron Phosphate Respihaler, Dalalone, Decadrol, Decadron, Decaject, Decameth, Demasone	Oral inhaler Solutions for injection	Adults: 300 µg (3 inhalations), tid or qid (*maximum daily dosage:* 1200 µg or 12 inhalations) Children: 200 µg (2 inhalations), tid or qid (*maximum daily dosage:* 800 µg or 8 inhalations) *IM* or *IV:* Adults: 0.5–24 mg/day; children 6–40 µg/kg or 0.235–1.25 mg/m², 1 or 2 times daily

All drugs in this table are in pregnancy risk category C, except cortisone (category D) and prednisolone (category B). See Appendix A. *Can* = Canadian trade name.

(continued)

Table 30-1. (Continued)

Drug Name	Preparation	Usual Dosage
Dexacen-4, Dexameth, Dexon, Dexone, Dezone, Gammacorten, Hexadrol, Savacort D, Solurex)	Topical cream (0.1%)	Apply sparingly and rub gently into affected area tid or qid.
diflorasone diacetate (Florone, Flutone)	Topical cream and ointment (0.05%)	Apply sparingly and rub gently into the affected area bid–qid.
flunisolide (Aerobid, Syntaric; Can: Rhinalar)	Aerosol inhalant	Use only twice a day.
fluocinolone (Fluronid, Flurosyn, Synemol)	Topical cream, ointment, and solution (0.01%, 0.025%)	Apply sparingly and rub gently into the affected area bid–qid.
fluocinonide (Lidemol, Lyderm, Lidex, Metosyn)	Topical cream, gel, ointment, and solution (0.05%)	Apply sparingly and rub gently into the affected area bid–qid.
fluprednisolone (Alphadrol)	Oral tablets	Adults: *Initial:* 2.5–30 mg/day, divided in 3 or 4 doses Children: *Replacement:* 0.07 mg/kg/day or 2 mg/m²/day, divided in 3 doses
flurandrenolide (Cordran, Drenison, Drocort, Sermaka)	Topical cream, lotion, and ointment (0.025%–0.05%) Dressing (4 µg/cm²)	Apply sparingly and rub gently into the affected area bid or tid. Apply to clean, dry affected area q12h.
halcinonide (Halog)	Topical cream, ointment, and solution (0.025%–0.1%)	Apply sparingly and rub gently into the affected area bid or tid.

Hydrocortisone (Cortisol)

Drug Name	Preparation	Usual Dosage
hydrocortisone (Bactine, Cetacort, Cortate, Cortef, Cortenema, Cortiment, Cortril, Dermacort, Emo-Cort, Hycort, Hydrocortex, Hytone, Prevex, Hydrocortone, Proctocort, Synacort, Texacort, Unidort)	Powder, oral tablets, suspension for injection	*Oral:* Adults: *Initial:* 10–320 mg/day, divided in 3 or 4 doses; children: 0.56–8 mg/kg/day or 16–240 mg/m²/day, divided in 3 or 4 doses *IM:* Adults: *Initial:* 15–240 mg/day, divided in 2 doses
	Topical cream, solution, ointment, powder, and lotion	Apply sparingly and rub gently into affected area 1–4 times daily.
	Topical aerosol spray	Spray each 10 cm² of affected area for 1–2 sec from a distance of about 15 cm bid or tid.
	Rectal suspension (100 mg/60 mL)	Adults: 100 mg nightly administered as a retention enema
	Rectal cream, ointment (0.5%–1.0%)	Apply creams and ointments externally to the anal area.
	Powder for suspension	Adults: 40 mg dissolved in 30–180 mL water, administered as a retention enema
hydrocortisone cypionate (Cortef Fluid)	Oral suspension	Adults: *Initial:* 10–320 mg/day, divided in 3 or 4 doses Children: 0.56–8 mg/kg/day or 16–240 mg/m²/day, divided in 3 or 4 doses
hydrocortisone acetate (Alocort, Cortocet, Corticreme, Fernisone, Lanacort, Can: Novohydrocort)	Suspension for injection	For intrasynovial, intrabursal, or intra-articular injection, 5–50 mg, q3–5d (for bursae) or q1–4wk (for joints); dosage varies with degree of inflammation and size and location of affected area.
(Cortifoam)	Rectal aerosol foam suspension (10%)	Adults: 90 mg (1 full applicator) 1 or 2 times daily
(Cort-Dome, Corticaine)	Rectal suppositories (10 mg, 25 mg)	Adults: 10–50 mg bid or tid
(Cortaid, Cortef, Pharm-Cort, Rhulicort)	Topical cream, lotion, ointment, and paste (0.5%–1%)	Apply sparingly and rub gently into affected area 1–4 times daily.
(CaldeCORT)	Topical aerosol spray (0.5%)	Spray each 10 cm² of affected area for 1–2 sec from a distance of 15 cm bid or tid.

All drugs in this table are in pregnancy risk category C, except cortisone (category D) and prednisolone (category B). See Appendix A.
Can = Canadian trade name.

(continued)

Table 30-1. (Continued)

Drug Name	Preparations	Usual Dosage
hydrocortisone sodium phosphate (Hydrocortone Phosphate)	Solution for injection	Adults: *Initial:* 15–240 mg/day, divided in 2 doses Children: 0.16–1 mg/kg or 6–30 mg/m², 1 or 2 times daily
hydrocortisone sodium succinate (A-hydroCort, Solu-Cortef)	Solutions for injection	Adults: 100–500 mg, q2–10h Children: 0.16–1 mg/kg or 6–30 mg/m², 1 or 2 times daily
Methylprednisolone		
methylprednisolone (Metastab, Urbason; *Can:* Medrate)	Oral tablets	Adults: *Initial:* 2–60 mg/day, divided in 4 doses Children: 0.117–1.66 mg/kg/day or 3.3–50 mg/m²/day, divided in 3 or 4 doses
methylprednisolone acetate (Duralone, Medrone, Mepred)	Suspension for IM, intra-articular, intralesional, or soft-tissue injection	Adults: 10–80 mg
(Medrol)	Powder for rectal suspension	40 mg dissolved in 30–180 mL water administered as a retention enema
(Medrol)	Topical ointment	Apply sparingly and rub gently into affected area 1–4 times daily.
methylprednisolone sodium succinate (A-methaPred, Solu-Medrol)	Solutions for IM or IV injection	Adults: 10–250 mg (may be repeated up to 6 times daily) Children: 0.03–0.2 mg/kg or 1–6.25 mg/m², 1 or 2 times daily
mometasone furoate (Elocon)	Topical cream and ointment	Apply only once a day.
paramethasone acetate (Alondra, Dilar, Haldrate, Haldrone, Monocortin, Stemex)	Oral tablets	Adults: *Initial:* 2–24 mg/day, divided in 3 or 4 doses Children: 0.058–0.8 mg/kg/day or 1.67–25 mg/m²/day, divided in 3 or 4 doses
Prednisolone		
prednisolone (Cortalone, Delta-Cortef, Hydeltra, Prelone, Tracortenol)	Powder Oral tablets	Adults: *Initial:* 5–60 mg/day, divided in 2–4 doses Children: 0.14–2 mg/kg/day or 4–60 mg/m²/day, divided in 4 doses
prednisolone acetate (Fernisolone, Meticortelone, Savacort; *Can:* Pred-Forte, Pred Mild)	Suspensions for IM, intra-articular, or soft-tissue injection	Adults: *Initial:* 4–60 mg/day, divided in 2 doses, administered at 12-hr intervals Children: 0.04–0.25 mg/kg/day or 1.5–7.5 mg/m²/day, 1 or 2 times daily
prednisolone sodium phosphate (Articulose, Hydeltrasol, solu-Predalone)	Solution for injection	Adults: *Initial:* 4–60 mg/dose Children: 0.04–0.25 mg/kg or 1.5–7.5 mg/m², 1 or 2 times daily
prednisolone tebutate (Hydeltra-T.B.A., Metalone T.B.A.)	Suspension for intra-articular, intralesional, or soft-tissue injection	Adults: 4–40 mg, q2–3wk; dosage varies with degree of inflammation and size and location of affected area.
prednisone (Cortan, Deltasone, Meticorten, Panasol, Prednicen-M)	Powder Oral tablets and solution	Adults: *Initial:* 5–60 mg/day, divided in 2–4 doses Children: 0.14–2 mg/kg/day or 4–60 mg/m²/day, divided in 4 doses
Triamcinolone		
triamcinolone (Apo-Triazo, Aristo-Pak, Traderm, Triamacort)	Oral tablets	Adults: *Initial:* 4–48 mg/day, divided in 1–4 doses Children: 0.117–1.66 mg/kg/day or 3.3–50 mg/m²/day, divided in 4 doses
(Azmacort)	Oral inhalation	2 sprays (200 µg)

All drugs in this table are in pregnancy risk category C, except cortisone (category D) and prednisolone (category B). See Appendix A.
Can = Canadian trade name.

(continued)

Table 30-1. (Continued)

Drug Name	Preparation	Usual Dosage
triamcinolone acetonide (Acetospan, Aristocort, Cenocort, Cinomide, Flutex, Kenaject, Kenalog, Tac-3, Triacet, Triam-A, Triam-onide, Tri-Kort, Trilog, Trymex)	Suspension for IM, intra-articular, intrasynovial, intralesional, sublesional, and soft-tissue injection Oral aerosol inhaler Topical aerosol spray Topical cream, lotion, ointment, and paste (0.025%–0.1%)	*IM:* Adults and children older than 12 yr: 60 mg q6wk; children 6–12 yr: 0.03–0.2 mg/kg or 1–6.25 mg/m² q1–7 days 200 µg (2 sprays) tid or qid Apply sparingly and rub gently into affected area 1–4 times daily. Apply sparingly and rub gently into affected area 1–4 times daily.
triamcinolone diacetate (Amcort, Aristocort, Cenocort, Cino, Kenacort, Triacort, Trilone)	Oral solution Suspension for IM, intra-articular, intrasynovial, intralesional, sublesional, and soft-tissue injection	Adults: *Initial:* 4–48 mg/day, divided in 1–4 doses Children: 0.117–1.66 mg/kg/day or 3.3–50 mg/m²/day, divided in 4 doses
triamcinolone hexacetonide (Aristospan)	Suspension for intra-articular, intralesional, or sublesional injection	*Intralesional:* up to 0.5 mg/square inch of affected skin *Intra-articular:* 2–20 mg/q3–4wk; dosage varies with size of affected area

All drugs in this table are in pregnancy risk category C, except cortisone (category D) and prednisolone (category B). See Appendix A. *Can* = Canadian trade name.

Physiologic and behavioral changes occur in clients on long-term therapy. The adrenal glands of these clients atrophy because pituitary corticotropin production is suppressed and the normal diurnal fluctuation of glucocorticoids is obliterated. The client becomes physically dependent on the hormone medications. Prolonged treatment may irreversibly damage the adrenals, resulting in permanent Addison's disease. Psychologic dependence on the euphoria produced by the hormones also may occur. Anaphylactoid reactions have been reported, possibly because of the corticosteroid base or the ester form of the preparation.

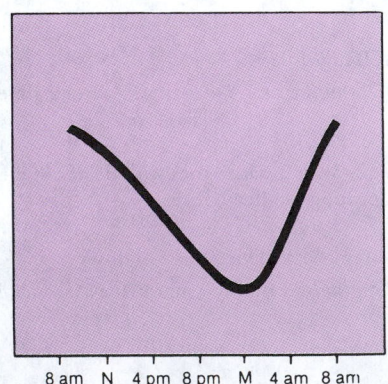

8 am N 4 pm 8 pm M 4 am 8 am

Figure 30-2. Spontaneous diurnal variation in 17-hydroxycorticoids in people with daytime activity schedule. Without stress, adrenal production of glucocorticoids reaches a maximum at about 6 AM, after which production gradually declines to the lowest level from early evening to midnight. The difference between maximal and minimal levels of active 17-hydroxycorticoids in the blood is twofold to fourfold in most people. The actual curve is not smooth; corticotropin is secreted intermittently by the pituitary in short bursts or boluses.

Drug Interactions. When used with other drugs, glucocorticoids may interfere with their therapeutic effects. Other drugs also may affect the action of the hormones. Some combinations increase the risk of adverse effects (Table 30-3).

Precautions and Contraindications. Whenever glucocorticoids are used for purposes other than replacement therapy, the potential benefits must be weighed against the risk of harmful effects and toxicity. The decision for or against therapy requires considering the expected progress of the condition, the severity of likely complications, the availability of alternative treatments, and the life goals of the client. Box 30-1 lists principles that influence the decision for or against glucocorticoid therapy.

Before long-term glucocorticoid therapy begins, a baseline electrocardiogram, blood-pressure evaluation, chest and spinal x-rays, glucose tolerance tests, and evaluations of hypothalamic-pituitary-adrenal axis function should be performed. Parameters that require monitoring during therapy include height, weight, blood pressure, growth rate in children, serum glucose levels, and signs and symptoms of infection. Periodically, chest and spinal x-rays, complete blood cell counts, blood chemistries (especially glucose and electrolyte levels), and ocular pressure should be assessed.

When glucocorticoid therapy is prescribed for clients with a history of active tuberculosis, isoniazid may be used to prevent recurrence of the disease. Anti-tuberculosis drugs are sometimes ordered also for clients with a positive skin test for tuberculosis, because glucocorticoids may reactivate dormant organisms in the body.

Table 30-2. Major Physiologic Effects of Glucocorticoids

Organ System/Mechanism of Action	End Result of Prolonged Excessive Hormone Action*
Nutrient Metabolism	
Favors the formation of glucose from nutrients that contain calories (increases gluconeogenesis)	Increased blood sugar, diabetes mellitus in susceptible people, increased severity of preexisting diabetes mellitus
Favors glycogenolysis	
Antagonizes the action of insulin	
Favors the breakdown of protein	Muscle wasting, osteoporosis
Inhibits protein synthesis	
Promotes lipolysis of triglycerides of adipose tissue	Abnormal fat distribution ("buffalo hump," "moon face")
Fluid and Electrolytes	
Promotes sodium and water retention	Edema, hypertension, increased intraocular pressure
Favors potassium excretion	Weakness, fatigability
Tissue Response to Injury and Infection	
Suppresses the immune response	Serious infections with few signs and symptoms, post-transplant lymphoma
Suppresses inflammation	
Gastrointestinal Tract	
(Mechanisms obscure)	Peptic ulcerations, pancreatitis
Central Nervous System	
Stimulates the brain (Mechanisms obscure)	Insomnia, euphoria, manic psychosis
	Blunting of the senses (pain, taste, smell, hearing)
	Dementia that resembles Alzheimer's disease (rare)
Musculature	
Protein depletion	Progressive weakness of the shoulder and pelvic girdles and muscles of the extremities
Endocrine Glands	
Inhibits adrenocorticotropin secretion by the pituitary	Adrenal atrophy (when administered as a drug)
Blood	
Increases red blood cell production	Polycythemia
Increases coagulability	Increased incidence of thrombi and emboli
Cell Reproduction	
Inhibits cell division	Growth retardation, dwarfism, poor healing

*Most likely with systemic treatment, but some are seen after topical use (eg, eye drops, skin preparations).

Table 30-3. Interactions Between Glucocorticoids and Other Drugs

Interacting Drug	Effects
Hepatic enzyme inducers (eg, barbiturates, phenytoin, rifampin)	Enhanced glucocorticoid metabolism (need to increase glucocorticoid dosages)
Estrogens	Potentiation of effects of glucocorticoids (need to decrease glucocorticoid dosages)
	Potentiation of electrolyte imbalances and hypercoagulation effects
Ulcerogenic drugs (eg, indomethacin, aspirin and other nonsteroidal antiinflammatory agents)	Increased risk of GI ulceration
Salicylates	Decreased serum concentration of salicylates
Potassium-depleting diuretics (eg, thiazides, furosemide, ethacrynic acid)	Pronounced hypokalemia
Anticholinesterase agents (eg, ambenonium, neostigmine, pyridostigmine)	Severe weakness
Vaccines and toxoids	Diminished response to toxoids or vaccines
	Potentiation of replication of attenuated vaccines
	Increased risk of neurologic reactions to vaccines
Oral anticoagulants	Increased blood coagulability and need for increased dosages of anticoagulant

After prolonged use, glucocorticoids must be withdrawn gradually. Abrupt withdrawal can cause cardiovascular collapse and death in adrenal crisis. The route of administration does not affect the need for weaning. Dosage of topical as well as systemic preparations should be tapered gradually. The rate at which dosages should be decreased and the length of time required for weaning vary with the dosage and the duration of hormone therapy. Some clients who have received large doses for prolonged periods may require a weaning period of up to a year.

Glucocorticoid drugs are not generally recommended for children or in pregnancy or lactation. An exception is therapy to prevent abortion in pregnant women with lupus erythematosus. When glucocorticoids are required for treating a life-threatening condition, the risk of fetal damage or growth retardation in children must be considered.

Glucocorticoids should be used with caution in clients with seizure disorders, renal insufficiency, osteoporosis, or viral infections (especially those that affect the eye). Caution is also required in clients tak-

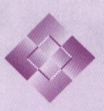

Box 30-1
Therapeutic Principles of Glucocorticoid Therapy

- Glucocorticoids should never be used unless the client's condition cannot be controlled by safer standard therapy.
- Each drug preparation has distinctive effects; the proper steroid should be carefully selected by the prescriber for each client. The appropriate dosage must be titrated for each client.
- The administration of glucocorticoid is palliative, not curative therapy.
- The prescriber should determine the smallest daily dose that will keep the client comfortable.
- The administration of massive doses of glucocorticoid for brief periods is virtually without harmful effects.
- When glucocorticoids are administered by a step-down dosage regimen (initial large dose and then reduction of dose each day for a week or two), there are rarely harmful effects.
- An individually tailored program may include alternate-day therapy or intermittent dosage schedules.
- When therapy is prolonged or the dosage is high, the incidence of potential disabling or lethal effects increases.
- Systemic glucocorticoid toxicity may be lessened by the use of locally acting drugs.
- Abrupt withdrawal of high dosage levels of glucocorticoids can result in acute adrenal insufficiency and may be life-threatening.

ing anticholinesterase or ulcerogenic antiinflammatory drugs.

Glucocorticoids are contraindicated in clients allergic to them. Because of the adverse reactions associated with glucocorticoids, many prescribers avoid such therapy except in life-threatening or permanently disabling situations.

◼ SUMMARY

Glucocorticoids are adrenal cortex steroid hormones that play a major role in the body's physical response to stress. They are used as replacement hormone therapy for Addison's disease and as drugs for the treatment of dangerous inflammatory conditions, acute allergy, serious autoimmune diseases, and certain cancers. Toxic and side effects are similar to the signs and symptoms of Cushing's disease and may be debilitating and life-threatening. Multiple preparations of both natural and modified hormones are available for use. Because their toxic potential is high, glucocorticoids are not prescribed unless the expected benefits clearly outweigh the risks.

❖ NURSING MANAGEMENT: CLIENT RECEIVING GLUCOCORTICOID THERAPY

The needs of the client who receives glucocorticoid therapy vary depending on the underlying illness, stage of disease, and therapeutic goals of nursing care. The nurse must assess the client's therapeutic response carefully, provide accurate and consistent administration of the drugs, minimize the incidence and severity of complications, and monitor the client for adverse reactions and toxic side effects. Education of clients and their families is vital.

NURSING PROCESS: HORMONE REPLACEMENT THERAPY

ASSESSMENT

Clients for whom replacement therapy is prescribed should be assessed to determine the effects of the hormone deficiency. In most cases, clients complain of fatigue, depression, weakness, and increased perception of pain. They may be prone to inflammatory or allergic conditions, such as arthritis or dermatitis. A history of circulatory shock or heat exhaustion is not unusual; tissue turgor is apt to be reduced. Clients or their relatives may have noticed a marked change in personality with clinical depression. If pituitary function is normal, the skin may appear bronzed. Abnormal pigmentation reflects excessive corticotropin production. The health history should describe the client before the onset of symptoms. Reestablishing the premorbid personality and level of function is a major goal of hormone therapy.

NURSING DIAGNOSIS

After hormone replacement therapy begins, nursing diagnoses reflect the client's risk for toxic reactions to the drug until optimal dosage is established. Diagnoses related to excessive medication may include:

- Constipation, related to hypokalemia secondary to glucocorticoid excess
- Fluid Volume Excess, related to sodium retention secondary to glucocorticoid excess
- Altered Body Image, related to metabolic changes secondary to glucocorticoid excess

Newly diagnosed clients also probably have:

- Knowledge Deficit, related to glucocorticoid deficiency and its treatment by hormone replacement

PLANNING

The long-range goal for treatment is to educate the client and family in managing the drug regimen to maintain proper hormone balance. Clients must learn how to administer the hormones for optimal effect, detect the signs and symptoms of both deficiency and excess of hormones, and adjust hormone dosages to meet the increased requirements of unusual stress. Short-range goals include reducing anxiety, pain, abdominal discomfort, and the number of stools, maintaining blood volume, restoring normal tissue turgor, and conserving limited energy.

INTERVENTION

At the time of diagnosis, clients need emotional support and assistance in accepting a chronic health condition that requires lifelong medication. The nurse helps the client through the grieving that precedes acceptance. Until the client resolves the conflicts inherent in this situation, therapeutic adherence may be poor.

Client Education. For the short time until medication restores hormonal equilibrium, the client should be taught measures to compensate for residual deficiency. Foods rich in potassium should be avoided so that blood levels of this electrolyte begin to decline. Foods should be nonirritating; any food known to cause abdominal cramping or diarrhea should be excluded from the diet. The client should continue to take extra salt and fluids to maintain blood volume. Extra rest and reduced stress help conserve energy. Higher-than-normal doses of analgesics may be needed to relieve common pain such as headache. These precautions need to be observed for only a few days until the medication regimen is well established.

The nurse must stress the importance of maintaining the drug regimen, because failing to do so can have life-threatening consequences. The client with a history of an acute shock may have no trouble understanding the importance of medication, but another client without such an experience may have a prolonged denial reaction.

The nurse also must explain the importance of carrying medical identification that names the client's hormone deficiency. A medical bracelet, tag, or wallet card alerts healthcare personnel to these needs even when the client cannot communicate.

Another area for teaching is identification of signs and symptoms that herald both hormone deficiency and excess. The full-blown syndrome of both imbalances should be described to clarify the differences between each extreme. The client should be advised to watch for mood changes (euphoria from excess glucocorticoids, dysphoria characterized by anxiety and depression from deficiency). A tendency toward hypotension occurs in deficiency, whereas the blood pressure rises with excesses; the client or a family member may be taught to monitor blood pressure as one indicator of hormone balance.

The client should understand the dosage schedule. Usually, a morning dose and an afternoon dose are ordered. The highest level of serum corticosteroids normally occurs during the hour before awakening; therefore, the morning dose should be taken immediately on arising. The client usually will feel "below par" until adequate blood levels of the hormone are restored. The second dose should not be delayed beyond early afternoon, because high blood levels of the hormone stimulate the brain and may prevent sleep at the normal bedtime if a dose is taken late in the day. The timing of drug administration is not set arbitrarily to certain clock hours but should be adapted to correspond with the client's normal activity patterns. Changes in routine, such as moving from day-shift work to night-shift work, require similar changes in drug schedules.

The prescriber's directions for increasing dosages in response to stress must be clearly delineated. Usually, doses are doubled for moderate stress, such as a common cold or a visit to the dentist, and tripled for severe stress, such as serious illness or surgery.

The nurse should emphasize that hormone balance is more easily achieved if the client maintains a consistent routine. Consistent routines for sleep and activity are particularly helpful. Techniques for controlling and managing stress can significantly improve the client's general condition.

OUTCOME EVALUATION

The success of short-term measures to alleviate the signs and symptoms of residual deficiency are evaluated by the client and reported to the healthcare professional. Anxiety, dysphoria, pain, and feelings of weakness and fatigue should subside. Diarrhea should decrease. Within a few days after initiation of the drug regimen, the signs and symptoms of corticosteroid deficiency should resolve completely. The nurse should assess blood pressure and tissue turgor as indicators of fluid volume.

The success of the teaching program can be evaluated on a short-term basis by asking the client to repeat facts learned (or demonstrate procedures taught) during the teaching sessions. Over the long term, the absence of signs and symptoms of hormone imbalance (either excess or deficiency) signify successful management of the drug regimen and imply adequate teaching. See the Example of Nursing Process for Hormone Replacement Therapy.

NURSING PROCESS: GLUCOCORTICOID THERAPY FOR DISEASE

ASSESSMENT

The initial assessment of clients for whom glucocorticoids are prescribed varies according to the condition for which the hormones are prescribed. Assessment should include an evaluation of how much adrenal secretion has compensated for the stress of illness or injury. An adequate response maintains homeostasis, whereas a marginal or inadequate response may result in hypotension, potassium retention, hypoglycemia, emotional depression, anxiety, and increased perception of pain.

Baseline data should include a history of allergy, infection, autoimmune disorders, hyperacidity or peptic ulcer disease, and usual sleep pattern. The physical examination should measure vital signs, blood chemistries

Example of Nursing Process for Hormone Replacement Therapy

The client is a 35-year-old housewife and mother with a history of hypophysectomy a year ago to remove a pituitary adenoma. Since the surgery, she has taken maintenance doses of cortisone, thyroid hormone, and estrogen for replacement therapy. Her husband spent 10 years in the army as a noncommissioned officer. Since leaving the service recently, he has had difficulty in securing steady work as a civilian.

The family is also being followed by a public health nurse since the 14-year-old daughter was hospitalized 6 months ago for acute asthma.

During today's visit, the nurse finds the daughter at home recovering from a cold accompanied by acute asthma. She has treated the asthma with bronchodilators and a glucocorticoid inhalant medication. She is much improved and states she plans to attend school the next day. The client, however, appears listless and depressed. She complains of feeling "like a dishrag."

On examination, the client's vital signs are T 37°C (PO), P 105 and somewhat weak, R 18, and BP 96/48. The mother feels that she might have caught her daughter's cold. When the nurse suggests that she take an extra dose of cortisone as prescribed for mild infections, the client apathetically explains that she ran out of that medicine 3 days ago and that they have not had the money to renew the prescription.

Assessment Data

Iatrogenic Addison's disease after hypophysectomy

Last dose of cortisone 72 hours ago

Blood pressure below normal limits, pulse rapid and weakened

Lack of energy

Emotional depression

Lack of glucocorticoid medication due to lack of money

Absence of concern regarding omission of hormone medication

Nursing Diagnosis	Intervention	Goals and Outcomes
Altered Tissue Perfusion: Hypotension related to fluid volume deficit secondary to hypocortism	**Advise** the client to take salty fluids immediately; prepare and administer a cup of hypertonic salt water (1 t salt in 6–8 oz water), bouillon, or commercially prepared soup. (If the soup is "low salt," add extra salt.) Encourage her to take fluids (both salted and unsalted) at frequent intervals.	The client's blood pressure will be maintained at or above the level found when first measured.
	Monitor the client's vital signs. If the client's blood pressure declines, contact the prescriber.	
	If the client develops serious shock, **call** for emergency medical assistance; inform them that the daughter has a glucocorticoid medication for asthma, should the prescriber wish to approve administering a dose to the client.	
	Remain with the family until the client's cortisone prescription is refilled and she has taken a double dose as prescribed for moderate stress.	
	When the client's condition is stabilized, **inform** her of the life-threatening nature of glucocorticoid deficiency. Stress the importance of taking this medication without interruption.	In the future, the client will give a high priority to maintaining hormone therapy, with the highest priority given to glucocorticoid medication.
	Prepare and implement a teaching plan to reinforce and supplement teaching carried out when the hormone replacement drug regimen was initiated.	

(continued)

Example of Nursing Process for Hormone Replacement Therapy (continued)

Nursing Diagnosis (continued)	Intervention (continued)	Goals and Outcomes (continued)
Ineffective Management of Therapeutic Regimen, related to apathy and economic difficulties	**Contact** the local office of social services to obtain financial help for the family so that medication can be obtained on an emergency basis.	In the future, drug therapy will be maintained without interruption.

(electrolytes and glucose), weight, fluid balance, and predominant mood and affect. The nurse should also note general appearance, body contours, and pattern of fat deposition and muscle mass.

NURSING DIAGNOSIS

Many clients who receive glucocorticoid therapy for more than a few days exhibit some degree of Cushing's syndrome. Nursing diagnoses are likely to include:

- Constipation, related to hypokalemia secondary to glucocorticoid excess
- Risk for Fluid Volume Excess, related to sodium and water retention secondary to glucocorticoid excess
- Risk for Infection, related to inhibited immune processes secondary to glucocorticoid excess
- Risk for Injury, related to muscle atrophy and decreased bone density secondary to glucocorticoid excess
- Sensory/Perceptual Alterations: Blunting of the senses secondary to excessive glucocorticoids
- Sleep Pattern Disturbance: Insomnia related to CNS stimulation secondary to glucocorticoid excess
- Body Image Disturbance, related to elation, mania, and cushingoid appearance secondary to glucocorticoid excess

Most clients also have:

- Knowledge Deficit, related to treatment with glucocorticoids
- Risk for Ineffective Management of Therapeutic Regimen (Individual), related to insufficient knowledge of drug therapy

Common collaborative problems to be differentiated from the nursing diagnoses include:

Potential Complication: Hypertension
Potential Complication: Hypokalemia

PLANNING

Anticipated outcomes include prevention or prompt detection and treatment of drug-induced constipation, hypertension, infection, injury, malnutrition, sensory deprivation, and insomnia. In addition, a positive image and sustained wound healing should be promoted. With prolonged treatment, a major goal of nursing care

is to educate the client in managing the drug regimen and making an optimal adjustment to the changes caused by glucocorticoid excess.

INTERVENTION

Glucocorticoid treatment of medical conditions is likely to begin during hospitalization. The nurse must monitor the client for therapeutic response to the regimen. Poor response is indicated by signs and symptoms forewarning shock, undiminished inflammation, or signs and symptoms of allergy. The neurologic client may develop increased intracranial pressure. The nurse must report to the prescriber data that indicate inadequate response, so that the hormone dosage may be increased as necessary.

Once treatment begins, nursing measures become important to protect the client from adverse drug reactions. Clients should be monitored for signs and symptoms of glucocorticoid toxicity.

Diet for most clients should be low in sodium, rich in potassium and fiber, moderate in calories, and free of irritating components. Low-sodium diets are harmful to some clients and should not be imposed indiscriminately. For example, sodium restriction is inadvisable for clients who lose electrolyte-rich fluids due to renal impairment or drainage from ileostomies or fistulas.

Clients who receive glucocorticoids must be protected from infection. Asepsis, both medical and surgical, should be meticulous. Occasionally, reverse isolation is necessary. Many physiologic defenses against pathogens (fever, increases in white blood cells, and changes in the differential count) are suppressed by these drugs. Infections tend to develop insidiously because the signs and symptoms of inflammation do not develop. The skin and mucous membranes should be inspected closely and regularly for changes. Complaints of pain and nausea, which may be the first symptoms of serious infection, must be reported and investigated. If a history of tuberculosis is discovered and antimycobacterial drugs are not ordered, the physician should be informed of the history. Prophylactic antituberculosis drug therapy is often required, because tuberculosis is likely to reactivate when glucocorticoid levels are high. Cough and hemoptysis may signal the development of active pulmonary infection.

Clients undergoing surgery may need an increase in cortisone dosage because their adrenocortical response to stress has been inhibited as a result of drug therapy. When clients with wounds receive glucocorticoids, wound healing is delayed. The wound should be monitored closely, and undue stress on surgical areas should be avoided. The removal of stitches may have to be delayed to prevent dehiscence.

Ambulatory clients require protection from hazards that increase the risk of falls. The weak muscles and fatigue that characterize glucocorticoid excess leave the client prone to accidents. Fractures are more likely because of weakened skeletal structures.

Clients may require stronger sensory stimuli than normal. Foods should be well flavored with essences, herbs, and spices; bright colors are appropriate for decor and clothing. The client is likely to use a high volume setting for the television, radio, or stereo.

Because clients may have difficulty sleeping at night, frequent rest periods and all possible nursing measures to promote sleep should be provided.

Clients may be prone to peptic ulcer, the early signs and symptoms of which include heartburn, epigastric pain (both of which are minimized in clients taking glucocorticoids), and bloody or coffee-ground emesis. The stools should be tested for occult blood, a sign of gastric bleeding.

Clients should be monitored for diabetes mellitus. The prescriber usually orders periodic fasting blood glucose tests. Finger-prick glucose tests for sugar are useful for more frequent testing.

Clients should be monitored for excess fluid volume. Visible edema or a general rise in blood pressure should be reported to the prescriber. The client should also be monitored for signs and symptoms of potassium deficiency (weakness, constipation, and increased tendency toward digitalis toxicity in clients who receive the cardiotonic drugs).

Mental and emotional changes may occur when glucocorticoids are administered in high dosages or over long periods. Clients should be monitored for changes in affect (euphoria, excitement) and for sleep disorders (insomnia). Clients should also be monitored for undesirable skeletal effects. The growth and development of children should be assessed and compared with normal values. Adults should be monitored for pathologic bone fractures and reduced height (often indicative of vertebral compression).

Other abnormal changes in body structure include pronounced changes in weight, rounding of the face, development of a fat pad between the upper shoulders, and atrophy of muscle of the extremities. Striae and acne-like skin eruptions may also occur.

Client Education. Clients who receive prolonged glucocorticoid therapy for a chronic medical condition are likely to manage their own treatment at home. For these clients, the nurse can provide instruction and support. Like hormone-deficient clients, these clients must learn to monitor their own condition, administer drugs, and consult the healthcare provider when necessary. Teaching content differs slightly. In these clients, a degree of toxicity from the drugs may be acceptable in return for the benefits of therapy. The client should understand exactly what symptoms to report to the prescriber, who can then adjust the drug regimen. The client also needs assistance in minimizing the severity and impact of adverse effects. Appropriate assessment techniques and control measures should be taught.

In addition, clients and families should be informed of the changes in appearance and emotional affect that commonly develop with the use of glucocorticoids. In some conditions, dosages are high enough to produce a frank cushingoid appearance. The face becomes round and somewhat puffy. The torso thickens; arms and legs become thinner. Abnormal fat deposits may appear high on the back. The client may complain of feeling jittery; some may feel depressed. The family or significant other should be asked to monitor psychologic status, because the client may be unable to assess this objectively. The client should be reassured that these changes are temporary. Soft-tissue changes and emotional status revert to normal once the drugs are withdrawn or the dosages reduced.

Because clients who receive hormones for their drug effects develop adrenal atrophy secondary to suppressed pituitary corticotropin secretion, the normal response to stress may not occur. Although hormone levels may be above normal, they are inadequate for extreme stress. The client needs help controlling stressors and managing stress, similar to clients on replacement therapy. The nurse should point out the benefits of wearing a medical identification device.

Public Education. Because glucocorticoid hormones are frequently used for medicinal purposes, public education regarding their use is needed. The importance of weighing the risks against the benefits of this type of drug therapy should be stressed. Considered by some to be miracle drugs, glucocorticoids may be requested with no regard to their danger.

The ruling by the federal Food and Drug Administration (FDA) that skin ointments and creams containing glucocorticoids may be purchased without a prescription poses a risk of abuse. The drugs are absorbed by the skin, and systemic effects may occur. The public should be cautioned against using these preparations too frequently or for prolonged periods. Clients should adhere to the recommended dosage and seek medical treatment for conditions that fail to respond to drug therapy within a few days.

OUTCOME EVALUATION

Data required for evaluation include the frequency and consistency of stools; serial blood-pressure measurements; evidence of infection (pus, pain, fever); loss of function; evidence of injury, glucose, sodium, and potassium levels; degree of wound healing (dehiscence or evisceration); quality and amount of sleep; and degree of sensory perception. The client's self-image should be reassessed by evaluating his or her statements related to self-concept.

The client's success in managing the treatment regimen while avoiding complications implies effectiveness of the teaching plan. Questioning the client about facts conveyed during teaching sessions provides short-term evaluation.

❖ CHECKLIST OF NURSING ACTIONS

When Glucocorticoids Are Prescribed

❑ Recommend using a medical identification device that names the drug regimen.
❑ Teach the client techniques for stress management to minimize fluctuations in hormone status.
❑ Monitor clients for evidence of glucocorticoid imbalance and for response to therapy.
❑ Teach clients to manage their drug regimens.

When Hormones Are Prescribed for Replacement Therapy

❑ Protect the client from stress until hormone balance is restored.
❑ Administer hormones on arising from sleep and about 6 hours later.
❑ Help the client through the grieving process related to altered body function.
❑ Emphasize the importance of adhering to the drug regimen.

When Glucocorticoids Are Prescribed for Diseases

❑ Determine if the client has been exposed to tuberculosis.
❑ Monitor the client carefully for signs and symptoms of cortisone toxicity.
❑ Consult the prescriber for definitive treatment to prevent or control complications of therapy when indicated.
❑ Protect the client from exposure to infection.
❑ Protect the client from undue stress.
❑ Promote rest and sleep.
❑ Recommend a low-sodium, high-potassium diet with controlled levels of carbohydrates and calories, unless contraindicated by complicating conditions.
❑ If the client is receiving digitalis, monitor closely for digitalis toxicity.
❑ Inform the client of side effects of the drug, identifying signs and symptoms that should be reported to the healthcare provider.
❑ Emphasize the need for continued health supervision during drug treatment.
❑ Warn the client not to discontinue the drug abruptly.

(See the detailed care plan for a client receiving prednisone in Chap. 3.)

Mineralocorticoids

As noted previously, the mineralocorticoids are adrenal cortex steroid hormones that exert their most pronounced physiologic effects on fluid and electrolyte balance. Several drug preparations are available to replace the natural mineralocorticoids in deficient clients. One is fludrocortisone acetate (Alfoflorone, F-Cortef, Florinef Acetate), the synthetic form of the natural hormone desoxycorticosterone. This preparation, which is in pregnancy category C, is marketed in oral tablet form. The usual adult dosage is 50 to 200 µg/day.

Pharmacodynamics. The mechanisms of action of the mineralocorticoids are poorly understood. Because a time lag (about an hour) exists between administration of the drugs and renal response, the hormones are believed to act by altering the concentration of enzymes that affect renal tubule reabsorption. Two theories have been proposed regarding these enzyme effects: 1) mineralocorticoids initiate transcription of RNA, which serves as a template for the synthesis of a protein that facilitates the transport of sodium ions across the renal tubule; and 2) mineralocorticoids activate enzymes involved in the sodium pump at the tubular serosal surface. The hormones increase sodium reabsorption and increase potassium excretion by the kidneys. Reabsorption of water and anions increases, extracellular fluid volume increases, potassium levels decrease, hydrogen ion concentration drops, and body pH tends to rise.

Given to clients with salt-losing adrenogenital syndrome, mineralocorticoids help correct abnormal levels of pituitary corticotropin. They do so by replacing one of the natural hormones that stimulates the pituitary when deficient. Given concurrently with glucocorticoids, mineralocorticoids inhibit corticotropin production just as natural hormones do. As body levels of corticotropin decrease, adrenal production of androgens and the signs and symptoms of the disease subside.

Pharmacokinetics. The synthetic hormone fludrocortisone acetate is not inactivated by digestion and can be administered orally. Desoxycorticosterone is ineffective when given orally; it is administered by intramuscular (IM) injection or surgical implantation in the tissues. All mineralocorticoids are distributed to the tissues by the blood. They are metabolized to inactive forms by most body tissues to some degree, but the liver is the primary site for degradation or conjugation. They are excreted in the urine.

Therapeutic Uses. The mineralocorticoids are used for partial replacement of hormones required by clients with deficient adrenal cortex function from Addison's disease or salt-losing adrenogenital syndrome. Additional glucocorticoids are usually needed for most clients affected by these syndromes.

Dosage and Administration. Desoxycorticosterone must be administered, at first daily, by IM injection. When dosage requirements have been established, a surgically implanted depot preparation that provides medication for a longer time may be used. In such cases, desoxycorticosterone acetate, or pivalate in oil, is administered about once every 4 weeks. Because relatively large volumes of the preparation are required, the drug should be injected into the upper outer quadrant of the buttocks. The liquid is viscous, and a 20-gauge or larger needle should be used. Implantation or IM injection sites should be monitored for irritation or inflammation indicative of allergic reaction. When allergy develops, it may be necessary to change the form of medication.

Fludrocortisone acetate, which can be administered orally, is sometimes used for treating adrenal corticosterone deficiency states. This preparation has glucocorticoid as well as mineralocorticoid activity.

Adverse Reactions. Overdose of mineralocorticoids produces signs and symptoms of hormone excess: edema, hypervolemia, hypertension, and cardiac enlargement and arrhythmia. Headache, arthralgia, and tendon contractures can occur. Congestive heart failure or cerebrovascular accident (stroke) may develop. As potassium depletion continues, weakness and intestinal atony may progress to ascending paralysis and paralytic ileus. Laboratory data usually indicate hypernatremia, hypokalemia, and alkalosis.

Allergic hypersensitivity to mineralocorticoid drugs sometimes develops. The first sign of allergy may be increasing irritation or inflammation at the injection site.

Precautions and Contraindications. Clients with Addison's disease are more sensitive to mineralocorticoids than are persons with adequate adrenocortical function. Dosage must be established cautiously during initial stages of treatment. Blood analysis of electrolyte levels is performed often. Clients must be watched for sudden weight gain or rise in blood pressure, edema, and cardiac enlargement. If toxicity is manifest, sodium intake must be restricted and potassium supplements administered.

If mineralocorticoid therapy is necessary during pregnancy, the newborn must be assessed for signs and symptoms of hypoadrenalism. Mineralocorticoids are contraindicated for clients with high levels of these hormones. They are not administered to clients who exhibit hypertension or edema. Clients who develop allergy to the drugs should be treated with a preparation to which they do not react, or should undergo a course of desensitization treatment.

Unless necessary, glucose tolerance tests are contraindicated for clients who receive mineralocorticoids because their marginal hormone levels make them vulnerable to severe hypoglycemia.

■ SUMMARY

Mineralocorticoids are drugs that exert physiologic effects similar to those of the adrenal cortex steroid hormones aldosterone and desoxycorticosterone. They act to increase renal reabsorption of sodium and water and to increase renal excretion of potassium and hydrogen ions. They are used as replacement therapy for clients who suffer from Addison's disease and salt-losing adrenogenital syndrome.

Mineralocorticoid toxicity is characterized by hypervolemia, hypertension, edema, and hypokalemia. Allergy to the drugs sometimes develops.

❖ NURSING MANAGEMENT: CLIENT RECEIVING A MINERALOCORTICOID

Detecting the hormone inadequacy is an important nursing function in treating adrenal corticosterone deficiencies, because the earlier the hormone inadequacy is diagnosed, the easier it is to treat. Clients with signs and symptoms that suggest adrenal cortex insufficiency should be referred to a physician, preferably an endocrinologist, for definitive diagnosis and treatment. When mineralocorticoid deficiency is diagnosed, hormone therapy is needed indefinitely. Clients must adjust to a chronic condition that requires regular health supervision and uninterrupted drug therapy.

NURSING PROCESS

ASSESSMENT

Early manifestations of mineralocorticoid deficiency are subtle, making the deficiency difficult to detect. When taking the history, the nurse should inquire specifically about episodes of fainting, shock, or heat exhaustion. Baseline physical data include vital signs, weight, fluid balance, electrolytes, and blood glucose levels. The nurse should be alert to signs and symptoms characteristic of the syndrome, such as weakness, fatigue, tendency toward hypotension, hypoglycemia, and abdominal discomfort. Affected clients may crave salt; they usually maintain a high sodium intake. Ambiguous genitalia in female newborns or virilization of female children or young adults are additional manifestations of adrenogenital syndrome. Laboratory data may reveal tendencies toward hyperkalemia, hyponatremia, and acidosis. Weak cardiac action, excessive intestinal peristalsis, poor tissue turgor, hypotension, and flaccid muscles may be detected on physical examination.

After the diagnosis, the client's knowledge about the disease and his or her emotional response to it should be assessed.

NURSING DIAGNOSIS

Once hormone therapy begins, the potential for hormone toxicity exists, particularly during the initial phase of treatment when dosages have not been established. Diagnoses related to mineralocorticoid excess include:

- Activity Intolerance, related to metabolic changes (hypervolemia and hypokalemia) secondary to mineralocorticoid excess
- Fluid Volume Excess, related to hypernatremia secondary to mineralocorticoid excess

In addition, most clients will have:

- Knowledge Deficit, relating to minearlocorticoid deficiency and its treatment

PLANNING

Initial nursing goals are to alleviate or eliminate anxiety, conserve the client's energy, increase blood volume and cardiac output, and eliminate the knowledge deficit. Other goals are to prevent or promptly detect and treat hypertension and hypokalemia due to hormone excess.

INTERVENTION

Clients need emotional support and assistance in accepting the diagnosis of a chronic incurable disease. They should be encouraged to express their feelings openly. Clients should be told that their condition can be controlled with medication and that, if treated, it should not become life-threatening. However, detailed teaching should be delayed until the client's initial shock and disbelief are resolved.

During initial treatment stages, the nurse should promote rest and relaxation to conserve the client's energy. Physical activity should be resumed gradually, as blood pressure rises and muscle strength improves.

Until hormone therapy is established, the client should be given ample sodium and water in the diet. Sodium intake should be tapered gradually as the client responds to medication. If the client has hyperkalemia, potassium intake should be restricted.

When treatment begins, daily doses of desoxycorticosterone are administered until optimal dosage is established. During this period, the client is monitored closely for signs and symptoms of drug toxicity. To avoid hypertensive crisis, the drug is started at low levels and increased gradually. Fluid and electrolyte balance are assessed carefully by means of body weights and blood electrolyte levels. The nurse should assess emotional affect, tissue hydration, muscle strength, and cardiovascular and intestinal function.

The client should be evaluated for hormone imbalance (either excess or deficiency) at each nursing visit. The nurse should take vital signs and assess emotional affect, muscle strength, and GI motility. Most importantly, the nurse should plan and implement a teaching program that helps clients manage the drug regimen and maintain hormone balance.

Client Education. Clients should take an active part in managing their disease and treatment regimen. To do so, they must know the signs and symptoms of **hormone** deficiency and excess and must be able to monitor themselves for signs of imbalance. Clients should learn the skills needed to assess blood pressure, pulse rate, tissue turgor, and body weight. If IM drugs are prescribed, clients must learn injection techniques to administer their own medications. When clients cannot care for themselves because of disability, a family member or other responsible person may need to perform these functions.

Response to hormone therapy is reduced somewhat by stress, particularly exposure to hot or humid environments that increase salt loss through perspiration. Clients should be warned to avoid sauna baths and similar situations that stimulate sweating.

Clients must understand how the adverse effects of hormone therapy can be reduced through dietary adjustment of electrolyte intake. The effects of mineralocorticoids are enhanced by increased sodium intake and decreased potassium intake. Clients should be instructed to increase sodium in the diet when signs and symptoms of hormone deficiency appear; potassium-rich foods should be avoided at these times. Conversely, when signs and symptoms of excess hormone levels are noted, sodium restriction and potassium increases are appropriate. Clients must be taught techniques for altering dietary intake of these electrolytes, such as the preparation of attractive and tasty low-salt dishes, methods for reducing potassium intake, and selection of foods rich in each mineral.

Clients should be cautioned to seek regular health-care supervision by qualified professionals. They should notify the prescriber when signs and symptoms of persistent progressive hormone imbalance occur; dosage regimens may need to be altered.

OUTCOME EVALUATION

Data required for evaluation include the absence or presence of restlessness, irritability, or other signs of anxiety, statements by the client indicating emotional tension or relaxation, duration of sleep and rest periods, serial blood-pressure readings, and tissue turgor, muscle strength, and activity tolerance. The success of the teaching plan is evaluated by the client's ability to maintain hormone balance over the long term. The client should also be tested to determine retention of facts and ability to perform procedures taught during the teaching program.

❖ CHECKLIST OF NURSING ACTIONS

- ❑ Refer clients with signs and symptoms of adrenocorticosterone deficiency or adrenogenital syndrome to an endocrinologist for definitive diagnosis and treatment.
- ❑ Monitor clients who receive mineralocorticoid therapy for signs and symptoms of fluid, sodium, potassium, and acid–base imbalances that indicate hormone imbalance.
- ❑ Administer mineralocorticoids in oily suspensions by deep IM injection in the upper outer quadrant of the buttocks, using a 20-gauge or larger needle.

❑ Provide complete perioperative nursing care for clients scheduled for surgical implantation of desoxycorticosterone pellets.

❑ Help clients adjust emotionally to the reality of a chronic endocrine illness that requires lifelong treatment.

❑ Teach clients who require injectable drug preparations to administer their own drugs.

❑ Teach clients how to monitor hormone balance and response to medication.

❑ Teach clients how to adjust sodium and potassium intake to reduce fluctuations in response to mineralocorticoid therapy.

❑ Caution clients to maintain regular care by qualified health professionals.

Male Sex Hormones

Androgens

Male sex hormones (androgens) are responsible for the differentiation, growth, and development of the male reproductive system, as well as the induction and maintenance of male secondary sex characteristics. They influence metabolism and sex drive in both sexes.

Androgens are produced by both the male and female, but in very different amounts. Normal adult males secrete 7 to 9 mg/day, maintaining a serum level of 0.2 to 1 μg/100 mL. Adult females secrete about 3 mg a day; their serum levels are half or less than half those of men.

Androgens are produced in large amounts by the testes and in smaller quantities by the adrenal cortex. Some also arise from the metabolism of other steroid hormones, such as estrogens and progestogens.

The differentiation of genital tissues in fetuses of both sexes is affected by male sex hormones. In the male, high levels of androgens stimulate the growth of the penis, the descent of the testicles, and the formation of normal male genitalia. Although the proportion of androgens to estrogens is much smaller in the female embryo, some male hormone appears necessary to her proper reproductive development also. However, excessively high levels of androgens in utero can masculinize the female fetus, producing an appearance of male gender in an otherwise normally functioning, potentially fertile female.

Shortly after birth, the production of androgens in males declines sharply and remains low until puberty. Male hormone levels peak at about 20 years of age and then decline gradually; in old age they may be reduced to one-fifth the maximum levels.

Androgens exert an anabolic effect on metabolism. They increase protein synthesis, bone density, bone marrow function (especially erythropoiesis), sodium retention, and low-density and very-low-density lipoproteins in the blood. A tendency toward gain in lean body weight is accompanied by a decrease in subcutaneous fat deposits.

Male sex hormones affect emotions and behavior also. They increase libido in both sexes. Rises in androgen levels are accompanied by a subjective feeling of well-being. In animals these hormones influence mating behavior and stimulate aggressiveness; indications suggest that similar but less potent influences affect humans. In the pituitary, metabolites of these compounds inhibit gonadotropin secretion.

Forms of Androgens

Among the natural androgens are several distinct compounds (Table 30-4). Testosterone is the most abundant and most potent. Both natural hormones and modified drug preparations are used as drugs. Among the synthetic preparations are danazol (Danocrine), fluoxymesterone (Halotestin), and methyltestosterone (Android). Combinations of androgens and estrogens, sometimes including nutrient minerals and vitamins, are also marketed.

Pharmacodynamics. Androgenic drugs interact with receptors within the cells; they influence cell physiology in ways similar to endogenous male hormones. They exert antiestrogenic, anabolic, and masculinizing actions on the body. Synthetic preparations have been modified chemically in ways that enhance anabolic and minimize androgenic properties, but complete separation of these functions has not been achieved.

Pharmacokinetics. Androgenic drugs are most often administered orally, buccally, sublingually, or IM. Natural hormone preparations are not very effective when administered orally due to metabolism of the drugs in the GI mucosa and on first pass through the liver. The synthetic androgens and anabolics are less extensively metabolized after oral administration.

After absorption, most androgens are highly bound (about 98%) to plasma proteins. This inactive tissue depot prevents rapid fluctuations in the serum level of free androgen. As the level of free hormone in the serum declines, hormone is released from the protein-binding sites and becomes physiologically active. As with most steroids, male sex hormones are deactivated by the liver and excreted in urine.

Therapeutic Uses. Androgens are most valuable for treating sex-hormone deficiencies in males. They restore normal sexual appearance and potency in males affected by castration or panhypopituitarism. They are sometimes helpful in delayed puberty, postpubertal cryptorchidism, oligospermia, and impotence.

Androgenic drugs are rarely used for long-term therapy in females because of their masculinizing effects. The drugs have been used to reduce the symptoms of breast cancer in women when the disease is considered to be hormone-dependent and the less toxic anabolic derivatives are ineffective. On a short-term basis, androgens have been used to prevent postpartum breast pain and engorgement by suppressing lactation.

The anabolic hormones are used in treating refractory or aplastic anemias and osteoporosis in both sexes. They promote a positive nitrogen balance, bone healing in fracture clients, and tissue regeneration and weight gain in debilitated or cachexic clients. They are preferred to the more masculinizing preparations in treating advanced breast cancer in women.

The anabolic hormones produce some growth in pituitary dwarves but also initiate bone maturation and closure of the epiphyses, thereby terminating growth. For this reason, they are used only after somatotropin therapy has been exhausted, or when this hormone is unavailable.

The misuse of androgens by athletes for enhancing muscle size and strength is well known.

Table 30-4. Male Hormones and Related Drugs

Drug Name	Preparation	Usual Adult Dosage	Pattern of Effects
Natural Hormones			
testosterone (Andro 100, Android-T, Histerone, Malogen, Testaqua, Testoject, T Pellets, Testopel Pellets)	Powder Pellets for subcutaneous implantation Suspensions for IM injection	For replacement of endogenous testicular hormone: *IM:* 10–25 mg, 2 or 3 times weekly; *subcutaneous (pellets):* 150–450 mg q3–6mo For palliative treatment of carcinoma of the breast in women: *IM:* 100 mg, 3 times weekly For prevention of postpartum breast pain and engorgement: *IM:* 25–50 mg/day, for 3–4 days For treatment of impotence and male climacteric: *IM:* 25–50 mg, 2 or 3 times weekly	Full range of androgenic and anabolic properties
testosterone cypionate (Andro-Cyp, Andronate, dep Andro, Depotest, Depo-Testosterone, Duratest, T-Cypionate, Testred)	Solution in oil for IM injection	For replacement of endogenous testicular hormone: 50–400 mg, q2–4wk For the development and maintenance of testicular function in oligospermia: 100–200 mg, q2–4wk For palliative treatment of carcinoma of the breast in women: 200–400 mg, q2–4wk For treatment of impotence and male climacteric: 200–400 mg, q3–4wk	Full range of androgenic and anabolic properties
testosterone enanthate (Andro L.A., Android-T, Andropository, Andryl, Anthatest, Delatestryl, Durathate, Everone, Malogen, Testate, Testostroval)	Powder Solution in oil for IM injection	For replacement of endogenous testicular hormone: 50–400 mg, q2–4wk For treatment of impotence and male climacteric: 200–400 mg, q4wk For treatment of oligospermia: to develop and maintain testicular function: 100–200 mg, q2–4wk; to suppress and produce rebound stimulation: 200 mg weekly for 6–12 wk For palliative treatment of carcinoma of the breast in women: 200–400 mg, q2–4wk For adjunctive treatment of postmenopausal women or senile osteoporosis: 200–400 mg, q4wk	Full range of androgenic and anabolic properties
testosterone propionate (Androlan, Malogen in Oil, Oreton, Perandren, Testex)	Powder Solution in oil for IM injection	For replacement of endogenous testicular hormone: 10–25 mg, 2 or 3 times weekly For palliative treatment of carcinoma of the breast in women: 50–100 mg, 3 times a week For the prevention of postpartum breast pain and engorgement: 25–50 mg/day for 3 or 4 days For treatment of impotence and male climacteric: *IM:* 10–25 mg, 2 or 3 times/weekly	Full range of androgenic and anabolic properties
Synthetic Androgens			
danazol (Danocrine, Ladogal, *Can:* Cyclomen)	Oral capsules	*Initial:* For endometriosis: 200–800 mg/day, divided in 2 doses (depending on severity of condition); for fibrocystic disease: 100–400 mg/day, divided in 2 doses; for hereditary angioedema: 400–600 mg/day, divided in 2 or 3 doses *Maintenance:* Dosage is gradually reduced until individual requirements are determined	Inhibition of pituitary secretion of gonadotropins Weak androgenic and anabolic properties

All drugs are in pregnancy risk category X; see Appendix A. *Can* = Canadian trade names.

(continued)

Table 30-4. Male Hormones and Related Drugs (Continued)

Drug Name	Preparation	Usual Adult Dosage	Pattern of Effects
fluoxymesterone (Halodrin, Halotestin, Ora-Testryl, Ultandren)	Oral tablets	For replacement of endogenous testicular hormone: 2–10 mg/day, divided in 1–4 doses For palliative treatment of carcinoma of the breast in women: 15–30 mg/day, divided in several doses For prevention of postpartum breast pain and engorgement: 2.5 mg administered when active labor begins, then 5–10 mg/day, in divided doses, for 4–5 days	Androgenic activity equal to that of testosterone Anabolic properties Promotion of recalcification of osseous metastases and decrease in urinary concentration of calcium in malignant neoplasms
methyltestosterone (Android, Metandren, Neo-Hombreol, Oreton-M, Orchisterone, Testred, Virilon)	Powder Buccal tablets Oral tablets and capsules	For replacement of endogenous testicular hormone: *Oral preparations:* 10–50 mg/day, in divided doses; *buccal tablets:* 5–25 mg/day, in divided doses For delayed puberty in males: *Oral:* 10 mg/day; *buccal:* 5 mg/day For treatment of carcinoma of the breast in women: *Oral:* 50–200 mg/day; *buccal:* 25–100 mg/day For prevention of postpartum breast pain and engorgement: *Oral:* 80 mg/day; *buccal:* 40 mg/day (duration of treatment: 3–5 days after parturition) For treatment of impotence and male climacteric: *Oral:* 10–50 mg/day; *buccal:* 5–25 mg/day	Androgenic and anabolic properties comparable to those of endogenous hormones

All drugs are in pregnancy risk category X; see Appendix A. *Can* = Canadian trade name.

For more information, see Focus On Androgens: Similarities and Differences.

Adverse Reactions. Both male sex hormones and their anabolic derivatives exert similar adverse and toxic effects. Although the masculinizing properties are less pronounced in the anabolic compounds, they are not absent. Evidence indicates that the masculinizing and anabolic actions of this class of drugs cannot be completely separated.

Masculinization is the most obvious and troublesome adverse reaction in clients for which this is not the desired therapeutic result. The type and degree of sexual change varies with the sex and age of the recipient. Because fetuses of both sexes become masculinized, the use of male sex hormones is contraindicated in pregnancy. Women who receive these drugs experience menstrual irregularities, excess hirsutism, a deepening and weakening of the voice, clitoral enlargement, an increased incidence of acne, and male pattern baldness if they possess this genetic trait. Structural changes of the larynx are irreversible, and early withdrawal of the drugs is required to reverse voice changes. Prepubertal males exhibit enlargement of the phallus, increased frequency of erection, precocious sexuality, and permanent closure of the epiphyses, which limits stature. In postpubertal males the effects of androgens are masked if male sexual development has been completed. The drugs inhibit testicular function and sperm production, causing fertility problems. Gynecomastia may also develop.

The administration of androgens to hormone-deficient males may cause prostatic hypertrophy and acute urinary retention. Priapism (pronounced and persistent penile erections) may occur early in treatment but tends to subside with reduced dosages. When given to sexually immature males, androgens may permanently impair fertility.

General effects in all recipients include nausea, fever, reduced secretion of pituitary gonadotropins, and increased incidence of acne, edema, and cholestatic jaundice. Problems in sexual function include changes in libido (increases or decreases), infertility, impotency, and orgasmic dysfunction.

Toxic effects of androgens are seen most often in athletes who abuse these drugs to promote muscle growth and to improve performance and strength. Short-term effects include sodium and water retention, tachycardia, hypertension, vertigo, headache, acne, nausea, vomiting, diarrhea, insomnia, chills, muscle cramps, changes in libido, and elevated blood levels of sodium, cholesterol, triglycerides, and glucose; (in men) gynecomastia, decreased sperm production, and difficulty in urinating; and (in women) hirsutism, breast shrinkage, and clitoral enlargement. Long-term effects include liver damage (including cancer); (in men) atrophy of the testicles, prostate enlargement, and hair loss; and (in women) impaired fertility and permanent voice changes (deepening and weakening). Mania (so-called 'roid rage) has been reported.

FOCUS ON

Androgens: Similarities and Differences

Similarities

Pharmacodynamics

These agents stimulate RNA polymerase activity and RNA synthesis, resulting in increased protein production and tissue building. They suppress gonadotropin-releasing hormone, luteinizing hormone, and follicle-stimulating hormone through a negative feedback system. They promote maturation of male sex organs and male secondary sex characteristics. They stimulate production of red blood cells by enhancing the production of erythropoietic-stimulating factors.

Pharmacokinetics

These agents are administered orally, buccally, sublingually, or IM. Solutions for injection are slowly absorbed. The natural hormones undergo first-pass metabolism after oral administration; the synthetic hormones undergo less metabolism after oral administration. These agents are metabolized by the liver and excreted by the kidneys.

Therapeutic Uses

These agents are used for the treatment of sex hormone deficiency in males. They are also used for the palliative treatment of breast cancer and for the treatment of refractory or aplastic anemia and osteoporosis in both sexes.

Adverse Reactions

These include: (CNS) headache, anxiety, mental depression, vertigo, insomnia; (CV) tachycardia; (GI) nausea, vomiting, constipation, change in appetite, weight gain, gastritis, cholestatic jaundice, hepatic dysfunction, elevated liver enzymes; (GU) bladder irritability, frequency; (REPRO) masculinization, change in libido, priapism, clitoral enlargement, increased frequency of erection, fertility problems, diminished sperm production, gynecomastia, impotency, orgasmic dysfunction, prostate enlargement; (SKIN) acne, male pattern baldness; (ENDO) decreased thyroid function test, fluid imbalance; (HEMA) bleeding tendencies, polycythemia; (OTHER) fever, elevated sodium, potassium, phosphorus, calcium, and cholesterol, deepening of voice.

Drug Interactions

Androgens antagonize the action of estrogens. In combination with anticoagulants, they increase the risk of hemorrhage.

Differences

- **Testosterone** and **fluoxymesterone** cause growth spurts in adolescents and terminate long bone growth. They promote the retention of calcium, nitrogen, phosphorus, sodium, and potassium.
- **Danazol** suppresses the pituitary-ovarian axis and inhibits the output of pituitary gonadotropins.

- The half-life of **fluoxymesterone** is 9 hours; the half-life of **methyltestosterone** is 2.5 to 3.5 hours; the half-life of **testosterone** is 10 to 100 minutes; the half-life of **testosterone cypionate** is 8 days.
- **Methyltestosterone** peaks in 1 hour after buccal administration and in 2 hours after oral administration.
- Some **testosterone** is excreted in feces.

- **Danazol** is used as palliative treatment of endometriosis and fibrocystic breast disease.

- **Danazol** may cause increased intracranial pressure, blindness, hypertension, visual disturbances, thrombocytopenia, muscle cramps, and sweating.
- **Fluoxymesterone** may cause testicular enlargement, oligospermia, epididymitis.
- **Methyltestosterone** may cause irritation of the oral mucosa with buccal administration.
- **Testosterone** may cause pain at the injection site and generalized paresthesia and induration and irritation with pellet administration.

(continued)

Androgens: Similarities and Differences (continued)

Similarities (continued)

Precautions and Contraindications

These agents should be used cautiously in children.

These agents are contraindicated in males with breast or prostatic cancer or symptomatic prostatic hypertrophy. They are also contraindicated in clients with known hypersensitivity, severe cardiac, renal, or hepatic dysfunction, abnormal genital bleeding, and in women who are pregnant or lactating.

Nursing Considerations

Instruct client in disease, treatment, drug therapy, regimen, adverse effects, and adherence; provide emotional support; monitor serum studies, including electrolytes and liver enzymes; assess fluid balance and intake and output frequently for changes; institute sodium restriction if necessary; assess for edema, especially in the lower extremities; check daily weights; encourage diet high in calories and protein if not contraindicated; instruct male clients to report signs of priapism, decreased ejaculation; instruct females to report signs of virilization.

Differences (continued)

- Some preparations of **methyltestosterone** and **fluoxymesterone** contain tartrazine dye and should be used cautiously in people with tartrazine hypersensitivity.
- **Danazol** should be used cautiously in clients with seizures and migraine headaches.
- **Testosterone** and **methyltestosterone** are contraindicated in clients with hyperuricemia and those who are easily sexually stimulated.

- Administer **testosterone** IM deeply into a large muscle; store IM preparations at room temperature.
- Encourage clients who take **danazol** for fibrocystic disease to examine breasts regularly. Instruct clients who take **danazol** to wash after intercourse and wear cotton-lined underwear to prevent vaginitis.

Danazol, a synthetic androgen, may elevate intracranial pressure, which can cause blindness. This begins with headaches and visual disturbances such as double vision. Danazol can also cause thrombocytopenia.

Drug–Drug Interactions. Episodes of bleeding can develop in clients who receive both anticoagulants and androgenic hormones. Male hormones and female hormones antagonize each other.

Drug–Laboratory Test Interactions. Because of the metabolic effects of the hormones, changes in the results of certain laboratory tests occur. Thyroid function test results tend to show a decline in thyroid function, and the glucose tolerance test curve changes. Serum levels of sodium, potassium, phosphorus, calcium, and cholesterol increase. Hypercalcemia, which occurs in 3% to 5% of recipients, can reach dangerous levels. Clotting factors II, V, VII, and X decrease, and the accompanying decrease in coagulability can cause episodes of bleeding in clients who receive both anticoagulants and androgenic hormones.

Precautions and Contraindications. Male hormones must be administered with caution to clients with cardiac, renal, or hepatic disease and seizure disorders. They are con-traindicated during pregnancy, nephrosis, or the nephrotic phase of nephritis, and in males who suffer from cancer of the prostate or breast. The drugs are not used in treating nonhormone-dependent breast cancer in women. They should be discontinued if the serum calcium concentration rises above normal in recipients with bone metastases. Clients receiving this drug must be carefully selected, because the administration of androgens may permanently impair fertility, especially in young males.

■ SUMMARY

Male sex hormones are steroids produced by the testes and the adrenal cortex that stimulate development of the reproductive system and secondary sex characteristics in the male and promote normal sexual function. Natural hormones are prescribed for replacement therapy and treating cryptorchidism. The anabolic properties of modified hormones are useful in the palliative treatment of tissue-wasting conditions and anemia. Male hormones are rarely used for prolonged treatment of females because of their masculinizing effects. Side effects include nausea, fever, acne, and changes in sexual function. They are contraindicated in pregnancy, cancer of the prostate, and nephrosis.

❖ NURSING MANAGEMENT: CLIENT RECEIVING MALE SEX HORMONE THERAPY

Clients diagnosed with hormone deficiency receive replacement medication. These clients may be in their late teens, and they may be late to mature because of a hormone deficiency. When providing care for male clients receiving hormones for sexual immaturity, the overall goals of therapy include initiation of puberty and stimulation of autogenous hormone production. For clients who have undergone orchiectomy or have other endocrine problems, outcomes may vary. Whatever the reason for drug therapy, the nurse must convey regard for the serious nature of the problem and ensure the client's right to privacy and confidentiality.

NURSING PROCESS: ANDROGEN THERAPY

ASSESSMENT

Male hormone deficiency in adults may be caused by trauma or disease that affects the testes or by a pituitary deficiency. The client may complain of a gradual decline in sexual potency or gonadal injury. He may have had orchiectomy. Diagnostic studies indicating below-normal blood levels of male hormones suggest a physiologic rather than psychologic etiology for impotence.

NURSING DIAGNOSIS

Nursing diagnoses related to male hormone replacement therapy may include:

- Knowledge Deficit, related to male hormone deficiency and replacement therapy
- Altered Tissue Integrity: Inflammation of oral tissues secondary to irritation by buccal or sublingual administration of hormone drugs
- Risk for Sexual Dysfunction, related to tissue damage secondary to excess male hormone levels
- Risk for Altered Urinary Elimination: Retention related to prostatic hypertrophy secondary to excess male hormone levels
- Altered Body Image, related to delayed maturation and possible infertility

PLANNING

Goals for all clients include enhancing self-concept and fulfilling appropriate role functions. As appropriate, goals of nursing care include increased sexual potency, improved self-image, elimination of knowledge deficit, and prevention or prompt detection and treatment of adverse reactions to the drugs.

INTERVENTION

Recipients of male hormone drugs are subject to their general metabolic effects. Consequently, they should be monitored carefully for adverse reactions to the drugs. In immature clients, development of secondary sex characteristics and sexual responsivity should be monitored.

When drugs are administered sublingually or buccally, the nurse should examine the mouth to detect oral lesions. A change to injection administration may be necessary. However, parenteral preparations are also irritating, and sites for injection or implantation should be monitored for inflammation.

The client should also be assessed for adverse effects such as nausea, fever, acneiform skin lesions, and jaundice. In addition, the nurse must monitor laboratory reports for abnormalities in thyroid function, glucose tolerance, and levels of creatinine, electrolytes, cholesterol, and clotting factors. Abnormal changes are reported to the prescriber. Marked deviations from normal do not usually occur when drugs are used for replacement, because tissue hormone levels seldom exceed those found with normal autogenous production.

Client Education. When hormone replacement is prescribed, the goal of teaching is to provide the client with the knowledge and skills needed to manage the drug regimen. The sexually immature client must know that hormone therapy is not always helpful and may cause serious side effects; therefore, even when failure of maturation is a recognized problem, drug therapy may not always be appropriate.

All clients and their families need information about the therapeutic and adverse effects of the drugs and the medical tests required for monitoring drug treatment. They should be informed that hormone therapy is likely to be intermittent to maximize the potential for resumption of normal hormone production. They should be fully informed by the prescriber of the probable course of treatment and the outcome.

The nurse must explain that when hormone therapy is initiated, the client must report instances of priapism promptly. If it occurs, medication is temporarily discontinued and reinstituted later at a reduced dose. Persistent priapism is associated with subsequent, sometimes permanent, impotence and must be avoided.

A reduced urine stream, urinary hesitancy, or other difficulty in voiding must also be reported. These symptoms of prostatic hypertrophy may interfere with urethral patency and are likely to occur when these male sex hormones are administered to deficient men.

The nurse may need to teach the client how to administer the prescribed drugs. If IM doses are required, the client must learn the injection technique.

Clients must also be taught the signs and symptoms indicative of therapeutic response and of hormone excesses, with specific instructions regarding data that must be reported to the healthcare team.

OUTCOME EVALUATION

Data needed for evaluation include development of secondary sex characteristics (beard, muscle size and strength, deepening of the voice) and the absence or incidence of adverse drug reactions and their severity. Reports from the client of improved sexual function indicate therapeutic response to the drugs. Improved self-concept may be manifested by an increase in positive comments about himself and a decrease in negative comments, improved personal grooming and dress, or a more erect posture and striding gait. The client's knowledge about his condition and treatment is reflected by his ability to discuss these knowledgeably and by his adherence to the drug regimen.

NURSING PROCESS: ANABOLIC STEROID THERAPY

ASSESSMENT

Clients who receive anabolic steroids usually have chronic or severely debilitating diseases such as cancer. The nurse must assess the client's status in relation to this condition and be particularly observant for tissue wasting and other evidence of malnutrition. Although the physician retains the primary responsibility for screening clients before prescribing male hormone therapy, the nurse must be alert to and report signs and symptoms of contraindications of which the physician may be unaware.

NURSING DIAGNOSIS

Diagnoses likely to be made for clients who take anabolic steroids include:

- Altered Tissue Integrity: Muscle wasting (emaciation, cachexia) related to increased catabolism secondary to a chronic debilitating disease
- Pain, related to nausea and fever from adverse drug reaction and also to renal calculi resulting from drug-induced hypercalcemia
- Risk for Sexual Dysfunction (in males), related to persistent priapism secondary to male hormone excesses
- Altered Urinary Elimination (in males): Retention related to prostatic hypertrophy secondary to male hormone therapy

A common collaborative problem that should be differentiated from the nursing diagnoses is:

Potential Complication: Hemorrhage

PLANNING

The goals of treatment are to increase muscle mass and to prevent or detect and treat promptly any adverse drug reactions.

INTERVENTION

If anabolic therapy is to succeed in rebuilding tissue, the client must have adequate nutritional intake. The diet should be high in protein, minerals (except calcium), and vitamins. The caloric content should be adequate to prevent metabolism of protein nutrients for energy. Stress should be minimized, because stress hormones are generally catabolic and reduce anabolic response to the androgenic hormones. Unnecessary environmental stressors should be eliminated and measures taken to promote rest and relaxation.

To monitor therapeutic response to the drugs, the nurse should regularly weigh the client and test muscle strength. In addition, the client should be monitored for signs and symptoms of adverse drug reactions. Significant laboratory data include decreased thyroid function, abnormal fasting blood glucose levels, increased creatinine levels, electrolyte imbalances (especially hypercalcemia), and reduced levels of clotting factors. The nurse must watch the client for signs of abnormal bleeding: petechiae, occult blood in the stool or urine, pink-tinged sputum after oral care, or nose bleeds. In males, urinary retention or priapism should be reported to the prescriber. Some degree of masculinization is expected in females; if this distresses the client, the prescriber should be consulted and alternative therapy considered. A glucocorticoid is sometimes ordered to control fever.

Client Education. Many clients with chronic debilitating diseases are cared for at home with the support of home nursing services, so it is important to teach the client and family the skills necessary to manage the drug regimen. Anabolic drugs are usually administered orally. The teaching program must address their toxic and side effects.

The client must understand that abundant fluids are needed to help eliminate excess calcium. Adequate fluid intake helps prevent obstipation and calcium stone formation in the urinary tract. Blood levels of calcium should be monitored regularly. Marked hypercalcemia must be reported immediately, because this can lead to cardiac arrest in systole, which responds poorly to resuscitation. Other reportable adverse reactions include fever and jaundice.

In diabetic clients who receive male sex hormones, diabetes tends to be unstable. These clients should be cautioned against loss of glucose control during anabolic therapy.

OUTCOME EVALUATION

Data required for evaluation include the absence or incidence of adverse drug reactions and their severity. Therapeutic response is indicated by increases in body weight, muscle mass, and muscle strength. Successful teaching is evaluated by the client's and family's ability to manage and adhere to the drug regimen. On a short-term basis, teaching can be evaluated by the ability of the client or family to repeat information conveyed during teaching sessions and to demonstrate proper techniques in performing procedures taught by the nurse.

❖ **CHECKLIST OF NURSING ACTIONS**

❑ Warn clients of the risks of inappropriate use of male hormones (eg, by athletes).

When Replacement Androgens Are Prescribed

- ❑ Monitor clients for response to treatment and evidence of toxicity.
- ❑ Monitor clients for tissue irritation at administration sites.
- ❑ When hormones are administered buccally or sublingually, promote good oral hygiene.
- ❑ Teach clients and their families about anabolic male hormone therapy, including expected therapeutic response (specific to the client's situation), administration of the drugs, and signs and symptoms of adverse drug reactions.
- ❑ Reinforce a masculine self-image in male clients.
- ❑ Warn the client to report priapism promptly.

When Androgens Are Prescribed for Anabolic Effects

- ❑ Assess the client for contraindications to treatment (pregnancy, and heart, liver, or kidney disease).
- ❑ Recommend a diet high in protein, minerals, and vitamins, adequate in calories, and ample in fluids.
- ❑ Protect clients from undue stress.
- ❑ Monitor serum calcium levels and report excesses promptly to the prescriber.
- ❑ Monitor diabetics for increased severity of disease.

Female Sex Hormones

Estrogens and progestogens are the hormones responsible for the normal development and function of the female reproductive system. Like androgens, these chemicals are produced by both men and women, but they are present in much greater amounts in the female, the ovaries and placenta being their primary natural sources. The amounts secreted vary with the rhythms of the menstrual cycle, pregnancy, and lactation. The relative proportions of and interplay between these two kinds of chemicals control the progressive changes in the body necessary to promote and sustain reproduction.

Estrogens

Estrogens are produced by the ovary, placenta, testes, and adrenal cortex and are also produced through peripheral conversion of testosterone and androstenedione. Production in the female fluctuates during the menstrual cycle, with daily secretion of 60 to 400 µg. During pregnancy, estrogen levels increase steadily, and near term daily production may reach 50 mg.

Estrogens are responsible for the normal maturation of the female genital tract and the development and maintenance of feminine secondary sex characteristics. Like androgens in the male, estrogens stimulate pronounced skeletal growth, while simultaneously promoting closure of the epiphyses.

Estrogens affect several metabolic processes in the body. They promote retention of calcium and phosphate and are used in forming bone. Protein synthesis is stimulated, especially in the uterus, breasts, bone, and fatty tissues, but the anabolic effect of estrogens is less pronounced than that of androgens. The metabolic rate rises slightly and the kidneys retain more sodium. In large amounts, estrogens inhibit glucose metabolism and favor the development of diabetes mellitus. The hormones also increase blood levels of high-density lipoproteins and decrease those of low-density and very-low-density proteins, probably by enhancing the excretion of cholesterol in the bile.

During childbearing years, estrogen levels fluctuate regularly in response to pituitary gonadotropins, which control the menstrual cycle. As the ovarian follicle develops and matures, the ovary secretes estrogen in increasing amounts. After ovulation, secretion drops slightly but is maintained at a relatively high level until the last week of the cycle, when it drops precipitously. The sequence of endometrial stimulation followed by withdrawal of estrogen induces menstrual flow.

Estrogens are produced in large quantities by the placenta. Many of the metabolic effects of these hormones favor the nurturing of the fetus. Estrogens increase serum levels of prothrombin and clotting factors VII, VIII, IX, and X, enhancing the coagulability of the blood. This effect is progressive, with the tendency toward clotting rising steadily during continuous or repeated exposure to high levels of the hormones. By the end of a normal-term pregnancy, the expectant mother has considerable protection against severe hemorrhage, which helps limit blood loss during delivery.

Some estrogens function in part as antiestrogens. For example, by occupying receptor sites and blocking the action of the more potent hormone estradiol, estriol can reduce total estrogen response in the body.

Forms of Estrogens

The natural forms of estrogens—estrone and estradiol—are mostly converted to estriol by the body. Estradiol, the most potent of these compounds, is secreted in large amounts by the ovary. It is available for drug use both in its natural form and as modified by esterification (Table 30-5). Several orally active nonsteroidal estrogens, such as diethylstilbestrol (DES), are also available. DES is used for prostate cancer. Although not a steroid, this chemical resembles the steroid nucleus topographically, and on radiographic analysis the molecular structure appears similar to that of estradiol. Estrogens that are used as drugs are marketed as tablets and capsules for oral use, injectable solutions, transdermal patches, vaginal creams and suppositories, and solid forms for subcutaneous implantation.

Pharmacodynamics. Estrogenic drug preparations produce all the physiologic changes produced by endogenous hormones. They stimulate or maintain the development of female sex characteristics (eg, well-developed genitalia, enlarged breasts, feminine fat deposition, hair

Table 30-5. Estrogenic and Antiestrogenic Drugs

Drug Name	Preparation	Usual Adult Dosage
Natural Hormones		
estradiol (Brevicon, Demulen, Estinyl, Lo-estrin, Norlestrin, Or-tho, Ovral, Triphasil)	Oral tablets	For replacement therapy in female hormone deficiency: 0.05 mg, 1–3 times daily for 2 wk followed by progesterone for 2 wk to complete an arbitrary theoretical menstrual cycle
		For management of menopausal symptoms: 0.02–0.05 mg/day in a cyclic regimen (21 consecutive days followed by 7 drug-free days)
		For palliative treatment of metastatic carcinoma of the breast in selected postmenopausal women: 1 mg, tid
		For palliative treatment of carcinoma of the prostate: 0.15–2 mg/day
estradiol (Estrace)	Oral tablets Vaginal cream	For replacement therapy in female hormone deficiency and for management of menopausal symptoms: 1–2 mg/day
		For palliative treatment of carcinoma of the breast in selected men and postmenopausal women: 10 mg, tid
		For palliative treatment of carcinoma of the prostate: 1–2 mg, tid
(Estraderm)	Skin patch	For management of menopausal symptoms: 0.05 mg twice weekly
estradiol cypionate (E-Cypionate, Estronol-LA)	Solution in oil for IM injection	For replacement therapy in female hormone deficiency: 1.5–2 mg q1mo
		For management of menopausal symptoms: 1–5 mg, q3–4wk
estradiol valerate (Deles-trogen, Dioval, Dura-gen, Estradiol L.A., Es-tra-L, Estraval, Gynogen L.A., Valergen)	Solution in oil for IM injection	For replacement therapy in female hormone deficiency and for management of menopausal symptoms: 10–20 mg, q4wk
		For prevention of postpartum breast engorgement: 10–25 mg at the end of the first stage of labor
		For palliative treatment of carcinoma of the prostate: 30 mg or more q1–2wk
polyestradiol phosphate (Estradurin)	Solution for IM injection	For palliative treatment of carcinoma of the prostate: 40 mg, q2–4wk
conjugated estrogens (C.E.S., Estrace, Prem-arin)	Oral tablets Solution for IM or IV injection Vaginal cream	*Oral:* For replacement therapy in female hormone deficiency: 2.5–7.5 mg/day for 20 consecutive days, followed by 10 days without the drug (an oral progestogen is added to the regimen the last 5 days of drug treatment); alternatively: 1.25 mg/day for 21 days, followed by 7 days without the drug
		For management of menopausal symptoms: 0.3–1.25 mg/day for 21 days, followed by 7 days without the drug
		For prevention of postpartum breast engorgement: 3.75 mg, q4h for 5 doses, or 1.25 mg, q4h for 5 days
		For palliative treatment of carcinoma of the breast in selected men and postmenopausal women: 10 mg, tid
		For palliative treatment of carcinoma of the prostate: 1.25–2.5 mg, tid
		IM or IV: For emergency treatment of abnormal uterine bleeding caused by hormone imbalance: 25 mg, q6–12h
		Vaginally: For treatment of atrophic vaginitis or kraurosis vulvae: 2–4 g of vaginal cream daily for 21 days, followed by 7 days without the drug
Estrone		
estrone (Bestrone, Es-trone, Estronol, Gyno-gen, Kestrin, Kestrone, Ogen, Theelin Aqueous, Wehgen-V) *Can:* Femogen	Suspension for IM injection	For replacement therapy in female hormone deficiency: 0.1–1 mg, q1wk
		For management of menopausal symptoms: 0.1–0.5 mg, 2 or 3 times weekly
		For palliative treatment of carcinoma of the prostate: 2–4 mg, 2 or 3 times weekly

All drugs listed are in pregnancy risk category X; see Appendix A.
Can = Canadian trade name.

(continued)

Table 30-5. (Continued)

Drug Name	Preparation	Usual Adult Dosage
Estrone (continued)		
esterified estrogens (Estratab, Menest, Menrium, *Can*: Climestrone, Estromed)	Oral tablets	For replacement therapy in female hormone deficiency: 2.75–7.5 mg/day for 21 days, followed by 7 days without the drug or 20 days followed by 10 days without the drug
		For management of menopausal symptoms: 0.3–3.75 mg/day for 21 days, followed by 7 days without the drug
		For palliative treatment of carcinoma of the breast in selected men and postmenopausal women: 10 mg, tid
		For palliative treatment of carcinoma of the prostate: 1.25–2.5 mg, 1–3 times daily
estropipate (Ogen)	Oral tablets Vaginal cream	*Oral:* For replacement therapy in female hormone deficiency: 1.5–9 mg/day for 21 days, followed by 8–10 days without the drug; for management of menopausal symptoms: 0.75–6 mg/day for 21 days, followed by 7 days without the drug
		Vaginally: For treatment of atrophic vaginitis or kraurosis vulvae: 2–4 g of 0.15% vaginal cream daily for 21 days, followed by 7 days without the drug
Synthetic Nonsteroidal Estrogens		
chlorotrianisene (TACE)	Oral capsules	For replacement therapy in female hormone deficiency: 12–25 mg/day for 21 days, followed by several days without the drug (dosage is resumed on the fifth day of induced uterine bleeding)
		For management of menopausal symptoms: 12–25 mg/day for 21 days, followed by 7 days without the drug
		For prevention of postpartum breast engorgement: 12 mg, qid for 7 days, or 50 mg, q6h for 6 doses, or 72 mg, tid for 2 days
		For inoperable advanced cancer of the prostate: 12–25 mg daily
dienestrol (DV, Estraguard, Ortho Dienestrol)	Vaginal cream and suppositories	For treatment of atrophic vaginitis or kraurosis vulvae: *Initial:* 6–12 g of 0.01% cream daily or 1 or 2 suppositories (0.7–1.4 mg)/day, for 1–2 wk, followed by half the initial dosage for 1–2 additional weeks; *maintenance:* 6 g of 0.01% cream or 1 suppository (0.7 mg), 1–3 times weekly
diethylstilbestrol (DES, *Can*: Honvol)	Oral tablets and enteric-coated tablets	For palliative treatment of carcinoma of the breast in selected men and postmenopausal women: 15 mg/day
	Vaginal suppositories	For palliative treatment of carcinoma of the prostate: *Initial:* 1–3 mg/day; *maintenance:* 1 mg/day
diethylstilbestrol diphosphate (Stilphostrol)	Oral tablets Solution for IV infusion	For palliative treatment of carcinoma of the prostate: *Initial (oral):* 50 mg tid; *(IV):* 0.5 g, followed by 1 g/day for 5 or more days; *maintenance (oral):* 200 mg or more, tid; *(IV):* 0.25–0.5 g, 1 or 2 times weekly

All drugs listed are in pregnancy risk category X; see Appendix A. *Can* = Canadian trade names.

distribution) and exert a weak anabolic effect. Metabolic effects include increased sodium and water retention, lowering of elevated serum concentrations of cholesterol and phospholipids, a moderate increase in anabolism, and increased coagulability of the blood. Estrogens also affect pituitary gonadotropins, inhibiting their secretion by a negative feedback system.

Pharmacokinetics. Natural unconjugated estrogens are inactivated in the GI tract and liver and are ineffective when administered orally. Drug preparations with altered chemistry (synthetic conjugated and nonsteroidal compounds) may be administered orally. Most estrogens are metabolized promptly and must be administered one or more times a day. Chlorotrianisene, however, has a prolonged duration of action due to its storage in fatty tissue. Implantations provide long-term

treatment with a single dose, but absorption is gradual and may be erratic. Withdrawal of the drug before the life of the preparation expires is rarely feasible because it requires removal of the solid remnants.

Topical applications are used when a local (usually vaginal) effect is desired. Estrogens are readily absorbed from the skin and mucous membranes, and systemic effects from such use are not uncommon. The choice of drug preparation depends on convenience, cost, and the client's reliability as much as it does on the therapeutic goal.

In the blood, estrogens are bound by sex hormone-binding globulin and albumin. They are metabolized by the liver, primarily by conjugation as sulfates and glucuronates. Some enter the enterohepatic circulation and thus are handled repeatedly by the liver. The end products of estrogen metabolism are excreted mainly by the kidneys.

Therapeutic Uses. Hormonal therapy is used to relieve deficiency of estrogens in adult women, to promote sexual maturation in female gonadal failure states, to promote contraception, to treat diseases and disorders such as endometriosis and dysfunctional uterine bleeding, and to suppress lactation.

Some women with deficient estrogen levels experience such symptoms as "hot flashes" (feelings of hyperthermia, flushing, inappropriate sweating), chilling sensations, and paresthesias that often take the form of formication (sensations of ants crawling on the skin). Although the exact causes of these phenomena are unknown, they are believed to be associated with hypersecretion of pituitary gonadotropins or gonadotropin/sex hormone imbalances. The more severe and abrupt the withdrawal of estrogens, the more pronounced the symptoms. Young women of childbearing age who are surgically castrated exhibit the most pronounced symptoms. Between 15% and 25% of women who undergo natural menopause experience discomfort severe enough to prompt a request for medical help or advice. Administration of estrogens relieves the symptoms promptly. Hormone therapy also prevents the loss of femininity experienced with extended estrogen deficiency. Estrogens have been administered to prevent the postmenopausal changes of aging that are associated with deficiency of these hormones. Because long-term estrogen therapy poses some health risks, this practice is controversial; see the Critical Thinking Challenge: Issues Analysis.

Estrogens are also administered to promote sexual maturation in girls who suffer from primary gonadal failure. In some of these girls, the estrogen deficiency is part of a more complex condition such as Turner's syndrome, which also involves dwarfism. Long-lasting injected forms of estrogen are often used in this type of treatment. The drugs induce full development of the reproductive tract and feminization. Unfortunately, significant growth may not occur before the epiphyses close and linear bone growth ceases.

Contraception is another use of estrogen. Estrogen/progestogen preparations are popular forms of contraception and are discussed in depth in Chapter 31.

Treatment of disease, such as dysmenorrhea, endometriosis, dysfunctional uterine bleeding, and acne, may be accomplished with estrogen preparations. For most conditions, the same preparations and schedules of administration can be used as for contraception. The drugs serve to regularize and control endometrial changes through the cycle, relieving discomfort and preventing excessive blood loss. Their benefits in acne appear to stem from their antiandrogenic effects. Given the risks of estrogen use, some prescribers are reluctant to use them in such conditions until other therapeutic approaches have been exhausted. When oral contraception is prescribed, however, the use of the drugs may simultaneously reduce problems of these types.

Excessive hirsutism in females may also respond to estrogen therapy. Treatment with cortisol is usually tried first, but if this approach is ineffective, a year's course of estrogen treatment is initiated. Terminating treatment too early limits therapeutic response.

Hormone-dependent cancers that respond to estrogens include cancer of the prostate in men. Estrogens are used to treat inoperable (metastatic) carcinoma in the breast in both postmenopausal women and in men (McEvoy et al., 1995). Combined hormone and antineoplastic regimens may be more effective than hormones alone. Estrogen treatment alone is palliative and may not prolong life.

Estrogens are also used to suppress lactation in postpartum women and in those in whom lactation persists during weaning. Only a short term of treatment is required to interrupt breast function and prevent the discomforts associated with other methods to terminate milk production.

Adverse Reactions. Estrogens are considered among the most toxic of hormone drugs. This may be the result of widespread use of the compounds for fertility control, which has provided many client-years of exposure to abnormally high hormone levels for observation of toxic and side effects. Because some effects of the drugs are life-threatening, their use even for therapeutic purposes tends to be much more cautious today than before the development of oral contraceptives.

When used for contraception in women, exogenous estrogens, added to endogenous supplies, produce body levels above those normally present in the nongravid woman. In these concentrations, the chemicals produce many of the changes characteristic of pregnancy. Estrogens also exert a carcinogenic and teratogenic effect. A history of prolonged or high levels of the hormones is associated with increased incidence of endometrial cancer in postmenopausal women. Although not yet impli-

---

CRITICAL THINKING CHALLENGE
Issues Analysis

1. Prepare arguments for and against estrogen replacement for menopausal women. What factors should be considered when therapy is contemplated for a client?
2. (For female students) Have you sought or would you seek hormone replacement for yourself?
   (For male students) Would you recommend replacement therapy for your mother (wife, sister)? Why or why not?
3. What can you do to minimize the influence your own bias for or against estrogen replacement therapy (as revealed by the above exercise) might have on your menopausal clients?

cated as a cause of other human cancers, the hormones are known to cause cancer in animals. They also stimulate the growth of most preexisting tumors that affect the female genital tract, including ovarian, cervical, and breast cancer. Teratogenic effects on the fetus include limb deformities, cryptorchidism, and masculinization of the fetus (caused by conversion of excess estrogens to androgens by metabolic processes). Among persons whose mothers were given DES to prevent abortion during gestation, the incidence of vaginal cancer in females and genital malformations in males is greater than in the nonexposed population.

Estrogens predispose the recipient to gallbladder disease, increasing the incidence of cholelithiasis and cholecystitis in both men and women. The hormone appears to increase the concentration of cholesterol in bile, favoring the formation of stones.

Because they increase levels of renin and angiotensin, estrogens favor sodium and water retention and cause tissue edema. They tend to increase the frequency and severity of migraine headaches, epilepsy, asthma, and renal and heart disease. When estrogen levels are high, the body's need for several nutrients (vitamin C, folate, and pyridoxine) rises. Folate absorption declines; the physiologic mechanisms that cause vitamin C and pyridoxine deficits are poorly understood.

Although estrogens induce a feeling of well-being when administered to deficient women, high levels tend to produce depression. In susceptible clients, this may progress to psychotic levels.

When estrogens are used alone in cyclical therapy to mimic the normal menstrual cycle, midcycle or breakthrough bleeding can occur. This has been attributed to excessive endometrial proliferation in response to the stimulus of the estrogens. Adding progesterone to the regimen often corrects this problem (see Chap. 31).

Males treated with estrogens experience reversal of secondary sex characteristics and impotence. The testes and phallus atrophy, the beard thins, and the breasts enlarge. Scalp hair may regrow in areas affected by male pattern baldness (the expression of this genetic trait depends on the influence of androgens, which are inhibited by estrogens). The body assumes feminine contours as fat deposits change to female patterns.

Drug–Drug Interactions. When estrogen is taken concurrently with corticosteroids, the effect of the corticosteroids is increased. Concurrent use of barbiturates, phenytoin, or rifampin may decrease serum levels of estrogen.

Drug–Laboratory Test Interactions. Liver function tests are altered by these drugs, and the risk of cholestatic jaundice is increased.

Precautions and Contraindications. Estrogen therapy is contraindicated during pregnancy and in women with a history of genital tract cancer. Because they are secreted in breast milk and tend to suppress lactation, estrogens are not prescribed during lactation. They must be used with caution when a history of cardiovascular disease (especially thromboemboli), liver or renal disease, migraine, epilepsy, or depression exists. Care must be exercised when treating immature females to minimize undesirable stunting of growth.

❖ SUMMARY

Estrogens are female sex hormones produced by the ovary, placenta, and adrenal cortex. They are necessary for normal female development and sexual function. Their metabolic effects include sodium and fluid retention, increased coagulability of the blood, and a moderate increase in anabolism. Numerous hormone preparations are on the market. They are prescribed for hormone replacement therapy, for contraception, and for the treatment of hormone-sensitive malignancies. Estrogen therapy increases the risk of gallbladder and thromboembolic disease, hypertension, cancer, and congenital defects in fetuses. Males who receive these drugs become feminized. Contraindications to their use include pregnancy, lactation, and cancer of the female genital tract.

❖ NURSING MANAGEMENT: CLIENT RECEIVING FEMALE SEX HORMONES (ESTROGEN)

When estrogens are prescribed, brochures concerning the risks of use must, by law, be packaged with the drugs. The principle that the consumer should be informed of potential risk appears to be gaining recognition, as similar regulations are now in effect for other drugs (estrogen was the first drug so regulated).

The decision to initiate estrogen replacement therapy requires careful assessment for evidence of hormone depletion and for risk factors for adverse reactions. The decision whether to use the drugs should be made by the woman with the help of her healthcare providers (see the Critical Thinking Challenge: Issues Analysis).

NURSING PROCESS

Hormone replacement therapy is discussed here; the nursing process for clients receiving oral contraceptives is discussed in Chapter 31.

ASSESSMENT

When hormone therapy is being considered, clients should be carefully assessed for the need for therapy and risk for adverse reactions. Both the client and the prescriber should weigh expected benefits against possible risks before deciding for or against treatment. The decision should be made early in the transition stages to menopause, however, before permanent damage occurs from hormone deficiency (Box 30-2).

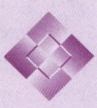

Box 30-2
Risk Factors for Osteoporosis and Heart Disease

In menopausal women at risk, hormone replacement therapy is believed to delay both osteoporosis and the onset of cardiovascular disease (due to its effect on high-density lipoprotein levels, which it increases).

Risk Factors for Osteoporosis

- Family history of blood relatives with "dowager's hump" or brittle bones
- Slight body build
- Smoking
- Excessive alcohol intake
- Lack of active weight-bearing exercise
- Inadequate lifetime calcium intake
- Repeated use of weight-reduction diets accompanied by acidosis and aciduria, which increases calcium loss in urine
- Dark complexion (because of reduced vitamin D synthesis)

The development of strong bone structure during childhood and its maintenance during the childbearing years is believed to reduce the risk of osteoporosis.

Risk Factors for Early Heart Disease

- Family history of cardiovascular disease in female members after menopause
- Diabetes mellitus
- Smoking
- Excessive alcohol intake
- Hypothyroidism
- High serum cholesterol levels
- Obesity

Not all menopausal women need hormones. Most women experience no noticeable distress from menopause. A few are plagued by frequent hot flashes or dyspareunia. Clients sometimes attribute emotional problems to menopause, but the degree to which hormonal imbalance is a factor is unknown. At this stage of life, women may experience many stressors that hormone therapy is unlikely to influence.

Hormone levels in menopausal women vary considerably. Evidence suggests that fat tissue plays a role in estrogen metabolism, and women with ample fat deposits appear to retain higher levels of these hormones than thinner women. This relative protection from estrogen deficiency is associated with an increased incidence of uterine cancer, hypertension, and diabetes.

Pregnancy must be ruled out before estrogens are prescribed. Other contraindications include a history of intravascular thrombosis (phlebitis, coronary thrombosis, cerebral thrombosis) and cancer of the female reproductive organs.

Surgical castration before menopause, premature menopause, and evidence of rapid or severe hormone depletion are indications for treatment. These clients are less likely than older clients to experience adverse drug reactions. The lowest effective dose is given to maintain femininity and prevent deficiency symptoms. For these women, the need for hormones is undisputed, and therapy should be continued without interruption at least until the normal age of menopause.

NURSING DIAGNOSIS
Clients are likely to have:

- Knowledge Deficit, regarding drug therapy with female sex hormones
- Risk for Injury, related to thromboembolic disease related to drug therapy
- Altered Self-Concept, related to sex hormone deficiency
- Fear, of degenerative body changes related to sex hormone deficiency

PLANNING
Goals of nursing care, depending on the purpose for which hormones are prescribed, may include avoidance of pregnancy, prevention of osteoporosis and cardiovascular degeneration, preservation of sexual function, and prevention or prompt detection and treatment of adverse reactions to hormone therapy (eg, malignant tumor growth, cholecystitis, intravascular clotting). An additional goal is to increase client knowledge by teaching about female reproduction and use of sex hormones.

INTERVENTION
During therapy, clients should be monitored for both therapeutic response and adverse reactions to the prescribed hormones. Most prescribers provide only a 6-month supply of hormones at a time, ensuring that the client returns for examination before the drug supply is renewed.

When vaginal atrophy is the only manifestation of estrogen deficiency, the use of an estrogenic vaginal cream often is effective. The drug exerts its greatest effect on the local tissues, and systemic effect is minimized. Absorption does occur, however, and systemic effects may be evident. Such creams cannot be used when estrogens are contraindicated, as in women with a history of genital cancer. When estrogens are to be applied topically, they should be administered at regular intervals.

Any woman who receives estrogenic drugs on a regular basis should be closely monitored for signs and symptoms of adverse reactions, including the development of breast or uterine masses, cholecystitis, and phlebitis. Because uterine (especially endometrial) cancer can occur late in life, regular Pap tests should be encouraged.

Regardless of the degree to which hormone depletion adds to emotional lability, the menopausal client needs support and encouragement. At this time, many women become acutely conscious of the effects that age has had on their physical appearance, energy levels, and life goals. Most children either have left home or soon will. The energy previously invested in nurturing the family must be diverted to other pursuits. In many families, menopause coincides not only with the "empty nest" but with a similar crisis in the other partner. The influences of hormone depletion on emotional balance simply add to the normally high stress level at this time.

The nurse can help the client and the family adapt to changed circumstances and promote healthy coping mechanisms and interpersonal relationships. When appropriate, referrals for counseling may be made.

Client Education. For women considering taking sex hormones, the nurse should provide the facts about the potential benefits and risks of therapy. The use of estrogens is often elective, and the client needs facts to help her make an informed decision.

For prepubertal girls, the nurse should explain that estrogens cause maturation of the reproductive tract and feminization, but—depending on the underlying condition—fertility may not be attained. If dwarfism is part of the clinical picture, estrogens do not ensure growth to normal adult stature; rather, they tend to terminate growth after an initial growth spurt because of closure of the epiphyses.

Postpubertal women who receive cyclic estrogen therapy also require a careful orientation to the effects of the drugs. The risk of adverse reactions is greatest in these clients, because the addition of estrogens to normal endogenous hormones raises the overall levels in the body. Alternatives to hormone therapy should be thoroughly explored, including other methods of contraception and the use of antibiotics and retinoic acid for acne.

Some women who desire hormone therapy may find that the healthcare provider opposes such treatment. In such cases, the client can be informed of the right to seek medical care from another provider.

Menopausal women for whom hormones are contraindicated and those who wish to avoid using medications may be taught strategies to minimize the effects of hormone deficiency.

Clients who receive estrogens need considerable education to understand the risks of such treatment as well as the benefits that can realistically be expected. They must remain under close medical supervision and should be taught the signs and symptoms of adverse reactions (eg, sudden weight gain, bloating, calf tenderness, pain on dorsiflexion of the foot, unusual vaginal bleeding) and the need to report these promptly. Diabetic women should be told that glucose tolerance may decline during estrogen use. Smokers should be warned of the high risks of cardiovascular disease posed by combined use of estrogens and tobacco. This risk is compounded in older women. Cessation (or at least a reduction) of smoking should be urged. If the client is receptive, referral to a smoking cessation program is appropriate.

Women for whom topical therapy is prescribed should be cautioned against using the agent for lubrication before intercourse. The hormones are absorbed by the surface of the penis and may reduce potency and cause some degree of feminization in the male partner. Applying the hormone after, not before, intercourse minimizes this effect. A water-soluble lubricant can be used before intercourse until vaginal secretion is restored by hormone replacement. The use of condoms prevents absorption of hormones by the male partner if intercourse is desired after applying the medication.

When estrogens are given to men, they are usually prescribed to treat cancer of the prostate. Because the purpose of hormone manipulation is to eliminate androgenic stimulation, some degree of impotence and feminization is expected. In fact, if this does not occur, or if it abates, further treatment to eliminate androgens (orchiectomy or adrenalectomy) may be required. The client and his partner may need help coping with this disruption of sexual function. Alternatives to genital intercourse are acceptable to some couples. For others, referral to a surgeon for implantation of a penile prosthesis may be helpful. Such a device provides an artificial erection, which allows intercourse.

❖ CHECKLIST OF NURSING ACTIONS

- Evaluate women who are to receive estrogens for contraindications and factors that increase the risk of complications (pregnancy, lactation, history of reproductive system cancers, phlebitis, hypertension, diabetes mellitus, and depression).
- Inform the client about the medication, the risks of treatment, and the expected benefits.
- For the client who declines hormone replacement therapy, help her develop health practices that reduce discomforts and risk of complications caused by hormone loss.
- When estrogen vaginal cream is prescribed, instruct the client in techniques to prevent exposing her sexual partner to the drug.
- When estrogens are prescribed for males, counsel the client and his partner about ways to preserve their sexual relationship.

Progestogens

Progesterone is the natural hormone that protects the embryo and maintains pregnancy. During and after ovulation, its production by the follicle and corpus luteum promotes secretion by the mucous membranes of the fallopian tubes and endometrium. These secretions sustain the zygote should an ovum be fertilized. The hormone also alters endocervical secretions from the watery fluid characteristic of estrogenic stimulation to a scanty viscid material that forms the mucous plug of pregnancy. If conception does not occur, the abrupt decline in progesterone levels that follows degeneration of the corpus luteum precipitates menstruation. When pregnancy does occur, the corpus luteum maintains progesterone levels until the placenta develops, at which time hormone production is taken over by this organ.

During gestation, progesterone suppresses uterine contractility and prevents immunologic rejection of the fetus by inhibiting the function of T lymphocytes. In conjunction with estrogen, this hormone stimulates proliferation of the acini of the breast in preparation for lactation. Both estrogens and progestogens inhibit the effects of prolactin, however, and lactation begins only after their levels drop after delivery.

Progesterone promotes a rise in body temperature of about 1°F during the secretory phase of the menstrual cycle. Detection of this change in basal temperature confirms ovulation and establishes the time of its occurrence. Progesterone increases renal sodium retention directly, but this effect is opposed by competitive inhibition of aldosterone, which results in a net effect of diuresis during short-term exposure. Progesterone tends to suppress pituitary gonadotropin production but does not prevent ovulation. It promotes tissue breakdown somewhat, having a catabolic effect similar to that of the glucocorticoids (Table 30-6).

Pharmacodynamics. Progesterone binds to a specific intracellular receptor protein. The progesterone/receptor complex then translocates to the nucleus, where it stimulates the synthesis of messenger RNA for ovalbumin, avidin, and other proteins. Because the number of progesterone cell receptor proteins fluctuates with estrogen levels, the effects of progesterone depend in part on adequate production of estrogen.

Pharmacokinetics. Natural progesterone is transported and metabolized rapidly. Its half-life in blood is only a few minutes. The chemical is held in tissue sites, where it continues to exert physiologic effects long after it has disappeared from the plasma. Compared to the low level during the follicular phase of the menstrual cycle, progesterone secretion and metabolism increase two- to fourfold during the secretory phase of the cycle and 50- to 70-fold by the end of pregnancy. Levels drop precipitously at menstruation and parturition.

Progesterone administered parenterally is rapidly absorbed and distributed in a manner similar to the handling of endogenous progesterone by the body. Oral administration is much less effective than parenteral because progesterone is promptly transformed by the liver. Most of the exogenous hormone is eliminated in the urine, but about 10% is excreted in the feces. The properties of synthetic and semisynthetic progestogens vary somewhat from those of progesterone; they are more effective when administered orally.

Therapeutic Uses. Progestogens are used therapeutically to treat dysfunctional uterine bleeding, reduce premenstrual tension and postpartum afterpains, suppress lactation, and prevent conception. They have been prescribed for toxemia in late pregnancy, for amenorrhea, and for the palliative treatment of some cancers. Progestogens help prevent abortion that is caused by inadequate luteal response to gonadotropin with inadequate progesterone secretion. This condition must be demonstrated by hormone assay, because the use of progestogens during pregnancy poses a high risk of fetal anomalies. In combination with estrogens, progestogens are used to prevent conception, regulate erratic menstrual cycles, relieve dysmenorrhea, and induce regression of endometriosis. Such combinations administered cyclically produce an anovulatory cycle that more closely resembles the natural menstrual cycle than does that produced by estrogens alone.

Adverse Reactions. The adverse reactions produced by progestogens are poorly differentiated from those of estrogens. Many studies that contribute to our understanding of these hormones involve combination contraceptives, so the individual effects of the two classes of hormones could not be distinguished. It is not surprising that the adverse reactions overlap to some degree because the physiologic effects of these hormones are similar in many respects. Both work together to regulate the menstrual cycle, promote fertility in the female, and prepare for lactation.

Progestogens, like estrogens, are teratogenic when administered during early pregnancy. Progestogen-related fetal abnormalities are more likely to affect the heart and limbs than estrogen-related abnormalities. Genital malformations are less likely to occur. Progestogens, like androgens, can cause masculinization of the female fetus. Because of these effects, progestogens are contraindicated during pregnancy, unless luteal production in response to gonadotropin is proven to be inadequate.

Progestogens are more likely to cause irregularities in vaginal bleeding than estrogens. Breakthrough bleeding is a common problem and causes a high dropout rate among users of progestogen contraceptives (the minipill). Mood changes, especially lethargy, loss of initiative, and fatigue, are more common with progestogens. Side effects related to sodium retention (hypertension, dizziness, weight gain) are less likely to occur than with estrogens but do develop with prolonged use of high doses. Breast engorgement and GI symptoms appear similar to those caused by estrogen.

Progesterone tends to increase a woman's energy needs slightly. It has also been suspected of contributing

Table 30-6. Progestogenic Drugs

Drug Name	Preparation	Usual Adult Dosage
hydroxyprogesterone (Delalutin, Duralutin, Gesterol L.A., Hydrosterone, Hylutin, Hyprogest, Hyproval, Pro-Depo)	Solution in oil for IM injection	For treatment of amenorrhea or abnormal uterine bleeding: 375 mg at 4-week intervals For adjunctive and palliative treatment of advanced endometrial carcinoma: 1 g or more, 1–7 times weekly
medroxyprogesterone (Amen, Curretab, Cycrin, Depo-Provera, Oragest, Provera)	Oral tablets Suspension for IM injection	For treatment of amenorrhea or abnormal uterine bleeding: 5–10 mg/day, PO, for 5–10 days beginning on the 16th to 21st day of the menstrual cycle For adjunctive and palliative treatment of endometrial or renal carcinoma: 400–1,000 mg/week, IM
norethindrone (Norlutin)	Oral tablets	For treatment of amenorrhea or abnormal uterine bleeding: 5–20 mg/day for 21 days (beginning on the 5th day of the menstrual cycle)
norethindrone acetate (Aygestin, Brevicon, Loestrin, Micronor, Norinyl, Norlutate, Ortho, Ortho-Novum; *Can:* Norlestrin)	Oral tablets	For treatment of endometriosis: 10–30 mg/day for 14 consecutive days (low dosages are used at first and may be increased with each cycle until maximum dosage is reached) For treatment of amenorrhea or abnormal uterine bleeding: 2.5–10 mg/day for 21 days (beginning on the 5th day of the menstrual cycle) For treatment of endometriosis: 5–15 mg/day for 14 consecutive days (low dosages are used at first and may be increased with each cycle until maximum dosage is reached)
progesterone (Femotrone in Oil, Gesterol, Progelan in Oil, Progest 50 Oil, Progestaject-50, Progestasert; *Can:* Progestilin)	Powder Solution in oil and suspension for IM injection	For treatment of amenorrhea: 5–10 mg/day for 6–8 days, beginning 8–10 days before the anticipated start of menstruation For treatment of abnormal uterine bleeding: 5–10 mg/day for 6 days (sometimes preceded by 2 weeks of estrogen therapy) or a single dose of 50–100 mg

All drugs listed are in pregnancy risk category X; see Appendix A. *Can* = Canadian trade name.

to the nausea of pregnancy, which may be associated with transient hypoglycemia.

Drug Interactions. Drug–drug interactions appear to be insignificant, but drug–laboratory test interferences include false results on hepatic and endocrine function tests.

Precautions and Contraindications. Progestogens, like estrogens, are generally contraindicated during early pregnancy, during lactation, and when a history of genital malignancy exists. Prolonged use should be avoided in clients with asthma, epilepsy, and migraine.

■ SUMMARY

Progesterone is the steroid hormone produced by the corpus luteum and placenta that promotes maintenance of pregnancy and preparation of the breasts for lactation. Synthetic and semisynthetic preparations of progesterone are available for therapy. They are prescribed for contraception and for treating various medical problems related to the female reproductive system. The hormones are carcinogenic, teratogenic, and masculinizing. They are contraindicated during pregnancy and lactation and when a history of genital cancer exists.

❖ NURSING MANAGEMENT: CLIENT RECEIVING PROGESTOGEN THERAPY

Because progestogens are potentially harmful, they are contraindicated during pregnancy, unless luteal production in response to gonadotropins is proven to be inadequate. To make an informed decision about treatment, clients need a careful explanation of the potential benefits and risks of drug therapy, as well as alternatives to drug therapy. The use of progestogens, like estrogens, is often elective. These drugs are used as components of oral contraceptives. Such combination contraceptives allow use of lower dosages of each active ingredient and may be administered in sequences that closely mimic the hormone fluctuations of normal menstrual cycles.

NURSING PROCESS

ASSESSMENT

Before progestogen therapy is instituted, clients should be screened for contraindications to treatment and risk factors for adverse reactions to the hormones.

NURSING DIAGNOSIS

Nursing diagnoses likely to be made for clients receiving progestogen therapy are:

- Fluid Volume Excess, related to sodium and water retention secondary to progestogen therapy
- Pain, related to altered comfort and nausea from transitory hypoglycemia secondary to progestogen medication

Common collaborative problems that should be differentiated from the nursing diagnosis include:

Potential Complication: Seizures
Potential Complication: Hyperglycemia

PLANNING

Goals for nursing treatment include preventing or reducing fluid volume excess and nausea, and maintaining blood glucose levels within normal limits.

INTERVENTION

Diets offered to clients who receive progestogens should be low in sodium; the caloric content should be limited to the level required for maintaining lean body weight. Complex carbohydrates are preferable to refined sugars. Carbohydrate snacks (eg, crackers, toast) help control nausea by relieving hypoglycemia.

Client Education. Clients should be fully informed of the potential benefits and risks of progestogen therapy, as well as alternatives to drug treatment. Women who elect to receive the drugs should be taught their effects, including the signs and symptoms of adverse reactions.

Fluid retention can be minimized if clients limit salt and sodium intake. Diabetic clients should be warned that progestogens can decrease glucose tolerance; the diabetic regimen should be followed conscientiously. Stress hormones have similar metabolic effects to those of progestogens—that is, they increase sodium and water retention and impair glucose tolerance. For this reason, clients should be taught stress management techniques.

When progestogen therapy is prolonged, the client should weigh herself at least twice a week and watch for signs of edema. Bloating, sudden weight gain, and frequent attacks of wheezing, headache, or seizures should be reported promptly.

Nursing care of clients who receive oral contraceptives is discussed in detail in Chapter 31.

OUTCOME EVALUATION

Data required for evaluation include fluid intake and output, tissue turgor, blood pressure, blood glucose levels, and reports from the client of nausea or bloating.

❖ CHECKLIST OF NURSING ACTIONS

- ☐ Assess the client for contraindications to treatment (pregnancy, lactation, history of genital cancer).
- ☐ Assess the client for the presence of medical conditions likely to be exacerbated by progestogen therapy (asthma, migraine, seizure disorder, diabetes mellitus).
- ☐ Explain the potential benefits and risks of progestogen therapy.
- ☐ Help the client develop health practices that minimize the discomforts and risks of progestogen therapy.

Steroid Hormone Antagonists

Spironolactone

Spironolactone, a potassium-sparing diuretic, antagonizes the action of most if not all corticosteroids (aldosterone, androgens, estrogens, and cortisone). It has been used to treat female hirsutism caused by excessive androgens and excessive estrogens associated with ovarian cysts. The drug can disrupt menstruation (causing metrorrhagia) and is best given only on days 4 through 24 of the menstrual cycle. Depression and hypotension have been reported as an adverse reaction, problems compatible with an antiglucocorticoid action. The most common use of spironolactone is for diuresis; it is the agent of choice when the potassium-wasting action of other diuretics is contraindicated. Spironolactone is discussed in detail in Chapter 27.

Male Hormone Antagonists

Except for female sex hormones and spironolactone, no male hormone antagonists are approved for medicinal use. However, substances that would inhibit or reverse the effects of male hormones could be useful in treating such conditions as virilization in women, precocious puberty, and cancer of the prostate. They might also function as male contraceptives. Such drugs could act by a number of mechanisms: inhibition of endogenous male hormone production, inhibition of pituitary gonadotropin, inactivation of free serum testosterone, or inhibition of tissue use of androgens.

Both estrogens and progestogens (and their analogs and derivatives) are natural antagonists of the male hormones. The estrogens appear to antagonize testosterone at the tissue level and also inhibit pituitary gonadotropin secretion. Their feminizing effects limit their clinical usefulness in males. One estrogen, chlorotrianisene, has been widely used for treating prostatic cancer, a disease that affects males in late maturity. The severity of the disease and the effectiveness of the drug in controlling tumor growth justify the use of this drug despite its effects on sexuality.

Antiestrogens

In addition to the antiestrogenic effects of the weaker estrogens themselves, progestogens and androgens exhibit mild antiestrogenic properties. By binding to cytoplasmic estrogenic receptors, they prevent the more potent estrogens from occupying these sites.

Two potent antiestrogens available for clinical use in the United States are tamoxifen and clomiphene. Because tamoxifen is used primarily as an antineoplastic agent, it is discussed in Chapter 47. Clomiphene is used in treating infertility and is discussed in Chapter 31.

Reference

McEvoy GK, ed. (1995). *AHFS '95 Drug information.* Bethesda: American Society of Health-System Pharmacists.

Bibliography

Anonymous (1990). A randomized, controlled trial of methyl-prednisolone or naloxone in the treatment of acute spinal-cord injury. *RN, 53*(7), 95.

Galandiuk S, Raque G, Appel S, Polk HC Jr. (1993). The two-edged sword of large-dose steroids for spinal cord trauma. *Ann Surg, 218*(4), 419–427.

*Peterson AP, Drass J. (1993). How to keep adrenal insufficiency in check. *AJN, 93*(10), 36–39.

*Raloff J. (1993). EcoCancers. *Sci News,* 144, 10–13.

*Raloff J. (1994). Gender benders. *Sci News,* 145, 24–26.

Scarfone RJ, Fuchs SM, Nager AL, Shane SA. (1993). Controlled trial of oral prednisone in the emergency department treatment of children with acute asthma. *Pediatrics, 92*(4), 513–518.

*Recommended for further reading.

For more information and sample tests and activities, refer to Chapter 30 in the Student Workbook for Clinical Pharmacology and Nursing Management, 5th edition, available through your bookstore.

31

Drugs That Affect Sexual Behavior and Reproduction

Conception occurs when a sperm fertilizes an ovum in the outer third of the fallopian tube, and their genetic information is integrated in the fertilized ovum. At the moment of fertilization, the blood type and tissue type, the hair color and eye color, and the general characteristics and body build of the person are established. The initial information about the baby's sex is also determined, depending on whether an X or Y chromosome is received from the sperm cell.

Despite the genetic input concerning gender that is present at fertilization, each human embryo starts life as a female. Males require the addition of fetal androgens to complete the process of sex determination. Even to the fetus, the presence or absence of sex hormones makes a difference.

Reproductive Systems

Once the baby is born, it relies on its own endocrine system to produce the hormones that add to gender identification. However, temporarily, the effects of maternal estrogens are still visible in some newborns. The baby's breasts may be enlarged and may produce a white discharge ("witch's milk"). Some female infants have vaginal bleeding, known as vicarious menstruation. These discharges cease as the maternal estrogen in the newborn disappears.

Growth and Development

Relatively low levels of sex hormones are produced by prepubertal children. At puberty, the pituitary gonadotropins stimulate the follicular hormone in the ovaries and testes, followed by maturation of sex organs. Production of sex hormones rises quickly. Estrogens, progestogens, and androgens are produced by both sexes but in different quantities.

In boys, high levels of androgens are associated with the development of male genitalia; the testes and phallus enlarge. Secondary sex characteristics become apparent: bone and muscle mass increases, the voice lowers, facial hair appears, and a final growth spurt (followed by epiphyseal closure) occurs. Nocturnal emissions of semen are normal, and penile erections may be difficult to control.

In girls, estrogens lead to the growth of female sex organs: the uterus lengthens to about 7.5 cm, and the labia minora, the labia majora, and the clitoris enlarge. Feminine body contour develops with enlargement of the breasts, increased fat deposits, and widening of the pelvis. Adult feminine voice pitch, pubic and axillary hair distribution, breast size, and skin texture evolve. Estrogens cause the cells of the myometrium and endometrium to multiply rapidly during the menstrual cycle. Estrogens also influence height by their effect on the growth of the long bones. An initial growth spurt is followed by epiphyseal closure, the end of bone growth, and transformation of cartilage into bone.

Adult Sexual Cycles

In males, hormone production is relatively stable, gradually declining from a peak in the late teens to reduced levels in old age. In females, on the other hand, hormone production varies cyclically.

Male Hormones and Sperm Production

Sperm production and testosterone levels are affected by the general level of the man's health, nutrition, immunology, exposure to drugs and chemicals, and stress. Sperm production is also influenced by testicular temperature (excessive heat suppresses spermatogenesis) and blood glucose levels (hypoglycemia impairs sperm production and motility). Normally, sperm production is constant, although it may progress more rapidly during sleep, when testosterone levels rise. As they accumulate, sperm and seminal fluid exert pressure on the male organs, stimulating the sex drive, until the semen is discharged during intercourse, masturbation, or nocturnal emission.

Female Hormones and the Menstrual Cycle

As the levels of hormones and other chemicals shift during the menstrual cycle, the female body is subjected to a series of changes. The sequence of the changes depends on the interactions of several hormones, the levels of which vary throughout the cycle (Fig. 31-1, Table 31-1).

The anterior lobe of the pituitary gland produces several hormones in the female. Follicle-stimulating hormone (FSH) initiates the development of the graafian follicle in the ovary. Luteinizing hormone (LH) is also known as the interstitial cell-stimulating hormone. Both FSH and LH stimulate the graafian follicle to mature and to produce estrogen. These effects result in ovulation and the formation of the corpus luteum.

The follicular hormone produced by the graafian follicle cells and the luteal hormone made by the corpus luteum are ovarian hormones or estrogens. They must exist in proper proportions for the normal development and activity of the reproductive system.

If pregnancy occurs, a third hormone, luteotropic hormone, also called lactogenic hormone or prolactin, activates secretory activity in the corpus luteum, resulting in progesterone production. Without luteotropic hormone, the corpus luteum disintegrates and does not supply progesterone. Whether or not pregnancy occurs, estrogen levels before ovulation can be expected to increase as the ovarian follicle develops. After ovulation, if fertilization and implantation of the ovum have not occurred, estrogen levels drop slightly, remaining at that level for over a week. During the last week of the cycle, estrogen levels drop precipitously. The withdrawal of estrogen results in menstruation.

Pregnancy and Lactation

The production of progesterone by the corpus luteum is essential in preparing and maintaining the uterine lining during pregnancy. Progesterone secreted during pregnancy also suppresses ovulation and enhances breast development, including the secretory action of the mammary glands in preparation for lactation.

The uterus must expand in many directions to allow room for the fetus, placenta, amniotic fluid, and umbilical cord. Maintenance of pregnancy depends on good muscle tone; this is assisted by estrogens, which stimulate protein synthesis in the uterus, and by androgens, which have a role in producing the proteins used for muscle development. The placenta produces a high level of estrogens in the maternal circulation during pregnancy. These nurture the fetus. Through another action of estrogen, serum levels of prothrombin and clotting factors VII, VIII, IX, and X increase progressively, providing protection against severe hemorrhage at parturition. These factors also increase the risk of thromboembolic disease, particularly during the postpartum period (see Chap. 30).

Human chorionic gonadotropin (hCG) is the luteotropic hormone produced by the placenta; it is not influenced by the pituitary. It apparently intensifies the action of the corpus luteum early in pregnancy, strengthening fetal and placental growth.

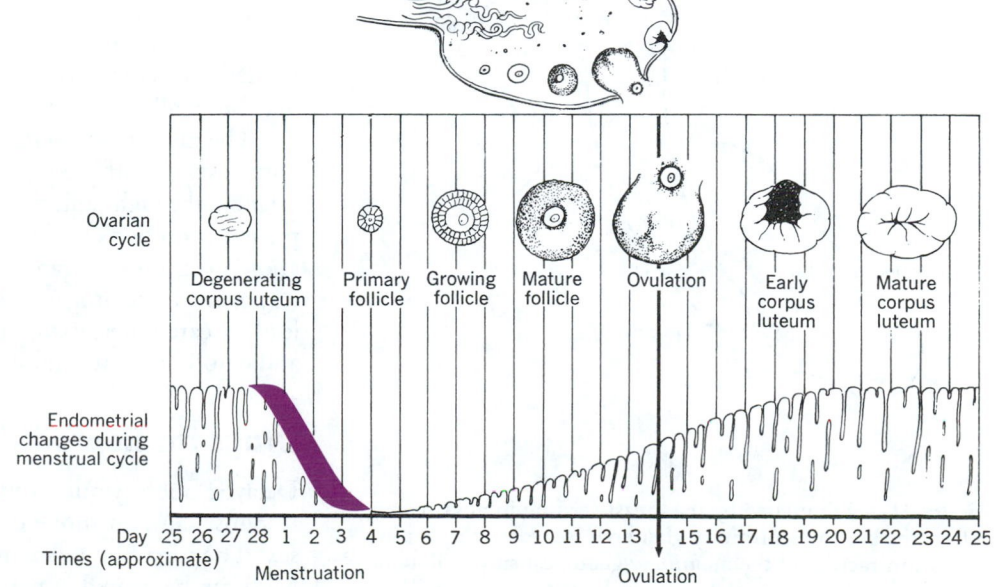

Figure 31-1. Schematic representation of one ovarian cycle and the corresponding changes in the thickness of the endometrium. The endometrium is thickest just before the onset of menstruation and thinnest just as menstruation ceases (compare with Table 31-1).

Table 31-1. Correlation of Hormonal Activities with Ovarian and Uterine Changes

Phase	Menstrual	Follicular	Ovulation	Luteal	Premenstrual
Days	1 2 3 4 5 6 7	8 9 10 11 12 13 14 15	16 17 18 19	20 21 22 23 24	25 26 27 28 1 2
Ovary	Degenerating corpus luteum; beginning follicular development	Growth and maturation of follicle	Ovulation	Active corpus luteum	Degenerating corpus luteum
Estrogen production	Low	Increasing	High	Declining, then a secondary rise	Decreasing
Progesterone production	None	None	Low	Increasing	Decreasing
FSH production	Increasing	High, then declining	Low	Low	Increasing
LH production	Low	Low, then increasing	High	High	Decreasing
Endometrium	Degeneration and shedding of superficial layer; coiled arteries dilate, then constrict again	Reorganization and proliferation of superficial layer	Continued growth	Active secretion and glandular dilation; highly vascular; edematous	Vasoconstriction of coiled arteries; beginning degeneration

Toward the end of pregnancy, the uterine contractions that mark labor may be stimulated by increased production of prostaglandins in the body. Oxytocin, a hormone produced by the posterior pituitary, also acts on the myometrium to stimulate uterine contractions.

Lactation, in a supplementary action, stimulates the uterus to contract by releasing neurohypophysial oxytocin. This speeds involution of the uterus after childbirth. Oxytocin continues to be released during the postpartum period when the lactating mother sees or hears her newborn's demands for feeding. This release results in the so-called milk let-down, a conditioned reflex in which smooth muscle in the breast contracts, releasing milk (Fig. 31-2).

Drug use during pregnancy and lactation is discussed in Chapter 10.

Changes in Aging

During middle and old age, sex hormone levels decline in both sexes. The decline is fairly rapid in women at menopause and more gradual in men, who may remain fertile to advanced ages. Lower hormone levels in both sexes place them at risk for tissue wasting (particularly muscles and bones) and a waning sex drive. In women, decreased serum levels of estrogens at menopause are often accompanied by decreased bone density, vaginal secretions, and size of breasts, mons pubis, and vagina.

Decreased testosterone levels in men tend to reduce the frequency, intensity, and duration of penile erection. These changes prolong the length of intercourse needed to achieve orgasm. The quantity of ejaculate may be smaller and propulsion less forceful.

The growth and state of the reproductive systems of both sexes are affected by many factors: nutrition (from infancy through adulthood), general health, environmental conditions (pollutants), health habits (rest, recreation, drug abuse, cigarette smoking), work environment (exposure to teratogens, abortifacients, substances that lead to carcinogenesis or mutagenesis), drug treatment, and emotional status (ability to cope with stress).

Drugs for Reproductive Abnormalities

Delayed puberty and failure to mature, impaired sexual response, and hormone deficiencies may occur in either sex. They may be particularly disturbing to the client. Most can be treated or managed with hormone therapies.

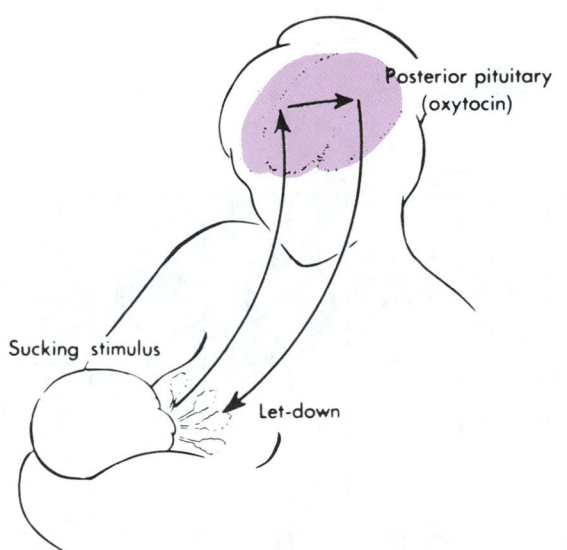

Figure 31-2. Stimulated by the breast-feeding infant's sucking reflex, the posterior pituitary gland releases oxytocin that induces contraction of the mammary gland, causing milk to be propelled through the nipples to the infant.

Delayed Maturation

In girls, delayed maturation usually is diagnosed as hypoestrogenic amenorrhea. It may be caused by rigorous sports activity or excessive exercise, excessive dieting, or disease. Certain congenital abnormalities, such as Turner's syndrome, are characterized by failure of sexual maturity. Calorie deprivation may delay or prevent menarche; a 17% level of body fat must be present for menarche to occur, and 22% fat must be present for maintenance of regular cycles.

Delay of menarche is not considered serious if breast development and the appearance of pubic and axillary hair have started by age 14 years. Medical care should be sought if menstruation has not started by age 16, and treatment usually begins by or before age 18. Hypoestrogenic amenorrhea may be complicated by bone loss, leading to osteoporosis and possible fractures, especially when it is accompanied by cigarette smoking and high caffeine or alcohol intake. Girls with delayed maturation tend to grow taller than normal due to delayed closure of the epiphyses. See the Critical Thinking Challenge: Case Analysis.

Treatment with sex hormones usually causes development of normal adult body conformation and sexual behavior. However, it may or may not result in normal fertility. Sexual development in boys tends to occur somewhat later than in girls.

Impaired Sexual Response

Impaired response in males may take the form of impotence (failure of or inadequate penile erection) or inability to ejaculate. Multiple factors may contribute to impotence: illness, injury, high stress levels, poor nutrition, nerve damage, exposure to pollutants (many of which have estrogenic properties), drug therapy, and psychogenic factors. Medications have been implicated in about 25% of impotent males. So many physical reasons for impotence are now apparent that authorities believe the incidence of psychogenic impotence was overestimated in the past. This diagnosis should not be made until physical causes have been ruled out. Ejaculatory failure may result from drug therapy or damage to the autonomic nervous system.

Impaired sexual response in women is poorly understood. Frigidity (failure of sexual arousal) is the female equivalent of impotence in men. Frigidity does not make intercourse impossible but does decrease its pleasure for both partners. Traumatic sexual experiences and abnormal fears may cause frigidity, but the degree to which physical factors (eg, testosterone deficiency) contribute is unknown. Interest in orgasmic failure (the female equivalent of male inability to ejaculate) has been limited.

Treatment of impaired sexual response begins with a search for physical causes. Improvement in general health, reduction of stress levels, and withdrawal from drugs known to impair sexual response may resolve the problem. If levels of sex hormones are low, replacement therapy may help. Psychologic counseling may be help-

CRITICAL THINKING CHALLENGE
Case Analysis

Jane, a 16-year-old student, is distressed that menarche has not yet occurred. She is finishing her third year of high school and expects to go college in about a year on a track scholarship. She is 5'6" and weighs 95 pounds.

1. What information about her health habits would you consider pertinent to her problem?
2. Formulate specific questions you would ask her to elicit this information.
3. What specific self-care measures would you suggest that could reduce the risk of continued amenorrhea?
4. What risks may Jane face if her situation does not change?

ful but should be used only as an adjunct unless physical causes have been ruled out.

Hormone Deficiency in Older Adults

Testosterone levels decline steadily but gradually as men age. Testosterone deficiency can produce growth of hair in men with male pattern baldness, tissue wasting (atrophy of the genitals and muscles and osteoporosis), and decreased potency and fertility. However, many men reach advanced age without signs and symptoms of adverse effects. Castration (surgical or traumatic) causes abrupt declines in hormones and more noticeable effects. Unless the client has prostate cancer, oral hormone therapy can correct the sexual dysfunction. When low testosterone levels are required for controlling cancer, potency may be restored via penile implants that provide an artificial erection.

Sex hormone levels drop much more rapidly in aging women than in men. Menopausal women experience a pronounced decline in estrogen with marked effects on the body. Increased production of pituitary gonadotropins, estrogen deficiency, and imbalances in estrogen and progesterone cause vasomotor instability, genital and breast atrophy, loss of calcium from bone, and loss of the protective effects of estrogens on the cardiovascular system. Menopause can cause "hot flashes" (vasodilation that causes flushing and a feeling of being very warm), sexual dysfunction and dyspareunia, osteoporosis and kyphosis ("dowager's hump"), and changes in blood lipids (decreased high-density lipoprotein levels, increased low-density lipoprotein and cholesterol levels). It also increases risks of bone fractures, atherosclerosis, heart attack, and stroke. Thin women are at higher risk than those with greater fat deposits, who appear to have higher estrogen levels after menopause; conversely, women with ample fat are at higher risk for endometrial cancer and diabetes.

Estrogen Replacement Therapy

Estrogen replacement therapy (ERT) has been used widely for relieving symptoms of menopause (see Chap. 30 for general information on estrogens). Among the most common products for restoring estrogen balance during menopause are oral estrogens and transdermal 17-beta-estradiol.

Pharmacodynamics. Estrogen replacement therapy raises the body level of estrogens toward the normal premenopausal level. It thereby reduces levels of gonadotropin, calcium loss, detrimental blood lipid changes (low levels of high-density lipoprotein, high levels of low-density lipoprotein, high levels of cholesterol), and other signs and symptoms of hormone deficiency.

Pharmacokinetics. Estrogen replacement may be carried out orally or by using a transdermal patch. Oral estrogens are initially metabolized within the intestinal wall, with the conversion of estradiol to estrone. They are carried to the liver by the portal circulation. Further metabolism then occurs, with the conversion of estrone to estrone sulfate and estrone glucuronide. A significant increase in estrone levels is noted after oral administration, with signs of estrogen retention after only three doses of oral estrogens.

Transdermal ERT produces levels of estradiol 24 hours after administration similar to oral ERT. The transdermal patch delivers drug directly to the blood, eliminating the first-pass effect in the liver. The use of a transdermal patch permits steady administration of the hormone. Serum levels of estradiol rise within 4 hours of application. Levels of estrone also increase slightly, remaining rather constant. Serum and urinary levels of estradiol conjugates appear to be typical of the early follicular phase in premenstrual women. Estrogens from local applications of estrogenic creams and suppositories are absorbed into the bloodstream.

Estrogens are stored in fatty tissues. They are degraded by the liver and excreted by the kidneys.

Therapeutic Uses. Estrogen replacement therapy reduces many signs and symptoms of menopause (hot flashes, dyspareunia from vaginal atrophy and dryness, emotional lability, thinning of the skin). When administered early, hormones help prevent osteoporosis and its effects (kyphosis, loss in height, pathologic fractures) and cardiovascular disease (heart attack, stroke). The Food and Drug Administration has approved the use of oral estrogens to retard bone loss in postmenopausal women.

Dosage and Administration. Drug preparations include oral conjugated equine estrogens (Premarin, 0.625 or 1.25 mg/day) and a micronized form of 17-beta-estradiol (Estrace). A transdermal 17-beta-estradiol patch (0.025, 0.05, or 0.1 mg/day) is applied as directed and left in place until changed, every third day (Fig. 31-3).

Although the doses of estradiol in the transdermal patches are lower than those given orally, 12 days of norethindrone may be ordered to prevent endometrial hyperplasia or the recurrence of menopausal symptoms

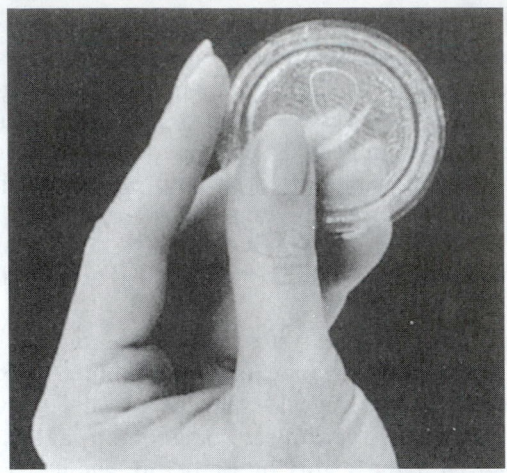

Figure 31-3. Low-dose estrogen skin patch, marketed as a transdermal drug delivery system. This estogen patch, available by the name of Estraderm (Estradiol Transdermal System) is transparent and about the size of a silver dollar. It contains 17-beta-estradiol, which is identical to the estrogen produced naturally before menopause. In releasing small amounts of estrogen directly into the bloodstream at a constant and controlled rate, the patch delivers the levels of estrogen produced by premenopausal women.

during treatment-free times. Low-dose progestogens produce a more acceptable bleeding pattern, ridding the uterus of the hyperplastic endometrial lining, regardless of the route of estrogen administration.

Adverse Reactions. Estrogens may increase the risk of endometrial cancer and stimulate the growth of other cancers of the reproductive organs (cancer of the cervix and breast). Recent studies indicate that endometrial cancer is slow-growing and can be easily diagnosed and cured before it causes a serious health threat. Overall death rate from all cancers seems to be no higher for estrogen users than for nonusers.

High levels of antithrombin III and renin tend to increase the risk of hypertension and thrombosis. The risk of gallbladder disease also rises.

The patch form of estrogen may cause topical side effects, such as itching, redness, rash, swelling, or dermatitis. Usually, these symptoms are mild to moderate and transitory. However, patch use should be discontinued if reactions are severe. Other symptoms, such as breast tenderness and breakthrough bleeding, are expected side effects, regardless of the administration route. Endometrial hyperplasia can also develop. Male partners who have contact with estrogenic vaginal creams may experience feminization, including some degree of impotence.

Drug–Drug Interactions. Estradiol increases the effects of concomitantly administered corticosteroids. Clients taking barbiturates, phenytoin, or rifampin may have decreased serum levels of estradiol.

Drug–Laboratory Test Interactions. Besides impaired glucose tolerance test values and decreased antithrombin

III, pregnanediol excretion, and serum folate concentrations, estrogens increase sulfobromophthalein retention; levels of prothrombin and factors VII, VIII, IX, and X; and levels of serum triglyceride, phospholipid concentrations, and thyroid-binding globulin, with increased protein-bound iodine.

Precautions and Contraindications. The risk of endometrial cancer can be reduced and possibly eliminated if ERT is prescribed in cycles of 3 weeks on and 1 week off, and if the drug is combined with progesterone during the last 7 to 13 days of each cycle. Regardless of the estrogen source for ERT, women should have semiannual checkups, including breast and pelvic examinations. Endometrial biopsies (before ERT) are recommended by some prescribers to determine the risk for endometrial carcinoma, as well as to determine the optimal dosage of progestin. Estrogen therapy is contraindicated in women with a history of endometrial or breast cancer, abnormal blood clots, strokes, coronary artery disease, severe migraine headaches, liver disease, or unexplained vaginal bleeding. Clients should be monitored for adverse reactions to the hormones.

Estrogen patches are commonly used on a cyclic schedule. They are usually replaced every 3.5 days (twice weekly). The usual starting dose is 0.05 mg, with adjustment possible to 0.1 mg. The 17-beta-estradiol in the patch is the same form of estrogen produced by premenopausal women. The patch must be applied to intact, hairless skin on the trunk of the body, preferably the abdomen.

❖ NURSING MANAGEMENT: CLIENT RECEIVING ESTROGEN

The use of ERT is controversial among healthcare professionals. Early research indicated that long-term estrogen therapy raised the risk of genital and breast cancer to a level considered unacceptable by many. However, these results are no longer credited by many experts because the subjects of the early studies were young women whose ovaries remained functional and whose estrogen dosage was higher than that used today. More recent studies with older women, taking smaller dosages of hormones, do not indicate risks as high as earlier studies. Estrogen has been shown to exert protective effects, particularly against heart disease and osteoporosis, that were not considered in the past (Carditz et al., 1994).

The public in general is also undecided about the benefits of ERT. However, many women feel that the health, cosmetic, and psychologic benefits of ERT are worth the seemingly low (to them) levels of risk. Women who wish to undergo therapy have the right to receive accurate information about the drugs and a voice in the decision regarding their use (see the Critical Thinking Challenge: Issues Analysis.)

NURSING PROCESS
ASSESSMENT
Women seeking treatment for hormone deficiency during menopause should be evaluated for risk factors for adverse effects from therapy, including past episodes of abnormal clotting (phlebitis, thrombotic strokes, coronary thrombosis), certain cancers (cervical, endometrial, or breast tumors characterized by estrogen receptors), obesity, serious depression, or other adverse reactions to estrogens in the past.

An evaluation of the risk of failure to treat should also be made. Women of slight build, with little adipose tissue, and those with a family history of osteoporosis (dowager's hump, vertebral compression fractures) are at increased risk of developing serious osteoporosis. Those with elevated serum levels of low-density lipoproteins, depressed levels of high-density lipoproteins, or a family history of hypercholesterolemia or heart disease are at high risk for developing cardiovascular disease.

Because hormone treatment is most effective if started early in menopause, clients should be counseled about ERT before menopause has begun, or very early in the process. The client's knowledge about menopause and its treatment should be evaluated also.

NURSING DIAGNOSIS
Nursing diagnoses for clients beginning treatment may include:

- Fear, related to adverse effects of estrogen therapy, unstable hormone levels, and menopause
- Body Image Disturbance, related to potential drug-induced physical changes
- Knowledge Deficit, related to estrogen therapy and its management in menopause

Collaborative problems for clients receiving hormone replacements include:

Potential Complication: Thrombi or thromboemboli
Potential Complication: Endometrial cancer

PLANNING
Desired outcomes of nursing care may include eliminating the knowledge deficit, preventing or minimizing degenerative changes related to estrogen deficiency, enhancing body image, eliminating fear of menopause, and preventing or promptly detecting and treating adverse reactions to hormone therapy.

INTERVENTION
A key nursing intervention is teaching the client how to weigh the benefits and risks of ERT to reach the best decision for her. Should the client desire hormone treatment, the nurse may refer her to a prescriber likely to recommend this therapy. Clients with serious risks of adverse reactions to treatment should be cautioned that these may contraindicate prescription of hormones.

When hormones are prescribed, the client needs teaching about the regimen. To help boost the client's

CRITICAL THINKING CHALLENGE
Issue Analysis

Should Menopausal Women Receive Estrogen Replacement Therapy?

Pros

Estrogens relieve vasomotor symptoms and vaginal atrophy in postmenopausal women.

They help prevent osteoporosis by enhancing absorption of calcium.

A positive effect of high-density to low-density lipoprotein cholesterol levels is found.

Women who receive estrogens appear to have increased feelings of well-being.

Cons

The risk of endometrial cancer may be increased.

Breast tenderness may occur.

Increased risk for high blood pressure and thromboembolic disease exists, especially in smokers, users of alcohol, and inactive women.

Breakthrough bleeding may occur.

The risk of gallbladder disease is increased.

Because you are a nursing student, one of your friends has asked you for advice. Your friend's mother at age 51 is experiencing irregular menstrual periods. She also has hot flashes that make her perspire profusely and wake her from a sound sleep. Generally good-natured, she has become grumpy and even agitated at times. The healthcare provider has suggested estrogen replacement therapy (ERT), but your friend's mother is afraid that the treatment will give her cancer. Review the above pros and cons of ERT and then:

1. Consider what advice you can offer your friend to help her mother make an informed decision about ERT.
2. Delineate and prioritize some risk factors the mother may want to investigate.
3. Propose some questions for the mother to ask her prescriber.

---

self-image, the nurse should offer warm acceptance and positive reinforcement when appropriate. The nurse's attitude should convey the acceptance of menopause as a natural event in adult growth and development that does not always cause major health problems.

Client Education. Clients who choose not to seek treatment, and those for whom hormone treatment is contraindicated, should be taught measures to decrease the severity of menopausal symptoms and should be reassured that vasomotor instability tends to decrease as the body adjusts to its new hormone status. These women should engage in active weight-bearing exercise and eat a diet low in fat, moderate in calories, and high in calcium (at least 1,200 mg daily).

Clients for whom hormones are prescribed should be advised to monitor their health status with yearly Pap smears to detect endometrial cancer and blood tests for cholesterol levels. They should watch for signs that might indicate cancer, especially lumps in the breast and abnormal vaginal bleeding. These clients must take measures to minimize the risk of phlebitis (use of support hose, avoidance of lengthy sitting)

When estrogen patches are prescribed, clients may need instruction in their use. Application sites should be rotated, and at least a week should be allowed before reusing the same site.

OUTCOME EVALUATION

Data required for evaluating nursing interventions include client statements regarding changes in body image and level of fear, absence or incidence of degenerative changes related to menopause, and absence or incidence

of adverse reactions to hormone therapy. The teaching program may be evaluated by assessing how much data the client has remembered and used, and whether health practices recommended by the nurse have been followed.

❖ CHECKLIST OF NURSING ACTIONS

- ❑ Assess clients for risk of degenerative changes of menopause and also for risks of adverse reactions to hormone therapy.
- ❑ Teach clients the risks of degenerative changes of menopause and also the benefits and risks of hormone replacement therapy.
- ❑ Refer clients wishing to receive ERT to an appropriate physician.
- ❑ Inform clients about self-care practices that minimize the degenerative changes of menopause and also those that minimize adverse effects of hormone therapy.
- ❑ Teach clients to report promptly to the healthcare professional any signs and symptoms of adverse reactions to hormone therapy.
- ❑ Promote an acceptance of menopause as a natural event in adult growth and development, with recognition that for some women it does present health risks and cause discomfort.

Premenstrual Syndrome

Women react differently to menses. For many, the cycle passes without symptoms or difficulty, but some women suffer premenstrual symptoms that range from mild to incapacitating. Premenstrual syndrome (PMS) is a condition characterized by mood swings, irritability, bloating, fluid retention, sore breasts, migraine-type headaches, anxiety, depression, loss of concentration, fatigue, food (carbohydrate) cravings, backache, lethargy, dizziness, heaviness in the legs, acneiform skin disorders, and general aches and pains. These symptoms may escalate under stress.

Most clinicians think that PMS has its basis in physiologic factors. The syndrome is thought to be related to the drop in progesterone levels that normally occurs before menstruation. The major diagnostic factor in PMS is that the symptoms present in a recurrent pattern after ovulation, occurring 1 to 14 days before or during the first few days of menstruation. The symptoms depend on ovarian rather than uterine function.

Premenstrual syndrome can develop at any time during the childbearing years but tends to affect women in their 30s and 40s. The syndrome is sometimes triggered by hormonal changes that develop after childbirth, after the discontinuation of oral contraceptives, after tubal ligation, or after removal of an ovarian cyst.

There are different reactions to PMS, including depression, anxiety, or anger. Mood swings are absent in 40% of women with PMS; 50% have mild mood swings, and 10% have moderate to severe problems.

Treatment for PMS varies and may include progesterone, mild diuretics 5 to 10 days before menses, oral contraceptives to prevent ovulation, vitamin B_6 (up to 500 mg daily), exercise, and high-protein snacks. Education and awareness appear to be helpful. (See Chap. 27 for information on diuretics.)

Progesterone Therapy

Progesterone is a female hormone associated with the secretory phase of the menstrual cycle and the maintenance of pregnancy. It inhibits uterine contraction. It is usually prescribed as medroxyprogesterone acetate (Provera) when used to treat PMS. (See Chap. 30 for basic information about progesterone.)

Pharmacodynamics. Progesterone, when administered orally to women with adequate endogenous estrogen, transforms proliferative endometrium tissue into secretory tissue.

Pharmacokinetics. Progesterone may be administered orally or intramuscularly (IM). It affects many organs throughout the body. It is degraded by the liver and excreted by the kidneys. Progesterone appears to cross the placenta, and detectable amounts have been found in breast milk.

Therapeutic Uses. In addition to treating PMS, oral progesterone is used to treat secondary amenorrhea and abnormal uterine bleeding not associated with organic pathology. It is often administered in combination with estrogen, primarily in oral contraceptives. It is also used in the adjunctive or palliative treatment of inoperable, recurrent, and metastatic endometrial or renal carcinoma.

Dosage and Administration. Oral doses vary from 2.5 to 10 mg. The IM dose varies from 100 to 400 mg.

Adverse Reactions. Administration of progesterone during pregnancy increases the risk of congenital anomalies (heart defects and limb reduction defects). When given with estrogen, as in oral contraceptives, it has been linked to a decrease in glucose tolerance. When given parenterally, progesterone inhibits gonadotropin production, which then prevents follicular maturation and ovulation, causing infertility (this is, of course, its therapeutic action in contraceptives).

The drug has been associated with abnormal clotting, pulmonary emboli, and fluid retention. Some skin problems may occur (urticaria, pruritus, generalized rash, acne, alopecia, and hirsutism). Breakthrough bleeding can also occur. The effects of prolonged use of progesterone on pituitary, ovarian, adrenal, hepatic, and uterine functions remain under study. Because it promotes fluid retention and tissue edema, progesterone increases the risk of illness in clients who suffer from epilepsy, migraine, asthma, or cardiac or renal dysfunction. It can also increase the severity of diabetes mellitus.

Drug–Laboratory Test Interactions. Use of progesterone can cause inaccurate test values for hepatic and endocrine function.

Precautions and Contraindications. Before using progesterone, a thorough physical examination with emphasis on the breast and pelvic areas should be carried out, including a Pap test and, if indicated, a pregnancy test. The drug should not be used if pregnancy or organic pathology is present. Pelvic examinations must be performed frequently to ensure that pregnancy has not occurred. Undiagnosed vaginal bleeding should be investigated immediately. Clients with epilepsy, asthma, migraine, depression, or heart or kidney disease should be monitored closely while taking progesterone.

❖ NURSING MANAGEMENT: CLIENT RECEIVING PROGESTERONE

In the past, most women believed they had to bear the discomfort of PMS in silence. They often were told that their complaints were based on emotional factors. Although emotional effects are among the symptoms of this disorder, biochemical imbalances have been identified as its source.

NURSING PROCESS
ASSESSMENT

The specific signs and symptoms experienced by the client should be determined. Charting the menstrual cycle and symptoms and keeping a dietary record and notations of stressful situations help determine whether the symptoms are really associated with the menstrual cycle or are due to other causes.

Before progesterone therapy begins, pregnancy should be ruled out. The client should also be evaluated for medical conditions that tend to worsen with progesterone therapy (epilepsy, migraine, asthma, cardiac or renal dysfunction, diabetes, and depression). The history should include specific inquiries about thrombophlebitis, thromboembolic disorders, cerebral apoplexy, liver dysfunction or disease, known or suspected breast or genital malignancy, undiagnosed vaginal bleeding, or known sensitivity to the drug.

NURSING DIAGNOSIS

Diagnoses likely to be made for women receiving progesterone to treat PMS may include:

- Knowledge Deficit, related to hormone therapy for PMS
- Risk for Injury, related to increased pathology (eg, asthma, epilepsy, diabetes, migraine, asthma, heart or kidney disease, abnormal clotting, clinical depression) secondary to progesterone therapy

PLANNING

Desired outcomes of nursing interventions include reducing the signs and symptoms of PMS, preventing or promptly detecting and treating adverse reactions to progesterone, improving the client's coping, and educating the client regarding therapy and self-care for optimal treatment response.

INTERVENTION

Before therapy begins, the prescriber should be informed of any elements in the history that indicate a high risk of adverse reaction to progesterone.

The client should be monitored for therapeutic and side effects of and adverse reactions to progesterone (breakthrough bleeding, abnormal clotting, changes in mood, undesirable skin changes, and worsening of epilepsy, migraine, asthma, diabetes, heart disease, or renal dysfunction).

The client should be treated in a warm, nonjudgmental manner. Social interaction should be encouraged. Referral to a self-help group may be helpful.

Client Education. A plan should be made and implemented for teaching the client how to manage the drug regimen and improve coping strategies. The client should be taught to recognize specific signs and symptoms that should be reported to the prescriber, including those signaling abnormal clot formation (tenderness of the legs, discomfort on dorsiflexion, angina-like pain, severe headache), breakthrough bleeding, skin outbreaks, and indications that conception may have occurred. The drug should be stopped if signs and symptoms of abnormal clotting or depression develop.

Diabetic clients should monitor blood glucose levels carefully and maintain them as close to normal as possible.

Clients should be advised to limit salt intake to minimize fluid retention. A wellness approach, including stress reduction, aerobic exercise, weight control, adequate nutrition, and limited alcohol, caffeine, and cigarette use seems beneficial.

OUTCOME EVALUATION

Data required for evaluation include changes in the signs and symptoms of PMS, the absence or incidence of adverse reactions to progesterone, and the absence or incidence of pregnancy resulting in congenital malformation in the infant. Teaching can be considered successful if the client promptly reports any critical information to the prescriber and makes lifestyle changes to promote wellness and minimize adverse reactions to progesterone. On a short-term basis, teaching may be evaluated by questioning the client to ascertain her understanding and retention of the facts presented during the teaching program.

Dysmenorrhea and Drug Treatment

Dysmenorrhea is a disorder in which painful cramps are experienced during menstruation. For some women, the condition is severe enough to be disabling. The cause of dysmenorrhea is believed to be release of prostaglandins in the uterus during menstruation. Nonsteroidal antiinflammatory drugs, which are thought to act by inhibiting prostaglandins, are recommended for symptomatic treatment of dysmenorrhea. These include aspirin, ibuprofen (Motrin), and mefenamic acid (Ponstel). See Chapter 36 for a discussion of nonsteroidal anti-inflammatory drugs.

Drugs That Affect Sexuality

Sexual behavior depends on the interweaving of many factors—physical, social, cultural, and emotional. Libido (erotic desire and the ability to enjoy sexual intercourse) is only one aspect of sexual behavior. The physiologic response (in men, erection, orgasm, and ejaculation; in women, lubrication of the vagina, tumescence, and orgasm) is another. Some pathologic conditions that affect other systems of the body may be important factors (Table 31-2) that affect the reproductive system and influence sexuality.

Libido and sexual response may be affected by drugs that alter the way the sex centers of the brain function or by medications that act on the peripheral nerves or blood vessels of the genitalia. Some agents are used to produce a direct modification of sexual behavior. More often, however, drugs are used for other medical purposes and influence sexual behavior only as a side effect (Table 31-3).

Aphrodisiacs

Aphrodisiacs are drugs used to stimulate the sex centers of the brain. Most substances used for this purpose are pharmacologically inactive but seem to have a placebo effect when used in a sexually provocative situation.

Historically, such substances have had symbolic significance based on male dominance and have included drugs made from rhinoceros horn and powdered lion penis.

Alcohol, frequently used as an aphrodisiac, acts on the brain centers in a sequence that first increases libido by decreasing inhibitions. However, continued alcohol intake acts as a general central nervous system depressant, which interferes with sexual performance. In fact, heavy or chronic use of alcohol may lead to sexual dysfunction. Therefore, clients who seek sexual therapy are told to limit alcohol consumption.

Marijuana (pot, grass) has an active ingredient, tetrahydrocannabinol (THC), that also seems to affect male sexual response in two phases. THC enters the bloodstream rapidly, with an almost immediate effect on the testes. This effect leads to instant testosterone production, with an increase in sexual arousal during and after smoking. In high doses, THC also results in an increase in LH manufactured by the pituitary. This increase occurs at the same time that testosterone is being produced by the testes, bypassing the usual sequence in which LH is produced by the pituitary about 20 minutes after sexual stimulation. Normally, LH would travel to the testes, where it is a factor in testosterone production. However, the testosterone level in the smoker's blood is higher than normal. This level causes a shutdown in the further production of testosterone, and the blood level is rapidly depleted to below normal within 20 minutes. This decreases sexual drive and, in heavy marijuana users, suppresses testicular activity.

Text continues on page 665.

Table 31-2. Disorders That Affect the Reproductive System and Sexuality

Systemic Illness	Anticipated Problems
AIDS	Weakness, debilitation, death
Alcoholism	Impotence with heavy use; fetal alcohol syndrome
Anorexia nervosa and bulimia	Amenorrhea; fetus small for gestational age
Cardiovascular disorders	Angina during and after intercourse; impairment of orgasmic response due to anxiety, depression, antihypertensive medications, or other prescribed drugs; effects of decreased maternal oxygenation on fetal development
Connective tissue disorders	Possibility of lupus erythematosus in offspring
Diabetes mellitus	Impotence caused by peripheral neuropathy that affects erection; impairment of orgasmic response due to neuropathy; effects of maternal diabetes on fetal development
Endometriosis	Pelvic pain; infertility
Infectious diseases	
Sexually transmitted diseases	Transmission of infection to fetus if acquired during pregnancy; fetal defects may occur; hydrocephalus, chorioretinitis, intracranial calcifications, microophthalmia, deafness; disease may not appear until infancy, childhood, or adulthood
Congenital toxoplasmosis	
Kidney disease and dialysis	Impotence due to arteriosclerotic changes in penis and pelvis; debilitation may preclude interest or ability to perform sexually; effects of maternal kidney disease on fetal development
Liver disease	Impotence that results from neutralization of androgens due to insufficient conjugation of estrogen; debilitation may lead to diminished desire or performance
Neurologic Disorders	
Brain	Sensations may be decreased; debilitation or confusion may lead to diminished desire or performance; effect of maternal anticonvulsive medication on fetal development
Peripheral nerves	Pain, urinary bladder or rectal difficulties, or alcoholic neuropathy may cause impotence or orgasmic problems; debilitation or paralysis of lower neural structures, particularly those that affect genital reflexes, may lead to impotence and lack of orgasm
Oncologic Diseases	Debilitation or pain may lead to avoidance of intercourse; impairment of orgasmic response due to anxiety, depression, physical state, chemotherapy, radiation therapy, or extensive surgery; effect of maternal oncology treatments on fetus; infertility
Endocrine Disorders	
Diabetes mellitus	See above
Thyroid deficiencies	May cause infertility in either sex; effect of maternal deficiency or medications on fetal development
Estrogen deficiency in females	Menopausal symptoms; atrophic vaginitis that causes dyspareunia; infertility
Testosterone deficiency in males or females	Loss of libido in both sexes; decreased penile erection or vaginal lubrication; decreased orgasmic response; infertility

Table 31-3. Effects of Drugs on Sexual Response

Drug	Actions	Responses Affected
Sedative–hypnotics		
alcohol and nontoxic doses of barbiturates and other similar agents (eg, ethchlorvynol, chloral hydrate, methaqualone)	General CNS depression. Effects are dose-related: in general, the higher the dose, the more interference with sexual performance. All these drugs affect the central state. Set and setting are very important. Expectation can override or alter pharmacologic effect. Most of these drugs potentiate one another. Alcohol with CNS depressants leads to greater CNS depression. In low doses, desire may be increased by reducing inhibition. In higher doses, all phases of sexual response are inhibited. Chronic alcoholism may result in permanent neurologic damage and consequent impaired genital functioning.	*Desire:* Increased in low doses in presence of inhibition; expectation may play a major role in this parameter; decreased in high doses *Excitation:* With low doses, excitement may be prolonged due to decreased sensitivity or to intimacy and shared feelings; impotence with high chronic intake of alcohol and barbiturates *Orgasm:* Delayed in high doses
Antianxiety Drugs		
Benzodiazepines (diazepam, chlordiazepoxide, chlorazepate), meprobamate	Action on limbic system and on internuncial neurons in the spinal cord	*Desire:* May enhance desire slightly if inhibited or avoided due to anxiety; diminished in high doses *Orgasm:* No effect in usual doses; in very high doses orgasm may be delayed
Narcotics		
morphine, codeine paragoric, D-propoxyphene, methadone	General depression of CNS and possible direct depression of sex centers; alteration of normal balance of biogenic amines in CNS	*Desire:* Absent in high doses *Excitation:* Impotence in high doses *Orgasm:* Inhibited by high doses
Antipsychotic Agents	Probably have no direct effect on the brain's sex centers (with the possible exception of haloperidol, which may affect the sexual response directly); may affect sexuality indirectly because of their favorable effects on the psychic state; in addition, some agents infrequently are reported to cause erectile and ejaculatory difficulties, probably because of their mild antiadrenergic or anticholinergic or antidopamine effects	
Phenothiazines (Stelazine, Mellaril, Thorazine)	Sexual response may be improved as by-product of recovery from mental illness; dry ejaculation may be caused by effects of internal vesical sphincter paralysis, causing semen to empty into bladder; often seen with thioridazine (Mellaril)	*Desire:* Decreased desire reported only in very high doses *Excitation:* Impotence reported with some agents (rare) *Orgasm:* Inhibition of ejaculation reported with thioridazine
Butyrophenones (Haldol)	Reported to reduce libido and potency and cause retarded ejaculations in some clients; mechanism unknown—may involve central or peripheral antiadrenergic or antidopamine activity	*Desire:* May be decreased *Excitation:* Impotence reported with some agents (rare) *Orgasm:* None reported
Antidepressants		
Tricyclics and monoamine oxidase inhibitors	No direct effects on sexuality; sex drive and performance may improve as depression lifts; antidepressants have some peripheral autonomic effects that rarely cause potency and ejaculatory problems in men	*Orgasm:* Some females reported delay of orgasm
Tricyclics (Elavil, Tofranil)	Anticholinergic side effects	*Excitation:* Impaired excitement
Monoamine oxidase inhibitors (Nardil, Marplan, Norpramin)	No reported effects on sexual response, except that sexual urgency may diminish manic activities	*Desire:* Urgency or desire may be reduced
lithium carbonate	No reported effects on sexual response, except that sexual urgency may diminish manic activities	*Desire:* Urgency or desire may be reduced

(continued)

Table 31-3. (Continued)

Drug	Actions	Responses Affected
Stimulants		
cocaine	General CNS stimulant; augments sympathetic CNS function	*Desire:* Reported to be enhanced *Excitation:* Reported to be enhanced; high doses may cause impotence *Orgasm:* May be enhanced; high doses may interfere with orgasm, more so in females
Amphetamines	General brain stimulation; in acute cases, reported to enhance libido; in chronic cases, diminishes libido and sexual functioning and causes general debility	*Desire:* Reported to be enhanced at low doses; diminished at high doses *Excitation:* Decreased in chronic doses *Orgasm:* May be enhanced; high doses may interfere with orgasm, more so in females
Hallucinogens		
LSD (lysergic acid diethylamide)	Vasoconstrictor; may be a central inhibitor of 5-hydroxytryptamine (5-HT)	*Desire:* Mixed effects reported *Orgasm:* Physiologically none; altered experience reported
DMT (dimethyltryptamine), mescaline	Disrupt neurotransmission in limbic system; reported by some to enhance libido and orgasm, by others to have no effect; some users report impaired sexuality	*Desire:* Mixed effects reported *Orgasm:* Mixed effects reported
THC (tetrahydrocannabinol)	May have some effects on muscle contractions; some reports of enhanced erotic feelings	*Desire:* Mixed effects reported *Excitation:* Mixed effects reported *Orgasm:* Enhanced orgasm reported
Miscellaneous CNS Agents		
L-dopa	Increased levels of dopamine centrally	*Desire:* Reports of increased desire in elderly male patients
p-CPA (parachlorophenylalanine)	Inhibitor of serotonin synthesis	*Desire:* Reports of increased desire
Hormones	Presumably stimulate the sex centers of the CNS and so increase libido and genital response; also maintain genital organs in a functional state	
androgens (eg, testosterone)	Stimulate sex centers of both genders; fetal androgen causes gender differentiation of behavior; also act on periphery to enhance the growth, development, and functioning of the male genitals and the clitoris	*Desire:* Stimulates sexual desire in both sexes *Excitation:* In males, may increase ability to have an erection in testosterone-deficient states *Orgasm:* In males, volume of ejaculate may be increased
estrogens (estriol, estradiol, estrone)	Do not increase libido; in fact, may decrease sexual interest; act on the cells of the female genitalia to enhance their growth, development, and functioning	*Desire:* In men, may decrease desire; in women, variable responses reported; increased desire may be due to decreased fear of pregnancy *Excitation:* May cause impotence in males *Orgasm:* Ejaculatory delay; volume of ejaculate decreased
progesterones (physiologic precursors to testosterone)	May decrease desire and excitement in males. Probably has no effect on females.	
thyroxine	Increased motor activity and augmented sympathetic nervous system activity; may decrease depression	*Desire:* Enhanced desire reported
cyproterone acetate	Antagonizes testosterone	*Desire:* Loss of libido in both genders *Excitation:* Impotence in males *Orgasm:* In males, volume of ejaculate may decrease; ejaculatory delay
adrenal steroids	Mechanisms unknown	*Desire:* May decrease libido in high doses

(continued)

Table 31-3. Effects of Drugs on Sexual Response (Continued)

Drug	Actions	Responses Affected
Antihypertensives		
Centrally acting (eg, alphamethyl dopa)	Block adrenergic nerves and innervated structures in periphery, causing disturbances in the hemodynamics of erection by various mechanisms; occasional inhibition of emission	*Desire:* Decreased *Excitation:* Decreased; impotence is major problem *Orgasm:* May be inhibited
Diuretics		
thiazides	Dilate blood vessel walls; decrease circulating fluid volume; disturb penile blood pressure	*Excitation:* May cause impotence
spironolactone	May block binding of testosterone at receptor site; gynecomastia due to action on breast tissue	*Desire:* Occasional loss of libido *Excitation:* May cause impotence
Ganglionic Blockers		
quaternary ammonium compounds	Block postganglionic nerves and innervated structures; disturb penile blood pressure; may inhibit sympathetic mediation of emission	*Excitation:* Often causes impotence *Orgasm:* May be inhibited
General Antiadrenergic Drugs		
phentolamine; phenoxybenzamine; ergot alkaloids		*Orgasm:* Inhibits emission in males
α-blockers (eg, clonidine)	Blocks α-adrenergic receptors—central and peripheral action	*Orgasm:* Block emission in males—dose-related
sympathoplegic drugs (eg, guanethidine, bretylium)	Deplete adrenergic nerves of norepinephrine	*Excitation:* Often cause impotence *Orgasm:* May be inhibited
β-blockers (eg, propranolol)	Blockade of β-adrenergic receptors of heart—central and peripheral action	*Desire:* Sometimes decreased *Excitation:* Sometimes decreased
Anticholinergic Drugs		
Banthine, Pro-Banthine, atropine, scopolamine, Cogentin	Block the nerves that control the smooth muscles and blood vessels of the genital organs involved in the sexual responses; inhibit the action of acetylcholine on structures innervated by postganglionic parasympathetic nerves; also have central anticholinergic action	*Excitation:* May rarely cause impotence
Aphrodisiacs		
Spanish fly (cantharides), amyl nitrite	Irritates genitourinary tract—causes priapism; may enhance vascular response of genitals; reported to improve orgasm	*Excitation:* Priapism, organic impotence
Miscellaneous Drugs		
disulfiram (Antabuse)		*Excitation:* Occasional impotence reported *Orgasm:* Delay of ejaculation
tryptophan	Increased CNS concentration of serotonin	*Desire:* Decreased *Excitation:* Decreased
ephedrine	α-adrenergic stimulator	*Orgasm:* Treatment of failure to ejaculate
cimetidine	Inhibits H_2 receptors; may cause lowered sperm count	*Desire:* Loss of libido and impotence reported
Neurotoxic Agents		
halogenated aromatic hydrocarbons	Neuropathy	*Desire:* Decreased *Excitation:* Decreased
carbon disulfide	Neuropathy and premature arteriosclerotic changes due to hyperlipidemia	*Desire:* Decreased *Excitation:* Decreased

The resultant lowered levels of testosterone lead to chronic reduction of sex drive. As with alcohol, limited use of marijuana may lead to increased arousal and stronger muscular contractions during orgasm. However, extended heavy use has the same negative effect as alcohol, with a resultant decrease in sexual function.

Other hallucinogens have an effect on the central nervous system, including the brain's sex centers. Hallucinogens cause the user to undergo intensified mental as well as auditory and visual awareness. Intercourse under these circumstances reportedly leads to a longer orgasmic response. Amphetamines and cocaine stimulate the brain centrally and are said to increase sexual drive and performance. Either drug may lead to habituation or addiction, with the probability that sexual drive and ability will eventually decrease significantly.

Androgen (the male sex hormone) increases sexual drive by acting directly on the brain's sex centers. This hormone is used by both men and women to enhance muscle development and athletic ability. However, it has undesirable side effects, such as faster growth of prostatic cancer in men, acne and hirsutism in women, and the possibility of cerebral or cardiovascular problems in either sex (see Chap. 30).

Cantharides (Spanish fly) acts as an irritant to the male bladder and urethra, resulting indirectly in sexual excitement and priapism (continuous penile erection). Its continued use may lead to permanent penile damage and impotence.

Antianxiety, antidepressant, and antipsychotic drugs may act as aphrodisiacs by lessening the person's negative self-image, thereby enhancing sexual interest and performance. However, their action is general and such drugs are not specific for sexual problems.

Clients beginning therapy for Parkinson's disease with levodopa sometimes experience a sudden, abrupt, temporary rise in libido.

Anaphrodisiacs

Anaphrodisiacs are drugs that impair sexual function. They include drugs that depress the action of the central nervous system (alcohol in large doses, barbiturates, hypnotics, sedatives, narcotics). Other drugs impair sexuality because of their peripheral effect on the genitalia, influencing either erectile or orgasmic responses. Hormones such as estrogen and hormone analogs such as leuprolide acetate (Lupron) used in treating some breast and prostate cancers can adversely affect sexual functioning.

Anticholinergic drugs, used to treat gastrointestinal and psychiatric disorders, may block the parasympathetic nerves that normally increase genital vascularization, thereby impeding erection. Antiadrenergic drugs (beta blockers) used to treat hypertension may block the nerves of the sympathetic division of the autonomic nervous system, leading to difficulty in ejaculation. Libido is not directly affected by either anticholinergic or antiadrenergic medications. However, repeated inability to respond favorably during sexual performance may lead to inhibitions and eventual withdrawal from sexual activity.

Some psychotropic drugs act as anaphrodisiacs. Haloperidol (Haldol), an antipsychotic drug used to treat Tourette syndrome, lessens libido and potency through a direct effect on the brain's sex centers. Lithium, an antidepressant used to treat bipolar depression, calms the manic phase and effectively lowers sexual activity.

Drugs That Treat Sexual Problems

Monoamine oxidase inhibitors are mood regulators sometimes used to treat premature ejaculation (see Chapter 20). These drugs help prevent panic attacks in clients with phobias concerning sexual activity. The person is usually more amenable to psychotherapeutic intervention after treatment. Antiandrogens lessen libido in either sex by antagonizing testosterone. Their use produces impotence in males and leads to reduced ejaculate. Cyproterone acetate is an experimental antiandrogen used to treat people with compulsive sexual disorders.

Because of the positive emotional responses they induce, some psychotropic drugs affect sexual response favorably. However, some of these drugs may also cause difficulties in erections or ejaculation because of their antiadrenergic or anticholinergic actions. Phenothiazines may improve sexual function as the mental state becomes healthier. However, one of these, thioridazine (Mellaril), may paralyze the internal vesical sphincter, causing semen to empty into the urinary bladder instead of being propelled through the penis. The possibility of a dry ejaculation should be explained to clients who take this drug.

Effects of Toxic Materials

Many chemicals used in industry and agriculture exert estrogenic effects on animals and people exposed to them. The high level of pollution by such substances is believed to underlie the steady worldwide decrease in sperm counts recently. Its ultimate effect could be to reduce human fertility to harmful degrees. Such effects on males are likely to persist, making prompt reversal unlikely should reproduction rates fall too far.

Women also are exposed to chemicals that can harm them and their unborn children. The number of women in the labor force is increasing yearly, particularly in jobs linked to exposure to toxic materials. Some of these women may be pregnant, and many are of reproductive age.

Employers are legally bound to make employees aware of these risks. In addition, employees are supposed to be made aware of substances known to be teratogens or abortifacients, as well as substances that lead to carcinogenesis or mutagenesis. Nurses, particularly those who work in operating rooms or radiology, oncology, or hematology departments, are at high risk because of their exposure to toxic substances.

Little has been done to identify substances that interfere with fertility. One substance, carbon disulfide, used in the production of viscose, has been documented as a cause of menorrhagia, amenorrhea, and sterility in women. Other industrial environments or wastes (eg, pesticides, mercury, polychlorinated biphenyl) are suspected of causing fetal damage or infertility.

Fetuses are at greater risk than mothers when exposed to toxic materials, because their tissues are more sensitive to substances that may be teratogenic at an early stage of fetal development or carcinogenic at a later point. One example is the synthetic hormone diethylstilbestrol (DES), which was used by women with threatened abortions. Daughters born to women who took DES during pregnancy are at high risk for vaginal adenosis and cancer and must be followed carefully during and after adolescence. Studies also show a higher than statistically expected incidence of varicocele and epididymal cysts in sons exposed prenatally to DES. They demonstrate a significantly lower sperm count and potential for decreased fertility. There is also the possibility of eventual malignancies, based on findings that males exposed to DES have an increased incidence of cryptorchidism and hypoplastic testes, which are risk factors for adult testicular carcinoma.

■ SUMMARY

Many factors (physical, social, cultural, and emotional) influence sexual behavior. Response may be affected by drugs that alter the function of the brain's sex centers, act on peripheral nerves, or act on genital blood vessels. Medications, pollutants, and recreational drugs can all directly or indirectly affect sexual response. Some drugs are used specifically for modifying sexual behavior; others are used for other medical purposes, altering sexual behavior as a side effect. Aphrodisiacs are drugs that stimulate sex centers of the brain, whereas anaphrodisiacs impair sexual functioning.

Increased exposure to chemicals threatens fertility of both sexes. Environmental pollutants tend to reduce sperm production in men and increase the risk of infertility, miscarriage, and sexual dysfunction in women.

❖ NURSING MANAGEMENT: CLIENT RECEIVING A DRUG THAT AFFECTS SEXUALITY

Because the subject of sexuality has been mired in secrecy, many taboos have developed. Even political and religious implications are involved in discussions of pregnancy and childbearing and the medications and techniques used to affect their outcomes. Small wonder that clients often hesitate to tell healthcare providers about changes in their sexual feelings that may be drug-related. Nurses who feel comfortable with their own sexuality will seem more approachable to clients who experience changes in sexuality related to chemical or drug exposure.

NURSING PROCESS

ASSESSMENT

Sexual behavior is not an independent issue: it may be affected by the client's physical status, emotions, or other factors, including medications. The nursing history should include inquiries about any drugs taken that may affect libido, performance, or orgasm. These include prescribed medications as well as self-administered preparations or recreational drugs. The nature of the sexual problem and the client's knowledge about the effects of chemicals should be explored.

NURSING DIAGNOSIS

Diagnoses may include:

- Knowledge Deficit, related to insufficient understanding of drug and the condition that it treats
- Ineffective Management of Therapeutic Regimen, Reduced Adherence, related to undesired adverse drug effects

PLANNING

Major goals for clients are optimization of sexual function through effective management of the therapeutic regimen. Therapy should maintain or increase self-esteem and self-acceptance regardless of the level of sexual performance. When sexual performance cannot be restored to normal, goals include separation of social identity from that of sexual performance, increased coping skills, return to a normal sense of power and hope, increased social interaction, and acceptance of sexuality with the ability to attain and give sexual satisfaction in ways other than intercourse.

INTERVENTION

Whenever possible, any chemical agent that affects sexuality adversely should be eliminated. The client should be counseled to avoid harmful toxins and to consult the prescriber regarding a change in medication if a therapeutic drug is involved.

The nurse should help the client develop a realistic appraisal of self and abilities that are not sexually oriented (eg, relationships with others, work or study success, bonds with family members, an interest in the outside world). The client should be encouraged to derive gratification from a loving relationship with caressing, kissing, and touching, and an interest in meeting the partner's needs.

Client Education. When teaching clients with sexual problems about drug effects, the nurse should remember that sexual dysfunction may be unacceptable to the client, even when his or her health is threatened by the use of chemicals or failure to adhere to the medication regimen. Clients have the right to determine what drugs to take or to refuse treatment if the adverse reactions are unacceptable.

Clients should be alerted if medications ordered for physical or emotional disorders may as a side effect alter sexual response. Clients who take medications to combat alcoholism or obesity may not realize that these drugs can cause temporary impotence. Clients should also be informed that some over-the-counter preparations (eg, sedatives, anticholinergics) can affect sexuality.

Clients taking medications ordered for sexual therapy may be unaware that self-prescribed substances can potentiate or lessen the effects of these medications. For example, clients who take monoamine oxidase inhibitors for treating premature ejaculation and who also take decongestants or eat foods high in tyramine or tryptophan may suffer hypertensive crises.

OUTCOME EVALUATION

Data needed for evaluation include adherence to the medication regimen and statements by the client that sexual performance or social relationships, emotional status, and coping ability have improved.

❖ CHECKLIST OF NURSING ACTIONS

- ❑ Become comfortable with your own sexuality and be accessible to clients who wish to discuss sexuality and sexual problems.
- ❑ Include information about drugs and pollutants that affect sexuality in the nursing history.
- ❑ Become familiar with the effects on sexual behavior of chemicals, including various medications.
- ❑ Inform clients about the possible sexual side effects of drugs they are taking.
- ❑ Inform clients about the possible sexual side effects of over-the-counter drugs.
- ❑ If a medication that affects sexuality must be taken, teach the client about alternative methods of lovemaking.

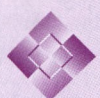

Box 31-1
Investigational Contraceptives for Men

Drugs under investigation for their usefulness as contraceptives for males include:

- **Gossypol,** a cotton-seed derivative used in China, reduces sperm formation and motility. Side effects include nausea, fatigue, decreased libido, hypokalemia, and high levels in the liver. About 25% of long-term users remained infertile after discontinuing gossypol.
- **Sulfasalazine** lessens sperm motility and density while increasing the percentage of abnormal sperm.
- **Phenoxybenzamine** causes azoospermia by paralyzing the ejaculatory system.
- **Tolnizamine** interferes with the maturation of sperm. Evidence of toxicity in the kidneys and marked reduction in testicular size in laboratory rats have been found. Researchers think that changing the dosage may decrease side effects without decreasing efficacy.
- The World Health Organization is supporting research on the development of a birth-control injection for men using a synthetic form of testosterone. The drug is being tested with weekly injections that keep the client's testosterone level at a high enough level to interfere with the pituitary gland's production of LH and FSH. This interference effectively stops the body's normal production of testosterone, preventing the production of sperm by the testes. A second synthetic testosterone would require injections only once every 3 months and would therefore be more acceptable. It is hoped that this method will have a lower failure rate than for condoms, which is about 17%.

Drugs That Prevent Conception

Contraceptives have been used since ancient times. Some methods have been more acceptable than others. Many factors influence the selection of a contraceptive: religious beliefs, political influence, economic power, cultural outlook, age, education, and convenience. Contraceptive techniques also vary in effectiveness and safety.

Male Contraceptive Measures

Besides coitus interruptus, which is reliable only if the man has total control and can ejaculate outside the vagina, and vasectomy, only condoms are available as male contraceptives. Condoms are 90% effective in preventing pregnancy. Additional protection can be attained by applying nonoxynol-9 or octoxynol-9 cream, jelly, or foam to the exterior of the condom before intercourse. These spermicidal agents act as surfactants and damage the cell walls of sperm. They can irritate the tissues of either sex partner. Spermicidal surfactants reportedly increase the risk of congenital defects if used during pregnancy. To date, there is no acceptable drug for reducing male fertility (Box 31-1). Clients using condoms with spermicide must understand that condoms provide "safer" rather than "safe" sex; they do not guarantee absolute safety, whether used as a contraceptive or in preventing the transmission of sexually transmitted diseases (STDs). Permanent male contraception can be provided by a vasectomy.

Female Contraceptive Measures

Pharmacologic contraceptive methods are summarized in Table 31-4. In addition to abstinence and tubal ligation, female contraceptive methods include nonpharmacologic

Table 31-4. Pharmacologic Contraceptive Measures for Women

Method	Rate of Pregnancy	Advantages	Disadvantages
spermicides	20%–25%	Kills sperm	Must be reintroduced before each attempt at intercourse; coital position may cause leakage from vagina; usage varies according to type and manufacturer's instructions
diaphragm	10.3%–57%	No systemic reaction	Must fit and be inserted properly; should be used with spermicidal cream or jelly; recurrent cystitis, allergy to latex; prolonged retention may increase risk of *Staphylococcus aureus* in lower genital tract (possible toxic shock syndrome)
cervical cap	8.1%–17.4%	Adheres to cervix by suction, can be left in place for 36 hr	Requires proper fitting; need for manual dexterity to replace; should be used with spermicidal jelly or cream; expensive; holds secretions against cervix as long as cap is in place, with possible relation to toxic shock syndrome and abnormal Pap smears; vaginal odor
intrauterine device (IUD)	5%	Convenient; high degree of effectiveness	Limited availability because of possibility of uterine perforation, with complications (eg, infection, intestinal obstruction); may cause ectopic pregnancy
oral contraceptives	4%–10%	High degree of effectiveness; useful for women with hypermenorrhea or endometriosis	Missing doses lessens effectiveness; possibility of thromboembolic disorders, gallbladder disease, mental depression, vaginal bleeding, visual disturbances, increase in size of fibroid tumors, infertility after discontinuation, cessation of milk supply during lactation, birth defects if used during pregnancy
Danazol	Experimental	Minimal side effects	Not always effective; breakthrough bleeding; occasional development of facial hair
Injectable contraceptives—medroxy-progesterone (Depo-Provera)		Injectable every 1–3 months	Same disadvantages as pill; need for injection every 3 months, weight gain; irregular vaginal bleeding
Implantable contraceptive (Norplant, with 35 mg levonorgestrel)	0.5%–2.6%	Protection after 24 h, lasting up to 5 yr Removal takes only about 15 min	Must be inserted beneath skin of forearm, upper arm, or scapular area; can be felt and sometimes seen; initial irregular vaginal bleeding; headaches; breast tenderness, mood changes, infection at implantation site; user must weigh <150 lb
Postcoital diethylstilbestrol (DES)	Depends on time elapsed since coitus (must be 72 hr or less)	Undesirable pregnancy (eg, rape, incest) can be aborted	Only effective if used within hours of intercourse. Side effects may be severe (eg, nausea, vomiting, headache, dizziness, abdominal pain); chance of thromboembolic disease; if already pregnant, may lead to vaginal adenosis in female offspring or epididymal anomalies in male offspring
Postcoital Ovral (estradiol and progesterone)	Investigational	Can abort undesired pregnancy; easy to use (2 tablets in morning, 2 tablets 12 hr later)	Must start within 24 hr; nausea, vomiting
Mifepristone (RU486)	Interrupts pregnancy in 85%–93% of cases	Eliminates need for surgical procedure in 60%–95% of cases	Legal concerns where abortions are illegal; at this writing is not available in U.S.; may need follow-up surgical procedure
Silastic vaginal ring	3.5%		
High dosage		Eliminates ovulation; can leave in place for 3 wk	Must be removed after 3 wk and replaced to prevent pregnancy; can be expelled spontaneously; may develop noninfectious discharge and/or vaginal erosion; irregular vaginal bleeding
Low dosage		Makes cervical mucus impermeable to sperm; can leave in place for several months	

(continued)

Table 31-4. (continued)

Method	Rate of Pregnancy	Advantages	Disadvantages
Tubal obstruction—silicone injected through uterus to block tubes	Experimental	Nonsurgical; 50%–80% chance of reversibility	Sometimes not reversible
Sterilization—banding or clipping of fallopian tubes	Almost 100%	50%–80% chance of reversal with microsurgery and drugs to prevent adhesions	May not be reversible

(natural), chemical, mechanical, and hormonal means. Nonpharmacologic methods include fertility awareness and avoidance of intercourse during fertile periods. Ways of determining ovulation include the basal body temperature method, the cervical mucus method, and the monoclonal antibody test. Mechanical contraceptives include the diaphragm, intrauterine device (IUD), cervical cap, and vaginal sheath (female condom). This chapter focuses on the chemical and hormonal agents women can use.

Chemical Methods

Chemical contraceptives are made up of two basic ingredients: a relatively inert vehicle that forms a barrier to delay progress of sperm and an active spermicidal agent that immobilizes or destroys the sperm biochemically (Table 31-5).

Spermicides are available as creams, jellies, foams, foaming tablets, and suppositories. High failure rates are probably due to inconsistent or improper use. Typical spermicides are nonoxynol-9 and octoxynol-9. They can cause irritation in the tissues of both partners. It has been reported that use of surfactant spermicides during pregnancy may increase the risk of birth defects. Spermicides must be used each time intercourse occurs, even if intercourse is repeated within a few minutes. Products must be inserted high in the vaginal vault, next to the cervix. Suppositories depend on body heat to melt them and to permit their spread over the cervix. Tablets require sufficient vaginal moisture to foam properly. To be effective, all spermicides must cover and remain in contact with the cervix during intercourse. Coital positions that result in leakage from the vagina may lead to contraceptive failure.

Oral Contraceptives

Female oral contraceptives are commonly referred to as the pill (see Chap. 30).

Pharmacodynamics. Oral contraceptives contain either progestogens alone (the minipill) or progestogen in combination with estrogen. (Progestogens, synthetic steroids related to progesterone, are combined with estrogen to prevent bleeding that might occur at odd times during the cycle.) The two types work differently: The combined pills suppress ovulation by inhibiting the secretion of FSH and LH in the anterior pituitary. In addition, the progesterone alone inhibits the transportation of the sperm and ovum and proliferation of the endometrium. Progestogen-only pills suppress ovu-

Table 31-5. Composition of Vaginal Chemical Contraceptives

Type of Product	Base Materials	Active Ingredients
Creams	Stearates	Nonoxynol-9
	Stearic acid	Octoxynol-9
	Glycerin	
Foam aerosol	Hydrocarbon and freon	Nonoxynol-9
	Polyethylene glycol	Benzethonium chloride
	Glycerin	
Foam tablets	Bicarbonate of soda	Nonoxynol-9
	Polyethylene glycol	Polysaccharide-polysulfuric acid ester
	Glycerin	Chloramine
	Tartaric acid	Sodium dichlorosulfamidobenzoate
Jellies and pastes	Polyethylene glycol	Diisobutylphenoxypolyethoxyethanol
	Gelatin	Polyoxyethylenenonylphenol
	Gum tragacanth	Phenylmercuric acetate
Suppositories	Cocoa butter	Nonoxynol-9
	Soap	Phenylmercuric borate
	Glycerin	Polysaccharide-polysulfuric acid ester

lation in only half the women who use them; combined pills provide the greatest effectiveness, with about a 4% to 10% pregnancy rate for the combination of estrogen and progestogen and a 5% to 10% pregnancy rate for progestogen alone.

The newer combined pills have fluctuating progesterone levels, thereby lowering unnecessary exposure to higher levels of progesterone throughout the menstrual cycle. They contain a higher level of progesterone to coincide with the expected time of ovulation, offering greater contraceptive protection at that time. These pills appear to have fewer side effects but offer a slightly lower level of efficacy. Oral contraceptives are listed in Table 31-6.

Therapeutic Uses. In addition to contraception, the pill can be used to treat hypoestrogenic amenorrhea, hypermenorrhea, or endometriosis. It may also protect against ovarian cysts, ovarian and uterine cancers, and benign breast disease. It provides the greatest safety when used by young women who are healthy, who do not smoke cigarettes, and who limit use to 10 years.

Birth-control pills may be prescribed for delayed maturation in girls; the combination of estrogen and progesterone helps convert the endometrium into a mature structure. The estrogen content in oral contraceptives also increases the body's ability to reabsorb dietary calcium from the intestinal tract before it is lost through the kidney tubules. This reabsorption decreases calcium loss from the bones, lessening the chance of osteoporosis and bone fractures, which may occur even in the young.

Dosage and Administration. The minipill is taken continuously, without interruption. The combined pill may be taken in a 21- or 28-day series. Women who use the 21-day series can expect menses to start 2 to 7 days after taking the last pill in the series. They are usually told to start a new pack on the fifth day, whether or not they are still bleeding, or to wait a week before starting a new series. Those on the 28-day series start a new pack as soon as the present pack is finished. (The additional pills are placebos, but they prevent the break in the daily pill-taking routine.) Forgotten doses should be taken as soon as remembered.

Adverse Reactions. The pill remains controversial because of its risks to the user. The biggest danger is increased mortality from thromboembolic disorders. Other potential problems include an increase in migraine headaches, mental depression, hypertension, disturbances in carbohydrate metabolism, elevated serum lipids, gallbladder disease, breakthrough vaginal bleeding, visual disturbances, impaired fertility after discontinuation, discolored skin areas, and an enlargement of fibroid tumors. After discontinuation of the pill, the risk of thrombotic strokes may persist for 6 years and that of myocardial infarction for 9 years.

Breakthrough bleeding may occur with either type of oral contraceptive. (The use of estrogen-only contraceptives has been abandoned, partly because of higher risk for breakthrough bleeding.) Oral contraceptives are believed to increase the need for certain vitamins, notably vitamin B complex and ascorbic acid.

Drug–Drug Interactions. Among the medications reported to interfere with the efficacy of oral contraceptives are the antituberculous drug rifampin (breakthrough bleeding and increased risk of pregnancy); anticonvulsants, including phenytoin, phenobarbital, and primidone; some antibiotics (ampicillin, tetracycline); analgesics (phenacetin); and the psychotropic drugs chlordiazepoxide and meprobamate. Clients who take anticoagulants may develop a higher circulating level of some clotting factors, particularly factor VII. Slower excretion of caffeine, diazepam, and prednisone may occur in women who take the pill. Vitamin plasma levels may also change, with an increase in vitamin A and decreases in vitamins B_2, B_{12}, and C, as well as folic acid.

Drug–Laboratory Test Interactions. Abnormal endocrine function findings may result with oral contraceptive agents; consult the package insert of the individual product.

Precautions and Contraindications. Women who smoke more than 15 cigarettes a day, who have vascular disease, cardiac problems, diabetes mellitus, breast or reproductive carcinoma, liver disease, hypertension, or obesity, or who are older than age 35 should not use oral contraceptives. Others who should seek different contraceptive methods are those with folic acid deficiency, epilepsy, fibrocystic breasts, infrequent or scant menses, or varicose veins. Using the pill during pregnancy is contraindicated (except to treat progesterone deficiency that threatens to cause miscarriage) because it may cause birth defects. Use during lactation may cause cessation of the milk supply. The effects on the infant of hormonal contraceptives used by the nursing mother have not been fully documented. Therefore, hormonal contraceptives should not be used during lactation. Dietary increases or supplements may be needed for women at risk—those who recently gave birth or who want to become pregnant shortly, adolescents, or those with poor diets.

Devices Used With Hormonal Contraceptive Methods

Silastic vaginal rings combine the convenience of a mechanical method with the greater efficacy of a hormonal contraceptive. They are available in two strengths, with differing actions. The high-dose ring contains 250 to 280 µg levonorgestrel with 180 µg estradiol. It acts by eliminating ovulation. It must be removed after 3 weeks and replaced a week later to prevent pregnancy. It can be expelled spontaneously, interrupting its contraceptive protection. It may cause a noninfectious vaginal discharge or vaginal erosion, as well as irregular bleeding. It releases a high level of estradiol. The low-dose

Table 31-6. Selected Combination and Microdose Progestin Contraceptives

Product	Manufacturer	Type	Estrogen	Progestin
Ortho-Novum 1/35–21	Ortho	Comb	0.035 mg ethinyl estradiol	1 mg norethindrone
1/35–28	Ortho	Comb	0.035 mg ethinyl estradiol	1 mg norethindrone
1/50–21	Ortho	Comb	0.05 mg mestranol	1 mg norethindrone
1/50–28	Ortho	Comb	0.05 mg mestranol	1 mg norethindrone
2 mg	Ortho	Comb	0.10 mg mestranol	2 mg norethindrone
Norinyl 1 + 35–21	Syntex	Comb	0.035 mg ethinyl estradiol	1 mg norethindrone
1 + 35–28	Syntex	Comb	0.035 mg ethinyl estradiol	1 mg norethindrone
1 + 50–21	Syntex	Comb	0.05 mg mestranol	1 mg norethindrone
1 + 50–28	Syntex	Comb	0.05 mg mestranol	1 mg norethindrone
Norlestrin-21 1/50	Parke-Davis	Comb	50 mcg ethinyl estradiol	1 mg norethindrone acetate
-28 1/50	Parke-Davis	Comb	50 mcg ethinyl estradiol	1 mg norethindrone acetate
Fe 1/50	Parke-Davis	Comb	50 mcg ethinyl estradiol	1 mg norethindrone acetate + 75 mg ferrous fumarate
-21 2.5/50	Parke-Davis	Comb	50 mcg ethinyl estradiol	2.5 mg norethindrone acetate
Fe 2.5/50	Parke-Davis	Comb	50 mcg ethinyl estradiol	2.5 mg norethindrone acetate + 75 mg ferrous fumarate
Nordette-21	Wyeth	Comb	0.03 mg ethinyl estradiol	0.15 levonorgestrel
-28	Wyeth	Comb	0.03 mg ethinyl estradiol	0.15 levonorgestrel
Ovral-21	Wyeth	Comb	0.05 mg ethinyl estradiol	0.5 mg norgestrel
-28	Wyeth	Comb	0.05 mg ethinyl estradiol	0.5 mg norgestrel
Demulen-1/50–21	Searle	Comb	50 mcg ethinyl estradiol	1 mg ethynodiol diacetate
-1/50–28	Searle	Comb	50 mcg ethinyl estradiol	1 mg ethynodiol diacetate
-1/35–21	Searle	Comb	0.035 mg ethinyl estradiol	1 mg ethynodiol diacetate
-1/35–28	Searle	Comb	0.035 mg ethinyl estradiol	1 mg ethynodiol diacetate
Brevicon-21	Syntex	Comb	0.035 mg ethinyl estradiol	0.5 mg norethindrone
-28	Syntex	Comb	0.035 mg ethinyl estradiol	0.5 mg norethindrone
Loestrin-21 1/20	Parke-Davis	Comb	20 mcg ethinyl estradiol	1 mg norethindrone acetate
-Fe 1/20 28	Parke-Davis	Comb	20 mcg ethinyl estradiol	1 mg norethindrone acetate + 75 mg ferrous fumarate
-21 1.5/30	Parke-Davis	Comb	30 mcg ethinyl estradiol	1.5 mg norethindrone acetate
-Fe 1.5/30 28	Parke-Davis	Comb	30 mcg ethinyl estradiol	1.5 mg norethindrone acetate + 75 mg ferrous fumarate
Lo/Ovral-21	Wyeth	Comb	0.03 mg ethinyl estradiol	0.3 mg norgestrel
-28	Wyeth	Comb	0.03 mg ethinyl estradiol	0.3 mg norgestrel
Modicon-21	Ortho	Comb	0.035 mg ethinyl estradiol	0.5 mg norethindrone
-28	Ortho	Comb	0.035 mg ethinyl estradiol	0.5 mg norethindrone
Ovcon-35–21	Mead Johnson	Comb	0.035 mg ethinyl estradiol	0.4 mg norethindrone
-35–28	Mead Johnson	Comb	0.035 mg ethinyl estradiol	0.4 mg norethindrone
-50–21	Mead Johnson	Comb	0.05 mg ethinyl estradiol	1 mg norethindrone
-50–28	Mead Johnson	Comb	0.05 mg ethinyl estradiol	1 mg norethindrone
Progestogens				
Micronor	Ortho	Prog		0.35 mg norethindrone
Nor-Q.D.	Syntex	Prog		0.35 mg norethindrone
Ovrette	Wyeth	Prog		0.075 mg norgestrel

Comb = Combination, Prog = progestogen

(continued)

Table 31-6. (Continued)

Product	Manufacturer	Type	Estrogen	Progestin
Fluctuating Progesterone Levels				
Ortho-Novum 7/7/7–21	Ortho	Comb	0.035 mg ethinyl estradiol	7–0.5 mg, 7–0.75 mg, 7–1 mg norethindrone
7/7/7–28	Ortho	Comb	0.035 mg ethinyl estradiol	7–0.5 mg, 7–0.75 mg, 7–1 mg norethindrone
10/11–21	Ortho	Comb	0.035 mg ethinyl estradiol	10–0.5 mg, 11–1 mg norethindrone
10/11–28	Ortho	Comb	0.035 mg ethinyl estradiol	10–0.5 mg, 11–1 mg norethindrone
Tri-Norinyl-21	Syntex	Comb	0.035 mg ethinyl estradiol	7–0.5 mg, 9–1 mg, 5–0.5 mg norethindrone
-28	Syntex	Comb	0.035 mg ethinyl estradiol	7–0.5 mg, 9–1 mg, 5–0.5 mg norethindrone
Triphasil-21	Wyeth	Comb	6–0.03 mg, 5–0.04 mg, 10–0.03 mg ethinyl estradiol	6–0.05 mg, 5–0.075 mg, 10–0.125 mg levonorgestrel
-28	Wyeth	Comb	6–0.03 mg, 5–0.04 mg, 10–0.03 mg ethinyl estradiol	6–0.05 mg, 5–0.075 mg, 10–0.125 mg levonorgestrel

Comb = Combination, Prog = progestogen

ring releases only 20 to 50 μg levonorgestrel and no estrogen. Ovulation, therefore, occurs. The low-dose ring is effective because it makes the cervical mucus impermeable to sperm. It can remain in place for several months.

Implantable Hormones

Levonorgestrel (Norplant) capsules are implanted during menstruation in a fanlike pattern in the medial aspect of the upper arm or in the scapular area. The procedure is carried out under local anesthesia by a physician. The capsules release 36 g of levonorgestrel and are effective after 24 hours for 5 years, with a failure rate of 0.5% to 2.6%. They can be removed (again, under local anesthesia) at any time. Although the initial expense is greater, the fact that no other contraceptive products need to be purchased equalizes the cost over time. Possible disadvantages include irregular vaginal bleeding that diminishes over time, ovarian cysts in 10% of the users (usually regressing within 6 weeks without intervention), irregular menstrual cycles, acne, headaches, breast tenderness, and infection at the insertion site. This method can be used only in clients weighing under 150 lb. The capsules can be felt and sometimes seen. They should not be used for women with acute liver disease or liver tumors, unexplained vaginal bleeding, breast cancer, or thrombophlebitis.

Postcoital Contraceptive

In emergency situations in which unprotected intercourse may lead to an undesirable pregnancy (rape, incest), a postcoital contraceptive may be the method of choice. DES is used to prevent (not terminate) a pregnancy by interfering with implantation of the fertilized ovum. A 25-mg tablet is given orally twice each day for 5 days. To be effective, the treatment should begin within 24 hours after intercourse and must be completed despite possible nausea, vomiting, headache, dizziness, abdominal pain, or other non–life-threatening side effects. Initiating treatment later than 72 hours after intercourse is probably ineffective.

The use of DES is contraindicated if the client is already pregnant, because it may lead to vaginal adenosis or cervical cancer in female offspring or to epididymal anomalies in male offspring. A blood test to detect pregnancy should be performed before administering the first dose. If the client is already pregnant, it is extremely unlikely that she ovulated again, and therefore DES is unnecessary. The treatment should be terminated if any signs of thromboembolic disease are present, because this condition can lead to death.

Oral contraceptives are also effective post-coital contraceptives. A triple dose must be taken within 72 hours of intercourse, followed by a similar dose 12 hours later.

■ SUMMARY

Contraceptive choices are influenced by the client's religious beliefs, knowledge, and socioeconomic level and by the method's effectiveness, esthetics, and safety, as well as other factors. Before choosing a method, couples must consider mutual comfort and motivation for success, as well as each partner's physical and emotional status.

Aside from abstinence or tubal ligation, oral contraceptives are the most effective female birth-control measure. However, the dangers of a thromboembolic incident have led many women to seek other methods. The IUD is infrequently prescribed because of physical dangers. Fertility awareness, diaphragms, and condoms are being used more widely because they are safer.

Men have fewer contraceptive choices. Researchers are studying the long-term effects of vasectomies and vas deferens intraluminal devices versus abstinence, coitus interruptus, or condoms as alternatives. Experiments with male contraceptive drugs are ongoing.

❖ NURSING MANAGEMENT: CLIENT USING A CONTRACEPTIVE AGENT

Sex is a very natural thing. If nurses can accept themselves as sexual beings and are comfortable discussing sexual matters, they can better serve their clients. It is particularly important for nurses who work in obstetrics, gynecology, and pediatrics (in hospitals, clinics, and doctors' offices), in the community health field, or in family planning clinics to be comfortable and skilled in discussing contraception and sexuality. However, all nurses probably will be asked some questions about sex and contraceptive measures, because most people are concerned about sexuality, sexual problems, family size, and family welfare. Contraceptive counseling requires knowledge, communication skills, and an ability to evaluate the background (religious, cultural, ethnic) of clients and their partners.

Both men and women should be provided with information about contraceptives, although women still bear the major responsibility for using contraception. Nurses can play an increasing role in the expanding field of women's health care, such as providing counseling and instruction in contraceptive practices.

The decision to prevent pregnancy is easy for some clients and difficult for others. The use or availability of contraceptives implies that sexual intercourse is anticipated. For some, acknowledgment of anticipated intercourse is too painful emotionally or too embarrassing, so unprotected intercourse becomes preferable. Men or women may spend a great deal of time rationalizing why they will or will not use specific contraceptive measures. The most important objective in family planning is finding a method that will be used. Even the "safest" methods are not safe if the client consciously or unconsciously wants to become pregnant. See the Example of Nursing Process for Oral Contraceptives.

NURSING PROCESS

ASSESSMENT

A history, physical examination, and laboratory work are important first steps in family planning. Discussions with the client and his or her partner provide information pertaining to lifestyle, values, priorities, religious and cultural feelings, and knowledge of and attitudes toward the body and contraceptive measures. Some methods may be eliminated as a result of this discussion, either for physical or personal reasons. Each method has

some drawbacks, and these should be discussed completely and honestly, along with the advantages. Only after open discussion of the facts can the couple make an intelligent choice about the method they prefer and the one with which they can comply.

NURSING DIAGNOSIS

Nursing diagnoses associated with contraceptive selection may include:

- Altered Sexuality Patterns, related to use of a contraceptive
- Spiritual Distress, related to use of contraceptives proscribed by religious beliefs
- Knowledge Deficit, related to genital anatomy or use of contraceptives

PLANNING

The desired outcome is to present knowledge to prevent pregnancy, including ensuring that the client knows how to use the contraceptive method correctly and is motivated to use it consistently. No side effects should be present. If they are, they should be corrected immediately, usually by selecting another method. If pregnancy occurs, contraceptive methods should be discontinued immediately (particularly oral contraceptives).

INTERVENTION

Some circumstances prohibit the use of certain types of contraceptives. For example, clients with physical disorders that might be affected by fluid retention (migraine, renal problems) and those with a history of genital or breast cancer or thromboembolic episodes are at high risk for adverse reactions to the pill. Oral contraceptives should be prescribed only after a complete evaluation of the client's physical status. Clients with pelvic abnormalities may not be able to be fitted properly for a diaphragm or cervical cap. Men with premature ejaculation may not be able to use a condom effectively.

Client Education. Education about the reproductive system, sexuality, and family planning should begin early so children learn it from a reliable source. It can be carried out at home, in school, in private practice, or in clinics. It may be taught or discussed in a group situation or on a one-to-one basis. Films, models, and other audiovisual equipment should be used.

After the client chooses a contraceptive, the nurse is responsible for giving further instruction on its use. This may include illustrations, models, demonstrations, and actual practice by the client. It may involve proper fitting, as with diaphragms, or advice on where to buy devices and supplies, such as monoclonal antibody tests for ovulation and thermometers and graphs on which to record information.

Skipping pills, particularly around the time of ovulation, decreases the effectiveness of the method, as does vomiting or diarrhea or the use of certain drugs. Other contraceptives should be added at such times. Missing

Example of Nursing Process for Oral Contraceptive

A 22-year-old woman has come to the clinic for her annual gynecologic checkup. Last year, she decided to take oral contraceptives, and after a thorough history and examination to rule out any contraindications, she received a prescription for a 28-day combination of estrogen and progestin. She returned to the clinic three times during the year, stating that she was taking the pills daily and offering no complaints. At the current examination, she stated that she had ended her relationship with her original boyfriend and was now taking the pills only when she was sexually active.

A review of the initial educational program demonstrated that at that time, she appeared to understand the need to take the pills consistently for efficacy. However, she saw no reason to continue them when she no longer was sexually active. Without seeking medical advice, she resumed their use when she developed another relationship. At this point, she was no longer consistent in her regimen, since her sexual activity was not as intense, and she assumed she did not require as much protection. She also resisted the use of condoms, saying they interfered with her pleasure and that she did not want her new friend to feel that she suspected him of having any STDs.

A new educational program was instituted so that the client would thoroughly understand the need for compliance to prevent pregnancy. Condoms were also discussed as a necessity so long as she did not have a monogamous relationship and had no assurance that neither she nor her partner had any STD.

Assessment Data

Inconsistent use of oral contraceptive medication

Nonuse of condoms

Termination of original sexual relationship and subsequent intermittent sexual activity

Nursing Diagnosis	Intervention	Goals and Outcomes
Knowledge Deficit, concerning oral contraceptive regimen	**Explore** the client's knowledge about the drug regimen; provide additional information and correct misinformation as required. **Stress** the need for consistency in dosage to achieve the desired result—suppression of ovulation.	The client will not become pregnant.
Risk for Infection: Sexually transmitted disease related to intercourse unprotected by condoms	**Discuss** with the client her present sexual practices to determine whether multiple partners are involved; if so, advise client of the increased risk of infection. **Explore** the client's knowledge related to STDs; provide additional information and correct misinformation as required. **Caution** the client that there is no vaccine for AIDS, which is believed to be 100% fatal. **Assist** the client in reassessing her sexual pattern and alternatives, such as abstinence and use of condoms. **Teach** the client signs and symptoms of sexually transmitted infection and caution her to report these promptly to her primary healthcare provider, so that she may be treated promptly.	The client will adopt sexual practices more likely to protect her from infectious disease. If infection develops, it will be promptly detected and treated.

three pills makes the method unreliable, and additional measures should be used through the rest of the cycle.

It is important for the client to learn to recognize any abnormal or adverse signs or symptoms related to the contraceptive method and to have them checked and, if indicated, treated immediately. These can include anything from a local irritation caused by a spermicidal agent to a thromboembolic incident, or a possible pregnancy.

Clients should be advised about signs and symptoms that can indicate problems with each type of contraceptive. The following information should be stressed to increase the effectiveness of each method:

- *Condoms:* If lubrication is desired, only a spermicide or a water-based product (eg, K-Y Jelly) should be used. Oil-based products (eg, petroleum jelly, cold cream, A and D Ointment) may weaken the condom. To be effective, condoms must cover the erect penis completely before insertion into the vagina. Condoms with holes or weak spots should not be used. Air must be removed from the condom before it is applied, and a half-inch space must be left at the tip to act as a reservoir for semen. The condom must be held firmly at the base of the penis during its withdrawal after intercourse, before the erection ends, to prevent leakage of the ejaculate into the vagina. Condoms are not reusable and should be discarded immediately after use.

- *Fertility awareness:* Client education is an important part of a successful fertility awareness program. The woman is unlikely to succeed if her cycles are irregular or if she or her partner is not motivated enough to remain abstinent during ovulation. Effectiveness increases when all four methods of ovulatory detection are used simultaneously.

- *Vaginal spermicides:* Spermicidal jellies, creams, foams, vaginal suppositories, or foaming tablets, with or without concurrent use of a condom, diaphragm, or cervical cap, all require proper application and timing according to manufacturers' instructions. Instructions for each type of spermicidal preparation must be followed carefully, because there are differences in insertion techniques, the time interval needed between application and intercourse, and the period of effectiveness. The client must check the product expiration date and store any remaining spermicide as directed by the manufacturer. Cans of foam must be shaken well before using, and suppositories or tablets must be removed from their wrappers before insertion. Using either of these methods requires some time, but not as much time as needed to insert a diaphragm. Spermicides can be adapted to foreplay and lovemaking.

- *Diaphragm:* Proper placement of a diaphragm requires instruction and supervised practice. Two teaspoonfuls of spermicide should be placed inside the diaphragm dome; an additional amount of spermicide should be used to cover the rim before insertion. The device may be inserted vaginally up to 6 hours before intercourse, with the flexible rim seated firmly from above the symphysis pubis over the cervix to the rear vaginal wall. Additional applications of spermicide may be advisable if more than 2 hours pass before intercourse, or when intercourse is repeated. The diaphragm must remain in place for 6 to 8 hours after intercourse. The diaphragm should be inspected for holes or tears, particularly under the rim, before and after each use. It should not be used if any holes or tears are found.

- *The pill:* Women who take oral contraceptives should be warned that breakthrough bleeding may occur, particularly during the first six cycles. The importance of reporting the following symptoms immediately should be stressed: abdominal pain (possible ectopic pregnancy); numbness, pain in legs (thromboembolic disorder); pressure or pain in chest, shortness of breath (embolus); visual disturbances with blurred vision, flashing lights, blind spots (cerebrovascular accident); and two consecutive missed periods (pregnancy). Clients should also be aware of possible changes in libido and of intolerance to contact lenses. Appetite or weight changes may occur. Clients should be encouraged to have annual gynecologic examinations as well as Pap smears at prescribed intervals to detect any problems as quickly as possible.

Clients should be encouraged to take oral contraceptives as advised, recognizing that missing a dose lessens the effectiveness of the method. Missed doses must be taken as soon as possible. If three or more pills are missed, the rest of the packet should be discarded and another method of contraception substituted entirely. A new pack of pills should be started on the fifth day of menstruation.

Women who receive oral contraceptives or progesterone should be cautioned against cigarette smoking, because smoking increases the risk of thromboembolic problems.

OUTCOME EVALUATION
Efficacy can be evaluated according to success (absence of pregnancy). Data indicating emotional acceptance of the method of contraception are also pertinent.

❖ CHECKLIST OF NURSING ACTIONS

- ❑ Become comfortable with your own sexuality and that of your client.

- Develop a knowledge base concerning reproductive systems, sexuality, and contraception.
- Develop an ability to assess, evaluate, and accept other backgrounds, lifestyles, and values.
- Use good communication skills when counseling clients.
- Take a careful history; obtain the results of a physical examination and appropriate laboratory work before discussing contraceptive methods.
- Present accurate information about each method of contraception. Discuss it honestly and provide precise instructions on its use.
- Become adept at using models and audiovisual materials in presenting methods.
- Provide printed material and advice on signs and symptoms of adverse reactions.

Infertility and Fertility Drugs

A diagnosis of infertility is made when couples who have engaged in frequent unprotected intercourse around the time of ovulation have not conceived in a year or longer. Multiple factors are present in 35% of the cases, with problems present in either or both partners. Treatment is based on the findings.

Among the treatment regimens available are cytotoxic therapy (in clients with certain autoimmune disorders) and immunization with vaginal suppositories derived from cell-free seminal plasma (in women with inappropriate alloimmune response to the fetus). Heparin and aspirin (in women with primary antiphospholipid antibody syndrome) are being investigated for their effectiveness in dissolving or preventing the formation of placental clots. Other techniques include intrauterine insemination, gamete intrafallopian transfer, in vitro fertilization (sometimes using a surrogate mother), and tubal ovum transfer.

Male Infertility

The inability of the male to procreate may be complicated by impotence, the inability to attain or maintain an erection firm enough for intercourse. Several factors (eg, disease, hormonal imbalance, side effects of medications, excessive alcohol or drug use, spinal cord injuries) have been implicated in impotence. A detailed history and physical examination must be carried out to determine the course of treatment.

Various medications have been used to overcome infertility in men. Testosterone may be helpful to men unable to produce it on their own. Tricyclic antidepressants may help reverse nerve damage to the penis caused by diabetes. Zinc supplements (100 mg daily) are needed for replacement for men undergoing kidney dialysis. Papaverine is no longer recommended for self-injection directly into penile erectile tissue because there are serious side effects, including priapism for up to 2 days. Occasionally, the reaction has been severe enough to require surgical intervention and has resulted in blood vessel scarring.

Menotropins

Menotropins (Pergonal) are used to treat infertile men diagnosed with hypogonadotropic hypogonadism. This condition, thought to affect one in 25,000 men in the reproductive age range, causes a low sperm count due to inadequate pituitary secretion of LH or FSH, both of which are needed for normal sperm production. In men, LH controls the testosterone-producing cells, whereas FSH is needed to transport testosterone to the sperm-producing cells. Inadequate amounts of either hormone interfere with the production of adequate numbers of sperm.

Intramuscular injection of menotropins stimulates testosterone production, leading to an increase in the sperm count. The injections may be given for 6 months to several years before pregnancy occurs in the treated male's partner.

Multiple births are not associated with Pergonal when administered to the male. Temporary breast enlargement has been the only side effect noted to date.

Female Infertility
Ovulatory Stimulants

Although most drugs that affect ovulation are used for contraceptive purposes, some are used to treat infertility caused by anovulation. The exact cause of this problem must be determined before proper treatment can be started.

Thyroid and adrenal gland activity may contribute to the lack of ovulation. Thyroid preparations to control hypothyroidism or hyperthyroidism may be appropriate. Cortisone, which increases the level of human gonadotropic hormones through suppression of the production of androgens and estrogens by the adrenals, is used in cases of adrenal insufficiency.

Menotropins

Menotropins are natural human gonadotropic hormones obtained from the urine of postmenopausal women. LH and FSH are present in equal proportions in menotropins.

Pregnancy occurs in about 20% to 45% of the women who receive menotropins within six series of treatments. Of these, about 25% of the clients abort and 17% to 50% have multiple births. LH and FSH, 75 IU of each, are given IM for 9 to 12 days to increase the growth and maturation of the graafian follicles. On the day after the last injection of LH and FSH, an injection of 10,000 U of human chorionic gonadotropin (hCG) is given to induce ovulation. In some instances, the doses of LH and FSH are doubled during the course of treatment.

Several uncomfortable side effects accompany administration of menotropins: fever, nausea, vomiting, diarrhea, and flatulence. More serious signs of adverse reactions include ascites, pleural effusion, hypercoagulation, oliguria, hypotension, and ovarian enlargement. If ovarian cysts rupture, intraperitoneal hemorrhage may occur, requiring abdominal surgery.

Human Chorionic Gonadotropin

Luteinized unruptured follicle syndrome is one of the ovulatory failures not commonly recognized. Diagnosis is made on the basis of low peritoneal fluid assays of progesterone and estradiol when other tests (serum progesterone, endometrial dating, and basal temperatures) appear to be normal after presumed ovulation. Ultrasound reveals this syndrome by showing a luteinized follicle that has not ruptured. Treatment is hCG, 5,000 U, given IM in the presence of a mature follicle. The follicle can be expected to mature within 24 to 36 hours.

Bromocriptine Mesylate

Bromocriptine mesylate (Parlodel) is used for infertility associated with amenorrhea in the presence of hyperprolactinemia not caused by a pituitary tumor (Forbes-Albright syndrome). It is given during the follicular phase and the preovulatory period to normalize prolactin levels, in the hope that it will lead to spontaneous ovulation.

One 2.5-mg tablet is given at mealtime on the first day. The dosage is increased to two or three tablets daily at mealtimes within the first week. Mechanical contraception should be used until normal cycles are established, and then contraception should be discontinued. The medication should be discontinued if menstruation does not occur within 3 days of the expected date, and a test for pregnancy should be performed. This drug should not be used once the client is pregnant.

Progesterone

Luteal phase defects are suspected when infertility is unexplained and when single or serial progesterone assays or endometrial biopsies carried out in two cycles during the midluteal phase demonstrate low progesterone levels. Decreased progesterone has been implicated in repeated early miscarriages. Progesterone in the form of vaginal suppositories (25 mg twice a day) or IM injections (12.5 mg) has been therapeutically successful.

Agents for Treating Endometriosis

Between 1% and 3% of women in their childbearing years have endometriosis. It may cause pain during menstruation, defecation, or intercourse and may be responsible for abnormal menses or hematuria. Endometriosis can prevent conception by causing ovarian adhesions that impede the release of ova, pressing against the fallopian tubes (preventing the ovum and sperm from meeting for fertilization), or blocking the passage of the embryo through the tubes to the uterus for implantation.

Diagnosis of endometriosis may be made by noninvasive tests (sonography or magnetic resonance imaging) but is usually made definitively through surgery, using a laparoscope. The degree of involvement is classified in stages. Stages I and II are milder; stages III and IV are considered serious, because they are more likely to interfere with fertility. Surgery to remove the areas of abnormal endometrial implantation may use electric or laser cautery via laparoscopy. The surgery is usually followed by a course of hormone therapy. Young women usually receive continuous low-dose oral contraceptives (referred to as a pseudopregnancy regimen) over several months.

Norethynodrel with mestranol (Enovid) may be used, beginning on day 5 of the menstrual cycle, starting with 5 to 10 mg/day for 2 weeks. This dosage is increased by 5 to 10 mg every 2 weeks up to 20 mg/day, for 6 to 9 months.

If this treatment is ineffective or if the client is an older woman, danazol (Danocrine), an oral androgen, may be prescribed. Danazol is used to inhibit the output of gonadotropins from the pituitary. The usual dosage is 400 mg twice daily, starting during menstruation and continuing without interruption for 3 to 6 months (possibly 9 months). If symptoms recur within a year, treatment can be restarted. This drug should not be used during pregnancy. Danazol causes weight gain, decreased breast size, hot flashes, muscle pains, changes in libido, or acne in about 85% of recipients.

Another drug, nafarelin, has fewer side effects and is administered as a nasal spray. It decreases estrogen production to cause a temporary menopause. Endometrial growth stops, and endometrial implants may regress. Its side effects mimic menopause (hot flashes, vaginal dryness, changes in libido, and about a 5% loss of existing bone mass), all of which end when the the drug is withdrawn.

Menopause brings an end to the signs and symptoms of endometriosis. Clients for whom drug therapy is ineffective may, however, elect surgery for relief. Laser destruction of endometrial tissue may be effective, but sometimes hysterectomy is required in addition.

Clomiphene Citrate

Clomiphene citrate (Clomid), another ovulatory stimulant, is a synthetic agent that resembles the synthetic estrogen chlorotrianisene (TACE). Its mode of action is not understood, but it seems helpful in treating amenorrhea that originates in the pituitary. Pregnancy occurs in 25% to 30% of the women who receive this drug, with multiple births occurring in 10%.

Clomiphene is usually started on the 5th day of the menstrual cycle, increasing the gonadotropins, hoping to produce one oocyte. (If in vitro fertilization is planned, clomiphene is started earlier so that more than one oocyte is available.) Dosage must be clinically tailored to the woman's needs, based on evidence of ovulation (temperature chart, endometrial biopsy), ovarian enlargement, and side effects. The FSH level should increase, stimulating normal follicular development with adequate LH receptors on granulosa cells. This process seems to promote an adequate luteal phase.

Clomiphene citrate may cause minor side effects, including nausea, vomiting, and hot flashes. Of greater concern is the possibility of ovarian enlargement or ovarian cysts and the possibility of teratogenic effects on the fetus if the client is pregnant.

■ SUMMARY

Fertility stimulants provide help for the infertile client. The drugs are used to stimulate ovulation or sperm production and to suppress endometriosis. Clients must be aware of possible adverse effects or side effects.

❖ NURSING MANAGEMENT: CLIENT RECEIVING FERTILITY DRUGS

Infertility is a field of health care in itself, and those who deal with it are specialists. However, nurses may help clients initially by recognizing problems of infertility, making assessments, and suggesting referrals to specialists. Any preliminary information the nurse can give the specialist is helpful.

The tests used to determine the cause of infertility and the treatments are time-consuming, expensive, and, in some cases, painful or embarrassing. Often no definite cause can be determined, and when intervention begins, no guarantee can be made that the woman will become pregnant. The entire experience is an emotional and (possibly) a financial drain on the family. Emotional support should be extended to the entire family, but especially to the woman who is undergoing assessment and treatment.

Women treated for infertility tend to be fairly depressed through the months of the treatment cycles. The injections are painful and expensive and the chance of success is less than 50%. In addition, sexual activity is determined by ovulation; therefore, sexual intercourse loses spontaneity.

NURSING PROCESS

ASSESSMENT

Determining the causes of infertility requires a complete history, including the timing of sexual intercourse versus the time of ovulation. Monoclonal antibody tests are used to help couples predict ovulation. Completion of the sex act with deposit of semen at the cervical orifice is important. Examinations of the semen to deter-

mine sufficient sperm motility and evaluation of the cervical environment are also necessary.

The histories of both partners must be examined to determine whether either has a physical condition or is taking medications that may interfere with initiating a pregnancy. Illicit drugs or alcohol may interfere with sperm production; douching may render the environment of the vagina detrimental to sperm.

NURSING DIAGNOSIS

Nursing diagnoses for clients taking fertility drugs may include:

- Sexual Dysfunction, related to changes in sexual practices secondary to the infertility treatment regimen
- Altered Family Processes, related to the precedence given to the requirements of the infertility treatment regimen
- Self Esteem Disturbance, related to the need for fertility drugs
- Hopelessness, related to drug regimen and repeated failures to conceive

Many clients with fertility problems have difficulty coping with the extreme pressure of regulating sexual activity to coincide with ovulation. The self-concept of each partner tends to go through extreme swings: up before each attempt to start a pregnancy, and down to the point of grieving if the attempt proves unsuccessful. Sexual dysfunction may result as each partner feels a sense of failure. Sexual avoidance may occur at the time of ovulation to avoid another defeat.

PLANNING

The reality of infertility treatment is that the failure rate is high. Treatment may be required for many months, or even years, without a promise of success. It is therefore important for the goal to be realistic. The primary goal is to attain pregnancy, but the important secondary goal is for the couple to retain a loving, trusting, supportive relationship that will survive the pressures of the testing and treatment process.

INTERVENTION

The couple needs help in maintaining a sense of priorities through the testing and treatment. They must be encouraged to continue other enjoyable activities to lessen the tension of the fertility program. Their other health needs should not suffer as they use time, energy, and often a great deal of money to achieve a pregnancy. Other avenues should also be explored: insemination with donor sperm, adoption, and, if no other choices are available, the possibility of surrogate parenthood or remaining childless.

OUTCOME EVALUATION

The ideal outcome is a successful pregnancy that leads to a healthy child and healthy parents. If that is impossible, an outcome that results in a continuation of a good marriage with the acceptance of adoption or childlessness should be regarded as a success.

References

Carditz GA, Giovannucci E, Colditz GA. (1994). Oral contraceptive use and mortality during 12 years of follow-up: The nurses' health study. *Ann Intern Med*, 120(10), 821.

Bibliography

Barrick B. (1990). Light at the end of a decade. *Am J Nurs*, *90*(11), 37–40.

Dunkin MA. (1991). Delivering hope. *Arthritis Today*, *5*(3), 20–24.

Hatcher RA, Stewart F, Trussell J. (1994). *Contraceptive technology*, 16th ed, p. 182. New York: Irving Publishers, Inc.

Organon's Humegon approved for infertility treatment. (1994). *FDC Reports, 56*(37), T&G-6.

Papazian R. (1991). Osteoporosis treatment advances. *FDA Consumer, 25*(3), 29–32.

Randal J. (1991). Trying to outsmart infertility. *FDA Consumer, 25*(4), 20–29.

*Return to fertility for anejaculatory men. (1991). *Am J Nurs, 94*(4), 18.

*RU 486: Headed for the United States? (1994). *Sci News*, 145(23), 367 (June 4).

Segal M. (1991). Norplant: Birth control at arm's reach. *FDA Consumer, 25*(4), 9–11.

Senanayake P, Potts M. (1995). *An atlas of contraception*. New York: Parthenon Publishing Group.

Shoupe D, Haseltine FP. (1993). *Contraception*. New York: Springer-Verlag.

*Suida S. (1990). The pill: 30 years of safety concerns. *FDA Consumer, 24*(10), 8–11.

*Recommended for further reading.

For more information and sample tests and activities, refer to Chapter 31 in the Student Workbook for Clinical Pharmacology and Nursing Management, 5th edition, available through your bookstore.

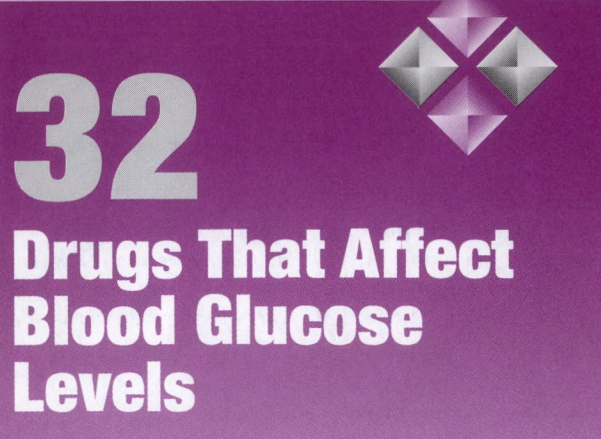

32

Drugs That Affect Blood Glucose Levels

nucleus, these hormones act more rapidly than steroid hormones.

Because most protein hormones have numerous peptide linkages, they are destroyed by the peptidases in the digestive tract and cannot be administered orally. Many are effective when applied topically to mucous membranes, which absorb them readily, but administration by injection is often required. Natural hormones usually are mobilized, distributed, and broken down rapidly by the body; they have a short duration of activity. Analogs (modifications of the natural compounds) are absorbed and metabolized more slowly, providing a longer duration of therapeutic activity.

Protein hormones are degraded at the receptor site by the target tissue and also, to a large degree, by the liver and kidneys. Both hormones and their metabolites are excreted primarily in urine.

Insulin

Insulin is a protein hormone secreted by the beta cells of the islets of Langerhans of the pancreas. Insulin is composed of two chains of amino acids held together by disulfide linkages. In comparison with inorganic substances, insulin, like most proteins, is a large molecule, with a molecular weight of 5,734.

Insulin and Normal Glucose Metabolism

Pancreatic secretion of insulin is stimulated by a rise in the blood glucose level and inhibited by a low blood glucose level. The hormone's physiologic effect is to enhance the body's metabolism of glucose and lower the concentration of blood glucose. Glucose–insulin interaction forms a stable negative feedback system that tends to return blood glucose levels to normal soon after the elevation that follows ingestion of carbohydrates.

Insulin increases the enzyme reactions involved in glucose metabolism and the active transport system by

Nonsteroidal hormones are usually proteins. They may be simple proteins, complex combinations of proteins and other substances, or amino acid derivatives. Insulin, glucagon, parathormone, and some pituitary hormones are simple proteins composed of chains of amino acids joined by the peptide link. Sulfide or other bonds may connect different chains or parts of a single chain.

Protein Hormones

Most protein hormones do not interact with the nuclei of body cells; instead, they interact with specific plasma membrane receptors linked with cellular enzymes (Fig. 32-1). The hormone/receptor complexes influence enzyme action and alter the synthesis of intracellular messenger proteins or electrolyte uptake. Because the primary site of action is the cytoplasm rather than the

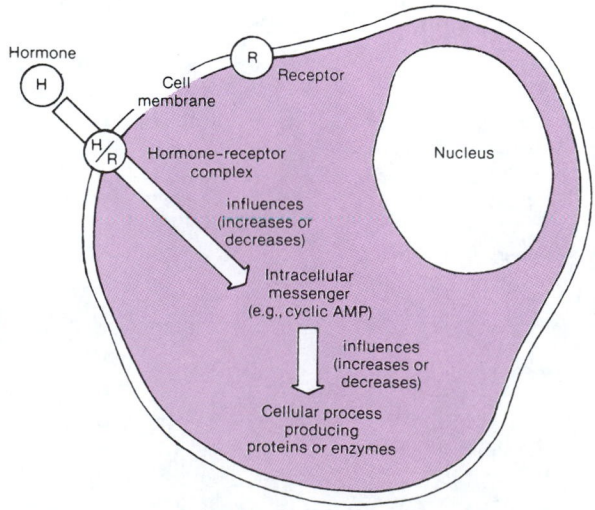

Figure 32-1. Mechanism of action of protein hormones. Protein hormones are believed to act in the cytoplasm.

which glucose crosses cell membranes. The hormone enhances glucose use by most body tissues, increases formation of glycogen in muscles and liver, promotes the oxidation of carbohydrates for energy by the muscles, and increases the synthesis of fats by adipose tissue.

Under the influence of insulin, formation of glucose and hepatic breakdown of glycogen decrease, and serum levels of glucose drop. Potassium and phosphate move from the serum into the cells, and the synthesis of protein and nucleic acid increases. Because it enhances energy production from carbohydrates, insulin spares both fat and protein from oxidation for energy. This prevents ketosis and promotes tissue growth and repair. Overall, insulin increases the movement of glucose from the blood to the intracellular compartment, where it is used for anabolic processes or energy production, or stored.

As yet, only a few factors have been identified as significant enhancers of glucose metabolism. Independent of insulin levels, vitamin C increases tissue use of glucose, apparently by a direct effect on cellular metabolism. Chromium is reported to enhance glucose metabolism and lower blood glucose; how this occurs is unknown. Also unknown is the mechanism by which exercise increases glucose use by skeletal muscle.

Insulin and Abnormal Glucose Metabolism

The significant impairment of glucose metabolism experienced by some people is known as diabetes mellitus. This disorder leads to unhealthful changes in body chemistry. Blood glucose levels rise, increasing the osmotic pressure of body fluids. When the renal threshold is exceeded, glucose is excreted in urine, carrying with it large amounts of water. At the same time, the body breaks down fats and proteins for energy metabolism, and the production of nitrogenous wastes increases. Blood lipid levels rise. Because fats cannot metabolize to completion in the absence of carbohydrate metabolism, intermediate products of fat metabolism (acidic ketone bodies) accumulate. The resulting dehydration, hyperosmolarity, and acidosis cause illness and, when progressive, coma and death. Treatment of diabetic ketoacidosis includes the use of insulin, carbohydrates, fluids, and electrolytes to reverse the disease process.

Blood glucose levels may be influenced by many substances other than insulin. Theoretically, the following could alter serum glucose levels:

- Rate of glycogen breakdown or glucose formation
- Use of glucose by peripheral cells
- Number of insulin receptors on peripheral cells
- Insulin antibody levels
- Secretion of other hormones that affect glucose metabolism, including glucagon, cortisone, epinephrine, and growth hormone

Abnormal insulin secretion may produce either excesses or deficiencies of the hormone. Insulin excess is less common than insulin deficiency, but it does occur intermittently in reactive hypoglycemia and chronically in insulin-secreting tumors (insulinomas). It can also develop when therapeutic insulin is given in excessive dosages. Hyperinsulinism is characterized by sudden drops in the blood glucose level. Because the brain depends on glucose for energy, a low blood glucose level (especially a rapid drop) causes loss of consciousness and can result in nerve cell death. Stroke may occur.

According to the "thrifty gene" theory of the cause of diabetes mellitus, the prediabetic period is characterized by some degree of hyperinsulinism. (This is consistent with results of glucose tolerance tests performed on nondiabetics at high risk for developing the disease.) Insulin increases growth in children and fat production in adults. During the transition to a diabetic state, erratic insulin production may produce alternating hyperinsulinism and hypoinsulinism. These fluctuations and changes in levels of insulin antibodies are reflected in blood glucose levels.

Inadequate insulin effect impairs glucose metabolism, the major clinical feature of diabetes mellitus. This condition is not always caused by an absolute deficiency of insulin; it may be related to antibodies that interfere with hormone action, or to a reduction of insulin receptors in the target tissues. Contributing factors include stress, obesity, lack of exercise, and vitamin C deficiency. The stress hormones, epinephrine and cortisone, antagonize insulin. Obesity is associated with the impaired ability of tissues to use glucose properly.

Exogenous Insulin Preparations

Until recently, the insulin used medicinally was derived solely from the pancreases of slaughtered cattle, pigs, and sheep. Animal insulin is not identical chemically to the human hormone but is physiologically active in humans. Porcine insulin most nearly resembles human insulin. A modified insulin, changed chemically to a form identical to endogenous human hormone, is now available. Human insulin is also produced by bacterial cultures using recombinant DNA techniques. These drugs are relatively expensive.

Although the purity of preparations has improved in recent years, insulin is still measured in units according to bioassay. Current preparations are more stable than previous ones, and the drug no longer requires constant refrigeration. Heat, light, and agitation are to be avoided because they destroy the drug.

Solutions for Injection

Insulin is marketed as solutions for injection containing 100, 200, and 500 U/mL. U-100 is recommended as the single concentration for all types of insulin and is the predominant form of insulin prescribed for newly diagnosed diabetics. Insulin with 200 U/mL is used by diabetic clients who require unusually large doses, and U-500 is reserved for clients requiring very large doses (200–500 U).

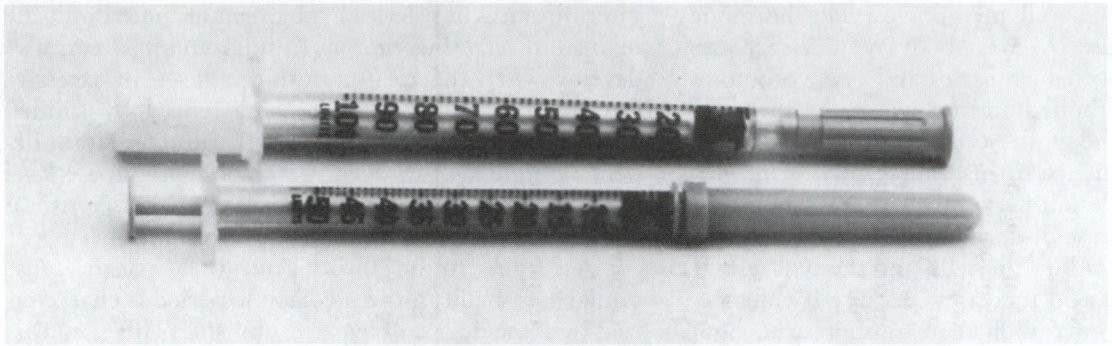

Figure 32-2. U-100 insulin syringes. The very short needle allows subcutaneous injection with a 90° angle of insertion. (*top*) Single-use, 1-mL insulin syringe. Note that the scale is in units with gradations of 2 units (equal to 0.02 mL) each. Odd numbers cannot be measured with precision with this syringe. Compare with the ½-mL syringe below and the tuberculin syrine in Figure 32-3. (*bottom*) Single-use, ½-mL insulin syringe has a narrower barrel and longer scale. Single-unit markings allow greater accuracy, but the capacity is 50 units. (Courtesy of Becton Dickinson and Company, Rochelle Park, NJ)

Syringes designed for use with U-100 insulin are scaled in units, with calibrations for every 1 to 2 U (Fig. 32-2). The system is compatible with the metric system, and a tuberculin syringe may be used for precise measurement of doses. Each 0.01-mL calibration on the tuberculin syringe measures 1 U of U-100 insulin (Fig. 32-3). When large doses of insulin are required, U-200 and U-500 insulin can be measured with a tuberculin syringe; 0.01 mL provides 2 U and 5 U, respectively, of these preparations.

Injectable insulins are divided into three categories according to rapidity of action: fast-acting, long-acting, and intermediate-acting. Time of onset, time of peak action, and duration of action differ for each group (Table 32-1 and Figs. 32-4 through 32-6).

Fast-Acting Insulins

Of the fast-acting preparations, insulin injection (crystalline zinc or regular insulin) is the only form of insulin suitable for intravenous (IV) administration. Its rapid action and prompt dissipation provide the most accurate control of blood glucose in labile clinical situations. Regular insulin dosage is often adjusted to blood glucose levels. When used in chronic management of the disease, it is administered about 20 minutes before each meal.

Long-Acting Insulins

Of the long-acting preparations, Ultralente and protamine zinc insulins (PZI) have the longest duration of action. PZI, a compound prepared by the reaction of insulin and zinc with protamine is no longer available in the United States.

Intermediate-Acting Insulins

Of the intermediate-acting preparations, isophane (NPH) insulin—a modification of the PZI combination—has a fairly rapid onset and moderate duration of action. The

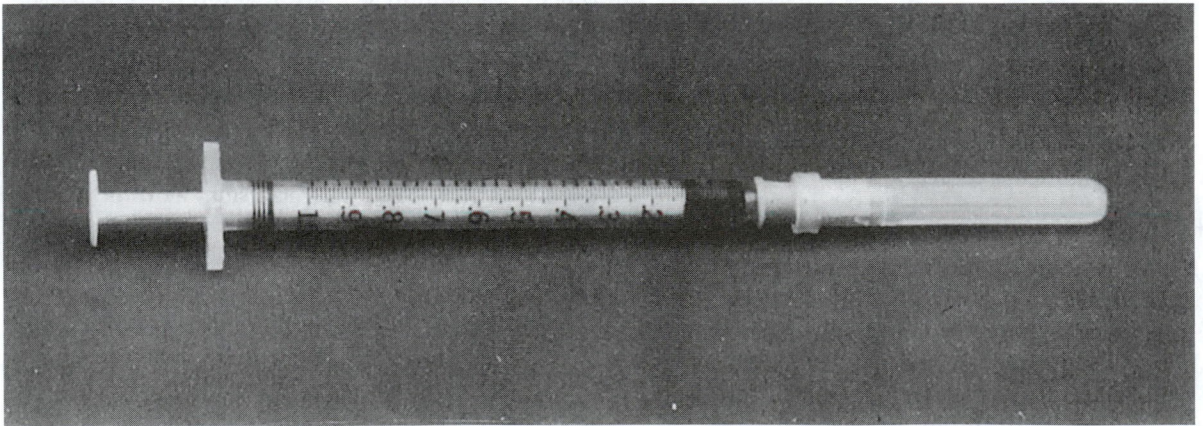

Figure 32-3. Calibrated tuberculin syringe. Note the scale graduated in hundredths of a milliliter. Insulin dosages of 1 unit to 100 units (of U-100 insulin) can be measured accurately, whether odd or even in number. (Courtesy of Becton Dickinson and Company, Rochelle Park, NJ)

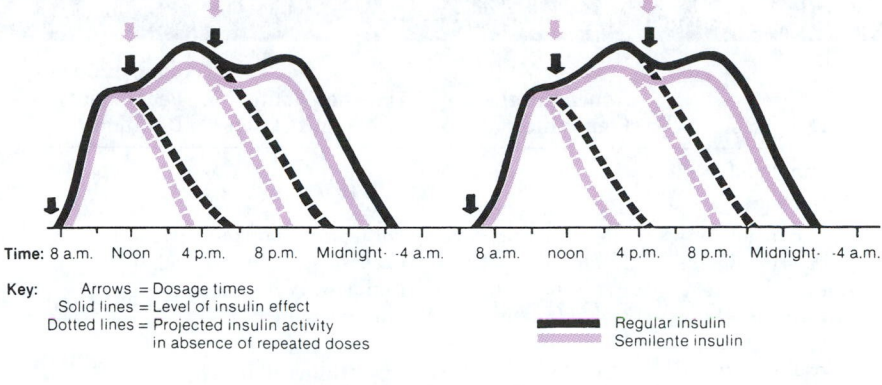

Figure 32-4. Level of drug action in fast-acting insulin preparations. When used alone, short-acting insulins must be administered several times a day to provide adequate activity at meal times (compare with Figs. 32-5 and 32-6).

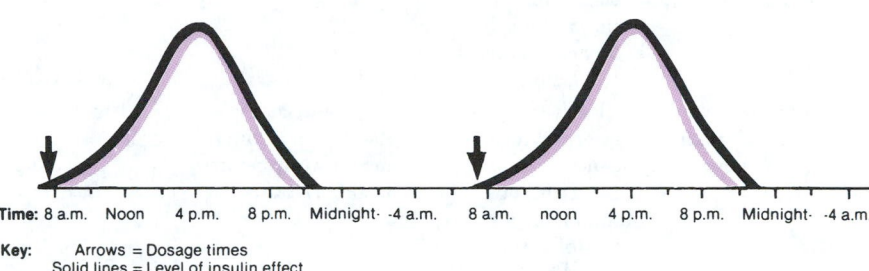

Figure 32-5. Level of drug action in intermediate-acting insulins. Reactions are most likely to occur in the late afternoon and early evening hours (compare with Figs. 32-4 and 32-6).

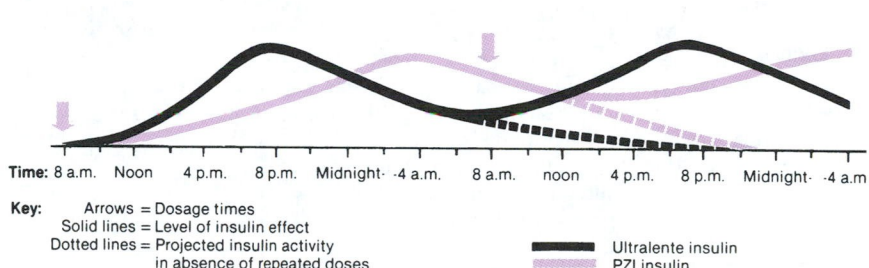

Figure 32-6. Level of drug action in long-acting insulin preparations. When administered in the morning, long-lasting insulins present the greatest risk of reactions during the night. Hyperglycemia is most likely after lunch.

letters *NPH* signify properties of the preparation and its origin: *N* denotes that the solution is neutral (pH 7.2), *P* stands for the protamine and zinc content, and *H* represents Hagedorn, the laboratory of origin.

Globin zinc insulin, a mixture of insulin, zinc, and the protein globin, has properties similar to NPH insulin but is not widely used.

The Lente insulins are prepared by precipitating insulin with zinc and resuspending the compound in an acetate buffer. The size of the crystals formed is influenced by the method of preparation; this in turn alters the duration and intensity of action. Extended (Ultralente) insulin contains large particles and produces effects similar to those of PZI. Prompt (Semilente) insulin contains smaller particles and has an action similar to that of regular insulin, but is somewhat longer-lasting. By mixing Ultralente and Semilente insulins, a preparation similar in effect to NPH insulin is produced (Lente insulin). Lente insulins are less allergenic than other animal preparations.

Intranasal Insulins

Intranasal sprays are prepared by combining insulin with lecithin, which enhances absorption and minimizes irritation of the mucous membranes.

Pharmacology of Insulin

Pharmacodynamics. Pharmacologically, insulin is an agonist that interacts with specific receptors on body cell membranes. Its presence on these receptors increases the movement of glucose into the cells, the use of glucose to produce energy, and the storage of energy as glycogen and fat. Its physiologic effects include a lowering of extracellular glucose concentrations, increased energy production, increased glycogen storage, and growth of fatty tissues.

Insulin increases the total quantity of protein in the body by at least three mechanisms: increased active transport of amino acid into the cells, faster translation of messenger ribonucleic acid (RNA) code by the ribosomes to form more protein, and increased transcription of DNA in the cell nuclei to form more RNA. Because it enhances the production of energy from carbohydrates, insulin also decreases the metabolism of amino acids for energy. Insulin is required for normal growth and development during childhood.

Pharmacokinetics. Insulin cannot be administered orally because peptidases in the digestive juices destroy the protein molecule. In most cases, the drug is injected

Table 32-1. Insulin Preparations

Drug Names	Appearance/ Preparation	Time and Route of Administration	Time of Onset/ Peak Action/ Duration	When Hyper- glycemia is Most Likely to Occur	When Hypo- glycemia is Most Likely to Occur
Animal Insulins **Fast-acting**					
insulin, regular in-sulin, crystalline zinc insulin, un-modified insulin (Actrapid, Iletin, Velosulin; *Can:* In-sulin-Toronto)	Clear solution/pork insulin in concen-trations of 100, and 500 U/mL; beef insulin in con-centration of 100 U/mL; mixed pork and beef insulins in concentrations of 100 U/mL	For treatment of ke-toacidosis: IM in-jection or IV infu-sion as required For maintenance: 15–20 min before meals, SC	1/2–1 hr 2–3 hr 5–7 hr	During sleep	2–3 hr after the lightest meal (usu-ally between 10 AM and noon if given before breakfast)
prompt insulin zinc (Semilente Insulin, Semilente Iletin, Semitard)	Cloudy suspen-sion/beef insulin in concentration of 100 U/mL; pork in-sulin in concentra-tion of 100 U/mL; mixed pork and beef insulins in con-centrations of 100 U/mL	For maintenance: 30–45 min before a meal (usually before breakfast), SC	1/2–1 hr 4–7 hr 12–16 hr	During sleep	Before meals, espe-cially before lunch if given before breakfast
Intermediate-acting					
isophane insulin (NPH Iletin, Ini-tard, Insulatard, Protaphane NPH)	Cloudy suspen-sion/beef insulin in concentrations of 100 U/mL; pork in-sulin in concentra-tion of 100 U/mL; mixed beef and pork insulins in concentrations of 100 U/mL	For maintenance: 1 hr before a meal (usually before breakfast), SC	1–2 hr 8–12 hr 18–24 hr	With daily doses, 5–6 h after admin-istration (at lunch if given before break-fast)	Before meals, 10 hr after administration (before the evening meal if given before breakfast)
insulin zinc (Lente Insulin, Lente Iletin)	Cloudy suspen-sion/beef insulin in concentration of 100 U/mL; pork in-sulin in concentra-tion of 100 U/mL; mixed beef and pork insulins in concentrations of 100 U/mL	For maintenance: 1 hr before a meal (usually before breakfast), SC	1–2 hr/8–12 hr/18–24 hr	With daily doses, 5–6 hr after admin-istration (at lunch if given before break-fast)	Before meals, 10 hr after administration (before the evening meal if given before breakfast)
Long-Lasting					
protamine zinc in-sulin (Protamine Zinc, Iletin, Prota-mine Zinc Purified)	Cloudy suspen-sion/beef insulin in concentrations of 100 U/mL; pork in-sulin in concentra-tion of 100 U/mL; mixed beef and pork insulins in concentrations of 100 U/mL	For maintenance: 1 hr before a meal (usually before breakfast), SC	4–8 hr/14–20 hr/36 hr	With daily doses, after administration to 5–14 hr later (lunch, supper, and bedtime specimens)	18–24 hr after ad-ministration (be-tween 2 AM and breakfast if given before breakfast)

All drugs listed are in pregnancy risk category B; see Appendix A. *Can* = Canadian trade name.

(continued)

Table 32-1. (Continued)

Drug Names	Appearance/ Preparation	Time and Route of Administration	Time of Onset/ Peak Action/ Duration	When Hyper- glycemia is Most Likely to Occur	When Hypo- glycemia is Most Likely to Occur
extended insulin zinc (Ultralente Insulin, Ultralente Iletin, Ultratard)	Cloudy suspension/beef insulin in concentration of 100 U/mL; mixed beef and pork insulins in concentrations of 100 U/mL	For maintenance: 1 hr before a meal (usually before breakfast), SC	4–8 hr/16–18 hr/36 hr	With daily doses, after administration to 5–14 hr later (lunch, supper, and bedtime specimens)	18–24 hr after administration (between 2 AM and breakfast if given before breakfast)
Human Insulins					
Rapid-acting					
insulin human, regular rDNA (Humulin R) semisynthetic (Novolin R; *Can:* Novolin-Toronto, Velosulin Human)	Clear solution/recombinant DNA origin in concentration of 100 U/mL; semisynthetic in concentration of 100 U/mL	For treatment of ketoacidosis: IM injection or IV infusion as required For maintenance: 15–20 min before meals, SC	1/2–1 hr/2–3 hr/5–7 hr	During sleep	2 hr after the lightest meal (usually between 10 AM and noon if given before breakfast)
Intermediate-acting					
human insulin zinc suspension, rDNA (Humulin L) Semisynthetic (Novolin L)	Cloudy suspension/semisynthetic in concentration of 100 U/mL	For maintenance: 1 hr before a meal (usually before breakfast), SC	1–2 hr/8–12 hr/18–24 hr	At lunch if given before breakfast	Before the evening meal if given before breakfast
isophane insulin human, rDNA (Humulin N), semisynthetic (Novolin N, Insulatard NPH Human)	Cloudy suspension/recombinant DNA origin in concentration of 100 U/mL	For maintenance: 1 hr before a meal (usually before breakfast), SC	1–2 hr/8–12 hr/18–24 hr	At lunch if given before breakfast	Before the evening meal if given before breakfast

All drugs listed are in pregnancy risk category B; see Appendix A. *Can* = Canadian trade name.

directly into the tissues; use of pumps and the intranasal route is uncommon. Because the onset and duration of action of plain (regular, crystalline) insulin are brief, the hormone has been combined with other substances to form complexes that must be broken down by the body before absorption can occur (see Table 32-1). This process delays the onset and prolongs the duration of action. Commercially available insulin preparations are classified as short, intermediate, or long-lasting in action. Absorption may also be delayed or decreased by the presence of insulin-binding antibodies, which tend to develop with advancing age, or as a result of exposure to exogenous (especially nonhuman) insulin.

After absorption, insulin is rapidly distributed throughout extracellular fluids. In healthy people, the hormone has a plasma half-life of a few minutes; however, its biologic half-life may be prolonged in diabetics, probably because of binding to antibodies. Insulin is rapidly metabolized, mainly in the liver but also in the kidneys and muscle tissue. The metabolites and a small fraction (less than 2%) of unchanged drug are excreted by the kidneys.

Therapeutic Uses. Insulin is widely used in treating diabetes mellitus, a disease characterized by an absolute or relative deficiency of insulin. When the pancreas cannot produce any insulin, the affected person is totally dependent on exogenous supplies of insulin. This condition, called insulin-dependent (type I) diabetes mellitus (IDDM), usually develops during childhood. Some evidence suggests that the inability to secrete insulin is caused by degeneration of the islets of Langerhans after a viral infection. Some older diabetics also develop IDDM, an indication that the pancreatic secretion of insulin has failed completely. Adequate insulin therapy corrects the metabolic abnormalities, normalizing glucose use for energy production, tissue repair, and the formation of glycogen. Insulin therapy eliminates excessive ketogenesis (although some ketosis normally develops in clients on weight-reduction diets) and corrects the negative nitrogen balance that occurs in ketoacidosis. The characteristic symptoms of IDDM (hyperglycemia, glycosuria, polyuria, polydipsia, polyphagia, muscle wasting, weight loss, and susceptibility to infection) subside.

Insulin is used also to treat acute ketoacidosis (diabetic coma), which requires intensive therapy in addition to IV fluids and electrolytes to correct body chemistry.

Occasionally, insulin is used to stimulate the appetite in cases of malnutrition. A small dose (about 5 U) of regular insulin is administered 20 to 30 minutes before a meal. The hormone is also given to control hyperglycemia in clients who receive large quantities of IV nutrients, as in total parenteral nutrition.

Dosage and Administration. Insulin is prescribed in doses adjusted to meet the body's needs. Most diabetic clients require 5 to 40 U per day. The need for very high doses indicates that some degree of drug resistance has developed. This may stem from insulin antibodies that inactivate the hormone, tissue resistance caused by a decrease in cell receptors, or an increase in biochemicals such as stress hormones that act as insulin antagonists.

Because insulin usually is administered by injection, it is preferable to reduce the number of doses needed daily. Most clients can be maintained with one injection daily of a sustained-release preparation. This is usually administered in the morning, before breakfast. Isophane (NPH) insulin is prescribed most often. Lente insulins are especially useful when allergic hypersensitivity develops.

Insulin therapy can be tailored to meet individual needs by altering the time of administration or by mixing various types of insulin. Occasionally, long-lasting insulin is administered before the evening meal rather than in the morning. Regular insulin may be mixed with the long-lasting forms or may be administered separately. The various Lente insulins may be mixed with each other. When used as the sole therapeutic agent, regular insulin must be administered before each meal.

Insulin can be administered subcutaneously (SC), intramuscularly (IM), or (if regular insulin) IV. The SC route is preferred when prolonged action is desired. IV administration is not as reliable as SC or IM injection because the drug adheres to the surfaces of solution bottles and tubing, preventing delivery of the entire prescribed dose. It may be necessary to administer the drug IV, however, in diabetic ketoacidosis when the client is in hypovolemic shock.

Adverse Reactions. When they contain foreign proteins, insulins can trigger antibody formation and allergic reactions (Box 32-1). Urticaria and edema at the injection site are early signs of allergy. These tend to subside with continued treatment. Changing the insulin prescription to a less antigenic preparation (pure porcine, a Lente insulin, or human insulin) may prevent allergic problems. Rarely, desensitization regimens may be needed. These are carried out on accelerated schedules (rapid desensitization) to prevent prolonged interference with diabetes treatment. A series of progressively larger doses of insulin are given until the therapeutic dose is achieved or the client experiences

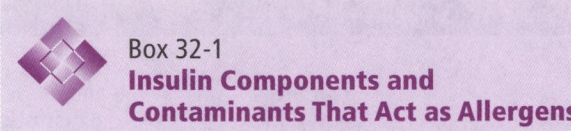

Box 32-1
Insulin Components and Contaminants That Act as Allergens

Allergen

Insulin of animal origin

Porcine proteins (contaminants)

Escherichia coli polypeptides (contaminants that amount to <4 ppm)

Protamine (derived from salmon sperm)

Insulin preparations

Bovine and porcine insulin

Semisynthetic human insulin

Biosynthetic human insulin (rDNA insulin)

NPH and PZI

---

an allergic reaction; desensitization usually is completed in less than 24 hours but must be restarted at a minimal dose if an allergic reaction occurs. Desensitization must be carried out if anaphylaxis occurs. Insulin allergy is most likely to develop when hormone use is suspended for a time and then resumed. Diabetics who use an insulin preparation that contains protamine (NPH or PZI) sometimes develop a silent allergy to protamine; this can cause an acute reaction if protamine is later used medicinally to neutralize heparin, as in hemodialysis.

Local effects of insulin at the injection site may cause deformation of fatty tissue (lipodystrophy). Either atrophy (pitting) or hypertrophy (swelling) may occur. The more frequently injections are administered in a given area, the more likely it is that lipodystrophy will develop. The injection of cold insulin also increases the risk. The mechanisms that underlie lipodystrophy are poorly understood but are undoubtedly related to the influence of insulin on fat metabolism. Paradoxically, additional injections of a pure insulin directly into atrophic areas can sometimes restore the normal contours of the area.

The introduction of insulin therapy for the treatment of newly diagnosed diabetes may coincide with a period of persistent visual blurring. This disturbance is caused by the rapid changes in fluid and electrolyte levels as metabolism is restored to normal.

High blood levels of insulin contribute to vascular degeneration. Insulin excesses are characteristic of both the prediabetic stage of non–insulin-dependent diabetes mellitus (NIDDM) and intensive insulin treatment for IDDM. Cardiovascular degeneration is a common complication of diabetes mellitus; not infrequently, it precedes the onset of frank diabetes. Excessive insulin levels can lead to insulin shock and coma (Box 32-2).

Insulin reactions develop much more rapidly than diabetic coma and are considered more dangerous. For this reason, labile diabetics are often advised to maintain a slightly elevated blood glucose level (100–110 mg/dL) to guard against frequent episodes of hypoglycemia. If it is uncertain whether the client is experiencing an insulin reaction or hyperglycemia, sugar should be given. Sugar can prevent severe hypoglycemia and permanent brain damage. The relatively small amounts of glucose added to the body are less likely to cause permanent damage, even in hyperglycemia.

Drug–Drug Interactions. The hypoglycemic effects of insulin increase when taken with monoamine oxidase inhibitors, beta blockers, salicylates, or alcohol. Altered insulin requirements in diabetics secondary to use of fenfluramine require cautious administration of insulin and regular monitoring of blood glucose levels. In addition, clients taking insulin concomitantly with beta-adrenergic blocking agents experience delayed recovery from hypoglycemic episodes and masked signs and symptoms. (Table 32-2 gives information on how to factor alcohol into diabetic diet exchanges).

Precautions and Contraindications. Except for hypoglycemia, no absolute contraindications to insulin therapy exist. Allergy to the drug may be controlled by using insulins with reduced antigenic properties or by rapid desensitization.

Because insulin accelerates cardiovascular degeneration, and because hypoglycemia poses a serious risk of permanent brain damage, the minimum amount of drug needed to restore normal metabolism should be used. Clients who respond to dietary management should avoid insulin therapy as long as possible. The practice of increasing insulin intake to compensate for increased food intake is dangerous: it promotes weight gain, which makes the diabetic condition more severe, and it exposes the client to higher insulin dosages than necessary, increasing the risk of vascular degeneration.

Once insulin therapy becomes necessary, it is best to maintain it without interruption. Soon after insulin therapy is started, an improvement in the diabetic condition is usually noted. This is associated with an improvement in general condition and cellular nutrition, which improves beta-cell function. The dosage of insulin should be decreased to minimize the occurrence of hypoglycemic reactions but should not be eliminated. In most cases, the improvement is temporary, with insulin needs rising after a short time. Interruption of insulin therapy during this temporary remission increases the risk of antibody formation and allergy.

Insulin may be discontinued when a marked decrease in obesity is followed by sustained improvement in the diabetes. These clients are considered to have reverted to the latent phase of diabetes. Over time, they may again experience overt diabetes if the disease progresses, during infectious illness, or if they again become obese.

Persistent hyperglycemia despite gradually increasing doses of insulin indicates the need for a careful evaluation for the Somogyi effect. The client may be experiencing undetected insulin reactions followed by rebound hyperglycemia. A reduction in insulin dosage may improve blood test results.

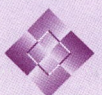

Box 32-2
Understanding Insulin Shock

Whenever the body's insulin level exceeds metabolic needs, the blood glucose level may drop below normal. The brain must have glucose for energy; it is essential for normal function. An abnormally low blood glucose level initially causes sympathoadrenal secretion of epinephrine. Headache and symptoms of CNS impairment follow. The faster the blood glucose level drops, the more severe the symptoms. Either hunger or nausea can occur.

In most people, a blood glucose level below 70 mg/dL results in signs and symptoms of sympathetic activity: perspiration, tachycardia, weakness, trembling, and anxiety. This release of catecholamines is compensatory, raising the blood glucose level by antagonizing insulin's effect. If the response is pronounced, a paradoxical hyperglycemia and glycosuria can follow (the Somogyi effect). Usually, however, insulin levels are insufficient to correct the hypoglycemia.

Diabetic clients who use sympathetic blocking agents (eg, beta-blocking drugs) do not exhibit these signs and symptoms. In such clients, the onset of hypoglycemia is signaled by severe headache, epigastric pain, diarrhea, nausea, vomiting, dizziness, lethargy, demoralization, or personality change. As hypoglycemia progresses, the brain is deprived of its sole source of energy and cannot function normally. Headache, confusion, and incoherent speech often develop. The client may exhibit bizarre behavior that resembles drunkenness. If the blood glucose level drops further, convulsions, coma, and death ensue. Permanent brain damage can occur in people who survive severe reactions. This can cause retardation, hemiparesis, ataxia, incontinence, aphasia, chorea, parkinsonism, or seizure disorder.

Emergency Care

The antidote to insulin toxicity is the immediate administration of sugar. If the client is conscious, sweetened orange juice, candy, or some other rapidly absorbed sweet is given. Most candy (except for chocolate) is appropriate to use. If the client resists taking the food (a result of brain malfunction) or is unconscious, parenteral therapy may be required. Either glucagon or IV glucose should be used. After regaining consciousness, the client should be fed, because continuing insulin activity may cause recurring hypoglycemia.

Table 32-2. Dietary Exchange Values for Alcoholic Beverages

Beverage	Approximate Measure	Substitute
Beer (average)	1 12-oz bottle	1 bread exchange and 2 fat exchanges
Brandy	1 brandy glass	1½ fat exchanges
Cordials	1 cordial glass	2 fat exchanges
Highball (with water)	1 glass	4 fat exchanges
Martini	1 cocktail	3 fat exchanges
Manhattan	1 cocktail	3 fat exchanges and ½ bread exchange
Rum	1 jigger (1½ oz)	2 fat exchanges
Tom Collins	1 cocktail	1 fruit exchange and 3 fat exchanges
Whiskey, rye	1 jigger (1½ oz)	3 fat exchanges
Whiskey, scotch	1 jigger (1½ oz)	2 fat exchanges
Wine, California sauterne	1 wine glass (4 oz)	½ fruit exchange and 1 fat exchange
Wine, California red	1 wine glass (4 oz)	1 fat exchange
Wine, port	1 wine glass (4 oz)	1 bread exchange and 2 fat exchanges
Gin, dry	1½ jiggers	2 fat exchanges
Champagne	1 wine glass (4 oz)	2 fat exchanges (3 glasses equals 1 fruit and 6 fat exchanges)

▪ S U M M A R Y

Insulin, a hormone produced by the pancreas, promotes glucose use by most body cells. Its secretion is highest when blood glucose is elevated, and it functions to reduce blood glucose to normal fasting concentrations. Insulin also promotes fat formation and body use of proteins for tissue building. Many body tissues cannot use glucose adequately without insulin.

Diabetes mellitus is a disease characterized by inadequate insulin effect, which causes serious metabolic disturbances. The administration of exogenous insulin helps correct these physiologic abnormalities and helps promote normal tissue nutrition.

Insulin has a relatively narrow safety margin. Inadequate dosage allows the pathology of diabetes mellitus to persist, whereas excessive dosage causes dangerous hypoglycemia. Because glucose metabolism is influenced by several extraneous factors, achieving and maintaining a steady state requires skillful manipulation of diet, exercise, and general hygiene, in addition to control with medication.

❖ NURSING MANAGEMENT: CLIENT RECEIVING INSULIN

Complications are a risk for diabetic clients who are critically ill. Diabetic coma and insulin reactions are medical emergencies. The nurse caring for a diabetic client must thoroughly understand diabetes mellitus and its effects on the body. When a diabetic suddenly becomes ill or the condition of a hospitalized diabetic worsens, accurate identification of the cause is critical.

Two common syndromes are hyperglycemia and hypoglycemia; a complicating condition is hyperventilation. Hypoglycemia, which may be difficult to distinguish from hyperglycemia or hyperventilation syndrome, develops within minutes and must be treated immediately to avert serious consequences. The nurse should be familiar with the signs and symptoms of all three conditions (Table 32-3). Few distinctive features differentiate hypoglycemia from hyperventilation. Both are characterized by hyperirritability of the nervous system; however, the hyperventilating client exhibits rapid, deep breathing not seen in hypoglycemia. The differences between hypoglycemia and hyperglycemia are generally more pronounced, but in some situations they may not be clear-cut. When in doubt, the safest course is to treat for hypoglycemia. This buys time for a definitive diagnosis of insulin reaction with little risk for clients with other conditions.

Diabetics may be admitted to general hospital units because of illnesses unrelated to the underlying metabolic condition or because of difficulty in maintaining metabolic balance. Any illness, including infections, increases the secretion of stress hormones that antagonize insulin's action. Careful assessment of glucose balance and the efficacy of the medical regimen is required.

Diabetics who normally are well controlled with insulin therapy may require larger dosages during other illnesses. Clients usually controlled by diet alone may develop hyperglycemia and require insulin. Fasting, which may be imposed for diagnostic or surgical procedures, further disrupts the diabetic regimen. When clients must fast, insulin medication may be delayed until just before the fast is broken. (However, in stressful situations, the insulin may be given despite fasting.) Regardless of the reason for hospitalization, diabetic control tends to be unstable in hospitalized clients and requires close monitoring.

Management of diabetic regimens may be difficult. When food intake is above the prescribed level, clients on insulin may take extra amounts to maintain glucose balance. Some healthcare providers allow some flexibil-

Table 32-3. Comparing Signs and Symptoms of Hypoglycemia, Diabetic Ketoacidosis, and Hyperventilation

	Hypoglycemia	Ketoacidosis	Hyperventilation
Usual history			
Onset	Sudden onset (within minutes)	Gradual onset (hours to days)	Sudden onset
Associated events (contributing factors)	Missed meal, unusual exertion, or (in labile diabetics and patients who experience remission) none	Unusual stress, febrile illness, missed doses of hypoglycemic medication, gradual weight gain, or (when disease has worsened) none	Stressful episode that culminates in a panic reaction
Presenting Complaints			
Reported problems	Feeling of weakness, anxiety, jitteriness	Feeling of sluggishness	Feeling of nervousness, worry, jitteriness, weakness
Behavior	Excited, "drunken," tremors	Lethargy, slowness	Excited, tremors
Headache	Present	Absent	Absent
Respirations	Normal to rapid and shallow; (in coma) stertorous	Kussmaul (rapid, deep), air hunger, acetone odor to breath	Rapid, deep breathing
Skin	Pale, cool, clammy	Warm, dry, flushed	Variable
Diaphoresis	Present (usually marked)	Absent	Variable, but rarely marked
Blood pressure	Normal to somewhat elevated	Low	Normal
Gastrointestinal	Hunger or (rarely) nausea	Nausea and vomiting	Nausea may occur
Central nervous system	Headache, hyperactive reflexes, increased alertness (before coma), demoralization, personality change, night sweats	Hypoactive reflexes, decreased level of consciousness	Increased alertness, hyperactive reflexes
Corroborating data			
Urine (fresh, double-voided specimen)	Negative for glucose	Strongly positive for glucose, low pH, positive for acetone	Usually positive for glucose, high pH
Blood	Low glucose	Elevated glucose	Glucose may be elevated

ity and encourage client control of diet and medication, especially for young insulin-dependent clients. The nurse should verify that the practice in question is indeed indicated by or contrary to the prescribed regimen. Careful addition of balanced amounts of insulin and carbohydrates may not significantly alter glucose balance, but imbalance can result from this practice. The chief danger may be that the additional intake of food and insulin promotes weight gain and adiposity, which eventually makes the diabetes worse. (See the Critical Thinking Challenge: Case Analysis for some thought-provoking considerations regarding insulin therapy.)

NURSING PROCESS

ASSESSMENT

Whenever a client with diabetes mellitus needs health care, his or her glucose balance should be determined and monitored. If the blood glucose level is within normal limits, no clinical or laboratory evidence of hyperglycemia or hypoglycemia should be present.

Inadequate insulin effect causes hyperglycemia and increased metabolism of fat and other tissue for energy. Over a period of hours to days, ketoacidosis and dehydration develop. The client is likely to appear flushed and may be lethargic or stuporous. Blood pressure tends to be low ("sugar shock") and respirations are rapid and very deep. Blood and freshly produced urine test posi-

tive for excessive glucose and ketones. If hyperglycemia and hyperosmolarity are severe, the client may be confused or show other signs of central nervous system (CNS) malfunction. Hyperglycemia and shock develop over a period of hours to days. They are more likely to develop in clients whose need for insulin has risen due to unusual stress, infection, or other illness, or to progressive declines in endogenous insulin production or use.

Excessive caloric intake (more than can be metabolized by the insulin available to the client) produces a syndrome called nonketotic hyperosmolar hyperglycemia. This condition is somewhat different from that of insulin deficiency. This client has sufficient insulin to meet basic needs for energy and growth, so the body does not burn extra fats or develop acidosis. However, no reserve insulin is available for tissue storage of excess calories, which tend to be converted to glucose. Blood glucose rises and body tissues become hyperosmotic. This condition is toxic to the tissues and stimulates osmotic diuresis and dehydration. The client with nonketotic hyperosmolar hyperglycemia exhibits signs and symptoms similar to those of insulin deficiency hyperglycemia, except that ketoacidosis does not develop. (This does not mean that overeating cannot lead to a true diabetic coma. If the client feels guilty about breaking the diet, the stress of this emotion may impair insulin function and cause ketoacidosis.)

CRITICAL THINKING CHALLENGE
Case Analysis

Mr. Mullen is a 36-year-old married man with two children, ages 8 and 10. He is a postal worker who delivers mail in an urban residential area. He entered the hospital recently to be treated for pneumonia. His fever has resolved and his lungs are nearly clear. However, he is undergoing diagnostic tests to determine the cause of pronounced fatigue and unexplained weight loss. Last night, he was told he had insulin-dependent diabetes mellitus. He received insulin before breakfast. When you first greet the client this morning, he asks abruptly, "How much will this disease shorten my life? Will I have to take insulin for the rest of my life?"

1. Identify the factor(s) you think contribute to this client's questions.
2. Identify at least two tentative nursing diagnoses pertaining to this client and his situation.
3. Explain what you can do to maximize the therapeutic regimen now and in your next contact with Mr. Mullen.

Excessive insulin (hypoglycemia, insulin shock) progresses much more rapidly than does hyperglycemia. This condition develops after an inadvertent overdose of insulin, unusual exercise, or missed feedings. Blood glucose decreases rapidly, depriving the brain of its only energy source. The client experiences apprehension, tremors, excitation, bizarre behavior (or other manifestations of CNS malfunction), perspiration, and severe headache. Blood tests show abnormally low blood glucose; freshly produced urine tests negative for glucose. Clients may lose consciousness and suffer brain damage if hypoglycemia is not corrected promptly.

Hyperventilation causes body changes that mimic in part both ketoacidosis and hypoglycemia. Like the client with ketoacidosis, the hyperventilating client breathes rapidly and deeply. In this case, however, the respiratory pattern is the cause of the syndrome rather than one of its effects. Rapid respirations increase the rate of carbon dioxide loss from the blood; respiratory alkalosis follows. Some signs and symptoms of alkalosis (apprehension, irritability, and tremor) resemble insulin reaction. Headache is usually absent.

If a client complains of episodes of apprehension, trembling, perspiration, and headache but has a high blood glucose level, the problem may be the Somogyi effect. These clients overreact to hypoglycemia by secreting excess glucagon, glucocorticoids, or epinephrine, all of which inhibit the effect of insulin and promote glycolysis and an increased blood glucose level. The Somogyi effect can be caused by excessive dosages of insulin and worsens if insulin dosages are increased in response to the hyperglycemia.

Clients with hyperglycemia should be closely assessed for signs and symptoms of infection, a frequent cause of hyperglycemia. Infection is more likely to develop when body fluids are rich in glucose because phagocytosis is inhibited and pathogens often feed on glucose.

NURSING DIAGNOSIS

Nursing diagnoses for clients receiving exogenous insulin may include:

- Anxiety, related to hypoglycemia secondary to insulin overdose (fasting, vigorous exercise)
- Pain: Headache related to hypoglycemia secondary to insulin overdose (fasting, vigorous exercise)
- Altered Thought Processes: Confusion, bizarre (aggressive) behavior, or coma related to hypoglycemia secondary to insulin overdose (fasting, vigorous exercise)

Most newly diagnosed diabetics and some clients with a longer history of disease exhibit:

- Knowledge Deficit, about diabetes mellitus and insulin therapy

PLANNING

Goals of nursing care related to insulin therapy include restoring homeostasis (normal blood levels of glucose, pH, and osmolarity and emergence from coma), promoting glucose metabolism, restoring tissue perfusion, preventing stroke due to hypoglycemia, reducing anxiety due to sympathoadrenal discharge or alkalosis, reducing hypoglycemic headache, preventing or promptly detecting and treating complications such as infection or decubitus, and eliminating knowledge deficits.

INTERVENTION

The initial nursing intervention for hypoglycemia is the immediate administration of sugar, orally if possible. A glass of skim milk or orange juice (to which 2 tsp of sugar may be added) can be offered to the client. If these are unavailable, candy or table sugar may be substituted. (Clients taking acarbose [Precose] must be given glucose; other sugars will not act quickly enough.) Some authorities recommend placing sugar or sugar gel under the tongue of the comatose client for absorption by the sublingual vessels; positioning the client to prevent aspiration is particularly important if this is done.

If response to the food is good, the client should eat a snack containing carbohydrate (preferably starch) and protein. These nutrients provide glucose over a period of time to counteract the continued action of insulin. The rise in blood glucose level from refined sugar tends to be temporary; therefore, hypoglycemia is apt to recur. More than one feeding may be necessary if the client is using a long-lasting insulin. If the client refuses to take food or is unconscious, parenteral treatment is required. Glucagon injections or IV infusions of dextrose are prescribed to correct serious hypoglycemia. Either can elevate blood glucose levels and restore brain function. After glucagon treatment, the client takes food. Clients who experience serious hypoglycemia must be observed for at least 24 hours for recurring episodes. If convulsions or coma have occurred, a careful assessment for CNS damage must be made.

Like hypoglycemia, severe diabetic ketoacidosis is a medical emergency. The client may be in a profound coma and hypovolemic shock. Restoration of fluid, electrolyte, and acid–base balance is of primary importance. Blood is drawn for chemical studies and IV therapy is begun. Initially, isotonic saline is infused rapidly to restore blood volume. Sodium bicarbonate may be added to the IV solution to offset acidosis. Insulin is administered IM or IV because SC injections are not absorbed efficiently during circulatory shock. As soon as a drop in the blood glucose level demonstrates response to the insulin, dextrose is added to the IV infusion; insulin administration is continued either in infusion solutions or by periodic IM injections. The electrolyte content of fluids is adjusted as needed. As the acidosis is corrected, serious hypokalemia develops and potassium levels must be maintained within normal limits to avoid life-threatening cardiac arrhythmia.

When the client's condition improves and glucose metabolism stabilizes, the usual diabetic regimen is reinstituted. The period of illness may have altered the diabetic status, however, and this regimen may now be inappropriate. Often the diabetes has worsened, and a higher dose of insulin is necessary. Occasionally, the client's immune status has changed. If insulin antibody levels have dropped, insulin dosages must be decreased.

Clients hospitalized specifically for adjustment of the diabetic regimen to reestablish control over the disease have orders for varying amounts of medication and diet until a satisfactory response occurs. During this period, the client's living conditions should be as normal as possible. Regular mealtimes and activity patterns should be maintained. Physiotherapy may be ordered to provide exercise. Excessive stress should be avoided. Because all these factors tend to alter insulin needs, the regimen established in the hospital will not prove satisfactory after discharge unless hospital conditions are comparable to those at home.

Insulin reactions can occur at any time but are more likely as the client's condition improves. The nurse must monitor clients for signs and symptoms of insulin reactions, particularly at times of peak action and when the client has not eaten for some time (see Table 32-1 and Figs. 32-4 through 32-6). Clients who receive long-lasting insulin in the morning are prone to hypoglycemia during sleep, especially if a bedtime snack has been omitted. Diaphoresis may be the only clue to hypoglycemia during sleep. The nurse must awaken the client and administer sugar if excessive perspiration is noted.

In acute care settings, blood glucose levels are routinely tested to determine the glucose level. Testing usually occurs before meals and at bedtime. In some chronic care settings, urine is tested for glucose and acetone. Urine tests are most reliable when double-voided specimens are collected. About 10 or 15 minutes after the bladder has been emptied, the client is asked to void again, and the second specimen is tested. Presumably, this urine has been freshly excreted by the kidneys and represents the current metabolic status. If tests indicate that the diabetic condition is stable, the usual diet and insulin regimen may be maintained. Monitoring should be continued, however, because changes of routine and stress levels affect metabolic status.

Often the hospitalized diabetic client exhibits an elevated blood glucose level. The prescriber may order regular insulin supplements to the medication regimen (termed "insulin coverage" or "sliding scale"). Typically, blood or urine is monitored periodically (every 4 hours, or before meals and at bedtime), and insulin is given according to the degree of glucose detected. Usually no insulin is given if urine tests show 0.25% glucose or less. For 0.5% glucose, a dose of 5 U of insulin is given; for 1% glucose, 10 U; and for 2% glucose, 15 U. When blood is monitored, coverage is about 1 U per 25 mg/dL glucose above 180 mg/dL. If the client is particularly unstable, long-lasting insulin may be discontinued temporarily and the client treated entirely with regular insulin.

Insulin by continuous infusion may be ordered for treating ketoacidosis or foot lesions. The inner surfaces of bottles, bags, and tubing absorb insulin. To ensure delivery of uniform dosages, the tubing may be flushed with a medicated solution before being connected to the IV line. (This is done by preparing 125% of the prescribed insulin solution and using the excess to flush the tubing.) This practice tends to saturate the tubing surface, preventing adsorption of insulin during the first part of the infusion. The nurse should follow the facility's written policies or standing orders regarding preparation of IV insulin solutions. In-line filters are not recommended for insulin infusions.

Before using any insulin preparation, the nurse must check the expiration date and inspect the contents for visible changes (solid clumps or deposits) that indicate deterioration of the drug. Because insulin has a narrow margin of safety, doses must be as accurate as possible. When possible, dosage should be verified by another nurse. Combinations of insulins should be prepared by drawing up regular insulin first, then adding the longer-lasting preparation; these doses should be administered without delay. Nurses should develop the habit of observing the appearance of insulin. Erroneous use of regular insulin in dosages prescribed for long-lasting preparations can cause severe and dangerous hypoglycemia. Regular insulin is clear; long-lasting insulins, which are suspensions, appear cloudy. Whenever the insulin being prepared is clear, the nurse should verify that regular insulin has been ordered. (Doses of regular insulin usually do not exceed 20 U.)

Client Education. Except during episodes of critical illness, the teaching needs of the diabetic client should assume high priority in nursing care. Comprehensive diabetic education is beyond the scope of this text except as it relates to insulin use. As always, sound teaching principles must be applied in the teaching plan.

In teaching about insulin administration, the nurse must cover:

- Proper injection technique
- Proper insulin-mixing technique
- How to store and handle insulin
- Signs and symptoms of insulin excess and deficiency
- Monitoring techniques
- Management of insulin reactions

Injection Technique. To provide safe self-care, clients must know how to administer insulin. It is usually administered SC using specifically designed disposable plastic syringes. These syringes are designed for one-time use, but some experts believe that disposable syringes may be used up to seven times without increased danger of infection, provided the needle is disinfected with alcohol after each use and recapped, and the syringe is refrigerated. (Such reuse can reduce the cost of syringes significantly.) With successive use, however, the needle dulls and eventually causes pain on insertion. Also, the longer the interval between initial use and final use, the greater the theoretical risk of infection. Keeping the syringe longer than 7 days is not recommended; some authorities limit use to three injections.

The client must learn to use good surgical asepsis when injecting insulin. Diabetics are unusually prone to infection, and infection in turn disrupts glucose balance, causing a rise in blood glucose. Imperfect asepsis, which would be harmless in people with normal metabolism, can cause abscesses in diabetics.

If an order for insulin is for an odd number of units, syringes must have gradations on the scale for 0.01 mL. Some insulin syringes and all tuberculin syringes allow accurate measurement of odd dosages.

When preparing insulin injections, the client must avoid air bubbles, because these alter the dose.

Whether or not the injection site should be massaged is controversial: massage causes local vasodilation and more rapid absorption.

The client should be instructed about using insulin syringes with short needles. This kind of needle should be inserted at a 90° angle to the skin. A 90° angle may also be used by obese clients when using ⅝" needles, but an oblique approach is necessary for thin clients. Aspiration to verify placement in SC tissue rather than in a blood vessel is recommended but is not always taught to children or adults who have difficulty mastering injection technique. If injection sites are properly chosen to avoid areas rich in blood vessels, inadvertent IV injection is unlikely. Clients who administer their own insulin are limited to injection sites within reach—mainly the arms, thighs, and abdomen (Fig. 32-7). If necessary, a family member may be taught to give injections to allow use of a greater range of sites. The latest recommendations for choosing injection sites are to use one anatomic region only (eg, the abdomen or the thighs) and to rotate sites within this region. This procedure promotes more uniform absorption of insulin.

Proper Insulin-Mixing Technique. When insulin prescriptions call for a mixture of insulins, the client should be taught how to prepare the doses (Box 32-3). Commonly, regular insulin and a long-lasting insulin are combined. When different types of insulin are mixed, they tend to interact to produce an effect somewhat different from the sum of their individual effects. For example, long-lasting preparations may contain an excess of material used to modify the molecules for slower absorption; these substances convert part of the regular insulin mixed with it to a long-lasting form. For consistency in effect, individual doses must be prepared in a regulated manner. The sequence used for drawing up the drug should be the same for each dose preparation. To preserve the purity of the regular insulin supply, the regular insulin is drawn up first, followed by the long-lasting insulin. The vial that contains the long-lasting preparation must contain positive pressure to eliminate suctioning the regular insulin from the syringe into the vial.

The composition of mixed insulins tends to change as the regular insulin combines with the excess complexing agent in the longer-lasting preparation. One way to maintain stability of dosage is to prepare a vial containing multiple doses of the mixture and allow the changes to proceed to the end point before use. (This practice must be started before the optimal dosage is determined.) If doses are prepared individually, they should be administered as soon after mixing as possible.

How to Store and Handle Insulin. Insulin deteriorates if exposed to excessive heat, light, or agitation. Constant refrigeration is not needed by the newer preparations, but clients should be instructed to refrigerate extra bottles until needed. Insulin must not be frozen. Insulin in current use should be kept at room temperature. Long-lasting insulins must be rolled to mix the suspen-

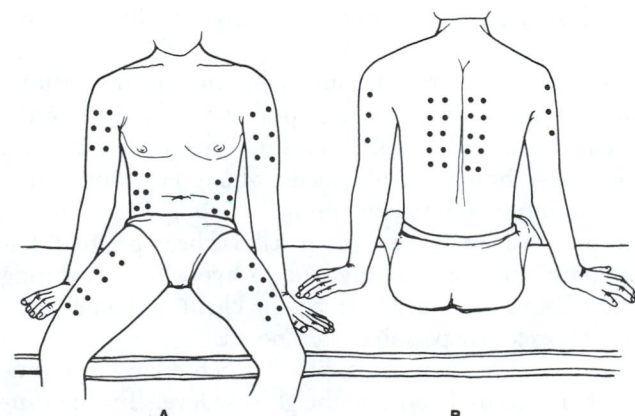

Figure 32-7. Sites for subcutaneous injections. **(A)** Usual sites for self-administration are in the outer aspects of the thighs. A systematic rotation of sites is important in insulin injections; it lessens irritation and improves absorption. **(B)** Family members or hospital staff can use posterior sites for a wider variety of sites.

Box 32-3
Preparing a Mixed Insulin Injection

To prepare an injection that contains both long-lasting and regular insulin, roll both vials of insulin to distribute the drug evenly throughout the solution. Then, using sterile aseptic technique, do the following:

1. Into the vial that contains the long-lasting insulin, inject a volume of air equal to the volume of long-lasting insulin required for the dose ordered.
2. Into the bottle that contains the regular insulin, inject a volume of air equal to the volume of the regular insulin required for the dose ordered; without withdrawing the needle, invert the vial.
3. Draw up the proper dose of regular insulin and withdraw the needle.
4. Invert the vial that contains the long-lasting insulin and insert the needle of the syringe through the rubber dam; do not allow the tip of the needle to protrude above the fluid level in the vial; allow the positive pressure in the vial to push the required volume of long-lasting insulin into the syringe.
5. Withdraw the needle from the vial. The volume in the syringe should be equal to the sums of the volumes of the two types of insulin ordered.

sion gently but thoroughly before drawing up the required dose. The bottle should never be shaken vigorously, because protein molecules are denatured by such whipping action. Frothing of the solution indicates the start of protein breakdown. Insulin should be protected from excessive heat or strong light. For convenience when traveling, insulin and equipment for administration are best carried in a compact kit of some kind; fitted containers are available commercially. Some kits have space for urine- or blood-testing equipment also.

Clients should be cautioned never to substitute one kind of insulin for another. The supply received from the pharmacist should conform exactly to that ordered by the prescriber. Substitution of a different concentration or type of insulin may cause errors in dosage and response. Because porcine, bovine, and human insulin differ antigenically, changing from one type to another requires close medical supervision.

Signs and Symptoms of Insulin Excess and Deficiency. Diabetics who receive insulin must be thoroughly familiar with the signs and symptoms of hypoglycemia and hyperglycemia. Many have developed hyperglycemia before the disease was diagnosed, and most experience one or more insulin reactions before a satisfactory medical regimen is achieved. The occurrence of such reactions provides a practical demonstration of the subjective symptoms of these conditions. The client should know the most likely times for hyper-

glycemia and hypoglycemia to develop and should be especially vigilant for symptoms at these times.

Because hypoglycemia may trigger socially unacceptable behavior, diabetics should always carry medical identification that indicates their disease and the hypoglycemic medication in use. If hypoglycemia is mistaken for drunkenness, the client is unlikely to receive timely treatment for this dangerous condition. Clients should also carry some form of sugar with them to take at the first sign of insulin reaction. Candy is a frequent choice, but cube sugar is preferable if the client craves sweets and is likely to eat the candy, a food allowed only in limited quantities in most diet regimens. Clients using acarbose (Precose) must use glucose instead of sugar or candy.

Monitoring Techniques. Blood testing is usually recommended for monitoring glucose balance. Most clients are instructed to test blood specimens before each meal and at bedtime. Urine tests are less frequently used, but when the renal threshold for glucose is normal, the occurrence and degree of hyperglycemia are reflected by the amount of glucose excreted by the kidneys in the urine. Urine tests are most reliable when double-voided specimens are used.

Testing is irrelevant if the client does not know what to do with the results. The record can be very useful for counseling and educating the client. Sometimes the prescriber wants the record of test results brought to the office for use in planning insulin and diet prescriptions. Absence of hyperglycemia and glycosuria is desirable in clients who have diabetes of adult onset and who are relatively stable. The more closely the blood glucose level approaches normal in these clients, the less likely it is that complications will develop (although strict control does not always ensure that complications will not develop). In labile diabetics or those subject to frequent insulin reactions, some degree of hyperglycemia or glycosuria may be desirable to minimize the risk of serious hypoglycemia. Glycosated hemoglobin (HbA$_1$C) is a blood test that is used to determine how well blood glucose levels have been controlled over the prior 3- to 4-month period. Normal is below 8%; diabetics usually are considered out of good control if it is above 11.5%.

Some clients have an abnormally low or high renal threshold to glucose. Because urine tests would not provide a reliable index to blood glucose levels, there is little purpose in monitoring the urine; instead, blood tests should be used.

Management of Insulin Reactions. Many clients omit insulin doses if they cannot eat. This practice is logical but not advisable if the inability to eat is caused by nausea or other symptoms of illness. During illness, blood glucose levels tend to remain high despite fasting, probably because of the additional stress. The regular dose of medication should be taken and the healthcare provider consulted for treatment of the illness. Nausea is one early sign of ketoacidosis, and many clients admitted to the hospital for treatment of this complication have omitted their regular dose of insulin, thus aggravating the condition.

OUTCOME EVALUATION

Data required for evaluation include records of blood glucose levels, insulin dosages, and diet, absence or incidence of hypoglycemic reactions, demonstration by the client of injection technique, statements by the client concerning the treatment regimen, and the presence or absence of diabetic complications.

❖ CHECKLIST OF NURSING ACTIONS

❑ Before drawing up insulin into a syringe, rotate the vial gently to mix it.

❑ Use special care in administering insulin. Be sure the proper drug preparation is used. When possible, have another nurse check the dosage for accuracy.

❑ When combining insulins, prepare individual doses immediately before injection.

❑ When preparing a mixture of regular and modified insulin, draw up the regular insulin first to avoid contaminating the vial of regular insulin with modified insulin.

❑ Rotate injection sites according to a regular plan that allows at least 1 month between injections at any one site.

❑ Monitor blood or urine glucose levels to assess therapeutic response.

❑ Monitor the client for signs and symptoms of hyperglycemia and hypoglycemia.

❑ Administer food or fluid containing sugar or glucose at the first sign of an insulin reaction and when in doubt about the nature of a reaction in an insulin-dependent diabetic.

❑ Teach clients how to manage the diabetic regimen, including insulin administration. Explain the factors that increase and decrease insulin requirements.

❑ Refrigerate reserve stocks of insulin but protect them from freezing. Keep bottles in current use at room temperature and protect them from heat and direct sunlight.

❑ Discard insulin whose expiration date has passed or in which solid clumps or deposits have appeared.

❑ Anticipate that insulin medication is likely to be delayed if the client must fast for testing procedures.

Oral Hypoglycemics

Two classes of drugs other than insulin have been used to control hyperglycemia: sulfonylureas and biguanides. Biguanides had been withdrawn from the U.S. market because they caused severe lactic acidosis; however, a new agent of this class appears to be safer and is now available for clinical use.

Sulfonylureas

These drugs are all arylsulfonylureas with substitutions on the benzene and urea groups. Second-generation sulfonylureas, such as glipizide, are more potent than first-generation agents (Table 32-4).

Pharmacodynamics. Sulfonylureas stimulate the pancreas to secrete insulin. They have no hypoglycemic effect in clients with an absolute deficiency of insulin due to pancreatectomy or total lack of insulin production. They lower blood glucose levels in clients with NIDDM. These agents also inhibit the release of catecholamines and may enhance the metabolic effect of insulin by limiting the secretion of these insulin antagonists. Some investigators believe that prolonged use of the drugs results in an increase in the number of insulin receptors, thus increasing tissue sensitivity to the action of endogenous hormone. Glyburide exerts a mild diuretic action and appears to inhibit platelet aggregation.

Pharmacokinetics. Sulfonylureas are well absorbed when administered orally. Onset of action, peak effect, and duration of effect vary with the preparation. The compounds that bind to serum proteins (tolbutamide, glipizide, and chlorpropamide) require several days of administration to achieve full effect. Elimination of the drugs is primarily through renal excretion. Metabolism by the liver is required for elimination of tolbutamide and glipizide and is involved in the action of acetohexamide and tolazamide by producing metabolites of varying physiologic potency. Chlorpropamide is excreted largely unchanged by the kidneys. A long-lasting (sustained-release) form of glipizide (Glucotrol X) was recently approved by the Food and Drug Administration.

Therapeutic Uses. Sulfonylureas are prescribed for the treatment of diabetes mellitus. They are recommended for use by clients who have not responded to dietary treatment and weight loss and who have difficulty managing insulin injection regimens. It is considered a treatment of last resort that carries a significant risk of shortened life expectancy.

Adverse Reactions. The overall risk of side effects from sulfonylureas is about 5%. The likelihood of adverse responses is related to potency, with reactions to chlorpropamide occurring four times more often than to tolbutamide. Some complications are most likely to occur within the first 2 months of treatment, whereas others develop only after prolonged treatment.

Because they stimulate endogenous insulin secretion, sulfonylureas can cause symptomatic hypoglycemia. Reactions tend to be less severe than with exogenous insulin but are more prolonged and may produce serious, even fatal, consequences. As with insulin, delayed meals or unusual exercise tend to precipitate such episodes. Hypoglycemia may occur at any time, even after months of trouble-free treatment.

Side effects include gastrointestinal (GI) distress, CNS malfunction, alcohol intolerance, skin eruptions,

Table 32-4. Oral Hypoglycemic Drugs

Drug Names	Approximate Time of Onset (Hours)	Peak Action (Hours)	Plasma Half-Life (Hours)	Duration of Activity (Hours)	Usual Adult Dosage	Pregnancy Risk Category*
Sulfonylureas						
acetohexamide (Dymelor; *Can*: Dimelor)	1	3	1.3 (4.5 for active metabolites)	12–24	250 mg–1.5 g daily, divided in 1 or 2 doses	D
chlorpropamide (Diabinese, Glucamide)	1	3–6	36	24+	100–500 mg daily, in a single dose	D
gliclazide (Diamicron)	NA	4–6	10.4	24	80–150 mg q12–24h	
glimepiride (Amaryl)	1	2–3	5.5–7	NA	*Initially:* 1–2 mg daily with breakfast or first meal of the day; *maintenance:* 1–4 mg once daily	B
glipizide (Glucotrol)	0.5	1–3	3–4.7	24	*Initially:* 2.5–5 mg once daily; *maintenance:* 2.5–40 mg daily	C
(Glucotrol XL)	2–3	6–12	NA (combined immediate and delayed action)	24+	5–10 mg daily, in a single dose	C
glyburide (Diabeta, Euglucon, Micronase)	0.5	1.5–3	1.4–1.8 (10 for active metabolites)	24	*Initially:* 1.25–5 mg daily, divided in 1 or 2 doses; *maintenance:* 1.25–20 mg daily, divided in 1 or 2 doses	B
tolazamide (Tolinase)	4–6	6–9	7	10	250 mg daily, divided in 1 or 2 doses	C
tolbutamide (Orinase; *Can*: Mobenol)	1	5–8	7	6–12	1 g daily, divided in 2 or 3 doses	C
Biguanide						
metformin (Glucophage)	Relatively slow	NA	Biphasic: 1.7–3 and 9–17	NA	500 mg tid	B
Glucosidase Inhibitor						
acarbose (Precose)	Acts locally in the gut to delay digestion of carbohydrate and absorption of glucose				200 mg tid with first bite of each main meal	

*See Appendix A.
NA = not available.
Can = Canadian trade names.

and syndrome of inappropriate antidiuretic hormone secretion. GI symptoms include heartburn, nausea, vomiting, abdominal pain, and diarrhea. CNS manifestations include confusion, vertigo, ataxia, paresthesia, weakness, tinnitus, headache, visual impairment, and intolerance of alcohol; a reaction that resembles that of disulfiram (Antabuse) may occur with alcohol intake. The most serious hematologic effect is agranulocytosis, but thrombocytopenia, pancytopenia, and hemolytic anemia also occur in rare instances. Jaundice is the cholestatic type. Excessive antidiuretic hormone secretion may be associated with hyponatremia. Agranulocytosis and jaundice are most likely to develop within the

first 2 months of treatment, but other complications may arise at any time. A significant risk of earlier death from cardiovascular problems is associated with the use of oral hypoglycemics. Administering large doses of sulfonylureas to animals results in increased congenital defects in the offspring.

Drug Interactions. Some sulfonylureas are highly bound to serum proteins. When used at the same time as other protein-bound drugs (eg, nonsteroidal antiinflammatory drugs, oral anticoagulants, hydantoin, sulfonamides), the combination tends to alter serum drug levels and response to treatment. Protein-bound drugs may enhance response to sulfonylureas, or their own action may be enhanced by sulfonylureas. In addition to its ability to displace sulfonylureas from plasma proteins, phenylbutazone also inhibits renal excretion of acetohexamide and the metabolism of tolbutamide. Other drugs that enhance hypoglycemic response include insulin, alcohol, and (for chlorpropamide and tolazamide) probenecid.

Clients treated with sulfonylureas may experience a disulfiram-like reaction (flushing, nausea, and vomiting) when drinking alcohol. The flush is particularly prominent with chlorpropamide, which also prolongs the duration of barbiturate action.

When beta-adrenergic blockers are administered concurrently with sulfonylureas, they tend to suppress some signs of hypoglycemia. The increases in pulse and blood pressure characteristic of sympathetic response to rapid decreases in blood glucose do not occur. (See Focus On Sulfonylureas: Similarities and Differences.)

Precautions and Contraindications. Sulfonylureas are contraindicated in IDDM, in clients with serious hepatic or renal disease, and during pregnancy. They are reserved for mild NIDDM with an onset at age 40 or later.

Because liver and kidney functions influence the metabolism and excretion of these drugs, and because these functions may be impaired in older clients, high loading doses are avoided. During the initial treatment, before the full effect of the drugs is achieved, insulin may be continued at reduced dosages, especially in clients who require more than 20 U daily. Metabolic status must be monitored closely with blood tests for glucose. Oral drugs may maintain normal blood glucose levels in clients with otherwise stable health. However, stressors such as infection, fever, surgery, or trauma increase the blood glucose level, and insulin therapy may be needed until the situation is resolved.

■ SUMMARY

Sulfonylureas act primarily by stimulating the secretion of endogenous insulin. They are effective only in mild NIDDM. Because sulfonylureas may increase the death rate from cardiovascular disease, insulin therapy is preferable if feasible. In addition to the usual toxic effects of insulin, sulfonylureas can cause GI, CNS, skin, liver, and hematopoietic symptoms. Periodic use of insulin is often required to control glucose metabolism during periods of illness in clients normally controlled by sulfonylureas.

❖ NURSING MANAGEMENT: CLIENT RECEIVING AN ORAL HYPOGLYCEMIC

Clients who receive oral hypoglycemics are likely to have had difficulty adjusting to the diabetic regimen, especially to insulin administration. They may need supervision, assistance, and teaching.

NURSING PROCESS

ASSESSMENT

Clients who receive sulfonylureas to treat diabetes mellitus must be monitored for glucose imbalance (hyperglycemia and hypoglycemia), just like clients who depend on insulin. The nurse should also assess the client for adverse reactions characteristic of these drugs. During the first 2 months of treatment, any evidence of agranulocytosis or jaundice is particularly significant. Frequent sore throats or other infections must be reported to the prescriber. Periodic blood tests should be ordered to monitor for hematologic changes. The client should be observed for jaundice using natural sunlight or incandescent light. Fluorescent light that lacks yellow tones masks jaundice, even when it is quite pronounced. The sclerae should be carefully examined for yellow discoloration to detect beginning jaundice. The client should be questioned about paresthesia, tinnitus, and visual changes to detect sensory/perceptual alterations.

Because sulfonylurea therapy increases the incidence of serious cardiovascular disease, clients receiving these drugs should be carefully and regularly assessed for such problems. The advisability of continued drug therapy should be reassessed if hypertension or cardiac arrhythmia develops.

NURSING DIAGNOSIS

Nursing diagnoses for clients taking sulfonylureas may include:

- Pain, related to altered comfort from nausea (vomiting, abdominal pain) secondary to sulfonylurea medication
- Risk for Infection, related to leukopenia secondary to bone marrow depression by sulfonylureas
- Body Image Disturbance, related to skin rash or jaundice secondary to adverse reaction to sulfonylureas
- Fluid Volume Excess, related to inappropriate secretion of antidiuretic hormone secondary to sulfonylurea medication
- Impaired Physical Mobility: Ataxia, vertigo, and weakness related to adverse reaction to sulfonylureas

Common collaborative problems that should be differentiated from the nursing diagnoses include:

Potential Complication: Hypoglycemia
Potential Complication: Anemia
Potential Complication: Bone marrow depression
Potential Complication: Cardiovascular degeneration
Potential Complication: Adverse reactions to sulfonylureas

PLANNING

The goals of nursing care include maintaining glucose balance and preventing or promptly detecting and treating adverse reactions to sulfonylureas.

FOCUS ON

Sulfonylureas: Similarities and Differences

Similarities

Pharmacodynamics

These agents stimulate the release of endogenous insulin for the pancreas, lowering blood glucose levels

Pharmacokinetics

These agents are rapidly and readily absorbed from the GI tract. They are distributed into the extracellular fluid. They are metabolized by the liver and excreted by the kidneys.

Therapeutic Uses

These agents are used to treat non–insulin-dependent diabetes mellitus.

Adverse Reactions

These include: (CNS) headache, weakness, confusion, paresthesia, ataxia; (EENT) tinnitus, visual impairment; (GI) nausea, vomiting, GI distress, anorexia, abdominal pain, heartburn, jaundice, altered liver function; (ENDO) hypoglycemia; (HEMA) blood dyscrasia, agranulocytosis, thrombocytopenia, hemolytic anemia, aplastic anemia, hyponatremia; (SKIN) urticaria, erythema, pruritus; (OTHER) disulfiram-like reaction, syndrome of inappropriate anti-diuretic hormone.

Drug Interactions

Some sulfonylureas are highly bound to serum proteins and may alter serum free drug levels of other protein-bound drugs (eg, NSAIDs, oral anticoagulants, hydantoin, sulfonilamides). The effect of sulfonylurea drugs may also be altered by these protein-bound substances. Hypoglycemic response is enhanced by insulin and alcohol. A disulfiram-like reaction can occur when alcohol is used with these drugs.

Precautions and Contraindications

These agents should be used with caution in clients with hepatic porphyria, women of childbearing age, and clients with impaired adrenal, pituitary, or thyroid function.

Differences

- **Chlorpropamide** has an antidiuretic action.
- **Glyburide** exhibits mild diuretic action and appears to inhibit platelet aggregation.

- **Chlorpropamide** is excreted unchanged in the urine.
- **Acetohexamide** has a half-life of 1 to 1.5 hours.
- **Chlorpropamide** has an onset of 1 hour, peaking in 2 to 4 hours, with a duration of 24 hours and a half-life of 36 hours.
- **Glipizide** has an onset of 15 to 30 minutes, peaking in 1 to 6 hours, with a duration of 24 hours and a half-life of 2 to 7 hours.
- **Glyburide** has an onset of 15 to 60 minutes, peaking in 2 to 8 hours, with a duration of 24 hours and a half-life of 10 hours.
- **Tolazamide** has an onset of 4 to 6 hours, with a duration of 10 hours and a half-life of 7 hours.
- **Tolbutamide** has an onset of 30 to 60 minutes, peaking in 3 to 5 hours, with a duration of 6 to 12 hours and a half-life of 7 hours.

- **Tolbutamide, tolazamide**, and **chlorpropamide** may cause photosensitivity.
- **Tolazamide** may also cause lethargy, dizziness, and vertigo.

- **Phenylbutazone** inhibits renal excretion of acetohexamide and the metabolism of tolbutamide. The effects of chlorpropamide and tolazamide are enhanced by probenecid. Chlorpropamide prolongs the duration of barbiturate action and causes a particularly prominent flush in disulfiram-like reactions to alcohol.

- **Chlorpropamide** should be used with caution in clients with impaired cardiac function and fluid retention.

(continued)

Sulfonylureas: Similarities and Differences (continued)

Similarities (continued)

Precautions and Contraindications (continued)

These agents are contraindicated in clients with insulin-dependent diabetes mellitus and in those complicated with ketosis, acidosis, coma, or other acute complication, such as major surgery, severe infection, trauma, or burns. They are also contraindicated in clients with severe hepatic or renal dysfunction and in those with a known hypersensitivity to sulfas, those who are pregnant, and those with nonfunctioning pancreatic beta cells.

Nursing Considerations

Instruct client in disease, treatment, drug therapy, regimen, adverse effects, and compliance; monitor blood glucose level and urine for glucose and ketones frequently; instruct client in how to check glucose levels; administer 30 minutes before breakfast daily or 30 minutes before breakfast and dinner for twice-daily regimen; assess for signs and symptoms of hypoglycemia and hyperglycemia; instruct client in all aspects of diabetes, including diet; warn clients to avoid alcohol; assess clients for signs of infection or stress, which may necessitate dosage changes; monitor serum studies, including blood counts and bilirubin levels, for changes.

Differences (continued)

- **Acetohexamide** is contraindicated in hyperglycemia and glycosuria with primary renal dysfunction.
- **Chlorpropamide** is contraindicated in clients with diminished thyroid function.
- **Tolazamide** is contraindicated in clients with uremia.
- **Tolbutamide** is contraindicated in clients with severe renal insufficiency.

- When administering **chlorpropamide,** monitor fluid balance closely; watch for signs of impending renal insufficiency, such as dysuria, anuria, and hematuria.

INTERVENTION

Clients who receive oral hypoglycemic drugs must adhere to a health regimen like that required of other diabetics. To maintain glucose balance, they must comply with the prescribed diet and medication, maintain a regular schedule of rest and activity, avoid infection, and avoid high stress levels.

The nurse should monitor the client for adverse reactions to drugs. These should be reported to the prescriber for adjustment of the drug regimen.

The nurse should ensure that institutionalized clients who take sulfonylureas are not served alcoholic beverages and that medicinal preparations containing alcohol are not administered to them. Concomitant use results in nausea and vomiting from a disulfiram-like reaction.

Client Education. Clients must know that the use of oral hypoglycemic agents may pose an increased risk of early death from cardiovascular complications. Without such information, consent for treatment is invalid because it is not fully informed. Clients who wish to discontinue oral hypoglycemic therapy need considerable assistance in undertaking insulin treatment. If the drug order is changed, intensive nursing care should be available to help the client cope with the new regimen.

Education is the cornerstone of treatment for all diabetics but is particularly important for the client receiving oral hypoglycemic agents. Control of diet and body weight is crucial to a successful therapeutic outcome. Blood glucose tests and monitoring for glucose imbalance are as important as for clients taking exogenous insulin.

Although many clients who receive sulfonylureas previously have not adjusted well to insulin therapy, the hormone may be needed periodically to maintain glucose balance during illness. Either the client or someone in the family should be able to administer insulin if it is needed.

In addition to the usual instruction in the detection of glucose imbalance, clients must be taught the signs and symptoms of adverse reactions to sulfonylureas that should be reported to the prescriber. Blood dyscrasias and jaundice are particularly dangerous. The client should immediately report infections, weakness, abnormal bleeding, or jaundice.

Example of Nursing Process for Tolbutamide Therapy

The client is an 80-year-old retired widowed printer who lives with his daughter, a part-time substitute teacher. Seven years ago, the client was told he had adult onset non–insulin-dependent diabetes mellitus. The condition was controlled by diet until last year, when the client was hospitalized for treatment of a severe episode of ketoacidosis. Until then, the client had lived alone in an efficiency apartment near his daughter.

After his recovery from ketoacidosis, the client required insulin to control hyperglycemia. He was unable to learn injection technique, however, and tolbutamide 325 mg tid was prescribed. He came to live with his daughter, who supervises his diet. On days she is called to work, the daughter leaves a cold lunch for the client in the refrigerator and his noon medication on the kitchen counter. When the public health nurse arrived for a visit at 2 PM today, she found the client wandering around the house, confused and incoherent. His lunch was still in the refrigerator, uneaten, but the medication container was empty.

Assessment Data

Prescription for tolbutamide

Confusion, incoherence

Apparent ingestion of noon dose of tolbutamide

Client's lunch had not been eaten

Client's failure to eat after taking hypoglycemic drug

Nursing Diagnosis	Intervention	Goals and Outcomes
Potential Complication: Hypoglycemia*	**Prepare** a small glass of sweetened orange juice; using a quiet, firm approach, try to persuade the client to drink it; if unsuccessful, call for emergency medical care. If the client drinks the orange juice and becomes more rational, **feed** him lunch.	The client's confusion will clear; he will become coherent and mentally alert.
Impaired Home Maintenance Management	**Inform** the daughter of the episode; suggest she put the client's medication with his lunch to ensure that he eats when he takes the drug.	Client will consistently take lunch with his noon dose of tolbutamide.
Knowledge Deficit, related to oral hypoglycemic drug and its relation to diet in the treatment of diabetes mellitus	When the client is mentally alert, **explore** his knowledge about tolbutamide and its function in the control of diabetes mellitus. **Explain** that, although tolbutamide is not a form of insulin, it does increase the level of insulin in his blood and can cause hypoglycemia, just as exogenous insulin does; stress the importance of eating the meals prescribed for his diet.	The client will accurately repeat to the nurse (or to the daughter) the information conveyed during teaching. The client will eat all the meals prescribed for his diet.

*Although potential complications generally are not included in the Examples of Nursing Process, in this situation the identification of this collaborative problem is critical to the outcome for this client and illustrates the broad range of nursing responsibilities.

Additional prescriptions for interacting drugs should not be accepted without reminding the prescriber that sulfonylurea therapy is in progress. If such drugs are prescribed, the client should understand that the risk of side effects is increased, and self-monitoring is critical.

Nonprescription drugs that contain salicylates and alcohol should be avoided while sulfonylureas are in use. Drinking alcoholic beverages, if tolerated, increases the likelihood of hypoglycemic reactions.

The public sometimes calls these hypoglycemic agents "oral insulin," but this term is inappropriate and may mislead clients about the nature of sulfonylureal actions. The drugs neither exert a hormone effect nor in any way replace insulin. Their stimulation of endogenous insulin secretion helps normalize glucose metabolism but appears to contribute to cardiovascular degeneration and may hasten total pancreatic failure and insulin dependency.

OUTCOME EVALUATION

Data required for evaluation include serial blood glucose levels, presence or absence of adverse drug reactions (depressed cell counts, overhydration, jaundice, infection), presence or absence of cardiovascular degeneration, and statements by the client relating to sensory perception, discomfort, and self-concept (see Example of Nursing Process for Tolbutamide Therapy on p. 699).

❖ CHECKLIST OF NURSING ACTIONS

When Sulfonylureas Are Prescribed

- ❑ Review with the client the prescribed diabetic regimen, stressing the importance of dietary control, regular exercise, good general hygiene, and monitoring practices.
- ❑ Provide the client with oral and written information about the sulfonylurea prescribed, including its action, toxic and side effects, and the amount and timing of the doses to be taken.
- ❑ Review all drugs used by the client to assess the risk of adverse drug interactions.

During the First 2 Weeks of Treatment

- ❑ Monitor closely for glucose imbalance.

During the First 2 Months of Treatment

- ❑ Monitor closely for infections (especially sore throats) and jaundice.

Throughout Treatment

- ❑ Analyze results of blood and urine tests to determine glucose balance.
- ❑ Assess client for symptoms of GI, CNS, hematopoietic, liver, and skin problems.
- ❑ Monitor cardiovascular function.
- ❑ Refer client to the prescriber for reassessment of the drug regimen when pertinent signs and symptoms are found.
- ❑ Caution the client that use of alcohol may cause an unpleasant (disulfiram-like) reaction.

Biguanides

Only one biguanide is available for clinical use: metformin (Glucophage).

Pharmacodynamics. Metformin increases the sensitivity of liver and muscle to the actions of insulin, resulting in decreased glucose formation by the liver and increased uptake and metabolism of glucose by muscles.

Pharmacokinetics. Metformin is administered orally. It is not appreciably bound to plasma proteins. Plasma half-life is about 6 hours. It is not metabolized but is excreted unchanged in the urine.

Therapeutic Uses. Metformin is used, with diet, in the treatment of NIDDM in clients who are not well controlled by diet and exercise alone.

Adverse Reactions. Metformin appears to decrease plasma insulin levels. It can cause lactic acidosis, but the incidence (about 10%) is lower than that seen with phenformin, a biguanide that was withdrawn from the market several years ago because of this complication. Renal and hepatic function may be adversely affected. The most common adverse reaction is GI upset, which tends to be self-limiting.

Drug Interactions. Concurrent use with cimetidine increases the risk of hypoglycemia. The risk of lactic acidosis increases if the client concurrently takes glucocorticoids or alcohol.

Precautions and Contraindications. Metformin should be avoided in clients with hepatic or renal impairment. The drug is temporarily withdrawn if the client cannot take oral fluids and foods. During treatment, renal and hematologic function should be assessed at least once yearly.

❖ NURSING MANAGEMENT: CLIENT RECEIVING METFORMIN

Nursing care of clients receiving metformin is similar to that for clients taking sulfonylureas, except for the differences in side effects. The risk of allergy and cardiovascular complications appears to be lower with metformin. However, clients should be assessed regularly for acid–base balance and renal and hepatic function.

Acarbose

Acarbose (Precose) is an oral alpha-glucosidase inhibitor that delays the digestion and absorption of ingested carbohydrates, thus lowering the postprandial rise in blood glucose. It reduces the insulin response to and weight-increasing effects of sulfonylureas, and reduces levels of glycosolated hemoglobin. It is used in the treatment of NIDDM, alone or with sulfonylureas.

Acarbose is presstribed in three daily doses of 200 mg each, to be taken with the first bite of each main meal.

Acarbose is contraindicated in clients with diabetic ketoacidosis, cirrhosis, inflammatory bowel disease, or colonic ulceration. Use of the drug can increase the production of gas in the gut and is contraindicated in those at risk for intestinal obstruction or adverse reactions to abdominal distention. Clients receiving acarbose should carry glucose tablets for the treatment of hypoglycemic reactions since sugar (sucrose) will not be absorbed promptly.

Hyperglycemics

Glucagon

Glucagon is a hormone secreted by the alpha cells of the islets of Langerhans of the pancreas. Its physiologic function is generally opposite to that of insulin. Glucagon, a protein hormone, is a single-chain polypeptide made up of 29 amino acids.

Normal Glucagon Metabolism

Glucagon stimulates glycogen breakdown into glucose, thereby increasing blood glucose levels. It also exerts a positive inotropic and chronotropic effect on the heart and relaxes the intestine. The main stimulus to glucagon secretion is a decrease in intracellular glucose concentrations, usually as a result of a drop in blood glucose levels. Increased intracellular glucose after a rise in the blood glucose level inhibits its production. Blood glucose and glucagon form a negative feedback mechanism that operates to restore blood glucose levels after a drop below normal, regardless of the cause. The effects of glucagon protect the body from tissue damage caused by a shortage of readily available energy. Most importantly, glucagon functions to maintain a steady supply of energy to the brain, retina, and germinal tissue, which are obligate users of glucose. Just as insulin functions to promote the storage of energy nutrients in tissue depots, glucagon functions to mobilize stored energy when needed by the body. Insulin is most active when the body has ample supplies of nutrients; glucagon is most active during starvation states and after injury, when body requirements for energy are not met by dietary intake. Glucagon secretion is the body's first line of defense against hypoglycemia.

Abnormal Glucagon Metabolism

Theoretically, disturbances in glucagon production could contribute to many problems in glucose metabolism. Excessive secretion could be a factor in the development of diabetes mellitus. High levels of glucagon have been found in diabetics, although glucagon has not been recognized as a cause of this disease. Glucagon excess could also be a factor in stress-related hyperglycemia and the Somogyi response to insulin reactions.

Erratic glucagon response may be a factor in the pronounced blood glucose fluctuations of clients with labile diabetes mellitus. Excessive glucagon tends to reduce the effects of insulin, whether endogenous or exogenous.

Deficient glucagon production makes a person susceptible to hypoglycemia. Anyone without a pancreas or functioning islet cells is prone to repeated and severe hypoglycemic reactions. This may be the reason why diabetics with IDDM are subject to wide fluctuations in blood glucose and are apt to experience frequent, severe hypoglycemic reactions.

The degree to which glucagon imbalance is actually involved in these situations is unknown. In clinical settings, the focus of medical treatment is the manipulation of insulin and glucose levels to achieve a metabolic equilibrium, with little attention paid to the possible roles of glucagon.

Exogenous Glucagon Preparations

The structure of glucagon appears to be identical in many species. Human, porcine, and bovine hormone are alike in molecular makeup. The hormone has been synthesized and is available for therapeutic use. The drug is measured in both units and milligrams, with 1 mg equaling 1 U.

Pharmacodynamics. Glucagon stimulates the synthesis of cyclic adenosine monophosphate (cAMP), especially in the liver and adipose tissue. It promotes the breakdown of fuels stored in the tissues to meet the body's energy needs. Glycogen breakdown and glucose formation increase, and the blood glucose level rises. In response to increased levels of cAMP, cardiac muscle contracts more strongly and more rapidly. The mechanism that underlies the hormone's relaxing effect on the intestinal musculature is unknown.

Pharmacokinetics. Glucagon cannot be administered orally because it is destroyed by proteolytic enzymes in the digestive tract. After absorption from parenteral sites, it circulates freely through the tissues. Peak hyperglycemic effect occurs within 30 minutes; relaxation of GI smooth muscle develops within 15 minutes. Duration of action is about 1 to 2 hours for the hyperglycemic effect and about 30 minutes for GI relaxation.

Glucagon is degraded at tissue-receptor sites and in the kidneys, liver, and plasma. Its plasma half-life (like that of endogenous insulin) is 3 to 6 minutes but may reach 19 minutes.

Therapeutic Uses. Glucagon is used to relieve hypoglycemia in clients not amenable to oral glucose. It is useful in treating diabetic clients prone to rapidly developing insulin reactions in which unconsciousness occurs with little warning and in treating clients in whom hypoglycemia causes behavioral disturbances characterized by resistance to treatment. Glucagon is also used to promote intestinal relaxation before radiographic examination. It is sometimes administered to strengthen heart function as an adjunct in treating shock.

Large doses of glucagon have been administered experimentally in treating cardiac disorders. Although such therapy has not proved effective, serious toxic or side effects from the glucagon were not reported.

Dosage and Administration. An initial dose of 1 U is administered by injection. Response to the drug (return to consciousness or improved behavior) should be evident in 5 to 20 minutes. After 20 minutes, the dose may be repeated if necessary. More than two doses are not recommended because succeeding doses have not proved to be effective. Clients who fail to respond to glucagon may have deficient glycogen stores.

Glucagon for medicinal use is supplied as hydrochloride salt. It is dispensed as a dry powder in 1- or 10-U ampules with diluent sufficient to make a solution that contains 1 U/mL. The solution should be freshly prepared and refrigerated if not completely used. The usual dose is 1 U (1 mg), administered SC, IM, or IV. The drug is ineffective when administered orally.

Adverse Reactions. Glucagon is a relatively safe substance. Nausea and vomiting can occur, although these reactions may also be caused by the hypoglycemia usually affecting the client. The drug can produce a pronounced hyperglycemia, but this is usually transitory because the glucagon is rapidly dissipated. Moreover, the rise in blood glucose level stimulates insulin secretion in some clients, which may correct the imbalance. In diabetics given the drug for insulin reactions, the hyperglycemia is also transitory, because continued insulin effect limits the body's response to glucagon and often causes recurrent hypoglycemia. If glucagon is administered to a ketoacidotic diabetic, the blood glucose level rises further, increasing the hyperosmolarity.

Drug Interactions. Concurrent glucagon and oral anticoagulant use increases anticoagulant effects and risks for bleeding.

Precautions and Contraindications. There is no absolute contraindication to the use of glucagon. Because of its life-saving potential in the treatment of severe insulin reactions, it is recommended for use even when the diagnosis of hypoglycemia is not firmly established. Prompt recognition of failure to respond to the drug is important, however, so that other treatment can be instituted. If the client is not conscious and cooperative after the first 30 minutes of glucagon treatment, IV dextrose is needed.

■ SUMMARY

Glucagon is a natural hormone secreted by the pancreas that mobilizes body stores of nutrient energy (ie, glycogen). Administered by injection, it causes a rapid but transitory hyperglycemia and is used most often for treating acute hypoglycemia.

❖ NURSING MANAGEMENT: CLIENT RECEIVING GLUCAGON

Because glucagon is generally reserved for use when sugar cannot be administered to terminate a hypoglycemic reaction, it is often given without the explicit consent of clients and sometimes in opposition to their immediate wishes. When a client is unconscious, the drug is clearly indicated as an emergency measure to terminate the coma. Questions of legal liability arise when the hypoglycemic client resists treatment. Because glucose deficiency impairs brain function, the client is subject to a temporary delirium and is truly mentally incompetent, but there is no time to establish this in any legal sense. Hypoglycemia is a medical emergency; treatment must be carried out quickly to prevent permanent brain damage. The safest course is immediate administration of glucagon, by force if necessary. This action poses a legal risk for the nurse, who may be accused of assault and battery if such a course is adopted. Clients who habitually exhibit resistive behavior while hypoglycemic (or their families) should be asked to sign a statement granting prior permission for treatment in such situations. This provides a measure of legal protection for healthcare personnel.

When forcible administration of medications is necessary for the client's safety, sufficient personnel should be mobilized to nullify resistance and prevent or limit conflict. A show of strength may prevent a physical struggle, which could cause serious injury to the client or staff. The staff should maintain an attitude of concern and helpfulness throughout the procedure. Successful treatment for the client is usually followed by a return to rational behavior.

NURSING PROCESS

ASSESSMENT

Glucagon is administered only when a client with acute hypoglycemia does not respond to or cannot be given oral carbohydrates. Diabetic clients who receive insulin or oral hypoglycemics and other clients with excess insulin secretion (eg, insulin-secreting tumors) should be monitored for signs and symptoms of low blood glucose: sympathoadrenal activity (apprehension, tachycardia, tremor, weakness, perspiration), bizarre behavior, and headache. Blood glucose levels may be tested by finger stick; a blood level of less than 60 mg/dL indicates hypoglycemia. However, the absolute blood level is not always a reliable indicator of the client's physiologic state. Treatment should not be delayed if blood glucose cannot be tested promptly, or if a normal level is inconsistent with the clinical picture. A client accustomed to an abnormally high blood glucose level may experience a hypoglycemic reaction while the blood glucose level is still in the high-normal range; a person who has become accustomed to a very low blood glucose level may appear, and be, normal with blood glucose levels below the normal range. The speed of decline seems to precipitate the reaction.

NURSING DIAGNOSIS

Nursing diagnoses likely in clients receiving glucagon include:

- Altered Thought Processes, related to hypoglycemia secondary to insulin or sulfonylurea toxicity (unusual exercise, fasting)
- Pain, related to altered comfort from headache (perspiration, apprehension) secondary to hypoglycemia resulting from insulin or sulfonylurea toxicity (unusual exercise, fasting)

PLANNING

The goal of nursing care is to eliminate the signs and symptoms of hypoglycemia by restoring and maintaining a normal blood glucose level.

INTERVENTION

If the client is conscious and cooperative, food containing sugar should be given orally. Skim milk, sweetened orange juice, hard candy (not chocolate), glucose, or sugar cubes are usually effective. Some practitioners believe that placing sugar or glucose gel under the tongue is therapeutic, through absorption from the mucous membrane. If this is done, the client should be positioned to prevent aspiration. As soon as the acute symptoms subside and the client is more comfortable, food should be given to prevent recurrent hypoglycemia.

If oral administration of carbohydrates is impossible or ineffective, glucagon should be administered. The medication must be reconstituted, using the diluent supplied in the package. The usual adult dosage is 0.5 to 1 mg (0.5–1 U) administered by IM or IV injection.

After glucagon is administered, the client should be monitored carefully for response to the drug. A return to consciousness or rational behavior may occur quickly. If response is inadequate or incomplete at the end of 20 minutes, a second dose should be administered. At the same time, preparations should be made for administration of IV dextrose in the event the second dose is also ineffective. If such treatment is unavailable, emergency medical care should be summoned immediately. No more than two doses of glucagon should be given for a single incident because response to further doses is unlikely. Such clients probably have little or no stored glycogen for the hormone to mobilize, and alternative treatment is imperative.

After response to glucagon therapy, the client should be fed promptly, because the effects of glucagon usually dissipate within 1 hour and hypoglycemia is likely to recur. The kind and time of feedings depend on the cause of the hypoglycemia. If the client is receiving exogenous insulin, a combination of sugar and starches, such as bread and jelly, is administered to provide quickly assimilable sugar and more slowly metabolized caloric nutrients. If the insulin has a prolonged action, a protein food may also be needed to provide material for glucose formation over a longer period. Clients who suffer from reactive hypoglycemia (inappropriate surges of endogenous insulin secretion) should not be given sugar because it tends to stimulate repeated insulin hypersecretion. Some starch with protein (food such as bread and meat, cheese, or peanut butter) is more appropriate.

Clients who suffer from insulin-secreting tumors require feedings at short intervals around the clock to maintain blood glucose levels. In this condition, insulin secretion is maintained at a steady high rate, relatively independent of nutrient intake. Each feeding should include rapidly assimilable sugars as well as more slowly metabolized caloric nutrients. Because feedings may be required as often as every 2 hours, these clients may experience sleep deprivation unless rest periods are provided during the day.

Client Education. Glucagon is used mainly to treat emergency situations. Because careful medical supervision is needed by clients subject to severe insulin reactions, the drug is not generally prescribed for use in the home by laypeople. Glucagon could be useful, however, for controlling rapidly developing hypoglycemia characteristic of IDDM. Relatives of insulin-dependent diabetics often learn to administer insulin injections; they could also manage glucagon therapy when necessary. Use of glucagon in the home could provide another resource in the therapeutic program and could possibly prevent serious CNS damage during the interval required for emergency medical care to reach the client's home.

Clients who experience rapidly developing hypoglycemic reactions may have no memory of the episodes. Because brain function is impaired at the onset of the incident, they are aware only of a lapse in time followed by waking up in the midst of physical ministrations by healthcare personnel. The nature of these episodes must be explained to the client and the importance of preventive measures stressed.

Clients with secreting tumors may have difficulty accepting the reality of their illness. The high insulin levels, combined with some degree of overnutrition, promote anabolism, including muscle hypertrophy. These clients feel and look healthy. With no conscious recollection of the hypoglycemic attacks, their subjective perception does nothing to validate the information healthcare personnel give them about their condition. To ensure active participation in treatment, the nurse must convince these clients that their illness is both real and serious; in fact, some of these tumors are malignant.

OUTCOME EVALUATION

Data indicating successful interventions include resolution of the hypoglycemia (return to consciousness, reduction of sympathoadrenal activity, resumption of normal behavior), increased blood glucose level, reports by the client that the headache and apprehension have ceased, and reports that he or she feels better.

❖ **CHECKLIST OF NURSING ACTIONS**

When Hypoglycemia Cannot Be Treated by Oral Sugar

- ❑ Administer 1 U of glucagon IM immediately.
- ❑ Monitor for response to the drug.
- ❑ After 20 minutes, administer a second dose of glucagon if response is incomplete or inadequate. Immediately prepare for administration of IV dextrose, or summon emergency personnel who can do so.

After the Client Responds to Glucagon

- ❑ Promptly administer oral feedings appropriate to the type of hypoglycemia.
- ❑ Monitor blood levels of glucose.
- ❑ Assess for CNS impairment.

When Glucagon is Prescribed

- ❑ Explore with clients their perceptions of the hypoglycemic episodes, explaining and clarifying as necessary.

When Clients' Past Behavior (While Hypoglycemic) in the Past Has Made Medication Difficult

- ❑ Obtain from clients (or their families) prior written consent for glucagon therapy despite resistance.

Miscellaneous Hyperglycemic Agents

Certain other drugs also act to elevate blood glucose levels. Many therapeutic agents cause hyperglycemia as a side effect. Of these, diazoxide and phenytoin have been prescribed therapeutically to control hypoglycemia caused by inappropriate endogenous insulin secretion. Both agents inhibit the secretion of insulin. Diazoxide also stimulates endogenous catecholamines, which further elevate serum glucose levels. These drugs are sometimes helpful in controlling hypoglycemia in clients with insulin-secreting tumors. (For more information on diazoxide, see Chap. 25; for phenytoin, see Chap. 19.)

Bibliography

Arbour R. (1994). Action stat! Acute hypoglycemia. *Nursing '94, 24*(1), 33.

*Atkinson MA, Maclaren NK. (1990). What causes diabetes? *Scientific American, 263*, 62–70.

Campbell PJ, Carlson MG. (1993). Impact of obesity on insulin action in NIDDM. *Diabetes, 42*, 405–410.

Clinical news: Diet's role in tight glucose control. (1993). *AJN, 93*(Dec), 10.

Clinical news: Restoring lost hypoglycemia awareness. (1994). *AJN, 94*(Nov), 10.

Cohen MR. (1994). Drug alert: Suffixes aren't afterthoughts. *Nursing '94, 24*(Oct), 15.

Deakins DA. (1994). Teaching elderly patients about diabetes. *AJN, 94*(Apr), 39.

Drug watch: Intranasal insulin plus lecithin: rapid action, fewer side effects. (1994). *AJN, 94*(Feb), 52.

*Kestel F. (1994). Are you up to date on diabetes medications? *AJN, 94*(Jul), 48–52.

Orci L, Vassalli J, Perrelet A. (1988). The insulin factory. *Scientific American, 259*, 85–94.

*Parker C. (1994). Emergency! Responding quickly to hypoglycemia. *AJN, 94*(Jun), 46.

Porterfield LM. (1994). What's new in drugs: Problem Rx; evaluating elevated blood sugar in diabetic patients. *RN, 57*(Nov), 87.

Porterfield LM. (1995). Drug news: Diabetics may benefit from longer-lasting form of glipizide. *RN, 58*(Feb), 79.

Swithers C. (1994). Avoiding hypoglycemia. *Nursing '94, 24*(Apr), 4–6.

Weakland BS. (1993). Administering insulin through an indwelling catheter. *Nursing '93, 23*(Nov), 58–61.

*Recommended for further reading.

For more information and sample tests and activities, refer to Chapter 32 in the Student Workbook for Clinical Pharmacology and Nursing Management, 5th edition, available through your bookstore.

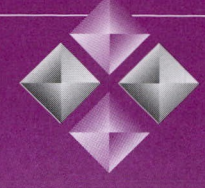

33

Drugs That Affect the Thyroid, Parathyroid, Pituitary, and Hypothalamic Glands

The hormones discussed in this chapter are proteins, polypeptides, or amino acid derivatives. Many protein hormones do not enter the nuclei of target cells but occupy receptors on the cell membrane. The hormone/receptor complex then influences enzyme action in the cytoplasm, altering the synthesis of intracellular messenger proteins or the uptake of substances from the extracellular fluid (see Fig. 32-1 on p. 680).

Physiology

Several related hormones, known as thyroid hormones, produced by the thyroid gland greatly affect body metabolism and energy production. Formed in the body by the conjugation of iodine and two molecules of tyrosine, these hormones are similar in structure and in their effects on the body. Iodinated thyroid hormones stimulate energy production, influence water and electrolyte balance, and promote cell differentiation and tissue growth. They also sensitize the central nervous system (CNS) and the heart.

Pathophysiology

Disorders caused by thyroid hormone imbalance are fairly common. Hyperthyroidism often affects young adults, causing signs and symptoms that reflect the stimulant properties of the hormones. Metabolism speeds up, causing nervousness, restlessness, and weight loss despite increased food intake. Body temperature rises and perspiration increases. Thyroid disorders are associated with enlargement of the gland (goiter).

Prolonged thyroid hormone deficiency in adults (myxedema) is less common than excess. Thyroid deficiency slows mental and physical processes, causing lethargy, sluggishness, weakening of the heart, memory defects, weight gain, dry skin, and intolerance to cold. Children who lack adequate thyroid hormone cannot develop normally. Without treatment, they become mentally retarded dwarfs (cretins).

High blood levels of dioxin in newborns are associated with disruptions of thyroid balance characterized by increased concentrations of thyroid-stimulating hormone (TSH, also known as thyrotropin) and thyroxine or T_4 (Adler, 1993).

Thyroid Hormone and Drugs Affecting Thyroid Function

Among the drugs affecting thyroid balance and function are iodinated thyroid hormones, iodine, and thyroid-stimulating hormone (TSH).

Iodinated Thyroid Hormones

In some respects, the iodinated hormones resemble steroids more closely than protein hormones. Like most steroids, thyroid hormone is not destroyed by the digestive process and is fully effective when taken orally. Its actions are not limited to cell membrane or cytoplasmic sites but involve some interaction with cell nuclei.

Pharmacodynamics. Thyroid hormones enter the nuclei of many cells, binding to certain sites where they influence cell function programmed in the genetic code. They stimulate production of many enzymes that affect protein synthesis. As a result, they promote cell differentiation and tissue growth throughout the body, including the brain.

Thyroid hormones increase the basal metabolic rate of all body cells. Energy use rises, with a pronounced increase in heat production. This effect may be influenced by the mitochondria; thyroid-binding sites have been described in these structures. Thyroid hormones enhance fat breakdown associated with catecholamines and other catabolic hormone actions. (See Chap. 16 for information on catecholamines.) They stimulate conversion of cholesterol to bile acids and increase the metabolic rate of carbohydrates for the production of energy. Both nervous and cardiac tissues become more responsive to other stimuli, such as catecholamines and xanthines (eg, caffeine).

Thyroid hormone inhibits pituitary production of TSH. This negative feedback system tends to keep thyroid hormone at normal levels in the body. Exogenous hormones also inhibit pituitary TSH and can cause atrophy of the thyroid gland.

Pharmacokinetics. Thyroid hormones are absorbed from the gastrointestinal (GI) tract in sufficient quantities to be clinically effective. Intestinal absorption can vary, and part of each dose is lost in feces. Parenteral forms of thyroid hormone may be administered subcutaneously (SC), intramuscularly (IM), or intravenously (IV). After absorption, regardless of the route of administration, the drugs remain latent for a while before effects are seen. Onset of action requires hours to days; peak effect occurs only after weeks or months of treatment. The drugs tend to be cumulative, and their effects persist for some time after administration stops.

After entering the circulation, the hormones bind to certain plasma proteins and are distributed widely throughout the body. Less than 1% circulates in the free state, but this small proportion is responsible for the hormone's physiologic effects. Certain factors can alter thyroid binding and the proportion of free hormone. For example, estrogen therapy or pregnancy raises the concentration of T_4-binding globulin and tends to lower the concentration of free hormone. The body responds by increasing thyrotropin secretion and stimulating thyroid secretion. The net effects include enlargement of the thyroid gland and increases in total and bound T_4 (the concentration of free T_4 remains relatively normal).

Thyroid hormone is degraded mainly in the liver by conjugation with glucuronic and sulfuric acids. These metabolites enter the enterohepatic circulation, where 60% to 80% of them are hydrolyzed and reabsorbed; the remainder is eliminated in feces.

Therapeutic Uses. Thyroid hormone is used for replacement in deficiency states, to prevent and treat cretinism and to correct myxedema. The drug is administered to clients with iatrogenic hypothyroidism caused by surgical removal of the thyroid or the pituitary gland or the destruction of these glands by radiation. Clients with mild hypothyroidism may benefit from treatment, and the hormones are also occasionally used for simple goiter that does not respond to iodine therapy. Except in myxedema coma, when the hormones are administered IV, thyroid hormone is usually administered orally. In severe deficiency, the initial dose is small to prevent a sudden rise in metabolism, which can be dangerous. Full doses are usually attained by 2 to 4 weeks. Significant response may not be observed for weeks, and maximal effect develops over months.

In the past, thyroid hormones were used to treat obesity, but this treatment is no longer considered good medical practice. Only when the obese client shows other signs and symptoms of hypothyroidism is thyroid hormone therapy indicated. The use of thyroid combined with such medications as digitalis and amphetamines in weight-reduction regimens is dangerous and has produced fatalities, usually from cardiac complications.

Levothyroxine (L-thyroxine) has been used as an adjunct to diet therapy to decrease elevated serum cholesterol and low-density lipoprotein concentrations in treating primary hyperlipoproteinemia. It exerts a pronounced hypocholesterolemic effect with less metabolic stimulation than other thyroxine preparations.

Drug Preparations. The first thyroid hormone used medicinally was made from dried animal thyroid glands. Taken orally, this drug effectively treated thyroid deficiencies for nearly a century. Refined and synthetic preparations have been developed that provide greater uniformity of dosage with decreased antigenicity (Table 33-1). The standard for measuring the strength of thyroid preparations is iodine content. Some preparations are also subject to bioassay and chromatographic analysis to ensure metabolic potency.

Table 33-1. Thyroid Hormone Preparations

Drug Name	Preparation	Usual Adult Dosage
levothyroxine sodium (Eltroxin, Synthroid, Levothroid, Levoxine)	Synthetic salt from the natural isomer of L-thyroxine (T_4) for oral use or injection	50–400 μg daily depending on client requirements; for children, 8 μg/kg/day PC: A
liothyronine sodium (Cytomel)	Synthetic salt of L-triiodothyronine (T_3) for oral use	25–75 μg daily PC: A
liotrix (Euthroid, Thyrolar)	Mixtures of sodium salts of T_3 and T_4 (a pure mixture that resembles the natural secretion) for oral use	60–180 mg thyroid equivalent daily PC: A
thyroglobin (Proloid)	Extract from porcine thyroids for oral use	60–200 mg daily PC: A
thyroid (S-P-T, Thyrar, Thyroid P.D., Thyroid Strong, Thyro-Teric, Westhroid)	Crude animal glands prepared by defatting and drying with alcohol for oral use	15–180 mg daily PC: A

KEY: PC = pregnancy risk category; see Appendix A.

Adverse Reactions. Toxic effects of the hormones mimic the signs and symptoms of endogenous hyperthyroidism, as seen in toxic goiter. The skin is flushed, warm, and moist. Heat tolerance declines. Muscle fatigability and tremor develop. Blood pressure, pulse rate, and pulse pressure rise, and the heart beats more forcefully. Appetite increases, but the client tends to lose weight despite increased food intake. The client experiences increased alertness, difficulty in sleeping, nervousness, and mood swings. Increased GI motility may cause diarrhea. Blood glucose levels rise, and serum cholesterol levels drop. Women may experience menstrual irregularity. In severe toxicity, mental disturbances, cerebrovascular hemorrhage, or congestive heart failure (CHF) may develop. Long-term L-thyroxine treatment is associated with decreased bone mass in menopausal and premenopausal women.

Signs and symptoms of mild thyrotoxicosis have been reported after the consumption of ground beef that contains bovine thyroid tissue. Toxic reactions to thyroid hormone resolve slowly over several weeks because the body stores large hormone reserves in tissue depots.

Some thyroid preparations contain yellow dye No. 5 (tartrazine), which can trigger allergic reactions.

Drug Interactions. Phenytoin affects thyroid hormone therapy by increasing the breakdown of triiodothyronine (T_3) and T_4, reducing the effect of the hormone drugs as much as 50%. Lovastatin also increases the elimination of thyroid hormone and, additionally, interferes with its absorption. Thyroid dosages must be increased when either of these drugs is given concurrently with thyroid medication.

Therapeutic doses of thyroid hormones enhance the physiologic effects of warfarin anticoagulants, apparently by increasing the breakdown of vitamin K-dependent clotting factors. The risk of bleeding increases, and anticoagulant drug dosages may have to be reduced. The hormones increase the insulin or oral hypoglycemic requirements of diabetics, and diabetes mellitus may first appear during thyroid hormone therapy. Thyroid hormone also increases the severity of hypoadrenalism and may cause an acute addisonian crisis in cortisone-deficient clients.

Precautions and Contraindications. Thyroid hormone is contraindicated in clients with normal or excessive endogenous thyroid hormone production and in clients who have had myocardial infarction and uncorrected adrenal insufficiency. Thyroid hormones are not recommended for treating obesity in the absence of other signs of thyroid deficiency. Caution must be exercised when the hormones are administered to clients with a history of hypertension or cardiac disease. Clients who require warfarin anticoagulant or catecholamine therapy must be monitored closely and generally receive reduced doses of these drugs when thyroid hormones are administered concurrently, because the effects of these drugs are potentiated by thyroid therapy. Diabetics who receive thyroid hormones require close monitoring of glucose balance and may need increased doses of hypoglycemic medications.

Thyroid therapy is started with small doses that are gradually increased over 2 to 4 weeks or more, especially in severe deficiencies, because sensitivity to the hormone is pronounced and the usual therapeutic doses are not well tolerated. Dosages for elderly clients are usually lower because the need for thyroid hormone appears to decrease with age.

Hormone replacement should be avoided if possible after partial thyroidectomy. Some degree of hypothyroidism is likely, but this often subsides as the remaining gland enlarges under the influence of pituitary thyrotropin. Administering thyroid hormone inhibits this pituitary response.

■ SUMMARY

Thyroid hormones stimulate metabolism and promote growth and development. Drug preparations of the hormones are used for replacement therapy. They are administered orally over long periods of time. Response to treatment is slow, requiring weeks to months for full effect to appear. The drug is cumulative, and toxic states tend to resolve slowly. The signs and symptoms of toxicity include hyperactivity, muscle tremor, nervousness, intolerance to heat, and hypertensive cardiovascular disease.

Antithyroid Drugs

Substances that inhibit the production and use of thyroid hormone include propylthiouracil and related thioamide compounds, and goitrogenic substances in water, food, and drugs. Chemicals may oppose or block the effects of thyroid hormone by reducing thyrotropin stimulation of the thyroid, interfering with thyroid hormone synthesis, blocking the release of thyroid hormone into the general circulation, altering the proportion of very active and less active forms of the hormone, or reducing their use by peripheral tissues.

Most antithyroid chemicals exert their action directly on the thyroid gland. They cause levels of thyroid hormone to drop; subsequently, pituitary production of thyrotropin increases. As thyrotropin levels rise, the thyroid enlarges, becomes more vascular, and increases its hormone production. A visible enlargement of the gland (goiter) develops. The increase in hormone production may be sufficient to maintain a euthyroid state (a state of balance), or some degree of hypothyroidism may occur. Whether or not the client becomes deficient in thyroid hormone, the gland may become large enough to be disfiguring and to exert pressure on the esophagus and trachea, causing difficulty in swallowing and breathing. These effects may occur secondary to dietary intake of goitrogens or as side effects of drug therapy for non–thyroid-related disease. A few antithyroid compounds stimulate autoimmune thyroiditis. All these agents tend to reduce the physiologic effects of thyroid hormone (Box 33-1).

Thioamides

Thioamide antithyroid drugs used medicinally include methimazole and propylthiouracil.

Pharmacodynamics. Thioamides reduce the formation of thyroid hormones. They interfere with the linking of iodine with tyrosyl residues of thyroglobulin and inhibit the coupling of these iodotyrosyl residues to form iodothyronine. In addition, propylthiouracil appears to reduce conversion of T_4 to the more potent T_3 by body tissues.

Box 33-1
Sources of Goitrogenic Substances

Foods

Foods that contain flavinoid pigments (red, yellow, blue)

Cabbage, turnips, rutabagas, peas, spinach, carrots, radishes

Soybeans, peanuts

Strawberries, peaches

Kale and milk from kale-fed cattle

Millet, especially cooked millet that has been stored for prolonged periods before consumption

Contaminants in Drinking Water

Resorcinol

Phthalates (which are converted by bacteria to dihydroxybenzoic acids)

Methoxyanthracene and bromoform (which stimulate autoimmune thyroiditis)

Drugs

Resorcinol, phenylbutazone, thiopental, dimercaptol, lithium

Analine derivatives (sulfonamides and salicylates)

Thioamides (methimazole and propylthiouracil)

Pharmacokinetics. Thioamide drugs are well absorbed by the GI tract. They are concentrated in the thyroid gland, their target tissues. They cross the placenta and are secreted in breast milk. Although the drugs act promptly, clinical response is not evident for a few days to 2 weeks or more. Only when body stores of thyroid hormones have become depleted over time do signs and symptoms of hyperthyroidism subside. Duration of action varies with half-life and dosage (Table 33-2). Excretion of the drugs and their metabolites is mainly by the kidneys.

Therapeutic Uses. Thioamides are used to treat and control hyperthyroidism. Administered alone over several months, they help maintain a normal metabolism until the natural course of the disease can produce a spontaneous remission. They also are used with radioactive iodine therapy to reduce thyroid toxicity, which can reach high levels when the damaged thyroid tissue is reabsorbed. Antithyroid treatment before thyroid surgery minimizes hormone toxicity and reduces the surgical risks posed by the toxic state. The drugs are also useful in treating thyroid crisis, an acute and severe form of hyperthyroidism. Because of its additional peripheral action, propylthiouracil is the drug of choice for this condition.

Table 33-2. Antithyroid Thioamides

Drug Name	Preparation	Usual Dosage
methimazole (Tapazole)	Oral tablets	Adults: Initial: 15–60 mg/day, divided in 3 doses, administered q8h (depending on degree of thyroid toxicity); maintenance (after about 2 months of therapy): 5–30 mg/day Children: Initial: 0.4 mg/kg/day; maintenance: 0.2 mg/kg/day PC: D
propylthiouracil (Propyl-Thyracil)	Oral tablets	Adults: Initial: 300–1200 mg/day, divided in 3–6 doses, administered q4–8h (depending on degree of thyroid toxicity); maintenance: (after about 2 months of therapy) 100–150 mg/day Neonates: 5–10 mg/kg/day Children 6–10 yr: Initial: 50–150 mg/day Children 10 yr and older: Initial: 150–300 mg/day or 150 mg/m^2 body surface Maintenance dosage in children depends on response to therapy PC: D

KEY: PC = pregnancy category; see Appendix A.

Drug Preparations. Propylthiouracil and methimazole (Tapazole) are the chief antithyroid drugs used in the United States. They are marketed only as oral tablets. Carbimazole, which is widely used in Great Britain, is converted by body metabolism to methimazole.

Adverse Reactions. Antithyroid drugs used to treat hyperthyroidism are relatively safe. The overall incidence of side effects varies from 3% to 7%. The most common reaction is skin rash, either a mild papular rash or urticaria. Sometimes purpura and pruritus are features of the skin reaction. Skin complications often subside spontaneously, whether or not the drug is withdrawn. Other side effects include nausea, vomiting, nasal stuffiness, epigastric distress, arthralgia, myalgia, paresthesia, headache, drowsiness, neuritis, vertigo, hair loss, and fading of skin pigmentation. Rarely, drug fever, hepatitis, and nephritis occur.

The most serious (but rare) complication of antithyroid therapy is agranulocytosis. When the condition is diagnosed early and the drug discontinued, recovery is usually spontaneous and complete.

Thioamide therapy tends to increase the vascularity and friability of the thyroid gland, an undesirable effect in clients about to have surgery. Propylthiouracil further increases the risk of hemorrhage by causing prothrombin deficiency.

High doses of antithyroid drugs can cause hypothyroidism.

Drug Interactions. Propylthiouracil increases the effects of warfarin anticoagulants. Phenylbutazone, thiopental, lithium, sulfonamides, and salicylates may increase the effects of thioamides.

Precautions and Contraindications. Thioamide drugs are contraindicated during lactation and pregnancy. The drugs cross the placenta and suppress thyroid function in the fetus. They also are secreted in breast milk. During gestation and for some time after birth, the brain normally grows rapidly. Thyroid deficiency during this critical stage of development causes retardation and permanently impairs intellectual capacity. When thioamide therapy must be given to a pregnant woman, thyroid hormone is also administered to prevent hormone deficiency in her and in the fetus.

Women who receive thioamide drugs must not breast-feed their infants.

When skin eruptions caused by the drugs do not subside with continued therapy, the drug should be discontinued and a different antithyroid preparation prescribed. This switch is usually effective because cross-sensitivity is uncommon.

The development of agranulocytosis requires immediate drug withdrawal. This reaction usually develops during the first few months of treatment.

Clients who have received thioamide drugs before surgical thyroidectomy are given iodine for 10 days to 2 weeks preoperatively to decrease the vascularity and friability of the gland caused by such treatment.

▪ SUMMARY

Several chemicals found in drugs and foods inhibit the synthesis of thyroid hormone and cause enlargement of the thyroid gland (goiter). Of these, thioamides (propylthiouracil and methimazole) are used therapeutically to treat hyperthyroid disease. When administered orally over long periods, they control toxic symptoms and restore normal metabolism. Excessive dosage can cause hypothyroidism. An infrequent but serious side effect of thioamide therapy is agranulocytosis, which requires immediate withdrawal of the drug.

Iodine

Iodine is an essential nutrient for proper thyroid function. When there is a deficiency of this mineral, the thyroid gland lacks materials to produce the usual amount of hormone. Low thyroid levels stimulate pituitary production of thyrotropin. As thyrotropin levels rise, the thyroid gland enlarges to produce more hormone, a condition known as simple goiter.

Goiter is prevalent in certain areas, mainly inland upland areas (mountains or high plateaus). The soil in these "goiter belts" is subject to the leaching action of rain and fresh water drainage and tends to be deficient in trace minerals, including iodine. (Pollutants from coal mines may include several antithyroid compounds that add to this effect.) The crops and animals in such areas are low in iodine content, and both animal and human populations tend to develop thyroid malfunction. The incidence of goiter rises unless supplementary iodine is provided in the diet. Other thyroid diseases (thyrotoxicosis, myxedema, and cretinism) also develop more frequently in people who do not ingest enough iodine.

To be nutritionally complete, the diet must contain sufficient iodine to meet the thyroid's need for hormone production. A daily dose of 35 to 150 μg is required, depending on the client's age, sex, and condition. Infants need the lowest amounts, followed by nongravid women, and men, in that order. Pregnant and lactating women need the highest amounts of iodine. The mineral is found in abundance in salt-water fish, seaweed, and vegetables grown in iodine-rich soils (generally near the seacoast). Adding iodine to the diet helps reduce the incidence of thyroid disease associated with deficiencies of this mineral. In the United States, the government subsidizes the addition of iodine to table salt. Since iodized salt has become widely available at the same cost as plain salt, simple goiter and cretinism have become rare in the United States.

Pharmacodynamics. Iodine not only provides a building block for thyroid hormone production but also promotes storage of this hormone and may antagonize the stimulating effect of thyrotropin on the gland. During iodine therapy, the follicular storage depots become saturated with hormone, excesses are released into the circulation, and blood levels return to a more normal level. In simple goiter, providing iodine in low doses is sufficient to correct the nutritional deficiency and restore thyroid hormone production to normal levels. The usual negative feedback mechanism that controls thyrotropin production is restored. Thyrotropin levels drop and the thyroid gland shrinks.

In large doses, iodine has different effects. When plasma concentrations approach 100 times the normal levels and intracellular levels of the mineral reach a critical level, most thyroid gland activities decrease. The rate of iodide trapping drops, the rate of thyroid hormone formation declines, the secretory activities of the thyroid cells decrease, and the rate of thyroid release from the gland drops. It is thought that some of these effects result from direct inhibition of the thyroid-stimulating effects of thyrotropin, but this remains unproven. Some of the effects subside after a few weeks. Circulating hormone levels rise when the storage depots of the thyroid follicles become saturated. Nevertheless, continued administration of high doses of iodine produces thyroid enlargement similar to the goiters caused by lack of iodine and by other thyroid inhibitors.

Pharmacokinetics. Iodine is well absorbed as iodides in the GI tract. It is taken up rapidly by the thyroid gland. Iodine is used to produce thyroid hormone molecules. It is stored for a time and is eventually secreted into the circulation. When the hormone is degraded, a portion of the iodine is reused by the thyroid. The remainder, with other excess iodide, is eliminated by the kidneys.

Therapeutic Uses. Iodine in small doses is used to supplement dietary sources in geographic areas where the soil is deficient in this mineral. Medicinal iodine preparations may be prescribed to treat simple goiter caused by dietary deficiency. To prevent this condition, the use of iodized salt is inexpensive and convenient. It is the most effective approach from a public health standpoint.

In treating thyroid disorders, iodine is prescribed before surgery on the gland to reduce thyrotoxicity and the size of the gland. Usually Lugol's solution or saturated solution of potassium iodide is prescribed for 10 days before the date of surgery. The inhibitory effect of the mineral on the thyroid peaks at the end of 10 days to 2 weeks. At this time, thyrotoxicity is at its lowest, and the gland is smallest and least vascular and friable. If surgery is delayed more than 2 weeks after iodine therapy is started, the effects decline; blood levels of thyroid hormone rise to, and often above, previous levels. The beneficial effects of iodine are lost, and the client may be at greater risk for toxicity than before treatment.

Before the development of thioamide drugs, iodine was the only drug available to decrease the severity of thyrotoxicity before thyroidectomy. Although improvement in the client's metabolic state was apparent, toxicity was not eliminated, nor was metabolism restored to normal. Surgery remained hazardous. Present treatment, which combines thioamide and iodine medication, greatly lowers toxicity before surgery. In most cases, a nearly normal metabolic state can be achieved, significantly reducing the risks of this type of surgery.

Iodides are also useful in treating thyroid crisis (thyroid storm, a sudden, life-threatening rise in thyroid toxicity). They are administered in combination with thioamides, propranolol, and other drugs as needed to stabilize the client's condition (Table 33-3).

Table 33-3. Selected Iodine Preparations

Drug Name	Preparation	Medicinal Use	Usual Adult Dosage
Iodized salt	1 part sodium or potassium iodine per 10,000 parts salt	Prevention of goiter	Add to food as ordinary salt
potassium iodine (Pima syrup, Iosol, Thyro-Block)	Solution (325 mg/5 mL or 1 g/mL)	Treatment of Graves' disease	60 mg tid
(Iosat, Thyro-Block)	Oral tablets	Prevention of thyroid irradiation during radiation emergencies	130 mg daily (children younger than 1 year: 65 mg daily; children older than 1 year: 130 mg daily) PC: D
strong iodine solution (Lugol's solution, compound iodine solution)	Iodine (50 mg/mL) and potassium iodine (100 mg/mL) in aqueous solution for oral administration	Induction of thyroid involution before surgery on the glands; treatment of thyroid storm; control of hyperthyroidism	3–5 drops q8h Neonates: 1 drop q8h PC: D
saturated solution of potassium iodide (SSKI)	Solution that contains potassium iodide 1 g/mL	Control of hyperthyroidism, induction of thyroid involution before surgery on the gland	50–100 mg daily or more, depending on client requirements PC: D
		Expectorant	300–600 mg, qid
iodinated glycerol (Iodrol, Iodur, Iophen, Organidin, R-Gen)	Oral solution that contains iodinated glycerol 60 mg per 5-mL dose	Expectorant	60 mg qid; dosage for children is half of this
tincture of iodine	Topical solution that contains 2% iodine and 2.4% sodium iodide in 46% ethyl alcohol	Topical antiseptic	Applied topically
povidone-iodine (Providine)	Detergent solutions, ointments, vaginal gel	Topical antiseptic	Strength and quantity vary with type of preparation
iopanoic acid (Telepaque)	Oral tablets that contain 500 mg of iopanoic acid	Radiopaque medium for cholecystography and cholangiography	3 g; for children, 50–150 mg/kg
diatrizoate sodium (Hypaque)	Solution and powder for preparing solutions for oral or rectal use Solution for injection Sterile solution for urogenital instillation	Radiopaque medium for various diagnostic procedures	Varies, depending on procedure and client requirements

KEY: PC = pregnancy category; see Appendix A.

Certain iodine compounds are used medicinally for other purposes. Iodine is a component of many antiseptics used for disinfecting utensils, linens, and the skin. Iodine salts are effective expectorants. They are occasionally used to promote resolution of granulomatous lesions, such as those that occur in leprosy, syphilis, and fungal infections. Iodine compounds are also contained in some contrast media for radiographic examinations (see Chapter 51). These uses are not pertinent to iodine's antihormone effects, except that clients who have been exposed to iodine in such situations may have become allergic to the element and therefore are at high risk for adverse reaction to any iodide therapy.

Adverse Reactions. Iodine administered orally is irritating to the gastric mucosa. The drug's expectorant properties are believed to derive in part from this property, which causes reflex stimulation of lung secretions. The drugs tend to produce anorexia, nausea and vomiting, diarrhea, and nasal congestion. Chronic adminis-

tration, especially in large doses, is associated with a metallic or brassy taste in the mouth, malaise, and depression. Allergy to iodine is not uncommon. Reactions may be immediate or delayed. Allergic effects include:

- Angioedema (anaphylaxis)
- Multiple skin hemorrhages or purpura
- Skin rash, including urticaria
- Reactions that resemble serum sickness with fever, arthralgia, lymph node enlargement, and eosinophilia
- Urticaria
- Thrombocytopenia
- Life-threatening periarteritis nodosa

Allergic reactions are more common and more serious with injected iodines.

Besides its role in treating thyroid disorders, iodine is used in germicides and in radiopaque contrast agents. Iodine poisoning requires immediate medical attention.

Activated charcoal may be administered to adsorb the chemical. The stomach is irrigated ("pumped out") to remove as much of the drug as possible before digestion can occur. Hospitalization is recommended to observe for and treat symptoms such as pulmonary edema and shock that arise from systemic absorption of toxic amounts. Iodine poisoning should be suspected when brown emesis has an odor of iodine. (Emesis may be tested for iodine by adding a small amount of starch, which turns blue when reacting with iodine.) Nausea, vomiting, diarrhea, burning sensations in the mouth and throat, thirst, and abdominal pain are further clues of iodine poisoning.

Precautions and Contraindications. Iodine therapy is hazardous to clients allergic to it. Adverse reactions are particularly likely when iodides are given by injection, as in diagnostic testing and imaging and in treating thyroid storm. When iodides are required for treatment despite a history of sensitivity, healthcare personnel must be prepared to treat allergic reactions, such as anaphylaxis, promptly and aggressively.

Because of their ability to break down granulomatous lesions, iodides are contraindicated in clients with a history of tuberculosis. Destruction of tubercles releases tubercle bacilli within the body and reactivates the infection.

Thyroid function must be monitored in any client who receives therapeutic doses of iodine over a period of time, because hypothyroidism is likely to develop. The use of supplemental iodine (even iodized salt) may be detrimental in some clients with acne, because iodine tends to aggravate this problem.

■ SUMMARY

Iodine is an essential nutrient required for normal thyroid function. In geographic areas where soils are deficient in this element, the use of iodized salt decreases the incidence of thyroid disease. Iodine and iodides are used medicinally as antiseptics, expectorants, and radiopaque contrast media, and in the prevention and treatment of thyroid disorders. The drugs are used to reduce thyroid toxicity and to reduce the size of the gland before thyroid surgery. Iodine is also used as one of several agents in treating acute thyroid toxicity. Allergic anaphylaxis, the most dangerous adverse reaction to drugs of this class, is most likely to occur when the drugs are administered by injection.

Radioactive Iodine

Radioactive iodine is produced by bombarding the element with high-velocity particles. The product of this process shares many properties with normal iodine but, in addition, emits nuclear particles, including alpha particles, beta particles, gamma rays, and conversion electrons. Because it can be measured easily and can be readily distinguished from normal iodine in the body, radioactive iodine is useful for diagnostic, therapeutic, and research purposes. In large therapeutic dosages, it delivers radiation to thyroid tissue without obvious damage to other body tissues.

Radioactivity is measured by the curie (Ci), a unit that indicates the rate at which a given number of atoms disintegrate in a given time. As in other metric scales, one thousandth of a curie is termed a millicurie (mCi); one millionth of a curie, a microcurie (μCi); and one trillionth of a curie, a picocurie (pCi).

Two radioactive isotopes of iodine are available for medicinal use (Table 33-4). Iodine-131 has been used most widely.

Pharmacodynamics. In small (tracer) doses, radioactive iodine has no detectable effect on cells or tissues. It can be traced by nuclear monitoring techniques for the study of physiologic processes by which iodine is used by the body. Radioactive iodine can also be used to monitor some aspects of thyroid function.

In large doses, radioactive iodine damages thyroid tissue by delivering toxic doses of gamma rays that have an effect similar to that of x-rays. In the thyroid gland, pyknosis and necrosis of the follicular cells develop. The colloid disappears and the gland becomes fibrous.

Pharmacokinetics. Radioactive iodine is handled by the body in exactly the same way as the nonradioactive element. It is concentrated by the thyroid, incorporated into thyroid hormone molecules, and stored in the gland follicles. Later, it is released to the tissues and eventually excreted in urine.

With a radiation half-life of about 8 days, the radioactivity of ^{131}I is 99% expended at the end of 56 days. Much of the drug is excreted from the body before that time. Half-life in the thyroid is normally 6 days and less in a hyperactive gland. Radioactive iodine may be administered orally or by IV injection.

Therapeutic Uses. Tracer doses of radioactive iodine (1–25 μCi) are used in diagnostic thyroid function evaluations. The amount of radioactive iodine that enters

Table 33-4. Radioactive Iodine Preparations			
Drug Name	Preparation	Half-Life	Type of Radiation
sodium iodide ^{131}I (Iodotope Therapeutic)	Solution for oral or IV administration; oral capsules	8 days	gamma rays,* beta particles
sodium iodide ^{123}I (for investigational use only)		13 hr	gamma rays*
*Similar in effect to x-rays.			

the thyroid gland (radioactive iodine uptake, or RAIU) provides an indirect measure of thyroid activity. A high RAIU is usually found in thyrotoxicity, a low RAIU in hypothyroidism. This test is inaccurate if iodine has been used in the diet or if antithyroid drugs have been taken for medicinal purposes, because further iodine uptake is suppressed by these substances.

The pattern of iodine uptake (and metabolic activity) is revealed by scanning the thyroid for radioactive emissions after the administration of a tracer dose of radioactive iodine. Metabolically active tissue shows up as "hot spots," inactive areas as "cold spots." Such areas often correspond to glandular lesions.

In therapeutic doses (1–200 mCi), radioactive iodine is used to treat thyrotoxicosis and selected thyroid cancers. Both normal and malignant thyroid cells are destroyed by the drug, provided they are active and capable of concentrating iodine.

When partial destruction of the gland is desired, as in thyroid toxicity, doses range from 4 to 10 mCi. These doses err on the low side to avoid excessive destruction of the gland and subsequent hypothyroidism. As a result, therapeutic response is delayed and tends to be incomplete. If required, a second or even third dose can be given at 3-month intervals. During the period before complete response to the drug, thioamide medication may be given to control symptoms of thyrotoxicity.

Radioactive iodine is a valuable treatment for thyroid toxicity in clients over age 50, especially those who are poor surgical risks, those with small glands or ectopic tissue, and those whose diseases recur after a course of antithyroid medication. Clients may receive ^{131}I as outpatients, avoiding the expense and trauma of surgery. The effect of radioactive iodine is fully evident about 8 to 10 weeks after administration.

Radioactive iodine is effective in treating thyroid cancer only when the malignant cells actively use iodine to produce hormone. Such tumors make up only a small fraction of thyroid neoplasms. However, when cancers are radiosensitive, the drug is effective in treating metastases as well as the primary lesion. Large doses (50–150 mCi) are required to treat cancerous lesions.

Radioactive iodine dosages are computed on the basis of gland size, RAIU, and the release rate of radioactive iodine from the gland. The amount of drug needed to deliver the required amount of irradiation varies with the age of the medicinal preparation, because nuclear disintegration continues during storage time. The drug loses half of its radioactivity for each half-life period that occurs after its manufacture. Therapeutic doses range from 7,000 to 10,000 rad/g of thyroid tissue.

Adverse Reactions. When used in tracer doses, radioactive iodine poses little radiation hazard. The dose of radiation is extremely low and of little physiologic significance. Like all exposure to radiation, however, this dose adds to the total accumulated during a lifetime and should be given only when a medical need exists.

Therapeutic treatment with radioactive iodine delivers toxic doses of radiation to the thyroid gland but appears to present a relatively low risk of damage to other body tissues. Concentration of the drug in the urinary tract can cause bladder inflammation. Exposure of other normal cells to radiation is inversely proportional to the square of their distances from the thyroid follicles in which iodine is stored. Theoretically, there is a risk of increased mutation in all exposed cells, and an increased risk of cancer at a future time. However, statistically significant increases in the incidence of cancer in throat structures have not been reported in the literature.

Adverse reactions to radioactive iodine may develop in clients allergic to iodine. Because the drug is usually administered orally, anaphylaxis is unlikely. Skin reactions have occurred, sometimes involving small isolated areas rather than a generalized rash. Although uncommon, tenderness and swelling of the thyroid gland have been reported. If swelling is severe, the trachea can be compressed. This symptom is more apt to occur with higher doses, as in cancer treatments.

The incidence of hypothyroidism 10 years after using radioactive iodine therapy is about 70% (Saha, 1992). In treating cancer, when high doses are administered, this symptom is probably an effect of the drug action. However, hypothyroidism in clients treated with lower dosages may be the normal final stage of thyroid disease. In Graves' disease, many authorities consider hypothyroidism to be the expected end result of the process, regardless of the method of treatment. The incidence of end-stage hypothyroidism in thyrotoxic clients who receive radioactive iodine does not correlate significantly with drug dosage.

Therapeutic use of ^{131}I could also cause a deficiency of calcitonin or parathormone.

Precautions and Contraindications. The use of radioactive substances, including radioactive iodine, is restricted to personnel with training and experience in the safe use and handling of radioactive pharmaceuticals. Radioactive therapy is available mainly in medical centers with departments of nuclear medicine. Special precautions are required to control radioactive emissions and to prevent harmful exposure of personnel and others to radiation hazards. Caution should be used if this drug is used for diagnosing or treating clients with a history of allergy to iodine. The healthcare team must be prepared to treat acute allergic reactions should they occur.

Because of the mutagenic and teratogenic potential of radioactive materials, therapeutic doses of radioactive iodine are relatively contraindicated for children and should be avoided in women of childbearing age. If radioactive drugs are used in lactating mothers, breast-feeding must be discontinued until the substances are eliminated from the body.

■ SUMMARY

Radioactive iodine is used to diagnose thyroid disease and to treat selected cases of hyperthyroidism and thyroid cancers. Tracer doses used for diagnostic studies are measured in microcuries and present no appreciable radiation hazard. Therapeutic (millicurie) doses deliver effective radiation to the thyroid gland without obvious damage to other body tissues. Because of the theoretical risk of genetic damage and malignant changes, the drug is not ordinarily used in these doses to treat children or women of childbearing age. Radioactive iodine treatment offers significant advantages in terms of safety and economy. Treatment does not involve hospitalization and often eliminates the need for thyroid surgery. The drug may cause allergic reactions in iodine-sensitive clients.

❖ NURSING MANAGEMENT: CLIENT RECEIVING THYROID DRUGS

Whenever drugs affecting thyroid balance or the function of the thyroid gland are prescribed, the client is likely to have a problem with hormone balance. Treatment is designed to correct the imbalance, but may overcorrect before the proper level is achieved. For this reason, assessment of thyroid hormone status must be ongoing. Nurses must recognize the signs and symptoms of thyroid imbalance so that clients may be referred for diagnosis and treatment (Table 33-5). For timely diagnosis and treatment, special attention should be given to early signs of imbalance.

Clients who show minimal signs and symptoms of thyroid imbalance, such as changes in body weight, may take measures to influence thyroid function and metabolism. Those who experience nervous tension and other signs and symptoms of hyperthyroidism should increase their consumption of foods that tend to inhibit thyroid secretion (see Box 33-1). They should stay warm and avoid chilling. Warm baths are recommended over showers. Clients who wish to increase thyroid function should avoid ingesting food, water, and drugs that contain goitrogens and should avoid overheating the body. Alternating hot and cold showers may stimulate thyroid secretion. Diet should be adequate in protein and iodine, but not excessively high in iodine.

Prompt diagnosis of thyroid deficiency in infants is particularly important, because even a short treatment delay results in some degree of permanent mental retardation. Blood tests for thyroid are the best screening procedure for infantile hypothyroidism, allowing diagnosis and treatment before brain damage occurs. Such tests are carried out routinely on all newborns in some medical centers. Nurses should support these programs and promote them where they have not been adopted. On the other end of the age spectrum, some elderly clients may require a higher level of serum T_4 and free thyroxine index (FT_4I) to sustain a euthyroid state.

When radioactive iodine is used in therapeutic settings, personnel and clients must be protected from undue exposure to radiation. Exposure is directly proportional to the time spent near the source of radiation and inversely proportional to the square of the distance from the source. Personnel who work regularly in departments of nuclear medicine are exposed repeatedly and must be trained in techniques to minimize exposure and reduce the hazard. Rubber gloves are worn when handling radioactive drugs, and special care should be exercised to avoid spilling medication. Monitoring devices (dosimeters or film badges) are carried by personnel at all times to measure exposure to radiation. The Nuclear Regulatory Commission considers maximum safe exposure levels to be 20 mrem/day, 100 mrem/week (0.1 rem), and 5 rem/year. Fetal expose must not exceed 550 mrem/year (Early and Sodes, 1995). Dosimeters are worn on clothing, where radiation is greatest. When exposure approaches maximum levels, personnel must be rotated to other areas of service until the designated period of time has elapsed.

Clients receiving radioactive substances may be quite fearful, as the toxic effects of radiation are well known, and the precautions taken to control exposure of personnel emphasizes the risk. Although the client who receives tracer doses of radioactive iodine runs little risk, the acknowledged aim of treatment with therapeutic doses is tissue destruction. Anyone receiving a radioactive medication needs considerable emotional support.

After administration of radioactive iodine, clients are generally not considered to be sources of dangerous radioactivity. When therapeutic doses are administered, radioactive iodine is excreted in urine. Dilution in a municipal sewage system provides adequate protection. Nevertheless, when clients are hospitalized for treatment, urinals and bedpans should be emptied promptly to eliminate this source of radiation from the immediate environment.

NURSING PROCESS: DRUG THERAPY IN HYPOTHYROIDISM

ASSESSMENT

In assessing clients for hypothyroidism (or goiter), the nurse reviews such risk factors as residence in inland upland regions (where soils are often deficient in iodine), exposure to groundwater pollutants, particularly from coal mines (resorcinol, phthalates, dihydroxybenzoic acids, methoxyanthracene, and bromoform), consumption of goitrogens, and a family history of thyroid disease.

The thyroid is palpated to determine the degree of enlargement, and the client is assessed for signs and symptoms of early hypothyroidism (see Table 33-5). When thyroid deficiency begins, its onset is subtle and

Table 33-5. Signs and Symptoms of Thyroid Imbalance

Degree of Imbalance	Hyperthyroidism	Hypothyroidism
Mild	Increased energy and alertness Increased bowel motility Nervousness, restlessness	Fatigue, muscle cramps Constipation Cold intolerance Paresthesias Memory deficits
Moderate	Insomnia, sense of nervous tension Weight loss despite increased food intake Abundant hair growth Increased peristalsis, diarrhea Increased body temperature with heat intolerance and perspiration Increased sensitivity to stimulant drugs, such as pressor amines and caffeine Onset or increased severity of diabetes mellitus Low serum cholesterol level Increased protein-bound iodine (PBI) Tachycardia and palpitations Hypertension, wide pulse pressure Dyspnea	Mental slowness, lethargy, sleepiness, slowed speech Weight gain despite loss of appetite and decreased intake Thinning of the hair; increased acne; dry, thickened, coarse skin Constipation and fecal impaction Continued cold intolerance Increased sensitivity to depressant drugs Increased insulin reactions in diabetics Hypercholesterolemia Decreased PBI values Decreased response to stress
Severe	Manic-type psychosis Cardiac enlargement or CHF, arrhythmias Cerebrovascular hemorrhage	Emotional depression; mental lethargy and apathy Slow, weak pulse Weakened cardiac contraction Enlarged tongue and periorbital edema (myxedematous facies), pretibial edema Occasionally, deafness

it may easily be overlooked. Infants deficient in thyroid hormone have puffy faces (especially around the eyes), excessive drooling, enlarged and protruding tongue, rough dry skin, coarse hair, potbelly, swayback, and an increased incidence of umbilical hernia.

Clients who receive thyroid replacement therapy should be assessed for therapeutic response and excess hormone levels as well as for deficiency.

Because some thyroid preparations contain tartrazine, clients should be questioned about allergic sensitivity to this substance. Any client with a history of asthma associated with nasal polyps and aspirin allergy is at high risk for adverse reaction to tartrazine. Serious reactions, such as anaphylaxis, may be difficult to treat because thyroid hormone alters the body's response to the drugs (cortisone and epinephrine) used in their treatment.

NURSING DIAGNOSIS

Nursing diagnoses for clients who receive thyroid hormone relate to the excessive hormone effects.

Many clients have:

- Knowledge Deficit, related to hypothyroidism and its treatment

A common collaborative problem that should be differentiated from the nursing diagnoses is:

Potential Complication: Cardiac failure

PLANNING

Goals for most clients who show signs and symptoms of hypothyroidism are proper diagnosis and treatment. For clients with goiter, the goals are to restore normal body appearance and enhance thyroid function. When hypothyroidism follows thyroid surgery or irradiation, the goal may be to stimulate gland function and avoid replacement hormone therapy. The goal for the client who receives hormone replacement therapy is to achieve or to remain in thyroid balance.

INTERVENTION

In iodine-poor areas, nurses should recommend using iodized salt. Case-finding and referral for treatment are critical and should be a priority, especially among nurses who provide primary health care. The client who exhibits signs and symptoms of thyroid deficiency should be referred to appropriate professionals for diagnosis.

The nursing needs of clients who receive thyroid hormone replacement therapy vary, depending on the degree of hypothyroidism. Severely deficient clients are at high risk for serious complications. In such instances, treatment begins in the hospital. The drugs may be administered IV, in which case only freshly prepared solutions should be used. The client should be watched closely for circulatory shock and other signs and symptoms of addisonian crisis (acute hypoadrenalism). Cortisone may be ordered to correct adrenal deficiencies before thyroid therapy is initiated.

Many myxedematous clients have weakened hearts and a tendency toward CHF. These clients are sensitive to thyroid hormones, and the heart can tolerate only small dosages of the drugs at first. Doses are advanced in small increments to promote strengthening of the heart before full dosages are administered. Clients diagnosed in the early stages of myxedema do not show advanced symptoms and may have little cardiovascular involvement. For these clients, drug therapy may be carried out on an outpatient basis.

Treatment is needed for long periods, often for life. It is important that the client remain under medical supervision. Regular blood tests to determine thyroid hormone levels are important, because signs and symptoms of hypothyroidism and hyperthyroidism develop insidiously and may not be recognized by clients or their families, even when pronounced. However, clinical status does not always coincide with blood test results in clients who have thyroid antibodies. Because the drug effects are delayed and cumulative, day-to-day adjustments in dosage are avoided. Dosage is changed when there is a clear trend away from hormone balance.

The client should be assessed for evidence of diabetes mellitus, because this disease can develop during thyroid hormone therapy. Previously diagnosed diabetics find their conditions more difficult to control and may require additional hypoglycemic medication.

If anticoagulants are prescribed during thyroid hormone therapy, clients should be monitored closely for abnormal bleeding. Dosages of anticoagulants may have to be reduced, because the action of these drugs is increased by thyroid therapy.

A product that does not contain tartrazine should be obtained for allergic clients.

Client Education. Simple (euthyroid) goiter can be prevented by dietary measures. Factors that increase the risk of goiter are a vegetarian diet high in goitrogenic fruits and vegetables and soybeans (see Box 33-1), very low or very high intake of iodine, use of milk from kale-fed cattle, and use of soybean infant formulas. To maintain optimal thyroid function, the diet should contain adequate amounts of protein and iodine and should be free of excessive amounts of goitrogenic foods. A varied diet without excessive intake of any one kind of food is recommended.

Clients with profound hypothyroidism cannot concentrate on or remember information; teaching should be delayed until treatment corrects the mental sluggishness and forgetfulness affecting the client.

The need for adherence to the drug regimen should be stressed. Obvious changes in body function or well-being do not occur when occasional doses are missed, and even complete omission of the drugs may not cause noticeable effects for several weeks. Failure to correct the hormone deficiency adequately, however, increases the risk of heart disease, by raising cholesterol levels in the blood and by weakening heart action.

The nurse must stress the need for regular medical care while thyroid drugs are used. This can rarely be avoided because the drugs are limited to prescription use, and most prescribers do not renew prescriptions repeatedly without reassessing the client. However, a client who does not accept the need for continued care is apt to discontinue therapy and delay seeing the prescriber.

Thyroid hormones should be taken on an empty stomach. Most preparations may be stored at room temperature.

Clients must learn the signs and symptoms of both hypothyroidism and hyperthyroidism and the need to report these to the prescriber. Hypothyroidism should subside gradually but steadily during the first months of treatment. Thereafter, hormone balance should be maintained steadily. Symptoms of imbalance may develop after many months of uneventful treatment, because the body requirements for thyroid hormone vary somewhat with the degree of stress and environmental temperatures to which the client is subjected. Because early changes tend to be subjective, the client should watch for them and communicate them clearly to the clinician.

Clients with hypothyroidism after partial loss of the thyroid gland need to learn measures to promote gland growth and shorten the recovery phase. Exercise and alternating hot and cold showers stimulate pituitary secretion of thyrotropin. As much as possible, high environmental temperatures should be avoided, because these inhibit the tropic hormone. The client should dress in layered clothing and wear the minimum necessary to avoid chilling. The diet should be of high quality and should contain adequate iodine and protein for thyroid hormone production. The need for iodized salt should be carefully weighed. In inland upland areas, this source of iodine may be needed to promote optimal thyroid function. However, in other areas, or when clients consume large amounts of seafood, iodized salt may raise intake of this mineral to levels that slow thyroid recovery. Caloric intake should be limited to avoid weight gain, a task made easier because appetite tends to decline. Excessive amounts of foods that contain goitrogens should be avoided. The latter include turnips, rutabagas, cabbage, carrots, kale, soybeans, peanuts (especially the skins), peaches, peas, strawberries, spinach, mustard seed, radishes, milk from kale-fed cattle, and millet, especially that which has been allowed to stand for several days after cooking. Drinking water contaminated by resorcinol or phthalates can also inhibit thyroid function.

OUTCOME EVALUATION

Data required for evaluation relate to thyroid balance or imbalance. Clients should be assessed regularly for signs and symptoms of hypothyroidism or hyperthyroidism. See the Critical Thinking Challenge: Case Analysis.

CRITICAL THINKING CHALLENGE
Case Analysis

Your client, a 22-year-old woman with a 2-year-old toddler, lives in Chicago. Her food budget is limited. She has read that iodine is essential for health and that the usual American diet is likely to be deficient in this element. She asks you, "Should I take kelp tablets?"

1. Where could you obtain the information needed to answer her question?
2. What factors would influence your advice?
3. Research this question and decide what advice you would give this client.

❖ CHECKLIST OF NURSING ACTIONS

❑ Promote the use of iodized salt in iodine-poor areas; recommend a varied diet adequate in protein.
❑ Be alert to early signs and symptoms of thyroid imbalance and refer affected clients for diagnosis and treatment.

When Hormone Therapy is Initiated for Severe Deficiencies

❑ Prepare parenteral solutions immediately before use and discard unused preparations.
❑ Assess the client frequently for cardiac decompensation and addisonian crisis; be especially alert for shock.
❑ Protect the client from stressors, including exertion.

During Maintenance of Long-Term Therapy

❑ Teach clients how to self-monitor hormone imbalance.
❑ Stress the long-term benefits of adherence to the drug regimen.

When Hormone Deficiency is Deemed Temporary
❑ Teach clients measures that stimulate thyroid function, as well as environmental factors that can inhibit it.

NURSING PROCESS: DRUG THERAPY IN HYPERTHYROIDISM

ASSESSMENT
During the physical examination, the nurse should palpate the thyroid gland and assess for signs and symptoms of hyperthyroidism (see Table 33-5), including client reports of nervousness, tension and irritability, and mood swings. Hand tremor, clumsiness, and weakness may be apparent. Women may complain of menstrual disturbances. The client's personal and family history should be checked for goiter, Graves' disease, or autoimmune thyroiditis (Hashimoto's disease). A tendency to lose weight is also pertinent.

If thioamide therapy is likely, examine the client for signs and symptoms of infection.

If iodine drugs are prescribed, the drug history must include specific questions about previous tolerance to iodine. Use of iodine or iodides as topical antiseptics, nutritional supplements such as iodized salt, expectorants, radiographic contrast media, cold remedies, or prescription drugs (expectorants or antithyroid medications) should be explored. Adverse and allergic reactions associated with such use should be noted.

NURSING DIAGNOSIS
Once antithyroid therapy begins, clients are vulnerable to hypothyroidism as well as adverse reaction to these drugs. Nursing diagnoses may include:

- Risk for Infection, related to bone marrow depression secondary to thioamide medication
- Pain, related to discomfort from nasal congestion from thioamide medication

Nursing diagnoses likely to be made for a client receiving iodine therapy include:

- Pain, related to discomfort of anorexia and nausea related to gastric irritation secondary to iodine therapy
- Ineffective Airway Clearance: Airway congestion related to reflex stimulation of nasal and bronchial secretion secondary to iodine therapy
- Fluid Volume Deficit, related to vomiting or diarrhea secondary to iodine therapy
- Sensory/Perceptual Alterations (Gustatory): brassy taste related to iodine therapy
- Risk for Impaired Tissue Integrity: Urticaria related to allergic reaction secondary to iodine therapy
- Altered Nutrition: Less Than Body Requirements, related to nausea and vomiting secondary to iodine therapy
- Diarrhea, related to iodine therapy

Most clients have:

- Knowledge Deficit, related to hyperthyroidism and its treatment

PLANNING
Goals of treatment include preventing or detecting and treating adverse effects of drug therapy, increased comfort, normal bowel elimination, and teaching the client to manage the drug regimen. The goal of teaching is an optimal response to the drug regimen.

INTERVENTION
Because desired effects of thioamide drugs cannot be expected for days to weeks, clients need care to help minimize the possible adverse effects of drug therapy

and toxic effects of hyperthyroidism. Until medication takes effect, clients with hyperthyroidism need light clothing and bed covers. The environment should remain cool and relatively humid. As much as possible, the nurse must promote rest to conserve the client's energy and minimize fatigue. Stimuli should be minimized. Elimination of noise and glare may be helpful, and healthcare staff should maintain a calm but efficient manner. The client's diet should be high in vitamins, minerals, and protein, with adequate calories to prevent weight loss. Frequent feedings are usually needed. Coffee, tea, and cola drinks are contraindicated, and foods with a laxative effect should be avoided. As the medications induce reduced thyroid toxicity, caloric intake should be reduced. If some weight gain is desired, this should be carefully controlled. A lean body mass may be beneficial if the cardiovascular system was adversely affected by the toxic state.

During drug therapy, the client's hormone balance should be monitored so that antithyroid medication can be decreased appropriately (by as much as 33%). Assessment is critical at this time, because either hyperthyroidism or hypothyroidism may develop before the client is stabilized on a maintenance dose.

Considerations for Thioamide Therapy. Should the client become pregnant, the prescriber must be notified at once. Thioamide therapy may be discontinued and alternative therapy (surgery) recommended. If the drugs are to be continued, thyroid hormone is added to the regimen and the client is observed closely to detect any evidence of hypothyroidism that would harm the fetus. Also, in clients receiving thioamide drugs, signs of infection, such as fever, sore throat, head cold, or malaise, are important indicators of possible leukocytopenia. In such cases, the drug should be discontinued, medical attention should be sought at once, and another treatment method should be started. Any existing infection needs vigorous treatment. Clients need protection from exposure to communicable diseases until their white blood cell counts return to normal.

Clients in thyroid crisis require intensive nursing care to maintain vital functions and to control the severe physical problems characteristic of this condition (fever, hypertension, dehydration, and hypocorticism). These clients receive thioamide drugs by injection. Because parenteral solutions are unavailable commercially, they are prepared in the healthcare institution, and quality control may not approach the level of the drug factory. Such preparations are likely to contain pyrogens or antigens not found in commercial solutions. The client should be watched closely for fever, chills, allergy, or other adverse reactions.

Both thioamide and iodine drugs cause nasal congestion. However, the thyrotoxic client must not use decongestants that contain stimulant substances. To reduce nasal stuffiness and bronchial congestion, air should be kept humid; during the winter, containers of water may be placed on top of radiators, near heating units, or in hot-air ducts. Persistent discomfort may be relieved by nasal irrigation with normal saline.

Considerations for Iodine Therapy. Clients receiving iodine must be monitored for allergy and other adverse reactions (skin eruption, anorexia, nausea, vomiting, diarrhea, and nasal congestion). Irritant foods should be excluded from the diet. Adult fluid intake of up to 3 L/day should be encouraged. If urticaria (hives) develops, iodine should be discontinued and the prescriber informed immediately. If the client has antiallergy medicine such as diphenhydramine (Benadryl), a dose may be taken. If none has been prescribed, the prescriber is likely to order one. To relieve itching, the client may take tepid baths with sodium bicarbonate or a strained oatmeal paste. The client should be kept comfortably cool and advised to press on any itching areas (to reduce the sensation) rather than scratching. Oral iodine or iodides should be given with meals and ample fluids. As implied by their use as antiseptics, concentrated iodine solutions tend to damage cells. Doses should be well diluted to prevent damage or irritation to the GI tract. Liquid preparations are mixed with milk or fruit juice and given through a straw to disguise the taste.

Iodine solutions are sensitive to light and are stored in light-resistant containers. Doses must be measured precisely. Because iodides are poisonous, they should be stored in locked cupboards to reduce the risk of accidental ingestion.

Clients who receive iodides for hyperthyroidism are likely to have some persistent signs and symptoms of thyrotoxicosis. These clients need rest, relief from stress and undue stimulation, and a high-quality and high-calorie diet. Their thyroid status should be monitored to assess response to medication. Clients scheduled for surgery need the usual preoperative preparation.

Client Education: Iodides. Nurses can do much to reduce the incidence and severity of thyroid disease by stressing early treatment and teaching clients about adequate nutrition and iodine. An essential element for normal thyroid function, iodine is contained in seafood, kelp, and fruits and vegetables grown in coastal areas. Nurses should promote the use of iodized salt in "goiter belt" areas known to have iodine-poor soils, particularly for families who raise much of their own food or who use local produce. In the continental United States, iodine-poor soils are found in most inland areas, including the Great Lakes basin.

Nurses should urge clients with goiter or signs and symptoms of thyroid imbalance to seek medical attention and undergo diagnostic testing promptly to help prevent severe disease and complications. In young women, prevention or treatment protects their future children also; the risk of cretinism rises if the mother-to-be has an iodine deficiency or other thyroid problems.

Clients who receive iodides in preparation for thyroidectomy need information about possible side effects. Rash, dyspnea, swelling or soreness of the parotid glands, fever, or irritation or swelling of the eyes should be reported promptly. Clients should be warned not to use over-the-counter (OTC) cold remedies that contain decongestants or other stimulants. It is best if no drugs are used without the knowledge and approval of the prescriber. Adherence to the drug regimen should be stressed. Missing doses reduces the effect of the iodine and results in greater toxicity and higher surgical risks; the rate of complications is higher for such clients. Because timing in relation to surgery is critical, the client should inform the prescriber immediately if there is a possibility that surgery will need to be postponed.

Clients allergic to iodine compounds should wear a medical identification device that warns of this condition.

Clients should also be informed about other side effects of iodine; for instance, excess iodine can worsen acne.

Client Education: Thioamides. Clients who take thioamide medications must know that they need to take the drugs for long periods. After the initial few weeks, their toxic symptoms usually subside and they feel well. However, drug treatment must continue even when no evidence of illness is present. Interruption of therapy is likely to cause renewed symptoms and may prevent permanent remission. Clients need help in devising an acceptable regimen that promotes a habit of regular and accurate medication.

Clients and their families must know that thioamide dosage must be controlled to maintain optimal hormone balance. Too little medication prolongs the period of thyrotoxicity; too much can cause hypothyroidism. Clients also must be taught to recognize the signs and symptoms of hormone imbalance (see Table 33-5). After the latent period of initial treatment, evidence of imbalance should be reported to the prescriber so that dosages can be adjusted. Teaching should also include the need to report any other illness, especially infections, because these may be early signs of adverse reaction to the drugs. Periodic blood tests may be required. Clients should understand the need for frequent medical follow-up throughout the lengthy treatment period.

General Client Education. Clients should be warned against taking OTC medications without the prescriber's approval. Many OTC remedies contain pressor amines (decongestants) that are poorly tolerated by hyperthyroid clients. Diarrhea remedies that contain kaolin may adsorb oral medications, reducing their absorption from the GI tract. These compounds could interfere with the effectiveness of the antithyroid drugs, causing recurrent thyroid toxicity. Remedies that contain aspirin delay clotting and should be avoided by clients taking propylthiouracil.

OUTCOME EVALUATION

Data required for evaluation include evidence of thyroid balance, presence or absence of infection, patency of nasal airways, blood cell counts, number and consistency of stools, client comments and behavior indicative of self-concept, and client reports related to nervous tension and tolerance to heat and cold. Success of the teaching program is judged by the client's ability to manage the drug regimen and to repeat to the nurse information conveyed during teaching sessions. See Example of Nursing Process for Methimazole Therapy.

❖ CHECKLIST OF NURSING ACTIONS

- ❑ While hyperthyroidism remains, prevent accidental injury, reduce environmental stressors, and promote rest.
- ❑ Encourage the client to take medications as prescribed.
- ❑ Discontinue thioamide medications and notify the prescriber at once if symptoms of infection occur.
- ❑ Teach the client to report any symptoms of infection to the prescriber immediately.
- ❑ Teach the client signs and symptoms of both hyperthyroidism and hypothyroidism. Instruct the client to report them to the prescriber.
- ❑ Recommend the use of iodized salt to clients who live in "goiter belt" areas.
- ❑ Warn clients with hyperthyroidism not to use OTC preparations containing decongestants.
- ❑ Refer persons with signs and symptoms of goiter or thyroid imbalance for medical diagnosis and treatment.
- ❑ Emphasize the importance of follow-up care throughout the period of drug treatment.
- ❑ Store methimazole and iodine in light-resistant containers. Instruct the client to keep these drugs in their original containers.
- ❑ Before administering iodides (including radiopaque contrast agents), inquire specifically about past adverse reactions to iodides.
- ❑ Protect iodine preparations from excessive heat.
- ❑ Store iodine preparations in secure areas.
- ❑ Monitor clients taking iodine drugs for symptoms of serum sickness syndrome, respiratory congestion, skin rash, and thyroid imbalance. Warn them not to use OTC medicines containing decongestants.
- ❑ Recommend the use of a medical identification device to all clients hypersensitive to iodides.

Example of Nursing Process for Methimazole Therapy

The client, a secretary, housewife, and mother, is 35. Ten weeks ago, she began treatment for hyperthyroidism with methimazole. She returns to the physician's office monthly for check-ups. During her last visit 2 weeks ago, she complained to the nurse of a head cold that she could not get rid of. At that time, the nurse informed her that this could be a side effect of the antithyroid medication and cautioned her not to use over-the-counter decongestants, because hyperthyroidism causes sensitivity to their stimulant effects.

Today the client telephones the office and tells the nurse, "That head cold must be going down. I have a sore throat today."

Assessment Data

Methimazole treatment for 10 weeks

Complaint of sore throat

Nursing Diagnosis	Intervention	Goals and Outcomes
Risk for Infection, related to bone marrow depression secondary to antithyroid medication	**Remind** the client that a sore throat can signal adverse reaction to the medication she is taking. **Direct** the client not to take any more drug until she is seen by the prescriber; make an appointment for her to see the prescriber as soon as possible.	The client will not develop life-threatening irreversible bone marrow depression and aplastic anemia.

NURSING PROCESS: CLIENTS RECEIVING RADIOACTIVE IODINE

ASSESSMENT

Many clients who receive radioactive iodine are affected by an imbalance in thyroid hormones. Those who receive tracer doses may have either a deficiency or an excess of these hormones. Clients who receive therapeutic doses often have thyrotoxicity. Initial assessment should include an evaluation of thyroid function. Laboratory tests for T_4 and T_3 are usually performed.

Before administering a radioactive iodine, a careful history should be taken of the illness and its treatment. If antithyroid drugs have been prescribed, the date of the last dose must be determined. These drugs affect iodine uptake and may alter response to radioactive iodine. Thiouracil or iodine taken within the preceding week invalidate diagnostic tracer tests, as does potassium thiocyanate taken within the preceding month. Medication taken within these time spans also reduces the effectiveness of therapeutic doses of radioactive iodine and increases exposure of normal tissue to radiation, because the radioactive element is not taken up by the thyroid at the usual rate. The radioactive iodine continues to circulate in the bloodstream and appears in the urine in higher-than-normal concentrations. The nurse should question the client specifically about past adverse reactions to iodine or iodinated medications, including contrast media used for radiographic imaging.

The nurse should determine the client's response to previous exposure to iodine, attitudes toward and emotional response to the use of radioactive substances, and knowledge of thyroid imbalances and their treatment. In addition, the sewage disposal method used in the client's home should be recorded.

NURSING DIAGNOSIS

Diagnoses likely to be made for clients who are to receive radioactive iodine include:

- Fear, related to exposure to radiation secondary to use of radioactive iodine
- Knowledge Deficit, concerning thyroid diseases and drug treatment
- Risk for Impaired Tissue Integrity: Skin rash related to allergic reaction to iodine

A common collaborative problem that should be differentiated from the nursing diagnoses is:

Potential Complication: Anaphylaxis, renal-urinary impairment, or metabolic problems

PLANNING

Goals for nursing care include reducing fear and promptly detecting and treating allergic reaction to iodine, radiation injury, and parathyroid imbalance. Goals for the teaching plan are increased client knowledge about thyroid disorders and the use of radioactive iodine in their diagnosis and treatment.

INTERVENTION

The nurse should foster the client's trust in the health-care personnel. Competence in medical procedures and expression of a warm concern for clients and their families establish initial trust. Honest explanations about the client's condition and the proposed treatment, including its risks, are essential. The nurse should clearly differentiate between a client's one-time or occasional exposure and the healthcare staff's cumulative exposure from daily contact with radioactivity.

If the client has a history of allergy to iodine, the nurse should immediately notify the physician. Before radioactive iodine is administered, equipment, supplies, and trained personnel must be available to treat any allergic reaction, including anaphylactic shock. After administration, the client should be monitored regularly.

Provide fluids before therapy, because clients should be as well hydrated as possible before receiving any radioactive substance. This helps prevent high levels of radioactive iodine in body tissues and the urinary tract.

Clients with hyperthyroidism require the same nursing care as any thyrotoxic person. After drug administration, they are likely to receive antithyroid medication to suppress toxic symptoms until the effects of radioactive iodine are well established. Long-term follow-up should include monitoring for parathyroid imbalance and hypothyroidism.

Client Education. Clients who receive tracer doses of radioactive iodine can be assured that the level of radiation is extremely low and does not pose a significant health hazard. The precautions exercised in the nuclear medicine department may be compared to those practiced in the radiology department, where personnel must be protected from even low doses of radiation because of the constant risk of exposure. After treatment, no special precautions need be taken by the client who receives low doses of radioactive iodine.

When therapeutic doses are administered, clients usually feel anxious. The nurse can explain that drugs potentially harmful to normal people are often helpful in disease conditions, that the client is exposed to radioactivity a limited number of times, and (when cancer is not involved) that doses are computed to err on the side of undertreatment. Except for clients treated for cancer, most experience no discomfort or other adverse reactions after receiving radioactive iodine.

If the client is treated as an outpatient, the nurse should discuss plans for self-care to evaluate the need for special instructions. Clients should not live alone or be isolated from emergency medical care during the 3 months after therapy. Although rare, tissue destruction can release sufficient hormone to produce a thyroid crisis. Thyroiditis can occur, with subsequent swelling of the gland, pressure on the trachea, and an acute respiratory emergency. Should either situation arise, the client needs immediate medical treatment. For the first week after treatment, the client should remain in a locale served by a multiple-dwelling sewage system to avoid the concentration of radioactive wastes in a septic system.

The nurse must teach the signs and symptoms of hypothyroidism and parathyroid imbalance. Signs and symptoms of hyperparathyroidism include increased flexibility of joints (double-jointedness), bone pain, mood swings, and abdominal pain due to renal calculi (kidney stones). Parathormone deficiency causes muscle irritability, cramps, and tetany. Any of these symptoms should be reported promptly to the prescriber. Clients should be encouraged to remain under continued health supervision so that serum levels of thyroid hormone and calcium can be monitored. These tests can alert the prescriber to abnormal changes before other signs and symptoms of disease develop. Hypothyroidism or parathormone imbalance can develop years after radioactive iodine therapy.

OUTCOME EVALUATION
Data required for evaluation include the presence or absence of fear in the client, the incidence and severity of allergic reaction or bladder inflammation, the long-term incidence and severity of hypothyroidism or parathyroid imbalance, and the long-term absence or incidence of radiation sickness. For short-term evaluation of the teaching plan, the client is questioned to test retention of material conveyed during teaching sessions. Success over the long term is judged by the client's maintenance of health supervision and prompt reporting of abnormal signs and symptoms to the primary care provider. See Example of Nursing Process for Radioactive Iodine Therapy.

❖ **CHECKLIST OF NURSING ACTIONS**

❑ Before administering radioactive iodine, determine whether the client received antithyroid medication in the preceding month and whether an iodine allergy exists. Report either finding to the prescriber.
❑ Assess the client for evidence of thyroid hormone imbalance.
❑ Explain the potential risks to clients in realistic terms.
❑ Handle radioactive substances with rubber gloves and minimize exposure to radiation by reducing the time spent in close proximity to the drugs.
❑ Be prepared to treat anaphylactic shock, should it develop.
❑ Provide emotional support to clients fearful of radiation.

When Therapeutic Dosages of Radioactive Iodine Are Prescribed

❑ Explain to clients the need for diluting body wastes for 1 week after treatment.
❑ Stress the need for long-term health care to detect thyroid and parathyroid imbalances, should they develop.

Example of Nursing Process for Radioactive Iodine Therapy

The client is a 45-year-old farm wife and writer who has come to the medical center to receive radioactive iodine therapy. She previously had 2 years of propylthiouracil treatment and a subtotal thyroidectomy. After each treatment, she remained euthyroid for several months but thyrotoxicity gradually recurred.

Comments by the client indicate that she is well informed about health care. She understands that the proposed treatment involves exposure to ionizing radiation in relatively large doses, but she prefers not to undergo additional surgery.

Assessment Data

Order for radioactive iodine therapy

Client's knowledge about health and health care related to previous therapies

Rural residence

Nursing Diagnosis	Intervention	Goals and Outcomes
Risk for Impaired Tissue Integrity: Dermatitis related to allergic reaction secondary to medication	**Ascertain** whether the client has a personal or family history of allergy, especially allergic reaction to iodine; report any positive findings. **Advise** the client to notify the office promptly if skin rash develops after the radioactive iodine treatment.	The client will not develop allergic reaction to radioactive iodine; if such a reaction does occur, it will be detected and treated promptly.
Knowledge Deficit, concerning some aspects of radioactive iodine therapy	**Explore** with the client her knowledge of radioactive iodine; ascertain her plans for care after the treatment. **Provide** the client with any information about radioactive iodine of which she is unaware; ensure that she knows she should remain in an area supplied with a central sewage plant for 1 week and should avoid living alone for 3 months after receiving the radioactive iodine.	The client will express confidence in relation to the radioactive iodine treatment. The client will make appropriate arrangements for aftercare.

Calcitonin

A hormone with physiologic functions that oppose those of parathormone is produced by the parafollicular C cells of many animals. Depending on the species involved, these cells may be found in the parathyroid, thymus, or (in humans) thyroid gland. This hormone, called calcitonin, lowers calcium levels in the extracellular fluid by inhibiting bone resorption and altering absorption and excretion of calcium by the body. Calcitonin does not block the actions of parathormone, but its effects tend to reverse those of parathormone.

Calcitonin is a single-chain polypeptide composed of 32 amino acids with two disulfide linkages. Its molecular weight is about 3,600. The hormone is highly potent, producing pronounced effects in small doses. Its presence is determined by radioimmunoassay.

Commercial preparations of calcitonin for clinical use include human calcitonin and salmon calcitonin (Table 33-6). After preparation as sterile solutions, the drugs must be refrigerated to maintain potency. They should be used within 6 hours.

Pharmacodynamics. Calcitonin is believed to increase cyclic adenosine monophosphate (cAMP) in bone cells other than those affected by parathormone. It decreases the activity of osteoclasts and their formation from mesenchymal stem cells. Its immediate effect on osteoblasts is enhancement of their activity, although this declines with continued exposure. Calcitonin increases renal excretion of calcium, phosphorus, and sodium. Some evidence suggests that it may inhibit intestinal absorption of calcium. The hypocalcemic effect of calcitonin is rapid but transitory; effects on bone metabolism are more long-lived.

Pharmacokinetics. Because its protein structure is destroyed by digestive enzymes, calcitonin must be administered by injection (SC, IM, or IV). When given IV, the onset of action is immediate and the duration of action is 30 minutes to 12 hours. After IM or SC administration, the onset of action is 15 minutes, peak action is seen at 4 hours, and the duration of action is 8 to 24 hours. Little is known about calcitonin's distribution. It is believed not to cross the placenta. Endoge-

Table 33-6. Medicinal Preparations of Calcitonin

Drug Name	Preparation	Therapeutic Uses	Usual Adult Dosage	Additional Information
calcitonin (human) (Cibacalcin)	Solution for injection	Paget's disease	SC: Initially: 0.5 mg/day; maintenance: up to 0.5 mg bid PC: C	Allergic hypersensitivity occurs infrequently.
calcitonin (salmon) (Calcimar, Miacalcin)	Solution for injection	Paget's disease	SC: Initially: 100 IU/day; maintenance: 50 IU 3 × weekly–100 IU/day	Allergic hypersensitivity to salmon calcitonin is more likely than to human calcitonin.
		Hypercalcemia	SC or IM: Initially: 4 IU/kg q12h, increased to a maximum of 8 IU/kg q6h when necessary	Calcium supplements are usually prescribed with calcitonin for the treatment of osteoporosis or osteogenesis imperfecta.
		Menopausal osteoporosis	100 IU/day	
		Osteogenesis imperfecta	2 IU/kg 3 × weekly PC: C	

KEY: PC = pregnancy category; see Appendix A.

nous calcitonin has been detected in human milk in concentrations 10 to 40 times that in serum. Calcitonin appears to be metabolized by the kidneys, in the blood, and in peripheral tissues. Its metabolites are excreted in urine.

Therapeutic Uses. Calcitonin is useful in treating hypercalcemia due to hyperparathyroidism, idiopathic hypercalcemia of infancy, vitamin D intoxication, osteolytic bone metastases, and hyperphosphatemia. Its use in treating postmenopausal osteoporosis is relatively recent. Calcitonin's major clinical use is treating Paget's disease of the bone, in which abnormal and excessive bone formation and resorption cause abnormal bone structure. Long-term parathormone therapy in this disease tends to correct its characteristic physiologic abnormalities (elevated levels of blood alkaline phosphatase and urinary hydroxyproline, increased blood flow in affected bone). The rate of bone turnover declines and a more normal bone structure is restored.

Adverse Reactions. Adverse reactions to calcitonin have been infrequent and mild; only occasionally have they been severe enough to discontinue the drug. The administration of calcitonin can cause flushing, urticaria, diuresis, or nausea and vomiting. Gastric acidity may decline. The drug can also cause a drop in the blood calcium level, with tetany and cardiac arrhythmias. Continued use can cause swelling and tenderness of the hands. After several months of therapy, antibodies may form, causing resistance to the drug and decreased therapeutic effect. Allergic reactions also can occur. High doses of calcitonin, or an exaggerated response to the drug, may cause acute hypocalcemia as well as nausea and vomiting.

Precautions and Contraindications. Calcitonin is contraindicated in pregnancy. Clients with a history of allergy should be monitored for reactions; these are most likely when salmon calcitonin is used. Before calcitonin treatment is started, a skin test for allergy should be performed. During the initial period of calcitonin treatment, calcium solutions for injection should be available for parenteral administration to correct hypocalcemia if it occurs. Clients who receive long-term therapy with calcitonin must be monitored for clinical response and hormone status; other treatment is prescribed if resistance to the hormone develops.

■ SUMMARY

Calcitonin is a hormone whose physiologic effects (hypocalcemia and decreased osteoclastic activity) generally oppose those of parathormone. The drug is used mainly for the long-term treatment of Paget's disease of the bone. It is given three to seven times a week by injection. Over time, immune bodies tend to develop and the effectiveness of the drug declines.

❖ NURSING MANAGEMENT: CLIENT RECEIVING CALCITONIN

Calcitonin therapy is relatively new, and little is known about its long-term effects. Clients should be regularly assessed for adverse reactions that have not been reported. Resistance to the medication may develop due to antibody formation. Return of symptoms should be reported to healthcare personnel so that another treatment can be prescribed.

NURSING PROCESS

ASSESSMENT

Before administering calcitonin, a broad data base should be established for comparison with the client's status during drug therapy. Additional assessment areas include allergic tendencies, cardiac status, visible bone deformities, and signs and symptoms of hypercalcemia (increased formation of dental plaque, constipation, emotional lability, lethargy, prolonged systole, calciuria, and abdominal pain caused by urinary calculi). The client's knowledge of and emotional reaction to the disorder and to the use of hormone medications should be assessed as well.

NURSING DIAGNOSIS

Nursing diagnoses likely to be made for clients receiving calcitonin therapy include:

- Body Image Disturbance, related to the need for calcitonin to treat skeletal deformities caused by disorders of bone metabolism (osteoporosis, osteogenesis imperfecta, Paget's disease)
- Pain: Abdominal, from urinary calculi secondary to hypercalcemia; nausea and vomiting and nerve and muscle irritability related to side effects of calcitonin
- Fluid Volume Deficit, related to diuresis secondary to calcitonin therapy

Most clients have:

- Knowledge Deficit, concerning calcitonin therapy

Common collaborative problems that should be differentiated from the nursing diagnoses include:

Potential Complication: Tetany, angioedema, cardiac arrhythmia, and allergic reaction

PLANNING

Goals of nursing care are improved self-concept and emotional stability, increased comfort, normal fluid and electrolyte balance, and prompt detection and treatment of adverse drug reactions.

INTERVENTION

Clients who receive calcitonin also receive close medical supervision. Injections are required three to seven times a week. When therapy begins in an acute care setting, the nurse administers the medication. Only fresh solutions (less than 6 hours old) should be used. The drug may be administered by IV infusion or by IM or SC injection. During initial treatments, calcium solutions for injection should be readily available in the nursing unit for use if the client develops signs and symptoms of hypocalcemic tetany (numbness and tingling or carpopedal spasm when the blood-pressure cuff is applied).

Long-term treatment is carried out in the community. Clients' responses should be closely monitored to detect previously unrecognized effects of the drugs. These should be reported to the federal Food and Drug Administration (FDA; see Chap. 2 for reporting procedure). Significant responses include dehydration due to diuresis and loss of sodium and water, abnormal blood calcium levels, and signs and symptoms of allergy. Therapeutic response should be assessed at each nursing visit. A return of symptoms may indicate development of antibodies to the medication and should be reported to the prescriber so that another treatment can be considered.

Skeletal deformities are not corrected by treatment. Clients should be praised and complimented for appropriate appearance and behavior whenever possible. The nurse's relationship to the client should be characterized by warm acceptance.

Client Education. Clients who receive calcitonin should be taught to report their health status in detail. They should know the identity of the drug they are receiving.

Clients should be advised that skillful design and fit of clothing may camouflage skeletal changes.

For clients who administer their own drugs after the dosage has been adjusted, instruction is needed in administration technique and in the specific signs and symptoms they should report to the prescriber. They must understand the general properties of the drug as well as the characteristics of the disease for which they are being treated. Regular medical supervision is needed indefinitely.

OUTCOME EVALUATION

Data required for evaluation include behavior or comments by the client indicative of self-image, emotional status, and comfort level, and the incidence or absence of adverse drug reactions (GI upset, dehydration, muscle irritability, skin rash, or cardiovascular collapse). Short-term evaluation of the teaching program may include questioning the client about facts conveyed during teaching sessions and observing the client's self-administration technique.

❖ CHECKLIST OF NURSING ACTIONS

When Calcitonin Therapy Is Initiated

- ❑ Administer drug doses as ordered.
- ❑ Watch for nausea, vomiting, and tetany.
- ❑ Have parenteral calcium gluconate available for immediate administration should tetany occur.
- ❑ Report tetany immediately and help administer IV calcium.

When Long-Term Calcitonin Therapy Is Planned

- ❑ Teach the person who is to manage treatment how to administer parenteral medication.
- ❑ Teach the signs and symptoms of adverse reactions to calcitonin, including reduced therapeutic response.
- ❑ Caution the client to remain under medical supervision and to report significant changes in health status to the primary care provider.

Throughout Calcitonin Therapy

- ❑ Monitor the client for signs and symptoms of allergy to the hormone.
- ❑ Monitor the client for continued response to the drug. Should signs and symptoms of the disease process recur, refer the client to the prescriber for

reassessment of the drug regimen and alternative therapy.

Whenever Calcitonin Is Prescribed

❑ Watch the client for previously unrecognized effects of the drug; report these to the FDA to facilitate collection of data related to calcitonin's toxic and side effects.

Parathyroid Hormone (Parathormone)

Parathyroid hormone (parathormone) is a polypeptide composed of 84 amino acids arranged in a single chain. Its molecular weight is about 9,500. The only form of parathormone available for clinical use is teriparatide acetate (Parathar), a synthetic preparation that contains 34 of the 84 amino acids of the natural hormone. This preparation exerts the physiologic actions of the hormone.

Physiology

Parathormone is produced by the parathyroid glands and acts to increase calcium levels in the blood. It is secreted by the chief cells in the gland in response to decreased calcium ion concentration in the extracellular fluid. Parathormone increases resorption of calcium from the bones, absorption of calcium and phosphorus by the gut, and reabsorption of calcium in the renal tubule. High levels of calcium in the extracellular fluid inhibit parathormone production.

Pathophysiology

Pathologic conditions associated with parathormone imbalance include primary excesses of the hormone caused by hypertrophy of the glands or hyperparathyroidism secondary to pregnancy, lactation, and rickets or other hypocalcemic conditions. Deficiencies of parathormone are usually a complication of neck surgery, when the glands have been inadvertently removed. When there is too little hormone, calcium ion levels in the extracellular fluid drop, causing tetany and cardiac arrhythmias. Excessive parathormone causes hypercalcemia, calciuria with formation of calcium calculi in the urinary tract, and bone demineralization.

Pharmacodynamics. Parathormone activates osteoclasts by increasing cAMP in these cells, stimulates formation of new osteoclasts from mesenchymal stem cells, and delays the conversion of osteoclasts to osteoblasts. These actions inhibit new bone formation and enhance bone resorption. At the same time, the hormone decreases kidney tubule reabsorption of phosphorus, sodium, potassium, and amino acid ions and increases reabsorption of calcium, magnesium, and hydrogen ions. Intestinal absorption of calcium and phosphorus also increases.

With continued exposure to the hormone, as seen in hyperparathyroidism, osteoblastic activity recovers somewhat as large numbers of osteoclasts are converted to osteoblasts. The bones can become significantly demineralized, however, with abnormal mobility of the joints and increased plasticity of the bones. Permanent skeletal deformities tend to develop.

Pharmacokinetics. Because the hormone is destroyed by peptidases in the intestinal tract, parathormone cannot be administered orally. The effects of the drug are prompt and continue for at least 2 hours. Parathormone appears to be degraded by the liver and kidneys.

Therapeutic Uses. Parathormone is not used in treating disease, but is used in a diagnostic test to determine the cause of hypocalcemia. Chronic hypoparathyroidism is managed with large doses of vitamin D, which has a physiologic effect similar to that of the hormone.

Adverse Reactions. Subcutaneous injections of parathormone often produce local inflammation. Allergic hypersensitivity accentuates this response. Administration of large doses of the drug causes anorexia, vomiting, diarrhea, and weakness. Cardiac arrhythmias may develop.

Precautions and Contraindications. Parathormone is contraindicated in hypercalcemia. It must be used with caution in renal or cardiac disease. Before administration, a skin test should be done for sensitivity; during the test, epinephrine must be available for treating anaphylactic or other allergic reactions.

▪ SUMMARY

Parathormone has limited clinical utility. It is used in a diagnostic test for pseudohypoparathyroidism. The drug must be injected, and allergic reactions may occur.

❖ NURSING MANAGEMENT: CLIENT RECEIVING PARATHORMONE

Parathormone is used only for diagnosing pseudohypoparathyroidism, a condition in which the target tissues for parathormone (mainly bone) are unresponsive to the hormone. The drug is administered to determine whether it will trigger a rise in the serum calcium level. Failure of response indicates that the tissue is refractory to the hormone. This procedure is not likely to produce adverse reactions unless the recipient is allergic to the hormone.

NURSING PROCESS

ASSESSMENT

When parathormone is to be used, the client should be questioned about previous use of the drug. If previous exposure to the hormone is suspected, a skin test for allergic hypersensitivity must be performed.

The client given parathormone usually has a low serum calcium level and should be assessed for signs and symptoms of pretetany (facial fasciculations where the skin over the facial nerve is tapped, or carpopedal spasm on inflation of a blood-pressure cuff on the arm). Hypocalcemia is also associated with nerve irritability; clients may be tense and apprehensive.

NURSING DIAGNOSIS

Nursing diagnoses likely to be made for clients who undergo a parathormone test include:

- Knowledge Deficit, concerning the diagnostic use of parathormone

A common collaborative problem that should be differentiated from the nursing diagnoses is:

Potential Complication: Tetany

PLANNING

Goals of nursing care are to detect and treat hypocalcemic tetany promptly (if it develops), to increase the client's comfort, to prevent or detect and treat promptly allergic reactions to parathormone, and to teach the client about the diagnostic test to be performed.

INTERVENTION

Clients who undergo parathormone testing procedures are likely to have low serum calcium levels. If they experience paresthesia and muscle and nerve irritability, they should be given a paper bag and instructed to breathe in and out of the bag several times in a row. Bag rebreathing increases the carbon dioxide load of the blood and lowers its pH. This effect increases the ionization and physiologic action of the calcium in the blood, temporarily reducing the signs and symptoms of calcium deficiency and delaying the onset of tetany. Sterile calcium solution should be available if IV doses are required.

The nurse may be responsible for coordinating the services needed for accurate diagnostic testing. Urine tests for calcium are collected before and at timed intervals after the administration of parathormone. The nurse may also be responsible for administering the hormone. Epinephrine should be available for treating acute allergic reaction to the drug if it occurs.

The site of hormone injection should be monitored for local inflammation, an indication of possible allergy. Because parathormone is a relatively new drug, the nurse should also watch for any unusual response by the client.

Client Education. Clients should be informed about the test, expected responses, and the need to report any unusual symptoms that occur during the procedure. The client is unlikely to experience recognizable changes when the drug is administered. Clients who do

respond have less nerve and muscle irritability as the serum calcium level rises.

Clients should be informed that they are receiving parathormone and should be advised to report this fact to healthcare personnel if the test is ever reordered in the future. Each exposure to the hormone increases the likelihood of allergic hypersensitivity.

OUTCOME EVALUATION

Data required for evaluation include the presence or absence of muscle fasciculations and tetany and client reports of changes in comfort level. Teaching may be evaluated by the client's ability to anticipate and adapt to procedures required for the diagnostic test.

❖ CHECKLIST OF NURSING ACTIONS

When Parathormone Is Used as a Diagnostic Tool

- ❏ Ask the client about previous exposure to parathormone and susceptibility to allergic hypersensitivity; if an allergic reaction is likely, arrange for a skin test to determine sensitivity to parathormone before the diagnostic test is performed.
- ❏ Have medication (epinephrine) available at the bedside for treating an allergic reaction; obtain an "as circumstances may require" (PRN) order for its use.

During the Test

- ❏ Monitor the client closely for anaphylaxis, nausea, weakness, and irregular heart rate.
- ❏ If anaphylaxis occurs, immediately follow protocols for administering epinephrine and summon medical help.
- ❏ Observe the client for any unusual change in status; record and report any changes, because they may indicate previously unrecognized effects of parathormone.

When Hypocalcemic Tetany Occurs

- ❏ Immediately institute paper bag or glove rebreathing to lower body pH.
- ❏ Prepare for the administration of IV medications, such as calcium.

Adenohypophyseal Hormones and Related Substances

The anterior pituitary produces several protein hormones that regulate the activity of various target tissues in the body. Hormones identified to date include growth hormone, prolactin, two gonadotropins, thyrotropin, and corticotropin. Similar protein hormones are produced by the human placenta. Some of these proteins closely resemble each other in structure, and a few share physiologic properties to some degree.

Because of their protein structure, pituitary tropic hormones are ineffective when administered orally, and they are not routinely used for hormone replacement in deficiency states. Instead, oral hormone preparations normally produced by the target glands (corticosteroids, thyroid and sex hormones) are prescribed to maintain normal body function. Notable exceptions are growth hormone, which is the only agent effective in treating pituitary dwarfism, and the gonadotropins, which are sometimes effective in restoring fertility to clients with pituitary hypofunction. Some anterior pituitary hormones are used in diagnostic tests to differentiate primary from secondary failure in relation to thyroid gland or adrenal cortex production. One tropic hormone, corticotropin, is used as a pharmaceutical agent in treating certain progressive degenerative autoimmune diseases.

Corticotropin

Corticotropin is a protein hormone produced by the chromophobic cells of the anterior lobe of the pituitary gland. It controls steroid hormone production by the adrenal cortex.

Medicinal preparations are produced mainly from the pituitaries of slaughtered animals, but some synthetic hormone is also available. Animal hormones differ from the human type by substitution of different amino acid residues at three positions on the protein chain. Animal hormones are physiologically effective in humans, however. Medicinal preparations of corticotropin include aqueous solutions for IV infusion and suspensions and gelatin solutions for IM or SC administration (Table 33-7). The latter are absorbed by the body at relatively slow rates and provide longer periods of treatment per dose.

Physiology

Corticotropin is a vital link in stress adaptation. It helps heighten circulation and produces the energy required to resist environmental stressors. This response begins when sensory impulses stimulate the brain. Excitation of the anterior hypothalamus increases production of corticotropin-releasing factor. Itself a protein hormone, this chemical is conveyed to the adenohypophysis (anterior pituitary), where it causes the tissues to produce corticotropin. Corticotropin, in turn, stimulates the adrenal cortex to produce steroid hormones, most notably the glucocorticoids. Undesirable variations in hormone response to stress are prevented by a negative feedback system: high blood levels of glucocorticoids inhibit corticotropin production in the anterior pituitary.

Pathophysiology

Excess corticotropin can be caused by a secreting tumor of the pituitary. When adrenal function is normal, this is followed by excess secretion of corticosteroids (glucocorticoids and sometimes adrenal androgens), a condition known as Cushing's disease. Treatment of Cushing's disease is directed at the pituitary problem.

Corticotropin deficiency may be one feature of complete pituitary failure with atrophy of the adrenals, the thyroid, and the gonads. In this condition, the most convenient treatment is replacement of hormones by the administration of oral hormones: cortisol, thyroid, and either estrogen or testosterone. If an underlying progressive pituitary problem exists, this must also be treated.

Pharmacodynamics. Corticotropin reacts with a specific hormone receptor on adrenal cell membranes, causing an increase in cAMP in these cells. This raises cholesterol levels (cholesterol is a building block for steroid hormone formation), cholesterol binding to cytochrome P-450, and cholesterol esterase activity. The cells of the zona reticularis, which produces glucocorticoid

Table 33-7. Drug Preparations of Corticotropic Hormone

Drug Name	Preparation	Usual Adult Dosage
corticotropin injection (Acthar, ACTH, Cortrophin)	Lipophilized powder for reconstitution for injection	40 U daily PC: C
repository corticotropin (ACTH Gel Repository, H.P. Acthar Gel, Corticotrophin Gel)	Highly purified corticotropin in gelatin solution for IM or SC injection	40 U daily PC: C
corticotropin zinc hydroxide suspension (Cortrophin-Zinc)	Purified corticotropin absorbed in zinc hydroxide, for IM injection	40 U daily PC: C
cosyntropin for injection (Cortrosyn)	Synthetic peptide with 24 amino acid residues that make up the active portion of the corticotropin molecule for IV or IM administration	0.25 mg (equivalent to 25 U) used for diagnostic testing PC: C

KEY: PC = pregnancy risk category; see Appendix A.

hormones, are the most affected. Weaker stimulation occurs in the zona fasciculata, where adrenal sex hormones are produced. The effect on the zona glomerulosa, which produces mineralocorticoids, is weakest of all, but the response of this part of the cortex to the primary stimuli of hyperkalemia and hypovolemia is enhanced.

Total absence of corticotropin produces partial atrophy of the zona glomerulosa and almost total atrophy of the rest of the cortex. Thus, corticotropin is a necessary factor for normal adrenal production of corticosteroids. If adrenal function is normal, the level of glucocorticoid production is directly proportional to corticotropin levels.

Pharmacokinetics. As a protein substance, corticotropin is destroyed by digestive enzymes and is ineffective when administered orally. It is rapidly absorbed parenterally and may be administered IM, SC, or IV. Like other protein hormones, corticotropin appears to be degraded by the tissues; the hormone does not appear in appreciable amounts in urine or other body excretions. Its half-life in plasma is 15 minutes, and the effects of a single dose are largely dissipated after 6 hours. Because repeated administration of the hormone causes enlargement of the adrenal cortex, increased secretion of corticosteroids continues for a time after tropic hormone levels have returned to normal.

Therapeutic Uses. Corticotropin is used diagnostically in corticosteroid deficiency states to determine the functional capacity of the adrenal cortex to respond to stimulation. If corticosteroid levels rise after administration of corticotropin, adrenal dysfunction is ruled out as a cause, and a search for pituitary disease begins. Failure of the adrenals to respond to stimulation indicates the likelihood of primary adrenal disease, rather than pituitary disease. The test involves measurement of 17-hydroxycorticoid levels in the urine over 24 hours, before and after the administration of corticotropin by IV infusion for 2 or 3 consecutive days. Production of 17-hydroxycorticoids should triple if adrenal function is normal. In primary adrenal corticoid deficiency, steroid production rises slightly on the first day, with no increase thereafter. In secondary insufficiency, steroid production rises higher with each succeeding dose of corticotropin.

Limited courses of corticotropin therapy also are used to produce temporary hypercorticism to produce remissions in certain progressive degenerative diseases. Therapeutic administration of corticotropin appears to be most useful in conditions that respond to glucocorticoid therapy, such as rheumatic disease, autoimmune conditions, myasthenia gravis, and multiple sclerosis.

Theoretically, persons with conditions characterized by remissions and exacerbations are most likely to benefit from corticotropin therapy. Although these conditions do improve when treated by oral glucocorticoids, long-term therapy involves a high risk of serious complications and is not recommended. Use of oral glucocorticoids causes atrophy of the adrenal cortex. When the oral drugs are withdrawn, the body cannot produce adequate hormones, and the resultant hypocorticism tends to exacerbate the disease. Administration of corticotropin increases endogenous steroid production, eases symptoms, and may trigger a lasting remission without the risk of cortisol deficiency when the drug is withdrawn.

Adverse Reactions. Corticotropin therapy is seldom continued over a long period; hence, hypercorticism is rare. Continued administration of the drug can cause iatrogenic Cushing's syndrome, a state characterized by glucocorticoid toxicity and by masculinization in the female. Although full-blown Cushing's syndrome is not seen in short-term corticotropin therapy, there is a tendency toward some of its effects: sodium retention, potassium depletion, hypervolemia, hypertension, ketosis, lipolysis, immunosuppression, and mood elevation. The dermal atrophy that may occur when steroids are given is not a feature of corticotropin therapy, presumably because of the anabolic effects caused by increased androgen secretion.

Immediately after administration of corticotropin, blood glucose is depressed; later, insulin resistance and a tendency toward hyperglycemia are apparent. When administered to clients capable of adrenal cortex response, corticotropin is both diabetogenic and ulcerogenic.

Allergy to animal preparations of corticotropin is not uncommon. Reactions vary from mild fever to anaphylaxis. Although allergy to synthetic preparations is less likely, it does occur. The usual dosage schedules—short terms of intensive therapy separated by long periods of drug withdrawal—favor the development of antibodies.

Precautions and Contraindications. When a history of previous exposure to corticotropin or adverse reaction to it exists, precautions should be taken to prevent or treat allergic reactions. Rapid desensitization may be attempted before beginning the therapeutic regimen. Drugs and equipment necessary for treating anaphylaxis should be available before administering the hormone.

Antituberculosis drugs are frequently prescribed for the period of therapy for clients with a history of this disease. Any infection occurring at this time should be aggressively treated with anti-infectives, because the body's immune and inflammatory response is suppressed during corticotropin therapy.

■ SUMMARY

Corticotropin, a protein hormone normally produced by the pituitary gland, stimulates the adrenal cortex to produce glucocorticoids and enhances production of mineralocorticoids and adrenal sex hormones. Because it can be administered only by injection, corticotropin is not used for replacement therapy in hypopituitarism. Instead, the cortisol normally secreted by the target glands is prescribed. Corticotropin is used diagnostically to differentiate between adrenal and pituitary causes of hypocorticism. It is also administered in therapeutic doses for short periods of time to trigger remissions in certain progressive degenerative diseases. Allergic reactions are the most common adverse reactions to such therapy. Continued administration can produce signs and symptoms of Cushing's syndrome.

❖ Nursing Management: Client Receiving Corticotropin

Clients who undergo diagnostic procedures that involve corticotropin administration are usually deficient in steroid hormones. They show various features of hypocorticism characteristic of Addison's disease: lack of energy, emotional depression, and a tendency toward shock. Their ability to adapt to stress is impaired. The period required for diagnosis is particularly trying because the nature of the underlying problem is unknown. Regardless of the specific disease process, the hormone deficiency is likely to be chronic. Therefore, the signs and symptoms of corticosteroid deficiency are likely to be unusually pronounced.

Clients who receive therapeutic doses of corticotropin usually have normal corticosteroid levels, but they commonly suffer from exacerbation of chronic progressive degenerative diseases. The nursing care required by clients during such a period of acute illness varies, depending on the underlying condition, but invariably clients require careful physiologic monitoring, continuing rehabilitation, and emotional support.

Corticotropin medication continues daily or several times a week until symptoms subside or it is apparent that no response will occur.

Nursing Process: Corticotropin in Diagnostic Testing

These clients need the same nursing care as do those with glucocorticoid deficiency (see Chap. 30). These clients also need considerable emotional support while waiting for diagnosis and treatment.

Client Education. Clients who undergo diagnostic procedures that involve corticotropin need careful explanations of the procedure to minimize the stress imposed by the test. The nature of the corticotropin test for adrenal function should be carefully explained. Twenty-four-hour urine specimens are collected before and during the period of corticotropin dosage. Clients must understand the need to collect all urine produced

during the testing period because loss of part of the specimen invalidates the test.

Clients should be instructed to drink ample fluids and increase sodium intake temporarily. The need for increased sodium is eliminated when the hormone deficiency is treated. Until that time, reduction of stressors and management of stress levels may be critical in preventing hypovolemic shock.

The nurse should teach stress management techniques. The ability to control stress also enhances the client's response to hormone replacement therapy if this is prescribed. Clients may need reassurance that definitive diagnosis of their condition can lead to effective treatment.

Nursing Process: Therapeutic Corticotropin

Assessment

Clients who receive corticotropin therapy usually have normal corticosteroid levels, but they commonly suffer from exacerbation of chronic progressive degenerative diseases. They should be assessed for signs and symptoms of the underlying illness. The data base should include a complete history of the disorder, with a detailed description of the course over recent weeks or months.

Before administering corticotropin, the nurse must carefully assess the client for infection, peptic ulcer disease, and diabetes mellitus. The severity of these conditions is likely to increase when corticotropin is given. The client should be questioned specifically about exposure to or history of tuberculosis.

The client's ability to manage stress and to maintain blood volume and adequate circulation under conditions of stress should be determined. Any tendency toward hypotension may indicate a reduced adrenal reserve. Hypertension may indicate an already high output of corticosteroids.

The client should be questioned about previous exposure to corticotropin and reaction to such exposure. The client's susceptibility to allergic reactions may be determined by gathering a personal and family history of allergic conditions.

Nursing Diagnosis

Nursing diagnoses likely to be made for clients receiving therapeutic doses of corticotropin include those appropriate for exacerbation of the underlying disorder. After corticotropin therapy is established, the client may have:

- Risk for Infection, related to immunosuppression secondary to high levels of corticosteroids
- Altered Thought Processes: Euphoria related to CNS stimulation secondary to excess glucocorticoids
- Impaired Tissue Integrity: Inflammation related to allergic reaction to corticotropin

Some clients may have:

- Knowledge Deficit, concerning the underlying disease and corticotropin therapy to induce remission

A common collaborative problem that should be differentiated from the nursing diagnoses is:

Potential Complications: Peptic ulcer, thrombi, hyperglycemia

PLANNING

Nursing goals include remission of the underlying disease and prevention or prompt detection and treatment of adverse drug reactions (infection, peptic ulcer, diabetes mellitus, intravascular coagulation, and acute allergic reaction). Teaching should provide the client with information about corticotropin, signs and symptoms of adverse reaction to corticosteroids, procedures for monitoring urinary or blood glucose levels, and methods for stress management useful to prevent overproduction of corticotropin. A final nursing goal is to maintain the client's motivation to participate in the treatment and rehabilitation regimen.

INTERVENTION

If there is a history of allergic reaction to corticotropin, or a strong personal or family history of allergic illness, a skin test for allergy to corticotropin should be done. Rapid desensitization may be carried out to reduce the allergic response before therapeutic doses of corticotropin are administered. The healthcare team must be prepared to treat promptly any allergic reaction that may occur, including anaphylaxis.

Corticotropin therapy may be carried out in the hospital to facilitate IV therapy, or it can be given on an outpatient basis when the IM route is used. Medication is given daily or several times a week until symptoms subside or it is apparent that no response will occur.

When preparing corticotropin medication, care should be taken to avoid rough handling. Proteins are degraded by agitation, and the potency of the medication can be impaired by shaking or repeated bubbling of air through the solution. The recommended solvent must be used when dissolving powders. Vials may be rolled gently to accelerate dissolution. Drug preparations should be protected from excessive heat and freezing temperatures.

Clients who receive therapeutic doses of corticotropin must be protected from exposure to contagious disease. Ambulation should be encouraged to promote circulation and decrease the risk of clot formation and phlebitis. To minimize the tendency toward diabetes, the diet should be low in concentrated carbohydrates, moderate in protein, and limited in calories to the level necessary to maintain a lean body weight. Clients known to have allergic reactions should be protected against exposure to any substances that trigger the reaction, because allergic reaction to one allergen lowers the threshold for allergic response to another (in this case, corticotropin).

Clients who receive repeated doses of corticotropin should be monitored for signs and symptoms of Cushing's syndrome, especially if the course of treatment is prolonged. They must be assessed regularly for pain and suppuration, which may be the only signs of infection, due to the antiinflammatory action of glucocorticoids. Urine tests or finger sticks for increased glucose levels should be performed regularly. Clients must also be monitored for signs and symptoms of hyperacidity, peptic ulcers, and abnormal clots. These adverse drug reactions should be promptly reported so they can be corrected.

Anti-infectives may be prescribed to control infection or prevent a recurrence of tuberculosis if a history of this condition exists. Medications to control peptic ulcer disease (histamine [H_2] receptor antagonists or antacids) may be ordered also. If the client develops hyperglycemia, insulin injections may be required.

Client Education. Clients who receive corticotropin therapy need explanations of the rationale for using the drug and instructions about its side effects. During and after treatment, clients should avoid exposure to infection, for which they are at high risk. The signs and symptoms of hypercorticism should be explained, and clients should be told to report any evidence of hypertension, increase in symptoms attributable to peptic ulcer or diabetes mellitus, or infection. Because the inflammatory response is suppressed by glucocorticoids, some of the usual warning signs of infection, such as fever, redness, and swelling, may be absent. Pain and loss of function may be the only indications of infection, and these should be promptly reported. Infections tend to progress rapidly when adrenal cortex function is high; prompt treatment is essential.

The client should understand that the feeling of well-being produced by increased blood levels of corticosteroids is drug-induced and may not correspond to the degree of remission induced. This euphoria must not be allowed to interfere with motivation to participate in the treatment and rehabilitation regimen.

Clients should avoid severe stressors. These can limit therapeutic response and reduce the chances of a full or lasting remission. If remission is achieved, subsequent exacerbations are more likely to occur when stress levels exceed the client's adaptive capacity. This produces a relative hormone deficiency state, which predisposes to recurrence of full-blown disease. Clients can benefit greatly by developing coping strategies and skill in managing stress.

OUTCOME EVALUATION

Data required for evaluation relate to the severity of signs and symptoms of the underlying disease, absence or incidence and severity of adverse reactions to corticotropin, increased knowledge of corticotropin therapy by the client, and increased ability of the client to manage stress (see Example of Nursing Process and Corticotropin Therapy).

Example of Nursing Process for Corticotropin Therapy

The client is a 31-year-old housewife and mother of two with a 5-year history of multiple sclerosis. At the time of diagnosis, she was pregnant; termination of the pregnancy produced a remission. She had no symptoms until yesterday, when she experienced difficulty walking due to a significant weakness in the left leg. The exacerbation coincided with a record-breaking heat wave.

The client has been admitted to the hospital for intensive treatment with IV corticotropin in an attempt to produce another remission. The client appears tense and apprehensive. She expresses fear that the treatment "won't work" and states, "I hate needles."

Assessment Data

Diagnosis of multiple sclerosis

Weakness of the left leg

Need for administration of medication by injection

Client's statement that she hates needles

Corticotropin therapy, involving stimulation of glucocorticoid secretion (glucocorticoids act as immunosuppressants)

IV therapy

Client statement that she is afraid the treatment might not work

Muscular tension and fearful facial expression

Heat wave coinciding with exacerbation of multiple sclerosis (increased stress can precipitate an attack of multiple sclerosis)

Nursing Diagnosis	Intervention	Goals and Outcomes
Impaired Physical Mobility, related to demyelinization secondary to multiple sclerosis	**Administer** IV corticotropin as ordered. **Eliminate** stressors that impinge on the client as much as possible. **Suggest** to the physician that the client receive physiotherapy while in the hospital. **Ensure** a comfortably cool environment for the client during her hospital stay.	Before leaving the hospital, the client will be able to walk with a normal gait.
Fear, of pain related to IV therapy venipuncture required for treatment of multiple sclerosis	**Explore** with the client previous experience with venipuncture; ascertain any special problems that relate to this procedure (eg, "poor veins") and relay this information to the person responsible for starting the IV infusion. **Request** special precautions to facilitate venipuncture (eg, use of topical nitroglycerin to dilate the vein in which the needle is inserted, use of a topical anesthetic to prevent pain from penetration of the skin, use of a heparin lock). **Inform** the client of measures taken to decrease the discomfort of venipuncture.	The client will state that the IV procedure was not as painful as she expected.
Risk for Infection, related to impaired skin integrity secondary to venipuncture and immunosuppression	**Maintain** strict sterile asepsis in relation to venipuncture, heparin lock, and IV infusion. **Caution** the client not to touch the infusion site or to get it wet.	The client will not develop redness, swelling, or pain at the site of injection or at the intubated vein. She also will not have chills and fever indicative of septicemia.

(continued)

Example of Nursing Process for Corticotropin Therapy (continued)

Nursing Diagnosis (continued)	Intervention (continued)	Goals and Outcomes (continued)
Fear, of continued or progressive disability	**Acknowledge** that multiple sclerosis sometimes progresses rapidly and can cause severe disability; stress that sometimes it remains arrested for years and causes little disability, and that occasionally the disease will not recur at all after one or two acute episodes.	The client will appear more relaxed. Client comments will indicate that she feels better or more in control in relation to her disease.
	Inform the client of measures she can take to reduce the risk of exacerbation (eg, management of stressors and prevention of high levels of stress, avoidance of acute infection).	
	Teach the client stress management techniques or refer her to a clinic or independent practitioner where instruction in stress reduction is offered.	
Knowledge Deficit, concerning relation of stress to exacerbation	**Explore** with the client her knowledge concerning the effects of stress on multiple sclerosis. Identify heat as a stressor likely to precipitate an exacerbation. Discuss with the client measures she can take to reduce the stress of high temperature (fans, air conditioning)	The client will not experience exacerbations during future periods of hot weather.

❖ **CHECKLIST OF NURSING ACTIONS**

❑ Before beginning treatment, assess the client carefully for infection and history of tuberculosis, peptic ulcer disease, diabetes mellitus, and allergic sensitivity to corticotropin; take action to prevent these complications.

❑ Protect corticotropin solutions from heat, freezing, and agitation to prevent denaturing the drug's protein molecule.

❑ Continue treatment of the client's underlying condition during corticotropin therapy.

❑ Monitor clients for evidence of hypercorticism.

❑ Teach clients to report symptoms that indicate infection, peptic ulcer disease, glucose imbalance, or hypercorticism.

❑ Teach clients techniques of stress management to promote long-term remission.

Growth Hormone

The hormone produced most abundantly by the anterior pituitary is growth hormone (somatotropin). This protein hormone is necessary for normal growth and development of the immature organism. Forms of biosynthetic human growth hormone available for therapeutic use include somatrem (Protropin) and humatrope. Both are products of recombinant DNA. A protein fragment of the molecule, TGF-beta, is reportedly helpful in treating macular degeneration (Adler, 1994).

Physiology

In adults, growth hormone appears to play a role in the adaptive response to stress, especially during the fasting state, and in the maintenance of muscle mass and strength.

Somatotropin is produced by specific acidophilic cells in the anterior pituitary known as somatotrophs. Secretion is not steady but tends to be intermittent or sporadic. In prepubertal children, somatotropin production is highest during sleep, especially the deep sleep stage, lending credence to the folk saying that children grow most rapidly during sleep. Somatotropin production at all ages is stimulated by emotional excitement, exercise, hypoglycemia, and other stressors.

Pathophysiology

Abnormalities of growth hormone production produce several disease conditions. During childhood, excessive production of somatotropin causes excessive growth or gigantism; hormone deficiencies impair growth, producing dwarfism characterized by delayed maturation and inadequate but symmetric growth. In the adult, somatotropin deficiencies appear to be rare but may underlie weakness in bones, muscles, and the heart. Excesses cause a thickening of bony and soft-tissue structures, a condition known as acromegaly. At any age, excesses of growth hormone eventually lead to musculoskeletal disorders and diabetes mellitus, and deficiencies predispose to hypoglycemia and reduce the hyperglycemic response to stress.

Pharmacodynamics. The specific mechanisms by which somatotropin stimulates cellular division and differentiation are unknown, but the hormone causes many metabolic changes in most tissues. In the liver, kidneys, and other tissues, somatotropin stimulates the production of somatomedins, substances that stimulate the incorporation of sulfate into tissues such as cartilage. Body levels of electrolytes such as sodium, chlorine, potassium, phosphorus, and calcium rise. All of these, except calcium, are reabsorbed by the kidneys at higher levels than normal; renal excretion of calcium increases but is offset by a distinct increase in calcium absorption by the intestines. The body's lipid energy reserves are mobilized, and levels of circulating free fatty acids rise. Energy production is switched from carbohydrate to fat fuel sources, and blood sugar levels rise. Growth hormone has anabolic effects similar to those of insulin but opposes the hypoglycemic action of insulin by decreasing tissue sensitivity to it. As would be expected when tissue growth is accelerated, the transport of amino acids into tissue cells and their incorporation into protein are increased. The production of urea and other nitrogenous wastes declines, and a positive nitrogen balance is established.

The metabolic effects of somatotropin appear not only to enhance tissue growth in immature organisms but also to protect persons of all ages from tissue breakdown during states that require increased use of stored energy because of stress or fasting. Somatotropin appears to reverse some of the effects of aging; it is known to increase muscle mass, increase bone strength, decrease fat deposits, and increase skin thickness in the elderly.

Pharmacodynamics. As a protein substance, somatotropin is degraded by proteases in the digestive tract and cannot be administered orally. It is administered only by injection. Once absorbed, somatotropin moves rapidly into the cells. Although the serum half-life of somatotropin is only about 20 minutes, the effect of a given dose lasts at least a week. The hormone appears to be degraded by both the liver and the kidney, which return the amino acid residues to the metabolic pool.

Therapeutic Uses. Somatotropin is indicated for treating pituitary dwarfism. In usual dosages (thrice-weekly IM injections of 0.1 mg/kg), it stimulates normal proportional growth in dwarves without stimulating sexual maturation or symptoms of hormone excess. Growth may be tripled the first year of treatment and doubled subsequently. Treatment is aimed at producing a height of at least 5 feet, considered the minimum necessary for normal function in modern society.

Somatotropin may become useful in maintaining muscle and cardiac strength in the aged and in body tissues under conditions of weightlessness (in which muscles and bones atrophy). It may also be useful as an adjunct in treating obesity.

Adverse Reactions. In the dosages used therapeutically to date, somatotropin toxicity has not been reported. High doses could produce gigantism or acromegaly. Theoretically, somatotropin could increase the growth rate of malignant tumors; it has been reported to double the risk of leukemia. It is diabetogenic.

Precautions and Contraindications. Clients who receive the drug should be monitored carefully in relation to growth and maturation. If sexual immaturity persists as height approaches adult proportions, replacement therapy with appropriate sex hormones may be needed.

■ SUMMARY

Somatotropin is the anterior pituitary hormone responsible for normal growth and development. It is approved for use only as replacement therapy for persons deficient in this hormone (pituitary dwarves).

❖ NURSING MANAGEMENT: CLIENT RECEIVING SOMATOTROPIN

NURSING PROCESS

ASSESSMENT

Before growth hormone therapy is begun, the client should be assessed for growth and development and for the emotional impact of growth retardation.

NURSING DIAGNOSIS

Diagnoses for the client receiving growth hormone may include:

- Altered Growth and Development: Physical growth less than normal related to growth hormone deficiency
- Body Image Disturbance, related to physical growth less than normal secondary to growth hormone deficiency

PLANNING

Goals of nursing care for the client receiving growth hormone include improved body image and resumption of physical growth. The long-term goal is attainment of a body size compatible with a normal lifestyle.

INTERVENTION

The nurse may promote an improved self-image by warm acceptance of the client and appropriate encouragement of physical appearance and personality traits. Clients need considerable emotional support, especially during the early phases of treatment.

Client Education. The nurse should promote hope of successful treatment but should realistically explain that the result may not fully satisfy the client's wishes regarding adult body size.

OUTCOME EVALUATION

Data required for evaluation include comments by the client indicative of self-image and measurements of body growth, especially height.

❖ CHECKLIST OF NURSING ACTIONS

- ❑ Assess body growth and development (especially height) each time the client is seen.
- ❑ Reinforce a positive self-image when interacting with the client.

Growth Hormone Antagonist

A mutant bovine hormone similar in structure to somatotropin has been reported to antagonize growth hormone. Its action may be that of competitive inhibition for cell receptors that normally respond to somatotropin. This substance may prove useful in treating gigantism (excess of somatotropin during childhood), acromegaly (excess of somatotropin in adults), or diabetic retinopathy (which appears to improve or stabilize when the pituitary is destroyed and endogenous somatotropin eliminated).

Thyrotropin

Thyrotropin is a glycoprotein produced by basophilic cells in the anterior pituitary. The rate of production is inversely proportional to circulating thyroid hormone levels, a negative feedback system that normally maintains thyroid hormone production within a narrow range. Bovine thyrotropin (Thytropar) is available for medicinal use.

Pharmacodynamics. Thyrotropin increases cAMP levels in thyroid cells. As a result, all phases of thyroid hormone synthesis and release are stimulated: iodine uptake, formation of organic iodides, and hormone synthesis. The pituitary hormone increases vascularity in the thyroid and produces glandular hypertrophy and hyperplasia. It may exert a protective role in reducing the risk of atrial fibrillation (Brooks, 1994).

Pharmacokinetics. Little information is available about the distribution or elimination of thyrotropin. As a protein substance, it must be administered by injection.

Therapeutic Uses. Thyrotropin is administered only to differentiate between primary thyroid hypofunction and hypothyroidism due to deficiency of pituitary thyrotropin. To carry out this diagnostic test, a dose of 10 U of thyrotropin is administered IM, followed 18 to 24 hours later by a tracer dose of radioactive iodine (^{131}I). After another 24-hour interval, RAIU is measured and compared with the baseline RAIU. If uptake has increased significantly, thyroid gland response to thyrotropin is demonstrated and pituitary hypofunction is indicated. This diagnostic test may eventually be replaced by direct measurement of endogenous thyrotropin levels by radioimmunoassay.

Adverse Reactions. Thyrotropin has caused cardiac arrhythmias (tachycardia, atrial fibrillation), GI problems (nausea, vomiting), headache, fever, and menstrual irregularities. Allergic manifestations include urticaria and anaphylaxis. In high doses, the drug can cause thyroid enlargement (goiter).

Precautions and Contraindications. Clients in an advanced state of myxedema can tolerate only minute increments of thyroid hormone, and a thyrotropin diagnostic test could induce cardiac failure. Diagnosis should be delayed until the acute hormone deficiency has responded to carefully graduated doses of thyroid hormone.

■ SUMMARY

Thyrotropin is the protein hormone of the anterior pituitary that stimulates the thyroid gland to produce thyroid hormone. It is used medicinally in a diagnostic test to differentiate pituitary from thyroid causes of hypothyroidism.

❖ NURSING MANAGEMENT: CLIENT RECEIVING THYROTROPIN

The client who undergoes diagnostic testing with thyrotropin is deficient in thyroid hormone. If frank myxedema or cardiac malfunction is apparent, the diagnostic test may be postponed until the client has received some thyroid hormone therapy and is in better condition to withstand the test.

When preparing thyrotropin doses, the vial must be handled gently. Bubbling air through the solution or shaking the vial may cause breakdown of the protein molecule, reducing the preparation's potency. The hormone should be stored in a part of the refrigerator that does not drop below freezing.

NURSING PROCESS

The client may exhibit various levels of thyroid deficiency and require the usual nursing care for this condition.

Client Education. At first, teaching should be limited to the facts needed to gain the client's cooperation in the nursing regimen and to refute the client's negative self-image. Before the diagnostic test, the procedure should be explained to the client, with simple instructions for participation. When hormone treatment improves memory and mental functioning, a teaching program appropriate for the final diagnosis can be carried out.

❖ CHECKLIST OF NURSING ACTIONS

- ❑ For clients undergoing a thyrotropin diagnostic test, provide nursing care appropriate to hypothyroidism, as well as emotional support.
- ❑ Before the test, assess the degree of hormone deficiency and cardiac status. Report frank myxedema or evidence of cardiac disease promptly.
- ❑ Teach hypothyroid clients only the information needed to cooperate with and accept the diagnostic procedure.
- ❑ To preserve drug potency, protect thyrotropin solutions from heat, freezing, and agitation.

Hypothalamic Hormones

In recent decades, scientists have discovered that the hypothalamus produces hormone substances that control secretions of tropic hormones by the anterior pituitary. The hypothalamus also produces the hormones previously believed to have been synthesized in the posterior pituitary. The hypothalamus lies near the pituitary and is connected to it by a major vascular pathway. This pathway transports brain hormones to the pituitary gland.

Releasing and inhibiting factors that control anterior pituitary function include thyrotropin-releasing hormone, corticotropin-releasing factor, growth hormone-releasing factor, growth hormone release-inhibiting factor (somatostatin), and various factors that control the release of pituitary gonadotropins (Box 33-2). Research into the properties of these substances and their potential therapeutic value is in progress. These substances are unavailable for therapeutic use, although nurses involved in research may encounter them in investigational procedures.

Two hormones long known to enter the blood from the posterior pituitary include antidiuretic hormone (ADH) and oxytocin. These hormones are synthesized by nerve bodies of the supraventricular or paraventricular nuclei of the hypothalamus. In normal persons, these chemicals are transported to the neurohypophysis, where they are stored until they are subsequently released into the bloodstream. Persons whose pituitaries have been damaged or destroyed by disease or trauma may still produce enough of these hormones, provided the adjacent hypothalamic structures have escaped injury.

Antidiuretic Hormone

Antidiuretic hormone (vasopressin) is a protein hormone produced in the hypothalamus and stored in and released by the posterior pituitary. Medicinal preparations of ADH include solutions (in both water and oil) of animal pituitary extracts and synthetic preparations (Table 33-8).

Physiology

Antidiuretic hormone maintains normal osmotic pressure and extracellular fluid volume by controlling water

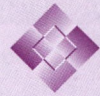

Box 33-2
Hypothalamic Hormones That Control the Release of Pituitary Hormones

Corticotropin-releasing factor

Thyrotropin-releasing hormone

Luteinizing hormone-releasing hormone and follicle stimulating hormone-releasing hormone (gonadotropin-releasing hormone)

Growth hormone release-inhibiting hormone

Growth hormone releasing factor

Prolactin release-inhibiting hormone

Prolactin-releasing factor

Melanocyte-stimulating hormone release-inhibiting factor

Melanocyte-stimulating hormone release factor

reabsorption in the renal distal tubule. Osmoreceptors and vascular pressure receptors in the higher cerebral centers react to increased osmolarity in the blood and reduced extracellular fluid volume by stimulating ADH production by the hypothalamic neurosecretory cells. Other factors that stimulate ADH secretion include decreased plasma volume, pain, stress, sleep, exercise, positive-pressure ventilation, and certain drugs (eg, nicotine, morphine, barbiturates, some anesthetics, vincristine). Released into the bloodstream, ADH promotes reabsorption of water in the medullary portion of the collecting duct of the nephron. This action tends to correct hyperosmolarity and inadequate extracellular fluid volume.

Pathophysiology

Hyposecretion of ADH is the disease syndrome known as diabetes insipidus. The deficiency may arise spontaneously as an idiopathic state or may occur as a result of brain trauma. After head injury or cranial surgery, diabetes insipidus tends to be a temporary malfunction that improves spontaneously as healing proceeds and brain function improves.

Excessive ADH is sometimes secreted by clients with tumors, head injury, meningitis, encephalitis, pulmonary infections, or other diseases. Excess ADH may be produced by secreting tumors or by drugs such as vincristine or cyclophosphamide, which stimulate endogenous production. Hypersecretion of ADH causes water retention and pronounced dilutional hyponatremia.

Pharmacodynamics. As with many protein hormones, the effects of ADH appear to be mediated by an increase in cAMP in the target cells. In the kidney, ADH is bound by receptors on the cell surfaces of the collecting duct. As a result, cortical and medullary segments of

Table 33-8. Medicinal Preparations of Antidiuretic Hormone

Drug Name	Preparation/Concentration	Uses	Usual Dosage
desmopressin acetate (DDAVP)	Clear liquid solution of synthetic peptide for intranasal administration; 100 μg/mL	Agent of choice for control of diabetes insipidus	Adults: 10–40 μg daily, divided in 2–4 doses Children: 0.05–0.3 mL daily, divided in 2–4 doses
	Solution for IV and SC injection; 4 μg/mL	Control of diabetes insipidus	Maintenance: 2–4 μg daily in accordance with response (divided in 2 doses)
		Management of excessive bleeding	0.3 μg/kg (by slow IV infusion) PC: B
lypressin (Diapid)	Solution for intranasal administration; 185 μg/mL	Control of diabetes insipidus	1 or 2 sprays (7–14 μg) in each nostril 4 times daily PC: B
vasopressin injection (Pitressin)	Aqueous solution of synthetic vasopressin for injection; 20 pressor U/mL	Treatment of diabetes insipidus	Adults: 0.25–0.5 mL q6–12h PRN PC: B
vasopressin tannate (Pitressin Tannate)	Peanut oil suspension of water-insoluble tannate of antidiuretic principle; 5 pressor U/mL	Second-choice agent for control of diabetes insipidus	Adults: 0.3–1 mL every 2–3 days Children: 0.25–0.5 mL every 2–3 days PC: B

KEY: PC = pregnancy risk category; see Appendix A.

the collecting duct become more permeable to water, and the water then diffuses passively across the membrane at a more rapid rate. High concentrations of ADH cause vasoconstriction and increased blood pressure. The net effect partially depends on the reactivity of pressure receptor reflexes. When the efficiency of this reflex is impaired (eg, during anesthesia), small amounts of hormone cause greater-than-usual responses. Normally, such effects are not seen because the doses necessary for them exceed those required to maintain water balance.

Pharmacokinetics. Drug preparations may be given by injection or intranasal spray. The plasma half-life of some preparations is as short as 10 minutes. Some of the hormone is destroyed by blood peptidases and some binds to receptors on smooth muscle, but 33% to 50% of a given dose reaches the receptors of the renal distal tubule, where it stimulates water reabsorption. Most of the hormone is degraded by target tissues, with less than 20% eliminated unchanged in urine.

Therapeutic Uses. Antidiuretic hormone is prescribed for hormone replacement in clients affected by diabetes insipidus. The treatment period is limited for clients who experience transient diabetes insipidus as a result of head injury or surgery, but treatment is lifelong for clients with idiopathic hormone deficiencies. The drugs of choice for chronic deficiency are desmopressin and lypressin, which are administered intranasally two to four times a day in accordance with the degree of polyuria. When these drugs are not effective or cannot be used, vasopressin tannate is prescribed. This preparation is administered every 2 to 3 days. Dosage schedules

are flexible and are determined by the duration of response to a given dose. When urine production rises above normal, another dose is administered.

Vasopressin is sometimes used to control hemorrhage by vasoconstriction or to elevate blood pressure in clients with vasogenic hypotension. It is also used in a diagnostic procedure to determine the ability of the kidneys to concentrate urine.

Adverse Reactions. Antidiuretic hormone is irritating to the tissues and can cause redness, swelling, and burning pain at the injection site. Nasal congestion and inflammation or itching can follow intranasal administration. Systemic effects of the medication include headache, nausea and vomiting, flushing or pallor, abdominal cramps and an urge to defecate, uterine cramps and vulval pain, and cardiovascular changes (angina pectoris, increased blood pressure). Large doses can produce hyponatremia and water intoxication, bradycardia, premature atrial contractions, heart block, myocardial infarction, and peripheral vascular collapse.

Allergy to ADH can develop regardless of the route of administration. Allergic reactions range from local inflammation in the nose when intranasal preparations are used to urticaria and anaphylaxis. Drug resistance may also develop.

Vasopressin tannate administration may result in sterile abscesses at the injection site. Large doses can produce peripheral vasoconstriction sufficient to cause gangrene.

Precautions and Contraindications. Clients with cardiovascular disease, especially coronary artery disease, should not receive vasopressin, except in minimal doses if required for the control of diabetes insipidus. Increased angina, decreased cardiac output, and increased peripheral resistance may precipitate serious cardiac complications, including arrhythmia and CHF. The heart action of clients who receive IV infusions of ADH should be continually monitored.

When ADH is administered to clients who do not have diabetes insipidus, fluid intake should be restricted to prevent water intoxication. Vital signs, urine volume, and urine specific gravity should be monitored.

Intranasal preparations should not be inhaled. The effect of a given dose in this form may be reduced by nasal congestion and hypersecretion, which impair absorption. Until the rhinitis subsides, doses should be taken more frequently, as required by frequency of micturition.

Antidiuretic hormone should be used with caution in treating diabetes insipidus in children. The drug should be administered intranasally. Special care should be taken to prevent water intoxication, which is likely to cause seizures in children.

The use of ADH is contraindicated in clients allergic to it and in those with type IIB or platelet-type von Willebrand disease.

Drug Interactions. Lithium, demeclocycline, heparin, alcohol, and large doses of epinephrine decrease the physiologic effect of ADH. Chlorpropamide, urea, fludrocortisone, and clofibrate enhance ADH action.

▪▪ S U M M A R Y
ADH, a protein normally produced by the hypothalamus, acts to control osmolality and volume of extracellular fluid by moderating water reabsorption in the renal distal tubule. Injectable or intranasal preparations are used to control the symptoms of diabetes insipidus and to treat shock caused by vascular hypotonicity or hemorrhage. Side effects of the drug include mild discomforts, such as intestinal hyperactivity or uterine cramps, and more serious complications, such as CHF and peripheral vascular insufficiency. The drug is rarely given to clients with cardiovascular disease.

❖ NURSING MANAGEMENT: CLIENT RECEIVING ANTIDIURETIC HORMONE

As with all protein preparations, ADH solutions must be protected from heat, freezing, and agitation. However, vasopressin tannate in oil must be warmed by immersion in heated water before it can be drawn up in a syringe. At room temperature, the solution is too viscid to pass through the bore of an IM needle.

NURSING PROCESS
ASSESSMENT
Before administration of vasopressin, the client's fluid and electrolyte balance and cardiac status should be carefully assessed. Clients with chronic deficiencies of ADH are relatively dehydrated despite intake of large amounts of fluids. Serum levels of sodium are likely to be elevated. Dehydration usually is not found in clients treated for vasogenic shock but may be apparent in clients with hemorrhage. The client's knowledge about and emotional reaction to the diagnosed medical condition and the use of vasopressin in its treatment should be explored.

NURSING DIAGNOSIS
Nursing diagnoses likely to be made for the client receiving vasopressin include:

- Risk for Fluid Volume Excess: Hyponatremic water intoxication related to excessive reabsorption of water by the kidneys secondary to vasopressin medication
- Knowledge Deficit, concerning the diagnosed illness and the use of vasopressin in its treatment

A common collaborative problem that should be differentiated from the nursing diagnoses is:

Potential Complication: Cardiovascular

PLANNING
Goals of nursing care include maintaining fluid balance, restoring circulation (by slowing hemorrhage, correcting vasodilation, or restoring fluid volume), and promptly detecting and treating adverse drug reactions. The goal of the teaching program for clients receiving ADH for hemorrhage or vasogenic shock is to supply specific information needed to adhere to the treatment regimen. Clients with diabetes insipidus must learn to manage long-term hormone therapy.

INTERVENTION
Preparations of ADH may be administered by SC, IM, or IV injection or nasal spray. Intranasal administration is preferred for the control of diabetes insipidus; for clients who cannot tolerate this form of medication, vasopressin tannate is usually prescribed.

Before using the nasal spray, the condition of the nasal membrane should be assessed. Redness, swelling, and discomfort or itching can develop. One or two sprays are administered, with subsequent doses used as needed (usually four times a day). If the frequency of micturition is not controlled, the amount of each dose should not be increased; rather, the drug should be taken more often.

To assess response to therapy, fluid balance must be monitored carefully. Inadequate hormone replacement causes excessive production of dilute urine and a return of the symptoms of diabetes insipidus. Excessive dosage causes fluid retention and dilution of electrolytes in body fluids. To prevent fluid and electrolyte imbalances, clients must be watched for low specific gravity of urine, polyuria and polydipsia (which denote ADH deficiency), and high specific gravity of urine and oliguria (which denote ADH excess). Sudden changes in weight and blood pressure indicate serious fluid imbalance.

When vasopressin is used for purposes other than hormone replacement, clients should be closely watched for signs and symptoms of water intoxication or cardiovascular malfunction. Vital signs and urine osmolality should be monitored regularly. Fluid intake should be carefully controlled. When vasopressin is administered IV, clients should be placed on cardiac monitors, and the peripheral circulation should be assessed frequently. Injection sites used for administration of vasopressin should be watched for signs of inflammation.

Client Education. Clients with chronic hormone deficiency need a comprehensive teaching program designed to provide the knowledge and skills needed to maintain hormone and fluid balance over the long term through the use of ADH medication. They face a lifetime of hormone therapy and may require considerable support to accept the treatment regimen. They must be taught techniques for administration of the drug by intranasal spray or injection. Dosage must be adjusted in accordance with the degree of polyuria. Clients should be taught the signs and symptoms of allergic reactions and urged to report these promptly.

OUTCOME EVALUATION

Data required for evaluation of the care of clients treated for diabetes insipidus include information pertinent to fluid balance (tissue turgor, urinary frequency, urine volume and osmolarity, thirst, and serum osmolality) and the absence or incidence of toxic or side effects. Evaluation of clients who receive vasopressin for its pharmacologic effect requires data about circulation (vital signs, color, warmth of extremities), intestinal motility, blood loss from hemorrhage, and absence or incidence of adverse drug reactions.

❖ CHECKLIST OF NURSING ACTIONS

When Vasopressin Is Used for Hormone Replacement

- ❑ To preserve the potency of drug preparations, protect solutions from excessive heat, freezing, and agitation; warm ampules of pitressin tannate in oil before drawing up the dose.
- ❑ Assess clients for local and systemic allergic reactions.
- ❑ Monitor administration sites for inflammatory changes.
- ❑ Teach clients with chronic diabetes insipidus to administer their own drugs and adjust dosage regimens in accordance with the volume of urinary output.
- ❑ Support client acceptance of lifelong drug therapy.

When Vasopressin Is Used for Other Purposes

- ❑ Monitor clients closely for water intoxication and cardiovascular complications (angina, myocardial

infarction, cardiovascular collapse, impaired peripheral circulation).
- ❑ Monitor injection sites for inflammatory changes.

Oxytocin

Oxytocin, another hormone produced by the hypothalamus, is involved in the stimulation of labor and postpartum lactation. It is used pharmacologically to induce labor. Because deficiency of this hormone is not recognized as a clinical problem, it is not used for replacement therapy. Oxytocin is discussed in detail in Chapter 10.

References

Adler T. (1993). Dioxins meddle with key thyroid hormone. *Science News, 144,* 391 (Dec. 11, 1993).

Adler T. (1994). New drug helps close macular holes. *Science News, 146,* 7 (July 2, 1994).

Brooks AC. (1994). Low TSH: An early warning for stroke. *Science News, 146,* 311 (Nov. 12, 1994).

Early PJ, Sodes DB. (1995). *Principles and practice of nuclear medicine,* 2d ed. St. Louis: CV Mosby.

Saha GB. (1992). *Fundamentals of nuclear medicine,* 3d ed. New York: Springer-Verlag.

Bibliography

*Angelucci PA. (1995). Caring for patients with hypothyroidism. *Nursing '95, 25*(May), 60–61.

Brody JE. (1995). Restoring ebbing hormones may slow aging. *New York Times,* July 18, C1–C3.

Erickson D. (1990). Big-time orphan: Human growth hormone could be a blockbuster. *Scientific American, 263*(3), 164–166.

Growth hormone in the elderly: Trying to balance dose and adverse effect. (1993). *Am J Nurs, 93*(3), 53.

Hussar DA. (1990). New drugs: Nafarelin acetate. *Nursing '90, 20*(12), 49.

Kortbawi P. (1990). Myxedema coma: Causes and symptoms. *Nursing '90, 20*(8), 90.

Langreth RN. (1990). Milk from engineered hormone: Udderly safe. *Science News, 138,* 372.

Mercer ME. (1990). Myths and facts: About diabetes insipidus. *Nursing '90, 20*(5), 20.

Weiss PL. (1990). Growth-gene mickey makes mice mini. *Science News, 138,* 20.

*Recommended for further reading.

For more information and sample tests and activities, refer to Chapter 33 in the Student Workbook for Clinical Pharmacology and Nursing Management, 5th edition, available through your bookstore.

X

Drugs Affecting the Immune System

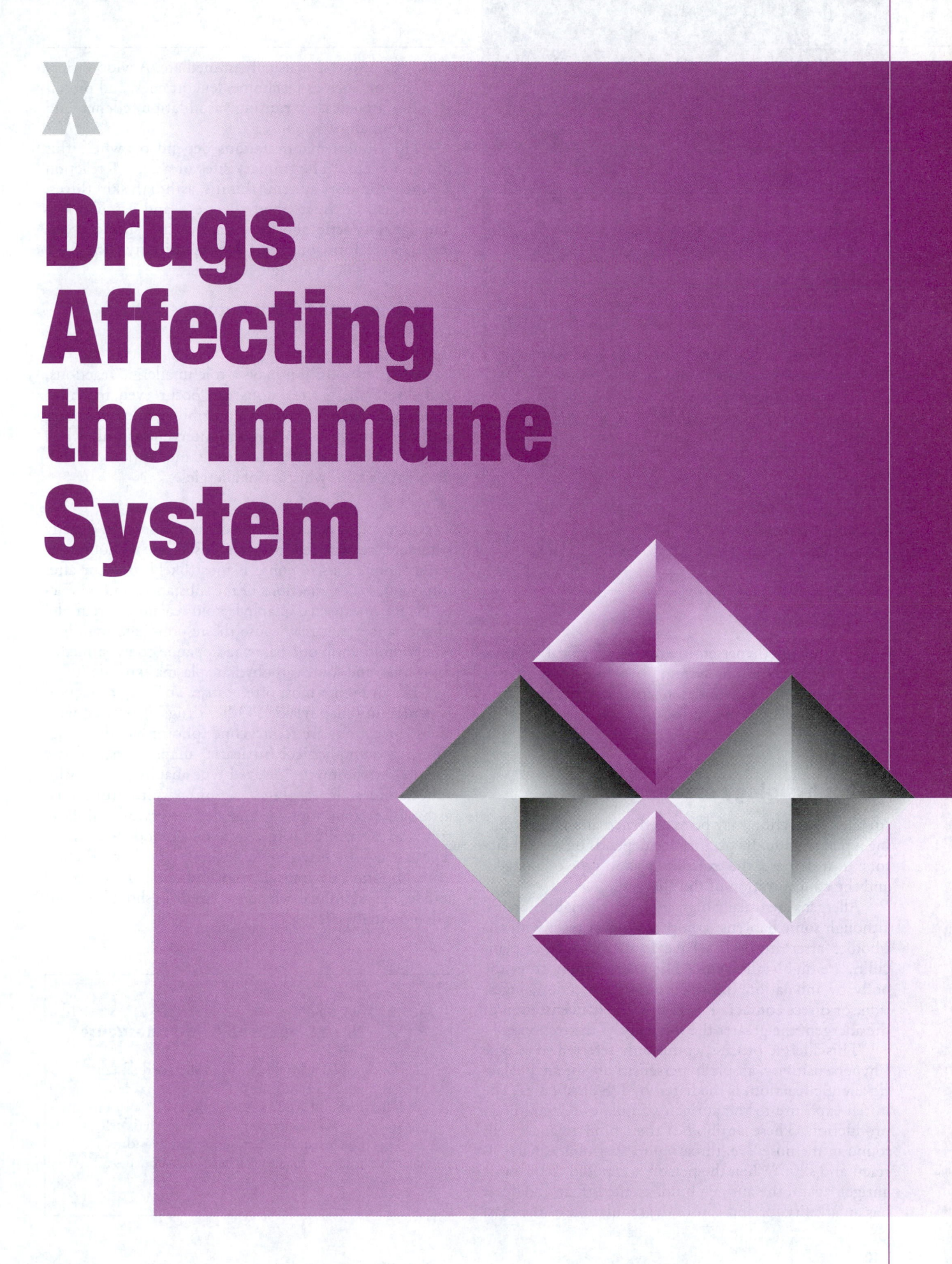

34

Drugs That Control Allergies

An allergy (hypersensitivity) is an atypical response of the immune system to a foreign substance (antigen) that under normal conditions causes no problems. About one in four Americans suffers from allergies.

Pathophysiology of Allergies

An allergic reaction may be exacerbated at any time during a person's life. Its occurrence depends on several factors: host defense, the exposure to and type of allergen, and the concentration of the allergen.

Allergens are usually high-molecular-weight proteins, although some haptens (compounds that react with antibodies after antibodies have formed), such as penicillin, are highly allergenic. The allergen may enter the body by inhalation (most common), injection, ingestion, or direct contact. The higher the concentration of the allergen, the greater the intensity of the response.

This allergic process, commonly referred to as type I hypersensitivity, atopic hypersensitivity, or anaphylactic allergic reaction, is mediated by IgE antibodies. The initial exposure to the antigen stimulates IgE antibody production. These antibodies then bind to mast cells found in the nose, eye, throat, lung, gastrointestinal (GI) tract, and skin. When the person is exposed to the same antigen again, the antigen binds to the IgE antibodies it has an affinity for and causes degranulation of the mast cells. The response is usually immediate. A wide variety of mediators such as histamine, leukotrienes, and prostaglandins are released, causing vasodilation, edema, and an inflammatory response.

The clinical manifestations depend on where this reaction occurs. The primary sites of a type 1 reaction are the respiratory system (rhinitis, asthma), skin (hives, dermatitis), GI tract (food allergies), and vascular system (anaphylactic shock). Anaphylactic shock is the most severe form of type I hypersensitivity. Box 34-1 lists the steps in an allergic response.

Components and Contributors to Allergic Reactions
Genetic Predisposition

Genetic predisposition plays a role in allergic reactions, and severe allergic reactions can occur even in childhood. Anaphylaxis is always a possibility, and healthcare providers should be prepared to intervene rapidly when administering vaccines or allergenic medications to children with a family history of allergies.

Drugs

Certain compounds, especially organic bases, can directly stimulate the mast cells to release histamine without prior sensitization. This response is most likely to occur after intravenous (IV) injections of the substances and may account for unexpected anaphylactoid reactions. Examples of substances that may cause the response are pyridium compounds, antibiotic bases, radiopaque contrast media, morphine, and some carbohydrate plasma expanders.

The drug that most often causes an allergic reaction is penicillin (anaphylaxis). Other drugs associated with allergic reactions are tetracycline (phototoxic skin reaction), chloramphenicol (urticaria, anaphylaxis, aplastic anemia), streptomycin (delayed-type anaphylactic shock), sulfonamides (fever, skin reaction), aspirin (urticaria, asthma), acetaminophen, and derivatives of aminopyrine and pyrazoline (skin, systemic, blood dyscrasias). These drugs are listed in Table 34-1. Local anesthetics, cephalosporins, dextrans, heroin, and radiopaque organic iodides are additional offenders. No drug should be considered totally safe.

Box 34-1
Three Steps in an Allergic Response

1. The specific antibody links to the allergen (antigen), which excites the cell membrane receptors.
2. The antibody is adsorbed by the specific receptor, which is thought to exist on the mast cell.
3. Histamine, leukotrienes, and prostaglandins are released, initiating the signs and symptoms of the allergic response.

Table 34-1. Drugs Most Likely to Cause an Allergic Response

Drugs	Allergic Responses
Penicillins	Urticaria, anaphylactic shock
Tetracycline	Phototoxic skin reaction
Chloramphenicol	Delayed skin allergy, urticaria, anaphylaxis, aplastic anemia
Streptomycin	Delayed-type anaphylactic shock
Sulfonamides	Fever, skin reaction
Aspirin	Urticaria, asthma, rhinitis, nasal polyposis
Aminopyrine, phenacetin, and pyrazolone derivatives	Skin reaction, systemic reaction, blood dyscrasia

Sulfites, Foods, Additives, and Dyes

Sulfiting agents, used as preservatives for fruit juices, wines, beers, soft drinks, potato chips, dried vegetables and fruits, and many commercially prepared or restaurant foods, can cause severe reactions, including airway constriction. At highest risk are people with asthma. To protect the public, the Food and Drug Administration (FDA) requires that the package insert for prescription drugs containing sulfites must include a warning about possible allergic reactions. Injectable sulfite-containing epinephrine has an alternate warning: epinephrine should still be used in the treatment of serious allergic or other emergency situations, even for sulfite-sensitive persons, because the benefits outweigh the disadvantages.

Dyes may also produce an allergic response. Prime offenders are tartrazine and yellow dye no. 5. In addition, other drugs, foods, additives, and some natural substances, such as salicylates, may also trigger allergic reactions. For instance, most food allergies in children result from cow's milk, soybeans, wheat, peanuts and other nuts, and hen's eggs.

In clients with a history of urticaria who take multiple medications, for instance, healthcare professionals usually suspect an allergy to a common ingredient or activity of the drugs. Over-the-counter (OTC) drugs used by the client should be assessed because they may contain, or act synergistically with, substances responsible for allergic reactions.

Insect Bites

The stings of yellow jackets, bees, wasps, and hornets are responsible for allergic reactions that can range in severity from acute anaphylactic shock (usually within 15 minutes) to transient swelling, pain, and redness. The peak of the reaction can be expected to appear within 48 to 72 hours and may last a week. Neurologic or vascular reactions or immune-complex disease may also be seen. Severe edema of the pharynx, epiglottis, and trachea is the major cause of death in sensitive persons.

Other

Other common triggers include pet dander, feathers, pollen, mold, dust, and other airborne agents, cold (eg, holding or eating cold substances), heat, pressure, and sunlight.

Allergic Signs and Symptoms

Allergic drug reactions can occur at the time of administration or be delayed up to 2 weeks after administration. Some reactions can last for weeks and produce symptoms that resemble those of immune-complex disease: neutropenia, eosinophilia, enlarged lymph nodes, fever, urticaria (hives), arthralgia, edema, diarrhea, vomiting, coughing, wheezing, tearing, itching or swelling of the eyes, itchiness of the ears, or a runny nose (clear, nonirritating fluid), sneezing, and nasal stuffiness.

Ingested allergens usually trigger urticaria, angioedema, or GI symptoms. Skin contact can cause urticaria as well, although internal symptoms, such as rhinitis or asthma, may also occur. Urticaria appears as an erythematous, sometimes pruritic, skin elevation that blanches with pressure; angioedema results in a swollen area, with the skin appearing normal. Both conditions may appear in acute (self-limiting) or chronic (lasting longer than 6 weeks) forms. Cutaneous reactions to drugs are described in Table 34-2.

Skin Symptoms

Eczema manifests itself by erythema and vesiculation of the skin in the acute stages and by scaling and thickened skin in the chronic stages. Atopic eczema, also called atopic dermatitis, is a pruritic form of eczema, frequently associated with asthma and allergic rhinitis. About 40% to 65% of clients with this disease have family histories of allergies. Most of them react to many common food and inhalant allergens by producing IgE antibodies.

Atopic eczema is found in children primarily on the cheeks or the antecubital or popliteal fossae, and in adults as a response to harsh chemicals or scratching. In adults, it is called neurodermatitis.

Extreme pruritus is present in all phases of eczema, possibly becoming worse on contact with rough fabrics or when the person is under stress.

Respiratory Symptoms

Respiratory symptoms may occur after the client inhales an allergen, such as dust, which can be expected to cause sneezing, coughing, or wheezing.

Allergic rhinitis (also known as hay fever) occurs on a seasonal basis, coinciding with the presence of airborne pollens or mold spores that trigger sneezing, congestion, nasal itching, tearing, and itchy eyes, throat, and ears. Triggers of the chronic form (perennial) of allergic rhinitis are dust, feathers, animal dander, and other antigens. Peptide leukotrienes, which are produced by the immune system in defense against the allergens, are thought to be the cause of the runny nose and eyes, sneezing, swelling, and itchiness.

Table 34-2. Cutaneous Reactions to Drugs

Disorder	Usual Precipitating Drug	Manifestations
Urticaria	Acute form: penicillin, sulfa, diuretics, sedatives, laxatives Chronic form: aspirin	Transient wheals, reddened papules
Angioedema	As above	
Maculopapular (exanthematous eruptions)	Varies with medication	Possible vesicles; toxic epidermal necrolysis (life-threatening)
Erythema multiforme	Sulfonamides, phenytoin barbiturates	Macules, papules, vesicles, bullae, target lesions on palms; 6–8 weeks to resolve
Toxic epidermal necrolysis	Allopurinol, sulfonamides, penicillin, phenylbutazone, anticonvulsants, barbiturates	Facial puffiness, bullae with yellow fluid; malaise, anorexia; 4 weeks to heal; 50% morbidity regardless of treatment
Fixed drug eruption	Tetracycline, phenolphthalein	Occurs at same site(s) as previous reactions (lips, genitalia, sacral area, palmar or plantar areas), pruritus, burning
Photosensitivity reactions	Thiazides, phenothiazines, psoralens, chlorpromazine	Urticaria; burning or tingling
Acneiform eruptions	Halogens, corticosteroids, iodine, testosterone, anticonvulsants, bromides	Comedones, papules, pustules, cysts
Pigmentary changes	Oral contraceptives, arsenic, phenothiazides	Hyperpigmentation or hypopigmentation
Allergic purpura	Sulfa drugs, penicillin, barbiturates, anticonvulsants	Palpable purpuric papules
Temporary burning sensations	Alcohol, as found in Rhus Tox antigen injection, used in the treatment and prophylaxis of dermatitis caused by poison ivy, oak, and sumac	No change

Ocular Symptoms

Allergies can affect the eyes, causing itching, redness, and tearing. As with other allergies, the ideal situation is prevention by avoidance of the allergens.

Other

When sensitized persons inhale certain organic dusts or animal proteins, hypersensitivity pneumonitis may occur. It more commonly affects farmers, pigeon breeders, and people in contact with drugs or certain low-molecular-weight industrial chemicals. Preventing sensitization depends on preventing inhalation of the antigen—for instance, compost should be wetted before handling or grinding, organic dust fibers should be sterilized, the water in humidifiers should be cleaned and changed, appropriate indoor ventilation systems should be used, and workers should wear protective face masks and clothing covers.

Clinical Manifestations

Allergic reactions to drugs may or may not result in specific antibodies or sensitized lymphocytes. For this reason, the recognition of clinical manifestations is of utmost importance. Some adverse allergic reactions related to drug therapy are presented in Table 34-3.

Anaphylactic Shock

The most serious manifestation of a drug allergy is anaphylactic shock, with acute cardiovascular collapse and hypotension occurring within 5 to 30 minutes of taking the offending substance. At the most extreme level, death from anaphylaxis may ensue within minutes. In its less severe form, anaphylaxis may cause malaise, vertigo, nausea, vomiting, hives, itching, or diffuse erythema. Bronchospasm, laryngeal edema, and hyperperistalsis may also occur. Cardiac arrhythmia, which may lead to myocardial infarction and sudden cardiac arrest, may also occur.

Hematologic Problems

Some drug allergies produce hematologic problems. This is known as a type II or cytolytic hypersensitivity reaction and is mediated by both IgG and IgM antibodies. These antibodies activate the complement system, which in turn targets the circulatory system cells for cytolytic reactions. Examples of a type II allergic reaction are penicillin-induced hemolytic anemia, quinidine-induced thrombocytopenia, sulfonamide-induced granulocytopenia, procainamide-induced systemic lupus erythematosus, and methyldopa-induced autoimmune hemolytic anemia. Fortunately, these autoimmune reactions to the drugs usually cease within 1 week to 1 month after the offending drug is withdrawn.

Hepatic Damage

Liver damage resulting from drug allergy may lead to intrahepatic biliary obstruction or hepatocellular damage and necrosis. The former is associated with chlorpromazine, thiouracil, propylthiouracil, and methyltestosterone. The latter usually results from the use of sulfonamides, erythromycin estolate, PAS, halothane, phenylbutazone, nitrofurantoin, and indomethacin.

Table 34-3. Clinical Manifestations of Drug Allergies

Condition	Usual Causative Agents
Anaphylactic shock	Penicillin, local anesthetics, streptomycin, tetracycline, cephalosporins, dextrans, heroin, radiopaque organic iodides
Thrombocytopenia	Quinidine, quinine, chloramphenicol, sulfonamides, thiouracil, meprobamate, phenylbutazone
Agranulocytosis	Aminopyrine, thiouracil, anticonvulsants, phenothiazines, tolbutamide, sulfonamides, chloramphenicol
Aplastic anemia	Chloramphenicol
Hemolytic anemia	Acetophenetidin, p-aminosalicylic acid (PAS), quinine, mesantoin, penicillin
Severe vasculitis	Penicillin, sulfonamides, tetracyclines, pyrazolone derivatives, thiazides, quinidine, allopurinol, thiouracil
Syndrome that resembles rheumatoid arthritis or lupus	Hydralazine
Intrahepatic biliary obstruction	Chlorpromazine, thiouracil, propylthiouracil, methyltestosterone
Hepatocellular damage and necrosis	Sulfonamides, erythromycin estolate, PAS, halothane, phenylbutazone, nitrofurantoins, indomethacin
Elevated fever levels	Sulfonamides, streptomycin, penicillin, quindine, iodine, thiouracil, antithyroid drugs, anticonvulsants, procainamide, PAS, mercurial diuretics
Rebound effect (nasal mucosa)	Phenylephrine HCL, oxymetazoline HCL, chlorpheniramine maleate, pseudoephedrine
Excitability (especially in children)	Beta$_2$ agonists, methylxanthines

Accompanying the hepatocellular damage are symptoms such as fever, lymphadenopathy, skin rash, blood eosinophilia, and infiltration of the liver with eosinophils, lymphocytes, or plasmacytes.

Fever

Fever is also a clinical sign associated with drug allergies. The usual offending drugs are sulfonamides, streptomycin, penicillin, quinidine, iodine, thiouracil, antithyroid drugs, anticonvulsants, procainamide, PAS, and mercurial diuretics.

Allergy Treatments

Treatment aims to relieve symptoms rather than to prevent the linkage of the antigen with the antigen-specific antibody found on the mast cells. Having the client avoid the offending substance is the preferred method of management. If that is impossible, medications may be necessary.

Some allergic reactions may be prevented by eliminating or minimizing contact with allergens. Because many types of mediators are released during an allergic reaction, drugs that act on only one mediator are usually ineffective. However, drugs used to treat allergic responses include epinephrine (to treat anaphylaxis), corticosteroids (to suppress the allergic response and inflammation), antihistamines (to ameliorate the signs and symptoms), and other palliative drugs, depending on the tissues and organs affected.

Treatment for urticaria and angioedema and related symptoms such as sneezing and wheezing usually involves removing the offending substance, whether it is a material with which the client has contact (eg, feathers, wool, dust), a food, or a drug. In selected cases, hyposensitization or desensitization can increase tolerance to the allergen.

Drug Therapy

Epinephrine in emergencies, as well as antihistamines and corticosteroids, may help relieve allergic manifestations. Desensitization therapy may be beneficial for some clients.

Epinephrine

Epinephrine (adrenaline) is a key drug for controlling severe allergic reactions such as anaphylaxis; a complete discussion of epinephrine is presented in Chapter 16.

Pharmacodynamics. In addition to its cardiovascular stimulant effects, epinephrine is thought to stop the release of histamine and leukotrienes from mast cells. It does this by activating the beta-adrenergic receptors in the mast cells that suppress the mediators' release.

Pharmacokinetics. By any route except the topical ophthalmic route, epinephrine has an onset of action within 10 minutes, a peak within 20 minutes, and a duration of action of 20 to 30 minutes. It is metabolized by the neurologic system, crosses the placenta, and passes into breast milk.

Therapeutic Uses. In allergic reactions, epinephrine is used primarily to reverse anaphylactic shock and to treat severe urticaria.

Dosage and Administration. For anaphylactic shock, a systemic injection of epinephrine 0.1 to 0.5 mL of 1:1,000 solution should be given immediately. It can be given intramuscularly (IM) or, in potentially fatal situations, diluted to 1 mL of 1:10,000 solution and administered IV. If the results are unsatisfactory, the injections should be repeated every 10 to 15 minutes. Also, 50 mg of diphenhydramine (an antihistamine) should be administered IV. Laryngeal obstruction may require tracheostomy and oxygen. Bronchospasm requires IV use of 200 to 500 mg aminophylline in a drip. IV saline solution may be needed to increase hydration, and cardiopulmonary resuscitation may be needed if cardiac arrest occurs. Other helpful drugs include antihistamines, oxygen, vasopressors, and, if the reaction is of long duration, corticosteroids.

To relieve urticaria, with or without angioedema, epinephrine may be injected (0.5 mL of 1:1,000 solution) subcutaneously (SC) every 15 minutes, up to three injections. Systemic steroids may also help but should not be used unless necessary. Topical corticosteroids are ineffective.

Adverse Reactions. Central nervous system (CNS) effects such as fear, anxiety, restlessness, dizziness, tremor, and convulsions are among the adverse effects. The need to reverse anaphylaxis, however, overrides the risk of adverse effects.

Antihistamines

Pharmacodynamics. Antihistamines compete with histamine for binding to histamine (H_1) receptor sites throughout the body. They do not displace histamine already bound to the receptor. Antihistamines cause smooth muscle relaxation, particularly in the bronchial tree. They prevent or reduce salivary, gastric, lacrimal, and bronchial secretion and reduce itching.

First-generation antihistamines, such as diphenhydramine (Benadryl), have lipophilic structures and bind both peripheral and CNS histamine (H_1) receptors. They also have anticholinergic effects and cross the blood-brain barrier. Consequently, more side effects—especially sedation—occur. Second-generation antihistamines, such as astemizole (Hismanal), block the effects of histamine at peripheral histamine (H_1) receptor sites, do not cross the blood-brain barrier, and have negligible anticholinergic properties. As a result, they have substantially fewer side effects and are nonsedating (Table 34-4).

Pharmacokinetics. Antihistamines can be administered orally as tablets, capsules, or elixirs. They are also available as topical ointments, nasal sprays, and injectables. They are readily absorbed from the GI tract. After oral administration, plasma concentration peaks in 2 to 3 hours. The effects of first-generation antihistamines usually last 4 to 6 hours, although some drugs have a longer duration. They are degraded in the liver and are almost completely excreted through the kidneys. Second-generation antihistamines are metabolized in the liver to active metabolites by the hepatic microsomal system and excreted in the urine. They have a longer duration of action, 6 to 24 hours. Antihistamines are well distributed, with the highest concentrations in the lungs. They have not been proved safe in pregnancy or lactation.

Therapeutic Uses. Antihistamines may be prescribed or purchased OTC to ease allergic reactions to food, inhalants, or contact allergens. Antihistamines may also be used to treat rigidity from parkinsonism or extrapyramidal symptoms caused by some psychotropic medications. Antihistamines are used to alleviate symptoms of seasonal allergic and vasomotor rhinitis, allergic conjunctivitis, urticaria, rashes, and other allergic manifestations. They are also used to relieve motion sickness and vestibular system disorders. Antihistamines may be combined with decongestants to dry secretions in the respiratory tract.

Adverse Reactions. Sedation and drowsiness is the side effect most characteristic of first-generation antihistamines. Other CNS side effects include vertigo, tinnitus, incoordination, blurred vision, nervousness, insomnia, and tremors. The next most common adverse effects involve the GI system and include anorexia, nausea, vomiting, epigastric distress, and constipation or diarrhea. The first-generation antihistamines also produce anticholinergic effects: dry mouth, urinary retention, constipation, and cardiovascular problems. These atropine-like side effects and sedation are not a problem with the second-generation antihistamines. Drug allergy may occur after oral ingestion of antihistamines but is more common when the drug is applied topically. Allergic dermatitis, drug fever, and photosensitivity may also occur.

Drug Interactions. The interaction of a first-generation antihistamine and a monoamine oxidase inhibitor may result in increased and prolonged anticholinergic effects. Alcohol taken concurrently with antihistamines has an additive effect on CNS depression. The second-generation antihistamine astemizole should not be used concurrently with erythromycin, ketoconazole, or itraconazole due to life-threatening cardiovascular problems such as ventricular arrhythmias and cardiac arrest.

Precautions and Contraindications. Antihistamines should be avoided by persons with a history of bronchial asthma, cardiovascular disease, increased intraocular pressure or narrow-angle glaucoma, hyperthyroidism, hypertension, stenosing peptic ulcer, pyloroduodenal obstruction, symptomatic prostatic hypertrophy, or bladder neck obstruction. They should not be taken concurrently with monoamine oxidase inhibitors or alcohol. The client taking a first-generation antihistamine should know about the possibility of CNS depression and should not operate dangerous equipment or perform functions that require alertness. Antihistamines should not be used during pregnancy or lactation. (See Focus On Antihistamines: Similarities and Differences.)

Decongestants

Antihistamines, with the possible exception of astemizole, have little effect on nasal congestion and are frequently used in combination with decongestants. The oral decongestants, for example, are adrenergic agents with alpha-adrenergic activity; an example is pseudo-

Table 34-4. Antihistamines

Drug Name	Trade Name	Route	Usual Adult Dosage
First-Generation Antihistamines			
Ethanolamides			
carbinoxamine	Clistin	PO	4–8 mg q6–8h
clemastine	Tavist	PO	1.34–2.68 mg q12h
diphenhydramine	Benadryl, others	PO, IV, IM, topical	25–50 mg q6–8h
dimenhydrinate	Dramamine	PO, IM, topical	50–100 mg q6–8h
Ethylenediamines			
pyrilamine	Nisaval	PO	25–50 mg q6–8h
tripelennamine	PBZ	PO	25–50 mg q4–6h
Alkylamines			
chlorpheniramine	Chlor-Trimeton, others	PO, IV, IM, SC	4 mg q4–6h
brompheniramine	Dimetane, others	PO, IV, IM, SC	4 mg q4–6h
dexchlorpheniramine	Dexchlor, others	PO	2 mg q4–6h
Piperazine			
azatadine	Optimine	PO	1–2 mg q12h
hydroxyzine	Atarax, Vistaril	PO, IM, IV	25–100 mg q12h
cyclizine	Marezine	PO, IM	50 mg q4–6h
meclizine	Antivert	PO	12.5–50 mg q12h
diphenylpyraline	Hispril	PO	5 mg q12h
Phenothiazine			
promethazine	Phenergan	PO, IV, IM, supp.	25 mg q6–12h
methdilazine	Tacaryl	PO	8 mg q6–12h
trimeprazine	Temaril	PO	2.5 mg q6h
Second-Generation Antihistamines			
Alkylamines			
acrivastine	Semprex	PO	8 mg q12h
Piperazine			
cetirizine HCL	Zyrtec	PO	5–10 mg q12h
Piperidines			
astemizole	Hismanal	PO	10 mg q24h
levocabastine	Livostin	topical	one drop q12–24h
loratadine	Claritin	PO	10 mg q24h
fexofenadine HCL	Allegra	PO	60 mg q12h

ephedrine (Sudafed, Afrin). Examples of inhalable decongestants are phenylephrine (Neo-Synephrine, Allerest Nasal) and desoxyephedrine (Vicks Inhaler).

Atropine, decongestants, and corticosteroids have also been used to relieve congestion. After they have been used for a time, however, they appear to be less effective. Decongestants relieve symptoms by promoting vasoconstriction; corticosteroids reduce inflammation. Excessive use of topical decongestants and corticosteroids may lead to a rebound effect, which involves temporary decongestion followed by increased congestion more severe than it was initially.

Cromolyn sodium can be used as a nasal solution to inhibit the release of mediators from mast and other cells. One spray in each nostril every 3 to 4 waking hours is the usual dose. When symptoms are less severe, administration can be decreased to every 5 to 6 waking hours.

Corticosteroids and Topical Preparations

A complete discussion of corticosteroids appears in Chapter 30. Systemic corticosteroids should be used for the shortest time possible. Prednisone may be prescribed at 5 to 60 mg/day for a short time, then reduced to every other day at the same dose. The dose should then be tapered down to the lowest possible amount to prevent symptoms. Periodically, attempts to discontinue the drug should be made, because spontaneous remission, which eliminates the need for medication, may occur.

Clients with skin allergies (eg, eczema) may benefit from topical corticosteroid creams or lotions, coal tar products, and supportive measures, such as wet dressings of Burow's solution or tap water. (See Example of Nursing Process for Topical Corticosteroid Therapy.)

Text continues on page 748.

FOCUS ON

Antihistamines: Similarities and Differences

Similarities

Pharmacodynamics

These agents compete with histamine for H_1 receptor sites on effector cells.

Pharmacokinetics

These agents are administered topically, nasally, or parenterally. They are well absorbed after oral or parenteral administration. They have an onset of action of 15 to 30 minutes, peaking in 1 hour, with a duration of 3 to 6 hours. They are well distributed, with highest concentrations in the lungs and lower concentrations in the spleen, kidneys, brain, muscles, and skin. They are metabolized by the liver and excreted in the urine.

Second-generation antihistamines do not cross the blood-brain barrier.

Therapeutic Uses

These agents are used in the symptomatic relief of allergy and as adjunctive therapy in anaphylaxis and laryngeal edema. They are also used in the management of nasal allergies, rhinitis, common cold, allergic dermatoses, and chronic idiopathic urticaria.

Adverse Reactions

First-generation antihistamines: (CNS) headache, sleepiness, decreased alertness, inability to concentrate, dizziness, sedation, incoordination, excitation; (CV) hypotension, palpitations, tachycardia; (RESP) thickening of bronchial secretions, wheezing, nasal stuffiness; (EENT) blurred vision; (GI): nausea, diarrhea, constipation, epigastric distress, dry mouth, cholestatic jaundice; (GU) urinary frequency, retention; (ENDO) early menses; (SKIN) urticaria; (HEMA) hemolytic anemia, thrombocytopenia, agranulocytosis; (OTHER) photosensitivity.

Second-generation antihistamines: low incidence of side effects; no sedation or atropine-like effect.

Differences

- **Diphenhydramine** inhibits the action of acetylcholine; it suppresses the cough reflex directly by its effect on the cough center; possesses significant antimuscarinic activity.
- **Pyrilamine** most specific H_1 antagonist.
- **Chlorpheniramine** is among the most potent H_1 antagonists.
- **Dimenhydrinate, diphenhydramine,** and **promethazine** diminish vestibular stimulation and depress labrynthine function.

- **Astemizole** is excreted unchanged; **fexofenadine** is the active metabolite of terfenadine.
- Second-generation antihistamines tend to have a longer duration of action; small amounts are distributed into breast milk. Half-life varies: **astemizole** has a half-life of 1.5 days; **azatadine** a half-life of 12 hours; **brompheniramine** a half-life of 25 hours; **carbinoxamine** a half-life of 10 to 20 hours; **chlorpheniramine** a half-life of 21 to 27 hours; **diphenhydramine** a half-life of 1 to 4 hours; **fexofenadine** has a half-life of 14.4 hours.
- **Dimenhydrinate** IM has an onset of 20 to 30 minutes; rectally, it has an onset of 30 to 45 minutes.
- **Clemastine** has a duration of 12 hours; **pyrilamine** a duration of 8 hours; **tripelennamine** a duration of 4 to 6 hours; **azatadine** a duration of 12 hours; **cyproheptadine** a duration of 8 hours.

- **Dimenhydrinate, diphenhydramine,** and **promethazine** are used in the treatment and prevention of nausea, vomiting, and vertigo of motion sickness.
- **Diphenhydramine** is used as a sleep aid and for the symptomatic treatment of parkinsonian and extrapyramidal reactions.
- **Diphenhydramine** and **tripelennamine** are used topically for the temporary relief of pruritus and pain of minor skin conditions.
- **Hydroxyzine** is widely used for skin allergies.
- **Fexofenadine** has replaced terfenadine as a nonsedating antihistamine.

- **Promethazine** may cause transient myopia; possesses considerable sedative and anticholinergic effects.
- **Trimeprazine** and **methdilazine** may cause extrapyramidal reactions, postural hypotension, tonic-clonic convulsions, and electrocardiographic changes.
- **Diphenhydramine** may cause hallucinations, fever, chest tightness, and anaphylaxis.
- **Chlorcyclizine** has comparatively low incidence of drowsiness.
- **Hydroxyzine** has considerable central depressant activity.
- Second-generation antihistamines do not cause drowsiness.
- **Pyrilamine** frequently causes GI problems and somnolence.
- **Astemizole** may cause weight gain and arthralgia.
- **Cyclizine** may cause tinnitus and dysuria.
- **Cyproheptadine** and **dexchlorpheniramine** may cause appetite stimulation, visual hallucinations, ataxia, and weight gain.

(continued)

FOCUS ON

Antihistamines: Similarities and Differences (continued)

Similarities (continued)

Interactions

Additive sedation when used in conjunction with other CNS depressants such as alcohol, antidepressants, narcotic analgesics, and sedative/hypnotics. MAO inhibitors prolong and intensify anticholinergic properties of antihistamines.

Precautions and Contraindications

These agents should be used cautiously in clients with increased intraocular pressure, hyperthyroidism, cardiovascular or renal disease, diabetes, hypertension, asthma, urinary retention, prostatic hypertrophy, bladder neck obstruction or stenosis, peptic ulcer disease, or closed-angle glaucoma, and in the elderly.

These agents should be used with caution in clients with hypersensitivity and in clients having an acute asthmatic attack.

Nursing Considerations

Instruct client in disease, treatment, drug therapy, regimen, adverse effects; assess cardiopulmonary status and vital signs frequently. If sedation occurs, institute safety measures to prevent injury; caution client about activities that require mental alertness until drug effects are known. Administer with food or milk to prevent GI upset; institute measures to relieve dry mouth, such as hard candy, ice chips; monitor blood studies for abnormalities; instruct client to avoid alcohol; do not crush extended-release tablets; evaluate for effectiveness of therapy.

Differences (continued)

Astemizole taken with erythromycin, ketoconazole, itraconazole or clarithromycin may cause potentially fatal cardiac arrhythmias; **dimenhydrinate** may mask signs and symptoms of ototoxicity in patients taking ototoxic drugs; both **methdilazine HCL** and **trimaprazine** increase likelihood of seizures when taken with metrazamide; decreased antihypertensive effect of guanethidine with **methdilazine; chorpheniramine** and anticholinergic drugs cause additive anticholinergic effects; food decreases absorption of **astemizole; loratadine** may cause false skin testing procedures. **Fexofenadine** does not cause QT prolongation or ventricular arrhythmias as occurred when terfenadine was used with other drugs affecting the microsomal enzymes.

- **Cyclizine** and **dimenhydrinate** should be used with caution in clients with GI obstruction.
- **Dimenhydrinate** should be used with caution in clients with seizure disorders.
- **Methdilazine, promethazine,** and **trimeprazine** should be used with caution in children with history of sleep apnea or Reye's syndrome.
- **Promethazine** and **trimeprazine** should be used with caution in clients with acute or chronic respiratory dysfunction.
- **Tripelennamine, methdilazine, diphenhydramine, dexchlorpheniramine, cyproheptadine, clemastine, chlorpheniramine, carbinoxamine, brompheniramine,** and **azatadine** are contraindicated in persons who have taken monoamine oxidase inhibitors in the preceding 2 weeks and in lactating or pregnant women.
- **Dimenhydrinate** is contraindicated in clients sensitive to theophylline.
- **Trimeprazine, promethazine,** and **methdilazine** are contraindicated in acutely ill or debilitated children.
- **Trimeprazine** and **promethazine** are contraindicated in clients with bone marrow depression, epilepsy, or coma and in neonates.
- **Tripelennamine** is contraindicated during lactation.
- **Hydroxyzine** is contraindicated in first months of pregnancy.
- **Astemizole** may cause cardiac arrhythmias if given concurrently with erythromycin, itraconazole, ketoconazole, and clarithromycin.

Administer **chlorpheniramine** IV slowly over 1 minute; do not give parenteral form intradermally. Instruct client that **buclizine** and **meclizine** tablets may be chewed, swallowed whole, or dissolved in water. Do not mix **cyproheptidate, diphenhydramine, promethazine,** or **dimenhydrinate** parenteral solutions with other solutions; they may be incompatible; administer 30 minutes before travelling for motion sickness and before meals and bedtime; undiluted IV solutions are irritating and may cause sclerosing. Rotate **promethazine** and **diphenhydramine** injection sites to prevent irritation; inject IM deep into large muscle. Protect IV **promethazine** from light; do not give SC because it may cause necrosis.

Example of Nursing Process for Topical Corticosteroid Therapy

The client is a 33-year-old woman who has had eczematous lesions on the fingertips and palmar surfaces of both hands for 10 years. Prior testing resulted in a medical diagnosis of allergic dermatitis, which has been kept under control with twice-daily applications of a topical corticosteroid. She is allergic to soaps, detergents, cleaning agents, and many household chemicals and avoids chores that involve their use. Her husband is very supportive and does the household cleaning to lessen her exposure to allergenic substances. She has been told to continue the medication and to undergo periodic testing for possible hypothalmic-pituitary-adrenal (HPA) axis suppression, which is negative at present.

Assessment Data

Eczematous lesions on fingertips and palmar surfaces of both hands; topical application of ointment that contains corticosteroids

Periodic testing for HPA axis suppression

Nursing Diagnosis	Intervention	Goals and Outcomes
Impaired Tissue Integrity: Delayed healing of eczematous lesions related to excessive absorption of corticosteroids through damaged skin	**Teach** the client to apply a thin coat of ointment to the lesions; caution client to avoid occlusive dressings, which tend to increase absorption of the drug. **Warn** the client that overmedication retards healing of lesions.	The client will demonstrate proper technique for applying the ointment.
Knowledge Deficit, concerning reversible HPA axis suppression, Cushing's syndrome, and other symptoms related to excessive absorption of corticosteroid drugs	**Teach** the client proper application and use of corticosteroid ointment as above. **Stress** the importance of periodic tests for adrenal function.	The client will not develop severe HPA axis suppression; if suppression does develop, it will be promptly reversed without causing symptoms of corticosteroid deficiency.

Pharmacodynamics. The efficacy of topical corticosteroids results from their antiinflammatory, antipruritic, and vasoconstrictor action. For chronic allergies, steroidal ointments and emollients counteract dermatitis and loss of skin moisture.

Pharmacokinetics. Topical corticosteroids are absorbed through normal intact skin. Absorption increases in the presence of inflammation, disease, or occlusive dressings. The addition of a solvent such as propylene glycol to the corticosteroid suspension contributes to drug dissolution, which also improves absorption. Corticosteroids are bound to plasma proteins, metabolized in the liver, and excreted by the kidneys and sometimes in bile.

Dosage and Administration. For adults, the dosage is one or two applications daily as directed. For children, the dosage is the same, but usually less potent corticosteroids are used.

Adverse Reactions. Topical corticosteroids can cause contact dermatitis, a burning sensation, skin dryness, itching, hypopigmentation, facial hirsutism, purpura, facial puffiness and swelling, and alopecia. Other adverse effects include possible skin infections or superinfections and even immunosuppression.

Precautions and Contraindications. When corticosteroids are applied topically to the perineal area, plastic or tight-fitting pants or diapers should not be used.

Cromolyn Sodium and Other Ophthalmic Solutions

For itchy, tearing eyes, a 4% ophthalmic solution of cromolyn sodium can be used. The dosage is one or two drops per eye four to six times a day or, when less serious, one drop per eye four times a day. There is transient stinging or burning on instillation.

Cromolyn sodium inhibits allergen-triggered release of histamine and leukotriene from mast cells. Other ophthalmic agents are also available to reduce the symptoms associated with allergic conjunctivitis. These agents include a nonsteroidal antiinflammatory drug, ketorolac (Acular); a mast cell stabilizer, lodoxamide (Alomide); antihistamines; and combination antihistamine/vasoconstrictors, such as naphazoline/antazoline (Vasocon-A) and naphazoline/pheniramine (Opcon-A). Table 34-5 compares drugs used in treating allergic rhinitis and ocular allergies.

Immunotherapy

Hyposensitization (also called desensitization) should be considered for adults who have had a systemic allergic reaction to an insect sting or for children who have

Table 34-5. Selected Antiallergy Drugs for Allergic Rhinitis and Ocular Allergies

Drug	Purpose	Adverse SideEffects/Additional Information
Antihistamines		
chlorpheniramine (Chlor-Trimeton,* Deconamine)	Block histamine effects	Drowsiness; ineffective with prolonged use
		Use caution with narrow-angle glaucoma, stenosing peptic ulcer, prostatic hypertrophy, bronchial asthma, and chronic pulmonary disease.
		PC: C
		PC: B
diphenhydramine (Benadryl*)	Blocks histamine effect without crossing the blood-brain barrier	Does *not* cause drowsiness
		Weight gain for 4% of clients
		Use caution with lower airway disease (asthma) and hepatic and renal impairment.
astemizole (Hismanal)	Treatment of seasonal allergic rhinitis	Efficacy drops 60% when taken with food.
		Risk of serious cardiac arrhythmias if taken with erythromycin, ketoconazole, itraconazole and clarithromycin
		PC: C
loratadine (Claritin)	Treatment of allergic rhinitis and allergic conjunctivitis	Nonsedating; take on empty stomach
		PC: C
fexofenadine HCL (Allegra)	Treatment of seasonal allergic rhinitis	Nonsedating
		PC: C
Decongestants		
phenylephrine (Neo-Synephrine* nasal spray)	Relieves nasal stuffiness and eustachian tube congestion; promotes vasoconstriction	Use only for severe congestion.
		Rebound congestion may occur if used more than twice a day or for more than 3 consecutive days.
		Insomnia, nervousness
		Decongestants may cause excessive dryness of mucous membranes (mouth, nose, vagina).
Oral		
pseudoephedrine (Novafed, Sudafed*; *Can*: Eltor, Robidrine))	Decongestion	Ephedrine-like reactions include tachycardia, headache, dizziness, nausea, anxiety, tremor.
		Clients older than 60 years may exhibit hallucinations, convulsions.
		Contraindicated in severe hypertension, severe coronary artery disease, monoamine oxidase inhibitor therapy, and for children younger than 12 years.
		PC: C
Combination Decongestant and Antihistamine		
(Actifed,* Brexin)	Relieves nasal congestion, tearing, itching	May react to either component as above.
		Impairment of mental and physical abilities
Intranasal Steroids		
beclomethasone (Beconase) flunisolide (Nasalide) triamcinolone (Nasacort) budesonide (Rhinocort) fluticasone (Cutivate)	Relieve allergic rhinitis without side effects of oral corticosteroids	Transient nasal irritation, burning, dryness, sneezing, headache; budesonide, triamcinolone, and fluticasone can be taken once a day.
		PC: C

*Over-the-counter
KEY: PC = pregnancy category; see Appendix A.
Can: Canadian trade name.

(continued)

Table 34-5. (Continued)

Drug	Purpose	Adverse SideEffects/Additional Information
Inhibitor of Sensitized Mast Cell Degranulation		
cromolyn sodium (Intal inhaler, Nasalcrom Nasal Spray)	Inhibits release of mediators histamines and leukotrienes from mast cells Preventive action—especially helpful before exercise or exposure to allergen (animal, cold, and so forth)	Throat irritation and dryness, bad taste, cough, wheeze, nausea, bronchospasm Overuse common Administer 10–60 min before exposure. PC: B
Ophthalmic Agents		
ketorolac (Acular)	Antiinflammatory action relieves redness, itching, tearing	Ocular irritation, allergic reaction PC: B
lodoxamide (Alomide)	Mast cell stabilizer	transient burning, stinging, pruritus PC: B
naphazoline + (Vasocon-A) antazoline	Combination antihistamine-vasoconstrictor	PC: B
pheniramine + (Opcon-A) naphazoline		PC: B
Immunotherapy	Builds up allergen antibodies	May require 100 or more injections over 3 years Possibility of anaphylaxis

*Over-the-counter
KEY: PC = pregnancy category; see Appendix A.

had a severe systemic reaction not limited to the skin. Clients who are allergic primarily to airborne allergens may also benefit from hyposensitization.

Because the treatment is based on clinical empirical evidence, it varies according to the practitioner. Most immunotherapy attempts to desensitize clients to ragweed, grass, and tree pollen allergens, as well as antigens from mold spores and house dust. Treatment is started by administering small doses of antigen SC in weekly injections that contain gradually increasing amounts of the antigen until a maintenance dose is reached, usually about 2,500 protein-nitrogen units (0.15 mg protein). The dosage schedule is then reduced to one injection every 2 weeks, later to one injection every 3 weeks, and finally to one every 4 weeks; injections are usually continued for 3 to 4 years. Immunotherapy may be limited to weekly or biweekly injections during or before the season in which the allergenic agent, such as pollen, is present.

The principal problems with injections for immunotherapy are cost, inconvenience (multiple visits to the prescriber), and the physical dangers, which include local reaction, malaise, nasal symptoms, bronchospasm, or anaphylactic shock.

SUMMARY

Allergic reactions may be due to environmental factors (pollens, dust, industrial pollutants), foods (cow's milk, wheat, eggs), drugs (penicillin, tetracycline, chloramphenicol, aspirin), or insect bites.

The body reacts to an allergen by producing specific antibodies that excite the membrane receptors on mast cells. This process leads to the release of histamine, serotonin, and other substances that also may be involved in the physical reactions recognized as allergic responses. Stress intensifies these responses. Treatment of allergies includes removal of the offending substance when possible, desensitizing procedures (allergen immunotherapy), preventive use of cromolyn, and symptomatic treatment with epinephrine, antihistamines, decongestants, and corticosteroids.

❖ NURSING MANAGEMENT: CLIENT RECEIVING DRUG THERAPY FOR ALLERGIC REACTION

Allergic reactions may involve any tissue or organ; therefore, their manifestations are varied and drug therapy may include epinephrine (for anaphylaxis), corticosteroids (to manage the inflammatory response characteristic of allergies), antihistamines (to control allergic symptoms), topical products (for hives or rashes), and other agents to control such symptoms as headache, indigestion, or joint pain as well as the more common dermatitis, rhinitis, and wheezing. Allergic symptoms often accompany an acute illness such as a cold or bronchitis. However, when symptoms such as cough persist after the illness resolves, the client may be showing signs of an allergy.

NURSING PROCESS

ASSESSMENT

The diagnosis of allergy should be made from the client's history or clinical observation and verified by specific allergy testing. Nurses play a vital role in initial case-finding. The history should include known and suspected allergens and the nature of allergic reactions. Then, any history of allergic reactions should be brought to the attention of the healthcare practitioner, who may refer such clients to their personal physicians or to allergists.

Triggers for allergic reactions are multiple. In acute care settings, for example, molds from air conditioning systems, volatile substances in the air, plastics, and latex may be offending allergens. In 1991, several clients died from anaphylactic reactions induced by allergies to the latex cuffs on enema tips, which were then recalled by the FDA. Healthcare professionals have also had allergic reactions to latex products, possibly due to repeated exposure to proteins in latex. For those who suspect sensitivity, or for those who have had an allergic reaction, plastic devices should be substituted for latex. Severe reactions to latex (or any other product, drug, or biologic substance) should be reported to the FDA via the Med-Watch Program.

As treatment is initiated, the nurse should assess the client's knowledge of the allergy and the prescribed treatment. Because the tendency to have allergies is inherited and related persons tend to have similar reactions, the client may be familiar with the particular condition (asthma, hay fever) but may not have accurate or complete information about it.

After treatment begins, the nurse must collect data related to the number and severity of recent allergic episodes, the current dosage of antiallergy drugs, therapeutic response to the drugs, adverse reactions to the drugs, and the client's general level of stress and coping skills.

NURSING DIAGNOSIS

Nursing diagnoses related to drug therapy for allergies may include:

- Risk for Injury, related to sedation from first-generation antihistamines or cardiovascular complications
- Knowledge Deficit, concerning allergy and its treatment

PLANNING

Goals of nursing care include decreasing the number and severity of allergic reactions and ensuring early detection and treatment of adverse reactions to treatment. Some short-term goals are resolving acute allergic reactions, minimizing client exposure to allergens, providing prompt detection and resolution of adverse drug reactions, helping the client reduce stress levels and integrate the treatment into his or her lifestyle, and educating the client about the allergy and its treatment.

INTERVENTION

Intervention for the most serious allergic reaction, anaphylaxis, requires emergency action. Epinephrine (adrenaline), the drug of choice, is administered by injection or aerosol inhalation. Bee-sting kits, for example, contain injectable epinephrine, a special syringe, and an oral antihistamine; the epinephrine syringe is designed for repeated administration of fractional parts of the contents. If an initial dose (0.1–0.5 mL of 1:1,000 solution) is not effective within 10 to 15 minutes, it is repeated and the antihistamine is administered. Successive doses are administered as needed every 10 to 15 minutes. If anaphylaxis occurs outside the healthcare center, emergency medical help should be summoned, because cardiopulmonary resuscitation may be required if cardiac arrest occurs.

Clients with acute dermatitis usually receive topical corticosteroids. Ointments should be applied sparingly in a thin layer because the active ingredients are absorbed readily by inflamed skin. Skin areas touched by poison ivy, sumac, or oak should be washed with cool water as quickly as possible. This action inactivates urushiol, the oily agent that evokes the allergic response that causes the itching rash and blisters. Soap should not be used, as it may spread the oil to other skin areas. Use of rubbing alcohol after the water helps remove oil absorbed by the skin. Steroids (oral or injected) can be helpful if administered before blisters form.

If the client is receiving treatment for an eye allergy, the nurse may need to administer cromolyn sodium eye drops initially and teach the client how to continue treatment. Before the drops are instilled, the nurse must confirm that the client is not wearing soft contact lenses: one of the drug ingredients, benzalkonium chloride, is contraindicated with soft lenses.

Throughout therapy, the nurse should evaluate the client for both therapeutic and adverse responses to the drug regimen. Signs and symptoms of adverse drug reactions should be recorded and reported promptly to the prescriber. (See the Critical Thinking Challenge: Case Analysis.)

Client Education. Avoiding allergens is a key to decreasing allergic reactions. To that end, the nurse must teach the client ways to avoid specific allergens. Offending foods may be removed from the diet. Allergenic fabrics, plastics, or cosmetics may be replaced with hypoallergenic substitutes. Inhaled allergens should be eliminated from the home as much as possible, and offending medications can be discontinued.

The nurse can advise clients who are allergic to pollens to stay in air-conditioned rooms or vehicles, with the windows closed and the air conditioning on when pollen counts are high. Air conditioner filters should be kept clean and replaced when necessary to decrease both the pollen and mold particles (from the air conditioner) in the atmosphere of the room or vehicle.

CRITICAL THINKING CHALLENGE
Case Analysis

As spring approaches, Ann complains of nasal congestion, runny nose (rhinorrhea), sneezing, and watery, itchy eyes. She tried an over-the-counter nasal spray for several weeks with no results. Her nurse practitioner diagnosed her with allergic rhinitis and ordered loratadine and budesonide nasal spray.

1. Why do you suppose the over-the-counter nasal spray did not work?
2. Generate a plan for teaching Ann about the beneficial actions and adverse effects of loratadine and budesonide.
3. Recommend some strategies for Ann to take to decrease her exposure to allergens.

Cleaning chores should be carried out by others when possible, and silicone-coated dust cloths should be used to decrease circulating dust particles in the air. The client who cannot delegate these tasks should wear a dust mask as appropriate.

Dust mites can be kept out of bedding by using plastic mattress and pillow coverings and by laundering covers, blankets, and pillows frequently. Feather pillows, a source of dander, may be replaced with washable pillows made of fiber or foam rubber.

Clients with dust allergies should avoid rugs. If carpets are used, they should have the shortest pile possible and should be vacuumed or washed frequently. Room temperature should be maintained below 70°F and humidity below 50% to provide an environment inhospitable to dust mites.

Pets are responsible for much of the dander found in homes. Clients who cannot part with their pets may be able to limit their access to certain rooms, such as the bedroom. Weekly bathing of cats and dogs removes dander and reduces their antigenicity.

Clients allergic to insect stings should wear drab or dark colors. Any cosmetics should be free of perfumes. Such clients should use insecticides and insect repellents when necessary. The nurse can teach them to use bee-sting kits and urge them to carry a kit at all times.

Clients allergic to sulfites must restrict their diets to fresh foods and must be sure that medications intended to lessen allergic reactions do not contain sulfites. Sulfiting agents include sodium sulfite, potassium or sodium bisulfite, sulfur dioxide, and potassium or sodium metabisulfite. Sulfites also form naturally in wines. Although sulfites help to keep foods looking fresh and prevent deterioration, the FDA prohibits adding sulfites to fresh fruits and vegetables. It also requires that labels of canned, prepared, or frozen foods identify sulfite contents when the concentration exceeds 10 parts per million. Clients allergic to sulfites must ask about the content of foods they order in restaurants. Very sensitive people should carry epinephrine with them for treating severe sulfite-related respiratory emergencies.

Clients with tartrazine sensitivity must check the labels on drugs and foods. Persons allergic to aspirin are also likely to be allergic to tartrazine.

Clients who use cromolyn sodium eye drops should be cautioned to use them as prescribed, without interruption, as the action is preventive. The agent is ineffective if an allergic reaction is allowed to develop.

OUTCOME EVALUATION

Data required for evaluation relate to the incidence and severity of allergic reactions, the absence or incidence of adverse drug reactions and the speed with which they are resolved, and the knowledge and skill with which clients manage their regimens and integrate them into their lifestyles.

❖ CHECKLIST OF NURSING ACTIONS

- ❑ Assess clients carefully for signs and symptoms of allergic reaction. Document specific substances associated with them.
- ❑ Provide emergency epinephrine therapy as prescribed and appropriate. Teach clients to carry and self-administer epinephrine for treating anaphylaxis.
- ❑ Apply topical corticosteroid preparations sparingly to minimize absorption of the hormone.
- ❑ Teach clients to rid their environments of specific substances associated with allergic reactions.
- ❑ Caution clients on long-term cromolyn therapy not to omit or discontinue doses without the advice of the prescriber.
- ❑ Teach clients how to minimize contact with allergenic substances.
- ❑ Teach clients about adverse reactions to drugs, including criteria for consulting the prescriber for a change in medication.
- ❑ Warn clients to clean air conditioners and home environments frequently to eliminate microbes, dust, and other allergenic organisms.

Bibliography

*Badhwar AK, Druce HM. (1992). Allergic rhinitis [review]. *Med Clin North Am,* 76, 789–803.

*Bernstein JA. (1993). Allergic rhinitis: Helping patients lead an unrestricted life. *Postgrad Med,* 93, 124–132.

Dockhorn RJ, Williams BO, Sanders RL. (1996). Efficacy of acrivastine with pseudoephedrine in treatment of allergic rhinitis due to ragweed. *Ann Allergy Asthma Immunol, 76*(2), 204–208.

Gordon BR. (1995). Future immunotherapy: What lies ahead? *Otolaryngol Head Neck Surg, 113*(5), 603–605.

*Recommended for further reading.

*Haldcroft C. (1993). Terfenadine, astemizole and loratadine: second-generation antihistamines. *Nurse Practitioner, 18*(11), 13–14.

Hardman JG, Limbird LE, et al., eds. (1996). *Goodman and Gilman's The Pharmacological basis of therapeutics,* 9th ed. New York: McGraw-Hill.

Hinriksdottir I. (1994). Allergic rhinitis and upper respiratory tract infections. *Acta Otolaryngol,* 515(suppl), 30–32.

Horak F, Toh J, Jager S, et al. (1993). Effects of H_1-receptor antagonists on nasal obstruction in atopic patients. *Allergy,* 48, 226–229.

*Howser RL. (1995). What you need to know about corticosteroid therapy. *AJN,* 8, 44–48.

Hussar D. (1995). New drugs. *Nursing '95,* 5, 62–64.

Kaliner M, Lemanske R. (1992). Rhinitis and asthma. *JAMA,* 268, 2807–2829.

Katcher M. (1996). Cold, cough and allergy medications. *Pediatr Rev, 17*(1), 12–17.

Lilley LL, Guanci R. (1995). Med errors: The new antihistamines. *AJN, 95*(5), 14.

Nacierio RM, Adkinson N, Creticos PS et al. (1993). Intranasal steroids inhibit seasonal increases of ragweed-specific immunoglobulin antibodies. *J Allergy Clin Immunol,* 92, 717–721.

———. (1995). New drugs. *AJN,* 3, 56–59.

———. (1993). OTC allergy products. *Nursing '93,* 9, 67–72.

*Ryhal BT, Fletcher MP. (1991). The second-generation antihistamines: What makes them different. *Postgrad Med, 89*(6), 87–94.

Sharkey P, Portnoy J. (1996). Rush immunotherapy: Experience with a one-day schedule. *Ann Allergy Asthma Immunol, 76*(2), 175–180.

*Smith LF. (1995). Diagnosis and treatment of allergic rhinitis. *Nurse Practitioner, 20* (10), 58–66.

*Recommended for further reading.

For more information and sample tests and activities, refer to Chapter 34 in the Student Workbook for Clinical Pharmacology and Nursing Management, 5th edition, available through your bookstore.

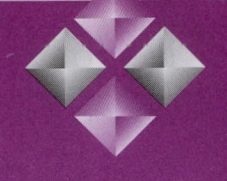

35

Drugs That Moderate the Immune System

The immune response was first recognized in 1798 by Edward Jenner, who differentiated the reactions of people who had received smallpox vaccinations from the reactions of those who had acquired immunity through the disease. In 1890, Robert Koch described the skin reaction (induration and swelling) that resulted from the subcutaneous injection of tuberculin into persons who had previously contracted tuberculosis. By 1919, this procedure, called the Mantoux test, was used for diagnostic purposes.

Physiology of the Immune System

The body's immune response is its third line of defense against microorganisms (the first includes the mechanical barriers of skin, mucous membranes, body hair, and body secretions; the second includes the inflammatory process). Immunity to disease exists when the body can produce specific substances (antibodies) that combat infectious agents (antigens) to which it is exposed. Invading organisms, or antigens, contain proteins and polysaccharides that stimulate the body's tissues to produce protective antibodies. This mechanism is specific—in other words, antibodies will bind only with the particular antigens that stimulated their formation. Figure 35-1 indicates sites where antibodies are produced.

Kinds of Immunity

Natural immunity, which is rare, is permanent immunity that is present at birth. Resistance to disease that develops as a result of exposure to the infectious agent, with subsequent production of antibodies in response to the exposure, is known as acquired immunity, which is not rare and which may persist for a lifetime. Acquired immunity may be obtained by invasion of the body with the infectious agent (active acquired immunity) or by use of antibodies obtained from an animal or another human immunized against the disease (passive acquired immunity).

Passive acquired immunity can also be obtained artificially through antiserum, antitoxin, and gamma globulin. The substance used for passive acquired immunity usually comes from a human or animal already actively immunized against the organism in question. The antibodies in the transferred agent temporarily provide the same protection afforded by an actively acquired immunity. However, unlike the continuing protection provided by active immunity, passively acquired immunity is lost within a few weeks, as the antibodies break down and are discharged from the body.

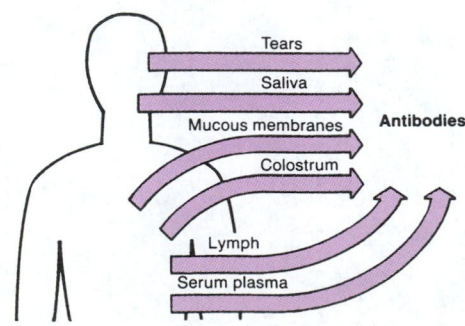

Figure 35-1. Body structures and sites in which antibodies are produced.

Antibodies transmitted through the placenta protect newborns against certain diseases to which their mothers have immunity. This is a type of passive acquired but also natural immunity. Thus, most infants are born with some natural immunity acquired from their mothers through an immunoglobulin (IgG). Additional protection is afforded by breast-feeding, because another specific immunoglobulin (IgA) found in colostrum can be absorbed through the newborn's intestinal tract.

Pathophysiology of the Immune System

Immunologic disorders include hypersensitivity states, autoimmune diseases, and immunodeficiency states. Organ transplants and cancer also involve immunity concepts.

Hypersensitivity

Hypersensitivity, an alteration in immune function, is a disorder that results from a specific antigen/antibody reaction or a specific antigen/lymphocyte interaction. The immune response in hypersensitivity is often inappropriate or excessive. There are four classes of hypersensitivity: type I hypersensitivity (atopic, anaphylactic), type II (cytotoxic or cytolytic), type III (immune complex/Arthus), and type IV (delayed).

Autoimmunity

Autoimmunity occurs when the immune system fails to distinguish a person's own cells (self) from foreign cells. Autoimmune diseases are the direct result of the reaction between self antigens and the immune system. Autoimmune diseases can be either organ-nonspecific and generalized or organ-specific and localized. An example of an organ-nonspecific autoimmune disease is systemic lupus erythematosus. Examples of organ-specific autoimmune diseases are myasthenia gravis and Hashimoto's thyroiditis. Other diseases associated with autoimmune processes are rheumatoid arthritis, multiple sclerosis, Crohn's disease, nephrotic syndrome, psoriasis, ulcerative colitis, pernicious anemia, and insulin-dependent diabetes.

Deficiencies

Primary deficiencies of immune function can be congenital, genetic, or acquired. Absence of stem cells in the marrow results in severe combined immunodeficiency disorder. Functional B and T lymphocytes are lacking, and infants with severe combined immunodeficiency disorder succumb to sepsis and opportunistic infections. Other types of primary immunodeficiency disorders include DiGeorge's syndrome, which is associated with total or partial loss of thymus gland function; chronic mucocutaneous candidiasis, which is due to abnormal T cells that cannot fight *Candida*; and Bruton's X-linked agammaglobulinemia or congenital hypogammaglobulinemia, which is a B-cell disorder.

Acquired deficiencies may be caused by infection such as the human immunodeficiency virus (HIV), which causes acquired immunodeficiency syndrome (AIDS). The key characteristic of AIDS is a decrease in CD4+ (T-helper) lymphocytes. B-cell responsiveness is decreased because of dependence on T-helper cell cytokines. Macrophages also have CD4+ receptors and are targets for HIV infection. With AIDS, the body cannot resist various infections and malignant growths.

Rejection Reactions

Organ transplantation has become an accepted therapeutic option for many types of end-stage organ disease. The introduction of genetically different organs and tissues affects the recipient's immune system in the same way as any other foreign body. If left to proceed uninterrupted, the immune system will attack and reject the foreign tissue. This rejection reaction will cause cell death, necrosis of the transplanted tissue, and failure of the transplanted organ. Therefore, in most cases, organ and tissue transplants cannot succeed unless immune system function is suppressed.

Cancer

Cancer is related to genetic damage. Full expression of cancer in a host is a multistep process described as initiation or genetic mutation, promotion, and progression. Usually cancer surveillance in the body is accomplished primarily by macrophages, natural killer cells, and lymphocytes. Persons with cancer often demonstrate deficits in immune system competence. For more information about cancer, see Chapters 46 and 47.

Immunopotentiators

Immunopotentiators are agents that induce active acquired immunity. They include vaccines and toxoids used in immunization procedures.

Vaccines and Toxoids for Children

Some vaccines are made from viruses, bacteria, or rickettsiae that have been inactivated (killed) by chemicals. Others are made from live microorganisms that have been treated to reduce their pathogenic or allergenic activity. For example, live virus vaccines prepared by growing viruses in cell cultures are essentially devoid of allergenic substances. Toxoids are detoxified by-products derived from organisms that induce disease primarily through the elaboration of exotoxins. During the preparation of toxoids, the toxin's pathogenic quality is destroyed but its antigenic quality remains, and therefore it stimulates specific antibody production. Active immunization induced through inoculation with vaccines and toxoids provides prolonged immunity because it is similar to the immunity acquired by a natural infection.

Table 35-1. Immunization Guidelines for Infants and Children

Vaccine	Birth	1 mo	2 mo	4 mo	6 mo	12 mo	15 mo	18 mo	4–6 yr	11–12 yr	14–16 yr
Hepatitis B[1,2]	HeP B-1										
			HeP B-2		HeP B-3					HeP B[2]	
Diphtheria, Tetanus, Pertussis[3]			DTP	DTP	DTP	DTP or DTaP at 15+ mo			DTP or DTaP	Td	
H Influenzae type b[4]			Hib	Hib	Hib[4]	Hib[4]					
Polio[5]			OPV[5]	OPV	OPV				OPV		
Measles, Mumps, Rubella[6]						MMR			MMR[5] or MMR[6]		
Varicella Zoster Virus Vaccine[7]						Var				Var[7]	

Recommended childhood immunization schedule, United States, January 1995. Approved by Advisory Committee on Immunization Practices, American Academy of Pediatrics, and American Academy of Family Physicians.

[1]Infants born to HBsAg-negative mothers should receive the second dose of hepatitis B vaccine between age 1 and 4 months, provided at least 1 month elapses since first dose. The third dose is recommended between age 6 and 18 months. Infants born to HBsAg-positive mothers should receive immunoprophylaxis for hepatitis B with 0.5 mL hepatitis B immune globulin (HBIG) within 12 hours of birth, and 0.5 mL of either Merck Sharpe & Dohme vaccine (Recombivax HB) or SmithKline Beecham vaccine (Engerix-B) at a separate site. In these infants, the second dose of vaccine is recommended at age 1 month and the third dose at age 6 months. All pregnant women should be screened for HBsAg.

[2]The fourth dose of DTP may be administered at age 12 months, provided at least 6 months elapse after third dose. Combined DTP-Hib products may be used when these two vaccines are to be administered simultaneously. DTaP (diphtheria and tetanus toxoids and acellular pertussis vaccine) is licensed for use for the fourth and/or fifth dose of DTP vaccine in children age 15 months or older and may be preferred for these doses in children in this age group. Td (diphtheria and tetanus toxoids for persons >7 years) is recommended at 11 to 12 years, provided at least 5 years elapse since the last dose of DTP or DT.

[3]Three H influenzae type b conjugate vaccines are available for infants: HbOC (HibTITER) (Lederle Praxis); PRP-T (ActHIB; OmniHIB) (Pasteur Merieux, distributed by SmithKline Beecham; Connaught); and PRP-OMP (PedvaxHIB) (Merck Sharp & Dohme). Children who have received PRP-OMP at ages 2 and 4 months do not require a dose at age 6 months. After the primary infant Hib conjugate vaccine series is completed, any licensed Hib conjugate vaccine may be used as a booster dose at age 12 to 15 months.

[4]The second dose of MMR vaccine should be administered either at age 4 to 6 years or at age 11 to 12, depending on state school requirements.

[5]Vaccines recommended in the second year of life (age 12–15 months) may be given at either one or two visits.

Pharmacodynamics. In most instances, both types of vaccines stimulate antibody production without inducing the disease.

Dosage and Administration. National immunization administration guidelines for children and adults are outlined in Tables 35-1 and 35-2. Boxes 35-1 and 35-2 define the standards for pediatric and adult immunizations. About 20 vaccines are available. They differ in their methods of preparation, recommendations for use, routes of administration, and conditions for storage (Table 35-3).

To reduce confusion over childhood immunization schedules, the two major recommending organizations (Advisory Committee on Immunization Practices of the Centers for Disease Control and Prevention [CDC] and the American Academy of Pediatrics Committee on Infectious Diseases) are now working together to provide a unified schedule. The current schedule represents a consensus of these two groups as well as the Food and Drug

Administration (FDA), the National Institutes of Health, and the American Academy of Family Physicians.

Several routine pediatric vaccines may safely and effectively be administered simultaneously at separate injection sites. This approach to vaccination is recom-

Table 35-2. Adult Immunizations

Immunization	Frequency
Tetanus-diphtheria (Td)	One booster every 10 years
Measles-mumps-rubella (MMR)	One booster if person was born after 1/1/57 and received only one shot
Influenza	Annual immunization for those at risk
Hepatitis B	Series of three shots for those at risk
Pneumococcal	One shot

mended if return of a vaccine recipient for a subsequent visit is doubtful.

Adverse Reactions. Vaccine antigens produced in systems containing allergenic substances (ie, embryonated chicken eggs) may cause hypersensitivity reactions, including anaphylaxis. Modern vaccines are otherwise generally safe and effective, but not completely so. Adverse events following immunization have been reported with all vaccines. These range from low-grade fever, swelling, and soreness at the injection site 12 to 24 hours

Box 35-1
Standards for Pediatric Immunization

1. Immunization services are readily available.
2. There are no barriers or unnecessary prerequisites to the receipt of vaccines.
3. Immunization services are available free or for a minimal fee.
4. Providers use all clinical encounters to screen and, when indicated, immunize children.
5. Providers educate parents and guardians about immunization in general terms.
6. Providers question parents or guardians about contraindications and before immunizing a child, inform them in specific terms about the risks and benefits of the immunizations their child is to receive.
7. Providers follow only true contraindications.
8. Providers simultaneously administer all vaccine doses for which a child is eligible at the time of each visit.
9. Providers use accurate and complete recording procedures.
10. Providers co-schedule immunization appointments in conjunction with appointments for other child health services.
11. Providers report adverse events following immunization promptly, accurately, and completely.
12. Providers operate a tracking system.
13. Providers adhere to appropriate procedures for vaccine management.
14. Providers conduct semiannual audits to assess immunization coverage levels and to review immunization records in the populations they service.
15. Providers maintain up-to-date, easily retrievable medical protocols at all locations where vaccines are administered.
16. Providers operate with client-oriented and community-based approaches.
17. Vaccines are administered by properly trained individuals.
18. Providers receive ongoing education and training on current immunization recommendations.

From Lukes E. (1995). Childhood immunizations. *AAOHN J, 43*(12), 624.

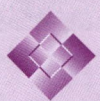

Box 35-2
Standards for Adult Immunization

1. The Standard encourages the promotion of appropriate vaccine use through information campaigns for healthcare practitioners and trainees, employers, and the public about the benefits of immunizations.
2. Encourages physicians and other healthcare personnel (in practice and in training) to protect themselves and prevent transmission to clients by ensuring that they themselves are completely immunized.
3. Recommends that all healthcare providers routinely determine the immunization status of their adult clients, offer vaccines to those for whom they are indicated, and maintain complete immunization records.
4. Recommends that all healthcare providers identify high-risk clients in need of influenza vaccine and develop a system to recall them for immunization each autumn.
5. Recommends that all healthcare providers and institutions identify high-risk adult clients in hospitals and other treatment centers and ensure that appropriate vaccination is considered either before discharge or as part of discharge planning.
6. Recommends that all licensing/accrediting agencies support the development by healthcare institutions of comprehensive immunization programs for staff, trainees, volunteer workers, and clients.
7. Encourages states to establish pre-enrollment immunization requirements for institutions of higher education.
8. Recommends that institutions that train healthcare professionals, deliver health care, or provide laboratory or other medical support services require appropriate immunizations for persons at risk of contracting or transmitting vaccine-preventable illnesses.
9. Encourages healthcare benefit programs, third-party payers, and governmental healthcare programs to provide coverage for adult immunization services.
10. Encourages the adoption of a standard personal and institutional immunization record as a means of verifying the immunization status of clients and staff.

From National Coalition for Adult Immunization. (1994). *AAOHN J, 42*(10), 515–516.

after immunization to rare, severe, systemic illness. The law requires the reporting of adverse reactions to the CDC and FDA (Table 35-4 and Fig. 35-2).

Precautions and Contraindications. Vaccines made with eggs should not be given to persons with known hyper-

Table 35-3. Vaccines and Toxoids

Bacterial Vaccines	Viral Vaccines	Toxoids
BCG vaccine (TICE BCG)	Hepatitis B vaccine, recombinant (Engerix-B, Recombivax HB)	Diphtheria toxoid, adsorbed (pediatric)
	Hepatitis A vaccine, inactivated (Havrix)	
Cholera vaccine	Influenza virus vaccines (Fluogen, FluShield, Fluzone, Fluvirin)	Diphtheria and tetanus toxoids, combined, adsorbed, pediatric
Haemophilus b conjugate vaccine (HibTITER, Pedvax HIB, ProHIBiT)	Japanese encephalitis virus vaccine (JE-VAX)	Diphtheria and tetanus toxoids, combined, adsorbed, adult
Meningococcal polysaccharide vaccine (Menomune-A/C/Y/W-135)	Measles (rubeola) virus vaccine, live, attenuated (Attenuvax)	Diphtheria and tetanus toxoids and whole-cell pertussis vaccine, adsorbed (DTwP) (Tri-Immunol)
Mixed respiratory vaccine (MRV)	Measles (rubeola) and rubella virus vaccine, live (M-R-Vax II)	Diphtheria and tetanus toxoids and acellular pertussis vaccine (DTaP) (Acel-Imune, Tripedia)
Plague vaccine	Measles, mumps, and rubella virus vaccine, live (M-M-R II)	Diphtheria and tetanus toxoids and whole-cell pertussis and *Haemophilus influenzae* type B conjugate vaccines (DTwP-HIB) (Tetramune)
Pneumococcal vaccine, polyvalent (Pneumovax 23, Pnu-Imune 23)	Mumps virus vaccine, live (Mumpsvax)	Tetanus toxoid, fluid or adsorbed
Staphage lysate (SPL-Serologic Types I and III)	Poliovirus vaccine, inactivated (IPV, IPOL, Poliovax)	
Typhoid vaccine (Vivotif Berna Vaccine, Typhoid Vaccine [H-P], Typhoid Vaccine [AKD], Typhim Vi)	Poliovirus vaccine, live, oral, trivalent (OPV, TOPV, Sabin; Orimune)	
	Rubella virus vaccine, live (Meruvax II)	
	Rubella and mumps virus vaccine, live (Biavax II)	
	Varicella virus vaccine (Varivax)	
	Yellow fever vaccine (YF-Vax)	

sensitivity. Some vaccines contain preservatives (eg, thimerosal) or trace amounts of antibiotics (eg, neomycin) and should not be given to clients hypersensitive to them.

Virus replication after administration of live, attenuated virus vaccines may be enhanced in persons with immune deficiency diseases or suppressed immune responses (eg, leukemia, lymphoma, generalized malignancy, or therapy with corticosteroids, alkylating agents, antimetabolites, or radiation). Live, attenuated virus vaccines must not be given to such clients, nor should such vaccines be given to a member of a household with a family history of congenital or hereditary immunodeficiency until the immune competence of the recipient is known.

Special immunization recommendations are used for persons infected with HIV. Persons with HIV infection or AIDS are theoretically at risk of disseminated infection after immunization with a live bacterial or viral vaccine. In general, immunization with an inactivated vaccine or toxoid poses no additional risk to persons with HIV infection or AIDS. However, these persons may be less likely to develop an adequate immune response to vaccination and may remain susceptible to the disease. Usually, immunization is recommended to confer at least partial protection. Optimally, the immunization of HIV-infected persons should be completed before they meet the criteria for AIDS.

Immunization of persons with severe febrile illnesses should generally be deferred until they have recovered.

Measles, mumps, rubella or oral polio vaccines may be safely administered to children of pregnant women. Experience to date does not reveal risks of polio vaccine virus to the fetus. However, live, attenuated virus vaccines are not generally given to pregnant women or to those likely to become pregnant within 3 months after vaccination. If a pregnant woman must be vaccinated, it is not done in the first trimester; waiting until the second or third trimester to minimize any concern over teratogenicity is a reasonable precaution. Tetanus and diphtheria toxoid should be given to inadequately immunized pregnant women (those who lack a primary series or who have had no booster within the past 10 years) because it affords protection against neonatal tetanus. Again, it is prudent to avoid vaccination during the first trimester.

Varicella Virus Vaccine

The newest vaccine is varicella virus vaccine (Varivax), which prevents chickenpox. Chickenpox, which is related to the herpes virus, causes illness in about 3.5 million people a year. Although complications develop in some young people with chickenpox, it is usually a benign

Table 35-4. Reportable Vaccine-Related Events

Vaccine/Toxoid	Event	Interval From Vaccination
DTP, P, DTP/polio combined	A. Anaphylaxis or anaphylactic shock	24 hours
	B. Encephalopathy (or encephalitis)*	7 days
	C. Shock-collapse or hypotonic-hyporesponsive collapse*	7 days
	D. Residual seizure disorder*	See aids to interpretation*
	E. Any acute complication or sequela (including death) arising from above events	No limit
	F. Events in vaccinees described in manufacturer's package insert as contraindications to additional doses of vaccine†(such as convulsions)	See package insert
Measles, mumps, and rubella; DT, Td, tetanus toxoid	A. Anaphylaxis or anaphylactic shock	24 hours
	B. Encephalopathy (or encephalitis)*	15 days for measles, mumps, and rubella vaccines; 7 days for DT, Td, and T toxoids
	C. Residual seizure disorder*	See aids to interpretation*
	D. Any acute complication or sequela (including death) of above events	No limit
	E. Events in vaccinees described in manufacturer's package insert as contraindications to additional doses of vaccine†	See package insert
Oral polio vaccine	A. Paralytic poliomyelitis in a nonimmunodeficient recipient; in an immunodeficient recipient; and in a vaccine-associated community case	30 days, 6 months, no limit
	B. Any acute complication or sequela (including death) of above events	No limit
	C. Events in vaccinees described in manufacturer's package insert as contraindications to additional doses of vaccine†	See package insert
Inactivated polio vaccine	A. Anaphylaxis or anaphylactic shock	24 hours
	B. Any acute complication or sequela (including death) of above event	No limit
	C. Events in vaccinees described in manufacturer's package insert as contraindications to additional doses of vaccine†	See package insert

*Aids to interpretation: Shock-collapse or hypotonic-hyporesponsive collapse may be evidenced by signs or symptoms such as decrease in or loss of muscle tone, paralysis (partial or complete), hemiplegia, hemiparesis, loss of color or turning pale white or blue, unresponsiveness to environmental stimuli, depression of or loss of consciousness, prolonged sleeping with difficulty arousing, or cardiovascular or respiratory arrest.

Residual seizure disorder may be considered to have occurred if no other seizure or convulsion unaccompanied by fever or accompanied by a fever of less than 102°F occurred before the first seizure or convulsion after the administration of the vaccine involved, AND, if in the case of measles-, mumps-, or rubella-containing vaccines, the first seizure or convulsion occurred within 15 days after vaccination OR in the case of any other vaccine, the first seizure or convulsion occurred within 3 days after vaccination, AND, if two or more seizures or convulsions unaccompanied by fever or accompanied by a fever of less than 102°F occurred within 1 year after vaccination.

The terms *seizure* and *convulsion* include grand mal, petit mal, absence, myoclonic, tonic-clonic, and focal motor seizures and signs. Encephalopathy means any significant acquired abnormality of, injury to, or impairment of function of the brain. Among the frequent manifestations of encephalopathy are focal and diffuse neurologic signs, increased intracranial pressure, or changes lasting at least 6 hours in level of consciousness, with or without convulsions. The neurologic signs and symptoms of encephalopathy may be temporary with complete recovery, or they may result in various degrees of permanent impairment. Signs and symptoms such as high-pitched and unusual screaming, persistent unconsolable crying, and bulging fontanel are compatible with an encephalopathy, but in and of themselves are not conclusive evidence of encephalopathy. Encephalopathy usually can be documented by slow wave activity on an electroencephalogram.

†The healthcare provider must refer to the Contraindication section of the manufacturer's package insert for each vaccine.

From *FDA Drug Bulletin*, October 1990.

disease for children under age 15 despite its highly contagious nature. The chickenpox virus remains in the body for life, entering nerve cells and migrating to the nerves in the spine. If the immune system is weakened later in life, the virus may emerge to cause shingles, a painful inflammation of a nerve. Signs and symptoms include a rash on the skin over a nerve pathway. Pain occurs along the nerve endings in the area of the rash, usually lasting a short time but sometimes persisting for years (postherpetic neuralgia). Shingles on the upper half of the face can involve the cornea (zoster keratitis) and can lead to blindness unless treated.

Hepatitis B Vaccine

The public—and in particular healthcare professionals (because of their exposure to contaminated blood and feces and other sources of the disease)—should be alerted to the seriousness of hepatitis B infections and to the importance of vaccinations.

It has been recommended that neonates at high risk for hepatitis B (those living in households with an infected person, children born to drug abusers or to immigrants from endemic areas such as Alaska, Southeast Asia, the Pacific islands, China) be given HBV (Recombivax-HB, Engerix B) at birth. Up to 50% of children

VACCINE ADVERSE EVENT REPORTING SYSTEM

24 Hour Toll-free information line 1-800-822-7967

Patient identity kept confidential

VAERS

For CDC/FDA Use Only
VAERS Number _____
Date Received _____

Patient Name: _____

Last   First   M.I.

Address
_____
_____
_____

City   State   Zip

Telephone no. (_____)_____

Vaccine administered by (Name): _____

Responsible
Physician _____
Facility Name/Address
_____
_____

City   State   Zip

Telephone no. (_____)_____

Form completed by (Name): _____

Relation to ☐ Vaccine Provider   ☐ Patient/Parent
Patient   ☐ Manufacturer   ☐ Other
Address *(if different from patient or provider)*
_____
_____

City   State   Zip

Telephone no. (_____)_____

| 1. State | 2. County where administered | 3. Date of birth ___/___/___ mm dd yy | 4. Patient age | 5. Sex ☐ M ☐ F | 6. Date form completed ___/___/___ mm dd yy |

7. Describe adverse event(s) (symptoms, signs, time course) and treatment, if any

8. Check all appropriate:
☐ Patient died   (date ___/___/___)
☐ Life threatening illness mm dd yy
☐ Required emergency room/doctor visit
☐ Required hospitalization (_____days)
☐ Resulted in prolongation of hospitalization
☐ Resulted in permanent disability
☐ None of the above

9. Patient recovered ☐ YES ☐ NO ☐ UNKNOWN

12. Relevant diagnostic tests/laboratory data

10. Date of vaccination
___/___/___
mm dd yy AM
Time _____ PM

11. Adverse event onset
___/___/___
mm dd yy AM
Time _____ PM

13. Enter all vaccines given on date listed in no. 10

	Vaccine (type)	Manufacturer	Lot number	Route/Site	No. Previous doses
a.					
b.					
c.					
d.					

14. Any other vaccinations within 4 weeks of date listed in no. 10

	Vaccine (type)	Manufacturer	Lot number	Route/Site	No. Previous doses	Date given
a.						
b.						

15. Vaccinated at:
☐ Private doctor's office/hospital   ☐ Military clinic/hospital
☐ Public health clinic/hospital   ☐ Other/unknown

16. Vaccine purchased with:
☐ Private funds   ☐ Military funds
☐ Public funds   ☐ Other /unknown

17. Other medications

18. Illness at time of vaccination (specify)

19. Pre-existing physician-diagnosed allergies, birth defects, medical conditions (specify)

20. Have you reported this adverse event previously?
☐ No   ☐ To health department
☐ To doctor   ☐ To manufacturer

Only for children 5 and under

22. Birth weight _____ lb. _____ oz.

23. No. of brothers and sisters

21. Adverse event following prior vaccination (check all applicable, specify)

	Adverse Event	Onset Age	Type Vaccine	Dose no. in series
☐ In patient				
☐ In brother or sister				

Only for reports submitted by manufacturer/immunization project

24. Mfr. / imm. proj. report no.

25. Date received by mfr. / imm. proj.

26. 15 day report? ☐ Yes ☐ No

27. Report type ☐ Initial ☐ Follow-Up

Health care providers and manufacturers are required by law (42 USC 300aa-25) to report reactions to vaccines listed in the Vaccine Injury Table. Reports for reactions to other vaccines are voluntary except when required as a condition of immunization grant awards

Form VAERS -1   P

Figure 35-2. Sample Vaccine Adverse Event Reporting System form. VAERS, PO Box 1100, Rockville MD 20849-1100.

infected with hepatitis B before their fifth birthday will become chronic carriers of the disease. Of those infected at birth, 90% will become chronic carriers.

To counteract the reluctance of adults to be immunized against hepatitis B, the Immunization Practices Advisory Committee of the Public Health Service recommends that children receive the hepatitis B vaccine at 2, 4, 6, and 15 months. This is suggested despite the fact that those affected by the disease are usually teenagers or adults. It is the first time that a program to prevent illness and possibly death in adults is being directed toward children. The effectiveness will not be apparent until the vaccinated children reach their teens or adulthood.

Immunizations for Adults

Some adults have been improperly or never immunized against vaccine-preventable diseases and may not have been exposed to these diseases as children. Therefore, medical histories taken from adults should include this information, with the idea of offering them a program of immunization, particularly if they are in a high-risk group or are pregnant.

Immunization for adults should be determined on an individual basis, taking into account age, physical status, and possible allergic reactions. For example, pertussis immunization is inappropriate because the risk of reactions to the vaccine outweighs the protection needed, particularly in older adults.

Flu vaccines have presented difficulties because a specific vaccine must be developed for each influenza virus. Again, past vaccines were not without risk, as was shown in the mass vaccination program against swine flu in 1976. Some recipients developed Guillain-Barré syndrome with paralysis, and some people even died. It is important to evaluate the medical risk for the client before administering any vaccine. Because the aged and infirm are usually at greater risk, they should be given the vaccine appropriate for the prevalent flu virus.

Pneumococcal Vaccine Polyvalent (Pneumovax 23, PN-Immune 23) is used for immunization against pneumococcal pneumonia and bacteremia caused by the types of pneumococci included in the vaccine. Adults with chronic illnesses, immunocompromised individuals, and institutionalized adults are considered at increased risk and should receive the vaccine. Those receiving the vaccine should be provided with a record of the immunization and should be cautioned not to receive another pneumococcal vaccine injection.

Rho(D) Immune Globulin

The immune system sometimes miscalculates when trying to protect itself, as when antibodies to an Rh-positive fetus develop in an Rh-negative mother. The fetus is perceived as an invader to be destroyed, a process that can be prevented or stopped with proper immunization treatment. Women who are already immunized should have monthly tests for antibodies through the 28th week of pregnancy and then twice a month. After the 22nd week of pregnancy, amniocentesis should be done if the antibody level exceeds 1.0 g/mL. Exchange transfusions are ordered for the fetus when appropriate.

Pharmacodynamics. Rho(D) immune globulin (RhoGAM) prevents sensitization in a subsequent pregnancy to the Rho(D) factor in an Rh-negative mother who has given birth to an Rh-positive infant by an Rh-positive father.

Therapeutic Uses. Prophylactic immunization with Rho(D) immune globulin prevents maternal production of anti-D antibodies to fetal blood cells. If antibodies are produced by the mother, they can cross the placenta and cause agglutination of the fetal red blood cells. This process may lead to hemolysis and loss of erythrocytes, with the possibility of fetal anemia, heart failure, and death.

Dosage and Administration. Rho(D) immune globulin is administered by intramuscular injection within 72 hours after delivery. Rho(D) immune globulin should also be given to any Rh-negative woman after accidental transfusion of Rh-positive blood, a chorionic villus biopsy, or an amniocentesis, particularly if the needle has gone through the placenta. The product is also available in microdose form (MICRhoGAM) to prevent maternal isoimmunization after miscarriage or abortion up to 12 weeks' gestation.

A supplement to the protocol has been developed using prenatal administration of Rho(D) immune globulin. This is particularly helpful if, for any reason, the Rho(D)-negative woman develops anti-D antibodies during the pregnancy. Because isoimmunization is unlikely to occur before the third trimester, the Rho(D) immune globulin is usually administered during the 28th week of gestation and again within 72 hours after delivery if the fetus is Rho(D)-positive.

Although the prenatal use of Rho(D) immune globulin is expensive, it is thought to lower maternal sensitization rates from 15% of all untreated women at risk to 1.5% to 2% for those treated.

Adverse Reactions. Maternal reactions to the immune globulin are infrequent and usually localized.

Antitoxins and Antivenins

Pharmacodynamics. Antitoxins are antibodies that combine with toxins and neutralize them. Antitoxins and antivenins are used for passive immunization.

Therapeutic Uses. Antivenin (*Crotalidae*) polyvalent is used to neutralize the toxic effects of venoms of crotalids (pit vipers) native to North, Central, and South America, including rattlesnakes, copperheads, and cottonmouth moccasins (Table 35-5). Rabies prophylaxis products are listed in Table 35-6.

Table 35-5. Antitoxins-Antivenins and Human Immune Serums

Antitoxins-Antivenins	Human Immune Serums
Antitoxins	
Botulism antitoxin	Cytomegalovirus immune globulin intravenous, human (CMV-IGIV)
Diphtheria antitoxin	Hepatitis B immune globulin (HBIG) (H-BIG, Hep-B-Gammagee, HyperHep)
Tetanus antitoxin	Immune globulin, intramuscular (IG, Gamma Globulin, ISG) (Gamastan, Gammar)
Antivenins	
Black widow spider species antivenin (*Latrodectus mactans*)	Immune globulin, intravenous (IGIV) (Gamimune N, Gammagard, Gammar-IV, Iveegam, Sandoglobulin, Venoglobulin-I)
Antivenin (*Crotalidae*) polyvalent	Lymphocyte immune globulin, antithymocyte globulin (equine) (LIG, ATG) (Atgam)
	Respiratory syncytial virus immune globulin intravenous (Human) (RSV-IGIV) (RespiGam)
Antivenin (*Micrurus fulvius*) (North American coral snake antivenin)	Tetanus immune globulin (Hyper-Tet)
	Rho(D) immune globulin (Gamulin Rh, HypRho-D, RhoGAM)
	Rho(D) immune globulin micro-dose (HypRho-D); mini-dose (MICRhoGAM, Mini-Gamulin Rh)
	Rho(D) immune globulin IV (human) (Win-Rho SD)
	Varicella-zoster immune globulin (human) (VZIG)

Adverse Reactions. Acute anaphylaxis or serum sickness may occur 7 to 12 days after administration. The incidence of serum sickness is 5% to 10%. Local pain or erythema and urticaria without systemic disturbance may occur 7 to 10 days after administration and may last about 2 days.

Precautions and Contraindications. Because some antitoxins or antivenins made from animals may cause allergic reactions, and because most antitoxins for human use are derived from horse serum, the client should be assessed for any previous reaction or exposure to horse serum. If the agent has been derived from animal products, even when lack of previous serum sensitivity has been established, epinephrine, corticosteroids, antihistamines, and oxygen must be available to manage any possible allergic response. Scratch, conjunctival, or intradermal tests are recommended to test for sensitivity before administering the product.

Immune Serums

Standard immune globulins contain about 16.5% gamma globulin. These products are obtained, purified, and standardized from pooled human plasma, either from donors in the general population or, in the case of immune globulins for specific diseases, from hyperimmunized donors.

Pharmacodynamics. Immune globulins provide antibodies to individuals.

Pharmacokinetics. Protection derived from immune globulins is of rapid onset but short duration (1–3 months).

Therapeutic Uses. Immune serums provide passive immunization to one or more infectious diseases. For example, immune globulin intravenous (IV) is used for maintenance treatment in clients who cannot produce sufficient amounts of IgG antibodies. Some clients with idiopathic thrombocytopenic purpura have shown an

Table 35-6. Rabies Prophylaxis Products

Agent	Notes
Antirabies serum, equine origin	Give on suspected exposure to rabies. May produce serum sickness, urticaria, local pain, and erythema.
Rabies immune globulin, human (RIG) (Hyperab, Imogam)	Give on suspected exposure to rabies. Used to provide rabies antibodies immediately. May produce fever and soreness at injection site; reduced risk of serum sickness compared to equine serum.
	Give 20 IU/kg; about half the dose should be used to infiltrate the wound and the remainder administered IM. Expect to give this and HDCV (see below); do not administer both medications at same site or in same syringe.
Rabies vaccine, human diploid cell cultures (HDCV) IM (Imovax)	Preferred prophylaxis product; may be used either pre- or postexposure. Postexposure use requires 5 doses (days 0, 3, 7, 14, and 28). Postexposure use should also include rabies immune globulin. May produce local reactions.

increase, albeit temporary, in platelet counts when this product is used. It is also used to prevent bacterial infections in clients with hypogammaglobulinemia or recurrent bacterial infections associated with B-cell chronic lymphocytic leukemia.

Cytomegalovirus (CMV) immune globulin IV is used to attenuate primary CMV disease associated with kidney transplantation. Specifically, the product is indicated for kidney recipients who are seronegative for CMV and who receive a kidney from a CMV-seropositive donor.

Immune globulin intramuscular (IM) may be used for prophylaxis when given before or soon after exposure to hepatitis A. It has been used to prevent or modify measles in a susceptible contact (one who has not been vaccinated, has not had measles previously, and was exposed less than 6 days previously).

Tetanus immune globulin is used for passive immunization against tetanus when the history of active immunization with tetanus toxoid is unknown or uncertain.

Hepatitis B immune globulin is used to provide postexposure prophylaxis (following, for example, an accidental needle stick or a pipetting accident involving hepatitis B antigen-positive materials such as blood, plasma, or serum). It is used as prophylaxis for infants born to mothers positive for the antigen.

Varicella zoster immune globulin (human) provides passive immunization of susceptible immunodeficient persons after significant exposure to varicella. There is no evidence that it modifies established varicella zoster infections.

Dosage and Administration. Except for immune globulin IV and CMV immune globulin IV, these serums are to be administered IM, not IV. IV injections can cause a precipitous fall in blood pressure and symptoms similar to anaphylaxis.

Adverse Reactions. Anaphylactic reactions, although rare, may occur. Local reactions include tenderness, pain, and muscle stiffness at the injection site. These effects may persist for several hours.

Drug Interactions. Live virus vaccines cannot be administered within 3 months of immune globulin administration because antibodies in the globulin preparation may interfere with the immune response to the vaccine. It may be necessary to revaccinate persons who received immune globulin shortly after live virus vaccination.

Precautions and Contraindications. Skin testing should not be performed, because intradermal injection of concentrated gamma globulin causes a localized area of inflammation that could be misinterpreted as a positive allergic reaction.

■ SUMMARY

Immunity to infectious diseases can be provided by administering immunizing agents to persons who have not been previously exposed. Passive immunity can be provided on a temporary basis through the use of antitoxins, antivenins, or immune sera. Active immunity can be provided by vaccines made from live or killed viruses, or from toxoids, which are manufactured from the poisons of some bacteria.

❖ NURSING MANAGEMENT: CLIENT RECEIVING IMMUNOPOTENTIATORS

Immunization is usually considered a safe procedure; in most cases, reactions are minor and pass in a few days. However, because there are some more serious risk factors, vaccines should always be given with caution. The nurse must monitor the client carefully for untoward reactions and educate the client and community about the purpose and expected outcomes of immunization.

NURSING PROCESS

ASSESSMENT

A complete immunization history, including reactions to any previous vaccinations and information about allergies (particularly to eggs and horse serum), and an assessment of the client's current health status help determine the proper immunization schedule.

NURSING DIAGNOSIS

Nursing diagnoses likely to be made for clients receiving immunizations include:

- Risk for Altered Body Temperature, related to response to immunizing antigen
- Knowledge Deficit, related to immunization agent

A common collaborative problem that should be differentiated from the nursing diagnoses is:

Potential Complication: Anaphylactic shock

PLANNING

Goals of nursing care are to alleviate or eliminate fever and inflammation, prevent severe reactions to immunizing medications, maintain vital functions during anaphylactic reactions, and teach the client (and public) about immunization.

INTERVENTION

No matter what the reason for vaccination, it is important to check the potency of the vaccine and be aware of how long it is expected to confer immunity. Vaccines must also be stored properly, according to the manufacturer's instructions, to ensure potency, and they must be used within the time limit set by the manufacturer and according to the manufacturer's recommendations.

When assessment of the client reveals contraindications for immunization, the nurse should alert the prescriber to the situation. After receiving the antigen, clients should be monitored for at least 30 minutes for an immediate reaction such as anaphylaxis. Emergency equipment and medications, such as epinephrine and antihistamines, must always be available for managing an anaphylactic reaction.

Accurate immunization records, including vaccine lot number, should be kept in the healthcare center. An immunization record should also be provided to the client or parents. Adverse reactions should be documented in both records and reported as required by law.

Client Education. Before giving an immunization, the nurse should inform the parents or the client about expected beneficial and possible adverse reactions. If a healthcare facility requires parents to sign informed consent papers, the nurse must explain the immunization procedure and help the parents and client understand it. The nurse should prevent undue alarm about signing consent papers.

Clients should be instructed to observe for adverse reactions and to contact the prescriber if they occur. Children should be instructed not to scratch or rub the site of injection; such an action may cause autoinoculation. To reduce itching, parents may apply cold compresses and instruct the child to press on the affected area. Acetaminophen may be recommended to control fever.

At the community level, nurses are actively involved in educating the public about the benefits and risks of immunizations. They must remain aware of changes in the agents used and the recommendations for their use as they evolve from new research findings. For example, in the early 1990s, a resurgence of measles occurred throughout the United States, due in large part to the ineffectiveness of the vaccine administered before 1957. In 1990, about 26,500 cases of measles were reported, with more children dying than any year since 1971. This illustrates the importance of immunization.

Another opportunity for community education relates to travel. The nurse should advise clients who plan to travel to contact the local health department or the CDC (www.cdc.gov) for current immunization requirements for the country they wish to enter.

OUTCOME EVALUATION

Data required for evaluation include immunization records of clients and populations, the presence or absence of adverse reactions to immunizations, and the speed and effectiveness of treatment for the adverse reaction.

❖ **CHECKLIST OF NURSING ACTIONS**

❑ Take a careful history to determine if any allergies are present that may be affected by the immunization.
❑ Inform clients or parents of expected beneficial and possible adverse reactions before starting immunization.
❑ Have clients or parents sign an informed consent form in accordance with the procedures of the healthcare facility.

❑ Before giving immunizations, consult package inserts and administer drugs according to the specific recommendations.
❑ Store vaccines properly to ensure potency.
❑ Give vaccines in the proper doses and according to the correct schedule.
❑ Have the client remain in the office for about 30 minutes after immunization so that you can observe for systemic reactions.
❑ Keep emergency equipment and medications available.
❑ Keep accurate immunization records in the healthcare facility and give a copy to the client.
❑ Advise clients or parents to observe for more serious adverse reactions and to report them to the physician. Advise clients how to treat minor adverse reactions.
❑ Report adverse reactions to vaccines as required by law.
❑ Advise clients who plan to travel to contact the local health department for current immunization requirements for the country they wish to enter.
❑ Do not give live virus vaccines to pregnant women or to children or adults infected with HIV (or those who are otherwise immunocompromised).

Biologic Response Modifiers

Biotherapy, the therapeutic use of biologic agents known as biologic response modifiers (BRMs), is developing as another modality in cancer therapy (joining surgery, radiation therapy, and chemotherapy). A BRM is any soluble substance that can alter or modify the immune system with either a stimulatory or a suppressive effect (Jassak, 1996). BRMs include the monoclonal antibodies (MoAbs), the cytokines (including interferons, colony-stimulating factors, and interleukins), and tumor necrosis factor (TNF). Much work with BRMs is still investigational.

Monoclonal Antibodies

One MoAb in current use is muromonab-CD3 (Orthoclone OKT3). Other MoAbs are investigational (eg, OKT4, BMA 031, ICAM-1, CD54). MoAbs are produced in the laboratory by injecting a laboratory animal with an antigen (eg, human cancer cells). The animal's lymphocytes recognize the antigen as foreign and produce antibodies. These antibodies are then removed from the animal's spleen and fused with other cells to form what is called a hybrid. The hybrid cells are screened for antibody production, and the resultant antibody is concentrated and purified. These cells can be continuously cultured and reproduced, so antibody can be produced in large quantities.

Pharmacodynamics. Muromonab-CD3 is an immunosuppressant agent that acts by specifically attacking all forms of the body's T cells, whether juvenile or mature, helper or suppressor. In clients receiving a kidney transplant, for example, the antibody attaches itself to the renal graft T-cell antigen, stopping the T cells from functioning at that time and moderating their future response so they no longer try to destroy the grafted tissue. MoAbs may be used alone (unconjugated) or in combination (conjugated) with radioisotopes or chemotherapeutic drugs to identify or destroy cells with specific antigens on their cell surface. The idea is to have the antibody carry the chemotherapeutic drug to the tumor site or sites.

Pharmacokinetics. The onset of action after muromonab-CD3 administration occurs within minutes. Action peaks within 2 to 7 days and the duration of action is 7 days. The agent is metabolized in the tissues, and it crosses the placenta.

Therapeutic Uses. Muromonab-CD3 is used to prevent acute rejection of kidney transplants; other uses for MoAbs are being studied. They have been researched as treatment agents against specific human tumor-associated antigens. They have also been investigated with acute lymphoblastic leukemia, chronic lymphocytic leukemia, B-cell lymphomas, and T-cell leukemias and lymphomas. Clinical responses have been noted in some clients. They can be used in vitro to deplete T cells from donor bone marrow before bone marrow transplantation. It is believed that MoAbs may eventually have a role in detecting cancer or metastases.

Dosage and Administration. These agents are usually administered by slow IV infusion over 1 to 2 hours.

Adverse Reactions. Because MoAbs are a new type of agent, some side effects remain undisclosed. The client must, therefore, be observed closely for any adverse reactions, which should then be reported and documented. Side effects that occur with the initial IV injection include fever, chills, dyspnea, tremor, and, less often, chest pain, nausea, vomiting, and wheezing. The symptoms usually occur within 45 to 60 minutes and are alleviated by the use of corticosteroids, antihistamines, and acetaminophen. There is usually better tolerance of subsequent doses.

Because mice are used in preparing most MoAbs, the possibility of an allergic response to mouse protein increases with each MoAb administration. The problem of hypersensitivity may eventually be eliminated when MoAbs are manufactured from human rather than mouse tissue. Allergic reactions are most likely to occur within 30 to 60 minutes after the IV infusion starts. Fever, hypotension, or an increase in heart rate or respirations may occur. Milder reactions (hives, urticaria) can be treated with 25 to 50 mg of diphenhydramine. For more serious responses (hypotension, bronchospasm, or anaphylactoid reactions), the infusion is discontinued immediately and an IV of normal saline solution is started. Epinephrine and resuscitative procedures may be needed.

Precautions and Contraindications. These agents should be administered cautiously to febrile clients (antipyretics are used to decrease fever before therapy). They should not be given if the client has an allergy to muromonab or any murine product or fluid overload (detected by chest x-ray). Because antibodies frequently develop, cautious use is advised if the client previously received the drug. The drug is contraindicated in pregnancy.

Although muromonab-CD3 treatment suppresses only the T cells, not the entire immune system, the risk of infection is the same as that incurred with administration of high-dose steroids. Therefore, measures to prevent or control infection are necessary.

Cytokines

Cytokines are substances released from activated immune system cells that affect the behavior of other cells (Table 35-7). They are basically immunopotentiators or immunostimulants. Recombinant DNA technology has made the production of purified cytokines possible. The cytokines include interferons, colony-stimulating factors, and interleukins. Some of these agents have investigational status, some as single agents and some in combination with antineoplastic drugs or cancer treatments. Table 35-8 summarizes their therapeutic indications.

Interferons

Interferons are a family of glycoproteins. Alpha-interferon is produced normally by B lymphocytes, T lymphocytes, macrophages, and null cells. Beta-interferon is produced normally by fibroblasts. Gamma-interferon is produced normally by T lymphocytes. Within the alpha class of human interferon, 14 different subclasses are known, each differing slightly in amino acid sequence (Box 35-3).

Several mechanisms are identified as typical of interferons: antiviral activity, antiproliferation, immunomodulation, and cytotoxicity.

First, in response to viral challenge, interferon is synthesized and released by infected cells. Interferon then binds to receptors on the infected cell's surface and induces enzyme production that damages the viral DNA strands; this interferes with intracellular replication of viral DNA. It protects neighboring cells from infection with a second virus (antiviral activity). Interferons also have antiproliferative activity. In *in vitro* studies, interferons slow the cycle of cell division of all cells; they interfere with the replication of DNA and protein synthesis. This effect is more pronounced with cancer cells.

Interferons also have immunomodulatory activities. They inhibit the expression of oncogenes, genes associated with the transformation of a normal cell into a malignant one.

Interferons exhibit cytotoxic activity and alter the body's immune defense system in several ways, includ-

Table 35-7. Effects of Selected Cytokines

Cytokine	Effect
Interferons	
interferon-alpha	Inhibits virus replication, toxic to cancer cells, stimulates leukocytes, facilitates killer cell activity, produces fever, increases B- and T-cell activity
interferon-beta	Inhibits virus replication, toxic to cancer cells, facilitates killer cell activity, produces fever
interferon-gamma	Inhibits virus replication, promotes antigen expression, activates macrophages, inhibits cell growth, induces myeloid cell lines
Interleukins	
interleukin-1	Stimulates T cells and macrophages, induces acute-phase reaction of inflammation, induces interleukin-2 secretion, produces fever
interleukin-2	Promotes growth of T cells, enhances function of natural killer cells, assists T-cell maturation in thymus
interleukin-3	Induces proliferation and differentiation of other lymphocytes, pluripotential stem cells, mast cells
interleukin-4	Promotes T-cell/B-cell interactions, promotes synthesis of IgE by B cells and T-cell growth, promotes mast cell and hematopoietic cell growth
interleukin-5	Promotes growth and differentiation of B cells to secrete IGA, induces differentiation of eosinophils
interleukin-6	Promotes immunoglobulin secretion by B cells, induces fever, promotes release of inflammation factors from liver cells, promotes differentiation of hematopoietic stem cells and nerve cells
interleukin-7	Stimulates B and T cells; synergistic with interleukin-2
interleukin-8	Chemotactic for neutrophils, B and T cells
interleukin-9	Promotes proliferation of mast cells
interleukin-10	Inhibits T cells
interleukin-11	Synergistic with interleukin-3
interleukin-12	Synergistic with interleukin-2
Colony-stimulating Factors	
granulocyte-macrophage colony-stimulating factor (GM-CSF)	Promotes bone marrow proliferation and activation of antigen-presenting cells

Adapted from Copstead LC. (1995). *Perspectives on pathophysiology.* Philadelphia: WB Saunders Co.

ing the stimulation of natural killer cells to attack and destroy tumor cells. They appear to increase tumor cell recognition by stimulating the expression of both human leukocyte antigens and tumor-associated antigens on tumor cell surfaces. After exposure to interferons, cancer cells have been observed to change in appearance and behavior so that they look and act more like normal cells.

Interferon Beta-1b

Interferon beta-1b (Betaseron) is a representative interferon. It is a purified, sterile, lyophilized protein product produced by recombinant DNA techniques. It is manufactured by bacterial fermentation of a strain of *Escherichia coli*.

Pharmacodynamics. Interferon beta-1b has antiviral, antiproliferative, and immunoregulatory activities. The mechanisms by which it exerts its actions are not clearly understood. However, it is known to interact with specific cell receptors on the surface of human cells. In binding to these receptors, it induces the expression of

products that are believed to be mediators of the biologic actions of interferon beta-1b.

Pharmacokinetics. Peak serum concentrations occur 1 to 8 hours after subcutaneous (SC) administration. Bioavailability is about 50%.

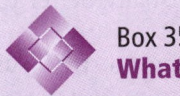

Box 35-3
What's Its Name?

In 1985 the World Health Organization (WHO) and United States Adopted Names Council (USAN) recommended a uniform nomenclature for the interferons.

Interferon-A is to be spelled *alpha* when used in scientific classifications and *alfa* in reference to the generic name of a special commercial product. The subclass is to be identified by number and subspecies by assigned letter (eg, Intron A is interferon alfa-2b, recombinant).

Table 35-8. Cytokines in Biotherapy*

Drug	Proposed Use
Interferons	
interferon alfa-2a (recombinant) (Roferon A)	Chronic myelogenous leukemia; with fluorouracil for advanced colorectal cancer & esophageal carcinoma; with teceleukin for metastatic malignant melanoma and renal cell carcinoma; AIDS-related Kaposi sarcoma
interferon alfa-2b (recombinant) (Intron A)	AIDS-related Kaposi sarcoma, acute hepatitis B, chronic myelogenous leukemia
interferon alfa-NL (Wellferon)	AIDS-related Kaposi sarcoma, human papillomavirus in severe resistant/recurrent respiratory (laryngeal) papillomatosis
interferon beta-1b (recombinant human) (Betaseron)	Multiple sclerosis, primary brain tumors, AIDS, acute non-A, non-B hepatitis
interferon beta (recombinant) (R-Frone)	Systemic treatment of cutaneous T-cell lymphoma, cutaneous malignant melanoma & metastatic renal cell carcinoma; intralesional/systemic treatment of AIDS-related Kaposi sarcoma; symptomatic clients with AIDS (including CD4 T-cell counts below 200 cells/mm^3)
interferon gamma-1b (Actimmune)	Chronic granulomatous disease
Interleukins	
interleukin-1 alpha (human recombinant)	Promotion of early engraftment in bone marrow transplantation; hematopoietic potentiation in aplastic anemia
interleukin-1 receptor antagonist, human recombinant (Antril)	Juvenile rheumatoid arthritis; prevention/treatment of graft-vs-host disease in transplant recipients
interleukin-2, IL-2 (Aldesleukin, Proleukin)	Alone or combined with lymphokine-activated killer cells to mediate regression of metastases in advanced cancers such as malignant melanoma, sarcoma, colon adenocarcinoma, bladder cancer, renal cell cancer; with tumor-infiltrating lymphocytes to mediate regression of metastatic tumors in metastatic melanoma; with other cytokines
interleukin-2, recombinant liposome encapsulated	Cancers of the kidney, renal pelvis; brain and CNS tumors
interleukin-3 human (recombinant)	Promotion of erythropoiesis in Diamond-Blackfan anemia/congenital pure red cell aplasia; with sargramostim to accelerate neutrophil and platelet recovery in clients undergoing autologous bone marrow transplantation for treatment of Hodgkin's disease or non-Hodgkin's lymphoma
Colony-stimulating factors	
erythropoietin (recombinant human) (Procrit)	Anemia related to HIV infection or treatment; anemia associated with end-stage renal disease; anemia of premature infants
granulocyte colony-stimulating factor (G-CSF)	Prevention of chemotherapy-induced neutropenia
granulocyte-macrophage colony-stimulating factor (GM-CSF)	AIDS clients with neutropenia due to the disease, zidovudine, or ganciclovir; myelodysplastic syndrome; aplastic anemia; to rescue bone marrow graft failure, to foster graft recovery after autologous bone marrow transplantation
macrophage colony-stimulating factor	Monocyte increase

*Some of these drugs are considered orphan drugs. The Orphan Drug Act defines an orphan drug as a drug or biologic product for the diagnosis, treatment, or prevention of a rare disease or condition. A rare disease is one that affects fewer than 200,000 persons in the United States or one that affects more than 200,000 persons but for which there is no reasonable expectation that the cost of developing the drug and making it available will be recovered from sales of that drug in the United States.

Therapeutic Uses. Interferon beta-1b is indicated for use in ambulatory clients with relapsing and remitting multiple sclerosis to reduce the frequency of clinical exacerbations. Efficacy beyond 2 years is unknown. Unlabeled uses include treatment of AIDS, AIDS-related Kaposi sarcoma, primary brain tumors, and some forms of hepatitis C.

Dosage and Administration. A typical dose is 0.25 mg or 8 mIU injected SC every other day. Reconstitution is carried out with the accompanying diluent; the product contains no preservatives and should be used within 3 hours of reconstitution. A vial is suitable for one use only. Before reconstitution, it is stored at 36° to 46°F. Clients must be taught appropriate reconstitution meth-ods and SC injection technique. Sites for self-injection include the arms, abdomen, hips, and thighs.

Adverse Reactions. Adverse reactions include injection site reactions, headache, pain, asthenia, abdominal pain, sinusitis, diarrhea, constipation, vomiting, mental symptoms (eg, depression, suicidal ideation), hypertonia, conjunctivitis, photosensitivity, dysmenorrhea, and metrorrhagia. Injection site reactions in general are transient and do not require discontinuation of therapy, but the nature and severity of reactions should be evaluated. The most common adverse reaction appears to be a flu-like syndrome that can include fever, chills, myalgia, malaise, fatigue, and sweating.

Drug–Drug Interactions. Interferon beta-1b administered concurrently with other agents that are potentially myelosuppressive may increase myelosuppression.

Drug–Laboratory Test Interactions. Elevated liver enzyme and bilirubin levels and blood urea nitrogen (BUN), calcium, and glucose levels have been reported. Neutropenia occurs.

Precautions and Contraindications. The use of beta-interferon is contraindicated in clients who are allergic to it or to human albumin or product components. It is contraindicated in pregnancy and lactation and must be used cautiously in clients with chronic progressive multiple sclerosis, suicidal tendencies, or mental disorders.

Interferon Gamma-1b

Pharmacodynamics. Interferon gamma-1b (Actimmune) has immunomodulatory, antiproliferative, and antiviral activities. Studies indicate that it enhances the oxidative metabolism of tissue macrophages, antibody-dependent cellular cytotoxicity, and natural killer cell activity.

Pharmacokinetics. Interferon gamma-1b is rapidly cleared after IV use and slowly absorbed after IM or SC injection. The mean elimination half-life after IV administration is 38 minutes; after IM and SC administration, it is 2.9 and 5.9 hours, respectively. Peak plasma concentrations occur about 4 hours after IM dosing and 7 hours after SC dosing.

Therapeutic Uses. Interferon gamma-1b is indicated for reducing the frequency and severity of serious infections associated with chronic granulomatous disease (the inherited disorder characterized by deficient phagocyte oxidative metabolism).

Dosage and Administration. A typical dosage for chronic granulomatous disease is 50 mcg/m^2 for clients with a body surface area of more than 0.5 m^2 and 1.5 mcg/kg for clients whose body surface area is 0.5 m^2 or less. It is administered SC three times weekly. A vial is suitable for a single use only; the product does not contain preservatives. Clients must be taught reconstitution methods and SC injection technique. The best injection sites are the right and left deltoid and the anterior thigh. Vials must be refrigerated at 36° to 46°F immediately on receipt to ensure optimal integrity. The agent must not be frozen or agitated. A vial of unopened drug can be left at room temperature for no more than 12 hours before use; after this time, the vial should be discarded.

Adverse Reactions. Common adverse effects include headache, rash, injection site erythema or tenderness, diarrhea, and nausea and vomiting. The most common adverse reaction appears to be a flulike syndrome of fever, chills, myalgia, malaise, fatigue, and sweating.

Drug Interactions. Caution should be exercised if this agent is administered concurrently with other agents that are potentially myelosuppressive.

Precautions and Contraindications. Contraindications include allergy to interferon gamma, *E coli*, or a component of the product; pregnancy; and lactation. This agent is given cautiously to clients with seizure disorders, compromised central nervous system (CNS) function, cardiac disease, and myelosuppression.

Interferon Alfa-2a

Interferon alfa-2a (Roferon A) is a protein product manufactured by recombinant DNA technology.

Pharmacodynamics. Interferon alfa-2a has antiviral, antiproliferative, and immunomodulatory activities.

Pharmacokinetics. Alfa interferons are totally filtered through the glomeruli of the kidneys and undergo rapid proteolytic degradation during tubular reabsorption. In healthy persons, interferon alfa-2a has an elimination half-life of 5.1 hours. After IM and SC administration, peak serum concentrations are reached at 3.8 and 7.3 hours, respectively. The apparent fraction of the dose absorbed after IM injection exceeds 80%.

Therapeutic Uses. Interferon alfa-2a is used for hairy cell leukemia and AIDS-related Kaposi sarcoma in clients 18 years and older. Unlabeled or investigational uses include renal cell carcinoma, metastatic malignant melanoma, advanced colorectal cancer and esophageal carcinoma, mycosis fungoides, and condylomata acuminata (by intralesional injection of the genital warts).

Dosage and Administration. Because interferon is a protein, it is destroyed by digestive enzymes and must be administered IM or SC. Interferons are supplied as powder in vials containing 3 to 50 million IU per vial. Each vial of interferon alfa-2a is packaged with a diluent that contains sodium chloride, albumin, and phenol. When the diluent is added during reconstitution, the vial should not be shaken but swirled gently to dissolve the contents.

For hairy cell leukemia, a typical dosage would be 3 million IU daily for 16 to 24 weeks as induction therapy, followed by maintenance therapy of 3 million IU three times a week. The maintenance dose may be halved if severe adverse effects occur.

For Kaposi sarcoma, induction therapy involves 36 million IU daily IM or SC for 10 to 12 weeks. Maintenance therapy is 3 million IU three times a week. The maintenance dose may be halved if severe adverse effects occur.

Clients should be treated for 6 months to determine the efficacy of therapy. Maintenance therapy may be continued for up to 20 months. Neutralizing antibodies to alfa-2a have been detected in 27% of clients, but the clinical significance has not been determined. Clients with platelet counts under 50,000/mm^3 should receive SC injections, not IM. Treatment may include premedication with acetaminophen to minimize the flulike syndrome and administration at night to minimize the persistent fatigue.

The lyophilized powder, the diluent, and the reconstituted solution should be refrigerated.

Adverse Reactions. Interferon alfa-2a should be used with caution in clients with cardiac disease. No direct cardiotoxic effect has been demonstrated, but it appears likely that acute, self-limited toxicities such as fever and chills may exacerbate preexisting cardiac conditions.

The problem of cognitive dysfunction associated with cancer and with treatments such as chemotherapy and radiation therapy has been clearly documented. The literature reports this as one of several manifestations of CNS toxicities associated with BRM therapy (Bender, 1994). The mechanisms underlying this adverse reaction are not clearly understood. Other CNS toxicities include exaggerated CNS function, dizziness, and, rarely, coma. Some abnormalities were reversible within days to weeks after dose reduction or discontinuation.

Drug–Drug Interactions. Caution should be exercised when administering interferon alfa-2a to clients in combination with other agents known to cause myelosuppression. Synergistic toxicity has been observed when the agent has been administered in combination with zidovudine (AZT).

Drug–Laboratory Test Interactions. Leukopenia and elevated hepatic enzyme levels have occurred frequently but have not been dose-limiting. Thrombocytopenia occurs, but less frequently.

Precautions and Contraindications. Contraindications include pregnancy, lactation, and allergy to interferon or any components of the product. The agent is used cautiously in clients with pancreatitis, hepatic or renal disease, seizure disorders, compromised CNS function, cardiac disease or history of cardiac disease, or bone marrow depression.

Colony-Stimulating Factors

Red bone marrow, the source of all blood cells, produces an immature, undifferentiated cell called a stem cell. The stem cell's maturation is mediated by certain glycoproteins called hematopoietic colony-stimulating factors (CSFs). CSFs regulate the proliferation and differentiation of hematopoietic progenitors; they also enhance the function of mature blood cells, promoting their survival and stimulating their activities.

Colony-stimulating factors are named for the target cells they affect. Thus, granulocyte-macrophage CSF (GM-CSF) targets both the granulocyte and macrophage lineages; granulocyte colony-stimulating factor (G-CSF) targets only granulocytes. Large quantities of purified CSFs can be produced by recombinant DNA technology.

Colony-stimulating factors are used in treating diseases in which anemia, thrombocytopenia, and myelosuppression prevail and limit therapeutic options. For example, they are used to prevent chemotherapy-induced myelosuppression after bone marrow transplantation. CSFs are thought to enhance the body's ability to manufacture blood, which has positive implications for blood donors, particularly for clients who wish to donate greater volumes of their own blood before surgery. Other uses of CSFs include treatment of anemia of malignant disease, cancers associated with neutropenia, infections in cancer clients, and certain other situations (eg, after radiation accidents).

Epoetin Alfa

Epoetin alfa, or human recombinant erythropoietin (Epogen, Procrit), is a hematopoietic CSF produced by mammalian cells into which the human erythropoietin gene has been introduced. It was the first CSF approved by the FDA.

Pharmacodynamics. Epoetin alfa stimulates red blood cell production by stimulating division and differentiation of erythroid progenitors in the bone marrow.

Pharmacokinetics. Onset of action of epoetin alfa is 7 to 14 days. In normal subjects, the half-life of epoetin alfa is about 20% shorter than its half-life (4–13 hours) in clients with anemia associated with chronic renal failure (CRF). After SC administration to clients with CRF, peak serum levels were achieved within 5 to 24 hours and were maintained for several hours. Epoetin alfa appears to be eliminated more rapidly after multiple than single doses.

Therapeutic Uses. Epoetin alfa is used to enhance autologous red blood cell donation before elective surgery. Treatment with epoetin alfa does not appear to correct anemia in clients who have undergone autologous bone marrow transplantation, but it does appear to accelerate recovery of red blood cells in allogeneic bone marrow transplant recipients. It elevates the hematocrit of clients with anemia and reduces the need for transfusion. Anemias treated with epoetin alfa include those secondary to CRF, those associated with zidovudine-treated HIV-infected clients, and those associated with certain cancers.

Clients with CRF typically have declining hematocrit values, probably from damage to the sites of renal erythropoietin production, and decreased red blood cell survival because of kidney damage. The anemia in cancer may be due to blood loss from mucosal surfaces, poor nutrition, or tumor infiltration of bone marrow. Chemotherapy (as with cisplatin) can be a major cause of anemia in cancer patients.

Dosage and Administration. Typically, epoetin alfa therapy begins with 50 to 100 U/kg three times a week IV or SC until the target hematocrit range of 30% to 33% is reached. (The hematocrit should not increase by more than 4 points in any 2-week period; a rapid increase in hematocrit increases the risk of more serious adverse reactions.) The dose may be increased in increments of 50 or more U/kg if the hematocrit has not increased 5 or 6 points after 8 weeks of therapy. For a child, a dosage of 150 U/kg three times a week initially may be given SC.

Adverse Reactions. Adverse reactions in clients with CRF include headache, hypertension, and arthralgia. In clients undergoing hemodialysis, adverse effects include clotting of the arteriovenous fistula. Adverse effects for clients with HIV infection include pyrexia, fatigue, headache, cough, rash, nausea, and respiratory congestion. Adverse reactions reported for cancer clients include pyrexia, diarrhea, nausea, edema, vomiting, and fatigue. SC administration of epoetin alfa may be accompanied by pain at the injection site. Hypertension occurs in up to 30% of clients who have end-stage renal disease and who have had long-term epoetin alfa therapy (Markham & Bryson, 1995). Seizures have occurred in clients receiving epoetin alfa, but seizure activity appears to relate to underlying pathology (eg, meningitis, cerebral neoplasm) rather than drug treatment.

Drug Interactions. No interactions have been reported.

Precautions and Contraindications. Epoetin alfa is contraindicated in clients with known hypersensitivity to human albumin. Epoetin alfa is not intended for clients with anemia caused by iron or folate deficiencies, hemolysis, or gastrointestinal bleeding.

Granulocyte Colony-Stimulating Factor

Filgrastim (Neupogen), a G-CSF approved by the FDA in 1991, is prepared by recombinant DNA technology with *E coli*.

Pharmacodynamics. The principal target cells for G-CSF are neutrophils.

Pharmacokinetics. After SC administration of G-CSF, peak serum concentrations occur within 2 to 8 hours. The elimination half-life is about 3.5 hours.

Therapeutic Uses. This agent is approved for chemotherapy-induced neutropenia. In a second use with transplant clients (when G-CSF is administered in the posttransplant regimen), platelet recovery occurs significantly earlier and neutrophil recovery also is accelerated.

Dosage and Administration. The starting dose of filgrastim is 5 mcg/kg/day for up to 14 days, administered SC or IV as a single daily injection. The preferred route of administration is the SC injection because of simplicity. If the drug is given IV, a short (15-minute to 1-hour) infusion is suggested. G-CSF is compatible only with dextrose. Doses may be increased in increments of 5 mcg/kg for each chemotherapy cycle.

This agent can be transported home unrefrigerated, but in hot weather it should shielded from the sun and sent home in a cooler. It should not be frozen but should be refrigerated at 36° to 46°F. The vial should not be shaken. A new vial is used for each injection; any vial that contains particulate matter or discolored liquid should be discarded.

Adverse Reactions. Adverse reactions may actually be consequences of underlying disease or cytotoxic chemotherapy. However, bone pain is generally reported as an adverse effect; the degree of this reaction appears to depend on the dose and route of administration (there is a higher incidence at higher doses and with IV administration). Bone pain, usually managed with nonnarcotic analgesics, may result from rapid expansion of cells in the bone marrow. Other adverse effects with long-term therapy may include subclinical splenomegaly and exacerbation of preexisting skin disorders (ie, psoriasis), alopecia, hematuria or proteinuria, thrombocytopenia, and osteoporosis.

Drug–Drug Interactions. No evidence of interaction of G-CSF with other drugs has been observed to date.

Drug–Laboratory Test Interactions. Elevations in leukocyte alkaline phosphatase, serum alkaline phosphatase, lactate dehydrogenase, and uric acid levels have been reported and have been reversible. These elevations may actually relate to the cytotoxic chemotherapy. Laboratory monitoring of the complete blood and platelet counts is important. White blood cell differentials demonstrate a left shift. Neutrophil monitoring is important to detect excessive leukocytosis. To avoid potential risks of excessive leukocytosis, filgrastim therapy is usually discontinued if the absolute neutrophil count surpasses $10,000/mm^3$ after the chemotherapy-induced nadir.

Precautions and Contraindications. Clients with preexisting cardiac conditions should be monitored closely because myocardial infarction and arrhythmias have occurred in a few clients receiving the drug (Box 35-4).

Granulocyte-Macrophage Colony-Stimulating Factor

Granulocyte-macrophage colony-stimulating factor (sargramostim [Leukine]) is prepared using recombinant DNA technology and yeast.

Pharmacodynamics. The principal target cells for GM-CSF are neutrophils, macrophages, and eosinophils.

Pharmacokinetics. This agent is readily absorbed from the SC injection site. Peak action occurs within 1 to 2 hours; the duration of effect is 5 to 10 days. The elimination half-life is 80 to 150 minutes.

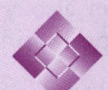

Box 35-4
Colony-Stimulating Factor Alert

No CSF should be administered within 24 hours before or after chemotherapy or within 12 hours before or after radiation therapy.

This time restriction is important because the cycling of the hematopoietic progenitor cells stimulated by a CSF will place more dividing cells at risk for destruction by the chemotherapy or radiation therapy, thereby producing an increase in cell kill instead of reducing the myelotoxicity of the therapeutic regimen.

Therapeutic Uses. This agent is approved for neutropenia associated with autologous bone marrow transplantation. It has been used for chemotherapy-induced myelosuppression as well.

Dosage and Administration. When used in clients having autologous bone marrow transplants, 250 mcg/m²/day are given for 21 days, SC or IV. Therapy begins 2 to 4 hours after bone marrow transfusion. When given IV (over 2–6 hours), GM-CSF is compatible only with normal saline solution. Between 250 and 500 mcg should be reconstituted with 1 mL of sterile water for injection without preservative. To avoid freezing before and after reconstitution, the drug should stored at 36° to 46°F. The vial should not be shaken. A new vial is used for each injection and should be administered within 6 hours of reconstitution.

This agent may be given SC for neutropenia at a dosage of 3 to 15 mcg/kg/day.

Adverse Reactions. Therapy with this agent produces a wider array of adverse effects than with G-CSF. Adverse reactions include hypotension, tachycardia, pleural or pericardial effusion, thrombocytopenia, bone pain, myalgia, arthralgia, fever, facial flushing, rash, and pruritus. Low-grade fever with chills may occur 4 to 6 hours after administration.

Clients with preexisting cardiac conditions should be monitored closely because of the potential for hypotension, tachycardia, arrhythmias, and pleural or pericardial effusion. If the client experiences dyspnea during administration, the IV rate should be halved; if respiratory symptoms persist, the infusion should be discontinued and the prescriber notified. The cause of reversible dyspnea seems to be rapid sequestration of neutrophils within the lung.

When administered SC, GM-CSF may produce a local skin reaction at the injection site. This reaction consists of a reddened induration persisting for 3 to 5 days after each injection.

Drug–Drug Interactions. No evidence of interaction of GM-CSF with other drugs has been reported.

Drug–Laboratory Test Interactions. To avoid potential risks of excessive leukocytosis, sargramostim therapy is discontinued if the white blood cell count surpasses 50,000/mm³ after the chemotherapy-induced nadir.

Precautions and Contraindications. Contraindications include hypersensitivity to yeast products and pregnancy. It must be used cautiously in clients with renal or hepatic failure, as well as during lactation. GM-CSF should not be administered within 24 hours before or after 24 hours after administering cytotoxic chemotherapeutic agents.

Interleukins

Interleukins are substances released by leukocytes that help control the behavior of other leukocytes. They act as autocrine, paracrine, and endocrine hormones and are involved in regulating normal and malignant cell growth and in recognizing and eliminating pathogens.

Interleukin-1

Interleukin-1 has an antiproliferative effect on tumor cells. It also induces cytokines that boost immune and antitumor activity. An example of its applications has been with carboplatin: for example, thrombocytopenia resulting from high-dose carboplatin administration was significantly less severe and of shorter duration after additional treatment with interleukin-1 than after chemotherapy alone (Aulitzky et al., 1994).

Interleukin-1 is highly toxic. Adverse events following systemic administration include fever, chills, abdominal pain, and hypotension.

Interleukin-2

Pharmacodynamics. The interaction of interleukin-2 (also called aldesleukin) with interleukin-2 receptors induces proliferation and differentiation of cells and stimulates a cytokine cascade that includes various interleukins, interferons, and TNF. The most common pharmacologic effects of interleukin-2 therapy appear to be acute lymphopenia followed by rebound lymphocytosis and induction of some T-cell activity (Aulitzky et al., 1994).

Therapeutic Uses. Interleukin-2 may be useful in promoting regression of some cancer cells. It has been used for treating some clients with metastatic renal cell carcinoma and metastatic malignant melanoma.

Dosage and Administration. Optimal dosages are still being identified. When used as a single agent, the maximum tolerated dose seems to be 1 million U/kg daily for a week via IV bolus or continuous IV infusion. It may be used for a 1- or 2-week cycle with 2- to 6-week intervals between cycles.

Adverse Reactions. Adverse effects include fever, nausea, vomiting, fatigue, malaise, and violent chills. Other effects include flushing, diarrhea, rash, edema, and hypertension. High doses can cause supraventricular tachycardia or lead to myocardial infarction. Chronic effects seem to be anorexia and depression. Adverse reactions seem to resolve rapidly with cessation of therapy and may be reduced with SC rather than IV administration.

Precautions and Contraindications. Contraindications include abnormal thallium stress test results, abnormal pulmonary function test results, organ allografts, and lactation. Cautious use is advised with renal, liver, or CNS impairment.

Interleukin-3

Interleukin-3 induces the growth and differentiation of early hematopoietic progenitors. In clients with primary and chemotherapy-induced pancytopenia, it has been found to promote megakaryocyte progenitor cell proliferation.

Tumor Necrosis Factor

In 1975, a factor was identified in mouse serum (after the animals were injected with a bacterial endotoxin) that induced hemorrhagic necrosis, growth inhibition, or regression in various human and mouse tumors, both in vivo and in vitro, with no effect on normal cells. This factor, TNF, is produced by endotoxin-activated macrophages.

Pharmacodynamics. Once produced in the body, TNF binds to designated receptors on cell membranes. The immediate effect on tumor cells is cytostasis, producing cell arrest in the G_2 phase of the cell cycle. Cell lysis is measurable after 7 hours and nearly complete after 24 hours. Some human cancer cell culture lines are extremely sensitive to the cytolytic effects of TNF, and others are resistant to it.

Therapeutic Uses. The therapeutic significance of TNF remains undetermined. Researchers believe a major role for this investigational agent will be in combination with other BMRs or antineoplastic agents to produce the highest possible destruction of malignant cells.

Dosage and Administration. Different routes of administration are being studied, including IV bolus, continuous IV infusion, and SC and IM injection. The optimal route and dosing schedule have yet to be established.

Adverse Reactions. Most clients experience adverse effects similar to those observed with the interferons and interleukins. The most common reaction is a flu-like syndrome of fever, chills, and tremors, headaches, and fatigue. Other effects include local tenderness, erythema, induration, and vesiculation at the SC or IM injection site. Most other adverse reactions appear to be dose-dependent and reversible, resolving within 48 to 96 hours after the drug is discontinued. TNF has also been identified as the primary mediator of endotoxic shock.

■ SUMMARY

Biologic response modifiers, the most recent modality in cancer therapy, include the monoclonal antibodies, the cytokines (interferons, colony-stimulating factors, interleukins), and tumor necrosis factor.

❖ NURSING MANAGEMENT: CLIENT RECEIVING A BIOLOGIC RESPONSE MODIFIER

Because of the many similarities in nursing care of clients receiving BRMs and immunosuppressants, general nursing management is discussed at the end of the section on immunosuppressants. For additional information, see the Example of Nursing Process for BRM Therapy.

Immunosuppressants

Immunosuppressants are used to treat several autoimmune diseases and to prevent transplant rejection. However, long-term preventive treatment with these agents poses high risks of infection. Immunosuppressive agents include azathioprine, cyclosporine, tacrolimus, MoAbs, antithymocyte globulin, cytotoxic drugs, glucocorticoids, and mycophenolate mofetil.

Azathioprine

Azathioprine (Imuran) is related to the antineoplastic antimetabolite 6-mercaptopurine.

Pharmacodynamics. Azathioprine alters antibody production; it interferes with nucleic acid metabolism at steps that are required for lymphocyte proliferation after antigenic stimulation.

Pharmacokinetics. Azathioprine is absorbed well when administered orally. It is moderately bound to serum proteins (30%) and is undetectable in urine after 8 hours. It is cleaved in vivo to 6-mercaptopurine. It is metabolized in the liver and erythrocytes. Conversion to inactive 6-thiouric acid by xanthine oxidase is an important degradative pathway.

Therapeutic Uses. Azathioprine is used as an adjunct for preventing rejection of renal homografts. It is also used in treating autoimmune disease (primarily adults with severe rheumatoid arthritis [RA] unresponsive to conventional treatment). Therapeutic response in RA occurs after 6 to 8 weeks of treatment; an adequate trial should be at least 12 weeks.

Dosage and Administration. Many current protocols use azathioprine in combination with steroids and cyclosporine. The initial oral dosage of azathioprine immediately after transplant is 3 to 5 mg/kg/day. If converted from an oral to an IV route, the IV dose should be 50% of the oral dose. Maintenance levels are 1 to 3 mg/kg/day. Because azathioprine is dialyzable, clients on dialysis should receive the drug after dialysis is completed. Those with oliguria may have delayed clearance and therefore require a lower dose.

Adverse Reactions. Chronic immunosuppression with azathioprine increases the risk of neoplasia. Because azathioprine affects rapidly proliferating cells indiscriminately, one of the most common adverse effects is bone marrow suppression. Severe leukopenia or thrombocytopenia, as well as macrocytic anemia, may occur. Hematologic toxicities are dose-related, may occur late in therapy, and may be more severe in renal transplant clients whose homograft is undergoing rejection. Serious, even fatal, fungal, viral, bacterial, or protozoal infections can occur and should be treated vigorously. Dosage may have to be reduced or even discontinued.

Adverse GI effects, such as nausea and vomiting, may occur within the first few weeks or months of ther-

Example of Nursing Process for BRM Therapy

The client is a 55-year-old man with carcinoma of the left kidney with metastasis to periaortic lymph nodes. Surgery is not an option. He is married and has three children. The family appears very supportive. His therapy includes subcutaneous aldesleukin (interleukin-2) 5 days a week, subcutaneous interferon alfa-2a 3 days a week, and IV fluorouracil. The therapeutic regimen involves administering the first 5 days of therapy in the outpatient clinic, then continuing therapy at home.

Assessment Data

Client started on BRM therapy

Client started on drugs that have been in use only recently

Nursing Diagnosis	Intervention	Goals and Outcomes
Risk for Injury related to BRM therapy	**Explain** importance of reporting apparent adverse reactions related to drug therapy.	The client will verbalize signs and symptoms of complications that must be reported.
	Monitor client for signs and symptoms of adverse reactions.	If signs and symptoms of adverse reactions develop, they will be promptly identified and alleviated, thereby reducing some related anxiety.
	Instruct in self-management of flulike adverse reactions.	
Knowledge Deficit, related to BRM therapy	**Explain** to the client/family the components of the treatment that has been ordered.	The client/family will state an understanding of the treatment plan.
	Teach proper storage techniques for interferon and interleukin.	
	Instruct in reconstitution techniques.	
	Instruct in self-administration techniques.	
	Observe client for reconstitution and self-administration techniques.	
	Teach proper disposal of used syringes and needles in puncture-resistant container.	
	Advise on record-keeping for drug administration documentation.	

apy. These reactions can be reduced by administering the drug in divided doses or after meals. Symptoms of GI toxicity reverse on drug discontinuation. The reaction can recur within hours, however, after rechallenge with a single azathioprine dose.

Other adverse reactions associated with azathioprine include hepatotoxicity, diarrhea, rash, arthralgia, drug fever, retinopathy, serum sickness, Raynaud's disease, alopecia, and pulmonary edema.

Drug–Drug Interactions. Azathioprine is degraded through conversion to inactive 6-thiouric acid by xanthine oxidase. Because allopurinol inhibits this conversion, the dose of azathioprine must be reduced about 25% to 33% of the usual dose for clients concurrently receiving allopurinol. Other drugs that affect leukocyte production may lead to exaggerated leukopenia when used concurrently with azathioprine (eg, angiotensin-converting enzyme inhibitors). Azathioprine may decrease the action of anticoagulants.

Drug–Laboratory Test Interactions. Azathioprine may be associated with elevated serum transaminase, alkaline phosphatase, and bilirubin levels.

Precautions and Contraindications. Allergy to azathioprine, rheumatoid arthritis previously treated with alkylating agents, and pregnancy are contraindications to therapy. Baseline blood counts should be performed before azathioprine therapy is initiated. Blood counts should be monitored throughout therapy.

Cyclosporine

Cyclosporine, discovered in 1972, is produced by the fungus *Tolypocladium inflatum gams* (Sandimmune) or *Beauveria nivea* (Neoral).

Pharmacodynamics. Cyclosporine's mechanism of action is incompletely understood. It binds with a protein called cyclophilin and then associates with an enzyme called calcineurin to inhibit calcineurin-stimulated events. This inhibition interferes with T-lymphocyte/ T-cell activation (T cells are important for killing foreign invaders). It also interferes with aldesleukin (interleukin-2) release. Aldesleukin normally promotes growth of T cells. Because aldesleukin release is disrupted, a result would be fewer T cells to contribute to the acute rejection response. Cyclosporine has no significant effect on T cells already present in peripheral blood. Thus, although it will help prevent the development of acute rejection with transplanted organs, it is ineffective in reversing an episode of acute rejection.

Pharmacokinetics. Cyclosporine is incompletely absorbed from the GI tract, with peak concentrations occurring in blood at about 3.5 hours. (However, during chronic use, absorption from the GI tract may be variable and erratic. Many factors, such as other drugs, diarrhea, vomiting, cystic fibrosis, and liver disease can increase or decrease absorption.) Cyclosporine is about 90% bound to proteins. It has a half-life of about 19 hours. It is extensively metabolized by enzymes in the liver (25 metabolites) and, to a lesser degree, in the GI tract and the kidney. Excretion is primarily biliary, with only 6% excreted in urine.

Therapeutic Uses. Cyclosporine is used for the prophylaxis of organ rejection in recipients of allogeneic kidney, liver, and heart transplants. It can be used to treat chronic rejection of transplanted organs in clients treated previously with other immunosuppressive agents. Its unlabeled uses include use with pancreas, bone marrow, and heart–lung transplants. It has also been used to treat various other disorders, such as Crohn's disease, multiple sclerosis, nephrotic syndrome, psoriatic arthritis, and pemphigus.

Dosage and Administration. Cyclosporine is available for oral administration in an olive oil–based liquid or in a gelatin capsule. The liquid is not soluble in water and should be mixed with a lipid solution such as milk. If mixed in carbonated beverages or other water-soluble liquids, precipitation and lower serum concentrations may result (Holmes, 1993). Sandimmune and Neoral are not bioequivalent—Neoral has increased bioavailability—so they cannot be used interchangeably.

The liquid is available in 50-mL bottles with a cyclosporine concentration of 100 mg/mL. Doses are measured via a syringe. A glass container is used to mix the drug to prevent adherence of the drug to plastic. Cyclosporine must be taken immediately after mixing to prevent loss of stability (because of the unpalatable taste, clients may wish to delay taking the drug). Food reduces absorption of the drug, so administration should be 1 hour before or 2 hours after food intake.

Oral gelatin capsules are available in 25 and 100 mg. The capsules have advantages: measuring is unnecessary and the problems with flavor are eliminated. The capsules can be taken with any liquid. However, because the capsules are available in only two strengths, adjustments can be made only in 25-mg increments. This may affect therapeutic effect and toxicity.

Intravenous administration of cyclosporine (sandimmune) eliminates the problems related to absorption and permits rapid concentration in the serum. The IV dose is about one-third the oral dose. The IV preparation is stable when diluted in either a normal saline or dextrose solution. Glass containers should be used. Methods of administering the IV preparation vary, but the manufacturer recommends infusion over 2 to 6 hours. Rapid infusion has been linked to intense burning and erythema of the palms and soles, particularly in bone marrow transplant clients with acute graft-versus-host disease and in those who received cytosine arabinoside as therapy before transplantation.

Adverse Reactions. The most common adverse reaction is nephrotoxicity. The mechanism is unclear, but most clients develop evidence of nephrotoxicity (rising serum creatinine and BUN levels, decreasing urine output, decreasing ability to concentrate urine manifested by lowered urine specific gravity and elevated urine sodium, and casts in the urine) regardless of the administration route. Cyclosporine damages the tubular cells. The result is a decrease in glomerular filtration and acute tubular necrosis.

Hemolytic uremic syndrome (hemolysis, thrombocytopenia, and symptoms of renal failure) has been reported in recipients of bone marrow and organ transplants (Holmes, 1993). Leukocytosis and altered clotting factors consistent with disseminated intravascular coagulopathy may also be present.

Hepatotoxicity, manifested by increased serum bilirubin levels, may occur. Because cyclosporine is metabolized in the liver, altered liver function may delay metabolism and elimination, thereby increasing other toxicity risks, such as nephrotoxicity.

Hypertension is common, and several neurologic symptoms may occur, including tremors, muscle weakness, headaches, ataxia, confusion, seizures, encephalopathy, and blindness. The severity of these symptoms seems to be correlated to the serum level of cyclosporine. There seems to be an association between the neurotoxicity and hypomagnesemia that occurs in relation to the nephrotoxicity.

Less common effects include significant hirsutism on the face and trunk, secondary lymphomas, GI disturbances, gingival hyperplasia, weight loss, joint pain, pancreatitis, and hyperlipidemia.

Drug–Drug Interactions. The concomitant use of other nephrotoxic drugs may potentiate cyclosporine's nephrotoxic effects. Some drugs (eg, metoclopramide) alter cyclosporine's intestinal absorption. Other drugs alter its bioavailability by either increasing the hepatic metabolism (eg, phenytoin) or decreasing its metabolism (eg, calcium channel blockers, ketoconazole). The effects of ketoconazole and calcium channel blockers have been used to lower significantly the required dose of cyclosporine.

Increases in cyclosporine levels can also result from concurrent administration of drugs such as erythromycin and methylprednisolone. A decrease in cyclosporine levels may be found in clients receiving rifampin, phenobarbital, phenytoin, and carbamazepine.

Clients receiving prednisolone, digoxin, lovastatin, and nifedipine may demonstrate a reduced clearance of these drugs while taking cyclosporine. As a result, severe digitalis toxicity has occurred within days after cyclosporine therapy has been instituted, myositis has occurred in clients on lovastatin, gingival hyperplasia in clients on nifedipine, and convulsions in clients on high-dose methylprednisolone.

Vaccines may be less effective when the client is receiving cyclosporine.

Drug–Laboratory Test Interactions. Elevated BUN and serum creatinine levels have been noted during therapy.

Precautions and Contraindications. Contraindications include allergy to cyclosporine or castor oil used in its oral preparation or pregnancy and lactation. Cyclosporine must be used with caution in clients with impaired renal function and malabsorption. Experts think that maintaining magnesium levels near normal may decrease the incidence of cyclosporine-associated neurotoxicity.

The use of live vaccines should be avoided in clients receiving cyclosporine. Potassium-sparing diuretics should not be used either, as cyclosporine may cause hyperkalemia.

Cyclosporine's immunosuppressive action increases the client's risk for infection and the possible development of lymphomas and other malignancies, particularly of the skin.

Tacrolimus

Tacrolimus (Prograf, FK506) is actually a macrolide antibiotic that was extracted from a fermentation broth of the soil microorganism *Streptomyces tsukubaenis* in 1984 (Hardman et al., 1996).

Pharmacodynamics. Tacrolimus, like cyclosporine, inhibits calcineurin-stimulated events and T-cell activation by binding to a protein, FKBP.

Pharmacokinetics. Studies of orally administered drug have demonstrated a wide variation in oral bioavailability (6%–56%). It appears to be metabolized extensively in the liver, with less than 1% being excreted unchanged. The reports on half-life have a wide range (11.7–21.2 hours).

Therapeutic Uses. The clinical uses of tacrolimus appear similar to those of cyclosporine. Tacrolimus is about 100 times more potent than cyclosporine.

Dosage and Administration. Tacrolimus can be administered IV (short or continuous infusion) or orally. The IV dosage range for adults is 25 to 50 mcg/kg/day; the oral dosage range for adults is 150 to 200 mcg/kg/day.

Adverse Reactions. Tacrolimus appears to have a spectrum of adverse reactions similar to those of cyclosporine, including nephrotoxicity and neurotoxicity.

Precautions and Contraindications. Contraindications include allergy to tacrolimus, hypersensitivity to castor oil used in oral preparation, pregnancy, and lactation. Cautious use is advised in clients with impaired renal function, hypokalemia, and malabsorption.

Monoclonal Antibodies

The use of MoAbs for immunosuppression was mentioned in the earlier discussion of biotherapy.

Antithymocyte Globulin

Antithymocyte globulin (Atgam), also called lymphocyte immune globulin, is a purified immunoglobulin (IgG) prepared commercially from hyperimmune serum of horse, rabbit, sheep, or goat following their immunization with human thymic lymphocytes.

Pharmacodynamics. Antithymocyte globulin binds to the surface of T lymphocytes found in the circulation, resulting in lymphopenia and impaired T-cell immune responses.

Pharmacokinetics. This agent is poorly distributed into lymphoid tissues such as the spleen and lymph nodes. Its half-life is about 6 days; about 1% of a dose is excreted in urine.

Therapeutic Uses. Antithymocyte globulin is used to prevent rejection and to treat allograft rejection during acute rejection episodes (kidney, heart, and others). It has also been used (unlabeled use) to treat aplastic anemia.

Dosage and Administration. It is available as a concentrate (50 mg/mL in a 5-mL ampule) for IV injection. It is diluted so that the final concentration in saline solution does not exceed 1 mg equine IgG/mL. It is usually administered through a large or central vein at a daily dose of 10 to 30 mg/kg in saline solution over 4 to 8 hours. Administration into high-flow veins decreases the potential for phlebitis and thrombosis. Ampules should be refrigerated and diluted solutions are refrigerated and kept no more than 12 hours. An intradermal skin test is usually performed before the drug is administered, although its predictive value is unproven. Therefore, the client must be observed carefully for allergic reaction.

Adverse Reactions. Major adverse effects result from the recognition of antithymocyte globulin as a foreign protein, which leads to serum sickness and nephritis. Other adverse reactions include chills and fever, leukopenia, thrombocytopenia, rash, and pruritus. Anaphylaxis occurs rarely. Antithymocyte globulin increases the client's susceptibility to viral infections; it may reactivate or support infection with CMV, herpes simplex virus, or Epstein-Barr virus.

Drug Interactions. Clients are usually receiving concomitant corticosteroids or other immunosuppressants, which increases the degree of immunosuppression.

Precautions and Contraindications. These are similar to those for cyclosporine.

Cytotoxic Drugs

Cytotoxic drugs are discussed in Chapter 46. The cytotoxic agent cyclophosphamide has been used successfully as a substitute for azathioprine in organ transplant recipients. Methotrexate has been used in the treatment of persistent acute rejection in heart transplant recipients. In addition, a few centers have added this agent to their prophylactic immunosuppressive regimens.

Glucocorticoids

Glucocorticoids are used alone or with other immunosuppressants for preventing transplant rejection and for treating autoimmune disorders. They may be used to reverse acute graft rejection or to prevent acute graft-versus-host disease. They may also be used to minimize the allergic reactions that may occur with the use of antilymphocyte globulin or MoAbs. The most common glucocorticoids used for these purposes are prednisone and prednisolone. The glucocorticoids (see Chap. 30) rapidly but briefly reduce lymphocytes in the peripheral blood. Recent studies suggest that glucocorticoids inhibit T-cell proliferation and the expression of genes encoding cytokines. Glucocorticoids also produce nonspecific antiinflammatory effects as well as antiadhesion effects (preventing the movement of inflammatory cells from the circulation into tissue) that may further contribute to immunosuppression.

Mycophenolate Mofetil

Pharmacodynamics. Mycophenolate mofetil (Cellcept) has an active metabolite, mycophenolic acid (MPA), that inhibits an enzyme critical in the synthesis of T and B lymphocytes. The drug suppresses lymphocyte proliferation and antibody formation by B cells and may also inhibit recruitment of leukocytes to inflammatory sites.

Pharmacokinetics. By the oral route, the onset of action varies, but peak action occurs within 45 to 60 minutes. The drug undergoes hepatic biotransformation. It crosses the placenta and is excreted in the urine.

Therapeutic Uses. Mycophenolate mofetil is approved for oral use after renal transplantation. Other uses are

under investigation. The initial dose should be given within 72 hours of transplantation.

Dosage and Administration. A dose of 1 g administered twice a day should be used in combination with cyclosporine and corticosteroids. It is rapidly absorbed after oral administration. MPA concentrations are increased in renal impairment, so doses greater than 2 g/day should be avoided in these clients.

Adverse Reactions. Hepatotoxicity is one of the more serious adverse reactions; others include tremors, insomnia, nausea, anemia, renal dysfunction, and nephrotoxicity.

Drug–Drug Interactions. Antacids decrease the absorption of this agent; cholestyramine reduces its plasma concentration.

Precautions and Contraindications. Contraindications include clients allergic to mycophenolate and those who are pregnant or lactating. Cautious use is advised in clients with impaired renal function.

■ **S U M M A R Y**

Several drugs are used for immunosuppressive purposes for the prophylaxis or management of organ rejection in clients who have received human kidney, liver, or heart transplants. Adverse reactions include the possibility of life-threatening infections and an increased risk of neoplastic disease.

❖ NURSING MANAGEMENT: CLIENT RECEIVING A BIOLOGIC RESPONSE MODIFIER OR IMMUNOSUPPRESSANT

Much work with BRMs can still be described as investigational, although work with several immunosuppressants is better established. The nurse must obtain accurate information on the specific agent to provide appropriate client care and teaching. The nurse's role centers on maximizing the safety of administration, identifying trends in toxicities, monitoring for unique complications and for adherence, and developing and testing interventions to decrease the severity and incidence of toxicities, while enhancing the client's adaptation and rehabilitation (Jassak, 1996).

NURSING PROCESS

ASSESSMENT

The nurse should assess the client for any history of conditions that may contraindicate the use of BRMs (eg, preexisting cardiac conditions) or immunosuppressants. Other factors to explore are whether the client is pregnant or has a condition requiring medication that may cause an interaction.

The assessment should include a physical examination and a review of pertinent laboratory values. Present symptoms should be evaluated in terms of onset, duration, frequency, location, setting, quality, quantity, aggravating and alleviating factors, and associated symptoms. The nurse should assess the client's support systems, functional coping mechanisms, and ability to accept self-care responsibility. The client's and family's economic concerns must also be explored.

NURSING DIAGNOSIS

Many clients receiving BRMs have cancer, CRF, or AIDS. Those receiving immunosuppressants may be undergoing organ transplant for CRF or other similar end-stage problems. Some nursing diagnoses that may apply to therapy with BMRs or immunosuppressants include:

- Anxiety, related to adverse effects of drug therapy and life-threatening disease
- Ineffective Individual Coping, related to debility or inability to fulfill expectations secondary to self-administering a BRM
- Risk for Infection, related to bone marrow suppression secondary to drug therapy
- Risk for Injury, related to drug therapy
- Knowledge Deficit, related to expected benefits of and adverse reactions to the prescribed BRM or immunosuppressant

PLANNING

Goals could include decreased anxiety; successful self-administration of drug; reduced potential for infection; reduced knowledge deficit; and prompt detection and treatment of adverse reactions. See the Critical Thinking Challenge: Case Analysis.

INTERVENTION

Frequently, BRM or immunosuppressant regimens combine an intensive inpatient regimen with a subsequent low-dose ambulatory regimen; the duration may exceed 6 months. Due to this extended time span and the unknown aspect of disease response, the nurse must take on the role of coach to the client and family, helping them to continue adhering to the drug administration schedule and fostering hope for disease response (Jassak, 1996).

Careful checks of the client for potential infection include monitoring temperature up to three times daily, inspecting any wounds once a shift for signs and symptoms of inflammation, culturing any wound if drainage is significant, and monitoring all culture reports.

The nurse must wash his or her hands before and after touching the client, who ideally should have a private room. Antibiotics may need to be ordered and administered. The environment should be kept as infection-free as possible when the client is on immunosuppressive therapy (fresh flowers may be restricted). Personnel and visitors with signs or symptoms of any infection should not be permitted near the client. Bacteria, viruses, fungi, and protozoa that are commonly resisted by normal persons may be infectious in immunosuppressed clients.

CRITICAL THINKING CHALLENGE
Case Analysis

Part 1: Acute Care

Mrs. Miller is a 68-year-old woman with metastatic melanoma. She has nodules in both lungs and enlarged mediastinal lymph nodes. She is currently receiving chemotherapy in the hospital, but she will be discharged soon. At home she will receive aldesleukin (interleukin-2) and interferon alfa-2a (Roferon A). Interferon will be self-administered.

Mrs. Miller's discharge is occurring earlier than it would have been had she been treated 1 year ago and had she not been receiving biotherapy. This has important implications for the working relationship between the cancer treatment staff and the home healthcare nurse.

1. Identify and discuss the prime concerns of both healthcare staffs.
2. What does the cancer treatment team need to know about the home healthcare staff?
3. What does the home healthcare nurse need to know about the client and the treatment regimen?
4. How can the home healthcare nurse best prepare for the initial home visit with Mrs. Miller?

Part 2: Home Care

You are visiting Mrs. Miller at home. Part of your care plan is based on the nursing diagnosis, Anxiety, related to anticipated adverse effects of drug therapy.

1. When Mrs. Miller tells you she cannot remember a thing the hospital nurses told her about her medications, what is your response?
2. Mrs. Miller asks you, "Why do I have to take two medicines? What good will they do me? I think they just make me feel sick." How do you phrase your explanation?
3. Identify the issues you want to be sure to discuss with Mrs. Miller. Explain why you think these are significant.

The client and family should be referred to social service agencies as indicated for economic concerns.

The client and family must be allowed time to face fears and anxiety. Emotional support should be provided.

Client Education. The client's and family's understanding of BRM and immunosuppressant therapy and the potential adverse reactions must be assessed. To teach effectively, the nurse must have information about the specific agent (predictable toxicities and contraindications) and the planned administration schedule, and effective ideas to promote the client's self-care. The nurse must know what the expected outcome of therapy is. The safe technique for self-administering BRM therapy must be conveyed to the client and family. The nurse also must discuss the treatment regimen clearly and thoroughly, explaining, for example, that frequent blood tests will be required to monitor liver and kidney function (other tests may be ordered, depending on the circumstances).

The nurse must organize the information in an efficient and effective manner to avoid information overload, distinguishing what is nice to know from what the client must know. Education must be individualized according to the client's needs, ability and readiness to learn, and prior experiences. Presentation of information should include one-on-one discussions, supplemented by visual and printed materials to reinforce and enhance information.

The possibility and the implications of infections should be explained. Clients must be informed of the importance of protecting themselves against infection by using self-care techniques (eg, thorough and frequent handwashing, avoiding crowds, recognizing early signs and symptoms of infection).

Outcome Evaluation

Careful records should be kept of the incidence or absence of, and reporting of, adverse reactions. Any changes (positive or negative) in the client's status should be reported and recorded. Teaching can be considered effective if the client understands the therapeutic regimen and drug administration techniques, manages predicted adverse reactions successfully, and notifies the healthcare team appropriately regarding questions and complications that arise.

❖ CHECKLIST OF NURSING ACTIONS

- ❑ Take a careful history to determine any condition that might contraindicate the use of a specific agent.
- ❑ List all drugs the client is taking; identify any that may interact with the BRM or immunosuppressant and report these to the prescriber.
- ❑ Consult package inserts for specific administration guidelines.
- ❑ Store the agent properly to ensure potency and safety.
- ❑ Inform the client and family of expected benefits and signs and symptoms of potential adverse reactions; specify those that should be reported to healthcare personnel.
- ❑ Keep accurate records.
- ❑ Report adverse reactions.

References

Anonymous. (1994). National Coalition for Adult Immunization. *AAOHN J, 42*(10), 515–516.

Aulitzky WE, Schuler M, Peschel C, Huber C. (1994). Interleukins. *Drugs, 48*(5), 667–677.

Bender CM. (1994). Cognitive dysfunction associated with biological response modifier therapy. *Oncol Nurs Forum, 21*(3), 515–523.

Hardman JG, Limbird LE, Molinoff PB, et al., eds. (1996). *Goodman and Gilman's The pharmacological basis of therapeutics*, 9th ed. New York: McGraw-Hill.

Holmes W. (1993). Cyclosporine immunosuppression: Clinical practice issues. *Curr Issues Cancer Nurs Pract, 1*(10), 1–7.

Jassak PE. (1996). Continuity of care: An integral concept for patients receiving biologic therapy. *Biotherapy: Considerations for Oncology Nurses, 1*(1), 1–3.

Markham A, Bryson HM. (1995). Epoetin alfa. *Drugs, 49*(2), 232–254.

Bibliography

Appelbaum FR. (1993). The application of hematopoietic colony stimulating factors (CSFs) in cancer management. *Curr Issues Cancer Nurs Pract Updates, 2*(2), 1–13.

Copstead LC. (1995). *Perspectives on pathophysiology*. Philadelphia: WB Saunders.

Jahansouz F, Kriett JM. (1993). Transplantation: A review of immunosuppressive agents. *Crit Care Nurs Q, 15*(4), 13–22.

Johnson HM, Bazer FW, Szente BE, Jarpe MA. (1994). How interferons fight disease. *Scientific American, 270*(5), 68.

Lancaster LE. (1992). Immunogenic basis of tissue organ transplantation and rejection. *Crit Care Nurs Clin North Am, 4*(1), 1–24.

Lukes E. (1995). Childhood immunizations: An update for occupational health nurses. *AAOHN J, 43*(12), 622–626.

Nichols GL. (1993). Update on biologic agents in home care of the cancer client. *Home Healthcare Nurse, 11*(5), 30–32.

Olin BR, ed. (1996). *Drug facts and comparisons*, 50th ed. St. Louis: Facts and Comparisons.

Sharts-Hopko NC. (1994). Current immunization guidelines. *Maternal Child Nursing J, 19*(2), 82–84.

Strannegard O. (1995). Recent advances in the treatment of human immunodeficiency virus infections with interferons and other biological response modifiers. *Advances in Pharmacology, 32*, 249–287.

For more information and sample tests and activities, refer to Chapter 35 in the Student Workbook for Clinical Pharmacology and Nursing Management, 5th edition, available through your bookstore.

36

Drugs That Treat Inflammation

Box 36-1
The Inflammatory Process

Purposes of Inflammation

To neutralize and destroy noxious agents at site

To prevent dissemination of noxious agents

To establish conditions necessary for repair and resolution

Stimuli That Initiate the Process

Thermal (heat or cold)

Chemical (foreign substances, organisms, drugs)

Mechanical (trauma)

Cardinal Signs

Redness *(rubor)*

Heat *(calor)*

Swelling *(tumor)*

Pain *(dolor)*

Loss of function *(functio laesa)*

The inflammatory process comprises multiple physiologic responses to a stimulus. It is not altogether undesirable; rather, it is a nonspecific defense to tissue injury and a protective mechanism essential for survival.

Physiology of Inflammation

As a protective mechanism, inflammation localizes infection and prevents the spread of pathogens. It also destroys pathogens and promotes tissue repair and healing. The affected person lacks adequate protection if the process is not sufficient to combat the stimulus. On the other hand, in certain situations the inflammatory process may cause harm.

Inflammation should not be confused with infection, although the two often coexist and normally infection is accompanied by inflammation (eg, otitis media, viral hepatitis). However, not all inflammation involves infection (eg, allergic rhinitis). Box 36-1 highlights information on the inflammatory process.

Diverse stimuli may initiate the inflammatory process, but the process is not individual to the stimulus. The stimulus may be thermal (heat or cold), chemical (foreign substances, foreign organisms, drugs), or mechanical (trauma and injury).

The cardinal signs of localized inflammation are redness, heat, swelling, pain, and loss of function (or, in Latin, *rubor, calor, tumor, dolor*, and *functio laesa*). Fever is an example of a systemic response that may accompany local inflammation, noninfectious or infectious.

Whenever tissues are injured, vascular and chemical responses occur. Immediately after injury, the vessels around the injured area constrict. This vasoconstriction lasts 2 seconds to 10 minutes and produces tissue hypoxia and acidosis. The amount of vasoconstriction depends on the degree of vascular injury (Copstead, 1995).

The chemicals involved in inflammation include histamines, prostaglandins, leukotrienes, cytokines, oxygen radicals, and enzymes.

Prostaglandins are arachidonic acids (unsaturated fatty acids) that play a significant role in inflammation and other processes, such as muscle relaxation and contraction, gastric acid secretion, and platelet aggregation. Prostaglandins exist in increased concentrations in inflammatory exudates; for example, they are highly concentrated in the synovial fluid of inflamed joints. Prostaglandins cannot be stored, and their release is dependent on biosynthesis. Arachidonic acid is released from phospholipids from injured cell membranes and is metabolized through two enzyme-mediated routes: the cyclooxygenase (or prostaglandin synthetase) and lipo-oxygenase pathways. The cyclooxygenase pathway results in the production of prostaglandins. With injury, prostaglandins sensitize nociceptors to mechanical stimuli and chemical mediators of nociception such as bradykinin. The prostaglandins lower the threshold of nociceptive fibers so that stimuli that would not evoke pain under normal circumstances now produce pain.

Evidently, various medications with an antiinflammatory action inhibit the conversion of arachidonic acid by inhibiting the release of prostaglandin synthetase or by interfering in some other way with the synthesis of prostaglandins. Individual medications have differing modes of inhibitory activity on prostaglandin synthetase. The inhibition of prostaglandin synthetase leads to a decrease in the inflammatory process and, subsequently, to relief of symptoms (fever and pain).

Pathophysiology of Fever

Under normal circumstances, the body's temperature remains between 98.0° and 100°F (36.5°–37.5°C). This range represents a dynamic equilibrium between the heat produced by cell metabolism and muscle activity and the heat lost by radiation, conduction, convection, and evaporation. Body temperature is regulated by a neuronal mechanism in the hypothalamus that adjusts heat-producing and heat-dissipating functions in response to changes in blood temperature.

Normal temperature varies from person to person and from time to time. Fever, an increase in body temperature above the normal range, is diagnosed whenever the temperature is 1° or 2° above the expected reading. Despite individual differences, fever is also diagnosed whenever oral temperature exceeds 100°F (37.8°C) or rectal temperature exceeds 101°F (38.4°C). In fever, the hypothalamic set point regulating body temperature is raised, and as a result thermoregulatory effectors are activated and mechanisms of heat production (increased muscle tone, chills) and heat conservation (vasoconstriction) predominate over mechanisms of heat loss until the temperature of the blood reaching the hypothalamus reaches the new setting.

When the hypothalamic thermostat is reset at a higher level through the influence of pyrogens (eg, viruses, bacteria), heat-dissipating mechanisms are inhibited and heat-producing mechanisms are activated: peripheral blood vessels constrict, perspiration decreases, and muscle tone increases. The affected person experiences a subjective feeling of cold and shivers uncontrollably. The skin is pale and dry. This syndrome, called a chill, usually persists until the body temperature rises to the level dictated by the new setting. At this point, the normal balance of control mechanisms is restored, the person feels comfortably warm and moist, and shivering subsides.

The resolution of fever may follow one of two patterns: crisis or lysis. In crisis, the hypothalamic thermostat reverts suddenly to a normal setting in response to a change in the disease process. Heat-dissipating mechanisms are stimulated. The person feels hot, and the skin is flushed and wet from perspiration. Body temperature drops rapidly to a normal level. Lysis is characterized by a more gradual decline in temperature: the thermostatic setting is readjusted by repeated small changes, causing a more erratic course in temperature decline.

Fever is a defensive response of the body that can generate both protective and harmful effects (Box 36-2). Protectively, fever seems to augment host defenses by increasing interferon production and enhancing its effects. Fever may also inhibit bacterial proliferation by interfering with iron metabolism in bacteria. Fever also promotes rest, because discomfort is less severe when activity decreases. An elevation in body temperature appears to be especially helpful during acute infectious illnesses, where complete suppression of fever is usually undesirable. In the years before antibiotics, fever was induced to treat some illnesses (eg, syphilis, gonorrhea).

Harmful effects of fever include increased stress on the heart. If the person has decreased cardiac output and the heart beats faster in response to fever, this may lead to decompensation and congestive heart failure. Increased heat production is accomplished by excessive consumption of calories. If nutritional intake is inadequate to meet the need for calories, protein catabolism is increased and body tissue is broken down, causing tis-

---

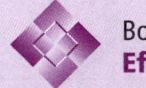

Box 36-2
Effects of Fever

Beneficial Effects

Promotion of rest in response to discomfort and weakness

Impairment or destruction of pathogens (eg, organisms that cause syphilis and brucellosis)

Increased production of immune substances

Improvement of inflammatory changes (eg, in uveitis, rheumatoid arthritis)

Detrimental Effects

Discomfort—headache, photophobia, malaise, muscle and bone soreness

Increased workload on the heart

Loss of water and sodium

Anorexia

Loss of body mass consumed for the production of energy—negative nitrogen balance

Stimulation of seizures

Tissue damage—local hemorrhage, parenchymal degeneration of cells

sue damage and possibly wasting. Very high fevers may be life-threatening. Rapid rises of temperature in children may lower their seizure threshold and often induce seizures. In adults, delirium is not uncommon. Prolonged or extremely high fever may produce severe dehydration. Very high temperatures (above 106°F [41°C]) appear to break down the body's enzyme systems and also seem to interfere with many critical life processes. Permanent brain damage, including the body's mechanism for temperature regulation, can occur. For these reasons, very high or prolonged fevers must be controlled to prevent serious injury.

Because body temperature is considered one of the cardinal signs of general physiologic status, it is an important diagnostic factor. Suppression of fever before diagnosis can make a definitive diagnosis difficult. For this reason, measures to reduce fever are often delayed or restricted until the basic pathologic process and appropriate therapy are determined.

Therapeutic Management of Fever

The aim of therapeutic measures to reduce fever is to prevent serious injury and reduce discomfort without eliminating the beneficial effects of the temperature elevation and without obscuring the diagnosis. Medication is only one method used to reduce fever. Nonpharmacologic relief measures include application of cool compresses, and use of hypothermia blankets (the latter are used in extreme cases or when brain trauma has impaired thermoregulatory mechanisms).

Drugs Used to Control Fever

Drugs that directly influence fever include quinine, dantrolene sodium, and nonsteroidal antiinflammatory drugs (NSAIDs) (Table 36-1).

Quinine

Quinine, currently used as an antimalarial agent, was the first, albeit weak, antipyretic drug. Although it is not used medically to reduce fever today, it still has value for advocates of folk or herbal medicine.

Dantrolene

Dantrolene (Dantrium) is a peripherally acting antispastic agent that has also been effective in treating malignant hyperthermia. It may be used prophylactically if this disorder is anticipated.

Malignant hyperthermia is a genetically determined rare syndrome usually precipitated by the administration of neuromuscular blocking agents and inhalation anesthetics during surgery. Signs and symptoms include rapid and dangerous increase in body temperature, tachycardia, tachypnea, metabolic acidosis, skeletal muscle rigidity, cyanosis, mottling of the skin, and signs and symptoms of renal failure. Apparently, the symptoms

are caused by an excessive release of calcium ions from the sarcoplasmic reticulum. The increase in calcium activates acute catabolic processes.

Therapeutically, dantrolene may interfere with the release of calcium from the sarcoplasmic reticulum to the myoplasm to reverse or relieve the crisis. Before dantrolene was used for this condition, the mortality rate for malignant hyperthermia was 50% to 70%.

Dantrolene is given by continuous rapid intravenous (IV) push. The beginning dose is 1 mg/kg, and administration continues until symptoms subside or the maximum dose (10 mg/kg) has been reached. Oral administration of dantrolene (1–2 mg/kg four times a day) may be necessary for 1 to 3 days to prevent recurrence of the symptoms.

Other Modalities for Fever and Related Pain

The goal of managing pain that accompanies fever is complete pain relief. If that is impossible, the goal is pain relief to a degree that the person can function comfortably. There are many pharmacologic and nonpharmacologic pain relief measures. Nonpharmacologic measures may include cutaneous stimulation, transcutaneous electrical nerve stimulation, surgical ablative procedures, heat and cold, relaxation, and distraction therapies. Pharmacologic therapies include nonopioid analgesia with NSAIDs, opioid analgesia, and local anesthetics. For an in-depth discussion of pain relief, see Chapter 18.

Drugs Used to Reduce Inflammation and Pain

Pharmacologic therapies for managing inflammation and related pain include NSAIDs, pyrazoles, para-aminophenol derivatives, gold compounds, drugs used in management of gout, and uricosurics.

Nonsteroidal Antiinflammatory Drugs

As a group, the NSAIDs have antiinflammatory, analgesic, antipyretic, and platelet-inhibiting action. They are classified by chemical group and include salicylic acid derivatives, anthranilic acid derivatives, indole and indene acetic acids, propionic acid derivatives or aryl-propionic acids, heteroaryl acetic acids, enolic acids or oxicams, and alkanones (Table 36-2).

Pharmacodynamics. These agents act by inhibiting prostaglandin synthetase activity. The mode of inhibition of the enzyme varies among the NSAIDs. Normally, prostaglandin synthetase catalyzes the conversion of arachidonic acid to create endoperoxides, some of which are prostaglandins. The inhibition of prostaglandin synthetase means a drop in the amount of one mediator of the inflammatory process (the prostaglandins) and thus a drop in inflammatory signs and symptoms (eg, pain).

Table 36-1. Antipyretic Drugs

Drug Name	Preparation	Usual Dosage	Adverse Reactions
Antispastic Agent			
dantrolene (Dantrium)	Oral IV	Prophylaxis: 4–8 mg/kg/day orally in 3 or 4 divided doses for 1–2 days before surgery OR 2.5 mg/kg 1¼ hr before anesthesia and infused over 1 hr; additional may be given during surgery OR when syndrome is recognized, give 1 mg/kg by continuous rapid IV push and continue until symptoms subside or a maximum cumulative dose of 10 mg/kg has been reached; following crisis, give 4–8 mg/kg/day orally in divided doses for 1–3 days to prevent recurrence PC: C	Drowsiness, dizziness, weakness, diarrhea; with IV use of drug during crisis, thrombophlebitis, urticaria, erythema, pulmonary edema
Salicylates			
aspirin, acetylsalicylic acid (Genuine Bayer Aspirin Tablets and Caplets, Aspergum, Norwich Aspirin, etc.)	Chewing gum Chewable tablets Enteric-coated tablets Timed-release tablets Controlled release tablets Suppositories	Adults: 0.5–1 g q4–6h as needed for fever; *maximum daily dose,* 4 g Children: 10–15 mg/kg q4–6h; *maximum daily dose,* 65 mg/kg PC: D	Not recommended for fever of viral etiology GI effects, ototoxic effects, asthma in association with hypersensitivity, increased bleeding tendency
Propionic Acid Derivatives			
ibuprofen	Tablets Suspension	Adults: 0.4 g q4–6h Children: 5–10 mg/kg q6–8h PC: B	GI effects, nephrotoxicity, many others occasionally reported
Para-Aminophenol Derivatives			
acetaminophen (Tylenol, Tempra, Panadol, etc.)	Suppositories Chewable tablets Granules Tablets Capsules Elixir	Adults: 0.5–1 g q4–6h as needed for fever; *maximum daily dose,* 4 g Children: 10–15 mg/kg q4–6h; *maximum daily dose,* 65 mg/kg PC: B	Usually negligible with recommended dosage; hepatotoxicity can occur with chronic use of alcohol; acute poisoning could occur
Enolic Acids or Oxicams			
piroxicam (Feldene)	Capsules (10–20 mg)	20 mg qd; may be given in 2 divided doses PC: B	GI effects, nephrotoxicity
Alkanones			
nabumetone (Relafen)	Tablets (500–750 mg)	Initially 1 g/day in 1 or 2 divided doses; max 2 g/day PC: B	GI effects

PC = Pregnancy risk category; see Appendix A.

Other processes apparently influenced by the NSAIDs include:

- Leukotriene synthesis (both diclofenac and indomethacin decrease the production of leukotrienes) and migration
- Superoxide generation (piroxicam, but not ibuprofen, inhibits the generation of hydrogen peroxide from neutrophils)
- Lysosomal enzyme release
- Neutrophil aggregation and adhesion
- Cell membrane functions (eg, enzyme activity, transmembrane anion transport, oxidative phosphorylation, uptake of arachidonate)
- Lymphocyte function
- Rheumatoid factor production
- Cartilage metabolism

Pharmacokinetics. Absorption, distribution, metabolism, and excretion processes depend on the individual

Table 36-2. Nonsteroidal Antiinflammatory Drugs

Drug Name	Preparation	Usual Dosage	Adverse Reactions
Anthranilic Acid Derivatives			
mefenamic acid (Ponstel)	Capsules (250 mg)	500 mg initially, followed by 250 mg q6h, max* 1 wk, PC: C	GI effects, nephrotoxicity
Indole and Indene Acetic Acids			
etodolac (Lodine)	Capsules (200–300 mg)	*Initially:* 800–1200 mg/day; *maintenance:* 600–1,200 mg/day in 2–4 divided doses, PC: C	GI effects, nephrotoxicity
indomethacin (Indocin)	Capsules (25–50 mg) Sustained-release capsules Oral suspension (25 mg/5 mL) Suppositories	25–150 mg/day in 2–4 divided doses, PC: B PC: D (3rd trimester)	GI effects, nephrotoxicity, hepatotoxicity
sulindac (Clinoril)	Tablets (150–200 mg)	150–200 mg initially, max 400 mg/day, PC: B	GI effects, nephrotoxicity
Propionic Acid Derivatives or Arylpropionic Acids			
fenoprofen (Nalfon)	Capsules (200–300 mg) Tablets (600 mg)	300–600 mg 3 or 4 times qd, max 3.2 g/day, PC: B	GI effects, nephrotoxicity
flurbiprofen (Ansaid)	Tablets (50–100 mg)	200–300 mg/day in 2–4 divided doses; max single dose 100 mg PC: B	GI effects, nephrotoxicity
ibuprofen (Advil, Motrin, Nuprin, Rufen, many others)	Tablets (200–800 mg) Suspension (100 mg/5 mL)	Varies widely by condition and client; for mild to moderate pain in adults, 400 mg q4–6h, PC: B	GI effects, nephrotoxicity
ketoprofen (Actron, Orudis, Oruvail)	Capsules (25–75 mg) Sustained-release capsules (200 mg)	12.5–25 mg q4–6h; max 75 mg/day PC: B	GI effects, nephrotoxicity
naproxen or naproxen sodium (Aleve, Anaprox, Naprosyn)	Tablets Delayed-release tablets (375–500 mg) Oral suspension (125 mg/5 mL)	200 mg q8–12h for 3 days (fever) or 10 days (pain) PC: B	GI effects, nephrotoxicity
oxaprozin (Daypro)	Caplets (600 mg)	600 mg–1.2 g once daily	GI effects, nephrotoxicity
Heteroaryl Acetic Acids			
diclofenac (Cataflam, Voltaren)	Tablets (50 mg) Delayed-release and enteric-coated tablets (25–75 mg)	May give 100 mg initially, 50 mg tid PC: B	GI effects
ketorolac (Toradol)	Tablets (used as continuation therapy after started with injections) Injection	30 mg IM or IV q6h; max 120 mg qd; use not to exceed 5 days PC: B	GI effects
tolmetin (Tolectin)	Tablets (200–600 mg) Capsules	600–1,800 mg/d in 3 divided doses, PC: C	GI effects, nephrotoxicity

PC = Pregnancy risk category; see Appendix A. *max = maximum of

drug. For the most part, NSAIDs have a rapid onset of action and provide relief for an adequate time.

Therapeutic Uses. With their antiinflammatory effect, NSAIDs are used primarily to treat musculoskeletal disorders such as RA, osteoarthritis, and ankylosing spondylitis. With their analgesic effect, they are effective against pain of low to moderate intensity, and they lack the unwanted effects of the opioids on the central nervous system (CNS).

These agents have a role in short-term perioperative management of surgically related pain. There is consid-erable interclient variability in relief of pain and inflammation with NSAIDs; this probably relates to pharmacodynamic actions and pharmacokinetic parameters. Preoperative administration of NSAIDs may appear logical but may increase the risk of bleeding. Postoperative administration of NSAIDs at fixed intervals, rather than in response to client demand, seems to provide better analgesia.

The release of prostaglandins by the endometrium during menstruation may cause severe cramps and other symptoms of primary dysmenorrhea. NSAIDs, particularly ibuprofen and naproxen, provide effective pain relief for these symptoms. Ibuprofen decreases elevated levels of prostaglandin in menstrual fluid and reduces resting and active intrauterine pressure, as well as the frequency of uterine contractions.

Dosage and Administration. The parenteral, rectal, and topical administration routes are associated with a reduced incidence of adverse effects and have been used with orthopedic, gynecologic, and abdominal surgery. One regimen is intramuscular (IM) ketorolac on the day of surgery, followed by oral ketorolac three times a day for 3 days.

Adverse Reactions. In addition to having similar therapeutic effects, the NSAIDs share several adverse effects, including gastrointestinal (GI) upset (dyspepsia, gastric erosion, peptic ulcer formation, perforation and hemorrhage, inflammation, and altered permeability of the intestine and lower bowel).

The NSAIDs induce a variety of renal side effects and can cause reversible impairment of glomerular filtration, acute renal failure, papillary necrosis, chronic renal failure, and acute tubular necrosis. Renal effects occur in up to 20% of high-risk clients and may occur within the first several days of use. Clients especially at risk for renal problems include those with hypovolemic states and preexisting renal impairment (eg, that due to atherosclerosis or hypertensive renal disease). The NSAIDs can decrease renal blood flow and the glomerular filtration rate (GFR) in clients with these disorders. Acute and chronic interstitial nephritis occurs rarely with NSAID use.

Sodium retention is the most common side effect of NSAID therapy. More than one mechanism may be involved. The prostaglandin PGE_2 normally directly promotes natriuresis (sodium excretion) by inhibiting tubular reabsorption of sodium and chloride and by inhibiting tubular responsiveness to vasopressin, thereby enhancing free water excretion. NSAID use reduces this inhibition and enhances tubular reabsorption of sodium chloride. Related factors in sodium retention include decreased renal plasma flow and increased capillary permeability, both of which may occur with NSAID use. In some clients, these effects may cause edema and may reduce the effectiveness of antihypertensive drug regimens. NSAIDs, except aspirin and sulindac, may increase blood pressure. NSAIDs also raise serum potassium levels, sometimes markedly (in excess of 6 mEq/L). This relates to the effects on sodium.

Between 15% and 20% of clients taking NSAIDs develop gastric or duodenal ulcer. About 3% of this group go on to experience hemorrhage or perforation. Therapy for NSAID-induced ulcers varies, depending on whether the goal is to prevent the ulcers or heal them. Agents used in such cases include histamine (H_2) antagonists (to reduce the incidence of NSAID-induced duodenal ulcers) and misoprostol (Cytotec), a synthetic PGE_1 analog (to reduce the incidence of gastric and duodenal ulcers). See Chapter 28 for more information about these agents.

The NSAID aspirin irreversibly acetylates prostaglandin synthetase. Platelets, lacking mitochondria, cannot synthesize more prostaglandin synthetase and remain dysfunctional for the rest of their lifespan (10–12 days). Nonaspirin NSAIDs affect platelet aggregation only for as long as the drug itself is active.

Toxicities can occur with NSAIDs that are more prostaglandin-independent. These include hepatic damage or hepatitis, photosensitivity or other skin disorders, cognition dysfunction or other neuropsychiatric changes, ocular changes (eg, retinal disorder, corneal deposition), and hematologic effects.

Physiologic changes of aging may also contribute to NSAID-related difficulties. For example, after menopause women no longer have the beneficial stimulating effect of estrogens and progestogens on gastric mucosa. This may contribute to NSAID-associated gastropathy in women age 75 and older. Another factor in adverse effects could be the decreased serum albumin concentration that occurs with aging; this increases the free drug fraction of NSAIDs (normally they are highly protein bound).

Drug Interactions. Table 36-3 lists the interactions that can occur between other drugs and NSAIDs. Because elderly people are the most likely to have multiple organ dysfunction and because NSAIDs are commonly used in this group, interactions are common in the elderly.

All NSAIDs reduce digoxin clearance, increase plasma digoxin concentration, and increase the risk of digoxin toxicity in clients with reduced renal function. If renal function is normal, there is no problem with this combination.

The NSAIDs (probably all except sulindac and aspirin) inhibit the renal excretion of lithium, increasing lithium concentration and the risk of toxicity. All NSAIDs probably reduce the clearance of methotrexate by an unknown mechanism, increasing plasma methotrexate concentration and the risk of toxicity. This interaction is seen with the antineoplastic dose levels of methotrexate but not with rheumatologic levels.

There is a reduction in the metabolism and renal clearance of NSAIDs when probenecid is used concurrently, causing a concomitant increase in the plasma concentration of the NSAID.

The NSAIDs (probably all except sulindac) reduce the antihypertensive effect of beta blockers and angiotensin-converting enzyme (ACE) inhibitors. This effect is probably related to inhibition of prostaglandin synthesis in the kidneys (producing salt and water retention) and blood vessels (producing increased vasoconstriction). NSAIDs should generally be avoided in clients receiving ACE inhibitors.

Interaction between NSAIDs (except possibly sulindac) and loop and thiazide diuretics reduces the ef-

Table 36-3. Drug Interactions Reported With NSAIDs

Drugs Potentiated by NSAIDs	Drugs Inhibited by NSAIDs
anticoagulants (Coumadin)	loop diuretics
hydantoins	thiazide diuretics
methotrexate (when used for cancer therapy)	beta-adrenergic blocking agents
lithium	angiotensin-converting enzyme (ACE) inhibitors
cyclosporine	
digoxin (with renal insufficiency)	
dipyridamole	
probenecid	
penicillamine	

fects of the diuretic, which may lead to an exacerbation of congestive heart failure in a client predisposed to such a complication. With potassium-sparing diuretics, potassium retention and consequent hyperkalemia may occur.

The use of NSAIDs should generally be avoided by clients on oral anticoagulant therapy, including warfarin (Coumadin) and dicumarol. The concurrent use of NSAIDs and anticoagulants increases the risk of GI bleeding because of direct damage to the GI tract mucosa, inhibition of platelet aggregation, displacement of the anticoagulant from plasma protein-binding sites with consequent potentiation of the anticoagulant action, and a tendency toward reduced plasma prothrombin levels. Enteric-coated aspirin preparations may minimize gastric erosions, but platelets are still inhibited.

Precautions and Contraindications. The GI complications related to NSAID use seem dose-related, but they also occur in clients with a history of peptic ulcer disease or GI bleeding. GI complications have occurred primarily in such high-risk groups as older adults, debilitated clients (particularly women), clients with hepatorenal dysfunction, and clients using alcohol or taking anticoagulants, high-dose NSAID therapy, combinations of aspirin and NSAIDs, or corticosteroids concomitantly with NSAIDs (Lanza, 1993).

Clients with conditions known to interfere with renal potassium excretion should use NSAIDs only under careful supervision. Clients at risk include those with spontaneous or drug-induced hypoaldosteronism, those receiving potassium-sparing diuretics, ACE inhibitors, or cyclosporine, and those with renal insufficiency.

A few asthmatics are sensitive to aspirin. All NSAIDs should be avoided in clients in whom aspirin induces asthma symptoms, urticaria, or other allergic-type reactions.

Use of indomethacin with triamterene potentiates the likelihood of nephrotoxicity, even in clients with normal renal function. This combination is contraindicated.

Salicylates

The medicinal effect of willow bark has been known to several cultures for centuries. Salicin, the active ingredient in willow bark, was discovered in 1827; acetylsalicylic acid (aspirin) was introduced in 1899. The word *salicylate* comes from the Latin name for willow tree, *salix*. The group of medications now known as the salicylates includes acetylsalicylic acid (aspirin), salsalate, sodium salicylate, salicylic acid, methyl salicylate, and diflunisal (Table 36-4).

Acetylsalicylic Acid

Acetylsalicylic acid (aspirin, ASA) has antiinflammatory, analgesic, antipyretic, antiplatelet, and antithrombotic properties. The name aspirin is said to have been derived from *Spiraea*, the plant species from which salicylic acid was once prepared.

Pharmacodynamics. The antiinflammatory action of aspirin results from its inhibition of prostaglandin synthetase. Aspirin also has an analgesic effect but is ineffective in noninflamed tissues. The salicylates relieve pain by both peripheral and CNS effects, but aspirin mainly acts peripherally in the inhibition of prostaglandin synthetase. The hypothalamus is believed to be the site of action of aspirin in the CNS. The antipyretic effect of aspirin results from its inhibition of prostaglandin biosynthesis within the brain. The antiplatelet effect of aspirin (see Chap. 26) is due to its effects on prostaglandin synthetase in platelets and results in an altered balance between thromboxane A_2 and prostacyclin (PGI_2). Thromboxane A_2 promotes platelet aggregation; prostacyclin inhibits it. After administration of aspirin, thromboxane A_2 synthesis does not recover until the affected group of platelets is replaced. For more information, see Focus on Salicylates: Similarities and Differences.

Pharmacokinetics. Aspirin taken orally is absorbed partly from the stomach but mostly from the upper small intestine. The rate of absorption depends on many factors, including dosage form, GI pH, gastric emptying time, and the presence of food in the stomach. There is little difference between the rates of absorption of pure and buffered aspirin. Food delays oral absorption. Rectal absorption is slower, incomplete, and unreliable.

Aspirin is distributed throughout most body tissues and can be detected in synovial, spinal, and peritoneal fluid, in saliva, and in human milk. It crosses the placental barrier readily and the blood-brain barrier slowly.

Biotransformation of aspirin occurs in the liver, where five metabolic products are formed. These are excreted mainly by the kidneys. Urinary pH has a significant effect on elimination: alkaline urine favors excretion.

Table 36-4. Salicylic Acid Derivatives

Drug Name	Preparations	Usual Dosage	Notes
aspirin, acetylsalicylic acid (Genuine Bayer Aspirin Tablets and Caplets, Aspergum, Norwich Aspirin, etc.)	Chewing gum Chewable tablets Enteric-coated tablets Timed-release tablets Controlled-release tablets Suppositories	Adults: 0.5–1 g q4–6h as needed; *maximum daily dose,* 4 g PC: D Children: 10–15 mg/kg q4–6h; *maximum daily dose,* 65 mg/kg	Not recommended for fever of viral etiology
choline salicylate (Arthropan)	Mint-flavored liquid	870 mg/5 mL; 870 mg q3–4h, up to 6 times/day PC: C	Fewer GI adverse reactions than aspirin
magnesium salicylate (Original Doan's, Magan, Mobidin)	Caplet Tablet	650 mg q4h or 1,090 mg tid, may increase to 3.6–4.8 g/day in 3 or 4 divided doses PC: C	May have low incidence of GI adverse reactions; possibility of magnesium toxicity in those with renal insufficiency
choline salicylate and magnesium salicylate (Trilisate)	Tablet Cherry-flavored liquid	Forms have 293–587 mg choline salicylate and 362–725 mg magnesium salicylate PC: C	
sodium salicylate	Enteric-coated tablets	325–650 mg q4h	Clients hypersensitive to aspirin may tolerate this; platelets not affected but prothrombin time increased. Each gram contains 6.25 mEq Na.
sodium thiosalicylate (Asproject, Rexolate, Tusal)	IM	*Gout:* 100 mg q3–4h for 2 days, then 100 mg/day until asymptomatic *Rheumatic fever:* 100–150 mg q4–8h for 3 days, then reduce to 100 mg bid until asymptomatic PC: C	Used in gout, musculoskeletal discomfort, rheumatic fever
salsalate (Amigesic, Disalcid, Argesic-SA, Salflex, Salsitab, Artha-G, MonoGesic)	Capsules Tablets	3,000 mg/day in divided doses PC: C	Not absorbed until reaches small intestine
diflunisal (Dolobid)	Tablets	500 mg–1 g followed by 250–500 mg q8–12h PC: C	Difluorophenyl derivative of salicylic acid, no antipyretic effects

PC = Pregnancy risk category; see Appendix A.

Therapeutic Uses. One systemic use for aspirin is antipyresis for clients in whom fever may be harmful. The use of aspirin does not influence the course of the disease that causes the fever. Aspirin is contraindicated for fever associated with chickenpox or influenza symptoms, as this administration has been associated with Reye's syndrome.

Aspirin is also used as an analgesic for low-intensity pain, such as headache, neuralgia, myalgia, dysmenorrhea, arthralgia, and other pain arising from integumental structures rather than viscera. Chronic use of aspirin for pain relief does not lead to tolerance or addiction.

Aspirin is used in rheumatic fever to suppress the acute inflammatory process of the disease. After 24 to 48 hours of therapy, there is considerable relief of pain, swelling, immobility, local heat, and redness of involved joints. Fever and pulse rate are lowered and the client feels better. Cardiac complications, chorea, encephalopathy, subcutaneous nodules, and other aspects of the disease are not prevented or relieved.

Aspirin is also used in RA to reduce inflammation in joint tissues and surrounding structures and to relieve pain. The analgesia produced allows for more effective exercise and, possibly, improved appetite and a feeling of well-being. If hypoalbuminemia occurs in RA, a higher level of salicylate is measured in plasma because the salicylate normally binds to albumin.

Many clinical trials have examined aspirin's antiplatelet effect (see Chap. 26). Given the available data, aspirin is advocated in a dose of 80 to 325 mg/day for clients with clinical manifestations of coronary artery disease.

Dosage and Administration. Aspirin is available in tablets of 81 to 500 mg and in rectal suppositories containing 120 to 600 mg. Chewable tablets, gum tablets, timed-release, controlled-release, and enteric-coated tablets are marketed.

The route of administration is oral or rectal. Oral doses should be taken with a full glass of water to mini-mize GI irritation. Absorption from enteric-coated tablets is sometimes incomplete. Preparations of aspirin containing alkali or buffer can be better tolerated, but these may alkalinize urine, which can shorten the plasma half-life of salicylates by enhancing excretion of the drug.

FOCUS ON

Focus on Salicylates: Similarities and Differences

Similarities

Pharmacodynamics

Acetylsalicylic acid (aspirin) and other salicylic acid derivatives are hydrolyzed to salicylic acid. They possess antiinflammatory, analgesic, and antipyretic effects. They act both peripherally and centrally and inhibit prostaglandin synthesis.

Pharmacokinetics

The salicylates are rapidly and completely absorbed after oral administration. Food decreases the rate but not extent of absorption. Rectal absorption is slower, incomplete, and unreliable. Protein binding is concentration-dependent; at low therapeutic concentrations about 90% is bound, and at higher plasma concentrations 76% is bound. Renal excretion of drug is affected by urine pH. The salicylates are metabolized in the liver.

Therapeutic Uses

The salicylates are used in the treatment of mild to moderate pain, especially low-intensity pain of nonvisceral origin, such as headache, myalgia, and neuralgia. They are also used to reduce fever and in the initial or long-term management of inflammatory conditions such as rheumatoid arthritis, osteoarthritis, and ankylosing spondylitis. They may be used with dysmenorrhea and in some postoperative pain situations.

Adverse Reactions

These include ototoxicity, GI effects such as dyspepsia, heartburn, epigastric distress, nausea, vomiting, anorexia, abdominal pain, and GI bleeding, nephrotoxicity, prolongation of gestation and labor, salicylism, and allergic reactions. Allergic sensitivity takes a variety of forms, but asthmatics who are aspirin-sensitive can experience severe respiratory complications if they receive aspirin. Evidence suggests an association between the use of aspirin to treat fever during the prodromal phase of varicella or influenza infections and subsequent development of Reye's syndrome.

Drug Interactions

Displace methotrexate from protein-binding sites and reduce its renal excretion by a second mechanism which increases serum level and potential toxicity. Share other potential interactions with other NSAIDs (see Focus on propionic acid derivatives).

Differences

- **Acetylsalicylic acid (aspirin)** more potently inhibits prostaglandin synthesis and irreversibly inhibits platelet aggregation.

- The salicylates differ in bioavailability, depending on dosage form, gastric emptying time, gastric pH, and possibly other factors. Bioavailability of some enteric-coated products may be erratic.
- **Aspirin** has a half-life of 15 to 20 minutes and **salicylic acid** has a half-life of 2 to 3 hours at low doses; at higher doses it may exceed 20 hours.

- **Aspirin** is used for reducing the risk of recurrent transient ischemic attacks in men due to fibrin platelet emboli. Aspirin is used to reduce the risk of death or nonfatal myocardial infarction in clients with previous infarction or unstable angina pectoris.
- **Salicylic acid** and **methyl salicylate** are used in topical preparations, not systemically.
- **Salicylic acid** is used for its keratolytic properties and **methyl salicylate** preparations are used as counterirritants for painful muscles and joints.

- **Diflunisal's** effect on platelet function seems reversible, lasting only about 24 hours after the drug is discontinued.

(continued)

FOCUS ON

Focus on Salicylates: Similarities and Differences (continued)

Similarities (continued)

Differences (continued)

Nursing Considerations

Instruct client in pathophysiology involved, drug therapy regimen, adverse reactions, and interactions. Administer with food or meals, milk, or antacids to minimize GI upset. Encourage client to take with full glass of water and remain sitting for 15 to 20 minutes afterward to ensure passage into the stomach. Do not crush enteric-coated tablets. Assess client's pain level before administering the drug; evaluate drug's effectiveness. Monitor laboratory studies for changes (see text). Assess for signs of ototoxicity. Watch for signs of bleeding complications. Instruct client in use of over-the-counter medications and possible interactions.

The usual dosage is 325 to 1,000 mg every 4 hours. In rheumatic fever and RA, higher doses are used. For antiplatelet effect, lower doses are used.

Adverse Reactions. Aspirin sensitivity is well documented. In asthmatic clients sensitive to aspirin, upper respiratory exacerbations occur and are of particular importance because of the potential for mortality and the crossover effect with all other NSAIDs that inhibit prostaglandin synthetase. Why asthmatics may have difficulty with aspirin remains unknown. Signs of aspirin intolerance in asthmatic clients range from rhinitis, with profuse watery secretions and urticaria, to laryngeal edema, bronchoconstriction, hypotension, shock, and complete vasomotor collapse. The asthmatic clients at highest risk are those 15 to 35 years old, those with a history of frequent sinusitis, and those with nasal polyps and anosmia.

In an asthmatic client who is having an acute response to aspirin or another NSAID, beta-adrenergic agonists are usually helpful. Acetaminophen is the drug of choice for persons with asthma who have experienced symptoms of aspirin sensitivity. Choline magnesium trisalicylate (Trilisate) also has been used satisfactorily. Propoxyphene, morphine, and codeine may generally be used in these clients. Desensitization is indicated in some aspirin-sensitive clients—for example, a client who needs aspirin for its antiplatelet effect.

Aspirin has been responsible for ototoxicity, including tinnitus, a feeling of fullness in the ear, and hearing loss. The mechanism of this reaction is not fully known, but it may be due to effects on the synthesis of prostaglandins, reduction of serum calcium levels, interference with membrane ion transport and with energy-demanding functions of hair cells, inhibition of oxidative enzymes in the cochlea, or increased labyrinthine pressure. The hearing loss is usually bilateral and is reversible within a few days after the medication is discontinued.

Epidemiologic evidence suggests an association between the use of aspirin to treat fever in children during the prodromal phase of varicella (chickenpox) or influenza B or A infections and the subsequent development of Reye's syndrome. Reye's syndrome is characterized by an inflammatory encephalopathy with fatty infiltration of the liver. In 20% to 30% of cases, the outcome is fatal. Survivors may have permanent brain damage. The incidence of Reye's syndrome has dropped sharply since 1985, due to strong professional and media recommendations not to use aspirin in such infections. Acetaminophen should be substituted for aspirin if an antipyretic effect is needed in children and adolescents with fever. Parents must check the label of over-the-counter (OTC) products for hidden aspirin or salicylates (eg, Pepto-Bismol). See Box 36-3 and Table 36-5 for combination products.

Like other NSAIDs, aspirin may also have a negative effect on GI and renal function. Moreover, because of the effect of aspirin on platelet function, its use should be avoided in clients with severe hepatic damage, hypoprothrombinemia, vitamin K deficiency, or hemophilia. Aspirin therapy should also be stopped at least 1 week before surgery.

Prolonged gestation and prolonged spontaneous labor have been demonstrated with aspirin. Prostaglandins of the E and F series are potent uterotropic agents. Their biosynthesis increases dramatically in the hours before childbirth, so it is hypothesized that they have a major role in the initiation and progression of labor and delivery. Inhibitors of prostaglandin biosynthesis have

Box 36-3
Products Containing Acetaminophen and Aspirin and Other Ingredients

Saleto Tablets (also salicylamide, caffeine)

Gelpirin Tablets (also caffeine [buffered])

Supac Tablets (also caffeine, calcium gluconate)

Buffets II Tablets (also caffeine, aluminum hydroxide)

Vanquish Caplets (also caffeine, magnesium hydroxide, aluminum hydroxide)

Extra-Strength Excedrin Caplets & Tablets (also caffeine)

Goody's Extra-Strength Headache Powders (also caffeine)

Toxicity Alert: Salicylates

Severe salicylate toxicity is characterized by CNS disturbances, skin eruptions, and marked alterations in acid–base balance. The CNS effects include an accentuation of the signs and symptoms seen in salicylism, as well as restlessness, garrulity, incoherent speech, apprehension, vertigo, tremor, diplopia, delirium, hallucinations, and convulsions. Fever may occur, especially in children. GI symptoms also occur and include epigastric distress, nausea, vomiting, and anorexia. Dehydration results from hyperpyrexia, sweating, vomiting, and the loss of water vapor during hyperventilation.

As poisoning progresses, CNS stimulation is replaced by CNS depression, manifested as stupor and coma. Cardiovascular collapse and respiratory insufficiency may ensue. Terminal asphyxial convulsions and pulmonary edema can occur. Death usually results from respiratory failure after a period of unconsciousness.

been shown to reduce contractions of the uterus in premature labor. Salicylates readily cross the placenta. By inhibiting prostaglandin synthesis, salicylates may cause untoward effects on the fetus (eg, increased incidence of intracranial hemorrhage in premature infants).

Because it is widely used in medicine and is easily available OTC, aspirin is connected with a high incidence of toxic reactions. The fatal dose varies, but death in adults has occurred after the ingestion of 10 to 30 g.

Mild salicylate intoxication, salicylism, usually occurs after repeated administration of large doses. This syndrome is characterized by headache, dizziness, tinnitus, decreased auditory acuity, dim vision, mental confusion, lassitude, drowsiness, sweating, thirst, hyperventilation, nausea, vomiting, and (occasionally) diarrhea.

Drug–Drug Interactions. Aspirin binds to plasma proteins, especially albumin, and thus may displace other drugs from binding sites. It is thought that aspirin displaces methotrexate from its protein-binding sites.

Table 36-5. Selected Combination Products

Preparation	Ingredients
Alka-Seltzer with Aspirin	aspirin 324 mg, sodium bicarbonate 1.9 g, citric acid 1 g, 567 mg sodium/tablet
Alka-Seltzer Plus Night-Time Cold Tablets	20 mg phenylpropanolamine bitartrate, 6.25 mg doxylamine succinate, 15 mg dextromethorphan Hbr, 500 mg aspirin, 16.2 mg phenylalanine, aspartame
Anacin	aspirin 400 mg, caffeine 32 mg
Ascriptin	aspirin 325 mg, magnesium hydroxide 75 mg, aluminum hydroxide 75 mg
BC powder	aspirin 650 mg, salicylamide 195 mg, caffeine 32 mg/powder packet
Bromo-Seltzer	acetaminophen 325 mg, sodium bicarbonate 2.781 g, citric acid 2.224 g, 761 mg sodium/capful measure
Bufferin	aspirin 324 mg, magnesium carbonate, aluminum glycinate
Comtrex	pseudoephedrine 30 mg, chlorpheniramine 2 mg, dextromethorphan 10 mg, acetaminophen 325 mg
Cope	aspirin 421 mg, caffeine 32 mg, magnesium hydroxide 50 mg, aluminum hydroxide 25 mg
Midol Caplets	aspirin 454 mg, caffeine 32.4 mg, cinnamedrine hydrochloride 14.9 mg
Midol PMS	acetaminophen 500 mg, pamabrom 25 mg, pyrilamine maleate 15 mg
Pamprin Maximum Cramp Relief	acetaminophen 500 mg, pamabrom 25 mg, pyrilamine maleate 15 mg
Pepto-Bismol	bismuth subsalicylate (2 tablets contain 204 mg salicylate, saccharine, mannitol) (30 mL contain 250 mg salicylate; 10 mg sodium, saccharine)
Sinutab II Maximum Strength No Drowsiness Formula	pseudoephedrine hydrochloride 30 mg, acetaminophen 500 mg

NSAIDs also reduce the renal clearance of methotrexate by an unknown mechanism. Thus, by two different mechanisms, the serum methotrexate level is increased. These interactions with methotrexate (in antineoplastic doses) increase the risk of methotrexate toxicity. Other drug interactions with aspirin were discussed in the introductory section on NSAIDs.

Drug–Laboratory Test Interactions. Salicylates compete with thyroid hormone for binding sites, resulting in increases in protein-bound iodine. Serum uric acid levels can be elevated or decreased with salicylate use. Salicylates interfere with urine glucose and ketone determinations by certain methods. Salicylates in the urine interfere with 5-HIAA and VMA (vanillylmandelic acid) determinations.

Precautions and Contraindications. Contraindications include allergy to salicylates or NSAIDs, allergy to tartrazine, hemophilia, bleeding ulcers, hemorrhagic states, blood coagulation defects, hypoprothrombinemia, vitamin K deficiency, impaired renal function, chickenpox, influenza, children with fever accompanied by dehydration, surgery scheduled within 1 week, pregnancy, and lactation.

Diflunisal

Diflunisal (Dolobid) is a difluorophenyl derivative of salicylic acid.

Pharmacodynamics. Diflunisal inhibits prostaglandin synthetase and thus produces antiinflammatory, analgesic, uricosuric, and antiplatelet effects. It has mild antipyretic properties.

Pharmacokinetics. Diflunisal is rapidly and completely absorbed from the GI tract and is highly bound to plasma proteins (99%). Its onset of action is within 60 minutes, with a peak in 2 to 3 hours and a duration of action of 8 to 12 hours. The plasma half-life is 8 to 12 hours; it increases in renal impairment. Diflunisal is not metabolized to salicylic acid. The agent is excreted in urine.

Therapeutic Uses. Diflunisal is used on an acute or long-term basis for mild to moderate pain. It is effective in the symptomatic management of osteoarthritis and RA. Diflunisal 500 mg is comparable in analgesic efficacy to aspirin 650 mg but produces longer-lasting responses. It is not recommended for antipyretic use.

Dosage and Administration. Administration with meals or milk is suggested. Tablets should be swallowed whole, not crushed or chewed. A typical dose for arthritis is 500 mg to 1 g daily in two divided doses.

Adverse Reactions. The most common type of side effect is GI, including nausea, dyspepsia, abdominal pain, and diarrhea. Diflunisal seems to cause fewer and less intense GI effects and antiplatelet effects than aspirin.

Other side effects include allergic reactions, peripheral edema, and tinnitus.

Drug–Drug Interactions. Administration of diflunisal with acetaminophen results in a 50% increase in acetaminophen plasma levels, but acetaminophen has no effect on diflunisal plasma levels. Interactions have been reported between oral anticoagulants, hydrochlorothiazide, indomethacin, and sulindac.

Drug–Laboratory Test Interactions. Borderline elevations in liver test results occur in up to 15% of clients. These abnormalities may progress, remain unchanged, or disappear with continued therapy. Severe hepatic reactions are rare but may occur. Thus, if abnormal liver tests persist or worsen, and if clinical signs and symptoms consistent with liver disease develop, the drug should be discontinued.

Precautions and Contraindications. Contraindications include allergy to diflunisal, salicylates, or other NSAIDs, pregnancy, and lactation. The agent must be used cautiously in clients with cardiovascular dysfunction, peptic ulcers, GI bleeding, and impaired hepatic or renal function.

Salsalate

Pharmacodynamics. Salsalate (Disalcid, Mono-Gesic) is a salicylate with antiinflammatory, analgesic, and antipyretic properties. It does not appear to inhibit platelet aggregation.

Pharmacokinetics. Salsalate is insoluble in gastric secretions and is not absorbed until it reaches the small intestine. It reaches its peak in 1.5 to 4 hours. It is hydrolyzed in the liver, GI mucosa, plasma, whole blood, and other tissues. It is excreted in the urine. A period of 3 to 4 days may be needed to establish a steady-state level.

Therapeutic Uses. Salsalate is used for mild to moderate pain associated with adult or juvenile RA and osteoarthritis.

Adverse Reactions. Evidence suggests that salsalate does not produce significant gastric irritation, and it has not been associated with sensitivity reactions in clients with asthma.

Drug–Drug Interactions. Interactions have been reported with other salicylates and with sulfonylurea preparations.

Drug–Laboratory Test Interactions. Hypoglycemia should be watched for if the client is diabetic and receiving a sulfonylurea preparation.

Precautions and Contraindications. Contraindications include allergy to salicylates or NSAIDs, bleeding disorders, impaired hepatic or renal function, GI ulceration, lactation, and pregnancy.

Salicylic Acid

Salicylic acid is a component of multiple topical products for external use only, including ointments, creams, lotions, liquids, gels, plasters, disks, strips, and transdermal patches. Trade name products include Dr. Scholl's Wart Remover Kit, Compound W, Wart-Off, and DuoFilm.

Pharmacodynamics. Salicylic acid produces desquamation of the horny layer of skin while not affecting the structure of the viable epidermis. It dissolves the intercellular cement substance. The keratolytic action causes the cornified epithelium to swell, soften, macerate, and then desquamate.

Therapeutic Uses. Salicylic acid is the only OTC product considered safe and effective by the Food and Drug Administration for use as a keratolytic agent for corns, calluses, and warts. With warts (in general), improvement should occur in 1 to 2 weeks and maximum resolution may be expected after 4 to 6 weeks. Salicylic acid preparations have also been used to treat dandruff, seborrheic dermatitis, tinea infections, and psoriasis.

Adverse Reactions. Local irritation of normal skin surrounding the affected area may occur from contact between the normal skin and the product. Prolonged use over large areas, especially in young children and clients with significant renal or hepatic impairment, could result in salicylism.

Methyl Salicylate

Methyl salicylate (also called sweet birch oil, wintergreen oil, gaultheria oil, and betula oil) is a colorless, yellowish, or reddish liquid found in gels, creams, ointments, or liniments. Trade name products include infraRUB Cream, Icy Hot Cream, Musterole Deep Strength Rub, Ben-Gay, Deep Down Rub, and Heet Liniment.

Pharmacodynamics. Methyl salicylate acts as a counterirritant to pain and muscle soreness.

Therapeutic Uses. Methyl salicylate is used externally as a counterirritant for painful muscles and joints.

Adverse Reactions. Poisoning with this salicylate has occurred when children have mistaken the aromatic oil for candy. In such a situation, the odor of the drug can be detected on the breath and in the urine and vomit.

Drug Interactions. An enhanced anticoagulant effect has occurred in some clients taking an anticoagulant and using a topical methyl salicylate preparation concurrently.

Precautions and Contraindications. Methyl salicylate should not be applied to irritated skin. It should not be used with an external source of heat (eg, a heating pad) because irritation or burning of skin may occur. Applying a tight bandage or wrap over these agents is not recommended, as increased absorption may occur. If pain persists for more than a week, a clinician should be consulted.

Anthranilic Acid Derivatives

This group of medications includes mefenamic acid. The anthranilic acid derivatives do not seem to have any clear advantages over other NSAIDs.

Mefenamic Acid

Pharmacodynamics. Mefenamic acid (Ponstel) has antiinflammatory, analgesic, and antipyretic properties (see Table 36-2).

Pharmacokinetics. Mefenamic acid is well absorbed after oral administration. Administration with food may minimize adverse GI effects. It reaches a peak in 2 to 4 hours, with a duration of 6 hours or less. It is partially metabolized in the liver. Its half-life is 2 hours, with 50% excreted in the urine and 50% in the feces.

Therapeutic Uses. Mefenamic acid is used to relieve moderate pain, such as that occurring with soft-tissue injuries and musculoskeletal conditions. It has also been used to manage dysmenorrhea.

Dosage and Administration. Mefenamic acid should not be used for pain relief for more than a week. With dysmenorrhea, the initial dose is 500 mg at the onset of bleeding and associated symptoms, and continued at 250 mg every 6 hours for 2 or 3 days. It may be administered with food or milk to reduce GI distress.

Adverse Reactions. Adverse reactions include nausea, vomiting, and abdominal pain. Diarrhea may be severe. GI bleeding or agranulocytosis would indicate the need to discontinue the drug.

Drug–Drug Interactions. Reported drug interactions have involved oral anticoagulants and heparin, lithium, phenytoin, and sulfonylureas.

Drug–Laboratory Test Interactions. The use of mefenamic acid may interfere with urinary bilirubin determinations.

Precautions and Contraindications. Contraindications include pregnancy and lactation. Cautious use is advised in clients with allergies and renal, hepatic, cardiovascular, and GI conditions.

Indole and Indene Acetic Acids

The drugs in this group include etodolac, indomethacin, and sulindac (see Table 36-2).

Etodolac

Pharmacodynamics. Etodolac (Lodine) has antiinflammatory, analgesic, and antipyretic properties. It inhibits prostaglandin synthesis.

Pharmacokinetics. The onset of analgesic action is 30 minutes, with a duration of 4 to 12 hours. It peaks at 1 to 2 hours and has a half-life of 7.3 hours.

Therapeutic Uses. Etodolac is indicated for osteoarthritis and mild to moderate pain.

Dosage and Administration. For osteoarthritis, initially 800 to 1,200 mg/day is administered in divided doses; then the dosage may be decreased. The maximum dose is 1,200 mg/day. For acute pain, typically the dose is 200 to 400 mg every 6 to 8 hours.

Adverse Reactions. Although adverse GI effects (especially diarrhea, dyspepsia, nausea, and abdominal pain) do occur, it has been reported to date that etodolac is safer for the GI system than other NSAIDs (Lanza, 1993). Several studies have documented this and have found no difference in efficacy between etodolac and the other agents tested.

Drug Interactions. See the discussion in the introductory section on NSAIDs.

Precautions and Contraindications. Contraindications include significant renal impairment, pregnancy, and lactation. Cautious use is advised in clients with allergies, impaired hearing, and hepatic, cardiovascular, and GI conditions.

Indomethacin

Indomethacin is one of the older NSAIDs.

Pharmacodynamics. Indomethacin has antiinflammatory, analgesic, and antipyretic properties. It is a methylated indole derivative and one of the most potent inhibitors of prostaglandin synthetase—it is considered more potent than aspirin. It appears to have both central and peripheral action. It also affects leukocyte migration, and it impairs platelet function.

Pharmacokinetics. Indomethacin is absorbed almost completely from the GI tract and has an onset of action within 30 minutes. The peak plasma concentration is attained within 2 hours but may be delayed when the medication is taken after meals. The concentration in synovial fluid is equal to the plasma concentration within 5 hours of administration. It is 90% bound to plasma proteins and is also bound to tissues. It is metabolized to more than one inactive metabolite. Indomethacin's half-life averages 3 hours. It is excreted in urine unchanged and as metabolites and in feces.

Therapeutic Uses. Indomethacin relieves pain, decreases the length of morning stiffness, increases grip strength, and reduces swelling and tenderness of joints with clients with ankylosing spondylitis, osteoarthritis, RA, and gout.

In treating gout, indomethacin seems to have efficacy equivalent to that of colchicine. A typical dose is 40 mg initially, followed by 25 mg three or four times a day. Pain is relieved in 2 to 4 hours, and swelling subsides in 3 to 5 days. The sustained-release form is not used with gout. Indomethacin has been used successfully with tendinitis, bursitis, and acute painful shoulder. A topical ophthalmic preparation has been used to treat cystoid macular edema. In addition, indomethacin has been used as an antipyretic in Hodgkin's disease when the fever has been refractory to other agents.

In an unlabeled use, indomethacin is an alternative to surgical ligation for pharmacologic closure of patent ductus arteriosus in infants, especially premature infants. A typical regimen is 0.1 to 0.2 mg/kg IV every 12 hours for three doses. It has been given IV, via retention enema, or via nasogastric tube. Indomethacin's greatest limitation is its potential renal toxicity. Therapy is stopped if the urine output drops to less than 0.6 mL/kg/hour. This use of indomethacin is thought to be contraindicated in renal failure, necrotizing enterocolitis, thrombocytopenia, or hyperbilirubinemia.

Dosage and Administration. A typical dose with RA is 25 to 50 mg two or three times a day. The total daily dose should not exceed 200 mg. If a dosage of 100 mg/day does not provide benefit in 2 to 4 weeks, other agents will probably be substituted. The medication should be given with food, immediately after meals, or with antacids to reduce GI irritation.

Sometimes indomethacin can be given at night and other better-tolerated NSAIDs can be used during the day. Administering the sustained-released form at bedtime with milk allows the client to sleep better and also reduces the morning stiffness associated with RA. Adverse effects seem better tolerated when the medication is given at night.

A rectal suppository and a flavored oral suspension are available.

Adverse Reactions. Up to 50% of persons taking indomethacin experience side effects, the most common of which is severe frontal headache. Adverse reactions appear to be dose-related in most clients. CNS side effects appear somewhat more prominent with this NSAID than with others. Dizziness, vertigo, lightheadedness, drowsiness, memory lapses, and confusion are common. Seizures and psychiatric changes (eg, severe depression, psychosis) have occurred. GI side effects include anorexia, nausea, abdominal pain, and diarrhea. GI bleeding, ulceration, and perforation have also occurred. Acute pancreatitis also has been reported.

Adverse hematologic reactions are rare. These include neutropenia, thrombocytopenia, and even aplastic anemia. Mouth sores, sore throat, fever, and chills should be reported. Hypersensitivity reactions manifested as rashes, urticaria, and asthma attacks have occurred.

Drug Interactions. Indomethacin antagonizes the diuretic and antihypertensive effects of furosemide and the antihypertensive effects of thiazide diuretics, beta-adrenergic blocking agents, and ACE inhibitors. The nephrotoxic potential of indomethacin appears to increase when triamterene is administered concurrently.

Indomethacin inhibits platelet aggregation like other NSAIDs; the effect appears dose-related and may be of shorter duration than that seen with aspirin. Indomethacin may also displace the anticoagulant from plasma binding sites. Concomitant administration of indomethacin and an anticoagulant should be carried out with caution. The ulcerogenic action of indomethacin may also complicate the interaction. Interactions with probenecid, lithium, and methotrexate have been documented.

Precautions and Contraindications. Clients sensitive to aspirin may exhibit cross-reactivity to indomethacin. Other contraindications for oral and rectal preparations include cardiovascular dysfunction, hypertension, GI bleeding, impaired renal or hepatic function, pregnancy, labor and delivery, and lactation. Contraindications to the IV preparation include bleeding, thrombocytopenia, coagulation defects, necrotizing enterocolitis, renal failure, and local irritation (if extravasation occurs). The sustained-release form of indomethacin should not be used with gouty arthritis.

Sulindac

Sulindac (Clinoril) was introduced in an attempt to find a less toxic agent than indomethacin. It appears to be less than half as potent as indomethacin.

Pharmacodynamics. Sulindac itself is apparently inactive; rather, it is a prodrug and its sulfide metabolite is responsible for its pharmacologic activity. The sulfide metabolite is more than 500 times more potent than sulindac as a prostaglandin synthetase inhibitor.

Pharmacokinetics. Sulindac is almost completely absorbed after oral administration and has an onset of action within 1 hour. Peak concentrations of sulindac are attained within 1 hour, those of the sulfide metabolite in about 2 hours. When taken with meals, absorption is delayed and peak plasma concentration is attained more slowly. Its duration of action ranges from 7 to 16 hours, and it is finally excreted in urine and feces.

Therapeutic Uses. Sulindac is used for clients with ankylosing spondylitis, osteoarthritis, and RA. It has also been used for gout and acute painful shoulder (acute subacromial bursitis/supraspinatus tendinitis).

Dosage and Administration. The drug is usually administered with food to reduce GI side effects. The maximum daily dosage is 400 mg. A period of about 7 to 14 days of therapy is usually adequate for acute painful shoulder.

Adverse Reactions. The incidence of GI adverse effects is higher than with many NSAIDs but lower than with indomethacin. This may be because the gastric or intestinal mucosa is not exposed to high concentrations of active drug during oral administration.

Sulindac is also considered a bit unusual because some studies indicate it does not alter renal function, perhaps because of the kidney's ability to regenerate sulfoxide from active sulfide metabolites. But if a "renal-sparing" effect exists, it must be seen as only relative, and caution is advised in administering this agent to clients with impaired renal function.

Drug–Drug Interactions. See the discussion under NSAIDs.

Drug–Laboratory Test Interactions. Alanine aminotransferase (ALT) and aspartate aminotransferase (AST) values should be checked periodically because abnormalities have occurred.

Precautions and Contraindications. Contraindications include pregnancy and lactation. Cautious use is advised in clients with allergies and renal, hepatic, cardiovascular, and GI conditions.

Propionic Acid Derivatives

The propionic acid derivatives include fenoprofen, flurbiprofen, ibuprofen, ketoprofen, naproxen and naproxen sodium, and oxaprozin (see Table 36-2). Outside the United States, investigational agents in this subgroup include fenbufen, carprofen, pirprofen, indobufen, and tiaprofenic acid.

The propionic acid derivatives seem comparable to aspirin for the control of signs and symptoms of arthritis, and the intensity of adverse reactions is less than with high doses of aspirin. Of the drugs in this group, naproxen may be best tolerated, followed by ibuprofen and fenoprofen. All are more expensive than aspirin.

See Focus on Propionic Acid Derivatives: Similarities and Differences.

Fenoprofen Calcium

Pharmacodynamics. Fenoprofen calcium (Nalfon) is an arylacetic acid derivative with antiinflammatory, analgesic, and antipyretic properties.

Pharmacokinetics. Fenoprofen is administered orally and is 85% absorbed (a lower absorption than others in this subgroup). Food in the stomach retards absorption and lowers peak concentrations in plasma, which are usually achieved within 2 hours. The onset of action is 2 hours, with a duration of 4 to 6 hours. It is almost completely bound to plasma albumin. It is metabolized in the liver. The half-life is 3 hours. Fenoprofen is excreted primarily in urine.

Therapeutic Uses. Fenoprofen is effective as initial therapy or as an alternative to aspirin in RA and osteoarthritis.

Dosage and Administration. For more rapid absorption, it is best taken on an empty stomach 30 to 60 minutes before or 2 hours after meals. However, if the client experiences GI disturbances, it may be given with meals or milk. The concomitant administration of antacids does not seem to alter the concentrations achieved. Tablets may be crushed or capsules emptied and the contents mixed with food.

Focus on Propionic Acid Derivatives: Similarities and Differences

Similarities

Pharmacodynamics

Propionic acid derivatives inhibit prostaglandin synthetase. Normally, prostaglandin synthetase catalyzes conversion of arachidonic acid to create the endoperoxides, some of which are the prostaglandins. The inhibition of prostaglandin synthesis means less of one mediator of the inflammatory process, the prostaglandins, and thus less of the inflammatory signs like pain.

Pharmacokinetics

These agents are rapidly and completely absorbed from the GI tract. They are mostly bound to plasma proteins and are metabolized by the liver and excreted in the urine. In general, food delays absorption but does not significantly affect the total amount absorbed. Administer these agents with meals to minimize GI effects.

Therapeutic Uses

The NSAIDs are basically used for analgesia or for their antiinflammatory effects. All agents in this Focus are indicated for rheumatoid arthritis, osteoarthritis, and mild to moderate pain. Analgesic action peaks in 2 hours and lasts 6 hours for most of the preparations. However, antiinflammatory action (as measured by reduced joint swelling, decreased duration of morning stiffness, increased mobility, and enhanced functional capacity) is evident at 7 to 14 days.

Adverse Reactions

The NSAIDs all can cause adverse GI effects, including nausea with or without vomiting and dyspepsia. By decreasing platelet adhesion and aggregation, NSAIDs can prolong bleeding time by about 3 or 4 minutes. The NSAIDs all can be nephrotoxic. Clients at greatest risk for renal effects include those with preexisting renal disease or compromised renal perfusion, the elderly, premature infants, those with heart failure, and those on diuretics.

Drug Interactions

All NSAIDs reduce digoxin clearance and increase the risk of digoxin toxicity in those with reduced renal function. Inhibit the renal excretion of lithium and increase the risk of toxicity. Reduce the clearance of methotrexate and increase the risk of toxicity. Reduce metabolism and renal clearance when probenecid is used concurrently. Reduce antihypertensive effect of beta-blockers and angiotensin-converting enzyme (ACE) inhibitors. Reduce effects of loop and thiazide diuretics. Increase potassium retention with potassium-sparing diuretics. Increase risk of adverse reactions if used with oral anticoagulants.

Differences

- Some sources consider propionic acids to be ibuprofen, ketoprofen, and oxaprozin and consider fenoprofen, flurbiprofen, naproxen, and naproxen sodium to be arylacetic acid derivatives. For purposes of this Focus, all seven agents are considered together.

- Time to peak levels is about 2 hours, except for **oxaprozin,** which peaks in 3 to 6 hours. Half-life ranges from 2 to 6 hours, except for **naproxen** (12 to 15 hours and up to 28 hours in the elderly) and **oxaprozin** (40 to 60 hours). **Fenoprofen** is the least completely absorbed of the group, at 85%.

- **Ibuprofen, naproxen,** and **naproxen sodium** are also indicated for primary dysmenorrhea.
- **Ibuprofen** is indicated for fever.

- **Fenoprofen** appears to be one of the three NSAIDs with the highest incidence of headache as an adverse reaction.
- Within this group, **ketoprofen** has the highest incidence of dyspepsia.
- **Ibuprofen** can cause ocular disturbances; if they occur, the drug should be discontinued.

- **Sulindac** may be an exception: may not inhibit lithium excretion, may not reduce effects of beta-blockers and angiotensin-converting enzyme inhibitors, and may not interfere with diuretic function.

(continued)

Focus on Propionic Acid Derivatives: Similarities and Differences (continued)

Similarities (continued)

Nursing Considerations

Instruct client in pathophysiology involved, drug therapy regimen, adverse reactions, and interactions. Administer with food or meals, milk, or antacids to minimize GI upset. Assess client's discomfort level before administering the drug; evaluate drug's effectiveness. Instruct client to avoid taking salicylates and alcoholic beverages while taking these medications due to drug–drug interactions (plasma concentrations of NSAIDs may be decreased by salicylates, and the combination may significantly increase the incidence of GI effects).

Differences (continued)

- Because **ibuprofen** is indicated for fever and widely available over-the-counter, advise clients not to take it for more than 3 days for fever or more than 10 days for pain. When such symptoms persist or worsen, a healthcare professional should be consulted.

Adverse Reactions. Adverse reactions include abdominal discomfort and dyspepsia, nausea, vomiting, anorexia, indigestion, and constipation. Other side effects include skin rash and CNS effects such as headache, blurred vision, tinnitus, and dizziness. Fenoprofen appears to be one of the three NSAIDs with the highest incidence of headache.

Drug Interactions. Interactions have been reported with oral anticoagulants and heparin, phenytoin, phenobarbital, and sulfonylureas.

Drug–Laboratory Test Interactions. Certain methods of measuring total and free triiodothyronine seem to be affected when the client is receiving fenoprofen (false elevations).

Precautions and Contraindications. Contraindications include significant renal impairment, pregnancy, and lactation. Cautious use is advised in clients with impaired hearing, allergies, and hepatic, cardiovascular, and GI conditions

Flurbiprofen

Pharmacodynamics. Flurbiprofen (Ansaid) has analgesic, antiinflammatory, and antipyretic properties. Besides inhibiting prostaglandin synthesis, it decreases the migration of leukocytes into inflamed tissues and depresses monocyte function.

Pharmacokinetics. Flurbiprofen is rapidly absorbed after oral administration. Peak plasma concentrations occur within 1 to 2 hours. Administration with food lowers the peak plasma concentration but does not change the total amount of drug absorbed. Almost all (over 99%) of the drug is bound to albumin. It is metabolized in the liver. Its half-life is 5.7 hours and it is excreted in urine.

Therapeutic Uses. Flurbiprofen is effective as initial therapy or as an alternative to salicylates or other NSAIDs for managing RA and osteoarthritis. A solution for ophthalmic use is also available.

Dosage and Administration. To decrease night pain, improve the quality of sleep, and decrease the duration of morning stiffness, 100 mg has been given at bedtime to clients with RA. Acute gout has been successfully treated with a 400-mg loading dose administered in the first 24 hours (eg, 100 mg every 6 hours), followed by 200 mg/day. This agent is under study for treatment of soft-tissue lesions, administered as a transcutaneous patch.

Adverse Reactions. The most frequent adverse reactions are GI disturbances.

Drug Interactions. Flurbiprofen has the potential for the NSAID interactions described above in the introduction to NSAIDs.

Precautions and Contraindications. Contraindications include significant renal impairment, pregnancy, and lactation. Cautious use is advised with impaired hearing, allergies, and hepatic, cardiovascular, and GI conditions.

Ibuprofen

Pharmacodynamics. Ibuprofen (Motrin, Advil, Nuprin, Children's Advil, Pedia-Profen, Rufen, Excedrin 1B, Midol 200, and many others) was approved in 1974 and has antiinflammatory, analgesic, and antipyretic properties. It was the first propionic acid to be widely used.

Pharmacokinetics. Ibuprofen is administered orally and is absorbed rapidly. It is highly bound to plasma proteins and freely crosses the placenta. It passes into the synovial spaces and seems to remain there after the concentration in plasma has declined. It reaches its peak action in 1 to 2 hours and has a duration of action of 2 to 4 hours. Ibuprofen is metabolized in the liver; its half-life is about 2 hours and it is excreted in urine.

Therapeutic Uses. Ibuprofen is as effective as aspirin and certain other agents in RA and osteoarthritis. It may be administered with maintenance doses of gold salts for additional symptomatic relief, and it may also be given with corticosteroids. It is also effective in treating the pain of dysmenorrhea. It is also useful in ankylosing spondylitis and gouty and psoriatic arthritis. It may be useful as an alternative in Reiter's syndrome.

The propionic acids are used for pain associated with soft-tissue injury, such as postpartum pain and pain that follows dental, ophthalmic, and other types of surgery. Acute tendinitis and bursitis have also been treated with propionic acids.

Dosage and Administration. Ibuprofen is widely available in prescription and nonprescription strengths. For RA and osteoarthritis, a typical dose is 300 to 800 mg four times daily. RA clients seem to require higher doses than ones with osteoarthritis. For primary dysmenorrhea, a dose of 400 mg every 4 to 6 hours is used. The drug may be taken with meals or milk to reduce gastric distress.

The drug may be used at doses of 30 to 40 mg/kg/day in three or four divided doses for juvenile arthritis. It is also widely used for fever reduction in children. The recommended dose for fever over 102.5°F is 10 mg/kg. The duration of fever reduction is generally 6 to 8 hours.

Adverse Reactions. The most common adverse reactions are GI effects such as epigastric pain, nausea, heartburn, and sensations of fullness. Other adverse effects include thrombocytopenia, rash, headache, dizziness, blurred vision, and (in a few cases) toxic amblyopia. Clients who develop ocular disturbances should stop using ibuprofen.

Drug Interactions. See the discussion of drug interactions under NSAIDs. Ibuprofen appears to be one of the safer NSAIDs for concurrent use with anticoagulants, if necessary. Concurrent use of ibuprofen and aspirin appears to reduce plasma concentrations of the propionic acid and decrease the effectiveness of the propionic acid. The protein binding of the propionic acid is decreased and its renal clearance is increased. Additional adverse GI effects may be noted when a propionic acid is used with aspirin, other NSAIDs, glucocorticoids, or alcohol.

Precautions and Contraindications. Contraindications include allergy to ibuprofen, salicylates, or other NSAIDs (more common in patients with rhinitis, asthma, chronic urticaria, or nasal polyps), cardiovascular dysfunction, hypertension, peptic ulceration, GI bleeding, pregnancy,

and lactation. The agent must be used cautiously in clients with impaired hepatic or renal function.

Ketoprofen

Pharmacodynamics. Ketoprofen (Orudis), one of the newer propionic acids, has antiinflammatory, analgesic, and antipyretic properties. Besides inhibiting prostaglandin synthesis, it apparently inhibits leukotriene synthesis and has antibradykinin activity and lysosomal membrane-stabilizing action.

Pharmacokinetics. Ketoprofen is rapidly absorbed after oral administration. The presence of food in the stomach delays the rate, but not the extent, of absorption. It is extensively bound to plasma proteins. Its usual peak action is reached in 2 hours. Its half-life is about 2 hours, and it is excreted in urine. Persons with impaired renal function eliminate the drug more slowly. There are no known active metabolites of ketoprofen.

Therapeutic Uses. Ketoprofen is effective for the treatment of RA, osteoarthritis, ankylosing spondylitis, and acute gout.

Dosage and Administration. The usual dosage for arthritis is 150 to 300 mg/day administered in three or four divided doses. The sustained-release preparation is recommended for chronic treatment in clients who receive therapeutic effect with a daily dose of 200 mg. For dysmenorrhea, the usual dose is 25 to 50 mg every 6 to 8 hours. Attempts to minimize GI effects have included administration of ketoprofen with meals, milk, or antacids.

Adverse Reactions. The most frequent side effects are GI. Upper GI symptoms are more common than lower GI symptoms. GI effects include dyspepsia, nausea, abdominal pain, diarrhea, and constipation.

Drug–Drug Interactions. See the discussion in the introduction to NSAIDs. Adding ketoprofen to diuretic therapy regimens increases the risk for renal failure. In addition, there is an increased risk of photosensitivity when ketoprofen is used with other agents known to be photosensitizing.

Drug–Laboratory Test Interactions. Ketoprofen can cause increased plasma concentrations of creatinine. This effect is more common in clients over age 60.

Precautions and Contraindications. Contraindications include significant renal impairment, pregnancy, and lactation. The agent must be used cautiously in clients with impaired hearing, allergies, and hepatic, cardiovascular, and GI conditions.

Naproxen

Pharmacodynamics. There are two preparations: naproxen (Naprosyn) and naproxen sodium (Aleve, Anaprox). Both have antiinflammatory, analgesic, and antipyretic properties. They are about 20 times more potent than aspirin.

Pharmacokinetics. Naproxen is administered orally and is completely absorbed. It has a peak action of 2 hours and a duration of action of 7 hours. It is highly bound to plasma proteins and is metabolized in the liver. The half-life is 12 to 15 hours, but in elderly clients the half-life may be increased up to 28 hours and the dosage may need to be adjusted. (Its longer half-life and its potency distinguish it from the others in this NSAID grouping.) It is excreted primarily in urine.

Therapeutic Uses. Naproxen and naproxen sodium relieve symptoms of RA, ankylosing spondylitis, osteoarthritis, and acute gouty arthritis, as well as dysmenorrhea. All NSAIDs inhibit the migration of leukocytes to some degree, and this property of naproxen may contribute to its efficacy in treating acute gout. Unlabeled uses include Paget's disease of bone and Bartter's syndrome. Naproxen (but not naproxen sodium) may be used for juvenile RA.

Dosage and Administration. Naproxen is available as tablets, delayed-release tablets, and an oral suspension. Naproxen sodium is available as tablets and caplets. Naproxen sodium generally contains 1 mEq/25 mg sodium per 250-mg tablet. The typical dose of naproxen, 250 to 500 mg twice a day (10 mg/kg), should be taken on an empty stomach because food in the stomach influences the rate, but not the extent, of absorption. Improvement in arthritis symptoms is usually clear within 2 weeks.

Adverse Reactions. The GI side effects of naproxen include anorexia, heartburn, and nausea. The CNS effects, which have about the same incidence as the GI effects, include drowsiness, dizziness, headache, fatigue, depression, and ototoxicity. GI bleeding or agranulocytosis would indicate the need to discontinue the drug.

Drug–Drug Interactions. The rate of naproxen absorption is delayed slightly by magnesium oxide and aluminum hydroxide and is accelerated by sodium bicarbonate. Naproxen is highly bound to plasma proteins and may displace albumin-bound drugs from their binding sites (eg, oral anticoagulants, sulfonylureas, hydantoins), so their actions are potentiated. Interactions with lithium, probenecid, and methotrexate have been reported.

Drug–Laboratory Test Interactions. Transient elevations in blood urea nitrogen (BUN) and alkaline phosphatase may occur. Naproxen may interfere with 5-HIAA and urinary 17-ketogenic steroid determinations. Naproxen should be withdrawn 72 hours before adrenal function tests.

Precautions and Contraindications. Contraindications include pregnancy and lactation and allergy to naproxen, salicylates, or other NSAIDs. Cautious use is advised in clients with asthma, chronic urticaria, cardiovascular

dysfunction, hypertension, GI bleeding, peptic ulcer, and impaired hepatic or renal function.

Oxaprozin

Pharmacodynamics. Oxaprozin (Daypro), approved for use in 1992, has antiinflammatory, analgesic, and antipyretic properties.

Pharmacokinetics. Oxaprozin is well absorbed orally, with peak plasma concentrations achieved in 3 to 6 hours. The drug is metabolized in the liver and primarily eliminated by urinary excretion. The half-life is 40 to 60 hours, and this increases with age.

Therapeutic Uses. It is approved for acute and long-term use in osteoarthritis and RA.

Dosage and Administration. Due to its long half-life, it can be given once daily. For arthritis, the typical dose is 1,200 mg once a day, but less may be given. The maximum daily dose is 26 mg/kg (about 1,800 mg/day).

Adverse Reactions. The most common adverse reactions are GI: nausea, diarrhea, constipation, and abdominal distress.

Drug Interactions. See the discussion in the introduction to NSAIDs.

Precautions and Contraindications. Contraindications include significant renal impairment, pregnancy, and lactation. Cautious use is advised in clients with impaired hearing, allergies, and hepatic, cardiovascular, and GI conditions.

Heteroaryl Acetic Acids

The drugs in this subgroup include tolmetin, ketorolac, and diclofenac (see Table 36-2).

Diclofenac

Pharmacodynamics. Diclofenac (Voltaren, Cataflam) is a phenylacetic acid derivative with antiinflammatory, analgesic, and antipyretic properties. It is more potent than some of the other NSAIDs. In addition, it appears to reduce intracellular concentrations of free arachidonate in leukocytes, perhaps by altering the release or uptake of the fatty acid. This probably contributes to its efficacy, but exactly how is unclear.

Pharmacokinetics. It is well absorbed from the GI tract after oral administration. Food in the stomach delays the rate, but not the extent, of absorption. Peak action is usually reached within 2 to 3 hours, with an action duration of 4 to 6 hours. It is approximately 99% bound to plasma proteins. It undergoes extensive metabolism on its first pass through the liver, so only 50% of it is available systemically. It accumulates in synovial fluid, which may explain why its duration of therapeutic effect is considerably longer than its plasma half-life (1–2 hours). It is excreted via bile (35%) and urine (65%).

Therapeutic Uses. Diclofenac has been used for RA, osteoarthritis, and ankylosing spondylitis. It may also be used for short-term treatment of acute musculoskeletal injury, acute painful shoulder (bicipital tendinitis and subdeltoid bursitis), postoperative pain, and dysmenorrhea. The ophthalmic solution may be used to reduce postoperative inflammation after cataract extraction.

Dosage and Administration. Diclofenac sodium (Voltaren) is available as delayed-release enteric-coated tablets. A typical dose is 100 to 200 mg/day in divided doses. Diclofenac potassium (Cataflam) is available as tablets.

Adverse Reactions. The adverse effects include GI effects and other effects typical of NSAIDs.

Drug Interactions. See the discussion in the introduction to NSAIDs.

Drug–Laboratory Test Interactions. Elevation of hepatic aminotransferase activities in plasma occurs in about 15% of clients. In some, these values may more than triple. The elevations usually are reversible, but rarely are associated with clinical evidence of hepatic disease. Aminotransferase activity should be evaluated during the first 8 weeks of therapy, and the drug should be discontinued if signs and symptoms of hepatic dysfunction develop.

Precautions and Contraindications. Contraindications include significant renal impairment, pregnancy, and lactation. This agent must be used cautiously in clients with impaired hearing, allergies, and hepatic, cardiovascular, and GI conditions.

Ketorolac Tromethamine

Pharmacodynamics. Ketorolac tromethamine (Toradol), approved in 1989, is a heteroaryl acetic acid derivative with antiinflammatory, analgesic, and antipyretic properties. It inhibits prostaglandin synthesis. Its analgesic effect is greater than its antiinflammatory effect.

Pharmacokinetics. Ketorolac is completely absorbed after oral or IM administration and begins to act in 10 minutes. The peak action is reached in 30 to 60 minutes, with a typical duration of up to 6 hours. It is extensively bound to plasma proteins. The half-life is 2.4 to 8.6 hours. Ketorolac is excreted in urine. The rate of elimination is reduced in older adults and in clients with renal failure.

Therapeutic Uses. Ketorolac is indicated for the short-term (up to 5 days) management of moderately severe acute pain that requires analgesia at the opioid level. Unlike opioid agonists, it is not associated with tolerance, withdrawal effects, or respiratory depression. It is generally used in the postoperative setting and for dental, orthopedic, and gynecologic surgery.

This agent has been used successfully with small samples of clients with acute migraine symptoms. Its antiinflammatory effects may inhibit the perivascular inflammation that is thought to cause the headache pain, nausea, and photophobia associated with migraine.

Topical ketorolac may be useful for inflammatory conditions in the eye and is approved for the treatment of seasonal allergic conjunctivitis.

Dosage and Administration. Ketorolac is one of the NSAIDs approved for parenteral administration. It is available in prefilled syringes of 15 mg/mL, 30 mg/mL (1 mL), and 30 mg/mL (2 mL). It may be given IV as a bolus over at least 15 seconds, or it may be given IM slowly and deeply into the muscle.

Oral ketorolac is indicated only as continuation therapy to parenteral ketorolac. The combined duration of use of IM/oral is not to exceed 5 days. For a client under age 65, 20 mg is given as a first oral dose after the client received a single dose of 60 mg IM, a single dose of 30 mg IV, or multiple doses (IV/IM) of 30 mg. After the initial oral dose, 10 mg would be given every 4 to 6 hours, not to exceed 40 mg/24 hours. The dosage should be adjusted for clients over age 65, clients weighing less than 50 kg or 10 lb, and clients with moderately elevated serum creatinine levels.

Adverse Reactions. Adverse reactions include drowsiness and GI effects such as nausea.

Drug Interactions. See the discussion in the introduction to NSAIDs.

Precautions and Contraindications. Contraindications include significant renal impairment, pregnancy, lactation, and use of soft contact lenses (for the ophthalmic preparation). The agent must be used cautiously in clients with impaired hearing, allergies, and hepatic, cardiovascular, and GI conditions. Ketorolac is contraindicated for intrathecal or epidural administration due to its alcohol content. Use in labor and delivery is contraindicated because it may adversely affect fetal circulation and inhibit uterine contractions.

Tolmetin Sodium

Pharmacodynamics. Tolmetin sodium (Tolectin) is a heteroaryl acetic acid derivative with antiinflammatory, analgesic, and antipyretic properties. It inhibits prostaglandin synthetase.

Pharmacokinetics. Administered orally, tolmetin is absorbed rapidly and almost completely. It is approximately 99% bound to plasma proteins. Peak action is reached in 0.5 to 1 hour, and its half-life is about 5 hours. Accumulation of the drug in synovial fluid begins within 2 hours and persists up to 8 hours after a single oral dose. A therapeutic response with arthritis can be expected within a week, and during succeeding weeks of therapy there should be progressive improvement. The drug is metabolized in the liver and excreted in urine.

Therapeutic Uses. Tolmetin is used in treating adult and juvenile RA, osteoarthritis, and ankylosing spondylitis.

Dosage and Administration. The adult dose for arthritis is 400 mg three times a day initially. The maximum dose is 2 g/day. Tablets contain 200 or 600 mg, capsules

400 mg. The medication may need to be taken with meals, milk, or antacids to minimize gastric irritation, but if an antacid is used it should not be sodium bicarbonate. Bioavailability and peak plasma concentrations are reduced when the drug is taken with food or milk.

Adverse Reactions. The most common side effects are GI: nausea, vomiting, diarrhea, epigastric pain, dyspepsia, and flatulence. Ulceration has occurred but less often than with aspirin. CNS effects seem less common than with indomethacin. Similarly, the incidence of tinnitus, vertigo, and decreased auditory acuity is less than with aspirin.

Drug–Drug Interactions. See the discussion in the introduction to NSAIDs.

Drug–Laboratory Test Interactions. Tolmetin metabolites in urine produce positive tests for proteinuria by one method, so other methods should be used.

Precautions and Contraindications. Contraindications include pregnancy and lactation. This agent must be used cautiously in clients with allergies and renal, hepatic, cardiovascular, and GI conditions.

Enolic Acids or Oxicams

Piroxicam (see Table 36-2) is the only drug in this class currently available in the United States, but other oxicams, including piroxicam prodrugs, are under study. The main difference between the oxicams and other classes of NSAIDs is the long action of the oxicams.

Piroxicam

Pharmacodynamics. Piroxicam (Feldene), introduced in the late 1970s, has analgesic, antiinflammatory, and antipyretic activity. It inhibits the synthesis of prostaglandins.

Pharmacokinetics. Chemically, piroxicam bears some resemblance to the pyrazoles (Olkkola et al., 1994). Piroxicam is well absorbed after oral administration. As a result of its long half-life (30 to over 70 hours), plasma concentrations of the drug increase gradually for about 7 to 12 days and then reach a steady-state level. Piroxicam is 99% bound to plasma proteins. It is metabolized by the liver and excreted in urine and feces.

Renal impairment does not appear to alter the elimination of piroxicam. In one study, its elimination was enhanced in clients with end-stage renal disease (because plasma protein binding is probably lower in these clients).

Therapeutic Uses. Piroxicam appears equivalent to other NSAIDs for long-term management of RA or osteoarthritis, and it may be better tolerated than aspirin or indomethacin. Piroxicam is also used in treating ankylosing spondylitis and acute gouty arthritis.

Dosage and Administration. Piroxicam is administered once a day. Improvement in arthritic symptoms should be noted in 7 to 12 days, with peak benefit at 2 to 3 weeks. It may be administered with food to decrease GI side effects: food slows the rate of absorption but does not affect bioavailability.

Adverse Reactions. The most common adverse reactions are GI disturbances. Hematologic changes have been observed, including reduced hemoglobin and hematocrit and (rarely, after long-term therapy) anemia, leukopenia, thrombocytopenia, and eosinophilia. Piroxicam interferes with the function of platelets.

Piroxicam is a hydrophilic substance, sparingly soluble in fat. Such substances penetrate the blood-brain barrier poorly, which may explain why oxicams produce a lower incidence of CNS effects than other NSAIDs, such as indomethacin.

Drug Interactions. See the information on interactions in the introduction to NSAIDs.

Precautions and Contraindications. Contraindications include pregnancy and lactation. Piroxicam must be used cautiously in clients with allergies and renal, hepatic, cardiovascular, and GI conditions.

Alkanones
Nabumetone

Nabumetone is a recently introduced NSAID and the first in this class.

Pharmacodynamics. Nabumetone (Relafen) has antiinflammatory, analgesic, and antipyretic activity. As a prodrug, it is a weak prostaglandin synthesis inhibitor, but it undergoes hepatic biotransformation to the active component, a more potent inhibitor of prostaglandin synthesis.

Pharmacokinetics. It reaches peak effect in 2.5 to 4 hours, and the active metabolite has a half-life of 22.5 to 30 hours.

Therapeutic Uses. Nabumetone is used for osteoarthritis, RA, and ankylosing spondylitis.

Dosage and Administration. Nabumetone is available as tablets. The recommended starting dose is 1,000 mg taken as a single dose with or without food. It might be given in two divided doses. The maximum dose is 2 g/day.

Adverse Reactions. Although adverse GI effects (especially diarrhea, dyspepsia, and abdominal pain) do occur, nabumetone is reportedly safer for the GI system than other NSAIDs. Several studies have documented this fact and have found no difference in efficacy between nabumetone and the other agents tested. As a prodrug, nabumetone apparently does not inhibit gastroprotective prostaglandins. In addition, it appears to have little or no effect on platelet aggregation, in contrast to some of the other NSAIDs.

Drug Interactions. To date, drug interactions are unidentified. It is assumed that the interaction profile would be similar to that of other NSAIDs.

Drug–Laboratory Test Interactions. Nabumetone can cause elevated serum creatinine, BUN, and liver enzyme levels.

Precautions and Contraindications. Clients who are at greater risk for renal or liver problems should be monitored closely. Other contraindications include pregnancy and lactation. This agent must be used cautiously in clients with impaired hearing, allergies, and hepatic, cardiovascular, and GI conditions.

Pyrazoles

This group includes phenylbutazone, a pyrazolone derivative.

Phenylbutazone

Because of potentially severe adverse reactions, phenylbutazone (Butazolidin, Azolid) is not used routinely. Its prominent antiinflammatory effects have been used to relieve pain in horses.

Pharmacodynamics. It has antiinflammatory and analgesic effects, shows mild uricosuric activity, and inhibits platelet aggregation. It is theorized that the antiinflammatory effect of this agent may be due to inhibition of prostaglandin synthesis and leukocyte migration, as well as the release or the activity of lysosomal enzymes (or both).

Pharmacokinetics. Phenylbutazone is absorbed rapidly and completely from the GI tract. Peak action is in 2.5 hours, but its duration of action is 3 to 5 days. Concentrations may remain in the joints up to 3 weeks after treatment is completed. The drug has a long half-life (50–100 hours), is metabolized in the liver to an active metabolite (oxyphenbutazone), and is excreted in the urine (60%) and feces (30%). Oxyphenbutazone as an active metabolite also is extensively bound to plasma proteins and has a half-life in plasma of several days. It accumulates significantly during long-term administration of phenylbutazone and contributes to the pharmacologic and toxic effects of the parent drug. Oxyphenbutazone was marketed as a separate agent but was withdrawn from the market by its manufacturer.

Therapeutic Uses. Phenylbutazone is used to treat acute gout and can usually control an attack within 36 hours. It appears to be more reliable than colchicine when gout treatment has been delayed. Phenylbutazone has also been used for acute exacerbations of RA, ankylosing spondylitis, and osteoarthritis.

Dosage and Administration. Phenylbutazone should be used only after a careful assessment of the risks involved, and then only for short periods (eg, 1 week). This medication is taken with meals, milk, or antacids to lessen gastric irritation. It is available in tablets and capsules. A typical dosage is 300 to 600 mg/day in three or four divided doses initially, then reduced to a maximum maintenance dose of 400 mg/day.

Adverse Reactions. From 10% to 45% of clients treated with phenylbutazone suffer side effects. Nausea and dyspepsia are the most common. Phenylbutazone causes a significant retention of sodium and chloride, a reduction in urine volume, and an increase in plasma volume. Because of these effects, edema, cardiac decompensation, and acute pulmonary edema have occurred. Peptic ulcer or its reactivation with hemorrhage or perforation, allergic reactions, renal failure, and fatal and nonfatal hepatitis also have occurred. Hematologic disorders, including bone marrow depression, are the most serious complications, and deaths have occurred from aplastic anemia and agranulocytosis. The side effects seem more severe in elderly clients, and its use in this group is not advised.

Drug–Drug Interactions. Phenylbutazone is highly protein bound, so other medications may be displaced from their protein-binding sites by phenylbutazone, resulting in increased pharmacologic or toxic effects of the displaced drug. Phenylbutazone causes an increased anticoagulant response when given concurrently with warfarin, and hemorrhagic crises have occurred. In this case, besides the displacement phenomenon, phenylbutazone also inhibits the metabolism of warfarin.

Phenylbutazone inhibits the metabolic inactivation of sulfonylurea drugs (oral hypoglycemic agents), an effect that can cause profound hypoglycemia. It can also increase the effect of insulin.

Administering phenylbutazone with phenytoin may increase the serum levels and toxicity of phenytoin by inhibiting the metabolism of phenytoin. Phenylbutazone can also increase methotrexate toxicity.

Microsomal enzymes that metabolize digitoxin in the liver are stimulated by phenylbutazone; this in turn lowers digitoxin levels.

Drug–Laboratory Test Interactions. Displacement of the plasma protein-bound thyroid hormone by phenylbutazone complicates the interpretation of thyroid function tests.

Precautions and Contraindications. Phenylbutazone is not considered the drug of choice for any condition and should be used only after other drugs have failed.

The combination of phenylbutazone and oral hypoglycemic agents should be avoided if possible, but if concurrent use is needed, the blood glucose level must be monitored closely.

Para-Aminophenol Derivatives

Para-aminophenol derivatives are used to relieve muscle aches and pains. Prototypical para-aminophenol derivatives are phenacetin and acetaminophen. Although about 80% of phenacetin is metabolized to acetaminophen, phenacetin is no longer marketed.

Acetaminophen

Pharmacodynamics. The analgesic and antipyretic properties of acetaminophen are significant, but acetaminophen is only weakly antiinflammatory. Acetaminophen can inhibit prostaglandin synthetase only in an environment low in peroxides (eg, the hypothalamus), and sites of inflammation usually contain high concentrations of peroxides generated by leukocytes. Therefore, acetaminophen does not inhibit prostaglandin synthesis peripherally.

Pharmacokinetics. Acetaminophen is absorbed rapidly and almost completely from the GI tract. Its plasma concentration peaks in 30 to 60 minutes. Binding of the drug to plasma proteins ranges from 20% to 50%. It is metabolized by hepatic enzymes and excreted through the kidneys.

Therapeutic Uses. Acetaminophen is a good analgesic or antipyretic substitute for aspirin when aspirin is contraindicated or when its side effects pose a significant disadvantage. It does not produce the gastric irritation of the salicylates, and it has no effect on platelets, bleeding time, or uric acid excretion.

Dosage and Administration. The usual adult oral dose is 325 to 1,000 mg; the total daily dose should not exceed 4,000 mg.

Adverse Reactions. Acetaminophen is usually well tolerated, but allergic reactions, including skin rashes, occur occasionally. See Toxicity Alert below.

Toxicity Alert: Acetaminophen

Hepatotoxicity may occur after ingestion of a single 10- to 15-g dose of acetaminophen. Doses of 20 to 25 g or more may be fatal. Clinical signs of hepatic damage occur in 2 to 4 days; 10% to 20% of clients die of hepatic failure. Chronic alcohol ingestion and other drugs, such as phenobarbital and phenytoin, increase the risk for toxicity because they stimulate the microsomal enzyme system, increasing the metabolism of acetaminophen to the toxic metabolite N-acetylbenzoquinoneimine. With excessive doses of acetaminophen, this metabolite forms in amounts that deplete glutathione, allowing the metabolite to bind to hepatic cells. Eventually liver necrosis and, possibly, death result. Early diagnosis is vital because hepatic lesions may be reversible in nonfatal cases. Vomiting should be induced or gastric lavage carried out preferably within 4 hours of ingestion. Some laboratory tests that compare acetaminophen levels over time may be used to predict the severity of hepatotoxicity.

Antidote

A sulfhydryl compound, such as N-acetylcysteine (Mucomyst, Mucosal) is given orally or IV to replenish hepatic stores of glutathione. Ideally, this drug should be administered less than 10 hours (but up to 36 hours) after ingestion of the toxic dose. Adverse reactions to N-acetylcysteine include rash, nausea, vomiting, diarrhea, and anaphylaxis.

Drug Interactions. Repeated doses of acetaminophen may slightly increase the hypoprothrombinemic response to oral anticoagulants, and an occasional client develops a more marked increase. However, unlike aspirin, acetaminophen neither inhibits platelet function nor causes gastric erosions. Thus, acetaminophen is probably safer than aspirin.

Precautions and Contraindications. Acetaminophen must be used cautiously in clients with impaired hepatic function, chronic alcoholism, pregnancy, or lactation.

Gold Compounds

First-line drug therapy for RA includes NSAIDs and corticosteroids; second-line therapy involves gold salts. Other drugs used for RA (discussed elsewhere) include antimalarial drugs, D-penicillamine, sulfasalazine, methotrexate, azathioprine, cyclophosphamide, and cyclosporine, among others.

Gold was first used for arthritis in the 1930s. The observation that gold in vitro inhibited *Mycobacterium tuberculosis* led prescribers to try it as a treatment for arthritis and lupus erythematosus, which were thought by some to be manifestations of tuberculosis. The benefits of gold therapy (or chrysotherapy) are still debated. A review of 17 studies suggests that gold treatment retards the progression of RA (Slotkoff & Katz, 1994). Gold appears to arrest disease progress and induce remission in some. The consensus may be that gold is beneficial in clients who can tolerate it over the extensive therapy period required, because it has a high toxicity and a high client dropout rate.

Pharmacodynamics. Gold compounds have many actions, but it remains unclear which actions are precisely responsible for a beneficial result in RA. Gold may reduce C-reactive protein (CRP), erythrocyte sedimentation rate, and rheumatoid factor and immunoglobulin levels and may partially inactivate the complement cascade. It also may block T-lymphocyte and monocyte functions, including cytokine production. It is thought to inhibit neutrophil chemotaxis, migration, and phagocytosis.

Pharmacokinetics. The two most widely used parenteral gold preparations are aurothioglucose and gold sodium thiomalate. Another triethylphosphine gold compound, auranofin, is reasonably well absorbed after oral administration. Initially, the gold is highly bound to albumin. Later, it is found in the synovial fluid and many body tissues. As further doses are given, the half-life lengthens to weeks and months. After a cumulative dose of 1 g of gold, about 60% of it is retained in the body.

Therapeutic Uses. Gold compounds may be most effective in early RA, but they are also useful in later-stage disease. Gold is also used to treat juvenile RA, palindromic rheumatism, psoriatic arthritis, Sjögren's syndrome, nondisseminated lupus erythematosus, and pemphigus.

Dosage and Administration. Gold compounds are available as gold sodium thiomalate (Myochrysine, Aurolate), gold thioglucose/aurothioglucose (Solganal), and the oral form, auranofin (Ridaura).

Injectable gold therapy is initiated in test doses of 10 mg the first week, followed by 25 mg the next week. Subsequent doses of 50 mg each week are given until a cumulative dose of 1,000 mg is attained. Maintenance therapy is generally 25 to 50 mg every 2 to 4 weeks indefinitely. Therapeutic effects occur slowly, and several weeks of therapy are usually required before improvement is noted.

Because Solganal is administered in a sesame oil vehicle, dosing may be inexact, lumps may occur at the injection site, and pain from large-bore needles (18-gauge, 1.5″–2″ needles) may be reported.

About 25% of an orally administered dose of auranofin is absorbed. A typical initial dose for adults is 6 mg daily, either as 3 mg twice daily or 6 mg once daily. Therapeutic response is achieved in 3 to 6 months. If the response is inadequate after 6 months, the dosage may be increased to 9 mg/day. If the response is still inadequate after 3 months on 9 mg/day, the drug should be discontinued.

Adverse Reactions. From 25% to 50% of clients receiving gold have adverse reactions. The most common are cutaneous lesions (ranging from erythema to exfoliative dermatitis) and lesions of the mucous membranes (eg, stomatitis, gingivitis, glossitis, pharyngitis, tracheitis, gastritis, colitis, vaginitis). Evidence of bone marrow suppression includes eosinophilia, thrombocytopenia, leukopenia, agranulocytosis, and aplastic anemia. Proteinuria is a common complication, occurring in 25% of clients receiving 50 mg of gold per week. Other severe reactions include encephalitis, peripheral neuritis, hepatitis, and pulmonary infiltrates.

Parenteral gold is associated with a vasomotor (nitritoid) reaction resembling an anaphylactoid effect. Symptoms are fainting, dizziness, hypotension, flushing, and perspiration. This response is usually more frightening than harmful, but it has been seen in up to 33% of clients after injection. Nitroid reactions are more often associated with gold sodium thiomalate.

In some studies, auranofin was found to be less toxic (in terms of mucocutaneous and hematologic complications) than parenteral gold preparations. However, auranofin is considered less effective and also causes more GI disturbances, such as frequent or loose stools, often associated with abdominal cramping, than do parenteral preparations.

Drug–Drug Interactions. Few drug interactions with gold preparations have been reported. Some prescribers report that coadministration of gold and phenytoin increases phenytoin levels.

Drug–Laboratory Test Interactions. Bone marrow depression may occur, evidenced by hemoglobin levels, red and white blood cell counts, and platelet counts.

Drugs Used for Gout

Gout is hyperuricemia accompanied by clinical signs and symptoms. It may be primary or secondary. Primary gout, or overproduction of uric acid, represents 10% of gout cases and includes a group of inborn metabolic disorders (inherited enzyme deficiencies). Secondary gout occurs in certain diseases characterized by increased breakdown of nucleic acids or in clients who have an interference with renal excretion. Undersecretion may be associated with renal insufficiency, hypertension, drugs such as thiazide diuretics or salicylates, diabetes mellitus, or alcohol abuse. Although the origins are different, hyperuricemia is the common denominator, and the end result is that monosodium urate crystals precipitate into tissue (eg, joints) because of supersaturation of extracellular fluid. A 24-hour measurement of uric acid helps determine whether the client is a uric acid overproducer or an undersecretor.

Acute gouty arthritis is a monoarticular or oligoarticular arthritis involving the joints of the lower limbs. The first metatarsophalangeal joint of the big toe is involved at some point in 75% of clients. Affected joints are usually red, swollen, and exquisitely tender. Chronic tophaceous gout is less frequently seen because of the drugs available but is characterized by gouty tophi (subcutaneous deposits of monosodium urate crystals). The tophi occur over the extensor surfaces of the forearms and the Achilles tendons and on the helix of the ear; they could be confused with rheumatoid nodules.

Renal calculi composed of uric acid represent 5% to 10% of renal stones. The risk of urolithiasis is much greater in people with asymptomatic hyperuricemia or gout. Calcium stones are also more common in people with gout, with uric acid serving as a nidus for the calcium crystals. The deposition of uric acid in the renal tubules can occur with the treatment of hematologic malignancies and is called urate nephropathy; in many cases, it can be prevented by the use of allopurinol.

NSAIDs, colchicine, allopurinol, uricosurics, and corticosteroids are used to treat acute gouty arthritis (Table 36-6).

Colchicine

Colchicine is an alkaloid of the autumn crocus (*Colchicum autumnale*). Benjamin Franklin, who had gout, supposedly introduced colchicine in the United States for gout therapy in 1763.

Pharmacodynamics. Colchicine is a unique medication because it is relatively selective for gout. It inhibits the migration of granulocytes into the inflamed area, reduces the release of lactic acid and proinflammatory enzymes that occur during phagocytosis, breaks the cy-

Table 36-6. Common NSAIDs and Dosages for Gout

Drug	Dosage
diclofenac (Voltaren)	50–75 mg tid
indomethacin (Indocin)	50 mg tid or qid
ketoprofen (Orudis)	50–75 mg tid
naproxen (Naprosyn)	500 mg bid or tid
tolmetin (Tolectin)	400–600 mg tid

cle that leads to the inflammatory response, and decreases the inflammatory response and hence the pain.

Pharmacokinetics. Colchicine is rapidly absorbed after oral administration, with a peak action within 2 hours. It has a plasma half-life of 20 minutes and a half-life in white blood cells of 60 hours. It is excreted in urine and feces. Large amounts of colchicine and its metabolites enter the intestinal tract in the bile and intestinal secretions; this may account for the intestinal manifestations of toxicity.

Therapeutic Uses. Colchicine is used to treat acute attacks of gout, as well as to prevent attacks. If colchicine is given promptly, pain, swelling, and redness will be relieved within 12 hours and will completely clear in 48 to 72 hours. Other conditions for which colchicine is used include familial paroxysmal polyserositis, amyloidosis, primary biliary cirrhosis, multiple sclerosis, psoriasis, and Behçet's syndrome.

Dosage and Administration. Tablets should be stored in special containers to protect them from exposure to light.

The dose of colchicine is 0.6 mg four times daily for 2 or 3 days, then twice a day for 1 to 2 weeks. Some recommend colchicine at 0.6 mg every 1 to 2 hours until symptoms improve or GI symptoms occur. The maximum dose should be 6 mg or 10 tablets over 24 hours, and then no further colchicine should be given for 7 days.

When given IV, a total dose of 4 mg should not be exceeded. The medication should not be repeated again for 7 days. The IV route may help prevent adverse GI effects or decrease their frequency, but the higher blood levels increase the possibility of bone marrow toxicity. Elderly clients should be given no more than 2 mg of IV colchicine per attack, with at least 21 days between courses of medication.

Colchicine may be used to prevent acute attacks of gout precipitated by surgery. A major illness may precipitate acute gout, but such clients may have compromised renal and hepatic function and may be taking multiple medications. In such a situation, if NSAIDs, colchicine, and uricosurics seem contraindicated, intra-articular corticosteroids may be used.

Adverse Reactions. Nausea, vomiting, diarrhea, and abdominal pain are common GI side effects of col-

chicine. These effects may be unavoidable during the client's first therapeutic use of the medication. Other reactions include volume depletion related to diarrhea, hyponatremia, hypocalcemia, seizures, renal failure, bone marrow suppression, and disseminated intravascular coagulation. Chronic use can cause a neuromuscular syndrome resembling polymyositis.

Colchicine metabolism and excretion are impaired in renal or hepatic disease (renal failure may occur), and cumulative toxicity occurs. IV colchicine can cause local phlebitis and skin sloughing.

Drug–Drug Interactions. The effects of colchicine are enhanced by alkalinizing agents such as sodium bicarbonate and inhibited by acidifying agents such as ascorbic acid. Prolonged use of colchicine may reduce GI absorption of vitamin B_{12}.

Drug–Laboratory Test Interactions. Decreased thrombocyte values may be obtained. Colchicine may cause false-positive results when testing urine for hemoglobin or red blood cells.

Precautions and Contraindications. Contraindications include allergy to colchicine, blood dyscrasias, serious GI disorders, liver, renal, or cardiac disorders, pregnancy, and lactation.

Allopurinol

Allopurinol (Zyloprim, Lopurin) inhibits the final steps of uric acid biosynthesis. If an acute attack of gout has occurred, prophylactic treatment may be in order. Prophylactic treatment should include weight and blood-pressure control, a low-purine diet, education about the disease and its complications, and information about avoiding precipitating factors. The choice for pharmacologic prophylactic treatment may be a xanthine oxidase inhibitor (allopurinol) or a uricosuric drug.

Pharmacodynamics. Uric acid is formed by the xanthine oxidase-catalyzed oxidation of hypoxanthine and xanthine. Allopurinol inhibits the xanthine oxidase, which thereby reduces the plasma concentration of uric acid and increases the plasma concentration and renal excretion of uric acid precursors. Allopurinol's action differs from that of uricosuric agents, which lower the serum uric acid level by increasing urinary uric acid excretion. Allopurinol, thus, avoids the hazard of increased renal uric acid excretion posed by uricosuric agents (potential for uric acid calculi).

Pharmacokinetics. Allopurinol is fairly well absorbed after oral administration. Peak action is within 2 hours, and its duration of action is 18 to 30 hours. It is excreted in feces and urine.

Therapeutic Uses. Allopurinol is used for treating primary and secondary gout. It is indicated for uric acid overproducers and clients with contraindications to uricosuric therapy. It may be used in preference to uricosuric agents because it is easy to administer. It can also be used in clients with renal insufficiency, but at a reduced dose.

Dosage and Administration. In gout, the objective is to reach a uric acid level of 6.0 mg/dL. Allopurinol use should not be started during an acute gout attack. Acute attacks can increase in frequency or severity during early months of treatment with allopurinol because urate is mobilized from affected joints. Colchicine may be used with allopurinol prophylactically or, if necessary, in therapeutic doses if an attack occurs.

Dosage must be reduced in clients with renal impairment. If the GFR is 10 to 50 mL/min, the usual dosage is halved (perhaps 150 mg/day).

To prevent hyperuricemia secondary to chemotherapy for neoplasms, the adult dosage is 600 to 800 mg/day for 2 or 3 days before initiation of therapy. For children, the dosage is 150 to 300 mg once daily.

Adverse Reactions. Allopurinol is well tolerated by most clients, but common adverse reactions are headache, dyspepsia, and diarrhea. A pruritic rash develops in about 5% of clients. In a few of these clients, a syndrome of allopurinol hypersensitivity occurs, with fever, acute renal failure, and toxic epidermal necrolysis, possibly caused by allopurinol's active metabolite, oxipurinol, and the drug's prolonged half-life in clients with impaired renal function. If a rash or fever (or both) develops in a client receiving allopurinol, therapy should be discontinued. An important factor in reducing the incidence of the syndrome may be reducing the drug dose in clients with renal insufficiency.

Drug–Drug Interactions. Because allopurinol is an enzyme inhibitor, it delays the inactivation of certain other drugs and leads to increased plasma levels of those drugs and possible toxicity from them (see Chap. 6). This interaction is of concern with oral anticoagulants, mercaptopurine, and azathioprine (derivative of mercaptopurine). Despite allopurinol's use in chemotherapy, with concurrent use of some of the drugs, there is an increased risk of toxicity—for instance, with cyclophosphamide there is an increased risk of bone marrow suppression.

Allopurinol may increase serum levels of theophylline and its toxicity because concurrent use leads to decreased theophylline clearance.

The rate of ampicillin-induced skin rash appears much higher with allopurinol coadministration. This interaction may apply to other penicillins as well.

Drug–Laboratory Test Interactions. Some clients with renal disease experience increased BUN levels during allopurinol administration.

Precautions and Contraindications. Contraindications include allergy to allopurinol and blood dyscrasias. Allopurinol must be given with caution to lactating clients and those with liver disease or renal failure. Clients must be well hydrated: fluid intake should be sufficient to maintain a daily urine volume of more than 2,000 mL. Alkalinization of the urine is also desirable. These actions minimize the risk of calculi formation during allopurinol therapy.

Uricosurics

Uricosuric agents increase the rate of uric acid excretion. The uricosuric agents discussed here are probenecid and sulfinpyrazone (Table 36-7). Clients who should not be given a uricosuric agent include those with a history of nephrolithiasis or poor renal function and those over age 60. After treatment with a uricosuric agent begins and after dose changes, the serum uric acid level should be checked periodically to help determine the optimal dose of the agent. The goal should be to reduce the serum uric acid level to the normal range.

Probenecid

Probenecid (Benemid) was developed as an agent to depress the normally rapid tubular secretion of penicillin, so the available supply of penicillin might be used more thoroughly by the body.

Pharmacodynamics. Probenecid inhibits the transport of organic acids across epithelial barriers, primarily in

---

Table 36-7. Uricosurics

Drug Name	Preparation	Usual Dosage	Adverse Reactions
probenecid (Benemid)	Tablets	2 g/day in divided doses for uricosuric effect; 1 g in single dose half hour before antibiotic when used for sexually transmitted diseases PC: C	GI effects (anorexia, nausea, vomiting), headaches, lightheadedness, sore gums, hypersensitivity, urate nephrolithiasis
sulfinpyrazone (Anturane)	Tablets Capsules	400 mg daily in 2 divided doses PC: C	GI effects (epigastric pain, nausea, vomiting, dyspepsia), blood dyscrasias, urate nephrolithiasis

PC = pregnancy risk category; see Appendix A.

the renal tubule. The only important endogenous compound whose excretion is increased by probenecid is uric acid. Probenecid increases the urinary excretion of uric acid by inhibiting its reabsorption.

Pharmacokinetics. Probenecid is rapidly absorbed after oral administration and reaches a peak action in 2 to 4 hours. When probenecid is used as adjunct therapy with penicillin, penicillin serum levels persist for 8 hours after a dose. It is excreted in urine.

Therapeutic Uses. Probenecid is used to treat gout and, as noted, as an adjunct to penicillin therapy. If penicillin and probenecid are given together, plasma concentrations of the antibiotic are higher and more prolonged than when penicillin is given alone. Probenecid has also been used as an adjunct with some of the cephalosporins. For example, with a client with pelvic inflammatory disease, 2 g of cefoxitin (Mefoxin), a second-generation cephalosporin, may be given IM, plus probenecid 1 g orally in a single dose. This interaction is important in treating sexually transmitted diseases such as gonorrhea, acute pelvic inflammatory disease, and neurosyphilis.

Dosage and Administration. Probenecid is usually started at 0.5 mg/day and increased to a maximum of 1 g two or three times daily, or until the target serum uric acid is reached.

Probenecid and colchicine may be used together. When probenecid is first used, acute attacks of gout may increase in frequency or severity because urates are mobilized. Colchicine may then be added to the regimen. A preparation called ColBenemid is available as tablets containing 0.5 g of probenecid and 0.5 mg of colchicine. The recommended dosage is 1 tablet daily for 1 week, followed by 1 tablet twice a day. ColBenemid can be used in treating chronic gout when it is complicated by frequent, recurrent acute attacks of the disease.

During the initial treatment stages of gout, renal calculi may develop from the mobilization of urates. To prevent this complication, a large amount of fluids should be given. In addition, uric acid tends to crystallize out of acid urine, so alkalinization of the urine is recommended and may be accomplished by the daily use of 3 to 7.5 g of sodium bicarbonate or 7.5 g of potassium citrate. Alkalinization should continue until the serum urate level returns to normal.

Adverse Reactions. Probenecid is usually well tolerated. In a few clients, particularly those receiving higher doses, GI side effects occur, such as anorexia, nausea, and vomiting. Headaches, lightheadedness, sore gums, and hypersensitivity reactions have also occurred. Urate nephrolithiasis may occur.

Drug–Drug Interactions. When probenecid is being used to treat gout, aspirin or any salicylate should not be used simultaneously. The net effect of simultaneous administration is a decrease in the elimination of uric acid.

Probenecid inhibits renal excretion and may increase plasma levels of acyclovir, allopurinol, barbiturates, benzodiazepines, clofibrate, dapsone, methotrexate, NSAIDs, penicillamine, sulfonylureas, and zidovudine. Probenecid can prolong the action of penicillins and cephalosporins, as described above.

Drug–Laboratory Test Interactions. Probenecid may inhibit the renal excretion of phenolsulfonphthalein, 17-ketosteroids, and sulfobromophthalein.

Precautions and Contraindications. Contraindications include allergy to probenecid, blood dyscrasias, uric acid kidney stones, acute gouty attack, and pregnancy. This agent must be used cautiously in clients with peptic ulcer, acute intermittent porphyria, glucose-6-phosphate dehydrogenase (G6PD) deficiency, chronic renal insufficiency, and lactation.

Sulfinpyrazone

Sulfinpyrazone (Anturane) is chemically related to phenylbutazone but lacks its antiinflammatory and analgesic properties.

Pharmacodynamics. Sulfinpyrazone decreases serum uric acid levels by inhibiting the renal tubular reabsorption of uric acid and subsequently increasing its urinary excretion. It also inhibits thromboxane synthesis, so it decreases platelet aggregation, and has been studied as an antithrombotic agent.

Pharmacokinetics. Sulfinpyrazone is well absorbed after oral administration and has a peak action of 1 to 2 hours. After a duration of action of 4 to 10 hours, it is excreted in urine.

Therapeutic Uses. Sulfinpyrazone is used in maintenance therapy for chronic gout and chronic gouty arthritis.

Dosage and Administration. A typical maintenance dose is 400 mg/day, given in two divided doses. A variety of doses are used from the initiation of therapy to the maintenance dose; the dosage is adjusted in accord with serum urate levels. Sulfinpyrazone is given with meals, milk, or antacids.

Adverse Reactions. The most common side effects are GI irritation, manifested as epigastric pain, nausea, vomiting, and dyspepsia. Because reactivation or exacerbation of peptic ulcer has been reported, the drug should be used cautiously in clients with a history of peptic ulcer. Blood dyscrasias have been reported as well, although rarely. Urate nephrolithiasis may occur.

Drug–Drug Interactions. Sulfinpyrazone may displace sulfonylureas from protein binding and increase the risk of hypoglycemia. The antiprothrombin activity of oral anticoagulants may be enhanced. Sulfinpyrazone's uricosuric effect may be reduced by concurrent use of niacin, salicylates, and some of the other NSAIDs. The clearance of theophylline and verapamil may be increased, thus lowering their plasma levels.

Drug–Laboratory Test Interactions. Sulfinpyrazone decreases urinary excretion of aminohippuric acid and phenolsulfonphthalein.

Precautions and Contraindications. Contraindications include allergy to sulfinpyrazone, phenylbutazone, or other pyrazoles, blood dyscrasias, and peptic ulcer or symptoms of GI inflammation. Sulfinpyrazone must be used cautiously in pregnancy and lactation. Increased fluid intake and alkalinization of the urine are recommended to minimize the renal deposition of urate during the first few weeks of therapy to prevent renal calculi. The drug should be used with caution in clients with impaired renal function or a history of renal calculi. It should not be used if the GFR is less than 50% of normal.

■ SUMMARY

The inflammatory process consists of multiple physiologic responses to a stimulus. Antiinflammatory agents are used to manage inflammation that has deleterious effects. At times, high body temperature or fever, as one of the components of the inflammatory response, may damage the body. For the most part, the agents discussed in this chapter have antiinflammatory, analgesic, and antipyretic properties. The primary mechanism by which they create their effects is the inhibition of prostaglandin synthesis. The main NSAIDs are the salicylates, anthranilic acid derivatives, indole and indene acetic acids, propionic acid derivatives or arylpropionic acids, heteroaryl acetic acids, enolic acids or oxicams, and alkanones. Related agents include paraaminophenol derivatives and gold compounds.

Gout, a disorder related to the deposition of urate crystals in joints, may be treated with colchicine, allopurinol, probenecid, or sulfinpyrazone.

Some of the agents used for inflammation, namely aspirin and acetaminophen, are easily available to the public. Because of their wide use, there is a high incidence of problems, ranging from adverse reactions to toxicity from overdosage.

❖ NURSING MANAGEMENT: CLIENT RECEIVING ANTIPYRETIC AND ANTIINFLAMMATORY DRUGS

Many agents discussed in this chapter have serious or toxic side effects. For example, most NSAIDs have two common adverse effects to a greater or lesser degree: disturbances of the GI and renal systems. (See the Example of Nursing Process for Gold Therapy.)

NURSING PROCESS
ASSESSMENT

Because of the potential for hypersensitivity reactions to NSAIDs, the nursing assessment must include a history of allergy or sensitivity to the prescribed medications or similar ones. Clients sensitive to aspirin, for example, may be sensitive to any of the NSAIDs. The nurse must also determine whether the client has a history of GI or renal complaints and must learn what other medications he or she is taking (eg, ulcerogenic drugs or drugs known to interact with the prescribed medication).

When the client is on prolonged drug therapy (eg, for a chronic disease such as arthritis), laboratory tests may need to be performed regularly. In some cases, salicylate levels may need to be checked. Clients receiving oral anticoagulants should expect to have frequent prothrombin time assessments when any NSAIDs are used. Likewise, clients with preexisting renal disease may need periodic renal function tests. Also, if a drug is known to cause bone marrow depression, determination of the client's hematologic profile (eg, white blood cell count, hemoglobin, hematocrit) is warranted.

The assessment of fever requires accurate and consistent monitoring of body temperature. Procedures used for measuring temperature should include safeguards for accuracy. For example, oral temperatures should not be taken immediately after the client ingests very warm or very cold foods or beverages. Similarly, rectal temperatures should not be taken immediately after the administration of enemas. Temperature records should denote the body site where the temperature was measured and the type of instrument used, as well as the time: these are all variables in temperature fluctuations.

NURSING DIAGNOSIS

Many clients receiving the antiinflammatory drugs featured in this chapter have osteoarthritis, RA, gout, or fever associated with infection. Nursing diagnoses that might apply to antiinflammatory or antipyretic drug therapy may include:

- Ineffective Individual Management of Therapeutic Regimen, related to potential adverse effects of NSAIDs
- Risk for Impaired Skin Integrity, related to possible photosensitivity or allergic skin reactions
- Impaired Tissue Integrity, related to potential for GI, renal, or hepatic impairment
- Knowledge Deficit, related to lack of exposure to drug therapy, disease process, and adverse drug effects

PLANNING

Goals for drug therapy may include diminished pain, decreased inflammation, increased mobility, satisfactory self-medication and self-care, prevention or reduction of complications from adverse drug effects, enhanced knowledge of therapeutic regimen, and prompt detection and treatment of adverse reactions.

Example of Nursing Process for Gold Therapy

The client is a 48-year-old housewife who has had rheumatoid arthritis for 15 years. She experiences fatigue and muscle pain and aching, as well as joint pain and stiffness. Her knees are severely involved, as are her feet, hands, and wrists. Her range of motion in the affected joints is decreased and she depends on a wheelchair whenever she is outside her home.

The client was maintained on aspirin until adverse reactions necessitated its discontinuation. She has been admitted to the hospital for reevaluation and is going to start weekly aurothioglucose injections.

The client and her husband live in a city apartment with their three children, aged 12, 15, and 18. Her husband has a new boss at work and seems more dissatisfied with his job now than before this management change. The children challenge their parents on a variety of age-related issues. The client has made reference to feeling overwhelmed at home.

Assessment Data

Diagnosis of rheumatoid arthritis for 15 years

No longer able to use ASA.

To be started on aurothioglucose injections.

Feels overwhelmed with family-related issues.

Nursing Diagnosis	Intervention	Goals and Outcomes
Knowledge Deficit, concerning introduction of new therapeutic agent	**Explain** that complete blood count and liver and renal function tests are obtained before first injection (and periodically thereafter) to detect evidence of complication.	The client will verbalize signs and symptoms of complications that must be reported. The client will have laboratory tests done before receiving gold injections initially and thereafter as ordered.
	Teach client to watch for a variety of complications, including dermatologic ones.	
	Explain that signs of infection need to be reported to the prescriber.	
	Suggest client avoid exposure to sunlight because dermatologic drug effects may be increased.	
	Explain importance of excellent oral hygiene to reduce risk of stomatitis and other mucous membrane adverse reactions.	
	Explain the nitritoid reaction and that first doses of the drug will be low to evaluate for reaction to the drug.	
Chronic Pain, related to inflammation of joints secondary to rheumatoid arthritis	**Assess** for factors that seem to alleviate and aggravate pain.	The client will experience decreased discomfort as evidenced by verbalizing that pain is tolerable and by exhibiting relaxed facial expression and body positioning.
	Provide nonpharmacologic measures for pain relief (eg, backrub, position change, warm and cold packs as ordered, relaxation techniques, restful environment, diversional activities).	
	Monitor for therapeutic and nontherapeutic effects of agents such as NSAIDs that are ordered.	
Family Coping, Ineffective, related to stress of chronic illness and situational stressors of family members	**Listen** empathetically.	
	Help client and significant others express their needs, fears, and feelings.	
	Assist client and significant others to identify community sources of support able to assist them with coping.	

INTERVENTION

Because of the adverse effects of NSAIDs on the GI system, certain nursing interventions are necessary. In general, medications should be given with milk or food, or immediately after meals. The client should report any GI complaints. The prescriber may reduce the dosage, change the prescription, or order antacids in certain cases.

Diabetic clients receiving some of these agents may require adjustment in the dosage of their insulin or oral hypoglycemic agent. These clients should perform glucose assessment tests daily and report any changes, as well as any episodes of hypoglycemia.

Clients who receive drugs to control fever should be observed closely and assessed carefully. These drugs suppress both the fever and also the inflammation and pain that accompany the febrile illness, so clients feel better than they actually are. It may be more difficult to prevent overexertion or inappropriate activity. Temperature should be checked 1 hour after administering antipyretic medication to assess the response to drug therapy.

Usually the client's baseline temperature is not known because the fever is established before the client enters the healthcare system. The nurse should consider the client's age when determining probable norms. In children, temperatures of 39°C (102.5°F) may be acceptable, because children normally have higher temperature peaks than adults. However, a child with a history of febrile seizures requires maintenance at a lower temperature to avoid triggering seizure activity. Clients or their relatives may know what the normal temperature is. It is usually undesirable to lower temperature to normal ranges, because this deprives the client of the beneficial effects of fever and makes it more difficult to determine remission of the febrile illness.

Client Education. Clients with arthritis must be advised that it may take several days or even weeks for the NSAID to produce its therapeutic effect (see the Critical Thinking Challenge: Case Analysis).

Clients must be informed of both the beneficial and the harmful effects of fever. The importance of a daily intake of at least 3,000 mL of fluids (for adults) should be stressed to prevent dehydration. Clients should also be advised to seek medical help without delay when standard antipyretic remedies do not produce prompt and lasting improvement. A temperature above 102°F (38.5°C) or an elevation that persists for more than 48 hours should be evaluated by a healthcare professional. Clients should be warned not to increase the dose of antipyretic analgesics above the recommended levels to try to manage fever, because toxicity may develop.

Acetaminophen, ibuprofen, and aspirin are commonly used nonprescription preparations and as such are not regarded as dangerous. The danger is that clients will misuse these preparations or use them inappropriately. Education can play a pivotal role in preventing misuse. Clients usually have misconceptions or questions about these products and their advertising claims. Because of the high incidence of toxicity with some of these agents, the nurse should take particular care in educating clients fully about this potential danger. Also, proper storage should be stressed to prevent small children from gaining access to them.

These medications frequently cause renal side effects. Adverse reactions are more likely to occur in clients with preexisting renal dysfunction. The nurse should explain the reason for any renal function tests ordered. The client should be advised to report any edema, dysuria, hematuria, or other urinary symptoms experienced while taking NSAIDs.

The client should learn to recognize the CNS side effects of NSAIDs. If such neurologic effects as drowsiness or dizziness occur, the client should avoid driving and other activities that require alertness.

OUTCOME EVALUATION

For the client being treated for fever, data required for evaluation include vital signs (especially temperature), perception of comfort or discomfort, and the presence or absence of seizures or other evidence of impaired tissue integrity related to hyperthermia. For the client with pain, data that would indicate drug efficacy include verbalization of pain relief, relaxed facial expression and body positioning, increased participation in activities, statements of feeling rested, and absence of frequent yawning and irritability. Examples of data that would indicate the drug was not causing adverse reactions include absence of diarrhea, nausea, vomiting, blood in the stool, and abdominal pain, as well as normal BUN, serum creatinine, white blood cell count, hemoglobin, and hematocrit.

CRITICAL THINKING CHALLENGE
Case Analysis

Mrs. Peters, age 70, has rheumatoid arthritis. She also has diabetes mellitus, for which she takes an oral hypoglycemic agent, and hypertension, for which she takes a thiazide diuretic and a beta-adrenergic blocking agent. She had been taking aspirin for the arthritis, but the prescriber is recommending a change to ibuprofen.

1. Mrs. Peters is hesitant to take ibuprofen and asks if she could take acetaminophen instead. How would you explain the mechanism of action of NSAIDs to help her understand why acetaminophen is not the drug of choice?
2. Mrs. Peters asks if she can still take aspirin when she has a headache. What should be your response, and why?
3. What problems may occur when Mrs. Peters begins to take ibuprofen regularly?

❖ CHECKLIST OF NURSING ACTIONS

- ❏ Assess clients for hypersensitivity or allergy to the selected NSAID or to any NSAID.
- ❏ Determine if the client has asthma, a history of GI problems, or a history of renal disease.
- ❏ Ascertain what other medications the client is taking, as many drugs interact with NSAIDs.
- ❏ Discuss adherence to the drug regimen, explaining that regular intake of the drug is necessary to sustain the antiinflammatory effects.
- ❏ Advise taking the NSAID with milk or meals to reduce gastric irritation.
- ❏ Advise the client that in many situations, the therapeutic effects of the NSAID will take weeks to be achieved.
- ❏ When an NSAID is ordered for antipyresis, monitor the client's temperature and general condition closely.
- ❏ Remind clients to tell other healthcare providers about the NSAID being taken to avoid drug interactions.
- ❏ Inform the client about possible adverse reactions.
- ❏ Advise the client to report any symptoms of GI irritation not relieved by the prescribed GI-protective protocol.
- ❏ Discuss the need for regular medical supervision so that the dosage can be adjusted on the basis of the client's condition and drug response. Certain laboratory tests should be performed regularly.
- ❏ Teach the client about the proper use of OTC NSAIDs. Discuss their advertising claims.

References

Brooks PM, Day RO. (1991). Nonsteroidal antiinflammatory drugs: Differences and similarities. *N Engl J Med, 324*(24), 1716–1723.

Cashman J, McAnulty G. (1995). Nonsteroidal anti-inflammatory drugs in perisurgical pain management. *Drugs, 49*(1), 51–70.

Copstead LC. (1995). *Perspectives on pathophysiology.* Philadelphia: WB Saunders Co.

Cryer B, Feldman M. (1994). Strategies for preventing NSAID-induced ulcers. *Drug Therapy, 7,* 25–32.

deLeeuw PW. (1996). Nonsteroidal anti-inflammatory drugs and hypertension. *Drugs, 51*(2), 179–187.

Hardman JG, Limbird LE, Molinoff PB, et al., eds. (1996). *Goodman and Gilman's The pharmacological basis of therapeutics,* 9th ed. New York: McGraw-Hill.

Konstan MW, Byard PJ, Hoppel C, Davis PB. (1995). Effect of high-dose ibuprofen in patients with cystic fibrosis. *N Engl J Med, 332*(13), 848–854.

Lanza FL. (1993). Gastrointestinal toxicity of newer NSAIDs. *Am J Gastroenterol, 88*(9), 1318.

Mullins MD, Murray JJ, Serafin WE. (1994). Severe bronchospasm: When aspirin's the cause. *Drug Therapy, 6,* 20–28.

Olkkola KT, Brunetto AV, Matilla MJ. (1994). Pharmacokinetics of oxicam nonsteroidal anti-inflammatory agents. *Clin Pharmacokinetics, 26*(2), 107–117.

Olin BR, ed. (1995). *Drug facts and comparisons.* St. Louis: Facts and Comparisons.

Rakel RE, ed. (1996). *Conn's current therapy.* Philadelphia: WB Saunders.

Sager DS, Bennett RM. (1992). Individualizing the risk/benefit ratio of NSAIDs in older patients. *Geriatrics, 47*(8), 24–31.

Slotkoff AT, Katz P. (1994). Approach to the patient with RA. *Adv Intern Med, 39,* 197–240.

Visentin M, Salmina M, Tacconi MT. (1995). Reye's and Reye-like syndromes, drug-related diseases? (Causative agents, etiology, pathogenesis, and therapeutic approaches). *Drug Metab Rev, 27*(3), 517–539.

Bibliography

Adam D, Stankov G. (1994). Treatment of fever in childhood. *Eur J Pediatr, 153,* 394–402.

Brien J. (1993). Ototoxicity associated with salicylates. *Drug Safety, 9*(2), 143.

Hoppman RA, Peden IG, Ober SK. (1991). Central nervous system side effects of nonsteroidal anti-inflammatory drugs. *Arch Intern Med, 151,* 309–313.

Sandler DP, Burr FR, Weinberg CR. (1991). Non-steroidal anti-inflammatory drugs and the risks for chronic renal disease. *Ann Intern Med, 115,* 165–172.

For more information and sample tests and activities, refer to Chapter 36 in the Student Workbook for Clinical Pharmacology and Nursing Management, 5th edition, available through your bookstore.

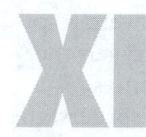

XI

Drugs Affecting Other Body Systems

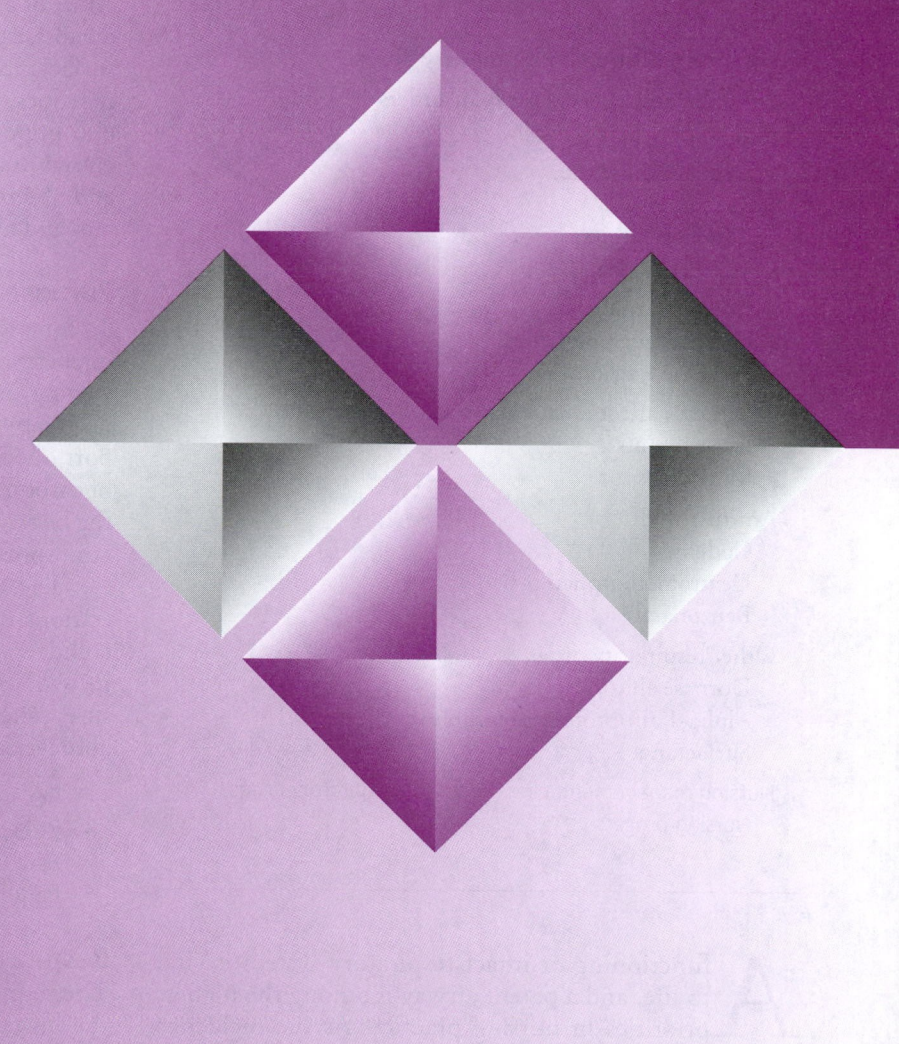

37

Drugs That Affect the Respiratory System

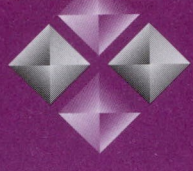

A functioning or intact respiratory system is vital to life, and a patent airway is among the highest priorities in nursing practice. As the incidence of respiratory disease continues to rise, more nursing functions are necessary for respiratory support. Moreover, as health care shifts from institutional to commu-nity settings, it is common for people with severe respi-ratory disease to be cared for at home with oxygen ther-apy and ventilatory support and other modalities.

The processes involved in respiratory disorders are complicated, diverse, and interrelated. For clients and their families, respiratory distress and failure are ex-tremely frightening. The client experiencing air hunger is usually in a panic, which increases the demand for oxygen. The situation may be life-threatening, and the nurse must respond quickly in a calm, efficient, and re-assuring manner. Psychological support is as important as physical care.

Physiology

The effort or cost of breathing is directly related to the elastic properties of the lung, the anatomy of the thorax, diaphragm, and abdomen, and the degree of pathology or resistance to air flow throughout the respiratory tract. This chapter presents the basic information needed to understand pharmacologic treatment and supportive res-piratory care for clients with chronic bronchitis, emphy-sema, or asthma. Drug agents discussed include broncho-dilators, expectorants, mucolytics, antitussives, aerosols, and surfactants. Antihistamines, corticosteroids, antibiotics, narcotics, muscle relaxants, and respiratory stimulants are also important drugs in respiratory therapy but are dis-cussed in depth in other chapters (refer to Chaps. 16, 34, and 35 for information about the autonomic nervous sys-tem and allergic and immune responses, respectively).

Purpose of Respiration

To function, the human body requires a constant source of energy. The energy comes from chemical reactions in-volving oxygen. A normal healthy respiratory system is necessary for this process. The process involves the trans-port of oxygen from the air to tissue cells and the export of carbon dioxide (CO_2) from the cells to the air outside the body. This exchange of oxygen and CO_2 between the atmosphere and the body's cells is called *respiration*.

The air that is exchanged contains varying concen-trations of different gases. Each gas has molecules that collide with molecules of other gases, and each gas exerts its own pressure on the remaining molecules. This pres-sure, called *partial pressure*, is abbreviated as P. Common abbreviations in respiratory terminology include:

- P_{O_2}: partial pressure of oxygen
- P_{CO_2}: partial pressure of carbon dioxide
- Pa_{O_2}: partial pressure of arterial oxygen
- Pa_{CO_2}: partial pressure of arterial carbon dioxide

Respiratory Structures

The respiratory system consists of the upper airway and the lower airway. Upper airway structures include the nose, mouth, pharynx, and larynx. Lower airway struc-tures include the tracheobronchial tree, consisting of the trachea, bronchi, and alveoli. The trachea and tracheobronchial tree are a series of bifurcating tubes that become smaller as they near the alveoli, which are tiny pocketlike air sacs (Fig. 37-1).

Filtration and Protection

Besides providing the passageway through which oxygen is exchanged for carbon dioxide, the airways warm and filter the air that enters the lungs. They also expel pathogens and other irritants from the airways. The bronchi and the respiratory tract are lined with a fine membrane and with brushlike cilia. These structures make up the mucociliary system. This system moves mucus and secretions up the tree toward the nasopharynx, where the secretions can be eliminated from the respiratory system by expectoration or swallowing. What controls the cilia is not fully known. They move at a rate set by their metabolic state—not by the nervous system, but by hormones and metabolic regulators. The rate is partially determined by the supply of adenosine triphosphate (ATP).

Goblet cells lie within the membrane (epithelium). They continually produce mucus to keep the respiratory tract moist. The composition of mucus is 84% to 94% water; other constituents include carbohydrates, lipids, and protein components. Normally, adults produce about 100 mL of mucus a day.

A layer of mucus covers the upper and lower airway as far as the terminal bronchiole. This mucus blanket, which has a sol layer and a gel layer, lines the trachea, bronchi, and larger bronchioles. The deeper sol layer is watery. Its low viscosity lets the cilia move freely, propelling material up to the overlying or surface gel layer, which is viscous and protects the cilia from dehydration, particles, and toxic gases. Smoke, infection, and pollutants decrease mucociliary transport, however.

Gas Exchange

The diffusion of gases occurs in the alveoli through the alveolar/capillary membrane. While oxygen passes through the membrane to the blood, waste CO_2 diffuses out.

Usually, respiration is passive and occurs involuntarily by way of pressure changes in the thoracic cavity. This allows air to enter and leave the respiratory tract by diffusing across the alveolar/capillary membrane. It also promotes a balance in the amount of oxygen consumed by the cells to meet energy demands and the amount of CO_2 given off by the cells. However, if the body's oxygen requirements change, respiration may become active and voluntary. This occurs by making an adjustment in the amount of oxygen supplied, which is accomplished by forceful active inspiration and expiration. For respiration to occur, the respiratory, neuromuscular, and circulatory systems must all be intact and able to interact. In addition, hemoglobin must be sufficient to carry the oxygen.

Pathophysiology

When disease strikes the respiratory system, the body's ability to maintain a supply of oxygen to meet energy demands may be impaired. The result could be *hypoxia* (decreased amount or availability of oxygen to the cells or tissues of the body) or *hypoxemia* (reduced oxygen in the body fluids, especially in the arterial blood). Disease may also affect the ability of the respiratory system to remove CO_2, resulting in *hypercapnia* (elevated levels of CO_2 in the body fluids, particularly at the cellular level). Much of respiratory therapy is directed at improving the exchange and movement of air by treating bronchoconstriction and promoting bronchodilation.

Bronchoconstriction

Bronchoconstriction occurs in various respiratory diseases (eg, asthma). The walls of the bronchi are mainly smooth muscle, and the walls of the bronchioles are almost entirely smooth muscle. Under normal conditions, air flows easily through these respiratory structures with little resistance. Direct control of the bronchioles by

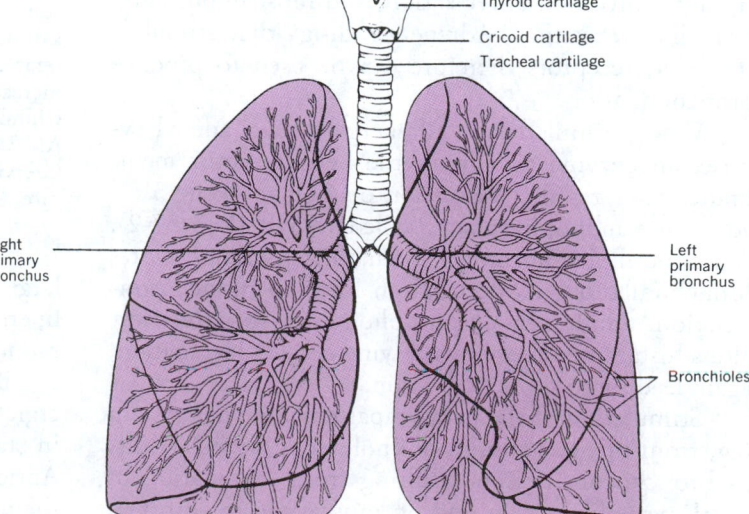

Figure 37-1. Anterior view of the larynx, trachea, and bronchial tree.

Thyroid cartilage
Cricoid cartilage
Tracheal cartilage
Right primary bronchus
Left primary bronchus
Bronchioles

sympathetic nerve fibers is weak. However, the bronchial tree is exposed to circulating norepinephrine and epinephrine, which are released by sympathetic stimulation of the adrenal medullae and produce bronchial dilation. On the other hand, some parasympathetic nerve fibers in the lung parenchyma secrete acetylcholine. When these nerves are activated, mild to moderate bronchial constriction occurs. Histamine and slow-reactive substance of anaphylaxis (SRS-A) are also formed in the lungs. These substances cause bronchoconstriction.

Irritants such as smoke, dust, smog, and sulfur dioxide can activate parasympathetic nerve reflexes, causing bronchoconstriction. In addition, certain respiratory diseases cause bronchoconstriction. Airway resistance increases as small bronchioles become occluded, and they constrict easily because they contain a high percentage of smooth muscle.

Bronchodilation

Bronchial smooth muscle tone is controlled by the tonic cholinergic (vagal) and the inhibitory (sympathetic) systems. The sympathetic nervous system plays a major role in determining the diameter of the bronchi. Sympathetic nerve endings secrete synaptic neurotransmitter substances. The endings that secrete norepinephrine are said to be *adrenergic*. (Drugs that mimic the action of sympathetic activity are called sympathomimetic or adrenergic drugs or catecholamines.)

Adrenergic activity affects two types of receptors: alpha and beta. Two types of beta-adrenergic receptors exist: $beta_1$ and $beta_2$. $Beta_1$-adrenergic receptors act chiefly at cardiac sites. $Beta_2$ receptors are present in the glands and smooth muscle and mucosal vessels of the bronchial tree. Adrenergic stimulation of $beta_2$ receptors results in bronchodilation.

Stimulation of alpha receptors produces vasoconstriction, smooth muscle contraction, intestinal relaxation, pilomotor contraction, and pupillary dilation. Stimulation of beta receptors leads to vasodilation in the muscles, cardioacceleration, increased myocardial strength, myometrial relaxation, and most importantly bronchial relaxation. Adrenergic drugs that stimulate the $beta_2$ receptors therefore can be used to produce bronchodilation.

When stimulated by adrenergic drugs, adenyl cyclase, an enzyme present in the $beta_2$-receptor membrane, catalyzes the conversion of ATP to cyclic $3',5'$ adenosine monophosphate, called cAMP (Fig. 37-2). An intracellular hormonal mediator, cAMP promotes bronchodilation; its destruction leads to bronchoconstriction. Inhibition of phosphodiesterases effectively alters histamine release by delaying cAMP degradation, again leading to bronchodilation.

Stimulation of the parasympathetic nervous system (eg, from noxious stimuli or cholinergic drugs) results in bronchoconstriction resulting from stimulation of vagal nerve fibers that end on muscarinic receptors in

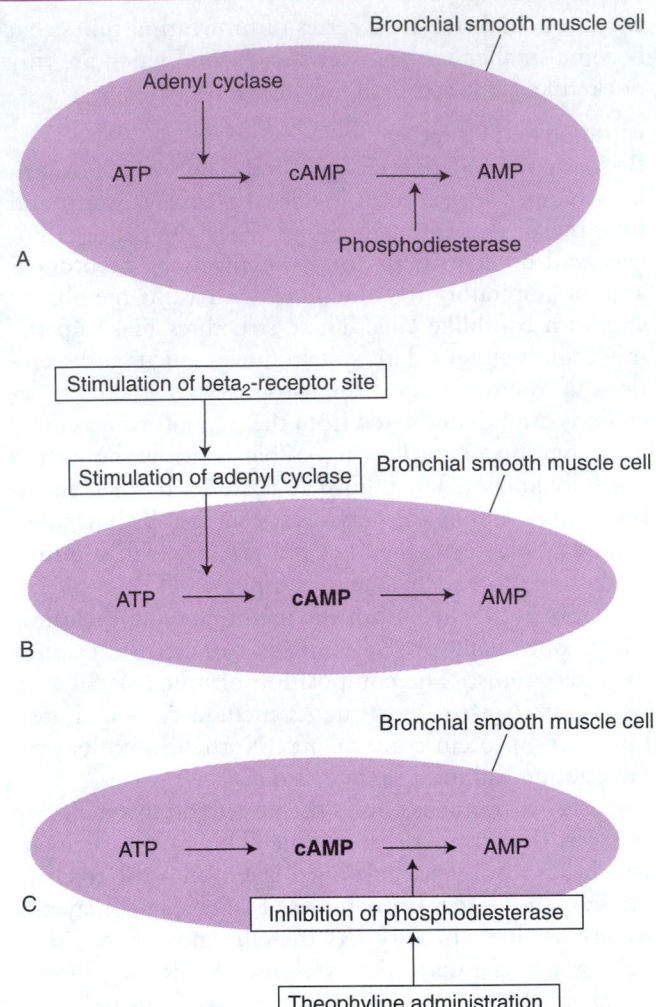

Figure 37-2. Factors in bronchodilation. **(A)** Sympathetic mechanisms controlling bronchial muscle tone. The enzyme adenyl cyclase is the catalyst for the conversion of ATP to cAMP. The enzyme phosphodiesterase breaks down cAMP into AMP. Increased levels of cAMP result in relaxation of bronchial smooth muscle. Decreased levels of cAMP lead to spasm of susceptible bronchial smooth muscle. **(B)** Bronchial muscle receptors are called $beta_2$-receptor sites. Stimulation of these sites results in stimulation of the enzyme adenyl cyclase. This, in turn, produces an increased level of cAMP, which results in bronchodilation. **(C)** Administration of the methylxanthine drug theophylline inhibits the enzyme phosphodiesterase. This inhibits the breakdown of cAMP and results in increased levels of cAMP and bronchodilation. ATP, adenosine triphosphate; cAMP, cyclic $3'5'$ adenosine monophosphate; AMP, adenosine monophosphate. (From: Barnhart MP, Czervinske MP. [1995]. Perinatal and pediatric respiratory care. Philadelphia: WB Saunders.)

large airway smooth muscle (Stimson, 1995). The cholinergic vagal effects are mediated by cyclic guanosine monophosphate (cGMP; Fig. 37-3).

Blockage of the cholinergic system with anticholinergic agents (eg, atropine, ipratropium bromide) results in stabilization of the mast cells and bronchodilation. Anticholinergic agents compete with acetylcholine at the muscarinic receptors. In the past, atropine was used

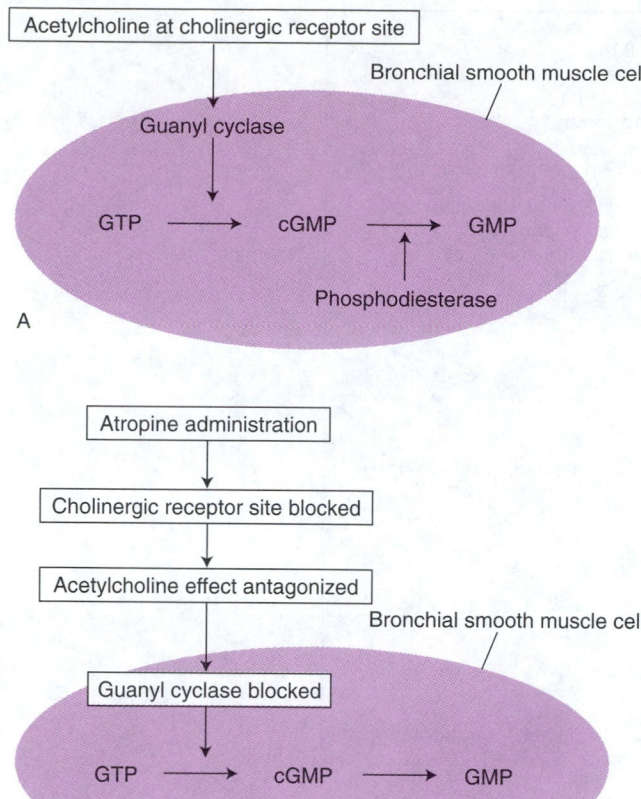

Figure 37-3. **(A)** Parasympathetic mechanisms controlling bronchial smooth muscle tone. Stimulation of the parasympathetic system causes the release of acetylcholine at the cholinergic receptor site. The acetylcholine stimulates the enzyme guanyl cyclase to convert GTP to cGMP. Phosphodiesterase then breaks down cGMP to GMP. High cGMP levels result in bronchoconstriction. **(B)** Administration of an anticholinergic drug (atropine) antagonizes the acetylcholine effect and prevents cGMP from forming. This relieves the bronchoconstriction. GTP, guanosine triphosphate; cGMP, cyclic 3'5' guanosine monophosphate; GMP, guanosine monophosphate. (From: Barnhart MP, Czervinske MP. [1995]. Perinatal and pediatric respiratory care: Philadelphia: WB Saunders.)

to treat asthma; however, its use was limited by unpleasant adverse reactions and the belief by some prescribers that the inhibition and drying of secretions in the upper and lower respiratory tract was potentially dangerous for clients with chronic bronchitis and emphysema. Continuing findings indicate that the bronchodilatory effect of inhaled or intravenous (IV) anticholinergics (atropine) is equal to and in some cases better than that of beta-adrenergic agents in chronic obstructive pulmonary disease (COPD) and some types of asthma.

Ipratropium bromide, a congener of methylatropine, is inhaled and produces bronchodilation through a local rather than systemic effect. It is a first-line agent in treating clients with COPD. It is as effective as the beta$_2$-adrenergic agonist albuterol in clients with chronic bronchitis, but albuterol is more effective in bronchial asthma.

In short, bronchodilation occurs through one of two mechanisms:

- Increased cAMP (the stimulation of cAMP production or the decrease and prevention of the destruction of cAMP), or
- Decreased cGMP (competitive inhibition of acetylcholine at muscarinic receptors in airway smooth muscle through local effect by ipratropium or systemic effects of atropine).

Disorders of the Respiratory Tract

Among the disorders that may respond to drug treatment are respiratory failure and COPD (chronic bronchitis, emphysema, and bronchial asthma).

Respiratory Failure

Respiratory failure is diagnosed if a client fails to maintain adequate oxygenation or experiences undue retention of CO_2. In respiratory failure, the Pa_{O_2} falls below 55 to 60 mm Hg; the Pa_{CO_2} may be normal or may exceed 50 mm Hg. The pH may be less than 7.25; however, this level may be misleading because kidney compensation in clients with long-standing lung disease may increase the pH. Early signs and symptoms of low Pa_{O_2} levels, or hypoxia, are irritability, hostility, headache, and altered mentation. Later signs and symptoms are tachycardia, dyspnea, muscle weakness, double vision, judgmental errors, loss of coordination, arrhythmias, apnea, cyanosis, and coma.

The symptoms of rising CO_2 levels may be difficult to differentiate from low levels of oxygen. CO_2 is a potent vasodilator, and the client's skin may assume a reddish hue. Clients also complain of headache, insomnia, and irritability. As the Pa_{CO_2} rises, the client cannot concentrate, becomes drowsy, appears intoxicated, and ultimately may become comatose.

Chronic Obstructive Pulmonary Disease

Chronic obstructive pulmonary disease occurs when the outflow of air from the lungs or the exchange of gases at the alveolar level is impeded. Obstruction and respiratory failure can result from changes in the airways, spasm within the airways, changes in the amount and viscosity of mucous secretions, or any combination of these factors: in short, increased airway and tissue resistance and decreased lung compliance.

Three common serious obstructive pulmonary diseases are chronic bronchitis, pulmonary emphysema, and bronchial asthma. Bronchitis (thick secretions, infections, and bronchospasm) or emphysema (overinflation of the lungs, collapse of airways, and dyspnea) rarely occur singly; they usually occur in combination.

Chronic Bronchitis

In chronic bronchitis, the expiratory air flow is impeded because of airway obstruction from mucous plugs and

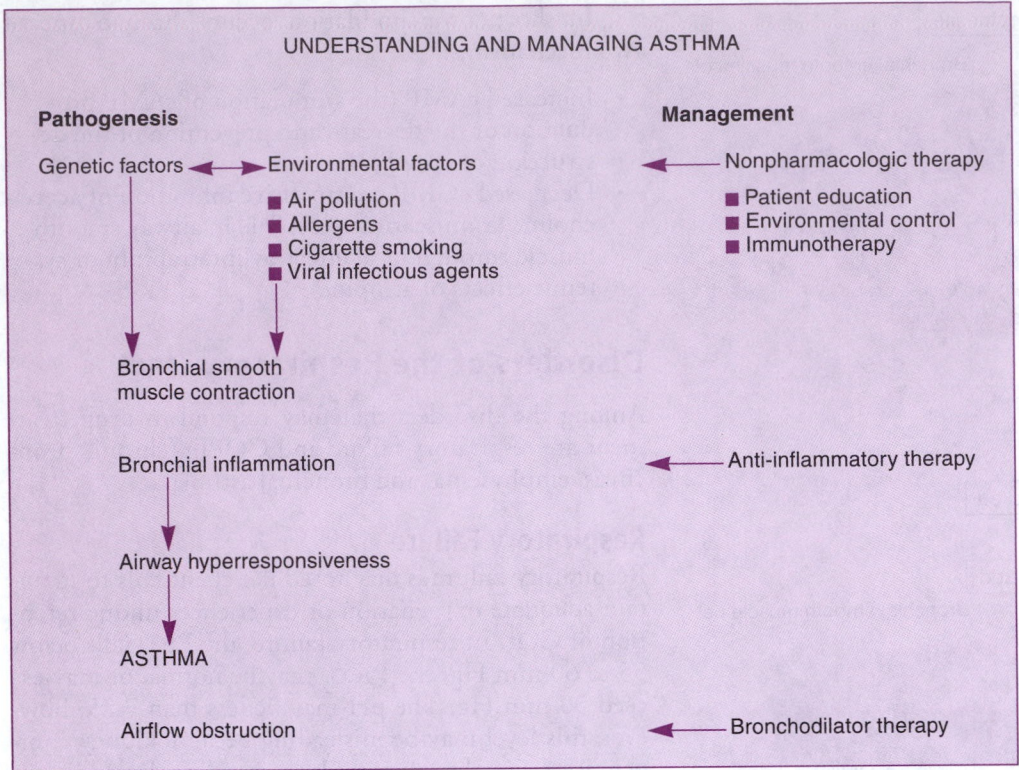

Figure 37-4. Overview of general approach to asthma management. Initial measures include identification of genetic and environmental triggers and avoidance if possible of allergens. Treatment aims include relieving bronchial inflammation with antiinflammatory drugs, such as corticosteroids, and easing air flow with bronchodilator drugs. (From National Institutes of Health, Expert Panel Report. National Asthma Education Program. [1991]. Guidelines for the diagnosis and management of asthma. Bethesda, MD: NIH publication No. 3042.)

excessive production of mucus. The client complains of a long-standing productive cough (at least 3 months a year over a 2-year period). Hypertrophy of the mucous glands occurs, and excessive mucous production results from infection or chemical irritation. Chronic inflammation and slowed ciliary function are characteristic. These decrease the client's ability to eliminate secretions.

Smoke, chemical irritants, dust, fumes, or cold air may contribute to bronchospasm, as does acetylcholine, serotonin, and histamine activity. Therapy involves removing the irritants (including cigarette smoke), rest, adequate hydration, antibiotics, bronchodilation, expectorants, and pulmonary hygiene.

Emphysema
Derived from Greek words meaning "to puff up," emphysema is marked by the enlargement and dilation of the air spaces distal to the terminal bronchioles. This phenomenon destroys the alveolar walls. The destruction of the elastic alveolar tissue leads to loss of elastic recoil, loss of tone, hyperinflation of the affected alveoli, and impaired two-way air flow. Air is trapped, and the lungs puff up as the residual volume increases. Affected clients have a barrel chest, use pursed-lip breathing, and are dyspneic. They use accessory muscles for inspiration. Movement of the chest and diaphragm de-

creases. Clubbing of the fingers and cyanosis may be apparent. Pulmonary hypertension with cor pulmonale may develop and lead to congestive heart failure. Hemoglobin and hematocrit values may rise in a compensatory mechanism as the PaO_2 decreases and the $PaCO_2$ increases.

Therapy is palliative and relies on improving air flow, eliminating respiratory tract infections and irritants (including cigarette smoke), removing secretions, and improving respiratory function with bronchodilator therapy.

Bronchial Asthma
Asthma affects 5% to 10% of the population, or an estimated 10 to 15 million people in the United States. It is the most common chronic illness in children, and African Americans are twice as likely as Caucasians to be hospitalized with asthma (Guidelines, 1991). Despite significant advances in treatment and therapy, the morbidity and mortality rates from asthma are rising and are unacceptably high. To determine the best treatment approaches (Figs. 37-4 and 37-5), consensus statements have been developed to provide guidelines for asthma treatment (National Asthma Education Program, 1991; National Asthma Education and Prevention Program, 1997; International Consensus Report, 1992).

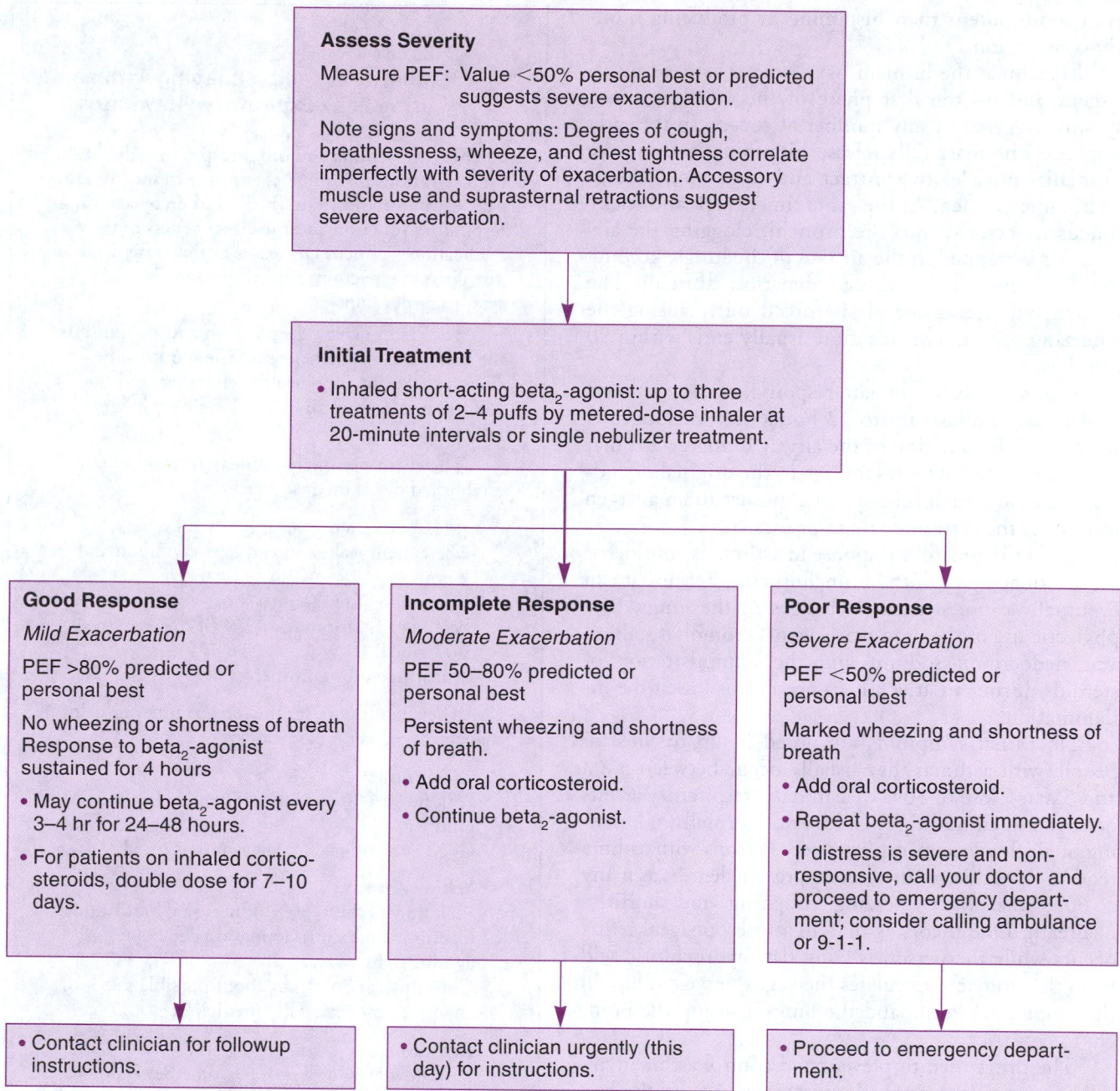

Assess Severity

Measure PEF: Value <50% personal best or predicted suggests severe exacerbation.

Note signs and symptoms: Degrees of cough, breathlessness, wheeze, and chest tightness correlate imperfectly with severity of exacerbation. Accessory muscle use and suprasternal retractions suggest severe exacerbation.

Initial Treatment

• Inhaled short-acting beta$_2$-agonist: up to three treatments of 2–4 puffs by metered-dose inhaler at 20-minute intervals or single nebulizer treatment.

Good Response

Mild Exacerbation

PEF >80% predicted or personal best

No wheezing or shortness of breath Response to beta$_2$-agonist sustained for 4 hours

• May continue beta$_2$-agonist every 3–4 hr for 24–48 hours.

• For patients on inhaled corticosteroids, double dose for 7–10 days.

Incomplete Response

Moderate Exacerbation

PEF 50–80% predicted or personal best

Persistent wheezing and shortness of breath.

• Add oral corticosteroid.

• Continue beta$_2$-agonist.

Poor Response

Severe Exacerbation

PEF <50% predicted or personal best

Marked wheezing and shortness of breath

• Add oral corticosteroid.

• Repeat beta$_2$-agonist immediately.

• If distress is severe and non-responsive, call your doctor and proceed to emergency department; consider calling ambulance or 9-1-1.

• Contact clinician for followup instructions.

• Contact clinician urgently (this day) for instructions.

• Proceed to emergency department.

Patients at high risk of asthma-related death should receive immediate clinical attention after initial treatment. Additional therapy may be required.

Figure 37-5. Management of Asthma Exacerbations: Home Treatment* (From: National Asthma Education and Prevention Program. [1997]. Expert Panel Report II: Guidelines for the diagnosis and management of asthma. Washington, DC: National Heart, Lung, and Blood Institute, National Institutes of Health. Internet www.nhlbi.nih.gov/nhlbi/nhlbi.htm)

Bronchial asthma typically occurs in people allergic or hypersensitive to a particular foreign substance (eg, ragweed, pollen, cat dander). The person forms an abnormal type of antibody (a protein, such as IgE) in response to the antigen (foreign substance). The antibodies attach themselves to mast cells beneath the bronchial epithelium in close association with the bronchioles and small bronchi. They are abundant in the airway structures.

When the antigen reacts with the antibody through a degranulation process, the cells swell and rupture, releasing histamine and SRS-A. Bradykinin, acetylcholine, serotonin, and prostaglandins are also released. SRS-A prolongs contraction of the smooth muscle in the bronchi. Histamine release then leads to bronchospasm, a significant increase in the production of mucus, and localized bronchial swelling and edema. SRS-A is composed of cysteinyl-containing leukotrienes, which are even more potent than histamine in producing bronchoconstriction.

In asthma, the bronchi have been sensitized by allergens and, in the first phase of the attack, go into spasms triggered by any number of causes. In the early response, the mast cells release histamine, causing the bronchial muscles to contract and the airway linings to become swollen. At the same time, thick and sticky mucus is secreted into the bronchi, clogging the airway. Air is trapped in the air sacs of the lungs, keeping the CO_2 there and making exhalation difficult. The bronchi vibrate as the air is forced out, causing the wheezing sound. This reaction usually ends within 90 minutes.

A second phase, the late response, occurs within 3 to 4 hours and lasts up to 12 hours or even longer. A sustained inflammation of the airway lining occurs that makes the tissue hyperresponsive to the original offending substance. Each subsequent exposure to an allergen intensifies the early and late responses.

The inflammatory response in asthma is considered more damaging than the bronchospasm, because it can eventually cause structural changes in the lungs. Prophylactic use of the preventive agents cromolyn sodium and nedocromil sodium and the administration of steroids during an attack help prevent or lessen the inflammation.

Nocturnal symptoms are noted in up to 90% of people with asthma; they usually occur between 3 AM and 5 AM. Close to 80% of asthmatic respiratory arrests occur between midnight and 6 AM. Normally, a lessening of air flow occurs during sleep. Persons with asthma tend to have this condition to a greater degree; as many as 60% wake with wheezing, coughing, and shortness of breath. One theory is that a gastroesophageal reflux occurs while the person is lying flat; hydrochloric acid from the stomach stimulates the vagus nerve endings in the esophageal lining and the lungs, causing the bronchi to constrict.

The drugs used to prevent and control asthma typically are used in a stepped approach to ensure the best outcome with minimal side effects. Management involves identifying asthma triggers, which may be allergy, exercise, cold, or sensitivity to viruses and bacteria in the airways. The 1997 guidelines for managing and treating asthma (National Asthma Education and Prevention Program, 1997) divide drugs used for asthma into two major classifications: those used for long-term control and those used for quick relief. Long-term control medications that are taken on a daily basis include corticosteroids (inhaled and systemic); cromolyn and nedcromil; long-acting beta$_2$ agonists; xanthines, and leukotriene modifiers. Quick-relief medications are used to reverse acute airway obstruction and to relieve bronchoconstriction; they include short-acting beta$_2$ agonists, inhaled anticholinergics, and systemic corticosteroids. Therapy is approached in a stepwise fashion, depending on the severity of the client's asthma. (Box 37-1).

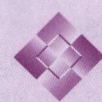

Box 37-1
Monitoring and Managing Asthma Using Peak Expiratory Flow Rates

Clients with asthma and other respiratory disorders can use various instruments at home to measure the peak expiratory flow rate (PEFR), thereby assessing respiratory function and the effectiveness of the medication regimen. Decreases in flow rates indicate airway restriction, sometimes even before symptoms develop.

The client takes a deep breath and then inserts the hand-held instrument into the mouth. The client exhales forcibly into the chamber, and the volume and force of air exhaled registers in a meter in liters per second.

The client personal best peak flow number is established by taking readings

-at least twice a day for 2 to 3 weeks
-when client wakes up and between noon and 2 pm
-before and after taking a short-acting inhaled beta$_2$ agonist for quick relief (if this is prescribed)
-as instructed by your prescriber

The client then uses the idea of zones to help manage his or her medications:

Green Zone:
Peak flow of 80 to 100% of personal best number:
Good control; take medications as usual

Yellow Zone:
Peak flow of 50 to 80% of personal best value
Caution: Take short-acting inhaled beta$_2$ agonist right away.
Consult with physician about possible need to change or increase daily medicines

Red Zone:
Peak flow 50% or less of personal best value
Medical alert: Take short-acting beta$_2$ adrenergic agonist right away.
Call doctor or emergency room and ask what to do, or go directly to the hospital emergency room

Adapted from: National Asthma Education and Prevention Program. (1997). Expert Panel Report II: Guidelines for the diagnosis and management of asthma. Washington, D.C. National Heart, Lung, and Blood Institute, National Institutes of Health. Internet: www.nhlbi.nih.gov/nhlbi/nhlbi.htm

Drug Therapy for Respiratory Disorders

Drugs that affect the respiratory system achieve their beneficial effects in different ways. Leukotriene modifiers inhibit the effects of leukotrienes on airway smooth muscle, mucous secretions, vascular permeability, and airway inflammation. Adrenergic drugs act by direct stimulation of cAMP through adenyl cyclase. Xanthine drugs act indirectly by inhibiting phosphodiesterase and may also act on bronchial smooth muscle by calcium sequestration and other mechanisms. Anticholinergics act by decreasing cGMP. Steroid drugs act through a variety of possible mechanisms. Cromolyn and nedocromil, although not bronchodilators, act prophylactically by stabilizing the membrane of the mast cells.

Bronchodilators

Bronchodilators act by reversing contraction of the smooth muscles in the airways. They include sympathomimetics, theophylline, and anticholinergics.

Sympathomimetics

Sympathomimetic drugs stimulate sympathetic nervous system activity (Table 37-1) and are used in treating bronchoconstriction.

Sympathomimetics act in several ways. Differences in actions are associated with the two main types of adrenergic receptors, alpha and beta. Norepinephrine, epinephrine, and isoproterenol are catecholamines used in bronchodilation. They act at the different receptor sites. Norepinephrine stimulates alpha receptors predominantly, isoproterenol stimulates both kinds of beta receptors, and epinephrine stimulates alpha, beta$_1$, and beta$_2$ receptors. The degree to which they are stimulated is dose-related or drug-related, because some sympathomimetic drugs are more beta$_2$-related. The latter is desirable because activation of beta receptors within smooth muscle leads to relaxation. Because receptors in bronchial smooth muscle are largely the beta$_2$ type, and because norepinephrine stimulates alpha receptors, norepinephrine has little effect on bronchial air flow (Hardman & Limbird, 1996). Beta-adrenergic drugs stimulate the production of cAMP.

Epinephrine

Pharmacodynamics. Epinephrine (adrenaline) is a potent bronchodilator because of its beta-receptor activity. Beta$_2$ receptors produce bronchodilation by the cAMP mechanism (see Fig. 37-2). Beta$_1$ receptors mediate the stimulation of cardiac muscle, which increases cardiac output, pulse rate, and palpitation. Beta-adrenoreceptor stimulants are direct smooth muscle relaxants that activate cell adenylate cyclase to convert ATP to cAMP. The beta$_2$-receptor agonists cause fewer beta$_1$ effects.

Epinephrine is a potent bronchodilator because it inhibits the antigen-induced release of histamine. Epinephrine is also a potent vasopressor through direct beta$_1$ myocardial stimulation, with positive inotropic effects leading to enhanced force of myocardial contraction and positive chronotropic action causing increased heart rate. The action of epinephrine on alpha-adrenergic receptors produces vasoconstriction in many vascular beds, thereby relieving congestion within the bronchial mucosa.

Therapeutic Uses. Epinephrine is used to relieve respiratory distress due to bronchospasm. It also produces rapid relief from hypersensitivity reactions.

Dosage and Administration. Epinephrine is not given orally because it is rapidly conjugated and oxidized in the gastrointestinal (GI) tract and liver and metabolized by catechol-O-methyl transferase (COMT). Norepinephrine and epinephrine are both destroyed by COMT, mainly in the liver.

Epinephrine injection 1:1,000, a sterile solution in water, is used for parenteral injection. The usual adult dose is 0.1 to 0.5 mL (0.1–0.5 mg) subcutaneously (SC). If symptoms do not abate in 15 to 20 minutes, another injection of the same dose may be repeated. It can also be administered slowly and with caution IV.

Epinephrine inhalation is a 1% aqueous solution that may be used in nebulizer, aerosol, or intermittent positive-pressure breathing (IPPB) form. This 1:100 solution must not be confused with the 1:1,000 solution.

Adverse Reactions. Many toxic and adverse reactions are associated with epinephrine. It increases rigidity and tremors in clients with Parkinson's disease. It increases glycogenolysis in the liver, reduces glucose uptake in tissues, increases glucose in the blood, and inhibits insulin release in the pancreas. As a result, hyperglycemia may occur (McEvoy, 1991). Nausea, vomiting, and sweating may also occur. Epinephrine has been known to cause syncope and loss of consciousness. Repeated injections can cause necrosis at the vascular site (as a result of vascular constriction) and in the extremities, kidneys, and liver.

Bronchial irritation and edema may result from oral inhalation of epinephrine. In some clients, rebound bronchospasm may also occur. The pharyngeal membranes may become dry from oral inhalation.

Toxicity Alert: Epinephrine

Signs and symptoms of epinephrine toxicity include fear, anxiety, restlessness, tension, tremor, palpitation, throbbing headache, pallor, ventricular arrhythmia, and tachycardia.

Drug Interactions. Concurrent use of epinephrine and tricyclic antidepressants increases the effects of the antidepressants. Concurrent use with propranolol, beta blockers, or furazolidone promotes excessive hypertension and decreases bronchodilation and cardiac activity. Concurrent use with guanethidine or methyldopa decreases the antihypertensive effects of these drugs. Epinephrine given with chlorpromazine or phenothiazines results in decreased vasopressor effects.

Table 37-1. Representative Sympathomimetic Bronchodilators*

Drug Name	Preparation	Usual Adult Dosage	Additional Information
albuterol, salbutamol (Proventil, Ventolin; *Can*: Volmax)	Oral tablets and solution	2–4 mg, tid or qid	Use with caution for patients on monoamine oxidase inhibitors or tricyclic antidepressants.
	Solution and powder for inhalation	0.5 mL (0.5% solution) PC: C	Dilute spray solution with 3 mL normal saline solution.
epinephrine (Adrenalin, EpiPen, Simplene, Asthma Nefrin)	Solution for injection	0.3–0.5 mL (0.3–0.5 mg) of 1:1,000 solution May be repeated 2 or 3 times at 20-min intervals PC: C	Do not use in clients with severe hypertension or a pulse rate more than 140 and with cardiac arrhythmia. Do not use with clients who have glaucoma or organic brain disease. Protect from light. Do not use if solution is brown or has precipitate. Do not administer in the buttocks. Client may report pounding in the chest and precordial distress.
(Bronkaid Mist, Primatene Mist)	Spray for inhalation	160–250 µg (once, or 2 doses at least 1 min apart) *Via IPPB:* 300 µg	Epinephrine may be destroyed by alkalies and oxidizers (eg, chlorine, chromate, bromine, iodine, nitrates).
isoproterenol, isoprenaline, isopropylnoradrenaline, isopropylarterenol (Aludrin, Isuprel, Isuprel-Neo Misthaler, Medihaler-Iso, Neoepinine, Norisodrine)	Sublingual tablets	10–20 mg sublingual, tid or qid (maximum of 60 mg/day)	Client may report similar feelings to above with pounding in chest.
metaproterenol (Alupent, Metaprel)	Tablets, syrup	10–20 mg, tid or qid PC: C	Therapy may start with 10-mg dose and increase to 20-mg dose after 2–3 weeks if indicated.
pirbuterol acetate (Maxaid)	Solution for inhalation	2 inhalations q4–6h	If drug fails to provide usual relief, client should seek medical advice.
terbutaline (Brethine, Bricanyl)	Solution for injection	0.25 mg injection SC repeated in 15–30 min PRN	Solution is sensitive to heat and light.
	Tablets	May repeat after 4 h 2.5–5 mg, tid or qid at 6-h intervals PC: B	Store at room temperature (15°–30°C).
	Solution for inhalation	2 inhalations separated by 1 min q4–6h	Solution should be clear. Do not use if discolored. Give SC in deltoid area; not used to initiate treatment because of delayed onset of action (30–60 min). Parenteral administration relatively contraindicated in cardiac disease. Produces systemic vasodilation with compensatory tachycardia. Tremors are common adverse effect.

*Use with caution in clients with cardiovascular disease, hypertension, hyperthyroidism, diabetes. Adverse reactions include palpitations, tremors, nervousness, tachycardia, nausea, vomiting, diaphoresis, anxiety, insomnia.
PC = pregnancy category; see Appendix A. *Can* = Canadian trade name.

Precautions and Contraindications. Epinephrine must be stored in tight light-resistant containers. Freezing should be avoided. Oxidation occurs if air is introduced into vials, turning the drug pink and rendering it unusable. Epinephrine should not be used if a precipitate is evident. Injections should be given with extreme caution in areas served by end arteries or otherwise limited blood supply (eg, fingers, toes, ears, genitals). Injections should not be given in the buttocks because gas gangrene may occur, possibly because epinephrine-induced vasoconstriction reduces tissue oxygen tension, thereby enabling anaerobic *Clostridium perfringens* (possibly present on the buttocks from the client's feces) to multiply (McEvoy, 1991).

Caution should be used if the drug is administered to clients with hyperthyroidism, hypertension, diabetes mellitus, cardiovascular disease (coronary artery disease [angina pectoris or myocardial infarction] and tachycardia), or susceptibility to adverse pressor reactions.

Beta-Adrenergic Agonists

Pharmacodynamics. Beta-adrenergic agonists are effective in preventing the immediate bronchostrictor response to challenge by allergens. Beta-adrenergic agonists used to treat asthma have greater effects (beta$_2$) on the heart.

Pharmacokinetics. Inhaled selective beta$_2$-adrenergic agonists (albuterol, terbutaline, fenoterol, and bitolterol) have a rapid onset of action and are effective for 3 to 6 hours. Salmetrol is longer-acting; it may be effective for more than 12 hours and therefore is useful in treating nocturnal symptoms. The oral route is used less frequently because of the increased incidence of side effects, but slow-release tablets may be used to prevent nocturnal asthma.

Dosage and Administration. It is important that clients use inhalers correctly to have full effect and to prevent overdosing from repeated use. The maximum daily dose should not be exceeded. If more than one inhalation per dose is required, the client should wait at least 1 full minute between inhalations (wait at least 3–5 min for isoproterenol and epinephrine; 2 min for metoproterenol). If GI upset occurs with orally administered doses, they can be taken with food.

Therapeutic Uses. Inhaled beta-adrenergic agonists are used for the short-term relief of bronchoconstriction and are the treatment of choice for acute exacerbations. They are also used for exercise-induced asthma. Isoproterenol and other nonselective beta-adrenergic agonists are used infrequently because of the high incidence of cardiovascular side effects.

Adverse Reactions. Beta blockers and beta agonists antagonize each other's effects. Regular use of inhaled beta agonists is thought to contribute to increased mortality from asthma. It is believed, however, that this is of little magnitude and may be restricted to the use of these drugs by nebulizer (Olin, 1995).

Drug Interactions. Increases in blood pressure may occur when beta adrenergic drugs are given with furazolidine, guanethidine, methyldopa, MAO inhibitors, rauwolfia alkaloids, oxytoxics, and tricyclic antidepressants. When given with theophylline, increased toxicity, especially cardiotoxicity, may occur. Albuterol may decrease serum levels of digoxin.

Drug–Laboratory Test Interactions. Isoproterenol may cause false increases in bilirubin.

Isoproterenol

Isoproterenol (Isuprel) provides powerful beta$_2$ stimulation, leading to relaxation of the bronchial tree.

Pharmacodynamics. Isoproterenol is the strongest sympathomimetic drug, acting almost exclusively on beta receptors. Isoproterenol increases cardiac output, lowers peripheral vascular resistance, relaxes smooth muscle, and inhibits antigen-induced release of histamine. Isoproterenol is used as a cardiac stimulant and as a bronchodilator to relieve bronchoconstriction.

Pharmacokinetics. Administered IV, isoproterenol acts immediately; by inhalation, it acts rapidly for about 1 hour. Isoproterenol is absorbed by the tissues; it crosses the placenta and enters breast milk. It is excreted in urine.

Therapeutic Uses. Besides relieving bronchospasm in bronchial asthma, emphysema, and bronchitis, isoproterenol may be used in managing shock and cardiac arrest, Stokes-Adams syndrome, ventricular tachycardia, and ventricular arrhythmias requiring increased inotropic activity for therapy.

Dosage and Administration. The drug is given parenterally or as an aerosol. It can be administered as a sterile injection: 1:5,000 equals 0.2 mg/mL. The infusion must be given slowly. Isoproterenol also can be given sublingually (10 mg repeated every 3 to 4 hours, to a maximum of 30 mg/day). Isoproterenol hydrochloride inhalation, an aqueous solution available in 1:100 or 1:200 solutions, may be administered in 1:200 strength by hand nebulizer or IPPB machine to relieve bronchoconstriction (as in asthma). (IPPB machines are used for aerosol therapy in clients who require high inspiratory pressures.) A dose of 0.5 mL of 1:200 solution diluted with 2.5 mL isotonic saline solution or water is given for 10 to 20 minutes four times daily with an IPPB machine. If administered by a hand-held nebulizer, the usual dose is five to 15 deep inhalations using a 1:200 solution (see the nursing management section for instructions on nebulizer use).

Isoproterenol metered-dose aerosols are available in solutions of 0.25%. One application equals five to seven inhalations from the hand-held nebulizer. This dose may be repeated up to five times daily at intervals of 3 to 4 hours. Initially, clients may complain of a sore throat from the alcohol content, but this symptom tends to subside.

Adverse Reactions. The toxic and adverse reactions of isoproterenol include palpitation, tachycardia, flushing of the skin, headache, tremor, anginal pain, nausea, dizziness, weakness, diaphoresis, bronchospasms, and cardiac arrhythmia.

Drug Interactions. Isoproterenol should not be administered with epinephrine or other sympathomimetics because of increased effects on the heart and possible cardiac arrhythmias.

Precautions and Contraindications. It is important to take the apical and radial pulse and to observe the electrocardiogram on the monitor when treating a client with isoproterenol.

Other Beta₂-Adrenergic Agonists

Because of beta₁ stimulation, with its resultant adverse reactions, prescribers tend to prefer medications with more selective beta₂-adrenergic stimulant action (agonists). Isoetharine is such a drug, as are other selective beta₂ stimulants that are not catecholamines and therefore less subject to COMT inactivation. Examples include metaproterenol (Alupent, Metaprel), terbutaline (Brethine, Bricanyl), pirbuterol (Maxair), and albuterol (Ventolin, Proventil). These drugs are used in treating bronchial asthma and reversible bronchospasm associated with bronchitis or emphysema. They reduce airway resistance and may be administered orally. The duration of action is 3 to 6 hours (Table 37-2).

Isoetharine

The bronchodilator isoetharine is available as a solution for nebulization (Bronkosol) and as a metered aerosol (Bronkometer). The onset of action is relatively rapid; the duration of action is 2 hours. Adverse reactions include tachycardia, nausea, anxiety, and restlessness. Isoetharine should not be given concurrently with epinephrine, although the drugs may be alternated.

Metaproterenol

Metaproterenol is an effective bronchodilator whether given by inhalation or orally. With a single oral dose of 20 mg, significantly improved airway function lasts about 4 hours. The effect is more variable if the drug is inhaled, but the duration of action may be 5 hours or longer. Adverse reactions include tachycardia, increased blood pressure, tremor, palpitation, nervousness, and nausea and vomiting. These adverse reactions seem to be less common than with catecholamines. Metaproterenol should be used with caution in clients with coronary artery disease, congestive heart failure, hypertension, diabetes, and hyperthyroidism.

Terbutaline Sulfate

Terbutaline sulfate, a synthetic sympathomimetic agent, is a selective beta₂ agonist and an effective bronchodilator. With oral administration, the onset of action occurs within 1 hour, but the effect lasts 4 to 8 hours. The onset of action for the inhaled product is more rapid (3–5 min), but the duration of effect is only 3 to 4 hours. If given SC, the onset of action is 5 to 15 minutes, with peak action at 30 minutes to 1 hour, and the duration is 4 hours. However, the SC administration of beta₂ receptors diminishes selectivity, and cardiovascular adverse effects are more common. Terbutaline may also lower the diastolic blood pressure.

Adverse effects include nervousness, muscle tremor, palpitation, tachycardia, diaphoresis, and nausea and vomiting. Effects usually are mild and often decrease as therapy continues.

In an unlabeled use, terbutaline may be given orally or IV to prevent premature labor.

Albuterol

Albuterol is known outside the United States as salbutamol, the name recommended by the World Health Organization (Stimson, 1995). Albuterol appears to induce less angina in asthmatics who have ischemic heart

---

Table 37-2. Representative Inhalants Used for Bronchodilation

Drug	Dose (Number of Inhalations)	Additional Information
Anticholinergics		
ipratropium bromide (Atrovent)	2 qid	Drug usually does not cause systemic anticholinergic effects, but can cause tachycardia.
Sympathomimetics		
albuterol (Brethine, Proventil)	2 q4–6h	
epinephrine (AsthmaHaler, Bronkaid, Primatene, AsthmaNefrin, Vaponefrin)	1–3 q4–6h	This OTC product should not be used without physician's recommendation for asthma (can cause tachycardia).
metaproterenol sulfate (Alupent, Metaprel)	2 or 3 q3–4h	
salmeterol (Serevent)	2 q12h	This drug has longer duration of effect; not appropriate for bronchodilation in acute situation when immediate bronchodilation is needed.
Corticosteroids		
triamcinolone acetonide (Azmacort, Aristocort, Aristo-Pak)	2 tid or qid	Medication reverses or prevents inflammation of bronchi; fewer systemic effects than oral steroids; may cause oral symptoms (hoarseness, dry mouth, irritated throat, oral candidiasis). Follow use with water or mouthwash to prevent oral fungus infection.

disease. Albuterol may be administered by inhalation or orally. Adverse reactions are similar to those of the other sympathomimetic agents. Although less common, other reactions may include tachycardia, palpitation, tremor, nervousness, nausea, vomiting, muscle cramps, angina, headache, vertigo, insomnia, and, rarely, dizziness. Blood pressure may increase or decrease. Some clients complain of an unusual taste in the mouth and of oropharyngeal symptoms such as cough, irritation, and dryness. This drug must be used cautiously in clients with hyperthyroidism, diabetes mellitus, hypertension, and cardiovascular disease. Albuterol also has been used to prevent premature labor.

Salmetrol

Salmetrol has a delayed onset of action (20 minutes) and a longer duration of action (12 hours) and therefore is not used to treat acute asthma symptoms. It should not be used more than twice a day (morning and evening) at the recommended doses. Use of larger-than-recommended doses can produce ventricular arrhythmias from prolongation of the Q-T interval. Clients receiving salmetrol also must have a short-acting inhaled beta agonist available for acute symptoms.

Xanthines

Another major drug class used to produce bronchodilation and treat bronchitis, emphysema, and asthma is the xanthine group. Theophylline, caffeine, and theobromine are closely related alkaloids chemically defined as methylated xanthines. Theophylline and various derivatives come in many preparations (Table 37-3), such as aminophylline and oxtriphylline. Dyphylline is structurally and pharmacologically similar to theophylline but chemically distant. Tolerance to these drugs rarely occurs. They can be used with the sympathomimetic agonists because they have different modes of action. Adrenergic drugs directly increase cAMP.

Theophylline

Pharmacodynamics. Theophylline directly relaxes the smooth muscle of the bronchi and pulmonary blood vessels. Until recently, this drug was a first-choice therapy, although its mechanism of action is not fully understood. Initially, it was thought to inhibit production of phosphodiesterase, thereby increasing the concentration of intracellular cAMP, which results in bronchodilation, although the amount of drug required to do this exceeds the therapeutic range. Other possible mechanisms of action include antagonism of adenosine receptors, inhibition of the intracellular release of calcium, stimulation of endogenous catecholamine release, or antiprostaglandin action. Theophylline may have anti-inflammatory action, however, and it has a synergistic effect with beta-adrenergic agonists. Slow-release preparations given in the evening help prevent nocturnal asthma. Other pulmonary effects include central respiratory stimulation, reduced pulmonary hypertension and alveolar CO_2 tension, and increased pulmonary blood flow.

Other actions include stimulation of the central nervous system (CNS), promotion of diuresis, increased secretion of gastric acid, and inhibition of uterine contractions. Cardiovascular effects include weak positive chronotropic and inotropic effects. Theophylline also enhances cardiovascular performance in clients with COPD. Theophylline improves both right- and left-sided heart systolic pump function and lowers pulmonary artery pressure and pulmonary vascular resistance. It also enhances mucociliary clearance.

Pharmacokinetics. Theophylline is well absorbed after oral administration, with peak concentration occurring in 1 to 2 hours. The oral route is preferred. Rectal absorption from suppositories is erratic, but if necessary rectal solutions administered by retention enema may be more rapidly absorbed. Food may slow drug absorp-

Table 37-3. Representative Theophylline Preparations		
Drug Name	**Preparations**	**Amount of Theophylline**
Aminophylline		
aminophylline	Oral solution (105 mg/5 mL)	90 mg/5 mL
	Tablets (100 mg, 200 mg)	79 mg, 158 mg
	Suppository (250 mg, 500 mg)	197.5 mg, 395 mg
Oxtriphylline		
Choledyl	Oral solution (100 mg/5 mg)	64 mg/5 mL
	Tablets (100 mg, 200 mg)	64 mg, 127 mg
Choledyl SA	Sustained-release tablets (400 mg, 600 mg)	254 mg, 382 mg
Theophylline anhydrous		
Slo-Phyllin	Syrup (80 mg/15 mL)	80 mg/15 mL
	Tablets (100 mg, 200 mg)	100 mg, 200 mg
Theo-Dur	Sustained-release tablets (400 mg, 450 mg, 600 mg)	400 mg, 450 mg, 600 mg

tion but does not affect bioavailability. A high-protein diet and a large volume of fluid accelerate absorption.

Enteric-coated tablets and sustained-release capsules may be absorbed unreliably. Clients must be monitored closely until the desired serum theophylline level is reached. The serum concentration necessary to produce bronchodilation is 10 to 20 μg/mL. The dosage needed to achieve this level differs from person to person. Once the client's dosage stabilizes, serum levels tend to remain constant.

With both theophylline and aminophylline, absorption is fastest using the IV route, with the desired level being achieved in 30 minutes.

Distribution is widespread, but not into fatty tissue. Theophylline crosses the placenta and is present in breast milk. Theophylline is metabolized in the liver and is essentially excreted by the kidneys. Many factors affect theophylline elimination, resulting in great variation. In adult nonsmokers, the plasma elimination half-life averages 7 to 9 hours; in smokers, it is 4 to 5 hours. Smokers, therefore, may require a larger dose and the interval between doses may be shorter, because smoking induces the hepatic metabolism of theophylline. In children, the half-life is reduced to 3 to 5 hours; for premature infants, it is 20 to 36 hours. Decreased plasma clearance also occurs in clients with heart failure, liver disease, pulmonary edema, and COPD. Prolonged high fever may decrease elimination, and various drugs affect clearance. The elimination of theophylline is increased by a high-protein, low-carbohydrate diet and the ingestion of charcoal-broiled beef. Conversely, elimination can be decreased by a low-protein, high-carbohydrate diet.

Therapeutic Uses. Theophylline is used to treat asthma and other obstructive airway diseases. Because it increases respiratory muscle strength, strengthens diaphragmatic contractions, and delays diaphragmatic fatigue, it is especially effective in clients who have chronic lung disease and who retain CO_2. It has also been used to treat apnea and bradycardia of prematurity.

Dosage and Administration. Dosages of theophylline are individualized because the amount required to achieve a therapeutic serum level varies. The dose is adjusted by monitoring serum levels and clinical response. To promote speedier absorption, the drug is taken with a glass of water on an empty stomach (30 minutes to 1 hour before meals or 2 hours after a meal). If the client complains of GI irritation, theophylline may be given with meals.

Parenterally, theophylline is not administered intramuscularly. For IV administration, a 25-mg/mL injection is used and may be further diluted with IV fluids. The medication must be administered slowly (no faster than 20–25 mg/min) to prevent hypotension and peripheral circulatory collapse. To initiate therapy, a larger loading dose is given, and maintenance doses follow.

Adverse Reactions. The margin of safety with theophylline is narrow, and the potential for toxicity is high, especially if the drug is administered too rapidly IV. Adverse reactions are uncommon with therapeutic serum theophylline levels, but at levels of more than 20 μg/mL, 75% of clients report GI symptoms such as nausea, vomiting, and diarrhea in addition to irritability, headache, and insomnia. At levels of more than 30 to 35 μg/mL, tachycardia, cardiac arrhythmia, hypotension, seizures, brain damage, and death may occur (see Focus on Xanthines: Similarities and Differences.)

Toxicity Alert: Theophylline

Because the therapeutic theophylline serum level is 10 to 20 μg/mL, serum levels must be monitored to avoid toxicity. The incidence of toxicity increases significantly at serum levels of more than 20 μg/mL.

- 20 to 40 μg/mL: sinus tachycardia and arrhythmias, nausea, vomiting, diarrhea, headache, insomnia, irritability
- More than 35 μg/mL: hyperglycemia, hypotension, tachycardia (>10 μg/mL in premature newborns), seizures, brain damage, death
- More than 40 μg/mL: Seizures and cardiopulmonary arrest can can occur but may also occur at concentrations as low as 25 μg/mL.
- In clients using sustained-release drug forms, toxic levels may occur up to 12 hours later and will not be prevented by earlier treatment.

Additional GI problems include dyspepsia, epigastric pain, rectal irritation if administered rectally, intestinal bleeding, and reactivation of peptic ulcers. CNS irritability, especially in children, may be observed as restlessness, lightheadedness, muscle toxicity, depression, speech disturbances, and hyperactivity. Occasionally, renal problems such as proteinuria and urinary retention occur in men with prostate enlargement.

Drug–Drug Interactions. Theophylline may antagonize the sedative effects of benzodiazepines and propofol. Lithium plasma levels may be reduced by theophylline, and theophylline may reverse the neuromuscular blockade of nondepolarizing muscle relaxants. Catecholamine-induced arrhythmias may result from the concurrent use of theophylline and halothane. Theophylline given concurrently with ketamine has resulted in extensor-type seizures. Probenecid may increase the pharmacologic effects of dyphylline by decreasing the renal excretion of dyphylline (Box 37-2).

FOCUS ON

Xanthines: Similarities and Differences

Similarities

Pharmacodynamics

These agents are believed to alter smooth muscle calcium ion concentration, inhibit the effects of adenosine receptors, and inhibit the release of histamine from the mast cells. They also directly stimulate the medullary respiratory center and directly relax smooth muscle of the respiratory tract. They also stimulate the vasomotor and vagal centers, relax all smooth muscles (with the respiratory smooth muscles as the most sensitive), and cause coronary vasodilation and cardiac, cerebral, and skeletal smooth muscle stimulation.

Pharmacokinetics

These agents are well absorbed after oral administration; absorption varies with the form used, and the rate of absorption varies with the size of the dose. These agents are rapidly distributed to the extracellular fluid and body tissues; they are also found in breast milk. They are converted to theophylline and metabolized in the liver to inactive compounds. They are excreted in the urine as theophylline and its metabolites. The half-life in adult nonsmokers is 7 to 9 hours.

Therapeutic Uses

These agents are used as bronchodilators in symptomatic treatment of acute and chronic asthma and reversible bronchospasm.

Adverse Reactions

These include: (CNS) restlessness, irritability, muscle twitching, headache, insomnia, dizziness, convulsions, reflex hyperexcitability; (CV) hypotension, palpitations, arrhythmia, ventricular tachycardia, sinus tachycardia; (RESP) tachypnea, respiratory arrest; (GI) nausea, vomiting, loss of appetite, diarrhea, dyspepsia; (GU) urinary retention, frequency; (HEMA) elevated aspartate aminotransferase; (DERM) urticaria.

Drug Interactions

Theophylline may antagonize the sedative effects of benzodiazepines and propofol. Lithium plasma levels may be reduced by theophylline. Tetracyclines may increase the incidence of theophylline adverse reactions. Theophylline may reverse the neuromuscular blockade of nondepolarizing muscle relaxants. Catecholamine-induced arrhythmias may result from concurrent use of theophylline and halothane. The use of theophylline with ketamine has resulted in extensor-type seizures.

Differences

- **Dyphylline** has only 10% of the bronchodilator effect of other drugs of this class.
- **Aminophylline** may help to reduce fatigability and increase contractility of the diaphragm in patients with chronic obstructive airway disease.

- Enteric and extended-release forms of **aminophylline, oxtriphylline,** and **theophylline** are unreliably absorbed.
- **Dyphylline** is rapidly absorbed, is not metabolized to theophylline, is excreted unchanged in urine, peaking within 1 hour, with a half-life of 2 to 2.5 hours; the half-life in smokers is 4 to 5 hours; in children, it is 3 to 5 hours, and in premature infants, it is 20 to 36 hours. Serum theophylline levels do *not* measure dyphylline.
- **Theophylline** (IM) is incompletely and slowly absorbed. Theophylline in oral and retention enema form peaks in 1 to 2 hours; enteric-coated theophylline peaks in 5 hours; extended-release theophylline peaks in 4 to 7 hours.

- **Aminophylline** and **theophylline** are used in the treatment of neonatal apnea and Cheyne-Stokes respirations, and to relieve periodic apnea and increase arterial blood pH.

- **Aminophylline** (rectal) can cause rectal irritation. Rapid IV administration of aminophylline can cause syncope, precordial pain, flushing, and profound bradycardia. IM aminophylline can cause local pain and tissue sloughing at the injection site.
- **Dyphylline** can cause hyperglycemia.

- Probenecid may increase pharmacologic effects of **dyphylline** by decreasing renal excretion of dyphylline.

(continued)

FOCUS ON

Xanthines: Similarities and Differences (continued)

Similarities (continued)	Differences (continued)
Drug Interactions (continued)	
Theophylline elimination is increased (and half-life shortened) by a high-protein, low-carbohydrate diet; it is also increased by ingestion of charcoal-broiled beef. Elimination would be decreased (and half-life prolonged) by a low-protein, high-carbohydrate diet. Food may affect bioavailability and pattern of absorption of sustained-release preparations. Rapid release (and toxicity) may occur when some sustained-release preparations are taken with food.	
Precautions and Contraindications	
These agents should be used with caution in young children and persons over age 55, neonates, and persons who are undergoing influenza immunization or those with active influenza infection; in persons with cardiac failure, COPD, cor pulmonale, renal or hepatic dysfunction, peptic ulcer, hyperthyroidism, glaucoma, diabetes, severe hypoxemia, hypertension, compromised cardiac or circulatory function, angina pectoris, or acute myocardial injury.	• Some **theophyllines** contain sulfites and should be used with caution in persons sensitive to sulfites.
These agents are contraindicated in persons who are taking other xanthines; those sensitive to theophylline, caffeine, or theobromine; and those with preexisting cardiac arrhythmia.	• **Aminophylline** is contraindicated in persons hypersensitive to ethylenediamine.
Nursing Considerations	
Instruct client in disease, treatment, drug regimen, adverse effects, and therapeutic adherence; administer with meals if GI irritation occurs; otherwise administer on an empty stomach with a full glass of water; monitor vital signs, especially pulse and blood pressure; assess pulmonary status, including respiratory rate and breath sounds; monitor serum levels of the drug and be alert for signs of toxicity; monitor intake and output; encourage fluids to liquefy secretions, institute safety precautions, especially for the elderly, if dizziness occurs; warn client about the use of over-the-counter drugs, which may contain ephedrine and cause excessive CNS stimulation.	• Warn clients not to crush, dissolve, or chew extended-release preparations of **theophylline**; administer "sprinkles" with soft food to children who cannot swallow.
	• Dilute IV **aminophylline** with dextrose and water to prevent burning and do not mix with any other drugs; administer IV push slowly at 25 mg/min. When administering aminophylline suppositories, give after the client has a bowel movement and instruct client to remain recumbent for 15 to 20 minutes after insertion.
	• Protect **dyphylline** from light and give only by the IM route.
	• Administer **oxtriphylline** after meals and at bedtime; protect elixir from light and protect tablets from moisture. Take sustained-release preparations of any xanthine drug on an empty stomach.

Drug–Food Interactions. Theophylline's elimination is increased and its half-life shortened by a high-protein, low-carbohydrate diet. It is also increased by ingestion of charcoal-broiled beef. Elimination is decreased and half-life prolonged by a low-protein, high-carbohydrate diet. Food may affect bioavailability and the pattern of absorption of sustained-release preparations. Rapid release (and toxicity) may occur when some sustained-release preparations are taken with food.

Precautions and Contraindications. It is helpful to administer oral theophylline with meals to avoid gastric irritation and GI upset. If the client is nauseated, the drug may be given after the meal.

With IV aminophylline, careful attention to infusion rate is required: if the drug is administered too rapidly, death may occur. Theophylline and other xanthines are commonly given with the sympathomimetic drugs and steroids. Clients with COPD typically complain of gas-

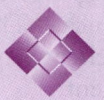

troesophageal reflux, which is thought to contribute to their disease. Theophylline can relax the lower esophageal sphincter; consequently, theophylline therapy may contribute to chronic respiratory disease as well as produce heartburn. This symptom can be minimized if the client sleeps with the head elevated rather than flat.

Anticholinergics

Anticholinergic drugs inhibit the action of acetylcholine or autonomic effects innervated by postganglionic cholinergic nerves (see Fig. 37-3). They produce bronchodilation by antagonizing cholinergic stimuli at muscarinic receptors, blocking cholinergic reflex constriction, and inhibiting vagal cholinergic tone. Although these drugs are also used as antispasmodics, the following discussion focuses only on their actions on the respiratory tract.

Atropine and ipratropium are representative agents. They are potent bronchodilators, especially in the large bronchial airways. They are effective if bronchoconstriction is the result of parasympathetic stimulation. They are effective in treating COPD and less effective in chronic asthma. However, they are effective for exercise-induced bronchospasm.

Although atropine can be administered orally, it is usually administered parenterally or by inhalation for respiratory effect. The effect is similar to that of isoproterenol. Onset of action is slower than that of inhaled isoetharine, but the duration of action is longer. Adverse reactions of atropine include dry mouth, blurred vision, tachycardia, urinary hesitancy, and constipation. Some clients complain of dizziness, weakness, nervousness, nausea, vomiting, and insomnia. Urticaria, rashes,

and anaphylaxis have been reported. These reactions are less common when the drug is administered by inhalation, although the drying of secretions has been a serious problem for people with COPD. Atropine sulfate is given 1.0 mg orally, 0.4 to 0.6 mg SC, or by inhalation 0.8 to 1 mg in 2 mL of saline solution. Onset of action occurs in 30 minutes and lasts 2 to 3 hours.

Ipratropium (Atrovent) is available only for inhalation; its anticholinergic effects, therefore, are primarily local in the lung. It has few of the adverse effects of atropine and is as effective as terbutaline. Ipratropium does not appear to affect the volume or viscosity of sputum. Dosage is two inhalations (36 µg) four times daily. Additional doses may be taken but should not exceed 12 inhalations in 24 hours. Clients should be cautioned to avoid contact of drug with the eye, which can cause eye pain, temporary blurred vision, and precipitation or worsening of narrow-angle glaucoma. Although systemic absorption is minimal, side effects can occur (eg, headache, bronchitis, dyspnea, coughing, upper respiratory infections).

Other Asthma Drugs

Corticosteroids

Corticosteroids are also used to treat clients with asthma. Several of the halogenated corticosteroids can be given by inhalation. They have selective topical effects, leading to improvement in respiratory status with minimal absorption in the blood. Inhalation helps avoid the associated adverse reactions of steroids and does not appear to suppress adrenal function. Corticosteroid aerosol products and dosages used for treating asthma include:

- Beclomethasone dipropionate (Vanceril, Beclovent): two inhalations (84 µg) three or four times a day
- Dexamethasone sodium phosphate (Dexacort Phosphate in Respihaler): three inhalations three or four times a day
- Triamcinolone acetonide (Azmacort): four inhalations (200 µg) three or four times a day
- Flunisolide (AeroBid): two inhalations (500 µg) twice daily

All oral steroids do essentially the same thing. Systemic administration of corticosteroids improves air flow in respiratory failure in clients with COPD. Clients who are being transferred from systemic to aerosol steroids may experience symptoms of adrenal insufficiency during and after transfer (eg, when exposed to trauma, surgery, or infections, especially gastroenteritis). These clients may require systemic steroids during these periods of stress.

Short-term use of high-dose steroids (a "burst of steroids") includes doses of 100 to 200 mg/day, or treatment may include 7 to 10 days of high doses such as 40 to 80 mg/day of prednisone, with subsequent dose tapering to withdrawal.

Some clients with severe uncontrolled asthma require chronic treatment with oral steroids. Corticosteroids suppress inflammation and block the steps necessary for late-phase reactions by inhibiting arachidonic acid metabolism. Until recently, corticosteroids were used when other bronchodilators were ineffective. With the current concept that a chronic inflammatory process plays a central role in the pathophysiology of asthma, antiinflammatory agents such as corticosteroids are being prescribed far more commonly, and sooner. Prophylactically, corticosteroids are useful in preventing the inflammatory response. They act by inhibiting the release of mediators from eosinophils and macrophages. Administered over a longer time (2–3 months), they also reduce bronchial hyperresponsiveness. Steroids that are given over a certain time also prevent exercise-induced asthma, reduce the response to allergens, reduce the number of mast cells in the airways, and reduce the formation of certain cytokines.

Steroid inhalants are available in high-dose (200 µg of steroid per puff) and low-dose (50 µg/puff) forms. The different steroid inhalers are similar in effectiveness. They are effective when used twice a day (a dosage schedule that improves therapeutic adherence), although some clients require therapy four times a day. Systemic steroids given orally may be indicated during periods of exacerbation. Oral steroids may be given for 5 to 10 days until the PEFR is stable or approaches the client's best or predicted values (see Box 37-1). Inhaled steroids are safe and reduce the need for the chronic use of oral steroids.

Adverse reactions to corticosteroid aerosols include sore throat and oropharyngeal and laryngeal infection with *Candida albicans*. Strict oral hygiene and proper inhalation techniques must be practiced, and antifungal medication may be necessary. See Chapter 30 for more information about corticosteroid therapy.

Leukotriene Modifiers

Leukotrienes are components of SRS-A, which is associated with bronchoconstriction in clients with asthma. A representative leukotriene modifier is zafirlukast (Accolate).

Pharmacodynamics. Zafirlukast is a selective and competitive receptor antagonist of leukotriene D4 and E4. It prevents or inhibits bronchoconstriction in asthmatic clients exposed to various allergens, such as grass, animal dander, ragweed, or cold air.

Pharmacokinetics. Zafirlukast is rapidly absorbed after oral administration, with peak plasma concentration in 3 hours and a half-life of about 10 hours. It is primarily excreted in feces; about 10% is excreted by the kidneys. It is biotransformed in the liver and inhibits certain P-450 microsomal enzymes.

Therapeutic Uses. Zafirlukast is used in the prophylaxis and treatment of chronic asthma in clients over age 12.

Dosage and Administration. A dose of 20 mg is given twice daily 1 hour before or 2 hours after meals. The dosage may need to be decreased in elderly clients and clients with cirrhosis and other liver impairment.

Adverse Reactions. Adverse effects include headache, infections (more common in clients over age 55), dyspepsia, nausea, vomiting, diarrhea, generalized pain, abdominal pain, back pain, asthenia, dizziness, myalgia, fever, and elevated SGPT levels. A pregnancy category B drug, zafirlukast should not be used by lactating women.

Drug–Drug Interactions. Zafirlukast can significantly increase the prothrombin time in clients on oral warfarin anticoagulant therapy. Plasma levels of zafirlukast may be decreased by erythromycin and theophylline and increased by aspirin. Because the drug inhibits certain microsomal enzymes, other drug interactions may occur but have not been studied.

Drug–Food Interactions. Food reduces the bioavailability of zafirlukast.

Precautions and Contraindications. This drug must be taken regularly as prescribed, even during symptom-free periods. It is not to be used to treat acute asthma episodes.

Preventive Agents

Cromolyn sodium and nedocromil sodium are two inhaled drugs used in preventing asthma. These drugs also are considered to be nonsteroidal antiinflammatory agents used in treating asthma.

Cromolyn Sodium

Cromolyn sodium, or disodium cromoglycate (Intal), is an antiasthmatic, antiallergenic, mast cell stabilizer. It has enabled some asthmatic clients to decrease their use of steroids. It is available as a nasal solution to prevent and treat allergic rhinitis (Nasalcrom) and is also used orally (Gastrocrom) to treat mastocytosis. It is being studied for possible use in treating food allergies.

Pharmacodynamics. Cromolyn sodium appears to act by stabilizing the cell membranes of mast cells, thereby preventing the release of asthmatic mediators that occurs when an allergen combines with immune globulin E (IgE) fixed to the cell surface. The precise action is not fully understood, but cromolyn indirectly blocks the calcium channels in mast cells and prevents mast cell degranulation by blocking phosphorylation of a membrane protein. Cromolyn interferes, therefore, with the release of allergic mediators from bronchial mast cells. It is used prophylactically to prevent the secretion and release of histamine and SRS-A, thereby reducing the stimulus for bronchospasm. Cromolyn may also act on macrophages and eosinophils.

Pharmacokinetics. Cromolyn is poorly absorbed from the GI tract. It is not metabolized and is excreted essentially unchanged.

Therapeutic Uses. Cromolyn prevents immediate and late-phase allergic reactions. It also prevents the late response seen in asthma and bronchial hyperresponsiveness.

Dosage and Administration. Cromolyn sodium is inhaled because it is poorly absorbed orally. It is available for inhalation as a dry powder in a gelatin capsule (20 mg), a solution for nebulizer use (20 mg), or an aerosol spray (880 µg per actuation). The drug has not shown the promise hoped for, however, because it is impractical to take and must be used four times a day. Bronchospasm has been a repeated problem, even though it is minimized somewhat by concurrent administration of an adrenergic bronchodilator.

Adverse Reactions. Adverse reactions include bronchospasm, wheezing, cough, nasal congestion, and pharyngeal irritation. Although rare, other effects are dizziness, dysuria, joint swelling, pain, nausea, headache, rash, and, rarely, laryngeal edema, angioedema, urticaria, and anaphylaxis. If eosinophilia pneumonitis develops, the drug should be discontinued.

Precautions and Contraindications. Cromolyn sodium is not used in acute attacks of asthma; it is effective only when given to prevent asthmatic attacks.

Nedocromil Sodium

Nedocromil sodium (Tilade) is an antiinflammatory agent used to prevent the development of early and late bronchoconstriction from inhaled antigens. It is similar to cromolyn in its effect and use. It inhibits the activation and release of mediators, including histamine, leukotriene C4, and prostaglandin D2. It is used as preventive maintenance therapy for clients with mild to moderate bronchial asthma. Nedocromil has no known systemic action when delivered by inhalation at recommended doses. It is generally well tolerated but may cause pharyngitis, coughing, bronchospasm, nausea, headache, chest pain, and an unpleasant taste. The usual dosage for adults and children over age 12 is two inhalations four times a day (14 mg/day). Effectiveness depends on proper inhalation technique.

■ SUMMARY

Drugs that affect the respiratory system achieve their beneficial effects through different mechanisms. Adrenergic drugs act by direct stimulation of cAMP through adenyl cyclase. Xanthine drugs act indirectly by inhibiting phosphodiesterase and may also act on bronchial smooth muscle by calcium sequestration and other mechanisms. Anticholinergics act by decreasing cGMP. Steroid drugs act through a variety of possible mechanisms, particularly as antiinflammatory agents. Cromolyn and nedocromil, although not bronchodilators, prevent asthma episodes by stabilizing the membrane of mast cells.

Drugs That Affect Mucus and Mucous Secretion

Expectorants and mucolytic agents are another group of drugs used to treat respiratory problems. These drugs affect mucus or the mucous blanket either by direct action on the mucus or by increasing the secretion of mucus. As discussed earlier, the mucous blanket is the mucous layer that covers the tracheobronchial tree. Mucus is moved up the tree by the motion of the cilia that line the respiratory tract. Ciliary function depends on the moisture and viscosity of mucus; dehydration and lack of humidification increase the viscosity of the mucus.

Expectorants, derived from the Latin for "out of the chest," stimulate the production of respiratory secretions and increase the amount of sputum. If the drug also stimulates mucous production, it is called bronchomucotropic. These drugs are administered systemically or by inhalation. If the amount of mucus produced must be decreased, a drug that inhibits the production of respiratory tract fluid is prescribed (an antibronchomucotropic agent).

Expectorants

Potassium iodide and guaifenesin are expectorants.

Potassium Iodide

Saturated solution of potassium iodide stimulates the respiratory mucosal glands by reflex stimulation of the gastric mucosa. Adverse reactions to the drug include GI upset with nausea, vomiting, and epigastric pain. The client may complain of a metallic taste, and skin rashes sometimes occur. Potassium iodide should not be used in clients with known allergies to iodine or in clients with hyperthyroidism. It is administered diluted in a glass of water and given orally, 300 to 650 mg, three or four times a day. Enteric-coated tablets are also available; the dosage is one or two tablets, three times a day.

Guaifenesin

Guaifenesin (Robitussin), formerly called glyceryl guaiacolate, is a frequently used expectorant. It is thought to stimulate secretions. It also inhibits platelet function in these doses and should be used with caution in clients taking anticoagulants. The usual dosage is 200 to 400 mg (10–20 mL), four times a day. The drug has been used as a mucolytic agent, but this action has not been adequately demonstrated. Although the drug is widely used, with few adverse reactions, there is little objective evidence that it actually produces bronchorrhea.

Mucolytics

Mucolytic agents act directly on mucus, helping to break down tenacious viscid secretions. Their action disrupts chemical bonds that hold segments of mucoproteins together. They loosen secretions and enable clients to raise sputum. Table 37-4 lists selected mucolytic agents.

Table 37-4. Representative Mucolytic Agents*

Drug Name	Preparation	Usual Adult Dosage	Additional Information
Mucolytic agents			
acetylcysteine alone or with isoproterenol (Mucomyst, Mucosil; *Can*: Airbron)	Solution (10% undiluted, 20% undiluted)	6–10 mL of 10% tid or qid 3–5 mL of 20% tid or qid	Observe for bronchospasm, stomatitis, rhinorrhea. If epistaxis or bronchospasm occurs, discontinue the drug. If bloody secretions occur, discontinue. Store in refrigerator. Use within 96 hours. Drug may corrode metal.
Expectorants			
potassium iodide	Tablets, solution Saturated solution (1 g/mL)	300–600 mg 5–10 drops if saturated solution	Observe for gastric distress, headache, acneiform skin rash. Use with caution in clients with thyroid disease. Do not use if client is sensitive to iodine products. Administer solutions well diluted in water or preferably in fruit juice.
theophylline 120 mg/15 mL iodinated glycerol 30 mg/15 mL, and alcohol 15% (Theo-Organidin)	Elixir	15–30 mL, q6–8h	Drug may cause drowsiness, rash. Use care with clients with thyroid disease and sensitivity. Use caution when using with other xanthine drugs.

*To decrease viscosity of secretions to liquefy tenacious sputum. Used in clients with pulmonary disease, cystic fibrosis, COPD, and atelectasis from mucous obstruction.
Can = Canadian trade name.

Acetylcysteine

Although it is irritating to tissue, acetylcysteine (Mucomyst) is the only true mucolytic drug available in the United States.

Pharmacodynamics. Acetylcysteine is a sulfhydryl compound that liquefies mucus and DNA through the process of mucolysis. Acetylcysteine breaks down the disulfide bonds of mucus protein. It also decreases the viscosity of mucus and is one of the most effective mucolytic agents. Liquefaction occurs within minutes after administration.

Pharmacokinetics. By inhalation, onset of action occurs in about 1 minute, peak action occurs in 5 to 10 minutes, and the duration of action is 2 to 3 hours. Tissue absorption is rapid; the drug crosses the placenta and enters breast milk. It is excreted unchanged in urine.

Therapeutic Uses. Acetylcysteine is used to mobilize mucous secretions. It is also used orally as an antidote in treating acetaminophen overdose. It is believed to protect the liver from damage by facilitating the detoxification of acetaminophen by maintaining or restoring glutathione levels or acting as an alternate substrate for its conjugation (Olin, 1995).

Dosage and Administration. Acetylcysteine is available in a 10% or 20% solution. A dose of 1 to 10 mL of 20%, or 2 to 20 mL of 10%, may be given undiluted three or four times a day by hand nebulizer, aerosol, or IPPB machine. The usual dose is 3 to 5 mL of 20% solution or 6 to 10 mL of 10% solution. Occasionally, it is administered directly into the trachea through an endotracheal or tracheostomy tube in doses of 1 to 2 mL of 10% to 20% solution.

When used as an antidote for acetaminophen overdosage, a loading dose of 140 mg/kg is given followed by a maintenance dose of 70 mg/kg; this can be repeated every 4 hours for up to 17 doses.

Adverse Reactions. The nurse must watch closely for bronchospasm. Because of this possibility, the drug is usually administered with or immediately after a bronchodilator. Should bronchospasm occur, the drug should be discontinued. Other adverse effects include a burning sensation in the back of the throat, stomatitis, nausea, rhinorrhea, and epistaxis. This drug has an unpleasant odor, similar to rotten eggs.

Drug Interactions. Acetylcysteine should not be mixed in the same solution as tetracycline, erythromycin, amphotericin B, or ampicillin.

Precautions and Contraindications. Acetylcysteine should not be put in a heated nebulizer, nor should it come in contact with iron, copper, or rubber, as these may affect the concentration. The drug is stored in the refrigerator and must be used within 96 hours. After opening the container, the nurse should initial it and write the date and time on it.

■ SUMMARY

Expectorants and mucolytic agents affect mucus or the mucous blanket. Expectorants reduce the viscosity of mucus and help remove it from the respiratory tract. Mucolytic agents work directly on mucus.

Antitussive Drugs

Antitussives control or bring relief from coughs. They are used to treat dry, nonproductive coughs. Most of the agents used as antitussives affect the cough control center in the medulla and suppress the cough reflex. Both narcotic and nonnarcotic preparations are used as cough remedies. Some of the preparations include combinations of antihistamines or sympathomimetic agents in addition to the antitussive. Ingredients must be checked carefully for each antitussive, and adverse reactions should be assessed for each client (Table 37-5).

Codeine

Codeine is an effective narcotic cough suppressant. Antitussives that contain codeine are usually obtained by prescription. The adult dose varies from 10 to 30 mg, but 15 mg four times a day is commonly used. (The adverse reactions to codeine are discussed in Chap. 18.)

Dextromethorphan

An equally effective but nonnarcotic drug is dextromethorphan. It is widely used in over-the-counter preparations. Adverse reactions are rare, although occasional GI distress and drowsiness have been reported. The dose is 15 to 30 mg four times a day.

Benzonatate

Benzonatate (Tessalon) is related to tetracaine; it reduces the cough reflex by anesthetizing the stretch receptors in the respiratory passages, lungs, and pleura. Capsules must be swallowed whole, because if they are chewed or dissolved, numbness of the oropharynx will occur. Adverse effects include sedation, headache, constipation, nausea, GI upset, hypersensitivity, and chest numbness.

Other Respiratory Drugs

Dornase Alfa

Dornase alfa (recombinant human deoxyribonuclease; Pulmozyme, DNase) is a genetically engineered enzyme that hydrolyzes DNA in the sputum of clients with cystic fibrosis. It is given in inhalations of an aerosol mist through a compressed-air nebulizer system. It reduces the incidence of respiratory infections in these clients.

The usual dose is one 2.5-mg, single-use ampule inhaled once a day. Once the ampule is opened, it must be used or discarded. Ampules must be stored in the refrigerator at 36° to 46°F (2°–8°C). They also must be protected from light and stored in their special foil pouch. Adverse effects are uncommon, but voice alteration, pharyngitis, rash, chest pain, and allergic reactions may occur.

Alpha-1 Antiproteinase Inhibitor

Alpha-1 antiproteinase inhibitor (Prolastin) is used to treat clients with panacinar emphysema who have alpha-1 antitrypsin deficiency. This deficiency is a chronic hereditary and usually fatal disease that traditionally manifests itself in the third or fourth decade of life. Em-

Table 37-5. Representative Cough Suppressants

Drug Name	Preparation	Usual Adult Dosage	Additional Information
benzonatate (Tessalon, Perles)	Capsules	100 mg tid (up to 600 mg daily) PC: C	Swallow whole to prevent numbing of oropharynx.
diphenhydramine 12.5 mg/ 5 mL (Benylin Cough Syrup)	Syrup	10 mL, q4h PC: B	Use with care in clients with narrow-angle glaucoma, stenosing peptic ulcer disease, prostatic hypertrophy, bladder neck obstruction. Observe for rash, drowsiness, increased viscosity, bronchial secretions, GI disturbance.
brompheniramine 2 mg/5 mL (Dimetane)	Elixir	10 mL, q4h	Same as above
hydrocodone 5 mg/5 mL, homatropine 1.5 mg/5 mL (Hycodan)	Syrup	5–15 mL, q4h	Take after meals. Observe for sedation, nausea, vomiting, constipation, CNS depression. Clients should not drive or operate dangerous machinery.
codeine 10 mg/5 mL, pseudoephedrine 30 mg/5 mL, chorpheniramine 2 mg/5 mL, alcohol 5% (Novahistine DH)	Liquid	10 mL, q4–6h	Use with caution in clients with coronary artery disease, hypertension, glaucoma, urinary tract obstruction, diabetes mellitus. All the same potential adverse reactions as sympathomimetics.
guaifenesin 100 mg/5 mL (Robitussin)	Liquid	10–20 mL PC: C	

KEY: PC = pregnancy category; see Appendix A.

physema occurs as a result of progressive degradation of elastin tissues. An imbalance between elastase and alpha-1 proteinase inhibitor (inhibitor of elastase) is believed to be the basis of the disease.

This agent is given IV once a week. Clients must be monitored closely for circulatory overload because this is a colloid solution. The drug is derived from pooled fresh human plasma and has been heat-treated to reduce the potential transmission of infectious agents. Clients should be immunized for hepatitis B before beginning therapy. Adverse effects are fever (may occur up to 12 hours after treatment), lightheadedness, dizziness, and transient leukocytosis.

Surfactants

Surfactants are used to treat newborns with infant respiratory distress syndrome (IRDS). In these infants, a deficiency of surfactant prevents reexpansion of certain alveoli—for example, those with smaller radii. This causes the alveoli with larger radii to enlarge. As a result, lung compliance decreases and inadequate pulmonary perfusion develops (Hall et al., 1995).

Two artificial surfactants are approved for current use: beractant (Survanta) and colfosceril palmitrate (Exosurf). Beractant is made from cow lungs and supplemented with DPPC, palmitic acid, and tripalmitin. Colfosceril palmitrate is not derived from animals. It also contains DPPC and other components of endogenous surfactant.

Pharmacodynamics. Surfactants lower the tendency of the alveoli to collapse by lowering the alveolar surface tension and stabilizing the alveolar volume.

Pharmacokinetics. Beractant and colfosceril are administered intratracheally. They are distributed and metabolized by lung tissues.

Therapeutic Uses. Surfactant is given in emergency situations to prevent IRDS at birth or before the onset of IRDS in newborns at high risk (eg, infants with gestational age under 32 weeks or birth weight under 1,300 g, or both). It is also given once IRDS has been diagnosed in any infant.

Dosage and Administration. Beractant is frozen and must be warmed before administration. Although beractant and colfosceril palmitrate seem equally effective, most prescribers think that neonatal nurseries should use only one of them because of the differences in administration, dose timing, and responses (Hall et al., 1995).

Administration is by instillation into the lung; the drugs are administered in a slightly different manner.

After thawing, beractant is given as a 4-mg/kg dose through a #5 French catheter placed with the tip just beyond the end of the endotracheal tube above the carina. Quarter-doses are administered while the infant is placed in various positions. After each quarter-dose, the infant is ventilated with positive pressure.

Colfosceril palmitrate is given as a 5-mg/kg bolus dose in small portions through a sideport adapter that fits into the endotracheal tube. The infant must be in the supine midline position for the first half of the dose. The infant is then turned 45° to the right for 30 seconds, returned to the midline position, given the second half of the dose, and then turned 45° to the left for 30 seconds.

Surfactants are administered by clinicians with specialized skills and expertise. Educational audiovisual materials detailing administration techniques are available from each drug's manufacturer.

Adverse Reactions. Surfactants can have adverse effects such as pulmonary and intracranial hemorrhage, hypotension, apnea, and barotrauma. Infants receiving surfactants have a higher incidence of patent ductus arteriosus. During surfactant administration, bradycardia and decreased oxygen saturation can occur. Endotracheal tube obstruction also may occur.

❖ NURSING MANAGEMENT: CLIENT RECEIVING RESPIRATORY DRUGS

Clients with respiratory disorders pose a special challenge to the nurse. Clients with chronic respiratory diseases are often hostile, uncooperative, anxious, dependent, restless, and irritable. Despite this, the nurse must remain calm, often in an emergency situation. The nurse must stay with the client who is having respiratory difficulty and keep the client informed of what will be done and what is expected of him or her. Most clients cannot talk much at this time, and the nurse must second-guess many needs while assisting with proper breathing, coughing, and positioning. The client's respiratory status must be assessed continually, and the client's cooperation must be encouraged. Cooperation of clients and their families is a necessary component of health care; without it, health goals will not be attained.

The aims of respiratory nursing care and drug therapy include improved respiratory function, relief from anxiety, adequate rest and conservation of energy, prevention of further complications, and optimal functioning. See the Example of Nursing Process for Aminophylline Therapy.

In addition to administering respiratory drugs to decrease airway resistance, relieve bronchospasm, reduce the viscosity of secretions, mobilize and remove secretions, and control bronchial secretions (with expectorants), the nurse must be prepared to establish a patent airway, provide oxygen therapy (when indicated), provide mechanical ventilatory support (when indicated), monitor gas exchange, provide adequate hydration and humidification, decrease anxiety, prevent or detect and treat superimposed respiratory infections,

Example of Nursing Process for Aminophylline Therapy

The client, 64, has smoked three packs of cigarettes a day for 40 years. He is restless, hostile, and breathing heavily. His color is pale and cyanotic and he exhibits air hunger and pursed-lip breathing. He has productive cough and green sputum. His chest is barrel-shaped. Vital signs are BP 162/95, P. 132 irregular, R. 32-grunting, T. 37.4°C. Blood gases are pH 7.47, PaO_2 50, $PaCO_2$ 95, AB, 31. On auscultation, there is a prolonged expiratory wheeze and decreased breath sounds, with rales noted at the lung bases.

The prescriber orders aminophylline IV 0.6 mg/kg/mL, Bronkosol 0.5 mL in 1.5 mL normal saline solution in IPPB and nasal O_2 1–2 L/min.

Assessment Data

History of emphysema

Decreased breath sounds and rales at lung bases

Prolonged expiratory wheeze

Barrel chest

Pursed-lip breathing

Air hunger

Abnormal blood gases

Aminophylline, Bronkosol, and oxygen ordered

Thick inspissated, greenish mucus

Hostility

Restlessness

Irritability

Nursing Diagnosis	Intervention	Goals and Outcomes
Impaired Gas Exchange, related to inadequate air flow in and out of alveoli secondary to poor lung compliance	**Administer** oxygen as ordered. **Monitor** respiratory rate and blood gases. **Monitor** vital signs. **Administer** medications as ordered. **Identify** if client is taking a drug that interacts with methylxanthine or sympathomimetic drugs. **Instruct** patient in proper respiration techniques.	Client's color will become less cyanotic and more pink. Depth of respiration will increase. Rate of respiration will decrease. Adverse reaction from medication will not develop.
Ineffective Airway Clearance, related to increased thick secretions	**Perform** percussion and vibration, followed by suction. **Observe** for adverse reactions. **Monitor** for therapeutic level of aminophylline. **Instruct** client in coughing technique. **Position** client to promote respirations.	Secretions will be thinner. Amount of secretion will decrease.
Anxiety, related to air exchange and poor aeration and possible CNS stimulation from aminophylline	**Remain** with client. **Instruct** client in breathing and relaxation techniques. **Check** serum theophylline levels and O_2 saturation.	The client will appear more relaxed. The frequency and intensity of hostile behavior will decline.

and teach coughing, deep-breathing, and new-breathing and self-medication techniques. Clearly, some of these are part of the medical regimen; however, the nurse is instrumental in administering the therapy and in evaluating the response.

NURSING PROCESS

ASSESSMENT

Nursing measures related to data collection for clients receiving medications for respiratory disorders must be comprehensive. Usually, assessment begins with baseline data on the client's respiratory status and vital signs. Then the nurse takes the client's health history and explores other diseases that may contribute to respiratory complications (eg, diabetes, thyroid disease, cardiovascular problems). The health history should identify smoking habits, degree of fatigue, and symptoms. Other notable data include allergy history, exposure to environmental pollutants, medication history, and any previous experience with ventilatory support.

Physical findings should cover weight loss, anorexia, dyspnea, gastroesophageal reflux disorder, peptic ulcer disease, or hiatal hernia, all of which may affect the diaphragm. Many clients with asthma have gastroesophageal reflux disorder. If sputum is present, its quantity, color, viscosity, and any change in character should be noted.

Other aspects of assessment include the client's ability to speak in full sentences (difficult with compromised respiratory status), level of consciousness, mentation, and irritability or confusion. Evaluate the client's positioning: is he or she sitting and leaning forward? using accessory muscles for breathing? breathing through pursed lips? Is breathing labored? Are the nostrils flared? Are intercostal or sternal retractions apparent? What is the inspiratory/expiratory ratio? What is the pulse rate, respiratory rate, and depth of respiration? Is chest expansion or chest excursion symmetric? Is there a barrel chest? Is there digital clubbing? Look for signs of congestive heart failure. Observe also for cyanosis of the lips, nostrils, or tip of the nose or, in a dark-skinned person, the cheeks or oral mucosa.

The nurse must also percuss and auscultate the chest to determine the presence of breath sounds, fine or coarse rales, rhonchi, or wheezes. Finally, the nurse must review the blood gas levels, blood cultures and counts, and any radiographic findings.

NURSING DIAGNOSIS

Some nursing diagnoses for clients receiving medications for respiratory diseases such as asthma, bronchitis, and emphysema include:

- Sleep Pattern Disturbance, related to CNS stimulation secondary to sympathomimetic and methylxanthine drug use
- Pain, related to nausea, vomiting, cramping, palpitation, nervousness, dizziness, angina, and tremor from use of stimulant drugs

- Ineffective Management of Therapeutic Regimen, related to adverse effects of drug therapy

Clients and families may also have:

- Knowledge Deficit, concerning the condition, drug therapy, and treatment regimen

PLANNING

Goals of nursing care and drug therapy focus on improving ventilation and tissue oxygenation, reducing airway resistance, preventing or curing infection, reducing and managing adverse drug effects, reducing mucous secretions and viscosity, improving hydration, promoting adherence to the therapeutic regimen, and educating the client about drug therapy and delivery devices (see the Critical Thinking Challenge: Case Analysis).

INTERVENTION

The nurse's first priority is maintaining a patent airway. To meet this goal, the nurse helps the client into semi-Fowler's position and turns the client's head to the side or hyperextends the neck if the client is drowsy and cannot be aroused. The client should be turned from side to side every 2 hours. Respiratory status must be continually observed, and emergency measures must be instituted for clients with respiratory failure.

When administering drugs to clients with respiratory disorders, the nurse should stay with the client initially to help relieve the client's anxiety (anxiety increases the need for oxygen), to assess the client's response, and to determine whether adverse reactions are occurring. Adverse reactions do not necessarily mean that drug therapy must be stopped, but in some cases it may need to be discontinued until an alternate drug can be prescribed. Because some of the adverse effects of medications mimic anxiety, the nurse must also assess precipitating factors in anxiety.

In general, medications are stopped if the client develops a tachyarrhythmia that continues or if a ventricular arrhythmia, such as frequent premature ventricular contractions, occurs, especially with the use of isoproterenol. Chest pain and bronchospasm are also indications that therapy must be discontinued in favor of another drug.

Administering Xanthines. When the client receives a xanthine such as theophylline, serum drug concentrations must be monitored closely, and the dosage must be reduced if the serum level nears the toxic level of 20 μg/mL. If toxicity develops, therapy must be stopped and emergency measures instituted.

Administering Bronchodilators. For bronchodilation, the selective beta$_2$-adrenergic stimulants and the local anticholinergic ipratropium produce fewer and less severe adverse reactions. For other agents (eg, epinephrine), the nurse must protect the medication from light and inspect it for any discoloration and crystals, which render the drug unusable. In addition, the nurse must monitor the client's response and reassure

CRITICAL THINKING CHALLENGE
Case Analysis

Mr. Thomas, 57, comes to the clinic complaining of a respiratory infection. He says he has been coughing for about 2 weeks, even though he has been taking Bactrim 80/400 bid. He has had increasing shortness of breath and wheezing. He says he sleeps only 3 or 4 hours in naps. He denies chest pain, palpitations, or headache. He has no problems with voiding or bowel elimination. He says he occasionally gets an upset stomach, which he attributes to the theophylline.

The physical examination reveals BP 162/94 (elevated from previous visit), apical pulse of 106 regular, wheezing on inspiration and expiration, and 2 to 3 +edema in the lower extremities.

The nurse asks him what medications he currently takes and compares this information to what has been prescribed:

Prescribed	Taken
Azmacort 2 puffs qid	Taking tid
Atrovent 2 puffs q4h	Taking as prescribed
isosorbide 20 mg qid	
metaproterenol 20 mg qid	
metaproterenol 2 puffs q4–6h	Not using regularly
nitroglycerin SL 0.4 mg PRN	Has not been needed
prednisone 4 5-mg tabs each morning	Taking 2 tabs in AM, 2 in PM
theophylline (Uniphyl) 400 mg hs	Taking in AM; also taking Slo-Bid in PM from a leftover prescription
Bactrim 80/400 tid	Has been taking for 2 weeks

1. Based on this information, what hypotheses do you have about the causes of Mr. Thomas's complaints of respiratory infection and cough? his insomnia? his upset stomach?
2. Based on the above information about his actual medication use, what are the main points you would cover in a teaching plan for Mr. Thomas?

the client that an initial effect of epinephrine may be an accelerated heart rate, often reported as a pounding in the chest. For additional nursing precautions, review Tables 37-1 through 37-5.

If the client suffers from bronchospasm, bronchodilators are administered to reduce airway resistance. The nurse must instruct the client in the proper use of inhaling aerosolized bronchodilators. The metered-dose inhaler is the most common administration device.

Administering Mucolytics. When expectorants or mucolytic agents are ordered for the client with scant inspissated (thick and dry) secretions, mucous plugs, and atelectasis, the nurse adds these medications to the nebulizer immediately before the client receives treatment. In some settings, respiratory therapists administer these treatments; in this case, the nurse ensures that the treatment is arranged and then evaluates the client's response, making sure the client uses all the medication. Using only some of the medication and saving the rest for later is an improper administration method.

In the client receiving acetylcysteine, bloody secretions are a reason to stop treatment. The symptoms should be reported to the prescriber.

Performing Pulmonary Hygiene. Percussion, vibration, and bronchial drainage may be needed to loosen secretions if the client cannot expel them by coughing. These treatments, called pulmonary hygiene,

pulmonary toilet, or chest physical therapy, are administered in sequence. First, bronchodilators or mucolytic agents are given as prescribed; humidification may be administered by aerosol or nebulizer devices. Coughing to expel secretions is called expulsive coughing. The routine may involve aerosol treatment for 10 to 15 minutes, followed by chest physical therapy for 10 to 20 minutes. If an inhaled steroid or anti-infective agent is prescribed, the nurse should administer it after the treatments. If it is given before the treatments, the client will eliminate the medication by coughing. This procedure seems so obvious that it does not warrant mentioning; however, often the schedule for these medications conflicts with the chest physical therapy.

Because coughing triggers the gag reflex and vomiting may occur, these treatments must be administered before meals. Ultimately, coughing, proper client positioning, ambulation, and exercise have the greatest effect on mucous clearance.

Administering Oxygen. When oxygen is prescribed, safety precautions must be instituted. The nurse should check the type of oxygen and percentage prescribed and ensure that the correct delivery device is ordered—for example, a low-flow oxygen device must be used for oxygen delivery below 6 L/min. During and after oxygen administration, the client's response must be monitored by assessing his or her respiratory effort (labored or easy), color (cyanotic or normal), and blood gas levels. CO_2 narcosis is a potential complication in a client with a high $PaCO_2$ level.

Promoting Rest, Energy, and Nutrition.

Respiratory drug therapy is most effective in a client who is well rested and well nourished. Procedures such as inhalation therapy, pulmonary hygiene, and even oxygen delivery require energy, which is a scarce commodity for clients with respiratory problems. The nurse must emphasize the need for rest to the client and family. One way to conserve energy is to adhere to a schedule of eating, performing daily activities, doing chest physical therapy, and resting. Uninterrupted rest and sleep periods are an important part of therapy. For the hospitalized client, the nurse can coordinate treatments, laboratory and diagnostic tests, and meals to avoid constant interruptions. Nutrition is an important component of energy. Because respiratory clients are often anorexic due to both disease and treatment, frequent small meals may be the answer to nutritional problems.

Preventing Complications.

To prevent complications, scrupulous aseptic technique is necessary for both the client and the healthcare staff. The client's secretions should be disposed of properly, and the client must learn how to do this. The client should be protected from or avoid contact with people with infections and colds. Dehydration should be prevented. All respiratory irritants, such as dust, smoke pollutants, and allergenic materials, should be removed.

Client Education.

Throughout respiratory drug therapy, the nurse must implement measures to complement the effects of medication. Foremost is client education to teach efficient breathing, coughing, and self-administration techniques.

Breathing Techniques.

Because proper breathing and coughing improve oxygen and CO_2 exchange, the client should be taught how to take slow, deep breaths. This is essential if the client is dyspneic and breathing in a rapid, shallow, and ineffective manner. The client should be urged to take at least six to eight deep breaths an hour. Clients should learn how to breathe diaphragmatically. This type of breathing can be practiced by placing the hands on the chest or abdomen and inhaling in such a way that the hands rise as the chest or abdomen expands.

Another method is for the client to place the hands on the rib cage, take a deep breath, and try to move the hands out by lateral chest expansion. The client should inhale slowly through the nose, hold the breath for up to 3 seconds, and then exhale slowly through the mouth.

The client with severe COPD may need to learn pursed-lip breathing, in which air is exhaled slowly through pursed lips. The diaphragm is exercised if the client inhales through the nose in short, quick sniffs and exhales through the nose the same way.

Coughing Techniques.

Proper coughing can be helpful in clearing the airway. An effective cough has three phases. First, the client must inhale deeply through the nose. Then, pressure behind the air must be built up by contracting the abdominal, accessory, and thoracic muscles. This promotes a pressure buildup by closing the glottis and trapping the air. Once the intrapulmonary pressure is increased, the client can exhale forcefully, opening the glottis. The air is then expelled at the speed of sound, carrying with it sputum and respiratory secretions.

The cough may be more effective if the client first takes several slow, deep breaths to build up the intrathoracic pressure before the cough. Another way to accomplish this is to take one deep breath and then expel the breath and undesired secretions with several coughs. The cough is most effective if the client is in a position that allows free movement of the chest wall. The client should be assisted to a sitting position and instructed to lean slightly forward.

Self-Medicating With Inhalants.

The nurse must also teach the client about humidification and proper self-medication techniques. The client must learn to assess the environment to determine whether the humidity is too low. If it is, the client should consider using a room humidifier or vaporizer. If it becomes necessary to administer increased humidity directly to the respiratory tract, the nurse can teach the client how to do so, possibly while instructing him or her on the use of an aerosol device such as a nebulizer or a metered-dose inhaler (Box 37-3).

The client should be urged to perform the treatment fully as prescribed rather than taking frequent short puffs throughout the day. Because most clients awake in the morning with congestion, the first treatment should be on arising. For information on various drug-delivery devices, see Home and Community Care: Kinds of Inhalers.

Some points to cover in teaching the client about proper inhalation techniques include:

- Mix the medication by shaking the inhaler.
- Breathe in and out slowly and normally.
- Follow the directions of the prescriber or those on the medication container.
- Implement the open-mouth inhalation technique by tilting the head back and holding the inhaler 2″ from the open mouth.
- Implement the closed-mouth technique by tilting the head back, placing the mouthpiece between the teeth and over the tongue, closing the lips tightly around the mouthpiece, inhaling slowly while activating the drug chamber, continuing to inhale as deeply as possible, and holding the breath (up to 10 seconds) so that medication settles deep in the airways, not in the mouth.
- Wait several minutes before taking another puff.
- Rinse the mouth with water to prevent oral dryness.
- A way to estimate the amount of drug remaining in the canister is shown in Figure 37-6.

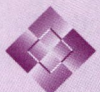

Box 37-3
Guidelines for Using a Metered-Dose Inhaler

Consult the directions below when teaching clients how to use a metered-dose inhaler correctly and effectively.

1. Remove the cap and hold inhaler upright.
2. Shake the inhaler.
3. Tilt the head back slightly and breathe out.
4. Position the inhaler in one of the following ways (A is optimal, but C is acceptable for those who have difficulty with A or B):

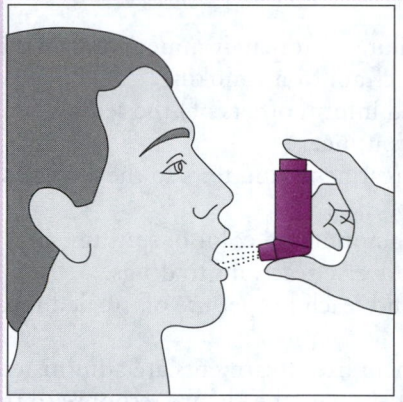
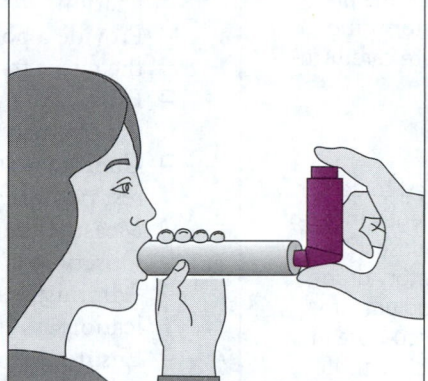
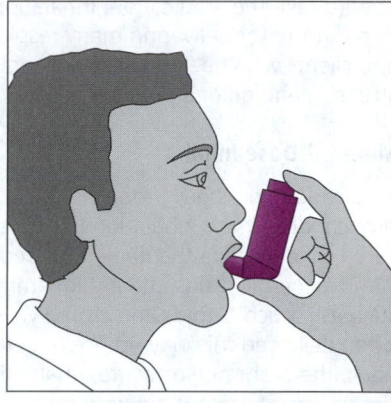

A. Open mouth with inhaler 1–2 inches away.

B. Use spacer (this is recommended especially for young children).

C. In the mouth.

5. Press down on inhaler to release medication as you start to breathe in slowly.
6. Breathe in *slowly* (3–5 seconds).
7. *Hold* breath for 10 seconds to allow medicine to reach deeply into lungs.
8. Repeat puffs as directed. Waiting 1 minute between puffs may permit second puff to penetrate the lungs better.
9. Spacers are useful for all patients. They are particularly recommended for young children and older adults and for use with inhaled steroids.

Note: Inhaled dry powder capsules require a different inhalation technique. To use a dry powder inhaler, it is important to close the mouth tightly around the mouthpiece of the inhaler and to inhale rapidly.
Adapted from National Institutes of Health, Expert Panel Report. National Asthma Education Program. (1991). Guidelines for the diagnosis and management of asthma. Bethesda, MD: NIH publication No. 3042.

The nurse can decide which points are appropriate to cover. Because much material needs to be taught, careful scheduling is needed. Demonstrations and return demonstrations by the client and family must be included. The nurse should remember that the client's intellectual capacity may be impaired when oxygen levels are disturbed. Showing the client how to monitor the adequacy of control using PEFR is an important focus of teaching (see Box 37-1).

OUTCOME EVALUATION
Data required for evaluation include:

- Are secretions decreased? Are they thinner?
- Are laboratory tests such as hematocrit and hemoglobin levels normal? Are cultures negative? Is the white blood cell count normal?
- When the chest is auscultated, are breath sounds present and adventitious sounds absent?
- Does the client report that dyspnea is reduced and that anxiety and fear have decreased?

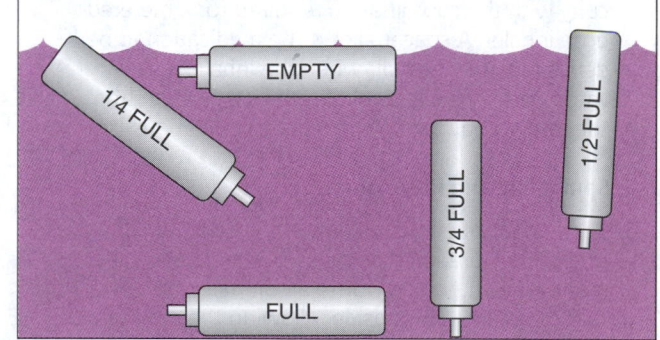

Figure 37-6. Estimating how much medication remains. Clients who use a metered-dose inhaler may benefit from the above tip on estimating how much medication remains in the inhaler. By doing so, they can renew the supply before it runs out. The client can place the canister in a container of water and observe the position it takes.* A full canister usually sinks; an almost empty canister usually floats. (From National Asthma Education Program. [1992]. Teach your patients about asthma: A clinician's guide. NIH publication No. 92-2737. Bethesda, MD, National Institutes of Health.) *This method does not work for all canisters.

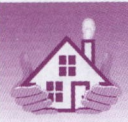

HOME AND COMMUNITY CARE

Kinds of Inhalers

Various inhaler devices are available for clients who need medications that relieve breathing problems quickly. All too often, clients who need inhalers receive a prescription but no instructions on why or how to take the medication. Inhalation is the preferred route for delivering many respiratory drugs, and clients who need these drugs require careful instruction and guided practice.

Metered-Dose Inhaler

Medication and a gas propellant are used to deliver bronchodilators by inhalation in consistently measured doses (hence the name metered-dose inhaler). Anticholinergic drugs and antiinflammatory drugs, such as corticosteroids and cromolyn sodium, are often delivered this way. To use a metered-dose inhaler, the client must start to inhale, then activate the device while continuing to inhale. This requires coordination.

Small-Volume Jet Nebulizer

This device operates with a compressed gas–air source with a sidestream method of nebulization. The medication and diluent are placed in a small reservoir; the air is driven by a small electrical compressor to deliver the medication.

Spacers

Spacers are tubelike attachments for nebulizers. They extend and enclose the space between the client's mouth and the drug source. They are used to deliver medication by inhalation to young children, older clients, and others who may have difficulty with the coordination required for a metered-dose inhaler. A spacer allows the medication to be deposited in a reservoir when the inhaler is activated. Then the client inhales the medication from the reservoir by taking slow, deep inspirations.

Spinhalers and Rotohalers

Some medications, such as cromolyn sodium and albuterol, are prepared as capsules that contain the medication in powder form. A spinhaler is a device that punctures the capsule, allowing the medication to be inhaled.

The presence or absence of adverse drug reactions directs the nurse as to whether therapy should be continued as indicated. The success of client education is evaluated by adherence to the therapeutic regimen, proper order of drug administration, and effective performance of inhalation, breathing, and coughing techniques.

❖ CHECKLIST OF NURSING ACTIONS

- ❑ Maintain a patent airway.
- ❑ Remain calm, especially in emergencies.
- ❑ Stay with the client in respiratory distress and keep him or her informed about procedures and expectations.
- ❑ Assess respiratory status and vital signs continually.
- ❑ Assess the client for dehydration.
- ❑ Assess the room environment for adequate humidification.
- ❑ Provide a pollutant-free environment and advise the client to refrain from smoking.
- ❑ Establish (and inform others of) the sequence of the planned routine.
- ❑ Coordinate treatments and tests so the client has rest periods.
- ❑ Measure the amount and color of sputum.
- ❑ Observe for adverse reactions to drugs.
- ❑ Administer and teach proper use of inhaled medications.
- ❑ Ensure that nebulizer treatments are administered properly, and evaluate the client's response to treatment.
- ❑ Wash the nebulizer and let air-dry after each use.
- ❑ Administer expectorants before meals.
- ❑ Ensure an adequate supply of oxygen.
- ❑ Secure oxygen cylinders so they will not fall.
- ❑ Ensure that electrical equipment is grounded and in good working order. Do not place oxygen supply near heat.
- ❑ Prohibit smoking when oxygen is being administered, particularly in the client's home. Post warnings on doors and at the client's bedside.
- ❑ Perform percussion, vibration, and drainage as ordered.
- ❑ Promote rest for the client.
- ❑ See that the client is properly nourished.
- ❑ Prevent further complications, especially from infectious diseases and colds.
- ❑ Instruct the client in breathing techniques and help him or her perform them. Teach the client to cough properly.
- ❑ Instruct the client on beverages to avoid when he or she is dehydrated.
- ❑ Accept clients and family members as an essential part of the healthcare team.

References

*Guidelines for the diagnosis and management of asthma. (1991). National Heart, Lung, and Blood Institute. National Asthma Education Program Expert Panel Report. *J Allergy Clin Immunol, 88*(Suppl. 2), 425–533.

*Recommended for further reading.

Hall W, Walter D, Barnhart SL. (1995). Surfactant replacement therapy. In Barnhart MP, Czervinske MP, eds. Perinatal and pediatric respiratory care. Philadelphia: WB Saunders, pp. 432–444.

Hardman JG, Limbird LE, eds. (1996). *Goodman and Gilman's The pharmacological basis of therapeutics.* New York: McGraw-Hill.

*International Consensus Report on Diagnosis and Treatment of Asthma. (1992). Washington, DC: NIH Publication No. 92-3091.

McEvoy GK, ed. (1991). *AHFS Drug Information '91.* Bethesda: American Society of Hospital Pharmacists.

*National Asthma Education Program. (1991). Expert Panel Report: Executive summary: Guidelines for the diagnosis and management of asthma. Washington, DC: NIH Publication No. 91-3042A.

National Asthma Education and Prevention Program. (1997). Expert Panel Report II: Guidelines for the diagnosis and management of asthma. Washington, DC: National Heart, Lung, and Blood Institute, National Institutes of Health. Internet: www.nhlb:.nih.gov/nhlbi/nhlbi.htm

Olin BR, ed. (1995). *Facts and comparisons.* St. Louis: Facts and Comparisons, Inc.

Stimson JM. (1995). Pharmacology. In Barnhart MP, Czervinske MP, eds. Perinatal and pediatric respiratory care. Philadelphia: WB Saunders.

*Recommended for further reading.

Borkgren MW, Gronkiewicz CA (1995). Update your asthma care: From hospital to home. *AJN, 95*(1), 26–35.

Clark NM, Evans D, Mellins RB, et al. (1992). Patient use of peak flow monitoring. *Am Rev Resp Dis,* 145, 722–725.

Dellinger RP. (1991). Acute life-threatening asthma. *Postgrad Med, 90*(3), 63–77.

Kaliner M, Lemanske R. (1992). Rhinitis and asthma. *JAMA,* 268, 2807–2829.

*National Asthma Education Program. (1992). Teach your patients about asthma: A clinician's guide. NIH Publication No. 92-2737.

Pedersen B. (1992). Home care management of the chronic obstructive pulmonary disease patient increases patient control and prevents rehospitalization. *Home Healthcare Nurse, 10*(2), 24–31.

Sittlington N, Tubman R, Halliday HL. (1991). Surfactant replacement therapy for severe neonatal respiratory distress syndrome: Implications for nursing care. *Midwifery,* 7, 20–24.

Stechschute DJ. (1990). Leukotrienes in asthma and allergic rhinitis. *N Engl J Med, 323*(25), 1769–1770.

Weiss KB, Gergan PJ, Hodgson TA, et al. (1992). An economic evaluation of asthma in the United States. *N Engl J Med,* 326, 862–866.

Bibliography

Ahrens RC. (1991). On comparing inhaled beta adrenergic agonists. *Ann Allergy, 67*(3), 296–298.

Barnhart MP, Czervinske MP. (1995). Perinatal and pediatric respiratory care. Philadelphia: WB Saunders.

38

Drugs That Affect the Musculoskeletal System

Physiology

Pathophysiology
  Peripheral muscle spasms
  Spasticity from central nervous system damage

Drugs that relax skeletal muscles and treat spasticity
  Skeletal muscle relaxants
  Antispasmodic agents

Nursing management: client receiving musculoskeletal agents
  Nursing process

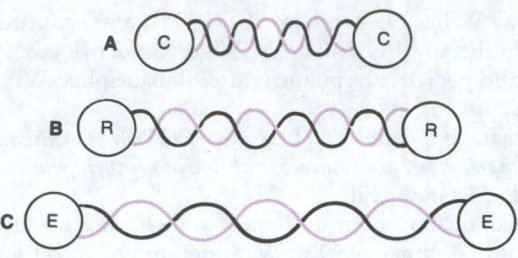

Figure 38-1. Sarcomeres perform the contraction (C) and the relaxation of muscles. **(A)** Muscle fibers shorten as they contract. **(B)** Muscle fibers at rest (R) in a semicontracted state in which they are ready for action. **(C)** Muscle fibers elongate (E) as they relax.

point called the motor endplate (Fig. 38-2). The action potential in the motor neuron releases acetylcholine at the motor endplate. Acetylcholine binds to receptors on the muscle cell membrane and triggers an action potential in the cell.

For contraction to occur, cytoplasm must contain sufficient calcium. Without calcium, tropomyosin covers binding sites on the actin filament and prevents cross-bridge formation. When calcium is bound to troponin, a regulatory protein, tropomyosin is moved to expose binding sites on actin. Calcium ions are stored in the sarcoplasmic reticulum and released into the cytoplasm when the muscle cell depolarizes during an action potential.

Bones, joints, ligaments, tendons, and muscles are the body tissues that make up the body's superstructure. They are the tissues that permit mobility and form a protective casing for the organs that conduct other body functions.

Physiology

Muscle tissue is characterized by contraction and relaxation, a process that moves bones around joints for locomotion and other body movements. The body contains more than 600 skeletal muscles, which, together with skeletal bones, support and move the body. Skeletal muscles are called voluntary because they are controlled by conscious commands, in contrast to cardiac and visceral muscles, which are involuntary (not commanded by conscious thought).

Muscle fibers can contract (shorten), relax (elongate), or rest (Fig. 38-1). Resting muscles are in a semicontracted state and are always ready for action. The fundamental unit of muscle contraction is the sarcomere, which consists of interdigitating thick and thin filaments. Muscle contraction occurs when myosin head regions bind to sites on the actin filament, forming cross-bridges.

The nerve impulse that a muscle fiber needs to receive to begin contracting is transmitted by a motor neuron to a muscle cell membrane at a communication

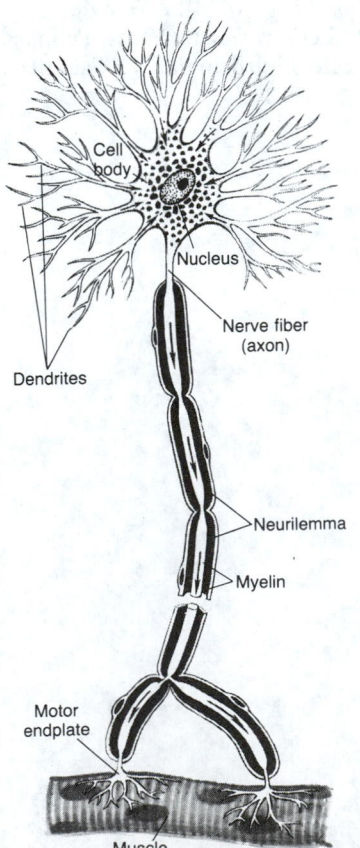

Figure 38-2. A typical motor neuron.

Pathophysiology

Spasticity, a muscle dysfunction characterized by spasmodic episodes, is difficult to define, probably because of the many questions that remain about the neurobiology of the motor system. Spasticity can be of peripheral or central origin.

Peripheral Muscle Spasms

Injury to peripheral muscle system structures, such as muscles, joints, tendons, or ligaments, can cause involuntary muscle contractions or spasms. Spasms are sudden, violent, and painful. Spasticity can make movement difficult, cause pain, increase fatigue, and interfere with sleep.

The injured muscle part sends sensory impulses to the spinal cord. The impulses are transferred by one or more connecting interneurons to the spinal motor neurons. The excessive number of motor impulses passing to the periphery from the spinal cord triggers the muscle spasms. Specific conditions that cause muscle spasms include whiplash injuries, cervical root syndromes, herniated vertebral discs, lower back syndromes, bursitis, myositis, neuritis, dislocations and fractures, muscle strains from excessive stretching or overuse, and sprains from wrenched joints with stretched or torn ligaments.

Although spasms are distressing, they are also a natural protective mechanism associated with injury. Treating the spasms without eliminating the cause would be counterproductive.

Spasticity From Central Nervous System Damage

Spasticity can also result from damage within the central nervous system (CNS) rather than in the peripheral structures. It can be caused by injury to nerve cells at any of the various CNS centers that control muscle tone and coordinate complex movements. Spasticity can result from an increase in excitatory influences or a de-

GRADE	DEGREE OF MUSCLE TONE
1	no increase in tone
2	slight increase in tone
3	more marked increase in tone, but affected part easily flexed
4	considerable increase in tone; passive movement difficult
5	affected part rigid in flexion or extension

Figure 38-3. The Ashworth Scale is an assessment tool for evaluating muscle tone. The score is calculated by summing the grades for hip flexion, hip abduction, knee flexion, and ankle dorsiflexion bilaterally and then dividing by 8. For example, if hip flexion and hip abduction scores were 5 in both hips and if the score for knee flexion in the right knee were 5 and in the left knee 3, and ankle dorsiflexion rated a 2 in both ankles, the sum of grades would be 32, or 4 on the Ashworth scale. A total of 5 on the scale indicates severely impaired muscle tone; a total score of 1 indicates mild impairment.

SCORE	REFLEX RESPONSE
0	no response
1	hyporeflexia
2	normal response
3	mild hyperreflexia
4	4 beats clonus
5	unsustained clonus, >4 beats
6	sustained clonus

Figure 38-4. The Reflex Scale is an assessment tool for evaluating the reflexes of the knee and the ankle. Scores are calculated by summing the grades assigned by the examiner to the right and left knee and ankle reflexes and then dividing by four. The highest score indicates hyperreflexivity; the lowest score suggests paralysis. (From: Lewis KS, and Mueller WM. [1993]. Intrathecal baclofen for severe spasticity secondary to spinal cord injury. *The Annals of Pharmacotherapy,* 27[6], 767–774.)

crease in inhibitory influences. It requires some time to develop after neural injury and varies in its severity during recovery from injury or during the progression of a disease. Some experts liken it to a complex of symptoms characterized by hyperactive tendon reflexes, hyperactive muscle stretch reflexes, abnormal spinal reflexes, and increased resistance to passive movement.

Specific conditions that cause spasticity include cerebral palsy, multiple sclerosis, poliomyelitis, hemiplegia, spinal cord injury (15%–60% of quadriplegics and paraplegics are affected by spasms), spinal tumors, and tetanus. In some situations, such as in multiple sclerosis, spasticity may increase significantly during an exacerbation or with a concurrent urinary tract infection. Treating the exacerbation or urinary tract infection often decreases spasticity.

Measuring the severity of spasticity is important. An assessment tool, based on the examiner's subjective assessment of the resistance experienced when muscles are passively lengthened, is the Ashworth Scale (Fig. 38-3). The Reflex Scale (Fig. 38-4) is also helpful (Lewis & Mueller, 1993).

Drugs That Relax Skeletal Muscles and Treat Spasticity

Drugs that can relax skeletal muscles and treat spasticity include neuromuscular blocking agents, local anesthetics, and spinal and general anesthetics (see Chap. 18). This chapter discusses skeletal muscle relaxants and antispasmodic agents that have more selective action than many other agents.

The drugs in this chapter are divided into two categories: skeletal muscle relaxants and antispasmodic agents. Although there is no completely satisfactory therapy for alleviating skeletal muscle spasticity, several drugs provide varying relief. A drawback to their overall usefulness is their adverse effects; therefore, doses must be carefully titrated. Overmedication for spasticity must be avoided in ambulatory clients, as these clients need a small amount of extensor spasticity for weight-bearing purposes.

Skeletal Muscle Relaxants

Mephenesin (Tolseram) is the oldest skeletal muscle relaxant but is not discussed here because it is no longer used clinically. Muscle relaxants that are similar to mephenesin include carisoprodol, chlorphenesin, chlorzoxazone, metaxalone, and methocarbamol (Table 38-1). Choosing one of these preparations over the others is a subjective decision, because no well-controlled studies compare their relative safety and efficacy. In addition, it remains debatable whether the beneficial effects of therapy are due more to the drug's muscle-relaxing properties or its sedating effects. Short-term use (less than 2 weeks) is generally recommended: drug studies have not demonstrated long-term efficacy, and tolerance may develop rapidly (especially with carisoprodol and its combination products). Prescribers generally agree that a skeletal muscle relaxant used with an analgesic drug provides greater pain relief than either drug used alone.

Pharmacodynamics. The mechanism of action of carisoprodol, chlorphenesin, chlorzoxazone, metaxalone, and methocarbamol is unclear. They appear to depress transmission through spinal and supraspinal polysynaptic pathways. Fasciculations and muscle stretch reflexes resulting from stimulation of areas in the reticular formation are depressed. These drugs cause drowsiness, possibly reflecting depression of neuronal activity in the medial reticular ascending system that is needed for wakefulness.

Pharmacokinetics. These drugs are generally well absorbed after oral ingestion. They have a rapid onset of action, generally within 30 minutes to 1 hour. Peak plasma concentrations of carisoprodol, for example, are reached within 2 to 4 hours. The drugs undergo biotransformation in the liver and are excreted primarily in urine as metabolites. They have varied half-lives and durations of action.

Therapeutic Uses. These drugs are used for pain relief and increased mobility of affected muscles in acute musculoskeletal disorders with spasticity as a component. They are used with nonpharmacologic interventions such as controlled physical activity and rest, spinal manipulation, physical therapy, behavior modification, relaxation and biofeedback techniques, and transcutaneous electrical nerve stimulation. They are not used to relieve the spasticity of cerebral palsy, multiple sclerosis, or spinal cord injury. Chlorphenesin is reportedly useful in treating trigeminal neuralgia.

Dosage and Administration. Dosage and administration data on these drugs appear in Table 38-1. Methocarbamol may be given orally or intramuscularly (IM).

Table 38-1. Representative Skeletal Muscle Relaxants

Drug Name	Preparation	Usual Dosage	Half-Life	Duration of Action
carisoprodol (Rela, Soma)	Tablets	Adults: 350 mg qid PC: C	8 hr	4–6 hr
chlorphenesin carbamate (Maolate)	Tablets	Adults: *initially,* 800 mg tid; *maintenance,* 400 mg qid PC: C	2.5–5 hr	No data
chlorzoxazone (Paraflex)	Tablets Caplets	Adults: 250–750 mg tid or qid PC: C Children: 125–500 mg tid or qid PC: C	1–2 hr	3–4 hr
cyclobenzaprine (Flexeril)	Tablets	Adults: 10 mg tid; *maximum dosage:* 60 mg qd PC: B	2–3 hr	4–6 hr
metaxalone (Skelaxin)	Tablets	Adults: 800 mg tid or qid PC:	1–2 hr	No data
methocarbamol (Robaxin)	Tablets Solutions for IM and IV use	Adults: *initially,* orally, 1.5–2 g qid for 48–72 hr; *maintenance,* 1 g qid; IV, 1–3 g qd at 3 mL/min; IM, 500 mg q8h PC: C	14 hr	4–5 hr
orphenadrine (Norflex)	Tablets Prolonged-release tablets Solutions for IM and IV use	Adults: orally, 100 mg bid; IM or IV, 60 mg bid PC: C	1–3 days	12–24 hr

PC = pregnancy risk category; see Appendix A.

The IM route is uncommon, and IM injections may cause pain. Subcutaneous injection is not recommended. Methocarbamol may be administered undiluted directly into the vein at a maximum rate of 300 mg (3 mL) per minute. It may also be administered as an intravenous (IV) infusion of 0.9% sodium chloride solution or 5% dextrose solution (1 g diluted in 250 mL). Overly rapid IV injection has been associated with syncope, hypotension, bradycardia, and convulsions. It is not recommended for use in clients with seizures.

Adverse Reactions. The most common adverse effect of this group of drugs is drowsiness. Other CNS effects include dizziness, blurred vision, confusion, hallucinations, agitation, and headaches. Reported gastrointestinal effects include anorexia, nausea, vomiting, and epigastric distress. Allergic reactions, including skin rash, pruritus, edema, and anaphylaxis, have also been observed. These drugs are generally not recommended for use in children or in pregnant or lactating women.

Carisoprodol has been responsible for occasional idiosyncratic reactions after initial administration (eg, extreme asthenia, transient quadriplegia or paralysis, ataxia, diplopia or temporary visual loss, agitation, confusion, disorientation).

Chlorzoxazone may color urine orange or purple-red.

A drug-associated hemolytic anemia has been reported with metaxalone. Like chlorzoxazone, hepatotoxicity has been reported. This effect is not as severe as that from chlorzoxazone.

Methocarbamol may darken urine that has stood for a period to brown, black, or green.

Drug–Drug Interactions. These drugs may enhance the effects of CNS depressants and alcohol.

Drug–Laboratory Test Interactions. Methocarbamol may cause a color interference in screening tests for urinary 5-HIAA and VMA. Metaxalone may cause a false-positive Benedict's test. Liver function tests (aspartate aminotransferase, alanine aminotransferase, and alkaline phosphatase) may be affected if hepatotoxicity occurs with chlorzoxazone or metaxalone.

Precautions and Contraindications. Because of their hepatic metabolism and renal excretion, these drugs should be used cautiously in clients with compromised hepatic or renal function.

Carisoprodol is a precursor of meprobamate (a schedule IV controlled substance), which is one of its three primary metabolites. Meprobamate dependency secondary to carisoprodol use has been reported. Carisoprodol's uncontrolled status and its availability through mail-order veterinary catalogs should warrant concern. Because of the potential for abuse, some prescribers recommend it only for acute conditions and for short time spans. It should be used cautiously or not at all in suspected or documented drug abusers.

Chlorphenesin contains FD&C Yellow No. 5 dye, containing tartrazine; tartrazine has produced allergic reactions in clients who have asthma or who manifest asthmatic symptoms after taking aspirin. A combination agent, Paragen Fortified Tablets (chlorzoxazone and acetaminophen), also contains tartrazine.

Chlorzoxazone, a benzoxazole derivative, is chemically distinct from the other skeletal muscle relaxants. Because hepatotoxic symptoms have been reported, clients receiving this drug should be monitored closely for signs of liver damage; it should be used cautiously in clients with a history of liver disease. The symptoms resemble those of viral hepatitis.

The injectable form of methocarbamol should not be administered to clients with known or suspected renal disease, because of the polyethylene glycol 300 in the vehicle. Polyethylene glycol 300 by itself may increase preexisting acidosis and urea retention in clients with renal impairment. If methocarbamol is used parenterally for more than 3 days, even if no known or suspected renal pathology exists, renal function should be monitored because of the nephrotoxicity of the polyethylene glycol 300. Care should be taken to avoid extravasation of the hypertonic solution, which may result in thrombophlebitis. The client should be in a recumbent position for 10 to 15 minutes after the injection to reduce the likelihood of fainting, syncope, or hypotension. Methocarbamol is contraindicated in clients with seizure disorders.

Cyclobenzaprine and Orphenadrine

Pharmacodynamics. Cyclobenzaprine and orphenadrine differ somewhat from other drugs in the skeletal muscle relaxant class. Cyclobenzaprine is structurally related to the tricyclic antidepressants (ie, amitriptyline), but its antidepressant effects are thought to be minimal. It acts neither at the neuromuscular junction nor directly on skeletal muscle. It acts at the level of the brain stem rather than the spinal cord, and it reduces motor neuron efferent activity.

Orphenadrine is an analog of diphenhydramine. It may reduce skeletal muscle spasm through action in the cerebral motor centers or medulla. It does not have direct skeletal muscle relaxant activity. It has some of diphenhydramine's antihistaminic and anticholinergic effects. Unlike the other skeletal muscle relaxants, it produces some independent analgesic effects that may contribute to its efficacy.

Pharmacokinetics. Cyclobenzaprine and orphenadrine are metabolized by the liver. They cross the placenta and enter breast milk. They are excreted in urine.

Therapeutic Uses. Therapeutic uses are basically the same as with other skeletal muscle relaxants.

Dosage and Administration. Dosages are reviewed in Table 38-1. Orphenadrine is also one of the skeletal muscle relaxants that is part of a combination product (Table 38-2).

Adverse Reactions. Like the tricyclic antidepressants, orphenadrine has anticholinergic properties and may cause dry mouth, blurred vision, increased intraocular pressure, urinary retention, and constipation in addition to other side effects of skeletal muscle relaxants. Rare instances of aplastic anemia have been reported. Anaphylactoid reactions have been reported after parenteral administration.

Drug Interactions. Cyclobenzaprine and orphenadrine may enhance the effects of CNS depressants and alcohol. Hyperpyretic crisis, severe convulsions, and death have occurred in clients receiving tricyclic antidepressants and monoamine oxidase inhibitors. Cyclobenzaprine may interact similarly because it is related to the tricyclic antidepressants. A few instances of tremors, confusion, and anxiety have been reported when orphenadrine and propoxyphene have been used together. Hypoglycemic reactions have developed when propoxyphene or a phenothiazine was given concurrently. Interactions have been reported between orphenadrine and amantadine and haloperidol.

Precautions and Contraindications. Orphenadrine should be used with caution in clients with glaucoma or prostatic hypertrophy. In addition, cyclobenzaprine is contraindicated during recovery from myocardial infarction or in clients with cardiac arrhythmias or heart block because of its cardiotoxic effects.

Antispasmodic Agents

As their class name implies, antispasmodic agents are used to treat muscle spasms. Antispasmodic agents may be centrally acting or peripherally acting (Table 38-3).

Centrally Acting Antispasmodic Agents

The principal centrally acting antispasmodic in current use is baclofen (Lioresal). Other drugs used for their centrally acting antispasmodic effect include the benzo-

Table 38-2. Combination Products

Drug Trade Name	Components
Chlorzone Forte, Paragen Fortified Tablets, Polyflex, Miflex, Blanex, Flexaphen, Lobac, Mus-Lax, Skelex	chlorzoxazone and acetaminophen
Robaxisal	methocarbamol and aspirin
Soma Compound, Sodol Compound	carisoprodol and aspirin
Soma Compound with Codeine	carisoprodol, aspirin, codeine
Norgesic, Orphengesic	orphenadrine 25 mg, aspirin 385 mg, caffeine 30 mg
Norgesic Forte, Orphengesic Forte	orphenadrine 50 mg, aspirin 770 mg, caffeine 60 mg

diazepine diazepam and the imidazoline derivative tizanidine.

Baclofen

Pharmacodynamics. Gamma-aminobutyric acid (GABA) is an inhibitory neurotransmitter, and baclofen is a derivative of GABA. Its mechanism of action is not completely understood, but it acts primarily at spinal cord level by binding to GABA receptors in the superficial layers of the dorsal gray matter. Baclofen is more lipophilic than GABA, but it is still essentially hydrophilic and only part of it crosses the blood-brain barrier. It appears to act presynaptically to reduce motor neuron excitability by inhibiting the release of excitatory neurotransmitters from large afferent fibers. Its effect is thought to be from depression of the voltage-sensitive calcium conduction channels (Lewis & Mueller, 1993).

Pharmacokinetics. The onset of this drug's action is variable. Peak action is at 2 hours, duration of action is 6 to 8 hours, and the half-life is 3 to 4 hours. Baclofen is excreted in urine and feces. Intrathecally administered baclofen must diffuse to its site of action and clinical effect may not occur for 6 to 8 hours, peaking 24 to 48 hours after the infusion has begun.

Therapeutic Uses. Baclofen is the drug of choice in spinal forms of spasticity: oral baclofen is effective in 70% to 80% of clients with spinal cord injury. It relieves involuntary flexor and extensor spasms and resistance to passive movements. Decreasing spasticity promotes improved self-care by increasing range of motion in the extremities, decreasing pain associated with spasms, improving bladder function, decreasing the incidence of decubitus ulcers, and promoting better sleep by decreasing nocturnal awakening due to spasms.

Tried over 3 to 48 months with a small group of clients with cerebral palsy, baclofen achieved desired outcomes (Albright et al., 1993). However, it is not useful for spasms that follow cerebrovascular accident or those that occur with Parkinson's or Huntington's disease. It has been used in clients with focal dystonic movements, including torticollis (wryneck). Other uses include Miege's syndrome (blepharospasm and oromandibular dystonia), stiff-man syndrome, and Moersch-Woltmann syndrome (predominant in men; characterized by muscular rigidity, paroxysmal painful spasms precipitated by physical and emotional stimuli, diaphoresis, and tachycardia).

Baclofen has been used for trigeminal neuralgia and intractable hiccups (daily hiccup episodes). Low-dose baclofen produced a prolonged antitussive effect in clients with persistent angiotensin-converting enzyme (ACE) inhibitor–induced cough. (Dicpinigaitis, 1996).

Dosage and Administration. By starting oral baclofen at a low dosage and gradually increasing it (5 mg three times daily for 3 days with an incremental increase of 5 mg/dose every 3 days), side effects may be minimized.

Table 38-3. Representative Antispasmodic Agents

Drug Name	Preparation	Usual Dosage	Adverse Reactions
Centrally Acting Agent			
baclofen (Lioresal)	Tablets	Adults: *initially,* 5 mg tid; dose increases based on client response; *maximum dosage,* 20 mg qid	Drowsiness, dizziness, confusion, weakness, fatigue, nausea, hypotension, headache
	Ampules for intrathecal use	Children: 1–1.5 mg/kg qd PC: C	
Peripherally Acting Agent			
dantrolene (Dantrium)	Capsules IV	Adults: *initially,* orally, 25 mg qd; dose increases based on client response; *maximum dosage,* 400 mg qd Children: 0.5 mg/kg bid; increased to a maximum of 3 mg/kg qid PC: C	Weakness in nonspastic muscles, drowsiness, dizziness, malaise, fatigue, diarrhea, photosensitivity, hepatotoxicity

PC = pregnancy risk category; see Appendix A.

In spasms resulting from spinal cord injury, oral baclofen fails to achieve the desired effects in 25% of clients. Intrathecal infusion via a subcutaneously implanted drug-delivery pump has been studied—with mixed results—for long-term treatment of clients in whom oral administration fails to control spasticity (in multiple sclerosis and with traumatic spinal cord lesions).

Adverse Reactions. Adverse CNS effects include drowsiness, dizziness, and confusion. Nausea, hypotension, and headache may also occur. In general, however, baclofen causes less sedation than diazepam and fewer serious adverse effects than dantrolene. Larger doses of baclofen may be needed when given orally because of its limited penetration of the blood-brain barrier. Once past the barrier, it penetrates both brain and spinal cord tissue, resulting in CNS symptoms that are poorly tolerated by most clients. When given intrathecally, small dosages of baclofen produce high local concentrations at the spinal cord level, considerably reducing the concentration of drug to which the brain is exposed (Lewis & Mueller, 1993).

In clients who receive baclofen intrathecally, overdose has occurred, producing excessive salivation, dizziness, nausea and vomiting, muscle hypotonia or flaccidity, mental confusion, and somnolence. As symptoms progress, respiratory depression or coma can occur. No antidote has been established. Drainage of the CSF by lumbar puncture and symptomatic treatment in the intensive care unit is recommended (Lewis & Mueller, 1993).

Drug–Drug Interactions. The effects of baclofen may intensify the effects of CNS depressants, such as alcohol and barbiturates.

Drug–Laboratory Test Interactions. Asymptomatic increases in aspartate aminotransferase, alanine aminotransferase, and alkaline phosphatase and serum glucose levels have occurred.

Precautions and Contraindications. Baclofen may be poorly tolerated by elderly clients, and low doses should be used for clients with impaired renal function. In ambulatory clients, baclofen dosage must be monitored and adjusted to prevent a decline in strength resulting from too much drug.

Baclofen should be used with caution when spasticity actually appears to sustain posture, balance, or function, because baclofen reduces the rigidity of flexor muscles at the same time that it lessens extensor muscle spasticity of the legs. The loss of this reflex response can reduce some clients' ability to walk, because they have greater difficulty balancing themselves while standing.

Sudden or abrupt withdrawal after long-term administration causes a rebound increase in flexor spasms. To discontinue baclofen, drug dosage should be reduced gradually over 1 to 2 weeks. Also, auditory and visual hallucinations, paranoid ideation, agitated behavior, and seizures (especially in clients with cerebral lesions) have occurred with abrupt withdrawal.

Benzodiazepines

This group of drugs includes diazepam (Valium). Diazepam has an antispasmodic action in addition to its antianxiety and anticonvulsant properties. It depresses the CNS, probably by potentiating GABA or GABA-mediated presynaptic inhibition at spinal and supraspinal sites. It probably produces skeletal muscle relaxation by inhibiting spinal polysynaptic afferent pathways.

Diazepam has been administered for many musculoskeletal problems that involve pain and muscle spasm. It has been used to relieve spasticity caused by spinal cord injury and cerebral palsy. However, its sedation, abuse potential, and dependence effects limit its long-term use. Because it does not relax peripheral muscles and cause weakness, it may be appropriate for clients with borderline muscle strength. In addition, it has been used in stiff-man syndrome, but it usually produces sedation at the doses required. When given IV, it is a useful adjunct in muscle spasms caused by tetanus toxin or strychnine. Its anticonvulsant property has made it useful in status epilepticus.

Diazepam is available as 2-, 5-, and 10-mg tablets; in solution and concentrated solution; in 2-mL ampules and 10-mL vials for injection; and in 15-mg sustained-release capsules (Valrelease). The pharmacokinetics, dosage and administration, adverse reactions, and nursing implications of the benzodiazepines are discussed in Chapter 20.

Imidazoline Derivatives

Tizanidine (Zanaflex), a central-acting agent, became available in 1996. It principally affects spinal polysynaptic reflexes. It has similarities to clonidine (Catapres), but its cardiovascular properties are mild.

Peripherally Acting Antispasmodic Agents

Dantrolene

Dantrolene (Dantrium), unlike the drugs discussed earlier in this chapter, exerts its effects directly on skeletal muscle tissue.

Pharmacodynamics. Dantrolene produces skeletal muscle relaxation by acting directly on excitation/contraction coupling within each muscle fiber. It sequesters or inhibits the release of calcium ions from the sarcoplasmic reticulum. The release of calcium is the fiber's usual response to excitation by nerve impulses and is necessary in activating the contractile response. Thus, dantrolene prevents activation of the contractile apparatus and diminishes the mechanical force of contraction.

Pharmacokinetics. Dantrolene is incompletely absorbed from the GI tract. Onset of action is 1 hour, action peaks between 4 and 6 hours, duration of action is about 8 hours, and the half-life is 9 hours. Significant amounts are reversibly bound to plasma proteins. It is metabolized by the liver. From 15% to 25% of this drug is excreted in urine.

Therapeutic Uses. Dantrolene is used to treat spinal cord injury, stroke, multiple sclerosis, and cerebral palsy. Clients whose functional rehabilitation is retarded by spasticity may benefit from dantrolene. It has significantly reduced spasticity and has sustained this reduction for most of the paraplegic and hemiplegic clients who have taken it. Mass reflex movements and abnormal resistance to passive stretch are reduced. About half the clients with athetoid cerebral palsy and some with multiple sclerosis have improved with dantrolene therapy. Tolerance to dantrolene's therapeutic effect has not been noted.

Dantrolene therapy can produce a greater ability to carry out activities of daily living (washing, dressing, or self-feeding), to exercise, to maintain posture and balance, and to use braces. However, dantrolene produces generalized weakness. In some clients, the ability to stay upright and maintain balance actually depends on certain muscles remaining in a spastic state. Therefore, dantrolene may be more useful in less ambulatory clients with spasticity.

Dantrolene has also been effective in treating malignant hyperthermia, the rare genetic disorder characterized by an excessive release of calcium ions from the sarcoplasmic reticulum. It may even be used prophylactically if this disorder is anticipated. The increase in calcium activates acute catabolic processes. Dantrolene may interfere with the release of calcium from the sarcoplasmic reticulum to the myoplasm to reverse or attenuate the crisis. Before dantrolene was used for this condition, the mortality rate for malignant hyperthermia was 50% to 70%. Dantrolene has also been used in neuroleptic malignant syndrome and in an investigational capacity in heatstroke and muscle rigidity from toxicity caused by cocaine use or carbon monoxide exposure.

Dosage and Administration. Dantrolene is available for oral use in capsules. It is available for IV use in vials that contain 20 mg dantrolene and 3,000 mg mannitol to be reconstituted with 60 mL sterile water for injection.

For spasticity, the recommended dose is 25 mg once daily, increasing to 25 mg two to four times daily, then incrementally by 25 mg up to 100 mg two to four times daily, if necessary. Each dosage level is maintained for 4 to 7 days to determine response. If benefits are not evident within 45 days, dantrolene should be discontinued.

For malignant hyperthermia, dantrolene is given by continuous rapid IV push. The drug is available as a powder for reconstitution with sterile water for injection. It is to be used within 6 hours after reconstitution. Reconstituted solutions may be stored at room temperature (59°–86°F). The starting dose is 1 mg/kg. Administration continues until symptoms subside or the maximum dose (10 mg/kg) is reached. This treatment is accompanied by discontinuation of all anesthetic agents and the use of 100% oxygen. Oral administration of dantrolene (1–2 mg/kg four times a day) may be necessary for 1 to 3 days after the crisis to prevent recurrence of the symptoms.

Adverse Reactions. The most common adverse effects of dantrolene are muscle weakness, drowsiness, dizziness, and malaise. Dantrolene may cause persistent weakness in nonspastic muscles, resulting in slurred speech, drooling, and enuresis. This weakness is probably an extension of its effect on skeletal muscle.

Diarrhea may be severe enough to require treatment, dose reduction, or even cessation of therapy. A gradual increase in dosage may help keep this and other adverse reactions under control. Photosensitivity may occur, and hepatotoxicity is a potential adverse reaction to dantrolene. Symptomatic hepatitis (fatal and nonfatal) has occurred (usually 3–12 months after initiation of therapy). The incidence is greater in clients who take more than 400 mg/day, in females, in clients over age 35, and in clients who are taking other medications (eg, estrogens).

Drug–Drug Interactions. Dantrolene may compound the effects of alcohol, barbiturates, and other CNS depressants. Other reported interactions include clofibrate and warfarin, where plasma protein binding of dantrolene may be reduced.

Drug–Laboratory Test Interactions. Liver function tests may be affected by this drug. If detected early, abnormalities may revert to normal when the drug is discontinued.

Precautions and Contraindications. Dantrolene must be given cautiously to clients with hepatic disease. Because hepatotoxicity is a potential adverse effect, baseline data on liver function (aspartate aminotransferase, alanine aminotransferase, and alkaline phosphatase) should be obtained and the studies repeated periodically during dantrolene therapy. The drug must also be used cautiously in clients who need some spasticity to maintain upright posture and ambulation.

Quinine

It may appear that including quinine in this chapter is an error, but the drug does have a role in one musculoskeletal condition. The bark of the cinchona tree of South America contains more than 20 alkaloids, chief among them quinine. The first written record of cinchona use appeared in 1633.

Pharmacodynamics. Quinine acts on skeletal muscle by increasing its refractory period through direct action on the muscle fiber, decreasing the excitability of the motor endplate region to acetylcholine, and affecting the distribution of calcium within the muscle fiber. It also has analgesic, antipyretic, and oxytocic effects.

Pharmacokinetics. Quinine is readily absorbed when given orally. Peak plasma concentrations occur within 1 to 3 hours, and the half-life is 4 to 5 hours. The subcutaneous and IM routes of administration are contraindicated because of the likelihood of local tissue damage (eg, pain, sterile abscess). Quinine is metabolized largely in the liver, and the metabolites are excreted mainly in urine. Small amounts are excreted in feces, bile, gastric juice, and saliva. If the urine is acidic, renal excretion is twice as rapid as when it is alkaline. Urinary alkalinizers may increase quinine blood levels and cause toxicity.

Therapeutic Uses. Until the 1930s, cinchona alkaloids were the only agents used for malaria. Today, synthetic antimalarial drugs are available that are less toxic and more effective. Quinine is still needed, however, to treat resistant strains of plasmodia. It is used as an adjunct with pyrimethamine and sulfadiazine or tetracycline to treat chloroquine-resistant *Plasmodium falciparum*. Quinine is also prescribed for clients with nocturnal leg cramps, including those associated with arthritis, diabetes, varicose veins, thrombophlebitis, arteriosclerosis, and certain foot deformities. These cramps occur at night when clients are recumbent. Some clients require only a brief period of quinine therapy to achieve long periods of freedom from leg cramps. However, in some cases, even large doses of quinine do not give relief.

Dosage and Administration. For leg cramps, the quinine dose is 260 to 300 mg before bedtime. This dosage may be increased if needed by adding one dose after the evening meal. For clients with chloroquine-resistant malaria, the usual oral dosage is 650 mg every 8 hours for 10 to 14 days. It is taken with food or after meals to decrease gastric irritation.

Adverse Reactions. Quinine produces many different adverse reactions. However, if only one or two tablets are used daily, these manifestations are unlikely to occur unless the recipient is hypersensitive to the drug. In a hypersensitive client, as little as 300 mg of quinine may produce tinnitus or other evidence of hypersensitivity. Other common signs and symptoms of hypersensitivity include extreme cutaneous flushing accompanied by intense pruritus, fever, gastric distress, dyspnea, and visual difficulties.

When quinine is given in full doses or over a period of time or when plasma levels exceed 10 to 12 g/mL, a cluster of symptoms called cinchonism occurs, including tinnitus and decreased auditory acuity, headache, visual disturbances, nausea, diarrhea, hematologic changes, and evidence of neurotoxicity. These signs and symptoms usually subside when the drug is discontinued.

Drug Interactions. Quinine interacts with digoxin, digitoxin, aluminum-containing antacids, neuromuscular blocking agents, warfarin, and urinary alkalinizers.

Precautions and Contraindications. Quinine must be used cautiously in clients with cardiac arrhythmias. It is contraindicated in clients who are allergic to it or who have G6PD deficiency, optic neuritis, tinnitus, or a history of blackwater fever. It is contraindicated in pregnancy and lactation as well. Pregnancy category is X.

Botulinum Toxin

Botulinum toxin (Botox, Dysport, Oculinum), the lethal agent in botulism, contributes in an unusual way to solving the problem of spasticity: it inhibits the release of acetylcholine from cholinergic nerves. It is used to cause prolonged but not permanent weakening or paralysis of the skeletal muscles that control rotation of the eye or other muscles in the ocular region. This effect is useful in treating severe or refractory blepharospasm (involuntary spasmodic eyelid twitching), other facial muscle spasms, and some cases of strabismus. The drug is injected with a specialized device that helps ensure the drug is placed directly into the desired muscle(s) and measures the effects of the drug on muscle function during administration.

Botulinum toxin has also been effective in treating spastic dystonia of cerebral palsy, and it is undergoing trials for use in other types of spasticity (eg, hemiplegia, multiple sclerosis). Injection into the endplate zone of muscles reduces or abolishes the release of acetylcholine from presynaptic motor axons and weakens the muscle. The effect develops over a few days and lasts several months. The toxin cannot be injected into all affected muscles, so the usefulness of this agent depends on treating a few crucial muscles (Young, 1994).

■ SUMMARY

No completely satisfactory therapy for relaxing skeletal muscles or treating spasticity exists. Sometimes it is unclear whether these drugs provide relief through their muscle-relaxing properties or through their sedative effects. Skeletal muscle relaxants include carisoprodol, chlorphenesin, chlorzoxazone, metaxalone, methocarbamol, orphenadrine, and cyclobenzaprine. Antispasmodic drugs include centrally acting agents (baclofen and benzodiazepines) and peripherally acting agents (dantrolene, quinine, and botulinum toxin).

❖ NURSING MANAGEMENT: CLIENT RECEIVING MUSCULOSKELETAL AGENTS

Clients with spasticity often require long-term nursing care and support despite drug therapy (see Example of Nursing Process for Antispasmodic Drug Therapy).

NURSING PROCESS

ASSESSMENT

The nurse should assess the client for underlying conditions that may create problems when taking skeletal muscle relaxants or antispasmodic agents and for a history of sensitivity to medication, because allergic reactions have occurred with carisoprodol, chlorphenesin, and chlorzoxazone. When conducting the physical examination, the nurse should assess the client's neuromuscular function—gait, coordination and strength, spasticity, posture, and ability to perform activities of daily living.

NURSING DIAGNOSIS

Many of the clients who receive skeletal muscle relaxants or antispasmodic agents are being treated for a her-

niated lumbosacral disc, multiple sclerosis, or paraplegia. Nursing diagnoses related to the use of these drugs include:

- Impaired Physical Mobility, related to spasticity
- Risk for Injury, related to drug therapy
- Self Care Deficit, related to spasticity
- Ineffective Management of Therapeutic Regimen, related to potential adverse effects of skeletal muscle relaxant or antispasmodic agent
- Knowledge Deficit, related to drug therapy and disease process

PLANNING

Goals may include eliminating constipation, attaining urinary continence, achieving maximum physical mobility, performing self-care activities within physical limitations, and managing the therapeutic regimen as effectively as possible (see the Critical Thinking Challenge: Case Analysis).

INTERVENTION

Clients require extra supervision because of the drowsiness and dizziness that may occur from therapy with muscle relaxants and antispasmodics. If the client is in a wheelchair, the nurse should provide adequate body support or use restraining methods to prevent the client from falling out of or tipping the wheelchair.

CRITICAL THINKING CHALLENGE
Case Analysis

You are the home care nurse for Robert Slattery, the client featured in the Example of Nursing Process for Antispasmodic Drug Therapy. He was discharged from the hospital and has been taking baclofen for about 14 days. For your first visit, you have developed a care plan based on the nursing diagnosis Knowledge Deficit, related to baclofen therapy. When you first meet with Robert at his home, the dog is barking loudly, the TV is on, and Robert's mother keeps offering you snacks while Robert nearly overwhelms you with conversation and questions. Some of his questions have to do with his medication and some do not.

1. What steps can you take to focus the interview on the goals you have identified in your care plan? What are these goals? What elements of Robert's situation may affect these goals?

2. Once you settle on discussing baclofen, Robert asks you what will happen if this drug does not control his spasms. What options are available to him?

3. Before the interview ends, Robert asks if some symptoms he has been experiencing are related to baclofen therapy. He volunteers that he has been thinking of stopping the medicine altogether, concluding, "After all, how much worse could I be?" Explain how you would approach his concerns while providing correct information about the adverse effects of this drug and the effects of discontinuing therapy.

Example of Nursing Process for Antispasmodic Drug Therapy

The client is Robert Slattery, age 24. He is being admitted to the hospital for treatment of a urinary tract infection and a trial of baclofen therapy. Two years ago, he sustained a complete spinal cord transection at the T9-10 level. He reports having increased difficulty with leg spasms, which are disrupting his exercise program and activities of daily living. He has been taking dantrolene for these spasms. He also has a neurogenic bladder and catheterizes himself every 6 hours.

Before admission, he took mandelamine 1 g four times a day and Dulcolax rectal suppositories every other morning. Now, mandelamine has been discontinued temporarily and a urine specimen obtained for culture. The client is started on an IV antibiotic every 6 hours.

It is August, and the client is scheduled to begin community college classes in September. He is fearful that this setback may interrupt his plans. He is irritable and angry. He speaks about having no control over his situation and expresses frustration over his inability to perform previously mastered activities.

Assessment Data

Complete transection of spinal cord at level T9-10 2 years ago

Increased spasticity in legs over last 2 months

Exercise program and daily activities disrupted

Was receiving dantrolene; will receive baclofen

Irritable

Expresses anger at staff

Speaks of having no control over his situation

Expresses frustration about loss of some abilities

Nursing Diagnosis

Risk for Injury, related to baclofen therapy

Powerlessness, related to hospitalization due to complications of spinal cord transection

Intervention

Administer baclofen as follows: 5 mg three times daily for 3 days with an incremental increase of 5 mg per dose for next 3 days as ordered.

Observe for drowsiness, dizziness, confusion, weakness, fatigue, nausea, hypotension, headache.

Encourage verbalization of concerns and feelings.

Assist in identifying factors that are controllable and those that are not.

Reinforce gains and achievements; provide positive feedback on active participation in self-care.

Provide opportunities for control (allow client to manipulate surroundings, discuss daily plan of activities and allow client to make as many decisions as possible about it).

Record client's specific choices on plan of care.

Sensitize staff and significant others to the importance of their reaction to client's situation.

Goals and Outcomes

The client will maintain normal range of motion.

The client will resume exercise program.

The client will participate as possible in self-care.

The client will experience decreased spasticity.

The client will participate in decision making about care.

The client will participate as possible in self-care.

The client will verbalize ability to control/influence situations and outcomes.

When giving methocarbamol or dantrolene IV, the nurse should follow the special instructions to avoid extravasation of the drug into subcutaneous tissues.

When methocarbamol is administered IV, the nurse should advise the client to remain in a recumbent position for 10 to 15 minutes after the injection to reduce the likelihood of fainting, syncope, or hypotension. The client should be helped with ambulatory activities (as allowed) for at least 2 hours after IV administration. If CNS effects are severe, the client should remain recumbent until the effects decrease.

If dry mouth is an adverse effect of the agent being administered (eg, cyclobenzaprine), relief may be obtained by sipping water, sucking ice chips or hard candy, or chewing gum.

Liver function tests (aspartate aminotransferase, alanine aminotransferase, and alkaline phosphatase) are performed before the onset of therapy with chlorzoxazone, metaxalone, and dantrolene and periodically thereafter during treatment. The nurse should monitor the results for evidence of hepatotoxicity.

Quinine may be given with the evening meal and a bedtime snack to minimize GI upset. Capsule contents should not be emptied or tablets crushed and added to food, because the drug has a bitter taste and is irritating to the stomach. An oral suspension is available if the client has difficulty swallowing the capsule or tablet.

Client Education. Mephenesin-related drugs, such as cyclobenzaprine, baclofen, and dantrolene, can cause drowsiness and dizziness. Nurses should tell clients about these effects and advise against driving a motor vehicle or performing potentially hazardous tasks, such as operating machinery, if such reactions occur. These effects should decrease or cease after the client has become accustomed to the medication.

Because these drugs may compound the effects of alcohol, barbiturates, and other CNS depressants, the nurse should advise clients to avoid such combinations, including the use of nonprescription preparations (eg, liquid cough medications) that contain alcohol.

Because clients who receive quinine may experience nausea, vomiting, and epigastric pain, the nurse should suggest taking the medication with food. Because some clients experience continued relief from nocturnal leg cramps after brief treatment with quinine, it may be appropriate to discuss the possibility of a quinine-free period with the prescriber and client as part of the program evaluation.

Sudden withdrawal of baclofen after prolonged administration may cause hallucinations and exacerbate spasticity. Therefore, if it has been determined that the drug should be discontinued because of its limited efficacy, withdrawal should be gradual.

OUTCOME EVALUATION

The nurse must evaluate the client to determine drug efficacy and to observe for evidence of adverse reactions. It is important to establish whether real benefit has been achieved. Data that indicate drug efficacy include client statements about pain relief, decreased frequency or severity of spasms, increased mobility, increased ability to carry out daily activities, decreased flexor spasticity on physical examination as compared with baseline, increased range of motion, decreased intensity or degree of nursing care required, and increased ease of positioning the client's extremities properly.

❖ CHECKLIST OF NURSING ACTIONS

- ❏ Assess clients for underlying conditions that may create problems with the administration of cyclobenzaprine, orphenadrine, baclofen, or dantrolene.
- ❏ Advise clients about possible drowsiness and dizziness related to muscle relaxants and antispasmodics, as well as the need to avoid potentially hazardous tasks.
- ❏ Watch for idiosyncratic reactions during the early period of carisoprodol therapy.
- ❏ Watch for allergic reactions with carisoprodol, chlorphenesin, and chlorzoxazone.
- ❏ Check that liver function tests are performed periodically during therapy with chlorzoxazone, dantrolene, or metaxalone.
- ❏ Take special precautions when assisting with IV administration of methocarbamol and dantrolene to avoid extravasation of the drug into subcutaneous tissues.
- ❏ Teach the client the benefits to expect from the drugs and the possible adverse reactions.

References

Albright AL, Barron WB, Fasick MP, Polinko P, Janosky J. (1993). Continuous intrathecal baclofen infusion for spasticity of cerebral origin. *JAMA, 270*(20), 2475–2477.

Dicpinigaitis PV. (1996). Use of baclofen to suppress cough induced by angiotensin-converting enzyme inhibitors. *Ann Pharmacother, 30* (11), 1242–1245.

Lewis KS, Mueller WM. (1993). Intrathecal baclofen for severe spasticity secondary to spinal cord injury. *Ann Pharmacother, 27*(6), 767–774.

Young RR. (1994). Spasticity: A review. *Neurobiology, 44*(suppl 9), S12–S20.

Bibliography

Caroff SN, Mann SC. (1993). Neuroleptic malignant syndrome. *Med Clin North Am, 77*(1), 185–202.

Coward DM. (1994). Tizanidine: Neuropharmacology and mechanism of action. *Neurobiology, 44*(suppl 9), S6–S11.

Dillin W, Gurvinder SU. (1992). Medications used in treatment of cervical disk degeneration. *Orthop Clin North Am, 23*(3), 421.

Elder NC. (1991). Abuse of skeletal muscle relaxants. *Am Family Physician,* 44, 1223–1226.

Hardman JG, Limbird LE, Molinoff PB, et al., eds. (1996). *Goodman and Gilman's The pharmacological basis of therapeutics,* 9th ed. New York: McGraw-Hill.

Littrell RA, Hayes LR, Stillner V. (1993). Carisoprodol (Soma): A new and cautious perspective on an old agent. *South Med J,* 86(7), 753–756.

Littrell RA, Sage T, Millwer W. (1993). Meprobamate dependence secondary to carisoprodol (Soma) use. *Am J Drug Alcohol Abuse,* 19, 133–134.

Mitchell G. (1993). Update on multiple sclerosis therapy. *Med Clin North Am, 77*(1), 231.

Philichi LM, Brunn V. (1990). Rhizotomy surgery to relieve spasticity in young children. *MCN, 15*(6), 657–670.

Ramirez FC, Gramah DY. (1992). Treatment of intractable hiccup with baclofen: Results of a double-blind randomized, controlled, cross-over study. *Am J Gastroenterol, 87*(12), 1789–1791.

United Kingdom Tizanidine Trial Group. (1994). A double-blind, placebo-controlled trial of tizanidine in the treatment of spasticity caused by multiple sclerosis. *Neurobiology, 44*(suppl 9), S70–S78.

Waldman HJ. (1994). Centrally acting skeletal muscle relaxants and associated drugs. *J Pain Symptom Manag, 9*(7), 434–441.

For more information and sample tests and activities, refer to Chapter 38 in the Student Workbook for Clinical Pharmacology and Nursing Management, 5th edition, available through your bookstore.

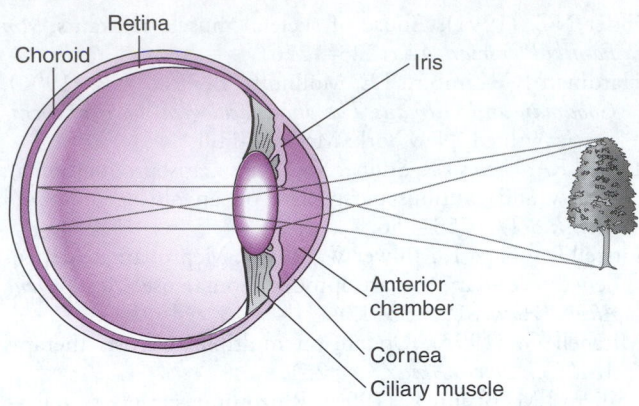

Figure 39-1. The pathway of light in the normal eye.

39

Drugs That Affect the Eyes and Ears

cused on the retina is produced by light that is refracted (bent) by the lens, the cornea, and the fluids of the anterior and posterior chambers. A person with a refractive error needs corrective lenses for proper focus.

The iris contains two separate smooth muscles. The constrictor muscle, activated by parasympathetic nerves from the third cranial nerve, makes the pupil smaller; the dilator, activated by sympathetic nerves, makes it larger (Fig. 39-2). Accommodation, the process of focusing for near or far vision, is accomplished by changing the shape of the lens. This is done by the ciliary muscle, which is also activated by the parasympathetic system from the oculomotor nerve (Fig. 39-3).

Drugs that activate the sympathetic (alpha-adrenergic) receptors or those that block the parasympathetic (cholinergic) receptors of the iris cause mydriasis, or pupillary enlargement. Drugs that block the sympathetic receptors or activate the parasympathetic recep-

Although many medications affect vision or hearing, this chapter deals specifically with medications directly applied to either the eyes or ears for a direct therapeutic effect on the local tissue. The eyes and ears are both sensory systems, but the structures of the eye are more accessible and complex; thus, the range of problems (and therefore medications) is broader for the eye.

Physiology of the Eye

In the simplest terms, the eye acts as a camera (Fig. 39-1). Light enters the focusing system (the cornea, anterior chamber, and lens), passes through the iris, which functions as an aperture, and falls on the retina—the film. The camera-like functions of the system are controlled by the autonomic nervous system. Muscles in and around the eye control the size of the pupil and the shape of the lens, thereby regulating how much light enters the eye and the focus of the image. The image fo-

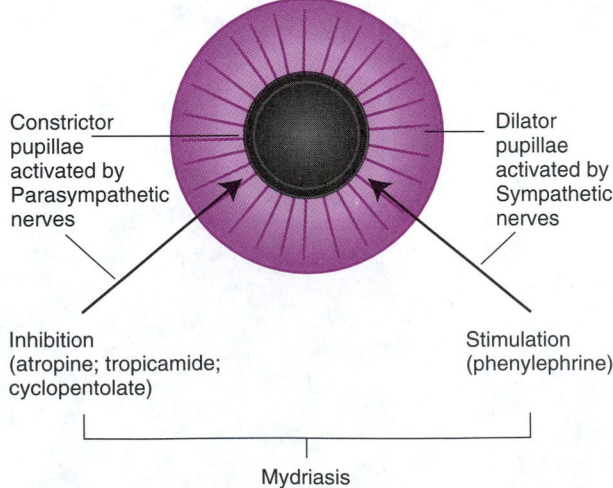

Figure 39-2. Muscles of the iris control pupillary size. Pupillary dilation is activated by the sympathetic nervous system; pupillary constriction is activated by parasympathetic mechanisms. A drug such as phenylephrine stimulates dilation, whereas drugs such as atropine, tropicamide, or cyclopentolate inhibit dilation.

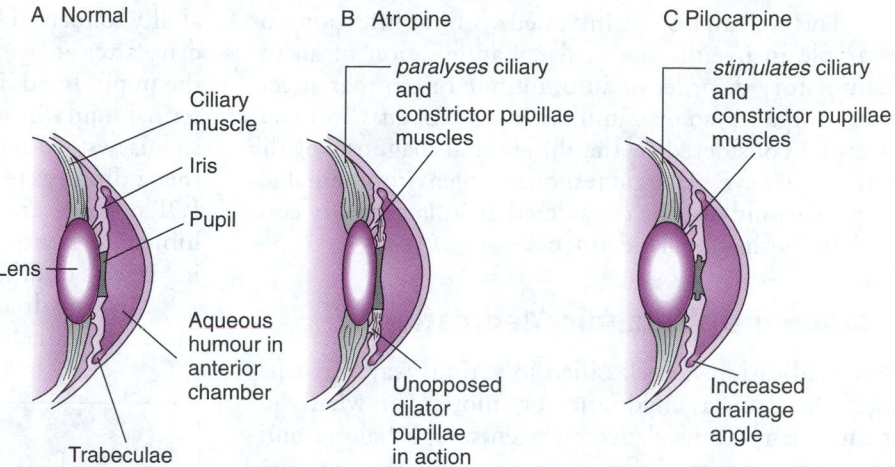

Figure 39-3. Sites of action of parasympathetic agents. (A) Normal eye. (B) Drugs, such as atropine, inhibit constrictor muscles, allowing light to flood the lens. (C) Drugs such as pilocarpine activate constrictor muscles, controlling the amount of light reaching the lens.

tors of the iris cause miosis, or pupillary constriction. Because the drugs that affect the cholinergic mechanisms of the eye act on both the receptors of the iris and the ciliary muscle, drugs with atropine-like effect paralyze accommodation, called cycloplegia. This results in the inability to focus for near vision, impairing reading ability. The tricyclic antidepressants, such as amitriptyline, are one group of medications whose atropine-like properties may have this side effect.

Aqueous humor, the fluid in the anterior chamber of the eye, is generated by the ciliary processes and normally drains through the canal of Schlemm (Fig. 39-4). This fluid generates a normal intraocular pressure (IOP) of 12 to 21 mm Hg. If drainage is impaired, IOP increases, eventually causing retinal damage. Elevated IOP is called glaucoma. This process is usually slow, progressive, and chronic, although it may occur suddenly. Acute glaucoma, presenting with severe eye pain, is a medical emergency. In either case, untreated glaucoma eventually leads to blindness from destruction of the ganglionic cells of the retina and atrophy of the optic nerve.

Because the problem is the presence of more aqueous humor than the system can drain, treatment consists of either slowing production or promoting drainage of the fluid, or both. This can be achieved with medications or surgical intervention. Surgery would be the choice for such conditions as congenital glaucoma, in which the aqueous fluid cannot reach the canal of Schlemm to drain, or post-traumatic glaucoma, in which displacement of the lens or fibrosis may impede drainage. Sometimes laser surgery is the treatment of choice.

Like any other part of the body, the eye is susceptible to infection and inflammation. The offending organisms can be viral, bacterial, or even fungal. The conjunctiva and cornea form a protective barrier, but because the eye is not highly vascular, topical treatments, rather than systemic, are more effective in treating infections. The tears that bathe the eye drain through the lacrimal duct into the nasopharynx and help prevent infections from establishing a foothold. Both medica-

tions and offending organisms can gain access to the entire body by this route through the nasopharynx, although the body has several defense mechanisms along the way, including the adenoids and tonsils. Altered tear flow can generate complaints and prompt clients to seek treatment. Dry eyes can be more susceptible to infection. Contact lenses can interfere with the flow of tears and can also be a source for infection if contaminated.

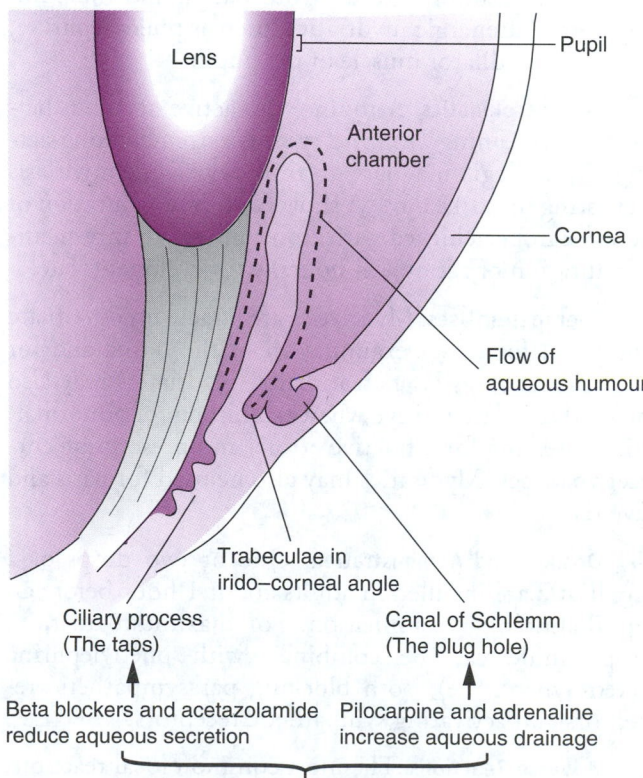

Figure 39-4. Drug actions affect the flow of aqueous humor in clients with glaucoma. Pilocarpine and epinephrine (adrenaline) increase the drainage of aqueous humor, whereas beta blockers and acetazolamide reduce the secretion of aqueous humor.

The eye can also be inflamed without infection, for example in uveitis, the ocular manifestation of an inflammatory disorder of autoimmune origin that affects many organ systems simultaneously. Uveitis must always be considered in the differential diagnosis of the painful red eye. Allergic responses to environmental allergens would also be considered as inflammatory conditions, with similar treatments.

Common Ophthalmic Medications

Eye medications are classified in various ways: by what they do, such as mydriatics or miotics, or what they treat, such as antiglaucoma agents, ophthalmic anti-infectives and antiinflammatories and other preparations. This chapter uses a combination of classifications.

Mydriatics and Cycloplegics

Atropine sulfate is usually considered the prototypical mydriatic agent. Other examples include cyclopentolate (Cyclogyl), epinephrine hydrochloride (Epifrin), homatropine, phenylephrine, and tropicamide (Mydriacyl).

Pharmacodynamics. Mydriatics produce cycloplegia. Anticholinergic mydriatics, such as atropine, block the actions of acetylcholine. In doing so, they relax the ciliary muscles, allowing the lens to flatten and the pupil to dilate. Adrenergic mydriatics, such as phenylephrine, contract the dilator muscle of the pupil.

Pharmacokinetics. Atropine, the active agent in belladonna (meaning *beautiful eyes*), is extremely long-acting. Cycloplegia may last up to 6 days, with mydriasis persisting up to 12 days. A short (2–6-hour) duration of action can be achieved with tropicamide, an intermediate duration of action (24 hours) with cyclopentolate.

Therapeutic Uses. Mydriatics are largely used to dilate the pupil for closer examination of the retina and for therapies such as laser treatments. Mydriatics may also be used to dilate the eye when examining for abnormalities, assessing for refractive errors, and prescribing corrective lenses. Mydriatics may also be used for iritis and uveitis.

Dosage and Administration. One or two drops of a mydriatic are instilled in adults about 1 hour before an ophthalmologic examination. For maximum dilation, tropicamide can be combined with phenylephrine (Neo-Synephrine), both blocking parasympathetic receptors and activating sympathetic receptors.

Adverse Reactions. The most common local reactions include blurred vision, discomfort on instillation, and photophobia. Systemic reactions may involve flushing, dry mouth, tachycardia, and irritability. See Box 39-1.

Precautions and Contraindications. The mydriasis and cycloplegia that occur are responsible for the client's in-

ability to focus. Hence, adults must be cautioned not to drive after an eye examination that includes dilation of the pupil. In addition, dilation of the pupil can lead to retinal injury in strong sunlight, so the client may need sunglasses with good ultraviolet protection. If anesthetic drops were used, as they would be for measuring IOP or for laser therapy, the corneal (blink) reflex is inhibited, presenting the risk of corneal abrasion from flying insects or other foreign bodies.

Most mydriatic drug products are contraindicated in clients with closed-angle (narrow-angle) glaucoma.

Box 39-1
Major Side Effects of Selected Ophthalmic Medications

Miotics

Twitching eyelids caused by increased cholinergic stimulation

Brow pain due to increased cholinergic stimulation

Headache due to vasodilation

Conjunctival pain from local irritation

Contact dermatitis caused by local irritation

Anticholinergics

Dry mouth due to decreased salivation

Flushing and fever resulting from central nervous system (CNS) effect

Blurred vision from pupillary dilation

Skin rash resulting from hypersensitivity

Tachycardia due to decreased vagal stimulation

Ataxia from CNS effect

Mydriatics

Brow ache, headache, and hypertension due to vasoconstriction

Blurred vision as a result of pupillary dilation

Tachycardia due to increased sympathetic stimulation

Carbonic anhydrase inhibitors

Diuresis due to increased excretion of sodium and water

Paresthesia from fluid and electrolyte imbalance

Nausea and vomiting due to gastrointestinal irritation

Osmotic agents

Headache due to cerebral dehydration

Nausea and vomiting from fluid and electrolyte imbalance

Antiglaucoma Agents

In practice, miotic agents are restricted to treating glaucoma, so these agents will be discussed along with the sympathomimetics, beta blockers, and other classes of drugs used to treat glaucoma. The two principal treatments for glaucoma are reducing the production of aqueous humor and promoting its drainage. These treatments, alone or together, lower the IOP in most cases. Among the drugs used for glaucoma treatments, pilocarpine hydrochloride (Isopto-Carpine, Pilopine HS, Ocusert-Pilo) is the prototypical miotic drug. Others include carbachol (Isopto Carbachol), physostigmine (Isopto Eserine), and demecarium (Humorsol).

Other drug classes used to treat glaucoma are the sympathomimetics (eg, epinephrine), beta blockers (eg, timolol maleate), and carbonic anhydrase inhibitors (eg, acetazolamide). These drug classes are discussed in Chapters 16, 25, and 27.

Pharmacodynamics. Miotics increase the outflow of aqueous fluid by constricting the pupil and increasing the drainage angle (see Fig. 39-4). Pilocarpine is a direct-acting agent that stimulates the ciliary and constrictor pupillae muscles, thereby increasing the drainage angle. Indirect-acting miotics, which function as cholinesterase inhibitors, include physostigmine and demecarium. They act by inhibiting the enzyme cholinesterase, prolonging the action of acetylcholine on the parasympathetic receptors of the constrictor pupillae muscle (see Fig. 39-2).

Sympathomimetics, such as epinephrine and dipivefrin (Propine), lower IOP by increasing uveal and scleral outflow. They also have some effect in decreasing the production of aqueous humor, thus working on both sides of the problem. Dipivefrin, a prodrug of epinephrine, is activated enzymatically after absorption into the anterior chamber and thus has fewer local and systemic side effects.

Beta blockers, such as timolol maleate (Timoptic) or betaxolol hydrochloride (Betoptic), decrease the secretion of aqueous humor and thereby lower IOP. Beta blockers can be supplemented, or perhaps replaced, by carbonic anhydrase inhibitors, such as oral acetazolamide (Diamox), for the same effect. Dorzolamide hydrochloride 2% ophthalmic (Trusopt) is a recently approved topical carbonic anhydrase inhibitor. Osmotic diuretics, such as mannitol, which reduces IOP rapidly, have an emergency use in acute glaucoma (see Chap. 27).

Pharmacokinetics. Although most miotics are applied topically, they can be absorbed systemically. Pilocarpine is available as an ocular insert system, gel, and solution. Onset of action is 10 to 30 minutes, peak action occurs in about 75 minutes, and duration of action is 4 to 8 hours.

Therapeutic Uses. Sympathomimetics (epinephrine and dipivefrin) are generally used as an adjunct therapy to miotics. However, because they do not cause pupillary constriction, they may be used as the primary treatment for glaucoma in patients who have central cataracts and whose vision may be impaired by miosis.

Dosage and Administration. Pilocarpine is available in strengths of 0.05% to 6%. Clients with heavily pigmented irises or advanced glaucoma may require higher concentrations. Carbachol is another miotic that may be used in higher concentrations to attain therapeutic effect.

Adverse Reactions. Some adverse effects of pilocarpine include blurred vision, ciliary spasm, conjunctival irritation, tearing, and brow pain and suborbital headache. Other agents used to treat glaucoma, such as topical dorzolamide, may induce systemic side effects common to carbonic anhydrase inhibitors, such as increased salicylate toxicity.

Drug Interactions. Indirect-acting miotics (physostigmine and demecarium) can potentiate the action of succinylcholine, which is often used during anesthesia. Both nurses and clients using cholinesterase inhibitors should be aware of this interaction and should discuss it during the preoperative assessment.

Ophthalmic beta blockers can potentiate the effects of oral beta blockers. Concurrent use of antiglaucoma agents and tricyclic antidepressants increases IOP.

Precautions and Contraindications. Pilocarpine should be administered with caution to clients with bronchial asthma or hypertension. It is contraindicated in clients allergic to the particular drug or other substances in the drug product and in clients with acute iritis, secondary glaucoma, or an acute anterior eye inflammation. Ophthalmic beta blockers may induce adverse effects in clients with asthma or heart failure.

Ophthalmic Anti-Infectives

Ophthalmic anti-infectives are used to fight infections in the eyes (Table 39-1). Typical ophthalmic anti-infective agents are antibacterial drugs such as chloramphenicol (Chloroptic), ciprofloxacin (Ciloxan), and sulfacetamide sodium (Bleph-10). Antiviral drugs include idoxuridine (Stoxil), trifluridine (Viroptic), and vidarabine (Vira-A).

Pharmacodynamics. Antibacterial anti-infectives are bactericidal or bacteriostatic, depending on the drug strength and the pathogen's susceptibility. Some interfere with the synthesis of folic acid, which is needed by bacteria to grow. Antiviral drugs appear to inhibit viral replication. One drug, natamycin, is an antifungal.

Pharmacokinetics. Ophthalmic solutions and gels penetrate the cornea. In general, absorption appears to be local, not systemic, and probably depends on the drug's concentration and frequency of application. Onset, peak, and duration of action depend on the specific drug preparation.

Table 39-1. Selected Ophthalmic Anti-infectives

Drug Name	Preparation	Precautions
Antibacterials		
chloramphenicol (Chloromycetin, Chloroptic)	1% oint., 0.5% soln.	Client may need supplemental systemic antibiotics. Generally reserved for organisms resistant to safer agents.
ciprofloxacin (Ciloxan)	0.3% soln. PC: C	Discontinue if rash occurs.
erythromycin (Ilotycin)	Oint (5 mg/g) PC: B	Not recommended for nursing mothers
gentamicin sulfate (Garamycin, Genoptic)	Soln. (3 mg/mL), oint (3 mg/g) PC: C	
ofloxacin (Ocuflox)	0.3% soln. PC: C	Not recommended for nursing mothers
sulfacetamide sodium (Bleph-10, Sulamyd)	10% soln., oint PC: C	Purulent exudate may inactivate drug. Ointment may retard corneal healing.
tobramycin (Tobrex)	0.3% soln., oint PC: B	Not recommended for nursing mothers
Antivirals		
idoxuridine (Stoxil, Herplex, IDU)	0.1% soln., 0.5% oint. PC: C	Indicated for herpes simplex keratitis; contraindicated in bacterial, fungal, or chlamydial infections
trifluridine (Viroptic)	1% soln. PC: C	Indicated for herpes simplex keratitis; contraindicated in bacterial, fungal, or chlamydial infections
vidarabine (Vira-A)	3% oint. PC: C	Indicated for herpes simplex keratitis; contraindicated in bacterial, fungal, or chlamydial infections
Antifungals		
natamycin (Natacyn)	5% soln. PC: C	Indicated for fungal conjunctivitis and keratitis.

Key: PC = pregnancy risk category (see Appendix A), oint=ointment, soln. = solution.

Therapeutic Uses. Topical anti-infectives treat such disorders as conjunctivitis, a bacterial or viral infection of the conjunctiva characterized by redness and purulent discharge, and keratitis, an infection that has the potential to ulcerate and scar the cornea.

With the increase in clients with compromised immune systems (eg, AIDS clients, organ transplant recipients), cytomegalovirus (CMV) retinitis is another eye infection of consequence. CMV infection is fairly common in the general population. Most victims experience a mild viral illness and then become quiet carriers of CMV. Organs from a donor who had CMV may be transplanted to a person who then receives antirejection therapy with immunosuppressive drugs. This may result in a flare-up of CMV and retinitis.

Adverse Reactions. Common adverse effects include sensitivity reactions, stinging, burning, itching, photophobia, and, in long-term use, bacterial or fungal overgrowth of nonsusceptible organisms.

Precautions and Contraindications. Anti-infective medications are not given to clients allergic to the drugs (see Table 39-1).

Ophthalmic Antiinflammatory Drugs

This group of drugs includes a wide range of antihistamines, corticosteroids, topical nonsteroidal antiinflammatory drugs (NSAIDs), and other ophthalmic agents. Some of the drugs listed in Box 39-2 can also be found in combination products. When prescribing antiinflammatory ophthalmic preparations, some practitioners avoid combination ointments and solutions because some clients tend to save medications and use them in the future for the wrong condition. This is particularly true of steroid combinations, which, if used in an unrecognized viral keratitis, can harm the client's vision.

Corticosteroids are also useful in treating uveitis, an inflammatory condition of autoimmune origin that can affect almost any part of the eye. Should the iris be affected, mydriatics may also be required to relax the muscles of the pupil and lens. Glaucoma can either arise from or be aggravated by the use of steroids and mydriatics. Although uveitis is uncommon, it is a problem that challenges the nurse's understanding of both the disease process and the actions of all potential medications needed.

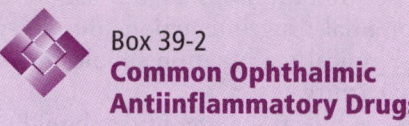

Box 39-2
Common Ophthalmic Antiinflammatory Drugs

Corticosteroids

dexamethasone (Ocu-Dex)

prednisolone acetate (Pred-Forte, AK-Tate)

Nonsteroidal antiinflammatory drugs

diclofenac sodium (Cataflam, Voltaren)

flurbiprofen sodium (Ocufen)

ketorolac tromethamine (Acular)

Ophthalmic Anesthetics

For certain procedures, such as tonometry to measure the pressure in the eye, the cornea must be anesthetized to tolerate having the tonometer rest on its surface. The cornea usually needs to be numbed for removal of a superficial foreign body, just to deaden the corneal blink reflex. The prototype ophthalmic anesthetic is cocaine. However, tetracaine or another short-acting synthetic is more likely to be available, if only because cocaine is a schedule II drug. See Home and Community Care: Eye Care After Topical Anesthesia.

A single drop of tetracaine applied to the cornea provides anesthesia to the sensory fibers of the third cranial nerve in less than 10 seconds. At the same time, the drug acts as a vasoconstrictor, which reduces the healing blood supply to the conjunctiva and thereby the cornea. A single drop is not a problem, but clients with corneal burns, not wishing to have the pain return, may plead for additional medication. Complying with the request can endanger the client's vision: misuse of a topical ophthalmic anesthetic may lead to severe infection with corneal scarring (Zagelbaum et al., 1994).

Other Ophthalmic Drugs

Various other drugs are used in treating or diagnosing eye problems; some are commercially available, and some are investigational (Box 39-3). Fluorescein sodium (Fluor-I-Strip) is a topical dye used to evaluate corneal injuries. It binds to defects in the smooth epithelial surface and fluoresces when exposed to ultraviolet light, clearly revealing the defect. This drug can also be given intravenously to trace the vascular system of the retina.

Lodoxamide tromethamine (Alomide) is a mast cell stabilizer. It inhibits increased permeability of ocular blood vessels in response to substances such as histamine

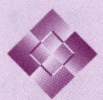

Box 39-3
New Horizons: Investigational Ophthalmic Therapies

Several drugs that hold promise for future treatment are in various stages of development and trial.

Botulinum Toxin

This substance is being studied for treating certain problems associated with muscles around the eye. Botulinum toxin is the protein produced by the anaerobic bacteria *Clostridium botulinum,* the organism responsible for death by flaccid paralysis after ingestion of improperly processed food. This toxin can induce the same paralysis in the eye muscles responsible for blepharospasm, an uncomfortable dystonic muscle contraction of the orbicularis oculi muscle that causes unilateral or bilateral eye closure. The toxin can also be used in evaluating strabismus. In this application, the toxin is used on the stronger muscle to allow the client to see what improvement in vision might result from surgery. For nonsurgical clients, paralysis of the stronger muscle for up to 12 weeks (the duration of one treatment) may be all the treatment needed. Finally, the toxin can be used to induce ptosis by paralyzing the levator muscle. This may be useful when healing of a corneal injury requires long-term eye closure. The toxin works by exhausting acetylcholine vesicles at the neuromuscular junction. This effect is permanent, and muscle function returns only when new neuromuscular junctions, sprouted from the presynaptic neurons, are created (Smith, 1995).

Healing Peptides

Recombinant DNA technology may allow the creation of an increasing number of endogenous growth regulatory proteins. These peptides have great potential use in ophthalmic wound healing, although there are many unanswered questions before these drugs enter clinical trials (Stromberg et al., 1994).

Drug Delivery Lenses

Soft (hydrophilic) contact lenses, because of their ability to absorb water, have the potential to absorb and deliver medications. This ability is most often used in dry eye conditions to increase lubrication, but it can also be used for treating corneal infections. Clients who are contact lens users should be aware of this possibility and advised appropriately.

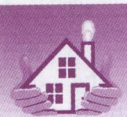

HOME AND COMMUNITY CARE

Eye Care after Topical Anesthesia

Nurses caring for clients who have had topical ophthalmic anesthetics must provide some instruction for eye care. Usually the client returns home while the eye still lacks feeling.

- Caution the client that the unfeeling eye is at risk for injury until the effect of the anesthetic wears off.
- Suggest wearing an eye patch until sensation returns as a way to protect the eye from injury.
- Warn the client without an eye patch not to rub the eye. Doing so could introduce a foreign body that would not be felt and could cause severe corneal abrasion.
- Topical ophthalmic anesthetics slow the healing process, so additional doses of such drugs should not be used and are not recommended even after emergency treatment of a painful corneal burn. The temptation to use a topical anesthetic is great because the pain relief from anesthetics is superior to that from an oral analgesic.

that are secreted in inflammatory conditions. It is useful in treating keratitis and keratoconjunctivitis.

Dapiprazole hydrochloride (Rev-Eyes), an alpha-adrenergic blocker, can be used to constrict the pupils after a mydriatic drug dilates them.

Artificial tears are various isotonic mixtures of salts and buffers used to lubricate dry eyes or contact lenses. They may also contain an agent to increase viscosity and thereby increase contact time with the eye. Most are available without prescription.

❖ NURSING MANAGEMENT: CLIENT RECEIVING OPHTHALMIC DRUG THERAPY

The use of medications for treating eye problems, particularly glaucoma, is generally a client self-care activity. The nurse's role is to be supportive and instructive. Similarly, clients receiving ophthalmic anti-infective or antiinflammatory drugs or other ophthalmic preparations need encouragement and careful instruction.

NURSING PROCESS

ASSESSMENT

In compiling the health history for the client receiving ophthalmic drugs to treat glaucoma, the nurse must rule out a known allergy to the medication prescribed. A complete medication history should be taken to en-

sure there are no contraindications to the use of any given agents or potential drug interactions due to systemic absorption. Physical examination should include vital signs and visual acuity.

In clients with eye infections, the nurse should obtain a specimen of the exudate or discharge for culture before drug therapy begins. Examination of the eye, with a careful description of the findings, is essential to monitor therapy. In addition, risk factors for spread of infection in the client's household must be investigated, because prevention is needed to stop the spread of these infections. In close quarters, such as families, acute care nursing units, and nursing homes, these infections can become epidemic.

NURSING DIAGNOSES

Some nursing diagnoses that may apply to clients receiving an antiglaucoma drug include:

- Sensory/Perceptual Alteration: Visual
- Risk for Injury, related to adverse effect of medication such as blurred vision
- Knowledge Deficit, related to therapeutic drug regimen and disease course

Nursing diagnoses that may be applied to clients receiving anti-infective, antiinflammatory, or other ophthalmic preparations may include:

- Sensory/Perceptual Alteration: Visual, secondary to effects of medication and disease
- Pain, secondary to infection and medication
- Knowledge Deficit, regarding proper use of medication

PLANNING

The goals of nursing care include promoting and preserving vision, monitoring the client's response to drug therapy, and most of all educating the client to adhere to the regimen and administer drug therapy correctly and effectively.

INTERVENTION

The nurse should monitor vital signs as needed and construct a care plan to meet the client's instructional needs. The nurse can help schedule follow-up appointments as recommended.

Client Education. The client should be shown how to use medications properly (Box 39-4). The nurse must explain the importance of keeping the tip of the drug applicator sterile—this means the applicator tip must not rest on a table top, nor should it come in contact with the eyelid or eyeball. Clients should be taught the signs and symptoms of problems and should report them to the prescriber.

The client receiving anti-infective, antiinflammatory, or other ophthalmic preparations should be instructed to apply warm compresses with a warm, damp washcloth to the affected eye for 5 to 10 minutes three or four times a day. Warm compresses promote circulation and vasodilation, which helps propel the body's healing mechanisms to the affected sites. Warm compresses also enhance comfort by soothing inflamed tissues.

The nurse must explain hygienic considerations as well. To prevent transmitting infections, the client must not share a washcloth or towel with anyone else. Potentially contaminated eye makeup must be discarded, as must any medication remaining after therapy concludes (bacterial contamination can produce strains of organisms resistant to the old medication, and the organism can be reintroduced to the eye with reuse).

Clients receiving miotic medications should be cautioned that the effects of the medication may impair their vision in low light conditions. This may present a problem for clients who drive at night, particularly those using pilocarpine.

Clients must understand that some of these drugs, such as ophthalmic beta blockers, may be absorbed systemically. Clients with glaucoma should avoid atropine-like mydriatics, or drugs with anticholinergic effects, such as tricyclic antidepressants. As shown in Figure 39-4, dilation of the pupil (mydriasis) decreases the angle for drainage and can lead quickly to increased IOP.

Other teaching points include showing the client how to store drug products safely. These medications are not benign substances: one report (Pfliegler & Palatka, 1995) cites a death caused by oral ingestion of pilocarpine, with 60 mg considered a lethal dose. As this medication is often stored in the refrigerator, access by children is possible.

Clients using these medications must tell any other healthcare providers that they are doing so, specifically anesthetists. Many of these medications can interact with drugs used to reverse neuromuscular blocking agents during surgery. The interaction can lead to prolonged intubation, hypotension, or even heart failure (Kelsey, 1992).

The nurse should inform the client that the duration of therapy will vary, depending on the drug. Topical medications tend to induce more side effects as the treatment course lengthens. The nurse can help the client work out a flexible schedule that offers the client some control. For instance, with bacterial conjunctivitis, therapy may continue for 2 days after the symptoms resolve. If the client has keratitis, a stricter treatment plan with frequent follow-up is needed because of the potential for a poorer outcome.

Clients should be discouraged from self-prescribing any anti-infectives, ophthalmic or systemic, as the selection of appropriate therapy is best left to a skilled prescriber. Incomplete or inappropriate therapy can produce resistant strains of organisms.

OUTCOME EVALUATION

Outcome evaluation involves monitoring the status of the infection and the progress of ongoing treatment and tests. In most instances, this is up to the client,

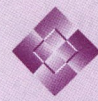

Box 39-4
Guidelines for Administering Ophthalmic Medications

How to Apply Ophthalmic Solutions

First, wash your hands. Of course, be sure you have the right drug, client, dose, route, and time.

Apply pressure over the medial canthus of the eye with the index finger to occlude the lacrimal duct.

Tilt the client's head back, and with the middle finger of the same hand, gently pull down on the lower lid to form a pouch. (Although more than one drop per application may be prescribed, the normal eye can retain only 10 microliters (µL) of fluid, and the normal drop is 25 to 50 µL. Thus, it is doubtful there is any value to more than one drop per application.)

Tell the client to look up, and then insert the number of drops ordered into the pouch and close the eye.

Maintain gentle pressure on the medial canthus for 3 to 5 minutes. This pressure inhibits drainage of the medication into the lacrimal duct, thereby limiting systemic absorption and possible side effects.

To maintain the sterility of the contents, be sure not to touch the tip of the bottle or the eyedropper.

How to Apply Ophthalmic Ointments or Gels

Pressure is not needed on the inner canthus, because the ointment does not quickly migrate down the lacrimal duct. Usually 1 to 1.5 cm of ointment is an adequate dose.

Do not touch the tip of the tube, as this may contaminate the sterile contents.

Instruct the client to close the eyelids gently and rotate the eye to spread the medication.

How to Apply Ophthalmic Inserts

Special instructions come with this dosage form and should be followed. For pilocarpine (Ocusert-Pilo), the insert is placed in the upper or lower lid pouch and is changed every 7 days. Advise the client to check that the insert is in the eye at bedtime and on arising.

who should contact the prescriber if progress is unsatisfactory. Having the client perform a return demonstration of drug administration will reveal any skills that need more practice. Assessing vital signs may reveal systemic effects of the medication. Visual acuity should remain stable, although some blurred vision may be expected initially after application of the medication.

❖ CHECKLIST OF NURSING ACTIONS

☐ Take baseline vital signs.

☐ Assess the client for a history of hypersensitivity to the ophthalmic drug or other contents in the drug solution.

☐ Monitor the client's response to drug administration.

☐ Teach the client proper technique for self-administering eye drops or ointment and maintaining drug sterility.

☐ Have the client perform a return demonstration of drug administration to verify effective and safe technique.

☐ Teach the client to recognize signs and symptoms of unsatisfactory progress that should be reported to the prescriber.

Topical Otic Medications

Because the acoustic and vestibular functions of the ear occur behind the eardrum, most drugs applied directly to the ear are intended to treat local conditions. Thus, otic preparations are truly topical medications, assuming the client has an intact tympanic membrane. Medications applied to the ear fall into several general categories: anti-infectives (with or without antiinflammatory properties), anesthetics, and ceruminolytics.

Pathophysiology

Anatomy, rather than physiology, determines what drugs are developed for ear problems. The major anatomic consideration is that the ear canal passes through a bony orifice in the skull. By limiting the size of the ear canal to the dimensions of the opening in the bone, any swelling that might occur in the tissues of the ear canal must be directed inward, constricting the patency of the canal. This problem—inflammation of the tissues of the canal—is called otitis externa (swimmer's ear) and can result in complete occlusion of the canal. Complete occlusion is rare but occurs suddenly. To deliver medication past the occlusion, a wicklike delivery system may be inserted. This allows successful topical treatment, although some clients may need systemic antibiotics as well.

Otic Anti-Infectives

Because the ear canal is not sterile, infections are usually opportunistic infections caused by normal skin flora. In swimmer's ear, water trapped in the canal provides an excellent medium for bacterial or fungal growth.

The most commonly used anti-infective is Cortisporin Otic (suspension or solution), which contains polymyxin B sulfate, neomycin, and hydrocortisone. Other topical anti-infectives include chloramphenicol otic solution (Chloromycetin Otic), and gentamicin sulfate otic solution (Garamycin). Used systemically, chloromycetin and gentamicin are associated with serious adverse effects—aplastic anemia for the former and ototoxicity and nephrotoxicity for the latter.

Other agents are solutions containing an acetic acid (vinegar). Acetic acid is an effective antibacterial and antifungal agent and is found in such solutions as Vosol, which contains 2% acetic acid (household vinegar is 5%) and 3% propylene glycol diacetate. It is also available as Vosol HC, with the addition of 1% hydrocortisone.

Pharmacodynamics. Cortisporin Otic produces an antiinflammatory effect to minimize swelling and also contains topical antibiotics.

Pharmacokinetics. Most otic solutions are not significantly absorbed from the ear canal. Onset, peak, and duration of action vary with the specific drug.

Therapeutic Uses. Cortisporin Otic is often used prophylactically after tympanostomy for aural tube insertion. It does not harm the middle ear (Welling et al., 1995) and is suitable for use with a perforated tympanic membrane.

Dosage and Administration. Five to 10 drops of the drug are instilled in the ear canal and should remain there for about 15 minutes. Treatment usually lasts 5 to 7 days, although some practitioners instruct the client to use the drug for 2 days after relief of symptoms. For a severe infection requiring wick insertion, the duration of therapy may be extended and systemic antibiotics may be added to prevent the spread of infection to the mastoid process.

Adverse Reactions. Local irritation, itching, burning, and swelling are the most common adverse effects. With prolonged use, superinfection may occur.

Precautions and Contraindications. When applied topically for local infections, the amount of drug that enters the systemic circulation does not approach the blood levels needed to produce severe side effects. However, otic drugs are available in dropper bottles that could be misused by children, so clients should store them safely away from children.

Otic Analgesics

Otic analgesics are a small group of medications with limited application. The primary use of a topical anesthetic for the ear is to treat the pain of otitis media, especially in children. With the pressure that can build behind the eardrum, children become very uncomfortable, crying inconsolably and pulling at the ear. The pain usually responds to oral analgesics such as acetaminophen (Tylenol) or the oral NSAIDs approved for use in children. The pain usually subsides after several doses of a systemic antibiotic. However, faster pain relief can be obtained with a topical anesthetic such as Auralgan, a combination of the anesthetic benzocaine and the analgesic antipyrine. (Auralgan is also instilled to provide local anesthesia before irrigating the ear canal to remove wax.)

Ceruminolytics

Ceruminolytics are agents that loosen impacted ear wax for easy removal. Carbamide peroxide 6.5% (Debrox) is available without a prescription; triethanolamine polypeptide 10% (Cerumenex) is a prescription medication. Both agents work by penetrating and softening the dried wax. Debrox can be used daily over several days before attempting ear wax removal; Cerumenex should not be allowed to stay in the ear canal more than 30 minutes before irrigation.

❖ NURSING MANAGEMENT: CLIENT RECEIVING OTIC DRUG THERAPY

The nurse must remember that the pain of otitis media is also relieved by rupture of the tympanic membrane. In using Auralgan or other otic anesthetics, a single dose should be applied in the office or clinic. Clients who use the drug at home must understand that pain relief alone does not indicate successful treatment of infection. Treating the pain only, without antibiotic therapy, gives the infection additional time to perforate the eardrum or invade internal structures.

NURSING PROCESS

ASSESSMENT

The client's history should be compiled and reviewed for conditions that contraindicate the use of otic agents. Baseline assessment should include a description of the ear infection or impacted ear wax.

NURSING DIAGNOSES

Possible nursing diagnoses for a client receiving otic agents may be:

- Risk for Infection, related to drug-induced overgrowth of nonsusceptible organisms
- Knowledge Deficit, related to use of medication

PLANNING

Nursing care objectives include controlling pain related to infection or impaction and increasing the client's skill in self-administering medications.

INTERVENTION

Before administering an otic solution, the nurse should have the client lie down or tilt the head so that the affected ear faces up. The earlobe is gently pulled up and back for adults, down and back for children, to straighten the ear canal. Next, the prescribed number of drops are instilled into the ear canal.

The client should remain with the ear facing up for 1 or 2 minutes to allow the medicine to come in contact with the entire canal and eardrum. A sterile cotton plug may be gently inserted into the ear opening to prevent the medicine from leaking out.

Client Education. For clients who are self-administering the otic medication, the nurse must teach the above procedure and have the client perform a return demonstration. The nurse also must teach the client how to keep the medicine as germfree as possible by not touching the applicator tip to any surface, including the ear. This is not, however, as important as with ophthalmic medications.

The client must understand the need to continue using the medication for the prescribed period, even though symptoms may resolve before therapy is scheduled to conclude.

OUTCOME EVALUATION

Data needed to evaluate the success of otic drug therapy include resolution of ear infection and symptoms, verification of proper drug administration techniques, and absence of adverse drug effects and superinfection.

❖ CHECKLIST OF NURSING ACTIONS

- ❑ Assess the client's response to therapy.
- ❑ Review test results, particularly culture and sensitivity tests, if done.
- ❑ Administer medications, and teach the client or a member of the client's family to administer medication safely and effectively.
- ❑ Be alert for possible adverse effects.
- ❑ Teach the client how to keep the drug solution free of contaminants.

References

Kelsey M. (1992). Ophthalmic medications, glaucoma, and the surgical patient. *J Postanesthesia Nurs, 7*(5), 312–316.

Pfliegler GP, Palatka K. (1995). Attempted suicide with pilocarpine eye drops. *Am J Ophthalmol, 120*(3), 399–400.

Smith H. (1995). The effects of botulinum toxin on ocular tissue. *Nursing Times, 91*(4), 41–43.

Stromberg K, Chapekar MS, Goldman BA, Chambers WA, Cavagnero JA. (1994). Regulatory concerns in the development of topical recombinant ophthalmic and cutaneous wound health biologics. *Wound Repair and Regeneration, 2*(3), 155–164.

Welling DB, Forrest LA, Goll F. (1995). Safety of ototopical antibiotics. *Laryngoscope, 105*(5), 472–474.

Zagelbaum BM, Tostanoski JR, Hochman MA, Hersh RS. (1994). Topical lidocaine and proparacaine abuse. *Am J Emerg Med, 12*(1), 96–97.

Bibliography

Barlow DW, Duckert LG, Kreig CS, Gates GA. (1995). Ototoxicity of topical otomicrobial agents. *Acta Otolaryngol, 115*(2), 231–235.

Brennan KM, Brown RM, Roberts CW. (1993). A comparison of topical non-steroidal anti-inflammatory drugs to steroids for control of post-cataract inflammation. *Insight, 18*(1), 8–9.

Cloutier AO. (1992). Ocular side effects of chemotherapy: Nursing management. *Oncol Nurs Forum,* 19(8), 1251–1259.

Cohen MR. (1995). Sound-alike ophthalmics: Eye-opening error. *Nursing '95, 24*(4), 15.

Company to develop and market drug implant system for CMV. (1993). *AIDS Weekly,* Jan. 25, p. 5.

Davidson TM, Neuman TR. (1994). Managing inflammatory ear conditions. *Physician and Sports Medicine, 22*(8), 56–60.

Hussar DA. (1994). Drug update '94. *Nursing '94, 24*(5), 57–63.

Kelly J. (1994). Nursing intervention in the treatment of cataracts. *Br J Nurs, 3*(12), 602–606.

Nurse practitioners' prescribing reference, summer 1996. New York: Prescribing Reference, Inc.

O'Brien TP, Reynolds LA. (1995). Basic ocular pharmacotherapy. *J Ophthalmic Nurs Tech, 14*(4), 174–175.

Plona RP, Schremp PS. (1992). Nursing care of patients with ocular manifestations of human immunodeficiency virus infection. *Nurs Clin North Am, 27*(3), 793–805.

Rohn GN, Meyerhoff WL, Wright CG. (1993). Ototoxicity of topical agents. *Otolaryngol Clin North Am, 26*(5), 747–758.

For more information and sample tests and activities, refer to Chapter 39 in the Student Workbook for Clinical Pharmacology and Nursing Management, 5th edition, available through your bookstore.

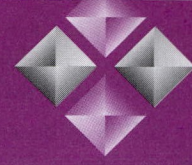

40

Drugs That Affect the Integumentary System

T he skin, the largest sensory organ, has many essential functions, including protection, thermoregulation, immune responsiveness, biochemical synthesis, and communication. As the largest organ of the body, the skin is the interface between the body's internal and external environments (Box 40-1). Integument is the term that denotes skin and its appendages (hair, nails, glands).

Box 40-1
Functions of the Skin

Prevents entry of microorganisms; dry external surface and acidic pH inhibit proliferation of microorganisms

Serves as a barrier against fluid and electrolyte losses; has low permeability to water and electrolytes

Detects sensations (pain, pressure, touch, temperature) through sensory nerve endings

Plays a role in vitamin D synthesis (photoconversion of precursor in epidermal malpighian cells produces vitamin D)

Stores glycogen and contributes to glucose metabolism

Regulates body temperature: evaporation of sweat secreted onto skin surface allows heat dissipation; cutaneous vascular dilation or constriction promotes or inhibits heat conduction from skin surface

Can express emotions (eg, shame, anger, fear)

Serves as a barometer of health and a sensitive reflection of the internal environment

---

Pathophysiology of Integumentary Disorders

Of the 2,000 known skin diseases, some of the most common are acne vulgaris, contact dermatitis, atopic dermatitis (eczema), seborrheic dermatitis, and psoriasis. Other skin disorders may result from trauma injury to the soft tissues or thermal injury (burns).

Acne Vulgaris

Acne vulgaris is a disease of specialized follicles known as sebaceous or pilosebaceous follicles, which are hair follicles that have large oil-producing glands. Lesions over these follicles may be papular, pustular, or nodular. Although it can occur in adults, acne typically affects adolescents and involves the face, neck, shoulders, and trunk. The disorder is characterized by open comedones (blackheads), closed comedones (whiteheads), papules, pustules, nodules, and cysts.

The exact cause of acne is unknown, but it is an interaction of several factors. Hormones (androgens) stimulate sebaceous follicles to produce larger amounts of sebum. The proliferation of follicular bacterium (*Propionibacterium acnes*) is assisted by use of sebum as a growth substrate. An inflammatory process occurs that results in shedding of epithelial cells that line the follicular lumen, and these accumulate and distend the follicle. The distended follicle wall subsequently ruptures.

Treatment may include topical treatment with benzoyl peroxide preparations, which have antibacterial action against *Propionibacterium acnes*. Local irritation is common and contact allergy can occur with this agent. Other treatments may involve acne-drying soaps and abrasive cleansers (which may be counterproductive because they may stimulate inflammation and reinforce the myth that acne is due to dirt and can be scrubbed away), topical retinoids (tretinoin or Retin-A), topical antibiotics (for mild acne), and systemic antibiotics such as tetracycline, erythromycin, minocycline, clindamycin, or trimethoprim/sulfamethoxazole (for severe acne).

Psoriasis

Psoriasis is a chronic, genetically influenced skin disorder that affects up to 3% of the world's population (Greaves & Weinstein, 1995). It is characterized by the periodic exacerbation of erythematous papules and plaques covered by prominent, thick silvery-white scales. Although the exact cause is unknown, it is associated with arthritis (psoriatic arthritis), skin injuries, and medication use, and in many cases a familial tendency is noted. The basic abnormality is a hyperproliferation of epidermis and inflammation of epidermis and dermis; these changes are due to T-lymphocyte–mediated dermal immune response to unidentified antigenic stimuli (Greaves & Weinstein, 1995). The classic distribution of the lesions includes the elbows, knees, and back. The lesion may or may not itch. Psoriasis can be divided into four categories: psoriasis vulgaris, pustular psoriasis, pustular psoriasis on the palms and soles, and erythrodermic psoriasis.

There is no cure for psoriasis, only suppressive therapy. Treatment aims to decrease the severity and extent of the disease to the point at which it no longer interferes substantially with the client's occupation, personal or social life, or well-being. Topical therapy includes topical corticosteroids, intralesional corticosteroid therapy, tars (usually used in combination with phototherapy), anthralin, salicylic acid, tretinoin (Retin-A), 5-fluorouracil cream (Efudex), calcipotriene, and combination therapy. The folic acid antagonist methotrexate (see Chap. 46) is effective for selected clients with psoriasis; the mode of action is the blockade of DNA synthesis, inhibiting cell proliferation in rapidly dividing tissues such as the hyperproliferative psoriatic epidermis. The presumptive involvement of T cells in psoriasis is leading to intense interest in immunotherapy (such as with anti-CD4 monoclonal antibody).

Atopic Dermatitis (Eczema)

Atopic dermatitis is often associated with a family or personal history of allergies or asthma. It is characterized by itchy, erythematous, edematous, moist and weeping skin during the acute stage and dryness, scaling, and lichenification (thickening and furrows) in the chronic stage.

Treatment of atopic dermatitis aims to relieve pruritus and the scratching that may promote complications. Treatment of mild irritation focuses on preserving skin moisture and preventing continued drying. In more severe cases, topical steroids are an important part of therapy. Intermittent secondary infection is a common feature, so treatment may include oral antibiotics or even hospitalization and intravenous (IV) antibacterial or antiviral therapy.

Wounds

Trauma to skin and to the underlying soft tissue results in disruption of the circulatory and lymphatic systems. Wound repair incorporates the inflammatory response, reepithelialization (granulation tissue formation), revascularization (matrix formation and remodeling), collagen accumulation, and wound closure or contraction. Wounds do not heal readily in the presence of tissue debris and purulent exudate, which promote the growth of infectious organisms and stimulate inflammation in adjacent tissues. Mechanical methods may be used to remove necrotic material from wounds (surgical debridement, whirlpool baths, irrigation, suction drainage, wet-to-dry dressings), or chemical agents (topical enzymes) may be used with or instead of mechanical means.

General Skin Treatment Principles

Therapy typically begins with topical therapy, with systemic therapy added if topical therapy is ineffective. Once the medication is prescribed, the next decision involves the vehicle—soaks, powders, lotions, solutions, creams, ointments, sprays, or pastes. One general rule is that acute lesions that are moist or oozing respond best to the effects of medication in aqueous, drying preparations, whereas chronic scaling lesions respond best to medication incorporated in moisturizing, lubricating preparations. In choosing a vehicle, the likelihood of therapeutic adherence is a consideration. For instance, an ointment may be the most effective vehicle, but if the client thinks it is too greasy and does not use it, nothing has been gained.

Preparations for Drying the Skin

Wet soaks are an easy, inexpensive method of drying an acute moist, oozing eruption. This method relies on drying by evaporation. Soaks can also be used to clean the skin, debride wounds, promote drainage of inflammatory cysts or abscesses, and combat infection.

Open soaks are applied for 20 minutes, three times a day; no occlusive dressing is applied. Closed soaks use occlusion (water-impermeable substance) over a wet soak. This method causes heat retention, which is excellent for debridement but may lead to maceration.

Closed soaks are applied for 1 to 2 hours two or three times a day. The material used for occlusion might be plastic wrap, gloves (for the hands or feet), a shower cap (for the scalp), or a vinyl or cloth exercise suit (for large areas such as the arms or legs). Continuous closed soaks (left in place for 24 hours) are best for thick crusts. The dressing is left in place but rewetted four or five times a day. To enhance the action of soaks, a medication can be added to the water in which the dressing is first soaked.

Burow's Solution

Burow's solution (Bluboro Powder, Boropak Powder, Domeboro, Pedi-Boro Soak Paks) contains 5% aluminum acetate. It is usually used in a 1:20 or 1:40 dilution. One packet of powder or a tablet of Domeboro (which contains both aluminum sulfate and calcium acetate) dissolved in 1 pint of water yields about a 1:40 dilution. This solution is nonstaining and nonirritating.

Acetic Acid

Acetic acid can be used in a final concentration of 0.1% to 1%. White (distilled) vinegar is 5% acetic acid; thus, in a 1:4 dilution it is about a 1% solution. Acetic acid has an antibacterial effect but may be irritating to the skin.

Potassium Permanganate

A 1:4,000 to 1:16,000 dilution of potassium permanganate can be used, but it stains the skin.

Powders, Lotions, Astringents, Pastes, and Sprays

Powders are commonly used in intertriginous areas to reduce friction and maceration and promote drying. Lotions were historically "shake lotions" or suspensions of a powder in water (before application, they must be shaken to place the powder in suspension). As the water in the lotion evaporates, a coating of powder is left on the skin, producing a drying effect. Calamine lotion (Calamox, Resinol, Calamatum), a preparation of calamine with other ingredients such as zinc oxide, glycerin, bentonite magma, and calcium hydroxide solution, is a commonly used shake lotion. Today other liquid emulsions and foams that are of thin, uniform consistency may also be referred to as lotions.

Astringents are solutions that usually consist of a combination of alcohol, water, and acetone. They are used as facial applications to obtain a drying effect and to produce a cooling sensation (due to rapid evaporation), but they can be irritating. In gel form, the active ingredient is dispersed in a transparent or opaque semisolid preparation (which commonly includes agar, gelatin, or pectin). The gel liquefies on contact with the skin and dries to a greaseless, nonocclusive film. Gels lack emollient and protective properties, and some clients experience burning or stinging when using a gel. A subclass of gels includes the jellies; these are used for application to mucous membranes or as lubricants for gloves, finger cots, and catheters.

Pastes are mixtures of powder in ointment. They tend to have a drying effect because the powder constitutes up to 50% of the paste. They provide a protective barrier and are suitable for treating areas of persistent maceration, such as diaper dermatitis.

Sprays or aerosols are used for topical therapy. Clients might like the spray because it can be applied without touching the skin lesion, but because significant quantities of the spray usually miss the target, this is usually a wasteful and expensive method of application.

Preparations for Moisturizing the Skin

Chronic, scaling lesions are most effectively treated with medication incorporated into a moisturizing, lubricating preparation.

A cream is an emulsion of oil in water. Creams are more complex than most ointments because they contain emulsifying agents and preservatives. Examples of oil-in-water emulsions include Lubriderm Cream, Neutrogena Emulsion, and Cetaphil lotion. (The manufacturer's designation of a product as a cream, ointment, or lotion does not always correlate completely with the product by pure analysis.)

Ointments are considered water-in-oil emulsions. In general, ointments are more effective hydrating agents, provide more lubrication and occlusion, and require less frequent applications; however, they are often too greasy for client acceptance. Creams are usually less greasy and more easily removed (water-washable).

Examples of water-in-oil emulsions include cold cream and Eucerin cream. Anhydrous lanolin is an example of a water-absorbent ointment base. White petrolatum is an example of an oleaginous or water-repellent ointment base.

Drugs to Manage Integumentary System Disorders

The drugs and modalities used to manage integumentary system disorders include glucocorticoids (see Table 30-1 in Chap. 30), retinoids, cytotoxic and immunosuppressive drugs, antimalarials, antimicrobials, antipruritic agents, antipsoriasis drugs, therapy with ultraviolet radiation, antiseptics and germicides, preparations for burn and wound therapy, soaps and shampoos, sunscreens, and miscellaneous agents.

Topical Glucocorticoids

Pharmacodynamics. The exact mechanism of antiinflammatory activity of topical glucocorticoids remains unclear, but vascular constriction and decreased leukocyte and lymphocyte function appear to play primary roles. Fluorination at the C_9 position of the molecule enhances all activities of the compound, so fluorinated agents are more potent than nonfluorinated agents.

Pharmacokinetics. Absorption and distribution depend on the specific drug, as do onset, peak, and duration of action.

Therapeutic Uses. Many inflammatory skin diseases respond to topical or intralesional administration of glucocorticoids.

Low-potency agents are best used for diffuse eruptions, those involving the face and occluded areas such as the axilla or groin, and chronic dermatoses. Medium-potency agents are appropriate for acute flare-ups of chronic dermatoses and acute self-limited eruptions. They should be used for short periods (14–21 days). High-potency agents are best used for acute localized eruptions for a short time (7–14 days). They are fluorinated compounds that have a specially formulated vehicle that enhances penetration. High-potency corticosteroids should be avoided on areas susceptible to increased penetration and adverse reactions (eg, face, intertriginous areas, perineum). Very-high–potency corticosteroids have more pronounced adverse reactions than high-potency agents. These drugs are indicated for chronic skin disorders resistant to less potent therapy. They should be used twice daily for no longer than 2 weeks to avoid toxicity.

Dosage and Administration. Often a more potent steroid is used initially, followed by a less potent agent. Twice-a-day application is sufficient; more frequent application does not appear to improve response.

Intralesional injection of glucocorticoids is usually done with insoluble preparations of triamcinolone acetonide (Kenalog) or triamcinolone hexacetonide; these agents solubize gradually and therefore have a prolonged duration of action. Kenalog is used in concentrations of 2.5 to 40 mg/mL. The lower concentrations are used on the face, where atrophy is undesirable, and higher concentrations are used for lesions such as keloids, where atrophy is desirable. In most cases, the total dose at one treatment should not exceed 20 mg. Intralesional steroids are particularly valuable if the inflamed area is in fat, as in an inflammatory scalp alopecia or panniculitis.

Abrupt discontinuation of mid- or high-potency corticosteroids may result in rebound flare-up of the disorder. It is best to taper the dosage gradually and then switch to a less potent agent. Topical corticosteroids can be alternated with emollients or other topical agents every 1 to 2 weeks.

Adverse Reactions. Local adverse reactions include atrophy, hypopigmentation, and telangiectasia. Striae that develop are permanent, particularly on the face and intertriginous areas, where the skin is thinnest and more susceptible. Erythema may appear initially, and purpura may affect the extensor surfaces of the forearms because of atrophic effects on the dermis. Perioral dermatitis, rosacea-like eruptions, and acneiform eruptions all have been described on the face, especially with the use of fluorinated corticosteroids.

Ocular complications include exacerbation of glaucoma and cataracts. Cutaneous infections (bacterial or fungal) and infestations (scabies or lice) have occurred (these agents help relieve inflammatory symptoms but must be used with topical or systemic antimicrobial therapy). *Candida* superinfection and miliaria are complications of topical corticosteroid therapy. Miliaria is observed primarily with the use of creams or ointments under occlusive dressings. Wound healing may be impaired by excessive use of corticosteroids.

Adverse systemic effects, identical to those associated with systemic corticosteroid therapy, may occur when systemic absorption is increased. The most serious effect is suppression of the hypothalamic–pituitary–adrenal axis.

Precautions and Contraindications. Caution should be used in applying topical corticosteroids because factors that increase systemic absorption and the risk of adverse effects include the amount of steroid applied, the extent of the area treated, the frequency of application, the length of treatment, the potency of the drug, and the use of occlusive dressings.

Systemic Corticosteroids

Systemic glucocorticosteroids are discussed in depth in Chapter 30. Their use in integumentary disorders is summarized here.

Pharmacodynamics. The mechanism of action of systemic corticosteroids is incompletely understood. However, the antiinflammatory effects probably result from decreased leukocyte accumulation and function, monocytopenia and eosinopenia, suppression of steps in histamine-mediated reactions, decreased complement components, and decreased passage of immune complexes through basement membranes. The immunosuppressive effects probably result from decreased immunoglobulin and complement levels in plasma and decreased lymphocyte and monocyte function.

Therapeutic Uses. Systemic glucocorticoid therapy is used for a number of severe dermatologic illnesses. Skin diseases that respond to short-term therapy include acute contact dermatitis, atopic dermatitis, lichen planus, exfoliative dermatitis, and erythema nodosum. Examples of diseases that require long-term therapy are pemphigus vulgaris, bullous pemphigoid, herpes gestationis, dermatomyositis, systemic lupus erythematosus, relapsing polychondritis, vasculitis, sarcoidosis, Sweet's disease, pyoderma gangrenosum, type I reactive leprosy, and capillary hemangiomas.

Dosage and Administration. A glucocorticosteroid such as prednisone is usually taken daily initially. Fewer adverse effects occur with alternate-day dosing, so prednisone should be tapered to every other day as soon as possible. It would be unusual to use the intramuscular route for a skin disease, although this route might be needed to ensure adherence. Pulse therapy with large daily doses of methylprednisolone sodium succinate might be used for pyoderma gangrenosum, pemphigus vulgaris, bullous pemphigoid, dermatomyositis, and organ-threatening systemic lupus erythematosus. The dose is usually 0.5 to 1 g given IV over 2 to 3 hours.

Adverse Reactions. Adverse reactions of systemic glucocorticoids are discussed in Chapter 30, as are drug interactions. Most adverse reactions are dose-dependent. Pulsed IV glucocorticoids can cause hypotension or hypertension, hyperglycemia, hypokalemia or hyperkalemia, anaphylaxis, acute psychosis, seizures, congestive heart failure, pulmonary edema, and death. After brief high-dose treatment, a steroid withdrawal syndrome can develop, with transient arthralgias, myalgias, and joint effusions.

Retinoids

Retinoids include the natural compounds and synthetic derivatives of retinol that exhibit vitamin A activity. The essential role of vitamin A in vision is well documented, and vitamin A also affects normal epithelial differentiation.

There are three generations of retinoids (first: retinol, tretinoin, isotretinoin; second: etretinate, acitretin; third: arotinoid). First-generation compounds include retinol and compounds that can be derived from it metabolically. Second-generation retinoids are synthetic analogs in which part of the molecule has been altered by the addition of an aromatic ring. Third-generation retinoids have undergone extensive modification.

Retinoids influence cellular proliferation and differentiation, immune function, inflammation, and sebum production. Retinoid actions are mediated through retinoic acid receptors, which bind to the retinoids and DNA. Isotretinoin and tretinoin are approved for use with acne, etretinate for psoriasis. Clinical trials indicate that retinoids have significant activity in reversing oral, skin, and cervical premalignancies and in preventing primary tumors of the head and neck, lung, and skin.

Isotretinoin

Isotretinoin (Accutane) was first studied for acne in 1971 and was approved for use in 1982.

Pharmacodynamics. Isotretinoin's actions include normalization of the keratinizing process of the follicular epithelium, reduction of sebaceous gland cell size, decrease of sebum synthesis, and reduced numbers of *P acnes*. It stimulates T-lymphocyte killer cells, enhances the tumoricidal effects of macrophages, and inhibits tumor promotion and oncogene expression.

Pharmacokinetics. Blood concentration peaks 1 to 4 hours after oral administration; the presence of food may double the amount absorbed. Isotretinoin is nearly 100% bound to plasma albumin at therapeutic concentrations. It has a mean elimination half-life of 10 hours, although its metabolites have a longer half-life.

Therapeutic Uses. Isotretinoin is approved for treatment of severe recalcitrant nodular acne, but it is often used for moderate acne unresponsive to oral antibiotics and acne that produces scarring. Other skin diseases responsive to isotretinoin include gram-negative folliculitis, hidradenitis suppurativa, the disorders of keratinization, and pustular psoriasis. Prolonged therapy or doses larger than those used in acne may be required in some of these disorders.

High doses of isotretinoin produce partial regression of multiple basal cell carcinomas but are more effective in suppressing new tumors, as demonstrated in clients with xeroderma pigmentosum. Isotretinoin also prevents second primary tumors in clients who have had a previous squamous cell carcinoma of the head and neck. Isotretinoin is also effective in treating premalignant lesions such as oral leukoplakia.

Dosage and Administration. Isotretinoin is taken orally at 1 to 2 mg/kg/day for 15 to 20 weeks. Lower doses are effective, but relapses are reportedly more common and occur sooner. Improvement usually continues for 6 months after the first course is terminated. About 40% of clients have a relapse, usually within 3 years of therapy, and may require retreatment (Hardman & Limbird, 1996).

Adverse Reactions. Effects on the skin and mucous membranes are the most common adverse reactions, and they seem dose-dependent. Cheilitis, dry mouth, nose, eyes, and skin, epistaxis, blepharoconjunctivitis, erythematous eruptions, and xerosis are common. Alteration of epidermal surfaces may account for *Staphylococcus aureus* colonization and at times subsequent infection. Headache occurs. Hair loss and dark adaptation dysfunction are more uncommon reactions.

Retinoids are photosensitizing agents, so their use must be accompanied by protection from the sun to prevent sunburn and induction by ultraviolet light of new lesions.

Long-term therapy may produce skeletal adverse reactions, including skeletal hyperostoses, extraskeletal ossification, and, in children, premature epiphyseal closure.

Drug–Drug Interactions. Topical agents such as benzoyl peroxide and tretinoin should be discontinued before starting isotretinoin therapy because they potentiate the drying effect of isotretinoin. Oral tetracycline and minocycline should also be discontinued because of an increased risk of pseudotumor cerebri. Vitamin A supplements should not be taken concomitantly.

Drug–Food Interactions. When taken with food or milk, the absorption of isotretinoin is increased.

Drug–Laboratory Test Interactions. Hyperlipidemia is common, with 25% of clients developing increased levels of triglycerides and, less often, increased levels of cholesterol and low-density lipoproteins and decreased levels of high-density lipoproteins. Obese clients, diabetics, and those with a history of excessive alcohol intake or a family history of lipid disorders are more susceptible to these effects. The changes are reversible.

Some clients experience hyperuricemia, hyperglycemia, increased creatine phosphokinase, proteinuria, or microscopic or gross hematuria. Transitory abnormal elevations occur rarely in serum transaminases and the erythrocyte sedimentation rate.

Precautions and Contraindications. The teratogenic effects of isotretinoin include central nervous system (CNS), cardiac, thymus, and craniofacial abnormalities. In the past, many deformed infants were born to mothers exposed to isotretinoin during pregnancy. Pregnancy is an absolute contraindication to the use of isotretinoin. Women of childbearing potential should not receive isotretinoin until pregnancy is excluded by a sensitive urine or serum pregnancy test within 2 weeks before initiating therapy. Two reliable forms of contraception must be used if the woman engages in sexual intercourse for at least 1 month before, during, and 1 month after discontinuation of therapy. Pregnancy tests should be repeated monthly. Clients receiving isotretinoin should not donate blood during treatment and for 30 days after treatment ends to avoid a possible teratogenic effect in a pregnant recipient of the blood.

Etretinate

Etretinate (Tegison) was approved for treating severe refractory psoriasis in 1986.

Pharmacodynamics. Etretinate probably normalizes the expression of keratins by epidermal cells. It also suppresses chemotaxis, decreases stratum corneum cohesiveness, and may interfere with cytokine function.

Pharmacokinetics. Because of high lipophilicity, etretinate is stored in adipose tissue. When treatment concludes, the drug continues to be released slowly from fat; the drug has been detected in plasma 2 to 3 years after therapy.

Therapeutic Uses. Skin diseases responsive to etretinate include acne, the disorders of keratinization, leukoplakia, psoriasis (especially the inflammatory types), and skin cancers. Etretinate has demonstrated efficacy in the treatment of premalignant lesions such as actinic keratoses. Cancers, such as cutaneous T-cell lymphoma, also have improved with etretinate therapy combined with the use of interferon-alfa.

Dosage and Administration. The recommended dose of 1 mg/kg/day may produce intolerable adverse effects, so 0.5 to 0.75 mg/kg/day is generally used. Response is rapid, with resolution of pustules in pustular psoriasis within 2 weeks and slower improvement of residual disease over 2 to 3 months. Etretinate does not produce prolonged remissions of psoriasis, and maintenance therapy often is necessary. Response rates in other forms of psoriasis may be slower. Combination therapy may be needed. Etretinate can be combined with psoralen–ultraviolet A (PUVA) photochemotherapy.

Adverse Reactions. The adverse effects of etretinate are similar to those of isotretinoin. However, conjunctival symptoms are less common, but hair loss, initial cutaneous exfoliation, sticky skin, easy bruising, and liver function abnormalities are more common with etretinate.

Precautions and Contraindications. Etretinate is teratogenic (see the precautions under isotretinoin). Because therapy with etretinate may be prolonged, hyperlipidemia and skeletal adverse reactions may be a consideration.

Tretinoin

Tretinoin (trans-retinoic acid/Retin-A) is a first-generation retinoid.

Pharmacodynamics. Tretinoin decreases the cohesiveness of follicular epithelial cells and increases epidermal cell mitosis and cell turnover. It has been suggested that increased turnover of follicular epithelium prevents blockage by keratinous plugs. Tretinoin reduces the hyperkeratinization that leads to microcomedone formation, the initial lesion of acne. Tretinoin also thins the stratum corneum, enhancing the penetration of other topical agents.

Therapeutic Uses. Tretinoin is approved for use with acne. Acne may be aggravated during the first 6 weeks of therapy, but good results are noted after 3 or 4 months in most clients. Tretinoin has demonstrated efficacy in treating premalignant lesions such as actinic keratoses and dysplastic nevi.

Dosage and Administration. Tretinoin is available in cream, gel, and liquid forms. The preparation should be applied to dry skin, preferably 15 to 30 minutes after washing. It is applied once daily before bedtime to minimize photodegradation. Maximal clinical response may take 4 months, and maintenance therapy is necessary.

An emollient cream form of tretinoin (Renova) is approved for treating premature aging caused by excessive exposure to the sun (photoaging). Treatment must be combined with sunscreens and sun avoidance.

Adverse Reactions. Even if used correctly, tretinoin is irritating, especially the liquid preparation, although client sensitivity varies. It causes erythema, peeling, burning, and stinging. These effects often decrease spontaneously with time. Photosensitivity occurs, with a greater potential for sunburn.

Drug Interactions. Concomitant use of keratolytic preparations (eg, salicylic acid and sulfur preparations) and benzoyl peroxide should be avoided. Because of possible interactions, the client should use cautiously any medicated or abrasive soaps and cleansers, any soaps and cosmetics with a strong drying effect, and products with high concentrations of alcohol, spices, or lime.

Precautions and Contraindications. Oral tretinoin is highly teratogenic, but the low blood levels associated with topical therapy have not been associated with teratogenicity.

Cytotoxic and Immunosuppressive Drugs
Cytotoxic and immunosuppressive drugs are discussed in detail in Chapters 35 and 46. Drugs in these categories that are also used in managing selected integumentary system disorders include methotrexate, azathioprine, fluorouracil, hydroxyurea and thioguanine, cyclophosphamide, mechlorethamine, carmustine, cyclosporine, vinblastine, and bleomycin. Their specialized use in skin problems is summarized in Table 40-1.

Antimalarials
Antimalarials, including chloroquine (Aralen), hydroxychloroquine (Plaquenil), and quinacrine (Atabrine), are used for their antiinflammatory effects in treating vascular and photosensitivity diseases.

Pharmacodynamics. The exact mechanism of action is unknown, but there are immunologic and antiinflammatory effects. In porphyria cutanea tarda, chloroquine mobilizes uroporphyrin stores in the liver and skin, forming a stable complex; this leads to marked porphyrin excretion in urine, with resulting disease remission. The drugs inhibit phospholipase A_2, increase pH, stabilize membranes, inhibit release and activity of lysosomal enzymes, inhibit phagocytosis, inhibit superoxide production, increase intracellular pH in cytoplasmic vacuoles (which leads to decreased stimulation of autoimmune CD4+ T cells), decrease cytokine release from stimulated monocytes, and inhibit antibody production.

Therapeutic Uses. These drugs are approved for use with systemic and discoid lupus erythematosus. They are used for polymorphous light eruption, porphyria cutanea tarda, and some other conditions.

Dosage and Administration. The usual doses are hydroxychloroquine 200 mg twice a day, quinacrine 100 mg/day, and chloroquine 250 mg/day. Dosing is adjusted for weight (chloroquine, 3 mg/kg/day or less; hydroxychloroquine, 6.5 mg/kg/day or less). Full clinical effects may take several months. If a positive response is obtained, dosage can often be reduced to alternate-day therapy. Clients with porphyria cutanea tarda require different dosage regimens because of adverse reactions.

Adverse Reactions. The occurrence of retinopathy leading to retinal degeneration and possible blindness is dose-related. The incidence of vision disorders from chloroquine and hydroxychloroquine is low when doses are within guidelines and the drug is used for less than

10 years (in clients with normal renal function). Quinacrine does not cause retinopathy. Ophthalmologic supervision includes eye examinations every 6 months after a baseline examination. Other adverse reactions include mental changes, headaches, convulsions, leukopenia, and thrombocytopenia.

Precautions and Contraindications. The possibility of teratogenicity exists, so these drugs should not be used in pregnancy. During therapy, complete blood count, blood urea nitrogen, creatinine, and liver function tests should be obtained every 3 to 4 months after a baseline examination.

Antimicrobials
Both systemic and topical antimicrobials are used for skin disorders. Table 40-2 summarizes the antibacterial and antifungal agents.

Antibacterials
Antibacterial agents are often used to treat acne vulgaris by reducing the growth of *P acnes,* which is correlated with improvement in the acne. In mild acne, topical antibiotics such as erythromycin, clindamycin (Cleocin T), or tetracycline can be used. Benzoyl peroxide has antibacterial action against *P acnes* as a result of potent oxidizing effects. A combined erythromycin/benzoyl peroxide gel (Benzamycin) is available.

Topical therapy may be used for impetigo, a superficial bacterial infection of the skin caused by *S aureus* and *Streptococcus pyogenes.* Mupirocin (Bactroban), produced by *Pseudomonas fluorescens,* is effective for such infections and acts by inhibiting protein synthesis. Its antibacterial activity is enhanced by the acid pH of the skin. Diffuse impetigo might require systemic therapy with erythromycin or, if erythromycin resistance exists, an oral semisynthetic penicillinase-resistant penicillin.

Topical therapy may be useful for prophylaxis of infections in wounds and injuries. Neomycin is active against staphylococci and most gram-negative bacilli.

Acne rosacea is a chronic eruption of the face with inflammatory papules and pustules. Metronidazole is available as a gel or cream and is used for topical treatment; it reduces papules, pustules, and erythema, but not telangiectasis.

If acne vulgaris is severe or resistant to topical therapy, systemic antibiotics such as tetracycline, erythromycin, minocycline, clindamycin, or trimethoprim/sulfamethoxazole can be used. Tetracycline has been used for more than 25 years and is the least expensive agent. It must be taken on an empty stomach. Benefits of therapy are seen in 3 to 4 weeks. Tetracycline must not be given to pregnant women because it can cause permanent discoloration of the teeth in the fetus; it cannot be given to children under age 8 years for the same reason. Tetracycline may promote vaginal infection with *Candida albicans.* Minocycline may be more effective, but it is more expensive. Clindamycin is associated with a

Table 40-1. Cytotoxic and Immunosuppressant Drugs Used for Integumentary Disorders

Drug Name	Indications	Typical Dosage	Additional Information
azathioprine (Imuran)	Pemphigus Bullous pemphigoid Cicatricial pemphigoid Systemic polyarteritis nodosa Polymyositis Behçet's disease Photoallergic eruptions	1–2 mg/kg/d in one or two divided doses; maintenance doses are reduced to half the starting dose	Can take 6–8 wk to see an effect Steroid-sparing agent (its use decreases the amount of steroid needed for control of the disease)
bleomycin (Blenoxane)	Warts Squamous cell carcinoma palliation	Applied intralesionally or by multiple-puncture technique using bifurcated vaccination needle	Associated with Raynaud's disease and local skin necrosis
carmustine (BCNU, BiCNu)	Cutaneous T-cell lymphoma	Applied in solution or in ointment form; solutions must be mixed daily and so are more expensive	Erythema, post-treatment telangiectasias (see mechlorethamine); more bone marrow suppression than mechlorethamine
cyclophosphamide (Cytoxan)	Pemphigus Bullous pemphigoid Cicatricial pemphigoid Systemic polyarteritis nodosa Polymyositis Advanced cutaneous T-cell lymphoma Wegener's granulomatosis Churg-Strauss angiitis Behçet's disease Scleromyxedema Cytophagic histiocytic panniculitis	2–3 mg/kg/d in divided doses; or monthly IV drug, 0.5–1.0 g/m^2 infused over 1 hr	Risk of secondary malignancy, bone marrow suppression Can take 4–6 wk to see an effect
cyclosporine (Sandimmune)	Psoriasis Lichen planus Pyoderma gangrenosum Eczematous dermatitides Epidermolysis bullosa acquisita Alopecia areata Pemphigus Bullous pemphigoid	3–4 mg/kg/d in a single dose or two divided doses	Potential permanent nephrotoxicity
fluorouracil (solution: 1% Fluoroplex; 2% or 5% Efudex; cream: 1% Fluoroplex; 5% Efudex)	Multiple actinic keratoses Superficial basal cell carcinomas Carcinoma in situ of vulva	Application is continued for 2–4 wk until inflammation responses progress from erythema to necrosis; there will be local sloughing of dead tissue before regrowth of healthy skin; after cessation of therapy, healing may take 6–8 wk and may include use of topical corticosteroid	Adverse reactions of burning or rashes; rare systemic adverse effect of nausea Minimize exposure to sunlight for 1–2 mo after treatment.
hydroxyurea (Hydrea)	Psoriasis		Used especially when methotrexate cannot be used because of liver disease, but hydroxyurea is not as effective

(continued)

Table 40-1. (Continued)

Drug Name	Indications	Typical Dosage	Additional Information
mechlorethamine (Mustargen)	Cutaneous T-cell lymphoma	Applied in solution or in ointment form; solutions must be mixed daily and so are more expensive	Monitor liver function tests and obtain complete blood counts because of systemic absorption.
methotrexate (Folex, Mexate)	Psoriasis Pityriasis rubra pilaris Reiter's disease Vasculitis Sarcoidosis Dermatomyositis Pityriasis lichenoides et varioliformis acuta Lymphomatoid papulosis Pemphigus vulgaris Systemic lupus erythematosus Chronic actinic dermatitis Polymyositis	*Psoriasis:* given weekly as a single dose or in split doses q12h for 24–36 hr; dose is increased as needed in increments of 2.5–5 mg weekly, with final doses ranging from 7.5–30 mg/wk	Adverse reactions include contact dermatitis, secondary cutaneous malignancies, pigmentary changes. Can cause hepatotoxicity, so baseline liver function tests and scans are needed and are repeated periodically Drug should not be used in those with liver disease or alcohol abuse.
vincristine (Oncovin, Vincasar PFS)	Kaposi's sarcoma Advanced cutaneous T-cell lymphoma	Has been used intralesionally, and iontophoresis has been tried	

severe adverse reaction of pseudomembranous colitis (first manifested by diarrhea) and is not commonly used. There is the potential for allergic reactions with trimethoprim/sulfamethoxazole. Oral antibiotics may also be used for acne rosacea and atopic dermatitis.

Antifungals

Fungal infections are among the most common causes of skin disease in the United States. Topical and oral azoles (subdivided into the imidazoles and the triazoles) and the allylamines are the most effective agents. New agents are undergoing evaluation for use with fungal infections (itraconazole, fluconazole, and terbinafine [Lamisil]). Terbinafine cream may allow briefer therapy than other agents because drug levels exceeding fungicidal concentrations are present in the skin 1 week after discontinuation of therapy.

Systemic therapy is necessary for treating fungal diseases when they are no longer localized. Oral griseofulvin is the drug of choice for tinea capitis, disseminated tinea corporis, and onychomycosis (fungal infections of the nails).

Tinea pedis (athlete's foot) encompasses three syndromes: interdigital toe-web infection, scaly hyperkeratotic moccasin disease, and inflammatory vesicular bullous eruptions. The interdigital toe-web infection begins as dry interdigital scaling and progresses to maceration complicated by bacterial invasion. Topical therapy with azoles and allylamines is effective for dry interdigital toe-web infection. Macerated interdigital toe-web disease requires the addition of antibacterial therapy. Agents that may be used include econazole nitrate (Spectazole), aluminum chloride, and gentian violet. In scaly hyperkeratotic moccasin disease, involvement of thick stratum corneum on the sole of the foot makes it difficult to achieve suitable drug concentrations. Oral griseofulvin would be needed, followed by long-term topical therapy with azoles and allylamines.

Onychomycosis can be caused by dermatophytes, molds, and *Candida*. Nails should be cultured before therapy, because some nail problems that appear to be onychomycosis are actually psoriasis or another condition. Onychomycosis serves as a reservoir for dermatophytes and contributes to treatment failure and recurrence of tinea pedis. Oral therapy is necessary for onychomycosis, although the agents available have limited efficacy.

Antivirals

Acyclovir is used to treat cutaneous herpes simplex, herpes zoster, and varicella (chickenpox) viruses (see Chap. 44).

Antipruritic Agents

Theoretically, pharmacologic inhibition of the pruritic signal can occur at several levels: inhibition of formation or release of pruritogenic mediators in the skin, inhibition at the receptor site, or inhibition of the nervous transmission in the CNS or the peripheral nerves (Hagermark & Wahlgren, 1995). General management of pruritus includes attempts to interrupt the itch–scratch cycle and may include topical therapy, transcutaneous electrical nerve stimulation, phototherapy, and systemic therapy. The key to treatment lies in identifying

Table 40-2. Topical Antimicrobial Agents

Drug Name	Indications	Additional Information
Antibacterial Agents		
bacitracin (Baciguent)	Gram-positive bacterial skin infections; inhibits staphylococci, streptococci, and gram-positive bacilli	For all antibacterial agents, the affected area should be cleaned before the medication is applied.
bacitracin, polymyxin (Polysporin)		Example of combination agent
chloramphenicol (Chloromycetin)	Superficial bacterial skin infections	Bone marrow hypoplasia, including aplastic anemia and death, has occurred after local application.
chlortetracycline hydrochloride (Aureomycin)	Superficial bacterial skin infections	
clindamycin phosphate (Cleocin T)	Inflammatory acne vulgaris	
erythromycin (Eryderm, Staticin, T-Stat, Erygel, Aknemycin, others)	Acne vulgaris	Ointment or gel
gentamicin sulfate (Garamycin)	Aerobic gram-negative and some gram-positive bacterial skin infections	Ointment, cream; possible photosensitization
mafenide acetate (Sulfamylon)	Adjunct therapy in second- and third-degree burns	
meclocycline sulfosalicylate (Meclan)	Acne vulgaris	
metronidazole (MetroGel)	Inflammatory papules, pustules, and erythema of acne rosacea	Significant improvement should occur within 3 weeks and continue for another 6 weeks; reduces papules, pustules, and erythema but not telangiectasias
mupirocin (Bactroban)	Impetigo caused by *Staphylococcus aureus,* beta-hemolytic streptococci, and *Streptococcus pyogenes*	Structurally unrelated to other topical antibacterial agents; produced by *Pseudomonas fluorescens;* antibacterial activity enhanced by acid pH of skin; a special use is in later therapy of burn wound infections due to resistant *S aureus*
neomycin sulfate (Myciguent)	Aerobic gram-negative and some aerobic gram-positive bacterial skin infections Secondary infections of dermatoses Traumatic lesions that are inflamed or suppurated from bacterial infection	Ointment, cream; chronic application to inflamed skin of allergic contact dermatitis and chronic dermatoses increases possibility of hypersensitivity reactions; ototoxicity and nephrotoxicity have occurred
neomycin sulfate, bacitracin, polymyxin (Mycitracin, Neosporin)		Example of combination agent
nitrofurazone (Furacin)	Surface infections Adjunct therapy in second- or third-degree burns Prevention of skin allograft rejection	
silver sulfadiazine (Silvadene)	Many gram-negative and gram-positive bacterial infections Prophylaxis or adjunct therapy for second- or third-degree burns in clients at risk for wound infection	
tetracycline hydrochloride (Topicycline)	Inflammatory acne vulgaris	Ointment; may stain clothing
Antifungal Agents		
amphotericin B (Fungizone)	Cutaneous and mucocutaneous candidal infections	Produced by strain of *Streptomyces nodosum;* comparable to nystatin; cream, lotion, ointment; all preparations have slight sensitizing potential
butoconazole nitrate (Femstat)	Vulvovaginal candidiasis (moniliasis)	
carbol–fuchsin solution (Castellani's Paint, Castaderm)	Tinea pedis, tinea cruris	Liquid; components of Castaderm are basic fuchsin, phenol, resorcinol, acetone, boric acid, alcohol; components of paint are basic fuchsin, phenol, resorcinol, acetone; paint available with alcohol and without basic fuchsin

(continued)

Table 40-2. (Continued)

Test	Advantage	Disadvantage
Antifungal Agents (continued)		
ciclopirox olamine (Loprox)	Tinea pedis, tinea corporis, tinea cruris, tinea versicolor Cutaneous candidiasis (moniliasis)	Cream, lotion; use for full treatment time even though symptoms may have improved; notify prescriber if no improvement after 4 wk
clotrimazole (Lotrimin, Mycelex)	Tinea pedis, tinea cruris, tinea corporis, tinea versicolor Cutaneous candidiasis	Cream, solution, lotion; use for full treatment time even though symptoms may have improved; notify prescriber if no improvement after 4 wk
econazole nitrate (Spectazole)	Tinea cruris, tinea corporis, tinea pedis, tinea versicolor Cutaneous candidiasis	Belongs to azole class; azole of choice for dry toe-web disease of tinea pedis; treat candida, tinea cruris, and tinea corporis for 2 wk and tinea pedis for 1 mo to reduce possible recurrence
haloprogin (Halotex)	Tinea pedis, tinea cruris, tinea corporis, tinea manuum, tinea versicolor	
ketoconazole (Nizoral)	Cutaneous candidiasis Seborrheic dermatitis	Cream, shampoo; therapeutic effect in seborrheic dermatitis and dandruff may be due to reduction of *Pityrosporum ovale*; when using shampoo, use it twice a week for 4 wk with at least 3 d between each shampooing
miconazole nitrate (Micatin, Monistat-Derm)	Tinea pedis, tinea cruris, tinea corporis, tinea versicolor Cutaneous candidiasis	Cream, powder, spray; early relief of symptoms in 2–3 d in most clients, but treat candida, tinea cruris, and tinea corporis for 2 wk and tinea pedis for 1 mo to reduce possible recurrence; there are also vaginal and systemic preparations
naftifine hydrochloride (Naftin)	Tinea cruris and tinea corporis caused by *Trichophyton mentagrophytes, Trichophyton rubrum, Trichophyton violaceum, Epidermophyton floccosum,* or *Microsporum canis*	Belongs to allylamine class; synthetic; cream, gel
nystatin (Mycostatin)	Cutaneous candidiasis	Cream, ointment, powder; very moist lesions best treated with powder; cream preferred in candidiasis involving intertriginous areas
oxiconazole (Oxistat)	Tinea pedis, tinea cruris, tinea corporis	Cream, lotion; treat tinea cruris and tinea corporis for 2 wk and tinea pedis for 1 mo to reduce possible recurrence
sulconazole nitrate (Exelderm)	Tinea versicolor, tinea cruris, and tinea corporis caused by *Trichophyton mentagrophytes, Epidermophyton floccosum,* or *Microsporum canis*	Imidazole derivative; cream, solution
terconazole (Terazol 7)	Vulvovaginal candidiasis	
tioconazole (Vagistat)	Vulvovaginal candidiasis	
tolnaftate (Aftate, Tinactin, Genaspor, Ting)	Tinea cruris, tinea corporis, tinea manuum, tinea pedis, tinea versicolor	Cream, solution, gel, powder, spray powder, spray liquid; treatment may be required for 4–6 wk
undecylenic acid and zinc undecylenate (Cruex, Desenex)	Minor skin rashes, such as diaper rash, prickly heat, chafing Tinea pedis, tinea cruris, tinea corporis	Desenex available as powder, ointment, cream, foam, soap; Cruex available as powder, cream; avoid inhaling powders

the cause of the pruritus (Box 40-2) and eliminating it when possible.

For many clients with pruritus, antihistamines are prescribed, although they do not relieve itch significantly. Antihistamines (H_1 and H_2 blockers) act by competitive inhibition of histamine at H_1 and H_2 receptor sites on target cells. Histamine-induced itch is mediated mainly by H_1 receptors. Urticaria is the only situation in which histamine is known to be the main mediator of itch; in urticaria, classical antihistamines (H_1 inhibitors) do relieve the itch. Sedation by antihistamines also does not seem to be associated with itch relief.

All H_1 blockers have anticholinergic and CNS effects as well as antihistaminic effects. Of the six

Box 40-2
Causes of Pruritus

Integumentary Disorders

Xerosis, scabies, pediculosis (lice), dermatitis herpetiformis, psoriasis, atopic dermatitis, prurigo nodularis, papular urticaria or arthropod bite reactions, pemphigoid, varicella, mastocytosis

Systemic Disorders

Hyperthyroidism, pregnancy, chronic renal failure, cholestatic or obstructive liver disease, polycythemia vera, paraproteinemia, iron deficiency, parasitic infestation, drug reaction, Hodgkin's disease, cutaneous T-cell lymphoma or mycosis fungoides, central nervous system tumors, psychogenic pruritus, senile pruritus

subgroups of H_1 blockers (hydroxyzines, terfenadines, phenothiazines, piperidines, alkylamines, and ethylenediamines), the first and second are most commonly prescribed for pruritus. Hydroxyzine hydrochloride (Atarax), hydroxyzine pamoate (Vistaril), and chlorpheniramine (Chlor-Trimeton) are the preferred H_1 blockers for pruritus. Combinations of H_1 blockers, such as cyproheptadine hydrochloride (Periactin) and hydroxyzine, are used occasionally. Combinations of H_1 and H_2 blockers have been tried to relieve itching.

The opioid antagonist nalmefene may relieve itch in some clients, such as those with liver disease, urticaria, and atopic dermatitis. Glucocorticoids and cyclosporine affect inflammatory skin diseases and the itching associated with them; they reportedly inhibit the release and production of cytokines. The itching of eczema might be due to cytokines released from the lymphocytes in the skin lesions.

Antipsoriasis Drugs
Anthralin

Chrysarobin, the active ingredient of Goa powder, was first used in 1877 for treating psoriasis. It was replaced in 1916 by the synthetic compound anthralin.

Pharmacodynamics. The anthralin molecule is unstable, leading to formation of degradation products that produce the characteristic violet-brown staining of skin and clothes. The mechanism of action is not well understood, but the agent inhibits cellular respiration by inactivating mitochondria (Hardman & Limbird, 1996).

Pharmacokinetics. Anthralin penetrates damaged skin faster and to a greater extent than normal skin.

Therapeutic Uses. Anthralin is used to relieve scaling and other manifestations of psoriasis.

Dosage and Administration. Anthralin is available as an ointment (Anthra-Derm) or a cream (Drithocreme). Anthralin can be used as a single agent or in combination with topical corticosteroid therapy or phototherapy. Therapy usually begins at low concentrations (eg, 0.1% Drithocreme). The cream is applied once daily for 10 to 30 to 60 minutes to affected areas and then washed off. If this lower concentration is tolerated without irritation, the concentration can be increased (0.25%, 0.5%, and 1% concentrations). Short-contact therapy may be used with higher concentrations. Treatment should be continued until psoriasis has cleared (plaques have flattened). This may take 6 to 8 weeks or longer.

Adverse Reactions. The primary adverse reactions are staining of skin, clothing, and bathroom fixtures and irritation of uninvolved skin. Anthralin-induced hyperpigmentation of treated areas resolves a few days after therapy is discontinued. No known systemic toxicity is associated with this drug.

Calcipotriene

Calcipotriene (Dovonex) is a vitamin D analog. It was noted incidentally that psoriasis improved in a client with osteoporosis who was receiving a form of vitamin D (Hardman and Limbird, 1996). This observation led to the development of a drug that might be specifically used for psoriasis.

Pharmacodynamics. Vitamin D has a role in many physiologic functions besides calcium homeostasis. The vitamin binds to an intracellular receptor, and this receptor/vitamin D complex binds to a specific gene in the DNA that modulates and controls transcription. The receptor is present in human epidermal keratinocytes, dermal fibroblasts, islets of Langerhans cells, macrophages, and T lymphocytes. It causes a decrease in the proliferation and an increase in the biochemical differentiation of keratinocytes.

Dosage and Administration. Calcipotriene is applied as an ointment twice daily to areas of psoriatic plaque. Some improvement occurs within 1 to 2 weeks, maximal improvement within 6 to 8 weeks. Maintenance therapy usually is necessary. In trials, the drug seems slightly more effective than a corticosteroid or short-contact anthralin treatment.

Adverse Reactions. This drug is less potent than the parent vitamin D_3 compound in causing hypercalciuria and hypercalcemia.

Precautions and Contraindications. Calcipotriene cannot be used on the face and should be used with caution in intertriginous areas, in which facilitated absorption results in irritation.

Coal Tar

Coal tar, a byproduct of coke and gas from bituminous coal, is extremely complex and variable in composition.

Pharmacodynamics. How coal tar works is unclear, but its efficacy may be related to suppression of epidermal cell DNA synthesis and mitotic activity, with restoration of normal rate of proliferation.

Therapeutic Uses. Coal tar is usually combined with ultraviolet B (UVB) phototherapy in the treatment of psoriasis.

Dosage and Administration. A typical treatment approach for severe unresponsive psoriasis is the Goeckerman regimen, in which 5% crude tar in hydrophilic ointment is applied in a heavy layer to the body at night. The client then dresses in a partially occlusive suit to cover the tar overnight. In the morning, the tar is removed in a bath containing coal tar bath oil (Balnetar), and the skin scales are lightly scrubbed off. UVB light is applied to the skin by a sunlamp equipped with special fluorescent bulbs. The dose of light is sufficient to produce mild erythema 12 hours later. The client undergoes this phototherapy every day of the week. The exposure time is increased to maintain a mild erythema. After each light exposure, involved areas are retreated with tar. A period of 2 to 3 weeks of treatment is needed, and remissions of up to 1 year may be achieved.

Modifications of the Goeckerman regimen include using salicylic acid to remove scale from plaques, corticosteroids with occlusive dressings, and anthralin.

Various tar preparations are available over the counter as body oils, gels, lotions, ointments, pastes, shampoos, and soaps. Prescription preparations include body oils (Balnetar 2.5%, Doak Oil 2%, Lavatar 25%, and Zetar Emulsion 30%), cream (Fototar 2%), gel (Estar 5%), ointment (Unguentum Bossi 5%), and soap (Packer's Pine Tar 5.87%).

Adverse Reactions. Folliculitis is the primary adverse reaction of coal tar and may occur with occlusive or excessive therapy. Irritation and allergic reactions are rare. Tars may have an unpleasant odor and stain skin, hair, and clothes.

Precautions and Contraindications. Clients should not be taking any extraneous photosensitizing medications (eg, phenothiazines, thiazides, sulfonylureas, tetracyclines, benzodiazepines).

Photochemotherapy

Photochemotherapy with psoralen-containing plant extracts was used in Egypt and India in 1500 B.C. for treating vitiligo (the loss of pigment from portions of the skin). In 1974, the combination of psoralen and UVA (PUVA) was first used.

The psoralens belong to a class of compounds that are derived from the fusion of a furan with a coumarin. They occur naturally in many plants, including limes, lemons, figs, and parsnips. Four psoralens are used in PUVA therapy: psoralen, 5-methoxypsoralen (bergapten), 8-methoxypsoralen (methoxsalen), and 4,5,8-trimethylpsoralen (trioxsalen).

Pharmacodynamics. The mechanism of photosensitivity production by PUVA is unknown. The therapeutic effects of PUVA in psoriasis may result from a decrease in DNA-dependent proliferation. Alteration in the immune system caused by PUVA may also play a role.

Pharmacokinetics. The psoralens are rapidly absorbed after oral administration. Photosensitivity peaks 1 to 2 hours after the ingestion of methoxsalen. Liquid formulations produce a more rapid, higher peak serum level. There is considerable first-pass elimination in the liver. Although 8-methoxypsoralen has a half-life of about 1 hour, the skin remains sensitive to light for 8 to 12 hours. It is widely distributed through the body but is activated only in the skin where the UVA penetrates.

Therapeutic Uses. This modality is used to treat vitiligo, psoriasis, cutaneous T-cell lymphoma, atopic dermatitis, alopecia areata, lichen planus, urticaria pigmentosa, and cutaneous photosensitivity.

Dosage and Administration. Methoxsalen is supplied in capsules (Oxsoralen, Oxsoralen-Ultra). The dose is 0.5 mg/kg taken 1.5 to 2 hours before UVA exposure. Treatment is administered three times weekly. Relapse occurs within 6 months after cessation of treatment in most clients.

Adverse Reactions. The major acute adverse reactions of PUVA include nausea, blistering, and painful erythema. PUVA-induced inflammation peaks 48 to 72 hours after exposure. Chronic effects include actinic keratoses, PUVA lentigines, photoaging, and nonmelanoma skin cancer. Squamous cell carcinomas occur at 10 times the expected frequency; the male genitalia are a very susceptible area.

Drug Interactions. Clients should not be taking any extraneous photosensitizing medications (eg, phenothiazines, thiazide diuretics, sulfonylureas, tetracyclines, benzodiazepines).

Photodynamic Therapy

Photodynamic therapy involves the combined use of photosensitizing drugs and light for the treatment of malignant or benign disease. Potential uses in dermatology include treatment of malignant cutaneous (and noncutaneous) lesions, psoriasis, alopecia, viral infections, and vascular malformations. Photodynamic therapy requires oxygen. Light, delivered to the skin, activates porphyrin molecules. These molecules transfer their energy to form cytotoxic oxygen, which results in lethal alteration of cellular membranes and subsequent tissue destruction. Porphyrin derivatives photofrin I and II are the photosensitizing drugs used for photodynamic therapy.

Antiseptics and Germicides

Agents such as iodine, povidone-iodine, thimerosal, triclosan, benzalkonium chloride, chlorhexidine gluconate, hexachlorophene, sodium hypochlorite, gluta-

Table 40-3. Antiseptics and Germicides

Agent	Examples	Indications	Additional Information
iodine	Iodine Topical; strong iodine (Lugol's Solution); Iodine Tincture, Strong Iodine Tincture	Used externally against bacteria, fungi, viruses, spores, protozoa, yeasts; may be used to disinfect skin preoperatively	Avoid contact with eyes and mucous membranes; highly toxic if ingested, and sodium thiosulfate is most effective antidote; iodine preparations stain skin and clothing; avoid occlusive dressings
povidone-iodine	Betadine (aerosol, antiseptic gauze pads, antiseptic lubricating gel, cream, vaginal gel, mouthwash/gargle, ointment, perineal wash concentrate, skin cleanser, foam skin cleanser, solution, surgical scrub, surgi-prep sponge brush, vaginal suppositories); Betagen, Aerodine, ACU-dyne, Iodex, others	In vitro, appears to completely inactivate HIV, but further study is needed	Water-soluble complex of iodine with povidone; retains bactericidal activity of iodine but less potent so causes less irritation to skin and mucous membranes; may use dressing
thimerosal	Mersol (1:1,000 solution, 1:1,000 with 50% alcohol tincture); Aeroaid (1:1,000 antiseptic spray)	Used externally preoperatively for antisepsis of skin and as first aid for cuts, scratches, lacerations, abrasions, wounds; sustained bacteriostatic and fungistatic activity	Contains 50% mercury; hypersensitivity reactions may occur; incompatible with potassium permanganate and iodine
triclosan	Septi-Soft, Septisol (solution); Septi-Soft is skin cleanser, not a surgical scrub	Used externally on clients for hand and body wash, shampoo, bathing; skin degermer for healthcare personnel	Bis-phenol disinfectant bacteriostatic against gram-positive and gram-negative bacteria
benzalkonium chloride	BAC, Benza, Zephiran; aqueous solution, disinfectant concentrate, tincture, tincture spray	Aqueous solutions in appropriate dilutions: antisepsis of skin, mucous membranes, wounds; preoperative preparation of skin; surgeons' hand and arm soaks; treatment of wounds; irrigation of eye, body cavities, bladder, urethra; vaginal douching; tinctures and sprays: preoperative preparation of skin, treatment of minor skin wounds	Can be bactericidal or bacteriostatic, depending on concentration, toward a variety of bacteria and some viruses, fungi, protozoa; rapidly acting and relatively long duration of action; inactivated by soaps or anionic detergents, so these should be thoroughly rinsed off skin before use; may be used for sterile storage of instruments and hospital utensils and if so, add antirust tablets
chlorhexidine gluconate	Hibiclens, Dyna-Hex, Exidine, Hibistat, Peridex	Surgical scrub; skin and wound cleanser; preoperative showering and bathing; healthcare personnel germicidal hand rinse; when hands are physically clean but need degerming and when routine handwashing is inconvenient or undesirable	Used twice daily as oral rinse (Peridex) for treatment of gingivitis; keep away from eyes and ears (deafness could occur if it reaches middle ear)
hexachlorophene	pHisoHex, Septisol	Surgical scrub and bacteriostatic skin cleanser; control of outbreak of gram-positive infection when other procedures are unsuccessful	Do not use with burns, open wounds, or on mucous membranes; rinse thoroughly; not intended for routine bathing of infants because they are likely to absorb it in significant amounts and systemic toxicity may be manifested as CNS stimulation
sodium hypochlorite	Dakin's	Applied topically to skin as antiseptic	Chemical burns can occur; avoid skin or eye contact
glutaraldehyde	Cidex	Germicidal agent for disinfection and sterilization of rigid and flexible fiberoptic endoscopes, plastic and rubber respiratory and anesthesia equipment, surgical and dental instruments and thermometers	Potent bactericidal, tuberculocidal, fungicidal, sporicidal, and virucidal activity; high degree of effectiveness retained even in presence of organic material (eg, blood, mucous, tissue)

(continued)

Table 40-3. (Continued)

Agent	Examples	Indications	Additional Information
oxychlorosene sodium	Clorpactin XCB, Clorpactin WCS-90; powder for solution	Used for treating localized infections, particularly when resistant organisms are present; to remove necrotic debris in massive infections or from radiation necrosis; to counteract odorous discharges; as a preoperative and postoperative irrigant and for cleansing and disinfection of fistulas, sinus tracts, wounds	If used for bladder/eye instillations, it may cause severe discomfort, so pretreat eye with topical anesthetic and for bladder use 0.1% concentration for first treatment

raldehyde, and oxychlorosene sodium are used for preoperative cleaning of the skin or for treatment of minor wounds or abrasions (Table 40-3).

Topical Wound Therapy Agents

Chemical agents may have a role in the treatment of wounds that do not heal readily in the presence of tissue debris or purulent exudate. The value of the adjunctive use of topical debriding enzymes such as collagenase (Santyl), fibrinolysin with desoxyribonuclease (Elase), and sutilains (Travase) is controversial (Table 40-4). They have been extensively advertised and are effective in degrading protein in vitro, but their effectiveness in vivo has been questioned for removing necrotic tissue, clotted blood, purulent exudates, or fibrinous accumulations resulting from burns, trauma, inflammation, infected wounds, or leg ulcers. They appear to be of value only when the wound base has yellowish necrotic connective tissue (mainly collagen) that must be removed before epithelialization can proceed. Once the wound base is clean, debriding enzymes should no longer be used and in fact may inhibit healing.

Occlusive biosynthetic dressings used in wound therapy include IntraSite Gel, DuoDerm Dressings, DuoDerm CGF (control gel formula), and Sorbsan. The advantages of moist wound healing with the use of occlusive biosynthetic dressings are:

- A wet wound environment promotes faster healing and better cosmetic results than a dry wound.
- An environment of relative anoxia is as good or better than one of normal or increased oxygen tension.
- Accumulation of wound exudate and detritus beneath an occlusive dressing is not necessarily harmful. Bacteria are excluded, and pain and healing time are significantly reduced in such an environment.
- Occlusion prevents the loss of drug from the skin, promotes skin hydration, and increases skin temperature. These actions also enhance the penetration of certain medications (as in psoriasis or leg ulcers).

The major disadvantages are that occlusive dressings may increase the number of silent or invisible infections and that therapeutic adherence is reduced because considerable amounts of serous or purulent foul-smelling exudate can accumulate under the dressing or seep from the wound. Occlusive dressings can cause overgrowth of bacteria and candidal organisms.

Absorbing beads or granules (eg, dextran polymers such as dextranomer [Debrisan Beads or Paste]) are not dressings but cleansing agents that absorb wound secretions and detritus so they will not interfere with wound healing. They can be used only during the wet exudative phase of healing; they are ineffective in dry wounds. The beads are 0.1 to 0.3 mm in diameter, so the material resembles a powder. Dextranomer is poured into wet surface ulcers or wounds, and the area is covered with a dry dressing closed on all sides. When saturated, it changes color. Removal is best achieved by irrigation (soaking or whirlpool). Highly porous and intensely hydrophilic, the beads act by physical absorption and capillary action to cleanse the wound surface continuously. The wound may appear larger during the first few days of treatment due to reduction of edema by the agent.

Substances with a molecular weight below 5,000 are absorbed by the beads, which can swell to four times their original size, resulting in the removal of plasma protein, fibrinogen, bacteria, and inflammatory exudates from the surface of the wound. Dextranomer is not an enzyme and does not debride.

Dextranomer is not absorbed systemically and appears to be nonantigenic, chemically inert, and free from toxic effects. Some clients experience mild discomfort when the dextranomer is applied because of its suction effect.

Topical Therapy for Burns

Thermal injury is common, and meticulous wound management is a key component of treatment. The wound is likely to be colonized by bacteria from the client; subsequently, septicemia may develop. Topical agents are initially used because systemic antibiotics cannot reach the wound due to the lack of blood supply in the burn eschar.

Mafenide

Mafenide (Sulfamylon) is available in the chloride or acetate form.

Table 40-4. Topical Enzymes

Drug Name	Preparation	Therapeutic Action	Additional Information
collagenase (Santyl)	Ointment; source is cultures of *Clostridium histolytica*	Digests collagen in the physiologic pH range and temperature to make it effective in removal of tissue debris; complete debridement in 10–14 d; used with burns, chronic dermal ulcers; active at pH 6–8	Proteolytic enzymes tend to be inactivated by extremes of pH; these enzymes are also inactivated by oxidizers such as hydrogen peroxide, by heavy metals such as silver and mercury, by detergents, and by iodine, nitrofurazone, and hexachlorophene. If any of these substances are used, they must be removed thoroughly by repeated flushings with normal saline before enzyme application. Cross-hatching thick eschar allows agent more surface contact with necrotic debris.
sutilains (Travase)	Ointment; apply moist dressing over ointment; source is cultures of *Bacillus subtilis*	Digests necrotic soft tissues by proteolytic action; dissolves and facilitates removal of necrotic tissues and purulent exudates; used with second- and third-degree burns, decubiti, peripheral vascular disease ulcers; active at pH 6–8	Enzyme activity may be impaired by other agents as described above; neomycin, mafenide, streptomycin, penicillin do not seem to interfere
fibrinolysin and deoxyribonuclease (Elase)	Lyophilized powder, ointment, ointment with chloramphenicol; ointment can be covered with petrolatum gauze or other non-adherent dressing; ointment can be used intravaginally; powder can be mixed with saline to soak a dressing for applying wet-to-dry dressing; powder can be mixed with saline to use as irrigating agent for wound; source is bovine plasma	Deoxyribonuclease attacks DNA; fibrinolysin attacks fibrin of blood clots and fibrinous exudates	Hypersensitivity reactions can occur; superinfection can occur with ointment preparation containing chloramphenicol; bone marrow suppression and death have been reported when using preparation containing chloramphenicol
papain and urea (Panafil White) or papain, urea, and chlorophyllin copper complex (Panafil)	Ointment; source is papaya fruit	Used for enzymatic debridement and promotion of normal healing; active at pH 3–12	Clean wound before application, but hydrogen peroxide may inactivate papain; chlorophyll derivatives control wound odor; urea is emollient and keratolytic
trypsin, Balsam Peru, castor oil (Dermuspray, Granulderm, Granulex, GranuMed)	Aerosol; source of trypsin is bovine pancreas	Trypsin used for enzymatic debridement and promotion of normal healing	Balsam Peru is an effective capillary bed stimulant intended to improve circulation to wound site; castor oil is used to improve epithelialization by reducing premature epithelial desiccation and cornification, and as a protective covering

Pharmacodynamics. The mechanism of action is unknown.

Pharmacokinetics. Mafenide diffuses through devascularized areas (ie, it penetrates eschar). It is quickly absorbed from the burn surface, so the amount on the wound is below effective antibacterial levels within 8 to 10 hours. It reaches peak plasma concentrations in 2 to 4 hours. It is rapidly metabolized and eliminated by the kidney.

Therapeutic Uses. Mafenide is used to prevent and treat sepsis in second- and third-degree burns. It is bacteriostatic against *Pseudomonas aeruginosa* and *Clostridia*. Its activity is not altered by changes in pH, and it is active in the presence of purulent material and serum. It has minimal activity against fungi. It has limited activity against *S aureus*, particularly the methicillin-resistant strains.

Mafenide has antifibrinolytic action by competitively inhibiting plasmin through interaction with its lysine site. The initial adherence of a skin graft to its prepared bed may be a result of fibrin deposition secondary to local coagulation. It is the fibrin bonding of the graft to the wound bed that may be important early after graft placement. Thus, mafenide may have a theoretical advantage in the prevention of early graft failure.

Dosage and Administration. Mafenide is applied to the clean and debrided wound twice a day. The client may be bathed in a whirlpool to aid debridement. The wound may be covered with a single layer of gauze or left open.

Adverse Reactions. Common adverse reactions are pain, burning, or stinging at the application site. Pain relief occurs 20 to 30 minutes after application; this timing correlates with the depletion of the drug in the cream layer closest to the skin.

Mafenide acetate is supplied in a cream containing sodium metabisulfite, which can cause allergic reactions, including anaphylaxis, and life-threatening episodes of asthma, especially in asthmatic clients.

A maculopapular rash often occurs, but treatment with antihistamines and continuation of the drug are usually recommended.

Mafenide and its metabolite inhibit carbonic anhydrase, which may result in metabolic acidosis. In a client with impaired renal function, high blood levels of mafenide and its metabolite may exaggerate the carbonic anhydrase inhibition.

Silver Sulfadiazine

Silver sulfadiazine (Silvadene, Thermazene, SSD Cream) is another burn therapy agent.

Pharmacodynamics. Silver is slowly released from the preparation in concentrations that are toxic to bacteria. Silver sulfadiazine reacts rapidly with DNA and releases sulfadiazine. The silver replaces the hydrogen bonding between strands of DNA and prevents replication. In addition, it can modify the cell membrane. Low solubility and large molecular size impair its absorption and facilitate relatively high concentrations in wound exudates.

Therapeutic Uses. Silver sulfadiazine is used for preventing and treating sepsis in second- and third-degree burns. It is bactericidal for many gram-negative and gram-positive bacteria such as *S aureus, Escherichia coli, Klebsiella, P aeruginosa, Proteus mirabilis* and *vulgaris, Enterobacter,* and *C albicans.*

Dosage and Administration. Silver sulfadiazine cream (10 mg/g in a water-miscible base) is applied to the clean and debrided wound once or twice daily. The client may be bathed in a whirlpool bath to aid debridement. Dressings are unnecessary but may be used. Generally, application is painless. The drug reacts with proteinaceous exudates in the wound, and if the drug is not removed adequately between dressings, a yellow-gray build-up appears that can be confused with a deeper tissue injury.

Adverse Reactions. Adverse reactions may include leukopenia, skin necrosis, skin discoloration, burning sensation, and rashes. Leukopenia associated with the drug's use is primarily characterized by decreased neutrophil count. Maximal white blood cell depression occurs within 2 to 4 days of initiation of therapy, with a rebound to normal leukocyte levels following 2 to 3 days later. Recovery does not seem influenced by continuation of therapy.

Drug–Drug Interactions. Silver may inactivate topical proteolytic enzymes if these agents are used concurrently. An increased incidence of leukopenia has been reported in clients treated concurrently with cimetidine.

Drug–Laboratory Test Interactions. Absorption of the propylene glycol vehicle may affect serum osmolality.

Nitrofurazone

Nitrofurazone (Furacin) is a synthetic nitrofuran with a broad antibacterial spectrum.

Pharmacodynamics. Nitrofurazone is bactericidal against a number of gram-negative and gram-positive bacteria, including *S aureus, Streptococcus, E coli, Clostridium perfringens,* and *Aerobacter aerogenes; Pseudomonas* and *Proteus* are often resistant.

Therapeutic Uses. Nitrofurazone is used as adjunctive therapy for clients with second- and third-degree burns when bacterial resistance to other agents is a real or potential problem.

Dosage and Administration. Nitrofurazone is applied directly to the burn or placed on gauze. It is available as a topical solution, ointment, and cream. Flushing the dressing with sterile saline facilitates removal.

Adverse Reactions. Varying degrees of contact dermatitis may occur, such as rash and pruritus.

Precautions and Contraindications. Nitrofurazone must be used with caution in clients with known or suspected renal impairment. The polyethylene glycol in the base can be absorbed through denuded skin and may not be excreted normally by a compromised kidney, leading to increased blood urea nitrogen and metabolic acidosis.

Soaps and Shampoos

Ordinary soaps are sodium or potassium salts of fatty acids. These cleansers emulsify fats, thereby promoting the removal of foreign particles from the skin. The pH of bar soaps varies in solution; some are alkaline (pH 8.8–10.5), including superfatted bar soaps. Superfatted soaps (eg, Camay, Neutrogena Glycerine Soap) contain unsaponified fat, unreacted fatty acids, or emollients (eg, lanolin, cold cream). Neutral soaps contain synthetic detergents or soap substitutes (eg, triethanolamine lauryl sulfate, sodium lauryl sulfate).

Soaps can be irritating, especially to persons with dry or already irritated skin and especially during the winter, when there is low humidity. Dry, irritated skin can be remedied by decreasing the frequency of washing with soap and water, using mild soap (eg, Dove), and applying moisturizing cream after washing.

Medicated soaps are available. Some abrasive soaps contain inert aluminum oxide, polyethylene, or sodium tetraborate decahydrate particles. Antimicrobial soaps (eg, Coast, Irish Spring, Dial, Safeguard) contain sufficient amounts of antiseptics to be effective deodorants or to be useful for preoperative preparation of the skin and for hand washing for healthcare personnel.

Shampoos are liquid soaps or detergents used to wash the hair and clean the scalp of scales. The detergent properties of special shampoos for use on dry, normal, or oily hair differ. Shampoos may also be used as vehicles for applying medication to the scalp for dandruff, seborrheic dermatitis, or psoriasis.

Sunscreens

Sunscreens provide either a chemical or physical barrier to sunlight. Chemical sunscreens absorb ultraviolet radiation in the UVB range, the spectrum of ultraviolet light most responsible for sunburns. Chemical sunscreens include benzophenones (oxybenzone, dioxybenzone), para-aminobenzoic acid and esters, cinnamates, salicylates, and other agents. Physical sunscreens reflect or scatter UVA, UVB, and visible light to prevent skin penetration. Physical sunscreens contain ingredients such as titanium dioxide, red petrolatum, zinc oxide, talc, magnesium oxide, kaolin, ferric chloride, and ichthammol. These agents are opaque and may be cosmetically unacceptable, but they are used in such areas as the nose.

The effectiveness of a sunscreen is usually indicated by its sun protection factor (SPF), which indicates the product's relative resistance to sunburning. For example, a SPF of 6 means the product offers six times the protection as the use of no sunscreen. Persons who tend to burn easily should use products with an SPF of 15.

A "water-resistant" sunscreen should continue to function after 40 minutes in water; a "waterproof" sunscreen withstands 80 minutes in water.

Contact dermatitis can develop with some sunscreens, particularly those containing PABA or its esters, benzophenones, and cinnamates. Contact with the eyes should be avoided.

Miscellaneous Agents
Minoxidil

Normal scalp hair growth (anagen phase) is relatively steady over a mean period of 3 years, and then the follicle enters a resting stage (telogen phase) for about 3 months. New growth then ensues, and the old hair is pushed out of the follicle. Most follicles continue this cycle throughout life, but in clients with pattern baldness, follicles in the area of hair loss become progressively smaller and produce thinner and less pigmented hair, then nonpigmented, fine vellus hair, and finally no hair.

Minoxidil is a direct-acting peripheral vasodilator (see Chap. 25) used to treat hypertension. During use for hypertension, it was noted to cause regrowth of body hair. From there, a topical preparation was developed for treating male hereditary androgen-dependent alopecia and female androgenetic baldness (diffuse hair loss or thinning of hair in frontoparietal areas).

Pharmacodynamics. Minoxidil (Rogaine) causes elongation and normalization of follicles in the area of alopecia; new follicles are not formed. It has no endocrine action. Topical application causes a dose-dependent increase in dermal blood flow. In androgenetic alopecia, minoxidil converts vellus hairs to terminal hairs, possibly by stimulating the enlargement and turnover of vellus follicles in early anagen phases.

Dosage and Administration. In androgenetic alopecia, younger persons with less hair loss over a shorter time (less than 5 years) respond best. Older persons with more than a 5-year history of hair loss and with a greater degree of hair loss would not be expected to respond in most cases.

A period of at least 4 months of twice-daily applications is generally required before evidence of hair growth can be expected. The preparation comes in a 2% solution in alcohol, propylene glycol, and water with either a metered spray or extender spray applicator or a rub-on applicator tip. The hair and scalp should be dry before application. One mL of solution is applied to the scalp twice a day. The beneficial effect of topical minoxidil ceases when therapy is discontinued, so lifelong treatment is recommended.

Adverse Reactions. A few cases of allergic contact dermatitis and folliculitis have been reported, but local reactions are minimal. Absorption is poor from normal intact scalp.

Drug Interactions. Minoxidil should not be used in conjunction with other topical agents, including topical corticosteroids, retinoids, and petrolatum, or agents known to enhance cutaneous drug absorption.

Precautions and Contraindications. The use of oral minoxidil to promote hair growth is not approved.

Capsaicin

Capsaicin is a naturally occurring substance derived from plants of the Solanaceae family. It appears to act by causing local depletion and preventing reaccumulation of substance P, an endogenous neuropeptide involved in the transmission of pain impulses. It is available as a cream in 0.025% (Zostrix) and 0.075% (Zostrix HP) strengths to be applied three or four times a day. It has been used for relieving postherpetic neuralgia (pain after herpes zoster or shingles), rheumatoid arthritis, osteoarthritis, and diabetic neuropathy.

Keratolytics

Keratolytics cause degeneration and sloughing of epidermal cells and are used to remove warts and excessive keratin in hyperkeratotic skin disorders. Keratolytic agents (Table 40-5) include salicylic acid, cantharidin, masoprocol, podofilox, podophyllum resin, and urea.

Pigmenting/Depigmenting Agents

Normal skin pigmentation results from melanocytes in the basal layer of the epidermis. These cells can form the pigment melanin by oxidation of tyrosine. There are several hyperpigmentation and hypopigmentation disorders.

Two psoralen compounds, methoxsalen (Oxsoralen, Oxsoralen-Ultra) and trioxsalen (Trisoralen), can facilitate repigmentation in clients with vitiligo, a disorder characterized by patchy areas of nonpigmented skin. Significant repigmentation may take 6 to 12 months and may occur in only 15% of cases. The psoralens are effective in enhancing pigmentation only when followed by exposure of affected skin areas to UV light.

The combination of methoxypsoralen and UVA was discussed in the section on the treatment of psoriasis.

Two agents are available for reducing hyperpigmentation of skin. Hydroquinone (Eldopaque, Esoterica Regular, Porcelana) usually produces a temporary lightening of skin areas. Principal uses for hydroquinone are for freckles, chloasma, melasma, or senile lentigines. Monobenzone produces irreversible depigmentation.

Scabicides and Pediculicides

Scabies is infestation of the skin with the *Sarcoptes scabiei* mite. It is acquired by close contact with an infected person. The inflammatory papulopustular eruption that develops is associated with severe pruritus.

Pediculosis is infestation of the skin by lice. Head lice (*Pediculus humanus capitis*)and body lice (*Pediculus humanus corporis*)are transmitted among persons who

---

Table 40-5. Keratolytics

Agent	Examples	Indications	Additional Information
salicylic acid	Dr. Scholl's Wart Remover Kit, Compound W, Wart-Off, DuoFilm, Freezone, Keralyt, Occlusal, Trans-Ver-Sal	Corns, calluses, common warts, plantar warts	With warts, improvement should occur in 1–2 wk, maximum resolution after 4–6 wk; irritation of normal skin surrounding affected area may occur from contact between normal skin and product; other salicylic acid preparations are used for acne vulgaris, seborrheic dermatitis, dandruff, psoriasis, other conditions
cantharidin (also known as Spanish fly or dried blister beetles)	Canthaerone, Verr-Canth	Warts, molluscum contagiosum	Affects epidermal cell membranes and leads to blister formation; do not apply to anogenital area because it is a strong irritant; application to skin results in tingling, itching, or burning within hours
masoprocol	Actinex	Actinic keratoses	Massage into areas where keratoses are present twice a day for 28 d; do not use occlusive dressing; transient burning can occur after application, and allergic contact dermatitis has occurred; can stain clothing
podofilox	Condylox	Condylomata acuminata (external genital warts) (these warts may resemble squamous cell carcinoma; accurate diagnosis is needed, as agent must not be used for squamous cell carcinoma)	Topical antimitotic drug; applied twice daily for 3 d, then withheld for 4 d; repeat cycle up to four times
podophyllum resin	Pod-Ben-25, Podocon-25, Podofin	Condylomata acuminata, other papillomas, verrucae, multiple superficial keratoses	Cytotoxic, produces degeneration of epithelial cells and mitotic arrest; powerful caustic and severe irritant; should not be used in diabetics or those with compromised circulation
urea	Aquacare, Carmol 10, Ureacin	Used to promote hydration and remove excess keratin in dry skin or hyperkeratotic conditions; may be used to remove dystrophic nails	Has a softening or moisturizing effect on stratum corneum and can facilitate solubilization of keratin

Table 40-6. Scabicides and Pediculicides

Drug Name	Indication	Additional Information
crotamiton (Eurax) (lotion, cream)	*Scabies:* apply from neck down and leave on for 24 hr; reapply 24 hr later without removing previous application; cleansing bath is taken 48 hr after final application *Pediculosis:* in treating head lice, apply Eurax to scalp, leave on for 24 hr, then shampoo; repeat in 7–10 d	Treat all family members and close contacts as well; often need retreatment because not as effective as lindane but considered less toxic so often used for young children; drug should not be applied to inflamed or denuded skin or to eyes or mouth; drug has antipruritic properties
lindane (G-Well, Kwell, Scabene) (cream, lotion, shampoo)	*Scabies:* apply cream or lotion from neck down, including all skin creases and between toes; leave on for 6 hr, then wash off *Head lice:* apply lindane shampoo, leave on for 5 min, then rinse and dry hair (do not use blow-dryer); use shampoo again in 7–10 d *Pubic lice:* follow suggestions for head lice	Treat all family members and close contacts as well; reapply if living lice detected 7 d later or if there are highly inflammatory crusted eruptions; fine-toothed comb may be used to comb nits out of hair; do not apply to face, open wounds; percutaneous absorption can result in CNS stimulation; in treating body lice, treat the clothing, not the client, because the lice reside in the clothing, not on the body; wash in hot water and dry in hot dryer
permethrin (Elimite, Nix)	Lice, mites, ticks, fleas *Head infestation:* shampoo with regular shampoo and towel-dry; saturate hair and scalp with permethrin cream rinse and leave in place for 10 min before rinsing off *Body infestation:* massage cream into skin and leave on for 8–14 hr before washing	Acts on nerve cell membranes of parasites to cause paralysis; adverse reactions may include itching and transient burning or stinging
pyrethrins (RID, R & C Shampoo), A-200 Shampoo (combined with piperonyl butoxide) (liquid, gel, shampoo)	*Pediculosis* *Head lice:* apply for 10 min, rinse out, let hair dry naturally; repeat in 7–10 d	Irritating to eyes and mucous membranes; synergistic action against head, body, and pubic lice

live in unhealthy, crowded conditions and share clothing or other personal articles. Pubic lice (*Pthirus pubis*) are most commonly transmitted sexually. Treatment preparations for scabies and pediculosis are summarized in Table 40-6.

▪ SUMMARY

Over 2,000 skin disorders are recognized. Among the agents discussed for the management of skin disorders and integumentary system disorders are drying and moisturizing preparations, retinoids, coal tars, psoralens, and various products used in phototherapy and wound and burn care.

❖ NURSING MANAGEMENT: CLIENT RECEIVING MEDICATION FOR A SKIN DISORDER

The many integumentary disorders that exist require expert and meticulous nursing care. Clients with these disorders are typically treated on an outpatient basis, so nurses must offer supervision and instruction to help the client perform the needed self-care.

NURSING PROCESS
ASSESSMENT

Assessment of a skin symptom begins with a history of the chief complaint, along with a health history and review of systems. Included should be details about the duration and onset of lesions, their relation to external events or seasons, and associated symptoms and any systemic symptoms.

The physical examination should note the client's general appearance and then details on the four main skin signs: the type, shape, arrangement, and distribution of lesions. Enhanced lighting and magnification help assess the detail of the lesions. The color and characteristics of tissue surrounding the lesions should be noted. Note any signs of secondary infection, excoriation, tissue erosion, scaling, crusting, or ulceration. Lesions should be measured and a drawing should be made to note the distribution and shape.

NURSING DIAGNOSIS

Nursing diagnoses that may apply to clients receiving drug therapy for a skin problem include:

• Impaired Skin Integrity, related to inflammatory process and to initial sensitivity to drug therapy

- Body Image Disturbance, related to skin lesions and unsightly appearance of some topical medications
- Knowledge Deficit, related to lack of experience with skin disorder and its management with medications

PLANNING

Goals are to promote skin integrity (relieving pruritus, preventing or managing secondary infection), enhance body image, and decrease knowledge deficit.

INTERVENTIONS

Nursing interventions depend on the therapeutic regimen prescribed to manage the skin disorder. Many interventions focus on client education. For example, the client with acne vulgaris should be taught what causes acne; myths about its cause and treatment should be dispelled (see the Critical Thinking Challenge). Common myths are that acne is caused by diet, that vigorous cleansing or scrubbing is helpful (actually, gentle, nonabrasive cleansing is less likely to increase the inflammatory process), that acne results from the client's failure to take care of himself or herself, and that it always resolves after adolescence (in reality, it may persist into adult life).

Client Education. The nurse should explain the pathophysiology of the integumentary disorder and the expected actions and possible adverse reactions of treatment. If topical treatment is included, it is important to tell the client not to apply anything to the rash or area being treated except water, the prescribed medications, or substances the prescriber has approved. Irritation of the treated area from allergy to the prescribed agent or from a home remedy or an over-the-counter preparation being used without the prescriber's knowledge could cause further difficulties and treatment failure.

It is important to teach the client how to apply the prescribed preparation and how much of it to use. One

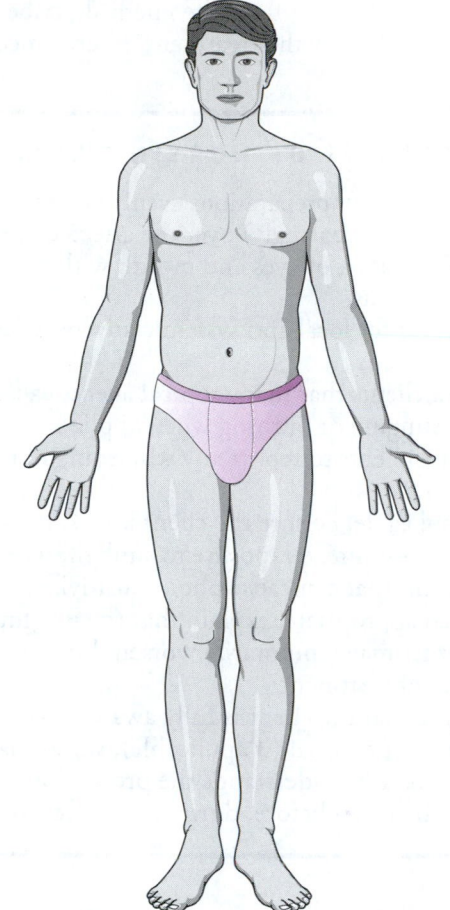

Figure 40-1. How much ointment the client needs to apply to the skin for treatment depends on several variables. As a rule, however, he or she will apply the drug with the fingertips (one fingertipful is a fingertip unit, or FTU). Usual FTU application measurements follow: For the face and neck, 2.5 FTU or 1.25 g of ointment; for the chest or back, 7 FTU or 3.5 g; for the arm, 3 FTU or 1.5 g; for one hand (both sides), 1 FTU or 0.5 g; for one leg, 6 FTU or 3 g; and for one foot, 2 FTU or 1 g. (Source: Habif TP. [1996]. Clinical Dermatology: A Color Guide to Diagnosis and Therapy. St. Louis: Mosby–Yearbook.)

rule of thumb is that about 35 g of cream is needed to cover the entire body, 10% less ointment than cream will cover the entire body, and about 50% more lotion than cream is needed to cover the whole body (Fig. 40-1). The client should be given specific written instructions on how to carry out the treatment.

OUTCOME EVALUATION

The nurse must evaluate the client to determine the efficacy of treatment and to observe for adverse reactions. Data that indicate treatment efficacy include maintenance of skin in the best possible condition, decreased itching and scratching, prevention of secondary infection, adaptation by the client to changes in appearance, and understanding by the client of etiologic factors, management, and his or her role in controlling the disorder. It

CRITICAL THINKING CHALLENGE
Case Analysis

Vicky Norris, 16, a high-school cheerleader and swimmer, comes to the clinic with a severe case of acne vulgaris. At her mother's insistence, she washes her face and hands at least six times a day because, her mother says, the problem is caused by sweating and wiping the dirt from her hands onto her face. Benzoyl peroxide is prescribed.

1. What can you tell Vicky about acne?
2. What can you tell her about the medication prescribed?
3. What printed materials can you supply for home reference?

ful to have the client describe or dem-
y how the treatment is performed.

CHECKLIST OF NURSING ACTIONS

- ❏ Spread topical preparations evenly and as prescribed (liberally or sparingly) over the affected area.
- ❏ Avoid contact of eyes and mouth with topical preparations.
- ❏ Monitor for local and systemic adverse effects of medications.
- ❏ Warn clients that many topical agents cause localized stinging or burning when applied.
- ❏ Advise clients to report any worsening of the condition.
- ❏ If applicable, be sure the client knows the steps to take to minimize exposure to sunlight when using an agent that can cause photosensitivity.
- ❏ When appropriate, explain that the integumentary disorder may temporarily worsen during early stages of treatment.
- ❏ Ensure that the client is fully aware of a drug's teratogenic potential (if applicable); verify that the client clearly understands the precautions that must be taken before, during, and after treatment.

References

Greaves MW, Weinstein GD. (1995). Treatment of psoriasis. *N Engl J Med, 332* (9), 581–588.

Hagermark O, Wahlgren CF. (1995). Treatment of itch. *Sem Dermatol, 14* (4), 320–325.

Hardman JG, Limbird LE, Molinoff PB, et al., eds. (1996). *Goodman and Gilman's The pharmacological basis of therapeutics*, 9th ed. New York: McGraw-Hill.

Bibliography

Allen TG. (1994). Common skin problems. *ADVANCE for Nurse Practitioners, 2* (11), 21–24.

Bondi EE, Jegasothy BV, Lazarus GS, eds. (1991). *Dermatology: Diagnosis and therapy*. Norwalk, CT: Appleton & Lange.

Division of Drugs and Toxicology. (1993). *Drug evaluations subscription*, v. 2. Chicago: American Medical Association.

Driscoll MS, Rothe MJ, Abrahamian L, Grant-Kels JM. (1993). Long-term oral antibiotics for acne: Is laboratory monitoring necessary? *J Am Acad Dermatol, 28*, 595–602.

Ekblom A. (1995). Some neurophysiological aspects of itch. *Sem Dermatol, 14* (4), 262–270.

Epstein E. (1994). *Common skin disorders*, 4th ed. Philadelphia: WB Saunders.

Greaves MW. (1995). Chronic urticaria. *N Engl J Med, 332* (26), 1767–1772.

Habif TP. (1996). *Clinical dermatology: A color guide to diagnosis and therapy*. St. Louis: CV Mosby.

Helm TN, et al. (1991). PUVA therapy. *Am Family Physician, 43* (3), 908–912.

Kumasaka BH, Odland PB. (1992). Acne vulgaris: Topical and systemic therapies. *Postgrad Med, 92* (5), 181–194.

Straus SE. (1993). Shingles: Sorrow, salves, and solutions. *JAMA, 269* (14), 1836–1839.

For more information and sample tests and activities, refer to Chapter 40 in the Student Workbook for Clinical Pharmacology and Nursing Management, 5th edition, available through your bookstore.

XII

Drugs Affecting Inflammation and Infection

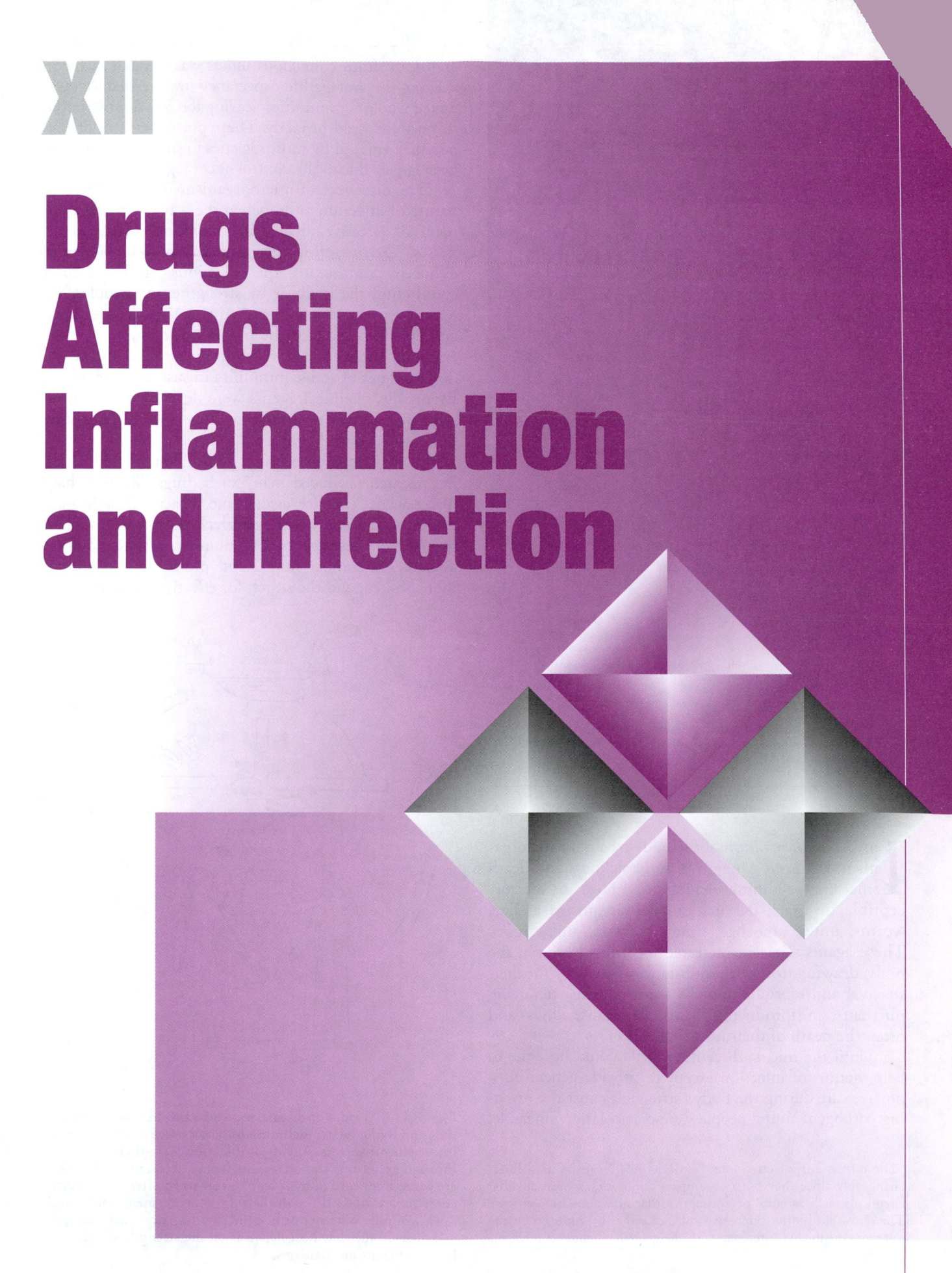

41

Antimicrobial* Drugs That Affect Bacterial Cell Wall Synthesis

Infection, or invasion of the body by a parasitic organism, has been a major cause of sickness and death since the beginning of humanity. Humans are susceptible to attack by such smaller organisms as lice, worms, mites, amoebae, fungi, bacteria, and viruses. These agents settle in preferred locations on or in the body, drawing from it the substances necessary for their survival and reproduction. By injuring cells, removing nutrients, and producing toxins, they cause illness and often the death of their host (Fig. 41-1).

Until the mid-19th century, little could be done to help victims of infection except to provide general supportive care during the body's struggle against the invading pathogen. Young people were particularly vulnerable,

*The terms "antiinfective" and "antimicrobial" can be used interchangeably since they both encompass antibiotics as well as other chemicals such as sulfa or antiseptics that affect microorganisms. The term "antibiotic" refers to a substance that is produced by one microorganism that interferes with the growth of another microorganism.

and death from contagious illness was a major factor in keeping the average life expectancy low. Epidemics decimated whole communities, leaving too few survivors even to bury the dead properly. The rapid increase in life expectancy enjoyed by most societies in the last century has been largely due to the control of contagious diseases.

The discovery of microorganisms revealed the true nature of infection and opened the way to the development of effective means of combating infectious illnesses. The first efforts attempted to prevent infection, either by eliminating the infectious agent before it could enter the body or by strengthening people's defenses against the pathogen. Antiseptics, disinfectants, and sanitizers reduced the number of organisms in the environment. Vaccines were administered to induce the development of active immunity in susceptible persons. Eventually, chemical agents were developed that could selectively inhibit or destroy pathogens within the body without harm to the host.

In the mid-20th century, well-organized, wide-ranging research produced many such drugs. We now have many agents effective against most bacterial pathogens; unfortunately, many pathogens have developed resistance to many of these agents. The number of systemic drugs available to combat fungal and protozoal infections is more limited, and the search for effective antiviral agents

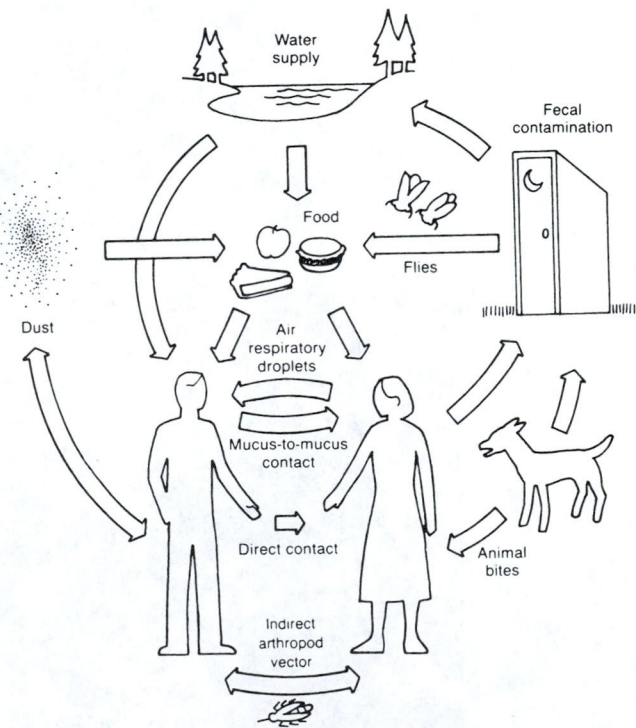

Figure 41-1. Modes of disease transmission. Inanimate materials and living hosts, including humans, serve as reservoirs of infectious organisms. Agents of infection leave their hosts through excretions and secretions (urine, feces, mucus). They are sometimes carried by insect vectors or fomites. They gain entry to new hosts through the skin, mucous membranes, and open wounds. Whether or not the invading organism can live and grow in the new host depends on the strength of that host's resistant mechanisms.

continues. The effort is a competitive one—an attempt to develop weapons in the fight against infection faster than pathogens can adapt through mutation to their presence.

Unlike most medicinal drugs, many anti-infective drugs are truly curative in that they correct the cause of the disease by killing or inhibiting the growth of pathogens. Most drugs cannot cure in this sense but instead alleviate symptoms, reverse pathologic processes, or support the body in its recuperative process.

Introduction to Antimicrobials

When it became widely accepted that microorganisms cause disease, medical scientists began searching for a "magic bullet"—a substance that would be lethal to pathogenic microorganisms without affecting the health of the host. They believed that for each disease, a chemical exists that would selectively destroy the causative microbe. (Although antitoxins do possess this kind of specificity, their usefulness is limited by their antigenicity as foreign proteins. Vaccines and antitoxins are discussed in Chap. 35.) Selectivity in antimicrobials depends on differences in structure and function between host and pathogen cells. Because most living organisms share the same basic characteristics, these differences are not sufficient to provide complete safety when antimicrobial chemotherapy is used. However, drugs have been found that exhibit both effectiveness and an acceptable therapeutic index.

Recently there has been increased awareness and appreciation of the role of humoral and cellular immunity in antibiotic therapy. If the client has an adequate immune system, bacteriostatic agents (those that arrest the growth of bacteria) may be used to treat infections because the client's defense mechanisms will then resolve the infection. Bactericidal agents (those that kill microorganisms) with rapid effectiveness are needed to treat infections in clients who are immunologically suppressed.

With the increased numbers of clients with immunosuppression (eg, clients with AIDS, clients receiving cancer chemotherapy, radiation therapy, or steroid therapy), the use of potent antibiotics to prevent or treat infections has increased; this is believed to contribute to the increasing problem of microbial resistance to antimicrobials.

Characteristics of the Ideal Antimicrobial

A perfect antimicrobial agent would destroy pathogens without harming host cells. It would be effective against large numbers of infectious organisms and would lose none of its action in the presence of such materials as exudates or tissue enzymes. The ideal antimicrobial agent would not promote the development of resistance by pathogens. It would distribute rapidly to all body fluids and tissues and would remain in the body for relatively long periods.

This ideal will probably never be achieved; indeed, some of the characteristics of the ideal anti-infective agent tend to be mutually exclusive. For example, a selective agent probably could not affect a wide variety of pathogens. Because pathogens vary in their characteristics, an agent chemically suited to damage a particular microorganism would affect similar organisms but not others that differ in nature.

Other problems exist as well. The ability to affect a wide variety of pathogens is a double-edged sword. Treatment agents with a broad spectrum of activity are apt to reduce the natural microscopic flora of the body to such a degree that the host is rendered vulnerable to superinfection or overgrowth of fungi and protozoa normally suppressed by this flora. Probably no chemical exists to which resistance cannot be developed. Microorganisms use several mechanisms to transfer the ability to resist a particular chemical agent. The rapid rate of reproduction of these small life forms favors the emergence of mutant strains. Microbes can transfer genetic material from one to another, a process that allows the resistant organisms to transfer their resistance to a large percentage of a pathogenic population.

It is not surprising, therefore, that with prolonged use, antimicrobials tend to become less effective, because susceptible pathogens have been replaced by resistant ones. Because they interact with living matter, antimicrobials also combine with many biochemical materials of the host. This decreases the therapeutic activity of the antimicrobials.

The Use of Antimicrobials

Many antibiotics are substances secreted by one microorganism that are toxic to other microorganisms; other antibiotics are synthetic or semisynthetic preparations. The best antimicrobials interfere with metabolic or growth processes that are specific to pathogenic microorganisms and not characteristic of host cells (Box 41-1). These mechanisms include:

- *Inhibition of bacterial cell wall synthesis.* Bacterial cell walls are generally thicker and more rigid than

Box 41-1
Actions of Antimicrobial Drugs

Mechanisms by which drugs affect microorganisms include:

- Inhibition of bacterial cell synthesis
- Inhibition of protein synthesis
- Interference with the cell membrane
- Interference with energy metabolism
- Interference with nucleic acid metabolism

membranes of mammalian cells. One important molecule responsible for this rigidity is mucopeptide. Certain antimicrobials interfere with the formation of mucopeptide, thereby producing deficiencies in the cell walls, which then function as semipermeable membranes. Because the interior of the cell is hypertonic, water enters the interior of the cell, swells it, and eventually causes lysis. Antimicrobials with this action are all antibiotics (ie, a metabolic product of one organism that can damage or kill another organism); they include penicillin, cephalosporin, novobiocin, bacitracin, cycloserine, and vancomycin.

- *Inhibition of protein synthesis.* Although the mechanism for protein synthesis is similar in both mammalian and microbial cells, differences in ribosomal number and structure permit relative selectivity in inhibiting protein synthesis. Among the antimicrobials that affect protein synthesis are aminoglycosides, tetracyclines, erythromycin, lincomycin, gentamicin, and chloramphenicol. As might be expected, these drugs—all antibiotics—are more toxic than agents that interfere with a system unique to pathogens.

- *Interference with the cell membrane.* Certain compounds attack microbial cell membranes by binding to the cell wall. Because the permeability of the membrane is thereby increased, assorted electrolytes and sugars leak from the cytoplasm. Examples of this type of antimicrobial are the polymyxins, nystatin, colistin, and amphotericin.

- *Interference with metabolism.* Bacteria that cannot use preformed folic acid, as mammalian cells do, synthesize it by using para-aminobenzoic acid (PABA) as the substrate. Antimicrobials, such as the sulfonamides, trimethoprim, and para-aminosalicylic acid (PAS), function as competitive analogs of PABA in the synthesis of folic acid. Because the molecules of folic acid that incorporate these drugs do not perform their metabolic function, the pathogen develops folic acid deficiency. Because various microbes use different biochemical pathways in producing folic acid, these antimetabolites have differing spectra of activity. A pathogen sensitive to one of the group may not respond to the others.

- *Interference with nucleic acid production.* Agents that block nucleic acid synthesis prevent reproduction of microbial cells. Rifampin, nalidixic acid, other quinolones, and griseofulvin appear to use this mechanism.

The mode of action of some antimicrobials remains unknown. Antimicrobials may either inhibit the growth of pathogens (bacteriostatic) or kill pathogens (bactericidal). Bacteriostatic agents rely on host defenses to eliminate pathogens. Treatment of infection in clients with inadequate resistance to infection requires bactericidal drugs.

Spectra of Activity

A drug's spectrum of activity refers to the number and type of organisms vulnerable to its action. Broad-spectrum antimicrobials injure a wide variety of pathogens, narrow-spectrum drugs only a few. Antimicrobials tend to affect pathogens with similar biochemical characteristics. One of the methods used to distinguish various microorganisms is to stain them with certain laboratory dyes. The characteristic ways organisms take the stain are associated with chemical differences in the cell membrane or intracellular components. Pathogens with similar staining properties tend to be sensitive to the same antimicrobials. A drug's spectrum of activity, therefore, may be described in terms of its effectiveness against gram-positive, gram-negative, or acid-fast bacteria. Morphology also influences a drug's efficacy because drugs vary in their effects on such groups as cocci, rods, spirochetes, and fungi. The spectra of some drugs appear to be unrelated to the ordinary systems of classification, and microbial strains susceptible to their action are listed individually.

Bacterial Resistance

One factor that limits the usefulness of antimicrobial agents is the propensity of pathogens to develop resistance to a drug's action. Resistance is the ability of a microorganism to live and grow in the presence of an antiinfective substance that usually exerts a bactericidal or bacteriostatic action on organisms of its species. Resistance, arising from chance mutation in one or more cells, allows the cell to survive in the presence of the antimicrobial.

This capacity may spread throughout the bacterial population by the mechanisms of selected reproduction (survival and multiplication of more resistant cells than nonresistant), transduction (transfer of genetic material from one microbe to another through a bacteriophage viral transducer), transformation (incorporation by one pathogen of genes from another that have been released into the environment), or conjunction (a flow of cytoplasmic genes from one organism to another through a corridor that connects two cells in conjugation). The mutant strain may produce an enzyme that breaks down the chemical structure of the drug. The cell wall may be so altered that it is less permeable to the drug, increased production of an endogenous antagonist to the drug may occur, or the critical target or receptor on the cell may be so altered that the drug cannot function.

The likelihood of drug resistance varies from microbe to microbe and from drug to drug. Mutation of microbes may occur if antimicrobials fall below therapeutic levels. Whether or not resistance develops is also directly related to whether an organism is exposed to nonlethal doses of the drug in question. The staphylococcal species has been notoriously proficient in developing resistance to penicillin by the production of the enzyme penicillinase. A common inhabitant of skin and environmental surfaces, resistant strains of this microbe often develop in healthcare institutions, where antimicrobials are in common use. Nosocomial infections result and can be difficult to eradicate. Not only are clients vulnerable, especially those who are debilitated or who have wounds, but infections due to resistant strains are an occupational hazard for employees and their families.

Adverse Effects

Antimicrobials are potentially harmful to the recipient, who can develop allergic sensitivity to the agent, alterations of body functions, or toxic tissue changes. The drug may damage body tissues or organs and interfere with the absorption or use of nutrients. Disruptions of the normal microscopic flora in the body may precipitate infection by overgrowth of nonsusceptible organisms.

Allergy

Every antimicrobial can stimulate antibody production in some people. The frequency of sensitivity varies greatly from one drug to another, depending on the antigenic properties of the chemical and how frequently the population is exposed to it. People who have never received drug therapy may have become allergic to antimicrobials due to exposure to environmental contamination from agricultural or industrial use of the chemicals. Reactions vary from minor to catastrophic, and succeeding reactions tend to increase in severity.

A personal or family history of atopic allergy indicates increased susceptibility to allergic drug sensitivity. The topical use of antimicrobials (especially application to open wounds) appears to stimulate antibody production and increase the incidence of allergy. Reactions are most likely if a drug is initially applied topically and then subsequently administered systemically. For this reason, topical agents are prepared from antimicrobials, such as bacitracin, that are not generally suitable for systemic use. Allergic responses to injected drug doses are generally more severe than to drugs given orally.

Toxicity

Theoretically, harmful effects on host cells should correspond to the drug's mechanisms of action. For example, rapidly dividing cells would be more likely to suffer toxic effects from chemicals that interfere with nucleic acid formation and protein synthesis because these two processes proceed at a rapid rate during reproduction. Clinical data indicate that drugs that affect nucleic acid production do not seem to damage rapidly dividing mammalian cells, whereas those that interfere with protein synthesis do. In other categories, the relation between biochemical action and toxic effects seems obscure, probably because we lack essential knowledge of biology at the molecular and chemical levels to explain them.

Antimicrobials can damage any part of the body. Symptoms of toxicity range from the trivial to the serious and vary depending on the agent. Nausea, vomiting, and diarrhea are fairly common. Liver malfunction, kidney damage, bone marrow depression, degeneration of nerves (eg, ototoxicity, neuropathies), and teeth and bone defects can occur. Damage to the rapidly dividing cells of the body causes symptoms related to alterations of bone marrow and intestinal mucosa. Leukopenia and agranulocytosis are usually reversible if they are detected early and drug treatment is discontinued. If the damage is allowed to progress to pancytopenia and aplastic anemia, it may be irreversible and fatal. Lesions of the gastrointestinal (GI) tract cause nausea and vomiting. Ulcerations may develop throughout the tract, and fulminating colitis can ensue.

The liver and kidneys are subject to damage by certain agents, especially when these organs are involved in the degradation and excretion of the drugs. The sulfonamides, which tend to crystallize in the urine, cause mechanical damage to the kidneys. Other agents precipitate renal shutdown, especially when administered concomitantly with diuretics. The kidneys are the major avenue for elimination of most antimicrobials. Initially, altered liver function may be characteristic of drug-induced cholestasis. Symptoms of hepatitis may occur. Some antibiotics affect both organs, placing the recipient in double jeopardy.

Manifestations of damage to the central nervous system (CNS) include nervousness, convulsions, paresthesia, ataxia, neuropsychiatric episodes, photosensitivity, peripheral neuritis, insomnia, encephalopathy, temporary blindness, and eighth cranial nerve toxicity. Fortunately, most of these effects are relatively rare. The most common is acoustic nerve damage, with initial symptoms of tinnitus, decreased perception of high tones, and eventual deafness. In some cases, loss of hearing is temporary, but it may be permanent.

Bone and tooth defects occur primarily from tetracycline therapy. The drug is deposited in developing teeth, producing permanent discoloration. The rate of bone growth is also affected by the drug. Because of these effects, tetracyclines are not administered during pregnancy or early childhood.

Interaction With Oral Contraceptives

Some antibiotics (eg, penicillins) decrease the effectiveness of oral contraceptives. Clients should be advised to use alternative forms of contraception when taking these antibiotics.

Superinfection

A superinfection is an infection that develops during antimicrobial treatment of another infection; thus, it is superimposed on the original infection being treated. The destruction of large numbers of normal microbial inhabitants of the body may alter the environment so as to enable the uncontrolled growth of nonsusceptible organisms. For example, yeasts and molds normally present in certain tissues do not reproduce rapidly because their growth is inhibited by bacteria also present in the normal flora. If the inhibiting bacteria are eliminated by an antimicrobial drug, these fungi can then multiply rapidly and cause symptoms of an infection (eg, inflammation of oral, vaginal, anal, and other tissues). Symptoms of superinfection can range in severity from annoying, non–life-threatening diarrhea or vaginal yeast infections to life-threatening ones such as septicemia.

Concomitant administration of an antifungal, such as nystatin, is often necessary to suppress such opportunistic mycotic infections in clients taking antimicrobial drugs. Superinfection commonly occurs with administration of broad-spectrum antimicrobial agents, combinations of antimicrobial agents, and second- or third-generation antimicrobials.

Any organism present in the body that is not susceptible to the systemic anti-infective administered may produce a superinfection. Common offenders are fungi of the *Candida* genus, which produce localized infections in the mouth and vagina; resistant strains of staphylococci, which can cause severe diarrhea; and gram-negative *Pseudomonas* organisms, which can cause the most serious superinfections. Such infections are most common in clients taking broad-spectrum antibiotics; they are most dangerous in debilitated clients or those receiving corticosteroids or antineoplastic treatments, which reduce the body's inflammatory or immune responses. *Clostridium difficile*, as well as staphylococci and *Clostridium perfringens* type C, may produce pseudomembranous colitis, which can be fatal if the characteristically profuse diarrhea is not treated.

Superinfection may require the administration of one or more antimicrobial drugs in addition to the primary agent prescribed for the original infection. The use of multiple drugs increases the risk of serious adverse reactions. Despite vigorous treatment, iatrogenic superinfection causes illness in some clients treated with antimicrobials and can cause death. Prescribers should use broad-spectrum antimicrobials conservatively because of the likelihood of causing superinfection and the risk of contributing to the emergence of resistant strains of virulent bacteria.

Treatment Failures

For drug therapy of infections to succeed, the pathogen must be susceptible to the action of the antimicrobial and the host's response to both the treatment agent and the invading organism must be adequate. Several factors may interfere with the recovery of the client treated for infection (Box 41-2).

The concentration of the drug in tissue fluids must be adequate. If the prescribed dose is too low or some doses are omitted, drug concentration will be inadequate. If the infection affects parts of the body with a poor blood supply, drug levels in these tissues may be too low to eliminate the microorganisms, despite a high blood level. Poor absorption and rapid metabolism or excretion of the drug can also depress blood levels.

The antimicrobial chosen must be able to inhibit or kill the microorganism involved. Results of culture and

Box 41-2
Factors Influencing Antimicrobial Treatment Failure

A failure of drug treatment may be due to:

- Inadequate blood levels of the drug
- Failure of antimicrobial to reach site of infection
- Too short a period of chemotherapy
- Selection of the wrong treatment agent
- Resistance to the antimicrobial by the pathogen
- Failure to use combination drug therapy when indicated
- Delay in treatment
- Inadequate body defenses within the host
- Concomitant or previous treatment by a drug antagonistic to the action of the antimicrobial
- Adverse reaction in the host, which requires discontinuation of treatment
- Failure to adhere to drug regimen

sensitivity tests of tissue specimens (needed to identify infecting organisms and appropriate drug treatment) require 2 to 3 days. Specimens for cultures must be taken before antimicrobial therapy begins. In the interim, drugs are prescribed in accord with the initial diagnosis based on clinical signs and symptoms. If the organism causing the illness is resistant to the drug prescribed, initial therapy will be ineffective.

Delays in treatment allow large populations of pathogens to establish themselves. Overwhelming infections tend to deplete the host's defenses—that is, the inflammatory response, antibody levels, numbers and activity of white blood cells, and the integrity of membrane barriers, such as skin and mucosa. Reduced resistance to infection may also be due to genetic defects, malnutrition, general debility, suppression of the immune response by disease (eg, AIDS) or medical therapy (eg, steroid therapy, cancer chemotherapy), or stress. Defenses fluctuate during the life cycle, with increased susceptibility to infection in the very young, the very old, persons under severe stress, and pregnant women.

If a drug antagonistic to an antimicrobial is in the host, the effectiveness of the antimicrobial is reduced. For example, bacteriostatic antimicrobials reduce the susceptibility of microorganisms to bactericidal drugs by slowing the rate of reproduction. Bactericidal drugs are most toxic to rapidly dividing organisms. Moreover, they are not very effective when used with or immediately after administration of a bacteriostatic agent. A drug that is compatible with the residual drug should be used.

Client nonadherence may be due to difficulty in remembering to take the correct number of doses at designated times, lack of money to purchase the prescribed amount, unwillingness to use limited funds for medication, unhappiness with side effects, or lack of information about the drug's importance. The most common nonadherence issue is a client who stops taking the medication because he or she feels better; therefore, the full prescription is not completed. Drug therapy may also be discontinued before the infection is completely resolved if the prescriber underestimates the time required for treatment or if severe adverse reactions occur.

■ SUMMARY

Antimicrobials are valuable agents for preventing and treating infections. They kill or inhibit the growth of pathogens with minimal risk to the host. Adverse reactions to these drugs include allergic reactions, damage to specific organs, and overgrowth of opportunistic organisms in the normal flora of the body. Widespread use of antimicrobials has resulted in the emergence of resistant strains of pathogens, especially in healthcare institutions. Resistant infections are a hazard for clients and staff alike in affected agencies.

❖ NURSING MANAGEMENT: CLIENT RECEIVING ANTIMICROBIAL THERAPY

Given the real dangers of antimicrobial therapy, the nurse's first obligation is to prevent the need for its use, whenever possible. Prevention entails nursing care designed to protect vulnerable clients from exposure to infectious agents and to maintain and increase their resistance to these pathogens.

Risk Factors. Those at risk for bacterial infections include persons whose normal body defenses against infection are impaired: the very young and the very old, malnourished or debilitated clients, clients with interruptions in skin integrity (eg, surgical incisions, traumatic wounds), and clients undergoing immunosuppressive therapy, cancer chemotherapy, or irradiation. In addition, any client subjected to prolonged or severe stress is likely to have reduced resistance due to hormone response (chiefly cortisone secretion) during the alarm and the subsequent exhaustion stages of stress adaptation.

Aseptic Measures. The general measures of cleanliness and hygiene adequate to control healthy clients' exposure to pathogens in the community are insufficient in healthcare institutions. The clients in hospitals and nursing homes are generally at high risk. The use of Standard Precautions or Transmission-Based Precautions (HICPAC, 1996) is needed to protect personnel and to prevent transfer of pathogens between clients. In addition to environmental and personal hygiene, barrier techniques must be used to restrict the mobility of pathogens. Housekeeping routines have been developed to control the level of infective microorganisms in the institutional environment. Specific techniques are beyond the scope of this discussion; the student is referred to texts that deal with basic nursing skills for details. Reverse isolation is employed to protect particularly vulnerable clients from the pathogens present in the normal institutional environment.

Prevention of Nosocomial Infections. To reduce the incidence of antibiotic nosocomial infection, it is vital to reduce the resident population of microorganisms, minimize contact between microbes and antibiotics, and eliminate the transmission of microorganisms from infected victims and carriers to healthy people. To accomplish these tasks, rigorous environmental cleanliness, careful handling of antibiotic drugs, and good medical asepsis are required.

Although environmental cleanliness in healthcare institutions is the responsibility of the housekeeping staff, the nurse shares responsibility for environmental safety. Staff should be summoned promptly when infectious material escapes into the environment. The nursing staff should work with the housekeeping staff to ensure adequate cleanliness.

Exposure of environmental microbial inhabitants to antibiotics occurs in two ways. Because some antibiotics may be present in the urine of clients who undergo treatment, it can reach the environment if excreta are not properly handled. Antibiotics may contact bacteria in the environment by being spilled or sometimes through ejection of excess amounts in a syringe into a sink. The more antibiotics are ordered and administered to clients, the greater the potential for environmental contamination and the development of resistant strains of bacteria.

General Considerations. Some of the factors used in selecting an anti-infective agent are the assessment findings of renal and hepatic function, allergies, and pregnancy and lactation status. Goals of treatment include alleviating or eliminating the signs and symptoms of infection, preventing adverse drug reactions, encouraging client adherence to the regimen, and ensuring the prompt detection and treatment of adverse reactions. Timing of administration is important to maintain the serum drug concentration at therapeutic levels. Drugs ordered for adminstration several times a day (bid, tid, qid) should be administered at equal intervals (q12h, q8h, q6h).

Agents Affecting Bacterial Cell Wall Synthesis

These agents selectively interfere with bacterial cell wall synthesis. They are most effective when bacteria are actively proliferating; their effectiveness is decreased by use of bacteriostatic agents, which slow bacterial cell division.

Beta-Lactam Antibiotics

Two major antibiotic families, penicillins and cephalosporins, share a structural component, the beta-lactam ring. The fact that penicillins and cephalosporins exhibit some cross-sensitivity (ie, persons allergic to penicillin are likely to exhibit allergic sensitivity to some cephalosporins) indicates that this shared component is clinically important. Drugs from both families are inactivated by an enzyme, beta-lactamase, that is produced by some resistant pathogens.

Penicillins

The era of antibiotic chemotherapy began with the development of penicillin during World War II. This natural product of a blue-green bread mold was remarkably effective in treating a wide range of infections. Although many pathogens have developed resistance to some penicillins, this family of drugs remains a valuable therapeutic agent for treating a wide range of infections.

Pharmacodynamics. Penicillins interfere with a number of enzymes and protein-binding activities involved in processes such as cell division and synthesis, as well as maintenance of cell walls. As a result, organisms fail to reproduce, and some die from cell lysis. Penicillins, therefore, are both bacteriostatic and bactericidal.

Pharmacokinetics. Many forms of penicillin are destroyed in the digestive tract. Other preparations are acid-resistant and consequently are unaffected by digestion. Penicillin is widely distributed in the body, but concentrations are highest in the plasma, where much of it is reversibly bound to plasma albumin. Protein binding provides some prolongation of biologic half-life but can cause interactions with other protein-bound substances due to competitive displacement. Most preparations penetrate the blood-brain barrier poorly, except when the meninges are inflamed or fever is present.

Penicillin is excreted from the body largely unchanged by metabolic processes. Most of the drug is eliminated by the kidneys, where it is actively secreted by the tubules. Urinary excretion of the drug may be inhibited by the concurrent administration of probenecid, resulting in higher plasma concentrations. Some drug is eliminated in bile and other body secretions.

Therapeutic Uses. Penicillin is one of the most important classes of antibiotics. Its derivatives are used in the treatment of many common infections. Penicillins can be classified according to their spectrum of antimicrobial activity (Table 41-1).

Dosage and Administration. Preparations of penicillin for oral, intravenous (IV), and intramuscular (IM) administration are available for clinical use (Table 41-2). IV (aqueous) solutions and IM suspensions must not be confused: the suspensions must never be administered IV. Topical applications and inhalation therapy are not recommended because they are not very effective and often induce allergic sensitivity.

Adverse Reactions. Some strains of microorganisms (notably staphylococci) readily develop resistance to penicillin. One form of resistance is the ability to produce an enzyme (penicillinase) that chemically degrades the penicillin molecule. When penicillinase-susceptible drugs are prescribed to treat infections caused by pathogens with this type of resistance, therapeutic response is absent or inadequate. Immunity to drugs caused by this or other inheritable traits can be transferred from one organism to another by several mechanisms that involve the exchange of chromosomal material.

Table 41-1. Penicillin Groups by Spectrum of Activity

Penicillin Group	Example	Usual Spectrum	Comments
Natural	penicillin G	Gram-positive and gram-negative cocci, gram-positive bacilli, spirochetes	Susceptible to inactivation by beta-lactamases
	penicillin V	Similar to penicillin G but not used for treating septicemia because of high doses needed to eliminate the infection	More acid-stable than penicillin G
Antistaphylococcal penicillins	cloxacillin dicloxacillin methicillin	Use restricted to treatment of penicillinase-producing staphylococci	Resistant to effects of penicillinase
Extended-spectrum penicillins	amoxicillin ampicillin	Less potent than penicillin G against gram-positive and gram-negative cocci; spectrum extends to gram-negative bacilli	Administration with beta-lactamase inhibitor (clavulanic acid or sulbactam) can protect from resistance developed through plasmid-mediated penicillinase.
Antipseudomonal penicillins	carbenicillin piperacillin ticarcillin	Effective against *Pseudomonas* infections and many gram-negative bacilli but ineffective against *Klebsiella*	
Acylureido penicillins	azlocillin mezlocillin	Also effective against *Pseudomonas aeruginosa* and many gram-negative organisms	

Harvey RA, Champe PC, eds. (1992). Lippincott illustrated reviews: Pharmacology. Philadelphia: JB Lippincott, pp. 274–276.

Table 41-2. Penicillin Preparations

Drug Name	Preparation	Usual Dosage
amoxicillin (Amoxil, Biomox, Polymox, Trimox, Wymox) *Can*: Apo-Amoxi, Novamoxin	Capsules, suspensions, chewable tablets, powders for oral administration PC: B	Adults and children who weigh 20 kg or more: 750 mg–1.5 g/day, divided in 3 doses, administered at equal intervals Children who weigh less than 20 kg: 20–40 mg/kg/day, divided in 3 doses administered at equal intervals
amoxicillin and potassium clavulanate (Augmentin)	Tablets, chewable tablets, and suspension for oral administration PC: B	Adults: "250" or "500" coated tablet every 8 hours. Note: Each "250" or "500" tablet contains same amount of clavulanic acid (125 mg as potassium salt); therefore, do not substitute two "250" tablets for one "500" tablet; "125" or "250" chewable tablet every 8 hours; "125" banana-flavored or "250" orange-flavored suspension
ampicillin (D-Amp, Polycillin, Totacillin, Unasyn, Omnipen, Principen, *Can*: Nu-Ampi, Penbriten)	Capsules and suspensions for oral administration Vials that contain powder for reconstitution for IM or IV administration PC: B	Adults: 1–2 g/day, divided in 4 doses, administered at equal intervals Children: 24–50 mg/kg/day, divided in 4 doses, administered at equal intervals For severe infection, larger doses may be required
ampicillin and sulbactam sodium (Unasyn)	Powder for injection	Adults: IV or IM: 1.5 g (1 g ampicillin and 0.5 mg sulbactam) to 3 g (2 g ampicillin and 0.5 g sulbactam) every 6 h (maximum of 4 g/day of sulbactam
bacampicillin (Spectrobid) *Can*: Penglobe	Tablets and powders for oral administration PC: B	Adults and children who weigh 25 kg or more: 800–1,600 mg/day divided in 2 doses, administered at equal intervals Children who weigh less than 25 kg: 25–50 mg/kg/day, divided in 2 doses, administered at equal intervals
carbenicillin indanyl sodium (Geocillin)	Oral Tablets PC: B	Adults: 1.5–3.0 g/day, divided in 4 doses
cloxacillin sodium (Cloxapen, Tegopen) *Can*: ApoCloxi, Novacloxin, NuClox, Orbenin	Capsules and solution for oral administration PC: B	Adults and children who weigh 20 kg or more: 1–2 g/day, divided in 4 doses, administered at equal intervals Children who weigh less than 20 kg: 50–100 mg/kg/day, divided in 4 doses
dicloxacillin sodium (Dycill, Dynapen, Pathocil)	Capsules and suspension for oral administration PC: B	Adults and children who weigh 40 kg or more: 0.5–1 g/day, divided in 4 doses, administered at equal intervals Children who weigh less than 40 kg: 12.5–25 mg/kg/day, divided in 4 doses
methicillin sodium (Staphcillin)	Vials that contain powder for reconstitution for IM or IV administration PC: B	Adults: 4–12 g/day, divided in 4–6 doses, administered at equal intervals Children: 100–300 mg/kg/day divided in 4 doses, administered as equal intervals (for severe infections, larger doses may be required)
mezlocillin sodium (Mezlin)	Vials and infusion bottles that contain powder for reconstitution for IM or IV administration PC: B	Adults: 75–300 mg/kg/day, divided in 4–6 doses, administered at equal intervals
nafcillin sodium (Nafcil, Nallpen, Unipen)	Capsules, solution, and tablets for oral administration Vials that contain powder for reconstitution for IM or IV administration PC: B	*Oral:* Adults: 1–6 g/day, divided in 4–6 doses Children: 20–50 mg/kg/day, divided in 4–6 doses *IM:* Adults: 500 mg q4–6h Children: 25 mg/kg twice daily *IV:* 3–6 g per 24 hr

KEY: PC = pregnancy category; see Appendix A.
Can: Canadian

(continued)

1-2. Penicillin Preparations (Continued)

Drug Name	Preparation	Usual Dosage
oxacillin sodium (Bactocill, Prostaphilin)	Capsules and solution for oral administration Vials that contain powder for reconstitution for IM or IV administration PC: B	Adults and children who weigh 40 kg or more: 2–3 g/day, divided in 4–6 doses Children who weigh less than 40 kg; 50 mg/kg/day, divided in 4 doses
penicillin G, benzathine (Bicillin, Permapen)	Suspensions for IM injection in multiple-dose vials, prefilled cartridges, and disposable syringes PC: B	*IM:* 300,000–2,400,000 U (dosage varies with indications)
penicillin G, potassium (Pentide, Pfizerpen) *Can*: Falapen, Megacillin, Novopen G	Tablets and solution for oral administration Vials that contain powder for reconstitution for IM or IV administration	Varies with age of recipient and severity of infection *Oral:* Adults and children more than 12 yr: 1,200,000–2,000,000 U/day, divided in 3 or 4 doses; children less than 12 yr: 25,000–90,000 U/kg/day, divided in 3–6 doses *Parenteral:* Adults: 5,000,000–20,000,000 U/day; children: 30,000–50,000 U/kg/day, divided in 4–6 doses (dosage varies greatly with indication and severity of infection)
penicillin G, procaine (Ayercillin, Crysticillin, Pfizerpen-AS, Wycillin)	Suspensions for IM injection in multi-dose vials, prefilled cartridges, and disposable syringes PC: B	Adults and children more than 12 yr: 600,000–1.2 million U/day Children: 50,000 U/day, given in a single dose (dosage varies greatly with indication)
penicillin V, potassium, (Beepen VK, Betapen VK, Ledercillin VK, Pen-Vee-K, Robicillin VK, V-Cillin K, Veetids) *Can*: Nadopen-V, Novopen VK	Tablets, powders, and solutions for oral administration (250 mg-400,000 U) PC: B	Adults and children more than 12 yr: 0.25–2 g/day, divided in 2–4 doses Children less than 12 yr: 15 mg/kg/day, divided in 3–6 doses
piperacillin (Pipracil)	Solutions for IM or IV injection PC: B	Adults: 6–18 g/day, divided in 4–6 doses; maximum adult dose: 24 g/day Children: 50–100 mg/kg/day divided in 6 doses, administered at equal intervals
ticarcillin (Ticar)	Vials that contain powder for reconstitution for IM or IV administration PC: B	Adults and children: 200–300 mg/kg/day, divided in 4–8 doses
ticarcillin disodium and clavulanate potassium (Timentin)	Vials that contain powder for reconstitution or premixed frozen vials for IV administration by direct infusion over 30 min or piggyback (discontinue other drugs temporarily during infusion) PC: B	Varies with weight of recipient, type and severity of infection Adults (>60 kg): moderate gynecologic infection—200 mg/kg/day (3.1-g vial) divided in 6 doses; severe gynecologic infection—300 mg/kg/day divided in 6 doses Adults (<60 kg): 200–300 mg/kg/day, divided in 4–6 doses

KEY: PC = pregnancy category; see Appendix A.
Can: Canadian

Allergic reactions to penicillin are relatively common. Initially, penicillin sensitivity may be manifested by local erythema and itching at the site of parenteral injection. Skin rashes, especially urticaria with pruritus, are common and occur after oral, as well as parenteral, administration. Anaphylactic shock, a rapidly developing syndrome characterized by dyspnea and hypotension, can be fatal. When penicillin is combined with procaine, an adverse reaction to the procaine component may take the form of a violent psychotic reaction. These reactions tend to resolve in 15 to 30 minutes.

Other adverse reactions to penicillin include neutropenia, hemolytic anemia, bleeding due to platelet malfunction, adult respiratory distress syndrome, superinfection, and CNS changes (seizures, psychoses). Superinfection tends to cause intestinal symptoms (sore mouth, nausea, diarrhea). Seizures are most likely in clients with meningitis, because inflammation of the meninges allows the drug to penetrate the blood-brain barrier in large amounts.

Drug Interactions. Penicillin reduces the effectiveness of oral contraceptives. When atenolol and ampicillin are administered concurrently, serum levels of the beta blocker reportedly drop. Penicillins may increase the bleeding time in clients also receiving anticoagulants, especially when the penicillins are given parenterally. The renal excretion of penicillin is decreased by probenecid; this interaction may be used therapeutically to maintain higher serum levels of penicillin.

Another beneficial drug interaction is the combined use of penicillin and an aminoglycoside to treat enterococcal infections. The intact cell wall of enterococci is impermeable to the aminoglycosides. Penicillin, as an inhibitor of cell wall synthesis, permits uptake of aminoglycosides. The combination of penicillin and gentamicin is used in enterococcal endocarditis and meningitis. Both natural and semisynthetic penicillins deactivate aminoglycosides in vitro and therefore should not be mixed in the same syringe.

Drug–Food Interactions. Food affects the absorption of most penicillins; penicillin V may be taken with food.

Drug–Laboratory Interactions. Testing for urine glucose using Clinitest, Benedict's solution, or Fehling's solution may result in false positive results.

Precautions and Contraindications. Any indication of developing sensitivity is reason for caution. Clients receiving the drug IV must be observed closely, as any systemic reaction will occur rapidly. The drug should be avoided if possible if the client has a history of respiratory distress, shock, or anaphylaxis after administration of penicillin. There may be cross-allergenicity between penicillins and cephalosporins. A urticarious rash may occur when ampicillin is used with allopurinol. If penicillin is prescribed for high-risk clients, rapidly eliminated forms are preferred.

Rapid desensitization with oral doses should be attempted if penicillin therapy is required for allergic clients. Doses are administered at 15-minute intervals, starting with very small doses and doubling the dose with each succeeding administration.

When some penicillins are prescribed for women who are taking oral contraceptives, an alternate method of contraception should be used for the duration of antibiotic therapy. The oral contraceptive regimen should be continued at the same time to preserve the anovulatory cycle.

■ SUMMARY

Penicillin and its derivatives are reliable agents for the treatment of many common infections. They exert primarily bactericidal effects on pathogens. Their action can be prolonged by the concurrent administration of probenecid. Allergic sensitivity can cause dangerous reactions.

❖ NURSING MANAGEMENT: CLIENT RECEIVING A PENICILLIN

The client's response to penicillin therapy must be closely monitored. With IV penicillin, there is a risk of electrolyte imbalance from either the sodium or potassium content. Excessive blood potassium can precipitate cardiac arrest. To prevent this problem, IV potassium salts should be administered slowly.

Because penicillin inactivates aminoglycosides, these two drugs should not be mixed in the same solution and should be administered at least 1 hour apart.

Anaphylactic reactions to penicillin require immediate treatment, including administration of epinephrine, antihistamines, and a corticosteroid. These drugs should be readily available when penicillin therapy is initiated.

NURSING PROCESS

ASSESSMENT

Whenever penicillin therapy is contemplated, the nurse must take a careful history to assess the risk of allergic reaction. The client should be questioned specifically about previous use of penicillin and any adverse reaction to it. Of particular significance are urticaria, skin rash, itching, or inflammation at sites of penicillin injection. Other drugs may be chosen if hypersensitivity to penicillin is present.

NURSING DIAGNOSIS

Diagnoses are concerned primarily with responses (therapeutic or adverse) to the drug regimen and may include:

- Pain: Abdominal discomfort related to antimicrobial medication
- Diarrhea, related to superinfection from antimicrobial medication
- Risk for Impaired Skin Integrity: Rash related to allergic reaction to antimicrobial medication
- Ineffective Individual Management of Therapeutic Regimen (Noncompliance): Stopping medication before full course has been taken, related to discomfort of adverse reactions to the drug, or omission of the drug related to inability to pay for the prescription
- Knowledge Deficit, related to antimicrobial drugs and the regimens for their administration

PLANNING

Goals of nursing care are to promote recovery from the infection and to reduce the risk and severity of adverse drug reactions.

INTERVENTION

Because clients may become sensitized to penicillin through environmental exposure, all clients who receive penicillin should be monitored for signs and symptoms of allergic reaction (skin rash, urticaria, dyspnea). Epinephrine should be readily available for treating serious reactions (anaphylaxis).

Client Education. Clients should not drink acidic beverages for an hour after taking penicillin G, or the effectiveness will be lessened. Some penicillins (particularly amoxicillin and clavulanate, azlocillin, mezlocillin, oxacillin, piperacillin) occasionally cause abdominal pain, dark urine, or jaundice, which should be reported to the prescriber immediately. Other penicillins (ampicillin, bacampicillin, penicillin V) may interfere with the effectiveness of birth-control pills that contain estrogen, requiring additional contraceptive measures.

Some form of lactobacilli (yogurt, buttermilk, or Bacid capsules) may be administered to help maintain a normal intestinal flora and reduce the risk of superinfection. These inoculants should not be administered for at least 1 hour after the oral dose of penicillin so that they are not inactivated by the drug. If white patches are seen on the tongue or oral mucosa (indicating a possible infection with a *Candida* organism), the prescriber should be asked to prescribe an antifungal drug, such as nystatin.

Clients who react allergically to penicillin must be informed that they are hypersensitive to such drugs. A medical identification device that lists this allergy should be recommended.

When penicillin is prescribed for clients in the community, the importance of completing the treatment regimen should be stressed. Many clients discontinue medication as soon as they feel well. Residual pathogens may cause a later recurrence, and due to their exposure to the antibiotic, the surviving organisms are more likely to be resistant, and the recurring infection will be more difficult to treat. Interrupting therapy also increases the risk of developing an allergy.

OUTCOME EVALUATION

Data required for evaluation include therapeutic response to the antibiotic regimen and signs and symptoms of adverse reactions.

❖ CHECKLIST OF NURSING ACTIONS

- ❑ When taking the drug history from a candidate for penicillin therapy, ask specifically about previous exposure to penicillin and adverse reactions to it, such as urticaria or skin rash.
- ❑ Avoid spilling penicillin solutions into the environment.
- ❑ Monitor clients receiving penicillin for signs and symptoms of allergic reaction.
- ❑ Advise clients who are allergic to penicillin to wear a medical identification device with this information.
- ❑ Encourage clients receiving penicillin to complete the course of treatment. If an adverse reaction occurs, the client should contact the prescriber for alternative therapy.

Cephalosporins

The first cephalosporins were produced by an organism cultured from sea water collected near a sewer outlet off the coast of Sardinia. Like penicillin, these compounds (and their semisynthetic derivatives) contain a beta-lactam structure in their molecules. Mechanism of action, renal excretion, and allergenicity resemble those of penicillin, and some cross-sensitivity exists between the two groups of drugs. Penicillin-resistant organisms that produce beta-lactamase also tend to be resistant to many cephalosporins.

The cephalosporins have been altered chemically to produce many different molecules with antibiotic properties. These are classified into "generations," based on when they were developed and their characteristics (Table 41-3). Each generation has slightly different spectra of activity and susceptibility to enzymes produced by resistant organisms.

Pharmacodynamics. The cephalosporins exert primarily bactericidal effects by inhibiting enzymes needed for mucopeptide synthesis in bacterial cell walls. As a result, defective cell walls are formed, and autolysis causes cell death.

Pharmacokinetics. Cephalosporins can be administered orally, IM, or IV (Table 41-4). Preparations vary in the extent to which they are absorbed from the intestinal tract, in their degree of plasma binding, and in their metabolism. After absorption, they are widely distributed except in the CNS; only a few penetrate the blood-brain barrier sufficiently to deliver therapeutic concentrations to the cerebrospinal fluid. Cephalosporins cross the placenta as well as the synovial and pericardial membranes. They penetrate the bile and aqueous humor but not the vitreous humor. Binding by serum proteins ranges from 6% to 86%, depending on the drug.

The cephalosporins and their metabolites are excreted by the kidneys, with the same tubular secretory

Text continues on page 899.

Table 41-3. Cephalosporin Generations

Generation	Spectrum of Activity
First	Good activity against gram-positive bacteria
	Relatively modest activity against gram-negative microorganisms
Second	Increased activity against gram-negative microorganisms
Third	Less active than first generation against gram-positive cocci; much more active against Enterobacteriaceae
Fourth	Greater spectrum than third generation
	Increased stability from certain beta-lactamases

Table 41-4. Cephalosporins

Drug Name	Preparation	Usual Dosage	Therapeutic Uses and Additional Information
First-Generation			
cefadroxil (Duricef, Ultracef)	Capsules, suspensions, and tablets for oral use	Adults: 1–2 g/day, divided in 2 doses Children: 30 mg/kg/day, divided in 2 doses PC: B	Treatment of susceptible infections caused by gram-positive cocci (staphylococci, streptococci) and some strains of gram-negative bacteria (*Klebsiella* organisms)
cefazolin (Kefzol, Zolicef) *Can*: Ancef	Vials that contain powder for reconstitution for IM or IV administration	Adults: 750 mg/kg/day, divided in 3 or 4 doses (maximum daily dosage: 12 g) Children 1 mo or older: 25–50 mg/kg/day, divided in 3 or 4 doses PC: B	Treatment of serious susceptible infections of the biliary tract, bones, joints, and respiratory tract
cephalexin (Biocef, Keflex) *Can*: Novalexin, Ceporex	Capsules, suspension, and tablets for oral use	Adults: 1 g/day, divided in 4 doses Children: 25–50 mg/kg/day, divided in 4 doses PC: B	Treatment of serious susceptible infections of the bones, respiratory tract, urinary tract, and skin
cephalothin (Keflin) *Can*: Ceparacin	Vials that contain powder for reconstitution for IM or IV administration	Adults: 2–6 g/day, divided in 4–6 doses (maximum daily dosage: 12 g) Children: 80–160 mg/kg/day, divided in 4–6 doses PC: B	Treatment of susceptible infections caused by gram-positive and gram-negative bacteria Perioperative prophylaxis in contaminated or potentially contaminated surgery
cephapirin (Cefadyl)	Vials that contain powder for reconstitution for IM or IV administration	Adults: 2–6 g/day, divided in 4–6 doses (maximum daily dosage: 12 g) Children 3 mo or older: 40–80 mg/kg/day, divided in 4 doses PC: B	Treatment of serious susceptible infections, including septicemia, endocarditis, and osteomyelitis Dosage adjustment required for clients with renal dysfunction
cephradine (Velosef)	Capsules, suspension, and tablets for oral use Vials that contain powder for reconstitution for IM or IV administration	Adults: 2–4 g/day, divided in 2–4 doses (maximum daily dosage: 8 g) Children 9 mo or older: 25–100 mg/kg/day, divided in 2–4 doses (maximum daily dosage: 4 g)	Treatment of susceptible infections, including otitis media and infections of the respiratory tract Dosage adjustments required for clients with renal dysfunction
Second-Generation			
cefaclor (Ceclor)	Capsules and suspension for oral use	Adults: 0.75–1.5 g/day, divided in 3 doses (maximum daily dosage: 4 g) Children 1 mo or older: 20–40 mg/kg/day, divided in 3 doses (maximum daily dosage: 1 g) PC: B	Treatment of susceptible infections caused by gram-positive cocci (staphylococci, streptococci), some strains of gram-negative bacteria (*Klebsiella* organisms and *Haemophilus influenzae*)
cefamandole (Mandole)	Vials that contain powder for reconstitution for IM or IV administration PC: B	Adults: 1.5–6 g/day, divided in 4 doses (maximum daily dosage: 12 g) Children 1 mo or older: 50–100 mg/kg/day, divided in 3 or 4 doses	Treatment of serious susceptible infections of the bones, joints, respiratory tract, biliary tract, as well as peritonitis and septicemia
cefmetazole sodium (Zefazone)	Sterile powder for IV use; reconstituted drug may be diluted in 0.9% normal saline, 5% dextrose solution, or lactated Ringer's solution	Adults: 2 g/day divided in 2–4 doses for 5–14 days PC: B	Treatment of susceptible infections caused by aerobic and anaerobic organisms, gram-positive and gram-negative organisms Resistant to beta-lactamases Treatment of lower respiratory tract, skin, urinary tract, and intra-abdominal infections, prophylactically before some surgeries

KEY: PC = pregnancy category; see Appendix A.
Can: Canadian

(continued)

Table 41-4. Cephalosporins (Continued)

Drug Name	Preparation	Usual Dosage	Therapeutic Uses and Additional Information
Second-Generation (continued)			
cefonicid (Monocid)	Vials that contain powder for reconstitution for IM or IV administration	Adults: 500 mg–2 g/day, given as a single dose PC: B	Treatment of lower respiratory, skin, bone, joint, and urinary tract infections and septicemia; perioperative prophylaxis
cefoxitin (Mefoxin)	Vials that contain powder for reconstitution for IM or IV administration	Adults: 3–8 g/day, divided in 3 or 4 doses (maximum daily dosage: 12 g) Children 3 mo or older: 80–160 mg/kg/day, divided in 4–6 doses PC: B	Treatment of serious susceptible infections, including bone and joint infections, lung abscess, pelvic inflammatory disease, and septicemia
cefotetan (Cefotan)	Vials that contain powder for reconstitution for IM or IV administration	Adults: 2–4 g/day, divided in 2 doses PC: B	Treatment of respiratory, urinary, skin, bone, joint, gynecologic, and intra-abdominal infections; perioperative prophylaxis
cefpodoxime proxetil (Vantin)	Tablets and granules for suspensions for oral use	Adults: 100–400 mg q12h PC: B	Treatment of upper respiratory infections, otitis media, and urinary tract infections
cefprozil (Cefzil)	Tablets for oral use	Adults: 250–500 mg in 24 hr in 1 or 2 divided doses PC: B	Treatment of pharyngitis, tonsillitis caused by *Streptococcus pyogenes*, otitis media, uncomplicated skin infections caused by *Streptococcus pyogenes* or *Staphylococcus aureus*
cefuroxime (Kefurox, Zinacef) *Can*: Ceftin	Vials that contain powder for reconstitution for IM or IV administration	Adults: 2.25–4.5 g/day, divided in 3 doses Children older than 3 mo of age: 50–100 mg/kg/day, divided in 3 or 4 doses PC: B	Treatment of lower respiratory, skin, and genitourinary infections, septicemia, and meningitis; perioperative prophylaxis
loracarbef (Lorabid)	Tablets and capsules for oral use	Adults: 200–400 mg q12h Children: 15–30 mg/kg/day in divided doses q12h PC: B	Treatment of upper and lower respiratory tract infections, urinary tract infections, and skin infections
Third-Generation			
cefixime (Suprax)	Tablets and suspension for oral administration	Adults: 400 mg/day in 1 or 2 divided doses Children: 8 mg/kg/day in 1 or 2 divided doses PC: B	Treatment of uncomplicated urinary tract infections caused by *Escherichia coli* or *Proteus mirabilis*, upper and lower respiratory tract infections, and gonorrhea
cefoperazone (Cefobid)	Vials that contain powder for reconstitution for IM or IV administration Frozen solutions for IV infusion	Adults: 2–4 g/day, divided in 2 doses (maximum daily dosage: 12 g) Children: 50–200 mg/kg/day, divided in 2 doses PC: B	Treatment of serious susceptible infections, including pelvic inflammatory disease, peritonitis, and septicemia
cefotaxime (Claforan)	Vials that contain powder for reconstitution for IM or IV administration Frozen solutions for IV infusion	Adults: 3–8 g/day, divided in 3–6 doses (maximum daily dosage: 12 g) Children 1 mo to 12 yr: 50–180 mg/kg/day, divided in 4–6 doses PC: B	Treatment of serious susceptible infections caused by gram-negative bacteria (*E coli, Klebsiella, Proteus, Shigella, Acinetobacter, Neisseria, Serratia,* and *Providencia* organisms) Dosage adjustment required for clients with renal dysfunction

KEY: PC = pregnancy category; see Appendix A.
Can: Canadian

(continued)

Table 41-4. (Continued)

Drug Name	Preparation	Usual Dosage	Therapeutic Uses and Additional Information
Third-Generation (continued)			
ceftazidime (Fortaz, Tazicef, Ceptaz, Pentacef, Tazidime) *Can*: Magnacef	Vials that contain powder for reconstitution for IM or IV administration Frozen solutions for IV infusion	Adults: 2–3 g/day, divided in 2 or 3 doses Children 1 mo–12 yr: 90–150 mg/kg/day, divided in 3 doses Maximum daily dosage: 6 g PC: B	Treatment of lower respiratory, skin, urinary tract, bone joint, gynecologic, central nervous system, and intra-abdominal infections; treatment of septicemia After reconstitution, solutions generate carbon dioxide gas and must be vented before use.
ceftizoxime (Cefizox)	Vials that contain powder for reconstitution for IM or IV administration	Adults: 2–6 g/day, divided in 2 or 3 doses (maximum daily dosage: 12 g) Children 6 mo or older: 150–200 mg/kg/day, divided in 3 or 4 doses PC: B	Treatment of serious susceptible infections, including those of the respiratory tract, urinary tract, and skin, including septicemia Dosage adjustment required for clients with renal dysfunction
ceftriaxone (Rocephin)	Vials that contain powder for reconstitution for IM or IV administration	Adults: 1–2 g/day, given in 1 or 2 doses (maximum daily dosage: 4 g) Children 12 yr or older: 50–75 mg/kg/day, divided in 2 doses (maximum daily dosage: 2 g) PC: B	Treatment of lower respiratory, skin, bone, joint, urinary tract and intra-abdominal infections; treatment of septicemia, meningitis, and gonorrhea; perioperative prophylaxis
Fourth-Generation			
cefepime (Maxipime)	Powder for injection	Adults: 0.5–2 g every 12h	Treatment of urinary tract infections, pneumonia, and uncomplicated skin and skin structure infections

KEY: PC = pregnancy category; see Appendix A.
Can: Canadian

mechanism as penicillin. As with penicillin, their elimination can be inhibited by the concurrent use of probenecid. Serum half-lives range from 21 to 132 minutes, depending on the preparation.

Therapeutic Uses. The cephalosporins are used for the treatment of septicemia and infections that involve the skin, soft tissues, bones, joints, and urinary and respiratory tracts caused by susceptible organisms, including streptococci, staphylococci, *Escherichia coli, Proteus mirabilis,* and *Shigella* organisms. Table 41-3 details the differences in spectrum of activity.

Adverse Reactions. The most common adverse reactions to the cephalosporins are nausea, vomiting, and diarrhea after oral administration, phlebitis in veins used for injection, pain with IM injection, superinfection, pseudomembranous colitis, and allergic reactions. Kidney damage, bone marrow depression, prolonged prothrombin time, and mild hepatotoxicity have also been reported. Intrathecal administration can result in CNS toxicity (hallucinations, nystagmus, seizures).

Allergic hypersensitivity to the cephalosporins resembles that to penicillin. It is manifested by a maculopapular rash, sometimes associated with fever; eosinophilia; and lymphadenopathy. Less commonly, anaphylaxis, bronchospasm, urticaria, or blood dyscrasia occurs.

Drug Interactions. Ingestion of alcohol during or within 72 hours after therapy with certain cephalosporins (ceftamandole, cefoperazone, cefotetan, and moxalactam) may cause a disulfiram-like reaction. Nephrotoxicity may be increased by concurrent use of cephalosporins and aminoglycosides; the nephrotoxic effects of colistimethate may be increased by cephalothin. The hypoprothrombinemic effects of anticoagulants may be increased by certain cephalosporins. Cephalosporin plasma levels may be increased and prolonged when used with probenecid.

Drug–Food Interactions. Food increases the absorption of cefpodoxime and cefuroxine.

Drug–Laboratory Interactions. Enzyme-based tests for urine glucose (eg, Clinistix, Tes-Tape) should be used to avoid diagnostic interferences. A false positive test for proteinuria may occur with acid and denaturization-precipitation tests. Cephalosporins may falsely elevate urinary 17-ketosteroid values. They also may cause a false–positive direct Coombs test.

Precautions and Contraindications. The cephalosporins should not be used in clients with a history of a recent, severe, immediate allergic reaction to either penicillin or cephalosporins. The drugs must be used with caution if previous reactions have been mild or far removed in time. Epinephrine should be available for emergency use.

To prevent phlebitis and the need for frequent changes of parenteral administration sites, cephalosporin solutions should be infused into veins slowly. Continuous, slow drip, or intermittent infusion is recommended. Bolus medication, if required, should be administered over a period of several minutes.

Because they are potential nephrotoxins, the cephalosporins should not be used concurrently with other nephrotoxic drugs. They should be used with caution in clients with a history of renal pathology, especially if kidney function is less than optimal.

■ SUMMARY

The cephalosporins are similar to penicillin in their mechanism of action, toxicity, and some aspects of molecular structure. They are sometimes effective against pathogens resistant to penicillin. Adverse reactions include allergic reactions, superinfections, and occasionally nephrotoxicity.

❖ NURSING MANAGEMENT: CLIENT RECEIVING A CEPHALOSPORIN

Solutions of cephalosporins for parenteral use should be freshly prepared. If solutions must be stored, they should be refrigerated. The labeling information packaged with each preparation provides data on stability and storage requirements.

NURSING PROCESS

ASSESSMENT

Candidates for cephalosporin therapy should be screened for renal impairment and allergic sensitivity to either cephalosporins or penicillins.

NURSING DIAGNOSIS

Diagnoses concern both therapeutic and adverse responses to medication and may include:

- Altered Nutrition: Less Than Body Requirements, related to nausea and vomiting
- Knowledge Deficit, related to drug regimens necessary for effective anti-infective treatment
- Ineffective Individual Management of Therapeutic Regimen: Noncompliance, related to knowledge deficit or to cost of drug prescriptions

A common collaborative problem that should be differentiated from the nursing diagnoses is:

Potential Complication: Renal toxicity
Potential Complication: Pseudomembraneous colitis

PLANNING

Goals of nursing care are to resolve the infectious process, to reduce the risk of adverse reactions, and to detect promptly and treat any adverse reactions. See the Example of Nursing Process for Oral Cephalosporin Therapy.

INTERVENTION

Doses given IV must be infused slowly, preferably over at least 30 minutes. Rapid injection causes pain and irritation of the vein. Pain at the site of IM injection may be minimized by applying ice packs to the site before and after the injection.

If cephalosporins are prescribed for clients in renal failure, the dose is reduced. Because the drugs are removed from the body by dialysis, they should be administered after each treatment.

If cephalosporins are prescribed for clients with a history of allergy to either these drugs or penicillin, an acute reaction could occur. Epinephrine should be available for emergency treatment.

Clients should be monitored closely for signs and symptoms of superinfection (diarrhea, sore mouth, vaginal itching or drainage). Diarrhea, the main sign of intestinal superinfection, is most common when oral preparations are used. Women sometimes develop vaginal yeast infections, manifested by itching, inflammation, and increased vaginal drainage. If signs and symptoms of superinfection develop, the prescriber should be consulted about the need for antimycotic medication.

Before cephalosporin therapy is begun, the prescriber should be informed of any history of allergic reaction to penicillin or cephalosporins. Clients who have an allergic reaction to cephalosporins should be informed that they are sensitive to these drugs. A medical identification device should be recommended.

Client Education. Clients should be cautioned not to discontinue medication prematurely, even though the signs and symptoms of infection have resolved completely. Adverse reactions, including sore mouth, diarrhea, vaginal irritation, or signs and symptoms of renal malfunction, should be reported to the prescriber promptly. An alternate antibiotic may be substituted to complete the regimen.

Oral cephalosporins should be taken on an empty stomach, not with meals. The client should minimize the use of foods that irritate the intestinal tract. The timing of meals and medicines can be a problem: the drug must be taken at least 2 hours after food intake, and food may not be taken for 1 hour after medication. Four doses of cephalosporins are usually ordered daily. To maintain a fairly normal schedule of meals, the first dose of medication should be taken before breakfast. Clients may need help planning a schedule of meals and medication to maintain proper nutrition and accommodate the drug regimen.

The use of buttermilk or yogurt containing active acidophilus cultures with every meal should be recommended to prevent intestinal superinfection.

Advise clients to avoid using alcohol during therapy and for 72 hours after therapy.

Example of Nursing Process for Oral Cephalosporin Therapy

The client, age 71, fell after having two glasses of wine on an empty stomach and suffered a serious hand injury that required surgical repair. Infection has occurred, for which oral cephalosporin has been prescribed. The client is to be treated as an outpatient. She lives in a rural area 25 miles from the nearest hospital; the local emergency medical unit is 15 minutes away from her home. She has a history of severe generalized skin rash during oral penicillin therapy.

Assessment Data

Order for cephalosporin for infected hand

History of severe generalized allergic reaction to oral penicillin (People with penicillin allergy are also likely to be allergic to cephalosporins, which are related drugs.)

Client's residence is 15 minutes or more from emergency medical care.

History of alcohol use.

Nursing Diagnosis	Intervention	Goals and Outcomes
Risk for Altered Tissue Perfusion, related to vasodilation secondary to allergic reaction on cephalosporin drug therapy	**Inform** the prescriber of the client's history of generalized allergic reaction to penicillin, as well as the inaccessibility of prompt emergency care in the area where she lives. If the antibiotic order is not changed to a non-beta-lactam drug, **advise** the client of emergency measures that may be needed should an allergic reaction occur (eg, cardiopulmonary resuscitation by a member of the family or neighbor and emergency medical personnel).	The client will not suffer an allergic reaction to cephalosporin drugs (because an alternate drug was prescribed). Should an allergic reaction to cephalosporin occur, the risk of permanent harm will be minimized by prompt emergency treatment.
Self Care Deficit, related to inability to use injured hand	**Teach** the client one-handed techniques for self-care. **Teach** a family member or significant other how to assist the client in self-care.	Good hygiene and grooming will be maintained throughout the period of disability.
Risk for Injury (disulfiram-like reaction), related to ingestion of alcohol during cephalosporin therapy	**Advise** the client not to ingest alcohol during cephalosporin therapy and for 72 hours after the drug is discontinued.	Client will not experience disulfiram-like reaction.

OUTCOME EVALUATION

Data required for evaluation include signs and symptoms that indicate resolution of the infectious process and indications of adverse reactions to the drug regimen. Clients should be monitored for GI upset, vaginitis, renal impairment, neutropenia, impaired clotting, and renal dysfunction.

❖ CHECKLIST OF NURSING ACTIONS

- Before initiating cephalosporin therapy, take a complete drug history to rule out allergic hypersensitivity to penicillin or cephalosporins.
- Assess the client for renal dysfunction and a history of kidney disease.
- Use fresh solutions for administration by injection.
- Administer IV cephalosporins slowly.

- Teach the client taking oral cephalosporins to schedule doses at least 1 hour before and 2 hours after meals.
- Advise the client to avoid alcohol during therapy and for 72 hours after therapy.
- Recommend taking buttermilk or yogurt with each meal during cephalosporin treatment.
- Monitor clients who receive cephalosporins for signs and symptoms of superinfection or renal impairment.
- If cephalosporins are prescribed for clients with a history of allergy to these antibiotics or penicillin, have epinephrine available for emergency treatment.

Miscellaneous Beta-Lactam Antibiotics

Other beta-lactam antibiotics are neither penicillins nor cephalosporins (Table 41-5).

Table 41-5. Miscellaneous Antimicrobials Affecting Bacterial Cell Wall Synthesis

Drug Name	Preparation	Usual Dosage	Therapeutic Uses and Additional Information
aztreonam (Azactam)	Powder for reconstitution for IM or IV administration	Adults: 500 mg–1 g q8–12h (maximum dose: 8 g/day) PC: B	Treatment of infections of lower respiratory tract, urinary tract, skin, abdomen
bacitracin (Baciguent, Baci-IM, Basitin, Topitracine)	Vials containing powder for reconstitution for IM administration	Infants weighing 2.5 kg or less: 900 U/kg/day, divided in 2 or 3 doses Infants weighing more than 2.5 kg: 1,000 U/kg/day, divided in 2 or 3 doses PC: C	Treatment of pneumonia and empyema in infants caused by susceptible staphylococci Antisepsis of the intestinal tract (using the oral route) Treatment of superficial wounds (applied topically)
imipenem–cilastatin (Primaxin)	Powder for reconstitution for IM or IV administration	Dosage recommendations represent amount of imipenem to be administered Adults and children over 40 kg: IV: 250–500 mg q6h	Treatment of serious infections of lower respiratory tract, urinary tract, abdomen, skin and skin structures, bones and joints; bacterial septicemia, gynecologic infections, endocarditis
vancomycin (Vancocin, Vancoled, Lyphocin)	Capsules and solutions for oral use Vials containing powder for reconstitution for IV administration	Adults: 2 g/day, divided in 2–4 doses Children: 40 mg/kg/day, in divided doses Newborn infants: 20 mg/kg/day, in divided doses PC: C	Treatment of staphylococcal and other infections caused by susceptible organisms that cannot be treated by other less toxic drugs Treatment of necrotizing enterocolitis caused by *Clostridium difficile* Dosage adjustment required for clients with renal dysfunction, elderly, or young infants Use cautiously for hearing-impaired clients or those on other ototoxic drugs.

PC = Pregnancy category, see Appendix A.

Imipenem resembles the penicillins in therapeutic action but is resistant to beta-lactamases. It is active against a wide range of gram-positive and -negative organisms. It must be administered parenterally (IM or IV) because it is not absorbed by the GI tract. Because it is rapidly hydrolyzed in the proximal tubule of the kidney by an enzyme (dehydropeptidase), the drug preparation of imipenem (Primaxin) also contains a dehydropeptidase inhibitor, cilastatin. Nausea and vomiting are the most common adverse reactions to Primaxin. CNS effects, such as confusion and seizures, may occur; generalized seizures may occur if used with ganciclovir. Cross-sensitivity may occur in clients with allergies to penicillin.

Aztreonam (Azactam) is a synthetic agent that is effective against Enterobacteriaceae and *Pseudomonas aeruginosa* but not against most anaerobic and gram-positive organisms. Its spectrum is more similar to that of aminoglycosides than the other beta-lactam antibiotics. Clients with allergy to penicillins or cephalosporins do not appear to react to aztreonam but nonetheless should be closely monitored for allergic responses.

Beta-Lactamase Inhibitors

Certain chemicals bind to and inactivate beta-lactamases, thus reducing the drug resistance of pathogens that produce beta-lactamase. One of these, clavulanic acid, has been combined with oral amoxicillin (Augmentin) and parenteral ticarcillin (Timentin) in preparations used to treat resistant infections. Such combinations have a synergistic effect, attacking both the bacteria and the beta-lactamase enzyme produced by the bacteria that are resistant to antimicrobials. GI effects have been noted in some children when the proportion of clavulanic acid has been increased. Sulbactam may be administered concurrently with beta-lactam antibiotics to increase their efficacy in treating resistant pathogens.

Other Antibiotics Affecting Cell Wall Synthesis

Other agents that affect bacterial cell wall synthesis but are not beta-lactam antibiotics are bacitracin, novobiocin, and vancomycin.

Bacitracin

Bacitracin, an antibiotic produced by *Bacillus subtilis*, has a polypeptide structure.

Pharmacodynamics. The action of bacitracin is bactericidal or bacteriostatic, depending on the concentration of the drug and the susceptibility of the pathogen. It inhibits bacterial cell wall synthesis, probably by interfering with the final dephosphorylation step in the phospholipid carrier cycle involved in the transfer of mucopeptide to the growing cell wall. Bacitracin also damages the bacterial plasma membrane. It is active against many gram-positive organisms and some gram-negative pathogens. Resistance to bacitracin seldom occurs in susceptible bacteria.

Pharmacokinetics. Bacitracin is not absorbed from the GI tract. After IM injection, it is widely distributed to body organs and fluids, including ascitic and pleural fluids. Only traces cross the blood-brain barrier, unless the meninges are inflamed. After oral administration, bacitracin is excreted in feces. After parenteral injection, most of the dose cannot be accounted for and may be destroyed in the body. About 10% to 40% is excreted in the kidneys by glomerular filtration.

Therapeutic Uses. Because of its potential to cause severe renal toxicity, the only role of systemic use (IM) of bacitracin is to treat infants with pneumonia and empyema caused by susceptible staphylococci that are resistant to penicillin. However, penicillin-resistant penicillin and cephalosporins are equally effective and less toxic. Oral bacitracin has been used to treat antibiotic-induced colitis. Over-the-counter bacitracin ointment is marketed for use in treating superficial wounds.

Adverse Reactions. The most serious toxic effect of bacitracin is renal tubular and glomerular necrosis. This reaction occurs less often in infants than in older persons. Pain and induration may occur at the site of injection. GI upset, superinfection, and respiratory paralysis have occurred. Allergic reactions include urticaria, fever, blood dyscrasias, eosinophilia, and anaphylaxis.

Drug Interactions. Concurrent use of neuromuscular blocking agents should be avoided. Use of bacitracin with aminoglycosides may increase the risk of respiratory paralysis and renal dysfunction. Bacitracin is not administered IV because it causes severe thrombophlebitis. Because of stability problems, bacitracin powder should be kept refrigerated.

Precautions and Contraindications. Renal function should be assessed before beginning parenteral bacitracin therapy and regularly during treatment. The drug is contraindicated in clients with renal impairment and should be discontinued if renal toxicity develops. Myasthenia gravis, pregnancy, and allergic sensitivity to bacitracin are other contraindications. Clients receiving bacitracin should be kept well hydrated and the urine pH should be kept at or above 6 to decrease renal irritation.

Novobiocin

Novobiocin is an antibiotic produced by *Streptomyces niveus* or *Streptomyces speroides*.

Pharmacodynamics. Novobiocin appears to interfere with bacterial cell wall synthesis and to inhibit protein and nucleic synthesis in pathogens. It is usually bacteriostatic in action. It is active against some gram-positive cocci and bacilli and certain gram-negative bacteria. Resistant strains can develop rapidly during therapy.

Pharmacokinetics. Novobiocin is well absorbed from the GI tract. Concentrations in pleural, synovial, and ascitic fluids are usually lower than concurrent serum concentrations. The drug does not cross the blood-brain barrier in significant amounts, even when the meninges are inflamed. Highest concentrations of novobiocin are found in the liver, small intestines, and bile. The drug is excreted primarily in bile and feces, with a small fraction eliminated by the kidneys.

Therapeutic Uses. Novobiocin is used only when other, less toxic agents are ineffective or contraindicated. It has been used to treat infections caused by *Staphylococcus aureus* and *Proteus*.

Drug-Laboratory Interactions. Novobiocin may interfere with the bromosulphalein test. Since novobiocin may cause a pseudojaundice, it may interfere with serum bilirubin and icterus index determinations.

Adverse Reactions. Allergic reactions are common in clients receiving novobiocin. GI reactions also occur but are rarely severe. Other adverse effects include hematologic changes, hepatotoxicity, and dizziness, drowsiness, and lightheadedness. Superinfection can also occur.

Precautions and Contraindications. Hepatic and hematologic systems should be assessed before and at regular intervals during novobiocin therapy. The drug should be discontinued if impairment of either system develops. It is contraindicated in clients allergic to the drug. Because the drug tends to cause hyperbilirubinemia, its use is contraindicated in neonates. Safe use during pregnancy has not been established.

Vancomycin

Vancomycin is a tricyclic glycopeptide antibiotic produced by *Streptococcus orientalis*, isolated from soil samples from India and Indonesia.

Pharmacodynamics. Vancomycin does not appear to be metabolized by the body. It is approximately 55% serum protein bound. It acts through inhibition of cell wall biosynthesis and alterations in bacterial cell membrane permeability and RNA synthesis. It is active against staphylococci, streptococci, *C difficile*, and diphtheroids. It is active primarily against gram-positive bacteria. There is no cross-resistance to other antibiotics.

Pharmacokinetics. Because it is poorly absorbed by the GI tract, vancomycin is administered orally only for treatment of staphylococcal enterocolitis and antibiotic-associated pseudomembranous colitis. It is administered IV for any other systemic infections. In the first 24 hours, about 75% is excreted in urine by glomerular filtration; that percentage may be reduced in the elderly. It diffuses poorly across normal meninges into the cerebrospinal fluid but does penetrate when the meninges are inflamed. Doses for young infants or low-birth weight infants must be lowered to prevent ototoxicity and nephrotoxicity.

Therapeutic Uses. Vancomycin is used in treating serious infections caused by beta-lactam–resistant staphylococci in penicillin-allergic clients or in clients with methicillin-resistant staphylococci or infections unresponsive to other antimicrobials. It also can be useful in treating clients allergic to penicillin and cephalosporins. It can be used in combination with an aminoglycoside for synergistic action against early-onset prosthetic valve endocarditis caused by *Staphylococcus epidermidis* or diphtheroids.

Adverse Reactions. Adverse reactions to vancomycin include transient or permanent ototoxicity, mostly in clients receiving excessive doses, those with an underlying hearing loss, or those taking another ototoxic agent. Reversible neutropenia may occur. Nephrotoxicity has become less common with improved dosing and assessment of renal function.

Drug Interactions. Because of its ototoxicity and potential for nephrotoxicity, caution should be exercised when vancomycin is administered concurrently with other ototoxic, neurotoxic, and nephrotoxic drugs, such as the aminoglycosides. Neuromuscular blockade may be increased when vancomycin is used with nondepolarizing muscle relaxants. Use with anesthetics has been associated with erythema and histamine-like flushing in children.

Precautions and Contraindications. Vancomycin should be used with caution in clients with renal insufficiency or renal dysfunction. The risk of thrombophlebitis can be minimized by slow administration and rotation of infusion sites. Hearing should be tested regularly, especially if other ototoxic drugs are administered concurrently.

Vancomycin is contraindicated in clients with a known hypersensitivity to this antibiotic. IV administration must take place over at least 60 minutes, using a dilute solution. Rapid infusion may result in sudden, profound hypotension, accompanied by an erythematous maculopapular rash ("red neck" or "red man's syndrome") that is not an allergy. Too-rapid administration may also lead to cardiac arrest. During infusion, blood pressure should be monitored. Renal function and hearing should be checked serially with prolonged vancomycin therapy. Pain and necrosis may result from extravasation.

Reference

Hospital Infection Control Practice Advisory Committee (HICPAC). (1996). Guidelines for isolation precautions in hospitals. Atlanta: Center for Disease Control and Prevention. Internet: http://wwwonder.ccd.gov

Bibliography

(1993). Antimicrobial prophylaxis in surgery. *Med Lett Drugs Ther, 35,* 91–94.

Davies J. (1994). Inactivation of antibiotics and the dissemination of resistant genes. *Science, 264,* 375–382.

Garret L. (1994). The coming plague. Newly emerging diseases in a world out of balance. New York: Penguin.

Goldman MP. (1995). Antibiotic prophylaxis in the critical care setting. *Crit Care Nurs Clin North Am, 7*(4), 667–674.

Hardman JG, Limbird LE, Molinoff PB et al. (1996). *Goodman and Gilman's The pharmacological basis of therapeutics,* 9th ed. New York: McGraw-Hill.

Levy SB. (1992). The antibiotic paradox: How miracle drugs are destroying the miracle. New York: Plenum Press.

Olin BR, ed. (1996). *Facts and comparisons.* St. Louis: Facts and Comparisons, Inc.

Swartz MN. (1995). Antibiotic use: The path of least resistance. *Harvard Health Letter, 20*(6), 6–7.

For more information and sample tests and activities, refer to Chapter 41 in the Student Workbook for Clinical Pharmacology and Nursing Management, 5th edition, available through your bookstore.

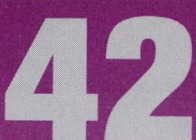
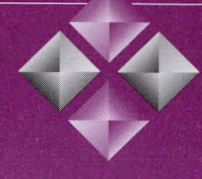

42

Antimicrobial Drugs That Affect Protein Synthesis

The drugs discussed in this chapter inhibit protein synthesis by bacteria. They act primarily by binding to the 30S or 50S subunits of bacterial ribosomes. Most are bacteriostatic; the aminoglycosides are usually bactericidal. In high doses these agents may also affect human ribosomes, with resulting toxicity.

General principles of antimicrobial therapy are discussed in Chapter 41, along with antimicrobials (penicillins and cephalosporins) that act by inhibiting bacterial cell wall synthesis. Antimicrobials for specific infections are discussed in Chapter 43.

Aminoglycosides

The first antibiotic to join penicillin and sulfanilamide in the struggle against infection was an aminoglycoside, streptomycin. Streptomycin was the first systemic antimicrobial effective against gram-negative pathogens. It was an excellent complement to penicillin, and combined therapy with the two drugs was often employed to achieve a broader spectrum of efficacy. Table 42-1 summarizes the aminoglycoside antibiotics.

Pharmacodynamics. Aminoglycosides contain two or more amino sugars in glycoside linkage with a hexose nucleus. They act as bactericidal agents against susceptible organisms by binding irreversibly to ribosomal subunits within the pathogens, thus preventing protein synthesis.

Pharmacokinetics. Aminoglycosides are highly polarized molecules that are poorly absorbed by the gastrointestinal (GI) tract. They are rapidly absorbed from intramuscular (IM) sites, producing a peak action in 30 to 90 minutes if tissue perfusion is good. After systemic administration, aminoglycosides are widely distributed in the extracellular fluid, accumulating in high concentrations in the renal cortex and the perilymph of the inner ear. They do not cross the blood-brain barrier when administered in therapeutic amounts. They bind to plasma proteins—in the case of streptomycin, about 35% is so bound.

Aminoglycosides are not metabolized and are excreted unchanged in urine, primarily by glomerular filtration. Although the drugs do enter the enterohepatic cycle, this is not an important route for elimination. Plasma half-life is 2 to 4 hours in normal adults. The drugs are readily removed by hemodialysis and, to a lesser extent, by peritoneal dialysis. When given orally, kanamycin and neomycin are excreted in feces.

Therapeutic Uses. Aminoglycosides are valuable therapeutic agents for controlling aerobic gram-negative bacterial infections. Each aminoglycoside varies in its properties and has advantages in certain clinical situations.

When administered by IM injection or intravenous (IV) infusion, aminoglycosides are effective against infections in most tissues except the central nervous system (CNS) and the eye. Intrathecal administration is required for CNS conditions. The drugs are also administered orally to reduce the microscopic flora in the intestinal lumen preoperatively, in acute intestinal infections, and in the treatment of hepatic encephalopathy. The drugs are sometimes nebulized and administered by inhalation or applied topically to the eyes.

Adverse Reactions. As often happens with new treatment agents, the dangers of the aminoglycosides were not recognized at first. Streptomycin was regarded as nontoxic until it was used for intensive therapy for tuberculosis, when its toxic properties became apparent. Ototoxicity and nephrotoxicity are the most serious adverse reactions to aminoglycosides. These effects are most common in the elderly, clients with preexisting renal dysfunction, and those receiving other drugs capable of producing ototoxicity and nephrotoxicity.

The aminoglycosides can cause irreversible damage to the eighth cranial nerve. In general, gentamicin and streptomycin primarily cause toxicity to the vestibular portion of the eighth cranial nerve. Kanamycin, amikacin, and netilmicin primarily cause cochlear toxicity.

Table 42-1. Aminoglycoside Antibiotics

Drug Name	Preparation	Usual Adult Dosage	Additional Information
amikacin sulfate (Amikin)	Solutions for IM and IV injection	15 mg/kg/day, divided in 2 or 3 doses Maximum daily dosage: 1.5 g Desired peak serum concentration: 15–30 μg/mL Desired trough serum concentration: 10 μg/mL PC: D	Monitor for ototoxicity and nephrotoxicity. Dosage adjustment required for clients with renal dysfunction
gentamicin sulfate (Garamycin, G-Myticin, Jenamicin) *Can:* Alcomicin, Cidomycin	Solutions for IM or IV injection Preservative-free solutions for intrathecal or intraventricular injection Ointments and creams for topical application Ointments and solutions for ophthalmic use	Adults: 3–5 mg/kg/day, divided in 3 or 4 doses, administered at equal intervals Children: 6–7.5 mg/kg/day, divided in 3 doses, q8h Desired peak serum concentration: 4–6 μg/mL Desired trough serum concentration: 2 μg/mL *Ophthalmic ointment:* 1 cm ribbon bid or tid *Ophthalmic solution:* 1–2 drops q4h PC: C (can cause deafness in child exposed in utero)	Dosage adjustment required for clients with renal dysfunction Inactivated by carbenicillin if mixed in same solution Sometimes administered intrathecally for treatment of gram-negative meningitis Monitor for ototoxicity and nephrotoxicity.
kanamycin sulfate (Kantrex) *Can:* Anamid	Capsules for oral use Solutions for IM or IV or aerosol administration	15 mg/kg/day, divided in 2 or 3 doses administered at equal intervals Maximum daily dosage: 1.5 g Desired peak serum concentration: 15–30 μg/mL Desired trough serum concentration: 5 μg/mL Oral dose to "sterilize" gut: 1 g every hour for 4 doses, then every 6 h for 36–72 h; 8–12 g/day, in divided doses for treatment of hepatic encephalopathy Aerosol: 250 mg 2–4 times a day PC: D	Oral preparations used for preoperative "sterilization" of the gut and in the treatment of hepatic encephalopathy; 1% solutions administered as retention enemas Rarely used IV; ineffective against *Pseudomonas* organisms Used to treat gram-negative urinary tract infections and tuberculosis resistant to other therapeutic agents Monitor for toxicity and nephrotoxicity. Dosage adjustment required for clients with renal dysfunction
neomycin sulfate (Myciguent) *Can:* Mycifradin	Oral tablets and solutions for ophthalmic and otic use Ointments and creams for topical application Sterile solution for preparation of irrigating solutions Powder for reconstitution for IM injection	Adults: 4–12 g daily, divided in 4 doses Children: 50–100 mg/kg divided in 6 doses, administered at equal intervals PC: C	Inhalation route used in cystic fibrosis Used orally to "sterilize" bowel Used as an adjunct in the treatment of hepatic encephalopathy
netilmicin (Netromycin)	Solutions for IM or IV administration	Adults: 4.0–6.5 mg/kg/day, divided in 2 or 3 doses Infants and children 6 wk–12 yr: 5.5–8.0 mg/kg/day, divided in 2 or 3 doses Neonates: 4.0–6.5 mg/kg/day, divided in 2 doses Desired peak serum concentration: 6–10 μg/mL Desired trough serum concentration: 0.5–2 μg/mL PC: D	Monitor for ototoxicity and nephrotoxicity. Dosage adjustment required for clients with renal dysfunction

KEY: PC = pregnancy category; see Appendix A.
Can: Canadian

(continued)

Table 42-1. (Continued)

Drug Name	Preparation	Usual Adult Dosage	Additional Information
paromomycin sulfate (Humatin)	Oral capsules	25–35 mg/kg/day, divided in 3 doses	Used as an adjunct in the treatment of hepatic coma Also used in the treatment of intestinal amebiasis Monitor for ototoxicity and nephrotoxicity.
streptomycin sulfate	Vials that contain solution for IM administration	Adults: 1–2 g/day, divided in 2–4 doses, administered at equal intervals Children: 20–40 mg/kg/day, divided in 2–4 doses, administered at equal intervals Desirable peak serum concentration: 5–25 μg/mL Desirable trough serum concentration: 5 μg/mL PC: D	Used in the treatment of serious infections that do not respond to other agents, such as bacterial endocarditis, tularemia, plague, and brucellosis; sometimes used in combination with penicillin or other antibiotics Monitor for ototoxicity and nephrotoxicity. Rarely administered IV because of ototoxicity Dosage adjustment required for clients with renal dysfunction Used in treating mycobacterial infections, tuberculosis (in combination with one or more other drugs), and leprosy
tobramycin sulfate (Nebcin)	Vials that contain powder for reconstitution for IM or IV administration Ophthalmic ointments and solutions	Adults: 3 mg/kg/day divided in 3 doses, q8h Children: 6–7.5 mg/kg/day divided in 3 or 4 doses Desired peak serum concentration: 4–10 μg/mL Desired trough serum concentration: 2 μg/mL *Ophthalmic ointment:* 1 cm ribbon bid or tid *Ophthalmic solution:* 1–2 drops q4h PC: B	Ineffective against mycobacteria; very effective against *Pseudomonas* organisms Monitor for ototoxicity and nephrotoxicity. Dosage adjustment required for clients with renal dysfunction

KEY: PC = pregnancy category; see Appendix A.
Can: Canadian

Tobramycin causes both types of toxicity. The degree of damage associated with aminoglycosides is somewhat dependent on the dose, length of therapy, renal function, and concomitant use of other potentially ototoxic drugs. There is a strong correlation between high trough levels and ototoxicity.

Acoustic nerve irritation is first indicated by abnormal (often ringing) sensations in the ear. Both vestibular and auditory functions are affected. Vertigo or tinnitus are indications of damage to vestibular function. Hearing loss begins with reduced perception of high tones, which can seriously impair comprehension of speech, even though deafness is not apparent. Nerve cell death is irreversible, and hearing loss is permanent.

Peripheral nerve toxicity is further manifested by neuromuscular blockade, which sometimes occurs when aminoglycosides are administered to clients immediately after surgery.

The incidence of acute renal failure in humans due to nephrotoxicants is about 15%. The most frequently cited cause of toxicant-induced acute renal failure is antibiotics, with aminoglycosides the most frequently mentioned antibiotic. The severity of aminoglycoside nephrotoxicity ranges from clinically trivial effects on tubular function to life-threatening acute tubular necrosis. Aminoglycoside nephrotoxicity is characterized primarily by various renal functional alterations, including enzymuria; tubular proteinuria; transport defects of amino acids, magnesium, and potassium; nephrogenic diabetes insipidus; and diminished glomerular filtration rate. The initial manifestation of aminoglycoside nephrotoxicity is enzymuria, which can occur as early as 24 hours after a single therapeutic dose. Aminoglycoside nephrotoxicity is related to the rapid uptake of the drug by the proximal tubular cells and subsequent active concentration of the drug within the renal cortex to some five to 50 times serum levels. Streptomycin is the least nephrotoxic aminoglycoside.

Although only small amounts of the aminoglycosides are absorbed from the GI tract, oral administration can produce systemic toxicity in clients with poor kidney function, in whom the drugs accumulate. Superinfections sometimes develop during therapy.

Aminoglycosides exhibit little allergic potential. However, allergy to these drugs may produce rash, urticaria, stomatitis, pruritus, generalized burning, fever, and eosinophilia. Agranulocytosis and anaphylaxis have rarely occurred. Persons who develop allergic sensitivity to one aminoglycoside sometimes exhibit cross-sensitivity to other drugs of this class.

Bacterial strains resistant to the action of the aminoglycosides arise when organisms acquire the ability to produce enzymes that break down the aminoglycoside molecule. Traits such as a cell transport mechanism less accepting of the aminoglycosides and ribosome structure with less affinity to the drug molecules can also cause resistance. Organisms resistant to one aminoglycoside are not necessarily resistant to all drugs of this class.

Drug Interactions. Aminoglycosides should not be administered concurrently with other ototoxic, neurotoxic, or nephrotoxic drugs, general anesthetics, muscle relaxants, or diuretics such as ethacrynic acid, furosemide, urea, and mannitol. Sequential use should also be avoided, because residues of the first drug may increase the toxicity of succeeding agents. Oral aminoglycosides potentiate the action of oral anticoagulants (warfarin) by decreasing bacterial synthesis of vitamin K in the intestine. The dose of anticoagulant should be reduced initially when these antibiotics are prescribed, and the prothrombin time should be closely monitored (see Focus on Aminoglycosides: Similarities and Differences).

Precautions and Contraindications. Kidney function in clients who receive aminoglycosides should be monitored closely. Doses of aminoglycosides must be reduced in clients with kidney damage to maintain serum concentrations below the toxic level. Drug serum levels should be monitored and dosage controlled to prevent excessive peak and trough serum concentrations.

Aminoglycoside therapy is contraindicated in clients with a history of toxic or hypersensitivity reactions to aminoglycosides. Oral doses are contraindicated in clients with intestinal obstruction. The drugs should be discontinued if tinnitus, hearing loss, oliguria, azotemia, or respiratory paralysis develops. Periodic audiometric and caloric stimulation tests are advised for clients who receive aminoglycosides over a long period.

■ SUMMARY

The aminoglycosides are the major antibiotics for use in gram-negative infections. When administered orally, they exert a local effect on the GI tract. Systemic effects require administration by injection. The aminoglycosides are often used with other antibiotics to achieve a broad spectrum of activity and to minimize the development of resistant strains. These drugs are ototoxic and nephrotoxic but not markedly allergenic.

❖ NURSING MANAGEMENT: CLIENT RECEIVING AN AMINOGLYCOSIDE

Aminoglycoside solutions are relatively unstable and should be used promptly. Solutions that must be stored should be refrigerated. Specific data regarding stability are available in the labeling information that accompanies the drug. Before the administration of each dose, the solution's expiration date should be checked.

NURSING PROCESS

ASSESSMENT

The renal function and hearing of clients about to receive aminoglycosides must be carefully evaluated before drug therapy begins. If these functions are marginal, alternative treatment may be considered.

NURSING DIAGNOSIS

Diagnoses relate to both therapeutic and adverse responses to aminoglycoside therapy and may include:

- Risk for Injury, related to nephrotoxicity or ototoxicity of aminoglycoside antibiotic drugs
- Sensory/Perceptual Alterations, related to loss of auditory input secondary to ototoxicity of drugs
- Knowledge Deficit, concerning need for adherence to regimen and recognition of adverse effects
- Ineffective Individual Management of Therapeutic Regimen: Noncompliance, related to adverse reactions or inability to pay for prescriptions

Common collaborative problems that should be differentiated from the nursing diagnoses include:

Potential Complication: Renal toxicity or ototoxicity

PLANNING

Goals of nursing care are to support the client's resistance to infection, reduce the risk of adverse drug reaction, and detect and promptly treat any adverse reaction.

INTERVENTION

Nursing interventions include implementing measures to enhance resistance to infection, administering the antibiotics, monitoring response to treatment, and consulting the prescriber if an adverse reaction occurs or if there is no therapeutic response.

Client Education. Clients should be taught the signs and symptoms of adverse drug reactions that should be reported to the prescriber (especially tinnitus, vertigo, hearing loss, or changes in urination amounts or pattern).

Text continues on page 911.

FOCUS ON

Aminoglycosides: Similarities and Differences

Similarities

Pharmacodynamics

These agents are bactericidal and appear to inhibit protein synthesis by irreversibly binding to the ribosomal subunits in susceptible bacteria.

Pharmacokinetics

These agents are rapidly absorbed after IM administration, and they are absorbed in significant amounts by body surfaces. They are poorly absorbed from the GI tract after oral administration. They are widely distributed into body fluids, primarily extracellular, and they diffuse poorly into the cerebrospinal fluid after IM and IV administration. They readily cross the placenta, and small amounts are found in bile, saliva, sweat, tears, sputum, and milk. The elimination half-life ranges from 2 to 4 hours in clients with normal renal function. They are not metabolized, and they are excreted unchanged in urine.

Therapeutic Uses

These agents are used in the short-term treatment of serious infections by gram-negative bacteria. They are also active against aerobic gram-negative and some aerobic gram-positive bacteria. They are also used in the treatment of serious recurrent urinary tract infections caused by gram-negative bacteria.

Adverse Reactions

These include: (CNS) peripheral neuropathy, eighth cranial nerve damage, vertigo, ataxia, paresthesia, headache, tremors, lethargy, numbness, tingling, muscle twitching, neuromuscular blockade; (CV) tachycardia, hypotension, myocarditis; (EENT) ototoxicity, nystagmus;

Differences

- **Kanamycin, paromomycin,** and **neomycin** also inhibit ammonia-forming bacteria in the GI tract.

- **Gentamicin** (intrathecal) has a half-life of 5.5 hours.
- **Amikacin** peaks in 45 minutes to 2 hours (IM) and over 1 hour (IV infusion).
- **Gentamicin** and **tobramycin** (IM and IV infusion) peak in 30 to 90 minutes.
- **Kanamycin** (IM and IV infusion) peaks in 1 hour.
- **Netilimicin** (PO and IM) peaks in 30 to 60 minutes; IV infusion peaks within 30 minutes.
- **Streptomycin** (IM) peaks in 1 to 2 hours.
- **Neomycin** (PO) is excreted unchanged in feces.
- **Neomycin** and **gentamicin** administered topically are best absorbed when the cornea is abraded (ophthalmic) and are readily absorbed through denuded areas of skin or through skin that has lost its keratin layer.
- **Neomycin** is also rapidly absorbed from the peritoneum, draining wounds, sinuses, and surgical sites.

- **Paromomycin,** active against protozoa, is used to treat intestinal amebiasis.
- **Streptomycin** is active against mycobacterium.
- **Gentamicin** is used intrathecally or intraventricularly to supplement IM or IV administration in the treatment of CNS infections.
- **Clindamycin,** in conjunction with an IM or IV aminoglycoside, is used for the treatment of mixed aerobic–anaerobic infections.
- **Gentamicin** and **neomycin** topical are used to treat superficial eye and skin infections and bacterial ocular infections.
- **Neomycin** topical is used to treat otitis externa, and it is combined with **polymyxin B** for urinary tract irrigation to prevent bacteremia and bacteriuria from use of an indwelling catheter.
- **Gentamicin** and **clindamycin** are used to treat pelvic inflammatory disease.
- **Kanamycin, neomycin,** and **paromomycin** (PO) are used as a retention enema as an adjuvant treatment for hepatic encephalopathy.
- **Kanamycin** and **neomycin** are used in combination for preoperative intestinal antisepsis.
- **Neomycin** (PO) is used as an adjunct for fluid and replacement treatment for severe diarrhea caused by *Escherichia coli.*

- **Gentamicin** (ophthalmic) may cause transient irritation, burning, or stinging.
- **Neomycin** (topical) may cause local irritation, dermatitis, erythema, rash, urticaria, and photosensitivity.

(continued)

Aminoglycosides: Similarities and Differences (continued)

Similarities (continued)

Adverse Reactions (continued)

(GI) nausea, vomiting, diarrhea; (GU) nephrotoxicity; (HEME) hemolytic anemia, transient neutropenia, leukopenia, thrombocytopenia; (OTHER) hypersensitivity, vein irritation, phlebitis, sterile abscess at injection site.

Interactions

Parenterally administered aminoglycosides should not be used with other drugs causing nephrotoxicity (especially cephalosporins, enflurane, methoxyflurane, vancomycin) or ototoxicity (eg, loop diuretics). Aminoglycosides act synergistically with penicillins. The effects of neuromuscular blockers may be enhanced by both oral and parenteral aminoglycosides. Concurrent use of oral and parenteral aminoglycosides with polypeptide antibiotics may increase the risk of renal dysfunction and respiratory paralysis.

Precautions and Contraindications

These agents should be used cautiously in clients with neuromuscular disorders, such as parkinsonism and myasthenia gravis, in premature and full-term neonates less than 6 weeks of age, in those with impaired renal function, and in the elderly.

These agents are contraindicated in clients with history of toxicity or hypersensitivity and in those receiving other ototoxic, neurotoxic, or nephrotoxic drugs.

Nursing Considerations

Instruct client in disease, treatment, drug regimen, adverse reactions, and adherence; obtain specimens for culture and sensitivity before initiating therapy; monitor vital signs, especially temperature and pulse, for changes that indicate improvement of infection; assess renal function studies, such as specific gravity, blood urea nitrogen, and creatinine levels before and periodically after the start of therapy for changes; encourage fluids and monitor intake and output for changes; assess hearing before and periodically during therapy for changes; assess for signs of hearing difficulties; obtain serum peak and trough levels and report abnormalities; do not mix with other drugs when giving parenterally; stop IV infusion of aminoglycoside if other drugs must be given and flush tubing with normal saline or dextrose and water afterward; administer IM deep into large muscle and rotate injection sites to prevent tissue injury; instruct client in signs and symptoms of possible superinfection and toxicity.

Differences (continued)

- Oral aminoglycosides may interfere with the absorption of dietary vitamin K resulting in increase in warfarin-induced hypoprothrombinemia. The absorption of methotrexate and digoxin may be decreased. Serum levels of retinol and carotene may be decreased when vitamin A is given with oral aminoglycosides.

- **Neomycin, kanamycin,** and **paromomycin** (PO) are contraindicated in clients with intestinal obstruction.
- **Streptomycin** is contraindicated in clients with labyrinthine disease.

- When giving **neomycin** preoperatively, administer a low-residue diet and cathartics as ordered. IM neomycin is not recommended because of the possibility of ototoxicity and nephrotoxicity. When given for tuberculosis, discontinue neomycin when client's sputum is negative. Watch for respiratory depression in clients with renal disease, hypocalcemia, and neuromuscular disease. Administer neomycin (otic) to a clean dry ear canal. Administer neomycin as a GU irrigant through a three-way indwelling catheter.
- Apply **gentamicin** or **neomycin** ophthalmic ointment to the conjunctival sac; apply topical ointment or cream gently to the clean affected area and cover with sterile gauze; protect hands when applying, because drug is irritating.

OUTCOME EVALUATION

Data required for evaluation include signs and symptoms of infection and signs and symptoms of adverse drug reaction.

❖ **CHECKLIST OF NURSING ACTIONS**

❑ Before administering the initial dose of aminoglycoside drugs, evaluate the client for renal dysfunction, hearing loss, allergy to aminoglycosides, and concurrent use of other ototoxic or nephrotoxic drugs.

❑ Verify that the client has been informed of the risks of treatment, especially the risk of hearing loss.

❑ Use only fresh solutions of aminoglycosides.

❑ Monitor clients receiving aminoglycosides for early signs and symptoms of ototoxicity or nephrotoxicity, such as ringing or a sense of fullness in the ears and changes in urinary excretion.

❑ Monitor the respiratory status of clients receiving aminoglycosides concurrently with neuromuscular blocking agents.

Tetracyclines

Tetracyclines are derivatives of the polycyclic chemical naphthacenecarboxamide obtained from cultures of *Streptomyces* organisms. They exhibit a wide range of activity against both gram-positive and gram-negative bacteria and other microorganisms not responsive to other drugs. Various preparations are available for clinical use (Table 42-2).

Pharmacodynamics. Like the aminoglycosides, tetracyclines interfere with protein synthesis by microbial ribosomes. Unlike the aminoglycosides, these compounds gain access to the interior of the cell by more

Table 42-2. Tetracycline Preparations

Drug Name	Preparation	Usual Dosage
demeclocycline (Declomycin)	Tablets and capsules for oral use PC: D	Adults: 600 mg daily, divided in 2–4 doses Children: 8 yr or older: 6–12 mg/kg/day, divided in 2–4 doses
doxycycline (Doryx, Doxy-Caps, Doxy-chel, Doxy-Lemmon, Doxy-Tabs, Vi-bramycin, Vibra-Tabs, Monodox) *Can:* Doxycin	Tablets, capsules, syrup, and suspensions for oral use Vials that contain powder for reconstitution for IV administration PC: D	Adults and children 8 yr or older and more than 100 lb: 100–200 mg/day, divided in 1 or 2 doses Children over 8 yr and less than 100 lb: 4.4 mg/kg divided into 1 or 2 doses on first day, then 2.2 mg/kg daily in 1 or 2 doses
methacycline (Rondomycin)	Capsules for oral use PC: D	Adults: 600 mg daily, divided in 2–4 doses Children 8 yr or older: 6–12 mg/kg/day, divided in 2–4 doses
minocycline (Minocin)	Tablets and capsules for oral use Vials that contain powder for reconstitution for IV administration PC: D	Adults: 200 mg daily, divided in 2–4 doses, administered at equal intervals Children 8 yr or older: 2 mg/kg/day, divided in 2 doses q12h
oxytetracycline (Terramycin, Uri-Tet)	Tablets, capsules, and suspensions for oral use Vials that contain powder for reconstitution for IV administration PC: D	*Oral:* Adults: 1–2 g daily, divided in 4 doses; Children 8 yr or older: 25–50 mg/kg/day, divided in 4 doses *IM, IV:* Adults: 250–300 mg daily, divided in 1–3 doses; Children 8 yr or older: 15–25 mg/kg/day divided into 1–3 doses (maximum 250 mg per single daily injection)
tetracycline (Achromycin, Nor-Tet, Pan-mycin, Robitet, Sumycin, Tetracap, Tetralan, Tetram, Topicycline) *Can:* Cefracycline, Medicycline, Neo-Tetrine, Novotetra, Tetralean	Tablets, capsules, and suspensions for oral use Ointment and suspension for ophthalmic use Vials that contain powder for reconstitution for IM or IV administration Powder for preparing topical solutions PC: D	*Oral:* Adults: 1–2 g daily, divided in 2–4 doses; Children 8 yr or older: 25–50 mg/kg/day, divided in 2–4 doses *IV:* Adults: 500 mg–1 g daily, divided in 2 doses, administered at equal intervals; Children 8 yr or older: 10–20 mg/kg/day *IM:* Adults: 250–300 mg/day; Children 8 yr or older: 15–25 mg/kg/day

KEY: PC = pregnancy risk category; see Appendix A.
Can = Canadian

than one mechanism, including passive diffusion. They affect only multiplying organisms but are both bacteriostatic and, in high concentrations, bactericidal.

Pharmacokinetics. Although not completely absorbed by the GI tract, tetracyclines produce adequate blood levels when given orally, the usual route of administration. Because the drugs react with polyvalent cations (calcium, magnesium, aluminum, iron), foods or medicines that contain these minerals chelate the tetracyclines and prevent absorption if ingested at the same time. Although they can be administered parenterally, tetracyclines are rarely injected. IM injection produces intense pain and is not recommended. The drugs are never injected intrathecally.

Tetracyclines are widely distributed in body tissues. They cross the blood-brain barrier gradually, eventually reaching therapeutic concentrations in the CNS. The ability of individual drugs to bind to plasma protein varies, ranging from 20% to 95%. Tetracyclines localize in and form stable complexes at sites of new bone and tooth formation. They readily cross the placenta and are distributed into breast milk in concentrations similar to maternal serum concentrations.

Both the liver and kidneys excrete tetracyclines, eliminating the drugs in both urine and feces. Much of the drug secreted in the bile is reabsorbed, contributing to the tendency of these drugs to persist in the body. Tissues that store the drugs in significant amounts include the liver, spleen, bone marrow, bone, and dentin.

Therapeutic Uses. Tetracyclines are useful therapeutic agents in treating infections caused by rickettsiae (Rocky Mountain spotted fever, Q fever), bacteria (brucellosis, tularemia), some *Mycoplasma* organisms that cause pneumonia, and *Chlamydia* organisms (lymphogranuloma venereum, psittacosis, trachoma). They also are used in managing acne and amebiasis. Since the introduction of tetracyclines, many pathogenic strains have developed resistance to tetracyclines, and their clinical use has diminished accordingly. Tetracyclines remain important agents for treating serious infections resistant to other antibiotics. Doxycycline is used to treat uncomplicated *Chlamydia trachomatis*, a prevalent sexually transmitted disease.

Adverse Reactions. Tetracyclines irritate the GI mucosa. When taken orally, nausea, vomiting, abdominal distress, distention, and diarrhea are common. Esophageal ulcers have been reported. Preparations administered IV are highly irritating to the veins and frequently cause phlebitis and thrombosis.

If administered during the period of tooth formation (while in utero during last half of pregnancy and during childhood to age 8), tetracyclines permanently discolor the teeth. Initially, the color changes to yellow, but with aging the enamel turns brown permanently. Minocycline colors not only teeth, but also bones, skin, fingernails, and the thyroid gland.

Tetracyclines should not be used during pregnancy because they retard skeletal development of the fetus.

Allergic reactions are rare but potentially serious. They include skin manifestations (rash, urticaria, fixed eruptions), asthma, fever, angioedema, and anaphylaxis. Cross-sensitivity is the rule: recipients allergic to one tetracycline are usually allergic to all.

Superinfections may develop due to alterations of the normal microbial flora. Enteritis caused by tetracycline-resistant bacteria can be life-threatening. Mycotic infections can affect the mouth, throat, or vagina. Even systemic infections can develop in immunosuppressed recipients and diabetics.

Adverse reactions, which vary with individual drugs, include phototoxicity, liver and kidney damage, and vestibular malfunction. Pseudotumor cerebri (benign intracranial hypertension) also may occur. The drugs exert a catabolic effect, producing a tendency toward negative nitrogen balance and weight loss. Blood dyscrasias and increased intracranial pressure have also developed during therapy.

As they age, tetracyclines tend to be degraded and become more toxic. Outdated preparations are thought to cause photosensitivity, a lupoid lesion of the face, and nephrotoxicity, including a form of Fanconi syndrome evidenced by nausea, vomiting, polyuria, polydipsia, proteinuria, acidosis, glycosuria, and aminoaciduria.

Drug–Drug Interactions. Drugs that contain bismuth salts, calcium, magnesium, aluminum, iron, or zinc prevent absorption of tetracyclines (Box 42-1).

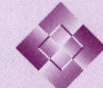

Box 42-1
Tetracycline Drug Interactions

Agents that Impair Tetracycline Absorption

Antacids, bismuth salts, cimetidine, iron salts, sodium bicarbonate, foods and drugs containing aluminum, calcium, magnesium, zinc

Agents that Decrease Tetracycline Serum Levels

Barbiturates, carbamazepine, hydantoins

Drug Serum Levels (or Effects) Increased by Tetracycline

Oral anticogualants, digoxin, insulin, lithium*

Drug Serum Levels (or Effects) Decreased by Tetracycline

Lithium,* oral contraceptives, penicillin

*Lithium levels may be increased or decreased.

Drug–Food Interactions. Often oral tetracyclines cause epigastric distress and are given with food. However, milk or dairy products or other foods containing calcium prevent absorption and should not be taken concurrently.

Precautions and Contraindications. Tetracyclines are contraindicated in pregnancy because of their potential for interference with fetal growth and for discoloring the developing teeth of the fetus. Also, gravid women are highly susceptible to tetracycline-induced hepatic damage. These drugs are not recommended for nursing mothers or children younger than 8 years. Most are also contraindicated in clients with renal insufficiency.

Because they are irritating to tissues, tetracyclines are rarely administered by injection. If IV use cannot be avoided, the drug should be well diluted and infused by slow continuous drip.

Diarrhea that occurs during tetracycline therapy must be carefully evaluated to rule out enteritis due to superinfection. When this potentially life-threatening condition is suspected, tetracycline therapy should be discontinued.

To minimize GI irritation, oral doses of the drugs may be administered with food, provided it is not milk or milk products.

If tetracyclines are administered for a long time, laboratory tests should be performed periodically to screen for blood dyscrasias and liver or kidney damage. Clients with a history of allergy should be monitored for hypersensitivity. Emergency treatment for severe reactions, such as anaphylaxis, must be available.

▪ SUMMARY

Tetracyclines are used to treat serious infections caused by strains of organisms that are resistant to other drugs but are susceptible to tetracyclines. They are usually administered orally. They are accompanied by many adverse reactions, the most serious of which are liver and kidney damage and life-threatening enteritis. Fetuses and children under age 8 develop permanent brown discoloration of the teeth when exposed to tetracyclines, so the drugs should not given to pregnant or nursing women or to children under age 8.

❖ NURSING MANAGEMENT: CLIENT RECEIVING A TETRACYCLINE

The expiration date of tetracycline preparations should be checked before use. Outdated preparations must never be used because the drugs are prone to degradation and may cause toxic reactions. Preparations marketed as sterile powders should be used promptly after reconstitution. IV solutions must be well diluted and administered by continuous slow drip. Orders for IM injections should be questioned because this route is seldom recommended. See the Critical Thinking Challenge: Case Analysis.

CRITICAL THINKING CHALLENGE
Case Analysis

Mrs. Jones, the mother of Johnny, age 3, is at the prenatal clinic for a checkup. She is expecting in 3 months. As you weigh her and ask how she's feeling, she tells you, "Gee, I had a bad cold last week, so I took that tetracycline that Dr. Smith prescribed for my infected finger last year. It really did the job. My cold went away after only a few doses, which is a good thing because it upset my stomach so much that I drank about a gallon of milk with it. Now I think little Johnny is coming down with my cold. Should I give him half a dose or a whole dose?"

1. Based on your knowledge of drug therapy, drug and food relations, and nursing, what issues does Mrs. Jones's conversation raise?

2. What points do you want to emphasize in responding to her?

NURSING PROCESS
ASSESSMENT

Clients who are to receive tetracycline drugs should be screened for allergic hypersensitivity to these drugs, renal impairment, pregnancy, and lactation. The age of children should be ascertained. Tetracyclines are not appropriate for pregnant or nursing women, children under age 8, or older children who show delayed or arrested growth and development.

NURSING DIAGNOSIS

Diagnoses consider the client's response to drug therapy, including therapeutic effects and adverse reactions and may include:

- Altered Urinary Elimination, related to nephrotoxicity from tetracycline therapy
- Risk for Fluid Volume Excess, related to increased need for fluids to prevent drug toxicity
- Diarrhea, related to superinfection from tetracycline therapy
- Altered Nutrition: Less Than Body Requirements, related to diarrhea secondary to tetracycline medication
- Ineffective Individual Management of Therapeutic Regimen: Noncompliance, related to adverse reactions to medication or inability to pay for prescriptions
- Knowledge Deficit, concerning antimicrobial medications, their adverse effects, and dosage schedules

PLANNING

Goals of nursing care are to promote therapeutic response to the antibiotics and to reduce the risk of adverse drug reactions.

INTERVENTION

Oral preparations of tetracycline should be administered with ample fluids (for adults, 2–3 L in a 24-hour period). To prevent irritation and possible ulceration of the esophagus, the dose must be propelled into the stomach. This is particularly important for clients with a history of hiatal hernia or gastroesophageal reflux disorder, who may have a malfunctioning lower esophageal sphincter.

If oral tetracyclines cause epigastric or abdominal distress, they can be administered with food, provided no milk or milk products are given. Drugs that contain calcium, magnesium, aluminum, or iron prevent absorption of these antibiotics and should not be administered at the same time.

Clients who receive tetracyclines should be monitored for signs and symptoms of adverse drug reactions, including intestinal upset, allergy, diarrhea, renal or hepatic impairment, and vestibular impairment.

Client Education. Clients often need help in establishing a regimen to provide optimal drug absorption with the least irritation to the intestinal tract. If possible, the drugs should be taken on an empty stomach and each dose should be taken with a full glass of water. They should be taken at least 1 hour before bedtime to prevent esophagitis. If the client experiences epigastric or abdominal discomfort, the antibiotics may be taken with selected food. The client should be in-structed not to ingest milk or dairy products or drugs that contain calcium, iron, magnesium, or aluminum with the antibiotic. Stools may become somewhat looser during the drug regimen. The client should be cautioned to report true diarrhea (liquid or loose stools accompanied by gripping or cramping pain) to the prescriber.

Clients should understand that exposure of young children to tetracyclines permanently discolors their teeth. The drugs can also cause hypersensitivity to sunlight, especially in persons with pale, lightly pigmented skin. The client should avoid direct sunlight and ultraviolet light.

As with all prescription drugs, tetracyclines should never be used by anyone other than the person for whom they were prescribed. Clients should check the expiration date on all tetracycline preparations. Unless the medication is discontinued by the prescriber, all the prescribed doses should be taken. If the prescriber advises that the drug be stopped, remaining doses should be discarded in accordance with agency or local regulations.

OUTCOME EVALUATION

Data required for evaluation include signs and symptoms that indicate reduction or elimination of infection and the absence or incidence of adverse reactions to the anti-infective drug (see Example of Nursing Process for Tetracycline Therapy).

Example of Nursing Process for Tetracycline Therapy

The client is a 19-year-old female being treated with tetracycline for acne. The client takes occasional doses of acetaminophen for headaches, a multivitamin daily. She currently takes an oral contraceptive but is planning to become pregnant soon.

Assessment Data

Prescription for tetracycline for treatment of acne

Plans for pregnancy

Use of oral contraceptive

Nursing Diagnosis	Intervention	Goals and Outcomes
Knowledge Deficit, concerning the effects of tetracycline on the teeth of a fetus exposed to it in utero	**Ask** the client the purposes for which the oral contraceptive has been prescribed. **Explain** to her the effect tetracycline has on the teeth of the fetus in utero; caution the client to consult her dermatologist for a change in medication before attempting conception and to request alternative treatment for acne should accidental pregnancy develop.	The client will not discontinue contraceptive medication without consulting her dermatologist for a change in medication. Should conception occur, the client will discontinue tetracycline immediately and consult her dermatologist for an alternative treatment for acne. If the client becomes pregnant, the child's deciduous teeth will be free of the yellow-brown discoloration characteristic of tetracycline exposure during tooth development.

❖ **CHECKLIST OF NURSING ACTIONS**

❑ Screen clients for pregnancy, lactation, incomplete skeletal development, renal or liver impairment, and allergic hypersensitivity before initiating tetracycline therapy.

❑ Administer oral tetracyclines with ample fluids (an 8-oz glass of water for adults).

❑ Use only fresh solutions for parenteral injection.

❑ Monitor clients for signs and symptoms of liver or renal malfunction, enteritis, superinfection, and bone marrow depression.

❑ For clients with a history of allergy, be prepared to give emergency care should an acute reaction occur.

❑ Do not give milk, dairy products, or drugs that contain calcium, magnesium, aluminum, or iron with oral tetracyclines. Nonmilk foods may be given with the drugs if they cause intestinal discomfort.

❑ Warn clients not to take outdated tetracyclines, nor to share their prescriptions with other people.

❑ Instruct clients to report adverse reactions, especially diarrhea, to the prescriber.

Macrolides

Erythromycin is a macrolide produced by *Streptomyces erythraeus*. It acts as a bacteriostatic agent but kills highly susceptible organisms, especially when used in large doses. The macrolide drug category includes not only erythromycin and its derivatives but also azithromycin, clarithromycin, and troleandomycin (Table 42-3).

Pharmacodynamics. Macrolides may be bacteriostatic or bactericidal, depending on the concentration. They inhibit protein synthesis in susceptible organisms by binding to ribosomal subunits, thereby inhibiting polypeptide synthesis. Other drugs that bind to these receptors on the ribosomal units include clindamycin, lincomycin, and chloramphenicol. Because they compete for sites of action, these drugs should not be used together.

Macrolides share a similar antibacterial spectrum and are effective against some gram-negative organisms (cocci and bacilli). Other gram-negative organisms (*Escherichia coli*, *Enterobacter*, *Klebsiella*, *Proteus*, *Pseudomonas*, *Salmonella*, and *Shigella* organisms), as well as viruses, yeasts, and fungi, are resistant to erythromycins. Erythromycins also are ineffective against anaerobes.

Pharmacokinetics. Macrolides differ in their pharmacokinetics. Erythromycin drugs are usually given by mouth. They are absorbed in the duodenum. Gastric acidity partially destroys the drug; oral preparations must be delivered in an enteric coating or buffered. The drug should be given a half-hour before or 2 hours after a meal; enteric-coated tablets can be taken with meals. Binding to serum proteins ranges from 73% to 93%. The drug is partially metabolized by the liver, and a portion enters the enterohepatic circulation. Serum levels of the drug are not significantly reduced by hemodialysis. The drug does not cross the blood-brain barrier readily.

Therapeutic Uses. Macrolides are often used in treating infections involving the respiratory tract, genital tract, and soft tissue. They are often used when beta-lactam antimicrobials or tetracyclines are contraindicated.

Erythromycin is used in treating mild to moderately severe streptococcal infections, especially in clients in whom penicillin is contraindicated. It is also used in treating impetigo contagiosa caused by group A beta-hemolytic streptococci and *Staphylococcus aureus*. It is considered the antibiotic of choice for the treatment of diphtheria. Erythromycin may also be used in the treatment of primary atypical pneumonia due to *Mycoplasma pneumoniae*.

Adverse Reactions. The most common side effects of systemic macrolide therapy are GI symptoms: abdominal pain and cramping, nausea, vomiting, and diarrhea. Clarithromycin tends to produce fewer GI side effects than do other macrolides. Pseudomembranous colitis has occurred.

Allergic manifestations include skin rashes, photosensitivity, angioedema, and (rarely) anaphylaxis.

Cholestatic hepatitis has been associated with the estolate salt of erythromycin (Ilosone), but not with other formulations. This hepatitis may occur when drug therapy lasts longer than 10 days or repeated courses are prescribed. The hepatitis is characterized by fever, abdominal cramps, an enlarged tender liver, hyperbilirubinemia, dark urine, eosinophilia, and elevated serum bilirubin and transaminase levels. Although the hepatitis usually occurs 10 to 20 days after initiation of therapy, it can occur within hours in a client who previously has had a reaction. The hepatitis is believed to be the result of both a hepatotoxic effect and a hypersensitivity reaction; this latter effect is reversible on withdrawal of the drug.

Erythromycin lactobionate has caused transient deafness, which is most likely to occur in persons with renal impairment.

Drug Interactions. Antacids decrease the absorption of most macrolides. Increased effects of anticoagulants and digoxin may occur if given with erythromycins or clarithromycin. Erythromycins and troleandomycin may increase levels of carbamazepine and triazolam. Erythromycins increase levels of astemizole, corticosteroids, theophylline, triazolam, valproate, alfentanil, bromocriptine, cyclosporine, and ergot alkaloids. Fatal arrhythmias have occurred when erythromycins have been given with astemizole or terfenadine; serious cardiac arrhythmias

Table 42-3. Erythromycin Preparations

Drug Name	Preparation	Usual Dosage*	Therapeutic Uses
azithromycin (Zithromax)	Capsules for oral administration	500 mg as single dose on first day followed by 250 mg PO on days 2–5 for a total dose of 1.5 g PC: B	Treatment of mild to moderate acute exacerbations of chronic obstructive pulmonary disease, pneumonia, pharyngitis/tonsillitis (as second-line therapy), and uncomplicated skin and skin structure infections
clarithromycin (Biaxin)	Tablets, suspension, and granules (for reconstitution) for oral administration	Adults: 250–500 mg q12h Children: 15 mg/kg/day in divided doses q12h PC: C	Treatment of pharyngitis/tonsillitis, otitis media, pneumonia due to *Mycoplasma pneumoniae* or *Streptococcus pneumoniae*; uncomplicated infections of skin and skin structure; infections due to *Mycobacterium avium* and *Mycobacterium intracellulare*
erythromycin* (Ak-Mycin, A/T/S, E-Mycin, Eryc, Eryderm, Erymax, Ery-Tab, Ilotycin, Robimycin, Staticin, T-Stat)	Capsules, tablets, and enteric-coated tablets for oral administration Ophthalmic ointments	*Oral:* adults: 1 g/day, divided in 3 or 4 doses, administered at equal intervals; children: 30–50 mg/kg/day, divided in 4 doses *IV:* adults: 15–20 mg/kg/day in continuous IV infusion or up to 4 g/day in divided doses q6h PC: B	Treatment of syphilis, gonorrhea, chlamydial infections during pregnancy, pertussis, and legionnaires' disease and pneumonia caused by *Mycoplasma pneumoniae* Alternative to penicillin in the prevention of streptococcal infections
erythromycin estolate (Ilosone, Novorythro)	Capsules, suspension, and tablets for oral administration		
erythromycin ethylsuccinate (E.E.S., E-Mycin, EryPed)	Suspensions, tablets, and chewable tablets for oral administration		
erythromycin gluceptate (Ilotycin Gluceptate)	Vials that contain powder for reconstitution for IV administration		
erythromycin lactobionate (Erythrocin Lactobionate)	Vials that contain powder for reconstitution for IV administration		
erythromycin stearate (Eramycin, Wyamycin-S)	Tablets for oral administration		
troleandomycin (Tao)	Capsules and suspension for oral use	Adults: 1–2 g/day, divided in 4 doses Children: 0.5–1 g/day, divided in 4 doses	Respiratory tract infections caused by susceptible staphylococci or streptococci when erythromycin is contraindicated or ineffective

*Erythromycin dosages expressed as erythromycin base
KEY: PC = pregnancy risk category; see Appendix A.

also have occurred when clarithromycin has been used with cisapride. Troleandomycin may increase levels of methylprednisolone and theophylline. Clarithromycin may increase levels of terfenadine, digoxin, carbamazepine, tacrolimus, triazolam, and theophylline and may decrease the effects of zidovudine.

Precautions and Contraindications. Erythromycin estolate is contraindicated in clients with hepatic disease or malfunction. Other erythromycins should be used with caution in clients with liver or biliary disease. Hepatic function should be monitored when large doses of the antibiotic are required. Clients receiving astemizole or terfenadine should not be given clarithromycin because of the danger of fatal arrhythmias.

Erythromycin is contraindicated in clients with a history of allergic reaction to this class of drugs. Safe use in pregnancy has not been determined.

■ SUMMARY

Macrolides are antibiotics with primarily bacteriostatic action used in the treatment of mild to moderate infection. They are especially useful in the treatment of clients who are allergic to penicillin or in whom beta-lactam antibiotics or tetracyclines are contraindicated. Macrolides are considered drugs of relatively low toxicity among antibiotics, but they can cause GI upset, skin rash, and cholestatic hepatitis.

❖ NURSING MANAGEMENT: CLIENT RECEIVING A MACROLIDE

NURSING PROCESS

ASSESSMENT

Before macrolide therapy is initiated, clients should be assessed for previous allergic response to this or other antibiotics, liver or biliary disease, and pregnancy.

NURSING DIAGNOSIS

Diagnoses address the client's response to drug therapy, both therapeutic and adverse, and may include:

- Altered Nutrition: Less Than Body Requirements, related to nausea and vomiting secondary to anti-infective drug therapy
- Diarrhea, related to superinfection secondary to anti-infective drug therapy

A common collaborative problem that should be differentiated from the nursing diagnoses is:

Potential Complication: Deafness

PLANNING

Goals of nursing care are to promote natural resistance to infection, reduce the risk of adverse drug reactions, and detect and treat promptly any adverse reactions.

INTERVENTION

Because macrolides are usually administered orally, orders for administration by other routes should be questioned. Clients who receive macrolides should be monitored for signs and symptoms of GI upset, skin rash, and hepatic impairment. Clients receiving astemizole or terfenadine should not receive erythromycin. Because macrolides are often prescribed for clients allergic to other antibiotics, recipients are often prone to allergic responses and should be monitored for signs and symptoms of developing allergy.

Client Education. The client should be instructed to report persistent abdominal discomfort, skin rash, yellowing of the skin or eyeballs, and signs and symptoms of allergic reaction. If erythromycin lactobionate is prescribed, changes in hearing should also be reported.

OUTCOME EVALUATION

Data required for evaluation are the signs and symptoms of therapeutic or adverse reactions to antibiotic therapy.

❖ CHECKLIST OF NURSING ACTIONS

- ☐ Assess clients who receive macrolide antibiotics for liver disease or impairment and allergic hypersensitivity to these drugs.
- ☐ Monitor clients who receive macrolides for signs and symptoms of GI irritation, skin rash, and liver impairment.
- ☐ Teach clients the symptoms of adverse reactions to macrolide antibiotics and caution them to report them if they occur.

Chloramphenicol

Chloramphenicol is a broad-spectrum antibiotic originally produced by a strain of *Streptomyces* organisms but now produced synthetically. Its molecular structure is unique among antibiotics: it contains a nitrobenzene structure.

Pharmacodynamics. Chloramphenicol inhibits protein synthesis by ribosomes of bacterial cells by binding to ribosomal subunits that catalyze peptide bond formation. Its action is usually bacteriostatic, but in high concentrations and against highly susceptible organisms, it is bactericidal.

Pharmacokinetics. Chloramphenicol salts must be hydrolyzed to free chloramphenicol before the drug can exert its pharmacologic action. When administered orally, hydrolysis occurs within the GI tract; after IV administration, hydrolysis occurs in the plasma. After absorption, the drug is widely distributed to most body compartments, including the cerebrospinal fluid. Plasma proteins bind about 60% of the drug. Chloramphenicol readily crosses the placenta and is secreted in breast milk.

Chloramphenicol is primarily deactivated by glucuronidase in the liver. The unchanged drug and the inactive metabolites are excreted in urine. A small fraction is eliminated in bile and feces after oral administration. Plasma half-life in normal adults is 1.5 to 3.5 hours, but it is much longer in persons with immature or inadequate liver function, reaching 24 hours or longer in neonates.

Therapeutic Uses. Because chloramphenicol causes serious and potentially fatal adverse reactions, and because few organisms have developed resistance to it, the drug is recommended as one of last resort for the treatment of life-threatening infections that are resistant to other antibiotics. The medical profession has proposed reserving systemic use for serious infections for which other treatment agents are ineffective. This policy is expected to reduce the incidence of serious toxicity and also to delay the development of resistance to chloramphenicol in virulent pathogens, thus prolonging the drug's usefulness.

Chloramphenicol is active against most gram-positive and gram-negative bacteria and *Rickettsia*, *Chlamydia*, and *Mycoplasma* organisms. It is inactive against fungi. Chloramphenicol is administered topically to treat eye and external ear infections.

Among the diseases for which this drug is used systemically are ampicillin-resistant typhoid fever, influenzal meningitis, pelvic and brain abscesses caused by anaerobic organisms, brucellosis, rickettsial disease in clients in whom the tetracyclines are contraindicated, and bacteremia caused by organisms resistant to other antibiotics. It is the drug of choice for treating typhoid fever (Table 42-4).

Adverse Reactions. The most important and serious adverse reaction to chloramphenicol is bone marrow depression. Two forms of bone marrow depression exist. The first is non–dose-related and is irreversible, leading to aplastic anemia, with a mortality rate of 50% or more.

This reaction may be a form of allergic hypersensitivity. There appears to be a genetic predisposition to this type of bone marrow depression; it is rare, with an estimated incidence of one in 40,000 or more courses of therapy. The more common type is dose-related and is usually reversible once the drug is discontinued. This type is seen commonly with plasma chloramphenicol concentrations of 25 µg/mL or more, or when the adult dosage exceeds 4 g/day. Neonates and recipients with hepatic dysfunction are at high risk, probably due to inadequate metabolism of the drug by their liver microsomal enzymes.

Table 42-4. Miscellaneous Antimicrobials Affecting Bacterial Protein Synthesis

Drug Name	Preparation	Usual Dosage	Therapeutic Uses
chloramphenicol (Chloromycetin)	Capsules for oral use, 0.5% ophthalmic solution, 1% ophthalmic ointment, 0.5% otic solution	50 mg/kg/day, divided in 4 doses (dosage should be kept as low as possible and must be reduced for clients with hepatic dysfunction)	Treatment of active typhoid fever; treatment of meningitis, bacteremia, or other serious infections caused by organisms resistant to other antibiotics
chloramphenicol palmitate (Chloromycetin Palmitate)	Suspension for oral use Ophthalmic ointment and solutions Otic solution	*Ophthalmic ointment:* small amount in lower conjunctival sac q3–6h *Ophthalmic solutions:* 1–2 drops q3–6h *Otic solution:* 2–3 drops tid PC: C (can cause gray syndrome in premature infants and normal neonates)	Treatment of superficial eye infections and otitis externa
chloramphenicol sodium succinate (Chloromycetin Succinate)	Powder for preparing solutions for IV administration Ophthalmic ointment and solutions Otic solution		
clindamycin (Cleocin)	Capsules and solution for oral use Solution for IM or slow IV injection	*Oral:* adults: 400–1,800 mg/day, in divided doses; children over 1 mo: 15–40 mg/kg/day divided in 3 or 4 doses PC: C	Treatment of septicemia, intra-abdominal infections, pelvic infections, serious infections affecting the skin, soft tissues, and respiratory tract, and bone and joint infections caused by susceptible anaerobes and staphylococci
lincomycin (Lincocin, Lincorex)	Oral capsules Solution for IV infusion	Adults: *Oral:* 1.5–2 g/day, divided in 3 or 4 doses; *IM:* 0.6–1.2 g/day, divided in 2 or 3 doses Children older than 1 mo: *Oral:* 30–60 mg/kg/day, divided in 3 or 4 doses; *IM:* 10–20 mg/kg/day, divided in 1 or 2 doses; *IV:* 10–20 mg/kg/day, divided in 2 or 3 doses PC: B	Treatment of serious respiratory tract, skin, and soft-tissue infections caused by susceptible cocci when other less toxic drugs are contraindicated
spectinomycin (Trobicin)	Vials containing powder for reconstitution for IM administration	Adults: 2 g as a single dose PC: B	Treatment of uncomplicated gonorrhea when penicillin and tetracycline are contraindicated and when resistant strains of pathogens fail to respond to other drugs

KEY: PC = pregnancy category; see Appendix A.

Less serious allergic reactions to chloramphenicol include macular or vesicular skin rashes, fever, and angioedema. All are uncommon. Other adverse reactions include nausea and vomiting, diarrhea, perineal irritation, and an unpleasant taste in the mouth after oral doses. Optic neuritis, superinfection, and inhibition of microsomal enzymes have also been reported.

Premature and newborn infants exposed to chloramphenicol in utero and infants who receive chloramphenicol therapy may develop a type of circulatory collapse known as the gray baby syndrome. Symptoms include failure to feed, abdominal distention, vomiting, pallor, cyanosis, and vasomotor and respiratory collapse. The syndrome usually develops 2 to 9 days after exposure to the drug. Death may occur within a few hours; however, the process may reverse completely if chloramphenicol is discontinued immediately when early symptoms appear. The cause of this toxic reaction is thought to be lack of enzymes for metabolizing the antibiotic and accumulation of drug to excessive blood levels. Inactive metabolites of chloramphenicol accumulate in the tissues of clients with renal insufficiency. The toxic potential of these substances is unknown.

Drug Interactions. Chloramphenicol may inhibit biotransformation and prolong the plasma half-lives of barbiturates, chlorpropamide, anticoagulants, iron salts, phenytoin, and sulfonylureas; dosages of these drugs may need to be reduced during concomitant chloramphenicol therapy. Chloramphenicol serum levels may be decreased by barbiturates. Decreased effects of vitamin B_{12} and cyclophosphamide may result when given with chloramphenicol.

Precautions and Contraindications. Systemic administration of chloramphenicol is contraindicated if alternative agents are available for the effective treatment of the infection. The drug is contraindicated in neonates and persons with a history of allergic hypersensitivity to it. Chloramphenicol therapy should be avoided in persons with anemia and during pregnancy and lactation. Reduced doses must be given to clients with impaired hepatic function, and to those receiving drugs that inhibit the liver microsomal enzymes. Complete blood counts should be carried out regularly during treatment to monitor bone marrow function. Prolonged therapy should be avoided.

∷ SUMMARY

Chloramphenicol is a drug of last resort for the treatment of serious infections that cannot be treated with other antibiotics. The most serious adverse reaction to this drug is bone marrow depression, which can lead to fatal aplastic anemia.

Spectinomycin

Spectinomycin is an antibiotic produced by *Streptomyces spectabilis.*

Pharmacodynamics. Spectinomycin appears to bind to 30S ribosomal subunits, thereby inhibiting bacterial protein synthesis. It acts against a wide variety of gram-positive and gram-negative bacteria but is used almost exclusively in the treatment of gonorrhea caused by penicillinase-producing strains of cocci. Drug resistance has been reported.

Pharmacokinetics. Spectinomycin is not absorbed from the GI tract. The drug is administered IM. It is unknown whether spectinomycin crosses the placenta or distributes into breast milk. Spectinomycin and its active metabolites are primarily excreted in urine by glomerular filtration.

Therapeutic Uses. Spectinomycin is used in the treatment of uncomplicated gonorrhea as an alternative to penicillin.

Adverse Reactions. The most common adverse effect of spectinomycin is pain at the injection site. Nephrotoxic, hepatotoxic, hematologic, and allergic reactions have been reported. Severe reactions are uncommon, however, and the drug is usually well tolerated.

Precautions and Contraindications. Before initiating spectinomycin therapy for gonorrhea, clients should be screened for syphilis. The drug is not an effective treatment for syphilis and may mask its symptoms. If syphilis is present, another agent effective against both diseases must be used.

Spectinomycin should be used with caution in clients with a history of allergies; hypersensitivity to the drug is a contraindication for its use. Safe use of spectinomycin during pregnancy or in infants and children has not been established.

Lincomycin

Lincomycin is an antibiotic produced by a variant of *Streptomyces lincolnensis.*

Pharmacodynamics. Lincomycin inhibits protein synthesis by binding to 50S ribosomal subunits. It is bacteriostatic or bactericidal, depending on the concentration of drug at the site of infection and the susceptibility of the pathogen. Its spectrum of activity is similar to that of clindamycin.

Pharmacokinetics. Lincomycin can be administered orally, although only 20% to 30% of the drug is absorbed from the GI tract. The presence of food both delays and decreases its absorption. The drug is also administered IV and IM. Distribution into body tissues and fluids is widespread. The drug diffuses into peritoneal fluid, pleural fluid, synovial fluid, bone, bile, and the aqueous humor of the eye. It crosses the blood-brain barrier only when the meninges are inflamed, and then only in low concentrations. Distribution into bone also is poor. Lincomycin readily crosses the placenta and appears in breast milk.

Lincomycin is partially metabolized by the liver. The drug is excreted in both urine and feces. A portion of drug is unaccounted for and may be destroyed in the body.

Therapeutic Uses. Lincomycin is used to treat serious coccal infections in persons in whom less toxic antimicrobials (eg, penicillin, erythromycin) are contraindicated.

Adverse Reactions. Adverse reactions to lincomycin resemble those to clindamycin. The drug has also caused hypotension and cardiac arrest.

Drug Interactions. The use of lincomycin with other drugs with neuromuscular blocking properties should be avoided. Concurrent use of kaolin with lincomycin interferes with absorption of the antimicrobial; absorption may be reduced to as little as 10% of a given dose.

Precautions and Contraindications. Lincomycin should be used with caution in clients with a history of GI disease (especially colitis), renal impairment, atopic allergy, and liver impairment. It is contraindicated in persons with allergy to either lincomycin or clindamycin. Safe use during pregnancy has not been established. The drug is not recommended for use in infants. Lincomycin has neuromuscular blocking properties and is used very cautiously in clients with myasthenia gravis.

Clindamycin

Clindamycin is a semisynthetic derivative of lincomycin.

Pharmacodynamics. Clindamycin appears to bind to 50S ribosomal subunits and inhibit peptide bond formation and protein synthesis. It is bacteriostatic or bactericidal, depending on the concentration of drug at the site of infection and the susceptibility of the pathogen. This drug is effective against most aerobic gram-positive cocci and several anaerobic and microaerophilic gram-negative and gram-positive organisms. Natural and acquired resistance to clindamycin and cross-resistance between clindamycin and lincomycin have been demonstrated.

Pharmacokinetics. Clindamycin is well absorbed from the GI tract. The presence of food may delay but does not appreciably decrease absorption. The drug is distributed into many body tissues and fluids but does not readily cross the blood-brain barrier, even when the meninges are inflamed. Clindamycin is distributed to synovial fluid and bone. It readily crosses the placenta and is distributed into breast milk.

Clindamycin is partially metabolized in the liver to both active and inactive metabolites. Excretion of metabolites and active drug is primarily through the kidneys, with a small fraction eliminated in feces. The drug is not dialyzable.

Therapeutic Uses. Clindamycin is used to treat septicemic disease and serious infections caused by susceptible organisms, including those found in skin and soft tissue, in the respiratory system, and in the intra-abdominal system. It is also used as an adjunct in the treatment of chronic bone and joint infections and acute hematogenous osteomyelitis caused by staphylococci.

Adverse Reactions. Adverse GI reactions to clindamycin (nausea, vomiting, diarrhea, abdominal pain) are common and may be severe enough to require termination of drug therapy. This reaction occurs with parenteral and oral administration. Fatal colitis has occurred.

Allergic reactions include generalized rash (the most common adverse reaction), fever, hypotension, polyarthritis, and anaphylaxis. A syndrome resembling Stevens-Johnson syndrome has also occurred.

Clindamycin is an irritating substance and can cause tissue damage when administered parenterally. Other adverse reactions include hepatotoxicity, blood dyscrasias, and superinfection.

Drug Interactions. Because of its nephrotoxic, neurotoxic, and neuromuscular blocking properties, the use of clindamycin with other drugs with these properties should be avoided. Its absorption may be delayed if given with kaolin-pectin.

Precautions and Contraindications. Clindamycin should be used with caution in clients with a history of intestinal disease, especially colitis. Renal and hepatic function should be monitored before and during therapy.

Clindamycin should be used with caution in clients with a history of atopic allergy; the drug is contraindicated in clients with a history of allergy to this drug. Clindamycin has neuromuscular blocking properties, and caution should be used when the drug is administered to clients with myasthenia gravis. Safe use of clindamycin during pregnancy has not been established.

Bibliography

Hardman JG, Limbird LE, Molinoff PB, et al. (1996) *Goodman and Gilman's The pharmacological basis of therapeutics,* 9th ed. New York: McGraw-Hill.

Harvey RA, Champe PC, eds. (1992). *Lippincott's illustrated reviews: Pharmacology.* Philadelphia: JB Lippincott.

Olin BR, ed. (1996). *Facts and Comparisons.* St. Louis: Facts and Comparisons, Inc.

For more information and sample tests and activities, refer to Chapter 42 in the Student Workbook for Clinical Pharmacology and Nursing Management, 5th edition, available through your bookstore.

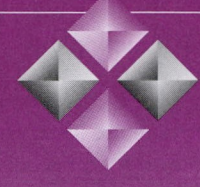

43

Other Antimicrobial Drugs

Until a few years ago, tuberculosis (TB) was considered essentially eradicated, and the time, money, and effort spent on controlling and eliminating it were significantly decreased. However, the presence of a large immunosuppressed population, due in part to the AIDS epidemic, contributed to a resurgence of TB. Persons infected with human immunodeficiency virus (HIV) have a 10% to 40% TB infection rate; those with full-blown AIDS have a TB incidence rate about 500 times that of the general population.

Pathophysiology of Mycobacterial Infections

Tuberculosis is caused by the tubercle bacillus, *Mycobacterium tuberculosis*, a gram-positive, acid-fast (meaning that mycobacteria do not lose their color in acid after staining) organism (Wiseman, 1995). There are about 30 members of the genus *Mycobacterium*. Certain characteristics of *M tuberculosis* are important to diagnosis and the subsequent treatment plan. The bacilli have a slower rate of reproduction than other bacteria, and it may take weeks of growth to produce a visible colony after incubation. This can delay diagnosis and the onset of treatment. The structure of the cell wall of the bacillus makes the organism hydrophobic or insoluble in water. This outer layer of the cell wall contributes to the slow growth rate and protects the organism from many antimicrobial agents. Body macrophages cannot destroy all invading bacilli because of the layer, and the organism may remain viable within macrophages; this is one reason why drug therapy for TB is prolonged.

A competent immune system can halt multiplication and spread of the bacilli within 2 to 10 weeks of initial infection. However, because viable bacilli remain in the host's macrophages in a dormant or latent state, reactivation of the disease is possible. Such hosts cannot transmit TB to others at this time, although they have a positive reaction to a purified protein derivative skin test. Persons with latent TB are at risk of developing active infections and symptomatic TB within their lifetime. Active TB must be considered in any client with an unexplained cough lasting more than 2 to 3 weeks (Leiner & Mays, 1996).

Another source of concern is the increased incidence of drug resistance. Multidrug-resistant TB is resistant to at least isoniazid and rifampin, presenting a major treatment dilemma.

Worldwide, about 12 million people are estimated to have leprosy. Leprosy (Hansen's disease) is similar to tuberculosis in that it is caused by a mycobacterium (*Mycobacterium leprae*), it is a chronic illness requiring years of treatment, and the causative organism tends to become resistant to therapeutic drugs. Although optimal drug combinations and dosages for treating leprosy have yet to be determined, a period of 3 to 5 years of treatment is recommended for active disease, with maintenance drugs given for life in many clients. Medical supervision is required indefinitely to verify that the disease remains arrested.

Other mycobacteria may cause disease in humans. The term "nontuberculous mycobacteria" describes mycobacteria that form colonies atypical of *M tuberculosis*. The prevalence rate has been found to be highest for *Mycobacterium avium* complex (MAC): up to 50% of AIDS victims are expected to have MAC infection at the time of autopsy (Division of Drugs and Toxicology, 1994).

Antimycobacterial Agents

Tuberculosis treatment may be for prevention, for active disease, or for drug-resistant strains. Certain basic principles apply to any drug regimen for TB: the appropriate drugs must be given at proper dosage intervals and for a period sufficient to eliminate all organisms. In 1994, the Centers for Disease Control and Prevention (CDC) recommended an initial drug regimen of at least four drugs: isoniazid, rifampin, pyrazinamide, and either ethambutol or streptomycin. These are considered the first-line TB drugs.

Second-line TB drugs include para-aminosalicylic acid, kanamycin, capreomycin, ethionamide, and cycloserine. Tuberculosis therapy is long term; clients must be monitored throughout treatment because antituberculosis drugs may be toxic and because client adherence needs constant attention.

Isoniazid

Isoniazid, also called INH (Laniazid, Nydrazid), is highly specific against organisms of the genus *Mycobacterium* (Table 43-1).

Pharmacodynamics. Isoniazid is bacteriostatic or bactericidal, depending on the concentration of the drug and the susceptibility of the pathogen. The exact mechanism of action is unknown, but the drug appears to interfere with bacterial metabolism. It changes the acid-fast characteristic of the bacteria, apparently by inhibiting cell wall mycolic acid synthesis. The drug is active primarily against dividing cells.

Pharmacokinetics. Isoniazid is administered both orally and by intramuscular (IM) injection. After absorption, it is distributed into all body tissues and fluids, including cerebrospinal fluid (CSF). Isoniazid readily crosses the placenta and appears in breast milk. Time to peak serum concentration is 1 to 2 hours. Protein binding is less than 10%. Isoniazid is inactivated in the liver primarily by acetylation, a process that is genetically determined. Slow acetylation or inactivation is an autosomal recessive trait that appears in about 50% of the U.S. population. Slow acetylators have a lower level of *N*-acetyl transferase. The rate of acetylation does not significantly affect the efficacy of isoniazid, but slow acetylation may lead to higher blood levels of the drug and thus to an increase in toxic reactions (Division of Drugs and Toxicology, 1994).

Most of the drug is excreted in urine, with small amounts appearing in saliva, sputum, and feces. Isoniazid is removed by both peritoneal dialysis and hemodialysis.

Therapeutic Uses. Isoniazid is used for treating clinical TB and for preventing TB in persons at risk.

Dosage and Administration. Fixed-dose combinations of isoniazid and rifampin (Rifamate) and of isoniazid, rifampin, and pyrazinamide are available (see Table 43-1).

Adverse Reactions. Isoniazid causes a relative deficiency of pyridoxine, evidenced most often by peripheral neuritis. The deficiency probably results from isoniazid's competing for the enzyme apotryptophanase. Concurrent use of pyridoxine (vitamin B_6) 10 to 25 mg can relieve the syndrome, which occurs most often in malnourished, alcoholic, or diabetic clients.

Evidence of liver dysfunction (increased AST level) is reported in 10% to 20% of clients receiving isoniazid. Advancing age and underlying liver disease are predisposing factors. Hepatotoxicity is reversible in most clients. Daily consumption of alcohol increases the risk of isoniazid-related hepatitis during therapy. The drug should be used with caution in patients with underlying liver dysfunction and in those receiving other hepatotoxic drugs.

Other adverse effects include optic neuritis, allergic hypersensitivity (fever, rashes, lymphadenopathy), vasculitis, hematologic reactions, and syndromes resembling systemic lupus erythematosus and rheumatic arthritis. Dry mouth, gastrointestinal (GI) upset, hyperglycemia, metabolic acidosis, urine retention, gynecomastia, seizures, and reversible psychotic episodes have also been reported.

Drug–Drug Interactions. Isoniazid is thought to affect the microsomal enzyme (cytochrome P450) system, so drugs that affect or are affected by this system may interact with isoniazid. There is evidence that inducers of cytochrome P450 (eg, carbamazepine, rifampin, phenobarbital, primidone, alcohol) increase the formation of hepatotoxic metabolites of isoniazid and the subsequent risk of hepatitis.

The use of ketoconazole, miconazole, and acetaminophen also may increase the potential for hepatotoxicity. Concomitant use of anticoagulants may result in enhanced anticoagulant effect due to inhibition of enzymatic metabolism of the anticoagulants. Isoniazid may decrease the hepatic metabolism of diazepam and impair the oxidation of triazolam. Isoniazid inhibits the metabolism of phenytoin, resulting in increased plasma levels, especially in slow acetylators. Concurrent use of these drugs may require a reduction in their dosage. Theophylline plasma concentrations may be increased if isoniazid is used concurrently.

Additive isoniazid-related central nervous system (CNS) effects (dizziness, drowsiness) occur when cycloserine or ethionamide is used with isoniazid. Alu-

Table 43-1. Antimycobacterial Agents

Drug Name	Preparation	Usual Dosage
Primary Antituberculosis Agents		
ethambutol (Myambutol)	Tablets and film-coated tablets for oral use PC: B	Adults: 15–25 mg/kg/day Not recommended for children younger than 13 yr
isoniazid (INH, Laniazid, Nydrazid) *Can:* Rimifan, Isotamine	Oral tablets Powder Solution for IM injection PC: C	Adults: *treatment:* 5 mg/kg/day; *prophylaxis:* 300 mg/day (maximum daily dosage: 300 mg) Infants and children: *treatment:* 10–20 mg/kg/day (maximum daily dosage: 500 mg); *prophylaxis:* 10 mg/kg/day (maximum daily dosage: 300 mg)
rifampin (Rifadin, *Can:* Rofact Rimactane)	Oral tablets Powder for reconstitution for IV administration PC: C	Adults: 600 mg/day Children older than 5 yr: 10–20 mg/kg/day (maximum daily dosage: 600 mg)
Other Antimycobacterial Agents		
Capreomycin sulfate (Capastat)	Vials containing powder for reconstitution for IM administration PC: C	Adults: 15 mg/kg/day (maximum daily dosage: 20 mg/kg/day) Safe use in children has not been established.
cycloserine (Seromycin)	Oral capsules PC: C	Adults: 500 mg–1 g/day, divided in 2 doses (maximum daily dosage: 1 g) Children: 10 mg/kg/day, divided in 2 doses (maximum daily dosage: 500 mg) (However, safe use in children has not been established.)
ethionamide (Trecator S.C.)	Oral tablets PC: D	Adults: 500 mg–1 g/day, divided in 1–3 doses (maximum daily dosage: 1 g) Children: 12–15 mg/kg/day, divided in 3 or 4 doses (maximum daily dosage: 750 mg)
para-aminosalicylic acid/aminosalicylate sodium (Sodium P.A.S.)	Oral tablets	Adults: 10–12 g/day, divided in 2 or 3 doses Children: 200–300 mg/kg/day, divided in 3 or 4 doses
pyrazinamide	Oral tablets PC: C	Adults: 20–35 mg/kg/day divided in 3 or 4 doses (maximum daily dosage: 2 g)
rifabutin (Mycobutin)	Oral capsules PC: B	Adults: 300 mg/day
Antileprosy Agents		
clofazimine (Lamprene)	Oral capsules PC: C	Adults: *for dapsone-resistant leprosy:* 100 mg/day with meals, combined with one or more antileprosy drugs for 3 years, then 100 mg/day; *for erythema nodosum leprosum reactions:* 200 mg/day, taper to 100 mg/day
dapsone/DDS	Oral tablets PC: A	Adults: 50–100 mg/day Children: 1–1.5 mg/kg/day

KEY: PC = pregnancy risk category; see Appendix A.
Can = Canadian

minum-containing antacids decrease the absorption of isoniazid. In addition, concurrent use of prednisolone and possibly other corticosteroids may increase their hepatic metabolism or excretion, resulting in decreased plasma concentrations and effectiveness.

Drug–Food Interactions. Isoniazid is closely related to monoamine oxidase inhibitors (MAOIs), so ingestion of certain fish, cheeses, or other foods containing tyra-

mine may induce a typical tyramine syndrome reaction (see Chap. 6).

Precautions and Contraindications. Vision and liver function should be monitored regularly during isoniazid therapy. Safe use during pregnancy has not been established. The drug should be used with caution in clients with liver dysfunction and in those receiving other neurotoxic or hepatotoxic drugs.

Rifampin

Rifampin (Rifadin, Rimactane), a semisynthetic derivative of rifamycin B, has a wide spectrum of action and is active against mycobacteria and many gram-positive and gram-negative bacteria.

Pharmacodynamics. Rifampin may be bacteriostatic or bactericidal, depending on the concentration of the drug and the susceptibility of the pathogen. It is most active against dividing cells but has some effect during the resting stage. It acts by binding to DNA-dependent RNA polymerase, inhibiting the attachment of the enzyme to DNA and resulting in a block of RNA transcription. Its action causes suppression of RNA synthesis and, therefore, protein synthesis.

Mycobacterial resistance can develop rapidly when the drug is used alone; combination therapy reduces its development. Bacterial resistance to rifampin results from production of an altered form of RNA polymerase.

Pharmacokinetics. Rifampin is administered orally and is widely distributed into most body tissues and fluids, including the CSF. The drug crosses the placenta and is secreted into breast milk. It is about 80% protein bound. Peak serum levels are reached in 1.5 to 4 hours. Rifampin is metabolized in the liver. The drug and its metabolite are excreted mainly in bile, and 60% to 65% of the dose appears in feces. Up to 33% of a dose is eliminated in urine as parent drug. Dialysis does not remove appreciable amounts of the drug.

Therapeutic Uses. Rifampin is used in treating active TB and other mycobacterial diseases. On an investigational basis, it is used to treat leprosy. Resistant strains of *M leprae* may appear in 3 to 4 years when rifampin is used alone, so it generally is part of a triple-drug treatment regimen (dapsone, rifampin, clofazimine).

Dosage and Administration. Oral and intravenous (IV) forms are available. For clinical TB, adults take 600 mg once daily. The dose for children is 10 mg/kg per day. The drug should be given in a single dose 1 hour before or 2 hours after a meal.

Adverse Reactions. The most common adverse reactions to rifampin are GI disturbances. Aching muscles and joints and leg cramps occur occasionally, especially early in treatment. Hypersensitivity reactions have been reported.

Jaundice with laboratory evidence of obstructive liver dysfunction may develop; it may be alleviated by reducing the dose. If symptoms and signs of hepatitis also occur, the drug should be discontinued. Hepatitis occurs less commonly with rifampin than with isoniazid. Daily use of alcohol may increase the incidence of rifampin-induced hepatotoxicity and the metabolism of rifampin.

Rifampin and its metabolites impart a reddish-orange color to urine, feces, saliva, sweat, and tears.

There may be permanent discoloration of soft contact lenses in clients taking this drug.

Intermittent treatment with large doses or interruptions in treatment have been accompanied by a serious reaction that may be immunologic in origin. The syndrome includes flulike symptoms with dyspnea, sometimes wheezing, purpura associated with thrombocytopenia, and leukopenia.

Drug–Drug Interactions. Rifampin is a potent inducer of microsomal enzymes, particularly cytochrome P450. It tends to increase dosage requirements of the interactant agent. Interactions have been reported with anticoagulants, oral contraceptives, methadone and other narcotic analgesics, nonopioid analgesics, sulfonylureas, barbiturates, glucocorticoids, quinidine, digoxin, digitoxin, theophylline, cyclosporine, chloramphenicol, beta blockers, verapamil, diltiazem, nifedipine, haloperidol, ciprofloxacin, diazepam, clofibrate, progestins, disopyramide, mexiletine, and phenytoin and other anticonvulsants. Clients should use an alternative contraceptive method while using rifampin if they have been taking oral contraceptives.

Blood levels of rifampin are increased by concurrent use of probenecid. With the usual dosages in short-term regimens, there appears to be no increased risk of hepatitis when rifampin and isoniazid are given together.

Drug–Food Interactions. Food interferes with the rate and extent of absorption.

Precautions and Contraindications. Clients receiving rifampin should be monitored for impaired liver function and symptoms resembling viral hepatitis. The daily dosage regimen must be maintained because the drug is not as effective when administered intermittently. Allergic hypersensitivity to rifampin or to any of the rifamycins is a contraindication to use of the drug.

Pyrazinamide

Pyrazinamide is a synthetic compound derived from niacinamide.

Pharmacodynamics. *M tuberculosis* strains susceptible to pyrazinamide produce the enzyme pyrazinamidase; the enzyme is absent in resistant strains. Pyrazinamide itself is inactive, but it is transformed by pyrazinamidase to the active compound. Its activity depends on unfavorable acidic conditions in the macrophages. It is bacteriostatic and can be used only in combination with other antituberculosis agents. Adding pyrazinamide to treatment regimens involving isoniazid and rifampin reduces the treatment period needed.

Pharmacokinetics. Pyrazinamide is administered orally and is well absorbed from the GI tract, reaching its peak effect in 2 hours. The drug is widely distributed into body tissues and fluids, including the CSF. Protein binding is low. The half-life is 9 to 10 hours, and excretion is primarily via the kidney. It is unknown if the drug crosses the placenta or enters breast milk.

Therapeutic Uses. Pyrazinamide is used in treating active TB.

Adverse Reactions. Hepatotoxicity may be a factor in pyrazinamide use, so liver function tests should be monitored before therapy and periodically during treatment.

The most common adverse effect is nongouty polyarthralgia. Pyrazinamide inhibits the renal excretion of urates and causes hyperuricemia. Baseline serum uric acid levels should be determined, and the drug should be discontinued if acute gouty arthritis develops. Other adverse reactions include hypersensitivity reactions, acne, photosensitivity, and GI disturbances.

Drug–Laboratory Test Interactions. Pyrazinamide reportedly interferes with Acetest and Ketostix urine tests to produce a pink-brown color.

Precautions and Contraindications. Liver function tests and uric acid levels should be monitored before pyrazinamide therapy begins and periodically during treatment. Caution should be used when the drug is administered to clients with renal failure or a history of gout, porphyria, or diabetes. Severe hepatic impairment is a contraindication for use.

Ethambutol Hydrochloride

Ethambutol (Myambutol) is a primary antituberculosis agent.

Pharmacodynamics. Ethambutol's exact mechanism of action is unknown, but the drug appears to inhibit the synthesis of cell metabolites, which inhibits cell metabolism and results in cell death. Its effects may be mediated through interference with RNA synthesis.

Pharmacokinetics. After oral administration, ethambutol is well absorbed from the GI tract, reaching peak effect in 2 to 4 hours. It is widely distributed into most body tissues and fluids. Protein binding is only 20% to 30%. The drug is secreted in breast milk.

Ethambutol is partially inactivated in the liver, with the unchanged drug and its metabolites excreted in urine. Unabsorbed ethambutol remaining in the GI tract is excreted in feces. The drug is removed by peritoneal dialysis and to a lesser extent by hemodialysis.

Therapeutic Uses. Ethambutol is used to treat active TB. It is especially useful in combination with other antimycobacterial agents for treating clients who may have contracted a resistant strain of *Mycobacterium* and for retreating clients whose initial course of medication did not fully arrest the disease.

Dosage and Administration. A typical dose is 15 to 25 mg/kg given once daily. The drug should be used cautiously and at lower doses in clients with impaired renal function.

Adverse Reactions. The most important adverse reaction to ethambutol is ocular toxicity, which appears to be dose-related. The visual changes, which generally are reversible, include decreased visual acuity, loss of color discrimination, and constriction of visual fields. A complete ophthalmologic examination might be recommended to establish a baseline before beginning treatment, but regular ophthalmologic examinations are unnecessary during treatment with lower doses unless the client complains of blurred or faded vision or other symptoms.

Other adverse effects of ethambutol include GI disturbances, rashes or more serious lesions, and CNS effects such as headache and mental acuity changes.

Drug Interactions. Absorption of ethambutol is decreased when drugs containing aluminum are given concurrently.

Precautions and Contraindications. Vision should be examined monthly during ethambutol therapy for clients receiving more than 15 mg/kg daily. Renal, hepatic, and hematopoietic function must also be monitored. The drug must be used with caution in persons with ocular defects and impaired renal function. Optic neuritis and allergic hypersensitivity are contraindications for use. Safe use during pregnancy has not been established.

Streptomycin

Streptomycin was the first chemotherapeutic agent of undisputed efficacy in treating TB. It must be administered parenterally. As an aminoglycoside, it is discussed in detail in Chapter 42. Streptomycin is often used in the initial treatment of TB in acute care settings. It is bactericidal for the tubercle bacilli, probably through action on the bacterial ribosome to inhibit protein synthesis. Ototoxicity is the most serious adverse reaction.

Rifabutin

In 1992, rifabutin (Mycobutin) was approved for use.

Pharmacodynamics. Rifabutin inhibits DNA-dependent RNA polymerase activity in susceptible strains of bacteria.

Pharmacokinetics. Rifabutin is absorbed after oral administration and reaches a peak of activity in 3.3 to 4 hours. It is excreted in urine (53%), primarily as metabolites, and in feces (30%). Clients with compromised renal function may have reduced drug distribution and faster elimination, resulting in decreased drug concentrations.

Therapeutic Uses. Rifabutin is used to prevent disseminated MAC disease in clients with advanced HIV infection. Rifabutin prophylaxis must not be administered to clients with active TB because it is likely to lead to TB that is resistant to both rifabutin and rifampin. Clients who need prophylaxis against both *M tuberculosis* and MAC may be given isoniazid and rifabutin concurrently.

Dosage and Administration. The typical dosage is 300 mg orally daily in single or two equal doses. It should be given on an empty stomach unless GI upset is severe.

Adverse Reactions. Adverse effects include anorexia, nausea, and other GI effects and hematologic effects such as eosinophilia, thrombocytopenia, and transient leukopenia. Like rifampin, rifabutin may color body fluids reddish-orange, and soft contact lenses may be permanently discolored.

Drug–Drug Interactions. Drug interaction has been reported between rifabutin and zidovudine and didanosine. Rifabutin does not appear to affect the inhibition of HIV by zidovudine, but it decreases plasma levels of zidovudine. Rifabutin, like rifampin, may decrease the efficacy of oral contraceptives. Rifabutin has liver enzyme-inducing properties but appears to be a less potent enzyme inducer than rifampin.

Drug–Food Interactions. High-fat meals slow the rate but not the extent of absorption.

Precautions and Contraindications. Rifabutin should not be given to clients who have active TB or an allergy to rifampin.

Kanamycin

Kanamycin, an aminoglycoside, is discussed in Chapter 42. In unlabeled use, it is part of a multiple-drug regimen for MAC.

Aminosalicylate Sodium

Aminosalicylate sodium is the sodium salt of para-aminosalicylate sodium (PAS).

Pharmacodynamics. PAS is thought to suppress the growth and reproduction of tubercle bacilli by competitively inhibiting the formation of folic acid. The drug is a highly specific agent, acting only against *M tuberculosis*, but it is much less effective than other antimycobacterial agents.

Pharmacokinetics. PAS is absorbed from the GI tract and distributed widely throughout the body, although it reaches low concentrations in the CSF. It exhibits low protein binding. The half-life is about 1 hour. It undergoes hepatic metabolism and is excreted in urine. Excretion is slowed in the presence of renal dysfunction. Small amounts of the drug are distributed into breast milk. It is unknown if PAS crosses the placenta.

Therapeutic Uses. PAS is used in treating clinical TB. When included in a regimen with isoniazid and rifampin, it may delay the development of resistance to these drugs.

Dosage and Administration. A typical dosage is 12 to 16 g/day in two or three divided doses. If powder or tablets, or solutions made with them, have a brown or purple tint, the product has deteriorated and should be discarded. Most of the GI effects are increased when the drug is taken on an empty stomach. Taking the drug after meals or with 10 or 15 mL of aluminum hydroxide may reduce GI irritation.

Adverse Reactions. The most common adverse effects of PAS are nausea, vomiting, diarrhea, anorexia, and abdominal pain. Hypersensitivity reactions may occur, usually between the second and seventh week of drug administration. Liver dysfunction, including hepatitis, may occur. A goiter may result from high-dose therapy.

Drug Interactions. Probenecid and sulfinpyrazone inhibit the renal tubular excretion of PAS; concomitant use of probenecid is not recommended, and the dose of PAS may have to be reduced during and after sulfinpyrazone therapy. The action of oral anticoagulants may be enhanced by this agent because of decreased hepatic synthesis of procoagulant factors.

Absorption of rifampin may be impaired by concurrent use of PAS, resulting in decreased serum concentrations of rifampin. The two drugs should be administered at least 6 hours apart.

Oral absorption of digoxin may be reduced, so digoxin doses may need to be increased.

The absorption of vitamin B_{12} from the GI tract may be impaired by concurrent use of PAS, and parenteral vitamin B_{12} may be required.

A cumulative effect of GI irritation occurs if PAS is administered with aspirin or aspirin-like drugs.

Precautions and Contraindications. Caution must be used when the drug is given to persons with renal or hepatic impairment or gastric ulcer. PAS contains considerable sodium (54.5 mg sodium per 500-mg tablet) and may not be tolerated by clients with congestive heart failure or other conditions requiring reduced sodium intake. Allergic hypersensitivity is a contraindication for its use.

Capreomycin Sulfate

Capreomycin (Capastat Sulfate) is an antibiotic derived from a strain of *Streptomyces capreolus*.

Pharmacodynamics. Capreomycin has a bacteriostatic action by an unknown mechanism. Its spectrum of activity includes *M tuberculosis*, *Mycobacterium bovis*, and *Mycobacterium kansasii*. It is less toxic and somewhat more bacteriostatic than kanamycin. It approaches streptomycin's therapeutic efficacy and is useful in clients with streptomycin-resistant tubercle bacilli.

Pharmacokinetics. Because it is not absorbed well from the GI tract, capreomycin is administered IM. Peak serum concentrations are achieved in 1 to 2 hours, and the half-life is 3 to 6 hours. It crosses the placenta but not the blood-brain barrier. An insignificant amount is metabolized, and the drug is eliminated unchanged in urine.

Therapeutic Uses. Capreomycin is used in treating clinical TB and other mycobacterial diseases. It is used when the primary agents cannot be used because of toxicity or the presence of resistant bacilli.

Dosage and Administration. Resistance may develop if the drug is used alone, so it is given with other antimycobacterial drugs. It is given by deep IM injection. A typical regimen is 15 mg/kg daily for 2 to 4 months, and then two or three times weekly for 6 to 12 months or longer. It takes 2 to 3 minutes for complete dissolution when preparing the solution from the powder. In clients with impaired renal function, capreomycin is cumulative, so reduced doses are required.

Adverse Reactions. The most serious adverse reactions to capreomycin are nephrotoxicity and ototoxicity. Both the auditory and vestibular portions of the eighth cranial nerve are affected. Prompt discontinuation of the drug usually results in reversal of these effects, but permanent deafness has occurred. Renal damage is manifested by elevated blood urea nitrogen levels, decreased creatinine clearance, albuminuria, and cylindruria. Renal abnormalities usually disappear on medication discontinuation.

Hypokalemia is a significant but uncommon adverse reaction. Eosinophilia often occurs during treatment. Occasionally leukocytosis, leukopenia, and thrombocytopenia are seen.

Local reactions at the site of injection may include pain, induration, and sterile abscess, especially if deep IM technique is not followed. Injection sites should be rotated.

Drug–Drug Interactions. The nephrotoxic or ototoxic effects of capreomycin could be enhanced by other nephrotoxic or ototoxic drugs (eg, aminoglycosides). Neuromuscular blockade may be enhanced, with resulting skeletal muscle weakness and respiratory depression or paralysis, if neuromuscular blocking agents are used concurrently with capreomycin.

Drug–Laboratory Test Interactions. Abnormal liver function tests have occurred in clients taking the drug along with other antimycobacterial agents. BSP and PSP excretion tests may be decreased.

Precautions and Contraindications. Caution should be used when administering capreomycin to clients with renal insufficiency or auditory impairment. Renal, auditory, and vestibular function should be monitored before and at regular intervals during therapy. Reduced dosage is required for clients with impaired renal function. Capreomycin is contraindicated in clients allergic to it; caution should be used in clients with a history of allergic reaction, especially to drugs. Safe use in children has not been established.

Cycloserine

Cycloserine (Seromycin) is a derivative of *Streptomyces* cultures and is also produced synthetically.

Pharmacodynamics. Cycloserine acts both as a bacteriostatic and bactericidal agent, depending on serum concentrations. It competitively inhibits an enzyme and interferes with an early step in cell wall synthesis.

Pharmacokinetics. Cycloserine is well absorbed from the GI tract and is widely distributed into body tissues and fluids (including CSF). Peak blood levels occur in 4 to 8 hours. About 66% of a dose is eliminated unchanged in the urine. The drug readily crosses the placenta and appears in breast milk.

Therapeutic Uses. Cycloserine is used in treating active pulmonary and extrapulmonary TB when treatment with the primary antimycobacterial drugs has been inadequate.

Dosage and Administration. The usual dose is 250 mg twice daily at 12-hour intervals for the first 2 weeks and then may be increased by 250 mg/day every few days as tolerated and required. Best results occur with peak serum concentrations of 25 to 30 mcg/mL; blood levels should be monitored during therapy. Serum levels above 30 mcg/mL have been associated with adverse reactions. Cycloserine should be administered with other effective antimycobacterial agents.

Adverse Reactions. Cycloserine is toxic to the CNS and causes neurologic and psychic adverse reactions. Pyridoxine has been administered concurrently, but its value has not been proved (as it has with isoniazid). Neurologic reactions vary from muscle twitching to seizures. Psychic disturbances range from nervousness to frank psychotic episodes. These psychic reactions are usually reversible, but close observation of the client is necessary because suicide has occasionally occurred during this drug-induced psychotic disturbance. Chlorpromazine has been used to treat psychotic disturbances.

Drug Interactions. Cycloserine should not be given with isoniazid or ethionamide because of potential additive CNS toxicity. Concurrent use of alcoholic beverages is contraindicated because alcohol can worsen CNS toxicity.

Precautions and Contraindications. Dosage should be reduced or the drug discontinued if symptoms of neurotoxicity appear. Administration of pyridoxine (100–300 mg) may prevent or alleviate these adverse reactions. Sedatives and anticonvulsants are useful in treating toxicity.

Cycloserine is contraindicated in clients with a history of mental depression, psychosis, anxiety reactions, or seizures. It should not be administered to persons who frequently drink alcohol, those with severe renal disease, and those who have an allergic hypersensitivity to it.

Ethionamide

Ethionamide (Trecator), a derivative of isonicotinic acid, is related chemically to isoniazid.

Pharmacodynamics. Ethionamide acts both as a bacteriostatic and bactericidal agent, depending on serum concentrations. It appears to inhibit peptide synthesis in mycobacteria.

Pharmacokinetics. Ethionamide is well absorbed from the GI tract and is widely distributed into body tissues and fluids (including the CSF). It crosses the placenta. Peak effect is reached in about 3 hours. Ethionamide is extensively metabolized to both active and inactive metabolites. It is excreted by the kidneys.

Therapeutic Uses. Ethionamide is effective against both *M tuberculosis* and *M kansasii* and is indicated in TB after therapeutic failure with the primary drugs. It is also used in treating leprosy on an investigational basis; for example, it may be substituted for clofazimine when dapsone, clofazimine, and rifampin are used for multibacillary leprosy.

Dosage and Administration. Ethionamide is administered orally and is rapidly absorbed from the GI tract. For TB, the usual dosage is 0.5 to 1 g daily in one to three doses after meals. Some prefer a single dose after the evening meal or at bedtime; if tolerated, therapeutic effect is more likely with this method because it results in higher serum concentrations.

Ethionamide is about 10% as active as isoniazid and should be administered with other effective antimycobacterial drugs. Its usefulness in TB has been limited because many clients cannot tolerate therapeutic doses.

Adverse Reactions. The most common adverse effects are GI disturbances, including anorexia, nausea, vomiting, diarrhea, salivation, and metallic taste. They are dose-related and are thought to be caused by CNS action rather than direct gastric irritation. Neurotoxic effects include peripheral neuritis; like isoniazid, ethionamide may act as a pyridoxine antagonist or increase the renal excretion of pyridoxine. Neurotoxic effects may be prevented or relieved by administering pyridoxine.

Hepatotoxic reactions include transient increases in hepatic enzymes and hepatitis. Hepatotoxicity is generally reversible if drug therapy is discontinued. Hepato-

toxicity is the major adverse effect of ethionamide in clients with leprosy.

Precautions and Contraindications. Liver function should be monitored before and regularly during treatment. The drug is contraindicated in clients with severe liver impairment and those allergic to it. Safe use during pregnancy and in children has not been established.

Dapsone

Dapsone is a synthetic sulfone.

Pharmacodynamics. Dapsone inhibits the synthesis of folic acid and is principally bacteriostatic in clients with leprosy. The mechanism of action in dermatitis herpetiformis has not been established.

Pharmacokinetics. Dapsone is well absorbed from the GI tract. Time to peak effect is 4 to 8 hours. The drug is 50% bound to plasma protein. It is distributed to most tissues and enters the enterohepatic cycle. It does not penetrate the eye well, a matter of concern because eye lesions can occur in leprosy. The drug is secreted in breast milk.

Therapeutic Uses. Dapsone, in conjunction with rifampin or clofazimine or both, is the drug of choice for treating leprosy. Other therapeutic uses are palliative treatment of dermatitis herpetiformis and treatment of malaria (in conjunction with pyrimethamine). Dapsone has recently been used alone or with trimethoprim for treating *Pneumocystis carinii* pneumonia.

Dosage and Administration. The usual dose is 1 to 2 mg/kg daily. It is usually given with other antileprosy drugs, commonly rifampin and clofazimine.

Adverse Reactions. Adverse reactions are usually mild at the doses used to treat leprosy. The major adverse reactions are dose-related hemolytic anemias. Many clients receiving 100 mg/day experience an increased rate of erythrocyte destruction. Complete blood counts should be performed weekly during the first month of treatment, monthly for 6 months, and periodically thereafter. Deaths from agranulocytosis, aplastic anemia, and other blood dyscrasias have occurred. Clients with glucose-6-phosphate dehydrogenase (G6PD) deficiency are most at risk for these problems; clients should be screened for G6PD deficiency before therapy begins.

A hypersensitivity reaction, called the sulfone syndrome, occurs rarely and begins 1 to 4 weeks after the onset of dapsone use. It is characterized by fever, malaise, exfoliative dermatitis, jaundice with hepatic necrosis, lymphadenopathy, methemoglobinemia, and anemia. The condition improves when dapsone is discontinued and corticosteroids are used.

Other adverse effects include peripheral neuropathy with paresthesias and phototoxicity.

Drug–Drug Interactions. Rifampin lowers dapsone levels by increasing its plasma clearance, so larger-than-usual doses of dapsone may be required. Oral probenecid decreases the urinary excretion of dapsone and its metabolites; when the two drugs are administered concurrently, the dosage of dapsone should be reduced to avoid toxicity.

Precautions and Contraindications. Pretreatment with ascorbic acid, folate, and iron helps prevent blood changes caused by the drug. If a reactional state is severe or accompanied by neuritis, the client is hospitalized and given corticosteroids. Erythema nodosum leprosum reactions include severe skin lesions and other symptoms and appear to result from the action of circulating immune complexes on locally sensitized tissues. They are treated with analgesics, steroids, and (in countries where the drug is approved) thalidomide. Dapsone is contraindicated in clients allergic to the drug or to other dapsone derivatives (eg, sulfoxone sodium).

Clofazimine

Clofazimine (Lamprene) is a dye that is effective against various mycobacteria.

Pharmacodynamics. The precise mechanisms of action of clofazimine are unknown, but it appears to bind preferentially to mycobacterial DNA and to inhibit mycobacterial replication and growth. In addition, it exhibits both antiinflammatory and immunosuppressive effects; it appears to enhance neutrophil and macrophage phagocytosis.

Pharmacokinetics. Clofazimine is retained in the human body for about 70 days, tending to be deposited in fatty tissue and cells of the reticuloendothelial system. It does not show cross-resistance with dapsone or rifampin.

Therapeutic Uses. Clofazimine is useful in treating leprosy, including dapsone-resistant disease. The World Health Organization recommends treating multibacillary leprosy with a regimen of dapsone, clofazimine, and rifampin. Clofazimine is also used for lepromatous leprosy complicated by erythema nodosum leprosum. It has also had some success in a limited number of clients with inflammatory or pustular dermatoses.

An unlabeled application is its use with other antimycobacterial agents in treating pulmonary and extrapulmonary MAC infections, including those in AIDS clients.

Dosage and Administration. Depending on the condition for which it is being used, the dosage is 50 mg once daily and 300 mg once monthly (multibacillary leprosy) or 100 mg one to three times daily (MAC infections).

Adverse Reactions. Clofazimine is usually well tolerated in dosages of 100 mg daily or less. However, crystals of the drug are distributed to and accumulate in tissues and fluids, particularly the skin, eyes, and GI tract. GI effects are the major dose-limiting adverse effects and appear dose-related. In clients receiving 300 mg or more daily, a syndrome has been noted that includes colicky abdominal pain, persistent diarrhea, and weight loss. Partial or complete bowel obstruction may then occur, exploratory laparotomies have been done, and fatalities have been reported.

Clofazimine discolors the skin (pink to red-brown to black) in 75% to 100% of clients. Skin discoloration usually is evident 1 to 4 weeks after therapy begins and gradually disappears within 6 to 12 months (or longer) after the drug is discontinued. During therapy, leprosy nodules may be replaced by scar tissue in the form of shiny, jet-black macules. Other effects include ichthyosis, dry skin, rash, and pruritus. Reversible, dose-related, red-brown discoloration of the conjunctiva, cornea, and lacrimal fluid may occur. Other ophthalmic effects include dryness, burning, itching, irritation, and watering of the eye, but visual acuity is seldom affected.

Drug Interactions. Concurrent administration of dapsone may inhibit the antiinflammatory activity of clofazimine, which may then adversely affect the efficacy of clofazimine in erythema nodosum leprosum reactions. Nevertheless, it is suggested that treatment with both drugs should continue. Concurrent use of clofazimine and isoniazid may result in increased plasma and urinary concentrations of clofazimine and decreased concentration of clofazimine in the skin.

Clofazimine decreases rifampin bioavailability, so clients should be monitored for decreased effectiveness when using rifampin and clofazimine concurrently.

Precautions and Contraindications. The client should be monitored for depression if skin discoloration occurs. It may take months or years before discoloration disappears.

▪ SUMMARY

Antimycobacterial anti-infective agents are used for controlling mycobacterial diseases such as TB and leprosy. To prevent resistance from developing in mycobacterial pathogens, the drugs are usually given concurrently in combinations of two or more. Treatment is prolonged. Antimycobacterial drugs are relatively toxic and may impair hearing or vision and cause hepatotoxicity, nephrotoxicity, and CNS changes.

❖ NURSING MANAGEMENT: CLIENT RECEIVING ANTIMYCOBACTERIAL ANTI-INFECTIVES

Successful treatment of both TB and leprosy hinges on the client's willingness to adhere to a lengthy and strict multidrug treatment regimen.

NURSING PROCESS

ASSESSMENT

Before antimycobacterial therapy begins, a complete history should be taken and a physical examination performed. Particular attention should be paid to factors indicating renal or liver impairment, cardiovascular disease, gastric ulcer, or chronic substance abuse. For women of childbearing age, reproductive status (pregnancy or lactation) should be determined. This information will help the prescriber select the safest agents for the drug regimen.

The physical examination should include assessment of respiratory status and characteristics of breathing. Any cough should be described in detail, and the color, amount, and consistency of secretions should be assessed. Sputum specimens should be obtained for culture and sensitivity studies. The client's admission weight is important, as are laboratory test findings that determine nutritional status (eg, serum albumin and protein, white blood cell count, glucose level).

A complete drug history must be taken, with specific attention given to any allergies to drugs and previous antimycobacterial therapy. All drugs currently used, including social drugs such as alcohol and nicotine, should be identified. Many medications interact with the antimycobacterial drugs. Smoking is harmful to clients being treated for TB because of its toxic effect on the lungs, the organs most often affected by the disease. Alcohol impairs liver function and potentiates the hepatotoxic and neurotoxic effects of some antimycobacterials.

The social circumstances of the client's life should also be evaluated. Treatment of mycobacterial infections generally requires lengthy therapy using multiple drugs. Consequently, the more stable the client's lifestyle, the more likely it is that therapy will be successful. Many people suffering from TB lack family or social support or are homeless or disadvantaged. Conditions of poverty contribute to active infection, reactivation of arrested infection, and treatment failure in both TB and leprosy. For some, the cost of medications is a barrier to treatment. All such issues must be addressed before clients are released from the acute care setting.

The nurse should explore the client's knowledge of and psychological reaction to the diagnosis, keeping in mind that some cultural groups attach a stigma to TB. Such a client may be blamed for the illness or labeled "unclean" or "sinful" and may experience periods of depression, denial, and isolation. This discouragement may be compounded by the responses of others who act out of fear or ignorance.

NURSING DIAGNOSIS
Diagnoses related to antimycobacterial drug therapy may include:

- Altered Nutrition, Less Than Body Requirements, related to GI complaints secondary to drug therapy, pyridoxine deficiency, and anorexia secondary to fever and coughing
- Anxiety, related to drug effects and diagnosis
- Ineffective Individual Management of Therapeutic Regimen: Noncompliance, related to complexity of drug regimen

- Knowledge Deficit, related to lack of familiarity with drug therapy and disease process

A common collaborative problem that should be differentiated from the nursing diagnoses is:

Potential Complication: Adverse effects of medication

PLANNING
Goals are to promote and maintain an effective breathing pattern, promote and maintain optimal nutritional status, reduce anxiety, encourage adherence to the treatment regimen, prevent spread of disease, increase the client's knowledge about therapy, reduce the risk of adverse reaction to medications, and detect and treat any adverse reactions promptly. See the Example of Nursing Process for Pyridoxine Deficiency from Isoniazid Therapy.

INTERVENTION
In the acute care setting, anyone suspected of having TB is assigned to a TB isolation room, which has negative pressure relative to other rooms in the facility (air flows into—not out of—the room when the door opens). The door must remain closed, and traffic into and out of the room must be minimized. A client with infectious TB may be discharged home after starting drug therapy. However, a client with multidrug-resistant TB may remain hospitalized and in isolation for longer periods.

At home, the client while contagious should have a separate room, away from others. He or she should eat, sleep, and remain in that room as much as possible. If it is not too cold outside, windows should stay open. Placing a fan in the window to blow air to the outside atmosphere helps decrease the number of TB bacilli floating in the room air. This decreases the risk of infecting others.

Optimal immune system function is a crucial factor in treating mycobacterial infections. The nurse should explore the client's health habits and help him or her enhance natural resistance to infection. Particular attention should be paid to nutrition, rest, and stress management. A high-protein, high-calorie diet and nutritional supplements are needed. Fluid intake should be encouraged to help liquefy secretions for easy expectoration. If isoniazid is prescribed, the prescriber should be consulted about supplementary pyridoxine, and the client should be monitored for early signs and symptoms of vitamin B_6 deficiency.

Clients with mycobacterial infections need emotional support during treatment. Historically, leprosy has been considered an incurable and loathsome disease and TB a scourge that has killed and incapacitated people through the ages. HIV-positive and AIDS clients justifiably fear the impact of these infections. Although antimycobacterial drugs have improved the outlook for these conditions, treatment requires years of medication. A return to health is only an arrest of the disease, not a cure. The microorganisms often remain in the

Example of Nursing Process for Pyridoxine Deficiency From Isoniazid Therapy

The client is a 45-year-old secretary. A month before this visit, she had been placed on a preventive regimen of isoniazid because of exposure to active TB and a positive tine test. (A tine test performed 5 years earlier had a negative result.)

The client is knowledgeable about TB and the hygienic measures necessary to support and enhance natural resistance to infection. She has had no signs or symptoms of active TB (cough, purulent sputum, fevers, fatigue).

The client has had some unusual sensations in her legs (prickling, mild pain), especially on weekends when she takes long walks.

Assessment Data

Isoniazid therapy
Leg pain and paresthesias

Nursing Diagnosis	Intervention	Goals and Outcomes
Pain: Leg pain and paresthesia related to pyridoxine deficiency secondary to isoniazid therapy	**Inform** the client that leg pains could be an adverse reaction to the isoniazid medication; advise her to report this symptom to the prescriber.	Within 1 month the client will no longer experience abnormal sensations, because additional B_6 will alleviate pyridoxine deficiency.
	Inform the client that isoniazid can cause such a reaction because it increases the body's need for pyridoxine (vitamin B_6).	
	Advise the client that pyridoxine supplements are usually prescribed to alleviate this type of reaction to isoniazid; recommend that she take additional vitamin B_6 while on isoniazid medication.	
Risk for Altered Health Maintenance, related to lack of knowledge of the TB disease process and the therapeutic regimen required to treat it	**Teach** the client the benefits of drug therapy, and the importance of therapeutic adherence.	The client will remain free of signs and symptoms of TB.
	Explain the adverse reactions that may occur, stressing the signs and symptoms that should be reported to the healthcare provider.	
	Help the client develop a drug dosage schedule that fits into her lifestyle.	

body, sealed off and inactive but capable of causing renewed infection should the host's defenses be depleted. When clients are hospitalized, anxiety is heightened, especially if isolation precautions are imposed. Stress levels must be controlled because undue stress impairs the immune and inflammatory responses.

The nurse or appropriate others must report all new or suspected TB infections to the local health department, which has the ultimate responsibility for ensuring that TB does not spread to others (Wiseman, 1995). Laws in every state require reporting TB cases, and laboratories must promptly report all positive TB cultures and smears, as well as all results of drug susceptibility tests. Clients then are interviewed by health department personnel; a list of contacts at risk is compiled, and the contacts are notified and interviewed. To promote adherence to the treatment regimen, the nurse may need to refer clients for the support services of social agencies and the health department, because the socioeconomic conditions that predispose many to TB infection also preclude adherence.

Hospitalized clients are likely to receive parenteral drugs. IV infusions should be closely regulated to control the rate and prevent rapid administration. IM injections are likely to cause acute discomfort at the site. Ice packs may be applied to prevent and relieve the pain, because cold has a numbing effect.

During treatment, clients must be closely supervised and evaluated for adverse reactions. Periodic monitoring of certain laboratory values is usually part of the evaluation for adverse drug reactions. If the client reports symptoms of adverse effects, further laboratory testing may be needed to ensure that the client is on the safest drug regimen possible.

Client Education. Most clients need careful instruction to manage their therapeutic regimens safely and effectively. When developing a teaching plan, the nurse should consider the client's knowledge of and feelings about the diagnosis. Misconceptions should be corrected. To protect family members or other close contacts, all must understand the principles of disease transmission and control. As long as clients require isolation, family members must be included in teaching to promote adherence to drug therapy and infection control and isolation measures. The nurse may even need to teach the client how to cover the nose and mouth with tissues while coughing or sneezing and how to dispose of tissues in appropriate receptacles. Some clients may need to learn how to apply and wear a surgical mask. The family must understand the reasons for infection control measures and the treatment regimen.

Close contacts of the client must understand the difference between infectiousness and noninfectiousness and their risk of contracting TB in each condition. Some contacts may feel angry or hostile, blaming the client if the contact has contracted TB. Nurses can evaluate these responses and help increase knowledge and decrease misunderstanding.

Nurses may be instrumental in explaining public health procedures. For example, all close contacts of clients with TB and leprosy will be screened. As long as clients are considered infectious, they must not go to work or school until it is determined that they cannot infect others. School officials and employers may need to be educated to ensure they know the reasons for clients' activity restrictions; the risks they personally may have resulting from contract with TB clients; and the follow-up, evaluation, and therapy that associates of the client may require. When care of TB clients is coordinated among personnel in healthcare and social support agencies, the chances of positive treatment outcomes are increased.

The nurse must emphasize the importance of adhering to the drug regimen. Interrupting or discontinuing treatment is likely to result in drug resistance, making successive treatment difficult. As needed, the nurse should help the client devise a system for maintaining the medication regimen. The client may pour all the drugs required for the day in the morning and check at night to be sure all have been taken. Whatever system is used, the drugs must be secured against accidental ingestion by others, particularly children.

If cost is a problem, the client should be referred to social service agencies for assistance. Many people are reluctant to take this step, and clients may need some persuasion to accept this kind of help. The nurse should point out that successful treatment of the infection as early as possible will shorten the time of dependence on financial aid.

The occurrence of an adverse drug reaction increases the chance that the client will omit doses of the offending medication or stop taking it entirely. Because most clients being treated for TB are on multidrug therapy, the risk is that they may not know which drug is causing the problem and may therefore stop taking all of them. To prevent this, client education is crucial and must cover each medication, the proper dose and times to take it, and the possible adverse reactions. Clients should be taught what symptoms to watch for, which ones must be reported, and to whom to report their symptoms. Written instructions should be provided.

OUTCOME EVALUATION

Data that indicate satisfactory treatment outcomes include diminished signs and symptoms of infection; satisfactory respiratory system function and blood gas values; increased weight, strength, and activity tolerance; absence of signs and symptoms of adverse drug reactions; and client statements that indicate lowered anxiety and an understanding of the disease and drug treatment.

❖ CHECKLIST OF NURSING ACTIONS

- ❑ Screen clients for contraindications to drug therapy and conditions that could increase the risk of adverse reactions.
- ❑ Assess clients frequently for therapeutic and adverse reactions; outpatients should be evaluated at least every 2 weeks.
- ❑ Monitor laboratory data for adverse drug effects; notify the prescriber promptly if these occur.
- ❑ Encourage the client to take all drugs as ordered; help him or her devise a system for ensuring adherence.
- ❑ Provide encouragement and emotional support throughout the long period of treatment.
- ❑ Teach clients to recognize adverse drug reactions and when to report them to the prescriber.
- ❑ Teach clients measures to improve nutrition, promote rest, and manage stress, all aimed at improving systemic resistance.

Miscellaneous Antimicrobials

The drugs discussed in this section are not used routinely because most are relatively toxic, newer drugs are more effective, or they are unsuitable for oral administration. They are useful for treating infections when the causative organisms are resistant to other less toxic agents or when the client is allergic to the usual treatment agents (Table 43-2).

Colistin

Colistimethate sodium or colistin sulfate (Coly-Mycin M), also known as polymyxin E, is an antibiotic produced by *Bacillus polymyxa* var. *colistinus*. It is structurally and pharmacologically related to polymyxin B.

Table 43-2. Miscellaneous Antimicrobials

Drug Name	Preparation	Usual Dosage	Therapeutic Uses and Additional Information
colistin (Coly-Mycin)	Powder for oral suspension Vials containing powder for preparing solutions for IM injection	5–15 mg/kg/day in 3 divided doses	Treatment of infections caused by susceptible strains of gram-negative bacteria when other anti-infectives are contraindicated or ineffective Dosage adjustment required for clients with renal dysfunction
colistimethate sodium (Coly-Mycin M)	Injection or powder for reconstitution for IM or IV administration	IM or IV: 2.5–5 mg/kg/day in 2–4 divided doses. PC: C	Treatment of acute or chronic infections of gram-negative bacilli Dosage adjustment required for clients with renal dysfunction
polymyxin B sulfate (Aerosporin)	Injection or powder for reconstitution for injection Solution for urogenital irrigation	Adults and children 2 yr or older: *IV:* 15,000–25,000 U/kg/day, divided in 2 doses; *IM:* 25,000–30,000 U/kg/day, divided in 4–6 doses Maximum daily dosage for infants: 40,000 U/kg/day Maximum daily dosage for adults: 2,000,000 U PC: B	Infection caused by organisms resistant to less toxic drugs Dosage adjustment required for clients with renal dysfunction IM route is not used routinely because of severe pain that occurs at the injection site 40 to 60 minutes after the injection.

KEY: PC = pregnancy risk category; see Appendix A.

Pharmacodynamics. Colistimethate sodium is inactive until hydrolyzed to colistin. It acts as a cationic detergent; it damages the bacterial cytoplasmic membrane, causing leakage of essential intracellular metabolites and nucleosides. It is active against many gram-negative bacteria but is inactive against gram-positive bacteria, fungi, and viruses. It is bactericidal. Complete cross-resistance occurs between colistin and polymyxin B, but cross-resistance to other anti-infectives has not been reported.

Pharmacokinetics. Colistin is not absorbed from the GI tract; the oral form, colistin sulfate, is no longer available in the United States. After IM or IV injection, colistin is widely distributed into body tissues. It is not distributed appreciably into synovial, pleural, or pericardial fluids. The drug tends to remain in body organs and muscles.

Colistin and its metabolites are eliminated primarily by the kidneys. The drug is only minimally removed by hemodialysis or peritoneal dialysis.

Therapeutic Uses. Colistin is used in treating gram-negative infections, but only when other more effective and less toxic anti-infectives are ineffective or contraindicated. It may be useful in treating urinary tract infections (UTIs) caused by *Pseudomonas aeruginosa* that are resistant to aminoglycosides and extended-spectrum penicillins.

Adverse Reactions. The most serious toxic reactions to colistin are nephrotoxicity and neurotoxicity. Acute tubular necrosis has been reported, not necessarily preceded by progressive renal impairment. Nephrotoxicity is usually reversible with discontinuation of the drug. Both mild and severe CNS effects, including paresthesias, dizziness, blurred vision, slurred speech, confusion, seizures, and coma, have been reported. Reducing the dosage may relieve the signs and symptoms of neurotoxicity; they generally disappear when the drug is discontinued.

Drug Interactions. Concurrent use of colistin and other nephrotoxic or neurotoxic drugs should be avoided. Colistin also increases the effects of neuromuscular blocking agents.

Precautions and Contraindications. Renal function should be monitored in clients receiving colistin. Dosage must be reduced for clients with renal dysfunction. If neurotoxicity occurs, the dosage should be reduced and the client observed closely. Clients should be warned that the drug may impair their ability to carry out activities requiring alertness or physical coordination. Colistin should be avoided in clients with myasthenia gravis. Should apnea occur, respiration must be assisted mechanically. Safe use in pregnancy has not been established.

Polymyxin B

Polymyxin B (Aerosporin) is an antibiotic produced by various strains of *Bacillus polymyxa*.

Pharmacodynamics. Polymyxin B binds to phosphate groups in the lipid portion of bacterial cytoplasmic membranes and acts as a cationic detergent, causing leakage of essential metabolites. The drug's spectrum resembles that of colistin (active against many gram-negative bacteria). Bacterial resistance to polymyxin B seldom develops. There is complete cross-resistance between colistin and polymyxin B.

Pharmacokinetics. Polymyxin B is not appreciably absorbed from the GI tract, so it is usually administered by IM or IV injection. After absorption, the drug is widely distributed into body tissues, although it does not appear in the CSF, even when the meninges are inflamed, and it does not cross the placenta or appear in synovial fluid or aqueous humor. The drug is not highly bound to serum proteins.

The serum half-life is 4.3 to 6 hours with normal renal function; with renal dysfunction, the serum half-life is prolonged. Polymyxin B is excreted primarily unchanged in urine (60%). It is not removed appreciably by hemodialysis or peritoneal dialysis.

Therapeutic Uses. Polymyxin B is useful in treating serious infections caused by pathogens resistant to other more effective and less toxic agents. Polymyxin B sulfate in combination with neomycin sulfate (Neosporin G.U. Irrigant) has been used for irrigation of the urinary bladder to prevent bacteriuria and bacteremia associated with the use of indwelling catheters. Its efficacy for this use is unclear. Polymyxin B also has some topical uses.

Dosage and Administration. A total of 500,000 units are dissolved in 5 mL sterile water for injection or normal saline solution to yield 100,000 U/mL. Then a single dose is withdrawn and further diluted in 300 to 500 mL of dextrose 5% in water and infused over 60 to 90 minutes. Polymyxin B may be reconstituted with 10 mL of normal saline solution for intrathecal use.

For continuous irrigation of the urinary bladder, 1 mL of the urogenital concentration is added to 1 L of 0.9% sodium chloride solution (normal saline solution) and administered via a three-way catheter at 1 L every 24 hours (about 40 mL/hour). If the client's urine output exceeds 2 L/day, the inflow rate may be adjusted to 2 L every 24 hours. Irrigation therapy should not exceed 10 days.

Adverse Reactions. Adverse reactions to polymyxin B resemble those to colistin, primarily nephrotoxicity and neurotoxicity. Neurotoxicity is manifested by facial flushing, dizziness, mental confusion, irritability, nystagmus, muscle weakness, drowsiness, giddiness, circumoral and peripheral anesthesia or numbness, blurred vision, slurred speech, ataxia, coma, or seizures.

Drug Interactions. Polymyxin B is believed to inhibit neuromuscular transmission. Parenteral polymyxin B may increase or prolong skeletal muscle relaxation produced by neuromuscular blocking agents or anesthetics if the antibiotic is administered during surgery, or it may reinstate neuromuscular blockade if administered parenterally after surgery. Nephrotoxic and neurotoxic effects may be additive with concurrent or sequential use of other drugs with similar toxic potential (eg, aminoglycosides, amphotericin B).

Precautions and Contraindications. Polymyxin B is contraindicated in persons with a history of allergy to any of the polymyxins. Before therapy, clients should be screened for renal impairment. During therapy, renal function should be monitored frequently. Safe use during pregnancy has not been established.

■ SUMMARY

The miscellaneous drugs discussed here are a heterogeneous group of agents; some have specialized uses and some have limited clinical usefulness.

Pathophysiology of Urinary Tract Infection

The most common causes of renal system infection are gram-negative bacteria. Several properties have been identified for one such organism, *Escherichia coli*, including the ability to adhere to uroepithelial cells. The organisms contain pili, or fimbriae, that allow attachment to host cell receptor sites (Leiner, 1995). It is thought that such properties and inherent weaknesses in the host defense play a more important role in UTIs than behavioral factors and hygiene habits about which healthcare providers have commonly counseled clients (eg, perineal cleansing, tampon use, bubble baths, douching, dietary factors [soda, coffee, alcohol], tight pants, cotton underwear, or pantyhose). It does seem that frequency of intercourse and the use of diaphragms with spermicide correlate with the occurrence of UTIs. It is believed that UTIs per se do not affect kidney function. Clients with both UTIs and chronic renal failure invariably suffer from contributory conditions such as vesicoureteral reflux, analgesic nephropathy, kidney stones, neurogenic bladder, diabetes, and obstruction.

Acute UTIs are treated with antimicrobial drugs. For clients with recurrent UTIs, continuous antimicrobial suppression may be used. Drug regimens have continued for long periods without the development of resistant organisms. The disadvantages of continuous prophylaxis are cost, the need to take medicine regularly, and the potential for adverse reactions with long-term therapy.

Asymptomatic bacteriuria is another entity. It is defined as bladder urine colonized with bacteria in a client who had no symptoms of UTI in the week before the urine sample was obtained (Melillo, 1995). The incidence of asymptomatic bacteriuria increases with age and is common in older adults, especially the very old and institutionalized. Asymptomatic bacteriuria is more common in women than men. In certain situations, antimicrobial treatment is recommended, but often no pharmacologic therapy is used.

Urinary Tract Anti-infectives

Urinary tract anti-infectives are a group of drugs given systematically for their local effect in the urinary tract. They lack significant systemic antibacterial action (Tables 43-3 and 43-4).

Quinolones

Quinolones are synthetic broad-spectrum antibacterial drugs. Three of them, nalidixic acid, norfloxacin, and cinoxacin, are used only to treat UTIs. Newer agents, fluorinated-4-quinolones (fluoroquinolones), have a much broader spectrum and use. Both quinolones and fluoroquinolones may cause CNS stimulation that results in tremor and (rarely) convulsions. They may also cause lightheadedness and confusion. Anaphylaxis has occurred after the first dose, requiring epinephrine and emergency measures.

Fluoroquinolones

Fluoroquinolones are synthetic broad-spectrum oral antibiotics that are generally well tolerated (see Table 43-3). Microbial resistance to them does not develop rapidly.

Pharmacodynamics. Fluoroquinolones interfere with DNA gyrase, an enzyme needed to synthesize bacterial DNA, and are therefore bactericidal.

Pharmacokinetics. When administered orally, fluoroquinolones are well absorbed from the GI tract, with peak serum levels occurring 1 to 3 hours after administration. They are widely distributed throughout the body in body secretions, lymph, peritoneal fluid, CSF, skin, bone, muscle, cartilage, and fat. Most are excreted in urine.

Therapeutic Uses. Fluoroquinolones are active against a wide range of gram-negative and gram-positive organisms. They are used to treat infections of the lower urinary and respiratory tracts, skin and skin structures, bones and joints, and prostate; infectious diarrhea; and sexually transmitted diseases.

Adverse Reactions. Fluoroquinolones may cause mild to moderate symptoms that usually abate without treatment soon after drug discontinuation. These include GI symptoms (pain, nausea, vomiting, discomfort), headache, and restlessness. Photosensitivity (which may occur even with use of a sunscreen or sun block), flushing, pruritus, and urticaria may occur, as well as disturbed vision and renal problems (nephritis, polyuria, urinary retention, renal failure). Rare adverse reactions include cardiovascular symptoms (palpitations, atrial flutter, syncope, myocardial infarction, cardiopulmonary arrest), respiratory symptoms, and leukopenia and eosinophilia.

Drug–Drug Interactions. Fluoroquinolones increase the effects of xanthines (theophylline, caffeine), predisposing the client to seizures. Sucralfate and antacids that contain magnesium hydroxide or aluminum hydroxide interfere with the absorption of quinolones and should be avoided. Probenecid interferes with the renal tubular secretion of fluoroquinolones.

The effects of anticoagulants may be increased. Nephrotoxicity of cyclosporine may be increased when given with fluoroquinolones. Nitrofurantoin may interfere with the antimicrobial effects of norfloxacin. The elimination of fluoroquinolones may be decreased by cimetidine. Bioavailability of enoxacin is decreased by bismuth subsalicylate.

Drug–Food Interactions. Food and dairy products reduce the absorption of ciprofloxacin. Food delays the absorption of lomefloxacin.

Precautions and Contraindications. Because fluoroquinolones cause arthropathy in immature animals, they should not be used during pregnancy or lactation or in children. They should be used with caution in clients with CNS disorders. Clients should not use machinery or perform activities that require alertness, as they may suffer from lightheadedness or confusion. Clients should be observed for signs of sensitivity to the drug. Maintaining an adequate fluid intake and avoiding alkalinization of the urine can prevent the development of crystalluria.

Methenamine

Methenamine is a synthetic chemical that decomposes in acid solution. Methenamine hippurate (Hiprex, Urex) contains about 44% methenamine and 56% hippuric acid. Methenamine mandelate (Mandelamine) contains about 48% methenamine and 52% mandelic acid.

Pharmacodynamics. The anti-infective effect depends on the release of formaldehyde from the drug. Formaldehyde is usually bactericidal and is effective against both gram-positive and gram-negative bacteria. The acid portions of methenamine salts (hippuric acid, mandelic acid) have some nonspecific bacteriostatic activity and may enhance the liberation of formaldehyde from methenamine by maintaining urinary acidity. When urine is acidic, methenamine is hydrolyzed to formaldehyde and ammonia; maximal hydrolysis occurs when urine pH is 5.5 or less. Resistance does not usually develop to methenamine.

Pharmacokinetics. Methenamine is administered orally. When administered as enteric-coated tablets, the percentage of the dose hydrolyzed in the GI tract and the rate of absorption are reduced. In the blood and in body tissues with pH levels above 7.0, little methenamine breakdown occurs.

The time needed to reach peak effect depends on the preparation; peak urine concentrations of formaldehyde are usually attained in 3 to 8 hours after a dose of methenamine as an enteric-coated tablet. The drug is excreted in urine. Methenamine crosses the placenta and is distributed in breast milk.

Table 43-3. Fluoroquinolones

Drug Name	Preparation	Usual Adult Dosage	Additional Information
ciprofloxacin (Cipro)	Oral tablets and solution for IV administration	Oral: 250–750 mg q12h IV: 200–400 mg q12h PC: C	Excretion is reduced by about 50% when given with probenecid. Can be taken without regard to meals If a skin rash develops, drug should be discontinued. Do not take with polyvalent cations (aluminum, calcium, iron, zinc). Avoid activities that require mental alertness or coordination.
enoxacin (Penetrex)	Oral tablets	200–400 mg q12h PC: C	Should be taken 1 hr before or 2 hr after meals. May cause increase in digoxin levels
lomefloxacin (Maxaquin)	Oral tablets	400 mg once daily PC: C	Can be taken without regard to meals Moderate to severe phototoxic reactions can occur in clients exposed to direct or indirect sunlight or sunlamps during or after lomefloxacin therapy.
nalidixic acid (NegGram)	Tablets and suspension for oral use	Adults: 4 g/day, divided in 4 doses Children 3 mo–12 yr: 55 mg/kg/day, divided in 4 doses PC: B	Kills urinary tract pathogens by inhibiting DNA synthesis
norfloxacin (Noroxin)	Oral tablets	400 mg bid (maximum dosage) PC: C	Not used in children Caution should be exercised in clients with CNS disorders. Taken with liberal fluids, 1 h ac or 2 h pc. Do not use antacids within 1 h before and 1 h after taking norfloxacin.
ofloxacin (Floxin)	Oral tablets and solution for IV administration	Oral and IV: 200–400 mg q12h PC: C	Do not take with food.

KEY: PC = pregnancy risk category; see Appendix A.

Therapeutic Uses. Methenamine is used for suppression or prophylaxis of recurrent UTIs, especially when long-term therapy is considered necessary. It should be used after the UTI has been eradicated by other appropriate anti-infectives.

Dosage and Administration. About 1 g of the hippurate preparation is administered twice a day; 1 g of the mandelate preparation is administered four times a day. The oral suspension preparation, which contains a vegetable oil base, should be administered with caution to debilitated clients because of the possibility of lipid (aspiration) pneumonia.

Generally, fluids are not forced, as copious amounts of fluid may increase diuresis, elevate urine pH, and dilute the formaldehyde concentration to subinhibitory levels.

The efficacy of methenamine therapy should be monitored by periodic urine cultures. Urine pH should be monitored during therapy; supplemental acidification of urine may be needed. Lowering the urine pH inhibits the growth of most common pathogens involved in UTIs. This may be achieved by dietary regulation or by concomitant administration of acidifying agents (eg, ammonium chloride, ascorbic acid, methionine). Acid-ash foods that can decrease urine pH include proteins, cranberry juice, plums, and prunes. The client should not ingest large amounts of alkali-ash foods (most fruits and vegetables). Supplementary acidification is particularly important when the causative organisms are urea-splitting strains of *Enterobacter, Proteus,* or *Pseudomonas,* which increase urine pH.

Several combination agents contain methenamine (eg, Trac Tabs 2X, Prosed, Urogesic, Uro-Phosphate, Uroqid-Acid No. 2, Urisedamine, Urised, Cystex). Additional ingredients may serve as analgesics or antispasmodics in the urinary tract.

Adverse Reactions. Adverse reactions are uncommon but include GI disturbances and rare hypersensitivity reactions. Bladder irritation, painful and frequent urination, albuminuria, and gross hematuria have oc-

Table 43-4. Miscellaneous Urinary Tract Anti-infectives

Drug Name	Preparation	Usual Dosage	Summary of Pertinent Information
cinoxacin (Cinobac)	Oral capsules	Adults: 1 g/day, divided in 2 doses PC: B	Not recommended for use by prepubertal children
methenamine (Hiprex, Mandelamine, Urex)	Tablets, enteric-coated tablets, and suspensions for oral use	Adults: 4 g/day, divided in 4 doses, administered pc and hs Children 6–12 yr: 0.5 g 4 times/day Children less than 6 yr: 0.25 g/30 lb (14 kg) 4 times/day PC: C	Releases formaldehyde in acid urine; avoid use of alkalinizing foods (milk products, citrus fruits) or medications (sodium bicarbonate)
nitrofurantoin (Furadantin, Macrodantin, Nitrofan) *Can:* Nephronex, Novofuran	Tablets and suspension for oral use	Adults: 200–400 mg/day, divided in 4 doses Children older than 1 mo: 5–7 mg/kg/day, divided in 4 doses PC: B	Rarely induces resistance in susceptible pathogens Antiseptic action enhanced in acid urine Turns urine brown Take with food or milk to reduce GI upset.
trimethoprim (Proloprim, Trimpex)	Tablets for oral use	Adults: 200 mg/day, divided in 1 or 2 doses Prophylactic dosage: 100 mg/day hs PC: C	Safety and efficacy in children younger than 12 years have not been established. Dosage adjustment required for clients with renal dysfunction
co-trimoxazole/sulfamethoxazole–trimethoprim combination (TMP-SMZ) (Bactrim, Cotrim, Septra)	Tablets and suspension for oral use Solutions for dilution for IV infusion	Drug combination is prepared in a fixed ratio of 5 mg trimethoprim to 25 mg sulfamethoxazole. Adults: *prophylaxis:* 40–80 mg trimethoprim (as co-trimoxazole) up to 7 times weekly; *treatment:* 320 mg/day trimethoprim (as co-trimoxazole), divided in 1 or 2 doses Children 2 mo or older: 15 mg trimethoprim (as co-trimoxazole)/kg/day, divided in 2 doses PC: C (D if near term)	See previous information for individual drugs. Dosage varies with type and severity of disease. Up to 720 mg/day may be used to treat severe infections in adults. Dosage adjustment required for clients with renal dysfunction

KEY: PC = pregnancy risk category; see Appendix A.C
Can = Canadian trade name

curred and probably result from higher-than-recommended dosages of methenamine and a high concentration of formaldehyde in the urinary tract. (Formaldehyde is a tissue irritant.) Methenamine's chemical reaction releases ammonia as a by-product, and this ammonia may increase the chemical imbalance in clients with hepatic impairment.

Drug–Drug Interactions. Drug interactions occur with sulfonamides, acetazolamide, and sodium bicarbonate. Formaldehyde and sulfonamides form an insoluble precipitate in acid urine. Sodium bicarbonate may prevent the hydrolysis of the drug to formaldehyde.

Drug–Laboratory Test Interactions. Methenamine interferes with certain procedures for determining urinary catecholamines, 17-hydroxycorticosteroids, and vanillylmandelic acid and may produce false high values. Transient elevations of AST and ALT concentrations have been reported with methenamine hippurate.

Precautions and Contraindications. Methenamine is contraindicated in clients with hepatic insufficiency. To avoid irritating the urinary tract, high initial treatment dosages should be reduced when the urine becomes sterile. Hiprex tablets contain tartrazine, to which some clients are hypersensitive. To avoid raising the urine pH, the client should not use commercial antacids containing sodium bicarbonate or sodium carbonate.

Nalidixic Acid
Nalidixic acid (NegGram) is a synthetic drug chemically related to cinoxacin.

Pharmacodynamics. Nalidixic acid is bactericidal and interferes with DNA synthesis in susceptible gram-negative bacteria.

Pharmacokinetics. Nalidixic acid is well absorbed from the GI tract. Except for serum proteins, to which the drug is 93% to 97% bound, nalidixic acid does not accumulate in the tissues. Nalidixic acid is partially metabolized by the liver and kidneys and is excreted predominantly in urine.

Therapeutic Uses. Nalidixic acid is used in treating UTIs caused by susceptible gram-negative organisms.

Adverse Reactions. Adverse effects include CNS effects (headache, dizziness, or more serious effects in persons with predisposing factors such as a history of seizures or cerebral arteriosclerosis), nausea, vomiting, diarrhea, and hypersensitivity reactions. Photosensitization may occur. A hemolytic anemia occurs rarely, both in those with inherited deficiency of G6PD and in those without this deficiency.

Drug–Drug Interactions. Nalidixic acid tends to displace warfarin from serum albumin-binding sites and thus enhances the effects of this oral anticoagulant. When the drug is administered concurrently with warfarin, the dosage of anticoagulant should be reduced.

Drug–Laboratory Test Interactions. Urinary metabolites of nalidixic acid liberate glucuronic acid and produce false-positive urinary glucose results with certain glucose test reagents. One method of ascertaining urinary 17-keto and ketogenic steroids is affected by nalidixic acid and produces falsely elevated results.

Precautions and Contraindications. Nalidixic acid is contraindicated in clients with known hypersensitivity to the drug, in clients with seizure disorders, and in infants under 3 months.

Nitrofurantoin

Nitrofurantoin (Macrodantin, Macrobid, Furadantin) is a synthetic, nitrofuran-derivative anti-infective agent.

Pharmacodynamics. Nitrofurantoin may inhibit an enzyme, interfering with bacterial carbohydrate metabolism. It may also disrupt bacterial cell wall formation, although development of resistance is rare. The drug may be bacteriostatic or bactericidal, depending on its concentration in tissues.

Pharmacokinetics. Nitrofurantoin is readily absorbed from the GI tract. Binding to plasma proteins is about 60%. It is rapidly metabolized by body tissues and excreted in urine. It crosses the placenta and is distributed in breast milk.

Therapeutic Uses. Nitrofurantoin is used in treating UTIs caused by susceptible organisms. Its spectrum of activity includes many gram-negative and some gram-positive organisms. It is generally inactive against most strains of *Proteus*, *Serratia*, and *Pseudomonas*.

Dosage and Administration. Nitrofurantoin is available as capsules (containing macrocrystals of the drug), dual-release capsules (containing macrocrystals and monohydrate forms of the drug), and a suspension (containing microcrystals of the drug). Administration with food may minimize GI upset.

The usual dosage of the capsules or suspension is 50 to 100 mg four times daily for at least 1 week. If used for long-term suppression therapy, the dosage should be reduced.

The usual dose of the dual-release capsules (Macrobid) is 100 mg every 12 hours for 7 days. The monohydrate component is contained in a powder blend that forms a gel matrix when in contact with gastric or intestinal fluids and slowly releases the drug over time.

Adverse Reactions. Nitrofurantoin often causes GI upset (nausea, flatulence, vomiting, diarrhea or constipation, anorexia). Headache is the most common adverse CNS effect. Peripheral neuropathy may become severe or irreversible; it may be life-threatening. Initial symptoms of neuropathy include paresthesias (usually of the legs), which may progress to muscle weakness and wasting. Severe neuropathy includes demyelination of peripheral nerve fibers. The neuropathy may be more severe in persons with predisposing conditions, such as diabetes mellitus.

Acute, subacute, or chronic pulmonary hypersensitivity reactions occur occasionally. Acute reactions usually develop within 8 hours of initiation of therapy. Early recognition of pulmonary reactions is important; the drug must be discontinued. Acute and subacute reactions usually resolve within 1 week to several months of discontinuing the drug.

Hepatotoxicity is thought to be an idiosyncratic hypersensitivity reaction and is rare. Renal function impairment carries an increased risk of toxicity because of impaired excretion. Hemolytic anemia has been reported, especially in those with G6PD deficiency. Severe dermatologic effects have been reported. Finally, nitrofurantoin may color urine a dark yellow or brown.

Drug–Drug Interactions. Uricosuric agents, such as probenecid or sulfinpyrazone, may inhibit the renal excretion of nitrofurantoin, which may increase its toxic potential. Concomitant administration of a magnesium trisilicate antacid may decrease the extent and rate of absorption of nitrofurantoin. Nitrofurantoin may antagonize the antibacterial activity of quinolone-derivative anti-infectives. Anticholinergic drugs increase nitrofurantoin's bioavailability by delaying gastric emptying and increasing absorption.

Drug–Food Interactions. The bioavailability of nitrofurantoin is increased by food.

Drug–Laboratory Test Interactions. A false-positive result for urinary glucose may occur with some urine glucose tests.

Precautions and Contraindications. Because serious adverse reactions to nitrofurantoin develop insidiously, clients should be monitored closely for signs and symptoms of drug reaction. The drug should be discontinued at the first sign of pulmonary reaction or neurotoxicity. Caution should be used in clients with renal impairment, asthma, diabetes mellitus, electrolyte imbalance, vitamin B deficiency, or general debility. Its use is contraindicated in infants younger than 1 month, in pregnant women at term, during labor and delivery, or when the onset of labor is imminent, because of the possibility of hemolytic anemia in the neonate secondary to immature enzyme systems.

Phenazopyridine

Phenazopyridine (Pyridium, Urodine) is an azo dye.

Pharmacodynamics. The exact mechanism of action of phenazopyridine is unknown. Although the drug acts as a weak inhibitor of the growth of microorganisms, it is most valued for its local, topical analgesic effect on urinary tract mucosa.

Pharmacokinetics. The pharmacokinetic properties of phenazopyridine remain undetermined. The drug is excreted mainly unchanged by the kidneys.

Therapeutic Uses. Phenazopyridine is used for relief of pain, burning, urgency, and frequency associated with infection, trauma, or instrumentation (eg, catheterization). It is compatible with urinary tract anti-infectives and may relieve discomfort before the anti-infective takes effect. It may be used on its own or together with the primary anti-infective (eg, Azo Gantrisin is a combination of sulfonamide and phenazopyridine).

Dosage and Administration. The usual dose is 200 mg three times a day after meals.

Adverse Reactions. Adverse reactions to phenazopyridine are relatively uncommon. Most effects are dose-related. Clients with renal impairment are at high risk. Phenazopyridine colors the urine orange or red. Stains on fabrics can be removed by soaking in a 0.25% solution of sodium dithionate or sodium hydrosulfite. Staining of contact lenses may also occur.

Drug Interactions. Because it is a dye, phenazopyridine may interfere with some urinalysis methods.

Precautions and Contraindications. Phenazopyridine is contraindicated in clients with glomerulonephritis, severe hepatitis, uremia, pyelonephritis, during pregnancy, or impaired renal function.

Trimethoprim

Trimethoprim is a synthetic compound available alone (Proloprim, Trimpex) or in fixed combination with sulfamethoxazole known as co-trimoxazole (Bactrim, Septra).

Pharmacodynamics. Trimethoprim inhibits the action of dihydrofolate reductase in the folic acid pathway. By inhibiting synthesis of the metabolically active form of folic acid, trimethoprim inhibits bacterial thymidine synthesis. It is slowly bactericidal. Given together, trimethoprim enhances the action of sulfamethoxazole, but it does work alone.

Pharmacokinetics. Trimethoprim is readily and almost completely absorbed from the GI tract. It is widely distributed into body tissues and fluids, including the aqueous humor, middle ear fluid, saliva, lung tissue, sputum, seminal fluid, prostatic tissue and fluid, vaginal secretions, bile, bone, and CSF. It readily crosses the placenta. It is metabolized in the liver and 80% is excreted unchanged in urine. It may be moderately removed by hemodialysis. Resistance may develop, more rapidly when trimethoprim is used alone than when it is used in combination.

Therapeutic Uses. Trimethoprim is used for acute UTIs caused by susceptible organisms, including *E coli*, *Proteus mirabilis*, *Klebsiella pneumoniae*, *Enterobacter*, and coagulase-negative staphylococci. The efficacy of trimethoprim in treating UTIs appears to be partly related to the suppression of normal vaginal and fecal flora. Unlabeled uses include treatment and prophylaxis of chronic and recurrent UTIs in both men and women, treatment (with dapsone) of *P carinii* pneumonia, and treatment of traveler's diarrhea.

Dosage and Administration. Typical dosage is 100 mg twice a day or 200 mg once a day.

Adverse Reactions. The most common adverse reactions to trimethoprim are skin rash and pruritus. Less commonly, hematologic changes related to its mechanism of action (eg, megaloblastic anemia), nephrotoxicity, and hepatotoxicity are seen. The incidence and severity of drug reactions are dose-related; reactions may subside with reduced dosage.

Drug–Drug Interactions. Trimethoprim may inhibit phenytoin metabolism, causing increased levels of phenytoin.

Drug–Laboratory Test Interactions. Trimethoprim interferes with certain methods of serum creatinine and methotrexate assay. In addition, elevations in AST, bilirubin, blood urea nitrogen, and serum creatinine levels have been reported.

Precautions and Contraindications. Trimethoprim must be used cautiously in clients with impaired renal or hepatic function or those with a folate deficiency or prone to such a deficiency (alcoholic, malnourished, elderly, or pregnant clients). The drug is not recommended for clients with a creatinine clearance of less than 15 mL/min. The drug is contraindicated in clients with allergic hypersensitivity to it.

Sulfonamides

The first effective systemic antimicrobial was a sulfonamide developed in Denmark and Germany in the 1930s. As a result of research that involved coal tar aniline compounds, Prontosil, a bright-red dye, produced dramatic improvement in clients with certain bacterial infections. This compound and its derivative, sulfanilamide, were used to treat coccal infections such as pneumonia, meningitis, and puerperal sepsis. In the absence of other effective treatment agents, use of the sulfonamides mushroomed, despite their relatively high cost. During World War II, sulfa powder sprinkled over the wounds of injured soldiers was credited with saving innumerable lives by suppressing infection.

Sulfonamides are structural analogs of PABA, a substance required by many microorganisms for producing folic acid. They are weak acids that are generally insoluble in water; most sodium salts of the drugs are strongly basic and readily soluble in water but deteriorate rapidly in solution (Table 43-5).

Modification of the sulfonamide drugs has resulted in the development of several other useful therapeutic drugs. These include the antituberculosis drug PAS, sulfones used to treat leprosy, carbonic anhydrase inhibitor diuretics, sulfonylurea hypoglycemics, and thiouracil antithyroid agents. The last three of these exploit side effects of the original sulfonamide group.

The emergence of resistant strains of pathogens has limited the usefulness of sulfonamides. Newer antimicrobials have superseded them in treating many infections caused by organisms likely to be insensitive to sulfonamides.

Pharmacodynamics. The sulfonamides are bacteriostatic rather than bactericidal. They prevent the growth of microorganisms by inhibiting the production of folic acid in bacterial cells through competition with PABA. Host cells (in mammals) are unaffected because they cannot synthesize folic acid but use the preformed vitamin.

Pharmacokinetics. Most sulfonamides (except sulfapyridine and sulfasalazine) are absorbed readily from the GI tract. Absorption from other mucous membranes and abraded skin is unreliable, but enough drug may reach the circulation to induce allergic hypersensitivity. Absorbable sulfonamides are lipid-soluble and distribute readily into body tissues and fluids, including the CSF, as well as the pleural, peritoneal, and synovial spaces. Most sulfonamides readily cross the placenta and are distributed in breast milk. Penetration is poor into bile, saliva, and prostatic fluid. Sulfonamides bind loosely to serum albumin and to a lesser degree to serum globulin. Within the body they are metabolized by acetylation and glucuronidation, mainly in the liver. Metabolites are inactive; the acetylated form is less soluble than the unchanged drug, particularly in acid media. Excretion is mainly through the kidneys. Solubility of these drugs in the urine and the rate of excretion are enhanced by alkalinization of the urine. Poorly absorbed sulfonamides remain in the GI tract and are eliminated in feces.

Therapeutic Uses. Sulfonamides are the agents of choice for treating UTIs and are useful secondary drugs for many other conditions, including shigellosis, nocardiosis, trachoma, and toxoplasmosis. In combination with trimethoprim, sulfamethoxazole is used to treat typhoid fever, *P carinii* infections, and brucellosis. Sulfasalazine is used in treating chronic ulcerative colitis. The drugs have a wide range of activity against both gram-positive and gram-negative organisms. Sulfonamides are also used prophylactically for traveler's diarrhea and otitis media.

Adverse Reactions. Because early sulfonamide preparations were poorly soluble, they tended to crystallize in the kidneys, causing serious renal impairment. Renal toxicity is less likely with current medications because more soluble salts have been developed and less soluble salts are used in combinations (eg, Triple Sulfa No. 2) that allow a lower dose of each component. Some potential for kidney damage remains, however. Other adverse effects of sulfonamides include allergic reactions, most commonly skin rashes and fever. Anaphylaxis, aplastic anemia, hemolytic anemia, and Stevens-Johnson syndrome seldom occur but can be life-threatening. Sensitivity is most likely to develop in clients with a history of topical treatment with sulfonamides.

Occasionally, sulfonamides cause hypoglycemia as a result of stimulating insulin release. The drugs can also suppress production of thyroid hormone, impair liver function, and reduce fertility in males.

When applied to denuded areas, sulfonamide creams cause a burning sensation. High doses of sulfasalazine may cause subclinical folate deficiency in persons with chronic colitis.

Long-term sulfonamide therapy can produce vitamin K deficiency because it inhibits microorganisms that normally synthesize this vitamin in the intestine. Hypoprothrombinemia and bleeding tendencies may result from the deficiency.

Drug Interactions. Sulfonamides increase the anticoagulant effects of warfarin and may cause bleeding when the drugs are used concurrently.

Precautions and Contraindications. Because sulfonamides easily cross the placenta and are excreted into breast milk, caution must be exercised when they are used during pregnancy and lactation. Sulfonamides are not used to treat newborns because they displace bilirubin from protein-binding sites, increasing the risk and severity of kernicterus.

Sulfonamide therapy is contraindicated in clients with a history of allergic reaction or anuria after use of a drug from this group.

When used concurrently with warfarin, the dose of anticoagulant should be decreased.

Before ophthalmic use of sulfonamides, crusts or discharge should be removed from the eyes with a new

Table 43-5. Sulfonamide Preparations

Drug Name	Preparation	Usual Dosage	Additional Information
sulfadiazine	Oral tablets	Adults: 2–4 g/day, divided in 4–6 doses Children older than 2 mo: 120–150 mg/kg/day, divided in 4–6 doses PC: B (D if near term)	Rapidly absorbed by the GI tract; rapidly excreted; less soluble than sulfisoxazole
sulfamethizole	Oral tablets	Adults: 1.5–4 g/day, divided in 3 or 4 doses Children older than 2 mo: 30–45 mg/kg/day, divided in 4 doses PC: C (Not to be used at term)	Rapidly excreted; use limited to treatment of UTIs
sulfamethoxazole (Gantanol, Urobak; *with trimethoprim:* Bactrim, Septra)	Oral tablets and suspension	Adults: 2–3 g/day, divided in 2 or 3 doses Children: 50–60 mg/kg/day, divided in 2 doses PC: B (D if near term)	More slowly absorbed and excreted, and less soluble than sulfisoxazole
sulfasalazine (Azulfidine)	Oral tablets and suspension	Adults: 1–4 g/day, divided in 1–4 doses Children older than 2 mo: 30 mg/kg/day, divided in 4 doses PC: B (D if near term)	Poorly absorbed in the GI tract; administered for local effect in the gut; used in the treatment of ulcerative colitis, regional enteritis, granulomatous colitis
sulfisoxazole (Gantrisin) *Can:* Novosoxazole	Oral tablets	Adults: 4–8 g/day in 4–6 divided doses Children older than 2 mo: 150 mg/kg/day, divided in 4–6 doses	Highly soluble; rapidly absorbed from the GI tract; rapidly excreted
trisulfapyrimidines (167 mg each of sulfadiazine, sulfamerazine, and sulfamethazine) (Triple Sulfa No. 2)	Oral tablets	Adults: 2–4 g initially, then 2–4 g daily in 3–6 divided doses Children: 75 mg/kg initially, then 120–150 mg/kg daily in 4–6 divided doses (not to exceed 6 g daily)	

KEY: PC = pregnancy category; see Appendix A.
Can = Canadian trade name

cotton ball and clean hands. Drops or ointment should be stored at room temperature and applied as prescribed, preventing contact between the dropper or tube tip and the eye. Clients with an infection should not use eye cosmetics nor share towels or washcloths.

■ SUMMARY

Urinary tract anti-infectives are given systemically for their local effect and are excreted by the kidneys. Fluoroquinolones are increasingly used as wide-spectrum antibiotics that are safe for most clients. Adverse reactions usually subside when the drug is discontinued. Norfloxacin is usually used only to treat UTIs or sexually transmitted diseases.

Methenamine, although not a primary drug for acute UTI, is useful in chronic suppressive treatment. Cinoxacin and nalidixic acid are effective against gram-negative bacteria. Phenazopyridine is most valuable for its analgesic property. Trimethoprim alone or in fixed combination with sulfamethoxazole (co-trimoxazole) is used for acute UTIs and several other purposes.

The sulfonamides are bacteriostatic antimicrobials that act by competitive inhibition of folic acid synthesis in the microbial cell. They are effective for treating UTIs and are useful adjuncts in treating many other infections. Their clinical usefulness is somewhat reduced by the development of drug-resistant strains of pathogens and allergic sensitivity in recipients. The sulfonamides have the potential to cause crystalluria-induced nephrotoxicity.

❖ NURSING MANAGEMENT: CLIENT RECEIVING A URINARY TRACT ANTI-INFECTIVE

These drugs are often used in recurrent infections. The nurse must help the client persevere with treatment.

NURSING PROCESS

ASSESSMENT

Because UTIs tend to recur in susceptible persons, a careful history of such infections and the anti-infective drugs used to treat them is needed before therapy begins. A complete history of other drugs is also required.

NURSING DIAGNOSIS

Nursing diagnoses related to drug therapy for a UTI may include:

- Altered Nutrition: Less Than Body Requirements, related to abdominal discomfort secondary to anti-infective medication
- Diarrhea, related to sulfonamide and other anti-infective drugs
- Ineffective Individual Management of Therapeutic Regimen: Noncompliance, related to discontinuation of medication before full course is completed secondary to adverse effects or relief of symptoms
- Risk for Infection, by resistant pathogens related to failure to complete course of medication
- Knowledge Deficit, related to UTIs, effects of medication, and need for adherence to drug regimen
- Pain, related to cystitis or to kidney damage secondary to adverse reaction to sulfonamides
- Anxiety, related to concern about recurrent UTIs and need for long-term drug therapy

A common collaborative problem that should be differentiated from the nursing diagnoses is:

Potential Complication: Adverse effects of drug therapy

PLANNING

Goals are to relieve discomfort, reduce anxiety, reduce the risk of recurrent infections, decrease knowledge deficit, reduce the risk of adverse reactions to medications, and detect and treat adverse drug reactions promptly.

INTERVENTION

Nursing actions include ensuring that urinalysis, urine culture and sensitivity, and any other diagnostic tests are done before, during, and after therapy as ordered. Measures should be taken to support and enhance normal resistance to infection (good nutrition, ample hydration, rest, and reduction of stress).

Risk factors for UTI should be reduced as much as possible. Bladder training programs should be instituted so that retention catheters can be discontinued. A bowel program can reduce fecal incontinence (incontinence increases the number of pathogens on the skin in the perineal area). Women using diaphragms with spermicide may try another method of birth control. The client should void within 15 minutes before and after sexual intercourse.

Management of the UTI may include dietary modification (eating more acid-ash foods and fewer alkaline-ash foods) or using urine acidifiers to lower the urine pH and inhibit the growth of pathogens in the urinary tract. Urine pH may be monitored during therapy.

Overhydration is helpful if tolerated (but not when methenamine is used). Volumes of fluid moving through the urinary tract wash out pathogens and reduce the population. For most normal adults, a goal of 3 L of fluid intake daily is appropriate. Amounts for children or adults with a reduced body mass should be adjusted accordingly. Forcing fluids to this degree may be difficult and should not be left to chance. Offering a glass of fluid hourly between meals during waking hours is usually sufficient. An accurate record of fluid intake and output should be maintained.

Client Education. Client instruction should include information about the drug regimen and specific instructions relative to the drug being used (eg, whether to take it with food or not). See the Critical Thinking Challenge: Case Analysis.

Clients should be counseled about the importance of hydration. Specific instructions should be given on the appropriate amounts and types of liquids to take. Acid-ash fruit juices (cranberry and prune) are usually preferable to citrus and vegetable juices, which are alkaline-ash. (If a UTI is associated with kidney stones composed of acidic materials such as oxalic acid, alkaline-ash foods are preferred to increase the solubility of the stones in urine.) Plain water is usually the most appropriate drink. If the quality of local water is poor, a little lemon juice may improve the flavor, or bottled water may be used.

When phenazopyridine or nitrofurantoin is prescribed, the client should be warned about the innocuous change in urine color.

OUTCOME EVALUATION

Data that indicate a successful outcome include decreased signs and symptoms of UTI; absence of UTI recurrence; relaxed facial expression and body movements; absence of signs and symptoms of adverse drug reactions; and client statements that indicate relief of anxiety and understanding of the UTI and its management.

CRITICAL THINKING CHALLENGE
Case Analysis

The client, a 31-year-old mother of two, has had three episodes of cystitis within the past 2 years. All have been treated successfully with sulfisoxazole. The client has a cystocele (a predisposing factor for cystitis) and a history of hay fever and asthma. There was no adverse reaction to previous courses of sulfonamides. She is leaving soon for a Caribbean cruise and will be continuing her sulfisoxazole medication.

1. What advice can you offer the client to help her adhere to drug therapy during her cruise?
2. Prepare written guidelines and a dosage schedule for her to follow to promote the beneficial effects of medication while preventing undesired adverse reactions.

❖ **CHECKLIST OF NURSING ACTIONS**

❑ Counsel clients regarding food and fluid intake to enhance hydration and maintain the desired urine pH.

❑ Advise clients of changes in urine color that will occur as a result of medication.

❑ Use nursing measures to avoid the use of catheters for continuous urinary drainage.

❑ Monitor clients receiving urinary tract anti-infectives for adverse reactions.

References

Division of Drugs and Toxicology. (1994). *Drug evaluations subscription,* v. 3. Chicago: American Medical Association.

Leiner S. (1995). Recurrent urinary tract infections in otherwise healthy adult women: Rational strategies for work-up and management. *Nurse Practitioner, 20*(2), 48.

Leiner S, Mays M. (1996). Diagnosing latent and active pulmonary tuberculosis: A review for clinicians. *Nurse Practitioner, 21*(2), 86.

Melillo KD. (1995). Asymptomatic bacteriuria in older adults: When is it necessary to screen and treat? *Nurse Practitioner, 20*(8), 50.

Wiseman KC. (1995). Tuberculosis: An old disease with a new face. *ANNA J, 22*(6), 541–555.

Bibliography

Brausch LM, Bass JB Jr. (1993). The treatment of tuberculosis. *Med Clin North Am, 77*(6), 1277–1288.

DiFerdinando GT Jr, Glassroth J, Hecht FM, Stover DE. (1993). TB and HIV: A deadly synergy. *Patient Care, 27*(14), 92.

Gantz NM, Kaye D, Weart CW. (1995). Antibiotics '95: Back to basics. *Patient Care, 29,* 68–72.

Hardman JG, Limbird LE, Molinoff PB, et al. (eds.) (1996). *Goodman and Gilman's The pharmacological basis of therapeutics,* 9th ed. New York: McGraw-Hill.

Hassay KA. (1995). Effective management of urinary discomfort. *Nurse Practitioner, 20*(2), 36.

Hospital Infection Control Practices Advisory Committee. (1995). Recommendations for preventing the spread of vancomycin resistance. *Infection Control Hosp Epidemiol, 16*(2), 105–113.

McEvoy GK. (1996). *American Hospital Formulary Service Drug Information.* Bethesda, MD: American Society of Health-System Pharmacists, Inc.

Stamm WE, Hooton TM. (1993). Management of urinary tract infections in adults. *N Engl J Med, 329,* 1328–1334.

Wolf L. (1995). A tuberculosis control plan for ambulatory care centers. *Nurse Practitioner, 20*(6), 34.

For more information and sample tests and activities, refer to Chapter 43 in the Student Workbook for Clinical Pharmacology and Nursing Management, 5th edition, available through your bookstore.

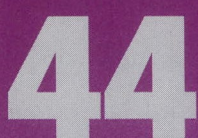
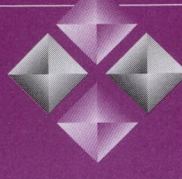

44

Agents That Treat Viral and Fungal Infections

Infections caused by viruses and fungi do not respond well to antimicrobial drugs. Viruses penetrate the cells of their hosts, and this intracellular location protects them from many anti-infective agents. Drugs capable of affecting viruses tend to be harmful to host cells. Fungi have a rigid cell wall in some stages of the life cycle, so they are unaffected by most antimicrobial drugs. In addition, the elimination of a host's natural microbial flora by broad-spectrum anti-infectives also allows fungi to grow without restraint. Fungi are often responsible for superinfection secondary to antimicrobial therapy.

Pathophysiology of Viral Infections

Viruses are either double-stranded or single-stranded RNA or DNA enclosed in a protein coat called a capsid (Hardman & Limbird, 1996). Some viruses also have a lipoprotein envelope that may contain antigenic proteins. Some viruses contain enzymes that initiate viral replication inside a host cell. Unlike other organisms, viruses do not have cellular structures, nor do they take in nutrients, produce and use energy through metabolism, excrete wastes, or propel themselves through the environment. Their reproduction is a parasitic process by which they use the mechanisms in a living cell to replicate themselves.

Typically, DNA viruses enter the host cell nucleus, except the pox virus, which replicates in the host cell cytoplasm. DNA viruses (and the diseases they cause) include pox viruses (smallpox), herpesviruses (chickenpox, shingles, herpes), adenoviruses (conjunctivitis, sore throat), hepadenaviruses (hepatitis B), and papillomaviruses (warts). RNA viruses (and the diseases they cause) include rubella virus (German measles), rhabdoviruses (rabies), picornaviruses (poliomyelitis, meningitis, colds), arenaviruses (meningitis, Lassa fever), arboviruses (yellow fever, arthropod-borne encephalitis), orthomyxoviruses (influenza), and paramyxoviruses (measles, mumps). Retroviruses are also one group of RNA viruses that are responsible for AIDS and T-cell leukemias.

The methods of viral replication are not fully understood. One strategy is for the virus to copy and incorporate within itself a gene that governs part of the host's immune system. The virus can then deactivate the host's immune cells that would fight the viral infection. At the same time, the host's cell can be transformed into a factory that quickly produces viral proteins and offspring, allowing rapid multiplication of the virus.

Antiviral Agents, Vaccines, and Interferons

The multiple stages of viral replication suggest the possibility for development of multiple classes of antiviral agents, with each class acting at a different stage. The search for chemicals that are selectively toxic to viruses requires an understanding and use of the differences between the replicative cycle of the viruses and that of the cells they invade. As yet, no safe, broad-spectrum antiviral drug has been discovered.

However, victims are not completely defenseless. A few compounds have been developed that are helpful in selected situations, and some substances under investigation show promise of broader usefulness. Antiviral agents in various stages of clinical development include nucleoside reverse transcriptase inhibitors, nonnucleoside reverse transcriptase inhibitors, protease inhibitors (including saquinavir [Invirase]), acyclic nucleoside phosphonates/nucleoside DNAp inhibitors, antisense oligonucleotides, receptor decoys, capsid-binding agents, and neuraminidase inhibitors.

Immunizing vulnerable populations against disease with vaccines has done much to reduce the ravages of certain viral parasites, such as those that cause rubeola, mumps, polio, rubella, varicella, and hepatitis (see Chap. 35).

Interferons offer another defense against viral infections. In 1957, a substance was isolated from chicken embryo cells that appeared to interfere with virus activity in cells; it was named interferon. Now many interferons have been identified and found to possess antiviral, antiproliferative, immunomodulatory, and cytotoxic actions (see Chap. 35).

Antiviral Anti-Infectives

The number of antiviral anti-infective drugs has increased dramatically in recent years (Table 44-1). Five of them will be discussed in more detail due to their unique contributions or representativeness: acyclovir, ganciclovir, amantadine, zidovudine, and ribavirin.

Acyclovir

Acyclovir (Zovirax) is an acyclic guanine nucleoside analog. Valacyclovir (Valtrex) is the newer prodrug of acyclovir (see Table 44-1).

Pharmacodynamics. Acyclovir is converted to the monophosphate derivative by herpesvirus thymidine kinase. Cells not infected by the virus convert little or no drug. The monophosphate form is further transformed into the diphosphate and triphosphate forms. Acyclovir triphosphate interferes with the virus DNA polymerase, blocking viral replication. It can also be incorporated into growing chains of DNA, thereby terminating further growth of the DNA chain. Resistant strains of viruses develop after exposure to the drug.

Pharmacokinetics. Oral bioavailability ranges from 10% to 20%. After absorption, acyclovir is widely distributed in body tissues and fluids, including vesicular fluid, aqueous humor, and the cerebrospinal fluid (CSF). About 9% to 33% of the drug is bound to plasma proteins. Acyclovir crosses the placenta and appears in breast milk. Excretion is primarily unmetabolized acyclovir by glomerular filtration and tubular secretion. The drug is removed by hemodialysis.

Therapeutic Uses. Acyclovir's use is limited to herpesviruses; it is useful in both immunocompetent and immunocompromised clients. Oral acyclovir can be used for initial genital herpes simplex virus (HSV) in-

fections and is more effective than the topical form. Neither approach reduces the risk of recurrent genital lesions. Oral acyclovir can be administered chronically to suppress recurring genital herpes, although HSV transmission to sexual partners may occur during suppression. Chronic suppression may be useful in persons with disabling recurrences of herpes whitlow or HSV-related erythema multiforme.

In clients with very localized labial or facial HSV infections, topical acyclovir may provide some benefits. However, immunocompromised clients with mucocutaneous HSV infection may receive intravenous (IV) or oral acyclovir. Recurrent infection is common and may require long-term suppression. In HSV encephalitis, acyclovir reduces mortality by more than 50%.

The use of IV acyclovir, started before transplantation and continuing for several weeks, prevents HSV disease in bone marrow transplant recipients.

If started within 14 hours of the onset of rash associated with varicella zoster virus infections, oral acyclovir has therapeutic effects. However, routine use in uncomplicated pediatric varicella is not recommended.

In older adults with localized herpes zoster, oral acyclovir reduces acute pain and healing time if treatment is initiated within 72 hours of rash onset. Valacyclovir may provide quicker relief of zoster-associated pain than acyclovir in acute herpes zoster of older adults. In immunocompromised clients with herpes zoster, IV acyclovir reduces viral shedding, healing time, and complications.

Acyclovir is ineffective in established cytomegalovirus (CMV) infections but has been used for CMV prophylaxis in transplant recipients.

In infectious mononucleosis, acyclovir is associated with transient antiviral effects but no clinical benefits. Epstein-Barr virus–related oral hairy leukoplakia may improve with acyclovir.

Adverse Reactions. The most common adverse effects of parenteral acyclovir are nephrotoxicity and central nervous system (CNS) adverse reactions. Preexisting renal insufficiency and high doses are risk factors for both.

Reversible renal dysfunction is related to high urine levels, causing precipitation of acyclovir in the renal tubules. Signs and symptoms of this nephropathy include nausea, vomiting, flank pain, and increasing azotemia. Rapid infusion and dehydration increase the risk. The nephrotoxicity usually resolves if the drug is discontinued and volume expansion occurs.

Signs and symptoms of CNS toxicity include lethargy, tremors, confusion, delirium, hallucinations, seizures, extrapyramidal signs, and coma. Local inflammatory reactions at the injection site occur, and phlebitis results from extravasation.

Oral acyclovir has been associated relatively infrequently with nausea, diarrhea, rash, or headache. Topical

Text continues on page 948.

Table 44-1. Antiviral Anti-Infective Drugs

Drug Name	Preparation	Usual Dosage	Additional Information
Antiherpes Agents			
acyclovir (Zovirax)	Tablets Capsules Suspension Powder for injection Topical	Adults: *parenteral:* 5 mg/kg infused IV over 1 h, q8h (15 mg/kg/d) for 7 d; *oral:* initial genital herpes: 200 mg q4h while awake (1,000 mg/d) for 10 d; typical oral dose for older adult with localized herpes zoster is 800 mg/d for 7 d; chronic suppressive therapy: 400 mg bid for up to 12 mo Children <12 yr: *parenteral:* 250 mg/m² infused IV over 1 h, q8h (750 mg/m²/d) for 7 d PC: C	Dosage adjustment necessary for clients with renal impairment
famciclovir (Famvir)	Tablets	Adults: 500 mg q8h PO for 7 d PC: C	Used for management of acute herpes zoster
foscarnet (Foscavir)	Injection	Adults: *induction:* 60 mg/kg q8h IV for 2–3 wk; *maintenance:* 90–120 mg/kg IV PC: C	Used for treatment of CMV retinitis in clients with AIDS
ganciclovir (DHPG) (Cytovene)	Capsules Lyophilized powder for injection	Adults: CMV retinitis: *initial dose:* 5 mg/kg given IV at a constant slow rate over 1 h, q12h for 14–21 d; *maintenance:* 5 mg/kg given by IV infusion over 1 h qd 7 d/wk or 6 mg/kg qd 5 d/wk; or 1,000 mg PO tid with food or 500 mg PO 6x/d q3h with food while awake. Prevention of CMV disease in transplant recipients: 5 mg/kg IV over 1 h q12h for 7–14 d, then 5 mg/kg/d qd for 7 d/wk PC: C	Dosage adjustment necessary for clients with renal impairment
idoxuridine (IDU) (Herplex, Stoxil)	0.1% solution for ophthalmic use	*Initially:* place 1 drop into infected eye(s) every hr during day & every 2 hr during night; continue for about 7 d until definite improvement, then reduce dosage to q2h during day & q4h during night for 3–7 d; maximum treatment period, 21 d PC: C	Used for herpes simplex keratitis
lamivudine (3TC) (Epivir)	Tablets Oral solution	Adults and children 12–16 yr: 150 mg PO bid in combination with zidovudine Children 3 mo–12 yr: 4 mg/kg PO bid; maximum, 150 mg bid PC: C	Dosage adjustment necessary for clients with renal impairment Used for treatment of HIV infection in combination with zidovudine when therapy is warranted based on evidence of disease progression
trifluridine (Viroptic)	1% solution for ophthalmic use	Instill 1 drop into cornea of affected eye(s) q2h while awake (maximum daily dose, 9 drops); after re-epithelialization has occurred, treat for 7 more days	Used for primary keratoconjunctivitis and recurrent epithelial keratitis due to herpes simplex virus types 1 and 2; epithelial keratitis that has not responded to idoxuridine; or when hypersensitivity to idoxuridine has occurred

KEY: PC = pregnancy risk category; see Appendix A.

(continued)

Table 44-1. (Continued)

Drug Name	Preparation	Usual Dosage	Additional Information
Antiherpes Agents (continued)			
valacyclovir (Valtrex)	Film-coated tablets	Adults: 1 g tid PO for 7 d; most effective if started within 48 h of onset of symptoms PC: B	Dosage adjustment necessary for clients with renal impairment Used for acute herpes zoster in immunocompetent adults
vidarabine (Vira-A)	3% ointment for ophthalmic use IV	Administer 0.5 inch ointment into lower conjunctival sac 5 times qd q3h; after re-epithelialization has occurred, treat for 7 more days at reduced dosage to prevent recurrence	Used for acute keratoconjunctivitis and recurrent epithelial keratitis due to herpes simplex virus types 1 and 2; superficial keratitis that has not responded to idoxuridine; or when hypersensitivity to idoxuridine has occurred
Antiretroviral Agents			
didanosine (ddI) (Videx)	Tablets Powder for oral solution, buffered	Adults: *tablets:* 125–200 mg PO bid; *powder:* 167–250 mg PO bid Children: tablets and powder dosages differ slightly; 125 mg/1.1–1.4 m² PC: B	Used for treatment of adults with advanced HIV infection who have received prolonged prior zidovudine therapy; treatment of adults and children over 6 mo with advanced infection who are intolerant to zidovudine
indinavir (Crixivan)	Capsules		
ritonavir (Norvir)	Capsules Oral solution		
saquinavir (Invirase)	Capsules	Adults and children >16 yr: 600 mg PO tid in combination with zidovudine or zalcitabine PC: B	Dosage adjustment necessary for clients with liver impairment Used for treatment of HIV infection in combination with zidovudine or zalcitabine in selected clients
stavudine (d4T) (Zerit)	Capsules	Adults: 40 mg q12h PO without regard to meals; <60 kg: 30 mg bid PC: C	Dosage adjustment necessary for clients with renal impairment Used for treatment of adults with advanced HIV infection who are intolerant to other therapies or who have experienced significant deterioration while receiving other therapies
zalcitabine (ddC) (Hivid)	Tablets	Adults: 0.75 mg PO q8h or 0.75 mg PO administered with 200 mg zidovudine PO q8h PC: C	Dosage adjustment necessary for clients with renal impairment Used for treatment of advanced HIV infection in combination with zidovudine
zidovudine, azidothymidine, AZT (Retrovir)	Capsules Syrup Injection	Adults: symptomatic HIV infection: *initially:* 200 mg q4h PO around the clock; asymptomatic HIV infection: 100 mg q4h PO while awake Maternal–fetal transmission: 100 mg PO 5×/d from ≥14 wk gestation to the start of labor Children 3 mo–12 yr: 180 mg/m² q6h PO or IV Infant born to HIV mother: 2 mg/kg q6h starting within 12 h of birth to 6 wk of age PC: C	In AIDS and ARC clients, associated with prolongation of survival, decreased opportunistic infections, weight gain, improved functional status, increased CD4 counts

KEY: PC = pregnancy risk category; see Appendix A.

(continued)

Table 44-1. (Continued)

Drug Name	Preparation	Usual Dosage	Additional Information
Other Antiviral Agents			
amantadine (Symadine, Symmetrel)	Oral	Adults: influenza A virus: *prophylaxis:* 200 mg/d PO or 100 mg bid PO for 10 d after exposure, for up to 90 d if vaccination is impossible and exposure is repeated; *treatment:* same as above, start as soon after exposure as possible, continue for 24–48 h after symptoms are gone; Parkinson's disease: 100 mg bid PO when used alone; reduce in clients receiving other antiparkinson drugs Children: influenza A virus: *prophylaxis:* 1–9 yr: 2–4 mg/lb qd PO in 2 or 3 divided doses; *treatment:* same dose and principles as for adult PC: C	Dosage adjustment necessary for clients with renal dysfunction or seizure disorders
ribavirin (Virazole, Viroptic)	Powder for reconstitution for aerosol	Dilute to 20 mg/mL and deliver for 12–18 hours/d for 3 to 7 d PC: X	Used for infants and children with respiratory syncytial virus of lower respiratory tract; other unlabeled uses in text Only for use in hospital because respiratory and cardiovascular function must be monitored during treatment
rimantadine (Flumadine)	Tablets Syrup	Adults and children >10 yr: *prophylaxis:* 100 mg/d PO bid; *treatment:* same dose, start treatment as soon after exposure as possible, continue for 7 d PC: C	Used for prophylaxis and treatment of illness caused by influenza A virus

KEY: PC = pregnancy risk category; see Appendix A.

acyclovir has a low order of toxicity. The most common reaction with topical use on lesions is mild pain, which may include burning and stinging.

Drug Interactions. Concurrent administration of probenecid inhibits renal excretion of acyclovir and prolongs the drug's effects. Extreme drowsiness occurs when it is given with zidovudine. There is increased nephrotoxicity if cyclosporine or other nephrotoxic drugs are given concurrently.

Precautions and Contraindications. Clients receiving parenteral acyclovir must be well hydrated. Because urine concentration peaks within the first 2 hours after infusion, urine flow should be sufficient during that period to prevent precipitation in renal tubules. IV dosages must be infused slowly over at least 1 hour. The drug must not be administered by IV bolus, intramuscularly (IM), or subcutaneously (SC). The nurse should consult the pharmacy for proper disposal of unused solution. Precautions are required for the disposal of nucleoside analogs.

Ganciclovir

Ganciclovir (DHPG) (Cytovene) is an acyclic guanine nucleoside analog similar in structure to acyclovir.

Pharmacodynamics. Ganciclovir is converted to the triphosphate form, which inhibits viral DNA synthesis by competitive inhibition of viral DNA polymerases. It can also be incorporated into viral DNA, resulting in termination of viral DNA elongation. Resistant strains of virus develop after exposure to the drug.

Pharmacokinetics. Oral bioavailability is less than 10%. After absorption, ganciclovir is widely distributed in body tissues and fluids, including the vesicular fluid, aqueous humor, and CSF. Only about 2% of the drug is bound to plasma proteins. Over 90% of ganciclovir administered IV is eliminated unchanged by renal excretion; oral doses are eliminated in feces.

Therapeutic Uses. Ganciclovir is approved for the treatment and chronic suppression of CMV retinitis in immunocompromised clients. Because of the high risk of relapse, AIDS clients with retinitis require suppressive therapy with the drug, and relapses may occur despite chronic suppression (sometimes due to ganciclovir resistance). Foscarnet therapy may benefit clients with ganciclovir-resistant CMV infections. Ganciclovir therapy may also benefit other CMV syndromes in AIDS clients. Ganciclovir has been used both for prophylaxis and for suppression of CMV infections in transplant recipients.

Adverse Reactions. Myelosuppression is the principal dose-limiting toxicity of ganciclovir. Neutropenia occurs in 15% to 40% of clients, thrombocytopenia in 5% to 20%. Neutropenia is usually observed during the second week of treatment and is usually reversible within 1 week of drug cessation. Fatal neutropenia has occurred. Oral ganciclovir causes neutropenia less commonly than the IV form. Recombinant granulocyte colony-stimulating factor may be useful in treating ganciclovir-induced neutropenia (see Chap. 35). CNS side effects affect 5% to 15% of clients and range in severity from headache to behavioral changes to convulsions and coma.

Drug–Drug Interactions. Interactions are reported with cytotoxic drugs, nephrotoxic drugs, probenecid, didanosine, and zidovudine. Zidovudine and probably other cytotoxic and nephrotoxic agents increase the risk of myelosuppression. Probenecid and possibly acyclovir reduce renal clearance of ganciclovir.

Drug–Laboratory Test Interactions. Abnormal liver function test results may be noted.

Precautions and Contraindications. Ganciclovir is very irritating to tissues and must not be given IM or SC. Oral doses should be given with food. This drug is contraindicated in clients with an absolute neutrophil count of less than 500/mm³ or a platelet count of less than 25,000/mm³.

Amantadine

Amantadine (Symmetrel) is a synthetic tricyclic amine with a structure unrelated to that of any other antimicrobial agent. Rimantadine (Flumadine) is its alpha-methyl derivative.

Pharmacodynamics. Amantadine and rimantadine exert two mechanisms of antiviral action. They inhibit the uncoating of virus particles, thereby preventing penetration of viruses into host cells. This leaves viruses stranded on the cell surface and vulnerable to attacks by host antibodies. A second action is theorized to be an altering of hemagglutinin processing. In the nervous system, amantadine has another action that may be useful in managing Parkinson's disease: it is thought to release dopamine from the intact dopaminergic terminals that remain in the substantia nigra in these clients.

Pharmacokinetics. Amantadine is administered orally and is well absorbed by the gastrointestinal (GI) tract. The drug distributes into saliva, nasal secretions, breast milk, and other body tissues. Amantadine is eliminated largely unmetabolized in urine. It is minimally dialyzable.

Therapeutic Uses. Amantadine is used to prevent and treat influenza A virus infections. For example, it might be started in conjunction with influenza A virus vaccine and continued for 2 weeks until protective immune responses to the vaccine develop. It also can be used early in the course of influenza A infection to treat and shorten the duration of viral symptoms. It is also used for symptomatic treatment of all forms of parkinsonism.

Adverse Reactions. Adverse reactions to amantadine include CNS disturbances (nervousness, lightheadedness, difficulty concentrating, insomnia). Higher amantadine plasma concentrations have been associated with more serious neurotoxic reactions, including hallucinations and seizures. Preexisting seizure disorders and psychiatric symptoms may be exacerbated. GI effects such as nausea, vomiting, anorexia, and dry mouth may occur.

Drug Interactions. Amantadine may exhibit additive atropine-like effects with concurrent use of anticholinergic drugs, tricyclic antidepressants, or antihistamines. Excessive CNS stimulation may occur if amantadine is combined with other CNS stimulants such as amphetamines or methylphenidate. Decreased urinary excretion of amantadine has occurred when hydrochlorothiazide and triamterene were administered concurrently.

Precautions and Contraindications. Dosage may need to be reduced in older adults and persons with renal impairment. When amantadine is used to treat Parkinson's disease, it should not be discontinued abruptly because symptoms may recur in an exaggerated form (parkinsonian crisis). Amantadine should be given cautiously to elderly clients, as they are more susceptible to adverse neurologic effects.

Zidovudine

Zidovudine (AZT; Retrovir) was formerly called azidothymidine and is a thymidine analog with antiviral activity.

Pharmacodynamics. Zidovudine competes with thymidine for incorporation into DNA or RNA molecules synthesized by the human immunodeficiency virus (HIV), the retrovirus responsible for AIDS. It inhibits viral RNA-dependent DNA polymerase (reverse transcriptase), which decreases viral DNA synthesis and viral replication. Resistance to the drug develops; the frequency and degree of resistance correlate with the stage of infection, CD4 count, and duration of therapy. Infection with resistant virus has occurred by sexual, percutaneous, and maternal–fetal transmission from treated persons.

Pharmacokinetics. Zidovudine is rapidly absorbed and exhibits 60% to 70% oral bioavailability. Absorption is decreased after food intake. It is 20% to 38% protein bound. It crosses the blood-brain barrier, enhancing its effect on the retroviruses in the brain. It is metabolized in the liver and excreted in urine.

Therapeutic Uses. The use of parenteral zidovudine is approved for managing HIV infection in adults with AIDS or AIDS-related complex (ARC) and a history of cytologically confirmed *Pneumocystis carinii* pneumonia or an absolute CD4 (T4 helper-inducer) lymphocyte count in the peripheral blood of less than 200/mm³ before therapy. Oral therapy is approved for managing clients with HIV infection and CD4 cell counts less than 500/mm³. It is also approved for preventing maternal–fetal HIV transmission and managing disease in HIV-infected children over 3 months old who have HIV-related symptoms or who are asymptomatic but have abnormal laboratory values indicative of HIV-related immunosuppression.

The drug is used palliatively; no cures have been reported in HIV-infected clients. In AIDS and ARC clients, the use of zidovudine is associated with prolonged survival, decreased opportunistic infections, weight gain and improved functional status, and increased CD4 counts. Treatment may benefit HIV-associated neurologic disease, thrombocytopenia, and lymphocytic interstitial pneumonia. In asymptomatic clients with CD4 counts of less than 500/mm³, the use of zidovudine decreases the risk of progression to AIDS-defining illness or death for about 2 years. The time-limited benefit has led to the increasing use of combination treatment strategies (Hardman & Limbird, 1996). The combination of zidovudine with zalcitabine or didanosine appears to be associated with greater and more sustained CD4 increases than monotherapy.

The efficacy of zidovudine for postexposure prophylaxis in transfusions or needle sticks is uncertain; failures occur. Treatment with zidovudine does not reduce the risk of transmission of the virus through sexual contact or blood contamination.

Adverse Reactions. Zidovudine suppresses bone marrow production in some recipients. The resulting anemia may require transfusions or the use of recombinant erythropoietin. Granulocytopenia has been managed with recombinant granulocyte colony-stimulating factor therapy. Hematologic indexes must be monitored every 2 weeks. The risk of hematologic toxicity increases with lower CD4 counts, more advanced disease, higher doses, and prolonged therapy.

Severe headache, nausea, vomiting, insomnia, and myalgia are common during the initiation of therapy, but these symptoms often diminish with continued use. Myopathy occurs with prolonged use and usually resolves slowly after the drug is discontinued.

Drug Interactions. Coadministration of zidovudine with bone marrow suppressive agents (e.g., ganciclovir, flucytosine, vincristine, adriamycin) may increase the risk of hematologic toxicity. Rifabutin and rifampin can induce hepatic microsomal enzymes and decrease plasma concentrations of zidovudine.

Precautions and Contraindications. Zidovudine should be used cautiously in clients with advanced symptomatic HIV infection, severe bone marrow depression, hepatomegaly, hepatitis, or renal insufficiency.

Ribavirin

Ribavirin (Virazole) is a purine nucleoside analog.

Pharmacodynamics. The exact mechanism of ribavirin's action is unknown. The drug is believed to interfere with the synthesis of such factors as guanosine triphosphate in viral particles by inhibiting enzymes necessary to these processes. Ribavirin has a wider spectrum of action than other antiviral drugs. It is active against both RNA and DNA viruses, respiratory syncytial virus, influenza A and B viruses, and HSV infections. The development of resistance has not been documented to date.

Pharmacokinetics. Ribavirin is usually administered orally or by inhalation. With inhalation, levels in respiratory secretions vary widely, and plasma levels increase with the duration of exposure. Oral ribavirin is rapidly absorbed, and oral bioavailability is 40% to 45%. It crosses the placenta and distributes into breast milk.

In a process believed to be essential to antiviral activity, ribavirin is phosphorylated by the liver and red blood cells. The drug and its metabolites are excreted mainly in urine. Ribavirin tends to persist in red blood cells, remaining in the body for weeks or longer after its use has been discontinued.

Therapeutic Uses. Ribavirin is used for treating hospitalized infants and children with severe lower respiratory infections caused by respiratory syncytial virus, such as bronchiolitis and pneumonia. An unlabeled use of the aerosol is treatment of some influenza A and B infections. Unlabeled uses of the oral preparation include treatment of acute and chronic hepatitis, herpes genitalis, and measles. The use of IV ribavirin has decreased mortality in Lassa fever and hemorrhagic fever with renal syndrome due to hantavirus infection. Ribavirin is under study in hantavirus-associated pulmonary syndrome.

Adverse Reactions. Aerosol ribavirin is generally well tolerated, although the mist is irritating and may cause mild conjunctival irritation, erythema of eyelids, and rash. Life-threatening reactions to the drug include worsening of respiratory function, cardiac arrest, and hypotension. The drug may cause dose-related anemia due to bone marrow suppression. In HIV-infected clients, chronic oral therapy is associated with dose-related lymphopenia and GI and CNS complaints, including headache, lethargy, insomnia, and mood alteration.

Drug–Drug Interactions. Use of ribavirin concurrently with digitalis can increase the possibility of digitalis toxicity.

Drug–Laboratory Test Interactions. Oral or parenteral administration may cause transient changes in liver function tests.

Precautions and Contraindications. Studies indicate that ribavirin is teratogenic, embryotoxic, and possibly gonadotoxic. Environmental exposure of healthcare workers is an issue; pregnant women should not directly care for clients receiving aerosolized ribavirin.

■ SUMMARY

The search for agents to combat viral infection has intensified in recent years. Most antiviral drugs have a narrow margin of safety. Because experience with many of the drugs is limited, knowledge of their adverse reactions and long-term toxicity is incomplete.

❖ NURSING MANAGEMENT: CLIENT RECEIVING ANTIVIRAL ANTI-INFECTIVES

Nursing management of clients receiving these drugs, which have such a short history, requires careful, complete health assessment.

NURSING PROCESS

ASSESSMENT

Because antiviral drugs are toxic, clients for whom they are prescribed tend to have serious infections or predisposing factors that reduce their natural defenses against infection. Before drug therapy is initiated, the client should be carefully assessed to determine his or her resistance to infection and general state of health. Women of childbearing age should be screened for pregnancy and lactation. Renal and hepatic function should be assessed. Clients' knowledge of their illnesses and proposed treatments and their emotional reaction to these should be assessed.

NURSING DIAGNOSIS

Nursing diagnoses for clients receiving antiviral anti-infective drugs may include:

- Impaired Tissue Integrity, related to phlebitis secondary to IV administration of antiviral medication
- Risk for Fluid Volume Excess, related to IV delivery of medication
  Anxiety, related to adverse effects of drug and to the diagnosis
- Knowledge Deficit, regarding the drug regimen and the disease process
- Risk for Injury, adverse reactions related to drug therapy

PLANNING

Goals are to promote tissue integrity, reduce anxiety, relieve discomfort, decrease knowledge deficit, reduce the risk of adverse reactions to medications, and detect and treat adverse drug reactions promptly.

INTERVENTIONS

Because there are no safe drugs for treating most viral infections, disease prevention remains of primary importance. The first way to prevent contagious diseases is by interrupting or eliminating contact between host and parasites. Resistance to infection can be promoted by eating a nutritious diet, getting adequate rest, and avoiding excessive stress.

Treatment of viral infections relies heavily on general supportive measures to help the body overcome the pathogenic agents. Hydration is important; fluid intake should be ample (up to 3 L/day for most adults) but not excessive. IV infusions of antiviral drugs require considerable dilution, and recipients must be monitored for fluid overload. Foods rich in vitamin C should be encouraged. The nurse should advise rest and control of stress.

Most people understand that viral infections are not as readily cured with medication as are microbial diseases. Therefore, clients with severe viral infections are likely to be anxious or fearful, especially those with compromised immune systems (eg, people with AIDS or organ transplants). They should receive consistent, personalized emotional support.

The nurse is responsible for monitoring the client's responses (both beneficial and detrimental) to the drug regimen. Any signs and symptoms of serious adverse reactions should be reported for possible modification of the drug regimen.

Client Education. An important nursing intervention is the development and implementation of a teaching plan to help the client understand the disease process and treatment regimen. The nurse can reassure clients that the treatment of viral infections has improved and that ongoing research continues to produce new treatment agents. Clients should be informed of the therapeutic and adverse effects of the drugs they are taking. They should know which signs and symptoms of drug response to report to healthcare personnel. Clients should be advised of interactions between this medication and others taken.

The nurse should teach the client about sanitary, hygienic, and aseptic measures needed to reduce infections. Teaching points may include a discussion of airborne pathogens and how to avoid unnecessary contact with persons who are sick and likely to transmit infection. Other teaching topics may include the importance of vaccines, especially for children and older adults, who are particularly vulnerable to viral pneumonia and influenza.

OUTCOME EVALUATION

Data that indicate a successful outcome include decreased signs and symptoms of infection, relaxed facial expression and body movements, absence of signs and symptoms of adverse drug reactions, and client statements that show decreased anxiety and increased understanding of the illness and its management. See the Example of Nursing Process for Ribavirin Treatment.

❖ CHECKLIST OF NURSING ACTIONS

- ❑ Urge parents to immunize their children against viral diseases, as recommended by public health authorities.
- ❑ Encourage good hygiene to promote general resistance.
- ❑ Give good supportive care to clients with active viral infections.
- ❑ Maintain appropriate fluid intake (up to 3 L/day for adults) in clients with viral infections.
- ❑ Report adverse reactions to new or experimental antiviral drugs.
- ❑ Inform the client of the expected benefits of medication and possible adverse reactions.

Pathophysiology of Fungal Infections

Infections caused by fungi are called mycotic infections or mycoses. Fungal infections may be superficial or systemic. Superficial mycoses, such as those caused by the dermatophytes (eg, tinea pedis), occur only on superficial tissue such as hair, epithelium, and nails. Fungi generally thrive in moist, warm environments. In tinea pedis (athlete's foot), infection occurs only in people who wear shoes.

Certain fungi live as normal flora in the body (eg, *Candida*) and become bothersome only when they are not kept in check by other body flora or by the immune system. For instance, because *Candida* often is part of the normal flora of the vagina, the newborn is likely to acquire the organism during birth. Newborns are highly susceptible to this organism, and epidemics develop quickly in the nursery if the infection is introduced. The first evidence often is the appearance of white patches on the tongue and mucous membranes of the baby's mouth (thrush). These patches resemble a thin layer of milk but adhere to the membrane and are not easily dislodged. The infection can spread to the skin, usually involving the diaper area. The affected skin becomes bright red, resembling the first-degree burns of a scald. Mothers of breastfeeding infants with thrush often develop candidal infection, manifested by sore or fissured nipples.

Once a fungus becomes established, it usually remains part of the natural flora of the skin or mucous membrane, ready to seize the opportunity for renewed growth when conditions are favorable. For this reason, fungal infections are often referred to as opportunistic. Conditions that predispose a person to an opportunistic fungal infection are AIDS, leukemia, cancer chemotherapy, organ transplantation with immunosuppressant therapy, alcoholism, substance abuse, and malnutrition. Opportunistic infections also thrive when the natural flora has been altered with antibiotics or when the environment contains more nutrients in which fungi can grow, such as the hyperglycemic blood of a diabetic.

Common systemic fungal infections include cryptococcosis, histoplasmosis, coccidioidomycosis, blastomycosis, and aspergillosis. These diseases usually affect the lungs, but can affect other tissues, causing peritoneal, ocular, urinary, and meningeal infections. The definitive diagnosis of such disorders is made by skin testing for antibodies against each organism.

Antifungal Anti-Infectives

Many victims of superficial fungal infections treat themselves using over-the-counter drugs. Only when an eruption fails to respond to these remedies, or when the infection is detected during medical appraisal for another condition, are these infections likely to be seen by a healthcare provider. Topical preparations for the more superficial fungal infections (eg, tinea pedis, tinea corporis, tinea cruris, tinea versicolor, cutaneous candidiasis) were discussed in Chapter 40.

Systemic therapy is necessary for treating fungal diseases when they are no longer localized or were systemic at the onset. The major drugs for systemic therapy are certain azoles (ketoconazole, itraconazole, fluconazole) and amphotericin B, flucytosine, and griseofulvin. Topical antifungal preparations include amphotericin B, clotrimazole, miconazole, and nystatin. Each antifungal drug has a distinct spectrum of activity and specific therapeutic uses (Table 44-2).

Clotrimazole

Clotrimazole (Lotrimin, Mycelex) is a synthetic antifungal imidazole derivative.

Pharmacodynamics. Clotrimazole binds with phospholipids in the fungal cell membrane, increasing permeability and causing loss of intracellular constituents. It inhibits or kills many fungi.

Pharmacokinetics. Clotrimazole's primary action is local; it binds to tissues in the skin or mucous membranes, from which it is released gradually. Only small amounts of the drug are absorbed systemically. After systemic absorption, clotrimazole is metabolized by hepatic microsomal enzymes.

Therapeutic Uses. Clotrimazole is used for the topical treatment of candidiasis, including oropharyngeal, skin, and vulvovaginal infections.

Adverse Reactions. Clotrimazole is usually well tolerated when administered topically, although local reactions (erythema, stinging, edema, blistering, pruritus, peeling, urticaria, general irritation) have occurred. When

Example of Nursing Process for Ribavirin Treatment

The client is 1 year old and has been diagnosed with lower respiratory tract infection with respiratory syncytial virus (RSV). The child has fever, elevated white blood cell count, decreased breath sounds over the affected area, and abnormal breath sounds. She is coughing intermittently. Ribavirin is prescribed.

Assessment Data

Fever
Elevated white blood cell count
Decreased and abnormal breath sounds
Cough
Diagnosis of RSV infection

Nursing Diagnosis

Risk for Injury, Adverse Effects, related to drug therapy

Intervention

Assess and record baseline data on client's status.

Use all possible nursing measures to promote natural resistance to infection.

Encourage fluid intake and intake of high-calorie, high-vitamin foods.

Reconstitute ribavirin powder with appropriate solution as indicated in package insert.

Discard solution if discolored or cloudy.

Administer ribavirin by aerosol, using Viratek Small Particle Aerosol Generator (SPAG). **Consult** manual for specific instructions.

Follow institutional guidelines for administration of aerosol. **Avoid** having pregnant women care for client and **involve** inhalation therapy department staff as appropriate.

Monitor client's cardiopulmonary status closely (worsening of respiratory function, cardiac arrest, and hypotension may occur).

Check blood pressure frequently.

Report any deterioration in cardiopulmonary status promptly.

Monitor hematologic studies closely for changes.

Goals and Outcomes

The client's airway will be free of secretions.

The client's gas exchange will be enhanced.

The client will be afebrile, and other signs of infection will clear.

The client will verbalize signs and symptoms of complications that must be reported.

Any adverse effects that occur will be promptly identified and alleviated.

---

administered intravaginally, local irritation can occur, as can abdominal cramps, urinary frequency, and burning or irritation in the sexual partner. Oral troches produce some systemic absorption of clotrimazole and may cause nausea and vomiting.

Drug Interactions. Minimally elevated liver enzyme studies have been reported in about 15% of the clients receiving the troche form of the drug.

Precautions and Contraindications. Clotrimazole should be avoided during the first trimester of pregnancy, regardless of the route of administration. Safe use in children younger than age 3 years has not been established.

Ketoconazole

Ketoconazole (Nizoral) is a synthetic antifungal agent.

Table 44-2. Antifungal Anti-Infective Drugs

Drug Name	Preparation	Usual Dosage	Additional Information
clotrimazole (Mycelex, Gyne-Lotrimin, Mycelex-G, Lotrimin)	Troche Vaginal preparations Topical preparations (cream, solution, lotion)	*Troche:* 1 troche 5 times a day for 14 consecutive days PC: C *Vaginal tablet:* insert 1 100-mg tablet intravaginally hs for 7 nights or 2 tablets for 3 nights or 1 500-mg tablet one time only PC: B *Vaginal cream:* one applicator hs for 7–14 consecutive days PC: B	Administer vaginal tablets at bedtime; if drug is administered at other times, the client must stay recumbent for 10–15 min.
miconazole (Monistat)	Parenteral Intrathecal Bladder instillation Vaginal suppositories or cream Topical preparations (cream, powder, spray)	Adults: 200–3,600 mg IV daily, depending on organism PC: B Children: 20–40 mg/kg IV as total dose; do not exceed 15 mg/kg per dose	For IV doses ≤2,400 mg/d, dilute in 200 mL of fluid and infuse at 2 hr/20-mL ampule.
nystatin (Mycostatin, Nilstat, Nystex)	Oral tablets Oral suspension Oral troche Vaginal tablets Topical preparations (cream, ointment, powder)	Adults: *tablets:* 500,000–1,000,000 U tid PC: A Adults and children: *oral suspension:* 400,000–600,000 U qid; *troches:* 200,000–4,000,000 U 4 or 5 times qd for up to 14 d; troche must be allowed to dissolve slowly in mouth	Continue treatment for at least 48 h after symptoms have subsided to prevent relapse.
amphotericin B (Fungizone)	Topical preparations (cream, lotion, ointment) Parenteral Intrathecal Intraventricular	Adults: 0.5–0.6 mg/kg qd; do not exceed total daily dose of 1.5 mg/kg PC: B	May load with 1 L of saline IV on day of administration; client may require supplemental potassium; several months of therapy usually necessary
itraconazole (Sporanox)	Oral capsules	Adults: 200 mg qd or bid PC: C	Take after full meal to ensure maximal absorption.
ketoconazole (Nizoral)	Topical preparations (cream, shampoo) Oral tablets	Adults: 400 mg daily PC: C Children: 3.3–6.6 mg/kg daily	Duration of therapy is 5 d for candidal vulvovaginitis, 2 wk for candidal esophagitis, and 6–12 mo for mycoses, such as blastomycosis.
fluconazole (Diflucan)	Oral tablets Oral suspensions Parenteral	Adults: 400 mg on first day, followed by 200–400 mg qd for 10–12 wk for acute cryptococcal meningitis; 150 mg orally as single dose qd for vaginal candidiasis Children: 6 mg/kg on first day followed by 3 mg/kg qd for 2 wk for oropharyngeal candidiasis; 12 mg/kg on first day followed by 6–12 mg/kg/d for 10–12 wk for cryptococcal meningitis PC: C	Dosage adjustment necessary for clients with renal impairment IV infusion is at maximum rate of 200 mg/hr. Dose or dosage interval should be changed if client has renal impairment.
griseofulvin (Fulvicin P/G, Grisactin, Grifulvin V)	Oral tablets and capsules Oral suspension	Adults: 500 mg microsize or 330–375 mg ultramicrosize–1 g microsize or 660–750 mg ultramicrosize in divided doses at 6-hr intervals PC: C Children: 10–15 microsize/kg qd	Several weeks to 1 year of therapy usually necessary to allow infected tissue to be replaced with normal tissue
flucytosine (Ancobon)	Oral capsules	Adult: 50–150 mg/kg/d in divided doses at 6-hr intervals PC: C	To reduce or avoid nausea and vomiting, take capsules a few at a time over 15 min.
terbinafine (Lamisil)	Topical Tablet	Adult: 250 mg/d PC: B	Dosage is adjusted for clients with renal insufficiency.

KEY: PC = pregnancy risk category; see Appendix A.

Pharmacodynamics. The action of ketoconazole is usually fungistatic. The drug blocks metabolic processes vital to cell membrane synthesis in fungi. The altered membrane cannot transport purines into the cell, and replication cannot proceed.

Pharmacokinetics. An acidic environment is required for the dissolution of ketoconazole. Plasma proteins bind 84% of the drug. The drug is metabolized in the liver, and the major pathway for elimination is the biliary tract to the feces, although smaller fractions are excreted in urine.

Therapeutic Uses. Ketoconazole is effective in blastomycosis, histoplasmosis, coccidioidomycosis, paracoccidioidomycosis, ringworm, tinea versicolor, chronic mucocutaneous candidiasis, candidal vulvovaginitis, and oral and esophageal candidiasis. Efficacy is poor in immunosuppressed clients and in meningitis. The slow response to therapy has made it inappropriate for clients with severe or rapidly progressive mycoses. Itraconazole has supplanted ketoconazole in many clients, although it is much more expensive.

Adverse Reactions. The most common adverse reactions are GI (nausea, vomiting, anorexia). An allergic rash and pruritus without rash may occur, and hair loss has been reported.

Ketoconazole inhibits steroid biosynthesis. Several endocrinologic abnormalities thus may be evident, including menstrual irregularities and gynecomastia and decreased libido in males.

Symptomatic drug-induced hepatitis is rare but potentially fatal. Hepatitis may occur after a few days of treatment or may be delayed for many months. The earliest symptoms are anorexia, malaise, nausea, and vomiting, with or without dull abdominal pain.

Drug–Drug Interactions. Bioavailability is decreased in clients taking histamine (H_2) antagonists. Simultaneous administration of antacids also may impair absorption. Induction of hepatic microsomal enzymes by rifampin and possibly phenytoin accelerates the metabolic clearance of ketoconazole and reduces its plasma concentration. Ketoconazole raises plasma cyclosporine concentrations; both drugs are metabolized by the microsomal enzyme system. Ketoconazole elevates terfenadine and astemizole blood levels, which can decrease cardiac conduction and potentially cause fatal torsades de pointes. Ketoconazole enhances warfarin's anticoagulant effect.

Drug–Laboratory Test Interactions. Mild, asymptomatic elevation of aminotransferase activity is common; these values usually revert to normal spontaneously.

Precautions and Contraindications. Taking the drug with food, at bedtime, or in divided doses may decrease GI effects. Ketoconazole should be used cautiously in clients with liver impairment or clients taking other hepatotoxic drugs.

Miconazole

Miconazole (Monistat) is a synthetic antifungal imidazole derivative.

Pharmacodynamics. At fungistatic concentrations, miconazole thickens fungal cell membranes and inhibits purine transport. At higher concentrations, it interferes with peroxisomal enzymes and causes necrosis of intracellular constituents, apparently because of peroxidase accumulation within the cell.

Pharmacokinetics. Absorption of miconazole varies depending on the route of administration. About 50% is absorbed from the GI tract. After absorption, miconazole is widely distributed into body tissues and fluids, including inflamed joints, the vitreous humor, and the peritoneal cavity. Little drug is found in sputum or saliva. The drug crosses the placenta and may be distributed into breast milk. Distribution into the CSF is unreliable, and the drug must be administered intrathecally to treat meningitis. Miconazole is 91% to 93% bound to plasma proteins. The drug is metabolized by the liver and excreted in urine.

Therapeutic Uses. Miconazole is used topically in the treatment of infections caused by susceptible fungi. It is also administered systemically in the treatment of serious systemic fungal infections, including coccidioidomycosis, candidiasis, cryptococcosis, and paracoccidioidomycosis.

Adverse Reactions. When applied topically, miconazole occasionally causes irritation and burning. The most common adverse reactions to IV administration are phlebitis at the infusion site and pruritus, with or without skin eruptions. Other adverse effects include GI disturbances (nausea, vomiting, diarrhea, anorexia) and febrile reactions.

Drug Interactions. Miconazole enhances the anticoagulant effect of warfarin and delays the metabolism of phenytoin. Amphotericin B and miconazole are antagonistic: the antifungal activity of the two drugs used together appears less than that of either drug used alone.

Precautions and Contraindications. Miconazole is dissolved in a vehicle that can cause an anaphylactoid reaction, so emergency resuscitative equipment should be on hand when the first dose is given. If the undiluted drug is given too rapidly IV, it may cause cardiac arrhythmias.

Fluconazole

Fluconazole (Diflucan) is a triazole.

Pharmacodynamics. Fluconazole binds to sterols in the fungal cell membrane, changing membrane permeability. It is fungicidal or fungistatic, depending on the concentration of drug and the organism involved.

Pharmacokinetics. Fluconazole is almost completely absorbed from the GI tract when administered orally.

Bioavailability is not altered by food or gastric acidity. Fluconazole diffuses readily into body fluids, including sputum and saliva. Concentrations in the CSF are 50% to 90% of the plasma values. About 12% of the drug is bound to proteins.

Therapeutic Uses. Fluconazole is used in oropharyngeal, esophageal, and vaginal candidiasis. It is the drug of choice to prevent relapse of cryptococcal meningitis in AIDS clients. Fluconazole has become the drug of choice for treatment of coccidioidal meningitis because it produces less morbidity than intrathecal amphotericin B. It is active against histoplasmosis, blastomycosis, sporotrichosis, and ringworm, but the response seems less than with itraconazole. Fluconazole does not appear effective in preventing or treating aspergillosis.

Adverse Reactions. Adverse reactions include nausea, vomiting, diarrhea, and abdominal pain. Headache is common. Hepatotoxicity and Stevens-Johnson syndrome have occurred. The incidence of adverse reactions to fluconazole is increased in clients with HIV.

Drug Interactions. Fluconazole increases plasma levels, and therefore the therapeutic and toxic effects, of phenytoin, cyclosporine, sulfonylureas, and warfarin. Rifabutin and rifampin plasma levels may be affected. It appears less likely to elevate terfenadine levels than does ketoconazole or itraconazole.

Precautions and Contraindications. The protective overwrap on the IV solution bag should not be removed until just before use. Also, the plastic container may look opaque from moisture absorbed during the sterilization process.

Itraconazole

Itraconazole (Sporanox) is a synthetic triazole approved for use in 1992.

Pharmacodynamics. Itraconazole inhibits the cytochrome P450–dependent synthesis of ergosterol, a vital component of fungal cell membranes.

Pharmacokinetics. Blood levels vary considerably among clients and are reduced by more than half in clients who are fasting, have reduced gastric acid, or have advanced AIDS. Itraconazole is more than 90% bound to serum proteins, and extensive binding to tissues also occurs. No detectable drug is found in the CSF. It is metabolized in the liver, and little or no intact drug appears in urine. It has one biologically active metabolite, to which many fungi are equally susceptible. Steady-state levels are reached only after several days, so a loading dose is often used for 3 days.

Therapeutic Uses. Itraconazole is approved for treatment of blastomycosis, histoplasmosis, aspergillosis, and onychomycosis in immunocompromised and immuno-

competent clients. Itraconazole is preferred over ketoconazole for treating nonmeningeal histoplasmosis. It is also the regimen of choice for maintenance therapy of AIDS clients with disseminated histoplasmosis whose disease has stabilized during amphotericin B therapy. To date, the drug has no value for the initial treatment of histoplasmosis in AIDS clients.

Unlabeled uses include treatment of oropharyngeal, esophageal, or vaginal candidiasis, as well as griseofulvin-resistant ringworm and extensive tinea versicolor.

Adverse Reactions. Nausea and vomiting are common. Occasionally hepatotoxicity has occurred. Profound hypokalemia has occurred in clients receiving 600 mg or more daily.

Drug–Drug Interactions. Multiple drug interactions are reported. Itraconazole concentrations are decreased by concomitant therapy with rifampin as well as with drugs that decrease gastric acidity (eg, histamine [H$_2$] antagonists, proton pump blockers). Simultaneous administration of itraconazole and didanosine should be avoided because didanosine is formulated with buffers that neutralize gastric acid. Itraconazole elevates plasma concentrations of drugs metabolized by the microsomal enzyme system, including digoxin, cyclosporine, and phenytoin. Ketoconazole inhibits the metabolism of astemizole, raising its serum concentration and possibly prolonging Q-T intervals, and it is likely itraconazole acts in a similar manner. Because increased serum levels of terfenadine, cisapride, and astemizole can lead to the potentially lethal torsades de pointes, coadministration is contraindicated.

Drug–Laboratory Test Interactions. Hypertriglyceridemia and increased serum aminotransferase levels occur.

Precautions and Contraindications. Itraconazole should be used cautiously in clients with hypochlorhydria, as they may not readily absorb the drug. Because itraconazole is bound to plasma proteins, it must be used cautiously in clients receiving other highly bound medications.

Griseofulvin

Griseofulvin (Fulvicin P/G, Grisactin, Grifulvin V) is effective against various species of the dermatophytes *Microsporum*, *Epidermophyton*, and *Trichophyton*. It has no effect on bacteria or other fungi.

Pharmacodynamics. Griseofulvin is fungistatic rather than fungicidal. It arrests cell division by disrupting the mitotic spindle. The presence of the drug in new keratin makes it resistant to fungal invasion. As nails and hair grow out, new growth becomes free of disease-producing organisms, and fungal cells are depleted as older growth is shed or cut off. Thus, griseofulvin eradicates from the body the reservoirs of infectious cells harbored at the base of the keratin layer.

Pharmacokinetics. Griseofulvin is administered orally. Because rates of dissolution have limited the bioavailability of griseofulvin, microsized and ultramicrosized powders are used in preparations. The bioavailability is said to be 50% greater for the ultramicrocrystalline preparation. Griseofulvin has a plasma half-life of about 1 day. It is excreted in urine, mostly in the form of metabolites. From the blood, the drug migrates to the skin, where it is deposited in keratin precursor cells. It has a special affinity for diseased skin but is also found in liver, fat, and skeletal muscle tissues.

Therapeutic Uses. Infections that respond well to this agent include infections of the hair (tinea capitis), ringworm of the glabrous skin, tinea cruris and tinea corporis, tinea of the hands and beard, and athlete's foot involving the skin and nails.

Adverse Reactions. Although multiple adverse reactions have been reported, they tend to be minor. CNS manifestations include headache (can be severe, but often disappears as therapy continues), peripheral neuritis, lethargy, confusion, fatigue, syncope, vertigo, and blurred vision. Dry mouth, heartburn, flatulence, nausea, vomiting, and diarrhea are common GI side effects. Skin eruptions and hepatotoxicity have been observed.

Drug–Drug Interactions. Griseofulvin induces hepatic microsomal enzymes, increasing the rate of metabolism of warfarin. The drug may reduce the efficacy of some oral contraceptives. Barbiturates decrease the absorption of griseofulvin from the GI tract. Combined use of griseofulvin and alcohol should be avoided because the effects of the alcohol tend to be augmented.

Drug–Food Interactions. Some studies have shown improved absorption when the drug is taken with a fatty meal.

Drug–Laboratory Test Interactions. Albuminuria and cylindruria occur, without evidence of renal insufficiency.

Precautions and Contraindications. Because very high doses of the drug are carcinogenic and teratogenic in laboratory animals, the drug should not be used to treat trivial infections that respond to topical therapy.

Blood studies should be carried out weekly during the first month of treatment to detect changes in hematopoietic function. Hematologic effects include leukopenia and neutropenia; these may subside with continued therapy.

Nystatin

Nystatin (Mycostatin, Nilstat) is an antifungal antibiotic produced by a strain of *Streptomyces*. It was discovered in the New York State Health Laboratory—hence its name.

Pharmacodynamics. Nystatin is both fungistatic and fungicidal. It acts by binding to sterols in the fungal wall, interfering with the integrity and function of the membrane. Loss of potassium and other intracellular constituents causes cell death.

Pharmacokinetics. Nystatin is poorly absorbed from the GI tract, skin, or mucous membranes. Whether taken orally or applied topically, it is used for local effect only. The drug passes through the GI tract unchanged and is eliminated in feces.

Therapeutic Uses. Nystatin is the main therapeutic agent for preventing and controlling infections caused by *Candida albicans*, including thrush (stomatitis) and diaper rash in children. Candidal infection in adults primarily affects persons rendered susceptible by deficient natural defenses, debility, or treatment with broad-spectrum antibiotics or immunosuppressants. Stomatitis and vaginitis are the most common manifestations. Nystatin is not indicated for the systemic mycoses.

Dosage and Administration. Oral nystatin is available as a suspension, troche, or powder for mixing with water. The dosage of nystatin suspension is 1 to 6 mL (100,000 U/mL), depending on the client's age, four times a day. When nystatin is ordered for fungal stomatitis, administration by "swishes" is usually specified. Clients should rinse the mouth thoroughly with the dose, gargle if necessary, retain it in the mouth as long as possible, then swallow it. This technique provides direct topical application of the drug to the affected area and has a prophylactic effect on the rest of the GI tract. Treatment should continue for 48 hours after clinical improvement is noted. The troche must be allowed to dissolve slowly in the mouth.

Topical preparations include ointments, creams, and powders (100,000 U/g). Powders are preferred for moist lesions. Combinations of nystatin with antibacterial agents or corticosteroids are also available. Vaginal tablets are available, but other agents appear more effective for vaginal candidiasis. An IV formulation is undergoing clinical trials with HIV clients.

Adverse Reactions. Adverse reactions to nystatin are rare and generally mild and transitory. Nausea, vomiting, and diarrhea occasionally develop from oral doses.

Drug Interactions. There are no known significant interactions.

Amphotericin B

Amphotericin B was discovered in 1956 by investigators studying a strain of *Streptomyces* from a river valley in Venezuela.

Pharmacodynamics. The antifungal activity of amphotericin B depends at least in part on its binding to sterols in the cell membrane of sensitive fungi. After this interaction, the permeability of the membrane increases, allowing leakage of various intracellular constituents (eg, potassium) from the cell. An additional mechanism of action may be oxidative damage to fungal cells. Resistance rarely develops.

Pharmacokinetics. Because amphotericin B is poorly absorbed from the GI tract, it must be given parenterally. In its formulation, it is complexed with the bile salt deoxycholate. In the bloodstream, the drug is released from its complex and remains in the plasma, largely bound to lipoproteins. Distribution is poorly understood but appears to be multicompartmental, although concentrations in many compartments are low (eg, CSF, pleural, pericardial, and synovial fluids, aqueous humor). Cross-placental transport has been reported. The metabolic fate of amphotericin B is unknown. Urinary excretion is the main pathway for elimination. Amphotericin B is not removed from the blood by dialysis.

Therapeutic Uses. Amphotericin B is used for the treatment of severe, life-threatening systemic infections caused by susceptible fungi and protozoa. It has useful clinical activity against *Candida, Cryptococcus neoformans, Blastomyces dermatitidis, Histoplasma capsulatum, Coccidioides immitis, Paracoccidioides braziliensis,* and *Aspergillus.* Other drugs are useful with blastomycosis, histoplasmosis, coccidioidomycosis, and paracoccidioidomycosis, but amphotericin B is preferred when those mycoses are rapidly progressive, occur in an immunosuppressed host, or involve the CNS.

Dosage and Administration. Intrathecal infusion of amphotericin B three times a week is necessary in clients with meningitis caused by *Coccidioides.* The drug can be injected into the CSF of the lumbar spine, cisterna magna, or lateral cerebral ventricle. Fever and headache are common reactions and may be decreased by intrathecal administration of 10 to 15 mg of hydrocortisone. Amphotericin B given once weekly has been used to prevent relapse in clients with AIDS who have been treated successfully for cryptococcosis or histoplasmosis.

Adverse Reactions. Most clients receiving amphotericin B experience adverse reactions; the most common are chills and fever. Sometimes hyperpnea and respiratory stridor or modest hypotension may occur, but true anaphylaxis is rare. The reaction tends to end spontaneously in 30 to 45 minutes. Pretreatment with oral acetaminophen or IV hydrocortisone at the start of the infusion decreases reactions. The mechanism of the febrile reaction is thought to be release of interleukin-1 and tumor necrosis factor from monocytes and macrophages (Hardman & Limbird, 1996).

Headache, nausea, vomiting, malaise, weight loss, and phlebitis at the infusion site are common. Amphotericin B usually causes azotemia and nephrotoxicity.

Hypochromic, normocytic anemia is usual. Decreased production of erythropoietin is the probable reason. Clients with low plasma erythropoietin levels may respond to administration of recombinant erythropoietin. Anemia reverses slowly after therapy.

Drug Interactions. Azotemia occurs in 80% of clients who receive amphotericin. Toxicity is dose-dependent and transient and is increased by concurrent therapy with other nephrotoxic agents, such as aminoglycosides or cyclosporine.

Precautions and Contraindications. To decrease the incidence of nephrotoxicity, 1 L of normal saline solution is administered IV on the day the drug is to be given. Amphotericin B is given only in the hospital setting under close supervision. An initial test dose is given with monitoring and emergency equipment available.

Flucytosine

Flucytosine (Ancobon) is a fluorinated pyrimidine and a relative of the antineoplastic drugs fluorouracil and floxuridine.

Pharmacodynamics. Within fungal cells, flucytosine is deaminated to fluorouracil. Fluorouracil is then metabolized and can be either incorporated into RNA or further metabolized to a substance that is a potent inhibitor of thymidylate synthetase. DNA synthesis is impaired as the result of the latter reaction.

Pharmacokinetics. Oral flucytosine is absorbed rapidly and well. It readily penetrates the blood-brain barrier to reach therapeutic levels in the CSF. Flucytosine is minimally bound to plasma proteins (2%–4%). Its half-life is 3 to 6 hours in clients with normal renal function. Flucytosine is minimally metabolized and is excreted almost entirely unchanged in urine. The drug is removed by hemodialysis and peritoneal dialysis.

Therapeutic Uses. Flucytosine is used only for the treatment of severe fungal infections caused by *Cryptococcus neoformans* and susceptible strains of *Candida.* Drug resistance may occur.

Adverse Reactions. Adverse reactions to flucytosine are similar to those of fluorouracil. It tends to cause bone marrow depression (causing anemia, leukopenia, and thrombocytopenia) and GI symptoms (nausea, vomiting, and diarrhea). Adverse reactions are more common when azotemia is present or when the client has AIDS.

Drug–Drug Interactions. The synergistic effects of amphotericin B and flucytosine can enhance toxicity.

Drug–Laboratory Test Interactions. Flucytosine raises the level of hepatic enzymes, but this effect is reversed when the drug is stopped.

Precautions and Contraindications. Flucytosine should be used cautiously in clients with bone marrow suppression or impaired renal or hepatic function.

Terbinafine

Terbinafine is an allylamine available as a topical preparation for tinea corporis, tinea cruris, and tinea pedis, among others. Outside of the United States, an oral preparation is being studied.

■ SUMMARY

Infections caused by fungi are called mycotic infections or mycoses and can be either superficial or systemic. Ketoconazole, itraconazole, fluconazole, amphotericin B, flucytosine, and griseofulvin are drugs used to treat systemic fungal infections. Because these drugs are relatively toxic, hospitalization is usually required for treatment. Amphotericin B, clotrimazole, miconazole, and nystatin are available as topical preparations for superficial fungal infections.

❖ NURSING MANAGEMENT: CLIENT RECEIVING ANTIFUNGAL ANTI-INFECTIVES

Clients receiving treatment for systemic fungal infections are seriously ill; these diseases can be life-threatening. Clients with systemic fungal diseases face a difficult and sometimes lengthy course of treatment. Not only is drug treatment uncomfortable and risky, but some clients with lung disease also eventually require surgery to remove infected tissue.

NURSING PROCESS

ASSESSMENT

Data required for assessment include a history of the client's illness; signs and symptoms indicative of the client's current condition; a full assessment of general health, particularly cardiovascular, neurologic, and renal function; an assessment of the client's emotional status; and information about the drugs being used currently. See the Critical Thinking Challenge: Case Analysis.

Clients at risk for fungal infection should be assessed for skin lesions (rough, itchy patches on the scalp or arms, itching and cracks between the toes, sore and reddened areas, sore and fissured nipples), mucous membrane lesions (white adherent plaques, sore and reddened areas), and abnormal drainage (thick, frothy vaginal drainage).

NURSING DIAGNOSIS

Nursing diagnoses for clients receiving antifungal anti-infective drugs may include:

CRITICAL THINKING CHALLENGE
Case Analysis

Your client, who has AIDS, was admitted with histoplasmosis, for which the prescriber has ordered amphotericin B. As a new nurse, this is the first time you will administer this drug.

1. What assessment and laboratory data will you need to study before administering this drug?
2. Discuss the significance of the laboratory findings. What effect do they have on medication administration?
3. Devise an explanation for the client of the benefits of the medication and adverse effects to anticipate. What can you do to help relieve these side effects?

- Body Image Disturbance, related to changes in skin appearance secondary to superficial antifungal medication
- Anxiety, related to the drug regimen and prognosis
- Knowledge Deficit, related to fungal infection and associated drug regimen
- Risk for Injury, adverse reactions related to drug therapy

PLANNING

Goals of nursing care are to lessen or eliminate symptoms of infection by administering medication correctly, to alleviate client anxiety, to reduce the risk of adverse drug reactions and to detect and treat promptly any that occur, and to increase the client's knowledge about the disease, its treatment, and self-care measures to reduce the incidence and recurrence of fungal infections.

INTERVENTION

General supportive measures (adequate diet and rest, management of stress levels) are important in promoting recovery by increasing the client's natural resistance to infection and ability to heal damaged tissue.

If thrush is detected among nursery newborns, vigorous measures should be taken to prevent contagion. The infection is less likely to develop in babies whose mouths are cleaned of milk after feeding. This can be done by rinsing the infant's mouth with water after every feeding.

In the hospital setting, the nurse is responsible for administering the prescribed drugs. Some IV preparations require precise methods of administration (eg, in-line filter, diluent, storage temperature for unopened containers and reconstituted drug, amount of time for infusion), and these must be followed carefully.

Some drugs may require additional supplements for safe administration. For example, because hypokalemia often develops with amphotericin B, foods high in potassium should be encouraged. Adequate sodium in-

Example of Nursing Process for Antifungal Drug Therapy

The client is a 53-year-old man who has AIDS and is considered malnourished. He has a central venous catheter as part of his treatment. Presenting symptoms included headache and stiff neck. He has been diagnosed as having cryptococcal meningitis. A regimen of amphotericin B (Fungizone) and flucytosine (Ancobon) is ordered.

Assessment Data

Headache and stiff neck

Diagnosis of cryptococcal meningitis, an opportunistic infection

Regimen of amphotericin B and flucytosine ordered

Diagnosis of AIDS and malnutrition

Nursing Diagnosis

Pain, related to fever secondary to use of amphotericin B

Risk for Infection, related to potential for additional opportunistic infections

Intervention

Assess and record baseline data on client's status: vital signs, CNS function.

Teach client about drug regimen and associated adverse reactions, advising client that treatment is going to be lengthy—possibly 4 to 8 weeks.

Premedicate client as ordered when he receives amphotericin B.

Be prepared to administer antipyretic or other agents during administration if fever and chills occur. Also, adjust thermostat and blankets.

Infuse IV amphotericin slowly and observe infusion site for signs of inflammation.

Administer capsules of flucytosine a few at a time over a 15-min period to minimize GI adverse effects.

Monitor laboratory studies of bone marrow, renal, and liver function (dysfunction may occur with either drug).

Monitor client for signs and symptoms of hypokalemia.

Wash hands before and after all contact with client, and teach client and others handwashing technique.

Assign client to private room, and **protect** client from others with infection.

Promote natural resistance to infection.

Encourage fluid intake and intake of high-caloric, high-vitamin foods.

Maintain meticulous aseptic technique during any invasive procedures.

Assess for and report signs and symptoms of additional opportunistic infection.

Obtain specimens for culture as ordered.

Goals and Outcomes

The client's infection will heal in a timely manner.

The client will be afebrile.

The client will participate in behaviors that reduce risk of infection.

take should also be maintained because sodium depletion increases the risk of renal toxicity.

Troches must be dissolved slowly in the mouth. Vaginal tablets should be inserted high into the vagina at bedtime. If bedtime administration is impossible, the client should remain recumbent for about 15 minutes after insertion. A sanitary napkin should be provided to protect clothing from stains.

Vaginal creams should be administered high into the vagina using the applicator supplied and should be administered for 7 to 14 consecutive nights, even during menstruation.

The client should be monitored carefully for signs and symptoms of adverse drug reactions, specifically for allergic reactions (including anaphylaxis) and renal or liver impairment.

Client Education. Clients subject to fungal infections should be instructed in special techniques of skin care to reduce the recurrence of active infection. Because the pathogens are usually part of the normal flora of the skin in such clients, it is crucial to prevent the moist, warm conditions that favor fungal growth. To suppress athlete's foot, for example, the feet should be kept clean and dry. Daily washing followed by thorough drying and the application of antifungal foot powder may be recommended. Care should be taken to distribute the powder or other medication to all areas, especially between the toes. Because conditions are ideal for fungal growth in intertriginous areas, lesions are most common there. Clients should be advised to avoid shoes made of plastic or synthetic material in favor of materials such as leather, which allow perspiration to evaporate. Socks should be changed daily and shoes rotated so that they dry thoroughly between wearings.

Oily preparations should never be applied to the feet if a fungal infection is suspected. By preventing evaporation of perspiration, oils promote fungal growth and may increase the irritation.

Before administering drugs to treat systemic fungal infections, the client should be informed about the expected beneficial and possible adverse reactions. Clients should contact the prescriber to report any unusual signs and symptoms. With nystatin, simple measures (bland food, avoidance of irritating drugs such as aspirin) may minimalize intestinal irritation. Clients receiving griseofulvin should report malaise, changes in urinary excretion, and photosensitivity or other neurologic symptoms. They should avoid drinking alcohol. During the first month of treatment with this agent, the client must report for weekly blood tests. The importance of completing the course of therapy should be stressed.

Clients treated with experimental antiviral or antifungal drugs must have full knowledge about the dangers involved. They may be required to sign an informed consent. They should be informed of their right to stop treatment at any time.

OUTCOME EVALUATION

Data that indicate a successful outcome include decreased signs and symptoms of inflammation, decreased anxiety, understanding by the client of the infection and its management and successful performance of self-care measures, and the absence of signs and symptoms of adverse drug reactions. See the Example of Nursing Process for Antifungal Drug Therapy.

❖ **CHECKLIST OF NURSING ACTIONS**

❑ Teach clients subject to fungal infections to keep their skin clean, cool, and dry.
❑ Provide good supportive nursing care to increase general resistance to the fungal infection.
❑ Monitor newborns for signs and symptoms of candidal infection. Institute early treatment and isolation to prevent epidemics in the nursery.
❑ Inform clients of beneficial effects and adverse reactions that can occur with prescribed medications.
❑ Warn clients receiving griseofulvin to avoid alcohol consumption.
❑ Assess clients completely on admission and periodically during treatment to detect adverse drug reactions promptly.

References

Clark JL, Tatum NO. (1995). Management of genital herpes. *Am Fam Phys, 51*(1), 175–182.

Hardman JG, Limbird LE, Molinoff PB, et al., eds. (1996). *Goodman and Gilman's The pharmacological basis of therapeutics,* 9th ed. New York: McGraw-Hill.

Olin BR, ed. (1995). *Drug facts and comparisons.* St. Louis: Facts and Comparisons.

Bibliography

Beutner KR, et al. (1995). Valacyclovir compared with acyclovir for improved therapy for herpes zoster in immunocompetent adults. *Antimicrob Agents Chemother, 39,* 1546–1553.

Dudley MN. (1995). Clinical pharmacokinetics of nucleoside antiretroviral agents. *J Infect Dis, 171,* S99–S112.

Englund JA, et al. (1994). High-dose, short-duration ribavirin aerosol therapy compared with standard ribavirin therapy in children with suspected respiratory syncytial virus infection. *J Pediatr, 125,* 635–641.

Kinoch-DeLoes S, et al. (1995). A controlled trial of zidovudine in primary human immunodeficiency virus infection. *N Engl J Med, 333,* 408–411.

McEvoy GK. (1996). *American Hospital Formulatory Service Drug Information.* Bethesda, MD: American Society of Health-System Pharmacists, Inc.

O'Maracaigh AS, Betcher DL. (1994). Amphotericin B and its lipid formulations. *J Ped Oncol Nurs, 11*(3), 125–127.

Rodriguez WJ, et al. (1994). Efficacy and safety of aerosolized ribavirin in young children hospitalized with influenza: A double-blind, multicenter, placebo-controlled trial. *J Pediatr, 125,* 129–135.

Smith MA, Brennessel DJ. (1994). Cytomegalovirus. *Infectious Dis Clin North Am, 8*(2), 427–438.

Stein DS, et al. (1994). The effect of the interaction of acyclovir with zidovudine on progression to AIDS and survival. *Ann Intern Med, 121,* 100–108.

Volberding PA. (1994). Perspectives on the use of antiretroviral drugs in the treatment of HIV infection. *Infectious Dis Clin North Am, 8*(2), 303–317.

Wagstaff AJ, Faulds D, Goa KL. (1994). Acyclovir: A reappraisal of its antiviral activity, pharmacokinetic properties and therapeutic efficacy. *Drugs, 47,* 153–205.

Wheat J. (1994). Histoplasmosis and coccidioidomycosis in individuals with AIDS: A clinical review. *Infectious Dis Clin North Am, 8*(2), 467–482.

White MH, Armstrong D. (1994). Cryptococcosis. *Infectious Dis Clin North Am, 8*(2), 383–398

For more information and sample tests and activities, refer to Chapter 44 in the Student Workbook for Clinical Pharmacology and Nursing Management, 5th edition, available through your bookstore.

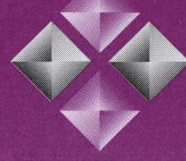

45

Drugs That Treat Parasitic and Helminthic Infections

presence of the vector, improper sewage disposal, lack of clean water, and consumption of contaminated food.

The immune system plays a crucial role in most protozoan/host relations, often limiting the pathologic consequences of infection. Thus, opportunistic infections with protozoa can affect infants, persons with cancer, transplant recipients, persons receiving immunosuppressive drugs, and persons with AIDS. *Pneumocystis carinii* is an opportunistic organism that is sometimes classified as a protozoan and sometimes as a fungus. Treatment of infection in immunocompromised clients is challenging, and the outcome is not as satisfactory as with persons whose immune system functions competently.

Rickettsia are parasitic organisms transmitted to humans from an infected arthropod. All rickettsial diseases cause fever, and most cause a rash resulting from rickettsial multiplication in cells of small blood vessels. The cells become swollen and necrotic, leading to lesions. Common diseases resulting from rickettsial infection include Rocky Mountain spotted fever, typhus fever, trench fever, and Q fever (Table 45-1). Rickettsial diseases are best controlled by suppressing the arthropods that serve as carriers. The drugs of choice for treating rickettsial diseases are the tetracyclines (discussed in Chap. 42).

Sometimes referred to as macroparasitic infestations, helminthic infections involve parasitic worms. The common intestinal helminths are divided into three groups: nematodes (roundworms), trematodes (flukes), and cestodes (tapeworms).

Ectoparasitic infestations are caused by parasites attached to the outer surface of the skin or situated beneath the skin of the host. The two most common ectoparasitic infestations are scabies and pediculosis. These infestations and the agents used to treat them were discussed in Chapter 40.

A vector is a carrier, and the term can refer to an arthropod that transfers an infective agent from one host to another. Arthropods can be insects such as ticks, mites, lice, and fleas. Organisms that can cause disease can multiply in the arthropod (the reservoir) without causing disease. Disease is transmitted to humans through the bite or feces of the infected arthropod.

Pathophysiology of Parasitic Infections

Protozoa are unicellular organisms that may lead parasitic existences; some protozoa cause disease in humans. These parasitic protozoa can be transmitted by vectors. Some of the more common human protozoal infections include malaria, trypanosomiasis, leishmaniasis, amebiasis, giardiasis, trichomoniasis, toxoplasmosis, and cryptosporidiosis. Multiple environmental factors contribute to the prevalence of parasitic infections, such as a hot, humid climate, overcrowded living conditions, the

Table 45-1. Diseases Caused by Rickettsia	
Disease	**Epidemiology**
Spotted fevers (*Rickettsia rickettsii;* Rocky Mountain spotted fever)	Multiply in nucleus and cytoplasm of infected cells of ticks and mammals; transmitted by bite of infected tick or through skin abrasions contacting tick feces or tissue juices
Typhus fevers (*Rickettsia prowazekii;* epidemic typhus)	Inhalation of dried lice feces; lice feces often rubbed into broken skin, as with scratching of bite
Rickettsia typhi (endemic typhus)	Transmitted by fleas
Q fever (*Coxiella burnetti*)	Inhalation of infected dust, ticks on body, and lice feces; sheep, goats, cows often infected
Trench fever (*Rickettsia quintana*)	Transmitted by body lice feces into broken skin
Scrub typhus (*Rickettsia tsutsugamushi*)	Transmitted by chigger bite

Lyme Disease

Lyme disease was first recognized in the United States in 1975, when an outbreak occurred in the small Connecticut town for which it was named. Since then, the disease has proliferated and is considered the most common vector-borne disease in the United States today. Lyme disease is caused by *Borrelia burgdorferi*, a spirochete form of bacteria transmitted to humans by the bite of deer ticks. These ticks are also found on birds, mice, dogs, cats, cows, horses, and raccoons. Lyme disease usually occurs during the late spring and early summer.

The disease process parallels the stages of untreated syphilis, also a spirochete disease. As with syphilis, treatment at the onset of Lyme disease usually prevents complications.

The most characteristic clinical symptom is a skin lesion, erythema migrans, that occurs at the site of the tick bite in 80% of affected persons. The lesion may be accompanied by such symptoms as intermittent fever, headache, fatigue, stiff neck, and migratory joint and muscle pain. If not treated, Lyme disease can progress in weeks or months to debilitating arthritis, cardiovascular disorders, and neurologic abnormalities.

Prevention of Lyme disease has included spraying insect repellent containing DEET on skin or permethrin on clothes and wearing protective clothing (long pants of light-colored fabric so ticks can be easily seen, long sleeves, pants tucked into long socks, closed shoes or boots). Insecticides might be used on lawns in areas where the ticks are prevalent. If lawns are sprayed, care should be taken to protect humans and pets by keeping them out of the area. Planting chrysanthemums, which appear to have a natural tick repellent, may also help. Natural methods of tick control have included the introduction of a small wasp that is an enemy of the tick but does not sting humans and the use of pheromones that attract ticks to insecticide traps. A gene-engineered vaccine has been developed to protect mice against Lyme disease; this research may lead to a vaccine for humans.

The drugs used to treat Lyme disease are a variety of antibiotics (eg, oral doxycycline or amoxicillin and intravenous [IV] ceftriaxone). If started promptly, the oral antibiotics usually shorten the period of symptoms and prevent cardiac, neurologic, and arthritic problems in the future. These drugs were discussed in earlier chapters of this textbook.

Protozoan Infections

Protozoa are among the most important causative agents of parasitic diseases. Especially prevalent in the underdeveloped tropical areas of the world, protozoa affect a large proportion of the world's population and are a major cause of morbidity and mortality.

Vector control and improved sanitation seem to be the most reliable methods of eradicating or controlling these illnesses. However, even massive international campaigns have been unsuccessful in achieving this goal. In some areas of the world, protozoan infections have been controlled for a time only to recur later.

As long as these protozoan diseases remain epidemic or endemic in large areas of the world, chemotherapy for their treatment is important. The agents used to treat protozoan diseases are not ideal drugs. In many cases, organisms have become resistant to previously effective drugs. As more people travel to areas where disease is prevalent, particularly the tropics, more healthcare professionals will need to become familiar with these diseases and able to diagnose and treat them. Travel medicine clinics are opening throughout the United States to counsel those going to areas where unfamiliar diseases may prevail. These clinics advise clients about health problems in the areas to be visited and are authorized to administer yellow fever vaccinations, which are required for entry into some countries. Clients should be referred to such a clinic or directed to tropical disease centers, epidemiology departments of hospitals, state health agencies, or Centers for Disease Control and Prevention (CDC) (http://www.cdc.gov) that can provide the information.

Malaria

Malaria, which is responsible for millions of deaths worldwide, is caused by four species of the protozoal genus *Plasmodium* (Table 45-2). The parasite is transmitted to humans through the bite of the female Anopheles mosquito. When an infected mosquito bites, malarial sporozoites, present in the saliva of the mosquito, are deposited under the skin and travel through the circulation to the parenchymal cells of the liver and other tissues, where they reproduce, forming schizonts. During this preerythrocyte phase of the disease, the victim remains free of symptoms. The schizonts later rupture, releasing spores (merozoites) that invade red blood cells, where they use hemoglobin as a nutrient. In all forms of malaria except infection with *Plasmodium falciparum*, some of the merozoites infect tissue cells, a stage of the disease that may continue for several years, causing relapses. The merozoites that infect red blood cells develop and reproduce, eventually bursting from the ruptured red cells. The liberated spores invade still more erythrocytes, reproducing once again. After several such cycles, the number of organisms is sufficient to destroy large numbers of red blood cells each time a new generation of merozoites is produced. The release of swarms of malarial organisms and of large amounts of cellular debris produces the chills and fever that mark the beginning of an exacerbation of the disease. The life cycle of the malarial parasite is shown in Figure 45-1.

Antimalarial Drugs

The oldest treatment for malaria was ingestion of a tea made from the bark of the cinchona tree of South America. The infusion contained several alkaloids, one of which (quinine) eliminated the symptoms of the dis-

Table 45-2. Malaria-Causing Plasmodia

Species	Form	Additional Information
Plasmodium falciparum	Malignant tertian* malaria, a frequently fatal form of the disease	By invading erythrocytes of any age, this species can produce an overwhelming parasitemia and fulminating infection in nonimmune persons. Rapid death may ensue.
Plasmodium vivax	Benign tertian* malaria	This species produces milder clinical attacks than those of *P falciparum*, but with a greater tendency to recur after treatment.
Plasmodium malariae	Quartan (4-day cycle) malaria	*P malariae* is common in localized areas in the tropics.
Plasmodium ovale	Rare mild form of tertian* malaria	This disease may be characterized by relapses, but it is more readily cured than *P vivax*.

*Tertian refers to the cycle characteristic of attacks, in which chills and fever occur at 3-day intervals.

ease. Until the third decade of the 20th century, quinine was the only available effective antimalarial agent. In 1930, the first antimalarial synthetic drug, quinacrine (Atabrine), was introduced. For a brief period it was the drug of choice, but because of its relative toxicity and therapeutic limitations, newer drugs replaced it.

Malarial strains that are resistant to all of the agents, including one of the most effective drugs, chloroquine, have emerged. Researchers are also finding a gene in resistant malaria parasites that is resistant to multiple drugs. As research continues, newer and better drugs may displace present drugs. Current drugs are listed in Table 45-3.

Quinine

An alkaloid derived from cinchona bark, quinine (Quinamm, others) is the antimalarial drug with the longest history of use (over 350 years). Although it has been synthesized, the procedure is complex; therefore, quinine is still obtained from natural resources. Cinchona contains more than 20 alkaloids, the most important being quinine, quinidine, cinchonidine, and cinchonine.

Pharmacodynamics. Quinine acts primarily as a schizonticide; it has little effect on sporozoites. Its action is not entirely clear; it may act by interfering with the function of plasmodial DNA. Quinine also relaxes skeletal muscles.

Pharmacokinetics. Because quinine is absorbed well by the gastrointestinal (GI) tract, it is administered orally. It reaches a peak plasma level in about 3 hours. Quinine is 70% bound by plasma proteins. About 95% of the drug is degraded by the liver and other tissues. The drug is excreted primarily by the kidneys. Renal excretion is enhanced with acidic urine. The half-life varies with the severity of malarial infection.

Therapeutic Uses. Quinine is used for treatment of severe illness due to chloroquine-resistant and multidrug-resistant strains of *P falciparum*. Quinine has also been used for the management of nocturnal leg cramps.

Dosage and Administration. A typical adult dose for a patient with malaria is 600 mg orally every 8 hours. The drug should be given with food or meals to decrease GI upset. There are several regimens for treatment and prophylaxis of malaria, depending on the species of *Plasmodium* responsible, the drug resistance in the region, and other factors. A parenteral preparation is available for use with acutely ill clients. Nocturnal leg cramps may be relieved by taking 200 to 300 mg before retiring.

Adverse Reactions. When quinine is given repeatedly at therapeutic doses, a typical dose-related cluster of symptoms occurs called cinchonism. This syndrome is manifested by tinnitus, vertigo, visual disturbances, and headache. Rare reactions include blood dyscrasias such as hypoprothrombinemia and leukopenia.

Drug–Drug Interactions. Absorption of quinine from the GI tract can be delayed by antacids containing aluminum. Quinine can delay the absorption and elevate plasma levels of digitalis preparations. Likewise, the

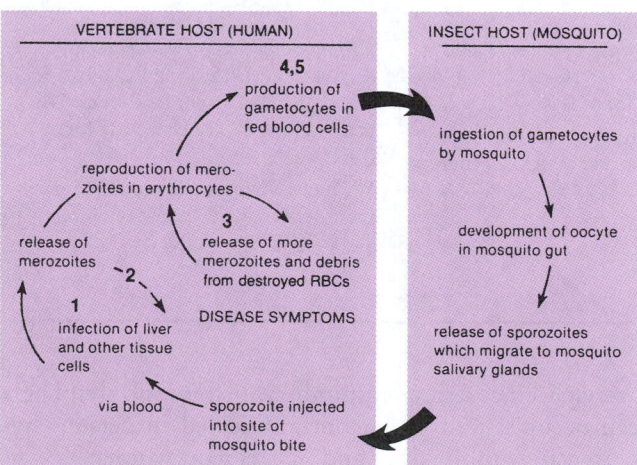

Figure 45-1. Life cycle of the malarial parasite. Points numbered on the illustration indicate the location in the malarial life cycle where specific drugs might be effective. (1) Chlorguanide, pyrimethamine, and primaquine used for causal prophylaxis. (2) Primaquine used to prevent relapses. (3) Agents against the erythrocytic phase: potent action—chloroquine, amodiaquine, quinine; limited action—pyrimethamine and chlorguanide. (4) Gametocidal drugs: primaquine. (5) Gametocyte sterilizing drugs: chlorguanide, pyrimethamine.

Table 45-3. Antimalarial Drugs

Drug Name	Preparation	Usual Dosage	
		Adults	Children
quinine sulfate (Formula Q, Legatrin, M-KYA, Quinamm, Quiphile, Q-vel)	Capsules Tablets	*Chloroquine-resistant malaria:* 650 mg q8h PO for 5–7 d *Chloroquine-sensitive malaria:* 600 mg q8h PO for 5–7 d *Nocturnal leg cramps:* 200–300 mg hs PC: X	*Chloroquine-resistant malaria:* 25 mg/kg per day given q8h PO for 5–7 d *Chloroquine-sensitive malaria:* 10 mg/kg PO q8h for 5–7 d
mefloquine (Lariam, Mephaquin)	Tablets	*Mild to moderate malaria:* 5 tablets (1,250 mg) PO as single dose *Prophylaxis:* 250 mg PO once weekly for 4 wk, then 250 mg PO every other week CDC recommends single dose taken weekly 1 wk before travel and for 4 wk after leaving the area; for prolonged stays in endemic area, take weekly for 4 wk, then every other week until traveler has taken 3 doses after return to a malaria-free area PC: C	*Prophylaxis:* starting 1 wk before travel and continued weekly during travel and for 4 wk after leaving such areas: 15–19 kg: 0.25 tab PO, 20–30 kg: 0.5 tab PO, 31–45 kg: 0.75 tab PO
chloroquine hydrochloride (Aralen)	chloroquine hydrochloride 50 mg is equivalent to 40 mg chloroquine base Tablets IM	*Suppression:* 300 mg base PO once a week on the same day for 2 wk before exposure and continuing until 6–8 wk after exposure *Acute attack:* 600 mg base PO initially; then 300 mg 6 hr later and on days 2 and 3 or 160–200 mg base IM initially and 6 hr later if needed; do not exceed 800 mg base/d PC: C	*Suppression:* 5 mg base/kg PO once a week on the same day for 2 wk before exposure and continuing until 6–8 wk after exposure *Acute attack:* 10 mg base/kg PO initially; then 5 mg base/kg 6 hr later and on days 2 and 3; or 5 mg base/kg IM initially and 6 hr later if needed; do not exceed 10 mg base/kg per day
primaquine	Tablets	Begin treatment during the last 2 wk of, or following, a course of suppression with chloroquine or a comparable drug; 26.3 mg (15 mg base)/d PO for 14 d PC: C	0.5 mg/kg per day PO (0.3 mg base/kg per day) for 14 d; maximum 15 mg base/dose
pyrimethamine (Daraprim)	Tablets	*Chemoprophylaxis of malaria* (adults and children over 10 yr): 25 mg PO once weekly for at least 6–10 wk With fast-acting schizonticides for treatment of acute attack: 25 mg/d PO for 2 d PC: C	*Chemoprophylaxis of malaria* (children 4–10 yr): 12.5 mg PO once weekly for 6–10 wk ; (children <4 yr): 6.25 mg PO once weekly for 6–10 wk With fast-acting schizonticides for treatment of acute attack (children 4–10 yr): 25 mg/d PO for 2 d

KEY: PC = pregnancy risk category; see Appendix A.

alkaloid may raise plasma levels of warfarin anticoagulants. The renal clearance of quinine can be decreased by cimetidine and increased by acidification of the urine.

Drug–Laboratory Test Interactions. Quinine interferes with results of 17-hydroxycorticosteroid determinations.

Precautions and Contraindications. Quinine cannot be used for clients with myasthenia gravis because it decreases the excitability of the motor endplate region, reducing responses to repetitive nerve stimulation and acetylcholine; serious respiratory distress and dysphagia can occur. The drug is contraindicated in persons hypersensitive to the drug and in pregnant women.

Mefloquine

Mefloquine (Lariam), taken alone, is recommended for the prevention and treatment of malaria caused by chloroquine-resistant and multidrug-resistant *P falciparum*. It can be used prophylactically for travelers who stay for only brief periods in areas where these infections are endemic. It may cause nausea, abdominal pain, diarrhea, and dizziness; these adverse reactions are dose-related and self-limiting. Mild or severe signs of central nervous system (CNS) toxicity (eg, dizziness, ataxia, headache, seizures, psychotic manifestations) occur but are usually reversible after drug withdrawal. Mefloquine is not recommended for pregnant women, persons using drugs that alter cardiac conduction, or persons with a history of epilepsy or psychiatric disorder.

Chloroquine

Pharmacodynamics. When used to treat amebiasis, chloroquine (Aralen) is a systemic amebicide because it concentrates in the liver and can eliminate trophozoites in liver abscesses. It is much less effective in intestinal forms of amebiasis because it is almost completely absorbed from the small bowel and reaches only low concentrations in the wall. There is no evidence that amoebas develop resistance to chloroquine.

Pharmacokinetics. Administered orally, chloroquine's onset of action varies: peak action occurs in 1 to 2 hours and duration of action is about 1 week. Onset of action after intramuscular (IM) administration is rapid: peak action occurs in 45 to 60 minutes and duration of action is about 1 week. The drug is metabolized by the liver and excreted in urine. Chloroquine crosses the placenta and enters breast milk.

Therapeutic Uses. Chloroquine's usefulness is declining because strains of *P falciparum* have developed resistance to it. Its advantages were that it was more potent and less toxic than quinine and needed to be given only once weekly. Chloroquine is also used in the therapy of amebiasis (discussed later in this chapter). It is used when treatment with metronidazole is unsuccessful or contraindicated.

Dosage and Administration. For amebiasis, a typical dose is 1 g/day for 2 days, followed by 500 mg/day for 2 to 3 weeks.

Adverse Reactions. Given by mouth or by injection, chloroquine is generally well tolerated, although it does cause pruritus and GI effects. It can cause toxic manifestations related to the heart.

Precautions and Contraindications. Because the drug is concentrated in the liver, it should be used with caution when hepatic disease is present. Chloroquine is one of the antimalarial agents that cause hemolysis in clients with glucose-6-phosphate dehydrogenase (G6PD) deficiency.

Primaquine

Primaquine destroys late hepatic stage and latent tissue forms of *Plasmodium vivax* and *Plasmodium ovale*. It also is effective against the gametocytic forms of all four plasmodia and destroys them in the blood or prevents them from maturing later in the mosquito. It causes marked hypotension after parenteral administration and therefore is given orally. Although it is fairly innocuous when given to most whites, the drug causes he-

molytic reactions in some blacks and in certain white ethnic groups (Sardinians, Sephardic Jews, Greeks, Iranians). These populations are deficient in G6PD. Clients should be tested for the deficiency before they receive primaquine.

Pyrimethamine

Pyrimethamine is generally used with sulfadoxine to treat uncomplicated chloroquine-resistant *P falciparum* infections. It inhibits plasmodial dihydrofolate reductase, which deprives the protozoa of tetrahydrofolate, a cofactor required in the biosynthesis of purines and pyrimidines. The low doses of each drug used in combination therapy are believed to be less conducive to the development of resistance in the malaria organism. Larger doses may produce a megaloblastic anemia resembling that caused by folic acid deficiency. Contraindications include G6PD deficiency. Pyrimethamine must be used cautiously in pregnant or lactating women.

■ SUMMARY

Antimalarial drugs include the natural alkaloid quinine and synthetic drugs. Certain systemic antibacterials with antimalarial properties are used as adjuncts in the treatment of malaria. Regimens for their use and objectives of treatment vary, depending on the status of the disease and whether or not malaria is endemic. Many drugs used in the past are no longer effective because of resistance developed by the malaria strains.

❖ NURSING MANAGEMENT: CLIENT RECEIVING ANTIMALARIALS

Nurses frequently have the opportunity to educate the public, and this is often the case in areas where vector-borne diseases such as malaria are prevalent. A primary concern in such areas is prevention and control of the disease. For prevention tips to benefit the community at large, see Home and Community Care: Preventing Malaria.

There is a 24-hour telephone information service available with detailed recommendations for the prevention of malaria. The Centers for Disease Control and Prevention malaria information number is (404) 332-4555.

NURSING PROCESS

ASSESSMENT

Clients who are to receive antimalarial medication should be assessed for contraindications and risk factors for adverse drug reactions. These factors include visual impairment, hearing impairment indicative of eighth cranial nerve damage, liver impairment, G6PD deficiency, and anemia (common in those infected with malaria). A careful assessment of general health is also required. The circumstances that mandate malaria treatment (existing disease, expectation of exposure, latent disease) should be delineated.

HOME AND COMMUNITY CARE

Preventing Malaria

In areas where mosquitoes breed and multiply, certain controls and precautions may help protect people from contact with the insects. Some prevention methods include:

- Put screens on windows and doors to exclude insect vectors from living areas.
- Treat damp basements to keep them as dry as possible, and moisture-proof dwellings; mosquitoes like to breed in damp areas.
- Cut weeds and grass, because long grass traps moisture and provides a good environment for mosquitoes to breed.
- Install canopies of netting around beds as a barrier to mosquitoes.
- Wear outdoor clothing that covers as much skin as possible and fits snugly at the wrists and ankles.
- Apply oil of citronella or other insect repellents to exposed skin. A minimum of repellent should be used because these chemicals may also be toxic.
- Use pesticides only when barriers and other methods fail to control vector populations. These toxic chemicals often disturb the ecology, poison beneficial life forms, and threaten human welfare. Wherever possible, natural predators (birds, frogs, toads, snakes, cats) should be used to combat vector populations.
- When using pesticides, handlers must protect themselves and others from contamination with the chemical. Certain toxic chemicals are reserved for use by specially trained and licensed applicators; others, however, are freely available to the public. Persons using these chemicals should read and heed warnings and precautions on the product label.

NURSING DIAGNOSIS

Nursing diagnoses likely to be made for clients receiving antimalarial drugs may include:

- Risk for Injury, related to potential adverse reactions to drug therapy
- Knowledge Deficit, concerning antimalarial drug regimen

PLANNING

Along with controlling disease symptoms, goals of nursing care are to alleviate discomfort, prevent adverse drug reactions (or detect and treat any that occur), and teach the client about the drug regimen and control of malaria.

INTERVENTION

Nursing measures to promote comfort and resistance to infection (ample fluids, good diet, adequate rest, reduced stress) are basic. Measures to prevent exposure to mosquitoes must be taken. If malaria is endemic to the area, the client could be infected by more than one strain of the *Plasmodium* species, making the infection more difficult to treat. If malaria is not endemic to the area, it could be established in the mosquito population if the infected client is bitten.

Antimalarial drugs must be secured to prevent accidental ingestion by children. Fatalities due to shock and respiratory arrest from antimalarial drug poisoning have been reported in children, who are particularly susceptible to the hypotensive and depressive effects of the drugs.

Because malaria is usually a chronic disease, treatment may be long-term or recurrent. Because antimalarial agents cause discomfort and are somewhat hazardous, clients need a great deal of encouragement to adhere to the medication regimen. The nurse should point out improvements and stress the benefits of suppressing or eradicating the disease. Clients should be informed that missed doses of medication may jeopardize the therapeutic result and may induce resistance in the malaria parasites. Clients may need help developing a system to minimize missed doses.

Acutely ill clients are usually treated in an acute care setting. The nurse is responsible for administering medications, which may be given parenterally at first. When given parenterally, quinine should be well diluted and administered by slow infusion. Because the drug is irritating to the veins, the injection site should be inspected regularly for signs of phlebitis. Clients must be assessed regularly for adverse reactions to antimalarial drugs. Selected laboratory tests should be monitored.

Client Education. Teaching plans should be developed and implemented for each client. The client should be taught self-care techniques to support and enhance natural resistance to infection and to ameliorate the debilitating effects of the illness. Clients should also be taught measures to prevent transmission of malaria to others and to prevent recurrences of active infection.

Clients should be taught to identify the early signs and symptoms of adverse drug reactions. They should report unusual auditory sensations (ringing or roaring noises and a sense of fullness in the ears).

Travelers should be instructed about special precautions to take. Immunization is usually recommended against diseases that are either epidemic or endemic to the area. Suppressant medication to prevent malaria is prescribed for those planning to visit malarial areas.

OUTCOME EVALUATION

Data that indicate a successful outcome include the absence of signs and symptoms of malarial infection and adverse drug reactions and the client's ability to relate

Example of Nursing Process for Chloroquine Therapy

The client is a 40-year-old Vietnam veteran with an exacerbation of malaria. Chloroquine has been prescribed. The client first contracted malaria during his service in Vietnam. He had one recurrence of symptoms 5 years ago, which was successfully treated. The client has no history of renal or hepatic impairment, but he has had several episodes of gastroenteritis over the past year. The client is unemployed, and he and his wife live in a beach house on a lake. The house is run down and poorly screened. Family income is limited to what the client and his wife can earn doing odd jobs.

Assessment Data

History of frequent episodes of gastroenteritis
Order for chloroquine therapy
House is poorly screened
Limited family income

Nursing Diagnosis

Risk for Injury, related to potential adverse reactions to drug therapy

Knowledge Deficit, concerning malaria and its control and management

Intervention

Determine if client is deficient in glucose-6-phosphate dehydrogenase before starting therapy.

Give chloroquine with or after meals to decrease GI irritation.

Observe for relief of symptoms and blood smears negative for plasmodia.

Explore client's episodes of gastroenteritis to determine what nutritional interventions might be helpful.

Discuss with the client and his wife their options regarding fixing their house so that it is screened to exclude insects, or moving to another home.

Refer the client to social services for assistance to obtain food needed during convalescence or appropriate housing changes.

Goals and Outcomes

The client, if not deficient in the enzyme, will be able to take chloroquine without developing hemolytic anemia.

The client will not experience nausea, vomiting, diarrhea, loss of appetite, or abdominal pain.

The client will exhibit blood smears that are negative for plasmodia within 48–72 hours.

The client and his wife will have a home that is screened to exclude insects, including mosquitoes.

The client and his wife will have adequate resources to supply them both with an adequate diet.

---

material conveyed during teaching sessions about the drug regimen. See the Example of Nursing Process for Chloroquine Therapy.

❖ CHECKLIST OF NURSING ACTIONS

- Teach safe and effective techniques for mosquito control.
- Monitor clients taking quinine for eighth cranial nerve irritation.
- Monitor clients taking synthetic antimalarial drugs or IV quinine for hypotension and respiratory depression.
- Dilute quinine solutions for IV use and administer by slow infusion.
- Monitor prothrombin time and complete blood count in clients taking quinine.
- Encourage clients taking antimalarial medication to adhere to the drug regimen.
- Warn clients that antimalarial drugs must be secured to prevent accidental ingestion by children.

Amebiasis

The cause of amebiasis is the protozoan organism *Entamoeba histolytica*. In most victims, the protozoa exist as trophozoites in the large intestine; cysts are produced, but otherwise there is little harm. In other victims, the parasites invade the intestinal mucosa, producing mild to severe colitis. In still others, the parasites invade extraintestinal tissues, chiefly the liver, producing amebic abscesses and systemic disease. Thus, the infection may be active in an acute or chronic form or harbored by carriers who remain asymptomatic. Transmission is by the anal–oral route: cysts excreted in the feces of hosts enter the environment and are ingested through contaminated food or water or are contracted from unclean hands (Fig. 45-2).

Amebicides

Drugs used to treat amebiasis can be categorized as luminal, systemic, or mixed amebicides (Table 45-4). Diloxanide furoate, a luminal amebicide, is active only against the trophozoite form of amebiasis. Systemic amebicides effective against the invasive forms of amebiasis include emetine and dehydroemetine or chloroquine. Metronidazole, a nitroimidazole derivative, is used against the parasite both in the intestine and in extraintestinal tissues.

Diloxanide Furoate

Diloxanide furoate (Furamide) is available only by special request from the Centers for Disease Control and Prevention in Atlanta. It is effective against cysts and is considered by some to be the drug of choice for treating asymptomatic carriers. It is of no value in the treatment of invasive or extraintestinal amebiasis. After oral administration, it is hydrolyzed in the intestinal mucosa, and it is about 90% absorbed. However, the unabsorbed drug is the active amebicide. Treatment must be carried out for 10 days. Diloxanide furoate appears to be nontoxic; only mild GI symptoms and increased flatulence have been reported.

Emetine and Dehydroemetine

Emetine, an alkaloid derived from ipecac, has been used since 1912. Dehydroemetine (Mebadin) has similar pharmacologic properties but is considered less toxic. Although both drugs have been widely used to treat severe invasive intestinal amebiasis and extraintestinal amebiasis, they have been largely replaced by metronidazole, which is as effective and far safer. Thus, these two drugs would not be used unless metronidazole is ineffective or contraindicated. Clients who receive emetine or dehydroemetine are hospitalized for treatment. Because both drugs are toxic to the heart, clients must be on complete bed rest for the duration of treatment (10 days for adults, 4–6 days for children). The drugs tend to accumulate in the tissues, and the risk of serious toxicity increases as treatment progresses. The heart is monitored by electrocardiography; therapy is discontinued if abnormalities appear.

Metronidazole

Metronidazole (Flagyl), a nitroimidazole introduced for treatment of infection with *Trichomonas vaginalis*, another protozoan infection, was soon recognized as a superior agent for the treatment of amebiasis. Other nitroimidazoles are available outside the United States.

Pharmacodynamics. Metronidazole is bactericidal and trichomonacidal, as well as amebicidal. It is effective against anaerobic cocci and both anaerobic gram-negative and anaerobic spore-forming gram-positive bacilli. Nonsporulating gram-positive bacilli are often resistant, as are aerobic bacteria. The mechanism of action has

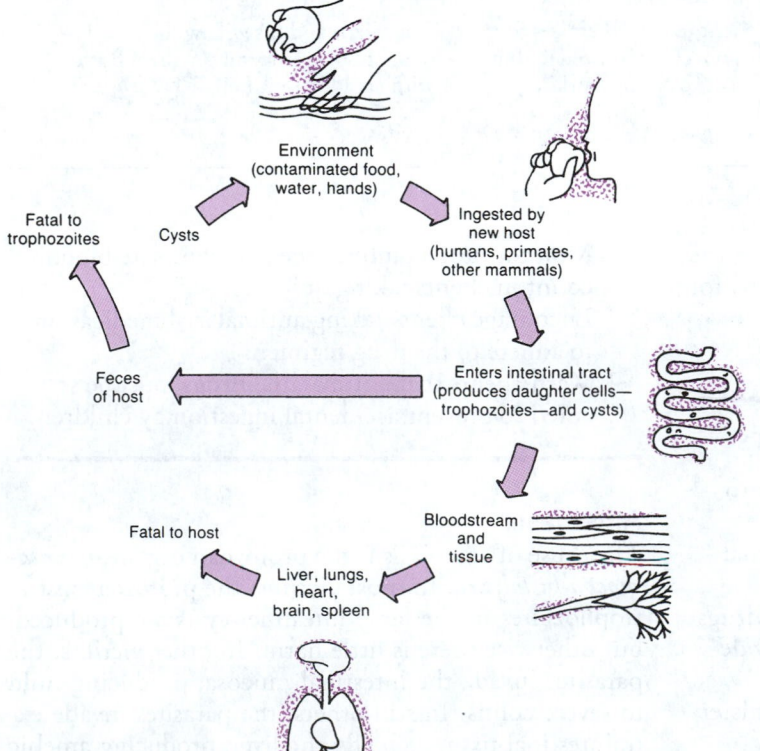

Figure 45-2. Life cycle of *Entamoeba histolytica*.

Table 45-4. Drugs Used to Treat Protozoa Infections

Drug Name	Preparation	Usual Dosage	Additional Information
diloxanide furoate (Furamide)	Oral	Adults: 500 mg tid for 10 d; children: 20 mg/kg/d in 3 divided doses for 10 d	Drug of choice for treating asymptomatic carrier of amebiasis Repeat in several weeks if necessary Available from Centers for Disease Control and Prevention*
metronidazole (Flagyl, Metizol, Protostat)	Tablets Capsules Powder for injection Injection, ready to use	Adults: *amebiasis:* 750 mg tid PO for 5–10 d; *trichomoniasis:* 2 g PO in one day or 250 mg tid PO for 7 d; *giardiasis:* 250 mg tid PO for 7 d Children: *amebiasis:* 35–50 mg/kg per day PO in 3 doses for 10 d PC: B	Agent of choice for amebiasis and giardiasis Avoid alcohol during and for 3 days after use.
paromomycin (Humatin)	Capsules	*Amebiasis:* 25–35 mg/kg/d in 3 divided doses with meals for 5–10 d PC: C	
quinacrine (Atabrine)	Tablets	*Giardiasis:* adults: 100 mg tid for 5–7 d; children: 7 mg/kg/d given in 3 divided doses after meals for 5 d	Examine stool 2 wks later and give repeat course if indicated. Bitter taste of pulverized tablets may be disguised in jam or honey.
pyrimethamine (Daraprim)	Tablets	*Toxoplasmosis:* adults: initially 50–75 mg daily with 1–4 g sulfa-pyrimidine; continue for 1–3 wk, depending on response and tolerance; then reduce dosage for each drug by one half and continue for additional 4–5 wk; children: 1 mg/kg/d divided into 2 equal doses; after 2–4 d reduce to one half and continue for about 1 mo; may give sulfonamide with it PC: C	Also used for malaria Other dosage schedules available Should be taken with food or meals
pentamidine (Pentam 300, NebuPent)	IM IV Aerosol	4 mg/kg qd for 14 d administered deep IM or IV Aerosol: 300 mg once every 4 wk administered via Respirgard II nebulizer PC: C	Used to prevent or treat *Pneumocystis carinii;* also used for leishmaniasis, trypanosomiasis IM/IV dose in renal failure must be individualized. Check written materials on drug and nebulizer for additional directions; must use freshly prepared solution; reconstitute with sterile water only
melarsoprol (Arsobal)			Used for trypanosomiasis; available from Centers for Disease Control and Prevention*
nifurtimox (Lampit)			Used for Chagas' disease; available from Centers for Disease Control and Prevention*
sodium stibogluconate (Pentostam)			Used for leishmaniasis
suramin (Fourneau 309, Bayer 205, Germanin, Moranyl, Belganyl, Naphuride, Antrypol, Naganol)	IV	1 g by slow IV injection weekly for 4–7 wk	Avoid extravasation during administration because severe pain may result. Used for trypanosomiasis, onchocerciasis; available from Centers for Disease Control and Prevention*

*Centers for Disease Control and Prevention can supply agents on request. May be requested from Drug Service, Division of Host Factors, Center for Infectious Disease, by calling 1-404-639-3670, 8 AM to 4:30 PM EST Monday through Friday; for emergencies call 1-404-639-2888. PC = pregnancy risk category; see Appendix A.

never been fully explained, but the drug is known to disrupt DNA structure and function. It is equally effective against dividing and nondividing cells. It can be considered a prodrug in the sense that it requires metabolic activation by sensitive organisms.

Pharmacokinetics. Taken by mouth, metronidazole is about 80% absorbed. Residues that remain in the intestinal tract eradicate the trophozoites in the large bowel. For these reasons, the drug is effective in treating both intraluminal and extraluminal amebiasis. After absorption, metronidazole is widely distributed into body tissues and fluids, including vaginal secretions, seminal fluid, saliva, cerebrospinal fluid (CSF), and cerebral and hepatic abscesses. Protein binding is less than 20%. The drug readily crosses the placenta and is distributed in breast milk. The plasma half-life of metronidazole is about 8 hours in normal adults. Plasma half-life is prolonged by hepatic impairment but not by renal impairment. The drug is metabolized by the liver and excreted in both urine and feces. Metronidazole is removed by hemodialysis but not by peritoneal dialysis.

Therapeutic Uses. Metronidazole is used in the treatment of trichomoniasis, amebiasis, and giardiasis. In amebiasis and giardiasis, it is the agent of choice. It is effective in anaerobic bacterial infections caused by *Bacteroides, Clostridium,* and *Helicobacter* species. It is also used to prevent postoperative anaerobic bacterial infection in clients undergoing intestinal surgery, in which contamination of the operative field by anaerobic bacteria is likely.

Metronidazole usually cures genital infections by *T vaginalis* in both females and males. Lack of satisfactory response may be due to chronic infection of the cervical or other glands, or to reinfection by an infected partner. In refractory cases, use of a topical gel or a 500- to 1,000-mg vaginal suppository increases the local concentration of the drug. Occasionally, treatment failure is due to the presence of metronidazole-resistant organisms.

Dosage and Administration. For amebiasis, the dosage is 750 mg three times daily for 5 to 10 days. The daily dose for children is 35 to 50 mg/kg, given in three divided doses for 10 days. Treatment with metronidazole is least effective in an asymptomatic passer of cysts; in this case, it is combined with a luminal amebicide. The IV dosage for anaerobic bacterial infections includes a loading dose (15 mg/kg) followed, starting 6 hours later, by a maintenance dose of 7.5 mg/kg every 6 hours, usually for 7 to 10 days.

Adverse Reactions. Metronidazole is relatively nontoxic. Even in large doses, it does not affect the cardiovascular or respiratory system. The most common adverse reactions are headache, nausea, dry mouth, and a metallic taste. Vomiting, diarrhea, and abdominal distress occur occasionally. Dizziness, vertigo, and rarely numbness, paresthesias of extremities, and convulsions are some of the neurotoxic effects that warrant discon-

tinuation of the drug. The compound may produce a disulfiram-like effect (unpleasant symptoms when alcohol is ingested). Neutropenia has been observed. Urine sometimes turns reddish-brown, because metronidazole contains metabolites that are water-soluble pigments. Superinfection by *Candida* organisms may occur.

Adverse Reactions. When metronidazole and warfarin are administered concurrently, prothrombin times must be closely monitored and the anticoagulant dosage adjusted accordingly. The concurrent use of metronidazole and disulfiram is not recommended because confusion and a psychotic state may occur. Enzyme inducers, such as phenobarbital, enhance the rate of metabolism of metronidazole; enzyme inhibitors, such as cimetidine, prolong its half-life.

Precautions and Contraindications. Caution should be used when metronidazole is administered to clients with CNS disease or hepatic impairment. If abnormal neurologic symptoms occur during therapy, withdrawal of the drug should be considered, because reversal of serious neuropathies may be slow or incomplete. Clients should avoid consuming alcohol during metronidazole treatment. White blood cell counts should be monitored before and during therapy because neutropenia has occurred. Metronidazole is contraindicated in persons with a history of allergic sensitivity to this and related drugs.

Paromomycin

Paromomycin (Humatin) is an aminoglycoside antibiotic with amebicidal properties.

Pharmacodynamics. Paromomycin exerts amebicidal effects against the intestinal forms of *E histolytica.* The exact mechanism of action is unknown, but aminoglycosides appear to inhibit protein synthesis in susceptible organisms.

Pharmacokinetics. Paromomycin is administered orally for its local effect on the GI tract. Its direct amebicidal action is probably due to the effects it has on cell membranes to cause leakage. The drug is poorly absorbed from the GI tract, but significant amounts may be absorbed if intestinal motility is impaired or if open lesions are present. Drug absorbed systemically is eliminated slowly in urine. Accumulation can occur in clients with renal impairment.

Therapeutic Uses. Paromomycin is used in treating intestinal amebiasis. It is used alone to treat mild cases and asymptomatic carriers and with other amebicides in acute or severe forms of the disease. Paromomycin is ineffective against extraintestinal forms of amebiasis. It is an alternative agent for the treatment of cryptosporidiosis.

Adverse Reactions. Paromomycin is relatively nontoxic. Adverse reactions are chiefly GI and include anorexia, nausea, vomiting, epigastric burning and pain, abdominal cramps, diarrhea, and pruritus ani. The drug can cause malabsorption similar to that caused by neomycin. Superinfection with *Candida* organisms can develop during paromomycin treatment. Like other aminoglycosides, paromomycin may cause nephrotoxic and ototoxic adverse reactions. Allergic reactions may also occur.

Precautions and Contraindications. Paromomycin is administered with caution to clients with ulcerative bowel lesions because the drug may be absorbed in large amounts. High doses of or prolonged therapy with the drug should be avoided. Paromomycin is contraindicated in persons allergic to it and in clients with impaired renal function.

■ SUMMARY

Clients receiving drugs to manage amebiasis require monitoring and good supportive care. The choice of drugs and regimen for treatment depend on the client's general condition, the previous course of the disease, and whether the infection involves extraintestinal tissues.

❖ NURSING MANAGEMENT: CLIENT RECEIVING AMEBICIDES

Clients who are to receive amebicides should be screened before treatment for risk factors that could influence the choice of treatment agent.

NURSING PROCESS

ASSESSMENT

The nursing history should include specific information about the client's nutritional status and kidney, liver, or cardiac impairment. In women of childbearing age, pregnancy should be ruled out. The client's general condition should be carefully assessed. Amebiasis can be debilitating, and poor physical condition increases the risk of drug therapy. The client's knowledge about amebiasis and its treatment should be assessed.

NURSING DIAGNOSIS

Nursing diagnoses related to drug therapy for amebiasis may include:

- Diarrhea, related to amebiasis or adverse reactions to medication
- Altered Nutrition: Less Than Body Requirements, related to diarrhea secondary to adverse effects of drug therapy
- Risk for Injury, related to potential adverse reactions to drug therapy
- Knowledge Deficit, related to drug therapy and disease

PLANNING

Goals of treatment include reducing the signs and symptoms of amebiasis, preventing or promptly detecting

and treating adverse drug reactions, and teaching clients about amebiasis and its treatment.

INTERVENTION

Nursing measures to support and enhance natural resistance to infection are essential. Because most amebicides cause anorexia, nausea, vomiting, and epigastric and intestinal distress, clients do not feel like eating. Good nutrition, however, is important, because many clients have become debilitated by the amebic infection. The nurse must employ every means available to provide inviting meals and to make mealtime enjoyable. The nurse should also take measures to promote rest and reduce stress.

Client Education. Clients who receive metronidazole must avoid alcohol, because the drug can cause a disulfiram-like reaction. They should be warned that their urine may turn reddish-brown. Clients who receive amebicides should be warned that nausea, vomiting, diarrhea, and intestinal discomfort are likely. They should be urged to eat a nourishing diet during the period of treatment to maintain general resistance to infection.

OUTCOME EVALUATION

Data that indicate a successful outcome include decreased signs and symptoms of amebiasis, absence of adverse reaction to drug therapy, and client statements that show knowledge about amebiasis and its treatment.

❖ CHECKLIST OF NURSING ACTIONS

- ❑ Screen clients who are to receive amebicides for malnutrition, major organ impairment, hypersensitivity, and pregnancy.
- ❑ Teach clients about amebiasis and the prescribed treatment regimen.
- ❑ Instruct clients who receive metronidazole to avoid alcoholic beverages.
- ❑ Reassure clients who receive metronidazole that the reddish-brown discoloration of urine is a normal, harmless result of the drug treatment.
- ❑ Stress the importance of maintaining good nutrition during treatment for amebiasis.

Miscellaneous Protozoan Infections

Trypanosomiasis (African sleeping sickness, Chagas' disease) and leishmaniasis (kala-azar) do not occur in the United States. Information about treatment of these infections can be obtained by writing to the Parasitic Disease Drug Service 8, Centers for Disease Control and Prevention, Atlanta, GA 30333. Trypanosomiasis is treated with melarsoprol, nifurtimox, pentamidine, and suramin. Leishmaniasis is treated with sodium stibogluconate.

Giardiasis

Giardiasis, an intestinal infection caused by *Giardia lamblia*, is characterized by diarrhea, malabsorption, and epigastric distress. It occurs frequently among people who travel abroad but is also seen in parts of the United States where the infection is endemic. As in amebiasis, the organism is transmitted as a cyst by the anal–oral route. It does not invade extraintestinal tissues. Once diagnosed, the disease should be treated whether or not the client has symptoms. One course of metronidazole is effective in most cases. If necessary, a second course, or quinacrine, can be given.

Trichomoniasis

Trichomoniasis is commonly manifested as vaginitis. The organism is often carried by infected males, most of whom are asymptomatic. Transmitted during sexual intercourse, the organism causes inflammation, itching, and burning of the vaginal mucosa and produces a greenish-yellow discharge. Oral metronidazole is effective in most cases. Both sexual partners must be treated at the same time.

Toxoplasmosis

Toxoplasmosis is a protozoan infection transmitted to humans from cats that excrete the organism in their feces. Infection in the adult generally produces few if any symptoms, but transmission from an infected mother to an infant in utero or at birth can severely damage the child's CNS. Treatment includes pyrimethamine and sulfisoxazole given simultaneously.

Cryptosporidiosis

Cryptosporidiosis is infection with protozoa of the genus *Cryptosporidium*, which may be associated with enteric disease in calves, lambs, foals, and piglets. In immunocompetent persons, the infection causes a self-limited diarrhea syndrome, but in immunocompromised clients, it is manifested as prolonged, debilitating diarrhea, weight loss, fever, and abdominal pain, with occasional spread to the trachea and bronchial tree.

Pneumocystis carinii

Pneumocystis carinii is an opportunistic organism, sometimes classified as a protozoan and sometimes as a fungus. It causes pneumonia in people whose immune response is depressed from debility, AIDS, or immunosuppressant therapy. It does not seem susceptible to antifungal drugs. Trimethoprim/sulfamethoxazole (Bactrim, Septra), dapsone, and pentamidine are three of the drugs that have been used to treat *P carinii* pneumonia (PCP).

Antiprotozoal Drugs

Pentamidine

The antiprotozoal activity of the diamidine family of drugs was discovered when the compounds were being investigated for their hypoglycemic effect. Pentamidine isethionate (Pentam 300, NebuPent) is the representative of the diamidines that is used clinically.

Pharmacodynamics. The mechanism of action is unknown. It may cause multiple effects on a given parasite and act by different mechanisms in different parasites. The diamidines bind to DNA, and pentamidine may inhibit an enzyme needed for the synthesis of RNA, DNA, and other materials needed by given organisms.

Pharmacokinetics. Pentamidine is fairly well absorbed from parenteral sites of administration. Drug accumulation in tissues occurs, especially in the liver, kidneys, adrenal glands, and spleen. It does not enter the CSF, which means it is ineffective against CNS infections. The drug is not metabolized and is excreted very slowly in urine.

Lungs contain intermediate but therapeutic concentrations after 5 daily doses of 4 mg of base per kilogram. Delivery of drug by aerosol results in little systemic absorption and less toxicity than with IV administration. The actual dose delivered to the lungs depends on both the size of particles generated by the nebulizer and the client's ventilatory patterns.

Therapeutic Uses. Pentamidine is indicated for the treatment of PCP, leishmaniasis, trypanosomiasis (in combination with suramin in this case), and other protozoan infections. Resistance can occur. It is ineffective against some trypanosomes, such as *Trypanosoma cruzi*.

Dosage and Administration. Fresh solutions are administered IM or as an aerosol. Pentamidine is given IV under some circumstances. With trypanosomiasis caused by *Trypanosoma brucei* or *Trypanosoma gambiense*, pentamidine can be given IM on days 1, 3, 5, 7, 13, and 17 and suramin is administered IV on days 1 and 13. Other approaches may also be used.

Prophylaxis against PCP is recommended for HIV-infected adults with CD4+ lymphocyte counts below 200/mm³. For prophylaxis, pentamidine is inhaled as an aerosol directly into the lungs to minimize systemic toxicity. The usual monthly dose is 300 mg of a 5% to 10% nebulized aqueous solution delivered over 30 to 45 minutes via a Respirgard II device. Clients may experience bronchospasm or cough with aerosolized pentamidine; in some cases, an inhaled bronchodilator is used before the pentamidine dose. In HIV-infected clients with CD4+ counts of 100 to 200/mm³, aerosol pentamidine is better tolerated than trimethoprim/sulfamethoxazole or dapsone and just as effective in preventing PCP. However, in more debilitated clients with lower CD4+ counts, pentamidine is less effective than trimethoprim/sulfamethoxazole. Some practitioners also prefer trimethoprim/sulfamethoxazole because it is less expensive than pentamidine.

For treatment of mild to moderate PCP, the usual dosage is 4 mg/kg given parenterally each day for 14 days. Pentamidine is used in PCP especially if the client has failed to respond to trimethoprim/sulfamethoxazole or if he or she is allergic to sulfonamides. Clinical improvement usually occurs 4 to 6 days after the first injection if therapy with pentamidine is successful.

Adverse Reactions. At therapeutic doses, pentamidine causes toxicity in about 50% of clients, whether or not they have AIDS. IV injection of pentamidine can be followed by dangerous reactions: breathlessness, tachycardia, dizziness or fainting, headache, and vomiting. These reactions probably relate to the sharp fall in blood pressure that follows too-rapid IV administration of the drug, and they may be due in part to the release of histamine.

If the IV drug form is not tolerated, IM injection is generally well tolerated, but the latter route is associated with discomfort and the formation of sterile abscesses at the injection site. Sites must be rotated, and warm compresses may need to be applied to the site for comfort.

Other adverse reactions include rashes, thrombophlebitis, and nephrotoxicity. Serious renal dysfunction may occur, possibly due to the drug's inhibition of an enzyme in the kidney. It is usually reversible on discontinuation of the drug.

Drug Interactions. No drug interactions have been clearly identified.

Precautions and Contraindications. Pancreatitis and hypoglycemia and, paradoxically, hyperglycemia and diabetes have been documented with pentamidine use. The client must be monitored closely for these reactions because hypoglycemia may be fatal if not recognized.

Pentamidine must be used cautiously in the presence of hepatic or renal dysfunction. Liver enzyme and renal function tests should be carried out periodically. Because hematologic effects have occurred, the client should be monitored for thrombocytopenia, anemia, and neutropenia.

The client should be in supine position if the drug is given parenterally in case blood pressure changes occur. When administered IV, it should be infused over 60 minutes. Emergency equipment and drugs, including vasopressors, must be available to treat hypotension should it occur. Blood pressure should be monitored at least every 15 minutes during IV infusion, and then every half hour for 2 hours after the infusion concludes.

Pentamidine is contraindicated in clients with a history of anaphylactic reaction to inhaled or parenteral pentamidine and in pregnancy and lactation.

Helminthic Infestations

Infestation by parasitic worms is the most common disease in the world. The prevalence is greatest in tropical regions, and simultaneous infestation with more than one type of helminth is common. There is a tendency toward a wider distribution of parasites because of easy, rapid long-distance travel and the mobility of migrating populations. As with other contagious diseases, helminthiasis is most common in areas with overcrowding, poverty, and limited sanitation.

Worm parasites may be classified into three groups: nematodes, trematodes, and cestodes (Table 45-5). These groups vary with respect to life cycle, bodily structure, development, physiology, location in the host, and susceptibility to drug therapy. Immature forms invade humans via the skin or GI tract and evolve into adult worms with characteristic tissue distributions. Most are visible to the eye in their adult form but are transmitted as microscopic ova or larvae. Effects on the host vary from minimal symptoms to lethal damage to vital organs. Many victims develop general debility, often with a severe anemia. Because they lower the energy level of affected populations, helminth infections are a serious impediment to economic and cultural well-being.

Anthelminthic Drugs

Anthelminthics are drugs that act locally to expel worms from the GI tract or systemically to eradicate adult helminths or developmental forms that invade organs and tissues (Table 45-6).

Ivermectin

Ivermectin (Mectizan), an investigational drug in the United States, is available on a compassionate-use basis from the manufacturer. It is a semisynthetic analog of an insecticide.

Pharmacodynamics. The drug immobilizes affected organisms by inducing a paralysis of the musculature. It seems to target the parasite's gamma-aminobutyric acid (GABA) receptors. Chloride efflux is enhanced and hyperpolarization occurs, resulting in paralysis of the worm.

Pharmacokinetics. Peak plasma levels are achieved within 4 hours after oral administration. Ivermectin is about 93% bound to plasma proteins. None appears in urine.

Therapeutic Uses. Ivermectin is used to treat onchocerciasis (river blindness), filariasis, strongyloidiasis, and other infections caused by intestinal nematodes.

Dosage and Administration. The drug is given orally. It does not cross the blood-brain barrier.

Adverse Reactions. Side effects usually are limited to mild itching and swollen, tender lymph nodes, which last a few days and are relieved by aspirin and antihistamines. Rarely, more severe reactions occur: high fever, tachycardia, hypotension, prostration, dizziness, headache, myalgia, arthralgia, diarrhea, and facial and peripheral edema (these may respond to therapy with glucocorticoids).

Drug Interactions. Interaction can be anticipated if benzodiazepines or barbiturates are taken concurrently because both of these drug classes act at GABA receptors.

Precautions and Contraindications. Although it does not cross the blood-brain barrier, ivermectin is contraindicated in clients with meningitis, since their blood-brain barrier is more permeable and CNS effects might occur. It is also contraindicated in pregnancy, lactation, and children younger than age 5.

Text continues on page 979.

Table 45-5. Characteristics of Selected Helminthic Infections

Infection	Transmission and Distribution	Signs and Symptoms	Prevention and Drug Therapy
Nematodes (roundworms)			
Ascariasis (*Ascaris lumbricoides*), roundworm disease infecting about one third of the world's population; common in indigent children in southern United States	Transmitted by the anal–oral route when ova shed in human or animal feces contaminate farm fields and ground water. Pets also may transmit infections to humans, especially children. Ingested eggs hatch into larvae in the small intestine, migrate to the lungs and then back to the stomach and intestine, where they grow to adult size. The infection remains intraintestinal unless perforation occurs.	Many clients have no symptoms. The infection is discovered when worms appear in the stools. Early signs and symptoms resemble a respiratory infection. Later, abdominal pain and distention may occur when worms are stimulated into migratory activity.	*Prevention:* water purification, thorough food cleansing (especially vegetables), composting of manure before use as fertilizer, careful handwashing after toileting and animal handling *Treatment:* pyrantel pamoate or mebendazole
Old World hookworm (*Ancylostoma duodenale*) and New World hookworm (*Necator americanus*), most common between latitudes 30°south and 40°north; organisms found in mines ("miner's disease") and in tunnels ("tunnel disease")	Transmitted by the anal–percutaneous route when ova shed in feces of hosts hatch into larva in the soil. The worms burrow into human skin, usually via the bare foot. They enter the bloodstream, which carries them to the lungs. They propel themselves up the trachea, are swallowed, and reach the intestines as adult worms. There they attach themselves to the intestinal mucosa and live on blood sucked from the host.	Fatigue and apathy resulting from iron deficiency anemia; fluid and electrolyte disturbances	*Prevention:* proper disposal of fecal waste; wearing of shoes *Treatment:* pyrantel pamoate or mebendazole
Strongyloidiasis (*Strongyloides stercoralis*), threadworm disease; most common in tropics and southern United States; occasionally found in mines, even in temperate climates	Transmitted by the anal–percutaneous route: larvae in soil enter the skin, usually via soles of bare feet. Once in the body, worms burrow beneath the mucosa of the small intestine, where the female lays many eggs that hatch into larvae able to penetrate all parts of the body.	Lightly infested victims may show no symptoms. Abdominal tenderness, epigastric pain similar to that of peptic ulcer, and diarrhea that resembles that of ulcerative colitis may occur. Extraintestinal effects depend on the area of the body invaded and may include bronchopneumonia or lung abscess. Can be fatal in immunocompromised clients.	*Prevention:* proper disposal of fecal waste; wearing of shoes *Treatment:* thiabendazole
Enterobiasis (*Enterobius vermicularis*), pinworm disease; most common helminthic infection in United States	Transmitted by the anal–oral route: ova shed in feces of infected hosts dry, becoming light enough to move easily in air currents. Ova are found in the dust of the environment where infected hosts live; ova under nails after scratching the pruritic anus may be ingested and travel to the large intestine, where they hatch into larvae. Worms migrate through the anus, especially at night, and may reach the genital tract in females.	Pruritus of the perianal and perineal regions is the most common symptom. Secondary infection, caused by scratching, may occur. Salpingitis and peritonitis are occasional complications in females.	*Prevention:* careful handwashing; wet mopping and disinfecting bathroom and bedroom floors; disinfecting toilet seats; fingernail care, including close trimming *Treatment:* mebendazole or pyrantel pamoate
Trichinosis (*Trichinella spiralis*), pork roundworm; worldwide distribution, common in North America and Europe; most common in areas where pigs are fed raw cabbage	Transmitted by ingestion of raw or inadequately cooked meat of animals infected with encysted larvae. Ingested larvae reach maturity in the intestinal tract. Fertilized females deposit larvae in the intestinal mucosa. Carried by the bloodstream throughout the body, the larvae penetrate skeletal muscles and other organs, evoking inflammatory reactions.	Skeletal muscle pain is common. Effects of damage to internal organs depend on the body areas involved and include pneumonia, heart failure, and encephalitis.	*Prevention:* thorough cooking of meats (animals other than pigs can carry the disease); cooking of cabbage used for feeding domestic animals; frequent thorough cleaning of utensils used to process raw meat or to prepare it for cooking *Treatment:* thiabendazole (only early in disease)

(continued)

Table 45-5. (Continued)

Infection	Transmission and Distribution	Signs and Symptoms	Prevention and Drug Therapy
Filariasis (*Wucheria bancrofti, Brugia malayi*), elephantiasis; common in central Africa, south-western Pacific, eastern Asia; also occurs in the West Indies and tropical South and Central America	Transmitted by flies, mosquitoes, and mites. Larvae are deposited in the host skin and develop into adults. Microfilariae produced by fertilized females migrate to the lymphatics and bloodstream and develop into worms, which lodge in lymphatic vessels and nodes.	Signs and symptoms of inflammation wherever living or dead worms are present—inflammation of the lymph nodes with temporary swelling in the affected area, red streaks along the extremity, pain, and tenderness. Obstruction of the lymphatic system leads to gross edematous enlargement of the arms and legs, scrotum, or breast.	*Prevention:* control of intermediate hosts *Treatment:* diethylcarbamazine
Trichuriasis (*Trichuris trichiura*), whipworm disease; occurs worldwide, especially in warm, humid climates	Transmitted in food contaminated with parasite eggs and distributed in the host intestine	Usually produces no symptoms, although abdominal pain, diarrhea, and flatulence may occur. Worms may lodge in appendix or penetrate bowel wall and cause peritonitis.	*Prevention:* thorough cleaning of food *Treatment:* mebendazole
Onchocerciasis (*Onchocerca volvulus*), river blindness; common in areas of tropical Africa, Mexico, South America	Transmitted by mosquitoes and distributed in the skin and eye	Characterized by subcutaneous nodules, pruritic skin rash, and ocular lesions often resulting in blindness	*Prevention:* mosquito control *Treatment:* ivermectin
Cestoda (flatworms)			
Taenia saginata, beef tapeworm; found worldwide	Transmitted in raw or inadequately cooked meat of infected animals. Most tapeworms remain intraintestinal. The scolex, or head, attaches itself to the intestinal wall and grows a variable number of segments, which may produce a worm several yards long. Segments of the worm break off and are passed in the feces.	Mild abdominal symptoms and weight loss are common. Discovery of worm segments in the stool often frightens the victim into seeking treatment.	*Prevention:* thorough cooking of meat before tasting *Treatment:* praziquantel and niclosamide
Taenia solium, pork tapeworm; found worldwide	Like the beef tapeworm, pork tapeworm is transmitted in raw or inadequately cooked meat of infested pork. The tapeworm produces larvae capable of extraintestinal invasion. They are carried by the bloodstream to muscles, liver, lungs, eye, or brain.	Signs and symptoms of extraintestinal infection vary with tissues involved.	*Prevention:* thorough cooking of meat before tasting *Treatment:* praziquantel
Diphyllobothrium latum, fish tapeworm; common in Europe; the Middle East and Asia, Siberia, northern Manchuria, Japan, and the lake regions of Canada and United States	Transmitted by eating infested fish (in the United States, pike is a common source); distributed in the intestine	Megaloblastic anemia (a deficiency of vitamin B_{12} results because the worm uses the vitamin)	*Prevention:* thorough cooking of fish before tasting *Treatment:* praziquantel or niclosamide
Hymenolepis nana, dwarf tapeworm			*Treatment:* niclosamide
Trematodes (flukes)			
Schistosomiasis (*Schistosoma haematobium, Schistosoma mansoni, Schistosoma japonicum*), blood flukes; common in South America, Caribbean islands, Africa, China, Philippines, Indonesia	Transmitted from snails to humans in contaminated bathing water. Larvae enter the skin and penetrate to the bloodstream or lymphatics and move to the lungs, then to the liver, where they mature in the portal veins. The mature adult worms mate and move to areas of the large and small intestines and bladder, producing eggs that are eliminated in feces and urine.	A pruritic rash, called swimmer's itch, develops as a reaction to larvae that die in the skin. About 1 to 2 months later, fever, chills, headache, and other allergic and inflammatory symptoms may occur. Heavy infestations cause abdominal pain and diarrhea. In chronic infections, engorgement of vital organs occurs from venous obstruction.	*Prevention:* control of snails; avoiding contact with contaminated water; avoiding fresh-water swimming; adding iodine or chlorine to water; filtering water with paper coffee filters *Treatment:* praziquantel

Table 45-6. Drugs Used in Treating Helminthiasis

Drug Name	Preparation	Usual Dosage	Additional Information
mebendazole (Vermox)	Chewable tablets	Adults and children: *trichuriasis, ascariasis, hookworm:* 1 tablet morning and evening on 3 consecutive days; *enterobiasis:* 1 tablet PC: C	Tablets may be chewed, swallowed, or crushed and mixed with foods; no special procedures (fasting, laxative) are indicated. If client is not cured in 3 wk, second course of treatment is advised.
niclosamide (Niclocide)	Chewable tablets	*Dwarf tapeworm:* adults: 4 tablets as single daily dose for 7 d; children 11–34 kg: 2 tablets on first day, then 1 tablet daily for next 6 d; children over 34 kg: 3 tablets on first day, then 2 tablets daily for next 6 d *Beef and fish tapeworm:* adults: 4 tablets as single dose; children 11–34 kg: 2 tablets as single dose; children over 34 kg: 3 tablets as single dose	Instruct client to chew thoroughly, then swallow tablets with a little water; for young children, crush tablets to powder and mix with small amount of water to form paste. No special dietary restrictions; take after light meal. Constipated clients may need laxative. Follow-up: examine stool after treatment to identify scolex; segments or ova of beef or fish tapeworm may be present in stool for up to 3 d after therapy. Persistent segments or ova on 7th d indicate treatment failure; give second course of treatment at that time.
pyrantel pamoate (Antiminth, Reese's Pinworm)	Oral suspension Liquid	Adults and children: 11 mg/kg (5 mg/lb) PO as single oral dose; maximum total dose of 1 g Safety and efficacy not established for children under 2 yr	Administer with milk or fruit juices. In case of pinworms, it is advisable to repeat treatment after 2 weeks.
praziquantel (Biltricide)	Tablets	Adults and children: *schistosomiasis:* give 3 doses of 20 mg/kg as 1-day treatment; interval between doses should be 4–6 hr; *clonorchiasis and opisthorchiasis:* give 3 doses of 25 mg/kg as 1-day treatment PC: B	Do not chew tablets; swallow tablets unchewed with some liquid during meals. Keeping tablets in mouth may reveal a bitter taste that can produce gagging or vomiting.
quinacrine (Atabrine)		*Dwarf tapeworm:* adults: 900 mg on empty stomach in 3 portions 20 min apart; on following 3 days take 100 mg tid; children 4–8 yr: 200 mg initially, then 100 mg after breakfast for 3 d; children 8–10 yr: 300 mg initially; then 100 mg bid for 3 d; children 11–14 yr: 400 mg initially, then 100 mg tid for 3 d *Tapeworm:* adults: 4 doses of 200 mg 10 min apart; give 600 mg sodium bicarbonate with each dose if desired to reduce nausea and vomiting; children 5–10 yr: 400 mg total dose, administered in 3 or 4 divided doses 10 min apart; children 11–14 yr: 600 mg total dose, administered in 3 or 4 divided doses 10 min apart	Tapeworm (beef, pork, fish): bland, semisolid, nonfat diet or milk diet day before medication, with fasting after evening meal; anticipate order for laxative before or after use of this medication; expelled worm is stained yellow to facilitate identification of scolex
thiabendazole (Mintezol)	Chewable tablets Oral suspension	Adults less than 150 lb: 10 mg/lb/dose; adults 150 lbs or more: 1.5 g/dose *Strongyloidiasis, ascariasis, uncinariasis, trichuriasis:* 2 doses/d for 2 successive days *Trichinosis:* 2 doses/d for 2–4 successive days PC: C	No special procedures (fasting, laxative)

KEY: PC = pregnancy risk category; see Appendix A.

Benzimidazoles

This group of broad-spectrum anthelminthic agents has both veterinary and human importance. Three compounds, thiabendazole (Mintezol), mebendazole (Vermox), and albendazole, have been used to treat human helminthic infections. Albendazole has become a drug of choice in certain situations, but it is not commercially available in the United States (although it is available on a compassionate-use basis from the manufacturer).

Pharmacodynamics. The benzimidazoles act by binding to and interfering with the synthesis of the parasite's microtubules and also by decreasing glucose uptake. Thiabendazole inhibits a helminth-specific enzyme named fumarate reductase.

Pharmacokinetics. Mebendazole is nearly insoluble in aqueous solution, and little of an oral dose (which is chewed) is absorbed by the body unless taken with a high-fat meal. The low systemic bioavailability (22%) is probably a result of poor absorption and rapid first-pass hepatic metabolism. Mebendazole is about 95% bound to plasma proteins and is extensively metabolized. Thiabendazole is administered orally and is readily absorbed from the GI tract. The drug is hydroxylated in the liver and excreted in urine. A small amount (5%) is excreted in feces.

Therapeutic Uses. These drugs are effective against both larval and adult stages of nematodes, and they are ovicidal in ascariasis and trichuriasis. Immobilization and death of susceptible parasites occur slowly. They may not completely clear the GI tract until a few days after treatment. They are expelled with feces. The benzimidazoles are effective in ascariasis, trichinosis, trichuriasis, enterobiasis, strongyloidiasis, and hookworm.

The usefulness of thiabendazole is compromised by its toxicity. If used in the early stages of trichinosis, it alleviates the symptoms (fever, tenderness, muscle pain). However, it has no effect on migrating or muscle-stage larvae. Thiabendazole is used topically in treating cutaneous larva migrans (creeping eruption).

Dosage and Administration. Thiabendazole comes in chewable tablets or as a suspension. The usual dose is 22 mg/kg if the client is 150 lb or less, 1.5 g if the client is more than 150 lb. Two doses per day are usually given, after meals. In topical treatment, 15% thiabendazole in a water-soluble cream base is applied to the affected area two or three times daily for 5 days.

With chewable mebendazole tablets, the typical dose is one tablet morning and evening for 3 consecutive days. For enterobiasis, one 100-mg tablet of mebendazole is given, and a second tablet is given after 2 weeks. For ascariasis, trichuriasis, and hookworm, 100 mg is taken morning and evening for 3 consecutive days. If the client is not cured 3 weeks after treatment, a second course is given.

Adverse Reactions. Because little of mebendazole is absorbed, the drug is relatively free of toxic effects, although clients may complain of abdominal pain and diarrhea. The adverse effects of thiabendazole include dizziness, anorexia, nausea, vomiting, and many others. CNS adverse effects include impaired alertness and coordination and occasionally hallucinations, sensory disturbances, and convulsions. Some clients excrete a metabolite that imparts an odor to the urine much like that occurring after ingestion of asparagus.

Drug–Drug Interactions. Carbamazepine and hydantoins may reduce the plasma level of mebendazole, possibly decreasing its therapeutic effect. Thiabendazole may compete with xanthines for sites of metabolism in the liver, thus elevating the serum level of the xanthine to a potentially toxic level. The xanthine serum level should be monitored and the dose reduced if necessary.

Drug–Laboratory Test Interactions. Liver function tests may become transiently elevated with thiabendazole.

Precautions and Contraindications. Mebendazole is contraindicated in pregnancy because it has been embryotoxic and teratogenic in experimental animals.

Caution should be exercised when thiabendazole is used in clients with hepatic or renal dysfunction. Clients should promptly report any skin rashes because among the cases of erythema multiforme and Stevens-Johnson syndrome reportedly caused by thiabendazole, there have been fatalities. The drug is contraindicated in clients allergic to it.

Pyrantel Pamoate

Pharmacodynamics. Pyrantel pamoate persistently activates the parasite's nicotinic receptors and inhibits cholinesterase, causing a spastic paralysis in parasitic worms. The paralyzed worm is then expelled from the intestinal tract.

Pharmacokinetics. Pyrantel pamoate is given orally and is poorly absorbed by the GI tract. Most of the dose remains in the GI tract and is eliminated in feces. Drug that is absorbed is partially metabolized in the liver and excreted by the kidneys.

Therapeutic Uses. Pyrantel pamoate is considered a broad-spectrum anthelminthic because it is effective against hookworms, roundworms, and pinworms. It is an alternative to mebendazole in the treatment of roundworms and pinworms. With pinworm, it is wise to repeat the treatment after 2 weeks.

Dosage and Administration. A single dose of 11 mg/kg is given (maximum total dose, 1 g). It may be taken with milk or fruit juice. It is available as an oral suspension (Antiminth) or liquid (Reese's Pinworm).

Adverse Reactions. Although pyrantel pamoate has a wide safety margin, nausea, vomiting, diarrhea, headache, dizziness, rash, and fever are occasionally reported.

Drug–Drug Interactions. Pyrantel pamoate and piperazine should not be given together because their actions are mutually antagonistic.

Drug–Laboratory Test Interactions. Liver function tests may become transiently elevated.

Precautions and Contraindications. Caution should be exercised in persons with liver dysfunction, malnutrition, or anemia. Safe use during pregnancy and in children younger than age 2 has not been established. The drug is contraindicated in persons with allergic hypersensitivity to it.

Praziquantel

Pharmacodynamics. Praziquantel (Biltricide) increases cell membrane permeability in susceptible worms, resulting in a loss of intracellular calcium, massive contractions, and paralysis of their musculature. The drug further results in disintegration of the schistosome.

Pharmacokinetics. Praziquantel is rapidly absorbed after oral administration and distributes into the CSF. High levels occur in the bile. The drug is extensively metabolized, resulting in a short half-life. The metabolites are inactive and are excreted primarily through urine.

Therapeutic Uses. Praziquantel is the drug of choice for the treatment of all forms of schistosomiasis and for some cestode infections.

Dosage and Administration. A typical dose is 20 mg/kg, with three doses administered in one day, 4 to 6 hours apart. The tablets should be swallowed unchewed with some liquid during meals. Keeping the tablets in the mouth may reveal a bitter flavor, which may induce gagging or vomiting.

Adverse Reactions. Common adverse effects of praziquantel include drowsiness, dizziness, malaise, and anorexia.

Drug Interactions. Drug interactions have been reported with dexamethasone, phenytoin, and carbamazepine. Cimetidine causes increased praziquantel levels.

Precautions and Contraindications. Praziquantel is not recommended during pregnancy or lactation or for children under age 4. Praziquantel appeared in the milk of lactating women in a concentration about 25% of that in maternal serum. Women should not breast-feed on the day of treatment or for the subsequent 72 hours.

Praziquantel is contraindicated for treating ocular cysticercosis: destruction of the organism in the eye may damage the eye.

Niclosamide

Pharmacodynamics. Niclosamide (Niclocide) seems to inhibit anaerobic phosphorylation of adenosine diphosphate (ADP) by the mitochondria of the parasite, which is normally an energy-producing process. Worms affected by the drug deteriorate: the scolex and segments may be partially digested and become unrecognizable. The drug is lethal for the cestode's scolex and segments of cestodes but not for the ova.

Pharmacokinetics. Very little niclosamide is absorbed from the GI tract. The drug does not change liver or kidney function, nor does it alter blood counts.

Therapeutic Uses. Niclosamide is the drug of choice for most cestode (tapeworm) infestations.

Dosage and Administration. The drug is given orally in a single dose, usually after a light meal. Constipated clients should first receive a laxative. The dose for an adult is 2 g. Tablets should be chewed thoroughly and washed down with a small amount of water. Providing a laxative 3 to 4 hours after the drug has been given helps clear the bowel of all dead worm segments. In the cestode cycle, after dead segments of the cestode have been digested, viable ova are liberated into the intestinal lumen. Giving the laxative, therefore, rids the bowel of all dead segments and precludes liberation of the ova.

Segments of the worm may be present in the stool for up to 3 days after therapy. If segments are still present 7 days after therapy, the treatment has failed and a second course of treatment should be given. A client is not considered cured unless the stool is negative for segments for at least 3 months.

In *Hymenolepis nana*, multiple infections occur, so the drug should be taken once daily for 7 days. Discharge of intestinal mucus can be promoted by administering sour fruit juices. Eliminating the mucus blanketing the worms leaves them unprotected from the effects of the drug.

Adverse Reactions. Niclosamide is almost free of undesirable effects, other than occasional GI upset.

Drug Interactions. No drug interactions have been identified.

Precautions and Contraindications. Safety for use during pregnancy, lactation, and for children under age 2 has not been established.

■ SUMMARY

Infestation by parasitic worms is the most common disease in the world. Worms are classified as nematodes, trematodes, and cestodes. Various anthelminthic drugs are used to treat these infestations.

❖ NURSING MANAGEMENT: CLIENT RECEIVING ANTHELMINTHICS

Treatment of helminthiasis has become considerably more simplified, as fewer agents are required and dosage schedules tend to be shorter. Although newer treatment agents tend to be less toxic than older drugs, many adverse reactions may still occur, and the client must be carefully supported during treatment. Often the client's general condition must be improved before anthelminthic agents can be administered safely.

Many of the diseases discussed here carry a stigma because of their association with poverty, squalor, and poor health practices. Nurses must strive to be nonjudgmental toward both victims and contacts of victims to promote adherence to healthcare recommendations. The dignity of the client must be respected, particularly when contagious illness occurs. Known or suspected carriers need encouragement because they are not ill and derive no personal benefit from treatment, except the knowledge that they are no longer capable of spreading the illness.

NURSING PROCESS

ASSESSMENT

Before anthelminthic therapy begins, clients must be carefully evaluated to determine if their general condition is good enough to withstand treatment. Anemia, fluid and electrolyte imbalances, and malnutrition as a result of the infestation are often present. Debilitated clients are at higher risk for adverse reactions to anthelminthic drugs. A period of general supportive care may be needed before treatment.

Because drug treatment is specific to the species involved, it varies with the class of worm. A definitive diagnosis, therefore, is required before treatment can be prescribed. If the infestation involves more than one organism, the order of treatment may be crucial. Roundworms are generally treated first, because some drugs used to treat other types of worms irritate roundworms, causing them to migrate actively from the intestines; invasion of the bile ducts and liver, intestinal obstruction, or intestinal perforation may result.

NURSING DIAGNOSIS

Nursing diagnoses for clients receiving anthelminthic drugs may include:

- Altered Nutrition: Less Than Body Requirements, related to anthelminthic medications or infestation
- Knowledge Deficit, concerning anthelminthic drugs and their effect on infestation

PLANNING

Goals of nursing intervention include preventing or promptly detecting and treating any adverse reaction to prescribed anthelminthics, as well as teaching the client about drug therapy for eliminating infestations.

INTERVENTION

Clients treated for helminth infestations require supportive care to enhance their natural resistance to disease. They may be debilitated by the disease. Drugs used as adjuncts in treating helminthic infections, but without specific anthelminthic effects, include corticosteroids, antihistamines, and analgesics. In addition, antipruritics, fluids, electrolyte solutions, blood, vitamins, and iron may be given to improve the client's general condition.

The client should be monitored carefully for adverse reactions to the prescribed drug. Among the signs and symptoms that may develop are GI upset (nausea, vomiting, abdominal pain, diarrhea), weakness and lethargy, blurred vision, CNS reactions, elevated liver enzymes, pruritus, and allergic reactions.

Pinworm infestations usually affect all members of a household, so treatment involves medication and education for all family members. Hygienic measures to eliminate the cysts from the environment are critical to prevent reinfestation. These cysts are light, move freely in the air, and permeate dust; hence, a thorough housecleaning is in order.

Client Education. While undergoing active treatment for disease, victims of contagion need help in managing their drug regimens. Specific instructions for administering the drug must be given. The teaching plan should cover precautionary measures to reduce the risk of any serious adverse reactions to the drug. Clients must be taught to recognize adverse reactions to the medications and should know when to contact the nurse, pharmacist, or prescriber for additional advice or treatment. Clients must also be instructed about the signs and symptoms of recurrence so they can obtain prompt medical attention when needed.

To teach clients about their disease, the nurse must be thoroughly familiar with it—for instance, its geographic distribution and environmental conditions associated with increased incidence. If the nurse does not have reliable information, consultation with public health nurses, public health authorities, or local physicians may help. The best prevention of contagious disease is to eliminate contact between host and parasites.

The nurse must also instruct clients about the sanitary, hygienic, and aseptic measures needed to reduce infections and infestations. Cleanliness alone may not be sufficient. Precautions for avoiding contaminated food and water are advisable. For example, tap water may be unsafe to drink in cities with aging sewage and water systems. Breaks in pipes or conduits often lead to cross-contamination. In countries where sanitation is poor or where fresh human wastes are used as fertilizer, raw fruits and vegetables often carry disease. Hot food that has been thoroughly cooked is usually safe; rare meat may transmit worms.

As appropriate, the nurse should discuss how to avoid overcrowding and how to protect oneself in the face of poor public sanitation. Proper disposal of human waste is of primary importance. No matter how human wastes are treated, sewage must be protected from access by flies, snails, and other disease carriers.

OUTCOME EVALUATION

Data required for evaluating the outcome of nursing interventions include changes in the signs and symptoms of helminthiasis, any signs and symptoms of adverse drug reactions, the degree of the client's adherence to the therapeutic regimen, and the client's ability to relate accurately the material covered in the teaching plan.

❖ CHECKLIST OF NURSING ACTIONS

- ❑ Before anthelminthic therapy, evaluate the client's fluid, electrolyte, and nutritional status.
- ❑ Verify the causative organisms through the laboratory reports.
- ❑ Recommend corresponding treatment for all family members affected by pinworms.
- ❑ Instruct clients in measures to interrupt the chain of reinfestation.

Reference

Hardman JG, Limbird LE, Molinoff PB, et al., eds. (1996). *Goodman and Gilman's The pharmacological basis of therapeutics,* 9th ed. New York: McGraw-Hill.

Bibliography

Masters EJ. (1993). Erythema migrans. *Postgrad Med, 94*(1), 133–142.

Olin BR, ed. (1995). *Drug facts and comparisons,* 50th ed. St. Louis: Facts and Comparisons.

For more information and sample tests and activities, refer to Chapter 45 in the Student Workbook for Clinical Pharmacology and Nursing Management, 5th edition, available through your bookstore.

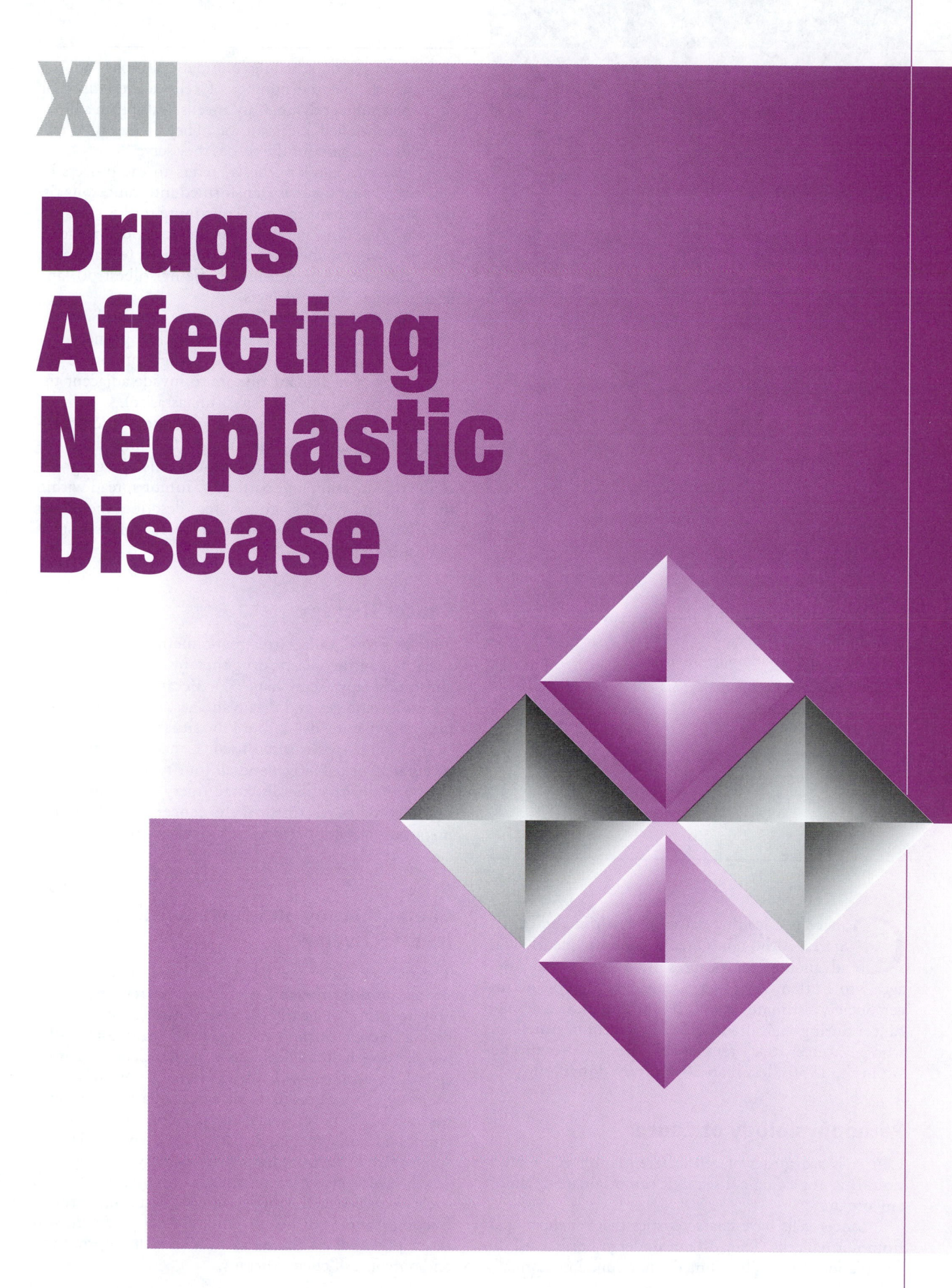

XIII

Drugs Affecting Neoplastic Disease

46

Chemotherapeutic Drugs: Alkylating Agents and Antimetabolites

and do not die on schedule. Normal cell proliferation is regulated so that the number of cells actively dividing equals the number dying. Cancer cells multiply in a disorderly, uncontrolled, incessant way. They divide and duplicate without regard for the tissues they serve.

The term "carcinogenesis" refers to the process by which a normal tissue is transformed into cancerous tissue. Many mechanisms may contribute to this transformation, including heredity, oncogenes and oncogenic viruses, chemical and physical carcinogens (eg, asbestos, vinyl chloride, cigarette smoke, diethylstilbestrol), and immunologic system defects.

The term "neoplasm" means new growth; both benign and malignant neoplasms exist. The primary difference between malignant and benign tumors is the propensity of malignant tumors to invade adjacent tissues and spread to distant sites (metastasize).

Tumor grading and staging are done to predict tumor behavior and to guide therapy. Grading is the histologic characterization of tumor cells. Staging describes the location and pattern of tumor spread within the host. The TNM staging system describes the *t*umor size, lymph *n*odes affected, and degree of *m*etastasis (Copstead, 1995).

Cancer Therapy

Four principal cancer treatment methods are surgery, radiation, antineoplastic drug therapy or chemotherapy, and biotherapy (see Chap. 35). Because each method has its advantages and disadvantages, choosing the appropriate therapy depends on the situation. A combination of modalities is often used. Cancer treatment can be curative or palliative, and all four types of treatment can be used with either intent. Surgery is considered the best method of treatment if the cancer is localized and metastasis has not occurred. Only chemotherapy is discussed here.

Chemotherapy and Factors Influencing its Effectiveness

The type of cancer greatly affects decisions about antineoplastic drug therapy. Some cancers respond favorably to drugs in nearly all cases; other types respond only a fraction of the time (eg, renal, pancreatic, colorectal, non-small cell lung carcinomas). Cancers that respond to antineoplastic drug therapy almost to the point that they can be considered cured are choriocarcinoma and Burkitt's lymphoma. Acute leukemias of childhood and Hodgkin's disease also have a high response rate to antineoplastic drug therapy.

The biologic characteristics of tumors, such as cell cycle concepts, cell kinetics, growth rate and growth fraction, tumor cell heterogenicity, tumor burden, and development of resistance, all influence the approach to and outcome of chemotherapy.

C ancer is a leading cause of death in the United States. Although it strikes more frequently with advancing age, it causes more deaths in children ages 3 to 14 than any other disease. The American Cancer Society estimates that 25% of Americans develop cancer during their lifetime. Forty percent of Americans who get cancer today remain alive 5 years after diagnosis; in the 1930s, less than 20% survived that long.

Pathophysiology of Cancer

Cancer is a disorder of cell differentiation and replication. It is not a single disease. It can originate in almost any organ.

Cancer cells have characteristics that set them apart from normal cells. They do not undergo normal cell differentiation and replication, do not function normally,

Host factors influencing response include the client's nutritional status, preexisting diseases other than cancer (eg, if kidney dysfunction exists, the antineoplastic drug may have increased toxic effects because kidney dysfunction affects the drug's excretion), level of immune function (immunocompetent persons respond more favorably to chemotherapy than immunocompromised ones), physical and psychological tolerance to specific drugs and regimens, and the availability and effectiveness of supportive therapies. Clients who have not received prior chemotherapy usually respond better to antineoplastic therapy than clients who have undergone chemotherapy previously.

Cell Cycle Concepts

To understand certain antineoplastic drugs, it is first necessary to understand the cell, the body's basic unit of tissue. There are three potential cell populations: those that are actively dividing (cycling cells), those that leave the cell cycle after a certain point and differentiate (destined to die), and those that temporarily leave the cell cycle, remaining dormant until they reenter the cycle (Groenwald et al., 1993).

Five phases exist in a cell's cycle of biochemical activity: G_1, G_2, S, M, and G_0. The cycle represents the interval from the midpoint of mitosis to the endpoint in mitosis in a daughter cell.

In G_1, the first postmitotic phase, DNA synthesis ceases, RNA and protein synthesis increases, and cell growth occurs. DNA molecules carry the genetic instructions or codes that control the activities of the cell and the construction of complex protein molecules. DNA molecules resemble a spiral ladder (Fig. 46-1). This phase has the greatest variability in length, from 2 to 3 hours to several days. Generally, a long G_1 phase reflects a slow-growing cell population and a short G_1 phase reflects a rapidly proliferating cell population.

G_2 is the time after cells complete DNA synthesis and are getting ready to enter mitosis, usually a brief period. There is premitotic synthesis of RNA.

In G_0, the resting or dormant phase, the cell performs all genetically assigned functions, such as synthesizing RNA and protein, except those related to cell reproduction. The time spent in G_0 varies according to the cell type. A biochemical stimulus probably triggers the cells to move from G_0 to the next phase.

The S (synthesis) phase is when DNA synthesis occurs, producing two separate sets of chromosomes (the DNA content of the cell doubles). This phase lasts about the same amount of time for all cells, 8 to 30 hours. This is a short period compared to the entire cell cycle; thus, drugs active in this phase affect only a fraction of cells for any given treatment.

The M (miosis) phase results in cell division and production of two daughter cells and includes the four

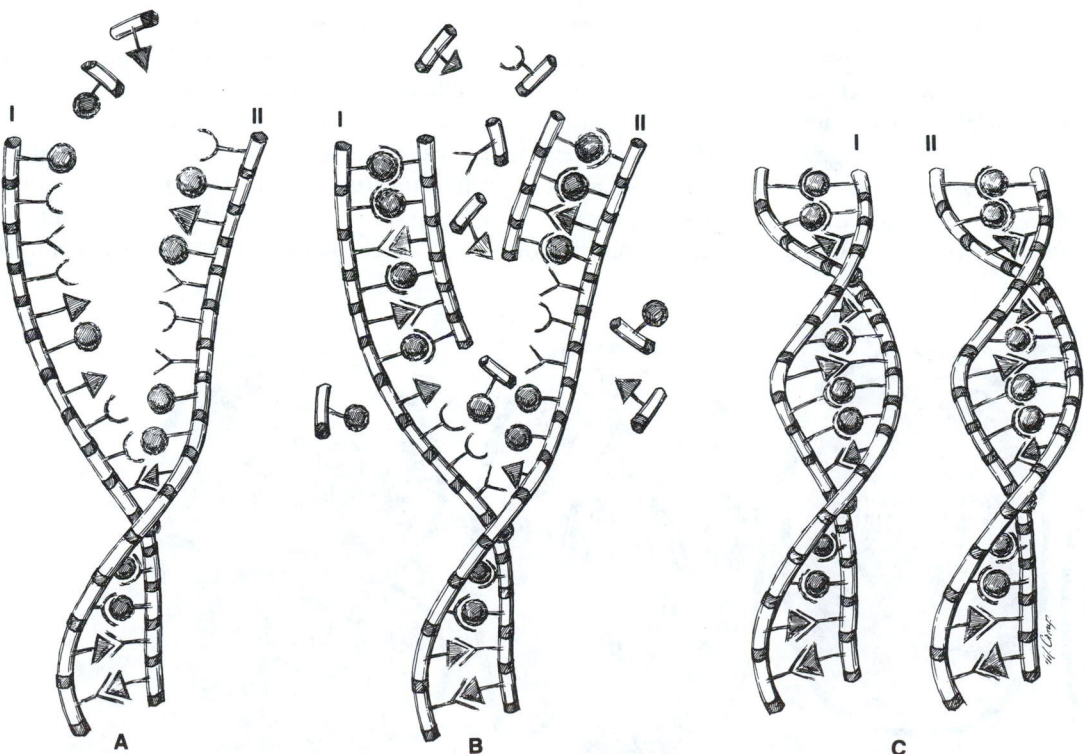

Figure 46-1. Schematic representation of the replication of DNA. **(A)** Before cell division, the bonds between the nitrogenous bases are broken, the two strands separate, and each strand takes with it the bases attached to its side. **(B)** The bases attached to each single strand attract free-floating nucleotide units and pair off, adenine with thymine, guanine with cytosine. **(C)** The end result is two exact replicas of the original DNA molecule, and the cell is ready to undergo division.

stages of prophase, metaphase, anaphase, and telophase (Fig. 46-2). During the M phase, RNA and protein synthesis diminish. After mitosis, a cell can reenter G_1 and continue to proliferate or enter G_0. It is a relatively short phase (30 to 90 minutes).

Several antineoplastic drugs are effective primarily during a specific phase of the cell cycle, and one way to classify the drugs is as cell cycle-dependent/cell cycle phase-specific or cell cycle-independent/cell cycle phase-nonspecific. The antimetabolites are particularly effective during the period when many tumor cells are in the S phase. Plant alkaloids are most effective during the M phase. Neither of these drug classes is as effective (on a relative dose basis) as the alkylating agents during the G_0 phase.

Cell Kinetics

Antineoplastic drugs do not kill every tumor cell; rather, they kill a constant fraction of cells rather than a fixed number (this concept also applies in antibiotic use). For instance, if the drug kills 99% of the cells, it reduces 1 million cells to 10,000, or 100,000 cells to 1,000. If the treatment kills 99.9% of cells in a tumor with 10^{10} cells, it reduces the tumor burden three logs, from 10^{10} to 10^7 (Fig. 46-3). Thus, some cancer cells remain even after antineoplastic agents have been used, and they may replicate. Combination chemotherapy is one way to deal with residual cancer cells.

Growth Rate and Fraction

Rapidly growing cancers are more susceptible to antineoplastic agents than slower-growing cancers. Growth fraction is the percentage of viable cells in active cell division. Tumors in which a large percentage of cells are actively making DNA and dividing over a short time span have a high growth fraction and are more susceptible to drug action than tumors in which only a few cells are making DNA and dividing. Unfortunately, normal cells, such as bone marrow, hair follicles, and cells of the gastrointestinal (GI) tract, also have a high growth fraction; this is why these tissues experience the most toxicity when antineoplastic drugs are used.

If tumors are small when therapy begins, the effectiveness of chemotherapy is enhanced. The doubling time of a tumor—the time it takes a tumor to double its volume—increases as the tumor volume increases. Therefore, larger tumors have longer doubling times and slower growth fractions. These principles provide the rationale for removing large tumors by surgery and following this action with chemotherapy—in other words, assuming that any remaining tumor cells will be stimulated into active division with the bulk of the tumor gone and thus will be more susceptible to chemotherapy.

Resistance

Resistance can be intrinsic or acquired. *Intrinsic* resistance is resistance to a specific drug without any prior exposure to that drug. *Acquired* resistance is resistance that occurs after the start of therapy and represents some type of change in the tumor cells themselves.

There are two major types of drug resistance, temporary (relative) and permanent. Factors related to temporary resistance include variations in drug bioavailability, metabolism, or elimination; tumor present in sanctuary sites; limited drug diffusion; alteration in cell kinetics; host toxicity; and tumor blood supply. These factors pose challenges, but strategies have been developed to overcome some of these barriers.

Permanent resistance is genetically based. Genetic changes in individual tumor cells that result in emergence of drug resistance appear to be the most significant factor in the failure of chemotherapy. Important in

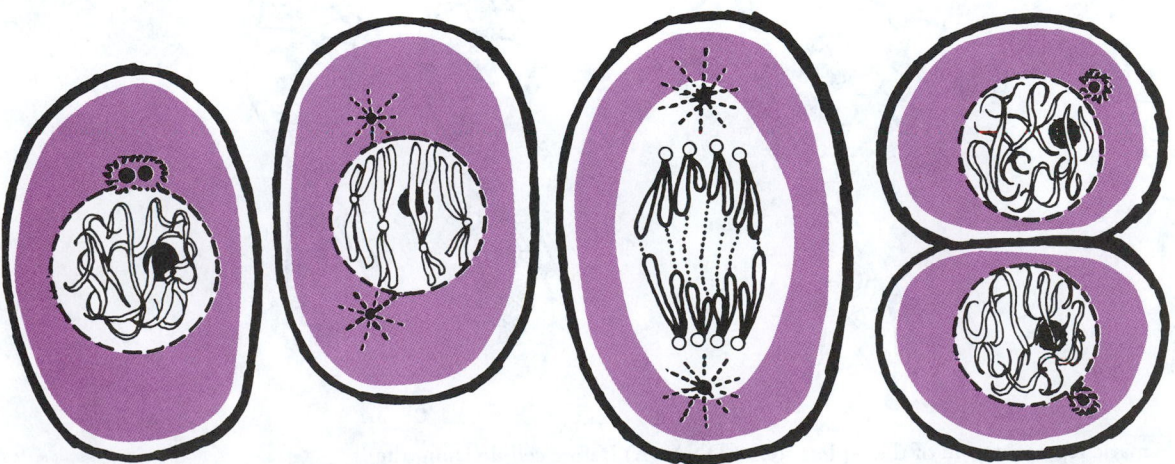

Figure 46-2. Simplified sequence of mitosis. The centrosome divides, the chromatin material of the nucleus changes into rod-shaped chromosomes, and two daughter cells form within the cell membrane.

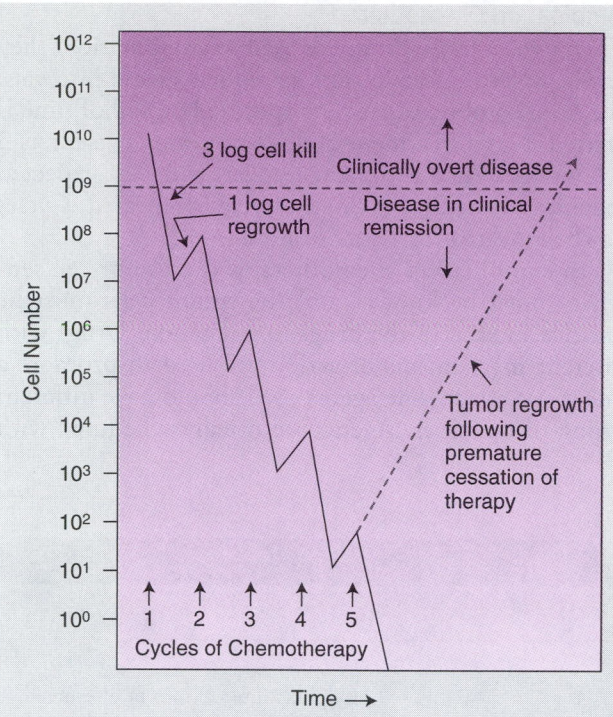

Figure 46-3. Relationship between tumor cell survival and chemotherapy administration. The exponential relationship between chemotherapy drug dose and tumor cell survival dictates that a constant proportion, not number, of tumor cells is killed with each cycle of treatment. In this example, each cycle of drug administration results in 99.9% (three-log) cell kill, and one log of cell regrowth occurs between cycles. The broken line indicates what would occur if the last cycle of therapy were omitted: Despite complete clinical remission of disease, the tumor would ultimately recur. (Source: Cooper MR, Cooper MR: Principles of medical oncology. In Holleb AI, Fink D, Murphy G (eds.): *Clinical Oncology.* American Cancer Society, Atlanta: 1991, pp. 47–68.)

permanent resistance is spontaneous genetic mutation; this theory proposes that all biologic systems have an inherent probability of undergoing genetic variation. If this theory is operating, drug-resistant cells, mutant cells, can develop. The probability of at least one resistant cell is the product of the mutation rate and the size of the tumor. Thus, increasing tumor size diminishes the chance for cure because it is almost certain that at least one resistant mutation has occurred.

Mechanisms of drug resistance include defective transport, defective drug metabolism, altered nucleotide pools, increased drug activation, altered DNA repair, gene amplification, altered target protein, and multidrug resistance. For example, some cancer cells can repair drug-induced DNA defects before the drug damage is lethal. The cancer cell may become better able to prevent drug activation, better able to deactivate the drug, better able to repair DNA damage, or less permeable to the drug's active form. When a tumor is large, greater heterogeneity in the tumor cell population increases the potential for drug resistance.

In multidrug resistance, exposure to a single drug is followed by cross-resistance to other drugs that are structurally unrelated and may have different mechanisms of action. The initial drug involved appears to be a natural product (see Chap. 47). Natural products vary widely in structure but appear to use a similar transport system, and drug transport appears to be the critical component in this resistance phenomenon. The drug binds to a factor called P-glycoprotein and is then actively pumped out of the cell. This energy-dependent drug efflux appears to be more efficient in resistant cells and results in less intracellular drug. The overexpression of P-glycoprotein is the predominant gene alteration responsible for multidrug resistance (Groenwald et al., 1993).

Toxicity

One of the greatest problems with antineoplastic drugs is their nonselective toxicity. The ideal antineoplastic drug would not be toxic to normal tissue, but no such drug exists. Bone marrow cells, with their high growth fraction, are very susceptible to antineoplastic drugs. The client must be monitored during and after antineoplastic drug therapy because bone marrow suppression is asymptomatic until severe damage has occurred.

The time of peak toxicity for a given adverse effect is called the nadir. For example, the nadir for bone marrow suppression with a given drug may be 10 days; that is, about 10 days after antineoplastic drug therapy is started, the client's hemoglobin, hematocrit, leukocyte count, and platelet count will reach their lowest values.

One of the most serious long-term consequences of cancer therapy is that it may contribute to a second malignancy. Therapy-related cancers generally have a poor prognosis, and treatment is often unsuccessful. Survival from the time of diagnosis of secondary malignancies may be brief. The mechanism for their development remains unclear, but several factors are probably involved. Lethal damage to the first neoplastic cells is the intent of chemotherapy; however, if cellular damage is not repaired in the normal cells, malignant transformation or mutation could occur (Groenwald et al., 1993). Long-term survivors of Hodgkin's disease who have received both chemotherapy and radiation have the highest incidence of secondary cancers. The alkylating agents (especially melphalan), nitrosoureas, and procarbazine are the agents most often implicated in chemotherapy-related cancers. Persons who receive alkylating agents, for instance, have a 1.5% to 2.3% risk of developing acute nonlymphocytic leukemia within 10 years.

Therapeutic Strategies With Chemotherapy

Types of Chemotherapy

An overall goal of chemotherapy is maximum cell kill with tolerable toxicity. The current understanding of mechanisms of resistance provides the rationale for treatment strategies, which include combination chemotherapy and adjuvant therapy.

Some clients with cancer obtain excellent results from a single antineoplastic agent, but most cancers must be treated with a combination of drugs (Table 46-1). Principles involved include selection of drugs that are active against the given tumor when used alone, that have different mechanisms of action (to minimize the possibility of drug resistance), and that have minimally overlapping toxicities. These principles allow administration of high doses to result in greater cell kill and administration of the drugs at consistent intervals (the narrowest intervals possible that still allow recovery of sensitive normal tissues such as the bone marrow).

Combination Chemotherapy

When two or more drugs are used in combination, they may be administered in varying sequences and intervals. The drug combination over a specified period of time is referred to as a treatment cycle. A common cycle lasts 3 to 6 weeks. When the client recovers from the expected toxicities of the first cycle, the cycle is repeated. Cycles may be repeated for 1 year or more.

In combination chemotherapy, the tumor cell sensitivity must be known, and the tumor cells must be sensitive to each of the drugs in a regimen. Drugs with different mechanisms of action are used to promote a synergistic effect. The agents used should have different timing of toxicities. Agents are usually scheduled with

Table 46-1. Selected Combination Regimens

Acronym and Drugs	Dosage	Uses
ABVD		
A—doxorubicin	25 mg/m² IV days 1 and 14	Hodgkin's disease (may be alternated
B—bleomycin	10 U/m² IV days 1 and 14	with MOPP)
V—vinblastine	6 mg/m² IV days 1 and 14	
D—dacarbazine	375 mg/m² IV days 1 and 14	
	Repeat every 28 days for 6–8 cycles	
CAV		
C—cyclophosphamide	500 mg/m² IV day 1	Non-small cell lung carcinoma
A—doxorubicin (Adriamycin)	50 mg/m² IV day 1	
V—vincristine	1.4 mg/m² IV day 1	
	Repeat every 28 days	
CAV		
C—cyclophosphamide	750 mg/m² IV day 1	Small cell lung carcinoma
A—doxorubicin (Adriamycin)	50 mg/m² IV day 1	
V—vincristine	2 mg/m² IV day 1	
	Repeat every 21 days	
CMF		
C— cyclophosphamide	100 mg/m² PO days 1–14	Node-positive breast cancer
M—methotrexate	40–60 mg/m² IV days 1 and 8	
F— fluorouracil	600 mg/m² IV days 1 and 8	
	Repeat every 28 days	
	Above age 60, reduce methotrexate dose to 30 mg/m² and	
	fluorouracil dose to 400 mg/m²	
MOPP		
M—mechlorethamine	6 mg/m² IV days 1 and 8	Hodgkin's disease
O—vincristine (Oncovin)	1.4 mg/m² IV days 1 and 8	
P— procarbazine	100 mg/m² PO days 1–14	
P— prednisone	40 mg/m² PO days 1–14	
	Repeat every 28 days for 6–8 cycles	
VAD		
V—vincristine	0.4 mg/day IV continuous infusion days 1–4	Multiple myeloma
A—doxorubicin (Adriamycin)	9 mg/m²/day continuous IV infusion days 1–4	
D—dexamethasone	40 mg PO daily, days 1–4	
VBP		
V—vinblastine	0.2 mg/kg IV days 1 and 2; repeat every 3 wk for 5 courses	Testicular carcinoma
B—bleomycin	30 U/week IV, 6 h after vinblastine on second day of each	
	week for 12 wk until total dose of 360 U	
P—cisplatin (Platinol)	20 mg/m² IV days 1–5, 6 h after vinblastine; repeat every	
	3 wk for 3 courses	

respect to tumor cell kinetics to potentiate the effect of each agent—that is, cell cycle-specific and cell cycle-nonspecific agents may be used together in a regimen to kill both dividing and nondividing cell fractions simultaneously. Intermittent rather than continuous daily therapy is generally helpful in decreasing drug toxicities.

The drug dose is related to the response of the tumor, and the therapeutic effect is compromised by inadequate dosing. Maximal tolerated doses must be administered at minimal intervals to prevent acquired drug resistance. The best way to determine the correct dose is by using a nomogram based on the client's body surface area in square meters (nomograms can be found in reference books). Blood levels of drug correlate better with drug doses on the basis of body surface area rather than on the basis of milligrams per kilogram.

Adjuvant Chemotherapy

Adjuvant therapy is the use of chemotherapy before, during, or after surgery or radiation therapy. The role of adjuvant chemotherapy is to eliminate micrometastasis. Adjuvant therapy has been successful in the treatment of some cancers. For example, clients have been followed for 20 years in one study in which adjuvant combination chemotherapy with cyclophosphamide, methotrexate, and fluorouracil was administered after radical mastectomy for breast cancer with axillary lymph nodes positive for metastasis. The long-term results show that the clients given the adjuvant combination chemotherapy had significantly better rates of relapse-free survival and total survival (Bonadonna et al., 1995).

Neoadjuvant chemotherapy is chemotherapy given before definitive local therapy with surgery or radiation. Its goal is to shrink advanced tumors so that they are amenable to therapy.

Routes of Drug Administration

Although a drug may be given by a variety of routes, careful selection of the route of administration, taking into account the drug and the specific cancer, may improve the drug's efficacy.

Cutaneous malignant lesions can be treated in various ways, including the topical application of antineoplastic agents. Examples include using nitrogen mustard for cutaneous T-cell lymphoma and fluorouracil for basal cell carcinoma and squamous cell carcinoma (topical application is discussed in greater detail under fluorouracil later in this chapter). Various antineoplastic agents are administered orally. Use of intramuscular (IM) and subcutaneous (SC) routes was uncommon until the development of the biologic response modifiers (eg, colony-stimulating factors are often given SC).

Intravenous (IV) delivery is the most common route for antineoplastic drug administration. Some of the specifics remain controversial, such as whether a large- or small-bore needle, or a stainless-steel needle or an over-the-needle catheter, should be used, whether the antecubital region should be used for access, and whether vesicants should be given first or last. The development of central venous catheters and long-term vascular access devices has assisted chemotherapy administration but has also added concerns and challenges. Device selection, client selection, maintenance procedures, and complication management continue to be refined by practice and research (Table 46-2).

Intra-arterial drug administration involves cannulation of the artery that supplies blood to the tumor. This increases the concentration of the drug to known areas of tumor and decreases the systemic drug concentration and thus the adverse reactions. The full strength of the drug reaches the tumor before it enters the general circulation. This route is used primarily in the hepatic artery for managing actual or potential metastasis of colon cancer to the liver.

The two methods of intra-arterial administration are external or internal. The external method involves placement of an arterial catheter. The catheter is usually advanced in the femoral artery, with placement guided by radiographic imaging. Then the catheter is connected to an external infusion pump for 3 to 7 days of drug delivery. The client must lie flat during the infusion. For long-term use, this method is uncomfortable, inconvenient, and costly.

The internal, or implantable, method involves the surgical placement of a totally implantable pump such as the Infusaid pump or the Synchromed Infusion System. The catheter is inserted into the appropriate artery and then attached to the pump, which is located in a surgically created subcutaneous pocket, usually in the lower abdomen or upper chest. The pump chamber is filled with the drug via a needle. This approach offers the client greater freedom and causes fewer complications than the external method, but it is expensive. However, the long-term cost of the external method may be greater due to the cost of disposable supplies.

Regional delivery of chemotherapy into the peritoneal space has been used for locally recurrent ovarian and colon cancers. Methods of gaining access to the peritoneal space include:

- Intermittent placement of temporary indwelling catheters (usually when short-term use is anticipated)
- Placement of a Tenckhoff external catheter
- Placement of an implantable peritoneal port.

The latter two methods are used when several months of therapy are planned and the treatment goal is cure. The procedures cause local side effects and the drugs cause systemic adverse reactions, but to a milder degree than with IV administration of the same drugs. In some situations, systemic adverse reactions can be minimized by infusing an agent IV to counteract the re-

Table 46-2. Selected Vascular Access Devices

Type	Description	Comments
Peripheral needle	Stainless steel	Excellent for short-term access (minutes to days)
Scalp vein	27–19 gauge	
Butterfly	Single lumen	
Peripheral catheter	Catheter over needle	Excellent for multiday therapy
Abbocath	Teflon or polyurethane	Provides greater client mobility—less likely to infiltrate
Insyte	Single or double lumen	
Streamline	26–14 gauge	
Nontunneled central venous catheter	Polyurethane or silicone	Excellent for emergency
Subclavian line	Single, double, or triple lumen	Inserted at bedside by physician
Arrow		High rate of trauma and infection compared to TCVC and port
Peripherally inserted central catheters (PICCs)	Silicone elastomer or other polymer	Excellent for continuous infusion (weeks or months)
C-PICs	Single or double lumen	Requires external site care and routine flushing
Per-Q-Cath	24–16 gauge	Requires adequate antecubital veins
Groshong PICC		Least expensive and most easily inserted long-term CVC
		Blood withdrawal difficult
Tunneled central venous catheter	Silicone catheter with Dacron cuff	Excellent for long-term, continuous, or intermittent therapy (months to years)
(TCVC)	Single, double, or triple lumen	Preferred for long-term TPN administration and vesicant infusion therapy
Hickman catheter		
Specialty Access Products		Requires external site care
Raaf Cath		Requires daily to weekly flushing/heparinization (Groshong design does not require heparin)
Groshong catheter		Blood withdrawal is easy
		External portion may accidentally be broken, punctured, cut
Implantable port*	Titanium, stainless steel, Silastic, or plastic portal attached to catheter	Excellent for long-term, intermittent therapy
Port-A-Cath		No site care required
Hickman Port	Single or double lumen	Surgical procedure required for removal
Lifeport	Access through skin with noncoring needle (allows 1,000–3,600 punctures per port)	Blood withdrawal is easy
		When not in use, flushed only monthly
		5 possible routes: venous, arterial, peritoneal, epidural, intrapleural
		Site selection for port is important

*There is also a port that combines properties of PICC and implantable port—the peripherally inserted port (PAS-Port); well accepted by clients due to placement near antecubital fossa
Adapted from Groenwald SL, Frogge MH, Goodman M, Yarbro CH, eds. (1993). *Cancer nursing: Principles and practice,* 3d ed. Boston: Jones and Bartlett Publishers.

actions through the venous system (eg, intraperitoneal cisplatin and IV sodium thiosulfate, which appears to decrease cisplatin's renal toxicity). Regardless of the drug used or the cancer treated, complications specific to this regional route include respiratory distress, abdominal pain, diarrhea, chemical irritation of the peritoneal space, infection, and electrolyte imbalances.

With a pleural effusion caused by malignant cells, treatment includes insertion of chest tubes, drainage of the fluid, and sclerosis of the pleural space, using an agent such as nitrogen mustard, to prevent recurrence of the effusion. The drug is injected into the chest tube and the tube is clamped for a specified time (eg, 24 hours). The procedure can be repeated daily for a few days as needed. Severe pleural pain can accompany this treatment, and a strong narcotic analgesic such as morphine may be administered via a pump for patient-controlled analgesia. Investigation continues on other agents and methods, such as insertion of small-bore percutaneously placed catheters instead of regular chest tubes.

The intravesical approach (direct instillation of an antineoplastic agent into the bladder) has been used for superficial bladder cancer. Instillation, which can be done weekly for 4 to 12 weeks, requires insertion of a urinary

Table 46-3. Alkylating Agents: Indications

Drug Name	Preparation	Usual Dosage	Therapeutic Indications
Nitrogen mustards			
chlorambucil (Chloraminophene, Leukeran)	Oral tablets (2 mg)	4–8 mg/m²/day × 3–6 wk	CLL and malignant lymphomas (including lymphosarcoma, giant follicular lymphoma, Hodgkin's disease), *breast cancer, hairy cell leukemia, multiple myeloma, and ovarian, testicular, and trophoblastic neoplasms*
cyclophosphamide (Cytoxan, Endoxan, Neosar)	Oral tablets IV	PO: 1–5 mg/kg/day or 60–120 mg/m²; adjust dose with renal dysfunction IV: 40–50 mg/kg in divided doses over 2–5 d; up to 100 mg/kg initially, then 10–15 mg/kg q7–10d or 3–5 mg twice weekly	Non-Hodgkin's lymphoma, Hodgkin's disease, myeloma, cutaneous T-cell lymphoma, neuroblastoma, adenocarcinoma of ovary, adenocarcinoma of breast, *ALL, ANLL, bladder, cervix, CML, endometrium, Ewing's sarcoma, head and neck, lung, osteosarcoma, testes, Wilm's tumor, sarcomas, prostate, rhabdomyosarcoma, retinoblastoma, trophoblastic neoplasms*
hexamethylmelamine (Altretamine, Hexistat, HMM)	Oral capsules (50 mg)	240–320 mg/m²/day	Single-agent use for persistent or recurrent ovarian carcinoma
ifosfamide (Ifex)	IV	1.2 g/m²/d for 5 consecutive days, administer over at least 30 min; repeat q3wk or after recovery from bone marrow suppression	Third-line therapy for germ cell testicular cancer, *ANLL, ALL, breast, Ewing's sarcoma, Hodgkin's and non-Hodgkin's lymphomas, lung, ovary, osteosarcoma, pancreatic, soft-tissue sarcoma, trophoblastic neoplasms*
mechlorethamine (Caryolysin, Cloramin, Erasol, Mustargen)	IV	*Hodgkin's disease:* 6 mg/m² on day 1 and 8 of a 28-d cycle; *other neoplasms:* 0.4 mg/kg given as single dose or in divided doses of 0.1–0.2 mg/kg/d; may repeat course in 3–6 wk	Hodgkin's disease, lymphosarcoma, CML, CLL, polycythemia vera, mycosis fungoides, bronchogenic carcinoma, palliative treatment of metastatic carcinoma resulting in effusion, *CML and brain tumors*
melphalan or L-sarcolysin (Alkeran)	Oral tablets	0.1–0.15 mg/kg/day × 2–3 wk; reduce dose with hepatic or renal impairment	Multiple myeloma, nonresectable epithelial carcinoma of ovary, *breast, testes, thyroid*
Ethylenimines and Methylmelamines			
triethylenethiophosphoramide/thiotepa (Thioplex)	IV Intracavitary Intravesical	0.3–0.4 mg/kg IV at intervals of 1–4 wk by rapid administration	Adenocarcinoma of breast or ovary, intracavitary effusions, superficial papillary bladder cancer, lymphoma, Hodgkin's disease, *lung cancer*
Alkyl Sulfonates			
busulfan (Busulphan, Mielucin, Myleran, Sulfabutin)	Oral tablets (2 mg)	4–12 mg/day for several wk	CML, *ANLL*
Nitrosoureas			
carmustine/BCNU (BiCNu)	IV	150–200 mg/m² every 6 weeks; give as single dose or divided daily injections (75–100 mg/m² on 2 successive days)	Brain tumors, multiple myeloma, Hodgkin's disease, non-Hodgkin's lymphoma, *melanoma, colorectal, stomach, liver cancers*
lomustine/CCNU (CeeNu)	Oral capsules (10–100 mg)	100–130 mg/m² every 6–8 wk)	Brain tumors, Hodgkin's disease (secondary therapy, in combination with other approved drugs), *breast, lung, colorectal, kidney, melanoma, myeloma, non-Hodgkin's lymphoma*
streptozocin (Zanosar)	IV	Daily: 500 mg/m² for 5 consecutive days every 6 weeks until maximum benefit OR weekly: 1,000 mg/m² weekly for 2 wk, then adjusted depending on response	Metastatic islet cell carcinoma of pancreas, *carcinoid tumors, Hodgkin's disease, pancreatic carcinoma*

Italicized indications were not FDA approved as of 1993.
Fischer DS, Knobf MT, Durivage HJ. (1993). *The cancer chemotherapy handbook*, 4th ed. St. Louis: Mosby-Year Book, Inc.
KEY: CLL, chronic lymphocytic leukemia; ALL, acute lymphocytic leukemia; ANLL, acute nonlymphocytic leukemia; CML, chronic myelogenous leukemia; AML, acute myelogenous leukemia

(continued)

Table 46-3. Alkylating Agents: Indications (Continued)

Drug Name	Preparation	Usual Dosage	Therapeutic Indications
Triazenes			
dacarbazine (DTIC-Dome)	IV	*Malignant melanoma:* 2–4.5 mg/kg/day IV for 10 days, repeated at 4-wk intervals *Hodgkin's disease:* 150 mg/m²/day for 5 days, with other drugs; repeat every 4 wk	Malignant melanoma, Hodgkin's disease, *islet cell carcinoma, neuroblastoma, soft-tissue sarcoma*
Platinum Complexes			
carboplatin (Paraplatin)	IV	360 mg/m² IV on day 1	Ovarian carcinoma, *cancers of head and neck, lung, and testes*
cisplatin (Neoplatin, Platinex, Platinol)	IV	Dosages vary depending on condition *Testicular carcinoma:* 20 mg/m²/day IV for 5 days q3wk for 3 courses, with other drugs	Testicular carcinoma, ovarian cancer, transitional cell bladder cancer, *cancers of brain, adrenal cortex, breast, cervix, endometrium, head and neck, esophagus, lung; melanoma; non-Hodgkin's lymphoma; osteosarcoma; prostate, stomach, uterus, trophoblastic neoplasms*

Italicized indications were not FDA approved as of 1993.
Fischer DS, Knobf MT, Durivage HJ. (1993). *The cancer chemotherapy handbook,* 4th ed. St. Louis: Mosby-Year Book, Inc.
KEY: CLL, chronic lymphocytic leukemia; ALL, acute lymphocytic leukemia; ANLL, acute nonlymphocytic leukemia; CML, chronic myelogenous leukemia; AML, acute myelogenous leukemia

catheter and retention of the drug for 1 to 2 hours with the catheter clamped. When the catheter is unclamped, the fluid that drains from the catheter must be sealed, labeled as cytotoxic waste, and disposed of properly.

The distribution of a drug within the body may influence the drug therapy chosen. Some drugs are excluded from certain areas of the body. For example, because of the blood-brain barrier, brain tumor cells and tumor cells in the cerebrospinal fluid (CSF) are inaccessible to most antineoplastic drugs. Most antineoplastic drugs, which are relatively insoluble in lipids, have limited access to the brain. Passage is restricted to molecules that are fat-soluble. Nitrosoureas and procarbazine are among the few antineoplastic drugs that cross the blood-brain barrier in sufficient amounts to be useful in treating brain tumors. In some cases, the CNS acts as a sanctuary for tumor cells, a fact that contributes to relapse in acute lymphocytic leukemia, for example.

Because most antineoplastic agents cannot cross the blood-brain barrier and enter the CSF in sufficient concentrations to kill cancer cells effectively, the agent may be injected into the intrathecal or intraventricular space. Agents used include methotrexate, cytarabine, thiotepa, and interferon. Administering drugs by the intrathecal route, via lumbar puncture, is relatively quick and easy, but the drug may not reach the area where it is needed. The intraventricular space may be better reached via a surgically placed Ommaya reservoir.

Specific Chemotherapeutic Agents

Chemotherapeutic or antineoplastic drugs are commonly classified into several pharmacologic groups. Alkylating agents and antimetabolites are discussed in this chapter; natural products, antibiotics, hormones, and miscellaneous agents are discussed in Chapter 47. Biologic response modifiers were discussed in Chapter 35.

Alkylating Agents

Two primary types of cytotoxic compounds are useful in treating cancer: ones that interfere with the synthesis of DNA precursors, and ones that interact with DNA itself. The alkylating agents interact with DNA itself. The major types of alkylators are the nitrogen mustards, the ethylenimines and methylmelamines, an alkyl sulfonate, the nitrosoureas, a triazene, and the platinum complexes. Dosages and therapeutic uses for the alkylating agents are summarized in Table 46-3, adverse reactions and interactions in Table 46-4.

Nitrogen Mustards

Nitrogen mustards were first synthesized in 1854 and were studied for use in chemical warfare during World Wars I and II. The nitrogen mustards include chlorambucil (Leukeran), cyclophosphamide (Cytoxan, Neosar), ifosfamide (Ifex), mechlorethamine (Mustargen, the first alkylating agent used clinically), and melphalan (Alkeran). See Focus on Nitrogen Mustards: Similarities and Differences.

Cyclophosphamide

Attempts to alter the chemical structure of mechlorethamine to increase its selectivity for neoplastic tissues led to the synthesis of cyclophosphamide.

Pharmacodynamics. The alkylating agents are cell cycle-independent and may act on cells at any phase of the cycle. Nevertheless, some do seem more cytocidal to cells in particular phases of the cycle (eg, nitrosoureas in G_1 or G_2).

Table 46-4. Alkylating Agents: Adverse Reactions and Interactions

Drug Name	Adverse Reactions	Interactions
chlorambucil	Nadir: 7–10 d Severe bone marrow suppression (BMS), slight nausea and vomiting, occasional dermatitis, abnormal liver function, pulmonary fibrosis with prolonged use, second malignancy, sterility	Anticoagulants, aspirin (increased risk of bleeding)
cyclophosphamide	Nadir: 7–14 d BMS, anorexia, nausea, vomiting, alopecia, hemorrhagic cystitis with gross or microscopic hematuria, amenorrhea, sterility	Mesna (decreased hemorrhagic cystitis); succinylcholine (increased neuromuscular blockade); probenecid or sulfinpyrazone (hyperuricemia, gout); may cause additive myelosuppression when used with other myelosuppressive drugs; live viral vaccines (increased adverse reactions to vaccine); doxorubicin (additive cardiotoxicity); insulin (increased hypoglycemia); anticoagulants (increased anticoagulant effect); thiazide diuretics (increased leukopenia)
hexamethylmelamine	Nadir: 21–28 d Acute liver toxicity is dose-limiting; nausea and vomiting are dose-related, mild BMS, abdominal cramping, diarrhea, peripheral neuropathies, agitation, confusion	
ifosfamide (Ifex)	Cerebellar dysfunction, seizures, altered mental status, nausea and vomiting, hemorrhagic cystitis, alopecia, BMS, cranial nerve dysfunction, reversible hepatic dysfunction; some differences in toxicity between cyclophosphamide and ifosfamide may relate to differences in their metabolism; for example, CNS toxicity is unique to ifosfamide	Acetylcysteine (decreased hemorrhagic cystitis), mesna (decreased hemorrhagic cystitis)
mechlorethamine	Anorexia, nausea and vomiting, BMS, menstrual irregularities, lacrimation, diarrhea, diaphoresis, vesication, thrombophlebitis, necrosis at injection site, hyperuricemia	Amphotericin B (blood dyscrasia), live viral vaccines (increased adverse reactions to vaccine), probenecid or sulfinpyrazone (hyperuricemia and gout)
melphalan or L-sarcolysin	Nadir: 10–18 d; nausea and vomiting usually mild, dermatitis, alopecia, abnormal liver function tests, hypersensitivity, stomatitis, mucositis, influenzalike syndrome	Cyclosporine (severe renal failure has occurred)
cisplatin	Nausea and vomiting, BMS, anaphylaxis, nephrotoxicity, ototoxicity, peripheral neuropathies, loss of taste, electrolyte disturbances	Aminoglycosides (potentiates nephrotoxicity and ototoxicity); loop diuretics (additive ototoxicity); phenytoin (decreased serum concentrations and effect); probenecid or sulfinpyrazone (hyperuricemia and gout); may cause additive myelosuppression when used with other myelosuppressive drugs; live viral vaccines (increased adverse reactions to vaccine)

The alkylating agents as a group affect a wide variety of cellular functions. They produce intermediates that readily form covalent bonds with negatively charged cellular substances. One reaction is alkylation of the 7-nitrogen of guanine in DNA, which can lead to miscoding and cross-linking between two DNA strands.

Alkylation of a single strand of DNA can often be repaired easily by the DNA repair system found in most cells. However, alkylating agents may attack DNA in double-stranded form, forming cross-links or chemical bonds between the strands. Because these strands must unwind and separate during replication, cross-linking blocks replication. Cross-linkages formed at low doses of these agents may also be corrected, but higher doses lead to the breakdown of DNA. Most of the agents in this group are considered polyfunctional alkylating agents because they contain more than one alkylating group.

Pharmacokinetics. Cyclophosphamide is absorbed after oral administration, or it may be given IV. It reaches a peak action in 1 hour, with a duration of action of 72 hours. Its half-life is 4 to 6 hours, and it is excreted in urine and feces.

Therapeutic Uses. Cyclophosphamide is probably the most commonly used antineoplastic drug. By itself, it has no alkylating activity; it is a prodrug that is metabolically activated in the liver by the enzymes before it can alkylate cellular components. Its first metabolite is hydroxycyclophosphamide, and its cytotoxic metabolites

FOCUS ON

Focus on Nitrogen Mustards: Similarities and Differences

Similarities

Differences

Pharmacodynamics

Nitrogen mustards are alkylating agents. Alkylating agents are cell cycle-nonspecific or independent because they may act on cells at any phase of the cycle. One reaction is alkylation of the 7-nitrogen of guanine in DNA, which can lead to cross-linking between two DNA strands. DNA is affected in double-stranded form and cross-links or chemical bonds are formed between the strands. Normally these strands must unwind and separate during replication, but cross-linking prevents this and blocks replication.

Pharmacokinetics

These agents are metabolized by the liver and excreted in urine.

- **Cyclophosphamide, chlorambucil, melphalan,** and **uracil mustard** may be given orally.
- **Mechlorethamine, melphalan, ifosfamide,** and **cyclophosphamide** may be given IV.
- **Cyclophosphamide** may be given as an oral solution by dissolving its injectable form in elixir.

Therapeutic Uses

- **Mechlorethamine** is indicated for palliative treatment of lymphosarcoma, CML, polycythemia vera, mycosis fungoides, lung carcinoma. It is part of the MOPP regimen for Hodgkin's disease. It has been used for control of pleural, peritoneal, and pericardial effusions caused by malignant cells via intracavitary administration with varying success.
- **Melphalan** has been used for palliative treatment of multiple myeloma and inoperable epithelial ovarian carcinoma.
- **Ifosfamide** has been used with other agents for testicular cancer.
- **Cyclophosphamide** is used for Burkitt's lymphoma, non-Hodgkin's lymphomas, multiple myeloma, breast cancer and small cell lung carcinomas, soft-tissue sarcomas, and pediatric solid tumors, such as embryonal rhabdomyosarcoma, Ewing's sarcoma, and neuroblastoma. It is also used as an immunosuppressant with organ transplant recipients.
- **Chlorambucil** is used for palliative treatment of CLL, lymphomas, and Hodgkin's disease.
- **Uracil mustard** has been used for palliative treatment in CLL, non-Hodgkin's lymphoma, and CML, polycythemia vera, mycosis fungoides.

Adverse Reactions

Leukemia and secondary malignancies have been observed. Nitrogen mustards can severely suppress bone marrow function. Nitrogen mustards have been shown to be teratogenic.

- **Mechlorethamine** is a vesicant.
- **Melphalan, cyclophosphamide,** and **ifosfamide** cause hemorrhagic cystitis, and **cyclophosphamide** causes secondary transitional cell carcinoma of bladder.
- **Chlorambucil** causes neurologic toxicity (from agitation and ataxia to seizures).

Drug Interactions

Nitrogen mustards may antagonize the effects of antigout medications by increasing uric acid levels, so dosage adjustments of antigout medications may be necessary.

- **Cyclophosphamide** interacts with succinylcholine, live viral vaccines, doxorubicin, insulin, anticoagulants, thiazide diuretics.
- **Melphalan** interacts with cyclosporine, nalidixic acid, and carmustine.

(continued)

FOCUS ON

Focus on Nitrogen Mustards: Similarities and Differences (continued)

Similarities (continued)	Differences (continued)
Nursing Considerations	
Instruct in disease, drug therapy regimen, adverse reactions, and interactions.	• Clients receiving **cyclophosphamide** or **ifosfamide** should be encouraged to drink plenty of fluids and to void frequently.
Assess for therapeutic and nontherapeutic effects of drug. Monitor laboratory studies.	

are probably phosphoramide mustard and *nor*-nitrogen mustard.

Cyclophosphamide is used in Burkitt's lymphoma, non-Hodgkin's lymphomas, multiple myeloma, breast cancer and small cell lung carcinomas, soft-tissue sarcomas, and pediatric solid tumors such as embryonal rhabdomyosarcoma, Ewing's sarcoma, and neuroblastoma.

Conditioning ("purging" of the bone marrow) regimens for bone marrow transplantation may use cyclophosphamide because of its potent immunosuppressive properties. It is also used in rheumatoid arthritis, in nephrotic syndrome in children, and in Wegener's granulomatosis because of these properties.

Dosage and Administration. Consult Table 46-3 for usual dosages.

Adverse Reactions. An unusual side effect is hemorrhagic cystitis, caused by the metabolite acrolein, which irritates bladder walls. The cystitis is particularly common in high-dose chemotherapy or with prolonged periods of oral therapy and may produce significant blood loss and inappropriate water retention. Systemic IV administration of 2-mercaptoethane sodium sulfonate (mesna) is proving helpful with this problem.

Cyclophosphamide also causes bladder fibrosis, hydronephrosis, hemorrhage and clot formation in the renal pelvis, vesicoureteral reflux, and secondary urothelial malignancies. Transitional cell carcinoma of the bladder occurs, generally in clients who previously developed hemorrhagic cystitis, and may not be detected for several years after treatment.

FD and C yellow no. 5 dye in cyclophosphamide preparations may cause allergic-type reactions, including asthma, most frequently seen in clients sensitive to aspirin.

More than 50% of clients who receive intensive or prolonged therapy with cyclophosphamide experience alopecia, usually reversible.

Cyclophosphamide causes dose-dependent hepatic injury, probably because of the impaired metabolism of acrolein. Signs include increased serum aminotransferase levels, which may be precipitated by prior exposure to azathioprine.

Drug–Drug Interactions. Increased bone marrow depression may occur if cyclophosphamide is given to a client also receiving other bone marrow depressants or radiation. A decrease in drug dosage may be indicated.

Hyperuricemia and gout may occur if cyclophosphamide is given with probenecid or sulfinpyrazone. The dosage of antigout medication may be adjusted. Allopurinol may increase the bone marrow toxicity of cyclophosphamide.

Increased risk of infection and further development of neoplasms exists when cyclophosphamide is given with immunosuppressant agents, including adrenocorticosteroids, azathioprine, chlorambucil, cyclosporine, and mercaptopurine.

Live viral vaccines should be avoided if possible when cyclophosphamide is used, to avoid a decrease in antibody response and an increase in adverse reactions.

Additive cardiotoxicity may be caused by concurrent use of doxorubicin. Concurrent use of cyclophosphamide with insulin increases hypoglycemia, with anticoagulants increases the anticoagulant effect, and with thiazide diuretics increases leukopenia.

Because cyclophosphamide is activated in the liver, its metabolism can be affected by drugs that induce (eg, phenobarbital) or inhibit (eg, allopurinol) enzymes of the mixed-function oxidase system. Although the half-life of cyclophosphamide is altered by such drugs, its antitumor activity does not change.

Drug–Laboratory Test Interactions. Cyclophosphamide suppresses positive reactions to *Candida*, mumps, trichophytons, and tuberculin PPD skin tests. Pap smears may be falsely positive.

Precautions and Contraindications. Cyclophosphamide should be used with caution in clients who have undergone radiation therapy or chemotherapy, have leukopenia, thrombocytopenia, or hepatic or renal disease, or have malignant cell infiltration of the bone marrow. Reconstitution and administration have been associated with carcinogenic, mutagenic, and teratogenic risks to personnel preparing this drug, who should follow precautions. Giving the drug at bedtime increases the chance of cystitis developing. With this drug, therapeutic effects are often coupled with toxicity.

Ethylenimines and Methylmelamines
This group of alkylating agents includes triethylenethiophosphoramide and the investigational agent hexamethylmelamine.

Alkyl Sulfonates
This group of alkylating agents includes busulfan.

Nitrosoureas
The nitrosoureas include carmustine, lomustine, and streptozocin. These agents cross the blood-brain barrier, unlike most other alkylating agents. Many nitrosoureas have been tried in attempts to improve the therapeutic index and decrease bone marrow toxicity. See Focus On Nitrosoureas: Similarities and Differences.

Carmustine (BCNU, BiCNu) was the first nitrosourea used. Carmustine undergoes spontaneous chemical degradation to a carbonium ion intermediate that alkylates DNA (DNA cross-linking occurs) and an isocyanate intermediate that carbamoylates proteins, such as DNA repair enzymes. RNA synthesis is also inhibited. Carmustine is considered cell cycle phase-nonspecific but shows a selectivity for cells in G_1 or G_2.

Streptozocin (Zanosar), a naturally occurring antibiotic, was originally derived from *Streptomyces achromogenes*. It is a nitrosourea, but because its structure differs from the others, its properties differ as well. Streptozocin has alkylating activity. Although it cannot cross-link DNA, it does inhibit precursor incorporation into DNA. It is cell cycle phase-nonspecific, but cells in the S phase seem the most sensitive.

Triazenes
This grouping includes dacarbazine (DTIC-Dome), an imidazole carboxamide derivative and a structural analog of a purine. Dacarbazine was originally considered to be an antimetabolite, but its alkylating activity now appears to be its most important action. The drug inhibits RNA and protein synthesis more significantly than DNA synthesis.

Platinum Complexes
The platinum complexes include cisplatin (Platinol) and carboplatin (Paraplatin). Cisplatin is a heavy metal compound that contains a central atom of platinum surrounded by two chloride atoms and two ammonia molecules. Carboplatin is a second-generation platinum analog.

Pharmacodynamics. Cisplatin's cytotoxic properties are similar to those of bifunctional alkylating agents; it produces interstrand and intrastrand cross-links in DNA and is probably cell cycle-nonspecific (although some cells seem more sensitive during G_1). The consequences of its action on DNA include changes in DNA conformation and inhibition of DNA synthesis. Carboplatin generates both interstrand and intrastrand cross-links in DNA. Cross-links appear more slowly after carboplatin than after cisplatin.

Pharmacokinetics. Cisplatin is administered IV. It has a biphasic half-life (25–49 minutes and 58–73 hours). It is excreted in urine.

Therapeutic Uses. Cisplatin is one of the most active antineoplastic drugs against testicular tumors. It is effective against disseminated seminomatous and nonseminomatous testicular cancer in combination with vinblastine and bleomycin (VBP regimen). It is used in metastatic ovarian carcinoma in a combination that includes cisplatin, doxorubicin, and cyclophosphamide. It also been used against bladder and cervical carcinoma, head and neck cancer, osteogenic sarcoma, non-small cell lung, esophageal, and gastric carcinomas, glioblastoma, and medulloblastoma (see Example of Nursing Process for Cisplatin and Paclitaxel in Ovarian Cancer). Direct intrapericardial instillation of cisplatin daily for 5 days for malignant pericardial effusion is well tolerated with only mild nausea. Constrictive pericarditis is not produced. Cisplatin has been administered by intraperitoneal instillation in clients with intraperitoneal malignancies such as ovarian cancer. Systemic toxicity can be prevented by simultaneous administration of sodium thiosulfate IV.

Cisplatin given by regional limb perfusion has been advocated for melanoma and soft-tissue sarcoma of the extremities.

Dosage and Administration. Because of its nephrotoxic potential, protocols of hydration and diuresis are used (acute damage can occur within 3 to 21 hours after cisplatin administration). Adequate hydration decreases drug exposure in the renal tubules. One approach is to precede cisplatin administration with a 4- to 6-hour period of prehydration in conjunction with the use of mannitol. Administering mannitol prevents the immediate platinum binding onto renal tubules. Furosemide has been used, but it can increase cisplatin toxicity (ie, ototoxicity). Mannitol and furosemide do not appear to alter cisplatin's pharmacokinetics. Another approach is to administer 250 mL of normal saline solution per hour for 12 hours before and 12 hours after cisplatin administration. Daily magnesium supplements are indicated during cisplatin therapy.

The protectant WR 2721 has been used in trials. Data suggest this compound protects against nephrotoxicity, ototoxicity, and neurotoxicity. It is administered as a 15-minute infusion before cisplatin is administered. Reported adverse reactions include flushing, nausea, vomiting, somnolence, and hypotension. Another compound being used as a protectant is diethyldithiocarbamate (DDTC), which reportedly removes tissue-bound platinum through chelation without reversing cisplatin's antitumor activity. DDTC is administered IV and can cause flushing, diaphoresis, chest discomfort, and uneasiness if given rapidly (Groenwald et al., 1993).

Focus on Nitrosoureas: Similarities and Differences

Similarities

Pharmacodynamics

Nitrosoureas are alkylating agents. Alkylating agents are cell cycle-nonspecific or independent because they may act on cells at any phase of the cycle.

Pharmacokinetics

These agents are rapidly metabolized and excreted in urine as metabolites. Small amounts are excreted via feces and the lungs. Unlike many antineoplastic agents, these cross the blood-brain barrier.

Therapeutic Uses

Two of these agents are widely used with brain tumors.

Adverse Reactions

Secondary malignancies have been observed with these agents. Nitrosoureas can produce a severe and delayed suppression of bone marrow function. Nitrosoureas have been shown to be teratogenic.

Drug Interactions

Bone marrow suppression common to the nitrosoureas would be potentiated by any other drug that usually causes bone marrow suppression.

Nursing Considerations

Instruct in disease, drug therapy regimen, adverse reactions, and interactions.

Assess for therapeutic and nontherapeutic effects of drug. Monitor laboratory studies.

Differences

- **Carmustine** undergoes degradation to a carbonium ion that leads to the DNA cross-linkages and to an isocyanate intermediate that carbamoylates proteins, such as DNA repair enzymes.
- **Lomustine** also leads to cross-linkages.
- **Streptozocin** is actually an antibiotic, and it does not lead to DNA cross-linkages; it inhibits precursor incorporation into DNA.

- **Lomustine** is administered orally and should be taken on an empty stomach just before bedtime.
- **Carmustine** and **streptozocin** are given IV.

- **Lomustine** is used for both primary and metastatic brain tumors and as secondary therapy with other drugs in Hodgkin's disease.
- **Carmustine** is used for both primary and metastatic brain tumors, in combination with prednisone for multiple myeloma, and as secondary therapy with other drugs in Hodgkin's disease.
- **Streptozocin** shows specificity for pancreas cells and is used for functional and nonfunctional islet cell carcinoma of the pancreas, as a single agent or with 5-FU.

- **Streptozocin** is associated with renal toxicity that is dose-related, cumulative, and possibly severe or fatal. Streptozocin is also associated with abnormalities of glucose tolerance that are generally reversible.
- **Carmustine** and **streptozocin** are irritating to the vein during drug administration.
- **Lomustine** and **carmustine** have been associated with reversible hepatotoxicity. Carmustine has been associated with ocular and lung toxicities.

- **Carmustine** interacts with cimetidine, digoxin, and phenytoin.
- **Streptozocin** should not be used with other nephrotoxic agents (such as aminoglycosides).

In contrast to cisplatin, renal tubular secretion of carboplatin has not been reported, which may account for its lower nephrotoxicity. Prehydration is not required. Carboplatin-induced nephrotoxicity is seen at high doses (more than 800 mg/m²) and after prior cisplatin therapy.

Adverse Reactions. Nephrotoxicity from cisplatin results from a direct toxic effect on the renal tubules.

Electrolyte abnormalities include hypomagnesemia and hypocalcemia. Any use of the drug in clients with renal dysfunction should be guided by kidney function evaluation. Some suggest that renal function must return to normal before any subsequent doses of cisplatin are given, as measured by a serum creatinine level of less than 1.5 mg/dL or a blood urea nitrogen (BUN) level of less than 25 mg/dL. Impaired renal function may last at least 6 months after treatment concludes.

Example of Nursing Process for Cisplatin and Paclitaxel in Ovarian Cancer

Mary Strom is a 63-year-old nulliparous woman diagnosed with cancer of the ovary with extension of the tumor to the uterus. She has had an abdominal hysterectomy and bilateral salpingo-oophorectomy, at which time the liver was biopsied and metastasis was identified. The first course of chemotherapy was ineffective. Ms. Strom will now undergo chemotherapy with cisplatin (Platinol) and paclitaxel (Taxol).

Assessment Data

Receiving cisplatin

Receiving paclitaxel

Nursing Diagnosis*	Intervention	Goals and Outcomes
Potential Complication: Nephrotoxicity	**Prehydrate** client with 1–2 L infused over 8 to 12 hours before administration of cisplatin. **Dilute** drug in 1–2 L 5% dextrose in 0.3% or 0.45% saline containing 37.5 g mannitol and infuse over 6–8 h. **Maintain** IV fluids as ordered during administration of cisplatin and for 24 hours after therapy. **Monitor** for therapeutic and adverse effects of mannitol. **Monitor** and **report** signs of renal dysfunction.	The client will maintain adequate renal function as evidenced by BUN less than 25 mg/dL, serum creatinine less than 1.5 mg/dL, and urine output at least 30 mL/h.
Potential Complication: Ototoxicity	**Assess** for evidence of cochlear toxicity—is client hearing ringing, roaring, or blowing noises, is client experiencing otalgia (ear pain) or aural fullness (full feeling in ear). **Perform** whisper test and ticking watch test. **Report** evidence of decreased auditory acuity.	
Potential Complication: Hypersensitivity reaction	**Pretreat** as ordered with protocol such as oral dexamethasone 20 mg administered about 12 and 6 hours before paclitaxel, diphenhydramine 50 mg IV 30 to 60 minutes prior, and 300 mg cimetidine or 50 mg ranitidine IV 30 to 60 minutes before. **Dilute** with 0.9% saline or other approved solution to a final concentration of 0.3–1.2 mg/mL as ordered. **Administer** soon after preparing (solutions are stable for 20 hours). **Use** a glass container for drug solution. **Administer** 135 mg/m² IV by infusion over 24 hours. **Assess** for evidence of hypersensitivity such as dyspnea, flushing, chest pain, and tachycardia.	The client will not develop evidence of minor or major hypersensitivity (eg, flushing, rash, hypotension/hypertension, dyspnea, tachycardia, chest pain).

*Although potential complications are not routinely addressed in these examples, in this situation the identification of such a collaborative problem is critical to the outcome for this client and illustrates the broad range of nursing responsibilities during chemotherapy.

Cisplatin is associated with a sensory peripheral neuropathy. It may be age-related, as it has not been recognized in children treated with cisplatin for neuroblastoma. It may be more likely to occur with prolonged treatment or high-dose therapy and may be reversible.

Cisplatin causes IgE-mediated hypersensitivity reactions, including flushing, pruritus, erythema, urticaria, dyspnea, bronchospasm, diaphoresis, vomiting, and hypotension. Pretreatment with antihistamines and corticosteroids may be warranted.

Ototoxicity, including tinnitus or high-frequency hearing loss, is common in very young and very old clients. Hearing loss may be unilateral or bilateral and tends to become more severe with repeated doses; it is irreversible. Audiometric analysis should be performed before and during therapy and may be an indicator for withholding subsequent doses.

Sexual function may be compromised in men after treatment with the VBP regimen, including diminished libido and ejaculatory dysfunction.

Cisplatin given by regional limb perfusion has resulted in compartment syndrome, necessitating fasciotomies with permanent loss of dorsiflexion. Local adverse effects also include cellulitis and wound infections and are probably secondary to the technique rather than to the drug itself.

Resistance to cisplatin develops, but its mechanisms are unclear. Platinum compounds are not cross-resistant with nitrosoureas or classic alkylating agents. The major advantage of carboplatin over cisplatin is its different toxicity: carboplatin appears less nephrotoxic, less ototoxic, less neurotoxic, and less emetogenic than cisplatin. A delayed type of myelosuppression is the primary toxicity with carboplatin. Thrombocytopenia is the predominant effect, with platelet nadirs occurring in 2 to 3 weeks and recovery by the 4th week after treatment. Leukopenia and anemia occur, but less commonly and to a lesser degree. The thrombocytopenia seems to be dose-related, to be more common in older clients, and to be more severe in clients with renal dysfunction or a history of antineoplastic therapy.

Drug Interactions. Cross-resistance exists between cisplatin and carboplatin. Concurrent use of other nephrotoxic drugs (aminoglycosides, amphotericin B, vancomycin) increases the nephrotoxicity of cisplatin and carboplatin. Ideally, administration of the drugs would be separated by 1 to 2 weeks. Use of aminoglycosides and furosemide increases the risk of cisplatin's and carboplatin's ototoxicity. Carboplatin is associated with decreased serum calcium, magnesium, potassium, and sodium levels and mild increases in liver function test values.

Precautions and Contraindications. Aluminum can react with cisplatin and carboplatin, resulting in precipitation and decreased potency. Thus, aluminum needles or IV sets with parts that contain aluminum cannot be used. Clients may need prolonged antiemetic therapy because delayed vomiting sometimes occurs 3 to 5 days after treatment with cisplatin. Carboplatin carries a greater risk of neurotoxicity in clients older than 65 years. Reconstituted carboplatin is stable at room temperature for only 8 hours, after which it must be discarded. Because of potential nephrotoxicity, protocols of hydration and diuresis must be used in conjunction with cisplatin.

■ SUMMARY

The alkylating agents as a group affect a wide variety of cellular functions. The basis for their therapeutic use against cancer is the process of alkylation, by which they cause interstrand and intrastrand cross-linkages in DNA, blocking replication. Alkylating agents are cell cycle phase-nonspecific, although in some cases cells appear more sensitive in one phase than another. The alkylating agents used as antineoplastic agents are the nitrogen mustards, the ethylenimines and methylmelamines, an alkyl sulfonate, the nitrosoureas, a triazene, and the platinum complexes. Of these, chlorambucil is the medication of choice for the management of chronic lymphocytic leukemia. Cyclophosphamide is probably the most widely used antineoplastic drug. Ifosfamide is a synthetic analog of cyclophosphamide. Mechlorethamine was the first alkylating agent used and is used in treating Hodgkin's disease. Busulfan provides palliation in chronic myelogenous leukemia. The nitrosoureas are lipid soluble and are used to treat various brain tumors. Cisplatin is one of the most active antineoplastic drugs against testicular tumors, and carboplatin is a cisplatin analog. All these drugs cause serious adverse reactions.

Antimetabolites

The antimetabolites include a folic acid analog, the pyrimidine analogs, and the purine analogs. Dosages and therapeutic uses for the antimetabolites are summarized in Table 46-5, adverse reactions and interactions in Table 46-6.

Folic Acid Analogs

Folic acid and its derivatives are critical to the metabolism of proliferating cells. Methotrexate is a representative folic acid analog.

Methotrexate

Pharmacodynamics. Methotrexate competitively inhibits dihydrofolate reductase, the enzyme that reduces dihydrofolic acid to tetrahydrofolic acid. Tetrahydrofolic acid is converted to various coenzymes required for several one-carbon transfer reactions. The reaction most sensitive to lack of a coenzyme is the conversion of 2-deoxyuridylate (dUMP) to thymidylate (dTMP), an es-

Table 46-5. Antimetabolites: Indications

Drug Name	Preparation	Usual Dosage	Therapeutic Indications
Folic Acid Analogs			
methotrexate sodium (Mexate, Folex, Rheumatrex)	Oral tablets IV IM Intrathecal	*Trophoblastic neoplasm:* PO: 15–30 mg/d for 5 d; repeat q12wk for 3–5 courses IM/IV: 15–30 mg/d for 5 d; repeat q12wk for 3–5 courses *Leukemia:* IM/IV induction: 3.3 mg/m²/d PO/IM/IV maintenance: 20–30 mg/m² 2 times/wk *Rheumatoid arthritis:* PO: 2.5–5 mg q12h for 3 doses each wk or 7.5 mg once/wk	Choriocarcinoma, hydatidiform mole, prophylaxis and treatment of meningeal lymphocytic leukemia, breast cancer, epidermoid cancers of head and neck, lung cancer, non-Hodgkin's lymphoma osteosarcoma, psoriasis (severe, recalcitrant, disabling), rheumatoid arthritis (second- or third-line treatment); *ANLL, bladder, brain, cervix, cutaneous T-cell lymphoma, esophagus, kidney, myeloma, ovary, prostate, rhabdomyosarcoma, stomach, testes*
Pyrimidine Analogs			
floxuridine (FUDR)	Intra-arterial	0.1–0.6 mg/kg/d	GI adenocarcinoma metastatic to liver (intra-arterial infusion of drug); *ANLL, ALL, bladder, brain, breast, cervix, gallbladder, head and neck, kidney, ovary, prostate*
fluorouracil/5-FU (Adrucil, Amethopterin)	IV	12 mg/kg/d for 4 consecutive days up to 800 mg or until toxicity develops or 12 days therapy; may repeat at 1-mo intervals If toxicity develops, 15 mg/kg once/wk can be given until toxicity subsides	Carcinoma of stomach, colon, rectum, breast, pancreas; *bladder, cervix, endometrium, esophagus, head and neck, islet cell, liver, lung, ovary, prostate*
fluorouracil (Efudex)	Topical cream	bid for 3–6 wk	Premalignant actinic keratoses and superficial skin cancers
cytarabine/cytosine arabinoside (Cytosar-U, Ara-C, Tarabine, Udacil)	IV SC Intrathecal	IV: 200 mg/m² over 24 hr Intrathecal: 5–75 mg q4d or once/d for 4 d	ANLL, ALL, CML, meningeal leukemia; *Hodgkin's and non-Hodgkin's lymphoma*
Purine Analogs			
mercaptopurine (Purinethol)	Oral tablets (50 mg)	80–100 mg/m²/day; reduce dose in presence of hepatic or renal dysfunction	Remission induction and maintenance therapy for ALL; *ANLL, CML, non-Hodgkin's lymphoma*
thioguanine (Lanvis)	Oral tablets (40 mg)	80–100 mg/m²	Remission induction, consolidation, and maintenance therapy for ANLL; *ALL, CML*

Italicized indications were not FDA approved as of 1993.
Fischer DS, Knobf MT, Durivage HJ. (1993). *The cancer chemotherapy handbook,* 4th ed. St. Louis: Mosby–Year Book, Inc.

sential component of DNA. Thus, as a result of the inhibition of dihydrofolate reductase, methotrexate causes an accumulation of cellular folates in the inactive oxidized form and leads to inhibition of dTMP, DNA, RNA, and protein synthesis. Methotrexate, and all the antimetabolites, are cell cycle-specific for the S phase.

Pharmacokinetics. Methotrexate may be administered orally, IV, IM, and intrathecally. Its half-life is 2 to 4 hours. It is excreted in urine.

Therapeutic Uses. Methotrexate is used in treating acute leukemia, for maintenance therapy and for CNS prophylaxis (used intrathecally and with cranial irradiation). It is an agent of choice in combination therapy with mercaptopurine.

Tumors sensitive to methotrexate include head and neck cancers, bone and soft-tissue sarcomas, trophoblastic neoplasms (choriocarcinoma, chorioadenoma destruens, hydatidiform mole), rhabdomyosarcoma, medulloblastoma, glioma, melanomas, testicular cancer, and bladder and cervical carcinomas. Methotrexate is a component of combination regimens used to treat non-Hodgkin's and Burkitt's lymphomas and breast and ovarian carcinomas.

Oral methotrexate has been used to treat psoriasis, a nonneoplastic skin disease characterized by abnormally rapid proliferation of epidermal cells. It is used also to

Table 46-6. Antimetabolites: Reactions and Interactions

Drug Names	Adverse Reactions	Drug Interactions
Folic Acid Analogs		
methotrexate sodium	Nadir: 7–10 d; nausea and anorexia, stomatitis and ulcerations can occur and are dose-limiting	Aspirin and NSAIDs (decreased renal elimination of methotrexate and increased toxicity), leucovorin (decreased methotrexate cytotoxicity), probenecid (increased methotrexate protein displacement and increased toxicity), sulfonamides (additive enzyme inhibition and increased toxicity)
Pyrimidine Analogs		
floxuridine	Anorexia, nausea and vomiting, diarrhea, inflammation of GI tract, dermatologic reactions, bone marrow suppression (BMS), elevated liver function tests, acute and delayed CNS toxicity	Dexamethasone (decreased floxuridine hepatotoxicity)
fluorouracil/5-FU	Anorexia, nausea and vomiting, diarrhea, inflammation of GI tract, BMS, alopecia, hyperpigmentation, acute and chronic conjunctivitis, excessive lacrimation, cerebellar dysfunction, hand–foot syndrome, myocardial ischemia	Allopurinol (decreased 5-FU cytotoxicity), cimetidine (increased 5-FU serum concentrations), interferon alfa, leucovorin, methotrexate, PALA (increased 5-FU cytotoxicity)
fluorouracil	Pain, pruritus, hyperpigmentation and burning at application site, allergic contact dermatitis, swelling, tenderness, suppuration, scaling, scarring	
cytarabine/cytosine arabinoside	BMS, nausea and vomiting, diarrhea, stomatitis, neurotoxicity at high doses (cerebellar and cerebral; ataxia, confusion, seizures), acute painful, swollen erythematous hands and soles, keratoconjunctivitis, pancreatitis in those treated earlier with asparaginase, pulmonary toxicity (ARDS), hepatotoxicity, alopecia, anaphylaxis, thrombophlebitis, cellulitis at injection site	Digoxin (may decrease serum digoxin levels)
mercaptopurine	Nadir 10–14 d; nausea and vomiting, mucositis, diarrhea, cholestatic injury and jaundice, pancreatitis, hepatic dysfunction, pulmonary toxicity/fibrosis with prolonged use	Allopurinol (inhibited mercaptopurine metabolism and increased toxicity), nondepolarizing muscle relaxants (decreased neuromuscular blockade), warfarin (potentiate or antagonize)
thioguanine	Nadir 7–28 d; stomatitis, diarrhea, hepatotoxicity	Myelosuppressants (increased risk of toxicity, bleeding and hepatotoxicity)

treat mycosis fungoides, rheumatoid arthritis (when refractory to other second-line drugs), and systemic lupus erythematosus. For these disorders, the drug is usually administered in a low dose of 7.5 to 15 mg weekly. Side effects of pancytopenia, GI toxicity, skin rash, headache, hepatotoxicity, and pulmonary toxic effects have all been reported at the low dose and are usually mild; the effects remain constant with prolonged use.

Methotrexate is used as an immunosuppressive agent to prevent graft-versus-host disease after allogeneic bone marrow transplantation.

Dosage and Administration. Consult Table 46-5 for usual dosages. The biochemical effects of methotrexate can be reversed by the administration of leucovorin calcium (or folinic acid or citrovorum factor). Leucovorin calcium is a folate coenzyme that does not need reduction by dihydrofolate reductase. When leucovorin calcium is supplied to cells, the methotrexate-induced block of tetrahydrofolic acid synthesis is bypassed. Using this res-

cue agent allows for recovery of normal tissues or reduction of toxicity to the bone marrow and GI epithelium. For example, side effects of mucositis, skin rashes, and altered taste sensation are reduced by the administration of leucovorin calcium, and renal failure may be prevented.

When using leucovorin calcium, serial methotrexate concentrations must be obtained to determine at what point it is safe to discontinue the leucovorin calcium. After 24 to 48 hours of methotrexate therapy, the methotrexate level is measured, and the leucovorin calcium is continued until the methotrexate concentration falls to less than 500 mmol/L. The cytotoxic effects of methotrexate are irreversible after 48 hours without adequate rescue.

A typical way to administer the methotrexate and leucovorin calcium (Jaffe regimen) is to give 50 to 250 mg/kg of methotrexate as an infusion over 6 hours. Leucovorin calcium administration begins 2 hours after the end of the drug infusion at a rate of 15 mg/m² IM every 6 hours for seven doses.

Due to the potential nephrotoxicity of methotrexate, adequate hydration and alkalinization of the urine (using sodium bicarbonate or acetazolamide) are recommended to enhance the excretion of methotrexate. Methotrexate is a weak dicarboxylic acid and precipitates in acid urine.

In the 12 hours before methotrexate treatment, the indicated prehydration regimen may include 1.5 L/m² dextrose 5% in water (D₅W) with 100 mEq bicarbonate and 20 mEq potassium chloride/L. The urine pH should be tested at the time of drug infusion to ensure it is 7 or more.

Adverse Reactions. Adverse reactions are listed in Table 46-6. Three distinct patterns of toxicity have been observed with intrathecal methotrexate. The acute form is a chemical arachnoiditis that begins shortly after the drug is administered and resolves in 1 to 5 days. The subacute form of toxicity develops over a few weeks and is characterized by motor dysfunction of the brain or spinal cord. This form is probably related to a continuously elevated level of CSF methotrexate, which may occur when clients receive multiple injections per week. The third form of toxicity is associated with months or years of intrathecal methotrexate. It is a necrotizing demyelinating leukoencephalopathy characterized by progressive neurologic deterioration, including dementia, dysarthria, ataxia, spasticity, seizures, and coma. Serial electroencephalograms in clients who receive high-dose methotrexate may be used to predict the leukoencephalopathy entity.

Chronic brain injury appears to occur in many children with acute lymphocytic leukemia who receive CNS prophylaxis with intrathecal methotrexate and cranial irradiation. In these children, computed tomography reveals intracerebral calcification, hypodensities, thinning of the cerebral cortex, and ventricular dilatation. Some studies indicate that reduced doses of methotrexate and cranial irradiation reduce CNS sequelae; others suggest using high-dose systemic methotrexate rather than intrathecal methotrexate.

Methotrexate may be distributed into the pleural and peritoneal cavities. If ascites or pleural effusion is present, these cavities may act as storage sites for methotrexate, subsequently releasing the drug and causing further adverse reactions. Therefore, pleural effusions and ascites should be evacuated before methotrexate administration.

Interaction with other drugs, renal impairment, or an idiosyncratic response may explain the pancytopenia that sometimes occurs with methotrexate. Hepatic dysfunction may occur as well. Elevated aspartate aminotransferase levels are common in clients on long-term methotrexate therapy. These may indicate liver fibrosis or cirrhosis. Liver biopsy is the most reliable method of documenting actual liver damage.

Acute life-threatening pneumonitis has been reported after using methotrexate to treat rheumatoid arthritis.

Resistance to methotrexate may develop as a result of more than one mechanism, including increased levels of dihydrofolate reductase, sequestration of dihydrofolate reductase in a site inaccessible to the drug, decreased sensitivity of dihydrofolate reductase to methotrexate, defective transport of methotrexate into malignant cells, or reduced conversion of methotrexate to active metabolites within malignant cells.

Drug Interactions. Cellular uptake of methotrexate is decreased by concomitant use of penicillin, hydroxyurea, mercaptopurine, neomycin, kanamycin, corticosteroids, bleomycin, and asparaginase.

Methotrexate may be displaced from plasma albumin by sulfonamides, salicylates, tetracyclines, chloramphenicol, and phenytoin. This displacement may result in greater methotrexate toxicity.

Salicylates and probenecid inhibit tubular secretion of methotrexate. Salicylates are contraindicated in clients receiving methotrexate because the methotrexate effect can be increased by two different mechanisms with this group of drugs.

Concurrent use of alcohol or hepatotoxic drugs with methotrexate increases the risk of hepatotoxicity; such combinations should be avoided if possible. Etretinate for psoriasis should also be avoided for this reason.

Concurrent administration of methotrexate and nonsteroidal antiinflammatory drugs may result in severe methotrexate toxicity and should be viewed as a possibly fatal interaction.

Oral aminoglycosides decrease the absorption of oral methotrexate.

Neurologic complications may occur with the combination of intrathecal methotrexate and acyclovir. Vincristine and vinblastine impair methotrexate elimination from the CSF.

Asparaginase may attenuate methotrexate toxicity if administration is correctly timed. Asparaginase should be given 9 to 10 days before or within 24 hours after the methotrexate.

Pretreatment with cytarabine may enhance methotrexate cytotoxicity because cytarabine increases the cellular uptake of methotrexate.

Administered before fluorouracil, methotrexate promotes the conversion of this drug to fluorodeoxyuridylate (FdUMP), its active metabolite. This conversion could enhance the cytotoxicity of fluorouracil, but to date this interaction has not been used to clinical benefit. Administered in reverse order, fluorouracil inhibits dTMP synthetase, which could inhibit methotrexate cytotoxicity.

Precautions and Contraindications. Because there are teratogenic, mutagenic, and carcinogenic risks associated with the preparation and administration of methotrexate, healthcare personnel should follow precautionary guidelines. This drug should be used cautiously in clients with peptic ulcer, ulcerative colitis, impaired renal or hepatic function, aplasia, leukopenia, thrombocytopenia, bone marrow suppression, or anemia. Once the drug has been administered, the client must be monitored for signs of bleeding and infection. To prevent drug precipitation in the urine, sodium bicarbonate may be administered to alkalinize the urine.

Pyrimidine Analogs

Included in the subgrouping of pyrimidine analogs are fluorouracil, topical fluorouracil, floxuridine, and cytarabine. See Focus On Antimetabolites: Similarities and Differences.

Fluorouracil

Fluorouracil (5-FU, Adrucil) is a fluorinated pyrimidine.

Pharmacodynamics. The cytotoxicity of fluorouracil is probably related to several of its biochemical actions. Fluorouracil was developed after scientists observed that certain tumor cells used uracil, a pyrimidine base, after it was converted to thymidine, for synthesis of DNA.

Metabolism of fluorouracil produces FdUMP. FdUMP inhibits dTMP synthetase, which catalyzes the methylation of dUMP to dTMP, an essential component of DNA. Thus, with this inhibition, a DNA precursor is unavailable, and DNA synthesis is prevented. Metabolism of fluorouracil also produces fluorouridine-5'-triphosphate, which is incorporated into RNA and interferes with its function.

FdUMP, dTMP synthetase, and $N^{5,10}$-methylene-tetrahydrofolate form a stable complex. Tumor sensitivity may correlate with the degree of inhibition of dTMP synthetase, which in turn correlates with the stability of the complex. This stability can be enhanced by exogenously adding reduced folates, such as calcium folinate; this concept has been used in treatment protocols to improve the efficacy of fluorouracil. Fluorouracil is cell cycle-specific for the S phase.

Pharmacokinetics. Fluorouracil has a half-life of 8 to 20 minutes. It is excreted in urine and via the lungs as carbon dioxide.

Therapeutic Uses. Fluorouracil is useful only in solid tumors. It is used in the palliative treatment of colorectal cancer. It is a component of the FAM regimen (fluorouracil, doxorubicin, mitomycin) used in the palliative management of gastric adenocarcinoma.

Fluorouracil is also a component of the CMF (cyclophosphamide, methotrexate, 5-fluorouracil) or CAF regimen (cyclophosphamide, doxorubicin [Adriamycin], fluorouracil) for breast cancer. It is also used in cancer of the ovary, bladder, cervix, endometrium, prostate, head and neck, pancreas, esophagus, and liver.

Dosage and Administration. Consult Table 46-5 for usual dosages. Colon cancer with liver metastasis or primary liver tumors may be treated by hepatic arterial infusion of fluorouracil or other agents (eg, cisplatin, mitomycin, doxorubicin).

Fluorouracil has been used in conjunction with leucovorin calcium (citrovorum factor, folinic acid, Wellcovorin) and levamisole (Ergamisol) (see Miscellaneous Agents, Ch. 47). Leucovorin calcium has been combined with fluorouracil in palliative treatment of colorectal cancer; however, toxicities may be more pronounced when both drugs are used.

Levamisole appears to restore depressed immune function. It has been used to treat clients with Dukes' stage C colon cancer, after surgical resection. One approach to its use would be levamisole 50 mg orally every 8 hours for 3 days, starting 7 to 30 days after surgery. Fluorouracil therapy is subsequently initiated no earlier than 21 days and no later than 35 days after surgery (450 mg/m²/day IV for 5 days concomitant) with a 3-day course of levamisole. The two drugs can also be combined for maintenance therapy.

Adverse Reactions. Acute and chronic conjunctivitis occur and may lead to tear duct stenosis and ectropion (everted eyelid). Discontinuing the drug may correct the acute inflammatory response, but if stenosis develops, surgical correction may be needed.

Gastrointestinal disturbances are common with fluorouracil. GI damage can occur at any level, and lesions similar to those seen with stomatitis can be seen in the stoma of colostomies. Repeated episodes of watery diarrhea for several days may lead to dehydration, sepsis, and death, so dosage adjustments are usually indicated when diarrhea occurs.

Cardiac toxicity has been increasingly reported with fluorouracil. One variation is constrictive anginal chest pain during infusion. Outcome is favorable if the drug is stopped. Reintroduction of the drug has been associated with death and is not recommended. Another example of cardiac toxicity is sudden death, apparently due to ventricular fibrillation. A syndrome of chest pain, serum enzyme elevations consistent with myocardial necrosis, and electrocardiogram findings consistent with myocardial ischemia has been identified.

Acute, painful, swollen, erythematous hands and soles have been reported after protracted fluorouracil infusion (palmar–plantar erythrodysesthesia). Fluorouracil also commonly causes other mucocutaneous effects, such as hyperpigmentation and multiple pigmented macules.

Cerebellar signs (including ataxia) may occur and may be dose-related. They may occur at any time during therapy, usually after several months, and may persist several weeks after discontinuing the drug.

Resistance to fluorouracil may result from deletion of enzymes required for its activation or from an increase in dTMP synthetase activity.

With hepatic artery chemotherapy with fluorouracil, systemic toxicity is mild, but other complications may occur (eg, catheter dislodgment, sepsis, local toxicity). If the catheter slips into the gastroduodenal artery, necrosis of the intestinal epithelium, hemorrhage, or

FOCUS ON

Focus On Antimetabolites: Similarities and Differences

Similarities

Pharmacodynamics

Antimetabolites are cell cycle-specific, exerting their effect during the S phase. This class primarily interferes with DNA and RNA synthesis by blocking enzymes necessary for synthesis or by being incorporated into DNA or RNA.

Pharmacokinetics

Some antimetabolites cross the blood-brain barrier. Most of the agents are metabolized in the liver and excreted by the kidneys. Some are unpredictably absorbed after oral administration and are given parenterally.

Therapeutic Uses

The antimetabolites have a wide range of uses. They are used with curative intent as well as palliative management. Several leukemias may be treated with antimetabolites.

Adverse Reactions

Secondary malignancies have been observed. Antimetabolites can produce a severe and delayed suppression of bone marrow function. GI adverse reactions such as anorexia, nausea, vomiting, and diarrhea are common.

Differences

- Folic acid analogs (**methotrexate**) competitively inhibit dihydrofolate reductase, an enzyme that reduces dihydrofolic acid to tetrahydrofolic acid, and tetrahydrofolic acid is converted to various coenzymes; the formation of one essential component of DNA is sensitive to the lack of one of the coenzymes.
- Pyrimidine analogs (**floxuridine, fluorouracil, cytarabine**) compete for an enzyme that is needed for synthesis of thymidine, an essential substrate of DNA, and thereby block DNA synthesis.
- **Mercaptopurine, thioguanine,** and **pentostatin** are analogs of natural purines; they are metabolized to active nucleotides that then interfere with the synthesis of the natural purines, thus preventing normal DNA synthesis.

- **Fluorouracil** is also partially eliminated by the lungs; it is usually given IV.
- **Floxuridine** is given intra-arterially.
- **Methotrexate** may be given orally, IM, IV, intra-arterially, or intrathecally.
- **Cytarabine** may be given SC, IV, or intrathecally.
- **Cytarabine** and **methotrexate** cross the blood-brain barrier.
- **Thioguanine** is given orally.

- **Fluorouracil** is indicated for palliative management of carcinoma of the stomach and pancreas and for treatment of breast, ovarian, cervical, and liver carcinomas. It is used with levamisole after surgery in Dukes' stage C colon cancer. It is used in combination with leucovorin in metastatic colorectal carcinoma.
- Topical **fluorouracil** is used for premalignant actinic keratoses of the head and neck and for treatment of superficial basal cell carcinomas.
- **Fludarabine** is used for CLL.
- **Methotrexate** is indicated for treatment of gestational choriocarcinoma, chorioadenoma destruens, hydatidiform mole, and for CNS prophylaxis with ALL and for maintenance therapy with ALL, and Burkitt's lymphoma. It is also used for psoriasis, mycosis fungoides, rheumatoid arthritis, and Crohn's disease.
- **Cytarabine** is used for AML in adults and children and treatment of certain other leukemias.
- **Mercaptopurine** is used for ALL, AML, and CML.
- **Thioguanine** is used for certain acute and chronic leukemias.

- **Fluorouracil** is also associated with alopecia, hyperpigmentation, acute and chronic conjunctivitis, excessive lacrimation, cerebellar dysfunction, hand–foot syndrome, and myocardial ischemia.
- Topical **fluorouracil** may cause pain, pruritus, hyperpigmentation, and burning at application site, followed by other skin changes.
- **Methotrexate** causes stomatitis and ulcerations and CNS disturbances.
- **Cytarabine** may cause stomatitis, cerebellar and cerebral neurotoxicity, palmar–plantar erythrodysesthesia, keratoconjunctivitis, pulmonary toxicity, alopecia, and anaphylaxis.

(continued)

FOCUS ON

Focus On Antimetabolites: Similarities and Differences (continued)

Similarities (continued)

Adverse Reactions (continued)

Differences (continued)

- **Mercaptopurine** is also associated with mucositis, cholestatic injury and jaundice, pancreatitis, and pulmonary toxicity.
- **Mercaptopurine, thioguanine,** and **methotrexate** cause hepatotoxicity.

Drug Interactions

Bone marrow suppression common to methotrexate and mercaptopurine would be potentiated by concurrent use of trimethoprim-sulfamethoxazole (Bactrim, Septra).

- **Fluorouracil** interacts with allopurinol, cimetidine, interferon alfa, leucovorin, methotrexate, PALA.
- **Methotrexate** interacts with aspirin and NSAIDs, leucovorin, probenecid, sulfonamides.
- **Mercaptopurine** interacts with allopurinol, nondepolarizing muscle relaxants, warfarin.

Nursing Considerations

Instruct in disease, drug therapy regimen, adverse reactions, and interactions.

Assess for therapeutic and nontherapeutic effects of drug. Monitor laboratory studies.

---

perforation may result. Signs of this complication include the sudden onset of epigastric pain or ileus. Duodenal ulcers (fatal in some clients) have been reported, appearing 5 to 7 months after initial administration of the fluorouracil. An erythematous blistering skin rash corresponding to the distribution of the selected artery has occurred with fluorouracil. It usually subsides 1 to 2 months after treatment stops, but residual pigmentation is left. Persistent neck and shoulder pain, which may be abolished by injecting a long-acting local anesthetic through the infusion catheter, has been reported. This pain is thought to be referred pain from the diaphragm.

Drug Interactions. Synergistic toxicity from the use of fluorouracil and cisplatin together has been manifested in acute dilated cardiomyopathy with left ventricular dysfunction. With drug discontinuation, recovery occurred.

The interaction between fluorouracil and methotrexate was discussed under methotrexate. The concurrent use of fluorouracil and allopurinol may decrease fluorouracil toxicity. The drug interactions described under cyclophosphamide in relation to bone marrow depressants and radiation may also occur if these agents are used with fluorouracil.

Precautions and Contraindications. Fluorouracil should be used cautiously in clients with impaired renal or hepatic function or bone marrow infiltration by the cancer. It should be used cautiously in clients who have undergone high-dose pelvic radiation or therapy with alkylating agents. Preparation and administration cautions include:

- Observe institutional policy to avoid carcinogenic, mutagenic, and teratogenic risks.
- Do not refrigerate prepared drug.
- Use household bleach to inactivate any drug spilled.
- Warm the solution if crystals form; do not administer cloudy solution.

The administration of any live virus vaccine during treatment with fluorouracil should probably be avoided. Fluorouracil suppresses normal defense mechanisms and thus may increase replication of the virus, causing adverse effects. Live virus vaccines should not be administered until months after chemotherapy has been discontinued. People in close contact with the client should not receive the oral polio vaccine, because the live virus is excreted by the person receiving it, and it can then be transmitted to the client.

Topical Fluorouracil

Therapeutic Uses. Topical fluorouracil is available as a solution at concentrations of 1% (Fluroplex) or 2% and 5% (Efudex) or as a cream at concentrations of 1% (Fluroplex) or 5% (Efudex). The 2% or 5% preparation is used on multiple premalignant actinic keratoses of the head and neck, the 5% preparation on keratoses of the body. For isolated lesions, curettage or cryosurgery is usually preferred.

In the 5% strength, fluorouracil can be used in treating superficial basal cell carcinomas when more usual treatment methods are impractical (eg, multiple lesions, difficult treatment sites). Carcinoma in situ of the vulva also has been treated successfully with a topical approach.

Dosage and Administration. The preparation is applied twice daily to the affected area. Mucous membranes, scrotum, eyes, and intertriginous areas should be avoided. Application is continued for 2 to 4 weeks until the inflammation response progresses from erythema to necrosis. The expected result is local sloughing of the affected area and eventual regranulization of normal tissue; thus, it is normal for the treated area to become red and tender, then to form a lesion that becomes necrotic, followed by superficial sloughing of the dead tissue and regrowth of healthy skin.

After cessation of therapy, healing may take 6 to 8 weeks. On the body, this healing phase can be accelerated by applying a topical corticosteroid, such as betamethasone valerate cream 0.1% (Valisone), twice daily to the affected area. On the face, 1% hydrocortisone cream can be used in the same manner.

With keratoses, little or no inflammation may develop. In this case, the treatment period may be prolonged, or concomitant therapy with 0.1% tretinoin cream may be used (the tretinoin cream appears to aid penetration by fluorouracil). With basal cell carcinomas, the treatment period may be 3 to 12 weeks.

Adverse Reactions. Systemic side effects are uncommon, but mild, delayed effects such as nausea have been reported. Adverse reactions such as severe burning or rashes may necessitate discontinuation of therapy or dose reduction.

Precautions and Contraindications. Tight occlusive dressings are probably not advisable, because their use is associated with irritation of the healthy tissue that surrounds the lesion. A loose gauze dressing may be used for cosmetic purposes. Clients need to know that treated areas may be unsightly during therapy and that lesions may not heal completely for 1 to 2 months after cessation of therapy. Restoration of skin color and texture is usually satisfactory, and scars usually do not occur.

Exposure to sunlight during and for 1 or 2 months after treatment should be minimized.

Gloves should be worn when applying the preparation. Cotton swabs may be used, but not a metallic applicator.

Cytarabine

Cytarabine (cytosine arabinoside; Ara-C) is one of several arabinose nucleosides first isolated from the sponge *Cryptothethya crypta*. Since its discovery, other similar preparations have been isolated or synthesized and tested as antitumor agents, but none are in general use. Two nucleosides (5-azacytidine/5-aza-C and 3-deazauridine)

have undergone clinical trials. For therapeutic uses, adverse reactions, and drug interactions, see Table 46-6.

Pharmacodynamics. Cytarabine's cytotoxic capabilities are due to its metabolite, arabinofuranosylcytosine triphosphate (ara-CTP), which blocks DNA synthesis by competitively inhibiting DNA polymerase. It is incorporated into DNA, leading to a marked slowing of the elongating chain of DNA and a defect in ligation of fragments of newly synthesized DNA.

Entry into cells is an important determinant of sensitivity to cytarabine. A strong correlation exists between the number of transport sites and the formation of the ultimate toxic metabolite (ara-CTP). Cytarabine penetrates cells best by a carrier-mediated process; it can also enter cells by passive diffusion, but this is a less efficient mechanism.

Cytarabine is subject to deamination by cytidine deaminase, an enzyme found in plasma and granulocytes. This deaminating enzyme is believed to be a factor in limiting drug action and possibly in the development of resistance. Cytarabine is cell cycle-specific for the S phase, but exposure of cells during other phases may lead to chromatid deletions and to a failure to repair strand breaks induced by other agents.

Pharmacokinetics. Cytarabine's onset and duration of action are undefined. Levels peak in 20 to 60 minutes after SC injection.

Precautions and Contraindications. Clients receiving high doses must be assessed for neurotoxicity, which may begin as nystagmus and progress to ataxia and cerebellar dysfunction. Nurses responsible for preparing and administering cytarabine must follow institutional policy to reduce carcinogenic, teratogenic, and mutagenic risks.

Purine Analogs

The purine analogs include mercaptopurine and thioguanine.

Mercaptopurine

Pharmacodynamics. Mercaptopurine (6-mercaptopurine, 6-MP; Purinethol) is a prodrug and an inactive compound in its native state. It is an analog of the purine hypoxanthine, and it requires activation to the nucleotide level by the enzyme hypoxanthineguanine phosphoribosyltransferase. The nucleotide inhibits purine biosynthesis at its first step and blocks the conversion of inosinic acid to adenylic or guanylic acid. Nucleotide metabolites are incorporated into DNA, a fact that may also be involved in the cytotoxic effects of the drug. Metabolites of the drug may also inhibit RNA synthesis. Mercaptopurine is cell cycle-specific for the S phase.

Pharmacokinetics. Mercaptopurine reaches its peak action in 2 hours, with a duration of 8 hours. Its half-life is 20 to 45 minutes. It is excreted in urine. Mercap-

Example of Nursing Process for Methotrexate and Mercaptopurine Maintenance Therapy in Acute Lymphocytic Leukemia

Jack is a 5-year-old boy with acute lymphocytic leukemia (ALL). He was considered to be one of the better-risk clients and was placed in a treatment program that in the induction phase combined vincristine, prednisone, asparaginase, and daunorubicin. He is now beginning the maintenance phase with oral doses of methotrexate 30 mg/m^2 twice a week and mercaptopurine 1.5 mg/kg/day.

Jack is one of two children (he has an identical twin) whose mother is studying for her baccalaureate degree in nursing. His father is a career Air Force officer and they live on the local air base. The twin has shown no signs of leukemia.

Assessment Data

Receiving methotrexate and mercaptopurine

Earlier use of vincristine, prednisone, asparaginase, and daunorubicin

Diagnosis of ALL

Nursing Diagnosis*	Intervention	Goals and Outcomes
Risk for Infection, related to bone marrow suppression secondary to cytotoxic drug therapy	**Monitor** results of complete blood cell count and differential. **Obtain** culture specimens as ordered. **Observe** for signs and symptoms of infection (skin, blood, sputum, urine). **Use** good handwashing technique, and teach client and family to do the same. **Maintain** optimal nutritional status. **Avoid** invasive procedures; if they are necessary, maintain meticulous aseptic technique. **Perform** actions to prevent respiratory infection as appropriate to condition. **Perform** actions to prevent urinary tract infection (teach client and parents proper perineal hygiene). **Place** client on protective precautions in private room.	The client will remain free of infection, as evidenced by absence of fever and chills, normal breath sounds, voiding without complaints of frequency, urgency, and burning, no complaints of increased weakness and fatigue, negative results of cultured specimens.
Potential Complication: Thrombocytopenia	**Monitor** coagulation test results (platelet count, prothrombin time, partial thromboplastin time). **Observe** client for evidence of unusual bleeding. **Avoid** parenteral injections or invasive procedures such as rectal temperatures. **Apply** prolonged pressure at venipuncture sites. **Instruct** client and family to try to avoid cuts, bruises, and falls. If hemorrhage occurs, **monitor** for therapeutic and nontherapeutic effects of agents that may be administered.	The client will not experience unusual bleeding or hemorrhage, as evidenced by skin and mucous membranes free of petechiae, purpura, ecchymoses, and active bleeding; absence of unusual joint pain; absence of frank and occult blood in stool, urine, and vomitus; vital signs within normal range for client; stable or improved hematocrit and hemoglobin.

(continued)

Example of Nursing Process for Methotrexate and Mercaptopurine Maintenance Therapy in Acute Lymphocytic Leukemia (continued)

Nursing Diagnosis* **(continued)**	**Intervention** **(continued)**	**Goals and Outcomes** **(continued)**
Risk for Altered Oral Mucous Membranes, related to cell injury secondary to methotrexate and mercaptopurine therapy	**Inspect** client's mouth daily for signs of stomatitis. **Reinforce** importance of, and assist client with, oral hygiene after meals and snacks. **Have** client rinse mouth with warm saline rinses and use soft-bristle toothbrush for dental care. **Encourage** client to use an artificial saliva product if his mouth is dry. **Lubricate** lips with lip-care product. **Maintain** optimal nutritional status with soft bland diet.	The client will maintain a healthy oral cavity, as evidenced by absence of signs and symptoms of inflammation; pink, moist, intact mucosa; no complaints of oral dryness and burning; ability to swallow without discomfort.

*Although potential complications are not routinely addressed in these examples, in this situation the identification of such a collaborative problem is critical to the outcome for this client and illustrates the broad range of nursing responsibilities during chemotherapy.

---

topurine is metabolized by two pathways. One involves methylation and the subsequent oxidation of methylated derivatives; the second involves oxidation by xanthine oxidase, which is present in large amounts in the liver. An attempt to modify this second pathway of metabolic inactivation led to the important development of allopurinol, a potent inhibitor of xanthine oxidase. Allopurinol is also used in several common medical situations.

Therapeutic Uses. Mercaptopurine is used to induce remission in adults and children with acute lymphocytic leukemia. Better results are obtained with combination regimens. The major role of mercaptopurine is maintenance therapy in acute lymphocytic leukemia, most often in combination with methotrexate. See Example of Nursing Process for Methotrexate and Mercaptopurine Maintenance Therapy in Acute Lymphocytic Leukemia.

Mercaptopurine and a derivative, azathioprine (Imuran), are used to suppress rejection of transplanted organs or to treat autoimmune diseases such as Crohn's disease, ulcerative colitis, and rheumatoid arthritis.

Dosage and Administration. Consult Table 46-5 for usual dosages. Therapeutic immunosuppression occurs at doses of 100 mg/day, a dosage that causes only a small decrease in the number of leukocytes.

Adverse Reactions. Mercaptopurine has been implicated in vascular liver disorders, peliosis hepatis, and hepatic venoocclusive disease. During therapy, determinations of serum bilirubin, serum alkaline phosphatase, and aspartate aminotransferase levels should be made.

With acute hepatic toxicity, elevations are seen in a pattern similar to that of cholestatic jaundice. The signs and symptoms of hepatotoxicity may appear 1 to 2 months after therapy is started, are reversible, and may occur more frequently with higher doses of the drug.

Bone marrow suppression is the major adverse reaction, but it usually develops more slowly with mercaptopurine than with folic acid analogs. Anorexia, nausea, and vomiting are common and affect adults more than children.

Hyperuricemia occurs commonly because of rapid cell lysis.

Biochemical resistance to mercaptopurine has been attributed to the absence of hypoxanthineguanine phosphoribosyltransferase in tumors. In human leukemic cells, resistance is also associated with an increased concentration of a degrading enzyme. Tumor cells resistant to mercaptopurine usually are cross-resistant to thioguanine.

Drug Interactions. Mercaptopurine is partly metabolized by xanthine oxidase to 6-thiouric acid. Because of allopurinol's ability to inhibit xanthine oxidase, the concurrent administration of allopurinol and mercaptopurine diminishes the catabolism of mercaptopurine and potentiates its cytotoxicity. If they must be given concurrently, the dose of mercaptopurine must be reduced to 25% of the usual dose. Interaction between mercaptopurine and cyclophosphamide was discussed under cyclophosphamide. Concurrent use of mercaptopurine and trimethoprim/sulfamethoxazole increases the risk of bone marrow suppression.

Precautions and Contraindications. The client's hepatic function should be assessed before drug administration begins, and signs and symptoms of dysfunction, as evidenced by liver tenderness, jaundice, clay-colored stools, and frothy dark urine, must be reported. Hepatic dysfunction is reversible once the drug is stopped.

■ SUMMARY

Antimetabolites are cycle-dependent antineoplastic drugs that are effective in phase S of the cell cycle. The antimetabolites include folic acid analogs, pyrimidine analogs, and purine analogs. Specific agents include methotrexate and mercaptopurine, which are significant in managing acute lymphocytic leukemia.

❖ NURSING MANAGEMENT: CLIENT RECEIVING AN ALKYLATING AGENT OR ANTIMETABOLITE

Antineoplastic drugs pose a potential occupational hazard to healthcare workers. The risks are related to the duration and frequency of exposure and may be short-term or long-term. All these agents should be considered carcinogenic. The primary routes of exposure are inhalation of droplets or particles of the drug and skin absorption. Aerosol generation of the drug is a prerequisite to inhalation, and withdrawing needles from vials, opening ampules, and expelling air from syringes are procedures that could result in aerosol generation. Measurable concentrations of anticancer drugs have been detected in areas where these drugs are prepared for client use. Dermal absorption can occur from direct skin contact, spillage, glove permeation, or contact with client excreta (Grajny et al., 1993). To prevent accidental ingestion, healthcare workers must not eat or drink in areas where drugs are mixed and administered. Eye contact with the drugs must also be avoided.

During preparation and administration, latex or double gloves, gowns, and face shields may be worn. In the home setting, any family member assisting with drug administration should wear protection. Spills must be handled with extra caution. Absorbent disposable pads should be used to wipe up liquid spills, and the contaminated area should be washed more than once. Any leftover drug or administration materials or materials used for cleaning up spills should be treated as hazardous wastes.

NURSING PROCESS
ASSESSMENT

The nurse must assess the overall physical status of each client before and during chemotherapy. The baseline data are essential for monitoring responses. The nurse should also determine whether the client is using other medications or herbs that may interfere with the chemotherapy program.

The nurse is responsible for monitoring the results of various laboratory tests. The tests needed depend on what drugs are being used. For example, if the drug is likely to cause bone marrow suppression, culture reports (eg, urine, vaginal, rectal, mouth, sputum, blood, skin), complete blood cell counts and differentials, and coagulation tests (eg, platelet count, prothrombin time, partial thromboplastin time) must be reviewed. Parameters to assess in clients receiving cardiotoxic drugs include heart sounds, venous pressure, intake and output, and weight, as well as electrocardiogram tracings. If the drug is likely to cause nephrotoxicity, the nurse must assess urine output and specific gravity and monitor the serum plasma concentration of urea, creatinine, uric acid, and the electrolytes (Na, K, Mg, Ca). For the client receiving a neurotoxic drug, the nurse assesses musculoskeletal and neurologic systems. For an ototoxic drug, the nurse must assess the client's ability to hear (eg, whisper test, watch test, Weber and Rinne tests). For the client receiving an hepatotoxic drug, the nurse monitors the results of serum bilirubin and alkaline phosphatase tests.

NURSING DIAGNOSIS

Most clients who receive antineoplastic agents have cancer. Because of the nature of neoplastic disease, almost any nursing diagnoses may apply. For the cancer client receiving chemotherapy, the most applicable diagnoses include:

- Anxiety, related to potentially life-threatening drug therapy and disease course
- Knowledge Deficit, related to the malignancy and its treatment with antineoplastic drugs
- Body Image Disturbance, related to alopecia, weight loss, and other body changes secondary to chemotherapy
- Anticipatory Grieving, related to need for chemotherapy for life-threatening disease
- Ineffective Individual Coping, related to debility (perceived threat to life, inability to fulfill role functions, anxiety) secondary to malignant disease or chemotherapy
- Pain, related to cancer or to tissue injury secondary to chemotherapy

Common collaborative problems that should be differentiated from the nursing diagnoses include:

Potential Complications: Bone marrow suppression, cardiotoxicity, GI toxicity, neurotoxicity, pulmonary toxicity, hepatotoxicity, nephrotoxicity, gonadal toxicity

PLANNING

Goals include decreased anxiety, increased understanding of the chemotherapeutic program, adaptation to changes in body appearance and function, progression through the grieving process, use of effective coping skills, decreased pain and discomfort, absence of injuries, absence of diarrhea or constipation, maximum physical mobility and activity tolerance, performance of self-care activities within physical limitations, maintenance of oral mucous membrane integrity, maintenance of optimal nutritional status, and maintenance of fluid and electrolyte balance.

INTERVENTIONS

Nursing interventions must be tailored for each client, but selected ones follow.

Coping With Hair Loss and Altered Body Image. The client receiving antineoplastic agents is at risk for alopecia, which usually alters his or her body image. Alopecia is a visible reminder of cancer and its treatment and makes it difficult to deny the reality of disease. The antineoplastic drugs associated with hair loss include cyclophosphamide, ifosfamide, mechlorethamine, hexamethylmelamine, busulfan, streptozocin, dacarbazine, methotrexate, fluorouracil, floxuridine, and cytarabine (discussed in this chapter), as well as bleomycin, daunorubicin, doxorubicin, etoposide, mitomycin, vinblastine, vincristine, and vindesine (see Chap. 47). Other drugs can also cause alopecia (eg, certain antibiotics, anticoagulants, anticonvulsants, hormones).

Antineoplastic agents damage the DNA of the stem cells, causing atrophy of the hair follicle and producing weak, brittle hair that either breaks at the surface of the scalp or is spontaneously released from the hair follicle. The dose and length of drug exposure determine the degree and duration of hair loss. Alterations in physiologic status (hormonal dysfunction, herpes zoster, pernicious anemia, protein malnutrition) can increase the degree and duration of alopecia.

Client Education: Alopecia. Clients must be informed that alopecia is probable and that it varies from thinning to partial or complete baldness. It affects all body hair. Hair loss usually occurs 2 or 3 weeks after chemotherapy begins; loss may be gradual or sudden.

Clients need to be reassured that when the antineoplastic agent is discontinued, the hair will grow again, but it may be of a different color and texture. Scalp hair usually grows about half an inch monthly. In the meantime, wigs or toupés, hats, scarves, and turbans may be used. Purchasing a wig before the hair falls out allows clients to match their own hair color and style. The client may be referred to the American Cancer Society, which in some regions provides hairpieces free of charge.

If a wig is not worn, the head must be protected from the sun to prevent sunburn and to prevent heat loss. A visit to a makeup artist or cosmetologist may help the client learn to apply eyebrows and eyelashes. Dark-rimmed eyeglasses may be worn to conceal the loss of eyebrows and eyelashes.

The client should be taught interventions that minimize hair loss, such as using a mild protein-based shampoo and conditioner and avoiding hair dryers, curling irons, electric curlers or bristly rollers, braids, ponytails, elastic bands, clips, barrettes, bobby pins, hair spray, hair dye, and permanent wave solutions.

To forestall alopecia, many techniques, such as scalp tourniquets, scalp sphygmomanometers, and various turbans and caps for scalp hypothermia, have been tried. Because the scalp is supplied by superficial blood vessels, these methods might minimize contact between the drug and dividing hair follicle stem cells by causing vasocontriction or reducing the amount of drug absorbed. Whether these methods offer any benefit remains controversial. Hypothermia caps in particular are suspect; the caps may prevent microscopic scalp metastases from receiving an adequate dose of chemotherapy. Thus, the commercial sale of the caps has been halted.

The client with alopecia should be encouraged to share concerns, fears, and perceptions of the impact of alopecia on his or her life, spouse, children, friends, and coworkers. Significant others must also have opportunities to share their feelings and fears.

Managing Potential Bone Marrow Suppression. Bone marrow suppression or myelosuppression in clients with cancer can result from tumor invasion of the bone marrow, chemotherapy, or radiation therapy. Anemia, thrombocytopenia, and neutropenia are the three most clinically significant complications that result from bone marrow suppression. Bone marrow suppression is the most common dose-limiting adverse reaction of chemotherapy and is potentially the most dangerous.

The prime function of neutrophils is phagocytosis; thus, neutropenia eliminates one of the body's prime defenses against bacterial infection. Microbial infections in neutropenic cancer victims are the most common cause of therapy-related mortality. The longer the neutrophil count remains low, the more susceptible clients become to infection from endogenous and exogenous microbial flora. Neutropenia typically develops 8 to 12 days after chemotherapy, with recovery in 3 to 4 weeks (Groenwald et al., 1993).

Because of the potential seriousness of any infection, attention recently has been focused on the use of colony-stimulating factors (CSFs) to augment neutrophil counts (see Ch. 35).

If a chemotherapy-induced infection occurs, the nurse will administer antibiotics, such as a broad-spectrum cephalosporin or penicillin in combination with an aminoglycoside. Other drug interventions may include more specialized drugs such as piperacillin/tazobactam (Zosyn). Antiviral agents such as acyclovir (Zoverax) and valacyclovir (Valtrex) are often needed.

Fluconazole or amphotericin B may be ordered for antifungal therapy, although fluconazole seems less toxic. Amphotericin B is associated with serious side effects, including nephrotoxicity, hepatotoxicity, and electrolyte imbalance. In clients with fungal infection, treatment may be prolonged. Some antibiotics and antineoplastic agents are incompatible; the client usually has one IV line for the chemotherapeutic agent and another for the antibiotic. Because early symptoms of fungal infection are not easily detected, the nurse must be alert for problems. If the client is still febrile and neutropenic, even with antibiotic therapy, an antifungal agent may be needed.

The neutropenic client with uncontrolled septicemia is at risk for septic shock. Again, the nurse must be alert for signs of early septic shock, such as fever with or without chills, warm, dry skin, confusion, tachypnea, and tachycardia. Late findings in septic shock include irritability and restlessness, cold, clammy skin, rapid, shallow breathing, thready pulse, and oliguria. Clients with septic shock are critically ill: unless treatment is immediate and aggressive, irreversible organ damage and death occur.

If hospitalized, the neutropenic client may be placed in a private room, and visitors and staff are screened to keep out infected or potentially infected persons. Sometimes a total protective environment is used, including a laminar airflow room, with sterilization of the entire room and its contents and of every item brought into the room.

Client Education: Infection.
Clients with neutropenia are often cared for at home because it is usually safer than the hospital in terms of infection. Education is necessary to make home care as effective as possible. The nurse must teach the client and family about white blood cells and normal immunologic function, neutropenia and its relation to the client's situation, signs and symptoms of infection, and measures to prevent or manage infection.

Clients should learn to take their temperature, maintain a record of the temperature, and report abnormal results. If necessary, the nurse should check the client's skill at reading a thermometer. Fever patterns may help identify the cause of infection. For example, a pattern of intermittent fevers is often seen with gram-negative septicemia; a slowly rising temperature that remains elevated may indicate a fungal infection. If the neutropenic client has two or three low-grade fevers (38°C) or a single elevation above 38.5°C, he or she should notify the healthcare provider for appropriate action.

Clients should practice strict handwashing procedures, particularly before eating and after using the toilet. Clients with neutropenia can get an infection from an organism being transferred from one part of their body to another (endogenous organisms). The client should limit contact with family and friends who are sick or who may be infected. Sources of environmental contaminants (eg, stagnant water, pet litter, potted plants, fresh flowers) should be eliminated. Specific measures should be used to prevent infection at common sites, such as performing pulmonary exercises (lungs); drinking copious fluids, voiding frequently, and avoiding douching and tampon use (genitourinary tract); performing aseptic contact lens care (eyes); maintaining an oral care regimen (mouth); using an-

timicrobial soap and avoiding injury (skin); and using meticulous care with existing wounds or at the sites of invasive devices.

Dealing With Potential Nephrotoxicity.
Several antineoplastic drugs pose a threat to the urinary tract, such as cyclophosphamide (severe hemorrhagic cystitis) and cisplatin, methotrexate, streptozocin, anthracyclines, nitrosoureas, and mitomycin. Nephrotoxicity is a dose-limiting adverse reaction for these drugs. Other treatment-related entities that indicate urinary tract damage and may lead to renal failure include radiation nephritis, hyperuricemic nephropathy, tumor lysis syndrome, and obstruction from ureteral or bladder tumors or retroperitoneal fibrosis.

Preventing nephrotoxicity involves close monitoring, aggressive hydration, urinary alkalinization, and diuresis (Table 46-7). Monitoring for nephrotoxicity may be difficult, because a 75% to 80% loss of renal function may occur before significant laboratory changes or symptoms develop. The nurse must monitor BUN and serum creatinine levels and the 24-hour creatinine clearance. Urine color, pH, specific gravity, urinary concentration and acidification capacity, and the presence of glucose, proteins, blood, or ketones are additional signs. The nurse can also compare current laboratory data with the initial assessment data, including any preexisting medical disorders and prescription or nonprescription medications that affect renal function. Allergic reactions to drugs, dyes, or blood components should also be noted, as they can result in renal damage.

Monitoring for nephrotoxicity includes evaluating fluid and electrolyte status by checking vital signs, fluid intake and output, weight, edema, skin turgor, and cognitive changes. Changes in vital signs can reveal dehydration or fluid overload, infection, and hypertension. Weight loss may be caused by dehydration, nausea and vomiting, or anorexia; weight gain in excess of 2.2 lb is a reliable indicator of edema. Other reliable signs of fluid overload include dyspnea, neck vein distention, elevated blood pressure, pitting edema, and periorbital edema. Cognitive changes such as decreased ability to concentrate, lack of coordination, and increase in fatigue can also be signs of renal impairment.

Providing Oral and Other Care.
Potential GI toxicity refers to effects from the beginning of the GI tract (mouth) to the end of the tract (anus). Any part can be damaged by chemotherapy. Xerostomia (dry oral mucosa from salivary gland dysfunction), dysgeusia (unusual or unpleasant taste perception), anorexia, diarrhea, nausea and vomiting, and constipation are all symptoms that may occur with GI toxicity.

Stomatitis, the inflammatory and ulcerative reaction that affects the mouth, is common with antineoplastics and some biologic response modifiers (interleukin-2). Cells in the oral mucosa have one of the highest proliferation rates in the body, making them more susceptible to chemotherapy than cells in other

Table 46-7. Nephrotoxicity and Antineoplastic Agents

Agent	Signs and Symptoms*	Risk Factors†	Mechanism of Damage	Protective/ Preventive Measures	General Management
nitrosoureas: cumulative dose of 1,200 mg/m2 for carmustine and lomustine	increased BUN, creatinine oliguria azotemia proteinuria decreased creatinine clearance hyperuricemia hypomagnesemia hypocalcemia	age dose of agent preexisting disease of kidneys nutritional status duration of cancer therapy concurrent aminoglycoside or amphotericin B therapy renal damage dehydration large tumor mass ileal conduits	direct cell damage in glomerulus chronic interstitial nephritis tubular atrophy can cause delayed renal failure months/ years after therapy	These 4 measures apply to all drugs: Monitor renal function tests Saline diuresis Hydrate client (3,000 mL/day) Decrease uric acid production with allopurinol	Substitute analog drug Hold dose for creatinine clearance 30–60 mL/min.
mitomycin: increased effect with vincristine and VM-26. Increased with cumulative dose of 100 mg or more after 6 mo of therapy			direct cell damage in glomerulus microangiopathic hemolytic anemia		Reduce dose 75% for creatinine clearance 30–60 mL/min
anthracyclines (1.5 g/m2/wk)			tubular atrophy diffuse tubulointerstitial nephritis		
streptozotocin: (>1.5 g/m2/wk)			tubulointerstitial nephritis tubular atrophy	Stop drug if creatinine does not return to baseline	
cisplatin: multiple doses (>50 mg/m2): Increased effect with cyclophosphamide			direct cell damage in proximal and distal tubules platinum metal chelates in tubules, damaging tubular basement membranes and leading to focal necrosis	Diuresis with mannitol (may prevent immediate binding of cisplatin onto tubules) Administer WR-2721 15 min before cisplatin administration Administer DDTC	Reduce dose 50% for creatinine clearance 30–60 mL/min

*Signs and symptoms with any of the drugs in this table.
†Risk factors with any of the drugs in this table.

(continued)

Table 46-7. (Continued)

Agent	Signs and Symptoms	Risk Factors	Mechanism of Damage	Protective/ Preventive Measures	General Management
methotrexate: high dose (>1 g/m2) Enhanced effect with cisplatin			precipitation of metabolites in acid environment of urine obstructive nephropathy	Maintain alkalinization of urine (pH>7) through administration of sodium bicarbonate or acetazolamide Administer leucovorin Avoid vitamin C	Reduce dose 50% for creatinine clearance 30–60 mL/min

Groenwald SL, Frogge MH, Goodman M, Yarbro CH, eds. (1993). *Cancer nursing: Principles and practice,* 3d ed. Boston: Jones and Bartlett Publishers.

kinds of healthy tissue. Normal mucosal cells live 10 to 14 days. The rate of cell formation stays the same, even if the rate of cell death increases. Younger cancer clients tend to have more oral complications than adults because the mitotic index of the oral mucosa is higher in younger people. When antineoplastic drugs are used, the oral mucosa shrinks and thins out. Minor trauma can disrupt the remaining thin layer of mucosa and produce ulceration. Damage to the oral mucosa reverses itself unless problems occur, such as secondary infection. Bone marrow suppression (as described earlier) increases the potential for secondary infection by opportunistic agents.

Candidiasis (thrush, moniliasis), the most common fungal infection, appears as cottage cheese–like white patches on the tongue and buccal mucosa. The first symptom of candidiasis may be a metallic taste. Herpes simplex, the most common viral infection, begins as painful, itching vesicles that rupture within 6 to 12 hours and become encrusted with exudate. Vesicles typically appear on the lips first. Gram-negative bacterial infections are common and appear as creamy, white, raised, shiny, nonpurulent, painful erosions on a reddened base. *Pseudomonas* organisms appear as raised, dry, nonpurulent, usually nonpainful lesions that are yellowish initially and progress to a dark necrotic core surrounded by a red halo. Gram-positive infections are also common. They appear as dry, raised, wartlike, yellowish-brown, round plaques (Dollar & Lawson, 1994).

Nursing care for these complications should start with assessment of usual oral hygiene practices, dental care, and history of alcohol and tobacco use. When examining the mouth, the nurse removes any oral prostheses. The status of the oral mucous membranes, including the lips, gingival tissue, tongue, palate, and pharynx, should be assessed. All mouth lesions should be cultured.

To prevent or treat candidiasis, nystatin oral suspension (500,000–1,000,000 U) may be swished around the mouth for 1 minute and swallowed; this process is repeated four to six times a day. Nystatin is active against *Candida albicans* and *Cryptococcus.* Popsicles or ice cups can be made from the suspension, nystatin vaginal suppositories or troches can be slowly dissolved in the mouth, or the powder can be reconstituted and frozen. Ketoconazole and clotrimazole may be used as antifungal agents. Acyclovir, an antiviral agent, is available for topical application in ointment form and for systemic administration in oral and IV forms. For bacterial infections, bacitracin, polymyxin B, and neomycin antibiotic ointments may be applied topically.

Client Education: Mouth Care. The nurse must teach the client to perform meticulous oral hygiene to help prevent oral mucosa complications. Teeth should be brushed within 30 minutes of eating and at bedtime with a soft-bristle, multitufted toothbrush and nonabrasive toothpaste. Dental floss should be used daily, but gently. A water pick may be used at a low setting.

Various agents can be recommended for oral care. Generally, the mouth should be rinsed three or four times a day, using normal saline solution or a nonirritating mouthwash containing 1/2 teaspoon each of baking soda and salt in 1 cup of warm water. Commercial rinses (eg, Listerine) that contain significant salt or alcohol (more than 6%) must be avoided. The use of hydrogen peroxide is controversial. It has been approved by the Food and Drug Administration as a safe and effective rinse. Because oxygen is released from peroxide, providing mechanical cleansing and exerting an antimicrobial effect, it is chemically active; however, it is also thought to cause overgrowth of filiform and foliate papillae of the tongue, thereby providing an excellent medium for candidiasis. If peroxide is used, a dilute preparation is recommended.

Lemon and glycerin swabs, although used in the past, have little value in cleaning or moisturizing the oral cavity. The citric acid of the lemon juice can irritate the oral mucosa and decalcify teeth. Glycerin is a trihydric alcohol that absorbs water and can be drying and irritating.

Water-soluble moisturizers such as K-Y Jelly can be recommended for the lips. Oil-based lubricants, including petroleum jelly, cocoa butter, or mineral oil, are effective on the lips but should be avoided inside the mouth when there is a danger of aspiration.

Agents such as topical allopurinol, sucralfate, prostaglandin E₂, and vitamin E have a potential role in protecting the integrity of the oral mucosa.

The client may be taught strategies to manage oral pain. Gargling 15 to 20 minutes before meals with a topical anesthetic solution such as Xylocaine Viscous 2% may help. Topical anesthetic solutions decrease the pain that occurs with swallowing, but only briefly. The taste is unpleasant to some people, and others dislike the feeling of numbness. Some agents could be painted on sore or ulcerated areas with a cotton-tipped applicator. Other anesthetics include benzocaine 20%, antacids, sucralfate, acetaminophen elixir, Benadryl elixir, and Zilactin (a medicated gel with an active ingredient of tannic acid).

If the oral mucosa is dry, water, saline solution, or artificial saliva may be sprayed on the mucous membranes as often as necessary. Artificial saliva is available by prescription.

Flossing and even brushing may need to be discontinued when thrombocytopenia exists. If the teeth cannot be brushed, the nurse, client, or a family member can clean the client's mouth with a 2″ gauze pad soaked in solution and wrapped around a tongue blade. Dentures, partial dentures, and orthodontic devices should be removed for cleaning twice a day; they may need to be removed entirely or for certain periods.

Coping With Anorexia, Nausea, and Vomiting.

Anorexia, nausea, and vomiting are common adverse reactions to chemotherapy and often produce a compromised nutritional status that can lead to debilitation. Nausea and vomiting may cause the treatment regimen to be altered or discontinued. Some agents have a higher likelihood of causing emesis than others; the onset and duration of emesis also vary (Table 46-8). The degree of nausea and vomiting may differ among persons and even in treatment courses in the same client.

The mechanism of chemotherapy-induced nausea and vomiting is not completely understood, although it is thought to reflect stimulation of various CNS and GI system receptors. There is no negative feedback loop in the emetic system, so even with an empty stomach, protracted, uncontrolled vomiting and retching can occur.

Nausea and vomiting can be classified as acute, delayed, or anticipatory. Acute nausea and vomiting occurs 1 to 2 hours after treatment and resolves within 24 hours. Delayed nausea and vomiting persists or develops 24 hours after chemotherapy, perhaps due to the

Table 46-8. Potential of Individual Chemotherapy Drugs to Cause Nausea and Vomiting

Incidence/Agent	Onset (h)	Duration (h)
Very high (>90%)		
cisplatin	1–4	12–96
cyclophosphamide*	6–8	8–24
cytarabine*	1–3	3–8
dacarbazine	1–2	2–4
mechlorethamine	1–3	2–8
High (60%–90%)		
streptozocin	1–3	1–12
carboplatin	2–6	1–48
carmustine	2–6	4–6
cyclophosphamide	6–8	8–24
dactinomycin	2–5	4–24
daunorubicin	1–3	4–24
doxorubicin	1–3	4–24
lomustine	2–6	4–6
Moderate (30%–60%)		
altretamine		
amsacrine		
asparaginase	1–4	2–12
azacitidine	1–3	3–4
epirubicin		
etoposide	3–8	—
idarubicin		
ifosfamide	2–3	12–72
mitomycin	1–2	3–4
mitoxantrone	4–6	6+
pentostatin		
plicamycin	4–6	4–24
procarbazine	24–27	variable
topotecan		
Low (0%–30%)		
bleomycin	3–6	—
busulfan		
chlorambucil	48–72	—
chlorodeoxyadenosine		
cytarabine	1–3	3–8
edatrexate		
5-fluorouracil	3–6	24+
floxuridine		
fludarabine		
hydroxyurea		
melphalan	6–12	—
menogaril		
methotrexate	4–12	4–12
mitoguazone		
paclitaxel		
piroxantrone		
mercaptopurine	4–8	—
taxotere		
thioguanine		
thiotepa		
trimetrexate	4–8	
vinblastine	4–8	
vincristine		
vindesine		
vinorelbine		

*high dose
Fischer DS, Knobf MT, Durivage HJ. (1993). *The cancer chemotherapy handbook,* 4th ed. St. Louis: Mosby–Year Book, Inc.

ongoing effect of the metabolites of the antineoplastic agent on the CNS or GI tract. If nausea is controlled within the first 24 hours after therapy, delayed patterns are less likely to occur.

When combinations of antineoplastic drugs are used, more than one emetic pathway may be stimulated simultaneously, resulting in more severe nausea and vomiting and the possibility of both acute and delayed symptoms.

Factors that affect the occurrence of nausea and vomiting include susceptibility to motion sickness, history of nausea or vomiting in response to stressful events, history of a nervous stomach, age 40 years or less, and previous experience with chemotherapy-related nausea or vomiting. Persons with a heavy alcohol intake seem to have a decreased occurrence of nausea and vomiting.

The best intervention for nausea and vomiting is prevention. A combination of antiemetic drugs with different mechanisms of action, higher doses, and round-the-clock administration are all more effective than single agents and as-needed dosage schedules (Table 46-9, Box 46-1). For example, the combination of ondansetron and dexamethosone has been found more efficacious than ondansetron alone.

Dietary adjustments do not seem to make any significant difference in the degree of anorexia, taste changes, nausea, and vomiting a client experiences. Clients may become conditioned to dislike certain foods as "sick" foods or dislike "reward" foods if these foods are consistently associated with nausea and vomiting. These are learned food aversions. So that a client does not develop an aversion to favorite foods, it may be wise not to offer them at the time of chemotherapy sessions.

Clients who report anorexia-related changes in taste perception may also report an aversion to foods with high amino acid levels, a decreased threshold for the bitter taste sensation, an increased threshold for the sweet taste sensation (more sugar is needed to achieve the preillness sweet taste sensation), an aversion to sweet foods, and a metallic or medicinal taste manifested continuously or intermittently, unrelated to food intake. These clients may prefer cold or room-temperature food to hot. Chicken or ham made into a salad, or roast beef in a sandwich, may be more acceptable, partly because the odor tends to be less potent than when served hot. Use of plastic rather than metal utensils may reduce the bitter taste. Meats can be marinated in soy sauce or fruit juice and cooked with fruit to improve their taste.

If the food aversion increases throughout the day, a high-protein breakfast should be encouraged. Eggs and cheese are usually not rejected.

If zinc therapy has been prescribed for the changes in taste sensation, the nurse should instruct the client to take the medication toward the middle of a meal and with a snack at bedtime to minimize potential GI symptoms.

Client Education: Diet and Nutrition. Many clients need dietary adjustments to ensure adequate nutrition. Usually, foods with citric acid are avoided because they cause the mucosa to burn. Pear and peach nectars, warm (not hot) tea, liquid gelatin, custards, and yogurt may be tolerated. Coarse foods and very hot foods should be avoided. Spicy foods that contain pepper, chili powder, and nutmeg may bother the mouth more than spices such as cinnamon, garlic, and oregano. Cold and frozen foods, such as water ice or sorbet, may be soothing. Noncarbonated beverages may be well tolerated. Sauces and gravies can be added to solid foods, and foods may be puréed. Cigarette smoking and drinking alcohol must be discouraged, as both irritate mouth tissues.

Table 46-9. Selected Antiemetic Combinations

Drug Regimen	Dosages	Comments
Regimen #1		
lorazepam (Ativan)	1–2 mg PO q6h beginning 24 h before morning of treatment	At hour of sleep:
diphenhydramine (Benadryl)	50 mg IV	lorazepam: 2 mg PO or SL
prochlorperazine (Compazine)	20 mg IV infusion over 30 min q3h × 2	diphenhydramine: 50 mg PO
dexamethasone (Decadron)	20 mg IV	prochlorperazine: 30 mg SR PO and 15 mg SR in morning and q12h prn
Regimen #2		
metoclopramide (Reglan)	1–3 mg/kg IV, 20 min before treatment and 90 min after treatment	
dexamethasone (Decadron)	20 mg IV 25 min before treatment	
lorazepam (Ativan)	1.5 mg/m² IV 30 min before treatment	Maximum dose 3 mg
diphenhydramine (Benadryl)	25–50 mg IV or PO	Repeated q4–6h prn ONLY for akathisia or dystonic reactions
ondansetron (Zofran)	0.15 mg/kg IV 30 min before and 90 and 120 min after treatment	Give over 15 minutes

SR = sustained-release

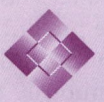

Box 46-1
Selected Antiemetic Agents

Serotonin Antagonists

Ondansetron (Zofran), an imidazole derivative related to 5-hydroxytryptophan, is a serotonin antagonist. It is extensively metabolized by the liver, is excreted in urine and feces, and has a plasma half-life of about 4 hours. Approved by the FDA in 1992, ondansetron administered IV a half-hour before chemotherapy prevents emesis after high-dose cisplatin in up to 40% of clients. Another serotonin antagonist, granisetron, may also prevent emesis for 24 hours. Adverse effects of these drugs include hypotension, headache, constipation, and sedation.

Corticosteroids

Steroids, such as dexamethasone (Decadron) and methylprednisolone (Solu-Medrol), decrease emesis. Steroids may be used IV before and during chemotherapy for acute emesis and orally after chemotherapy for delayed and persistent nausea and vomiting. These drugs are thought to inhibit prostaglandin synthesis. Side effects include insomnia, euphoria, anxiety, hypertension, and edema. These drugs are usually given with other antiemetics.

Anxiolytics

The benzodiazepines lorazepam (Ativan) and diazepam (Valium) are used because of their anterograde amnesic properties (ie, dose-related memory loss) and sedative effects. They decrease the response of the true vomiting center to a variety of afferent stimuli. They also reduce anticipatory nausea and vomiting. Besides sedation and amnesia, confusion may result. These drugs are used with caution in clients with hepatic or renal dysfunction.

Butyrophenones

Butyrophenones, such as droperidol (Inapsine) and haloperidol (Haldol), have sedative and antiemetic effects. Droperidol also produces a mild alpha-adrenergic blockade and peripheral vascular dilation and reduces the pressor effect of epinephrine, resulting in hypotension and decreased peripheral vascular resistance. Extrapyramidal effects, which are common with these drugs, may be prevented with diphenhydramine.

Cannabinoids

Dronabinol (Marinol) may be difficult to obtain, so it is not generally used as a first-line antiemetic. It suppresses pathways to the vomiting center. Side effects include dysphoria, sedation, dizziness, dry mouth, disorientation, impaired concentration, orthostatic hypotension, and tachycardia.

Phenothiazines

Phenothiazines, such as prochlorperazine (Compazine), promethazine (Phenergan), chlorpromazine (Thorazine), and perphenazine (Trilafon), block dopamine receptors and inhibit vomiting by blocking autonomic afferent impulses via the vagus nerve. Side effects include sedation, orthostatic hypotension, and extrapyramidal symptoms. These drugs, too, may be used as second-line antiemetics.

The client may need to chop meat or dry food that is difficult to swallow and serve it with gravy or broth. Salad dressings or mayonnaise may be added to vegetables to make them easier to swallow. The client may try adding substances to foods to increase the value of what is eaten. For example, nonfat dry milk powder may be added to milk, condensed soups can be diluted with milk instead of water, and extra sugar may be put on cereal.

Clients should avoid greasy foods because they take longer to leave the stomach. Carbohydrate-containing foods (eg, noodles, rice) leave the stomach more quickly. The volume in the stomach can be reduced by avoiding liquids at mealtime, drinking them 1 hour before or after eating. If the client craves a certain food, it should be provided if possible, because most people seem to tolerate foods they crave.

Because cooking odors may contribute to anorexia and nausea, clients may let someone else prepare the food, staying in another room or taking a walk while it is being cooked. Seeing food can decrease the appetite, so foods should be kept out of sight except when eating. Other factors that upset the appetite should be avoided as well. For example, bedpans and urinals should be put out of sight at mealtime, and ostomy care, dressing changes, and other unpleasant treatments should not be scheduled close to mealtime.

A liquid diet may be helpful if the client has anorexia, taste changes, nausea, or vomiting. Liquids such as apple juice, cranberry juice, lemonade, fruit ades, broth, Gatorade, ginger ale, gelatin, tea, or cola are usually well tolerated. Liquids should be sipped slowly.

Sour foods such as lemons, sour pickles, hard sour candy, or lemon sherbet may be tried. The client can rinse the mouth with a mixture of lemon juice and water (if stomatitis is not present). Sugar-free mints or sugar-free gum may be used to mask unpleasant tastes.

Various eating patterns can be used. Chemotherapy-associated nausea is usually not consistent throughout the day—it may be intermittent and more severe at one time of day than another. Food can be given when nausea is least severe, even if it is not consistent with the usual dietary routine.

Some clients avoid eating or drinking for 1 to 2 hours before and after chemotherapy. Some follow a clear liquid diet for 1 to 12 hours before chemotherapy and for 1 to 24 hours afterward. Some eat a large meal 3 to 4 hours before therapy and then eat lightly for the rest of the day. Some eat frequent light meals throughout the day and find it helpful if hospital trays are not laden with food. Trays should be simplified, containing smaller servings and even smaller dishes. Six small meals are better than the usual three average-sized ones, with the three in-between meals containing high-calorie, high-protein foods.

A semi-Fowler's or high Fowler's position accommodates digestion. Mouth care before meals may help increase appetite by eliminating unpleasant tastes. Washing the hands and face before mealtime is important. Having company (family members or a group of clients or friends) makes mealtime more pleasant and normal, which may help increase food intake. Distractions such as enjoyable music or a favorite television program may help. Using relaxation techniques, with or without positive visual imagery, may help as well.

Client Education: Disease and Treatment. The nurse should provide the client and family with information and literature about the specific type of cancer and the antineoplastic drugs being used. The anticipated results of chemotherapy should be explained, as well as possible adverse reactions (see the Critical Thinking Challenge). With the drugs discussed in this chapter, alopecia, bone marrow suppression (with anemia, thrombocytopenia, and neutropenia), nephrotoxicity, stomatitis, anorexia, taste changes, and nausea and vomiting are likely adverse reactions. Clients should know how and when to contact the healthcare provider to report adverse reactions or to ask questions.

Some clients must take additional medications (eg, antiemetics). Details of the protocol must be explained to the client and family. The importance of complying with all aspects of the therapeutic regimen should be stressed.

With some antineoplastic drugs, the client must be monitored with various laboratory tests. The client and family must know when and where they need to go for the laboratory work. The results of the laboratory tests may need to be explained to the client and family.

The client and family should be told about local cancer support groups and their functions and should know how to contact them.

OUTCOME EVALUATION

The nurse must evaluate the client to determine drug efficacy and to observe for evidence of adverse reactions. Data that indicate efficacy include reduced fear and anxiety, understanding of the chemotherapeutic program, prompt reporting of any signs or symptoms of

CRITICAL THINKING CHALLENGE
Case Analysis

Part 1

Larry Nelling, 43, has been diagnosed with a lymphocytic lymphoma/non-Hodgkin's lymphoma. Treatment involves combination chemotherapy with ifosfamide (Ifex) IV and mesna (Mesnex).

Using a reference such as BL Gahart's Intravenous medications (St. Louis: Mosby-Year Book, 1996), answer the following.

1. You are a nurse on the chemotherapy team. What is the correct dose of ifosfamide for Mr. Nelling, who weighs 81.8 kg and is 180 cm tall (the usual dose is 1.2 g/m²/day)?
2. Where is ifosfamide stored?
3. What diluent will you use if you are starting with a vial of powder for reconstitution? How many 1-g vials of drug will you need?
4. What is the correct rate of infusion? How much diluent would be used to facilitate this rate of infusion?
5. Can ifosfamide and mesna be mixed? Why or why not? As an inexperienced nurse, how could you get help in making this decision? Who would you consult, and why?

Part 2

You are visiting Mr. Nelling at home after discharge. He will be coming to your clinic every 3 weeks to receive additional ifosfamide therapy.

1. What assessments will you make of Mr. Nelling in terms of his diagnosis and therapeutic regimen?
2. What goals would you have for your visit that relate to the diagnoses Knowledge Deficit and Potential Complication: Bone marrow suppression?
3. Mr. Nelling complains of fatigue and says the nurse at the hospital told him to get more rest. Read "Fatigue and the cancer experience" (Oncology Nursing Forum, 1994). Why might you suggest that he keep a journal about this complaint?
4. What other complaints might he have that will help you differentiate fatigue from depression?
5. Identify several interventions that may alleviate his fatigue.

adverse drug reactions, adaptation to changes in body appearance and function, verbalization of feelings about the cancer diagnosis and chemotherapy, expression of grief, use of available support programs, identification of stressors and ways to cope with them, and participation in self-care measures recommended to reduce complications of chemotherapy. Other factors are absence of diarrhea, constipation, bone marrow suppression, cardiotoxicity, nephrotoxicity, neurotoxicity, and ototoxicity, maintenance of an optimal level of physical mobility and an increased tolerance for activity, increased ability to carry out activities of daily living, maintenance of healthy gums and oral mucous membranes, relief of discomfort, maintenance of weight within normal range, and normal skin turgor.

❖ **CHECKLIST OF NURSING ACTIONS**

❑ Monitor laboratory data for evidence of adverse reactions (eg, neutropenia, thrombocytopenia, anemia, hepatotoxicity, nephrotoxicity).

❑ Teach clients about the drugs, the possible adverse reactions, and what actions to take if adverse reactions occur.

❑ Follow suggested nursing interventions if adverse reactions occur.

❑ Inform the client if alopecia is expected. Help the client find a wig or contact a beauty consultant, if applicable. Inform the client if financial assistance is available for buying a wig. Teach the client how to minimize hair loss.

❑ If neutropenia occurs, monitor laboratory data, obtain physical assessment data, teach handwashing procedures, advise the client how to minimize the risk of infection, carry out infection precautions, and administer antibiotics and other antimicrobial agents as ordered.

❑ If nephrotoxicity is likely, monitor laboratory data, obtain physical assessment data, and carry out hydration protocols as ordered.

❑ If stomatitis occurs, obtain physical assessment data using the designated assessment instrument, encourage meticulous oral hygiene, help the client perform oral care as ordered, and adjust the diet appropriately.

❑ If anorexia, taste changes, nausea, or vomiting occurs, carry out the antiemetic protocol as ordered and adjust the diet to facilitate appropriate intake.

References

Beck SL. (1992). Prevention and management of oral complications in the cancer patient. *Current Issues in Cancer Nursing Practice Updates, 1*(6), 1–12.

Bonadonna G, Valagussa P, Moliterni A. (1995). Adjuvant cyclophosphamide, methotrexate, and fluorouracil in node-positive breast cancer. *N Engl J Med, 332*(14), 901–906.

Copstead L-E. (1995). *Perspectives on pathophysiology.* Philadelphia: WB Saunders.

Dollar BM, Lawson GC. (1994). Protocol for nursing assessment and management of stomatitis. *Home Healthcare Nurse, 12*(2), 25–27.

Grajny AE, Christie D, Tichy AM, Talashek ML. (1993). Chemotherapy: How safe for the caregiver? *Home Healthcare Nurse, 11*(5), 51–58.

Groenwald SL, Frogge MH, Goodman M, Yarbro CH, eds. (1993). *Cancer nursing: Principles and practice,* 3d ed. Boston: Jones and Bartlett Publishers.

Rostad ME. (1991). Current strategies for managing myelosuppression in patients with cancer. *Oncol Nurs Forum, 18*(suppl 2), 7–15.

Bibliography

Anderson B, Holmes W. (1993). Altered mental status: An algorithm for assessment of delirium in the cancer patient. *Current Issues in Cancer Nursing Practice Updates, 2*(5), 1–10.

Berman A, Chisholm L, deCarvalho M, Piemme JA, Gorrell CR. (1993). Programmed instruction: Cancer chemotherapy; Intravenous Administration. *Cancer Nursing, 16*(2), 145–160.

Charette JL. (1995). Contemporary approaches of chemotherapy. *Crit Care Nursing Clin North Am, 7*(1), 135–142.

Chisholm L, Berman AR, deCarvalho M, Gorrell CR. (1993). Programmed instruction: Cancer chemotherapy; Alternative administration routes. *Cancer Nursing, 16*(3), 237–246.

Cleri LB. (1995). Serotonin antagonists. *Oncol Nurs, 2*(1), 1–19.

DeCicco M, et al. (1993). Parenteral nutrition in cancer patients receiving chemotherapy: Effects on toxicity and nutritional status. *J Parenteral Enteral Nutr, 17*(6), 513–518.

DeVita VT Jr, Hellman S, Rosenberg SA. (1993). *Cancer: Principles and practice of oncology,* 4th ed. Philadelphia: JB Lippincott.

Dose AM. (1995). The symptom experience of mucositis, stomatitis, and xerostomia. *Semin Oncol Nurs, 11*(4), 248–255.

Fischer DS, Knobf MT, Durivage HJ. (1993). *The cancer chemotherapy handbook,* 4th ed. St. Louis: Mosby–Year Book, Inc.

Fuerst ML. (1996). Multidrug resistance. *Cope, 12*(2), 34–35.

Graydon JE, Bukela N, Irvine D. (1995). Fatigue-reducing strategies used by patients receiving treatment for cancer. *Cancer Nursing, 18*(1), 23–28.

Holland JF, Frei E III, Bast RC Jr, Kufe DW, Morton DL, Weichselbaum RR. (1993). *Cancer medicine,* 3d ed. Philadelphia: Lea & Febiger.

Holleb AI, Fink DJ, Murphy GP. (1991). *American Cancer Society textbook of clinical oncology.* Atlanta: American Cancer Society.

Lake T, Jenkins J. (1993). Programmed instruction: Cancer chemotherapy; Clinical trials. *Cancer Nursing, 16*(6), 486–497.

Levy W, Meadows BS, Quint-Kasner S, Carroll R, Gorrell CR. (1993). Programmed instruction: Cancer chemotherapy; Chemotherapy agents: Part I. *Cancer Nursing, 16*(4), 321–336.

Madeya ML. (1996). Oral complications from cancer therapy: Parts 1 and 2. *Oncol Nurs Forum, 23*(5), 801–821.

Pratt WB, Ruddon RW, Ensminger WD, Maybaum J. (1994). *The anticancer drugs,* 2d ed. New York: Oxford University Press.

Prescott LM. (1996). New approaches combat neutropenic infections. *Cope, 12*(2), 14–15.

Pui C-H. (1995). Childhood leukemias. *N Engl J Med, 332*(24), 1618–1630.

Quint-Kasner S, Chisholm L, deCarvalho M, Piemme J, Zimmerman K, Berman A. (1993). Programmed instruction: Cancer chemotherapy; Basic principles. *Cancer Nursing, 16*(1), 63–78.

Quint-Kasner S, Levy W, Meadows BS, Carroll R, Gorrell CR. (1993). Programmed instruction: Cancer chemotherapy; Chemotherapy agents: Part II. *Cancer Nursing, 16*(5), 398–418.

Rhodes VA, Johnson MH, McDaniel RW. (1995). Nausea, vomiting, and retching: The management of the symptom experience. *Semin Oncol Nurs, 11*(4), 256–265.

Rhodes VA, McDaniel RW, Johnson MH. (1995). Patient education: Self-care guides. *Semin Oncol Nurs, 11*(4), 298–304.

Saba MT, Magolan JM. (1991). Understanding cerebral edema: Implications for oncology nurses. *Oncol Nurs Forum, 18*(3), 499–505.

Winningham ML, Nail LM, Burke MB. (1994). Fatigue and the cancer experience: The state of the knowledge. *Oncol Nurs Forum, 21*(1), 23–36.

For more information and sample tests and activities, refer to Chapter 46 in the Student Workbook for Clinical Pharmacology and Nursing Management, 5th edition, available through your bookstore.

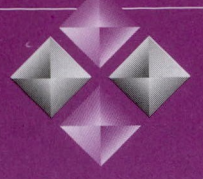

47

Other Anticancer Drugs: Natural Products, Hormones, and Antineoplastics

Natural Products

Natural products used in antineoplastic therapy include topoisomerase I and II inhibitors (anthracycline antibiotics, podophyllotoxin derivatives, and others), mitotic inhibitors, antitumor antibiotics, enzymes, and taxanes.

Topoisomerase Inhibitors

Topoisomerase I and II are enzymes critical for DNA function and cell survival; these enzymes are targets for several antineoplastic drugs. These nuclear enzymes are responsible for controlling, maintaining, and modifying the structures (topology) of DNA during replication and translation of genetic materials. To perform these functions, they normally induce transient cuts in one or both strands of DNA, allowing strands to pass through the nick, and then rejoining the nicked strand to DNA. During this function, a linkage is formed between topoisomerase and DNA. Topoactive drugs stimulate and stabilize this complex, causing strand scission and inhibition of DNA function.

There are common functions of the two enzymes, but there are also differences. Topoisomerase I is not a cell cycle-specific enzyme, thus making it a more desirable cellular target for antineoplastic drug action. Topoisomerase I induces only single-strand breaks, whereas topoisomerase II induces both single- and double-strand breaks. Topoisomerase I's function is independent of ATP, whereas ATP is required for the function of topoisomerase II (Sinha, 1995). Topoisomerase inhibitors are listed in Table 47-1.

Topoisomerase I Inhibitors

Plant extracts from *Camptotheca accuminata* have antitumor activity; camptothecin is the active component. Analogs of camptothecin, topotecan and irinotecan (CPT-11), are undergoing clinical trials. Topotecan has shown encouraging activity against refractory colorectal cancer, cancers of the head and neck, and malignant glioma. The adverse reaction of neutropenia has been significant, and other reactions included vomiting and diarrhea. Studies indicate that irinotecan has significant activity against colon and breast cancer, small cell lung cancer, and leukemia. Neutropenia and diarrhea are the major adverse reactions.

Topoisomerase II Inhibitors

Topoisomerase II inhibitors include anthracycline antibiotics (daunorubicin, doxorubicin, idarubicin), podophyllotoxin derivatives (etoposide, teniposide), and miscellaneous agents (amsacrine, mitoxantrone hydrochloride).

Anthracycline Antibiotics

Daunorubicin (Cerubidine) is produced by a strain of *Streptomyces coeruleorubidus*, and doxorubicin (Adriamycin) is isolated from cultures of *Streptomyces peucetius* var. *caesius*. Idarubicin (Idamycin) is a synthetic anthracycline, an analog of daunorubicin.

Pharmacodynamics. These antibiotics are classified as topoisomerase II inhibitors because their intracellular target is topoisomerase II. These compounds can intercalate between strands of the DNA double helix. DNA intercalation appears to trigger DNA cleavage by topoi-

Table 47-1. Topoisomerase Inhibitors

Drug Name	Preparation	Usual Dosage	Adverse Reactions
Topoisomerase I Inhibitors			
topotecan	Powder for preparing solutions for IVPB, IVCI		Diarrhea lasting 2–5 d, rash, nausea and vomiting, bone marrow suppression, flulike symptoms, mucositis, alopecia, cystitis, microhematuria
irinotecan			Neutropenia, diarrhea
Topoisomerase II Inhibitors			
Anthracycline Antibiotics			
doxorubicin (Adriamycin)	Powder for preparing solutions for IVP, IVS, IVCI Intra-arterial Intraperitoneal	20 mg/m²/wk	Cardiotoxicity (acute and delayed), leukopenia, thrombocytopenia, stomatitis, esophagitis, nausea, vomiting, alopecia, facial flushing, conjunctivitis, lacrimation, "Adriamycin flare," hypersensitivity reactions; vesicant
daunorubicin (Cerubidine)	Powder for preparing solutions for IVP, IVS	30–60 mg/m²/d for 3 d; repeat at 3- to 6-wk intervals	Leukopenia, thrombocytopenia, stomatitis, alopecia, GI disturbances, cutaneous toxicity, cardiotoxicity; vesicant
idarubicin (Idamycin)	Powder for preparing solutions for IVS, IVCI	*Induction therapy in adults with AML:* 12 mg/m² daily for 3 d by slow IV injection in combination with cytarabine	Nausea, vomiting, alopecia, stomatitis, cardiotoxicity
Podophyllotoxin Derivatives			
etoposide (Vepesid)	Oral IVPB	50–100 mg/m²/d IV for 5 d	Leukopenia, thrombocytopenia, nausea, vomiting, stomatitis, diarrhea, alopecia, hypersensitivity reactions, peripheral neuropathy
teniposide (Vumon)	IVPB	165 mg/m² in combination with 300 mg/m² cytarabine twice weekly for 8 or 9 doses	Somnolence, fatigue, nausea, vomiting, anorexia, diarrhea, alopecia, bone marrow suppression
Miscellaneous II Inhibitors			
amsacrine	IVCI	100–150 mg/m²/d for 5 d, diluted in 500 mL 5% D/W	Bone marrow suppression, acute and chronic cardiotoxicity, mucositis, alopecia, nausea, vomiting, diarrhea, hepatic dysfunction
mitoxantrone hydrochloride (Novantrone)	IV solution	*For induction with ANLL:* 12 mg/m²/d on days 1–3, with cytarabine given as IVCI over 24 h on days 1–7	Bone marrow suppression, cardiotoxicity, headache, nausea, vomiting, diarrhea, abdominal pain, GI bleeding, stomatitis, dyspnea, cough, alopecia

AML = acute myelogenous leukemia; ANLL = acute nonlymphocytic leukemia; IVCI = intravenous continuous infusion; IVP = intravenous push; IVPB = intravenous piggyback; IVS = intravenous side arm.

somerase II. Single- and double-strand breaks occur; this DNA damage interferes with replication and transcription. Peak toxicity occurs during the S phase of the cell cycle, but these agents are not considered cell cycle-specific.

Other mechanisms have also been proposed to help explain the antineoplastic activity of anthracycline antibiotics. Cytochrome P450 reductase, xanthine oxidase, and cytochrome B-5 reductase all can reduce daunorubicin and doxorubicin to free radicals that, in turn, can react with molecular oxygen to yield superoxide, hydrogen peroxide, and the hydroxyl radical. This process kills human breast cancer cells in vitro.

Pharmacokinetics. Anthracyclines are poorly absorbed orally and are administered intravenously (IV). Distribution is rapid and widespread. They are extensively tissue-bound and do not cross the blood-brain barrier. Much of each dose is metabolized in the liver. They are excreted predominantly in bile and also in urine as unchanged drug and metabolites.

Therapeutic Uses. Doxorubicin is active against a wide variety of tumors, including solid tumors. It is indicated for Hodgkin's and non-Hodgkin's lymphomas. Doxorubicin is part of several combination chemotherapy regimens used with acute lymphocytic and acute myelogenous leukemias. Doxorubicin has been helpful with osteogenic sarcoma, Ewing's sarcoma, and rhabdomyosarcoma. It may be the best agent for managing metastatic thyroid carcinoma. It is used with carcinomas of the endometrium, ovary, testes, prostate, stomach, lung, pancreas, and bladder, as well as neuroblastomas and Wilms' tumor.

Daunorubicin is indicated for acute lymphocytic and acute myelogenous leukemias. It is not used to treat solid tumors.

Idarubicin is used for acute myelogenous leukemia.

Dosage and Administration. Anthracyclines generally are administered via continuous IV infusion. Extravasation should be avoided. The drugs are never given intramuscularly (IM) or subcutaneously (SC).

Daunorubicin is available as a powder for reconstitution. Doxorubicin is available as a red-orange powder and as a solution for injection. Because the renal clearance of anthracyclines is minor, dosage decreases are unnecessary with renal dysfunction.

Adverse Reactions. Anthracyclines typically cause nausea and vomiting soon after administration. Clients should be advised that daunorubicin and doxorubicin turn the urine red or pink; this color may also affect sweat and tears. Anthracyclines cause bone marrow suppression, with the nadir around the tenth day; this is often the dose-limiting factor. Leukopenia is usually more significant than thrombocytopenia. Stomatitis occurs. Alopecia occurs, often suddenly after 3 to 4 weeks of therapy, but is usually reversible. Regrowth of hair is usually complete 2 to 5 months after treatment ends.

Extravasation of any anthracycline produces profound local tissue damage. Erythema and pain usually develop within 24 hours and can progress over weeks, resulting in deep ulceration that can reach tendon and bone. The lesions heal slowly and are difficult to skin graft. The allergic or "flare" reaction seen with doxorubicin or daunorubicin can be mistaken for extravasation. The flare includes a raised red streak that occurs within minutes, most commonly along the vein line of infusion. The client usually experiences itching, not pain. The red streak usually disappears in 30 to 90 minutes after drug infusion. It is considered a localized, benign allergic reaction.

One of the most unusual aspects of the anthracyclines is their ability to cause cardiomyopathy. Free radical formation seems to contribute to this toxicity. Heart tissue can activate doxorubicin to a free radical at multiple sites, including the mitochondria and sarcoplasmic reticulum. It is believed that free radical-induced cardiac injury results from the reaction between doxorubicin, iron, and peroxide. In addition, heart tissue has low levels of catalase, an enzyme needed in the detoxification of hydrogen peroxide. Doxorubicin also destroys

glutathione peroxidase activity, a major mechanism of peroxide removal.

Two forms of cardiac toxicity occur: acute and delayed. Acute toxicity is characterized by electrocardiographic abnormalities, including ST-T wave alterations and arrhythmias. The acute toxicity may be limited to 2 weeks. Delayed toxicity is manifested by congestive heart failure unresponsive to digitalis. The delayed form is related to the total cumulative dose of the drug. The risk of delayed toxicity increases significantly as the cumulative dose rises above 550 mg/m².

A cardioprotective agent, dexrazoxane (Zinecard), has been developed (Table 47-2). It is administered before the anthracycline. There are adverse reactions, but it is difficult to know if they are due to dexrazoxane or the anthracycline.

Drug Interactions. Doxorubicin may cause a recurrence of radiation-induced skin reaction and exacerbates tissue changes due to irradiation in mucous membranes and in the liver. Previous or concurrent cyclophosphamide, doxorubicin, or chest irradiation potentiate the cardiotoxicity of daunorubicin and doxorubicin. Increased bone marrow depression may occur if doxorubicin is given to clients receiving either other bone marrow depressants or radiation. A decrease in dosage may be indicated.

Hyperuricemia and gout may occur if doxorubicin is given with probenecid or sulfinpyrazone. Live viral vaccines should be avoided if possible when doxorubicin is used.

Doxorubicin may decrease plasma levels of digoxin. Concurrent use of doxorubicin and mercaptopurine increases the risk of hepatotoxicity, and concurrent use of doxorubicin and barbiturates increases the plasma clearance of doxorubicin.

Precautions and Contraindications. Daunorubicin and doxorubicin should be used with caution in clients with hepatic or cardiac dysfunction or those with myelosuppression. Dosages of daunorubicin and doxorubicin should be decreased with hepatic dysfunction because of the liver's role in their metabolism. Preparation and administration guidelines should be followed to reduce the risk of teratogenic, mutagenic, and carcinogenic effects. With both drugs, therapeutic effects are often coupled with toxicity.

Podophyllotoxin Derivatives

Podophyllotoxin, an extract of the mandrake plant (*Podophyllum peltatum*), was used as a folk remedy by Native Americans and early colonists for various purposes, including catharsis, conception promotion, and treatment of poisoning, parasites, and warts. It was found to have antitumor properties, but it was too toxic for clinical use. However, two semisynthetic derivatives, etoposide (Vepesid) and teniposide (Vumon), have important

Table 47-2. Adjunct Medications for Use With Antineoplastic Drugs

Drug Name	Preparation	Usual Dosage	Adverse Reactions	Indications
allopurinol (Lopurin, Zyloprim)	Oral	200–800 mg/d for 2–3 d or longer	Agranulocytosis, aplastic anemia, bone marrow suppression	Secondary hyperuricemia, which occurs with several antineoplastic drugs
dexrazoxane (Zinecard)	Powder for preparing solution for IV use	Dosage ratio of dexrazoxane: doxorubicin, 10:1 (eg, 500 mg/m² dexrazoxane, 50 mg/m² doxorubicin); dexrazoxane is given first, and 30 min from the onset of dexrazoxane, doxorubicin is given	Difficult to know if adverse reactions are due to dexrazoxane or doxorubicin; alopecia, nausea, vomiting, fatigue, malaise, anorexia, stomatitis	Prevention of cardiomyopathy associated with doxorubicin
leucovorin calcium (Wellcovorin)	Oral IM IV	10 mg/m² followed by 10 mg/m² q6h for 72 h; further doses based on serum methotrexate concentrations	Hypersensitivity reactions, thrombocytosis	Rescue therapy with methotrexate (see Chap. 46); used with fluorouracil (see Chap. 46)
levamisole hydrochloride (Ergamisol)	Oral tablets	Initially, 50 mg q8h for 3 d starting 7–30 d after surgery; maintenance, 50 mg q8h for 3 d every 2 wk for 1 year	Nausea, vomiting, diarrhea, taste perversion, altered sense of smell, bone marrow suppression, arthralgia, myalgia, pruritus, skin discoloration, rash, alopecia	Used in combination with fluorouracil as adjuvant therapy to treat Dukes' stage C colon cancer, after surgical resection
mesna (Mesnex)	IV	With ifosfamide, give dose equal to 20% of ifosfamide dose; give at time of ifosfamide administration and 4 and 8 h after	Bad taste in mouth, soft stools, nausea, vomiting	Used with drugs that cause hemorrhagic cystitis or nephrotoxicity, such as ifosfamide (see Chap. 46)

antineoplastic applications. These derivatives differ only in a single structural substitution and have many similarities.

Pharmacodynamics. These agents interact with topoisomerase II by forming a covalent topoisomerase II/drug/DNA complex and inducing DNA strand breaks.

Pharmacokinetics. Etoposide is highly (94%) bound to serum proteins. Despite its high lipid solubility, it does not readily cross the blood-brain barrier. Concentrations of etoposide in cerebrospinal fluid range from 1% to 10% of the plasma value. Etoposide is eliminated predominantly in urine, largely as unchanged drug (40%) but also as metabolites.

Therapeutic Uses. Etoposide is used mainly for the treatment of refractory testicular tumors. It is used with cyclophosphamide and vincristine for small cell lung carcinoma. It is also being investigated for use with Kaposi sarcoma.

Teniposide has been found to be about 10-fold more active than etoposide, probably due to the higher cellular uptake of teniposide. It has been used for refractory acute lymphoblastic leukemia in children.

Dosage and Administration. Etoposide is available as a solution (20 mg/mL) for IV administration and as 50-mg liquid-filled capsules for oral use. Oral capsules must be refrigerated. When given orally, the dose should be doubled; the oral form is not indicated for testicular tumors. Dosage by any route should be reduced in proportion to reductions in creatinine clearance.

When given IV, the drug should not be given by IV push but should be administered slowly via a 30- to 60-minute infusion (diluted in 5% dextrose injection or 0.9% sodium chloride injection) to avoid hypotension and bronchospasm. These reactions are believed to be due to solvents used in the drug's formulation.

Adverse Reactions. Bone marrow suppression is the major adverse reaction. Leukopenia is the dose-limiting feature, with a nadir of 10 to 14 days and recovery by 3 weeks. Thrombocytopenia occurs less frequently and is less severe. Other adverse reactions include alopecia, nausea, vomiting, and diarrhea. Fever, chills, and allergic reactions, including anaphylaxis, have also been observed.

Mild peripheral neuropathy occurs with etoposide, but it may be severe and cumulative in clients previously treated with a neurotoxic agent such as vincristine.

Secondary leukemias have developed within 10 years of using these agents.

Drug Interactions. No significant drug interactions have been identified with podophyllotoxin derivatives.

Precautions and Contraindications. Administration of teniposide is contraindicated in those known to be hypersensitive to the polyomyethylated castor oil component of the vehicle used in teniposide preparation. These agents have been linked to carcinogenic, teratogenic, and mutagenic risks for healthcare personnel.

Miscellaneous Topoisomerase II Inhibitors

Amsacrine

Amsacrine intercalates between strands of DNA and leads to DNA cleavage by topoisomerase II. Cytotoxicity is greatest during the S phase of the cell cycle, when topoisomerase II levels within the cell peak. Amsacrine is active against acute myelogenous leukemia, but severe toxicity limits its use.

Mitoxantrone Hydrochloride

Mitoxantrone hydrochloride (Novantrone) was originally synthesized as a structural analog of doxorubicin.

Pharmacodynamics. Mitoxantrone is a topoisomerase II inhibitor.

Pharmacokinetics. Mitoxantrone is rapidly and extensively distributed in tissues after administration, but distribution to the brain, spinal cord, cerebrospinal fluid, and eyes is low. It is highly bound to plasma proteins. The drug is excreted through both feces (via bile) and urine. Its half-life is 12 to 15 minutes and 1 to 2 days (the latter probably reflects release of the drug from tissue-binding sites).

Therapeutic Uses. Mitoxantrone is used in combination regimens for acute nonlymphocytic leukemia and other leukemias in adults. It also has produced some response in clients with metastatic breast cancer and malignant lymphoma (primarily non-Hodgkin's).

Dosage and Administration. The drug comes in an aqueous solution that must not be frozen. It is diluted before use with at least 50 mL of either 5% dextrose injection or 0.9% sodium chloride injection. The diluted solution is introduced into a freely running IV infusion of 5% dextrose or 0.9% sodium chloride over 3 minutes. Care should be taken to avoid extravasation, although mitoxantrone does not appear to be a vesicant. It should not be mixed in the same infusion as other drugs—for instance, precipitation may occur if mixed in the same syringe with heparin.

Adverse Reactions. Mitoxantrone may color the urine, sclera, and skin greenish-blue for 24 hours after therapy. Sometimes the vein used for administration develops a bluish discoloration, but this resolves within a few hours. Painful onycholysis has occurred. Blue discoloration of nails and reversible loss of fingernails have been reported.

Rapid lysis of tumor cells may cause hyperuricemia and may require concurrent administration of allopurinol.

Myelosuppression is the major adverse reaction. The nadir occurs in 1 to 2 weeks, and recovery is noted by the third week. The major effect is leukopenia, with anemia and thrombocytopenia occurring less frequently.

Cardiovascular reactions that resemble those seen with daunorubicin or doxorubicin may occur, including ST-T wave changes, decreased ejection fraction, arrhythmia, myocardial infarction, and congestive heart failure.

Drug Interactions. No significant drug interactions have been identified with mitoxantrone.

Precautions and Contraindications. Mitoxantrone should be used cautiously in clients previously exposed to cardiotoxic drugs or anthracyclines and those with significant myelosuppression.

Mitotic Inhibitors or Vinca Alkaloids

The mitotic inhibitors include four vinca alkaloids: vincristine (Oncovin), vinblastine (Velban), vindesine (Eldisine), and vinorelbine tartrate (Navelbine) (Table 47-3). These agents bind to tubulin, inhibiting the formation and assembly of the microtubular components of the mitotic spindle and leading to arrest of mitosis in metaphase. The microtubules are the filaments that move chromosomes during cell division; in the absence of microtubules, distribution of chromosomes to daughter cells becomes random and leads to cell death. These agents are considered cell cycle-specific.

The properties of the periwinkle plant (*Vinca rosea*) have been described in medicinal folklore. Due to the purported hypoglycemic effects, the plant was studied in the laboratory, but no significant ability to lower glucose could be documented. However, it was discovered that the plant suppressed bone marrow function. This information led to the development of the four vinca alkaloids. Structurally, they are very similar; for example, the only difference between vinblastine and vincristine is that vinblastine substitutes a methyl group for the formyl group in vincristine. However, the tumors they are active against and their adverse reactions differ.

Pharmacodynamics. The vinca alkaloids are mitotic inhibitors.

Pharmacokinetics. These agents are poorly absorbed when given orally, so they are only given IV. They are extensively bound to tissues or plasma proteins but either do not penetrate the blood-brain barrier or do so poorly. Multiphasic plasma clearance occurs. For vincristine, the elimination half-life is 10 to 155 hours; for vinblastine, the elimination half-life is about 24 hours. Both are partially metabolized in the liver and excreted primarily in feces, with some in urine.

Therapeutic Uses. Because it does not produce serious bone marrow suppression, vincristine is used in many combination regimens: COAP (cyclophosphamide, vin-

Table 47-3. Mitotic Inhibitors, Antitumor Antibiotics, Enzymes, Taxanes

Drug Name	Preparation	Usual Dosage	Adverse Reactions
Mitotic Inhibitors or Vinca Alkaloids			
vinblastine (Velban)	Powder for preparing solutions for IVP, IVS, IVCI	IVCI, 2 mg/m²/d for 5 d; or as part of VBP regimen, 4–8 mg/m² days 1 and 2; repeat cycle q21–28 d	Myalgia, nausea and vomiting, leukopenia, mucositis, stomatitis, glossitis, alopecia, Raynaud's phenomenon, neurotoxicity; vesicant
vincristine (Oncovin)	solution for IVP, IVS, IVCI	Adults: 0.4–1.4 mg/m² q7d as single dose Children: ≥10 kg: 1.5–2 mg/m² IV q7d as single dose	Neurotoxicities (eg, decreased DTRs, paresthesia, ataxia, slapping gait, footdrop, cranial nerve deficits; constipation, abdominal pain, paralytic ileus, bowel obstruction), SIADH, alopecia; vesicant
vindesine (Eldisine)	IVP, IVS, IVCI		Nausea, vomiting, diarrhea, parotid and jaw pain, rash, bone marrow suppression, paresthesias, peripheral neuropathy, stomatitis, alopecia, constipation, abdominal pain, paralytic ileus; vesicant
vinorelbine tartrate (Navelbine)	IVP, IVS	30 mg/m² as single IV dose, given once a week; may use with cisplatin	Neurotoxicity, but less common than with other vinca alkaloids; bone marrow suppression, headache, GI disturbances, increased liver enzymes; vesicant
Antitumor Antibiotics			
bleomycin (Blenoxane)	Powder for preparing solutions for IVBP, IVCI IM SC Intra-arterial Intrapleural	10–20 U/m² once or twice weekly for total dose of 300–400 U IM, IV, SC IV infusion: 15 U/m²/d over 24 h for 4–5 d Intra-arterial infusion for squamous cell carcinoma of head, neck: 30–60 U/d over 1–24 h Intrapleural approach for malignant pleural effusion: 15–120 U in 100 mL 0.9% sodium chloride, allowed to dwell for 24 h	Pulmonary toxicity, cutaneous toxicity (eg, erythema, pruritus, thickening, desquamation, hyperpigmentation, hyperesthesia, ulceration), alopecia, stomatitis, Raynaud's phenomenon, hypertension, hypersensitivity reactions, idiosyncratic reaction in lymphoma clients
dactinomyin (Cosmegan)	Powder for preparing solutions for IVS	Adults: 0.01–0.015 mg/kg/d IV for 5 d every 4–6 wk or 0.5 mg/m² IV once a week for 3 wk Children: 0.01–0.015 mg/kg/d IV for 5 d or a total dose of 2.5 mg/m² IV in divided doses over 7 d; may repeat every 4–6 wk	Leukopenia, thrombocytopenia, anorexia, nausea, vomiting, abdominal pain, diarrhea, stomatitis, cheilitis, glossitis, proctitis, GI ulceration, cutaneous toxicity, alopecia, hypersensitivity reactions; vesicant
mitomycin (Mutamycin)	Powder for preparing solutions for IVP, IVS Intra-arterial Intravesical	IV: 10–20 mg/m² as single dose repeated every 6–8 wk or 2 mg/m²/d IV for 5 d, skip 2 d, and repeat 2 mg/m²/d for 5 d; cycle may be repeated every 6–8 wk	Bone marrow suppression, anorexia, nausea, vomiting, stomatitis, alopecia, skin rashes, pulmonary toxicity, cardiomyopathy, nephrotoxicity
pentostatin (Nipent)	IVP IVCI	4 mg/m² every other week	Bone marrow suppression, CNS depression and toxicity, nausea, vomiting, rash, fever, infection, nephrotoxicity
plicamycin (Mithracin)	Powder for preparing solutions for IVPB, IVCI	*Hypercalcemia and hypercalciuria:* 0.015–0.025 mg/kg/d for 3–4 d; may repeat at 1-wk intervals	Bleeding syndrome, anorexia, nausea, vomiting, diarrhea, stomatitis, fever, hyperpigmentation, acneiform rashes, drowsiness, lethargy, malaise, headache, depression, abnormal liver function tests, abnormal renal function tests

DTRs = deep tendon reflexes; IVCI = intravenous continuous infusion; IVP = intravenous push; IVPB = intravenous piggyback; IVS = intravenous sidearm; SIADH = syndrome of inappropriate secretion of antidiuretic hormone.

(continued)

Table 47-3. (Continued)

Drug Name	Preparation	Usual Dosage	Adverse Reactions
Enzymes			
asparaginase (Elspar)	Powder for preparing solutions for IVP, IVPB, IVCI IM	Example of regimen: *asparaginase:* 1,000 IU/kg/d IV for 10 d starting day 22; *vincristine:* 2 mg/m² IV once a week on days 1, 8, 15; *prednisone:* 40 mg/m²/d in 3 divided doses for 15 d, then 20 mg/m² for 2 d, 10 mg/m² for 2 d, 5 mg/m² for 2 d, 2.5 mg/m² for 2 d	Hypersensitivity reactions ranging from urticaria to anaphylactic shock, neurotoxicity (reversible encephalopathy), thrombosis or hemorrhage, pancreatitis
pegaspargase (Oncospar)	IM IV	2,500 IU/m² q14d, generally as part of regimen	Pancreatitis, bone marrow suppression, nephrotoxicity, fatal hyperthermia, nausea, vomiting, anorexia, rash, urticaria, arthralgia
Taxanes			
paclitaxel (Taxol)	IV	135 mg/m² IV over 24 h every 3 wk or 175 mg/m² IV over 3 h every 3 wk	Bone marrow suppression (primarily neutropenia), cardiotoxicity, hypersensitivity reactions, peripheral neuropathy, alopecia
docetaxel (Taxotere)	IV	60–100 mg/m² IV over 1 h every 3 wk	Neutropenia

DTRs = deep tendon reflexes; IVCI = intravenous continuous infusion; IVP = intravenous push; IVPB = intravenous piggyback; IVS = intravenous sidearm; SIADH = syndrome of inappropriate secretion of antidiuretic hormone.

cristine [Oncovin], cytarabine, prednisone), COP (cyclophosphamide, vincristine, prednisone), COPP (cyclophosphamide, vincristine, procarbazine, prednisone), VAD (vincristine, doxorubicin [Adriamycin], dexamethasone), and MOPP (mechlorethamine, vincristine, procarbazine, prednisone). When vincristine is combined with prednisone, complete remissions are induced in up to 90% of children with acute lymphocytic leukemia (ALL). Other uses of vincristine include Hodgkin's disease, Burkitt's lymphoma, rhabdomyosarcoma, lung, breast, and cervical carcinoma, neuroblastoma, and Wilms' tumor.

Vinblastine is used in many combination regimens, such as VBP (vinblastine, bleomycin, cisplatin [Platinol]); see the Example of Nursing Process for VBP Therapy). VBP is the regimen of choice for testicular cancer. ABVD (doxorubicin [Adriamycin], bleomycin, vinblastine, dacarbazine) is an effective alternative to MOPP in the treatment of Hodgkin's disease (see Chap. 46). Vinblastine is also used for breast cancer, neuroblastomas, histiocytosis X (Letterer-Siwe disease), and Kaposi sarcoma. It has been effective with lymphomas refractory to alkylating agents and choriocarcinomas refractory to methotrexate.

Vindesine is used for malignant melanoma and colon and lung cancers.

Vinorelbine may be used with cisplatin for unresectable advanced non-small cell lung cancer.

Dosage and Administration. The vinca alkaloids may be administered by continuous IV infusion or by IV push. Dosage is decreased with hepatic dysfunction be-

cause of the liver's role in vinca alkaloid excretion. A reduction of 50% is recommended in clients with bilirubin levels of more than 3 mg/100 mL. No reduction is needed for clients with impaired renal function.

Adverse Reactions. All vinca alkaloids are vesicants. Vincristine's adverse reactions are primarily neurologic, affecting the peripheral, central, and autonomic nervous systems. Neurotoxicity is significantly greater than with vinblastine, possibly because of vincristine's longer half-life, which prolongs its contact with nerve tissue that contains high concentrations of tubulin. Loss of the Achilles tendon reflex is usually the first sign of peripheral neuropathy. Other manifestations of peripheral neuropathy include a decrease in other deep tendon reflexes, paresthesia of the upper and lower extremities, ataxia, slapping gait, and foot drop. The primary muscle groups involved are the dorsiflexors of the hands and the extensors of the feet. More advanced neurotoxicity may include cranial nerve deficits (eg, ptosis, diplopia, abducens nerve palsy, vocal cord paralysis). Optic atrophy and blindness have been reported.

At higher doses, involvement of the autonomic nervous system causes constipation, obstipation, abdominal pain, paralytic ileus, and bowel obstruction.

The syndrome of inappropriate secretion of antidiuretic hormone (SIADH) has also been observed with vincristine use. Fluid overload, hyponatremia, and hemodilution can result. Alopecia occurs. Mild bone marrow suppression may occur, with recovery by day 7.

With vinblastine, early adverse reactions include jaw pain, constipation, fever, anorexia, and headache.

Example of Nursing Process for Vinblastine, Bleomycin, and Cisplatin (VBP) Therapy

The client is a 30-year-old man with a diagnosis of advanced-state testicular nonseminoma. His symptoms include a testicular mass and a feeling of heaviness. The VBP program is as follows: (vinblastine 0.2 mg/kg IV days 1 and 2 and repeat every 3 weeks for five courses, bleomycin 30 U/week IV, 6 hours after vinblastine on the second day of each week for 12 weeks until total dose of 360 U, cisplatin 20 mg/m² IV days 1 through 5, 6 hours after vinblastine, and repeat every 3 weeks for three courses.

   The client has been married for 3 years; he and his wife have recently started thinking about having a family.

Assessment Data

Receiving vinblastine, bleomycin, and cisplatin

Married for 3 years; had considered starting a family

Nursing Diagnosis*	Intervention	Goals and Outcomes
Potential Complication: Fibrosis and inflammation of lung tissue*	**Monitor** for signs and symptoms of inflammation (eg, dry, hacking, persistent cough; tachypnea; dyspnea; rales).	The client will not experience signs and symptoms of pulmonary inflammation and fibrosis; if they occur, they will be promptly detected and treated.
	Monitor blood gas values, chest x-ray reports, and pulmonary function studies. If signs and symptoms of inflammation and fibrosis occur, **be prepared** to administer antibiotics, corticosteroids, and bronchodilators.	
	Carry out interventions to improve gas exchange (eg, positioning, coughing, and deep breathing, inspiratory exercises).	
Knowledge Deficit, concerning adverse effects of chemotherapy	**Monitor** for therapeutic and nontherapeutic effects of the three antineoplastic drugs.	If the client experiences adverse reactions related to the antineoplastic agents, they will be promptly detected and reported.
	Inform client of possible side effects and urge him to report any evidence of them immediately.	
	Allow time for questions and clarification.	
	Stress importance of keeping appointments for laboratory tests that monitor for possible adverse reactions.	
Self-Esteem Disturbance: Expected infertility related to chemotherapy	**Clarify** physician's explanation about fertility.	The client will demonstrate adaptation to changes in body functioning as shown by realistic comments that indicate acceptance of alternative plans for parenthood.
	Provide information about possibility of sperm banking and testicular implants.	
	Discuss alternate methods of parenthood.	
	Include wife in discussion and encourage her continued support of client.	

*Although potential complications are not routinely addressed in these examples, in this situation the identification of such a collaborative problem is critical to the outcome for this client and illustrates the broad range of nursing responsibilities during chemotherapy.

Later ones include mild paresthesias and peripheral neuropathies, stomatitis, depression, seizures, gonadal suppression, amenorrhea, and azoospermia. Alopecia occurs but is less common than with vincristine, and it is reversible. Bone marrow suppression occurs. Leukopenia is usually dose-limited, with the nadir occurring in 5 to 10 days and recovery in 12 to 24 days. With higher doses, the white blood cell count may not return to normal for 3 weeks. Thrombocytopenia and anemia are less common and have a nadir of day 10, with recovery by day 17.

Early adverse reactions to vindesine include mild nausea and vomiting, diarrhea, parotid and jaw pain, and rash with myalgias and fever within 48 hours of drug administration. Later adverse reactions include moderate bone marrow suppression, mild paresthesias and peripheral neuropathies, stomatitis, mild alopecia, constipation, abdominal pain, and paralytic ileus.

Adverse reactions with vinorelbine include headache, gastrointestinal (GI) toxic reactions, and increased liver enzyme levels. Neurologic adverse reactions are less common than with other vinca alkaloids. Bone marrow suppression occurs.

Drug Interactions. Concurrent use of vinblastine, vincristine, or vinorelbine with mitomycin has resulted in acute pulmonary reactions such as severe bronchospasm and shortness of breath. Concurrent radiation therapy to the lung with vindesine use may result in pneumonitis or local fibrosis.

The use of phenytoin with vinblastine or vincristine decreases the effect of the phenytoin. Use of calcium channel blockers with vincristine results in increased accumulation of vincristine in cells. Vincristine decreases the plasma levels and effect of digoxin.

When asparaginase and vincristine are given concurrently, asparaginase decreases the liver clearance of vincristine, and increased neurotoxicity from vincristine may result. Asparaginase should be administered after vincristine to reduce the possibility of increased vincristine neurotoxicity.

Concurrent use of vincristine with doxorubicin and prednisone has resulted in an increase in bone marrow depressant effects; this combination should be avoided.

Concurrent use of vincristine with probenecid or sulfinpyrazone may result in hyperuricemia and gout. Live viral vaccines should be avoided if possible when vincristine is used.

The combination of bleomycin and vinblastine may produce signs of Raynaud's disease in clients treated for testicular cancer.

There is increased bone marrow suppression if vinorelbine tartrate and cisplatin are used concurrently.

Precautions and Contraindications. Intrathecal administration of vincristine is absolutely contraindicated because it has been known to cause coma, seizures, and death. All the vinca alkaloids should be used cautiously in clients with hepatic dysfunction. Because of the neurologic complications, vincristine should be used with caution in clients with preexisting neuromuscular disease (eg, Charcot-Marie-Tooth disease, Friedreich's ataxia), in combination with other neurotoxic drugs, and in clients predisposed to neurologic complications (eg, those with diabetes or peripheral vascular disease). In some clients with Charcot-Marie-Tooth disease, quadriplegia has occurred with vincristine use. Vinorelbine should also be used cautiously in clients whose bone marrow has been suppressed or compromised from previous therapies.

Acute uric acid nephropathy has occurred with vincristine. Allupurinol may be used to try to prevent this complication.

Antitumor Antibiotics

Several antibiotics, natural products of certain soil fungi, are used in chemotherapy. They produce their effects by forming complexes with DNA, thereby inhibiting DNA activities. They generally are cell cycle-nonspecific. The antibiotics used in chemotherapy include bleomycin, dactinomycin, mitomycin, and plicamycin. Other antibiotics were discussed in the section on topoisomerase inhibitors. See Focus on Antitumor Antibiotics: Similarities and Differences.

Bleomycin

Bleomycin (Blenoxane) was first isolated in 1962 from *Streptomyces verticillus* obtained from a soil sample in a Japanese coal mine.

Pharmacodynamics. Bleomycin first binds to DNA. Ferrous iron is bound to nitrogen-containing groups of bleomycin. The bleomycin/ferrous iron complex catalyzes the reduction of molecular oxygen to superoxide or hydroxyl radicals, causing DNA strand breaks and inhibition of DNA synthesis. There seems to be some inhibition of RNA and protein synthesis as well. Bleomycin seems most active during the G_2 and M phases of the cell cycle.

Pharmacokinetics. Bleomycin is not absorbed orally and therefore must be administered parenterally. It concentrates particularly in the skin, lung, kidney, peritoneum, and lymph nodes but does not enter the cerebrospinal fluid. The half-life is 2 hours, and 60% to 70% is recovered in urine as parent compound.

Deactivation of bleomycin is apparently due to the enzyme bleomycin hydrolase, which is found in normal and most malignant cells of certain tissues and is especially prominent in the liver. The enzyme, however, is found in low concentrations in the lung and skin.

Therapeutic Uses. Because it does not produce serious bone marrow suppression, bleomycin is used in several combination regimens. VBP is a combination of choice in disseminated nonseminomatous testicular cancer and is also effective with disseminated seminomatous

FOCUS ON

Focus On Antitumor Antibiotics: Similarities and Differences

Similarities

Pharmacodynamics

Most antitumor antibiotics are cell cycle-nonspecific and interfere with DNA structure, synthesis, and function.

Pharmacokinetics

These agents are poorly absorbed orally and are therefore administered IV. They are metabolized by the liver and excreted in urine and bile.

Therapeutic Uses

The antibiotic antineoplastic agents have a wide range of uses.

Adverse Reactions

Most of these agents are vesicants or irritating to veins. Dose-limiting toxicity for most of the agents is bone marrow suppression.

Drug Interactions

Concurrent use of dactinomycin or mitomycin with doxorubicin potentiates doxorubicin's cardiotoxicity.

Differences

- **Bleomycin** seems most active in G_2 and M phases.
- **Dactinomycin** is most active in G_1 and inhibits RNA synthesis.
- **Mitomycin** is a prodrug that is converted to active form within cells; after activation it functions as an alkylating agent. It appears most active in late G_1 and early S phases.
- **Pentostatin** inhibits an enzyme and thereby suppresses DNA synthesis.
- **Plicamycin** shows some selectivity for S phase and inhibits RNA synthesis.

- **Bleomycin** may be administered IM, IV, or SC and has been used intra-arterially and intrapleurally.
- **Mitomycin** is used IV and has been administered by intra-arterial and intravesical routes.

- **Bleomycin** is used for squamous cell carcinoma of head and neck, testicular carcinoma, Hodgkin's disease, carcinoma of skin, penis, cervix, and vulva.
- **Dactinomycin** is used for Wilms' tumor, rhabdomyosarcoma, Ewing's sarcoma, osteosarcoma, Kaposi sarcoma, and advanced choriocarcinoma.
- **Mitomycin** is used for adenocarcinoma of stomach and pancreas and others.
- **Pentostatin** is used for hairy cell leukemia.
- **Plicamycin** is used for testicular carcinoma and hypercalcemia and hypercalciuria associated with advanced cancers.

- **Bleomycin** is not a vesicant and causes minimal bone marrow suppression. Bleomycin is known for its pulmonary toxicity, which is unpredictable but is usually considered to be age- and dose-related. Many clients receiving bleomycin experience some form of skin toxicity.
- Cutaneous reactions are also seen as a problem with **dactinomycin.**
- **Mitomycin** is associated with renal failure.
- **Pentostatin** causes CNS depression and other evidence of neurotoxicity.
- A dose-related bleeding syndrome is a serious toxicity with **plicamycin.**

- Cisplatin inhibits renal elimination of **bleomycin.** Bleomycin may decrease plasma levels of digoxin and phenytoin.
- If radiation therapy is used with **dactinomycin,** skin and GI reactions are potentiated.
- Acute respiratory distress and pneumonitis may occur when vinca alkaloids are used in clients who had previously or simultaneously received **mitomycin.** Mitomycin potentiates doxorubicin's cardiac toxicity.

(continued)

*FOCUS **ON***

Focus On Antitumor Antibiotics: Similarities and Differences (continued)

Similarities
(continued)

Nursing Considerations

Instruct in disease, drug therapy regimen, adverse reactions, and interactions. Follow specified administration guidelines. Follow guidelines for preventing or managing extravasation.

Differences
(continued)

---

testicular cancer. ABVD is an effective alternative to MOPP (see Chap. 46) in the treatment of Hodgkin's disease. Bleomycin has been used for squamous cell carcinomas of the head and neck (eg, buccal mucosa, tongue, tonsil, pharynx). It is also indicated in carcinoma of the skin, penis, cervix, and vulva.

Dosage and Administration. Bleomycin is available in vials as a powder. For IM or SC use, the vial contents are dissolved in 1 to 5 mL of sterile water for injection, sodium chloride injection, or 5% dextrose injection. For IV use, the vial contents are dissolved in 5 mL or more of sodium chloride injection or 5% dextrose injection and administered slowly over 10 minutes (IV bolus method).

A unit of activity is defined as 1 mg. A typical dose is 10 to 20 U/m^2 once or twice weekly to a total of 300 to 400 U. Dosage modifications (decreases of 50%–75%) are required in clients with impaired renal function.

Clients with a lymphoma-like non-Hodgkin's lymphoma appear to be at risk for an idiosyncratic reaction when bleomycin is used, and some have recommended that the client receive a test dose of 1 to 2 U before the therapeutic dose.

The intracavitary dosage for malignant pleural effusion is 15 to 240 U diluted in 100 mL of normal saline, with instillation after thoracostomy tube drainage. Intra-arterial infusions have been used for squamous cell carcinoma of the head and neck. Intraperitoneal instillations with 24-hour dwell times have also been used.

Adverse Reactions. As mentioned above, the lung tissue contains low concentrations of bleomycin hydrolase, which deactivates bleomycin. The low concentrations of this enzyme can result in dose-limiting pulmonary toxicity. Clients especially at risk for this toxicity are those age 70 or older, those receiving a total of 400 U or more of bleomycin, those who have received pulmonary or mediastinal irradiation, and those with underlying lung disease. Toxicity can occur at a dose lower than 400 U in clients treated with combination therapies, such as bleomycin and cyclophosphamide (which can independently cause pulmonary toxicity).

The development of pulmonary toxicity is usually delayed and may occur 4 to 10 weeks after initiation of therapy. Symptoms include cough, dyspnea, and fever. The first signs are insidious and include fine rales, rhonchi, and occasionally pleural friction rubs. These signs and symptoms often precede changes identifiable by radiography.

The radiographic appearance is typical of interstitial pneumonitis and may progress to that of pulmonary fibrosis. Identifiable damage often includes bibasilar pulmonary infiltrates. Computed tomography scans and gallium scans may detect drug-induced effects before chest radiographs do. The drug should be discontinued immediately if a lung reaction is detected.

Pulmonary toxicity can be potentiated by oxygen administration. After bleomycin use, lung damage can occur at oxygen concentrations usually considered safe.

When bleomycin therapy is discontinued, pulmonary abnormalities may or may not resolve. One percent of clients treated with bleomycin have died of this pulmonary toxicity.

The skin also lacks significant amounts of bleomycin hydrolase, so bleomycin frequently produces skin reactions. About 50% of clients develop erythema or pruritic erythema, thickening and desquamation of fingers and palms (peeling), and hyperpigmentation of skin creases, with a general darkening of the skin. The changes may begin with swelling and hyperesthesia of the hands or ulcerating lesions over the elbows, knuckles, and other pressure areas.

Bleomycin causes minimal bone marrow suppression and minimal nausea and vomiting.

Less common side effects include alopecia, stomatitis, Raynaud's phenomenon, and hypertension. Hypersensitivity reactions may occur.

A peculiar idiosyncratic reaction has been observed in clients with lymphomas that is characterized by hypotension, mental confusion, fever, chills, and wheezing. It does not appear to be a classic anaphylactic reaction and may be related to the release of an endogenous pyrogen. This has occurred in about 1% of lymphoma clients and has been fatal.

Drug Interactions. Bleomycin may decrease plasma levels of digoxin. Phenytoin serum concentrations may be decreased.

Precautions and Contraindications. Clients receiving bleomycin should have baseline pulmonary function studies done before therapy starts to help detect any pulmonary adverse effects that may occur.

Dactinomycin

Dactinomycin or actinomycin D (Cosmegan) is derived from *Streptomyces parvullus*. It is the only member of a large class of similar drugs with a significant clinical use.

Pharmacodynamics. This antibiotic intercalates between adjacent base pairs in DNA and becomes bound to DNA. The intercalation process distorts DNA structure. Because of this structural distortion, RNA polymerase cannot use DNA as a template, and the synthesis of RNA is inhibited. The drug is cell cycle-nonspecific, but activity may be highest in G_1.

Pharmacokinetics. Dactinomycin is poorly absorbed orally and thus is administered IV. Clearance of the drug from the plasma is initially rapid, but the terminal half-life is 36 hours because of slow release from tissue stores. Most of the drug is excreted unchanged in bile and urine. Dactinomycin does not cross the blood-brain barrier or enter the cerebrospinal fluid.

Therapeutic Uses. The most important use for dactinomycin is the treatment of Wilms' tumor. Effective therapy of this pediatric cancer requires multiple approaches, including surgery, radiation therapy, and combination chemotherapy with dactinomycin and vincristine. Dactinomycin is also used to treat rhabdomyosarcoma, Ewing's sarcoma, osteosarcoma, and Kaposi sarcoma. Advanced choriocarcinoma has also been sensitive to dactinomycin. Dactinomycin has been helpful with chlorambucil and methotrexate in metastatic testicular carcinoma, but this combination is not as satisfactory as the VBP regimen. It has been investigated to manage acute organ rejection in kidney and heart transplants.

Dosage and Administration. Dactinomycin is supplied as a powder for reconstitution. One schedule is 10 to 15 µg/kg IV for 5 days. If no toxic manifestations occur, additional courses may be given at intervals of 3 to 4 weeks. Daily injections of 100 to 400 µg have been given to children for 10 to 14 days. Another regimen is 3 to 6 µg/kg for a total of 125 µg/kg and weekly maintenance doses of 7.5 µg/kg. It is best to inject the medication into the IV tubing of a flowing infusion because of its vesicant property.

Adverse Reactions. Bone marrow suppression (leukopenia, thrombocytopenia) is the most common dose-limiting toxicity. The nadir is usually 2 to 3 weeks after a course of the drug, and thrombocytopenia is often seen first. Anorexia, nausea, and vomiting usually occur 4 to 5 hours after the drug is administered. Abdominal pain and diarrhea may occur. Stomatitis, cheilitis, glossitis, and proctitis are common and may be dose-limiting. GI ulceration may develop. Cutaneous reactions include dactinomycin folliculitis (an acneiform eruption), erythema, desquamation, and hyperpigmentation. Alopecia may occur 7 to 10 days after treatment and continuing 2 to 4 weeks. Anaphylactic reactions have also been reported. Dactinomycin is a vesicant.

Drug Interactions. If a client receiving dactinomycin receives radiation as well, skin or GI reactions from the radiation are potentiated (or could be reactivated if the radiation was used before the drug). Erythema, progressing sometimes to necrosis, has been noted in areas of skin exposed to radiation therapy before, during, or after administration of dactinomycin.

Precautions and Contraindications. The dose of dactinomycin is reduced in clients receiving concomitant treatment with other chemotherapy or radiation.

Mitomycin

Mitomycin (Mutamycin) is an antibiotic that was first isolated from *Streptomyces caespitosus* in 1958.

Pharmacodynamics. Mitomycin is a prodrug that is converted to active form within cells. Mitomycin's molecular structure differs from that of the alkylating agents described in Chapter 46; however, after intracellular activation, mitomycin basically functions as an alkylating agent. It can cause interstrand and intrastrand cross-linking of DNA, which results in inhibition of DNA synthesis. In high doses, it also decreases RNA and protein synthesis. It is cell cycle-nonspecific but appears to be most active in the late G_1 and early S phases.

Pharmacokinetics. Mitomycin is not absorbed orally, making parenteral administration necessary. Clearance of the drug is rapid after IV administration. The drug is widely distributed throughout body tissues, except the central nervous system (CNS). It is metabolized primarily in the liver.

Therapeutic Uses. Mitomycin is used in the palliative treatment of various solid tumors. It is part of the FAM (fluorouracil, doxorubicin [Adriamycin], mitomycin) regimen used in gastric adenocarcinoma. It is also approved for pancreatic cancer. Other uses include carcinoma of the colon, rectum, esophagus, lung, breast, cervix, and bladder. In these cases, responses to the drug are usually brief and complicated by adverse reactions. Intraperitoneal mitomycin has been suggested for use with relapsed gynecologic cancers that involve the abdomen. Mitomycin is also used intravesically for treatment of superficial bladder cancer.

Dosage and Administration. Mitomycin is available as deep blue-violet crystals in vials for reconstitution. It is administered through the tubing of a flowing IV infusion because of its vesicant nature. A typical dosage is 20 mg/m² given in a single dose.

Adverse Reactions. The major dose-limiting toxicity of mitomycin is myelosuppression, both delayed and cumulative. The client must be reevaluated before any repetition of therapy 6 to 8 weeks after the first therapy. Leukopenia usually persists 1 to 2 weeks, thrombocytopenia 2 to 3 weeks, with recovery of the blood count in about 74% of clients within 8 weeks. Another dose should not be administered until the leukocyte count has returned to 3,000 and the platelet count to 75,000.

Anorexia, nausea, vomiting, and stomatitis are common. Alopecia, skin rashes, and discoloration of fingernails occur.

Renal failure, often associated with microangiopathic hemolytic anemia, can occur in a syndrome called the hemolytic uremic syndrome. Both hemolysis and renal failure appear to be precipitated by renal vascular endothelial injury from the drug. This syndrome seems to be dose-related and seems more likely to occur when mitomycin is used with fluorouracil.

Glomerular sclerosis has been reported after several months of therapy and is manifested by increased levels of blood urea nitrogen and serum creatinine and often severe hypertension.

Mitomycin is a vesicant.

Drug Interactions. Pulmonary fibrosis occurs occasionally and can be severe. It manifests as interstitial pneumonitis, presenting with dyspnea, nonproductive cough, and fever. The incidence of this toxicity is higher in clients receiving both mitomycin and a vinca alkaloid or doxorubicin. Mitomycin potentiates doxorubicin's cardiac toxicity.

Precautions and Contraindications. Mitomycin should be used cautiously in clients with impaired renal function, myelosuppression, pregnancy, and lactation.

Pentostatin

Pentostatin (Nipent) was approved in 1991. It was isolated from fermentation cultures of *Streptomyces antibioticus*.

Pharmacodynamics. Pentostatin inhibits the enzyme adenosine deaminase and thereby suppresses synthesis of DNA.

Pharmacokinetics. When given IV, the onset is rapid and the peak occurs in 11 minutes. It is metabolized in the liver, distributed across the placenta and into breast milk, and excreted in urine.

Therapeutic Uses. The only approved indication is for hairy cell leukemia refractory to interferon alfa.

Dosage and Administration. Administration is by IV push or IV infusion. The dosage is 4 mg/m² every other week. The product contains 50 mg mannitol per each single-dose vial. Hydration with 5% dextrose in 0.5% normal saline or an equivalent is required before and after the drug is given.

Adverse Reactions. The major dose-limiting adverse reactions are bone marrow suppression and nervous system toxicity. Other adverse effects are nausea, vomiting, rash, fever, infection and nephrotoxicity. Anorexia, nausea, vomiting, and stomatitis are common. Alopecia, skin rashes, and discoloration of fingernails occur.

Drug Interactions. When pentostatin was used in combination with fludarabine phosphate (an analog of adenosine), clients had severe or fatal pulmonary toxicity, so this combination is not recommended.

Precautions and Contraindications. Pentostatin is contraindicated in pregnancy and lactation. It should be used cautiously in clients with myelosuppression or impaired renal function.

Plicamycin

Plicamycin, also known as mithramycin (Mithracin), is produced by *Streptomyces plicatus*, *Streptomyces argillaceus*, and *Streptomyces tanashiensis*.

Pharmacodynamics. Plicamycin inhibits RNA synthesis more than it affects DNA synthesis, although it binds tightly to DNA in the presence of magnesium or other divalent cations. It is cell cycle-nonspecific but shows some selectivity for the S phase. Plicamycin affects calcium metabolism and decreases blood calcium by blocking the effect of vitamin D, acting on osteoclasts that normally liberate calcium from bone and preventing the action of parathyroid hormone.

Pharmacokinetics. Plicamycin is poorly absorbed after oral administration, making parenteral administration necessary. The drug crosses the blood-brain barrier and is cleared rapidly from the blood. It concentrates in liver cells and renal tubular cells and along formed bone surfaces.

Therapeutic Uses. Lower doses have been helpful in severe hypercalcemia and hypercalciuria when associated with advanced or metastatic cancer that involves bone or produces parathyroid hormone-like substance. Its effects in this type of situation last 7 to 21 days. In most cases, specific therapy against the neoplasm is necessary to achieve permanent control of the serum calcium level.

The major antineoplastic use of plicamycin is in testicular tumors, but it is a secondary drug because it is toxic and other effective drugs are available (eg, the VBP regimen).

Dosage and Administration. Plicamycin is available in vials as a powder for reconstitution. For antineoplastic therapy, it is given IV in doses of 25 to 30 µg/kg/day for 8 to 10 days. It is diluted in 1 L of 5% dextrose in water and administered by IV infusion over 4 to 6 hours.

More rapid administration is associated with a higher incidence and greater severity of GI side effects. In responsive tumors, some degree of regression is usually seen within 3 to 4 weeks of initial therapy. Additional courses of therapy can be given at monthly intervals.

For hypercalcemia and hypercalciuria refractory to conventional treatment, doses of 25 µg/kg are given daily for 3 or 4 days. This treatment may be repeated at weekly intervals, or a single dose may be given each week; the latter schedule is associated with reduced toxicity.

Adverse Reactions. The most important form of toxicity is a dose-related bleeding syndrome manifested by thrombocytopenia, prolonged prothrombin time, and depression of clotting factors II, V, VII, and X. The first symptom may be an episode of epistaxis that may or may not progress to further symptoms. Death has occurred. Other adverse reactions include anorexia, nausea, and vomiting, which may begin 1 to 2 hours after initiation of therapy and persist for 12 to 24 hours. Diarrhea, stomatitis, fever, rash, drowsiness, lethargy, malaise, headache, depression, abnormal liver function tests, and abnormal renal function tests (eg, proteinuria, increased serum creatinine, increased blood urea nitrogen) occur occasionally.

A reversible flushing reaction has been seen in clients who receive multiple courses of the drug. Diffuse head and neck erythema progresses to edema and coarsening of facial features.

Drug Interactions. No significant drug interactions have been identified with plicamycin.

Precautions and Contraindications. Plicamycin is contraindicated in clients with thrombocytopenia or coagulation disorders, electrolyte imbalance, pregnancy, or lactation. It should be used cautiously in clients with hepatic or renal impairment.

Enzymes
Asparaginase

Asparaginase (Elspar) is an enzyme derived from cultures of either *Escherichia coli* or *Erwinia carotovora* (a plant parasite). Its mechanism of action differs from that of other antineoplastic agents, based on the concept of nutritional deprivation.

Pharmacodynamics. Asparaginase catalyzes the hydrolysis of the amino acid asparagine to aspartic acid and ammonia, thus depleting the amount of asparagine available to tumor cells. Most normal tissues synthesize whatever asparagine they need. The lymphoblast in ALL appears to lack asparagine synthetase and cannot convert aspartic acid to asparagine, but it does require asparagine for growth purposes. The asparagine-depleting action interferes with the synthesis of protein, DNA, and RNA in tumor cells. Asparaginase is probably cell cycle-specific for the G_1 phase.

Leukemic cells can become resistant to asparaginase because of the emergence of strains that make asparagine synthetase or produce a mutated form of the enzyme.

Pharmacokinetics. Asparaginase is not absorbed from the GI tract and must be administered IM or IV. The plasma half-life is 8 to 30 hours and varies among preparations and clients, but it is usually stable in a single person. Most of the drug is confined to the vascular system because of the large molecular size. It does not cross the blood-brain barrier. Asparaginase is probably inactivated by the immune and reticuloendothelial systems.

Therapeutic Uses. Asparaginase is usually used with vincristine and prednisone to induce remission in pediatric ALL.

Dosage and Administration. Asparaginase is available in vials as a powder for reconstitution. The preparation contains 80 mg of mannitol. For IM use, 2 mL of sodium chloride injection is added; for IV use, 5 mL of sterile water for injection or sodium chloride injection is added. When administered IV, it should be injected into the tubing of a flowing infusion of sodium chloride injection or 5% dextrose and water over a period of 30 minutes.

For a child, the dose schedule is 1,000 IU/kg/day for 10 successive days, beginning on day 22 of the treatment cycle, or 6,000 IU/m² on days 4, 7, 10, 13, 16, 19, 22, 25, and 28.

Adverse Reactions. It was originally thought that asparaginase exploited a unique difference between normal and leukemic cells, but now it is known that many normal tissues are sensitive to asparaginase. Thus, various adverse reactions to asparaginase may occur.

As a foreign protein, asparaginase is antigenic. About 66% of clients experience immediate side effects, including nausea, vomiting, chills, and fever.

Hypersensitivity reactions ranging from urticaria to anaphylactic shock occur in up to 40% of clients and can be fatal. The incidence of anaphylactic reactions is greater with IV administration than with IM administration. An intradermal skin test with 2 U of drug is recommended before the initial dose and before each subsequent dose if a week or more has elapsed (although allergic reactions have followed negative skin test results).

The neurotoxic reactions are believed to be caused by the inhibition of protein synthesis in the brain. About 25% of clients exhibit a reversible encephalopathy with manifestations ranging from confusion to coma.

Both thrombosis and hemorrhage have occurred with asparaginase. Pancreatitis has been observed and may progress to severe (even fatal) hemorrhagic pancreatitis. Biochemical evidence of hepatic dysfunction occurs (eg, elevation of liver enzyme levels), but these abnormalities are usually reversible with discontinuation of therapy. Acute renal insufficiency, which can be fatal, has been reported.

The drug does not cause alopecia or stomatitis. It is rarely associated with bone marrow suppression.

Drug Interactions. Vincristine and asparaginase interact, and asparaginase decreases the liver clearance of vincristine. Asparaginase should be administered 12 to 24 hours after vincristine to reduce the possibility of increased vincristine neurotoxicity.

When asparaginase and methotrexate are used concurrently, the effect of methotrexate is diminished, so this combination is not recommended.

When used with prednisone, the toxicity of asparaginase is increased, but administering asparaginase after prednisone may reduce this effect.

Precautions and Contraindications. Asparaginase should be used cautiously in clients with hepatic dysfunction, bone marrow suppression, pancreatitis or a history of pancreatitis, or lactation.

Pegaspargase

Pegaspargase/PEG-L (Oncaspar), a modified version of the enzyme asparaginase, was approved in 1994 for the treatment of clients with acute lymphoblastic leukemia who are hypersensitive to asparaginase. It is administered IM (preferred route) or IV and is available as a single-use vial containing 750 IU/mL in a phosphate-buffered saline solution. A typical dose in combination therapy is 2,500 IU/m^2 every 14 days.

Taxanes

The taxanes are a newer class of antineoplastic drugs. Paclitaxel (Taxol) was discovered as part of a National Cancer Institute program in which extracts of thousands of plants were screened for anticancer activity. In 1963 an extract from the bark of the Pacific yew *Taxus brevifolia*, a scarce and slow-growing evergreen found in old-growth forests of the Pacific Northwest, was found to have cytotoxic activity. In 1971 paclitaxel was identified as the active constituent of the extract.

The limited supply of paclitaxel has stimulated collaborations between private industry and government. Supplies of paclitaxel can be derived from parts of the tree other than the bark, semisynthetic materials, cultivated ornamental *Taxus* species, and plant-tissue cultures. The semisynthetic process uses a readily available precursor derived from the needles of more abundant yew species.

A paclitaxel analog, docetaxel (Taxotere), can be synthesized from the precursor process. Docetaxel was approved in 1996 for the treatment of breast cancer in clients whose disease has progressed; in those women, it seems to show a greater response rate than paclitaxel.

Pharmacodynamics. The function of microtubules is the formation of the mitotic spindle during cell divi-

sion, and they are also involved in other interphase functions. Microtubules are composed of tubulins. Paclitaxel promotes the polymerization of tubulin, inhibiting the disassembly of microtubules. The microtubules formed in the presence of paclitaxel are very stable and dysfunctional, thereby causing the death of the cell by disrupting the normal microtubule dynamics required for cell division and interphase processes. This mechanism of action is considered unique; other antineoplastic agents, such as vinca alkaloids, *induce* the disassembly of microtubules.

Pharmacokinetics. The drug is 89% to 98% protein bound. Renal clearance accounts for only 1% to 8% of total clearance, so dosage modifications do not appear necessary in clients with renal dysfunction. Hepatic metabolism, biliary excretion, fecal elimination, or extensive tissue binding appears to be responsible for most of the systemic clearance. It is thought to be metabolized in the liver.

Therapeutic Uses. Paclitaxel was approved in 1992 for treating advanced ovarian cancer. Through a National Cancer Institute program, it was initially provided to women whose ovarian cancers had progressed after treatment with three regimens of chemotherapy. Twenty-two percent of the first 1,000 clients had major responses despite poor prognostic characteristics (Rowinsky & Donehower, 1995). Further study has demonstrated the benefits of administering paclitaxel and cisplatin together in the treatment of such cancer.

In 1994 paclitaxel was approved for the treatment of breast cancer. Paclitaxel has also been evaluated in advanced non-small cell lung cancer, squamous cell carcinoma of the head and neck, and other cancers.

Dosage and Administration. There have been two approaches to paclitaxel administration: 135 mg/m^2 IV over 24 hours every 3 weeks for ovarian carcinoma and 175 mg/m^2 IV over 3 hours every 3 weeks for metastatic breast cancer. Premedication for hypersensitivity is used; it typically includes oral dexamethasone 20 mg administered about 12 and 6 hours before paclitaxel, diphenhydramine 50 mg IV 30 to 60 minutes before paclitaxel, and cimetidine (300 mg) or ranitidine (50 mg) IV 30 to 60 minutes before paclitaxel. Courses of paclitaxel are not repeated unless the neutrophil count is at least 1,500/mm^3 and the platelet count is at least 100,000/mm^3. If there is severe neutropenia or peripheral neuropathy, subsequent dosages might be reduced by 20%.

Contact of the undiluted drug with plasticized polyvinyl chloride (PVC) equipment or devices is not recommended, as the plasticizer DEHP may be leached from PVC infusion bags or sets. To minimize client exposure to this plasticizer, diluted paclitaxel solutions should be prepared and stored in glass or polypropylene bottles or polypropylene or polyolefin plastic bags. It should be administered through polyethylene-lined administration sets, and because the drug may contain fibers, there should be a 20- to 22-μm in-line filter at the client end. Solutions are stable for up to 27 hours. Unopened vials must be refrigerated in the original package.

Adverse Reactions. Bone marrow suppression (primarily neutropenia) is dose-dependent and is the major dose-limiting toxicity. Neutropenia is generally rapidly reversible, but it starts on day 8 to 10 of treatment. Recovery is usually complete by day 15 to 21. Neutropenia is not cumulative. In some trials the granulocyte colony-stimulating factor is given to prevent neutropenia. The severity of neutropenia appears related to the length of the infusion. One recommendation is a 20% reduction in dose for subsequent courses of paclitaxel for clients who develop severe neutropenia (less than 500/mm³ for a week or longer). Neutropenia with docetaxel seems more severe than that with paclitaxel.

Cardiotoxicity occurs. Severe conduction abnormalities (eg, bradycardia, heart block, myocardial infarction, atrial arrhythmias, ventricular tachycardia) have been documented. Cardiac monitoring may be used; drug treatment of the abnormality may be needed.

Hypersensitivity reactions to the Cremophor EL or polyoxyethylated castor oil used in paclitaxel's formulation occur. Although these reactions could be caused by paclitaxel itself, the vehicle was thought to be responsible, partly because other drugs formulated in the vehicle (eg, cyclosporine, vitamin K) have been associated with similar reactions. Premedication regimens are used, and minor symptoms of hypersensitivity do not require interruption of therapy; however, severe reactions require paclitaxel discontinuation.

Peripheral neuropathy is common and is characterized by sensory symptoms such as numbness and paresthesia in a glove-and-stocking distribution. Symptoms may begin as soon as 24 hours after treatment with higher doses or after multiple courses at conventional doses. Dose reduction may be recommended if peripheral neuropathy is severe. Motor and autonomic dysfunction may also occur, especially at high doses and in clients with preexisting neuropathies caused by diabetes mellitus and alcoholism. Almost all clients experience alopecia. Liver function can be affected seriously by docetaxel; it should not be used in clients with elevated liver enzyme levels.

Drug Interactions. Paclitaxel interacts with cisplatin and ketoconazole. Paclitaxel metabolism may be inhibited in clients receiving ketoconazole. The concept of sequence-dependent interactions is a factor in the paclitaxel–cisplatin interaction. Bone marrow suppression is more profound when paclitaxel is given after cisplatin than when paclitaxel is given before cisplatin. When given after cisplatin, paclitaxel's clearance is decreased. Sequence-dependent interactions have also been identified in studies of paclitaxel–doxorubicin and paclitaxel–cyclophosphamide regimens.

Precautions and Contraindications. Paclitaxel is contraindicated in clients with hypersensitivity to drugs formulated with polyoxyethylated castor oil, bone marrow suppression, severe neurologic toxicity, pregnancy, or lactation.

■ SUMMARY

Natural products used in antineoplastic drug therapy include topoisomerase inhibitors, mitotic inhibitors, antitumor antibiotics, enzymes, and taxanes. Daunorubicin and doxorubicin both may cause cardiotoxicity, acute or delayed. Vincristine's toxic effects are largely neurologic, affecting the central, autonomic, and peripheral nervous systems. Bleomycin may cause pulmonary toxicity that may be fatal. Mitomycin may cause two types of kidney damage, among other adverse reactions. Plicamycin may cause a bleeding syndrome. Asparaginase has a unique mechanism of action and may also induce serious adverse reactions. Taxanes are the newest natural products and are used for ovarian, breast, and other cancers.

Hormones

Hormones used in antineoplastic therapy include adrenocorticosteroids, androgens, estrogens, antiadrenal agents, antiandrogenic agents, antiestrogenic agents, progestins, estrogen/nitrogen mustard, and gonadotropin-releasing hormone analogs (Tables 47-4 and 47-5).

Adrenocorticosteroids

The adrenocorticosteroids are a group of steroid hormones produced by the adrenal cortex. They have a similar chemical structure but varied physiologic effects. Chapter 30 provides an in-depth discussion of this group of hormones. The major adrenocorticosteroids used in antineoplastic therapy are dexamethasone (Decadron) and prednisone.

The precise mechanism of action of the adrenocorticosteroids is not fully understood. However, in some cancers (eg, breast, lymphoid), the effectiveness of adrenocorticosteroids involves specific steroid receptor proteins in the cytoplasm or nucleus of the tumor cells. For the adrenocorticosteroid to act on lymphoblasts, the hormone must bind to the receptor. The adrenocorticosteroid interferes with mitosis in lymphocytes and lymphoid proliferation and induces cell death. This may result from glucose deprivation. Adrenocorticosteroids are cell cycle-specific and are active in phase G_1. They are used to induce remission in children with ALL, to relieve complications of treatment (eg, hemorrhagic thrombocytopenia), and as components of various chemotherapy regimens, such as MOPP for Hodgkin's

Table 47-4. Hormonal Agents

Drug Name	Preparation	Usual Dosage	Adverse Reactions
Adrenocorticosteroids			
dexamethasone (Decadron)	Oral tablets Elixir Oral solution IM IV	4–16 mg/d in divided doses	Vertigo, headaches, euphoria, insomnia, mood swings, depression, hypertension, fluid and electrolyte disturbances, amenorrhea, irregular menses, myopathy, suppression of hypothalamic–pituitary–adrenal axis, impaired wound healing, masking of signs of infection, petechiae and ecchymoses, thin and fragile skin
prednisone	Oral tablets Oral solution Syrup	Example of regimen: 60 mg/m² PO qd for 4 wk, then taper dose between weeks 5–7	See above
Androgens			
fluoxymesterone (Halotestin)	Oral tablets	*Inoperable breast cancer:* 10–40 mg qd in divided doses; continue for 1 mo for a subjective response and 2–3 mo for an objective response	Fluid retention, hypercalcemia, masculinization (clitorial enlargement, hirsutism, deepening of voice, increased libido, acne), alopecia, erythrocythemia, cholestatic jaundice (with oral therapy), hepatocellular neoplasms (long-term therapy), increased appetite and weight gain (or anorexia, nausea, vomiting at high doses)
methyltestosterone (Android, Oreton, Testered, Virilon)	Oral tablets Oral capsules Buccal tablets	*Breast cancer:* 50–200 mg/d orally; 25–100 mg buccal	See fluoxymesterone
testolactone (Teslac)	Oral	*Palliation in advanced disseminated metastatic breast cancer in postmenopausal women:* 250 mg qid	Paresthesias, nausea, vomiting, anorexia, glossitis
testosterone enanthate (in oil) (long-acting) (Andro L.A. 200, Andropository, Delatestryl, Durathate-200, Everone 200)	IM	*Palliation of inoperable breast cancer in women:* 200–400 mg q2–4 wk	See fluoxymesterone
testosterone cypionate (in oil) (long-acting) (depAndro 100/200, Depotest, Depo-Testosterone, Duratest-100/200)	IM	*Palliation of inoperable breast cancer in women:* 200–400 mg q2–4 wk	See fluoxymesterone
testosterone (short-acting) (Testandro, Histerone, Tesamone)	IM	*Palliation of breast cancer:* 50–100 mg three times a week; short-acting usually preferred to long-acting	See fluoxymesterone
Estrogens			
estrone (Aquest, Estrone 5, Kestrone)	IM	*Inoperable progressing prostatic cancer:* 2–4 mg 3 times/wk, give for 3 mo to evaluate for response; *inoperable progressing breast cancer in appropriately selected men and postmenopausal women:* 5 mg 3 times/wk	Sodium and water retention, nausea, vomiting, thromboembolic complications, hypertension, congestive heart failure, hypercalcemia, changes in libido, anxiety, insomnia *In women:* aggravation of chronic cystic mastitis, uterine fibroids, endometriosis, migraine, breast tenderness, pigmentation of nipples and areola, stress incontinence, uterine bleeding (with high doses or on withdrawal of drug), sensitization to the drug's oil carrier *In men:* feminization, as evidenced by gynecomastia and testicular atrophy, impotence

(continued)

Table 47-4. (Continued)

Drug Name	Preparation	Usual Dosage	Adverse Reactions
Estrogens (continued)			
estradiol (Estrace)	Oral tablets	*Prostatic cancer (androgen-dependent, inoperable, progressing):* 1–2 mg tid *Breast cancer (inoperable, progressing):* 10 mg tid for at least 3 mo	See estrone
estradiol valerate in oil (Delestrogen, Dioval XX, Estra-L 20/40, Gynogen LA, Valergen 20/40)	IM	*Prostatic carcinoma:* 30 mg or more every 1–2 weeks	See estrone
conjugated estrogens (Premarin)	Oral tablets	*Palliation in breast carcinoma:* 10 mg tid for at least 3 mo *Palliation in prostatic carcinoma:* 1.25–2.5 mg tid	See estrone
esterified estrogens (Estratab, Menest)	Oral tablets	*Inoperable, progressing prostatic carcinoma:* 1.25–2.5 mg tid *Inoperable, progressing breast cancer in appropriately selected men and postmenopausal women:* 10 mg tid for at least 3 mo	See estrone
ethinyl estradiol (Estinyl)	Oral tablets	*Inoperable, progressing breast cancer in appropriately selected postmenopausal women:* 1 mg tid *Inoperable, progressing prostatic carcinoma:* 0.15–2 mg/d	See estrone
diethylstilbestrol (DES)	Oral tablets	*Inoperable, progressing prostatic carcinoma:* 1–3 mg/d initially, increased in advanced cases *Inoperable, progressing breast cancer in appropriately selected men and postmenopausal women:* 15 mg/d	See estrone
chlorotrianisene (Tace)	Oral capsules	*Inoperable, progressing prostatic carcinoma:* 12–25 mg/d	See estrone
polyestradiol phosphate (Estradurin)	IM	*Inoperable, progressing prostatic cancer:* 40 mg IM q2–4 wk or less frequently	Hypertension, nausea, fluid retention, leg cramps, thromboembolic disorders
Estrogen/Nitrogen Mustard			
estramustine phosphate sodium (Emcyt)	Oral capsules	*Palliative treatment of metastatic or progressive carcinoma of prostate:* 10–16 mg/kg/d in 3 or 4 divided doses	Nausea, vomiting, anorexia, diarrhea, lethargy, emotional lability, insomnia, headache, anxiety, breast tenderness and enlargement, cutaneous reactions, cardiotoxicity
Progestins			
medroxyprogesterone acetate (Depo-Provera)	IM	*Adjunctive therapy and palliative treatment of inoperable, recurrent, and metastatic endometrial carcinoma:* 400–1,000 mg/wk IM	Breakthrough bleeding, spotting, change in menstrual flow, amenorrhea, rash with or without pruritus, acne, fluid retention, edema, increase or decrease in weight
megestrol acetate (Megace)	Oral suspension	*Palliative treatment of advanced carcinoma of breast or endometrium:* 400–800 mg or 10–20 mL/d *Anorexia, cachexia, weight loss in AIDS:* 400–800 mg or 10–20 mL/d	Diarrhea, impotence, rash, flatulence, headache

disease and CVP (cyclophosphamide, vincristine, prednisone) and CHOP (cyclophosphamide, doxorubicin [Adriamycin], vincristine, prednisone) for non-Hodgkin's lymphoma. They are sometimes used in radiation therapy to reduce radiation edema in the mediastinum, brain, and spinal cord. Adrenocorticosteroids may also be indicated for specific complications, such as hypercalcemia and nausea and vomiting, and for palliation and symptom relief because they can decrease pain and fever and increase appetite, strength, and sense of well-being. If the client's general physical condition improves, additional antineoplastic drug therapy may proceed.

A typical daily dosage of prednisone is 10 to 100 mg. For the regimen used in treating ALL, the daily

Table 47-5. Antihormonal Agents

Drug Name	Preparation	Usual Dosage	Adverse Reactions
Antiadrenal			
aminoglutethimide (Cytadren)	Oral tablets	250 mg qid	Drowsiness, rash, nausea, anorexia
Antiandrogen			
flutamide (Eulexin)	Oral capsules	*Metastatic prostatic carcinoma, in combination with LHRH analog:* 2 capsules 3 times a day at 8-hour intervals for total daily dosage of 750 mg	Diarrhea, nausea, vomiting, body pain, hot flashes, anemia, leukopenia, impotence, loss of libido, rash, gynecomastia
bicalutamide (Casodex)	Oral tablets	*Advanced prostate cancer, in combination with LHRH analog:* 50 mg tablet once daily, morning or evening, same time each day	See flutamide
Antiestrogen			
tamoxifen citrate (Nolvadex)	Oral tablets	20 mg/d	Nausea, vomiting, hot flashes, vaginal discharge, irregular menses, thrombophlebitis, weight gain or loss, fluid retention, skin changes, diarrhea, depression
Gonadotropin-Releasing Hormone Analogs			
leuprolide acetate (Lupron)	SC IM	*Advanced prostate cancer:* 1 mq qd; Depot 7.5 mg IM monthly; Depot–3 Month 22.5 mg q3mo	Disease flare, peripheral edema, hot flashes, impotence, decreased libido
goserelin acetate (Zoladex)	SC implant	Monthly 3.6-mg SC implant, or 10.8-mg SC implant q12wk	Hot flashes, impotence

prednisone dosage is typically 60 mg/m² orally for 4 weeks; the dose is tapered between weeks 5 and 7 to minimize the likelihood of complications (eg, infections, acute adrenocortical insufficiency). Prednisone is eventually discontinued in most cases.

Dexamethasone is used when an adrenocorticosteroid is combined with radiation therapy. The drug may be given orally, IM, or IV. The usual dosage is 4 to 16 mg/day in divided doses.

Some adverse reactions to adrenocorticosteroids with short-term use include sodium and water retention, potassium loss, psychosis, and exacerbation of diabetes. Adverse effects with prolonged use may be myopathy, osteoporosis, aseptic necrosis of bone, peptic ulceration, pancreatitis, pseudotumor cerebri, glaucoma, cataracts, hypertension, obesity, hyperlipidemia, immunosuppression, impaired wound healing, infection, striae of the skin, growth failure, amenorrhea, and suppression of the hypothalamic–pituitary–adrenal axis.

Androgens and Estrogens

A detailed discussion of estrogens and androgens is found in Unit IX; the discussion in this chapter is confined to the use of estrogens and androgens in antineoplastic therapy. The rationale for using estrogens and androgens is that some tumors (eg, breast, prostate) are hormone-sensitive. Neoplastic processes can be changed to some degree by changing the hormonal environment of such tumors.

Androgens

Androgens can be used in the palliative management of estrogen receptor-positive metastatic breast carcinoma in postmenopausal women. Androgens have induced objective responses in up to 50% of such clients, and these responses have lasted 12 to 14 months. Soft-tissue metastases are the most responsive, followed by bone metastases. Metastases to the viscera are the least responsive.

The most common adverse reaction to androgen therapy is masculinization: hirsutism, deepening of the voice, acne, clitoral enlargement, increased libido, and amenorrhea. The extent of virilization is related to the specific androgen, the dose, and the duration of treatment. Testolactone (Teslac) seems to produce the least masculinization.

Androgens may also produce fluid retention, cholestatic jaundice, hypercalcemia, alopecia, and erythrocythemia. If hypercalcemia develops, the androgen should be discontinued immediately (see discussion under estrogen therapy and hypercalcemia). Androgens have also caused a rare condition called peliosis hepatis (blood-filled cysts in the liver), hepatic adenomas, and hepatomas.

Estrogens

Pharmacodynamics. Estrogen is used for breast cancer in postmenopausal women and for prostatic cancer in men to change the hormonal environment of the tumor. Estrogen receptor and progesterone receptor determinations should be made on all breast cancer clients. If the breast cancer is positive for receptors for both estrogen and progesterone, the chances of response to hormonal manipulation are greater.

Pharmacokinetics. Estrogens are well absorbed from the GI tract after oral administration. They are metabolized in the liver. They are primarily excreted in urine, although small amounts are also eliminated through the bile in feces.

Therapeutic Uses. Estrogens provide palliative management of estrogen receptor-positive metastatic breast carcinoma in postmenopausal women and of advanced carcinoma of the prostate.

Estrogen may produce positive responses in metastatic breast disease of soft tissues and bone that may last 6 to 12 months or even years. It may take 8 to 12 weeks before the effectiveness of the hormonal therapy can be gauged. If hormonal therapy is beneficial, it should be continued until symptoms recur. At the time of exacerbation, discontinuing the hormone may produce another remission. Despite this positive discussion of estrogen use, the antiestrogenic compound tamoxifen citrate is often used instead of an estrogen preparation.

Estrogens and orchiectomy remove 90% of circulating testosterone in prostate cancer, the most common male cancer in the United States. Diethylstilbestrol (DES) is often the agent of choice to change the hormonal environment of the prostatic tumor. It is inexpensive and effective by oral administration, and its rate of activation is relatively slow, allowing small doses to be given once a day. If the client is older than age 75, another endocrine therapy may be used because DES is associated with cardiotoxicity.

Dosage and Administration. Dosages and routes of administration for estrogens and androgens are summarized in Table 47-4. Several are given orally.

Adverse Reactions. Severe fluid retention, especially in clients with cardiovascular, liver, or renal disease, is an adverse effect of estrogen in clients with cancer. Death has occurred from cardiac complications. The liver inactivates estrogens, so toxic effects may be more severe in clients with hepatic damage.

Gynecomastia occurs often in males. In rare instances, carcinoma of the breast has occurred in men given estrogen for prolonged periods. The combination of hormone and bone metastasis may result in significant hypercalcemia, which can cause renal calculi, polyuria, neurologic changes, and cardiac arrhythmias.

Drug Interactions. There are no known significant drug interactions.

Precautions and Contraindications. Because of the possibility of hypercalcemia, plasma calcium levels should be routinely monitored during estrogen therapy. If an elevated serum calcium level is found, a high fluid intake should be maintained, and the hormone may be discontinued until hypercalcemia resolves.

Estrogen therapy for breast cancer is contraindicated in premenopausal women because estrogen in these clients may accelerate the neoplastic process. Clients should be at least 5 years postmenopausal before they receive estrogen therapy.

Estramustine Phosphate Sodium

Estramustine phosphate sodium (Emcyt) contains an estrogen (estradiol) and nitrogen mustard.

Pharmacodynamics. The intact molecule of estramustine phosphate sodium acts as a weak alkylating agent by promoting microtubule disassembly, and after hydrolysis the released estrogen exerts an antigonadotropin effect.

Pharmacokinetics. The drug is absorbed from the GI tract and reaches a peak action in 2 to 3 hours. It is metabolized in the liver and excreted in feces.

Therapeutic Uses. Estramustine phosphate sodium is used for palliative treatment of metastatic or progressive carcinoma of the prostate. Effects may not be apparent for several weeks, so the drug must be administered for 30 to 90 days before deciding if the effects are therapeutic or not.

Dosage and Administration. The dosage is 10 to 16 mg/kg/day in three or four divided doses. It is available as oral capsules that should be refrigerated (although they are stable for up to 48 hours out of the refrigerator if necessary).

Adverse Reactions. Adverse reactions include nausea, vomiting, anorexia, and diarrhea, as well as lethargy, emotional lability, insomnia, headache, anxiety, breast tenderness, and mild to moderate breast enlargement. Dermatologic reactions include rash, pruritus, dry skin, and peeling skin or fingertips. Cardiovascular effects include edema, dyspnea, leg cramps, elevated blood pressure, thrombophlebitis, myocardial infarction, pulmonary emboli, and congestive heart failure.

Drug Interactions. No significant interactions have been identified.

Precautions and Contraindications. This drug should be used cautiously in clients with coronary artery or cerebrovascular disorders, epilepsy, migraines, impaired renal or hepatic function, metabolic bone disease with hypercalcemia, and diabetes. It is contraindicated in clients with an allergy to estradiol or nitrogen mustard, active thrombophlebitis, or thromboembolic disorders.

Progestins

About 80% of localized endometrial cancer is cured by surgery and radiation therapy. Clients with more widespread inoperable disease or those with recurrent disease after local treatment are often treated with progestins. About 35% of these clients respond positively with remissions in pulmonary, bone, hepatic, intra-abdominal, and pelvic metastases. Some remissions last for years. Progestin therapy also helps relieve pain and promotes a sense of well-being. It appears that response to progestins depends on the presence of progesterone receptors in the tumor. Treatment continues until the disease recurs.

Several progestins are available, but the primary ones used in cancer therapy are medroxyprogesterone acetate (Depo-Provera) for endometrial carcinoma and megestrol acetate (Megace), which is also used for treating anorexia, cachexia, or an unexplained, significant weight loss in clients with AIDS. Medroxyprogesterone acetate is usually given at a dosage of 400 to 1,000 mg/week IM. The recommended adult dosage of megestrol acetate, in oral suspension, is 20 mL/day. The container must be shaken well before use.

Adverse reactions to progestins are usually minimal. They may cause menstrual irregularities, edema, weight gain or loss, rash with or without pruritus, and diarrhea.

Antihormonal and Antiadrenal Agents

Antihormonal agents are summarized in Table 47-5. They include agents such as the antiadrenal drug aminoglutethimide. They reduce the synthesis of steroids.

Aminoglutethimide blocks the enzymatic conversion of cholesterol to pregnenolone at the first step in adrenal corticosteroid biosynthesis. It inhibits an enzyme that converts androstenedione to estrone and estradiol in extra-adrenal tissues. Because the adrenal gland is the principal source of estrogens in postmenopausal women, aminoglutethimide lowers plasma estrogen levels and is as effective as surgical adrenalectomy in the treatment of postmenopausal women with estrogen receptor-positive advanced breast cancer. It is sometimes used as an alternative to tamoxifen therapy. Durations of response average 14 to 30 months and occur primarily in soft-tissue and bone metastases. In this situation, aminoglutethimide is given with replacement hydrocortisone to prevent reflex ACTH hypersecretion from overcoming adrenal inhibition.

Aminoglutethimide is also used to suppress adrenal function in some clients with adrenal adenoma, adrenal carcinoma, and ectopic ACTH-secreting tumors. The drug does not affect the underlying disease, so if therapy stops, excess production of adrenal corticoids will begin again.

Antiandrogenic Compounds

Flutamide (Eulexin) and bicalutamide (Casodex) are antiandrogenic compounds.

Pharmacodynamics. Flutamide acts either to inhibit the uptake of androgen or to inhibit the nuclear binding of androgen in target tissues. Bicalutamide competitively inhibits the action of androgens by binding to cytosol androgen receptors in the target tissue. Thus, the effect of androgen in androgen-sensitive tissues is decreased.

Pharmacokinetics. Flutamide and bicalutamide are absorbed through the GI system after oral administration. Flutamide is highly bound to plasma proteins and rapidly metabolized in the liver, and its metabolites are mainly excreted in urine. Bicalutamide and its metabolite are excreted in urine and feces.

Therapeutic Uses. Flutamide and bicalutamide are used in combination with leuprolide acetate (see below) to treat metastatic prostatic carcinoma. Treatment must be initiated simultaneously with both drugs for maximum benefit.

Dosage and Administration. Flutamide is available as 125-mg capsules; the usual dosage is two capsules every 8 hours, for a total daily dose of 750 mg. Bicalutamide is available as 50-mg tablets, and one tablet is taken daily (morning or evening) with or without food. It should be taken at the same time each day.

Adverse Reactions. Because these agents and leuprolide acetate are given concomitantly, it is difficult to distinguish which side effects are due to which drug. However, diarrhea seems more attributable to flutamide and bicalutamide. Nausea, vomiting, body pain, hot flashes, anemia, leukopenia, impotence, loss of libido, rash, and gynecomastia occur.

Drug Interactions. Bicalutamide can displace coumarin anticoagulants from their protein-binding sites, increasing the anticoagulant effect.

Antiestrogenic Compounds

Tamoxifen citrate (Nolvadex) is a nonsteroidal antiestrogen first designed for use as a contraceptive. It was first used to treat advanced breast cancer in the early 1970s. Analysis of 10 years of data on 30,000 women with breast cancer from 40 different trials has shown that the administration of tamoxifen for 1 to 2 years results in a 17% reduction in the chance of death (Varricchio & Johnson, 1993). The data also show a 35% decrease in the occurrence of contralateral breast cancer in clients who received tamoxifen when compared with clients in the control group. It is the most widely prescribed endocrine agent for treating breast cancer in the United States. See the Critical Thinking Challenge: Research Analysis.

Pharmacodynamics. The discovery of estrogen receptors as a biochemical marker for the hormonal dependence of many breast tumors led to the use of estrogen receptor assays to predict tumor response. The absence of the estrogen receptor in a breast tumor predicts that it is less likely to respond to hormone therapy than is a tumor with a higher estrogen receptor content.

CRITICAL THINKING CHALLENGE
Research Analysis

Read WW Crabbe's 1996 article, "The tamoxifen controversy," in Oncology Nursing Forum, and consider these questions.

1. Should tamoxifen be used to treat breast cancer when it seems to cause another type of cancer (endometrial) in a few persons? Can you find other examples of this controversy in the literature?

2. You are caring for a client receiving tamoxifen. She tells you that she saw a television program about tamoxifen and cancer risk and is thinking of discontinuing the drug. What is your role in this situation? What would you say to her?

3. You were a participant in the Breast Cancer Prevention Trial that is using tamoxifen, and at the end of the study you were told you had received a placebo, not the drug. Five years after the end of the study, you are diagnosed with breast cancer. How would you feel?

Tamoxifen's effects appear to be related to its ability to compete with estradiol for binding to estrogen receptors on the cancer cell membrane, thus interfering with the cell's use of estrogen needed for cell proliferation (tumor growth). Laboratory data show that estrogen receptor-positive tumors treated with tamoxifen are arrested in the G_0/G_1 phase of the cell cycle, immediately after mitosis (Rich, 1993).

Tamoxifen may inhibit replication by additional mechanisms as well. It inhibits the production of several important growth factors that stimulate tumor cell growth, including growth factor-alpha, epidermal growth factor, and insulin-like growth factor. Tamoxifen also enhances the production of transforming growth factor-beta, an inhibitor of breast tumor cell growth. Other antiproliferative effects from tamoxifen may arise from an inhibition of protein kinase C[27] or a change in calmodulin function.

Tamoxifen may act as pure antiestrogen or as an estrogen, depending on the target organ and other factors. Its estrogen-antagonizing effects seem to be tissue-specific to the breasts, suggesting that tamoxifen might be a chemopreventive agent against breast cancer in women who are at increased risk for the disease. In addition, the estrogen-agonistic effects of tamoxifen are thought to offer some protection against osteoporosis and cardiovascular disease in postmenopausal women.

In organs such as the uterus, tamoxifen can have a stimulatory or estrogenic effect. Circulating estrogen levels reportedly increase in premenopausal women treated for advanced breast cancer. Uterine cancer is a known but uncommon complication of tamoxifen therapy (about 0.3% of women taking tamoxifen 40 mg/

day). The incidence of the endometrial cancer is not altogether clear because estimates vary from study to study; also, additional studies are needed to evaluate the impact of dose and duration of therapy on its incidence (Barakat, 1995). The increased risk of endometrial cancer does not appear to outweigh the advantage tamoxifen confers by controlling breast cancer. However, the issue is less clear for the chemopreventive trial, where tamoxifen is used in healthy women to try to prevent breast cancer. For postmenopausal women with a natural absence of ovarian function, treatment with tamoxifen proceeds without an increase in serum estrogen levels.

Pharmacokinetics. Tamoxifen is absorbed after oral administration. Peak concentration in the blood occurs in 3 to 6 hours. After metabolism in the liver, tamoxifen's metabolites are slowly excreted in bile and feces. The half-life varies but seems to be about 7 days. Small amounts are eliminated in urine, but excretion does not seem to be affected by decreased renal function.

Therapeutic Uses. Tamoxifen is used for advanced breast cancer in premenopausal and postmenopausal women. In 1992, work began on the first Breast Cancer Prevention Trial, sponsored by the National Surgical Adjuvant Breast and Bowel Project. The trial's primary objective is to evaluate the role of long-term tamoxifen therapy in preventing breast cancer in high-risk women. The trial will study 16,000 women for 5 years.

Dosage and Administration. Tamoxifen is administered orally at a standard dose of 20 mg/day. Measurable responses may occur in 4 to 10 weeks or may be further delayed in clients with bone metastases.

Adverse Reactions. Adverse reactions are less common and are milder with tamoxifen than with estrogens or androgens. The most common reactions are nausea and vomiting and hot flashes. One small study found that the hot flashes began 3 days to 4 weeks after the beginning of tamoxifen therapy and lasted a few seconds to 30 minutes. Occurrence varied from only at night to eight to 10 times a day. Hot flashes interfered with activities of daily living (McDaniel et al., 1995).

Vaginal discharge, irregular menses, and thrombophlebitis occur. Transient decreases in platelet and white blood cell counts have been noted. Other side effects include weight gain or loss, fluid retention, skin changes, diarrhea, and depression.

Rare ophthalmic effects (corneal changes, macular edema, optic neuritis, retinopathy) have been reported. A few cases of serious retinal or corneal damage have been reported and seem related to the use of large doses (120–160 mg twice a day for more than a year).

The estrogenic effects of tamoxifen may be implicated in a decrease in circulating levels of antithrombin III, predisposing the client to an increased risk of thromboembolic disorders. It may be that women with a history of thromboembolic disorders should not receive long-term tamoxifen therapy. The reduced levels of antithrombin III are rarely out of the normal range. This phenomenon is similar to that seen with women using oral contraceptives.

A rare complication is hepatotoxicity. Two cases of hepatocellular carcinoma have been reported in tamoxifen users, during a period when the clients were taking 40 mg of tamoxifen daily.

Studies indicate that tamoxifen helps maintain bone density in postmenopausal women, with the possibility of a small increase in bone density.

Drug Interactions. An interaction between tamoxifen and warfarin has been identified, occasionally resulting in life-threatening bleeding episodes. This interaction is probably related to the displacement of warfarin from protein-binding sites by tamoxifen. Prothrombin times must be closely monitored when this combination is used. There also may be an increase in bilirubin and aminotransferase levels.

Precautions and Contraindications. Tamoxifen is contraindicated in pregnancy and lactation.

Gonadotropin-Releasing Hormone Analogs

Leuprolide acetate (Lupron) and goserelin acetate (Zoladex) are synthetic analogs of luteinizing hormone-releasing hormone (LHRH). They are an alternative treatment for prostate cancer. They are more potent than natural LHRH. Leuprolide and goserelin reduce the amount of testosterone available for conversion, thereby inhibiting the growth of prostate cancer.

Pharmacodynamics. Initial doses of leuprolide or goserelin increase the production of luteinizing hormone (LH) and follicle-stimulating hormone (FSH) in the pituitary gland, resulting in transient increases in testosterone and dihydrotestosterone in males. With prolonged administration, LH and FSH receptors are down-regulated in the pituitary gland, thereby eventually decreasing gonadotropin secretion and ultimately decreasing testosterone to castration levels, which persist up to 3 years. These agents are considered as effective as surgical removal of the testicles (orchiectomy) in lowering testosterone levels.

Therapeutic Uses. Leuprolide and goserelin are effective in the palliative treatment of advanced prostate cancer when alternative treatment (eg, orchiectomy, estrogen) is not indicated or is unacceptable to the client.

Other uses for leuprolide include endometriosis, central precocious puberty, and uterine leiomyomata (fibroids). Goserelin is being evaluated in conjunction with radiation therapy for the treatment of early prostate cancer and for disease that involves the pelvic lymph nodes. It has also been used in advanced breast cancer and endometriosis.

Dosage and Administration. Leuprolide is available as a solution for injection; 1 mg as a single daily SC injection is the usual dose. Leuprolide is also available in depot preparations.

Goserelin is available in preloaded, single-use, disposable syringes. There are two depot preparations, one given monthly and the other given every 3 months. Goserelin is actually a dry drug pellet that is implanted in the soft tissue of the abdomen via SC injection. There, it gradually dissolves over 28 days. The injection process can include injection of a local anesthetic bleb (eg, lidocaine) to minimize discomfort, because the needle is large (16-gauge).

Adverse Reactions. Initial stimulation of gonadotropin release and sex steroid production may cause the disease to flare up during the first weeks of therapy. Hot flashes are common, but they decrease over time.

◼ SUMMARY

Various hormones are used in antineoplastic therapy. Adrenocorticosteroids are used in combination with other agents or alone to treat complications or for palliation. Estrogens and androgens are used to change the hormonal environment in prostate and breast carcinomas. Progestins may be beneficial with endometrial cancer. An antiestrogenic agent, tamoxifen citrate, is the drug of choice for palliative treatment of advanced breast cancer in premenopausal and postmenopausal women. Other newer agents include antiandrogenic agents, an estrogen–nitrogen mustard combination, and gonadotropin-releasing hormone analogs that are being used in various ways as antitumor agents.

Biologic Response Modifiers

The therapeutic use of biologic agents is emerging as the fourth modality of cancer therapy (joining surgery, radiation therapy, and chemotherapy). Biologic response modifiers (BRMs) include the monoclonal antibodies, cytokines (interferons, colony-stimulating factors, interleukins), and tumor necrosis factor. Much work with BRMs remains investigational.

Biologic response modifiers are immunomodulating agents; that is, they can enhance or suppress the body's immune responses. Certain disorders may be responsive to this approach, including cancer, immunodeficiency diseases, some types of viral and fungal infections, and certain autoimmune disorders. These agents work on the cellular or humoral immune aspects, or both. They tend to be more effective when the disease entity or tumor mass is quantitatively small. For this reason, although some are being studied for use as single agents, some are believed to have the greatest potential in combination with other antineoplastic agents or cancer treatment modalities. The BRMs are discussed in detail in Chapter 35.

Miscellaneous Agents

Several antineoplastic agents that do not fit into the established categories are listed as miscellaneous agents: analog of somatostatin, anastrozole, cladribine, hydroxyurea, mitotane, procarbazine, and retinoic acid all-trans. Table 47-6 lists these preparations and their dosage and adverse reactions.

Analog of Somatostatin

Pharmacodynamics. Octreotide acetate (Sandostatin) is a hormonal agent with effects similar to those of the natural hormone somatostatin. It acts on the anterior pituitary to inhibit growth hormone and thyrotropin and on the pancreas to inhibit insulin and glucagon. It inhibits the release of serotonin and gastrin from the GI tract, decreases GI blood flow, motility, and carbohydrate absorption, and increases water and electrolyte absorption.

Therapeutic Uses. Octreotide is used in metastatic carcinoid tumors to suppress or inhibit the associated severe diarrhea and flushing episodes. It is also indicated for the treatment of the profuse watery diarrhea associated with vasoactive intestinal polypeptide tumors (VIPomas). It has demonstrated activity in pancreatic neoplasia and GI and pancreatic fistulas.

Dosage and Administration. Administration should be by SC injection, but it may be given IV as a bolus in an emergency. The initial dosage is 50 µg once or twice a day. For carcinoid tumors, 100 to 600 µg is given daily

Table 47-6. Miscellaneous Antineoplastic Drugs

Drug Name	Uses	Usual Dosage	Adverse Reactions
anastrozole (Arimidex)	Nonsteroidal aromatase inhibitor for treatment of advanced breast cancer in postmenopausal women with disease progression after use of tamoxifen	1 mg PO once daily	Nausea, vomiting, headache, hot flashes, pain, dyspnea, cough, diarrhea or constipation
cladribine (Leustatin)	Hairy cell leukemia, investigational uses	0.09 mg/kg in 500 mL 0.9% sodium chloride, infused IV continuously for 24 h; repeat for 7 d	Neutropenia, fatigue, nausea, rash, headache, bone marrow suppression
hydroxyurea (Hydrea)	Chronic myelocytic leukemia, malignant melanoma, metastatic or inoperable cancer of ovary, with radiation therapy in carcinomas of head and neck	*Intermittent therapy:* 80 mg/kg as a single oral dose q3d *Continuous therapy:* 20–30 mg/kg as single daily dose *Concomitant therapy with irradiation:* 80 mg/kg as single dose q3d	Bone marrow suppression, drowsiness
octreotide acetate (Sandostatin)	Carcinoid tumors, vasoactive intestinal polypeptide tumors (VIPomas)	50 µg qd or bid initially, usually SC, then for carcinoid tumors 100–600 µg qd in 2–4 doses for 2 wk or for VIPomas 200–300 µg in 2–4 doses for 2 wk	Nausea, vomiting, dizziness, headache, diarrhea, abdominal pain, weakness
mitotane (Lysodren)	Palliation of inoperable carcinoma of adrenal cortex	2–6 g/d orally in divided doses tid or qid	Depression, sedation, lethargy, vertigo, dizziness, nausea, vomiting, diarrhea, anorexia, rash, adrenal insufficiency
porfimer sodium (Photofrin)	Selected cases of esophageal or bronchial cancer	IV dosage, followed by laser light treatment	Photosensitivity, constipation
procarbazine (Matulane)	Advanced Hodgkin's disease (MOPP regimen), primary and metastatic brain tumors, small cell lung cancer	2–4 mg/kg/d PO for first wk, maintain dose at 4–6 mg/kg/d until white blood cell count falls below 4,000 mm³ or platelets below 100,000 mm³, then stop drug and allow for hematologic recovery; may then resume treatment	Severe nausea and vomiting, pleural effusion, cough, coma, bone marrow suppression, infection
tretinoin (Vesanoid)	Acute promyelocytic leukemia	PO 45 mg/m²/d given as 2 evenly divided doses until complete remission is documented	Headache, nausea, vomiting, bone and joint pain, dry lips and skin, nasal congestion, rash

in two to four divided doses for the first 2 weeks. For VIPomas, 200 to 300 μg is given daily in two to four divided doses for the first 2 weeks. Ampules should be stored at 36°F to 46°F, but letting the solution reach room temperature before injection decreases the incidence of pain at the injection site.

Plasma clearance is reduced in clients with renal dysfunction, and dosage reduction is recommended.

Adverse Reactions. Octreotide can cause various adverse reactions, but they are generally mild to moderate. The most common side effects are nausea, vomiting, dizziness, headache, diarrhea, abdominal pain, and weakness.

Drug Interactions. Octreotide has various effects on endogenous hormones, so clients who receive therapy for diabetes or thyroid conditions must be monitored carefully. It seems to interfere with diazoxide, insulin, beta-adrenergic blocking agents, and sulfonylureas.

Precautions and Contraindications. Octreotide should be used cautiously in clients with renal impairment, diabetes mellitus, or thyroid disease and in pregnancy and lactation.

Anastrozole

Anastrozole (Arimidex) is a nonsteroidal aromatase inhibitor that lowers the serum estradiol concentration but has no detectable effect on the formation of adrenal corticosteroids or aldosterone. In postmenopausal women, the principal source of estrogen (primarily estradiol) is conversion of adrenally generated androstenedione to estrone by aromatase in peripheral tissues, such as adipose tissue, with further conversion of estrone to estradiol. Many breast cancers have estrogen receptors, and growth of the tumor can be stimulated by estrogens. This drug can decrease a source of estrogen. It is indicated in the treatment of advanced breast cancer in postmenopausal women with disease progression after tamoxifen therapy. Anastrozole is generally well tolerated. The principal adverse reaction is diarrhea.

Cladribine

Cladribine (Leustatin) is a synthetic antineoplastic agent approved in 1993. It inhibits both DNA synthesis and repair. It is phosphorylated and then accumulates intracellularly and is converted to triphosphate deoxynucleotide. Cells containing high concentrations of deoxynucleotides cannot properly repair single-strand DNA breaks. There is also evidence that triphosphate deoxynucleotide is incorporated into the DNA of dividing cells, resulting in impaired DNA synthesis. Cladribine is used to treat hairy cell leukemia. Typically, an IV infusion of 0.09 mg/kg/day is given for 7 consecutive days. Investigational uses include cutaneous T-cell lymphoma, chronic lymphocytic leukemia, non-Hodgkin's lymphoma, acute myeloid leukemia, autoimmune hemolytic anemia, and mycosis fungoides. Adverse reactions include neutropenia, fatigue, nausea, rash, and headache. Bone marrow suppression may be severe but reversible. Infections occur. Clients receiving cladribine are at risk for nephrotoxicity and neurotoxicity.

Hydroxyurea

Hydroxyurea (Hydrea) inhibits the enzyme ribonucleoside diphosphate reductase. This enzyme normally catalyzes the conversion of ribonucleotides to deoxyribonucleotides. In the absence of deoxyribonucleotides, DNA cannot be made. The drug is specific for the S phase of the cell cycle. Hydroxyurea is used for managing myeloproliferative disorders, primarily chronic myelocytic leukemia. It has produced temporary remissions with malignant melanoma and metastatic or inoperable ovarian carcinoma. Because cells are highly sensitive to irradiation in the G_1 phase of the cell cycle, combinations of hydroxyurea and irradiation cause synergistic toxicity in vitro. Thus, hydroxyurea has been used in combination with radiation therapy in carcinomas of the head and neck. Myelosuppression is a major adverse reaction, but bone marrow recovery is prompt after stopping therapy. This feature distinguishes hydroxyurea from busulfan, which is also used to manage chronic myelocytic leukemia.

Levamisole

The mechanism of action of levamisole hydrochloride in combination with fluorouracil is unknown. Levamisole has complex effects on the immune system and appears to restore depressed immune function. It can stimulate formation of antibodies to various antigens, enhance T-cell responses by stimulating T-cell activation and proliferation, potentiate monocyte and macrophage functions, including phagocytosis and chemotaxis, and increase neutrophil mobility, adherence, and chemotaxis. Levamisole has been used in combination with fluorouracil (see Chap. 46) as adjuvant therapy after surgical resection to treat Dukes' stage C colon cancer. Adverse reactions include nausea, vomiting, diarrhea, taste perversion, and altered sense of smell. Bone marrow suppression, arthralgia, myalgia, pruritus, skin discoloration, rash, and alopecia occur.

Mitotane

Mitotane (Lysodren) is a structural analog of two insecticides: DDD and DDT. The drug is selectively toxic to cells of the adrenal cortex, but normal cells and tumor cells are both damaged. Mitotane is used in the palliative management of inoperable carcinoma of the adrenal cortex. The mean duration of response is about 10 months. This drug is administered orally at 2 to 6 g/day, given in divided doses three or four times a day. If no clinical benefits occur after 3 months, the drug is discontinued. The drug is metabolized by the liver, excreted in urine and bile, and stored in tissues (primarily fat). Therefore, the active drug remains in the body for weeks after administration. The primary adverse effects of mitotane are depression, sedation, lethargy, vertigo, and dizziness, as well as nausea, vomiting, diarrhea, anorexia, and rash. Adrenal insufficiency is likely to develop because of mitotane's action on the adrenal cortex, and adrenal steroid replacement therapy may be necessary. The drug must be administered cautiously to clients with impaired liver function because drug metabolism might be impaired and the drug would accumulate at toxic levels. Mitotane does not cause the common antineoplastic adverse reactions of bone marrow suppression and GI inflammation.

Porfimer Sodium

Porfimer (Photofrin) is a photosensitizing agent used in the photodynamic therapy of tumors. The antitumor actions of porfimer are light- and oxygen-dependent. Photodynamic therapy with porfimer is a two-stage process. The first stage is the IV injection of porfimer. Clearance of porfimer from many tissues occurs over 40 to 72 hours, but tumors retain porfimer for a longer period. Illumination with a laser light is the second stage of therapy. The porfimer is activated by the light and causes cellular damage to the tumor.

This therapy has been used for a select group of clients with esophageal or bronchial cancer, including those with small, early cancers who are considered inoperable for medical reasons and those with multiple small tumors. This therapy does not eradicate tumors that have metastasized to lymph nodes. Systemic adverse reactions include photosensitivity and mild constipation. Clients must avoid sunlight and bright indoor light.

Procarbazine

The mechanism of action of procarbazine (Matulane) is unclear, but it appears to be a prodrug that requires activation; the end product is an alkylating agent. The drug appears to inhibit DNA, RNA, and protein synthesis. It seems to be activated by the cytochrome P450 mixed-function oxidase system of the liver to several metabolites. Procarbazine is cell cycle-nonspecific. Its primary use is in advanced Hodgkin's disease as part of the MOPP regimen. Procarbazine has also shown activity in primary and metastatic brain tumors and small cell lung cancer. It has been used as an immunosuppressant in clients with systemic lupus erythematosus and for suppression of graft-versus-host disease in bone marrow transplantation. Adverse reactions include severe nausea and vomiting, bone marrow suppression, and peripheral neuropathy.

Ingestion of alcohol along with procarbazine can result in a disulfiram-like response. Procarbazine also may enhance the effects of CNS depressants. Because procarbazine inhibits monoamine oxidase, the consumption of tyramine-containing foods may precipitate a hypertensive crisis (see Chap. 6).

Tretinoin

Tretinoin (trans-retinoic acid, Veasnoid) was approved in 1995 and is related to retinol (vitamin A). Vitamin A and its analogs (retinoids) are essential for epithelial cell differentiation. In animal models, retinoids have delayed the appearance, retarded the growth, and caused regression of cancers of the skin, GI tract, breast, and other tissues. One use of tretinoin is to treat premalignant lesions such as actinic keratoses and dysplastic nevi. This agent decreases the proliferation of acute promyelocytic leukemia (APL) cells and is used in the induction phase of treatment for APL. About 25% of clients with APL treated with this agent have experienced the retinoic acid–APL syndrome, characterized by fever, dyspnea, weight gain, pulmonary infiltrates, and pleural or pericardial effusions. This syndrome is sometimes accompanied by impaired myocardial contractility and hypotension and death.

❖ NURSING MANAGEMENT: CLIENT EXPERIENCING EXTRAVASATION OF AN ANTINEOPLASTIC AGENT

The nursing management and client education principles discussed in Chapter 46 also apply to clients receiving the drugs discussed in this chapter. The management of extravasation of antineoplastic drugs is discussed here because the number of antineoplastic vesicants is significant and several are discussed in this chapter (eg, vinca alkaloids, anthracycline antibiotics). Extravasation of an antineoplastic agent can be a serious problem, as vesicants can cause significant soft-tissue damage, loss of function, infection, and tissue necrosis requiring surgery.

NURSING PROCESS

ASSESSMENT

Early detection of extravasation is most likely to minimize soft-tissue damage. Common signs and symptoms of extravasation are swelling (most common); stinging, burning, or pain at the injection site (not always present); redness (seldom seen initially); and lack of blood return (not always indicative of extravasation). The signs of extravasation may not be immediately evident but may be noted several hours later.

NURSING DIAGNOSIS

One nursing diagnosis that applies to several agents discussed in Chapter 46 and a few discussed in this chapter is:

* Impaired Tissue Integrity, related to irritation and sloughing secondary to extravasation of vesicant drugs

PLANNING

In preparing a care plan for a client receiving a potential vesicant, one desirable outcome is absence of extravasation.

INTERVENTION

Prevention of injury from a vesicant drug begins with correct administration of the drug (Box 47-1). Continuous infusions may be best administered through a central line. Vascular access devices may be an appropriate alternative (Wood & Gullo, 1993). In push chemotherapy, the agent is given via IV push over less than 30 minutes. This procedure includes establishing a running IV line with 5% dextrose and water or normal saline solution (as specified in the printed information on the particular agent) and assessing the IV site for patency, infiltration, and phlebitis. The vein's patency may be checked by instilling 5 to 7 mL of normal saline solution. The vesicant drug is administered via the side arm of the running IV. The nurse must check for infiltration and patency with every 1 mL of drug infusion. The tubing is flushed after completion of the drug infusion with 5 to 10 mL of normal saline solution. The drug must be administered at the specified speed to prevent untoward sensations.

If extravasation occurs, the infusion must be stopped. Each institution has its own set of subsequent procedures. Some interventions that may be specified include attempting to aspirate any remaining drug from the needle, injecting an appropriate antidote, using a specific topical ointment, and applying heat or cold to the site. A photograph of the site may be ordered as a reference to evaluate progression or resolution of the extravasation. Careful documentation in the chart is important.

Specific antidotes are recommended for certain agents. For example, 10% sodium thiosulfate is recommended as the antidote for mechlorethamine extravasation. If the 10% solution is not immediately available, the 25% solution may be used or diluted to a 10% solution. For mitomycin extravasation, pain and necrosis may be diminished with local injection of pyridoxine. With the vinca alkaloids, local infiltration of hyaluronidase and warming of the area of infiltration are recommended. With daunorubicin or doxorubicin, topical application of dimethylsulfoxide is suggested.

OUTCOME EVALUATION

The nurse must evaluate the client for signs or symptoms of extravasation and, if extravasation occurs, for evidence of its progression or resolution. The effect of any antidote or treatment used should be noted.

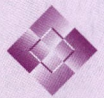

Box 47-1
Minimizing the Risk of Extravasation: A Guideline for IV Antineoplastic Therapy

Because many antineoplastic drugs are vesicants, the nurse must infuse them with particular care to prevent extravasation and subsequent tissue injury and pain.

Some common vesicants include dactinomycin, daunorubicin, doxorubicin, estramustine phosphate sodium, idarubicin, mitomycin, mechlorethamine, teniposide, vinblastine, vincristine, vindesine, and vinorelbine tartrate.

Some common irritant drugs include carmustine, dacarbazine, etoposide, plicamycin, and streptozocin.

The following guidelines are intended to minimize the risk of extravasation:

- Learn to recognize clients at increased risk for extravasation. Risk factors include:

    inability to communicate or report pain from extravasation
    elderly or debilitated condition or general vascular disease
    fragile veins
    lymphedema associated with mastectomy
    premedication
    peripheral neuropathy

- In general, never infuse vesicants over joints, bony prominences, or the antecubital fossa of the arms (little protective fat). The best site is usually the forearm.

- Dilate veins by wrapping arm or leg in warm towels.
- Do not use a tourniquet in elderly or frail clients.
- Avoid puncturing the same vein more than once. If no other vein is accessible, select an insertion site proximal to the previous insertion site in the same vein.
- Consider using a vascular access device (although extravasation can still occur).
- Avoid giving vesicant drugs in areas of poor venous or lymphatic circulation (eg, same side as a mastectomy, area of superior vena cava syndrome, or irradiated area).
- Make sure the peripheral IV site is fresh (less than 24 hours old).
- Assess for brisk blood return and easy fluid flow before administering vesicants by any IV needle or catheter (peripheral or central).
- Observe the needle or catheter insertion site continuously. Never leave the client unattended when administering a vesicant peripherally.
- Give vesicants by a steady, even flow, checking frequently for blood return. Check for blood return gently to avoid excessive pressure in the vein.
- Administer a vesicant ordered as an infusion through a central line, checking the line every 1 to 2 hours in the healthcare facility and every 2 to 4 hours in the client's home.
- If administering more than one drug, follow agency policy for sequencing the drugs.

❖ CHECKLIST OF NURSING ACTIONS

- ❏ Monitor laboratory data for evidence of adverse reactions (eg, leukopenia, thrombocytopenia, anemia, hypercalcemia).
- ❏ Teach the client about the drug, including the signs and symptoms to report and what to do if adverse reactions occur.
- ❏ For adverse reactions, follow suggested nursing interventions for the given problem.
- ❏ With vincristine, observe for early symptoms of central, autonomic, and peripheral nervous system toxicity so that steps may be taken to prevent more serious adverse reactions.
- ❏ With vincristine, take actions to prevent or control hyperuricemia.
- ❏ When helping with the IV administration of vesicants, take precautions to avoid extravasation of the drug into subcutaneous tissues.
- ❏ Advise clients who receive daunorubicin and doxorubicin that their urine will be red for 8 to 48 hours after drug administration. Clients who receive mitoxantrone may experience greenish-blue urine, sclera, skin, or nails for 24 hours after drug administration.
- ❏ Observe for signs and symptoms of cardiotoxicity with doxorubicin, daunorubicin, mitoxantrone, and amsacrine.
- ❏ With asparaginase, observe for signs and symptoms of allergic reaction.

References

Barakat RR. (1995). The effect of tamoxifen on the endometrium. *Oncology, 9*(2), 129–139.

Crabbe WW. (1996). The tamoxifen controversy. *Oncol Nurs Forum, 23*(5), 761–766.

Groenwald SL, Frogge MH, Goodman M, Yarbro CH, eds. (1993). *Cancer nursing: Principles and practice*, 3d ed. Boston: Jones and Bartlett Publishers.

McDaniel RW, Rhodes VA, Nelson RA, Hanson BM. (1995). Sensory perceptions of women receiving tamoxifen for breast cancer. *Cancer Nursing, 18*(3), 215–221.

Rich SE. (1993). Tamoxifen and breast cancer—from palliation to prevention. *Cancer Nursing, 16*(5), 341–346.

Rowinsky EK, Donehower RC. (1995). Paclitaxel (Taxol). *N Engl J Med, 332*(15), 1004–1014.

Sinha BK. (1995). Topoisomerase inhibitors: A review of their therapeutic potential in cancer. *Drugs, 49*(1), 11–19.

Varricchio CG, Johnson KA. (1993). The use of tamoxifen in the prevention and treatment of breast cancer. *Current Issues in Cancer Nursing Practice Updates, 2*(6), 1–10.

Wood LS, Gullo SM. (1993). IV vesicants: How to avoid extravasation. *Am J Nurs, 93*(4), 42–46.

Bibliography

Berman A, Chisholm L, deCarvalho M, Piemme JA, Gorrell CR. (1993). Programmed instruction: Cancer chemotherapy: Intravenous administration. *Cancer Nursing, 16*(2), 145–160.

Chisholm L, Berman AR, deCarvalho M, Gorrell CR. (1993). Programmed Instruction: Cancer chemotherapy; Alternative administration routes. *Cancer Nursing, 16*(3), 237–246.

DeVita VT Jr, Hellman S, Rosenberg SA. (1993). *Cancer: Principles and practice of oncology*, 4th ed. Philadelphia: JB Lippincott.

Fischer DS, Knobf MT, Durivage HJ. (1993). *The cancer chemotherapy handbook*, 4th ed. St. Louis: Mosby–Year Book, Inc.

Holland JF, Frei E III, Bast RC Jr, Kufe DW, Morton DL, Weichselbaum, RR. (1993). *Cancer medicine*, 3d ed. Philadelphia: Lea & Febiger.

Holleb AI, Fink DJ, Murphy GP. (1991). *American Cancer Society textbook of clinical oncology*. Atlanta: American Cancer Society.

Jenkins J, Wheeler V, Albright L. (1994). Gene therapy for cancer. *Cancer Nursing, 17*(6), 447–456.

Lake T, Jenkins J. (1993). Programmed instruction: Cancer chemotherapy; Clinical trials. *Cancer Nursing, 16*(6), 486–497.

Levy W, Meadows BS, Quint-Kasner S, Carroll R, Gorrell CR. (1993). Programmed instruction: Cancer chemotherapy; Chemotherapy agents: Part I. *Cancer Nursing, 16*(4), 321–336.

Pratt WB, Ruddon RW, Ensminger WD, Maybaum J. (1994). *The anticancer drugs*, 2d ed. New York: Oxford University Press.

Quint-Kasner S, Chisholm L, deCarvalho M, Piemme J, Zimmerman K, Berman A. (1993). Programmed instruction: Cancer chemotherapy; Basic principles. *Cancer Nursing, 16*(1), 63–78.

Quint-Kasner S, Levy W, Meadows BS, Carroll R, Gorrell CR. (1993). Programmed instruction: Cancer chemotherapy; Chemotherapy agents: Part II. *Cancer Nursing, 16*(5), 398–418.

For more information and sample tests and activities, refer to Chapter 47 in the Student Workbook for Clinical Pharmacology and Nursing Management, 5th edition, available through your bookstore.

XIV

Miscellaneous Drug Families

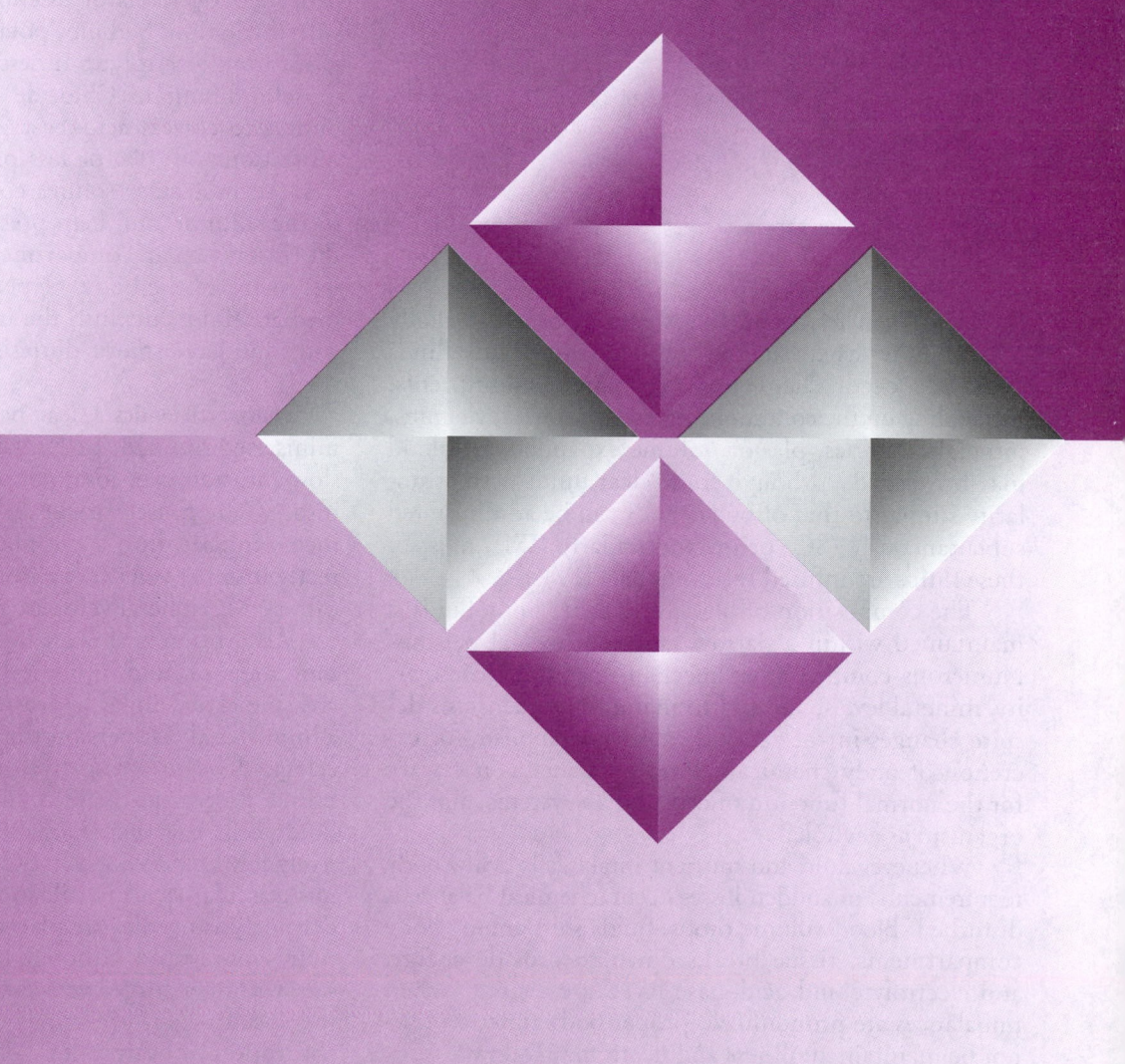

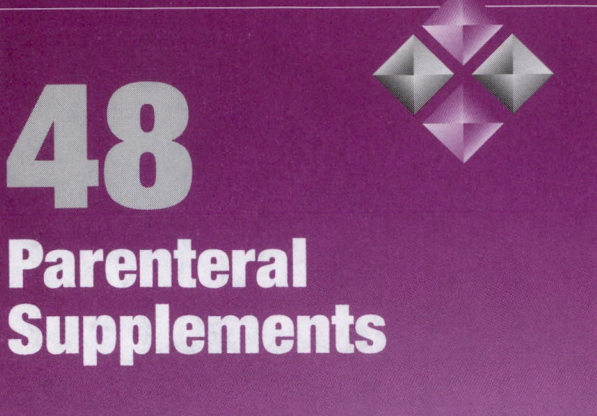

48

Parenteral Supplements

When food and fluids cannot be taken orally or when sudden large losses of body fluids occur, clients may need parenteral nutrients. Depending on the condition, water, electrolytes, vitamins, minerals, calories, plasma volume expanders, or blood may be needed. Although some clear fluids with osmolarity similar to that of body fluids can be administered subcutaneously (SC) or intramuscularly (IM), most of these fluids are infused intravenously (IV).

The composition of blood and other body fluids is maintained within a narrow range in normal persons. Numerous compensatory mechanisms adjust osmolarity, mineral levels, and pH to maintain homeostasis despite changes in the rate of intake, metabolism, or excretion of body chemicals. Proper balance is necessary for the normal function of cells, organ systems, and the organism as a whole.

Whenever fluid and nutrient intake falls below body requirements, or sudden losses occur, chemical balance is disturbed. Blood volume drops, fluids shift among body compartments, tissue breaks down to provide energy, and electrolyte and acid–base levels are altered. When imbalances are pronounced, proper body function cannot be maintained: illness and death may follow.

Parenteral Fluids

Parenteral fluid therapy is the major treatment for maintaining a proper chemical environment in the body until the underlying disruption can be corrected. The degree of correction required and the duration of therapy depend on the severity of the problem and the client's response to treatment. If the underlying condition cannot be corrected, parenteral solutions are administered palliatively to maintain hydration, nutrition, and the best possible level of function and comfort for as long as possible.

Clear Solutions

Clear solutions for parenteral administration contain several components in various combinations for use in appropriate clinical situations. Water is the solvent for all solutions. Solutes include salts of sodium, potassium, calcium, and ammonia; sugars; and synthetic carbohydrate polymers (Table 48-1).

Pharmacodynamics. Parenteral fluids maintain or replenish body levels of essential chemicals. Water provides hydration. Sodium, potassium, and calcium maintain cation electrolytes necessary for normal nerve and muscle function. Chloride and bicarbonate act as buffers to correct acid–base imbalance. Sugars in concentrations of 10% or less provide carbohydrate calories. All molecular solutes contribute osmotic tonicity to the solution and help preserve proper osmolarity in the intravascular compartment and other fluid compartments of the body. Hypertonic solutions cause immediate fluid shift into the intravascular compartment and stimulate osmotic diuresis.

Pharmacokinetics. Clear parenteral solutions are administered SC, IM, or IV. Large volumes are given by slow infusion over long periods. They may be injected into SC or muscle tissue via hypodermoclysis equipment, infused into a peripheral vein, or delivered directly into the vena cava through a central venous (CV) catheter. Peripheral veins are most commonly used.

Absorption is slowest by the SC route because the movement of fluid through the tissues is opposed by increasing extracellular hydrostatic pressure as the fluid is administered. Dispersion through the tissues can be accelerated by injecting hyaluronidase, an enzyme that breaks down the tissue cement (hyaluronic acid) that binds cells together. However, because there are relatively few blood vessels in SC tissue, movement into the intravascular space is still somewhat slow. When hypodermoclysis needles are placed in muscle tissue, absorption is more rapid, although increasing hydrostatic pressure within engorged vessels remains a limiting factor to the speed of absorption. Poor local perfusion reduces absorption by both routes.

Table 48-1. Clear Solutions Commonly Used for Parenteral Therapy

Solution	Administration and Dosage*	Mechanisms of Action	Therapeutic Uses
Isotonic			
saline			
0.9% NaCl in water (also called normal saline solution)	IV infusion; 90–125 mL/hr	Helps maintain osmotic pressure in extracellular fluid; helps maintain blood volume; sodium is necessary for impulse transmission in nerves and muscles; chloride buffers alkaline chemicals in the body and tends to lower pH	Replaces sodium, chloride, and water losses; prevents sodium, chloride, and water deficits in persons experiencing vomiting or nasogastric suction
dextrose (D-glucose)			
5.0% dextrose in water (D_5W)	IV, SC, or IM infusion; 90–125 mL/hr (maximum dose 650 mL/hr)	Provides fluid and calories for energy (200 calories/L of D_5W)	Maintains fluid levels when electrolytes are not needed or are contraindicated; provides calories to those unable to eat
2.5% dextrose in half normal saline	IV, SC, or IM infusion; 90–125 mL/hr	Provides fluid, electrolytes, and calories for energy	Treats shock due to diabetic ketoacidosis
Ringer's solution			
0.86% NaCl, 0.03% KCl, and 0.033% $CaCl_2$ ($2H_2O$) in water	IV infusion; 90–125 mL/hr	Provides fluid and the actions of saline; calcium modifies impulse transmission in nerves and muscles and promotes cardiac systole; potassium helps maintain intracellular osmotic pressure, is necessary to impulse transmission in nerves and muscles, and promotes cardiac diastole	Maintains or restores levels of fluid, sodium, chloride, potassium, and calcium in persons with actual or potential deficits of moderate degree (potassium concentration is inadequate to correct severe hypokalemia)
lactated Ringer's solution			
0.6% NaCl, 0.03% KCl, 0.02% $CaCl_2$ ($2H_2O$) and 0.31% Na lactate in water	IV infusion; 90–125 mL/hr	Provides the actions of Ringer's solution listed above plus lactate, which is metabolized in part to bicarbonate, which buffers acid in the body, raises the pH, and alkalinizes urine; the remainder of the lactate is metabolized to glycogen, which provides carbohydrate calories for energy	Maintains or restores fluid and electrolytes; treats dehydration accompanied by mild acidosis (especially ketoacidosis); alkalinization of urine in sulfonamide therapy
Hypotonic			
saline			
0.45% NaCl in water (also called half normal saline solution)	IV infusion; 90–125 mL/hr	Provides fluid	Restores normal osmolarity in clients with dehydration and hemoconcentration
Hypertonic			
saline			
3.0% NaCl in water	IV infusion; up to 80 mL/hr	Helps maintain osmotic pressure in extracellular fluid; helps maintain blood volume	Treats hypovolemic shock due to addisonian crisis or severe sodium depletion
5.0% NaCl in water	IV infusion; up to 50 mL/hr		
dextrose (D-glucose)			
10% dextrose in water	IV infusion; 45–65 mL/hr	Provides calories with minimal fluid intake	Treats persons needing extra calories who cannot tolerate fluid overload
20% dextrose in water	IV infusion; 90–125 mL/hr	Raises intravascular osmotic pressure and induces osmotic diuresis	Promotes fluid loss through osmotic diuresis
5% dextrose in 0.9% NaCl; 5% dextrose in 0.45% NaCl	IV infusion; 90–125 mL/hr	Provides fluid, electrolytes, and calories for energy; increases osmotic pressure in the intravascular compartment	Treats shock. Replaces fluid loss

*Dosage is the usual adult dosage.

(continued)

Table 48-1. (Continued)

Solution	Administration and Dosage*	Mechanisms of Action	Therapeutic Uses
Hypertonic (continued)			
fructose 10% fructose in water	IV infusion; 90–125 mL/hr	Provides energy without the need for insulin to promote intracellular use of the sugar	Replaces or supplements food and water
potassium chloride 0.15% KCl in D$_5$W 0.3% KCl in D$_5$W	IV infusion, diluted in 500–1,000 mL of electrolyte or dextrose solution for IV infusion; up to 20 mEq/hr (potassium concentration in IV fluids should not exceed 40 mEq/L)	Provides the actions of chloride and potassium listed above.	Maintains or replenishes potassium levels in adequately hydrated persons with good renal function, especially surgical clients and those experiencing fluid losses from the lower intestinal tract
ammonium chloride 2.14% NH$_4$Cl	IV infusion; in accordance with chloride deficit as calculated from carbon dioxide combining power	Provides the actions of chloride listed above; ammonia is metabolized by the liver and excreted as urea, which stimulates osmotic diuresis and helps mobilize edema fluid	Treats metabolic alkalosis, tetany due to metabolic alkalosis and chloride depletion
bicarbonate 5% NaHCO$_3$ in water	IV infusion; in accordance with plasma CO$_2$ levels or dyspnea and hyperpnea due to acidosis	Buffers acids in the body and raises pH	Treats severe acidosis accompanied by dyspnea and hyperpnea
synthetic carbohydrate polymers 10% dextran 40 with 0.9% NaCl (or with 5% dextrose) in water (Rheomacrodex) 6% dextran 70 with 0.9% NaCl (or with 5% dextrose) in water (Macrodex) 6% hetastarch with 0.9% NaCl in water	IV infusion; 30–60 g/d, depending on degree of fluid volume loss and hemoconcentration	Increases the osmotic pressure of circulating blood, causing a fluid shift into the intravascular compartment; increases blood volume and reduces hematocrit; may coat red blood cells, reducing bonding forces and aggregation; may reduce red blood cell rigidity, facilitating movement through small blood vessels	Restores circulation in hypovolemic shock due to burns, hemorrhage, or sepsis; priming solution for plasmapheresis procedures

*Dosage is the usual adult dosage.

With IV administration, the solution is delivered directly into the vascular compartment. Absorption is virtually instantaneous and complete. Distribution of water, the solvent of IV solutions, depends on their osmolarity. Isotonic solutions (those with osmotic pressures equal to those of body fluids) trigger the least movement of water from the intravascular compartment into or out of the interstitial and intracellular compartments. The administration of hypotonic solutions causes water to leave the intravascular compartment and enter, successively, the interstitial and intracellular compartments. Hypertonic solutions draw water from the interstitial and intracellular compartments into the intravascular space. Solute components of clear solutions are widely and rapidly distributed throughout the body.

Distribution and metabolism of specific components vary (Table 48-2). The kidneys are the major excretory organs for most components of parenteral solutions, including the fluid content.

Adverse Reactions. Rapid infusion of IV fluids can produce toxicity from excesses of any or all of the constituent chemicals. Fluid excesses produce circulatory overload and hypertension. Congestive heart failure and pulmonary edema may result. Excesses of individual chemicals produce characteristic signs and symptoms (Table 48-3).

Rapid infusion of solutions by hypodermoclysis or extravasation of IV fluids produces painful local tissue swelling. If interstitial hypertension is pronounced and prolonged, local tissue perfusion is impaired, and tissue damage can occur.

Tissue cells can be irritated or injured by several other mechanisms during IV therapy. Unless solutions

Table 48-2. Distribution, Metabolism, Storage, and Excretion of Components of Parenteral Solutions

Component	Distribution	Metabolism/Storage	Excretion
sodium	Distributes widely in the extracellular fluid compartment (interstitial and intravascular spaces)	Remains primarily in the extracellular compartment	Mainly through the kidneys and sweat glands
potassium	Moves quickly through the extracellular space and is actively transported into cells	Dextrose, insulin, and oxygen facilitate movement of potassium into cells.	Primarily renal, by active secretion in the distal tubule, a process stimulated by corticosteroid hormones secreted by the adrenal cortex; small amounts excreted by the skin
calcium	Binds to plasma proteins; crosses the placenta and appears in fetal circulation in higher concentrations than in maternal blood	Ions in excess of normal blood levels are stored in bony structures. (Nonionized calcium compounds in the blood are physiologically inactive.)	Excesses are excreted largely in feces by way of bile and pancreatic juices: kidney excretion is proportional to serum concentration of ionized mineral, parathyroid hormone, and vitamin D; also secreted in breast milk and by sweat glands
chloride	Distributes widely in body tissues	Combines with alkaline salts, reducing base reserve.	Kidneys and sweat glands
dextrose	Distributes widely in the extracellular space	Dextrose requires insulin for use by most body cells; it is oxidized for energy, producing water and carbon dioxide.	Excesses excreted by the kidneys
fructose	Distributes rapidly throughout the tissues	Fructose does not require insulin for use by the cells; it is oxidized for energy.	Excesses excreted by the kidneys
lactate	Distributes widely throughout the tissues	The levo form is oxidized to bicarbonate; the dextro form is converted to glycogen and stored.	Excess salts excreted by the kidneys
ammonium	Distributes widely throughout the tissues	Ammonia is metabolized by the liver to urea with release of hydrogen ions, which combine with bicarbonate to produce water and carbon dioxide.	Water eliminated through the kidneys, carbon dioxide through the lungs
bicarbonate	Distributes widely throughout the tissues	Combines with hydrogen ions to produce water and carbon dioxide	Water eliminated through the kidneys, carbon dioxide through the lungs
dextrans	Remain in the intravascular compartment initially (about 70% of dextran 40 and 50% of dextran 70 are excreted within 24 hours)	Molecules of molecular weight greater than 15,000 are degraded slowly to glucose and are metabolized for energy.	Molecules of molecular weight less than 15,000 are rapidly excreted by the kidneys; small amounts are excreted in feces by the bile.
hetastarch	Remains in the intravascular compartment initially (about 40% of hetastarch is excreted within 24 hours)	Molecules of molecular weight greater than 50,000 are slowly degraded to smaller molecules; some are metabolized as glucose.	Molecules of molecular weight less than 50,000 are excreted by the kidneys.

have an osmotic tonicity like that of normal body fluids or are rapidly diluted, cells are likely to be injured. Hypotonic fluids cause swelling and lysis of cells; hypertonic fluids crenate or shrink them (Box 48-1). With IV infusion, the cells most often affected are the erythrocytes. If such solutions are administered by clysis or infiltrate from an IV line, extravascular cells are vulnerable. Tissue necrosis and sloughing can result.

Solutions containing electrolytes in concentrations greater than normal serum levels are irritating to the tissues or veins into which they are introduced. Phlebitis may occur. If the solutions infiltrate, local tissue damage is likely.

Some clients develop an allergy to dextrans, hetastarch, or nickel, a contaminant in some solutions. Nickel also tends to increase coronary artery resistance and has an oxytoxic effect.

The injection or infusion of parenteral solutions breaches the natural barriers against microbial invasion and predisposes to infection. This is a particularly serious complication with IV infusions because the invading organism is introduced directly into the blood. Septicemia with chills, fever, and septic shock can develop.

Precautions and Contraindications. Intravenous infusions must be monitored closely to maintain proper flow rate and placement of the needle or access catheter. If the infusion infiltrates, it should be discontinued and restarted in another vein.

Table 48-3. Adverse Effects of Parenteral Fluid Components

Component	Toxic Effects	Treatment of Toxic State
sodium	Hypervolemia and fluid overload; edema Cellular dehydration with weakness and disorientation indicative of hypernatremia Excessive potassium loss by the kidneys with distention, anorexia, nausea, and depressed respirations Oliguria and increased blood urea nitrogen may develop	Discontinuation of sodium solutions; supportive care until excess sodium is eliminated; administration of diuretics
potassium	Locally, tissue irritation; causes smooth muscle spasm and vasoconstriction; can compromise circulation Nausea, vomiting, cramping abdominal pain, prolonged cardiac diastole, and reduced response to the stimulus of cardiac pacemakers indicative of hyperkalemia	Administration of dextrose and insulin or bicarbonate to stimulate movement of extracellular potassium into the cells; in extreme toxicity, administration of calcium salts to restore normal cardiac function
calcium	Locally, tissue irritation; phlebitis or extravascular tissue necrosis With rapid administration, vasodilation, hypotension, bradycardia, cardiac arrhythmias, syncope, and cardiac arrest With excessive doses, increased risk of calcium renal stone formation	Administration of fluids to promote dilution of urine and diuresis; in extreme toxicity, administration of potassium to restore normal cardiac function
chloride	Hyperchloremic acidosis as shown by acid urine, dyspnea, and hyperpnea, and by a reduction in body fluid pH Hyperkalemia and depletion of intracellular potassium	Administration of lactate or bicarbonate to increase alkaline reserve
dextrose	Hyperglycemia, glucosuria, and hyperosmolar nonketotic coma	Slowing of infusion rate; administration of insulin to promote metabolism of glucose
fructose	Hyperosmolarity, especially with rapid administration	Slowing of infusion rate; administration of hypotonic solutions
lactate	Metabolic alkalosis; tetany	Bag rebreathing and administration of calcium to relieve tetany; administration of chlorides to reduce alkaline reserve
ammonia	Hyperammonemia as shown by CNS abnormalities (headache, tremor, hyperreflexia, confusion, electroencephalogram changes, stupor alternating with excitement and coma) Azotemia, metabolic acidosis, and hyperkalemia if kidney function is impaired Depletion of intracellular potassium Skin rash	Discontinuation of infusion; supportive care; hemodialysis for severe toxicity
bicarbonate	Metabolic alkalosis; tetany	Bag rebreathing and administration of calcium to relieve tetany; administration of chlorides to reduce alkaline reserve
synthetic carbohydrate polymers	Increased bleeding time and hemorrhage Hypervolemia, hypoproteinemia, and congestive failure Allergic reactions (urticaria, nasal congestion, wheeze, mild hypotension, and rarely anaphylaxis), especially with dextran In dehydrated persons, renal tubular stasis, tubular obstruction, renal failure	Measures to control bleeding; transfusion if blood loss is severe Slowing or discontinuation of polymer infusion; administration of diuretics and digitalis Discontinuation of polymer infusion; administration of epinephrine, antihistamines, and glucocorticoids Diuresis or hemodialysis

Parenteral fluids must be administered with careful regard for fluid, electrolyte, and acid–base status so that treatment does no harm. Caution is required when sodium solutions are administered to clients with circulatory insufficiency, liver disease, kidney dysfunction, hypoproteinemia, and ongoing corticosteroid therapy. These conditions are risk factors for circulatory overload, edema, and chemical instability. Clients receiving dextrose solutions must be monitored for hyperglycemia and glucosuria.

Before administering potassium solutions, hydration and adequate renal function must be ensured. Dextrose 5% in water or in another solution low in electrolytes is commonly given before potassium solutions are infused. Renal function should be assessed carefully during this hydration phase. Once potassium solutions are started, the rate of administration should be kept at less than 20 mEq of potassium hourly; elderly persons or clients with renal impairment should receive 25% to 50% as much per hour. The serum potassium level should remain less than 6 mEq/L.

Before ammonium chloride solutions are administered, acid–base balance must be determined. Carbon dioxide combining power should be measured before fluid therapy is begun and again after half the solution has been administered. Ammonium chloride solutions must be administered slowly because they tend to deplete base bicarbonate and lower blood pH. Clients should be watched for signs and symptoms of potassium imbalance. Temporary hyperkalemia can result from displacement of intracellular potassium by hydrogen ions. This potassium raises serum levels and is excreted by the kidneys, resulting in a net loss of the electrolyte.

In general, only clients with severe or refractory acidosis require bicarbonate solutions. During treatment, blood gas levels are monitored to guide therapy. Clients receiving bicarbonate should be watched for signs and symptoms of alkalosis (shallow respirations, paresthesia, cramps) because overcorrection of the acid–base disorder can develop quickly. Caution must be exercised when bicarbonate solutions are administered to persons with congestive heart failure or edema because these fluids contain considerable sodium.

Adequate hydration and renal function should be established before plasma expanders are administered.

During therapy with dextran or hetastarch, urine output and urine specific gravity must be monitored. Both should increase as elimination of the solution is established. If the volume and density of urine do not rise, the polymer solution should be discontinued. However, the IV line must be maintained because further parenteral medication will probably be required.

Monitoring CV pressure is recommended when plasma volume expanders are administered. The infusion should be slowed or discontinued if CV pressure exceeds normal.

Coagulation or bleeding time should be evaluated before therapy with a plasma expander begins. These solutions should be given with caution to persons at risk for hemorrhage because synthetic polymers increase the risk of bleeding.

Infusions of large amounts of fluid are contraindicated in persons with circulatory overload or edema, as in cardiac, renal, or liver failure. Potassium must be given cautiously when urinary excretion is impaired. Liver or renal impairment is a contraindication for ammonium chloride administration. Clients with pulmonary edema or allergic hypersensitivity to components in the solutions should not receive dextran or hetastarch.

SUMMARY

Clear parenteral fluids are life-saving when administered to maintain or restore fluid, electrolyte, and acid–base balance. They also provide minimal carbohydrate calories for energy. Usually these solutions are administered by IV infusion, but they are sometimes delivered to SC or muscle tissue by hypodermoclysis. Solutions infused directly into the vascular system enter the systemic circulation directly and are distributed rapidly. Overdosage (or overcorrection of imbalances) must be avoided because once the medication enters a vein, the dose cannot be retrieved and absorption cannot be delayed.

Parenteral therapy can cause toxic responses, such as excess fluid, high serum concentrations of sodium, potassium, calcium, ammonia, and glucose, or acid–base imbalance (metabolic acidosis or alkalosis). Dextran and hetastarch can cause allergic reactions.

❖ NURSING MANAGEMENT: CLIENT RECEIVING A PARENTERAL SOLUTION

During parenteral therapy, the client is vulnerable to infection, extravasation, and other complications of infusion. The order in which solutions are administered is important: preparations must be given in succession as specified by the prescriber. Often a client must be hydrated to establish good renal function before solutions containing potentially toxic components can be administered. Changing the order of administration can have disastrous consequences. For example, giving potassium salts to a dehydrated client with poor renal function may cause cardiac arrest.

Nurses must be alert for alterations in certain laboratory test values as a result of dextran in the blood. During therapy with this type of plasma expander, blood glucose levels, blood cross-matching by proteolytic enzymes, and bilirubin assays using alcohol are unreliable.

Nurses responsible for parenteral therapy must understand physiology thoroughly, especially in relation to fluid, electrolyte, and acid–base balance. They must be able to evaluate the risks of such therapy and recognize the early signs and symptoms of adverse reactions. Considerations relative to specific components of common solutions are outlined in Table 48-4. Although nurses do not prescribe fluid therapy or change the medical regimen outlined by the prescriber, they may discontinue treatment judged to be detrimental to the client. They must be able to judge when to consult the prescriber for a change in orders.

NURSING PROCESS

ASSESSMENT

Before initiating treatment with IV fluids, the nurse should assess the client to determine cardiac and renal function, as well as fluid, electrolyte, and acid–base balance. The client's emotional reaction to the ordered therapy should also be assessed. Anxiety or fear can predispose to hypervolemia by activating hormone-regulated mechanisms of sodium and fluid retention. The very old, the very young, clients with small body size, and those with renal impairment are at increased risk for complications.

NURSING DIAGNOSIS

Nursing diagnoses for clients receiving IV solutions could include:

- Fluid Volume Deficit, related to inadequate oral intake secondary to nausea and vomiting, to excessive fluid losses secondary to diarrhea, or to loss of plasma secondary to burn wound
- Risk for Fluid Volume Deficit, related to cessation of oral intake and surgery

Common collaborative problems that should be differentiated from the nursing diagnoses include:

Potential Complications: Pulmonary edema, cardiac arrest, metabolic acidosis (alkalosis)

PLANNING

The goal of nursing care is to restore and maintain homeostasis, including fluid, electrolyte, and acid–base balance.

INTERVENTION

Parenteral fluid therapy may be initiated by the nurse if fluids are to be administered by hypodermoclysis, or if the nurse is qualified to perform venipuncture.

Clients receiving parenteral fluids must be monitored carefully for early signs and symptoms of circulatory overload, a serious complication of parenteral therapy. To prevent hypervolemia, fluid administration must be controlled to prevent excessive rates of flow. Volume-controlled infusion pumps deliver measured doses reliably. Clients should be assessed at least every 4 hours, more often if their condition is unstable.

If pumps or mechanical flow monitors are unavailable, the infusion should be checked three or four times hourly and adjusted as necessary to ensure an appropriate rate of flow. Solutions containing components that are hazardous at high serum levels are best administered with a small-bore needle into a large vein to prevent rapid rates of infusion and to promote rapid dilution. The client's general condition and respiratory function are noted with each contact. Output and specific gravity of urine should be measured regularly. If glucose solutions are used, blood or urine is tested for glucose also.

If fluid flow is impeded and the rate of administration is below that specified in the order, the client must never be flooded with solution in an attempt to catch up. If the client's condition indicates that more rapid administration could be needed, the prescriber should be consulted for a change in the rate ordered. Excessive flow rates can be especially dangerous for clients with cardiac or renal impairment and with solutions containing ammonium, potassium, magnesium, or calcium salts.

Clients under treatment for heat exhaustion or hypovolemic shock due to a sodium and water deficit could have an underlying corticosteroid deficiency. If blood pressure does not stabilize at an adequate level, the prescriber should be notified promptly so that hormone therapy can be considered.

The nurse should carefully evaluate laboratory data from blood studies. Electrolyte, blood glucose, blood gas, and blood urea nitrogen values are all significant. Movement of these values toward normal usually indicates a positive response to treatment.

Client Education. Parenteral fluid therapy is an invasive procedure that stimulates stress and anxiety in most clients. Immediately before infusion, the client should be told about the procedure; informing the client too early causes anxiety levels to rise. Information offered should describe what the client will experience, the expected benefits of therapy, and the alternatives to this method of treatment.

Clients should be instructed to keep the dressing over the insertion site dry and to avoid manipulating the tubing. The nurse should caution clients against putting pressure on the tubing or sharp flexion of the involved extremity, which could impede solution flow. The client is encouraged to ambulate with assistance and to maintain as many activities of daily living as possible.

Table 48-4. Implications of Administering Parenteral Solution Components

Solution Component	Factors Increasing the Risk of Therapy	Signs and Symptoms of Complications	Precautions and Corrective Treatment
sodium	Cardiac or renal impairment	Hypertension, edema, cough, or dyspnea indicative of circulatory overload Elevated serum sodium levels	Place client in high Fowler's position to facilitate breathing. Administer diuretics when ordered to eliminate sodium and fluid.
chloride	Acidosis	Hyperpnea and dyspnea indicative of acidosis Elevated serum chlorine levels	Administer lactate or bicarbonate when ordered to raise pH.
dextrose	Hyperglycemia; diabetes mellitus	Hyperglycemia; glucosuria	Slow infusion rate and administer insulin when ordered to reduce serum glucose.
potassium	Dehydration	Oliguria	Mix potassium additives thoroughly with diluting solutions.
	Renal impairment with oliguria, anuria, or azotemia	Elevated serum potassium levels	Administer solutions slowly (20 mEq potassium or less per hour).
	Recent crush injury	Elevated serum potassium levels	Limit potassium content of solution to 40 mEq/L.
	History of hyperkalemic familial periodic paralysis	Decreased serum calcium levels	Administer dextrose and insulin, bicarbonate, or Kayexalate as ordered to reduce serum potassium.
	Heat cramps	Weak cardiac contraction Cardiac arrhythmias	Administer digitalis as ordered to strengthen cardiac contraction.
calcium	Digitalis therapy	Cardiac arrhythmias	Administer solutions slowly.
	Renal or cardiac impairment	Elevated serum calcium level	Maintain good respiratory function.
	Sarcoidosis	Lethargy	Administer potassium when ordered to restore cardiac function.
	Cor pulmonale		
	Respiratory acidosis		
	Respiratory failure		
	Hypercalcemia		
lactate	Alkalosis	Shallow respirations	Bag rebreathe to relieve paresthesias or tetany.
	Low serum calcium	Paresthesias, tetany	
bicarbonate	Alkalosis	Elevated base excess	Administer chlorides when ordered to relieve alkalosis.
	Hypertension	Alkalosis	
	Cardiac or renal impairment	Edema Hypertension	Reduce the flow rate of infusions
ammonium	Pulmonary insufficiency	Abnormal CNS function (confusion, lethargy alternating with excitement, coma)	Have carbon dioxide combining power measured before initiating therapy and when half the ordered solution has been administered.
	Cardiac or renal impairment		
	Pronounced hepatic impairment	Elevated serum levels of ammonia or urea	Administer solutions very slowly.
synthetic carbohydrate polymers	Pregnancy	Hypertension	Observe client closely for first half-hour of treatment.
	History of allergic reaction to the solution ordered	Dyspnea, cough	
	Dehydration	Abnormal bleeding	Have epinephrine available for prompt treatment of allergic reactions should they occur.
		Hematocrit less than 30%	
		Elevated CV pressure	

For some clients, parenteral nutrition is a treatment that will be needed for life. For others, it is a temporary measure to sustain them through a limited period when eating and drinking are proscribed. As soon as gastrointestinal (GI) function resumes, the nurse should encourage these clients to resume oral intake, stressing the need for beverages and foods rich in electrolytes and other nutrients. Ice chips, tea, or ginger ale are usually tolerated better than is plain water. The usual progression is from clear liquids to full liquid, then to a soft diet and a full diet, as tolerated.

Clients on long-term parenteral therapy may need to manage their own therapy at home. These clients or their families need detailed instruction in techniques for preparing and administering parenteral solutions.

OUTCOME EVALUATION

Data required for evaluation include information related to fluid, electrolyte, and acid–base balance. Teaching success may be evaluated by the client's ability to cooperate with procedures related to the infusion and by the client's adherence to the instructions and cautions conveyed during the teaching session. (See the Example of Nursing Process for Adverse Effect of IV Therapy.)

❖ CHECKLIST OF NURSING ACTIONS

- ❑ Inform clients about parenteral therapy shortly before initiating infusions.
- ❑ Carry out strict surgical asepsis to minimize the risk of infection in clients receiving parenteral fluids.
- ❑ Maintain the infusion flow rate as prescribed.
- ❑ Administer solutions in the order specified.
- ❑ Monitor clients receiving parenteral solutions for circulatory overload and symptoms of toxicity from the solutes being administered.
- ❑ Monitor clients' therapeutic response to treatment.
- ❑ Administer solutions containing potassium, calcium, ammonium, or bicarbonate at a slow rate.

Total Parenteral Nutrition

The parenteral solutions previously described cannot provide all the nutrients needed to produce energy and build tissue. Therefore, clients who cannot take oral nourishment continue to break down body tissues to meet these needs. To reverse this catabolic state, sufficient calories, proteins, and fats must be supplied to sustain metabolism and tissue repair.

Preparations

Total parenteral nutrition (TPN) sufficient to provide for normal metabolism, tissue growth, and weight gain requires preparations containing concentrated sugars, amino acids, and lipids. Few feeding formulas contain all necessary nutrients, because certain combinations tend to be unstable. Sometimes lipid emulsions and combinations of dextrose, amino acids, vitamins, and minerals are infused at different times or through different venous lines because of compatibility problems. Formulas are tailored to meet individual needs, using a combination of ingredients (Table 48-5).

Pharmacodynamics. Nutrients administered IV replace those that normally would be absorbed from the GI tract.

Pharmacokinetics. Nutrients administered IV are introduced directly into the blood vessels and are subsequently metabolized and degraded, just like nutrients normally absorbed from the GI tract.

Therapeutic Uses. Parenteral nutrition aims to stabilize and improve the condition of cachectic or debilitated persons who cannot take adequate oral nutrition. It is used also to prepare such clients for surgery. These preparations can restore full nutrition to persons with severe intestinal malfunction. Parenteral nutrition may

---

Example of Nursing Process for Adverse Effect of IV Therapy

The client, age 45, has been in the recovery room for 2 hours after a hysterectomy. An IV infusion is running in her left forearm at 100 mL/hr. Examination of the infusion site reveals swelling of the tissues and increased luminosity of the site as compared with the corresponding tissues in the right arm.

Assessment Data

IV infusion running at 100 mL/hr

Swelling and increased luminosity of tissues at infusion site

Nursing Diagnosis	Intervention	Goals and Outcomes
Altered Tissue Perfusion at the infusion site, related to extravascular infiltration of parenteral fluids	**Discontinue** IV infusion; apply a dry sterile dressing to the venipuncture site.	The swelling will decrease and disappear; signs and symptoms of inflammation or tissue necrosis will not develop.
	Elevate the affected limb.	
	Apply warmth to the site.	
	Encourage the client to exercise the affected limb.	
	Monitor the site for signs and symptoms of inflammation or tissue necrosis.	

Table 48-5. Components of Solutions Used for Parenteral Nutrition

Component	Composition	Usual Concentration and Calorie Content	Osmotic Tonicity	Usual Adult Dosage
protein hydrolysates (Amigen, Aminosol, Hyprotigen, Parentamine, Travamin)	Amino acids and short-chain peptides that reflect the nutritive value of the natural protein (casein, lactalbumin, plasma, fibrin, or others) from which it is derived by hydrolytic processes, sometimes modified by partial removal or addition of specific amino acids	Concentration and calorie content vary with preparation	Hypertonic	50–100 g in 5–6 hr (1 g/kg/day)
amino acids (Aminosyn, Branchamin, Freamine, Travasol, Veinamine)	Approximately 15 amino acids in varying proportions. Both essential and nonessential amino acids	Concentration and calorie content vary with preparation	Slightly hypertonic (can be administered in a peripheral vein)	1 g/kg/day
essential amino acids (Nephramine)	Eight essential amino acids in a solution virtually free of electrolytes		Hypertonic (must be diluted with hypotonic glucose for administration in a peripheral vein)	Individualized in accordance with renal function (the preparation is used in the treatment of patients with renal failure)
vitamins	Injectable preparations of essential vitamins	Concentration depends on diluent. Calorie content: 0	Dependent on tonicity of diluent	Equal to or greater than the recommended daily allowances, depending on degree of deficiency present
minerals	Injectable preparations of electrolytes and trace minerals	Concentration depends on diluent. Calorie content: 0	Dependent on tonicity of diluent	Equal to or greater than the recommended daily allowances, depending on degree of deficiency present
fat Intralipid	Soy bean oil, egg yolk phospholipids, and glycerin	Calorie content: 450 per 500 mL	Isotonic	500 mL/day (maximum of 2.5 g/kg of ideal weight)
safflower oil	Safflower oil	Calorie content: 450 per 500 mL	Isotonic	500 mL/day

be a temporary measure to improve the prognosis of debilitated clients who need corrective therapy, such as surgery, or a long-term measure for maintaining clients with chronic debilitating intestinal malfunction.

Parenteral formulas containing sugars and amino acids are concentrated and cannot be infused into peripheral veins because their high osmotic tonicity would damage erythrocytes and other cells, as well as the vessels themselves. To provide rapid dilution to normal tonicity, these fluids are infused directly into the largest veins, such as the vena cava, via a CV catheter.

Adverse Reactions. Air embolism may occur during insertion of a CV catheter. Amino acid and protein hydrolysate solutions tend to aggregate and form solid particles that can cause emboli. Lipid emulsions can also form emboli if the emulsion separates, forming fat globules.

Metabolic imbalances that can develop during TPN include hypophosphatemia, hyperammonemia, and trace mineral deficiencies. Glycosuria occurs commonly when therapy is initiated but tends to subside with continued administration as endogenous insulin response is reestablished. Although solutions for parenteral nutrition are formulated to provide complete nourishment, they do not always meet individual needs completely. Optimal levels of some nutrients and variations in individual needs cannot always be determined accurately. Administration of lipid emulsions sometimes causes nausea.

Parenteral nutrition induces gallstones in some children; it can be hepatotoxic for premature infants. Long-term TPN is associated with a crippling bone disease affecting the weight-bearing joints. Parenteral nutrition solutions are rich media for microbial growth, and infection is a serious complication.

Precautions and Contraindications. To prevent air embolus and pneumothorax, special precautions are required during insertion of the CV line and whenever the system must be opened to air. Strict surgical asepsis is required to maintain sterility of tubing and solutions. Because the infusion rate must be carefully controlled, IV pumps should be used for administration. High-nutrient solutions containing amino acids are administered via lines with microscopic filters, to eliminate solid particles. Fat emulsions should be administered through tubing that has a low phthalate concentration in the plastic, because fat may extract this chemical from the tubing. Medications are not administered through the hyperalimentation port because they tend to be incompatible with hypertonic solutions.

■ SUMMARY

Total parenteral nutrition involves administering hypertonic solutions through a CV line and lipid solutions through either a central or a peripheral venous line. These solutions can support anabolic metabolism, tissue repair, and weight gain. They are used to build up debilitated clients and to maintain nutrition in those who cannot absorb nutrients via the intestinal route. Complications include infection (most common), electrolyte imbalance, trace mineral deficiencies, and emboli of air, fat, or protein aggregates.

❖ NURSING MANAGEMENT: CLIENT RECEIVING TOTAL PARENTERAL NUTRITION

Parenteral nutrition through CV lines presents some risks not inherent in the usual IV therapy. Air or fat embolism may occur, and septicemia is more likely to develop. Clients are completely dependent on parenteral nutrients and usually ingest little or no food or fluids.

NURSING PROCESS

ASSESSMENT

Before parenteral nutrition is instituted, the client should be assessed for fluid, electrolyte, acid–base, and nutritional status. The nurse should also assess the client's and family's knowledge about this treatment, as well as their emotional reaction to it.

NURSING DIAGNOSIS
Nursing diagnoses may include:

- Altered Nutrition: Less Than Body Requirements, related to nausea and vomiting, malabsorption, or inability to eat secondary to GI obstruction, or related to malabsorption secondary to inflammation of the small intestine

Nursing diagnoses arising from hyperalimentation therapy include:

- Risk for Infection: Septicemia related to introduction of pathogens through a CV line
- Altered Nutrition: Less Than Body Requirements, trace mineral deficiency related to inadequate intake or absorption
- Anxiety, related to inability to ingest or absorb nutrients and to parenteral nutritional therapy
- Knowledge Deficit, concerning hyperalimentation therapy

Common collaborative problems that should be differentiated from the nursing diagnoses include:

Potential Complications: Pulmonary embolism, lipid embolism, protein aggregation embolism, hyperglycemia, hyperammonemia

PLANNING
Goals of nursing care include improvement of nutrition; maintenance of fluid, electrolyte, acid–base, and trace mineral balance; prevention or prompt detection and treatment of complications (eg, embolism, septicemia); emotional acceptance of the therapy by the client and family; and client and family education about parenteral nutrition and the procedures required for its administration.

INTERVENTION
Before parenteral nutrition is initiated, the client should be informed about the procedure. Clients and their families should be encouraged to ask questions about the therapy and to express their feelings about its implications.

Usually, CV lines are used to introduce solutions into the vena cava through jugular or subclavian veins. For long-term parenteral nutrition, the line and a sealed reservoir may be implanted surgically. Temporary lines enter the vein transdermally.

To prevent aspiration of air into the circulation, the CV line is established with the client in Trendelenburg position. When the vein is entered, the client is instructed to perform a Valsalva maneuver to increase intrathoracic pressure. If air embolism occurs despite these precautions, the client should be placed immediately on the left side, trapping air in the right ventricle. The physician may attempt intracardiac aspiration or cardiac massage to remove or disperse the air bubble.

Whenever the system must be opened for tubing changes, the client should perform a Valsalva maneuver to minimize the risk of air entering the system. Tubing changes should be completed quickly.

Central venous catheters are anchored with a stay suture to prevent displacement. Normal saline solution is infused initially until proper placement of the catheter has been confirmed by imaging equipment. Fluids are administered through implanted lines by a special needle shaped at a 90° angle and terminating with a heparin lock. This is inserted into the reservoir transdermally and remains in place for several days. Solutions are commonly infused during sleep, with the tubing removed from the heparin lock for the rest of the day. When a transdermal CV line is used, infusions are often continuous.

Parenteral nutrient solutions containing amino acids may form microscopic aggregates in the bag, bottle, or tubing that can cause massive emboli if allowed to enter the vein. To prevent infusion of such material, microscopic filters are required in the IV tubing. These filters cannot be used when lipid emulsions are administered because the fat molecules are too large to pass through them. Lipid preparations are best administered through a double-lumen Hickman catheter in a central vein or by infusion into a peripheral vein. They are usually not mixed with other solutions. Lipid preparations are isotonic and can be safely administered peripherally.

When infusion of fat emulsions is begun, the rate should not exceed 1 mL/min for adults. Children should receive 0.1 mL/min. For the first 30 minutes, the client should be observed closely for dyspnea, cyanosis, allergic reaction, headache, flushing, nausea, vomiting, or pain in the chest and back. Should these reactions occur, the infusion should be discontinued and the prescriber notified.

Fat emulsions should be handled carefully to minimize the risk of separation. The container should never be agitated. The fluid should appear cloudy but uniform in color and density. Fluids that have separated or are not homogeneous in appearance should not be used.

Infusion of a daily dose of lipids requires 4 to 6 hours. Administration must be scheduled for a time when blood need not be drawn for analysis for at least 4 hours after completion of the infusion, because high lipid levels in the serum can alter some blood values. Usually, fat infusions are begun immediately after early-morning blood specimens have been collected.

Because rapid administration of hypertonic solutions does not allow dilution to normal tonicity, the rate of administration of such fluids must be carefully controlled. Signs and symptoms and laboratory data must be monitored closely to detect metabolic imbalances early and to guide adjustments in the formulation of succeeding solutions for infusion. If hyperammonemia develops, the nitrogenous (amino acid) content of the solution is reduced. Hyperglycemia is controlled with insulin injections to prevent excessive water loss through osmotic diuresis. Phosphate should be administered when parenteral therapy is prolonged.

Medications are not administered in the CV line used for these solutions because they tend to be incompatible with TPN formulations. Lipid emulsions are also administered without the addition of other drugs, but the peripheral line used for lipid administration is available for long periods of time for the administration of other substances because only a few hours are required for the infusion of the daily allotment of this solution.

Because concentrated solutions used for parenteral nutrition are good media for microbial growth, precautions to prevent contamination of the solutions and equipment are particularly important. Strict surgical asepsis must be maintained throughout the duration of parenteral nutrition to reduce the risk of infection. Once exposed to room temperatures, solutions must be infused within 24 hours or discarded. Microfilters remove most particulate matter and bacteria for a day, but rapid bacterial growth may occur if the solution is continued beyond that period. Additives should be mixed with solutions using strict surgical asepsis. This procedure is best carried out under a laminar flow hood by personnel wearing surgical masks. In many institutions, the pharmacist is responsible for preparing the solutions.

If the solution is significantly colder than room temperature when administered, multiple small bubbles tend to form in the tubing, some below the microfilter. To prevent this, solutions should be exposed to room temperatures for 30 to 60 minutes before infusion. If bubbles form in the tubing, the equipment should not be agitated to coalesce them because they cannot be forced back through the microfilter. Instead, the tubing should be disturbed as little as possible. Small bubbles tend to adhere to the tubing and, therefore, do not usually coalesce or move into the client's vascular system.

Clients receiving parenteral nutrition should be monitored for signs and symptoms of fluid, electrolyte, acid–base, and trace mineral imbalances, infection (especially septicemia), and nutritional status. Weight should be monitored daily. Blood specimens are collected periodically to verify homeostasis. The physician should be informed of abnormal laboratory data, rapid changes in weight, fever, or other signs and symptoms indicating inadequate therapeutic response or adverse reaction.

OUTCOME EVALUATION

Data required for evaluation include signs and symptoms of fluid, electrolyte, acid–base, or trace mineral balance or imbalance; absence or incidence of signs and symptoms of infection; client participation in procedures required for the treatment; the ability of the clients and family to manage parenteral nutrition therapy at home; and emotional acceptance of the treatment by the client and family. See the Example of Nursing Process for Parenteral Nutrition.

❖ CHECKLIST OF NURSING ACTIONS

- Provide emotional support for clients and their families during parenteral nutrition.
- Explain parenteral nutrition to the client and family before initiation.
- Position clients in the Trendelenburg position for insertion of a CV catheter; instruct them to perform

Example of Nursing Process for Parenteral Nutrition

The client is a 67-year-old retired railroad engineer who had had metastatic stomach cancer for 7 months. He has been hospitalized because of a progressive inability to eat, dehydration, and weight loss. His physician has ordered 1 L of D_5W at the rate of 120 mL/hr, to be followed by 1 L of dextrose in saline solution. He plans to order supplemental potassium according to electrolyte levels. A permanent CV catheter will be surgically implanted when the client's condition is stabilized; parenteral nutrition will be administered indefinitely. The client and his family will be informed about the requirements for treatment.

Assessment Data

Diagnosis of metastatic stomach cancer

Inability to eat

Order for parenteral nutrition of indefinite duration by implanted CV catheter

Nursing Diagnosis

Knowledge Deficit, concerning parenteral nutrition and the equipment and procedures required for its administration

Intervention

Explore with the client and family their knowledge about and emotional reaction to the proposed treatment.

Prepare and implement a teaching plan that covers the benefits to be derived from the treatment; sterile aseptic technique as it applies to IV infusions; thorough explanation of parenteral nutrition and the procedures necessary for its administration; supervised practice in the procedures required for administration of this therapy; and signs and symptoms of adverse reaction to the treatment, specifying those that require notification of healthcare personnel.

Refer the client and family to a community nursing service that offers care to clients receiving parenteral nutrition; inform this nursing service of the care plan used during the hospital stay and the response of the client and family to it.

Goals and Outcomes

The client and family will be able to demonstrate proper technique when carrying out procedures required for administration of parenteral nutrition.

The client and family will state that nursing care and support have continued without interruption during the illness.

---

a Valsalva maneuver during insertion of the catheter.

- If air enters the CV catheter, place the client immediately on the left side in the Trendelenburg position and inform the physician.
- Use IV tubing with in-line microfilters to administer concentrated solutions containing amino acids or protein hydrolysates.
- Use low-phthalate tubing without microfilters to administer fat emulsions.
- To minimize the risk of separation, do not agitate containers of fat emulsions.
- Inspect fat emulsions for homogeneity before administration.
- Begin infusion of fat emulsions slowly and monitor the client closely for the first half-hour of treatment for signs and symptoms of adverse reaction.

- Use strict aseptic technique when handling equipment used for parenteral nutrition.
- Monitor clients receiving parenteral nutrition for fluid, electrolyte, acid–base, and trace mineral balance.
- Monitor clients for changes in nutritional status.
- When parenteral nutrition is administered at home, teach the client and family how to manage the therapy.

Blood

Blood is the ideal nutrient because it contains all the constituents necessary for maintaining homeostasis in circulation: cells, proteins, electrolytes, and nutrients.

Because blood is a natural liquid tissue, transfusions are a kind of tissue transplant. Infusions of blood or blood components can restore homeostasis in many conditions not amenable to other therapeutic approaches.

The recipient of blood and blood products is at high risk for serious, life-threatening reactions, some of which cannot be ruled out for 2 years after treatment. For this reason, there is renewed interest in developing synthetic substances that can perform some or all of the functions of blood.

Physiology

To maintain a proper chemical milieu in the tissues, blood contains water, electrolytes, plasma proteins (albumin, globulins, and fibrinogen), nutrients, respiratory gases, hormones, antibodies, enzymes, clotting factors, red blood cells, white blood cells, and platelets. This mixture performs many vital functions in the tissues. It transports oxygen and nutrients to the cells and removes carbon dioxide and other metabolic wastes. It distributes hormones and enzymes throughout the tissues and conveys antibodies and white blood cells to sites of infection, injury, or inflammation. Its viscosity and volume contribute to the hydraulic factors that sustain adequate circulation.

Pathophysiology

The need for blood arises because of hemorrhage, accelerated destruction of certain constituents, or inadequate replenishment of components lost through normal attrition. In addition, in certain diseases, harmful components accumulate in the blood, and large proportions of the circulating blood must be replaced by fresh blood to prevent permanent injury or death.

Pharmacodynamics. Transfusions of whole blood or its components usually act to replenish blood constituents deficient in the client. Occasionally, blood is administered to replace large volumes of the client's blood, which are removed to eliminate one or more dangerous components, such as antibodies. In addition to the physiologic components unique to blood, transfusions provide calorie nutrients, electrolytes, vitamins, minerals, amino acids, and buffer salts.

The life span of transfused erythrocytes is somewhat less than the life span (averaging 120 days) of normal red blood cells produced by the client's bone marrow.

Pharmacokinetics. Blood and blood derivatives are administered by injection. Whole blood, packed cells, plasma, platelets, and albumin are infused directly into the venous vascular system. Clotting factors and gamma globulins may be injected IM; they are absorbed into the circulation from these sites and eventually enter the systemic circulation. Blood components are handled by the body just like the corresponding constituents of the client's blood; they are eventually metabolized or eliminated from the body.

Therapeutic Uses. Transfusions are used as therapy for several clinical conditions that are not amenable to treatment by other parenteral fluids (Table 48-6). Blood or blood products can temporarily correct deficiencies in erythrocytes, white blood cells, platelets, clotting factors, plasma proteins, and antibodies. They are used to treat such conditions as bone marrow depression, hemolysis, protein wasting by the kidneys or intestines, impaired liver function, and clotting disorders. Blood is also used to prime heart–lung machines for bypass perfusion.

Table 48-6. Therapeutic Uses of Blood and Blood Components

Blood or Blood Component	Disease or Condition	Therapeutic Effect
whole blood	Hemorrhage	Restoration of blood volume
replacement transfusion of whole blood	Erythroblastosis neonatorum	Removal of maternal antibodies from the baby's circulation and substitution of Rh-negative blood for Rh-positive blood with consequent reduction in hemolysis due to antigen–antibody reaction
packed cells	Anemia	Replenishment of erythrocytes
leukocyte-poor packed red blood cells	Anemia in persons with high levels of antibodies against white cells	Replenishment of erythrocytes without administering cells with antigens to which the recipient's antibodies will react
platelets	Platelet deficiency, as in aplastic anemia, leukemia, lymphomas, infection, drug toxicity, antineoplastic chemotherapy, consumptive coagulopathy, or immune destruction of platelets	Provision of platelets to promote coagulation
blood plasma	Nephrosis, protein-wasting intestinal disease	Replenishment of blood proteins
specific clotting factors	Clotting disorders such as hemophilia	Provision of clotting factors to promote coagulation
gamma globulins	Potential infection due to known exposure, such as contact with hepatitis virus	Provision of temporary passive immunity, which will prevent development of active infection

Adverse Reactions. Several adverse effects are associated with blood transfusions (Box 48-2). Among them are componential imbalances, allergic reactions, infectious diseases, and incompatibility reactions (Table 48-7). The incidence of adverse reactions can be reduced by careful screening of potential donors. Blood should not be accepted from persons who are acutely ill, are taking drugs (whether therapeutic or nonmedicinal), or have a history of jaundice. Blood collected from volunteers is generally safer than that purchased from professional donors.

Precautions and Contraindications. Numerous precautions are taken to ensure the safety of banked blood.

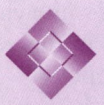

Box 48-2
Adverse Reactions to Blood

Componential Imbalances

Components of blood can produce excesses in the client. Hyperkalemia is most likely to develop because potassium from banked blood is gradually released from the erythrocytes into the plasma. Circulatory overload can also develop, particularly if multiple units of whole blood are given. Banked blood tends to lower calcium serum levels, and hypocalcemic tetany may result. In addition, banked blood may prolong coagulation time because citrate is added to it to prevent clotting. Citrate binds calcium, changing it from the ionic form to a physiologically inactive salt.

Allergic Reactions

Allergic reactions to blood arise because of antibodies in the donor blood. Initial signs and symptoms of an allergic reaction to blood include urticaria, itching, and wheals and sometimes laryngeal edema or bronchospasm. Symptoms can be controlled by treatment with antihistamines, epinephrine, and corticosteroids. If possible, the infusion should be stopped and another unit of blood be used. Allergic reactions are as likely to occur with the administration of plasma as with whole blood. Anaphylaxis can occur.

Infectious Disease

Blood can transmit disease present in the donor at the time of donation. Banking of blood eliminates the risk of some diseases (eg, syphilis, cytomegalovirus infection) because the causative organisms cannot survive prolonged exposure to refrigeration. The transmission of most other diseases by blood is rare. Rare but major exceptions are hepatitis, which accounts for most instances of transfusion-transmitted infection, and AIDS.

Incompatibility Reactions

A serious complication of blood therapy comes from antigen–antibody reactions resulting from tissue incompatibility. Although there are several antigenic systems characterizing blood types, most do not cause significant clinical problems. The ABO and Rh systems can induce serious reactions, however.

Blood types of the ABO system are inherited as single autosomal traits. Antigen A, antigen B, or both may be present on the erythrocytes of a person, giving rise to four different blood types: A, B, AB, or O (the absence of both antigens). Antibodies against these antigens are present naturally in any person whose erythrocytes lack them. Persons receiving a blood type that differs from their own are at risk for an antigen–antibody reaction. The most common type of reaction is hemolysis, which can disrupt circulation and damage organs, especially the kidneys. The severity of the reaction is influenced by the degree of mismatching and by the source of the antibodies (donor or recipient).

The most serious reactions occur when the plasma of the recipient contains antibodies against the antigens of transfused erythrocytes. The plasma in donated A, B, or O blood contains small amounts of antibodies that react with B, A, or AB antigens, respectively, if they are present on the recipient's erythrocytes. Such reactions are normally minor and produce no clinical signs or symptoms. With repeated or massive transfusions, however, a clinically significant, cumulative effect may occur. The risk of such a complication can be reduced by removing most of the plasma from donated blood and administering it in the form of packed cells.

Although persons with type AB blood are considered universal recipients and those with type O are considered universal donors, some degree of antigen–antibody reaction occurs whenever transfused blood is not identical to that of the recipient.

Another complication associated with incompatibility involves the Rh factor and erythrocyte antigens designated as D antigens. Inheritance of these traits is determined by three pairs of autosomal genes. There appears to be more than one type of D antigen, with varying degrees of potency in producing allergic reactions. One D antigen (Du) reacts with some anti-D sera but not others. The person with this type of blood must be treated as Rh-negative when receiving blood but Rh-positive when donating. Antibodies against D antigens do not occur naturally but arise as a result of a sensitizing exposure of Rh-negative persons to Rh-positive blood, through either transfusion or transplacental passage of red cells from an Rh-positive fetus. These antibodies can cause hemolysis if a second transfusion of Rh-positive blood is attempted. They also cross the placenta during subsequent pregnancies and can cause hemolytic disease in the Rh-positive fetus.

Table 48-7. ABO Antigens Occurring Naturally in Plasma

ABO Blood Type	Antibodies Contained in Plasma
A	B antibodies
B	A antibodies
AB	No antibodies of ABO type
O	Both A and B antibodies

These include testing blood for hepatitis B organisms and HIV. Blood is also tested for compatibility with the blood of the potential recipient. These tests involve typing for both ABO and Rh systems. Samples of donated blood of a suitable type are then mixed with the recipient's blood and observed for abnormal changes. If no adverse reaction occurs, the blood is considered suitable for the person tested. When the transfusion is begun, care must be taken to verify that the unit of blood given is identical to the unit tested and approved for administration to the recipient.

Diphenhydramine (Benadryl) is sometimes injected into the IV tubing before blood is infused. This tends to reduce the incidence and severity of allergic reactions to transfusions.

Blood should not be transfused through a CV line unless large amounts of blood are required quickly. The injection of cold blood directly into the heart can cause cardiac arrhythmias, especially in neonates.

Whenever possible, autotransfusions should be used. When the need for blood or a blood component can be predicted, many clients are now encouraged to bank their own blood. The required components may be separated from the blood unit and the remainder reinfused into the client. The generation of blood cells may be accelerated in between donations by administration of a bone marrow stimulant.

Blood containing ABO or Rh antigens (A, B, AB, or Rh-positive types) should never be administered to clients whose blood contains specific antibodies to these antigens (eg, O or Rh-negative types).

■ SUMMARY

Transfusions of blood or blood components are administered to maintain or replenish blood constituents that cannot be duplicated or provided by synthetic substitutes. Blood is also used to replace blood that must be removed from the body to eliminate one or more toxic elements and to prime heart–lung machines before bypass perfusion. Although blood transfusions provide unique therapeutic benefits, adverse reactions can be catastrophic. Because of its dangers, blood should never be administered unless necessary, and precautions designed to reduce its risks must be strictly observed.

❖ NURSING MANAGEMENT: CLIENT RECEIVING BLOOD

Blood is highly perishable and must be kept refrigerated until it is administered. It should not be allowed to freeze. Blood or platelets to be warmed should be removed from the refrigerator and allowed to stand at room temperature for up to 1 hour before using. Never attempt to warm it by any method that could warm any part of it above body temperature.

NURSING PROCESS

ASSESSMENT

When a transfusion is to be administered, the client's general condition should be assessed and the condition mandating transfusion identified.

Clients must give informed consent for the procedure. Some clients will not accept transfusions for religious reasons; others fear blood-borne infection. As with any other treatment, clients have the right to refuse therapy.

The client who is to receive IV blood or blood products should be assessed for allergy or systemic infection resembling transfusion reaction. These symptoms should be recorded as accurately and quantitatively as possible so that they will not be mistaken for transfusion reaction. Any increase in these symptoms should be interpreted as possible transfusion reaction until proven otherwise.

NURSING DIAGNOSIS

Nursing diagnoses for the client receiving blood products include:

- Fluid Volume Excess, related to IV administration of large volumes of blood
- Risk for Injury, related to potential allergic reaction to donor blood

Common collaborative problems that should be differentiated from the nursing diagnoses include:

Potential Complications: Cardiac arrest, hyperkalemia, tetany, anaphylaxis, or hemolysis

PLANNING

Goals of nursing care are to prevent administration of mismatched blood, to correct the condition for which blood is used, and to prevent or detect and treat promptly any adverse reactions to blood or blood products.

INTERVENTION

The nurse should verify that the designated unit of blood matches the client's blood type, in accord with institutional protocols, because the administration of the wrong type of blood can be fatal. Each unit of blood is identified by a multicopy label bearing the name and number of the donor, the blood expiration date, the ABO and Rh types, the results of tests for the presence of infectious pathogens, and the name and address of the blood bank that processed the unit. When a client's blood is matched, one copy of this information from each unit of blood used is placed in the client's chart. Before initiating the transfusion, two nurses (or a nurse and a physician) should verify independently all identifying information, matching the label attached to the blood container with its copy in the chart and the client's identification band. Unless all information corresponds, the blood must not be used and should be returned to the laboratory.

Blood must be administered through tubing with a special blood filter and a large-bore needle (18-gauge or larger). The system is primed with normal saline or other solution compatible with blood. Dextrose is not used because it promotes cell aggregation. Medication must not be administered in the system containing blood because drugs might injure the red cells.

The infusion should be started at a slow flow rate (1 mL/kg per hour or less). During transfusion, the recipient must be monitored carefully for signs and symptoms of circulatory overload, hyperkalemia, hypocalcemia, abnormal bleeding, or transfusion reaction. Early signs and symptoms of transfusion reaction include anxiety, restlessness, chest or back pain, flushing, and increased pulse and respirations. These reactions may be followed by shaking chills, fever, and cyanosis.

Should a transfusion reaction occur, the infusion must be stopped immediately. The IV line must be kept open because emergency treatment may be needed if the reaction is severe. To prevent the absorption of even small amounts of additional blood, the infusion bottles should be lowered below the level of the infusion site to induce a flashback. The tubing can then be disconnected at the injection site, flushed with priming solution, and reconnected to restore the flow of priming solution through the IV needle. The prescriber must be notified immediately when any reaction to blood occurs. The nurse should be prepared to institute measures to treat the reaction, including administering any medications ordered.

All transfusion reactions must be thoroughly investigated to determine the cause. The blood container and fresh samples of blood from the client are sent to the laboratory with a description of the reaction. The most common cause of such reactions is the administration of blood to the wrong person, underlining the importance of accurately matching the blood to the client at the time of administration.

The client with urticaria should be instructed to press on itching sites and to avoid scratching. Excessive clothing or bedding should be removed so that the client is comfortably cool, because heat increases itching.

Client Education. The client (or a family member, if the client is incompetent) must be informed of the plan for transfusion before blood is administered. Although written permission for the procedure is not always required, the use of blood is forbidden by some religions (notably Jehovah's Witnesses), and fear of blood-borne disease has increased since the risk of HIV transmission has been recognized. An opportunity must be provided for refusal of treatment.

The need for a transfusion often provokes anxiety, because most people know that using blood is somewhat hazardous, that blood is scarce, and that it is not used unless necessary. Therefore, transfusion implies that the illness is grave. The need for blood therapy should be explained to the client or family in as reassuring a manner as possible.

During the initial period of transfusion, when constant monitoring of the client is necessary, the nurse should maintain a calm, matter-of-fact demeanor. Productive use of time with the client for nursing care will deemphasize the critical nature of this interval. Before leaving, the nurse should instruct the client to report promptly any discomfort.

OUTCOME EVALUATION

Data required for evaluation relate to the incidence or absence of signs and symptoms of adverse reaction to the transfusion. The client should be assessed for fluid, potassium, and calcium balance, as well as for circulation and tissue perfusion.

❖ **CHECKLIST OF NURSING ACTIONS**

❑ Before initiating a transfusion, assess the client for signs and symptoms of conditions that resemble transfusion reaction.

❑ Inform the client about the transfusion and verify that the treatment is acceptable to him or her.

❑ Verify with another health professional that the unit of blood to be used is properly matched with the recipient.

❑ Observe the client continuously for signs and symptoms of adverse reaction until at least 50 mL of blood have been absorbed.

❑ Administer blood slowly.

❑ If signs and symptoms of adverse reaction develop, discontinue the transfusion immediately; maintain a patent IV line for administration of medications.

❑ When a transfusion reaction occurs, save the blood container and send it to the laboratory for tests to determine the reason for the reaction.

Bibliography

Adler T. (1995). Debugging blood: Protecting people from tainted blood. *Sci News, 147*, 92–93 (Feb. 11).

———. (1996). Blood transfusions: Playing it safe. *Nursing, 26*, 50–52 (Apr).

*Bohony J. (1993). Nine common IV complications and what to do about them. *AJN, 93*, 45–49 (Oct).

*Carroll PA. (1994). When you should—and shouldn't—give bicarb. *RN, 57*, 62 (Apr).

*Carroll PA. (1995). When a Jehovah's Witness refuses a transfusion. *Nursing, 25,* 60–61 (Aug).

*Harovas J, Anthony H. (1993). Managing transfusion reactions. *RN, 56,* 32–37 (Dec).

Hastings-Tolsma M, Yucha C. (1994). IV infiltration: No clear signs, no clear treatment? *RN, 57,* 34–39 (Dec).

Held JL. (1995). Correcting fluid and electrolyte imbalances. *Nursing, 25,* 71 (Apr).

*Hennessey B, FitzGerald A, Graham D. (1993). Venous air embolism: Keeping your patient out of danger. *AJN, 93,* 54–56 (Nov).

*————. (1994). KCl injection: Don't get pushy. *Nursing, 24,* 15 (Dec. 1994).

Kresevic DM. (1990). Understanding therapeutic plasma exchange. *Nursing, 20,* 68 (Apr).

Levins TT. (1996). Central intravenous lines: Your role. *Nursing, 26,* 48–49 (Apr).

Mathews LE. (1994). Preparing your patient for home infusion. *Nursing, 24,* 28 (Oct).

*McCormac M. (1990). Managing hemorrhagic shock. *AJN, 90*(8), 22.

*Metheny NM. (1990). Why worry about IV fluids? *AJN, 90*(6), 50–57.

Sansivero GE. (1995). Why pick a PICC? *Nursing, 25,* 35–42 (Jul).

Smith RA, Smith RN, Fallentine J, Keffel F. (1995). Autotransfusion. *Nursing, 25,* 52–54 (Mar).

Viall C. (1995). Taking the mystery out of TPI (Part 1). *Nursing, 25,* 34–43 (Apr).

Viall C. (1995). Taking the mystery out of TPI (Part 2). *Nursing, 25,* 57–59 (May).

*Vonfrolio LG. (1995). Would you hang these IV solutions? *AJN, 95,* 37–39 (Jun).

*Recommended for further reading.

For more information and sample tests and activities, refer to Chapter 48 in the Student Workbook for Clinical Pharmacology and Nursing Management, 5th edition, available through your bookstore.

49

Oral Nutritional Supplements

Nutrition and the detection and correction of nutritional deficiencies have always been a major concern of nurses. With improvement in food supplies and education of the public to the risks of undernutrition, deficiency states have become uncommon. However, health food fads and the marketing of supplemental nutrients have provoked an increasing incidence of toxicity. Many clients can benefit from counseling regarding these products. Clients with unusual nutritional needs or severe nutritional imbalances should be referred to a nutritionist for expert diagnosis and treatment. The nurse may, however, screen clients for nutritional problems and advise them on diet and the use of nutritional supplements. Nurses who function as primary healthcare providers often become knowledgeable about nutrition and can diagnose and treat a variety of nutritional problems.

Nutritional Agents

Several therapeutic agents are administered to prevent or correct nutritional deficiencies. These include vitamins, minerals, injectable fluids, energy nutrients, and blood. Although these agents are substances used by or produced in the body naturally during normal functions, they can cause adverse reactions, especially when administered in high dosages.

This chapter discusses the preventive and therapeutic uses of vitamins, minerals, and health food products. These substances are not classified as drugs and are not controlled by the Food and Drug Administration. The labels on these product packages rarely inform the consumer about use, safe dosage, or adverse reactions.

Vitamins

Vitamins are organic chemicals found in foods. They are essential in small quantities for growth, health, and life and perform vital functions in many biochemical processes of the body. Vitamins do not resemble each other chemically. Some are water-soluble, some fat-soluble. Their molecules do not share common structures that are characteristic of vitamins as a group. They are distinguished only by the fact that deficiencies cause impaired health, delayed growth, or disease.

Chemicals are classified as vitamins because they cannot be manufactured by the body and, hence, must be present in the diet for normal function. Chemicals required by specific species vary: a vitamin necessary to humans may be synthesized readily by other animals. Generally, a given vitamin is not required in a single chemical form. Rather, several similar molecules can be used by the body to produce the required biochemical. Synthetic vitamins do not differ significantly from vitamins contained in "natural" sources.

Role of Vitamins

Most vitamins are necessary to metabolic processes that transform food into tissue or energy. They are used by the body to synthesize cofactors or coenzymes that participate in essential metabolic processes in the body (Table 49-1).

Although much is known about the physiologic functions of vitamins, this area is still poorly understood. Vitamins are known to be necessary for normal growth, development, and body maintenance, but the degree to which they may enhance health in people who

Table 49-1. Physiologic Functions of Vitamins

Vitamin	Metabolic Function	Physiologic Effects
vitamin A (retinol, retinaldehyde, retinoic acid, retinyl esters)	Promotes mucin production in epithelial cells by an unknown mechanism	Essential in the growth, development, and maintenance of epithelial tissue
	May play a role in cell membrane regulation as an enzyme cofactor; may function as an enzyme cofactor in steroid and mucopolysaccharide synthesis	Essential in growth and reproduction
	Enhances resistance to carcinogenesis, possibly by destabilizing lysosomes, enhancing antitumor immunity, or direct cytotoxic action on abnormal cells	Reduces susceptibility to carcinogenesis
	Retinol is a component of the photosensitive pigments of the eye, rhodopsin and iodopsin.	Essential for normal function of the retina
vitamin B complex: thiamine (vitamin B$_1$)	Functions as a coenzyme (thiamine pyrophosphate) in Krebs' cycle	Essential for energy metabolism, especially that involving carbohydrates
	Plays a role in the transmission of impulses on nerve membranes, possibly by promoting sodium influx	Essential for normal nerve function
riboflavin (vitamin B$_2$, vitamin G)	Is a constituent of two coenzymes, flavin mononucleotide and flavin adenine dinucleotide	Essential for the completion of several reactions in the energy cycle that produces ATP
	Is a component of amino acid oxidases and xanthine oxidase	Involved in the oxidation of amino acids and hydroxy-acids to alpha-keto acids and the oxidation of a number of purines
niacin (nicotinic acid, nicotinamide)	Is a constituent of two coenzymes, nicotinamide-adenine dinucleotide and nicotinamide-adenine dinucleotide phosphate, which act as hydrogen acceptors in many metabolic reactions	Essential for the synthesis of fatty acids and the conversion of phenylalanine to tyrosine
vitamin B$_6$ (pyridoxine, pyridoxal, pyridoxamine)	Is a constituent of pyridoxal phosphate, a coenzyme for many metabolic reactions involved in amino acid metabolism	Serves an important role in amino acid metabolism, including decarboxylation, transamination, transulfuration, and conversion of tryptophan to niacin
		Required for glycogenolysis, synthesis of hemoglobin, and formation of antibodies
		May be required for conversion of linoleic acid to arachidonic acid
		Needed for formation of norepinephrine, epinephrine, tyramine, dopamine, serotonin
folacin (folic acid, pteroylglutamic acid)	Forms coenzymes known as tetrahydrofolates involved in one-carbon transfers in metabolism	Essential for DNA synthesis
		With cyanocobalamin, regulates the formation of red blood cells in the bone marrow
pantothenic acid (calcium pantothenate, dexpanthenol)	Is a constituent of coenzyme A, which serves as a cofactor for reactions involving transfer of acetyl (two-carbon) groups	Required for oxidative metabolism of carbohydrates, gluconeogenesis, synthesis and degradation of fatty acids, and synthesis of sterols, steroid hormones, and porphyrins
vitamin B$_{12}$ (cyanocobalamin, hydroxocobalamin, extrinsic factor)	Is a constituent of coenzymes involved in the demethylation of methylfolate and the maintenance of sulfhydroxyl groups of enzymes in a reduced state, the conversion of homocysteine to methionine and the maintenance of methyl-malonate-succinate isomerization	Required for DNA synthesis in bone marrow; with folacin, regulates the production of red blood cells
		May be essential for maintenance of metabolic activity of folacin
biotin	Is a constituent of a coenzyme for carboxylation and deamination reactions	Required in the synthesis of fatty acids, generation of tricarboxylic acid cycle, and formation of purines
vitamin C (ascorbic acid, ascorbate)	Functions as a cofactor in hydroxylation reactions	Needed for formation of collagen, conversion of tryptophan to serotonin, and conversion of cholesterol to bile acids
	Functions as an antioxidant	Protects vitamins A and E and polyunsaturated fatty acids from excessive oxidation
		Inhibits oxidation of crystallins (proteins in the eye lens), thereby delaying formation of cataracts
		May play a role in resistance to carcinogenesis and malignant tumor growth
		Promotes absorption and use of iron
		Converts folacin to its active metabolite, folinic acid

(continued)

Table 49-1. (Continued)

Vitamin	Metabolic Function	Physiologic Effects
		By as yet unknown mechanisms, is involved in clotting, synthesis of adrenocortical hormones, and resistance to infection
vitamin D (cholecalciferol, calcitriol, dihydrotachysterol, ergocalciferol, viosterol)	Is a constituent of a calcium-controlling hormone, calcitriol	Necessary for proper metabolism of calcium and phosphorus; promotes intestinal absorption of calcium and phosphorus, stimulates renal reabsorption of phosphate, stimulates release of calcium from bone tissue and bone resorption
vitamin E (tocopherols of several types)	Functions as a biologic antioxidant	Has no proven function in normal humans
		May oppose pathologic conditions characterized by increased oxidation, particularly by free radicals (cellular aging, oxygen toxicity, damage from air pollutants, other degenerative biochemical transformations)
vitamin K (menadione, phytonadione)	Is the lipid cofactor for membrane-bound peptide carboxylase	Essential for formation of prothrombin and other clotting proteins by the liver
		May participate in oxidative phosphorylation in tissues

show no overt signs or symptoms of deficiency remains controversial.

The dietary need for vitamins appears to assume a normal distribution. Requirements for most people lie within a fairly narrow range, but some people need dosages that deviate markedly from this norm.

Vitamin preparations exert the same nutritional effects as do the same nutrients ingested in food. They serve as replacement therapy for people who have deficient diets or whose needs for vitamins are exceptionally high.

Vitamin Deficiencies

Vitamins were discovered because of their ability to reverse the signs and symptoms of disease states caused by severe nutritional deficiencies. Diseases stemming from severe vitamin deficiencies include xerophthalmia, beriberi, pellagra, pernicious anemia, scurvy, rickets, osteomalacia, infantile hemolytic anemia, and hemorrhagic disease in the newborn (Table 49-2). Moderate deficiencies also produce symptoms of impaired health. The degree to which subtle deficiencies may contribute to minor problems, such as discomfort or fatigue, in people whose health appears normal has not been established.

Individual requirements for specific vitamins can be influenced by both genetic and environmental factors. Resistance to the effects of certain vitamins can be inherited. Some people do not absorb these nutrients readily. Hormone balance, growth, disease processes, stress, and drugs can influence the function of vitamins, as well as the dietary requirement. It is important that the nutritional requirements of people with unusual nutritional needs be met.

Vitamin deficiencies are relatively rare in the United States. When they do occur, they usually involve multiple rather than single deficiencies. For example, vitamin B deficiencies usually involve inadequate levels of all the nutrients in this group. Special circumstances usually underlie single deficiencies (eg, pellagra in corn-eating populations, pernicious anemia after gastrectomy, scurvy in older adults who subsist on soft foods, such as milk, bread, and eggs, and who do not eat citrus fruits). Most often, poor dietary habits involve an inadequate intake of many nutrients, including all vitamins.

Kinds of Vitamins

As constituents of the diet, vitamins enter the body normally through the digestive tract. They are widely distributed in the tissues and are found in high concentrations in the liver. Some are destroyed by the metabolic processes in which they participate; others are transformed and subsequently excreted in urine or feces. Because they are handled differently by the body, fat-soluble and water-soluble vitamins are discussed separately (Box 49-1).

Fat-Soluble Vitamins

Natural forms of fat-soluble vitamins require digestible fat and bile salts for absorption in the small intestine. Conditions in which fat absorption is decreased, such as diarrhea or steatorrhea, reduce absorption of these nutrients. Nondigestible fats in the tract, such as mineral oil or olestra (a noncaloric fat substitute), carry the fat-soluble vitamins out of the body in feces. Synthetic forms of fat-soluble vitamins that are water-miscible are available. These preparations do not require fat or bile salts for absorption but may be incompletely absorbed if peristalsis is excessive.

Vitamin D binds to a specific alpha-globulin known as vitamin D-binding protein. Vitamin E in the bloodstream is associated with plasma lipoproteins. These

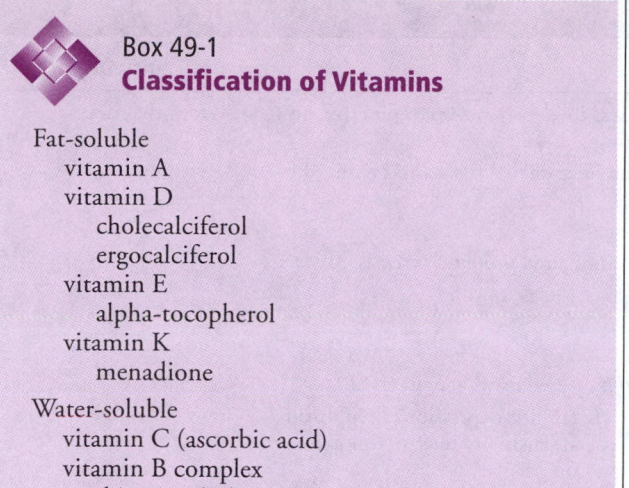

Classification of Vitamins

Fat-soluble
  vitamin A
  vitamin D
    cholecalciferol
    ergocalciferol
  vitamin E
    alpha-tocopherol
  vitamin K
    menadione
Water-soluble
  vitamin C (ascorbic acid)
  vitamin B complex
    thiamine (B_1)
    riboflavin (B_2)
    niacin (nicotinic acid)
    pyridoxine hydrochloride (B_6)
    pantothenic acid
    biotin
    choline; inositol; para-aminobenzoic acid
    folic acid
    cyanocobalamin (B_{12})

complexations serve to prevent renal excretion of the vitamin molecules. Transport of vitamin A from body depots is dependent on the globulin carrier, and deficiency of the vitamin associated with protein deficiency cannot be corrected by administering the vitamin alone.

Vitamins A and D tend to accumulate in the liver. (Animal livers are excellent dietary sources of these nutrients, and commercial preparations are derived from fish livers.) Some vitamin A is also deposited in the kidneys, lungs, adrenals, retinas, and intraperitoneal fat. Additional storage of vitamin D uses fat depots in the body. Vitamin K is not stored in large quantities in the body. Except in infants, vitamin E is widely distributed in large quantities in the tissues. The plasma tocopherol concentrations in newborns is only about 20% that of their mothers.

The precursors of vitamins A and D (beta-carotene and 7-dehydrocholesterol, respectively) accumulate in the skin. High levels of carotene in the skin impart a yellow or orange tinge that may be pronounced but appears to be physiologically harmless. The whites of the eyes are not affected by this color change. Precursors are transformed to active vitamin forms within the body. Beta-carotene is transformed to vitamin A in the wall of the small intestine. Vitamin D is produced by ultraviolet irradiation of 7-dehydrocholesterol. The deposition of this chemical in the skin is fortuitous because conversion occurs only in body tissues exposed to ultraviolet light.

Vitamins A, E, and K are metabolized by the liver and enter the enterohepatic circulation. Eventually, metabolites are excreted in both feces and urine. Calcitriol is transformed in the kidneys and is excreted mainly in bile and feces.

Water-Soluble Vitamins

Most of the water-soluble vitamins are well absorbed by the gastrointestinal (GI) tract. Niacin, pyridoxine (vitamin B_6), pantothenic acid, and vitamin C are absorbed readily from all areas of the GI tract and are widely distributed in the tissues. Folic acid and thiamine cross the intestinal membrane by active transport systems in specific areas of the small bowel. Adequate absorption of vitamin B_{12} requires hydrochloric acid and a specific gastric glycoprotein (intrinsic factor) for transport across the ileal mucosa. Passive diffusion of this vitamin is inadequate to maintain body stores unless concentrations in the intestinal lumen are extremely high.

Plasma binding of water-soluble vitamins appears to be minimal—only folic acid and vitamin B_{12} are bound to a significant degree.

Vitamins of the B complex are stored in the liver to variable degrees. Although high concentrations of vitamin C are found in tissues such as the adrenals, there appear to be no significant depots of this nutrient, and regular daily intake is considered essential to good health.

Thiamine used by the body is completely degraded in the tissues. Other water-soluble vitamins are metabolized by the liver. All are excreted by the kidneys. Vitamin B_{12} also participates in the enterohepatic cycle, an important avenue for body losses when reabsorption is inadequate. This vitamin may be present in feces in large amounts.

Therapeutic Uses

Vitamins are used to prevent and treat deficiency states. Because the underlying causes of deficiency in most clinical situations—inadequate dietary intake or malabsorption—affect most nutrients, attention must be given to total nutrition rather than to levels of individual nutrients. For this reason, vitamin supplementation usually involves administering multivitamins.

In some situations, individual needs for specific vitamins can be unusually high due to inborn errors of metabolism or to environmental factors that increase tissue needs. In these cases, vitamin dosage must be tailored to meet these needs. Occasionally, as in pernicious anemia, a single vitamin is needed.

Preparations

Multivitamin preparations for dietary supplementation are marketed in two strengths: maintenance and therapeutic. A daily dose of most maintenance preparations contains vitamin doses approximating the recommended daily allowances (RDA; Table 49-3). Vitamin A doses rarely exceed this allowance. Slight excesses of

Table 49-2. Physiologic Manifestations of Vitamin Deficiencies

Vitamin	Signs and Symptoms of Deficiency	Deficiency Disease
vitamin A	Changes in the eyes progressing from night blindness to xerosis of the conjunctiva, xerosis of the cornea, loss of corneal substance, scarring	Xerophthalmia
	Shrinking, hardening, and progressive degeneration of epithelial tissues and reduced resistance to invasion by infectious organisms	Keratomalacia
	Overgrowth of the bones with resultant nerve lesions	
	Growth retardation characterized by osteoblastosis, impaired protein synthesis, loss of appetite	
	Vague apathy	
	Dry, rough skin	
	Increased risk of lung and GI infections leading to increased death rate in children	
thiamine	Mild deficiency: fatigue, weakness, lack of interest, irritability, depression, sleep disturbance, restlessness, emotional instability (aggressiveness, sensitivity to criticism, poor impulse control, mood swings), anorexia, weight loss	Beriberi
	Moderate deficiency: pallor, apathy, indigestion, constipation, headaches, nightmares, bruxism, insomnia, sweating, tachycardia after moderate exercise, muscle cramps, paresthesias	
	Pronounced deficiency: muscle degeneration due to peripheral neuropathy, cardiomyopathy with congestive failure, emaciation, confusion, loss of memory. In infants: pallor, facial edema, irritability	
	Abdominal pain, vomiting, loss of voice, and convulsions	
riboflavin	Moderate deficiency: cheilosis, glossitis, greasy dermatitis (seborrhea) in skin folds (nasolabial, scrotal, vulval), asthenia, vascularization of the cornea, growth retardation in the young	
niacin	Early signs: fatigue, muscle weakness, lassitude, depression, headache, backache, anorexia, indigestion, weight loss, mild skin eruptions, loss of memory	Pellagra
	Late signs: asthenia, beefy-red glossitis, cheilosis, abdominal discomfort, nausea, vomiting, diarrhea, dermatitis (most pronounced in exposed areas), dementia; in children, growth retardation	
vitamin B$_6$ (pyridoxine)	In adults: seborrheic dermatitis, peripheral neuritis, impaired immunity	
	In children: anemia, impaired immunity, vomiting, ataxia, weakness, abdominal pain, nervous irritability, convulsive seizures	
	During pregnancy or use of oral contraceptives: possibly carbohydrate intolerance, depression, hypertriglyceridemia	
folic acid	Pallor, asthenia, megaloblastic leukopenia and macrocytic anemia, reduced platelet levels, possibly glossitis and diarrhea; during pregnancy, increased risk of spina bifida in the offspring	
pantothenic acid	Malaise, vomiting, burning cramps, fatigue, tenderness in the heels, insomnia, diarrhea	
vitamin B$_{12}$	Lemon-yellow pallor, asthenia, anorexia, vomiting, diarrhea, hand and foot paresthesias, signs and symptoms of psychosis, megaloblastic macrocytic anemia, progressive neuropathy due to progressive demyelinization	Pernicious anemia
biotin	Dermatitis, glossitis, lassitude, hyperesthesia, pallor, anorexia, nausea, loss of sleep, depression, muscle pains, hypercholesterolemia	
vitamin C	Early signs: intermittent joint pains, gum disease, dry skin, irritability, anemia, shortness of breath, poor wound healing, increased susceptibility to infection, petechiae due to increased capillary fragility; in children, growth retardation	Scurvy
	Late signs: anorexia, pain, tenderness and swelling of the joints, rough skin with dingy brown color, gingivitis, loss of teeth, anemia, petechial hemorrhages (progressing to spontaneous ecchymoses), muscle and cartilage degeneration	
	In infants: pallor, fever, diarrhea, vomiting, enlargement of the ends of the long bones, disinclination to move, crying when handled	
vitamin D	Unexplained cochlear deafness in middle age, demineralization of the teeth and bones with skeletal deformity, pretetany, bone pain	In adults: osteomalacia
	In infants: delayed closure of the fontanelles, softening of the skull, bossing of the forehead, enlargement of the ends of the long bones, bowing of the legs, enlargement of the costochondral junction ("rachitic rosary"), pigeon breast, scoliosis, narrowing of the pelvis, poorly developed muscles, weakness, restlessness, irritability, delayed dentition, malformed teeth, retarded growth	In children: rickets
vitamin E	Increased hemolysis of red blood cells, macrocytic anemia, increased capillary fragility	Hemolytic anemia in low-birth weight infants
vitamin K	Petechiae, ecchymoses, bleeding into the joints or muscles, GI bleeding, asthenia	Hemorrhagic disease in newborns

Table 49-3. Comparison of Vitamin Dosages

Vitamin	Recommended Daily Allowance*	Maximum Dosage Recommended for Correction of Deficiencies
vitamin A	1,400–6,000 IU (one IU = 0.3 µg retinol; one retinol equivalent = 3.33 IU)	30 mg retinol (100,000 IU) daily, in a single dose
thiamine	0.3–1.5 mg	90 mg daily in divided doses
riboflavin	0.4–1.8 mg	10 mg daily
niacin	5–20 mg	500 mg daily
vitamin B$_6$	0.3–2.5 mg	100 mg daily
folic acid		1,000 µg daily
Infant 6 mo–1 yr	35 µg	
Child 4–6 yr	75 µg	
Child 11–14 yr	150 µg	
Pregnant woman	400 µg	
Lactating woman (first 6 months)	280 µg	
Menstruating female	180 µg	
Adult male	200 µg	
pantothenic acid	10 mg	No recommendation available
vitamin B$_{12}$		100 µg daily
Child 4–6 yr	2.5 µg	
Child 11–14 yr	3.0 µg	
Pregnant woman	4.0 µg	
Lactating woman	4.0 µg	
Menstruating female	3.0 µg	
Adult male	3.0 µg	
vitamin C	60 mg (100 mg for smokers)	500 mg daily
vitamin D	400 IU (one IU = 0.025 µg pure crystalline vitamin D)	50,000 IU (malabsorption) 1,000 IU (uncomplicated deficiencies)
vitamin E	4–15 IU (one IU = 1 mg alpha-tocopherol)	100 mg daily
vitamin K	No recommendation available (estimated minimum daily requirement is 0.03 µg/kg or about 1.8–3 mg for adults)	10 mg daily

*As established by the Food and Nutrition Board, National Academy of Sciences–National Research Council (specific recommendations vary with age, sex, and reproductive status).

water-soluble vitamins may be included. Therapeutic formulas have much higher doses and are used for treating existing deficiencies and for preventing deficiencies in persons considered at high risk for deficiencies because of increased nutrient needs. Special formulations are marketed for specific groups who have a greater need for certain vitamins (eg, smokers, pregnant women). Children's vitamins also differ from adult formulations.

Adverse Effects

Theoretically, all vitamins can produce adverse reactions. The margin of safety for water-soluble vitamins is wide, and toxic symptoms are rare. Fat-soluble vitamins are more toxic.

Hypervitaminosis A is the most common toxicity. Symptoms may be due, at least in part, to retinyl esters associated with plasma lipoproteins that act as surfac-

tants. Dosages as low as twice the RDA may produce toxicity if continued over time. Signs and symptoms include malaise, nausea, desquamation, corneal opacities or erosion, decalcification of bones, early epiphyseal closure, bone tenderness, lethargy, increased intracranial pressure, and coma. Death may occur. The vitamin is teratogenic, and congenital malformations are likely to develop in embryos exposed to high levels.

Vitamin E toxicity in preterm infants is characterized by respiratory distress, renal failure, liver disease, ascites, and thrombocytopenia.

Vitamin D toxicity may develop at dosages 12 times the RDA. Signs and symptoms include weakness, fatigue, lassitude, headache, nausea, vomiting, diarrhea, renal impairment, or hypertension. Calcification of soft tissues tends to develop; this is most dangerous in the kidneys. High calcium serum levels characteristic of vitamin D toxicity are especially dangerous to persons receiving digitalis because calcium excess increases the risk of toxicity of this medication.

In children, vitamin D excess may cause cessation of growth for up to 6 months, and some permanent stunting of stature may result. Persons who have experienced this toxicity may retain permanent hypersensitivity to normal doses of the vitamin.

Although vitamin K is nontoxic in usual doses, large doses may cause problems in adults, and children are sometimes affected by moderate dosages. The drug can cause hemolytic anemia, hyperbilirubinemia, and kernicterus in infants. It is irritating to skin and respiratory tract tissues. Rapid intravenous (IV) administration may cause flushing, dyspnea, chest pains, and, rarely, death. Administration of vitamin K to persons with severe hepatic disease may aggravate the liver disease.

In the past, toxic syndromes were not considered to be a problem with most water-soluble vitamins. However, some toxic reactions have been recognized with pharmacologic doses, and several additional syndromes have been described recently.

Among the B-complex vitamins, niacin in large doses produces vasodilation, flushing, and increased peristalsis. Vitamin B_6 overdose causes neurologic problems characterized by paresthesias, numbness, and ataxia. Large doses of folic acid have caused recurrence of seizures in persons using anticonvulsants with antifolate properties (eg, phenytoin, phenobarbital, primidone). They are also associated with increased risk of miscarriage. Vitamin B_{12} toxicity is characterized by polycythemia vera and peripheral vascular thrombosis. Very large doses are required for these effects.

Exposure to high doses of vitamin C may speed up the metabolism and excretion of this chemical. Abrupt withdrawal then causes a temporary deficiency, despite seemingly adequate dietary intake. Rebound scurvy may occur; infants are particularly vulnerable. Vitamin C is also excreted as oxalate and can cause oxalate renal calculi.

Allergy to some vitamin preparations may represent reactions to extraneous chemicals in the preparations (eg, tartrazine). However, some allergic reactions appear to be true allergy to the vitamin molecule. Allergy may cause itching, diarrhea, or anaphylaxis.

Drug–Vitamin Interactions

Simultaneous use of thiazide diuretics and calcium and vitamin D supplements may result in hypercalcemia. Vitamin D enhances GI absorption of calcium, and thiazide diuretics reduce its excretion by the kidneys. Vitamin C may block the effect of copper, causing anemia. Vitamin B_6 opposes the action of levodopa, vitamin K that of warfarin, and folic acid that of antifolate anticonvulsants.

Precautions and Contraindications

Vitamin supplements and pharmacologic doses of vitamins should be discontinued if signs and symptoms of toxicity develop.

Large dosages of vitamin A are contraindicated during pregnancy. The dosage of vitamin D and calcium supplements should be reduced or discontinued in clients receiving thiazide diuretics.

The daily dose of vitamin B_6 used for premenstrual tension should not exceed 100 mg. Clients taking supplements should be warned to report any signs or symptoms of neuropathy, such as numbness or unusual sensations.

Hypervitaminosis or allergic sensitivity contraindicates the use of the particular vitamin or vitamins involved. Prolonged use of large dosages should be avoided unless there is a demonstrated need for abnormally high doses. The fat-soluble vitamins are particularly dangerous.

Intravenous doses of vitamins should be given slowly to avoid acute reactions.

To prevent toxicity, plasma levels of vitamin E used to treat premature infants should not exceed 3.5 mg/dL. The daily dose of folic acid supplements during pregnancy should not exceed 1 mg. This will prevent folate deficiency, even in persons taking antifolate anticonvulsants.

▪ SUMMARY

Vitamins are organic chemicals found in food that are essential in small quantities for health and normal growth. They cannot be synthesized by the body. Most are converted to metabolic coenzymes or cofactors by the body.

Although a well-balanced diet provides adequate vitamins for most people, supplements may be needed by persons at high risk for developing deficiencies because of inadequate diet, malabsorption, or increased tissue needs.

Water-soluble vitamins have a wide therapeutic margin of safety. Fat-soluble vitamins, especially A and D, are more apt to cause toxicity.

❖ NURSING MANAGEMENT: CLIENT TAKING VITAMIN SUPPLEMENTS

Vitamins are among the most commonly used nutritional supplements. Nutritionists have decried the waste of money spent on unneeded vitamin preparations, contending that a well-balanced diet furnishes all the vitamins needed by most consumers. It is now apparent, however, that dietary practices in developed countries may not provide optimal levels of nutrients. Because of aging populations and labor-saving technology, the need for calories has diminished, decreasing the amount of food (and vitamins) ingested. In addition, food processing tends to lower the vitamin content of food. There is growing recognition that the use of vitamin supplements may be a wise and cost-effective measure to ensure adequate intake.

NURSING PROCESS

ASSESSMENT

Basic assessment includes dietary analysis and physical assessment for signs and symptoms of nutritional deficiency or excess.

To determine dietary practices, clients should be questioned about their usual food intake. A listing of all foods consumed over the previous 24 hours often is revealing. It may corroborate the general diet history or raise questions about its accuracy.

Physical assessment should address the signs and symptoms of vitamin deficiency—abnormalities of skin and mucous membranes, delayed or abnormal skeletal development, defects in vision (eg, night blindness), low energy levels, emotional lability, mental aberrations, poor resistance to infection, poor color, anorexia, bleeding gums, or petechiae. The presence of such symptoms in a person with good dietary habits may indicate malabsorption or a condition in which tissue needs for nutrients are abnormally high (see Table 49-2).

The health history may disclose conditions that place the person at high risk for vitamin deficiencies. Pregnancy, use of oral contraceptives, smoking, habitual use of alcohol, rapid growth, and hyperthyroidism increase metabolic needs for vitamins. Dietary intake is apt to be reduced in elderly persons and in persons on rigorous weight-reduction regimens. A history of sprue, ulcerative colitis, or any other condition characterized by malabsorption may indicate that the person cannot assimilate normal amounts of nutrients. People who have undergone gastric surgery or who have serious gastric disease are at high risk for pernicious anemia. Malignant neoplasms, acute infections, and other tissue-wasting diseases increase the need for vitamins. Vitamins can also be lost from the system through dialysis or diuresis.

Detecting hypervitaminosis is as important as detecting deficiencies. Excessive vitamin intake is most common in children. Parents may administer toxic doses of vitamins by mistake. Sometimes they are overzealous in their attempts to provide optimal nutrition. Typically in such situations, various fortified foods are offered to children, in addition to vitamin supplements. Fortified foods are dietary products to which have been added vitamin doses in excess of the nutrients that may have been destroyed or removed during the processing of the food. They contain, therefore, higher levels of vitamins or other nutrients than do the natural foods from which they were made. Dairy products (milk, margarine, cheese), cereal products, and syrups for flavoring milk drinks are sometimes fortified with vitamins A and D. Ingestion of large quantities of such products, especially if a multivitamin supplement is used, can lead to hypervitaminosis.

Signs and symptoms of hypervitaminosis from fat-soluble vitamins include lethargy, fatigue, skeletal abnormalities, bone tenderness, headache, nausea, vomiting, diarrhea, increased urine output, and soft-tissue calcification, as shown by palpable lumps. In infants, the fontanelles may bulge or the cranial bones may soften. Coma may develop in very severe overdosage.

NURSING DIAGNOSIS

Nursing diagnoses may identify vitamin deficiencies, vitamin toxicity, or adverse reactions to pharmacologic doses of vitamins. Examples include:

- Altered Nutrition, Less Than Body Requirements: Vitamin C deficiency, related to inadequate dietary intake of foods rich in ascorbic acid
- Altered Nutrition, Less Than Body Requirements: Pyridoxine deficiency, related to increased need for vitamin B_6 during the premenstrual period
- Altered Nutrition, Less Than Body Requirements: Multiple vitamin deficiencies, related to malabsorption due to ulcerative colitis
- Altered Nutrition, More Than Body Requirements: Hypervitaminosis A, related to concurrent use of high-dose vitamin supplements and vitamin A fortified foods
- Altered Nutrition, More Than Body Requirements: Hypervitaminosis D, related to simultaneous intake of calcium and vitamin D supplements and thiazide diuretics
- Knowledge Deficit, related to vitamin nutrients

PLANNING

Goals for nursing care are specific to the nutritional problem diagnosed. For the diagnoses just listed, appropriate goals might include increasing intake of deficient vitamins, reducing intake of vitamins causing toxicity, and educating the client regarding vitamin nutrition.

INTERVENTION

When hypovitaminosis is suspected, the client may need referral to a specialist for definitive diagnosis and prescription. Clients under treatment for medical conditions contributory to nutritional problems should discuss this problem with the physician. When faulty health habits pose a risk for vitamin deficiency, however, the nurse may advise the client regarding correction of these habits.

If underlying health practices cannot be corrected immediately, specific suggestions may be made to reduce the risk of frank vitamin deficiencies. Smokers have an increased need for vitamin C and may need a multivitamin formula containing extra ascorbic acid.

Oral contraceptive use or pregnancy increases tissue needs for vitamins C, B_6, B_{12}, and folic acid. Vitamin formulas specially prepared to meet these needs are available.

The ingestion of alcohol increases the body's needs for B-complex vitamins. Clients with an alcohol problem should be advised to take high-potency B-complex vitamins. (Of course, vitamin therapy will not prevent all harmful effects of excessive alcohol use and will not eliminate the need to address and treat the problem of alcoholism.)

Weight-reduction regimens should be analyzed to determine which nutrients are likely to be deficient. If carbohydrate allowances are low, as shown by a restricted allowance for "cereal" exchanges, B-complex deficiency is likely. A very low allowance of fat exchange may predispose to vitamin A and D deficiencies.

Clients deficient in intrinsic factor need supplementary doses of cyanocobalamin. If some gastric function remains, high oral doses of B_{12} may suffice. Some preparations contain powdered intrinsic factor from animal tissues that enhances their effectiveness. These tend to become less effective over time due to the development of antibodies to the foreign intrinsic factor. Persons who cannot maintain adequate levels of B_{12} with oral supplementation need parenteral injections of this nutrient. (Injectable vitamin preparations cannot be purchased without a prescription. Even though a prescription is needed, the cost is usually not covered by insurance prescription plans because it is a vitamin.)

When oral vitamin preparations are prescribed, they should be administered with food. This will ensure secretion of adequate bile to promote absorption of fat-soluble vitamins. In addition, food will dilute the vitamin preparation. This may reduce the appetite-depressing effect experienced by some persons after ingesting vitamin preparations. (Some vitamin preparations contain fish-liver oils and concentrated yeasts, which have strong odors and flavors. These can cause anorexia or nausea, particularly if eructation occurs after the tablet or capsule has dissolved.)

If frank symptoms of vitamin toxicity are present, the client should be referred for medical care. Vitamin supplementation and the use of fortified foods should be discontinued immediately.

Vitamin Storage. Vitamin preparations are generally stable. However, ascorbic acid tablets are sensitive to light, heat, and moisture and should be stored in dry, cool environments. Darkened tablets are safe to use, but a vinegar odor to the tablet or container indicates that the vitamin molecule has been chemically broken down.

Client Education. Nurses are often asked for advice on the use of vitamin supplements by persons with good dietary habits and normal health. This is a controversial question. Few people argue with the basic nutritional principle that a varied, balanced diet is the best source of nutrients, including vitamins. However, actual dietary practices by many persons do not provide such a diet. Grocery stores carry many highly processed and high-calorie foods that are relatively deficient in important nutrients. Because personal preference and emotional conditioning influence food selection, many people do not eat highly nutritious diets; even concerned people with considerable knowledge of nutrition may not eat them consistently. The idea of using supplemental vitamins as "insurance" against deficiencies is not devoid of merit.

Another question that remains unresolved is the issue of optimal nutritional levels. Current RDAs were derived in part from older "minimal daily requirements." The latter represented the amount of nutrient that was sufficient to eliminate overt signs and symptoms of frank deficiency. For the most part, RDAs are only slightly higher than these levels. The eminent biochemist Linus Pauling believed that optimal levels may be considerably higher for many nutrients.

In some instances, vitamin supplements may be less expensive than the food items required to provide a specific nutrient. For example, the cost of an ascorbic acid tablet is usually considerably lower than the price of an orange. The fruit contains other nutrients that may be important, but if the orange is purchased solely for its vitamin C content, the pure vitamin may be a more prudent purchase. Persons on a severely restricted food budget may find that they can provide better overall nutrition by using part of that money to buy vitamin supplements.

In counseling clients regarding the use of vitamin supplements, the nurse should point out the importance of maintaining a good diet. Clients need information that will enable them to make a reasonable decision. This includes facts about the risks of hypervitaminosis. The difference between dosage levels of maintenance and therapeutic formulas should be explained clearly.

Conserving Nutrients. Clients may need instruction in techniques for conserving the nutrients in food. Proper refrigeration or storage is important to prevent breakdown of nutrients before food is cooked and eaten. High temperatures destroy vitamin C in low-acid foods. Copper also catalyzes the destruction of vitamin C. Cooking in copper utensils or using water that has absorbed copper from plumbing pipes is enough to lower vitamin levels. If the water system contains copper pipes, running a faucet long enough to flush out standing water before drawing water to be used in preparing food will prevent the destruction of vitamin C. Dietary sources of vitamin C require care in handling to ensure that the nutrient content is not compromised.

Water-soluble vitamins tend to leach from food if large amounts of water are used in cooking. Steaming with small amounts of liquid may be recommended. If boiling is preferred, the pot liquor (the liquid remaining after cooking) should be used in preparing soups or sauces so that the nutrients will not be lost.

Other Nursing Considerations. Clients who habitually consume mineral oil are at high risk for fat-soluble deficiencies, because this indigestible lipid carries these nutrients through the tract in an indigestible form. Mineral oil is used to prevent or relieve constipation. Unless the medication has been prescribed for a sound medical reason, the nurse should attempt to substitute an alternative regimen to maintain fecal elimination. Clients who are self-medicating may benefit from instruction in health practices designed to promote bowel function. In consultation with the prescriber, alternatives should be explored. If the mineral oil regimen cannot be changed, clients should be advised to take vitamins and oil at different times to minimize interaction in the gut. Higher-than-normal doses of fat-soluble vitamins may be needed because it may be impossible to schedule mineral oil administration so that it will not interact with either food or vitamin supplements.

Certain vitamins interfere with the therapeutic effect of specific drugs prescribed for the treatment of disease. In such situations, the dosage of the drug is adjusted to compensate for normal vitamin levels. Clients should be warned to maintain consistent levels of vitamins in such situations. They should not be told to avoid the vitamins or the foods containing them, because deficiencies could then develop. The most common interactions of this type involve levodopa and vitamin B_6, and coumarin anticoagulants and vitamin K.

Megavitamin Therapy. Some clients believe in the value of megavitamin therapy and consume large amounts of these nutrients. Although the risk of hypervitaminosis from water-soluble vitamins does not appear great, large doses of fat-soluble vitamins are dangerous. This risk should be clearly explained. Vitamin preparations should be assessed for total fat-soluble vitamin content. If dangerous levels are being consumed, specific suggestions may be made to moderate vitamin A and D consumption. Clients should be reminded that exposure to sunlight increases vitamin D levels in the body by converting biochemicals in the skin to the vitamin.

Clients consuming large amounts of vitamin C should be advised not to discontinue such dosages abruptly. A temporary vitamin C deficiency can occur in such situations due to the enhanced metabolism and excretion of that chemical after prolonged use of large doses. Weaning from megavitamin doses of vitamin C is advisable during pregnancy to avoid vitamin C deficiency in the fetus and newborn. Large doses of vitamin A are also undesirable in women of childbearing years because this vitamin is teratogenic.

Nurses working with clients who persist in using megavitamins may contribute to the ongoing investigation of the effects of such therapy. Careful client records may provide important data about the long-term health effects of such regimens (see the Critical Thinking Challenge: Case Analysis).

Nutritional therapy sometimes masks the symptoms of medical conditions. Clients who rely on vitamins or other nutrients to treat multiple symptoms should be advised to seek definitive diagnosis of any underlying condition that may be the cause of these symptoms. A 4- to 6-week holiday from vitamin use may be needed to reveal the baseline condition so that proper diagnostic and medical treatment measures can be taken.

CRITICAL THINKING CHALLENGE
Case Analysis

Nancy Klein, your new prenatal client, is a 23-year-old, well-developed, well-nourished white female. Her hematocrit and hemoglobin are slightly below normal limits. History showed no significant illnesses. She had chickenpox as a child and received the usual childhood immunizations. Her rubella titer is adequate.

Ms. Klein states she has always been interested in diet as a way of improving health. She avoids eating red meat but does eat chicken and fish. She has been taking high-dose (therapeutic level) multivitamins and minerals and additional vitamin C (2 g/day) since age 15. She uses fortified cereals (Total, Product 19) to enrich her diet further.

1. Do any of the nutrients this client is taking have the potential for harming her unborn child? If so, which ones?
2. How should Ms. Klein change her vitamin and mineral intake? Should she increase her iron intake to bring her hematocrit and hemoglobin levels up to normal range? Why or why not?
3. What advice would you give Ms. Klein regarding appropriate diet and dietary supplements during her pregnancy?
4. What would you teach Ms. Klein about diet and nutritional supplements for her family after her baby is born?

OUTCOME EVALUATION

Data required for evaluation include the absence or incidence of signs and symptoms of nutritional imbalance, and signs and symptoms of the health benefits of optimal nutrition.

❖ **CHECKLIST OF NURSING ACTIONS**

❑ Assess nutritional practices and the general health of clients to determine the risk of vitamin deficiency.
❑ Promote good dietary nutrition as the best source of vitamin nutrients.
❑ Teach clients about vitamins to enable them to make rational decisions about the use of vitamin supplements.
❑ Caution clients about the risks of toxicity from high doses of vitamins A and D.
❑ Monitor clients using megavitamin doses for toxic signs and symptoms.
❑ Advise clients taking large doses of vitamin C to wean themselves off these dosages rather than discontinue them abruptly.
❑ Advise women of childbearing age not to use extremely large doses of vitamin A or C.

❑ Refer clients with signs and symptoms of frank vitamin deficiency for medical care.
❑ Administer oral vitamin preparations with meals.
❑ Protect vitamin C preparations from air, light, heat, and contact with copper.
❑ To reduce the risk of fat-soluble vitamin deficiency, help clients dependent on mineral oil to find alternative measures to promote bowel function.
❑ Advise clients receiving coumarin anticoagulants to maintain a steady dietary intake of vitamin K.
❑ Advise clients receiving levodopa to maintain a steady dietary intake of vitamin B_6.

Minerals

Minerals are inorganic chemicals used by the body for essential physiologic functions. They are ingested in the form of salts in the diet. Certain minerals—sodium, potassium, calcium, magnesium, phosphorus, and chlorine (chloride)—are electrolytes; that is, in solution, their salts dissociate into two charged particles or ions, which perform vital physiologic functions (eg, in the transmission of impulses). Other minerals function as components of enzymes and complex proteins such as hemoglobin. Certain minerals, called trace minerals, are needed only in very small amounts. These trace minerals include cobalt, chromium, copper, fluorine (fluoride), iodine, iron, manganese, molybdenum, selenium, and zinc.

Role of Minerals

Minerals are involved in a wide variety of physiologic functions (Table 49-4). In the form of salts, they serve as structural materials in such tissues as bone, teeth, cell membranes, and connective tissue. They are components of biochemicals necessary for vital functions such as impulse transmission, oxygen transport in the blood, and cellular respiration. They are incorporated in many biologic enzymes. The electrolyte minerals also function to maintain osmotic pressure in the fluid compartments of the body and to buffer strong acids and bases.

Mineral metabolism is extremely complex. Many elements affect each other in both pharmacokinetics and pharmacodynamics. They sometimes compete with each other for absorption, biologic activity, and excretion. Two or more may be required to complete a physiologic function. For example, moderation of nerve and muscle impulses requires both calcium and magnesium; cholesterol metabolism is influenced by zinc and copper; and the production of red blood cells requires iron, copper, and cobalt (in the form of vitamin B_{12}).

Mineral nutrition is a rapidly expanding field of study, characterized by extensive research and a proliferating knowledge base. Only minerals for which dietary recommendations have been developed are discussed here. Other minerals known to play a role in physiology include silicon, cadmium, and nickel—even the deadly poison arsenic has been found in certain bioenzymes. The student would be well advised to keep abreast of developments in this area because they are likely to affect future developments in nutritional therapy.

Mineral Imbalances

Inappropriate mineral nutrition is emerging as a serious health problem. Iron deficiency is a common cause of anemia. Lack of calcium (especially in postmenopausal women) also is common. The incidence of trace mineral deficiencies is unknown but is suspected to be significant. These may arise from the use of highly processed foods from which many mineral constituents have been removed. Enrichment and fortification replace only some of these elements. Malabsorption and unusually high physiologic requirements for minerals may also lead to deficiencies.

Recommended daily doses have not been established for most minerals. Daily dietary intake estimated to be safe and effective has been designated for some minerals for which RDAs are not yet available. However, methods for assaying mineral content have not been standardized, and optimal levels are still unknown.

The diagnosis of deficiency states requires analysis of dietary habits, urine or serum mineral levels, mineral content of hair, and a complete history and physical examination. Serum levels are often of questionable value because tissue reserves may be seriously depleted before blood levels decline. For some minerals, specific diagnostic procedures provide important data (eg, hemoglobin level to detect iron-deficiency anemia, x-ray examination to reveal bone thinning due to calcium deficiency).

Mineral toxicity can also be a problem. Minerals are constituents of many metallic and organochemical environmental pollutants. Some people ingest high doses of mineral supplements in an attempt to enhance nutritional status. The requirement for specific minerals is often extremely low, and there is a narrow margin of safety between therapeutic and toxic doses. The body's ability to eliminate these chemicals is limited, and harmful levels may accumulate within a short time.

Physiologic effects of mineral imbalance vary with different elements (Table 49-5). In general, deficiencies impair growth and development, lead to tissue breakdown, or interfere with vital functions, such as circulation, oxygen transport, nerve and muscle function, or hormone balance. Symptoms of toxicity also vary with the specific chemicals involved.

Mineral Actions

Nutritional supplements of mineral nutrients replenish body stores and promote normal function. They correct many signs and symptoms of deficiency diseases but cannot reverse structural changes such as bone deformities or scarring of organs due to tissue damage.

Mechanisms of action of pharmacologic doses vary with the mineral involved (Table 49-6). For example,

Text continues on page 1084.

Table 49-4. Physiologic Functions of Minerals

Mineral Element	Representative Functions
sodium (Na)	Maintains osmotic pressure in the intravascular and extracellular fluids
	Plays an essential role in ion movement across cell membranes, which generates impulses in nerves and muscles
potassium (K)	Maintains osmotic pressure in intracellular fluid
	Plays an essential role in ion movement across cell membranes, which generates impulses in nerves and muscles
	Required for relaxation of cardiac muscle
	May exert a protective role in preventing blood vessel damage by hypertension
calcium (Ca)	Structural component of bone and teeth
	Functions as an activator of certain enzymes (eg, coagulation factors)
	With magnesium, plays a role in the moderation of nerve and muscle impulses
	Required for contraction of cardiac muscle
	Component of intracellular cement and cell membranes
	Blocks intestinal absorption of lead
	May play a role in preventing hypertension
magnesium (Mg)	Is second only to potassium in concentration in intracellular fluid
	With calcium, moderates the transmission of stimulant impulses in nerves and muscles
	Component of many enzymes (eg, transfer enzymes)
	Aids in bone growth and regulation of the heart rhythm
	May play a role in preventing hypertension, especially during pregnancy
phosphorus (P)	Aids bone growth and mineralization of teeth
	Is a component of molecules such as ATP that are essential for energy metabolism
	Maintains structural integrity of cells
	Plays a part in cellular immunity
chlorine (Cl)	Is important to normal fluid shifts, normal pH of the blood, and the production of hydrochloric acid in the stomach
iron (Fe)	Is a component of heme-containing enzymes (eg, cytochromes, catalase, peroxidase) and metalloproteins (eg, transferritin, xanthine oxidase, hemoglobin)
copper (Cu)	Plays a role in the production of red blood cells
	Component of microsomal enzymes (eg, ferroxidase, cytochrome oxidase, tyrosinase)
	Plays a role in the function of mitochondria, collagen metabolism, and melanin formation
	May help protect the heart from cardiomyopathy and angiopathy
	Acts as a cofactor in the use of iron by red blood cells
iodine (I)	Component of thyroid hormones, which control the rate of metabolic oxidation in cells
fluorine (F)	Essential component for normal formation of dentin and tooth enamel
	Keeps skin, hair, and nails healthy
	May help prevent osteoporosis in older people
zinc (Zn)	Essential component of many enzymes (eg, alcohol dehydrogenase, DNA polymerase, retinol dehydrogenase)
	Plays a role in healing, acuity of taste and smell, growth (especially of the immune system in utero), and sexual development
	May help protect the heart from cardiomyopathy and angiopathy
manganese (Mn)	Component of enzymes (eg, pyruvate carboxylase)
	Plays a role in oxidative phosphorylation, fatty acid metabolism, and mucopolysaccharide synthesis
	Required for normal bone growth and development, reproduction, and cell functions
cobalt (Co)	Component of vitamin B_{12}, a coenzyme necessary to red blood cell production
	Plays a role in biologic methylation
chromium (Cr)	Component of glucose tolerance factor, which mediates insulin effects on cell membranes
selenium (Se)	Component of enzymes (eg, glutathionine peroxidase)
	Appears to protect the body from toxic effects of mercury and cadmium
	Complements vitamin E to fight cell damage by oxygen
molybdenum (Mo)	Component of flavoenzymes (eg, xanthine oxidase)
	Plays a role in xanthine and hypoxanthine metabolism

Table 49-5. Physiologic Requirements for Minerals and Effects of Imbalances

Mineral	Nutritional Requirements/PC	Effects of Deficiencies	Toxic Effects
sodium	115–3,300 mg daily* Normal serum level = 136–145 mEq/L PC: C	Hypotension and tendency to develop circulatory shock If hydration is maintained, weakness and debility	Hypertension due to hypervolemia Thirst In dehydration, irritability, delirium, convulsions
potassium	350–5,625 mg daily* Normal serum level = 3.5– 5.0 mEq/L PC: A (C for potassium acetate)	Weakness or paralysis of muscles Abdominal distention, paralytic ileus Prolongation of cardiac systole, cardiac arrest	Smooth muscle spasm, intestinal colic Skeletal muscle weakness Prolongation of cardiac diastole, cardiac arrest Increased secretion of glucagon Locally, vascular constriction
calcium	360–1,200 mg daily† Normal serum levels = 4.5–5.5 mEq/L or 9–11 mg/dL (increased in persons with high intake of caffeine and alcohol, and in heavy smokers) PC: C	Osteoporosis, periodontal disease Rickets in children When serum levels decline, tetany or convulsions	Anorexia, nausea, vomiting Headaches, seizures, coma Muscle weakness, lethargy, coma Calcification of soft tissues Renal lithiasis Prolongation of cardiac systole, cardiac arrest Locally, irritation to tissues Constipation Kidney stones and gallstones Weight loss Slowed mentation Inappropriate behavior Bone pain Thirst Joint pain; exacerbation of rheumatoid arthritis
phosphate	800–1,200 mg daily Normal serum levels: 2.7–4.5 mg/dL	Muscle weakness Encephalopathy Cardiomyopathy with congestion Hemolytic anemia Ventilatory collapse GI and skin hemorrhages	Tachycardia Nausea, diarrhea Abdominal cramps Muscle weakness Hyperreflexia
chloride	1,700–5,100 mg daily Normal plasma levels: 100–110 mEq/L or 350–390 mg/dL	Metabolic alkalosis	Increased risk of atherosclerosis Metabolic acidosis
magnesium	50–450 mg daily† Normal serum levels = 1.5–2.5 mEq/L PC: B	Increased muscle tone, irritability, convulsions	Flaccid paralysis Cardiac arrest in diastole Increased congenital defects in exposed embryos

iron
   Infant 6 mo–1 yr
   Child 4–6 yr
   Child 11–14 yr
   Pregnant woman
   Lactating woman
   Menstruating female
   Adult male
	
	 15 mg
	 10 mg
	 18 mg
	 30–60 mg supplement
	 30–60 mg supplement*
	 18 mg
	 10 mg
	 PC: A
		Iron-deficiency anemia	Hematemesis, diarrhea, hypotension, coma
			 Cellular damage; organ dysfunction

*Estimated safe and effective daily dietary intake recommended by the Food and Nutrition Board, National Academy of Sciences–National Research Council.
†Recommended daily allowance as established by the Food and Nutrition Board, National Academy of Sciences–National Research Council (specific recommendations vary with age, sex, and reproductive status).
KEY: PC = pregnancy risk category; see Appendix A.

(continued)

Table 49-5. (Continued)

Mineral	Nutritional Requirements/PC	Effects of Deficiencies	Toxic Effects
copper	0.5–3.0 mg daily* Normal serum levels = 114 ± 14 µg/100 mL PC: C	Anemia, leukopenia, neutropenia	Damage to liver, kidneys, other organs Possible mutagenesis or carcinogenesis
iodine	40–200 µg daily† PC: C	Goiter, thyroid imbalances	Goiter, thyroid imbalances
fluorine	0.1–4.0 mg daily* PC: C	Abnormal dentin formation; soft tooth enamel	(During tooth formation) permanent discoloration of teeth Abnormal bone and tooth structure
zinc	50–200 µg daily PC: C	Retarded wound healing Growth retardation Hypogonadism Night blindness nonresponsive to vitamin A therapy Decreased acuity of taste Decreased resistance to infection Increased risk of heart disease During pregnancy, toxemia and increased incidence of fetal distress and congenital anomalies	Possible increase in the incidence of congenital anencephaly Decrease in high-density lipoproteins and increased risk of myocardial infarction
chromium	Unknown PC: C	Impaired glucose tolerance Diabetes mellitus characterized by high levels of circulating insulin	Hyperemia, emphysema, bronchitis, cancer of the respiratory tract (inhaled)
cobalt	0.3–4.0 µg daily (as vitamin B$_{12}$)	Macrocytic (pernicious) anemia	Polycythemia
lithium	None available	Accelerated atherosclerosis and coronary artery disease Pronounced mood cycles	Polydipsia, polyuria, nephrogenic diabetes insipidus Allergic dermatitis and vasculitis Goiter Nausea, vomiting, diarrhea Ataxia, fine tremors, hyperreflexia Confusion, sedation Tremor, convulsions, coma, death Increased incidence of cardiac anomalies in exposed embryos
manganese	0.5–5.0 mg daily* PC: C	Defective growth Reproductive dysfunction Collagen problems CNS disorders	Possible mutagenesis or carcinogenesis
molybdenum	0.03–0.5 mg daily*	Growth retardation (in animals) Dental disease	Molybdenum deposits in bone and soft tissue
selenium	0.01–0.2 mg daily* PC: C	Poor wound healing Growth retardation, hypogonadism Uremic impotence	Weakness, lethargy, tremors, anorexia, nausea, vomiting, abdominal pain, profuse diaphoresis, garlicky breath Fatigue, irritability Nail changes

*Estimated safe and effective daily dietary intake recommended by the Food and Nutrition Board, National Academy of Sciences—National Research Council.
†Recommended daily allowance as established by the Food and Nutrition Board, National Academy of Sciences–National Research Council (specific recommendations vary with age, sex, and reproductive status).
KEY: PC = pregnancy risk category; see Appendix A.

Table 49-6. Mineral Preparations Used as Drugs

Mineral Preparation	Usual Adult Dosage/PC	Pharmacologic Effects and Therapeutic Uses	Method of Administration
sodium			
sodium chloride (table salt)	Sodium equivalent to 1–2 tsp of table salt daily	Increases blood volume; prevents hypovolemia in excessive perspiration, Addison's disease, and excessive sodium losses, such as ileostomy	Increase the amount used in cooking. Ingest plain table salt. Use electrolyte solution as beverage.
bicarbonate of soda (baking soda)	1 tsp	Increases blood volume, increases base buffer; prevents and treats metabolic acidosis	Dissolve in 3–4 oz water; sip slowly; do not take on a full stomach.
saline solutions	50–150 mL/hr PC: C	Maintains blood volume; prevents and treats dehydration	Administer orally or IV.
potassium (Kaochlor, Kay Ciel, Kaon, K-Dur, K-Lyte, K-Lor, Slow-K)			
flavored effervescent tablets containing potassium citrate and bicarbonate (K-Lyte)	25 mEq potassium once or twice daily	Replenishes potassium, prolongs diastole of the heart; prevents or treats hypokalemia, prevents digitalis toxicity due to hypokalemia	Dissolve tablet completely in 3–4 oz water and administer while still effervescing.
potassium chloride solutions for oral use	20–100 mEq potassium daily in divided doses		Dilute well and administer orally; give with meals.
potassium gluconate solution for oral use (Kaon)	20–100 mEq potassium daily in divided doses		Dilute well and administer orally; give with meals.
potassium chloride tablets	20–100 mEq daily, in divided doses PC: A		Administer orally; direct client to swallow tablet whole without chewing or dissolving tablet.
potassium chloride for injection	20–100 mEq daily, in divided doses		Infuse slowly IV.
calcium (Apo-Cal, Cal-trate, Citracal, Os-Cal)			
calcium chloride for oral use	6–8 g daily in divided doses	Replenishes calcium; treats calcium deficiency (osteomalacia)	Administer orally.
dibasic calcium phosphate with vitamin D	One wafer (equal to 0.35 g calcium) tid	Replenishes calcium losses; treats calcium deficiency (rickets)	Instruct client to chew wafers before swallowing; give with meals.
calcium gluconate solution (10%) for injection	1.5–3.0 mL (equal to 7–14 mEq calcium); for tetany, up to 20 mL	Reduces nerve and muscle irritability; treats hypocalcemic tetany	Infuse slowly IV.
calcium carbonate for oral use (eg, Tums)	1–2 g PC: C	Replenishes calcium; manages renal failure, weight reduction regimens, and other conditions with high potential for hypocalcemia	Administer orally with meals.
magnesium (magnesium gluconate)			
antacid magnesium salts	Variable	Buffers gastric acid and reduces gastric acidity; promotes fecal elimination by saline catharsis; counteracts the constipating effects of drugs such as aluminum or calcium antacids	Administer orally.
laxative magnesium salts	Variable	Same as above	Administer orally.
magnesium sulfate solutions for injection	0.5–3.0 g daily	Replenishes magnesium; prevents magnesium deficiency	Add to total parenteral nutrition solutions.

KEY: PC = pregnancy risk category; see Appendix A.

(continued)

Table 49-6. (Continued)

Mineral Preparation	Usual Adult Dosage/PC	Pharmacologic Effects and Therapeutic Uses	Method of Administration
magnesium sulfate 10% solution for injection	Up to 4 g magnesium sulfate (40 mL)	Reduces muscle and nerve irritability; terminates convulsions of eclampsia of pregnancy	Administer slowly IV infusion (1.5 mL/min or less).
magnesium sulfate 20%, 25%, or 50% solutions for injection	4–5 g magnesium sulfate PC: B	Same as above	Administer IM injection q4h.
iron (Femiron, Feosol, Fergon, Fer-In-Sol, ferrous gluconate, Mol-Iron)			
ferrous sulfate enteric-coated tablets for oral use	100–1,000 mg/day in divided doses	Provides iron for hemoglobin formation; treats iron-deficiency anemia	Administer orally with fruit juice.
iron–dextran solution for injection (0.05%)	50–500 mg	Same as above; treats iron-deficiency anemia when rapid response is required or iron cannot be taken orally	Inject IM, using Z-track technique.
ferrous sulfate elixir for oral use	1–2 mL (equal to 220–440 mg ferrous sulfate) tid	Same as above; treats iron-deficiency anemia when rapid response is required or iron cannot be taken orally	Mix with water or juice (*not* milk or alcoholic beverages), and administer by placing a straw well back in the mouth; avoid contact between solution and teeth.
copper			
copper sulfate solutions for injection (no commercial preparations available)	Up to 0.05 mg/kg (injected)	Replenishes copper; prevents or treats copper deficiency in clients on chronic total parenteral nutrition	Infuse as directed by the pharmacist.
iodine			
iodide solution for oral use (Lugol's solution)	0.1–0.3 mL tid	Replenishes iodine; treats simple goiter	Dilute and administer orally.
		Promotes storage of thyroid hormone and reduces vascularity of thyroid gland; prepares client for thyroidectomy	
saturated solution of potassium iodide	0.3 or 0.6 mL (equal to 300 mg KI) 3 or 4 times daily	Stimulates sputum secretion; treats respiratory infections	Dilute and administer orally.
radiopaque dyes containing iodide	Varies with preparation	Blocks x-rays to outline structures on x-ray film; diagnoses organ pathology	Inject IV or administer orally.
Fluorine (EASYgel, Fluorinse, Fluoritab, Fluorodex, Pediaflor, Thera-Flur)			
Can: Fluotic			
sodium silicofluoride	1 ppm in water supplies	Promotes formation of normal dentin and strong tooth enamel in children; prevents dental disease (caries)	Add to water supply.
sodium fluoride tablets for oral use	1.1–2.2 mg/day (depending on age)	See above	Administer orally.
stannous fluoride (toothpaste)	QS for oral hygiene	See above; desensitizes tooth enamel	Use in place of nonmedicated toothpaste.
zinc			
zinc sulfate capsules and tablets for oral use (Zinc-220)	220 mg/day (equivalent to 80 mg elemental zinc)	Replenishes zinc; promotes the healing of wounds in zinc deficiency	Administer orally with meals or milk.

KEY: PC = pregnancy risk category; see Appendix A.
Can = Canadian trade name

(continued)

Table 49-6. (Continued)

Mineral Preparation	Usual Adult Dosage/PC	Pharmacologic Effects and Therapeutic Uses	Method of Administration
cobalt			
cyanocobalamin solution for injection	100 µg/week	Promotes formation of red blood cells; treats pernicious anemia	Administer subcutaneously or intramuscularly.
lithium (Lithane, Lithobid, Lithotabs)			
lithium carbonate tablets and capsules for oral use	300–600 mg tid (individu- alized to produce a serum level of 1.0–1.5 mEq lithium/L)	Alters sodium transport in nerve and muscle cells; treats and pre- vents manic episodes of bipolar psychosis, treats severe recurrent unipolar psychosis	Administer orally.

KEY: PC = pregnancy risk category; see Appendix A.

potassium and calcium oppose each other's effects on myocardial contractility. Magnesium reduces nerve cell irritability and may play a role in the inhibition of toxin production by bacteria responsible for toxic shock syn- drome. Iodine stimulates respiratory secretion, causing production of a more dilute sputum that is easier to raise and expectorate.

Pharmacokinetic Parameters

Normally, mineral salts are ingested in food. Their ab- sorption in the intestine is affected by binding and chelat- ing agents that either inhibit or facilitate their transfer across the intestinal membrane. Absorption may also be altered by other minerals, vitamins, hormones, and the oxidative state (valence) of the mineral (Table 49-7).

Except for the electrolytes, most minerals are protein bound in the serum. In some cases, the protein is specific

to one mineral (eg, transferrin, which binds iron, and ceruloplasmin, which binds copper). Protein deficiency can increase the loss of such minerals in urine because the unbound form is readily excreted in the kidneys. Minerals are distributed widely in tissues. Potassium uptake by the cells is enhanced by insulin. Most minerals also cross the placenta and appear in the milk of nursing mothers.

Minerals are stored in many tissue depots. Bone con- tains large amounts of calcium, magnesium, phosphorus, zinc, and fluorine. High levels of iron and cobalt are found in the liver; iodine is concentrated in the thyroid, copper in the intestinal mucosa, and iron in the spleen. Many metallic compounds are deposited in the kidneys.

Electrolytes and fluoride are excreted by the kidneys. Although high potassium levels do increase the release of this mineral by the gut and its elimination in feces, urine is the major route for elimination of potassium. Adrenal

Table 49-7. Factors Affecting Pharmacokinetics of Selected Minerals

Mineral	Interacting Factors	Effect on MIneral Levels
calcium	Parathormone and vitamin D	Increase intestinal absorption and renal reabsorption
	Lactose	Increases intestinal absorption
	pH of body fluids	Alters ionization of calcium (relation is inverse)
	Protein	In excess, reduces calcium levels in the body
	Weight-bearing	Increases calcium deposition in bone
	Stress	Increases renal loss of calcium
	Phytates and oxalates	Bind calcium, reducing intestinal absorption
	Fluoride	Reduces calcium levels
iron	Vitamin C and other acids	Increase intestinal absorption
	Cobalt, antacids, phytates, tannates, clay (geophagia), ethylenediaminetetraacetic acid (EDTA), tea	Decrease intestinal absorption
copper	Zinc	Displaces copper, reducing its absorption and increasing its excretion
	Iron	Decreases copper absorption in infants
fluoride	Copper, iron	Decrease absorption
zinc	Vitamin B$_6$	Increases absorption
	Copper	Decreases absorption
manganese	Copper, phosphorus, iron	Decrease absorption
	Soy supplements	Decrease absorption

corticoids control renal elimination of sodium and potassium, stimulating sodium reabsorption and potassium excretion. Calcium loss in urine is inversely related to parathormone and vitamin D levels.

Other minerals are excreted largely as metallic salts of bile acids. They participate in the enterohepatic cycle and are partially reabsorbed, thus conserving body supplies. Eventually, they are eliminated in feces. Excessive concentrations of these minerals stimulate their renal excretion. Urinary elimination also may be increased by diuresis, injury, infection, and other stressors. Minerals present in the body in high concentrations are eliminated also by the sweat glands.

Iron is poorly excreted by the body. When iron supplies are ample, intestinal absorption decreases, helping to maintain proper balance. However, adults who do not lose blood regularly (men and nonmenstruating women) are at high risk for iron toxicity.

Therapeutic Uses

Physicians prescribe minerals to replenish body supplies for the treatment of deficiency states. In addition, parenteral or oral preparations are used for many therapeutic purposes. Electrolyte solutions are given to maintain hydration and proper chemical composition of body fluids in persons suffering excessive losses or in those unable to maintain adequate oral intake. Sodium is used to treat lithium toxicity and heat exhaustion.

The dangerous cardiac effects of high concentrations of calcium may be reduced by administration of potassium salts, and vice versa. In addition, potassium can be used to reduce the toxic effects of high doses of digitalis. Parenteral calcium salts are administered to relieve the painful muscle spasms of tetany. Oral calcium is used in the treatment of osteoporosis.

Magnesium sulfate is the treatment of choice for convulsions due to eclampsia of pregnancy. Iodine salts are components of stimulant expectorants and radiopaque dyes. Zinc salts are administered to debilitated clients to promote the healing of decubiti and other wounds. Iron is used to treat anemia characterized by low levels of hemoglobin.

Preparations

Mineral salts are incorporated in many nonprescription nutritional supplements, often with vitamins. Many "one-a-day" preparations contain mineral doses equal to the RDA or estimated safe and effective daily dietary intake, in addition to RDAs of vitamins. Preparations are available that contain iron, iron with vitamins, dicalcium phosphate with vitamin D, and various other combinations. In addition, proprietary preparations of less highly refined mineral sources are available, such as dolomite or kelp (see the following section on health food supplements).

The therapeutic dose of iron is calculated according to the amount of elemental iron the preparation contains. Ferrous sulfate yields 20% elemental iron, so one 300-mg ferrous sulfate tablet contains 60 mg of elemental iron. A typical total daily dosage would be 300 to 1,200 mg in divided doses. Preparations of minerals usually used for medical therapy are given in Table 49-6.

Adverse Effects

The margin of safety for mineral preparations is much narrower than for other nutritional components. Toxic signs and symptoms often appear with dosages only slightly above the recommended range. Persons with impaired liver or kidney function are likely to develop toxic reactions while receiving normal dosages.

Unless balanced by water intake, sodium excess leads to hyperosmolarity of body fluids and a rise in concentration of the sodium ions. Hyperirritability of nerves and muscles follows. As toxicity increases, delirium, convulsions, and death can ensue. Sodium excess in the presence of ample fluids causes hypervolemia and hypertension. This is the most common form of mineral toxicity in developed countries.

Excessive levels of potassium stimulate smooth muscle contraction and prolong cardiac diastole. Hyperkalemia is characterized by colicky abdominal pain, diarrhea, paresthesias, weakness, and cardiac arrhythmias. The cardiac effects are most dangerous because ventricular fibrillation may occur. In addition, excessive potassium may stimulate the secretion of glucagon and raise blood glucose levels. Local concentrations of the electrolyte may compromise circulation by causing pronounced vasoconstriction, leading to infarction.

Initially, high serum levels of calcium cause some degree of lethargy and muscle weakness. The electrolyte is excreted by the kidneys, and high levels in urine predispose to renal calculi. Prolonged hypercalcemia often causes inappropriate calcification of soft tissues. Very high concentrations cause calcium rigor of the heart, a condition characterized by prolonged systole and inadequate filling time. Cardiac arrest in systole may develop.

Magnesium excesses cause decreased muscle contractility; flaccid paralysis or cardiac arrest in diastole may develop. The mineral is mutagenic and can cause anomalies in exposed embryos.

Iron overload is characterized by iron deposition in body tissues, including vital organs. This causes widespread damage to the liver, heart, pancreas, and other organs. Iron supplements are not recommended for use during the first trimester of pregnancy because they can cause congenital malformations.

Copper excess is damaging to the liver, kidneys, and other organs. This mineral is suspected of being both mutagenic and carcinogenic.

Iodine excess, like iodine deficiency, inhibits thyroid function. Enlargement of the thyroid (goiter) may develop in response to this effect. Acute poisoning by iodine solutions causes severe damage to the exposed tissues of the GI tract. (Concentrated iodine is a protoplasmic poison.) Circulatory collapse and death may occur. Chronic iodism is characterized by increased secretions of the respiratory tract, a brassy taste, soreness of the oropharyngeal tissues, eye irritation, and GI irritation. Signs and symptoms include soreness of the teeth and gums, coryza, sneezing, swelling of the eyelids, enlargement and tenderness of the parotid and submaxillary glands, bloody diarrhea, fever, anorexia, and depression. Iodine allergy is a common problem, particularly in relation to organic preparations such as those used as radiopaque contrast media. Hypersensitivity reactions are characterized by rash, angioedema, bronchospasm, thrombocytopenic purpura, or symptoms resembling those of serum sickness (fever, joint pain, lymph node enlargement).

Acute fluoride toxicity causes local symptoms similar to those of iodine: salivation, nausea, abdominal pain, vomiting, and diarrhea. Hyperirritability of the nervous system follows, with paresthesias, hyperactive reflexes, and tetany. Hypoglycemia and convulsions can occur. Systemic symptoms may be delayed for several hours. Shock, cardiac failure, or respiratory paralysis may lead to death. Chronic fluoride toxicity is characterized by increased density and calcification of bone (osteosclerosis) and by mottling of tooth enamel that is in the process of formation.

Medicinal preparations of zinc are irritating to the stomach and may act as emetics in high doses. Zinc may cause birth defects (anencephaly). The introduction of zinc is fairly recent, and there undoubtedly are toxic effects that have yet to be reported.

Manganese is suspected to have mutagenic or carcinogenic properties.

Massive doses of cobalt (as vitamin B_{12}) overstimulate bone marrow production of red blood cells and lead to polycythemia.

Few adverse reactions have been reported as a result of selenium or molybdenum therapy, probably due to their limited use to date.

Precautions and Contraindications

Precautions required during parenteral treatment of fluid and electrolyte imbalances are discussed in detail in Chapter 48. Solutions containing concentrations of minerals greater than those normally found in body fluids should be administered with great caution to avoid toxic responses.

Oral preparations of minerals are best administered with food or diluted with large amounts of fluids. Salt tablets are highly irritating to the gastric mucosa and are no longer recommended. Adding table salt to food is the safest and easiest way to provide additional sodium for the few people who require high amounts of this mineral.

Potassium salts are usually administered in liquid form and should be well diluted. High concentrations in the intestinal vasculature must be avoided because they produce vasospasm and intestinal infarction. Administration of potassium supplements with food provides further dilution. Slow-release forms of potassium

salts have recently been introduced. Clients receiving these preparations should be monitored closely for abdominal symptoms.

Although iron is most efficiently absorbed when administered on an empty stomach, it is very irritating, and administration with meals may be necessary to control intestinal symptoms such as nausea and diarrhea. Because total absorption may be reduced when the drug is given with food, dosages may have to be increased.

Allergic sensitivity is a relative contraindication for mineral therapy. Allergy is most common in relation to iodine.

All mineral preparations should be secured to prevent accidental ingestion, especially by children. They have a high toxic potential and can cause serious poisoning.

■ SUMMARY

Minerals are inorganic chemicals that greatly influence fundamental physiologic processes such as internal respiration, impulse transmission, membrane transport, and enzymatic reactions. They are used medicinally to prevent and treat deficiency states and for selective treatment of certain diseases. Mineral preparations generally have a narrow therapeutic index and can cause serious poisoning.

❖ NURSING MANAGEMENT: CLIENT TAKING MINERAL SUPPLEMENTS

Much of nursing care for clients taking mineral supplements involves careful assessment and thorough client teaching.

NURSING PROCESS

ASSESSMENT

An important nursing responsibility in relation to mineral deficiencies or toxicities is case finding and referral for treatment. Assessment for mineral imbalances begins with the history, which is important for identifying risk factors and symptoms. Physical examination should include observation to identify or rule out signs indicating imbalance (see Table 49-2). Imbalances may be substantiated by analysis of mineral levels in serum, urine, and hair samples.

Detecting Mineral Deficiencies. Iron-deficiency anemia is the most common cause of anemia (Box 49-2). Hallmarks of anemia include weakness, fatigue, headache, palpitations, tachycardia, and pallor. These may progress to shortness of breath and cardiac enlargement. The distinctive signs of iron deficiency include GI symptoms and koilonychia (spoon-shaped nails). In many clients with iron-deficiency anemia, the fingernails become brittle and flat and develop longitudinal ridges. About half the clients with iron deficiency have papillary atrophy of the tongue; some have fissures at the corners of the mouth, the mouth may be sore, and difficulty in swallowing may occur. Laboratory findings

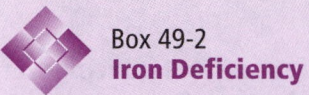

Box 49-2
Iron Deficiency

Iron deficiency may result from several situations, including:

    inadequate dietary supply
    increased requirements
    postgastrectomy
    excessive blood loss (eg, hemorrhage)
    infestation of GI tract with hookworm
    malabsorption syndromes (eg, chronic diarrhea, sprue, celiac disease, steatorrhea)

include a low hemoglobin level, a reduced or increased red blood cell count, a low hematocrit, a low serum iron level, and a low transferritin level.

Calcium deficiency is a common mineral deficiency. At risk are both the very young and the very old: children because they have a high need for calcium for skeletal growth, and older adults because they absorb calcium poorly and may ingest less in their diets. Postmenopausal women are especially vulnerable.

Sodium deficit is most likely to occur in warm environments because of excessive loss in perspiration. Susceptible persons include those engaged in strenuous physical exercise, persons with ileostomies, those with draining fistulas, and those undergoing surgery (during the postoperative period). Persons taking diuretics and those with marginal or inadequate production of corticosteroids are also at risk. Sodium loss is accompanied in most cases by fluid loss. Hypovolemia results in hypotension, weakness, syncope, and general malaise. Such dehydration is usually accompanied by mild metabolic acidosis.

Potassium deficiencies are most likely to develop in persons subject to increased stress, those receiving potassium-wasting diuretics, and those losing large amounts of intestinal fluids as a result of diarrhea or ileostomy or fistula drainage. Hypokalemia is particularly dangerous to clients receiving digitalis because potassium is the main physiologic antagonist to the action of this drug.

Risk factors for magnesium deficiency include alcoholism and diuresis. Hypomagnesemia is common in hospitalized clients but is not always diagnosed. Levels of this mineral are not usually measured by automated analyses of blood. Because magnesium is lost with other electrolytes, it should be measured whenever low serum levels of sodium, calcium, or phosphate are detected. Magnesium depletion may be a contributing factor in the development of eclampsia during pregnancy.

Inadequate levels of trace minerals may be associated with an environmental deficiency. For example, communities with fluoride-poor water show a higher incidence of dental caries (a condition associated with

fluoride deficiency) than do communities with naturally or artificially fluoridated water. Inland uplands tend to have poor levels of iodine in the soils, and iodine-deficient diseases (goiter and thyroid imbalances) are common unless iodine is added to the diet.

Trace mineral deficiencies are most likely to develop in persons whose diet is sharply limited, especially those relying entirely on parenteral fluids. Persons with intestinal malabsorption are at risk because ingested minerals may remain in the gut and be excreted in feces. Vegetarians may also develop mineral deficiencies unless care is taken to include mineral-rich foods in the diet.

Detecting Mineral Toxicities. Sodium chloride excess is the most common mineral toxicity. The average intake of table salt among persons in developed countries is at least 10 times greater than physiologic need. Excess salt predisposes to hypertension and edema.

Clients at highest risk for developing iron toxicity are those receiving multiple transfusions of whole blood or packed cells. Excesses also may develop in clients taking high-potency iron supplements, especially men and nonmenstruating women.

Hyperkalemia (potassium excess) is much less common than hypokalemia. In most cases, this problem is related to disease (renal impairment, inadequately treated Addison's disease, crush syndrome) or the use of potassium-sparing diuretics.

Excess blood levels of calcium often indicate loss of calcium from the bone and depletion of body stores. Rarely, hypercalcemia is caused by excessive dosages of parathyroid hormone or calcium and vitamin D supplements.

Persons at risk for magnesium excess are those with renal impairment who cannot excrete the mineral efficiently. These clients may develop high blood levels of many minerals unless intake is controlled carefully.

NURSING DIAGNOSIS
Nursing diagnoses are specific to the mineral imbalance; examples include:

- Fluid Volume Excess, related to excess intake of sodium chloride
- Altered Nutrition, Less Than Body Requirements: Calcium deficiency, related to impaired absorption secondary to postmenopausal estrogen deficiency
- Altered Nutrition, Less Than Body Requirements: Iron deficiency, secondary to blood loss and iron-poor diet
- Altered Nutrition, Less Than Body Requirements: Hypokalemia, related to glucocorticoid medication (or use of potassium-wasting diuretics)
- Altered Nutrition, More Than Body Requirements: Hyperkalemia, related to use of potassium-sparing diuretics
- Impaired Gas Exchange (or Altered Oral Mucous Membrane), related to anemia secondary to iron deficiency

- Fatigue (or Altered Thought Processes), related to impaired gas exchange secondary to iron-deficiency anemia

Many clients have a:

- Knowledge Deficit, concerning mineral nutrition and self-care measures to enhance supply and use of mineral nutrients

PLANNING

The nursing goal is to reduce or eliminate mineral imbalances.

INTERVENTION

Managing Deficiencies. Sodium and water depletion produce dehydration and may proceed to hypovolemic shock, a medical emergency. If the dehydrated client can take oral fluids, a solution of sodium salts in water may be given as a first-aid measure (Box 49-3). As an alternative, a saline solution may be administered IV. If the signs and symptoms do not subside promptly with fluid replacement, emergency medical aid should be summoned. If kidney function is normal, solutions administered in such situations should contain potassium salts in addition to the sodium compounds (Box 49-4). Oral mixtures may be mixed with fruit juices for better flavor.

Many clients maintain adequate potassium levels by dietary means alone. Foods of animal origin (meat, milk), orange juice, and bananas are rich sources of this mineral. Clients using potassium chloride as a salt substitute ingest extra potassium from this preparation also.

Medicinal preparations of potassium are prescribed for persons who cannot maintain normal levels of this mineral by dietary means. These medications must be administered with ample fluids to dilute them thoroughly. They are best given with meals. Concentrated potassium in the intestine is highly irritating and causes smooth muscle spasm. If absorbed rapidly, concentrations in the intestinal blood vessels may reach toxic levels, causing vascular spasm that can compromise circulation and produce infarction.

Potassium solutions have a strong, brassy taste. Administration in fruit juices or milk may reduce but cannot completely disguise this. Effervescent tablets containing potassium chloride (K-Lyte) must be dissolved in water just before administration and given while still effervescing. This preparation is colored and flavored.

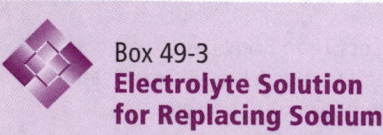

Box 49-3
Electrolyte Solution for Replacing Sodium

1 teaspoon sodium chloride (table salt)

½ teaspoon sodium bicarbonate (baking soda)

Water to make 1 quart of solution

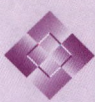

Box 49-4
Electrolyte Solution for Replacing Sodium and Potassium

1 teaspoon sodium chloride (table salt)

½ teaspoon sodium bicarbonate (baking soda)

⅓ teaspoon potassium chloride (salt substitute such as Lite Salt)

Water or fruit juice to make 1 quart of solution

Potassium solutions must be used cautiously in persons with renal impairment because excess potassium is not eliminated efficiently, and hyperkalemia may develop. They must also be used with caution in clients deficient in corticosteroids, who tend to retain potassium.

The treatment of iron deficiency requires, first, the correction of abnormal blood losses or exposure to environmental toxins that may underlie the anemia. For this reason, anemic clients should be referred for medical diagnosis. When anemia is diagnosed and the cause addressed, iron and vitamins (folic acid, vitamin B_{12}) may be prescribed. Anemic clients are cold-sensitive and should wear warm clothing. An elevated room temperature increases comfort and promotes vasodilation, which increases peripheral circulation. Clients do not tolerate exercise or high levels of activity.

Iron is marketed in tablet and solution forms. Liquid preparations can stain the teeth and should be placed on the back of the tongue with a dropper, or administered in well-diluted form through a straw. Drops may be mixed with fruit juices to improve their taste. Iron should not be given with antacids, tea, or coffee, which tend to impair its absorption. If possible, iron preparations should be administered while the client is fasting. Iron preparations may cause GI upset (either diarrhea or constipation). If the medication is tolerated only with food, the prescriber should be informed, as the dosage may need to be increased.

Treatment of calcium deficiency requires adequate intake of calcium plus vitamin D necessary for its absorption, and sufficient protein and phosphate for remineralization of body structures. Children are given additional milk when possible. An adequate diet is an important part of the treatment. When therapeutic minerals and vitamins are needed, multivitamin and mineral preparations high in calcium are often prescribed. Dicalcium phosphate with vitamin D or calcium-containing antacids, such as Tums, may be used for selected clients. Absorption and use of calcium are enhanced by weight-bearing exercise.

Calcium salts tend to be constipating, and clients should be monitored for difficulties with fecal elimination. The supplements must not be administered concurrently with drugs that form nonabsorbable complexes with divalent cations, such as tetracycline. Calcium solutions are injected IV to alleviate acute hypocalcemia characterized by tetany.

Zinc tablets are most often prescribed to promote healing of wounds such as decubiti. They should be given with food.

Deficiencies of trace minerals are best treated by ingestion of a variety of high-quality foods. Whole-grain cereals and vegetables (especially their peels) are good sources of most minerals. Because these salts dissolve in water, pot liquors should be used to make soups or gravies so they are not lost from the diet. Hard water contains significantly more minerals than soft water and is preferable for drinking and cooking.

Managing Toxicities. Treating toxic states requires controlling exposure to metallic pollutants and promoting excretion of these substances from the body. For some minerals, fecal excretion can be increased by oral administration of ion exchange resins or chelating agents that prevent the reabsorption of minerals secreted in bile or intestinal juices. If renal function is adequate, diuretics may be given to promote urinary excretion. In severe or refractory toxicity, dialysis may be necessary to reduce serum levels rapidly.

Client Education. The nurse can inform clients that cooking utensils may influence the mineral content of food significantly. Cast-iron utensils add some iron to the food cooked in them, especially when acid substances are present. Glass and enameled metal (if unchipped) appear to be inert and add nothing to the food prepared in them. According to recent reports, stainless-steel utensils may release nickel into the food cooked in them.

The degree to which aluminum leaches into food is unknown, but the obvious erosion of the metal with prolonged use implies that significant amounts of the metal may be consumed. Aluminum is under suspicion as a toxin because excessive accumulations in brain tissue have been associated with degenerative brain diseases, such as Alzheimer's disease. Aluminum utensils have been widely used for cooking for many years. Why only a small proportion of the people exposed to this metal develop brain damage is unknown; possibly their bodies cannot detoxify and excrete aluminum efficiently. Caution in the use of aluminum cooking materials and medicine containing aluminum would seem reasonable until the origin of such conditions is better understood.

Environmental pollution with mineral chemicals imposes a heavy burden of metallic salts on exposed persons. Those with renal impairment are most vulnerable to trace metal poisoning because they cannot eliminate metals efficiently. Certain populations are exposed to high levels of pollution from mining and smelting operations or industrial processes involving metals. Whenever mineral poisoning is suspected, assessment

for mineral levels should be carried out, including laboratory analysis of urine, serum, and hair.

Teaching About Sodium. High levels of dietary sodium are the most common mineral excess in developed countries. High sodium intake poses an increased risk of hypervolemia, hypertension, and cardiovascular disease, and it is important to educate the public about this health risk. Educational campaigns should stress the importance of controlling use of sodium compounds, such as table salt, baking soda, baking powder, and monosodium glutamate.

Processed food labels should be read carefully because large amounts of sodium compounds are used as preservatives and flavoring agents in most such products. To enhance the flavor of unsalted food, herbs and other low-sodium condiments should be used.

Persons at high risk for hypertension may need help developing low-sodium diets acceptable to them. Suitable flavoring agents for specific dishes favored by the client may be suggested. Cookbooks that address cooking with herbs contain helpful suggestions. The client may be referred to a nutritionist or dietitian for help with difficult problems. Adherence to a low-sodium regimen is unlikely unless it is tasty and satisfying.

Persons at high risk for sodium deficiency should be taught how to prepare an electrolyte solution for use as a beverage. Liberal use of table salt should be encouraged. Ileostomates or others losing large amounts of liquid feces should take some of their sodium as the bicarbonate to restore base bicarbonate. Some advise the use of 1 teaspoon of baking soda in water once a week. Because sodium bicarbonate reacts with hydrochloric acid in the stomach to produce carbon dioxide gas, this solution should be sipped slowly to prevent rapid generation of gas and gastric distention.

Teaching About Potassium. Clients at high risk for hypokalemia should be advised to increase their dietary intake of sources rich in this mineral. Fruits are recommended rather than meat to minimize calorie and fat intake. One banana a day provides an adequate supplement for many people. Orange juice and apricots are also good sources of the mineral. Citrus fruits other than oranges do not contain high levels of potassium.

Clients receiving potassium supplements should be instructed to take these preparations with meals, with a full glass of water, to prevent GI complications. If urinary output diminishes, the client should discontinue potassium dosage and seek immediate medical attention.

Teaching About Stress Management. Clients experiencing high stress levels need to learn stress management skills to minimize potassium wasting induced by high levels of corticosteroids. The nurse should help the client develop effective coping strategies, including relaxation techniques.

Teaching About Other Minerals. The use of medications containing calcium or aluminum compounds is likely to result in constipation. Unless medically contraindicated, the nurse should recommend a

Example of Nursing Process for Estrogen Replacement Therapy With Calcium Supplement

The client, age 50, complains of having intermittent pain in the thoracic vertebrae and hips for the last 3 months. Her last menstrual period was a year ago. She states she has experienced no hot flashes or other signs and symptoms of menopause.

During the history, the client states that none of the older women on her mother's side of the family developed spinal curvature but that all of her father's sisters (and her father, also) had typical "dowagers' humps" in their older years.

A chest x-ray reveals osteoporosis with moderate kyphosis. The physician has prescribed estrogen replacement therapy and supplemental calcium with vitamin D.

The client has led a sedentary life for years. When younger, she enjoyed swimming and bicycling. The client does not have dentures; most of her teeth are intact.

Assessment Data

Menopause

Family history of "dowager's hump"

Diagnosis of osteoporosis and moderate kyphosis

Orders for estrogen replacement and calcium supplement

Nursing Diagnosis	Intervention	Goals and Outcomes
Knowledge Deficit, concerning decreased calcium absorption resulting from estrogen deficiency secondary to menopause	**Explore** the client's knowledge of nutrition, especially calcium nutrition. **Develop** and implement a teaching plan that covers: 1) recommendations for administering calcium with food, taking divided doses to promote absorption; 2) cautions regarding excessive vitamin D intake, which promotes calcium loss by bones; 3) self-care practices to prevent constipation, which is likely to develop with high calcium intake. **Recommend** that the client undertake a gradually accelerated program of exercise that involves weight-bearing activities (walking, bicycling, workouts with weights); inform the client that although excellent exercise, swimming is not a weight-bearing activity and will not promote recalcification of bone.	The client's bone pain will decrease and disappear. The kyphosis will cease to progress.
Risk for Constipation, Colonic, secondary to high calcium intake	**Recommend** an active lifestyle, including daily exercise. **Recommend** a high fluid intake (at least 10 glasses daily). **Recommend** high fiber intake in the diet (or a bulk laxative daily).	The client will not develop constipation.
Risk for Impaired Tissue Integrity: Stomatitis related to excessive plaque formation secondary to high calcium concentrations in saliva	**Recommend** meticulous oral hygiene and professional cleaning every 3 months.	The client will not develop stomatitis.

daily fluid intake of 2,400 to 3,000 mL, regular exercise, a high-fiber diet, use of laxative foods (eg, pears, prunes), prompt response to the defecatory impulse, and regular daily fecal elimination. Taking a glass of warm liquid (lemon juice or coffee) before the usual time of defecation tends to stimulate mass peristalsis. Tea should be avoided, as it is constipating. If difficulty in fecal elimination develops, the prescriber should be consulted to determine if a less constipating preparation can be substituted. See the Example of Nursing Process for Estrogen Replacement Therapy with Calcium Supplement.

Clients taking medicines containing magnesium may have loose stools. If diarrhea becomes a problem, they should consult the prescriber for a change in prescription. If over-the-counter remedies, such as antacids, are involved, the client should substitute calcium salts for part or all of the dosage.

When iron supplements are prescribed, the client should be informed that stools will turn black or gray. Bowel habits may also change, and the client should be taught measures to minimize both constipation and diarrhea because either can occur. Taking iron with vitamin C or orange juice increases its absorption. To minimize GI irritation, the iron preparation may be taken with meals. If this is not the schedule recommended by the prescriber, he or she should be informed of the change because the dosage of iron may need to be increased to compensate for reduced overall absorption. Bloody stools or persistent abdominal discomfort should also be reported to the prescriber. See the Example of Nursing Process for Iron Deficiency.

Client teaching relevant to iodine medication is discussed in Chapter 33. The use of iodine solutions as dietary supplements without prescription should be discouraged. The amounts used (usually one drop in a glass of water per day) are difficult to measure accurately and may raise the total intake of the mineral to toxic levels, especially if iodized salt and multimineral preparations are taken at the same time. Persons living in iodine-poor geographic areas ("goiter belts") should use iodized salt.

Growing children should use fluoride toothpaste. Nonprescription fluoride dietary supplements should not be used unless the fluoride content of drinking water is clearly inadequate and other sources of fluoride are ruled out.

Zinc lozenges may relieve the symptoms of and shorten the duration of the common cold. The use of zinc supplements by healthy persons should be discouraged. This is particularly important in women of childbearing years, because the mineral is suspected of increasing the incidence of congenital anencephaly in exposed embryos.

Minimizing Mineral Toxicity. To promote appropriate mineral intake and minimize the risk of mineral toxicity, the nurse may recommend the use of glass, stainless-steel, enameled, or ceramic cooking utensils. (Despite isolated reports of leaching of nickel, stainless steel is generally considered safe.) Ceramic dishes used for food must be made with lead-free pigments and glazes.

Clients receiving relatively new medications (those developed within the last 10–20 years) should be advised to report any unusual signs, symptoms, or change in health status because they could represent previously unrecognized side effects or toxic effects.

OUTCOME EVALUATION

Data required for evaluation relate to the incidence or absence of signs and symptoms of mineral deficiency or toxicity, including laboratory tests for mineral serum levels, red blood cell counts, and hemoglobin, hematocrit, and transferritin levels. Client education may be evaluated over the short term by the client's ability to relate accurately material conveyed during the teaching sessions.

❖ **CHECKLIST OF NURSING ACTIONS**

❑ Assess clients for signs and symptoms of mineral deficiency or excess.

❑ If signs and symptoms of mineral imbalance are present, refer the client for definitive diagnosis and treatment.

❑ Advise clients that a high-quality diet containing whole-grain cereals, low-fat dairy products, adequate protein, and vegetables provides the best source of adequate mineral intake.

❑ Discourage the use of high-potency mineral preparations as dietary supplements by healthy people.

❑ Administer iron supplements with fruit juice; schedule drug doses between meals unless GI irritation occurs.

❑ If iron supplements cause abdominal distress, give the medication with meals; consult the prescriber regarding the need to increase dosage to compensate for decreased absorption.

Health Food Products

The health food industry offers many nutrient concentrates for the lay public. In most cases, these substances are marketed as single-ingredient preparations, but combinations are also available. In addition to various vitamin and mineral formulations, substances such as single amino acids, phospholipids, fatty acids, flavor essences, vinegar, and kelp are marketed. These products are not classified as drugs under control of the Food and Drug Administration. Directions for their use, including recommended dosages (which tend to be generous), usually do not appear on the labels but are available from salespersons or in promotional leaflets. For the most part, there is little or no scientific proof of the efficacy of these substances, nor is there controlled testing for adverse effects. Selected health food products are discussed below as examples.

Amino Acids

The effects of specific amino acids cannot be achieved by increasing dietary intake of protein because amino acids compete for transfer across the blood-brain barrier. Only an increase in the proportion of a single

Example of Nursing Process for Iron Deficiency

The client, Jackson Pale, is an 80-year-old man who had a subtotal gastric resection for a peptic ulcer when he was 60 years old. At the time of his ulcer surgery, he was a mechanical engineer for a large manufacturing company. He has had no recurrence of ulcer symptoms since his surgery. He has been on a regular diet, although he by choice did not eat highly spiced foods.

Currently, he exhibits lassitude, weakness, and fatigue. He complains of headaches, dizziness, palpitations, and a sore tongue. On examination, he was pale and had a rapid pulse, and his tongue was smooth and redder than normal. His hematocrit is 20, the serum level of vitamin B_{12} is 100 pg/mL, and the serum level of folic acid is 4 ng/mL. He is anorexic and has lost weight; currently he is 5′10″ and weighs 154 lbs.

A diagnosis of deficiencies of iron, vitamin B_{12}, and folic acid is made. He will be receiving ferrous sulfate 325 mg tid, cyanocobalamin 30 mcg/d intramuscularly for 10 days (followed by 100 mcg/month), and folic acid 1 mg/day.

Mr. Pale's wife died 2 years ago. They had been married 51 years and lived alone in their own home. They had three children, only one of whom lives in the city where they reside. Mr. Pale has been apathetic and irritable lately. He has no interest in the future and has withdrawn from friends and neighbors. He often behaves as if his wife died yesterday. In the past, he was busy every day on some task of maintenance of their home but has done no work on the house since her death. His children are beginning to feel nursing home placement might be more appropriate than living alone, but Mr. Pale is opposed to this idea.

Assessment Data

Has lost weight; is under the normal weight for his height

Has a sore tongue

Exhibits other symptoms of anemia

Exhibits laboratory data consistent with diagnosis of anemia

Lassitude, weakness, and fatigue

Dizziness

Diagnoses of deficiencies of iron, vitamin B_{12}, and folic acid

Apathetic—no work on home maintenance in 2 years; no interest in the future and has withdrawn from friends and relatives

Anorexia and weight loss

Wife died 2 years ago; had been married 51 years

Often behaves as if his wife died yesterday

Nursing Diagnosis

Altered Nutrition: Less Than Body Requirements (iron and folate), related to inadequate intake of nutritious foods and (vitamin B_{12}) gastrectomy

Intervention

Monitor percentage of meals eaten.

Serve small portions of nutritious foods and fluids that appeal to the client.

Allow adequate time for meals; reheat food if necessary.

Instruct and assist the client to select foods and fluids high in iron, vitamin C, vitamin B_{12}, and folic acid.

Administer ferrous sulfate, cyanocobalamin, and folic acid as ordered and monitor for therapeutic and nontherapeutic effects.

Carry out interventions relating to improving nutritional status.

Goals and Outcomes

The client will have an improved nutritional status as shown by a decrease in the signs and symptoms of iron deficiency.

(continued)

Example of Nursing Process for Iron Deficiency (continued)

Nursing Diagnosis (continued)	Intervention (continued)	Goals and Outcomes (continued)
Activity Intolerance, related to altered nutritional status	**Encourage** progressive activity and increased self-care as allowed and tolerated.	The client will demonstrate an increased tolerance for activity.
	Instruct client in energy-saving techniques such as shower chair for showering and sitting to do other parts of personal hygiene such as brushing teeth, combing hair.	
	Provide adequate rest periods between periods of activity.	
Dysfunctional Grieving, related to loss of wife	**Permit** and encourage review of life's achievements and experiences.	The client will experience less or no dysfunctional grieving.
	Support past achievements, current strengths, and coping skills.	
	Use active listening and encourage exploration of feelings and thoughts about wife.	
	Work through emotional reaction (apathy, hopelessness).	
	Encourage client to seek assistance from friends, relatives, professionals, or self-help groups.	

amino acid to other amino acids will produce therapeutic levels in the brain.

The amino acid L-tryptophan was used for a time as a natural sleep aid. It is found in abundance in milk and milk products and is believed to be the sedative agent in milk taken warm at bedtime. There is considerable evidence that this substance does indeed promote sleep. Some physicians prescribed it for insomnia, especially insomnia associated with autoimmune diseases such as rheumatoid arthritis and scleroderma. L-tryptophan has been withdrawn from the United States market because a serious neuromuscular disorder, eosinophile myalgia, developed in some recipients. Adverse effects included paralysis and death.

L-glutamine is sold as a brain stimulant and cognitive aid. Although these properties are substantiated by some medical reports of mania from its use, L-glutamine is not recognized as a therapeutic drug by the medical profession.

Tyrosine, a precursor of the neurotransmitters norepinephrine and dopamine, has been used successfully in the treatment of depression when other therapies fail.

Lipids

Linoleic acid is an essential fatty acid recommended by health food proponents for preventing cardiovascular degeneration. This acid plays a role in biomembrane structure and the production of prostaglandins. It has been found helpful in delaying and ameliorating relapses in the early stages of multiple sclerosis. Linoleic acid is unproved, however, as a cardiovascular protectant. It has the same caloric value as other fatty acids.

Lecithin, according to health food advocates, is also believed to protect the cardiovascular system. Lecithin is a phospholipid with a high linoleic acid content. Studies have not substantiated its purported hypocholesterolemic effect. Preliminary evidence suggests that it does improve the HDL:LDL ratio in the blood, especially in women. High doses of either linoleic acid or lecithin can significantly increase calorie intake.

Unrefined Products

One flavoring element available in capsule form is garlic, which is under study for hypotensive effects. Perhaps some component of this substance will eventually be accepted as a helpful drug. However, its pharmacologically active component appears to be removed during processing; the capsules are reported to exert no helpful pharmacologic effects.

Kelp is available in concentrated form from drugstore counters and health food stores. This substance is rich in iodine but has no other known pharmacologic agent.

Vinegar is another component of certain supplement capsules. Ingested vinegar is not accepted as a medicinal substance and has no known therapeutic effect. Like the iodine in kelp, the main ingredient in vinegar, acetic acid, is available in foodstuffs (eg, pickles, salad dressings).

Shark cartilage is recommended for the treatment of rheumatoid arthritis. A rationale for its use is emerging in the "oral tolerance" theory for the treatment of autoimmune disorders (Richardson, 1995). According to this theory, the ingestion of proteins stimulates the production of T cells capable of inhibiting the production of antibodies to that protein (and similar proteins). Long-term oral tolerance therapy should cause a decline in autoimmune bodies and improvement of the autoimmune condition. Improvement may occur from several days to several months after therapy is begun. Shark cartilage is marketed in capsules containing 750 mg of medication, and the usual adult dosage is two capsules a day.

■ SUMMARY

Most concentrated nutrients marketed by the health food industry are not controlled by the Food and Drug Administration. These products generally contain no instructions or cautions on their labels. Instructions for their use are disseminated by word of mouth, in anonymous printed material, or in publications largely supported by advertisements featuring proprietary preparations of these products. Some products have been recognized and used by the healthcare system, but others have no proven value, and some have proved to be toxic.

❖ NURSING MANAGEMENT: CLIENTS AND HEALTH FOOD PRODUCTS

To advise clients on the merits of health foods, the nurse must have some knowledge of nutritional research. By studying the literature in this discipline, the nurse can advise clients knowledgeably and specifically about individual products. In the absence of expertise in this area, the nurse should caution clients about the pitfalls of using unproven products not controlled by the Food and Drug Administration.

References

Richardson S. (1995). Teaching tolerance to T cells. *Discover, 1991, 16*(7), 35 (July).

Bibliography

*Blanchard DS. (1990). What women can do to protect against osteoporosis. *RN, 53*(10), 60–64.

Broun ER, Greist A, Tricot G. (1990). Excessive zinc ingestion. A reversal cause of sideroblastic anemia and bone marrow depression. *JAMA, 264*(11), 1441–1443.

Dagnelie PC, van Staveren WA, van den Berg H. (1991). Vitamin B$_{12}$ from algae appears not to be bioavailable. *Am J Clin Nutr, 53*, 695–697.

Food and Nutrition Board, National Academy of Sciences. (1990). *Nutrition during pregnancy*. Washington DC: National Academy Press.

*Garlic fights nitrosamide formation. (1994). *Sci News, 145*, 90.

Hallberg L, Brune M, Erlandsson M, Sandberg A-S, Rossander-Hulten L. (1991). Calcium: Effect of different amounts on nonheme- and heme-iron absorption in humans. *Am J Clin Nutr, 53*, 112–119.

*Marino G. (1994). Update on intake: Calcium consumption low. *Sci News, 145*, 390.

*Pauly-O'Neill S. (1990). Critical questions (number 1). *AJN, 90*, 94 (Sept).

*Perez A. (1995). Hypokalemia. *RN, 58*, 33 (Dec).

Picciano MF, Stokstad EL, Gregory JF, eds. (1990). *Folic acid metabolism in health and disease*. New York: Wiley-Liss.

*Raloff J. (1995). Enzyme error behind neural tube defects. *Sci News, 147*, 53.

*Rosenfeld I. (1995). *Doctor, what should I eat?* New York: Random House.

Rossander-Hulten L, Brune M, Sandstrom B, Lonnerdal B, Hallberg L. (1991). Competitive inhibition of iron absorption by manganese and zinc in humans. *Am J Clin Nutr, 54*, 152–156.

*Seachrist L. (1995). Excess vitamin A causes birth defects. *Sci News, 148*, 244.

*Recommended for further reading.

For more information and sample tests and activities, refer to Chapter 49 in the Student Workbook for Clinical Pharmacology and Nursing Management, 5th edition, available through your bookstore.

50
Diagnostic Drugs

Pharmacologic agents are often used in diagnostic procedures to determine the underlying cause of illness. These agents fall into four general categories:

- Radiopaque contrast media for x-ray imaging
- Markers that can measure the concentration, volume, or rate of flow of body fluids
- Provocative agents that stimulate measurable body responses indicating the presence or absence of disease
- Dermal reactivity agents used to detect antibodies.

Although these agents are not given for curative effects, they exert drug actions and can cause toxic effects

and side effects. Before diagnostic tests are performed, the potential risks and benefits of the tests are assessed. Then the tests are conducted in a way that ensures that reliable diagnostic data will be generated with the least risk to the client.

Ionizing Radiation

Although the benefits of radiography are undeniable, radiography is not without risk. Exposure to ionizing radiation has a cumulative effect over a person's life span. Ionizing radiation is associated with an increased risk of birth defects and malignant neoplasms, infertility, and tissue changes characteristic of aging. Although the body's repair processes seem capable of reversing some of the effects of radiation, no standards have been established for safe levels of exposure, and many authorities believe there is no "safe" level. For this reason, diagnostic radiography should be kept to a minimum and should never be used unless necessary.

❖ NURSING MANAGEMENT: CLIENT UNDERGOING RADIOGRAPHY

Modern radiographic equipment is designed to minimize exposure to ionizing rays. Low-voltage emissions, narrow beams, and shielding screens help confine radiation to the target area and keep it at a low level. Nevertheless, each image adds to the cumulative x-ray load.

NURSING PROCESS
ASSESSMENT
An attempt should be made to assess total exposure to radiation before the planned test. A history of exposure to radiation and radioactive drugs or tracers, as well as nonmedicinal exposure to ionizing radiation, should be taken. The reproductive status of female clients should be determined. The client's knowledge about the procedure and his or her emotional reaction to it should be explored.

NURSING DIAGNOSIS
Probable diagnoses for clients about to undergo diagnostic tests involving ionizing radiation include:

- Knowledge Deficit, related to exposure to radiation and its use in diagnostic procedures
- Anxiety, related to the threat of radiation exposure

  One possible collaborative problem is:

  Potential Complication: Damage to the fetus related to exposure to irradiation

PLANNING
Goals of nursing care are to prevent excessive exposure to ionizing radiation, to reduce anxiety, and to educate clients about the role of radiation in diagnostic testing.

INTERVENTION

The prescriber and radiologist should be notified if the client is pregnant or has a history of radiation sickness or frequent exposure to ionizing radiation. Tests performed on women of childbearing age should be scheduled for the first half of the menstrual cycle, when the likelihood of pregnancy is minimal.

Clients undergoing diagnostic tests should be given emotional support. Without giving false assurances, the nurse should encourage trust in healthcare personnel and should express hope for a favorable outcome.

Client Education. Clients should be discouraged from requesting diagnostic x-rays for trivial reasons. They should be fully informed of the health risks of exposure to ionizing radiation and radiographic agents. They should always be involved in the decision-making process when studies requiring radiation are contemplated.

Clients need information specific to the planned procedure and instructions regarding actions they can take to promote accuracy in test results.

During radiographic studies, care is taken to shield body areas that do not require exposure to the x-ray beam, especially the gonads before and during the reproductive years. The client should be encouraged to cooperate with safety measures, such as draping with lead covers. Such drapes are heavy and may be uncomfortable but usually are required only briefly.

OUTCOME EVALUATION

Data required for evaluation include the incidence or absence of adverse effects attributable to excessive radiation. Client teaching is evaluated according to the incidence or absence of signs and symptoms of anxiety, the client's ability to cooperate with technicians and other staff during the procedures, and client statements indicating an awareness of the risks and benefits of testing.

❖ **CHECKLIST OF NURSING ACTIONS**

❑ Assess the client's cumulative exposure to ionizing radiation before radiographic studies. Report excessive or unusual exposure promptly.
❑ Determine the reproductive status of women of childbearing age about to undergo diagnostic tests involving ionizing radiation.
❑ For women of childbearing age, schedule tests involving exposure to radiation for the period immediately after menstruation.
❑ Provide emotional support to clients undergoing diagnostic tests.
❑ Act as an advocate to ensure client involvement in the decision-making process.
❑ Tell the client what to do to facilitate the test procedure.

❑ Instruct the client about safety measures used to reduce exposure to radiation.
❑ Teach clients to include a history of exposure to ionizing radiation in their personal health records.

Radiopaque Contrast Media

Although plain x-rays disclose the shape, density, and integrity of dense tissues such as bone, the shadows cast by soft tissues are difficult to interpret. Some structures, such as blood vessels, cardiac chambers, and ductal systems, are not revealed at all. Visible organs generally project only a vague outline. Radiopaque chemicals inside such structures add contrast so that internal silhouettes can be clearly outlined. When used with fluoroscopy or cinematography, contrast agents allow the study of the kinetic function of specific organs. Data from such studies are crucial for correct medical diagnoses.

Barium Sulfate

Barium sulfate is an insoluble, nonabsorbable, opaque powder that is also radiopaque. It must not be confused with other salts of barium (barium sulfide, barium sulfite), which are soluble, readily absorbed, and highly toxic.

Pharmacodynamics. The function of barium sulfate depends on its distribution and concentration in the organs to be studied. Barium casts a shadow on radiographic films capable of outlining the lumen of structures in the gastrointestinal (GI) tract. Space-occupying lesions in the tract show up on films as filling defects, and ulcerations or discontinuities of the mucosa appear as outward deviations of the lumen.

Pharmacokinetics. Barium sulfate is administered orally or rectally as an aqueous suspension. It is not absorbed and passes through the GI tract to be eliminated in feces.

Diagnostic Uses. Barium sulfate is commonly used as a contrast medium in radiographic examinations of the esophagus, stomach, duodenum, and colon (barium swallow, upper GI roentgenogram, and barium enema). As orally administered material progresses through the tract, serial films can be taken for a complete study of the small intestine.

Adverse Reactions. The most common side effect of barium sulfate is constipation. The substance produces a hard stool. Obstipation and intestinal obstruction have occurred after its use. Barium can remain in the appendix and promote the formation of fecaliths; acute appendicitis with rupture can follow. Although practically inert within the GI tract, barium sulfate is irritating to peripheral tissues. Leakage outside the tract through perforations or fistulas can cause inflammation and symptoms of peritonitis or mediastinitis.

The elderly are at increased risk for adverse reactions such as fluid imbalance, hypotension, and changes in mental states.

Anaphylactic reactions have been reported during barium studies; these appear to be caused by hypersensitivity to latex rubber contained in tubes and cuffed enema tips. To prevent such reactions, most equipment is now made of synthetic materials (which may also trigger allergy in some people).

Precautions and Contraindications. Barium sulfate should not be administered to clients with known intestinal obstruction, GI perforations or fistulas, or allergy to materials used in administering barium contrast media.

■ SUMMARY

Barium sulfate is a chemical used as a radiopaque contrast medium in radiography of the GI tract. It is not absorbed systemically. It is contraindicated for clients with perforations or fistulas because it is irritating to the tissues. Barium produces a hard stool and can cause serious constipation.

❖ NURSING MANAGEMENT: CLIENT RECEIVING BARIUM SULFATE

Barium studies are among the most frequently used diagnostic tools. They are helpful in identifying abdominal strictures, obstructions, ulcers, polyps, and tumors.

NURSING PROCESS

Clients who are to undergo barium studies should receive the nursing care outlined above for everyone undergoing x-ray examinations.

ASSESSMENT

Clients scheduled for barium studies should be carefully assessed for history of allergy, particularly sensitivity to materials used in administration equipment, and for signs and symptoms of intestinal obstruction or perforation (eg, abdominal pain, rigidity, pronounced distention). Bowel status should be evaluated to determine the relative need for poststudy catharsis.

NURSING DIAGNOSIS

Nursing diagnoses for clients undergoing barium studies may include:

- Risk for Constipation (obstipation or obstruction), related to barium ingestion (or barium enema) secondary to diagnostic studies
- Knowledge Deficit, related to diagnostic procedures involving barium preparations

One possible collaborative problem is:

Potential Complication: Anaphylaxis related to allergy to materials in administration equipment

PLANNING

Nursing care goals are to prevent complications such as hypotension, constipation, obstipation, or obstruction, to detect and treat promptly any adverse reactions to barium, and to ensure the client's cooperation with laboratory personnel conducting the procedure.

INTERVENTION

Physicians and radiologists should be notified of risk factors identified in the initial nursing assessment. The need for and safety of barium studies can then be reevaluated. If barium is inadvisable, another contrast medium or test may be used.

Ample hydration before the procedure reduces the risk of hypovolemia and hypotension.

After studies involving ingested barium, the client's bowel status must be monitored carefully and measures taken to promote bowel elimination and prevent constipation. Laxatives such as milk of magnesia may be ordered.

Client Education. The client should be instructed to fast the night before the GI barium study. However, water should be taken freely before the test. The specifics of the bowel-cleansing regimen (laxative or enema), usually required the morning of the procedure, should be explained. If preparation is inadequate, films may be of poor quality and the test may have to be repeated.

Clients having upper GI studies should be informed that they will be asked to swallow a suspension resembling a thick milkshake. Clients scheduled for colon studies need to know that an enema will be administered in the x-ray department. Barium enema solutions may be drained from the colon after radiographic studies are completed, and the client is encouraged to defecate immediately to eliminate as much of the residual suspension as possible.

Various positions are used for serial exposures; clients must hold their breath when exposures are made. Clients who have been adequately informed are likely to make fewer errors during the procedure, reducing the need for repeated exposures. They will also experience less anxiety than poorly prepared persons.

After the studies are completed, the nurse should encourage the client to consume ample fluids to reduce the risk of constipation. The client should be informed that barium colors the stools a pale claylike gray. Stools should be monitored until the barium has passed and normal fecal color is resumed. Unless contraindicated, a laxative should be recommended to clients subject to constipation.

OUTCOME EVALUATION

Data required for evaluation include the incidence or absence of hypotension during the test and of constipation, obstipation, obstruction, or inflammation of parenteral tissues after the test. Client teaching can be evaluated by the effectiveness of bowel cleansing (when conducted by the client), the client's ability to cooperate with technicians and healthcare personnel during the procedure, and statements by the client that he or she felt well prepared for the procedure.

❖ CHECKLIST OF NURSING ACTIONS

❏ Before barium studies, assess the client for intestinal perforation, fistula, or obstruction, tendency toward constipation, and allergy to test materials and equipment.

❏ Instruct the client to fast but to take ample amounts of water before the test.

❏ Instruct the client regarding the bowel-cleansing regimen, when ordered.

❏ Follow protocols for diagnostic studies carefully to ensure accurate results without the need for repeated studies.

❏ Instruct the client about procedures to follow during the study.

❏ Monitor the client closely during studies for hypovolemia, hypotension, and mental changes such as confusion.

❏ Warn the client that stools containing barium will be clay-colored.

❏ After barium studies, administer laxatives as required by test protocols or the prescriber's order, or recommend a laxative to clients prone to constipation.

Iodinated Contrast Media

Various iodine compounds with radiopaque properties are used in diagnostic radiographic procedures. The function of these contrast agents depends on their distribution, concentration, and excretion within the body, rather than on their pharmacologic effects; therefore, pharmacologic effects of iodinated contrast media are considered side effects.

Pharmacodynamics. Contrast media are opaque to x-rays and cast shadows on x-ray film. These substances can be injected into the body to produce images that illustrate the distribution and flow of body fluids such as blood, bile, and urine. Their presence in tissues also enhances the images produced by computed tomography (CT scans).

Pharmacokinetics. Routes of absorption, distribution, and excretion vary with different preparations and are related to their diagnostic uses (Table 50-1). Oral preparations not readily absorbed by the GI tract are used for radiographic examinations of this tract. (However, variable amounts of these preparations are absorbed systemically.) Preparations readily absorbed in the GI tract and subsequently concentrated and excreted by the biliary or urinary tracts are used in examining these systems. Injectable solutions are often administered directly into the structures to be studied (eg, arteries, veins, cardiac chambers, joints) and must be absorbed

systemically before elimination. Most radiopaque compounds are excreted mainly by the kidneys, with lesser amounts eliminated in bile and feces.

Diagnostic Uses. Iodinated contrast media are used to produce or enhance images in many diagnostic studies (Box 50-1). When sufficiently concentrated in body fluids, they outline the structures (eg, blood vessels, joints, cerebrospinal space) in which they are contained or the ducts and tubules (urinary or biliary) by which they are excreted.

Dosage form and route of administration are chosen according to the area to be visualized, as well as the equipment and method used. Dosage and concentration are individualized and proportional to the size of the area to be studied, the anticipated dilution, and the degree of contrast required.

Adverse Reactions. Side effects from iodinated contrast media can affect many systems of the body and can range in severity from mild to life-threatening. Some effects are transitory, others permanent.

Vasomotor reactions affect up to half the clients receiving contrast media. Allergic reactions are common as well (Table 50-2). Treatment includes vasopressors, intravenous (IV) fluids, oxygen, antihistamines, and steroids. Pretreatment (with glucocorticoids and antihistamines) of clients at high risk may reduce the severity of the reaction.

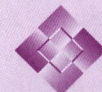

Toxicity Alert:
Iodinated Contrast Media

The toxicity of iodine contrast media is influenced by many factors. The type of cation in the molecule is significant; for example, meglumine salts are better tolerated than sodium salts. Factors directly related to toxicity include osmolarity, volume, concentration, viscosity, and rate of administration. The route of administration affects the type of reaction likely to occur. For example, neurotoxic reactions are most likely to occur in cerebral angiography when the drugs are delivered directly to the brain by injection into the carotid artery. Reactions are most likely with repeated tests over a short time and in clients who are dehydrated.

Precautions and Contraindications. Iodinated contrast media are contraindicated for clients with a history of severe reaction to any of these drugs. Other contraindications depend on the type of test. For example, cerebral angiography is contraindicated if cranial subarachnoid hemorrhage is suspected or if the client has an active migraine headache; IV urography is contraindicated in anuria.

Table 50-1. Iodinated Contrast Media

Drug Name	Preparation	Usual Adult Dosage	Diagnostic Uses/Additional Information
Aqueous Injectable Agents			
diatrizoate meglumine (Cardiografin, Cystografin, Hypaque-Cysto, Hypaque Meglumine, Reno-M)	Solutions for injection or instillation (30%, 60%, 76%, 85%)	Varies with the test to be done	Diatrizoate meglumine is employed in various procedures including angiography, phlebography, cardiography, IV and retrograde urography, direct cholangiography, and enhancement of CT of the brain.
diatrizoate sodium (Hypaque)	Solutions for injection or instillation (25%, 41.66%, 50%) Solutions for instillation (20%, 41.66%)	Varies with the test to be done	Diatrizoate is employed in various procedures including hysterosalpingography. It is used in preference to barium for GI radiography when perforation or obstruction is suspected.
iodamide meglumide (Renovue)	Solutions for injection (24%, 65%)	Varies with the test to be done	Iodamide is employed for IV urography and contrast enhancement of CT of the brain.
iodipamide meglumine (Cholografin Meglumine)	Solutions for injection or instillation (10.3%, 52%)	Varies with the test to be done	Iodipamide is employed for IV cholecystography and cholangiography.
iophendylate (Pantopaque)	Solution for intrathecal injection (305 mg iodine/mL)	Varies with the test to be done	Iophendylate is employed in myelography, especially in the lumbar region. It is usually aspirated from the cerebrospinal fluid after the procedure.
iothalamate meglumine (Conray, Cysto-Conray)	Solutions for injection or instillation (30%, 43%, 60%) Solutions for instillation (17.2%, 60%)	Varies with the test to be done	Iothalamate meglumine is employed in various procedures including IV urography, cerebral arteriography, peripheral arteriography, and venography.
iothalamate sodium (Angio-Conray, Conray-400)	Solutions for injection (54.3%, 66.8%, 80%)	Varies with the test to be done	Iothalamate sodium is employed in IV urography, angiocardiography, contrast enhancement of CT of the brain, and aortography; it is not suitable for cerebral angiography.
metrizamide (*Can:* Amipaque)	Solutions for instillation	Varies with the test to be done	Metrizamide is employed in myelography, cisternography, and ventriculography.
Oils			
ethiodized oil (Ethiodol)	Oil containing 370 mg iodine/mL for instillation or intralymphatic injection	Varies with the test to be done	Ethiodized oil is employed in lymphography and hysterosalpingography; it is not suitable for administration intravenously, intra-arterially, intrathecally, or by way of the bronchial tree.
propyliodone (*Can:* Dionosil)	Suspension for instillation	Varies with the test to be done	Propyliodone is employed in bronchography and laryngography.
Oral agents			
iocetamic acid (Cholebrine)	Tablets for oral use	3–4.5 g	Iocetamic acid is employed in oral cholecystography; it may be used for children older than age 12 years.
iopanoic acid (Telepaque)	Tablets for oral use	3 g	Iopanoic acid is employed in oral cholecystography.
ipodate (Oragrafin, Bilivist)	Capsules and powder for preparing suspension for oral use	3 g	Ipodate is employed in oral cholecystography; suspensions should be prepared with lukewarm water and used promptly because they are unstable. Both calcium and sodium salts are available.
tyropanoate sodium (Bilopaque)	Capsules for oral use	3 g	Tyropanoate is employed in oral cholecystography.

KEY: *Can* = Canadian trade name.

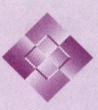

Box 50-1
Tests That Use Radiopaque Contrast Agents

Angiography, venography, lymphography

Cardiography, aortography

Urography (IV and retrograde)

Arthrography, discography, myelography

Cholecystography (direct, IV, and oral)

Gastrointestinal radiography (when barium is contraindicated)

Hysterosalpingography

Computed tomography (especially cerebral)

Table 50-2. Adverse Reactions to Contrast Media

Type of Reaction	Signs and Symptoms
Idiosyncratic/allergic	Anaphylaxis* Anaphylactoid reactions*
Vasomotor	Flushing, warmth, tingling†
Cardiovascular	Increased osmolarity in fluid compartments, hypotension or hypertension, bradycardia or tachycardia, hemodynamic shifts and thrombophlebitis, (rarely) shock, fibrillation, cardiac arrest, disseminated intravascular coagulation
Respiratory	Rhinitis, dyspnea, cough, sneeze, bronchospasm, laryngospasm, pulmonary edema, cyanosis, (with oil lymphography) pulmonary embolism*
GI	Metallic taste,† salivation, salivary gland swelling, nausea,† vomiting, retching
Neurologic	Restlessness, confusion, apprehension, anxiety, headache, dizziness, tremor, agitation, visual disturbances, convulsions,* stroke,* coma,* paraplegia,* permanent visual field defects*
Dermatologic	Pain at injection site† Urticaria, pruritus, rash, edema, pallor, petechiae, diaphoresis; necrosis has been reported after extravasation during injection
Hematopoietic	Neutropenia
Renal	Acute renal failure, oliguria, anuria, proteinuria
General	Chills, fever, flushing, warmth

*Most serious
†Most frequent

Caution must be used with clients who have a history of mild reaction to these agents, a history of migraine, or a personal or family history of allergy, especially asthma.

Several medical conditions increase the risk of adverse reactions because they slow elimination of the agents or predispose the client to injury to specific organs. Caution should be used when giving contrast media to persons with renal or hepatic impairment, hemocystinuria, congestive heart failure, multiple myeloma, thrombosis, phlebitis, ischemia, or diabetic nephropathy. Extreme caution is required if pheochromocytoma is known or suspected because severe hypertension may occur. Serial studies within a short time increase the risk of reaction.

Before studies using these agents are undertaken, clients should be well hydrated. Vasopressor drugs should not be given before the test. When the drugs are injected, care should be taken to deliver them to the desired site. Blood vessels should be flushed immediately after injection with an IV solution.

Support personnel and equipment must be immediately available to treat serious reactions, such as anaphylaxis.

■ SUMMARY

Radiopaque iodine compounds are used as contrast media in many diagnostic radiographic studies, including CT scanning. Dosage, route, and time of administration vary, depending on the test. Although serious adverse reactions are uncommon, these drugs can produce many toxic effects and side effects.

❖ NURSING MANAGEMENT: CLIENT RECEIVING IODINATED CONTRAST MEDIUM

Although x-ray personnel are responsible for administering some radiopaque agents, the nurse is usually responsible for preparing clients and monitoring them for delayed adverse reactions.

NURSING PROCESS

ASSESSMENT

Clients receiving iodinated contrast media should be assessed carefully for hypersensitivity to iodine, especially for a previous reaction to contrast media. Previous exposure to iodine contrast media should be documented.

The client's knowledge about the procedure and emotional reaction to it should be explored as well. Before the procedure, the client should be screened for fluid imbalances and liver and kidney impairment.

NURSING DIAGNOSIS

Nursing diagnoses for clients receiving iodinated contrast media may include:

- Pain, related to flushing, warmth, nausea, vertigo, dyspnea, apprehension, and restlessness induced by reaction to contrast medium
- Knowledge Deficit, concerning iodinated contrast agent and its effects
- Anxiety, related to contrast medium infusion and test procedure

One possible collaborative problem is:

Potential Complication: Allergic reactions (anaphylaxis, skin rash) to the contrast media

PLANNING

Nursing goals for clients receiving iodinated contrast media include preventing adverse reactions, promptly detecting and treating adverse reactions should they occur, reducing anxiety, and educating the client about the procedure and contrast agent.

INTERVENTION

The prescriber and radiologist should be informed promptly of the following assessment data: history of recent use of iodine compounds, excessive exposure to radiation, previous reaction to iodinated contrast media, or signs and symptoms of kidney or liver impairment. If the client is not well hydrated, an IV infusion should be requested to ensure adequate hydration.

Throughout contact with the client, the nurse should provide emotional support, promote trust in the healthcare team, and, without giving false assurances, encourage hope for a favorable outcome.

Protocols for test procedures must be followed carefully to ensure accurate results without repeated studies. Fasting is often required. Bowel cleansing is necessary before most abdominal studies. Sedation may be ordered for clients undergoing procedures that require instrumentation such as cystoscopy. Oral radiopaque drugs administered before the test must be timed correctly to ensure optimal results.

After diagnostic tests, clients should be monitored for adverse drug reactions such as skin rash, changes in vital signs, or dyspnea. (Because pretesting for sensitivity can produce severe reactions, it is generally not recommended.) Reactions are most likely to occur after parenteral administration of the contrast agent. Nurses should be prepared to treat anaphylaxis with sympathomimetic vasopressors such as epinephrine or to treat vagal reactions with atropine. Oxygen may also be required. Clients should be monitored for 30 to 60 minutes after the procedure to ensure that recurring symptoms are detected.

Client Education. Clients scheduled for diagnostic studies involving radiopaque dyes should be encouraged to drink ample water before the test. They should be informed about the usual procedure for the test and what will be expected of them during the procedure.

Clients who are to receive parenteral preparations should be told that they will feel a sensation of warmth when the contrast medium is injected. They should be instructed to report any unusual response, especially faintness or difficulty in breathing.

Clients who have had adverse reactions to contrast media should be instructed to report this whenever radiographic studies are proposed involving similar agents. If the reaction was anaphylactic, a medical identification device should be carried warning of allergy to iodinated contrast media.

OUTCOME EVALUATION

Data required for evaluation include the absence or incidence of signs and symptoms of anxiety, the promptness of detection and treatment of any adverse drug reactions, and the absence or incidence of serious effects from exposure to radiopaque contrast media. Client education can be evaluated by the client's ability to cooperate during the test and by client comments indicating he or she felt well prepared for the experience. (See the Example of Nursing Process for Managing Adverse Reaction to Contrast Agent.)

❖ CHECKLIST OF NURSING ACTIONS

- Before radiographic studies involving iodinated contrast media, assess the client for allergy to the agent, previous exposure to ionizing radiation, recent use of iodine compounds, tissue hydration, and kidney and liver function.
- To reduce anxiety and promote valid test results, explain procedures to clients.
- Provide emotional support to clients undergoing diagnostic testing.
- Promote adequate hydration before the study.
- Follow test protocols carefully to ensure valid test data without repeated studies.
- Be prepared to treat serious adverse reactions, including anaphylaxis, should they occur.
- Tell clients they will feel a sensation of warmth when the contrast medium is injected.
- Monitor clients carefully for adverse reactions after administration of iodine contrast media.
- Urge clients who have had adverse reactions to contrast media to carry a medical identification device.

Agents Used for Volumetric Testing

Chemicals with characteristic distribution and excretion patterns can be used to assess physiologic processes by which they move through the body. Rates of uptake, distribution, storage, and excretion reflect the function

---

Example of Nursing Process for Managing Adverse Reaction to Contrast Agent

The client, a 43-year-old man with a history of headaches and changes in visual fields, has been admitted to the hospital for a series of diagnostic studies. This morning a brain scan was performed. A radiopaque dye containing iodine was injected IV. In the early afternoon, he tells the nurse that his lower back and hips are itching. The affected skin is covered with various-sized wheals; several scratch marks are present.

Assessment Data

Complaint of itching
Urticaria
Scratch marks

Nursing Diagnosis

Impaired Tissue Integrity: Skin rash, possibly related to allergic reaction to radiopaque contrast agent

Intervention

Bathe the affected area with cool water; apply a soothing lotion.

Advise the client to keep the area cool to reduce itching.

Advise the client to apply pressure to itching areas rather than scratching.

Take measures to reduce the client's stress level to minimize the allergic reaction.

Report the adverse reaction; request antiallergy medication such as an antihistamine.

Provide the client with diversion to distract his attention from the itching stimuli.

Goals and Outcomes

No new scratch marks will appear on the affected area.

The rash will gradually fade and disappear.

---

of organs involved in their pharmacokinesis and can be used to measure flow rates, diffusion, and volumes of various body fluids. Chemicals that are relatively inert pharmacologically are preferred in such diagnostic studies because they induce minimal side effects and adverse reactions. The compounds used must be measurable by chemical assay, colorimetric analysis, or radioactivity monitoring.

Nonradioactive Compounds

The processes by which chemicals and fluids are distributed, metabolized, and excreted by the body can be monitored by tracer chemicals whose presence can be detected and measured. Once norms are established for a process, diagnostic tests can be developed to detect an impairment or abnormality.

Nonradioactive diagnostic agents are substances that can be detected by chemical or color measurements. They include polysaccharides and dyes (Table 50-3).

Pharmacodynamics. The use of volumetric diagnostic agents depends on the ways in which the compounds are distributed, metabolized, and excreted rather than on their pharmacologic activity.

Pharmacokinetics. Most volumetric agents are administered by IV injection and enter the extracellular fluid compartment. They are poorly or only temporarily bound to plasma proteins. They are usually taken up rapidly by the specific organ whose function is under study. Most are excreted by the liver or kidneys.

Diagnostic Uses. Polysaccharides, phenolsulfonphthalein, and aminohippurate are used to assess kidney function. Indigotindisulfonate locates the ureteral orifices and marks abnormal fluid passage from damaged ureters. The sulfobromophthalein test is a sensitive indicator of early liver impairment.

Adverse Reactions. Side effects of polysaccharides include increased circulatory volume and diuresis secondary to the osmotic effects of these compounds. Aminohippurate is administered in such large doses that hypervolemia usually occurs when the drug is first given. Large doses of indigotindisulfonate impart a temporary blue discoloration to the skin.

Among the adverse reactions to these agents are nausea, vomiting, urticaria, pruritus, malaise, fever, hypotension or hypertension, and bronchoconstriction (Box 50-2). Allergic reactions, including anaphylaxis, may occur. These

Table 50-3. Substances Used for Volumetric Testing

Drug Name	Preparation	Tissue Distribution	Usual Adult Dosage/PC	Diagnostic Use
Polysaccharides				
mannitol (D-Mannitol, *Can:* Isotol, Osmitrol)	Solutions for injection (5%, 10%, 15%, 20%, 25%)	Freely filtered by kidney glomeruli	200 mg/kg PC: C	Measure glomerular filtration rate
inulin (Alantin, Starch Alant, Dahlin)	Solution for injection (100 mg/mL in 0.9% NaCl)	Freely filtered by kidney glomeruli	50 mg/kg (priming dose); 18.8 mg/m² body surface area per minute (following priming dose)	Measure glomerular filtration rate
Dyes				
indigotindisulfonate (Indigo Carmine)	Solution for IM or IV injection (8 mg/mL)	Excreted by the kidneys, appearing in urine	40 mg IV; 50–100 mg IM	Localize ureteral orifices during cystoscopy and ureteral catheterization Identify severed ureters and fistulous communications
indocyanine green (Cardio-Green)	Powder for preparing solution for IV injection	Highly bound to plasma proteins Excreted unchanged in bile	0.5–5 mg/kg	Measurement of cardiac output Test of hepatic function and measurement of hepatic blood flow
phenolsulfonphthalein (Phenol Red, PSP)	Solutions for IM or IV injection	Partially bound to plasma proteins Excreted primarily by kidneys	6 mg	Evaluate renal blood flow Assess urinary retention and total kidney function
sulfobromophthalein (Bromsulphalein, BSP)	Solution for IV injection	Rapidly taken up and stored by liver parenchyma	5 mg/kg to maximum of 500 mg	Detect cirrhosis, acute hepatitis, and liver cell damage
Miscellaneous				
aminohippurate sodium (sodium paraaminohippurate, PAH)	Solution for IV infusion (200 mg/mL)	Rapidly excreted from kidneys by proximal tubular secretion and (to some extent) glomerular filtration	2 g; adjusted in accordance with plasma concentration	Estimate effective renal plasma flow Assess tubular secretion
sodium dehydrocholate (Decholin)	Solution for IV injection	Circulated by the blood to the tongue, where it stimulates taste buds	3–5 mL of 20% solution	Measure arm-to-tongue circulation time by counting seconds between injection and taste sensation
D-xylose (wood sugar)	Powder for oral administration	Absorbed in the GI tract and subsequently passed through the blood to kidneys, where it is excreted	25 g	Assess intestinal absorption and diagnose malabsorptive states

KEY: PC = pregnancy risk category; see Appendix A.
Can = Canadian trade name.

compounds tend to be irritating, and extravasation during administration may cause tissue necrosis. Aminohippurate can also induce cramps and a desire to void or defecate; D-xylose can cause abdominal bloating, cramping, abdominal discomfort, and diarrhea.

Precautions and Contraindications. These agents are contraindicated in clients with a history of hypersensi-

tivity to them and during pregnancy, especially in the early stages. They should be administered with caution to asthmatic and allergic clients. Equipment, supplies, and trained personnel must be available to treat allergic reactions, including anaphylaxis. Compounds used for kidney function tests should be avoided when renal function is severely impaired or when the recipient is dehydrated. Polysaccharides and aminohippurate are

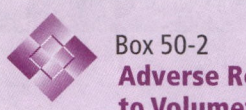

Box 50-2
Adverse Reactions to Volumetric Tests

Most Common Reactions

Hypervolemia (polysaccharides), abdominal cramps, micturition, defecation, GI discomfort (D-xylose)

Most Serious Reactions

Anaphylaxis, tissue necrosis (after extravasation of drug solutions)

not given when pulmonary edema or active intracranial bleeding is present. These drugs must be administered with caution to clients with limited cardiac reserve because they increase blood volume.

■ SUMMARY

Nonradioactive volumetric diagnostic agents are used to measure the concentration and movement of chemicals through the body and to ascertain volumes, flow, and diffusion of body fluids and organ function. They are commonly used to assess kidney and liver function. Serious reactions, including anaphylaxis, may occur during such tests. These agents are not used for clients with a history of adverse reaction to them. Staff must be prepared to deal with serious adverse reactions.

❖ NURSING MANAGEMENT: CLIENT RECEIVING SUBSTANCES USED IN VOLUMETRIC TESTING

NURSING PROCESS

ASSESSMENT

Before beginning volumetric diagnostic tests, a careful history should be taken to determine whether the client has been exposed previously to the agent. Adverse reaction to such exposure is particularly significant. A history of allergy, especially asthma, is also pertinent. The client should be evaluated for circulatory homeostasis and cardiac and kidney function. The client's knowledge about the test and emotional reaction to it should be explored.

NURSING DIAGNOSIS

Nursing diagnoses for the client scheduled to receive an agent used in volumetric testing may include:

- Anxiety, related to the effect of the agent used in the test
- Pain: Nausea, vomiting, itching, malaise, vertigo, dyspnea, abdominal cramping related to adverse reaction to the volumetric diagnostic agent
- Diarrhea, related to adverse reaction to D-XYLOSE
- Knowledge Deficit, concerning volumetric agents and their use in diagnostic procedures

A common collaborative problem that should be differentiated from the nursing diagnoses is:

Potential Complications: Anaphylaxis, hypervolemia, hypotension, tissue necrosis at the site of drug administration

PLANNING

Nursing goals include maintaining fluid balance, reducing anxiety, increasing comfort, maintaining normal bowel elimination, preventing adverse drug reactions, promptly detecting and treating adverse reactions should they occur, and increasing the client's ability to cooperate during the test.

INTERVENTION

The prescriber and radiologist should be notified of any risk factors apparent during the initial nursing assessment. This information may include previous exposure and adverse reaction to the diagnostic agent, history of asthma or other allergy, dehydration or circulatory overload, and cardiac or renal impairment.

The nurse should provide emotional support to the client and promote trust in the healthcare team. Without giving false assurances, the nurse should foster hope for a favorable outcome.

If the drug preparation contains crystals, it should be warmed and agitated gently until the crystals completely dissolve. Test protocols must be followed precisely. The reliability of test results depends on accurate dosage and timing of specimen collection. If a specimen collection is inadvertently delayed, the exact time it is obtained must be recorded so that proper adjustments may be made in the test calculations.

Extravasation of solutions from IV sites must be avoided. Should it develop, the infusion should be interrupted immediately and the swollen tissues gently compressed to encourage the fluid to seep from the tissues of the injection site onto sterile absorbent materials, such as gauze pads.

Blood pressure and respirations should be monitored during the test when agents that affect circulatory volume are used. Central venous pressure should be monitored for undesirable increases when polysaccharides or aminohippurate are used. The test should be discontinued if central venous pressure rises. Equipment, supplies, and trained personnel must be readily available to treat anaphylaxis, should it develop during the test.

The nurse should monitor for a reaction to the diagnostic agent for at least 1 hour after the test concludes.

Client Education. To allay anxiety, clients should be informed about the test in terms of what they will perceive. The client's cooperation should be sought to ensure accurate completion of the test. Clients whose skins turns bluish after receiving indigotindisulfonate should be reassured that this is temporary.

OUTCOME EVALUATION

Data required for evaluation include the absence or incidence of fluid imbalance (either hypovolemia or hypervolemia), diarrhea, urticaria, hypotension, soft-tissue necrosis, and signs and symptoms of anxiety. Client education can be evaluated by the client's ability to participate in the procedure and by comments indicating that he or she knew what to expect during the procedure.

❖ CHECKLIST OF NURSING ACTIONS

❑ Assess the client for increased risk of adverse reactions to the drug agent—history of adverse reaction to the compound, allergy (especially asthma), or cardiac or kidney impairment.

❑ Assess the client's fluid balance and report any evidence of dehydration or circulatory overload.

❑ Describe to clients what they will experience during the test.

❑ Provide emotional support to clients undergoing diagnostic tests.

❑ Follow test protocols precisely to ensure accuracy and test reliability.

❑ Discontinue infusions that have extravasated; promote drainage of drug solutions from the tissues.

❑ In clients receiving agents that affect circulatory volume, monitor for evidence of altered circulation.

❑ Monitor clients for adverse reactions during and after the procedure.

Radioactive Tracers

Radioactive drugs are compounds containing atoms that disintegrate by emission of electromagnetic radiation. They may be naturally occurring radionuclides or substances prepared in particle accelerators. They are useful diagnostic agents because their movements through the body can be traced by methods that reveal or measure radioactivity.

Levels of radioactivity can be defined in several ways, depending on the attribute or effect in question. Terms used in measuring radiation are defined in Box 50-3.

The body handles chemicals in characteristic ways, transporting, storing, metabolizing, and excreting them so as to provide substrate for vital life processes and to eliminate toxic substances. Radionuclides allow some of these biochemical processes to be studied. Abnormalities in the distribution and concentration of radioactive chemicals reflect pathologic changes in the functions of organs containing them.

The choice of the specific chemical used is influenced by the biochemistry of the organ or system studied. For example, radioiodine is used to study the thyroid gland because this element is used by the gland in

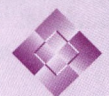

Box 50-3
Terms Used in Measuring Radiation

curie: the quantity of radioactivity emitted from a radionuclide equal to 3.7×10^{10} transformations per second

roentgen: the quantity of X radiation or gamma radiation in air

rad: the dose of any ionizing radiation absorbed per unit of mass of material

rem: roentgen equivalent (in) man; the estimated biologic effect relative to a dose of 1 roentgen of x-ray

MPL: maximal permissible limit; the recommended limit of accumulated exposure to ionizing radiation at any age

large amounts. The concentration and distribution of radioiodine in thyroid tissue, as measured by scintigraphy, provide useful information about the organ's size, integrity, and function.

Diagnostic radionuclides include several classes of compounds used medicinally in nonradioactive forms. These may be diuretics, vitamins, dyes, or iodides (Table 50-4). Dosage is measured in curies, which are units of radioactivity. Because radioactive substances are constantly decaying (losing radioactivity), the dosage must be computed according to the drug's age. The volume or mass of drug required for a given dose of radioactivity increases as the preparation ages.

Pharmacodynamics. Radioactive tracers emit energy particles that can be detected or measured by photography, scintiscopy, scintigraphy, monitoring with Geiger counters, or other methods.

Pharmacokinetics. Radioactive compounds are handled by the body in the same way as nonradioactive compounds. They are administered orally or parenterally. Distribution, storage, metabolism, and excretion are identical to the compound in its nonradioactive form. Radiation effects at any given time depend not only on the tissue concentration but also on the residual radioactivity in the drug. The tissue concentration of the chemical depends on the compound's distribution and biologic half-life. It decreases as the compound is deactivated and excreted by the body. At the same time, radioactive decay reduces the ionizing activity of the drug residues as time elapses. Radioactivity declines in inverse proportion to the chemical's radioactive half-life.

Diagnostic Uses. Radionuclides are used as radioactive tracers in three types of diagnostic procedures: biochemical concentration, dilution techniques, and flow or diffusion measurements. Concentration, commonly measured by scintiscope or scintigraphs of the body area

Table 50-4. Radioactive Tracer Compounds

Drug Name	Preparation/ Usual Adult Dosage	Physical Half-Life	Whole Body Radiation Exposure (for Adult Male of 70 kg)	Diagnostic Uses
Mercurial Diuretics				
chlormerodrin Hg^{197} (Neohydrin-197)	Solution for IV injection /For kidney imaging: 100–150 μc For brain imaging: 10 μc/kg to a maximum of 1,050 μc	64.8 hours	17 mrad/μc administered	Assess the anatomic and functional integrity of the kidneys Localize brain tumors
chlormerodrin Hg^{203} (Neohydrin-203)	Solution for IV injection /For brain imaging: 10 μc/kg to a maximum of 700 μc	46.6 days		Assess the anatomic and functional integrity of the kidneys Localize brain tumors
Vitamins				
cyanocobalamin Co^{57} (Rubratope-57) (Racobalamin-57)	Capsules and solutions for oral use /0.5 μc Solution for IM or SC injection	270 days	9.6 mrad/μc administered	Assess GI absorption of cyanocobalamin Differentiate pernicious anemia from other causes of cyanocobalamin malabsorption Assess liver uptake of cyanocobalamin
Dyes				
rose bengal sodium I^{131} (Radio-iodinated Rose Bengal, Robengatope)	Solution for IV injection /For nonscanning liver studies: 5–25 μc	8.08 days	1.47 mrad/μc administered	Assess liver function Detect biliary obstruction
Iodides				
iodinated I^{125} serum albumin (Albumotope I^{125}, Risa^{125}, IHSA I^{125}	Solution for IV injection / 5–60 μc	60 days	0.4 mrad/μc administered	Measure blood or plasma volume
sodium iodide I^{125} (Iodotope I^{125})	Capsules and solution for oral use /For thyroid uptake study: 50–100 μc Solution for IV injection /For protein-bound iodine study: 25–50 μc	60 days	0.39 mrad/μc administered	Assess thyroid function
iodinated I^{131} serum albumin (Albumotope I^{131}, IHSA I^{131}, Risa^{131})	Solution for IV injection /For blood and plasma volume determinations: 5–60 μc For placenta location: 5–10 μc	8.08 days	1.7 mrad/μc administered	Measure blood or plasma volume Placenta location
iodinated I^{131} serum albumin, macroaggregated (Albumotope-LS, MAAI^{131}, Macroscan^{131})	Solution for IV injection / 150–300 μc	8.08 days	0.67 mrad/μc administered	Assess arterial perfusion of lungs
iodohippurate sodium I^{131} (Hippuran I^{131}, Hipputope-131)	Solution for IV injection /For nonimaging renal function: 1–30 μc For kidney imaging: 200–300 μc	8.08 days	0.03 mrad/μc administered	Assess kidney function
sodium iodide I^{131} (Radio-caps-131, Tracervial-131)	Capsules and solution for oral use /For thyroid uptake test: 1–25 μc Solution for IV injection /For thigh–neck clearance test: 10–50 μc For protein-bound iodine and conversion ratio studies: 25–50 μc For thyroid imaging: 50–100 μc	8.08 days	0.5 mrad/μc administered	Assess thyroid function Localize thyroid tissue or tumors

(continued)

Table 50-4. (Continued)

Drug Name	Preparation/ Usual Adult Dosage	Physical Half-Life	Whole Body Radiation Exposure (for Adult Male of 70 kg)	Diagnostic Uses
Miscellaneous				
sodium pertechnetate Tc 99m (Pertechtin, Pertscan-99m)	Generators for producing solutions for oral or IV administration/For brain imaging: 5–15 mc For cardiac blood pool imaging: 3–5 mc For salivary gland imaging: 1–5 mc	6 hours	0.013 mrad/mc administered	Locate intracranial lesions Assess salivary gland function Assess cardiac blood pool
sodium phosphate P^{32} (Phosphotope)	Capsules and solution for oral use Solution for IV injection/250–1,000 μc	14.3 days	1 mrad/μc administered during the first 3 days; after this time, exposure varies with the tissues involved	Locate ocular tumors Locate cerebral tumors when other agents or techniques are unsuitable
technetium sulfide Tc 99m (technetium sulfide Tc 99m colloid, technetium sulfur colloid Tc 99m)	Generator for producing solutions for IV injection Solutions for IV injection/1–3 mc	6 hours	16.7 mrad/mc administered	Produce images of the liver and spleen
sodium chromate Cr^{51} (Chromitope Sodium, Rachromate-51)	Solution for in vitro labeling of red blood vessels and subsequent IV administration/For estimating red blood cell volume: 15–20 μc For estimating red blood cell survival time: 100 μc For estimating GI blood loss: 150–200 μc	27.8 days	0.24 mrad/μc administered	Measure red cell or total blood volume, red cell survival time, and GI loss
thallium	Solution for injection/2 mc (given in conjunction with dipyridamole)	Not available	Not available	Detect the presence and assess the severity of coronary artery disease

being studied, reflects organ or tissue function. Dilution techniques are used to determine the volume of whole blood, total body water, red blood cells, or other components. Cardiac output, pulmonary ventilation, and peripheral vascular circulation are among the measures taken by flow or diffusion tests.

Adverse Reactions. Although they have the same potential for producing toxic effects and side effects as their nonradioactive counterparts, diagnostic radionuclides are administered in such small doses that adverse reactions are unlikely except with iodides, which can trigger allergic responses in some recipients.

The radioactivity of these compounds is potentially toxic. Radiation emitted includes beta and gamma particles. Because of their high radiation and low penetrating ability, substances emitting alpha particles are not used medicinally.

There is no evidence that clients incur measurable harm from the doses usually given in diagnostic procedures. However, each exposure to ionizing radiation adds to the cumulative lifetime load. Excessive exposure is associated with an increased risk of malignant neoplasms, congenital defects in offspring, and premature

aging. Rapidly dividing cells are most vulnerable to the harmful effects of radiation.

Precautions and Contraindications. Precautions pertinent to the nonradioactive form of the drug in use are appropriate (see the previous discussion on iodides). In addition, special precautions to control radioactive exposure are required. All radiobiologic products are controlled by the Division of Biologic Standards of the United States Public Health Service. In Canada, radiopharmaceuticals are controlled by the Atomic Energy Control Board. Persons and institutions wishing to use radioactive substances in the United States must be licensed by the Atomic Energy Commission.

When radionuclides are used, precautions must be taken to control exposure of everyone in the area. The dosage of ionizing radiation is proportional to the time spent in proximity to the source of emissions and inversely related to the distance between the subject and the source. Shielding with lead barriers decreases exposure.

Clients most vulnerable to radiation damage are those with rapidly dividing cells (high growth rates). To prevent exposure of embryos, tests performed on women of childbearing age should be scheduled for the first half of the menstrual cycle. Testing of children and nursing mothers is avoided whenever possible (radioactive chemicals may be secreted in breast milk after the test).

Clients receiving tracer doses experience minimal exposure, and neither their bodies nor their excreta are considered significant sources of radiation. No special precautions need to be taken by persons undergoing diagnostic tests with radionuclides. (This does not apply to recipients of therapeutic doses, which involve much larger amounts of radiation.)

Personnel working in nuclear medicine units are at greater risk than clients because they spend more time near radioactive materials. Operating procedures are designed to minimize exposure of personnel. All workers wear devices that measure radiation exposure. When individual exposure levels approach maximal permissible levels, the person is assigned to other work until an appropriate time has elapsed without further exposure.

■ SUMMARY

Radioactive tracers are radionuclides used in small doses to assess the function of body organs or tissues and to measure fluid volume, flow, or diffusion. Although they emit beta and gamma radiation, these compounds add little to the cumulative radiation load of the client undergoing just one test. Clients exposed to repeated tests and personnel in nuclear medicine units receive greater doses. Use of radiopharmaceuticals is limited to personnel and institutions licensed by the Atomic Energy Commission.

❖ NURSING MANAGEMENT: CLIENT RECEIVING A RADIOACTIVE COMPOUND

The duration of radioactive emissions in the body is influenced by two variables: the compound's biologic half-life and its physical half-life. Biologic half-life varies and depends on metabolic and excretory function. For this reason, clients with liver or kidney impairment receive more radiation than those with normal organ function. Physical half-life reflects the rate of decay of the radionuclide and is the same in all clients. Radioactivity declines by 50% in each half-life period. After seven half-lives have elapsed, the radioactivity of any remaining material is less than 1% of its original radioactivity.

During procedures involving radionuclides, protocols for handling radioactive compounds must be followed carefully. Nurses working in nuclear medicine units must be trained in radiation control techniques.

NURSING PROCESS

ASSESSMENT

Clients undergoing diagnostic tests should be assessed for risk of adverse reactions to the chemical to be used. If an iodide is to be administered, a history of past responses and adverse reactions should be reported to the prescriber. Previous exposure to ionizing radiation should also be documented. The client's knowledge of and emotional reaction to the proposed diagnostic test should also be explored.

NURSING DIAGNOSIS

Nursing diagnoses for clients undergoing tests with radioactive tracers may include:

- Anxiety, related to exposure to irradiation secondary to diagnostic procedure using radioactive tracers
- Pain, related to risk for nausea, vomiting, itching, or diarrhea from adverse drug reaction

PLANNING

Nursing care goals include reducing anxiety and preventing or promptly detecting and treating adverse drug reactions.

INTERVENTION

The prescriber and radiologist should be notified of any history of adverse reaction to the chemical to be used or of unusual exposure to ionizing irradiation.

Clients need emotional support during diagnostic procedures involving radionuclides. Not only are they threatened by an as yet unidentified disease process, but they are also often acutely aware of the risks inherent in exposure to ionizing radiation. Anxiety may be heightened by the protective measures taken by personnel in the nuclear medicine unit.

The nurse should take measures to support the client and reduce discomfort from such reactions as nausea, vomiting, itching, or diarrhea.

At the conclusion of the procedure, the nurse should ensure that radioactive compounds are stored in lead containers to control ionizing emissions. In addition, storage must be appropriate to the chemical nature of the substance. For example, radiocyanocobalamin must be refrigerated; solutions may darken with time, but this does not alter their efficacy.

Client Education. Clients undergoing diagnostic studies involving radioactive tracers should be reassured that exposure to ionizing radiation in such tests is comparable to that in x-ray procedures. Although repeated exposure is undesirable, isolated or limited testing involves little risk. No undesirable effects have been detected as direct effects of tracer doses. No special precautions are required for the client undergoing such a study. Clients should be told that the precautions taken to protect personnel from radiation are necessary because of their more frequent exposure.

OUTCOME EVALUATION

Data required for evaluation include the incidence or absence of adverse reactions, the incidence or absence of serious effects following adverse reactions, and reports from the client indicating that anxiety and discomfort were reduced by the nursing care given.

❖ **CHECKLIST OF NURSING ACTIONS**

❑ Assess the client's risk of adverse response to the chemical substance being used (eg, allergy to iodides).

❑ Assess the client's exposure to ionizing radiation; report unusual histories.

❑ Provide emotional support during the procedure.

❑ Reassure clients that tracer doses of radionuclides carry no demonstrable risk of physical harm.

Provocative Agents

Drugs used in provocative diagnostic tests are administered to induce a measurable response in the body, the magnitude of which is medically significant. Most drugs fall into one of two categories: secretagogues and agents that influence endocrine secretion or activity. Secretagogues stimulate exocrine secretion, such as production of gastric acid, pepsin, and pancreatic enzymes, as well as contraction of the gallbladder. Agents affecting endocrine function include autocoids (eg, tropic hormones, histamine), hormone inhibitors (eg, metyrapone), competitive inhibitors of hormones (eg, saralasin), and chemicals that influence endocrine activity by as yet unknown mechanisms.

Provocative agents are usually administered parenterally. Dosages vary but tend to be very small for autocoids. (These physiologic constituents are produced in minute amounts by the body and are very potent.) Because they tend to be unstable, many injectable solutions must be refrigerated. Some are marketed in powder form and are reconstituted at the time of administration (Table 50-5).

Pharmacodynamics. Many secretagogues and tropic hormones stimulate organ functions by the same mechanism as natural autocoids. Mechanisms of action of other drugs in this group vary. Metyrapone inhibits adrenal cortex production of cortisol, triggering the negative feedback mechanism that stimulates pituitary secretion of adrenocorticotropin. Anticholinesterases oppose the breakdown of acetylcholine by the enzyme cholinesterase, inducing a rise in tissue levels of the neurotransmitter. Saralasin decreases physiologic response to angiotensin II by competitive inhibition at its receptor site on the smooth muscle of blood vessels.

Pharmacokinetics. Most provocative agents are administered systemically. After absorption into the circulation, they move to the target organ or tissue, where they induce a characteristic alteration of physiology. Metabolic deactivation, especially with autocoids, occurs rapidly.

Diagnostic Uses. See Table 50-5.

Adverse Reactions. Because most secretagogues influence multiple body processes, they tend to produce multiple side effects. Pentagastrin increases GI motility, stimulates pancreatic and biliary secretion, inhibits water and electrolyte absorption from the ileum, and promotes sodium and chloride diuresis. It may produce cramping pain, nausea and vomiting, and borborygmi. Secretin stimulates duodenal and intestinal secretion, pepsinogen release in the stomach, and insulin release.

Secretagogues also affect the cardiovascular system. Side effects of pentagastrin include hypotension, palpitation, dizziness, faintness or lightheadedness, and a feeling of tightness in the chest. Both this drug and betazole tend to produce tachycardia and a subjective feeling of warmth. Betazole also can induce flushing and diaphoresis. Drowsiness, blurred vision, fatigue, and headache have been reported with pentagastrin.

Secretagogues can produce acute symptoms of GI disease. Gallbladder stimulation tends to move stones into the common bile duct, where they can obstruct the flow of bile. Heightened secretion of gastric acid and pepsin aggravates the symptoms of peptic ulcer. Stimulation of pancreatic secretion increases symptoms of pancreatitis. As a result, tests may be followed by abdominal pain, nausea or vomiting, and increased risk of complications such as hemorrhage, perforation, and shock.

The most common adverse reactions to secretagogues are GI discomfort, vasomotor changes, and allergic reaction. The most serious adverse reactions are bile duct obstruction (gallbladder stimulants), circulatory shock, anaphylaxis, and cholinergic crisis (edrophonium). The sudden increase in hormone production induced by endocrine stimulants can produce toxic symptoms. Such reactions are most likely in clients being evaluated for excess hormone production. For example, a histamine test is likely to produce a severe hypertensive reaction in clients with pheochromocytoma. By their very nature, provocative tests tend to produce exaggerated responses that can reach serious proportions.

Adverse reaction to saralasin is rare. Headache, hypotension, lightheadedness, nausea, and discomfort at the injection site have been reported. Clients who are severely sodium-depleted before the test may have an exaggerated depressor response, as well as signs and symptoms of circulatory shock.

Allergic reactions to provocative agents are fairly common. Some agents are proteins derived from animal material and are highly antigenic. Allergic manifestations include pruritic rashes, bronchospasm, and anaphylaxis.

Precautions and Contraindications. Secretagogues that increase gastric acid secretion are contraindicated in clients with acute peptic ulcer disease. They should be used with caution in clients with pancreatic, hepatic, or biliary tract disease.

Table 50-5. Provocative Agents Used for Diagnostic Tests

Drug Name	Preparation	Mechanism of Action	Usual Adult Dosage/PC	Diagnostic Use
Secretagogues				
pentagastrin (Gastrodiagnost, Paptavlon)	Solution for SC injection	Stimulation of gastric acid secretion	6 µg/kg	Evaluation of gastric acid secretion
betazole hydrochloride (Histalog)	Solution for IM or SC injection	Stimulation of gastric secretion of hydrochloric acid	0.5 mg/kg	Testing of gastric secretory capabilities
secretin	Powder for preparing solutions for IV infusion	Stimulation of pancreatic secretion	1 C.H.R. unit*/kg over 5 min	Diagnosis of chronic pancreatic dysfunction
sincalide (C8-CCK, Kinevac, OP-CCK)	Powder for preparing solutions for IV injection	Stimulation of gallbladder contraction and evacuation / Stimulation of pancreatic secretion	0.02 µg/kg	Assessment of gallbladder function in conjunction with cholecystography or bile aspiration / Assessment of pancreatic exocrine function
Stimulants to Endocrine Secretion				
corticotropin (ACTH, Acthar, adrenocorticotropin hormone, Cortrophin)	Gel or solution for IM or IV injection	Stimulation of adrenal cortex secretion of glucocorticoids	10–40 units PC: C	Diagnosis of adrenocorticoid insufficiency
cosyntropin (Syn-Cortrosyn, Synacthen, Tetracosa-peptide, tetracosactide, tetracosactrin)	Powder for preparing solutions for IM or IV injection	Stimulation of adrenal cortex secretion of glucocorticoids	250 µg PC: C	Diagnosis of adrenocorticoid insufficiency
thyrotropin (Thytropar, T.S.H.)	Powder for preparing solutions for IM or SC injection	Stimulation of thyroid secretion of iodinated hormones (thyroxine and others)	10 IU	Differential diagnosis of primary thyroidal myxedema from pituitary myxedema
histamine	Solutions for IV injection	Stimulation of catecholamine release	10 µg of histamine base† initially	Diagnosis of pheochromocytoma
metyrapone (Metopirone)	Tablets for oral use	Stimulation of pituitary secretion of ACTH by inhibiting hydrocortisone secretion by the adrenal cortex	Orally, 750 mg q4h for 6 doses PC: C	Evaluation of hypothalamic pituitary function in the diagnosis of hypopituitarism / Differential diagnosis of primary from secondary Cushing's syndrome
sodium tolbutamide (Orinase Diagnostic)	Powder for preparing solutions for IV injection	Stimulation of insulin secretion by beta cells of the pancreatic islets	1 g PC: C	Diagnosis of mild diabetes mellitus, pancreatic carcinoma, acute pancreatitis, and functional pancreatic islet-cell tumor
arginine hydrochloride (R-Gene 10)	Powder for preparing solutions for IV injection	Stimulation of pituitary secretion of growth hormone	30 g infused over 30 min as a 10% solution / In children, 500 mg/kg	Evaluation of pituitary growth hormone reserve
Anticholinesterase				
edrophonium chloride (Enlon, Tensilon)	Solution for IV, IM, or SC injection	Inhibition of cholinesterase and subsequent accumulation of acetylcholine	10 mg PC: C	Diagnosis of myasthenia gravis / Differentiation of cholinergic crisis from myasthenic crisis

*Crick-Harper-Raper unit
†1 mg histamine base is equivalent to 2.75 mg histamine phosphate.
KEY: PC = pregnancy risk category; see Appendix A.

(continued)

Table 50-5. (Continued)

Drug Name	Preparation	Mechanism of Action	Usual Adult Dosage/PC	Diagnostic Use
saralasin (Sarenin)	Solution for IV infusion	Competitive inhibition of angiotensin II at the receptor site	18 mg over 20–30 min *or* 0.05 μg/kg/min, increased by 5, 10, and 20 μg/min at 10-min intervals	Assess the function of endogenous angiotensin II in the regulation of blood pressure
Cholinergic				
methacholine	Metered-dose inhaler	Bronchoconstriction	Five breaths	Diagnosis of asthma in the absence of clinically obvious asthma
Nutrient				
glucose	Flavored solution for ingestion	Hyperglycemia and insulin secretion	75 g	Diagnosis of diabetes mellitus and reactive hypoglycemia

*Crick-Harper-Raper unit
†1 mg histamine base is equivalent to 2.75 mg histamine phosphate.
KEY: PC = pregnancy risk category; see Appendix A.

With endocrine function tests, the healthcare team must be prepared to treat toxic reactions characterized by sudden increases in hormone levels. Adrenergic blocking agents, such as phentolamine, are used to treat hypertensive crises following administration of histamine.

Edrophonium can cause cholinergic crisis, respiratory paralysis, or cardiac arrest. Although infrequent, such reactions must be treated vigorously. Before administration of edrophonium, atropine is often administered to clients over age 50 to prevent muscarinic side effects. Atropine sulfate should always be available as an antagonist when edrophonium is used.

Although mild sodium depletion increases the blood pressure response to saralasin, clients scheduled to undergo a saralasin infusion test should not be severely sodium-depleted. If hypotensive shock occurs during the test, the saralasin infusion is discontinued and normal saline solution administered IV. Blood pressure is monitored every 15 minutes for 3 hours to detect continued hypotension or rebound hypertension.

Provocative agents are administered with caution to clients with a history of allergy, especially asthma. Skin tests may be administered before the test to detect allergic hypersensitivity. Equipment, supplies, and personnel trained in the treatment of acute allergic reaction such as anaphylaxis should be available during provocative tests.

■ SUMMARY

Provocative diagnostic agents include secretagogues and stimulants of endocrine secretion. They are used in tests to diagnose GI and endocrine disease and myasthenia gravis. Because they manipulate physiologic processes, provocative tests carry an inherent risk. Exaggerated responses can be life-threatening. Tests designed to exaggerate symptoms characteristic of disease are most likely to produce severe reactions. Provocative agents tend to be allergenic. Allergic reactions range from skin rashes to anaphylaxis.

❖ NURSING MANAGEMENT: CLIENT RECEIVING A PROVOCATIVE AGENT

The risk of toxic reaction depends on the suspected disease and the physiologic response to the drug agent. Whenever a provocative test is intended to increase signs or symptoms of the suspected disease, the risk of a serious reaction is high.

NURSING PROCESS

ASSESSMENT

Before beginning provocative tests, the client should be assessed for increased risk of adverse reaction. A history of previous exposure and reaction to the drug agent and a history of allergic disease (personal and family) should be taken. The client's knowledge of and emotional reaction to the test should be explored.

Clients scheduled for tests involving secretagogues that increase hydrochloric acid secretion should be screened for peptic ulcer disease or other conditions associated with gastric hyperacidity. When a saralasin infusion test is planned, sodium balance should be determined; mild sodium depletion is desirable.

NURSING DIAGNOSIS

Nursing diagnoses appropriate for clients receiving provocative test agents include:

- Pain, related to itching and other side effects of provocative agents
- Anxiety, related to effects of provocative test agent and undiagnosed health problem

- Knowledge Deficit, concerning the provocative agent and the diagnostic test
- Risk for Injury: Falls related to dizziness or loss of consciousness secondary to use of saralasin

PLANNING

Nursing goals for the client undergoing provocative diagnostic tests are to increase comfort, to prevent adverse drug reactions, to detect and treat adverse drug reactions promptly should they occur, to reduce anxiety, and to educate the client about provocative agents and their use in diagnostic procedures.

INTERVENTION

The nurse should report any risk factors revealed during the initial nursing assessment. If a history of allergy is found, a skin sensitivity test should be ordered to rule out allergic hypersensitivity to the test agent.

Clients undergoing provocative diagnostic tests are uncertain of the outcome and are understandably apprehensive that serious disease may be discovered. Their anxiety is compounded by the nature of many tests, which often involve parenteral injections and precise timing. By working competently and expressing a warm concern for the client, the nurse promotes trust in the healthcare team, thus reducing the client's anxiety.

Before the test begins, chemical antidotes, personnel, and equipment for treating adverse reactions must be readily available.

The nurse helps administer the provocative agent and accurately observes the results. To yield reliable data, provocative tests must be conducted with meticulous attention to detail. Drug dosage must be accurately measured. Syringes or IV tubing should be rinsed and the washings administered to ensure delivery of a complete dose. The timing of drug administration and specimen collection is also crucial. If either is delayed, the exact times must be reported so that calculations can be adjusted accordingly and misinterpretations of data avoided.

During and after the test, clients should be closely monitored for signs and symptoms of toxicity or adverse reactions. After a saralasin test with a positive result, clients should be monitored for rebound hypertension. After a methacholine test, a beta-adrenergic agonist may be ordered to reverse bronchoconstriction.

Client Education. Tests should be explained to clients in terms appropriate to their level of intellectual capacity and education. The subjective perceptions and sensations likely to occur should be described. Although the risks of the procedure must be explained, the client should be reassured that serious reactions are uncommon and that skilled medical treatment is available.

OUTCOME EVALUATION

Data required for evaluation include the incidence or absence of adverse reaction, the incidence or absence of serious effects, and comments by the client indicating reduced discomfort and anxiety. Client education can be evaluated by the client's cooperation during the procedure.

❖ **CHECKLIST OF NURSING ACTIONS**

- Assess the client for previous exposure or adverse reaction to the drug used and for allergy; report significant findings promptly.
- Explain the test procedure in terms of the subjective sensations and perceptions the client will experience.
- Ensure that equipment, supplies, and personnel to treat adverse reactions are readily available.
- Follow test protocols exactly to ensure the accuracy of test results.
- Monitor the client closely to detect adverse reactions promptly.
- Provide emotional support to the client throughout the procedure.

Dermal Reactivity Indicators

Dermal reactivity indicators are substances used to determine the presence of antibodies by means of skin tests for hypersensitivity. Antigenic preparations used for skin testing include concentrates derived from microbial cultures and extracts from antigenic materials. They are marketed as solutions for patch, scratch, or intradermal tests. Testing materials for sensitivity to some pathogens are also marketed in the form of solution-coated tines for multipuncture skin tests. These preparations should be protected from heat because most are proteinaceous. Materials for tine testing are not refrigerated, however, because moisture within the sealed package may condense, causing a loss in potency.

Pharmacodynamics. Antigenic material induces an antigen–antibody reaction, producing local inflammation proportional to the client's degree of hypersensitivity. The substance is applied to the skin or injected intradermally; the area of erythema or induration is measured after a specified time. Skin tests for sensitivity to infectious pathogens require hours (up to 2 days) for the reaction to appear. Test results of allergic sensitivity are ready within minutes.

A positive response to microbial extracts indicates previous exposure to the pathogen but does not necessarily mean that active infection is present. Positive reactions indicate the need for further diagnostic studies to rule out active disease. A negative response does not rule out disease in symptomatic clients: severe infections can overwhelm the body's immune defenses, depleting antibody titers to levels too low to produce a skin reaction.

Pharmacokinetics. Dermal reactivity indicators are applied to the skin, where they induce a local response. The material is absorbed systemically and sometimes reacts with antibodies in the tissues. The antigen–antibody complexes are assimilated by phagocytosis.

Diagnostic Uses. Table 50-6 lists the diagnostic tests specific to each dermal reactivity indicator.

Adverse Reactions. Local reactions to allergen skin tests include ulceration and necrosis in response to microbial extracts and itching after skin tests for allergy. Systemic allergic reactions can also occur, although these are rare because of the low doses used. The most common adverse reactions are minor allergic ones, such as itching at the test site. The most serious are anaphylaxis (with allergy tests) and tissue necrosis at the test site (in tests for bacterial sensitivity).

Precautions and Contraindications. Using dermal reactivity indicators to diagnose infectious disease is contraindicated in clients who have previously exhibited a severe local reaction to the specific antigen. For example, no client who has developed tissue breakdown after an old tuberculin test should be subjected again to skin testing for tuberculosis. When a high degree of sensitivity is suspected, an initial test with extremely dilute solutions should be used. Healthcare personnel involved in such tests must be prepared to treat both systemic and local reactions if they occur (see the Critical Thinking Challenge: Issues Analysis).

CRITICAL THINKING CHALLENGE
Issues Analysis

You have been hired as manager of nursing care in the office of a newly qualified allergist. The physician expects to develop office policies and protocols collaboratively with you.

1. What protocols would you suggest for clients undergoing allergy testing in this setting?
2. What medications should be stocked for treatment of adverse reactions to diagnostic testing?
3. Develop an outline for taking a nursing history during the initial interview with clients undergoing allergy testing.

■ SUMMARY

Dermal reactivity indicators are allergenic materials used in skin tests to assess the client's sensitivity to infectious pathogens or allergenic substances. They are applied to the skin by patch, scratch, or intradermal techniques. The development of local inflammation indicates a positive response. The reaction is proportional to antibody levels.

Table 50-6. Dermal Reactivity Indicators Used in Skin Tests

Drug Name	Preparation	Usual Adult Dosage	Diagnostic Test
Microbial Extracts			
coccidioidin	Solution for intradermal injection (1:100 and 1:10)	0.1 mL of 1:100 dilution	Sensitivity to the organism that causes coccidioidomycosis or to assess the status of cell-mediated immunity
histoplasmin	Solution for intradermal injection (1:100) Tine test (1:100)	0.1 mL 1 dosage unit	Sensitivity to the organism that causes histoplasmosis or to assess the status of cell-mediated immunity
tuberculin (old tuberculin [OT])	Tine test (multipuncture device)	1 dosage unit	Sensitivity to the tubercle bacillus
purified protein derivative (PPD)	Solutions for intradermal injection—1 TU*/0.1 mL, 5 TU/0.1 mL, 250 TU/9.1 mL Tine test (multipuncture device)	0.1 mL (of 5 TU/0.1 mL) 1 dosage unit	Sensitivity to the tubercle bacillus
mumps skin test antigen	Suspension for intradermal injection	0.1 mL	Sensitivity to the mumps virus or to assess the status of cell-mediated immunity
Allergenic Extracts			
Extracts of material from virtually any allergenic substance can be prepared for skin testing purposes. Common extracts used for allergy testing include ragweed, grasses, molds, animal danders, and food substances.	Suspensions for intradermal injection of varying dilutions	0.1 mL	Allergic sensitivity to foreign antigens

*Tuberculin units

Systemic allergic reactions can occur following skin tests, although they are rare and tend to be mild because of the low doses used. Local reactions may be severe in highly sensitive clients, producing ulceration or necrosis.

❖ NURSING MANAGEMENT: CLIENT RECEIVING A DERMAL REACTIVITY INDICATOR

Because skin testing for allergy can precipitate an acute systemic allergic reaction, medical treatment, directed by the prescriber, should be immediately available.

NURSING PROCESS

ASSESSMENT

A history of previous skin testing and reactions to allergenic substances should be taken before dermal reactivity indicators are administered. Any systemic or severe local reaction should be reported. An initial test with a dilute solution (commonly 10% of the usual concentration) may be desirable.

NURSING DIAGNOSIS

Nursing diagnoses appropriate for the client receiving a dermal test agent may include:

- Pain: Discomfort and itching related to antigen–antibody reaction secondary to exposure to allergenic extracts
- Anxiety (especially in children), related to invasive procedures (intradermal injection of agent)

A collaborative problem that should be differentiated from the nursing diagnoses is:

Potential Complication: Tissue necrosis at site of skin test for antibodies against infectious organisms, or Anaphylaxis related to exposure to antigenic material

PLANNING

Nursing goals for the client undergoing skin testing are to alleviate anxiety, to prevent or promptly detect and treat adverse reactions to the allergens used, to relieve itching, and to restore tissue perfusion.

INTERVENTION

The nurse should report risk factors revealed during the nursing assessment. An initial test using a very dilute (usually 1:10) solution of antigen may be ordered if the client's history indicates likelihood of an exaggerated response to the usual preparation.

Skin testing for sensitivity to infectious pathogens is commonly performed by nursing personnel, often in a public health agency or other community setting. Systemic reactions to these solutions are unlikely. The tine test is increasingly used because of its convenience and low level of trauma.

When intradermal tests are ordered, care must be taken to avoid piercing the internal layers of the skin; sub-cutaneous penetration may produce a false-positive reaction. Tuberculin syringes are used for such tests because the volumes to be administered are very small (0.01–0.1 mL).

The nurse should provide emotional support and comfort for anxious clients (especially children) who fear skin testing.

Clients undergoing skin tests for allergy must be observed for systemic reactions. Signs and symptoms include sneezing, rhinorrhea, itching in areas other than the test site, and difficulty in breathing. Anaphylaxis may (rarely) occur. Epinephrine and antihistamines should be readily available to treat such reactions.

Client Education. Before skin tests are performed, the nature of the test should be explained to the client. The possible results and their significance should also be described. To relieve discomfort, clients should be advised to apply pressure or cold compresses to test sites that itch.

OUTCOME EVALUATION

Data required for evaluation include the incidence or absence of signs and symptoms of adverse reaction, the incidence or absence of serious effects from adverse reactions, and comments by the client indicating that itching was promptly relieved.

❖ CHECKLIST OF NURSING ACTIONS

- ❑ Question clients who are to undergo skin sensitivity tests about previous tests of this nature and their responses to them; report systemic or severe local reactions.
- ❑ Provide emotional support for anxious clients.
- ❑ Measure doses of dermal reactivity indicators in tuberculin syringes for greater accuracy in dispensing small volumes.
- ❑ Avoid piercing the inner layers of the skin when performing intradermal tests.
- ❑ Observe clients receiving allergenic extracts for signs and symptoms of systemic reaction.
- ❑ Explain tests and the significance of the results to clients undergoing skin tests.
- ❑ Advise clients to apply pressure or cold compresses to skin sites that itch after the test.

Bibliography

McEvoy GK, ed. (1995). *Drug information '95*. Bethesda, MD: American Society of Health-System Pharmacists.

For more information and sample tests and activities, refer to Chapter 50 in the Student Workbook for Clinical Pharmacology and Nursing Management, 5th edition, available through your bookstore.

Appendix A
FDA Pregnancy Risk Categories

Category	Degree of Risk	Description
A	*Remote risk for fetal harm*	Controlled studies in women fail to demonstrate a risk for harm to the fetus in the first trimester. There is no evidence of risk in later trimesters.
B	*Slightly more risk for fetal harm than category A*	Animal studies show no risk to fetus, but controlled studies have not been done in women . . . or . . . animal studies demonstrate a risk for fetal harm, but controlled studies in women fail to show a risk in the first trimester. There is no evidence of risk in later trimesters.
C	*Greater risk than category B*	Animal studies show a risk for fetal harm, but no controlled studies have been done in women, or studies have been done in women or animals
D	*Proven risk for fetal harm*	Studies in women prove that drug harms the fetus, but the potential benefits of use during pregnancy may be acceptable despite the risks (*eg,* treatment of life-threatening disease for which safer drugs are ineffective). A statement identifying risk appears in the "WARNINGS" section of drug labeling (package insert).
X	*Proven risk for fetal harm*	Studies in women or animals show definite risk for fetal abnormality, or adverse reaction reports indicate evidence of fetal risk. The risks clearly outweigh any possible benefit. A statement identifying risk appears in the "Contraindications" section of drug labeling (package insert).

Appendix B

MEDWATCH
THE FDA MEDICAL PRODUCTS REPORTING PROGRAM

For **VOLUNTARY** reporting
by health professionals of adverse
events and product problems

Page ____ of ____

Form Approved: OMB No. 0910-0291 Expires:12/31/94
See OMB statement on reverse

FDA Use Only **[DAVIS]**

Triage unit
sequence #

A. Patient information

1. Patient identifier	2. Age at time of event:		3. Sex	4. Weight
In confidence	or _____ Date of birth:		☐ female ☐ male	____ lbs or ____ kgs

B. Adverse event or product problem

1. ☐ Adverse event   and/or   ☐ Product problem (e.g., defects/malfunctions)

2. Outcomes attributed to adverse event
(check all that apply)
- ☐ death _____ (mo day yr)
- ☐ life-threatening
- ☐ hospitalization – initial or prolonged
- ☐ disability
- ☐ congenital anomaly
- ☐ required intervention to prevent permanent impairment/damage
- ☐ other: _____

3. Date of event (mo day yr)	4. Date of this report (mo day yr)

5. Describe event or problem

6. Relevant tests/laboratory data, including dates

7. Other relevant history, including preexisting medical conditions (e.g., allergies, race, pregnancy, smoking and alcohol use, hepatic/renal dysfunction, etc.)

PLEASE TYPE OR USE BLACK INK

C. Suspect medication(s)

1. **Name** (give labeled strength & mfr/labeler, if known)
#1
#2

2. **Dose, frequency & route used**	3. **Therapy dates** (if unknown, give duration) from/to (or best estimate)
#1	#1
#2	#2

4. **Diagnosis for use** (indication)
#1
#2

5. **Event abated after use stopped or dose reduced**
#1 ☐ yes ☐ no ☐ doesn't apply
#2 ☐ yes ☐ no ☐ doesn't apply

6. **Lot #** (if known)	7. **Exp. date** (if known)
#1	#1
#2	#2

8. **Event reappeared after reintroduction**
#1 ☐ yes ☐ no ☐ doesn't apply
#2 ☐ yes ☐ no ☐ doesn't apply

9. **NDC #** (for product problems only)

10. **Concomitant medical products** and therapy dates (exclude treatment of event)

D. Suspect medical device

1. **Brand name**

2. **Type of device**

3. **Manufacturer name & address**

4. **Operator of device**
- ☐ health professional
- ☐ lay user/patient
- ☐ other:

5. **Expiration date** (mo day yr)

6.
model # _____
catalog # _____
serial # _____
lot # _____
other # _____

7. **If implanted, give date** (mo day yr)

8. **If explanted, give date** (mo day yr)

9. **Device available for evaluation?**   (Do not send to FDA)
☐ yes   ☐ no   ☐ returned to manufacturer on _____ (mo day yr)

10. **Concomitant medical products** and therapy dates (exclude treatment of event)

E. Reporter (see confidentiality section on back)

1. **Name, address & phone #**

2. **Health professional?** ☐ yes ☐ no

3. **Occupation**

4. **Also reported to**
- ☐ manufacturer
- ☐ user facility
- ☐ distributor

5. If you do NOT want your identity disclosed to the manufacturer, place an " X " in this box. ☐

FDA

Mail to: MEDWATCH
5600 Fishers Lane
Rockville, MD 20852-9787

or FAX to:
1-800-FDA-0178

FDA Form 3500 (6/93)   Submission of a report does not constitute an admission that medical personnel or the product caused or contributed to the event.

1116

ADVICE ABOUT VOLUNTARY REPORTING

Report experiences with:
- medications (drugs or biologics)
- medical devices (including in-vitro diagnostics)
- special nutritional products (dietary supplements, medical foods, infant formulas)
- other products regulated by FDA

Report SERIOUS adverse events. An event is serious when the patient outcome is:
- death
- life-threatening (real risk of dying)
- hospitalization (initial or prolonged)
- disability (significant, persistent or permanent)
- congenital anomaly
- required intervention to prevent permanent impairment or damage

Report even if:
- you're not certain the product caused the event
- you don't have all the details

Report product problems – quality, performance or safety concerns such as:
- suspected contamination
- questionable stability
- defective components
- poor packaging or labeling

How to report:
- just fill in the sections that apply to your report
- use section C for all products except medical devices
- attach additional blank pages if needed
- use a separate form for each patient
- report either to FDA or the manufacturer (or both)

Important numbers:
- 1-800-FDA-0178 to FAX report
- 1-800-FDA-7737 to report by modem
- 1-800-FDA-1088 for more information or to report quality problems
- 1-800-822-7967 for a VAERS form for vaccines

If your report involves a serious adverse event with a device and it occurred in a facility outside a doctor's office, that facility may be legally required to report to FDA and/or the manufacturer. Please notify the person in that facility who would handle such reporting.

Confidentiality: The patient's identity is held in strict confidence by FDA and protected to the fullest extent of the law. The reporter's identity may be shared with the manufacturer unless requested otherwise. However, FDA will not disclose the reporter's identity in response to a request from the public, pursuant to the Freedom of Information Act.

Appendix C
Enzymes and Drugs Affecting Enzymes*

Drug and Its Therapeutic Uses	Description	Nursing Management
Enzymes are biologic proteins catalysts that initiate or speed up specific organic chemical reactions. They are produced by plants, animals, and human tissues. Enzyme drugs have various uses, most involving the breakdown of specific biologic proteins. Except for digestive enzymes, most enzyme drugs must be administered parenterally. Enzymes are useful in treating digestive enzyme deficiencies, intravascular thrombi, and a few cancers. In the future they may be more useful in treating cancer and genetic errors of metabolism, once the problem of intracellular distribution is solved. Because enzyme drugs are antigenic, repeated use may cause serious allergic reactions. Other adverse effects include damage to body organs resulting from inhibited protein synthesis.		
alglucerase (Ceredase) and imiglucerase Provides palliative therapy for Gaucher's disease (which is rare). Early treatment may prevent some manifestations of the disease.	Hydrolyzes certain glycolated compounds, ie, glucocerebroside Stays in liver and other tissues	Administer IV. Tailor dosage to client. Monitor for adverse effects (*alglucerase:* fever, chills, nausea and vomiting; inflamed injection site; *imiglucerase:* dizziness, itching, rash, mild hypotension; abdominal discomfort and nausea) Monitor for allergic reactions (both drugs are antigenic). If allergy develops to one enzyme, client may be switched to other enzyme. Recommend self-care measures to control discomfort of adverse drug reactions. Report signs and symptoms of drug allergy to prescriber. File a report with the FDA if signs and symptoms of a previously undocumented adverse reaction develop.
chymopapain (Chymodiactin) Dissolves herniated lumbar intervertebral disks in procedure known as chemonucleolysis Because of increase in reported adverse reactions, use of chemonucleolysis is declining	Binds to protein molecules at the spinal injection site. If a small portion escapes into systemic circulation, it appears to be inactivated by globulins in plasma. Only small amounts of the drug appear in urine.	Assist as appropriate with intervertebral injection. Teach client that drug is likely to induce allergic hypersensitivity, so it can be used only once and not at all if client is allergic to papaya. Monitor for allergic reaction: anaphylaxis, erythema, rash, urticaria, conjunctivitis, rhinitis, piloerection, and GI upset.

*For more information on specific enzyme drugs, refer to the following: Chapter 26 (streptokinase and urokinase); Chapter 29 (pepsin, pancreatic enzymes, including trypsin, chymotrypsin, lipase, and amylase); Chapter 37 (dornase); Chapter 40 (collagenase, deoxyribonuclease, papain, sutilains, trypsin, and fibrinolysin). For further information on specific enzyme inhibitors, refer to Chapter 20 (monoamine oxidase inhibitors); Chapter 23 (angiotensin converting enzyme inhibitors); Chapter 36 (allopurinol).

(continued)

Drug and Its Therapeutic Uses	Description	Nursing Management
Also acts as a debridement agent when applied topically.	Comes from plant substance known as papaya latex	Monitor for adverse effects: back pain, stiffness and soreness, nausea, paralytic ileus, urinary retention, headache, dizziness, paresthesia (hypalgesia or numbness), weakness, muscle spasm in the back or legs, and sacral burning.
		Use nursing measures to control pain after chemonucleolysis; administer analgesics liberally. Provide emotional support.
hyaluronidase (Diffusin, Hyazyme, Infiltrose, Wydase)	Hydrolyzes hyaluronic acid, a viscous polysaccharide that helps bind soft tissue cells.	Because the drug is antigenic, assess clients for previous exposure to hyaluronidase and for allergic hypersensitivity.
Acts as dispersal agent to promote absorption of fluids given subcutaneously (may be injected into tubing used for hypodermoclysis)	Acts locally and is metabolized like other proteins	As indicated, perform an intradermal sensitivity test before administering the drug, which is usually injected.
During hypodermoclysis, prevents pain due to local edema and increased hydrostatic pressure in tissues		Avoid injecting drug into or around infected, acutely inflamed, or cancerous tissues to avoid spreading infection or metastases.
Diffuses local anesthetics, particularly those used in nerve blocks		Inject into distal clysis tubing so that drug enters the tissues before appreciable amounts of fluid are infused.
Decreases intraocular pressure during eye surgery		Monitor blood pressure. If the infusion is absorbed rapidly, intravascular pressure may rise abruptly. In such cases, slow the fluid flow rate to maintain desirable blood pressure.
		Even though the drug is well tolerated, monitor for adverse effects, such as fluid volume excess from rapid absorption of infused fluids, increased blood pressure, or damage to liver, pancreas, CNS, and kidneys from inhibited protein synthesis.
		Explain reason for using the drug, and advise client to report signs and symptoms of inflammation around the injection site.
pegademase bovine (an orphan drug)	Replaces deficient enzyme adenosine deaminase, which plays a role in antibody production during the inflammatory response (ie, initiating and sustaining antibody production and immune function)	Assess family history to detect potential client allergy to drug.
Treats the rare genetic disorder known as severe combined immunodeficiency disease (SCID).		Educate family and explain that weekly injections will be needed.
Children so treated have fewer infections and grow more rapidly than untreated children with SCID.	Is metabolized in same way as autogenous enzymes	Monitor for therapeutic response and for adverse drug effects, which are rare because the drug is seldom used. Reported effects include pain at the injection site and minor headaches.
		Recommend cold applications to relieve pain at the injection site.
		Store and handle vials of enzyme carefully to preserve drug potency. Because pegadamase is a protein, refrigeration helps prevent denaturing of the drug.
		Report signs and symptoms indicative of adverse drug reaction to the prescriber and the FDA.

Enzyme inhibitors interfere with enzyme action. They decrease the effect of one or a class of enzymes in the body and increase the level of substrate normally degraded by the enzyme. Toxicity can follow use, especially if foods or beverages that further increase the substrate are ingested. In addition, enzyme inhibitors may affect the hepatic microsomal enzyme system, which normally metabolizes drugs into less active or inactive metabolites that are excreted by the kidneys. Microsomal enzyme inhibitors can delay their own elimination, as well as that of other drugs taken concurrently. Other enzyme inhibitors, such as anticholinesterase inhibitors, are sometimes the active agents in insecticides and nerve gas. Enzyme inhibitors are used therapeutically to treat gout, emphysema, hypertension, cancer, alcoholism, depression, complications of renal disease, and jaundice in newborns.

disulfiram (Antabuse)	Prevents conversion of acetaldehyde acetate during normal alcohol catabolism.	Provide extensive patient education because the client needs to consent to and adhere to treatment. Never administer disulfiram otherwise.
Treats chronic alcoholism by discouraging alcohol consumption.		
Drug produces a disulfiram-alcohol interaction marked by flushing, throbbing headache, dyspnea, and hyperventilation, nausea and vomiting, palpitations and chest pain, confusion, anxiety, and blurred vision.	Consequent accumulation of acetaldehyde causes unpleasant symptoms when alcohol is consumed.	Explain that the disulfiram–alcohol reaction occurs from small amounts (15 mL) of alcohol and will persist as long as alcohol remains in the blood. Although most reactions are self-limiting and not life-threatening, others can be serious and deaths have occurred.

(continued)

Drug and Its Therapeutic Uses	Description	Nursing Management
disulfiram (Antabuse) con't.	The drug is administered orally and is rapidly but incompletely absorbed from the GI tract. Onset of action occurs in 3–12 hours. Disulfiram is metabolized in the liver and excreted mainly in urine. The drug has a long half-life; drug effects may persist for 1 to 2 weeks.	Inform client about possible adverse effects: drowsiness or insomnia; confusion, irritability, disorientation, delirium; abnormal gait; slurred speech; polyneuritis; optic neuritis; seizures; personality changes, psychoses; skin changes (dermatitis or acne); hepatitis, and blood dyscrasias. Explain that disulfiram interacts with many drugs degraded by the liver and therefore may increase drug concentration in the blood and the risk of toxicity from barbiturates, warfarin, paraldehyde, and phenytoin. Clients receiving disulfiram concurrently with metronidazole, isoniazid, or amitriptyline are at increased risk for additional adverse effects. Warn client to avoid alcohol in any form—beverages, medications, skin lotions, and foods. Also warn against using disulfiram to treat alcohol intoxication because a life-threatening reaction could ensue. Advise the client to have blood counts monitored regularly to detect blood abnormalities early.

Enzyme activators instigate enzyme activity. Many therapeutic drugs are microsomal enzyme inducers. They decrease serum levels of other drugs that are metabolized by the liver, when taken at the same time. One therapeutic drug, pralidoxime chloride, acts as an enzyme reactivator.

pralidoxime chloride (Protopam Chloride)* Treats poisonings caused by anticholinesterase drugs and pesticides; usually given on emergency basis	Reactivates cholinesterase and also detoxifies certain organophosphates directly, possibly interacting with cholinesterase to protect it from the effects of organophosphate compounds. Is given by mouth or injected but parenteral route (IM or IV) is more reliable than oral route for achieving therapeutic plasma level of 4 µg/mL or more. Drug does not bind to plasma proteins. Distributed throughout the extracellular compartment after absorption; pralidoxime and metabolites are excreted in urine Has reported serum half-life from 1.8 to 2.7 hours.	Prepare to implement emergency and general supportive measures (assisted respiration, seizure precautions, family reassurance) in addition to pralidoxime therapy. Monitor for adverse effects according to drug form: Oral route—anorexia, malaise, nausea, vomiting, and diarrhea; parenteral routes—IM, mild pain at the injection site; IV, hypertension, tachycardia, laryngospasm, muscle rigidity, and transient neuromuscular blockade. Possible additional effects include excitement, confusion, manic behavior, dizziness, blurred vision, diplopia and impaired accommodation, rash, and muscular weakness or rigidity. Anticipate possible drug interactions including atropine toxicity. Monitor vital signs, particularly blood pressure, to detect abnormal increases. Be sure to have phentolamine mesylate on hand to treat pralidoxime-induced hypertension. Administer cautiously to client with renal impairment or myasthenia gravis (drug may induce myasthenic crisis). Do not give to clients taking respiratory depressants, succinylcholine, theophylline, and aminophylline. Because pralidoxime is unstable, use solution within a few hours of preparation and administer slowly. Reduce environmental stimuli to minimize risk of nausea and confusion from pralidoxime and seizures from anticholinesterase toxicity. Develop a poison prevention and education program.

*For more information on specific enzyme drugs, refer to the following: Chapter 26 (streptokinase and urokinase); Chapter 29 (pepsin, pancreatic enzymes, including trypsin, chymotrypsin, lipase, and amylase); Chapter 37 (dornase); Chapter 40 (collagenase, deoxyribonuclease, papain, sutilains, trypsin, and fibrinolysin). For further information on specific enzyme inhibitors, refer to Chapter 20 (monoamine oxidase inhibitors); Chapter 23 (angiotensin converting enzyme inhibitors); Chapter 36 (allopurinol).

Glossary

absorbent Capable of reception by molecular or chemical action

absorption The movement of a substance into body fluids and tissues by passage through some entry. Except for direct injection, absorption involves passage through some surface or membrane barrier such as the skin or gastrointestinal mucosa

abuse (of drugs) Persistent inappropriate use of drugs

acid A molecule or ion that acts as a proton or hydrogen ion donor; a substance that ionizes in solution to form hydrogen ions; any substance that contains hydrogen capable of being displaced by basic radicals

acidifier, systemic A drug used to lower internal body pH

acidifier, urinary A drug used to lower the pH of urine

acidosis A physiologic state characterized by a shift in chemical balance toward acidity; a relative reduction in base buffers, a relative increase in acid salts, or an actual reduction in the pH of body fluids

acupuncture Therapeutic insertion of needles

addiction A behavioral state characterized by loss of power to control a drive or craving for a substance; also see *dependence*

addition Summation; when two drugs, acting simultaneously, elicit the same mechanism of action, and their combined effect is equal to the added sum of both drugs

adrenergic A drug whose effect on living systems is similar to that of epinephrine (Adrenalin) or the stimulation of sympathetic nervous tissue

adrenergic blocking agent A drug that inhibits responses to adrenergic nerve stimulation and to sympathomimetic drugs

adsorbent An agent that binds chemicals to its surface

adsorption Adhesion of a substance to the surface of a solid

aerosol A colloidal solution that is dispensed in the form of a mist

affinity A measure of the effectiveness of the interaction of a drug and its receptor; the greater the affinity of the drug, the greater its propensity to bind with its receptor and the smaller the concentration of drug needed to produce a given response

agent of choice The drug preparation generally regarded by physicians as the best choice for treatment of a given clinical condition

agonist A substance having a specific cellular affinity that produces a predictable response; a chemical capable of stimulating a cell membrane receptor

agranulocytosis A marked reduction in the number of granular leukocytes

akathisia Extreme restlessness, mental turbulence, and increased motor activity

akinesia Impaired or absent motor function

alkalizer, systemic A drug used to raise internal body pH

alkaloid One of a class of basic nitrogenous organic chemicals occurring in natural materials

alkalosis A physiologic state characterized by a shift in chemical balance toward alkalinity; a relative increase in base buffers, a relative decrease in acid salts, or an actual rise in pH of body fluids

allergen A substance that can elicit a specific immunologic response; an antigen

allergenic extract A suspension of antigenic chemicals prepared from the natural substance to which a person is allergic and which is administered to that person in gradually increasing doses for the purpose of decreasing the allergic response on subsequent exposure

allergic response An adverse response to a chemical due to the presence in an organism of immune bodies whose production was stimulated by previous exposure to that chemical

alopecia Loss of hair, baldness

amblyopia Dimness of sight

amebicide A drug used to destroy *Entamoeba histolytica,* the organism that causes amebic dysentery

ampules Sealed glass containers for powdered or liquid drugs

anabolic An agent that promotes body processes of repair and growth; a drug that promotes anabolism

anabolism Constructive metabolism; the building up of body tissue

analeptic A potent central nervous system stimulant, especially one that stimulates respiration and wakefulness

analgesic An agent that relieves pain without producing loss of consciousness

anaphylactoid reaction An immediate and serious physiologic response characterized by bronchospasm, vasospasm, and severe hypotension; usually fatal unless treated promptly

androgen A hormone that stimulates and maintains male secondary sex characteristics

androgenic Producing or promoting masculine characteristics

anesthetic An agent that causes reversible loss of feeling or sensation

anesthetic, general An anesthetic that not only causes loss of sensation but also loss of consciousness

anesthetic, local An anesthetic which causes loss of sensation only in the particular area where it is applied, by blocking out nerve impulses from the affected area

angioneurotic edema Large hives due to reflex nervous vasodilation

anhydrotic A drug that checks perspiration flow systemically; an antiphoretic

anodyne A medicine that relieves pain

anorexia Loss of appetite

anorexiant A drug that reduces appetite

antacid A substance that neutralizes acids; a drug taken to counteract symptoms caused by gastric hydrochloric acid produced in excessive amounts or present in an inappropriate body location, as in esophageal reflux

antagonism An interaction between two drugs in which the combined effect of the two agents is less than the sum of the effects of the drugs acting separately

antagonist A drug that reduces the physiologic effect of another drug, often a chemical that can occupy a cell membrane receptor without stimulating it and thereby block the action of agonists that interact with that receptor

anthelmintics Drugs used to rid the body of worms

antiadrenergic A drug that prevents response to sympathetic nervous system stimulation and adrenergic drugs; sympatholytic or sympathoplegic drugs

antiarrhythmic A drug used in the prevention and treatment of disorders of cardiac rhythm

antibacterial A drug that kills or inhibits pathogenic bacteria

antibiotic A chemical substance or metabolic product of living cells of molds, bacteria, or other plants that destroys or prevents the growth of microorganisms

antibodies Substances in the tissues or fluids of an organism that act to antagonize specific foreign bodies and are produced by the immune system in response to an initial exposure to the specific foreign body or antigen

anticholesteremic A drug that lowers blood plasma cholesterol level

anticholinergic A drug that decreases the activity of cholinergic nerve fibers or the physiologic effects of cholinergic nerve activity; parasympatholytic, parasympathoplegic

anticoagulant A drug that decreases blood coagulability and reduces the extension of blood clots already present but does not dissolve clots already formed

anticonvulsant A drug that selectively prevents epileptic seizures

antidepressant A psychotherapeutic drug that elevates mood

antidiarrheic A substance that reduces the production of frequent, watery stools and the intestinal cramping that accompanies diarrhea

antidote A chemical agent used to overcome the action or the effects of another chemical agent

antiemetic A drug that decreases nausea and vomiting

antigen A substance that can elicit a specific immunologic response; an allergen

antihistamine A drug that prevents response to histamine, including histamine released by allergic reactions

antihypertensive A drug that reduces blood pressure

anti-infective A drug used to treat infections

anti-inflammatory A drug that reduces the inflammatory response

antimuscarinic A substance that blocks the stimulating effect of muscarinic autocoids and drugs on the postganglionic receptors of the parasympathetic nervous system

antineoplastic A drug used to reduce the size of or the growth rate of a malignant tumor

antiplatelet A substance (drug) that delays coagulation by inhibiting platelet aggregation

antipruritic A drug that prevents or relieves itching

antipsychotic A drug used in the treatment of psychoses

antipyretic A drug used to reduce an abnormally high body temperature

antirheumatic A drug that alleviates inflammatory symptoms of arthritis and related connective tissue diseases

antiseptic A chemical agent that inhibits the growth of microorganisms but does not necessarily kill them

antisialogogue A drug that diminishes the flow of saliva

antispasmodic A drug that reduces the spasms of muscles, especially involuntary smooth muscle

antitoxin A biologic drug containing antibodies against the toxic principles of a pathogenic microorganism and used for passive immunization against the associated disease

antitussive A drug that suppresses coughing

anuria Lack of urinary output

aphasia Loss or impairment of speech

aplastic anemia Anemia due to impairment of the bone marrow

astringent A mild protein precipitant that diminishes secretions and toughens tissue

ataxia Lack of normal muscular coordination, especially the inability to coordinate voluntary movements

atomizer A device that breaks drugs into comparatively large particles for inhalation

atopy An allergy (usually manifested by bronchial asthma, vasomotor rhinitis, and chronic urticaria) for which there is a genetic predisposition

autocoid A chemical compound that occurs naturally in the body

bactericide An agent capable of rapidly killing microorganisms; disinfectant; germicide

bacteriostatic A substance that arrests the growth of bacteria

base A molecule or ion that acts as an acceptor of protons or hydrogen ions; a substance that ionizes in solution to form hydroxyl ions; any substance that has the property of neutralizing acids to form salts; any substance that can replace the hydrogen of an acid

binders Substances that give adhesiveness to a powdered drug

bioassay A procedure for determining the quantitative relationships between a dose of a drug and the intensity of the biologic response it evokes; used to determine the relative potencies of more than one drug or used as a standard of purity for the preparation of drugs

bioavailability The rate and extent to which a drug enters the circulation and reaches the site of action; the rate and extent to which the active drug ingredient is absorbed from a pharmacologic product and becomes available at the site of drug action (as defined by Federal Drug Administration [FDA] regulations)

bioavailable dose A dose available to an organism by virtue of the concentration of drug in the blood or at the active site

bioequivalent drug products Pharmaceutical equivalents, that is, drugs whose rate and extent of absorption do not show a significant difference when administered at the same molar dose under similar experimental conditions

biofeedback A process by which biologic changes normally unsensed by a person are converted to stimuli that provides sensory information about these changes

biotransformation Chemical changes in drugs that occur by virtue of physiologic processes in the body; metabolism

biotransport The translocation of a solute from one side of a biologic barrier to the other side

bronchodilator A drug that can dilate the lumina of air passages in the lungs

buffered Containing a substance that tends to preserve a proper hydrogen ion concentration

capsule A gelatin case for administering drugs in oral doses

capsule, time-release Capsule containing small beads of the active drug, some of which are treated to delay absorption by the gastrointestinal tract

carcinogenic Capable of causing cancer

cardiotonic A drug that increases the force of the heart muscle's contraction; a cardiac stimulant

carminative An aromatic or pungent drug that mildly irritates the gastrointestinal tract and is useful in the treatment of flatulence and colic

catecholamine A compound characterized by a catechol molecule combined with the aliphatic portion of an amine that mimics the effects of sympathetic nervous system stimulation when administered as a drug

cathartic A drug that causes defecation, usually by enhancing peristalsis or by softening or lubricating feces

caustic A topical drug that destroys tissue on contact and is suitable for removing abnormal tissue growth

ceiling effect The maximum intensity of a specific effect that can be produced by a given drug, no matter how large a dose is administered

central depressant A drug that decreases the functional state of the central nervous system

central stimulant A drug that increases the functional state of the central nervous system

chemical name A name that indicates the actual chemical composition of a drug, often designating the chemical atoms or radicals in the molecule and their placement in the drug molecule

chemotherapy The use of chemical agents that have a toxic effect on the disease-causing agent; specifically the use of drugs capable of destroying invading organisms or malignant tumor cells without destroying the host

cholagogue A drug that stimulates the emptying of the gallbladder and the flow of bile into the duodenum

cholinergic A drug that enhances the response of or the physiologic effects of cholinergic nerve fibers; parasympathomimetic

chrysotherapy Treatment (as in arthritis) by injection of gold salts

CNS Central nervous system

coagulant A drug that replaces a deficient blood factor necessary for coagulation; clotting factor

compartment A kinetically distinguishable pool in the body in terms of drug concentration profile

compendium A collected body of information on drugs, especially their strength, purity, and quality

compliance The degree to which advice (including prescriptions) is followed accurately and completely by the client

compounding The preparation of a medicinal substance by combining two or more ingredients

concomitant Associated with; taking place at the same time

concurrent Taking place at the same time

congener A drug that belongs to a group of chemical compounds having the same parent compound

contraceptive A drug used to prevent pregnancy

contraindication A condition or fact that makes a course of action, such as the use of a drug, inadvisable

corticoid A substance, natural or synthetic, that has actions similar to hormones of the adrenal cortex

counterirritant An agent that irritates the part to which it is applied and thereby produces vasodilation and an increase in blood supply in that part

cycloplegic A drug that paralyzes accommodation of the eye

cytotoxic A drug used to treat tumor growths; antineoplastic

deaggregation Dispersal of the particles of a whole

decongestant A drug that reduces congestion caused by an accumulation of blood

demulcent An agent that soothes and protects

dependence A condition in which the user of a drug has a compelling desire to continue taking the drug, either to experience its effects or to avoid the discomfort of its absence

dependence, physical An altered or adaptive physiologic state produced in a person by repeated administration of a drug (formerly termed *addiction*)

dependence, psychologic An emotional or mental drive, characterized by a compulsion to continue taking a drug (formerly termed *habituation*)

depressant A drug that temporarily slows some functional activity or process

detergent An emulsifying agent useful for cleansing wounds, ulcers, or skin

diaphoretic A drug used to increase perspiration; hydrotic; sudorific

diffusion The movement of molecules from a region of high concentration to one of lower concentration. Movement across the membrane may occur because the substance dissolves in its lipid portion, or because it attaches to a substance in the membrane which transports it to the opposite side (*facilitated diffusion*) where it is released

diffusion gradient The relative difference between concentrations of molecules from one region to another, which is directly related to the rate of diffusion

digestant A drug that promotes the process of digestion in the gastrointestinal tract

diluent A substance used to increase the bulk of a drug

disinfectant An agent capable of rapidly killing pathogenic microorganisms; especially used for killing microorganisms on inanimate objects; germicide

disintegrator A substance, such as starch, added to a dry drug to facilitate dissolution of the finished tablet in water

dissolution Solution in a liquid substance

distribution The movement of a chemical through the fluids and tissues of the body, usually in characteristic patterns and concentrations

diuretic A drug that promotes renal excretion of electrolytes and water, thereby increasing urine volume

dosage The regulated administration of doses expressed in terms of a quantity per unit of time

dose The quantity of drug to be administered at one time or the total quantity to be administered

drug Any chemical agent that affects living organisms, especially one used in the treatment, diagnosis, or prevention of disease, or one that poses a high risk of harmful effects

ecology The branch of biology dealing with the relations between organisms and their environment

eczema An inflammatory disease of the skin with infiltrations, watery discharge, scales, and crusts

effector Organ or cell that responds in a characteristic manner to a stimulus

effervescent Bubbling, sparkling, giving off gas bubbles

elixir An aromatic, sweetened, alcoholic preparation

emetic A drug that induces vomiting, either locally by gastrointestinal irritation or systemically by stimulating receptors in the central nervous system

emollient A topical drug, especially a fat or oil, used for its local protective or softening action

empiric Dependent on experience or observation alone without regard to science or theory

emulsion Suspension of fats or oils in water with the aid of an emulsifying agent (surface tension reducer), often stabilized by acacia or gelatin

endorphins See *enkephalins*

enkephalins Autogenous peptides that act as agonists on opioid receptors in the body; endorphins

enteral, enteric Pertaining to the intestinal tract

enteric coating A layer of material placed on the outer surface of a tablet or capsule to prevent dissolution in the stomach. Enteric coating may be used to protect the drug from the effect of gastric secretions or to protect the stomach from irritation by the drug

environmental medicine That branch of medicine dealing with the effect of the environment, especially pollutants, on the health of humans

enzyme A protein produced by living cells that accelerates biochemical reactions

equipotency The property of having equal strength, force, or power

essence A concentrated alcoholic solution of a volatile substance; spirits

estrogen A hormone that stimulates female secondary sex characteristics and functions in the menstrual cycle to promote uterine gland proliferation

excipient An inert substance used to give a pharmaceutical preparation a suitable form or consistency

excretion The physiologic elimination of substances from the body

expectorant A drug that increases secretion of respiratory tract fluid, making it less viscous, reducing its cough-inducing irritancy, and promoting its ejection

extracellular compartment The sum of the fluid-filled spaces of the body that are outside cell membranes (include both *interstitial* and *intravascular* compartments)

extracts A concentrated preparation of pharmacologic substances obtained from vegetable or animal materials by dissolving the active ingredients of the drug in a suitable solvent, then evaporating all or part of the solvent

extravasation The leakage of fluid into surrounding tissue, especially that of a vesicant or irritant drug, resulting in necrosis, pain, and tissue sloughing

fibrolytic A drug that dissolves the fibrin of blood clots

fluidextracts Alcoholic liquid extracts of vegetable drugs in 100% strength (*ie*, 1 ml of fluidextract contains 1 g of drug)

folk remedy A traditional familial practice related to health beliefs and customs in a specific cultural group, which has been passed on from generation to generation

forensic medicine The branch of medicine dealing with legal questions arising from illness, such as homicide, suicide, or accidental injury

galactorrhea Excessive flow of breast milk; inappropriate production of milk not associated with childbirth and nursing

galenical A medicinal prepared by extracting one or more active constituents of a plant

gels Aqueous suspensions of insoluble drugs in hydrated form

generic name A name indicating the origin of a drug; a name established by an authority, such as the Committee on International Nonproprietary Names (of the World Health Organization) to designate a single drug that may be marketed under various trade names

germicide Disinfectant; an agent capable of rapidly killing pathogenic microorganisms, especially one used for killing microorganisms on inanimate objects

glucocorticoid One of a class of hormones produced by the adrenal cortex, which exerts pronounced effects on the body's metabolism of carbohydrates by increasing gluconeogenesis

habituation See *dependence, psychologic*

half-life (t1/2) The time it takes for one half of an observed change to occur; serum half-life is the time it takes for one-half of a drug to disappear from the serum, or the time it takes for serum concentration to drop by half. (Serum half-life may be characterized by distinct phases: [1] the distribution phase during which the drug leaves the blood and enters the tissues, including tissue depots, [2] the phase during which the drug is simultaneously undergoing excretion and also moving from tissue depots to the blood, and [3] the elimination phase during which drug levels are influenced only by excretion; when serum half-life is termed *triphasic* figures are given for all three phases, when it is termed *biphasic,* figures are usually reported for the distribution and elimination phases.)

Radioactive half-life is the time it takes for the loss of one-half of the radioactive particles emitted by a radionuclide, or the time required for the radioactive emissions of the radionuclide to decline by half.

hapten A relatively simple compound that, although not itself a stimulant of antibody formation, reacts with specific antibodies after they have been produced

hematinic A medicine that promotes hemoglobin formation by supplying a factor essential for its synthesis

hematopoietic A drug that stimulates formation of red blood cells, especially by supplying deficient vitamins

hemostatic A locally acting drug that arrests hemorrhage by promoting clot formation

herb A plant with a soft stem containing little wood, especially one that contains aromatic constituents used as flavoring agents or medicines

herbal medicine The practice of using plants that contain active constituents known to be useful in the prevention or treatment of an illness

homeostasis The maintenance of the body's optimal internal environment

hormone A specific chemical substance secreted by cells in one part of a living organism that influences the growth, development, or behavior of other cells remote from the source of the hormone

hydrolysis a chemical reaction in which a compound is cleaved by the addition of a molecule of water

hyperglycemic A drug that elevates blood glucose level, especially for the treatment of hypoglycemic states

hyperosmotic Pertaining to solutions that have a higher osmotic pressure than a reference standard (usually physiologic fluids) and that cause a reduction of cell volume; hypertonic

hyperresponsivity Hypersensitivity

hypersensitivity A state in which a drug dose produces a response qualitatively greater than usual for that dose; hyperresponsivity

hypersensitivity, allergic A state characterized by the presence of antibodies that react with a given substance to produce an allergic reaction

hypertonic See *hyperosmotic*

hypnotic A drug that induces a clinical state resembling sleep

hypnosis A condition or state of consciousness that can be artificially induced and is characterized by strong susceptibility to suggestion and loss of sensation

hypodermic Beneath the skin, as in a hypodermic injection, which delivers drugs to the subcutaneous tissue

hypodermoclysis The introduction of large amounts of fluid into subcutaneous tissue

hypoglycemic A drug that promotes glucose metabolism and lowers the blood sugar level

hyposmotic Pertaining to solutions that have a lower osmotic pressure than a reference standard (usually physiologic fluids) and that increase cell volume; hypotonic

hypotensive A drug that diminishes pressure or tension to lower blood pressure

hypotonic See *hyposmotic*

hypovolemia Diminished blood supply in the body

iatrogenic Arising from or caused by medical treatment

idiosyncratic response An abnormal response to a drug that takes the form of extreme sensitivity to low doses, extreme insensitivity to high doses, or a response that is qualitatively different from the usual response

immune serum A biologic drug containing antibodies for a pathogenic microorganism; useful for passive immunization against a disease

immunity Resistance to disease by the presence of antibodies

immunizing agent, active An antigenic preparation (toxoid or vaccine) used to induce the formation of specific antibodies against a pathogenic microorganism, thus providing delayed by permanent protection against a disease

immunizing agent, passive A biologic preparation (antitoxin, antivenom, or immune serum) containing specific antibodies against a pathogenic microorganism

infection The presence of living organisms within the tissues

inflammation A local response to cellular injury, protective in nature, characterized by capillary dilation, leukocyte infiltration, swelling, heat and pain

inhaler A device used to spray liquid or powder in a fine mist into the lungs during inhalation

inscription The part of a prescription that states the name of the drug, the drug's dose form, and the amount of the dose

interstitial compartment The sum of the fluid-filled spaces of the body that are outside cell membranes and also outside blood vessels

intra-arterial Into an artery, as in an intra-arterial injection, which delivers drug to the blood in the arterial circulation

intracellular compartment The sum of the fluid-filled spaces inside cell membranes

intradermal Intracutaneous, as in an intradermal injection, which is made into the upper layers of the skin

intramuscular Into the muscle, as in an intramuscular injection, which introduces a drug into muscle tissue

intraperitoneal Into the peritoneal space

intrapleural Into the pleural space

intrathecal Into the spinal fluid, as in an intrathecal injection; the introduction of a drug into the spinal fluid, usually by means of a lumbar puncture (not administered by nurses unless they have received special training in the technique, as in the case of nurse-anesthetists)

intravascular compartment The sum of the fluid-filled blood vessels (including the heart chambers, arteries, capillaries, and veins)

intravenous Into a vein, as in an intravenous injection, which delivers drug into the blood of the venous circulation

ionic bond The chemical bond formed between two atoms by the outright transfer of one or more electrons from one atom to the other

ionizing radiation Forms of radiant energy that tend to dissociate compounds into their constituent ions

irritant Property of a drug whose administration causes pain and may be accompanied by inflammation

isotonic Pertaining to solutions that have the same osmotic pressure as the reference standard (usually physiologic fluids) and that do not cause any volume changes in cells; iso-osmolar

keratolytic A drug that softens the superficial keratin-containing layer of skin to promote exfoliation

laxative A gentle purgative medicine; a mild cathartic

lichenification Leathery hardening of the skin

liniments Liquid suspensions or dispersions intended for external application, often containing oil, soap, alcohol, or a rubefacient in addition to one or more active ingredients

lipid A broad term used to include all the ethersoluble, water-insoluble substances obtained from plant and animal sources; included are esters of fatty acids and alcohols (fats, oils, waxes, phospholipids, glycolipids, fatty acids, glycerols, sterols, and alcohols)

lipotropic factor A drug that prevents the abnormal accumulation of fat in the liver by promoting the transportation and utilization of fats

lotions Liquid suspensions or dispersions intended for external use

lozenges Flat, round, or rectangular preparations held in a cavity (mouth or vagina) until they dissolve, liberating the drug or drugs involved; troches

lubricant A substance added to a dry drug to prevent the formed tablet from sticking to the tablet-making machinery; a drug that acts by reducing friction

lysis Cellular destruction

magmas Bulky suspensions of insoluble preparations in water

materia medica The substances used in the composition of remedies for the treatment of disease; also the branch of medical science that deals with the sources, nature, and properties of drugs

median effective dose The smallest dose required to produce a stated effect in 50% of a population; ED_{50}; also median therapeutic dose (TD_{50})

median lethal dose The smallest dose required to produce death in 50% of a population; LD_{50}

medication The administration of drugs for the purpose of treating illness

medicine A substance administered for the purpose of treating illness

metabolism The changing of a substance by chemical processes in the body

metabolite A substance produced as a result of chemical transformation of another substance in the body. A given chemical often gives rise to a number of different but related metabolites

mineralocorticoid One of a class of hormones produced by the adrenal cortex with marked effects on metabolism of minerals, such as sodium and potassium

miotic (myotic) A substance that constricts the pupils

mists Medications administered in the form of cloudlike aggregations of minute particles

misuse (of drugs) The occasional inappropriate use of drugs, including nonmedical use, inappropriate medical use, or appropriate use in improper doses

mixture A solid material suspended in a liquid; also any preparation of several drugs for internal use

mucolytic A drug that reduces the thickness and stickiness of pulmonary secretions (usually administered by aerosol inhalation)

muscarinic A substance that, like muscarine, stimulates the postganglionic receptors of the parasympathetic nervous system

mutagenic Capable of causing genetic mutation

mydriatic A drug that dilates the pupils

narcotic A drug that induces sleep or stupor; legally: marijuana, cocaine, or a drug with morphinelike properties

narcotic analgesic A drug with both an analgesic and a sedative action

nebulizer A device for producing a fine spray or mist

neuroeffector junction A junction between a neuron and an effector organ or cell, such as smooth muscle or a gland cell

neuromuscular junction A function between a somatic motor neuron and a skeletal muscle fiber

nonpolar compound A substance whose molecular centers of positive and negative charges almost coincide, so that no permanent dipole moments are produced (nonpolar molecules do not ionize or conduct electricity)

nonprescription drug A medicine that is sold without a prescription; over-the-counter drug

nosocomial Acquired during hospitalization; of, or pertaining to, a hospital

nucleic acids A group of complex compounds of high molecular weight that occur in all plant and animal cells and in viruses; the chemical compounds that form deoxyribonucleic acids (DNA) and ribonucleic acids (RNA)

official drugs Preparations listed in pharmacopeiae that have been adopted by a government as pharmaceutical standards

ointments Semisolid preparations of medicinal substances in a base, such as petrolatum or lanolin, intended for application to the skin or mucous membranes

ointments, ophthalmic Sterile ointments for use in the eye

opiate A derivative of opium; a drug obtained from the opium poppy, *Papaver somniferum*

opioid A drug that resembles opium or morphine in its properties

osmotic effect The net movement of water across a semipermeable membrane when it separates two solutions of unequal concentration of solutes, or unequal osmotic pressure

over-the-counter (OTC) drug Nonprescription drug; a medicine sold directly to the public without requiring a prescription; usually a well-known substance of mixture taken for minor symptoms that is judged safe for use without medical supervision

oxidation A chemical reaction in which oxygen is added to a compound or the proportion of oxygen in a compound is increased by the removal of other groups

oxytocic A drug that selectively stimulates uterine motility and is useful in obstetrics

palliative A drug used for the control, rather than the cure, of a disease; suppressant

paradoxical reaction A physiologic response to a drug opposite to that which is usually seen (*eg*, restlessness and wakefulness following the administration of a hypnotic)

parasympatholytic A substance that tends to decrease the action of parasympathetic nerves or their effect on the body; anticholinergic

parasympathomimetic See *cholinergic*

parenteral Pertaining to the administration of drugs into any part of the body other than the gastrointestinal tract; although including topical applications and inhalation administration, in common usage applies only to administration by injection

paste A stiff ointmentlike preparation suitable only for external application

patent medicine A proprietary drug whose process of manufacture is controlled by patents granted to the developer; in common usage, used primarily to designate drugs advertised for self-use by the public

pathognomonic Indicative or characteristic of and specific to a disease

pharmaceutical chemistry The science dealing with the synthesis of new drugs either as modifications of older or natural drugs or as entirely new chemical entities

pharmacodynamics The science and study of the actions and effects of chemicals on living material

pharmacogenetics The science and study of genetic factors that account for individual differences in responses to drugs

pharmacognosy The science that deals with natural (animal and plant) sources for drugs

pharmacokinetics The science and study of the factors that determine the amount of a pharmacologic substance present at biologically effective sites at various times after its application to a biologic system

pharmacology The science and study of all aspects of the interactions of chemicals and living organisms

pharmacopeia A book, especially one published by an authority, that lists drugs and medicines and describes their preparations, properties, and uses

pharmacotherapeutics The use of drugs in the prevention, treatment, or diagnosis of disease and their use in the conscious alteration of normal functions

pharmacy That branch of pharmacology concerned with the preparing, compounding, and dispensing of drugs

pills Mixtures of a drug or drugs with a cohesive material, subsequently molded into globular, oval, or flattened bodies convenient for swallowing

pinocytosis The process whereby a particle is enveloped by the outer layer of a membrane, encased in the sac so formed, and transported to the inner layer of the membrane where it is released from the sac (the sac then merges with the inner layer of membrane)

placebo An inert substance used in place of a drug for its psychological effect and the physiologic changes that are triggered by the psychological response

placebo effect An actual biologic response to an inert substance believed to be caused by the power of suggestion

plasma The liquid part of blood or lymph

plasma clearance (renal) The volume of plasma needed to supply the amount of a specific substance excreted in urine in 1 minute

plasters Solid preparations that serve as simple adhesives or counterirritants

poison Any substance that impairs health or destroys life, especially one that exerts these effects in small doses

polar compound A compound that exhibits polarity, or local differences, in electrical properties; included are all electrolytes, most inorganic substances, and many organic ones

polarity The existence of opposing qualities; in relation to chemicals, the existence of electrical charges on a molecule or ion

pollutant An impurity

polypharmacy The concurrent use of two or more drugs

population A collection of items defined by a common characteristic

potency A comparative expression of drug activity measured in terms of the dose required to produce a particular effect of given intensity relative to a given or implied standard; strength, force, power

poultices Soft, moist preparations applied to the skin to exert osmotic pressure on fluids in the tissues (or to supply moist heat when warmed)

powders Finely divided solid drugs or mixtures of drugs for internal or external use

prescription A written formula given to the pharmacist by a physician, dentist, veterinarian, or other person legally permitted to prescribe medicine

prescription drug A drug whose purchase requires a prescription, because it has been judged to be unsafe for use except under supervision; a legend drug

prophylactic A remedy that prevents disease

proprietary drugs Preparations whose use is protected by patent or trademark to allow secrecy and monopoly in their manufacturing and sale

protectant A topical drug that remains on the skin and serves as a physical barrier to the environment

proteolytic enzyme An enzyme used to liquefy fibrinous or purulent exudates

psychoactive See *psychotropic*

psychoprophylaxis A technique of psychophysical training aimed at modifying the perception of painful sensations associated with normal childbirth

psychosomatic Pertaining to the interrelationship of the mind and body

psychotherapeutic A drug or interaction that modifies the behavior and emotional state of a person

psychotropic Affecting behavior, experience, or the function of the mind; psychoactive

purgative An agent that causes watery evacuation of the intestinal contents

rad Acronym for *radiation absorbed dose;* the quantity of ionizing radiation absorbed per unit mass of matter

radionuclide Atoms that disintegrate by emitting electromagnetic radiation

receptor A specialized area on a cell membrane that interacts with a drug substance

reduction A chemical reaction in which oxygen is removed from a compound or in which the reaction leads to a decrease in the proportion of oxygen in a compound

relaxant, muscle A drug that reduces muscle tension, especially in voluntary muscles

rem Acronym for *roentgen equivalent* (in) *man;* the estimated biologic effectiveness of one roentgen of radiation

resistance (In a host) the capability of an organism to counteract or destroy harmful agents or processes; a state of decreased response or a complete lack of response to drugs that ordinarily produce a biologic response

roentgen Unit for describing exposure dose of x or y radiation, with one unit representing the liberation of ions carrying positive and negative charges of 2.58×10^{-4} coulombs per kilogram of air

rubefacient A drug that reddens the skin; a counterirritant that increases circulation of blood in a specific part of the body

safety margin The relative distance between therapeutic and toxic doses of a given drug

sanitizer An agent that promotes health by its cleansing action

sciences, physical The fields of knowledge dealing with material phenomena

sciences, social The fields of knowledge dealing with psychosocial phenomena

scintiphotograph A graphic record of the scintillations emitted by radioactive tracers used to determine the outline and function of organs and tissues in which the radionuclide collects or by which it is secreted

sclerosing agent An irritant suitable for injection into varicose veins to induce their fibrosis and obliteration

secretagogue A chemical that simulates secretion by glandular organs

sedative A drug that exerts quieting or soothing effects

selectivity The capacity of a drug to produce one particular effect instead of multiple effects

semisynthetic Of or pertaining to a substance that is produced by a combination of natural and artificial processes or materials, often a natural substance that is chemically manipulated to modify its pharmacologic properties

sensitivity The ability of a member of a population, in comparison with other members of the same population, to respond in a qualitatively normal fashion to a particular drug dose

serum The clear, pale-yellow liquid that separates from the clot in the coagulation of blood; containing all the constituents of plasma except those involved in clot formation

side effect Any physiologic effect other than that for which a given drug is administered

signature The part of the prescription that gives directions for its use to the client who is to take the medicine

skeletal muscle relaxant A drug that inhibits contraction of voluntary muscles, usually by interfering with their innervation

smooth muscle relaxant A drug that inhibits contraction of involuntary (eg, visceral) muscles, usually by acting on their contractile elements

solution A homogeneous dispersal of one substance in another without chemical change, usually that of a solid in a liquid

solution, true Nonvolatile substances dissolved in water

spasmolytic An agent that relieves spasms and involuntary contraction of a muscle; an antispasmodic

specificity The capacity of a drug to manifest its effects by a single mechanism of action; selectivity

spinnbarkeit Ability to spin cervical mucus into a long thread at the time of ovulation

spirits Concentrated alcoholic solutions of volatile substances; essences

standard safety margin The percentage by which the dose effective in virtually all (99%) of the population has to be increased to produce a lethal effect in a minimum percentage (1%) of the population

sterilization The elimination of all life forms

stereoisomers Two substances of the same composition and constitution that differ in the relative spatial position of their constituent atoms or groups in that one is the mirror image of the other

stimulant A drug that temporarily quickens some vital process or functional activity

stomachic A drug used to stimulate appetite and gastric secretion

subcutaneous Within the tissue lying between the skin and muscle, as in a subcutaneous injection, which is the introduction of a drug by hypodermic into the subcutaneous tissue or the pocket between subcutaneous and muscle tissue

sublingual Beneath the tongue

subscription The part of a prescription that contains the directions to the pharmacist

summation The simultaneous action of two drugs that is the algebraic sum of their individual effects

superinfection An infection developing during antimicrobial treatment of another infection. The secondary infection is often caused by an organism that is resistant to the treatment agent and that grows more readily in the absence of the organisms suppressed by the treatment agent

superscription The part of the prescription that includes the client's name, age, and address; the date; and the symbol Rx (an abbreviation for "recipe," meaning "take thou")

suppositories Mixtures of a drug with a firm base that can be molded into shapes suitable for insertion into a body cavity, melting at body temperature to release the drug

suppressant See *palliative*

surfactant A surface active agent that decreases the surface tension between two miscible liquids

suspension A combination of a solid and a fluid in which the particles of the former are mixed with but not dissolved in the latter

sympatholytic A drug that decreases the activity of the sympathetic nervous system, or the physiologic effect of sympathetic nervous activity

sympathomimetic A drug that produces a physiologic effect similar to that of sympathetic nervous activity

synapse The junction between two neurons

synergism When the combined effects of two drugs acting simultaneously are greater than the sum of the individual effects of these drugs

synthetic Of or pertaining to a substance that is produced by an artificial rather than a natural process or material

syrup Aqueous solution of sucrose (85%) used as a vehicle and preservative for drugs

tablet A preparation of powdered drug that is compressed or molded into small disks; usually containing in addition to the drug a diluent, a binder, a disintegrator, and a lubricant

tachyphylaxis A significant decrease in effectiveness of a drug following repeated administration

teratogen A substance that induces abnormal fetal development when administered to a pregnant animal

teratogenic Property of developing abnormal structures in an embryo resulting in fetal deformities

therapeutic index The ratio between the median lethal dose and median effective dose; computed according to the formula: $T1 = LD_{50}/ED_{50}$

therapeutics The treatment of disease

threshold dose The dose of a drug barely sufficient to produce any preselected intensity of effect

tinctures Alcoholic or hydroalcoholic solutions of the active principles of drugs

tocolytic A drug used to inhibit uterine contractions

tolerance A condition of decreased responsiveness acquired after a single or repeated exposure to a given drug or one closely allied in pharmacologic activity

tonic An agent used to restore tone to muscle tissue; to laymen, a remedy that improves general body function

toxic effect A drug effect that is deleterious to the organism, especially an effect characteristic of high doses

toxicology The study of the toxic or harmful effects of chemicals as well as the mechanisms and conditions under which these harmful effects occur

toxicology, economic The study of the toxic effect of chemicals intentionally administered to a living organism to achieve a specific purpose; including therapeutic agents, food additives, cosmetics, insecticides, and herbicides

toxicology, environmental The study of toxic agents that influence health and safety in the work environment, in the atmosphere, and in ingested nutrients; the effects of these toxic elements on the human organism

toxicology, forensic The study of poisoning (intentional and accidental) and the legal aspects of the relationship between exposure and the harmful effects of chemicals

toxoid A modified bacterial toxin, less toxic than the original form, used to induce active immunity to bacterial pathogens

tracer A radioactive isotope that can be incorporated into compounds whose course through the body can be followed or traced by measuring the radioactivity of body tissue or fluids

tranquilizer A drug that reduces mental and emotional tension

transport Movement or transfer of substances in a biologic system; especially across cell membranes

transport, active Transfer of a substance across a membrane by means of carrier systems that require energy for their function; active transport systems often move substances against the diffusion gradient, from areas of low concentration to areas of high concentration

transport, passive Diffusion

troches Flat round or rectangular preparations that are held in a cavity (the mouth or vagina) until they dissolve, liberating the drug or drugs involved; lozenges

uricosuric A drug that increases the excretion of uric acid in the urine (useful in treating gout)

vaccine A suspension of either attenuated or killed microorganisms administered for the prevention of infectious diseases by the induction of active immunity

vasoconstrictor A drug used to constrict blood vessels and reduce tissue congestion

vasodilator A drug that relaxes vascular smooth muscles, especially for the purpose of improving peripheral or coronary blood flow

vasopressor A drug used systemically to constrict blood vessels and raise blood pressure

vehicle A drug component that is instrumental in transporting drug to site of action

vertigo Dizziness, giddiness

vesicant An agent that causes blistering and the formation of vesicles when applied to the tissues

vesiculation Formation of small sacs filled with fluid

vials Glass containers with rubber stoppers containing one or more doses of a drug

waters Solutions (saturated unless otherwise stated) of volatile oils or other aromatic substances in distilled water

Index

NOTE: A *t* following a page number indicates tabular material, an *f* following a page number indicates an illustration, a *b* following a page number indicates boxed or specially formatted material, and a *g* following a page number indicates a definition in the glossary. Insofar as possible, drugs are listed in bold face type under their generic names. Drug trade names are listed in capital letters and the reader is referred to the generic name. Combination drugs are listed under their trade names.

Selected Internet Sites Related to Pharmacology and Drug Therapy

Name of Site	Internet Address	Comments
Pharmacology Glossary: Boston University School of Medicine	http://med-amsa.bu.edu/Pharmacology/Programmed/glossary.html	Information on symbols and terms used in pharmacology
Glaxo Wellcome Pharmacology Guide	http://www.glaxowellcome.co.uk/netscape/science/phguide/index.htmlh/	Quick reference guide to most of the important terms and concepts of pharmacology.
PharmWeb	http://www.pharmweb.net/	Provides links by subjects to other pharmacology-related information sites for health professsionals and patients
PharmInfoNet	http://pharminfo.com/	Drug information and links to publications and disease centers
"Virtual" Pharmacy Center: Martindale's Health Science	http://www.sci.lib.uci.edu:80/-martindale/Pharmacy.html#CPT	Variety of types of information about pharmacology and pharmacy around the world
NP Web	http://www.unh.edu/npract/index.html	
NIH	gopher://gopher.nlm.nih.gov:70/11/alerts	Clinical alerts from clinical trials
Drug FAQ: Frequently Asked Questions about Drugs: PharmInfo	http://pharminfo.com/drugfaq/	Gives information about drugs, links to related articles and resources about the drug, plus questions from patients and health professionals and the answers.
U.S. National Library of Medicine	http://text.nlm.nih.gov/ftrs/gateway	Links to AHCPR guidelines; AHCPR Technology Assessments and Reviews; NIH Consensus Development Program; NIH Clinical studies
Doctor's Guide to New Drugs or Indications	http://www.pslgroup.com/NEWDRUGS.HTM	Information about new drugs or new indications in US and worldwide
Drug InfoNet	http://www.druginfonet.com/	Information about drugs, diseases, questions to experts, and links to other sites; names, addresses and phone numbers for many pharmaceutical manufacturers
Farmaweb	http://www.farmaweb.com/	Information about drugs in Spanish and English
Pharmacokinetics	http://jeffline.tju.edu/CWIS/OAC/pharmacology/pharm_guide/menu.html	Learning module on pharmacokinetics from Thomas Jefferson University
Center Watch	http://www.centerwatch.com/	Information about clinical trials in US and worldwide; also has information about newly approved drugs
Health A to Z-Pharmaceuticals and Drugs	http://www.healthatoz.com/categories/PC.htm	Information and links related to drug therapy
Antibiotic Use Guidelines (University of Wisconsin)	http://www.biostat.wisc.edu/clinsci/amcg/amcg.html	Data on antibiotics by drug name, drug class, organism, empiric therapy by site, and antimicrobial treatment if HIV-infected patient
Food and Drug Administration	http://www.fda.gov/	Access to information related to drugs and regulation of drugs

Is This Site Reliable? Evaluating Health Information on the Internet

FDA staff and others familiar with Internet medical offerings suggest asking the following questions to help determine the reliability of a Web site:

Who maintains the site?

Government or university-run sites are among the best sources for scientifically sound health and medical information. Private practitioners or lay organizations may have marketing, social, or political agendas that can influence the type of material they offer on-site and to which sites they link.

Is there an editorial board or listing of the names and credentials of those responsible for preparing and reviewing the site's contents?

Can these people be contacted by phone or through E-mail if visitors to the site have questions or want additional information?

Does the site link to other sources of medical information?

No reputable organization will position itself as the sole source of information on a particular health topic. Links alone, however, are not a guarantee of reliability, since anyone with a Web page can create links to any other site on the Internet—and the owner of the site that is "linked to" has no say over who links to it. A person offering suspect medical advice could conceivably try to make his or her advice appear legitimate by creating a link to FDA's Web site. What's more, health information produced by FDA or other government agencies is not copyrighted; therefore, someone can quote FDA information at a site and be perfectly within his or her rights. By citing a source such as FDA, experienced marketers using careful wording can make it appear as though FDA endorses their products.

When was the site last updated?

Generally, the more current the site, the more likely it is to provide timely material. Ideally, health and medical sites should be updated weekly or monthly.

Are informative graphics and multimedia files such as video or audio clips available?

Such features can assist in clarifying medical conditions and procedures. Bear in mind, however, that multimedia should be used to help *explain* medical information, not *substitute* for it. Some sites provide dazzling "bells and whistles" but little scientifically sound information.

Does the site charge an access fee?

Many reputable sites with health and medical information, including FDA and other government sites, offer access and materials for free. If a site does charge a fee, be sure that it offers value for the money. Use a searcher to see whether you can get the same information without paying additional fees.

*Adapted from: Larkin, M. (1996). Health Information On-Line. *FDA Consumer Magazine* (June 1996).

The *Lippincott's Pharmacology Review* Disk Instructions

System Requirements

A PC compatible computer with an Intel 386 or better processor
Windows 3.1 or later
4 Megabytes RAM (minimum), but recommend 8 MB RAM on Windows 3.1
8 Megabytes RAM (minimum), but recommend 12 MB RAM on Windows 95
3 Megabytes of available hard disk space.

Installation

Installing Pharmacology Review for Windows

1. Start up Windows.
2. Insert the disk into the floppy disk drive.
3. From the Program Manager's File Menu, choose the Run command.
4. When the Run dialog box appears, type a:\setup (or b:\setup if you're using the B drive) in the Command Line box. Click OK or press the Enter button.
5. The installation process will begin. A dialog proposing the directory "CPNM" on the drive containing Windows will appear. If the name and location are correct, click OK. If you want to change this information, type over the existing data, then click OK.
6. When the *Pharmacology Review* setup routine is complete, a new group called "Lippincott's Pharmacology Review" will appear on your desktop.
7. Start the *Pharmacology Review* program by double-clicking on its icon.

Lippincott's Pharmacology Review Disk Program

Lippincott's Pharmacology Review consists of two modes: Test Mode and Study Mode.

Test Mode

To begin a test, click the Start Over button with your mouse cursor. As a result, the first question will appear on the screen. If you decide to stop the test before you complete it, your answers will be saved. You can resume the test by selecting the Resume button from the Main Menu screen. You may clear your answers for a test at any time by clicking on the Start Over button.

Lippincott's Pharmacology Review Toolbar

The Toolbar contains a series of buttons that provide direct access to all test program functions. When you move the cursor over a button, an explanation of its function displays in the Status Bar, which is immediately above the Toolbar.

From left to right, the Toolbar buttons are:

Program Help	Prior Question Arrow (go to the previous question in the test)
Pause	Next Question Arrow (go to the next question in the test)
Mark Question	Last Question Arrow (go to the last question in the section)
Table of Contents	Stop
First Question Arrow (go to the first question in the section)	

To get help at any time during the test, choose the Program Help button. Program Help reviews basic functions of the program. To close the Program Help window, click on the Program Help button again. Answer each question by clicking on the oval to the left of an answer selection or by selecting the appropriate letter on the keyboard (A, B, C, or D). When an answer is selected, its oval will darken. If you change your mind about an answer, simply select that choice, by mouse or keyboard, again.

To register your answer selection and proceed to the next question, click on the Next Question Arrow button or press the Enter key.

If you are unsure about an answer to a particular question, the program allows you to mark it for later review. Flag the question by clicking on the Mark Question button. To review all marked questions for a test, click on the Table of Contents button, which is immediately to the right of the Mark button. This will open the Table of Contents window.

The Table of Contents window lists every question included on the test and summarizes whether it has been answered, left unanswered, or marked for later review. Click on an item in the Table of Contents window and the program will move to that test question. Or, use the Arrow buttons to move to the first, previous, next, or last question. To close the Table of Contents window, click on the Table of Contents button again.

At any time during the test or when you are finished taking the test, click on the Stop button. If you wish, you may return to the session at a later time without erasing your existing answers by selecting the Resume button.

After taking the test you may receive your score by clicking the Results button on the Main Menu Screen.

Study Mode

After taking the test and receiving your score you may wish to enter the Study Mode. This mode supplies you with the test questions, the answers that you chose, and the rationale for correct and incorrect answers. To enter the Study Mode, click the Study Mode button with your mouse cursor. You will not be able to modify the answers you have given, however, you can select any of the answer choices for an explanation of that answer. You may also wish to use the Table of Contents button to show you which questions you marked for review. Each of these windows may be closed by clicking again on their respective buttons.

To exit *Lippincott's Pharmacology Review* program, click the Exit button on the Main Menu.